The
Grey House
Performing Arts
Directory

2003

The Grey House Performing Arts Directory

Third Edition

- Dance
- Instrumental Music
- Vocal Music
- Theatre
- Series & Festivals
- Facilities
- Artist Management
- Information Resources

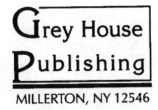

Grey House Publishing

MILLERTON, NY 12546

PUBLISHER:	Leslie Mackenzie
EDITOR:	Richard Gottlieb
EDITORIAL DIRECTOR:	Laura Mars-Proietti
EDITORIAL ASSISTANT:	Pamela Michaud
PRODUCTION MANAGER:	Karen Stevens
ASSISTANT TO PRODUCTION:	Cecilia Fletcher
PRODUCTION ASSISTANTS:	Vicki Barker, Debra Giordano, Gail Kusek, Jana Martin, Melissa Valyou
COMPOSITION:	David Garoogian
MARKETING DIRECTOR:	Jessica Moody

Grey House Publishing, Inc.
185 Millerton Road
Millerton, NY 12546
518.789.8700
FAX 518.789.0545
www.greyhouse.com
e-mail: books @greyhouse.com

While every effort has been made to ensure the reliability of the information presented in this publication, Grey House Publishing neither guarantees the accuracy of the data contained herein nor assumes any responsibility for errors, omissions or discrepancies. Grey House accepts no payment for listing; inclusion in the publication of any organization, agency, institution, publication, service or individual does not imply endorsement of the editors or publisher.

Errors brought to the attention of the publisher and verified to the satisfaction of the publisher will be corrected in future editions.

First edition published 2000
Third edition published 2002

Printed in the USA

ISBN 1-930956-87-8   softcover

The Grey House Performing Arts Directory
Table of Contents
Third Edition

The Grey House Performing Arts Directory
Introduction
Third Edition

Welcome to the third edition of *The Grey House Performing Arts Directory* – a comprehensive resource of performing arts organizations, their staff, structure, and business data. This work offers unequaled coverage of major performance categories, as well as resources for performers and managers alike. Chapters include **Dance, Instrumental Music, Vocal Music, Theatre, Series & Festivals, Facilities, Information Resources** and a brand new chapter on **Artist Management.**

The Grey House Performing Arts Directory contains more than 9,500 listings. The performing organizations are arranged first by performance category, then by state, and then by city, making it easy to research organizations by both category and location. In addition to performing organizations, the Directory contains comprehensive chapters on the business side of the industry. **Performance Facilities** range from Carnegie Hall to Giant Stadium, including university, library and outdoor venues, **Industry Resources**, include detailed information on hundreds of Arts Associations, Periodicals, Directories & Databases, Trade Shows & Conferences, and Web Sites. The chapter on **Artist Management** – NEW to this edition – includes agents, consultants and marketing professionals, and is designed to offer another avenue of business support to this eclectic and competitive industry.

This major work provides current, critical information for those who are studying, teaching, and performing in dance, theatre, instrumental and vocal music, as well as those who provide management and communication services to the industry.

Chapters One – Five: Performing Organizations

Each of these chapters focuses on a specific, major performing arts category, and includes both world renown performers, such as the Boston Symphony Orchestra at Tanglewood, and smaller ensembles in more intimate surroundings, such as the McHyden Theatre in rural New York. For each record, researchers will find contact information – name, address, phone, fax, web site, and e-mail – and lists of key staff members, both artistic management and business titles. A clear, concise mission statement defines the group's purpose, and is followed by the type of facility the group performs at, affiliations, performance season, annual attendance, income sources, and founding year.

As we are reminded during our update process for *The Grey House Performing Arts Directory*, the performing arts industry is not especially easy to track. Organizations often change locations, artists move around, performance spaces are sometimes far from business offices, and seasons are often only a few months long. Despite these challenges, our extensive update strategy continues to be successful. We utilize fax, telephone and particularly valuable e-mail campaigns, giving each listee several opportunities to update their entry. During this effort, we deleted many organizations no longer in operation.

In addition to updating thousands of existing records and deleting those that are out of business, we added nearly 200 new listings. The 9,511 listings in this third edition include 7,865 fax numbers, 5,680 e-mails, 6,275 web sites and 8,800 key contacts, making it easier than ever to reach the places and people who are important to you.

Chapter Six: Performance Facilities
This section comprises more than 2,500 facilities that host the performing arts. Many are multi-purpose, and listings often include facility manager, seating capacity, and type of stage. This chapter is also organized by state, and then city. We concentrated much of our update efforts for this edition on facilities, developing an especially strong chapter.

Chapter Seven: Artist Management
This section is new to this edition. It was developed largely to address the needs of previous users, who tell us they are looking for one reference tool that includes not only all the major performing categories, but all of the supportive industries as well. This newest chapter includes 200 agents and managers nationwide that represent the performing arts industry. Listings include address, phone, fax, web site and a key executive.

Chapter Eight: Information Resources
Drawn from our widely acclaimed, and recently updated, *Business Information Resources Directory*, and extensive independent research, this section lists nearly 1,000 resources for the performing arts industry. There are Associations, Newsletters, Magazines, Journals, Trade Shows, Directories, Databases, and Web Sites, all designed to give users the direction they are looking for, and their choice of media, within the performing arts industry.

Five Indexes
Again this year, *The Grey House Performing Arts Directory* has five indexes to make it easy for researchers to locate the exact organization, group or location they need.

Entry Name Index: An alphabetical listing of every performance organization and artist management company.

Executive Name Index: An alphabetical listing, by last name, of the key executives associated with performance organizations and artist management companies.

Facilities Index: A combined alphabetical listing of both the performing arts facilities that appear in the Facilities chapter, and those that may appear within each organization's individual listing.

Geographic Index: Every performing arts organization, artist management company and facility, listed by state, with city included.

Information Resource Index: An alphabetical listing of performing arts associations, periodicals, conferences and web sites.

As always, we look forward to your comments and are committed to providing an annual directory that continues to address the needs of this dynamic industry. To broaden its availability, *The Grey House Performing Arts Directory* is also available online.

User Guide

Descriptive listings in *The Grey House Performing Arts Directory* are organized into 8 major chapters: Dance, Instrumental Music, Vocal Music, Theatre, Series & Festivals, Facilities, Artist Management, and Information Resources. Listings within the first seven chapters are organized by state, then city.

Below is a sample listing illustrating the kind of information that is or might be included in a performing category. Each numbered item is described on the following page.

---

1 → **1234**

2 → **M&J Dance Company**

3 → **46 Sharon Road**
   Sharon, CT 06069

4 → **Phone:**   068-364-1234
5 → **Fax:**   068-364-1235
6 → **Toll Free:** 068-364-1236
7 → **E-Mail:**   info@M&JDance.com
8 → **Website:**   www.M&JDance.com

9 → *Management:*
   Executive Director: Jonathan Miller
   Production Manager: Marie Carren
   Conductor: Brian Burke
   Director of Touring and Education: Franco Petrell

10 → *Officers:*
   Chairman of the Board: William Thompson
   Vice Chairman: Steve Chapman
   Secretary: Joan Parker
   Treasurer: Sally Forbes

11 → **Mission:** To create, produce and maintain a repertorie of outstanding dance, strengthen and broaden the understanding and appreciation of ballet and modern dance, and provide increasing access and exposure to dance through development of informative, educational programs for children.

12 → **Founded:** 1996

13 → **Specialized Field:** Ballet; Modern Dance

14 → **Status:** Professional; Non-Profit

15 → **Income Sources:** Council; Ticket Sales; Donations

16 → **Performs At:** Sharon Civic Hall

17 → **Paid Staff:** 6

18 → **Volunteer Staff:** 25

19 → **Paid Artists:** 2

20 → **Budget:** $1.2 Million

21 → **Organization Type:** Performing; Touring; Resident; Educational

User Key

1 ➤ **Record Number**: Entries are listed alphabetically within each category and numbered sequentially. The entry number, rather than the page number, are used in the indexes to refer to listings.

2 ➤ **Company Name:** Formal name of company or organization. Where company names are completely capitalized, the listing will appear at the beginning of the section.

3 ➤ **Address:** Location or permanent address of the company.

4 ➤ **Phone Number:** The listed phone number is usually for the main office of the company, but may also be for the sales, marketing, or public relations office.

5 ➤ **Fax Number:** This is listed when provided by the company.

6 ➤ **Toll-Free Number:** This is listed when provided by the company.

7 ➤ **E-Mail:** This is listed when provided, and is generally the main office e-mail.

8 ➤ **Web Site:** This is listed when provided by the company and is also referred to as an URL address. These web sites are accessed through the Internet by typing http:// before the URL address.

9 ➤ **Management:** Lists key artistic executives of the company.

10 ➤ **Officers:** Lists key business executives of the company.

11 ➤ **Mission:** A brief description of the company and its purpose and services it offers.

12 ➤ **Founded:** Year company was founded.

13 ➤ **Specialized Field:** Lists the type of dance (or music, or theatre) the company focuses on.

14 ➤ **Status:** Indicates the company's status within the industry.

15 ➤ **Income Sources:** Indicates where the company's revenue is derived.

16 ➤ **Performs At:** Where the performances take place.

17 ➤ **Paid Staff:** Number of paid employees.

18 ➤ **Volunteer Staff:** Number of non-paid staff.

19 ➤ **Paid Artists:** Number of paid artists.

20 ➤ **Budget:** Annual budget.

21 ➤ **Organization Type:** Defines the types of activity the organization participates in, or sponsors.

Alabama

1 ALABAMA BALLET
2726 1st Avenue S
Birmingham, AL 35233
Phone: 205-322-4300
Fax: 205-322-4444
e-mail: alabamaballet@earthlink.net
Web Site: www.alabamaballet.org
Officers:
President: Katherine Mitchell
Executive President: Dudley Reynolds
Secretary: Susan Driggers
Treasurer: Joe Lassiter
VP Fundraising: Lia Rushton
Management:
Artistic Director: Wes Chapman
Ballet Master: Roger Van Fleteren
Music Director/Conductor: Leslie Fillmer
External Affairs Director: Alice C Cox
Assistant to the Director: Tamara Byrd
Bookkeeper: Ginny Cockrell
Mission: To promote and foster the development of classical and contemporary ballet through high-quality performances, dance education, and community outreach.
Founded: 1981
Specialized Field: Ballet
Paid Staff: 16
Paid Artists: 19
Non-paid Artists: 15
Income Sources: Ticket sales; donations; grants
Performs At: Civic Center Concert Hall; Alys Stephans Center
Organization Type: Performing; Touring

2 SOUTHEAST ALABAMA DANCE COMPANY
111 N St. Andrews Street
PO Box 125
Dothan, AL 36302
Phone: 334-702-7139
Fax: 334-702-7139
Web Site: www.snowhill.com/~seadac/
Management:
Director: Tracy Soloman
Founded: 1978
Specialized Field: Dance

3 HUNTSVILLE BALLET COMPANY
800 Regal Drice
PO Box 373
Huntsville, AL 35804
Phone: 256-539-0961
Fax: 256-539-1837
e-mail: david.herriott@communityballet.org
Web Site: www.communityballet.org
Officers:
President: Thomas F Craig
First VP: Dannye Drake
Second VP: Bruce Epps
Treasurer: Joe Ansley
Management:
Artistic Director: David Herriott
School Administor: Keren Gibb

Office Manager: Lori Lindstrom
Mission: Through our school, company, and professional touring company presentations, CAB/Huntsville Ballet Company enriches and educates people in the Tennessee Valley region.
Founded: 1964
Specialized Field: Ballet; Modern; Jazz; Tap
Status: Semi-professional; Nonprofit
Paid Staff: 20
Volunteer Staff: 100
Paid Artists: 20
Non-paid Artists: 100
Organization Type: Touring; Resident

4 ALABAMA DANCE THEATRE
Armory Learning Arts Center
1018 Madison Avenue
PO Box 11327
Montgomery, AL 36111
Phone: 334-241-2590
Fax: 334-241-2504
e-mail: ADTDance1@aol.com
Web Site: www.tfn.net/ADT
Management:
Artistic Director: Kitty Seale
Ballet Master: Haynes Owens
Jazz: Janie Allen Alford
Ballet: Emily Caruso
Modern: Jenny Letner
Tap/Ballet: Betsy Shedd
Ballet: Kate Robertson
Founded: 1986

5 MONTGOMERY BALLET
6009 E Shirley Lane
Montgomery, AL 36117
Phone: 334-409-0522
Fax: 334-409-2311
e-mail: montgomeryballet@yahoo.com
Web Site: www.montgomeryballet.com
Management:
Artistic Director/CEO: Priscilla Crommelin-Ball
Ballet Master: Oskar Antunez
Mission: To present a high quality dance program to large and small communities. The affordability of the Ballet's touring fees combined with the ability to adapt to a variety of performing spaces make the program possible for many communities.
Founded: 1958
Specialized Field: Ballet
Status: Semi-Professional; Nonprofit
Paid Staff: 4
Volunteer Staff: 5
Paid Artists: 55
Budget: $200,000-$500,000
Income Sources: Southeast Regional Ballet Association
Organization Type: Performing; Educational

Alaska

6 ALASKA DANCE THEATRE
2602 Gambell Street
Anchorage, AK 99503
Phone: 907-277-9591
Fax: 907-274-3078
e-mail: adt@gci.net
Web Site: www.alaskadancetheatre.com
Management:
  Artistic/School Director: Alice Bassler Sullivan
  Associate Artistic Director: C Noelle Partusch
  Executive Director: Kathleen Cline
Founded: 1981
Specialized Field: Dance
Status: Nonprofit Organization
Paid Staff: 25
Volunteer Staff: 5
Paid Artists: 5
Non-paid Artists: 30
Budget: $500,000
Income Sources: Grants; Donations; Tuition
Performs At: Alaska Center for the Performing Arts

7 NORTH STAR BALLET
PO Box 73486
Fairbanks, AK 99707
Phone: 907-451-8800
e-mail: nsdf@polarnet.com
Web Site: www.ptialaska.net/~nsdf/
Officers:
  President: Paul Kennedy
  VP: Bruce Gordon
  Secretary: Freddie Black
Management:
  Artistic Director: Norman Shelburne
  Administrative Director: Iris Lindsey
Mission: To promote the art of dance in Alaska through education and performance.
Founded: 1984
Specialized Field: Ballet
Status: Non-Professional; Nonprofit
Paid Staff: 26
Performs At: Bering Auditorium
Organization Type: Performing; Touring; Resident; Educational

Arizona

8 CROSSROADS PERFORMANCE GROUP
1870 W 5th Place
Mesa, AZ 85201
Phone: 480-969-6683
Fax: 480-962-4584
e-mail: crossroadsduo@yahoo.com
Management:
  Co-Artistic Director: Step Raptis
  Artistic Director: Lisa R Chow
Founded: 1989
Specialized Field: Interdisciplinary-Music and Dance Collaboration

9 BALLET ARIZONA
3645 E Indian School Road
Phoenix, AZ 85018
Phone: 602-381-0184
Fax: 602-381-0189
Toll-free: 888-322-5538
Web Site: www.balletarizona.org
Officers:
  Chairman: Jenny St John
  Vice Chairman: Robert Barnard
Management:
  Artistic Director: Ib Andersen
  Executive Director: Sherry New
  Marketing Director: Deanne Poulusger
Mission: To create and develop a professional dance institution that produces world class dance performances, nurtures its artists, and serves its communities through superior educational programs.
Founded: 1986
Specialized Field: Ballet
Status: Professional; Nonprofit
Paid Staff: 14
Paid Artists: 29
Budget: $2,700,000
Income Sources: Arizona Commission on the Arts; City of Phoenix; Corporate Support; Individual Donors; Ticket Sales
Annual Attendance: 70,000
Facility Category: Performing Arts
Organization Type: Performing; Touring; Resident; Educational

10 GROUNDING POINT DANCE COMPANY
4909 E McDowell Road
Suite 100
Phoenix, AZ 85008
Phone: 602-685-9607
Fax: 602-685-9608
e-mail: carrie.m@worldnet.att.net
Management:
  President/Artistic Director: Carrie A Miller
Mission: To educate students in the different forms of dance and its history. By creative teaching of self-expression, the power of symbolism and non-verbal communication, our students will gain a deeper understanding of themselves and others. GPDC creates workshops for grades K-12 promoting healthy lifestyles, creative problem solving, a sense of community, and artistic expression.
Specialized Field: Modern Dance

11 DESERT DANCE THEATRE
PO Box 25332
Tempe, AZ 85285-5332
Phone: 480-962-4584
Fax: 480-962-4584
e-mail: desertdancetheatre@yahoo.com
Web Site: www.DesertDanceTheatre.com
Management:
  Co-Artistic Director/Company Mgr: Lisa R Chow
Mission: To create and present dance theatre for all ages, providing classes, lecture demonstrations and performances.
Founded: 1979

All listings are in alphabetical order by state, then city, then organization within the city.

Specialized Field: Contemporary Dance Theatre
Notes: 4-10 dancers

12   YUMA BALLET THEATRE
PO Box 1275
Yuma, AZ 85366
Phone: 520-314-1925
Fax: 520-726-5911
e-mail: vscott@digitaldune.net
Web Site: www.yumaballet.org
Management:
    Artistic Co-Director: Jon Cristofori
    Artistic Co-Director: Kathleen Sinclair
    Business Manager: Carmen Feriend
    Technical Director: David Campbell
    Costume: Stephanie Jones
    Sound: Tom French
Mission: To encourage and promote the excellence of dance in Yuma and Arizona by nurturing the highest artistic and moral values in our dancers
Founded: 1979
Specialized Field: Ballet
Status: Non-Professional; Nonprofit; Regional Honor Company
Paid Staff: 40
Income Sources: Regional Dance America; Honor Company
Performs At: Snider Auditorium
Organization Type: Performing; Educational

Arkansas

13   FOUNDATION OF ARTS
115 W Monroe
PO Box 310
Jonesboro, AR 72403-0310
Phone: 870-935-2726
Fax: 870-933-9505
e-mail: foa@insolwwb.net
Web Site: www.insolwwb.net/-foa
Officers:
    Executive Director: Sherri Greuel
    Marketing Director/Box Office: Danita Martin
    Education Director: Lara Shelton
    Technical Director: Brett Kellett
Management:
    Music Director: Dr. Neale King Bartee
    Executive Director: Margaret Peacock
    Education Director: Lara Shelton
    Marketing/Box Office: Danita Martin-Wilkins
Mission: Education, Community Theatre Workshops, Guest Directors, etc. to conduct workshops. Emphasis on youth, but offered to all ages.
Founded: 1978
Paid Staff: 5
Budget: $35,000-$100,000
Income Sources: Box Office; Grants; Private Donation; Class Tuition
Annual Attendance: 25,000
Facility Category: Theatre
Type of Stage: Proscenium
Seating Capacity: 670
Year Built: 1940

Year Remodeled: 2000
Rental Contact: Executive Director Sherri Greuel
Resident Groups: Nea Symphony; Theatre on the Ridge; Act Experience; Jonesboro City Ballet

14   BALLET ARKANSAS
7509 Cantrell Road
Little Rock, AR 72207
Phone: 501-664-9509
Fax: 501-664-9509
Management:
    Executive Director: Philip Quick
    Artistic Director: Oliver Munoz
Mission: To provide for and promote the art of dance throughout the state of Arkansas.
Founded: 1978
Specialized Field: Ballet
Status: Semi-Professional; Nonprofit
Paid Staff: 13
Income Sources: Southwest Regional Ballet Association; National Association for Regional Ballet
Performs At: Robinson Center Music Hall
Organization Type: Performing; Touring; Educational; Sponsoring

California

15   ARTE FLAMENCO DANCE THEATRE
27 W Main Street
Suite B
Alhambra, CA 91801
Phone: 626-458-1234
Fax: 626-458-0113
e-mail: arteflamenco@earthlink.net
Web Site: www.clarita-arteflamenco.com
Management:
    Managing Director: Art Jauregui
Founded: 1990
Specialized Field: Cultural Dance
Status: Nonprofit
Paid Artists: 15

16   ANAHEIM BALLET
280 E Lincoln Avenue
Anaheim, CA 92805-3226
Phone: 714-520-0904
Fax: 714-520-0914
e-mail: anaheimballet@earthlink.net
Web Site: www.anaheimballet.org
Management:
    Director Ballet Master: Lawrence Rosenberg
    Director/Ballet Mistress: Sarma Lapenieks Rosenberg
    Administrator: Stephanie Balmer
Mission: To enlighten and entertain audiences with classically rooted programming and contemporary presentation. Provides quality performances to audiences of balletomanes as well as novice ballet-goers and acts as a haven to talented Southern California artists and as a magnet to international talents.
Founded: 1985
Specialized Field: Ballet

17 CRASH, BURN AND DIE DANCE COMPANY
259 Rio Del Mar Boulevard
Aptos, CA 95003
Phone: 831-688-3371
e-mail: gdzlla@aol.com
Web Site: www.ferrucci.com/crash
Management:
   Artistic Director: Leslie Swaha
Mission: To provide cutting edge dance performances.
Founded: 1982
Specialized Field: Post-modern Dance
Status: Professional; Nonprofit
Organization Type: Performing; Touring
Notes: Live/taped music

18 BAY AREA REPERTORY DANCE COMPANY
University of California
101 Dwinelle Annex
Berkeley, CA 94720-2560
Phone: 510-642-1677
Fax: 510-643-9956
e-mail: dolder@uclink4berkeley.edu
Management:
   Company Manager: Carol Egan
   Artistic Director: Christopher Dolder
   General Manager: Marni Thomas
   Stage Manager: Barbara Codd
Mission: To serve the community through various projects coordinated with arts education programs; to offer young dancers opportunities for performance experience.
Founded: 1970
Specialized Field: Modern
Status: Non-Professional; Nonprofit
Paid Staff: 15
Performs At: Zellerbach Playhouse, UC
Organization Type: Performing; Educational

19 BERKELEY BALLET THEATER
2640 College Avenue
Berkeley, CA 94704
Phone: 510-843-4687
Fax: 510-843-2606
Web Site: ww.berkleyballet.org
Management:
   Art Director: Ann Fisher
Budget: $200,000-$500,000

20 BERKELEY CITY BALLET
1800 Dwight Way
Berkeley, CA 94703
Phone: 510-841-8913
Fax: 510-841-0546
Web Site: www.berkeleycityballet.org
Management:
   Artistic Director: Elizabeth Godfrey
Mission: To provide training in dance and present quality dance performances in the Bay Area.
Founded: 1974
Specialized Field: Ballet
Status: Nonprofit

Performs At: Zellerbach Hall; Berkeley Community Theater
Organization Type: Performing; Educational

21 OMEGA WEST DANCE COMPANY
2838 Grant Street
Berkeley, CA 94703
Phone: 510-540-7227
Fax: 510-540-7254
e-mail: carlart@jong.com
Web Site: www.geocities.com
Management:
   Director: Carla Desola
Mission: Omega West Dance Company is a voice in the sacred dance movement, invoking and serving a vision of hope, healing, peace and community through the embodied spirituality of dance
Specialized Field: Liturgical Dance
Paid Artists: 5

22 SUHAILA DANCE COMPANY & SUHAILA SCLIMPAIR SCHOOL OF DANCE
Landscape Station
PO Box 8612
Berkeley, CA 94707
Phone: 510-526-4344
Fax: 510-526-4344
e-mail: suhalia@earthlink.net
Web Site: www.suhailaa.com
Management:
   Artistic Director: Suhaila Salimpout
   Executive Producer/Manager: Andre Khaury
Paid Staff: 4
Volunteer Staff: 10
Paid Artists: 45
Non-paid Artists: 50

23 DANIEL STEIN
PO Box 677
Blue Lake, CA 95525
Phone: 707-668-1844
Fax: 707-668-5665
e-mail: paupaulu@aol.com
Management:
   Director: Daniel Stein
Founded: 1978
Specialized Field: Performance

24 SHA SHA HIGBY - DANCE IN SCULPTURAL COSTUME
PO Box 152
Bolinas, CA 94924
Phone: 415-868-2409
Fax: 415-868-2409
e-mail: shasha@shashahigby.com
Web Site: www.shashahigby.com
Management:
   Artistic Director: Sha Sha Higby
Founded: 1983
Specialized Field: Dance Puppetry in elaborate sculpured costume
Paid Staff: 1

Volunteer Staff: 3
Paid Artists: 2
Non-paid Artists: 0

25   KARPATOK HUNGARIAN FOLK ENSEMBLE
4377 Park Carona
Calabasas, CA 91302
Phone: 818-363-2219
Fax: 818-363-1349
Management:
    Artist Managment: Mary Beth Treen
    Artistic Director: Janos Zsolt Olah
Mission: To familiarize audiences with the rich and exciting beauty of Hungarian folk dances through performances and concerts.
Founded: 1965
Specialized Field: Folk
Status: Professional; Nonprofit
Organization Type: Performing; Touring; Educational

26   CHANNEL ISLANDS BALLET
1 University Drive
Camarillo, CA 93013-8599
Mailing Address: PO Box 6395, Oxnard, CA. 93030-6395
Phone: 805-384-8558
Fax: 805-384-8559
e-mail: info@ciballet.com
Web Site: www.ciballet.com
Management:
    Artistic Director: Yves de Bouteiller
    Assistant Artistic Director: Kirsten Oakley
Founded: 1979

27   LA DANSERIE
9759 Mason Avenue
Chatsworth, CA 91311
Phone: 818-341-0525
Fax: 818-831-3884
e-mail: momnc@aol.com
Web Site: www.ladanserie.com
Management:
    Artistic Director: Patrick Frantz
    Company Manager: Lisa K Lock
    Artistic Coordinator: Patricia Davis
Mission: Contemporary Ballet Company
Founded: 1997
Paid Staff: 4
Volunteer Staff: 8
Paid Artists: 10
Non-paid Artists: 6

28   BALLET MONTMARTRE
2790 Harbor Boulevard
Suite 210
Costa Mesa, CA 92626
Phone: 714-241-1442
Fax: 714-241-1847
Officers:
    President: Maria Elva Sifuentes
Management:
    Artistic Director: Stela Viorica

Mission: To encourage children in the community to nurture the artistic side of themselves and to enhance the emotional and creative quality of their lives through an understanding and appreciation of dance.
Founded: 1972
Specialized Field: Modern; Ballet; Jazz
Status: Semi-Professional; Nonprofit
Paid Staff: 18
Organization Type: Performing; Resident

29   DUNAJ INTERNATIONAL DANCE ENSEMBLE
2332 Minuet Way
Costa Mesa, CA 92628
Phone: 714-641-7450
Fax: 714-641-7450
e-mail: dancetraditions@msn.com
Officers:
    President: Kenneth J Wenzel
Management:
    Artistic Director: Richard Duree
Mission: Research, reconstruct and perform traditional ethnic dances of Europe and the United States with the purpose of teaching the significance of traditional cultures through dance, costume and music.
Founded: 1978
Specialized Field: Ethnic Dance
Volunteer Staff: 100
Budget: $20,000
Income Sources: Public & Private Grants; Contributions
Affiliations: Folk Dance Federation of California
Annual Attendance: 2,000-5,000

30   WINIFRED R. HARRIS' BETWEEN LINES
5995 S Sepulvena Boulevard
Suite 206
Culver City, CA 90230
Phone: 310-313-1647
e-mail: wrhbl@aol.com
Web Site: www.betweenlines.org
Officers:
    Founder/Artistic Dir./Choreographer: Winifred R Harris
Mission: Multi-cultural contemporary company performing the choreography of Winifred Harris.
Founded: 1991
Specialized Field: Modern Dance

31   SAMAHAN FILIPINO AMERICAN PERFORMING ARTS
1441 Hillsmont Drive
El Cajon, CA 92020
Phone: 619-444-7528
Fax: 619-444-7528
e-mail: lindsay.carter@sdsu.edu
Officers:
    President: Dina B Ellorin
    VP: Violeta Aguilar
    Secretary: Irene Almoite
    Treasurer: Maria Teresa Abalos
Management:
    Executive Director: Lolita D Carter PhD

Artistic Director: Ruby Pearl B Chiong
Music Coordinator: Juanita Caccam
Mission: Dedicated to the preservation, development and presentation of the cultural performing arts of the Philippines.
Founded: 1974
Specialized Field: Ethnic; Folk
Status: Semi-Professional; Nonprofit
Paid Staff: 2
Volunteer Staff: 38
Paid Artists: 29
Income Sources: Grants; Admissions; Individual Contributions; Fundraisers; Classes
Affiliations: San Diego Culture & Dance Alliance
Facility Category: Theaters, informal spaces
Organization Type: Performing; Touring; Educational; Sponsoring

32 REDWOOD CONCERT BALLET

426 F Street
Eureka, CA 95502-0680
Phone: 707-443-4390
e-mail: rcb@reninet.com
Management:
  Director: Virginia L Niekrasz
  Ballet Master/Res Choreographer: Danny Furlong

33 AMERICAN REPERTORY THEATRE BALLET

969-G Edgewater Boulevard
Suite 753
Foster City, CA 94404
Phone: 650-342-4332
Fax: 603-251-5389
e-mail: info@artb.org
Web Site: www.artb.org
Mission: Professional performing arts company
Founded: 1997
Specialized Field: Ballet

34 CENTRAL CALIFORNIA BALLET

1752 W Bullard Avenue
Fresno, CA 93711
Phone: 559-222-3129
Fax: 559-222-1977
e-mail: livelyartsm@aol.com
Web Site: www.livelyartsfoundation.com
Management:
  Artistic Director: Diane K Mosier
Mission: To enhance the San Joaquin valley's cultural life.
Founded: 1988
Specialized Field: Dance; Performing Arts
Volunteer Staff: 35
Paid Artists: 6
Non-paid Artists: 25

35 CHOOKASIAN ARMENIAN CONCERT ENSEMBLE

2511 W Browning Avenue
Fresno, CA 93711-2508

Phone: 559-449-1777
Fax: 559-432-6666
e-mail: chook3@qnis.net
Management:
  Armenian Ensemble Director: John Chookasezian
Mission: To present, promote, and preserve the classical, folkloric, and troubadour songs and dances of Eastern & Western Armenia, to the world, through our traditional Armenian concert programs
Founded: 1995
Specialized Field: Traditional songs and dances of Eastern and historic Western Armenia; played on acoustic instruments indigenous to Armenia
Status: Professional Musicians
Paid Artists: 12

36 FRESNO BALLET

1401 N Wishon
Fresno, CA 93728
Phone: 559-233-2623
Fax: 559-233-2670
Web Site: www.fresnoballet.org
Officers:
  President: Wendy Swenson
Management:
  Artistic Director: Christopher Doyle
  Production Director: Cindy Lindstrom
  Media/Development Director: Shirley Raun
  Ballet Mistress: Francoise Thouveny Doyle
Mission: To produce and present dance and enrich the arts environment of central California.
Founded: 1967
Specialized Field: Classical, Contemporary Ballet
Status: Professional; Nonprofit
Paid Staff: 6
Paid Artists: 6
Performs At: William Saroyan Theatre
Organization Type: Performing; Touring; Educational; Sponsoring

37 JOHN CHOOKASIAN INTERNATIONAL FOLK ENSEMBLE

2511 W Browning Avenue
Fresno, CA 93711-2508
Phone: 559-449-1777
Fax: 559-432-6666
e-mail: chook3@qnis.net
Management:
  Performing Director: John Chookasian
Mission: To promote the folk music, folk dance and folk instruments of the Middle East, including Armenian, Arabic, Greek and Persian traditions. Available for festivals, concerts, and films, etc.
Founded: 1964
Specialized Field: Near and Middle Eastern Music
Status: Professional; Nonprofit
Paid Staff: 12
Paid Artists: 12
Income Sources: Churches; Institutions; Organizations; Individuals; Corporations; Colleges
Annual Attendance: 4,000 - 10,000
Organization Type: Performing; Touring; Educational

38 BACH DANCING AND DYNAMITE SOCIETY GROUP
Mirmar Beach
Half Moon Bay, CA 94018
Mailing Address: PO Box 302, El Granada, CA 94018
Phone: 650-726-4143
Fax: 650-712-0506
e-mail: bachsociety@aol.com
Web Site: www.bachddsoc.org
Management:
   President/Concert Manager: Pete Douglas
   Operations: Jeremy S Foster
   Secretary/Tresurer: Linda Goetz
   Fundraising/Publicity: Viviana Guzman
Mission: To offer classical chamber music and all jazz forms.
Founded: 1964
Specialized Field: Vocal Music; Instrumental Music; Headliner; Jazz
Status: Professional; Nonprofit
Volunteer Staff: 2
Income Sources: Half Moon Bay
Performs At: Douglass Beach House
Organization Type: Presenting

39 DIAVOLO
PO Box 2463
Hollywood, CA 90078
Phone: 310-312-1648
Fax: 310-479-3388
e-mail: LiebermanD@aol.com
Web Site: www.diavolo.org
Officers:
   Chairman: Jordan Peiner
   Secretary: Carmel Boemer
Founded: 1992
Specialized Field: Modern Dance

40 LOLA MONTES & HER SPANISH DANCERS
1529 N Commonwealth Avenue
Hollywood, CA 90027
Phone: 323-664-3288
Fax: 323-663-7742
Management:
   President/Artistic Director: Lola Montes
Mission: To perserve and present the culture of Spain and Hispanic America. The company presents a colorful panorama of performances.
Budget: $40,000-$100,000

41 LULA WASHINGTON DANCE THEATRE
609 Venice Way
Inglewood, CA 90302
Phone: 323-678-6250
Fax: 310-671-4572
e-mail: luladance@aol.com
Officers:
   President: Todd Reznik
Management:
   Executive Director: Erwin Washington
Mission: To explore the Black experience through high-quality dance.

Founded: 1980
Specialized Field: Modern; Jazz; Ethnic; Dance
Status: Professional; Nonprofit
Income Sources: Black Dance Companies Association
Organization Type: Performing; Touring; Educational; Sponsoring

42 BALLET PACIFICA
1824 Kaiser Avenue
Irvine, CA 92614
Phone: 949-851-9930
Fax: 949-851-9974
e-mail: balletpacifica@earthlink.net
Web Site: www.balletpacifica.org
Officers:
   Board President: Janet Ray
   VP: Peter Yeung
   VP: Barbara Kennedy
   Treasurer: Dennis Keith
   Secretary: Gayle Bullock
Management:
   Artistic Director: Molly Lynch
   Conservatory Director: Gillian Finley
   General Manager: Patricia de Luna
   Development Director: Barbara Grady
Mission: To provide entertainment and enhance enjoyment of ballet for all ages.
Founded: 1962
Specialized Field: Ballet
Status: Professional; Nonprofit
Paid Staff: 15
Paid Artists: 15
Budget: $1,000,000
Income Sources: Forum Theatre
Facility Category: Studio
Year Built: 1995
Organization Type: Performing; Touring; Resident

43 ANCIENT FUTURE: #1 NET WORLD MUSIC ENSEMBLE
PO Box 264
Kentfield, CA 94914
Phone: 415-459-1892
e-mail: info@ancient-future.com
Web Site: www.ancient-future.com
Management:
   Music Director: Matt Montfort
Founded: 1978

44 SAPPHIRA
PO Box 264
Kentfield, CA 94914
Phone: 415-459-1892
e-mail: sapphira@ancient-future.com/sapphira.html
Web Site: www.anicent-future.com

45 BODYTALK
3130 Montrose Avenue
Suite 116
La Crescenta, CA 91214

Phone: 818-248-9502
Fax: 818-248-9502
e-mail: lwkearns@bodytalkdance.org
Web Site: www.bodytalkdance.org
Officers:
   Board Member: Christopher Winslow
   Board member: Gail M Kearns
   Board Member: Paul Watson
   Board Member: Joseph Sullivan
Management:
   Artistic Director: Lauren W Kearns
   Company Manager: Sally E Lambert
Mission: Choreographer Lauren Winslow Kearns uses autobiography as a jumping off point to create movement taspestries of full-bodied technique, quiet gesture and athletic partnering; creating emotionally and kinesthetically charged dance metaphors.
Founded: 1999
Specialized Field: Modern Dance/Contemporary
Status: California nonprofit
Paid Staff: 2
Volunteer Staff: 10
Paid Artists: 11
Budget: $25,000
Income Sources: Grants; Ticket Sales; Donations
Type of Stage: Black Box
Seating Capacity: 75-250

46   TOM BOZIGIAN

14615 Greenworth Drive
La Mirade, CA 90638-2918
Phone: 310-941-0845
Fax: 310-941-0845
Specialized Field: Armenian-Lebanese Dance

47   ANTELOPE VALLEY BALLET

2763 W Avenue L
Suite 152
Lancaster, CA 93536
Phone: 661-722-9702
Web Site: www.avballet.com
Officers:
   VP: Dr. Bradford M Boyd
   Secretary: Gina Rossall
   Treasurer: Dr. Mark Mewborne
Management:
   Artistic Director: Kathleen Burnett
   Executive Director: Lara Arnaiz
Mission: To provide dancers from across the Antelope Valley region with professional quality performance opportunities in a company setting. To provide high quality performances locally and regionally, stimulating interest in and appreciation for dance as a performing art. To be a positive force in the cultural climate of the Antelope Valley and the state of California.
Founded: 1998
Specialized Field: Ballet
Status: Nonprofit organization

48   RUTH FENTROY

3959 Manhattan Beach Boulevard
Lawndale, CA 90260

Phone: 310-675-7275
Fax: 310-675-7275
e-mail: rfentroy@worldnet.att.net
Management:
   Principal/Soloist: Ruth Fentroy

49   REGINA KLENJOSKI DANCE COMPANY

1441 E Poinsettia Street
Long Beach, CA 90805
Phone: 562-728-6496
e-mail: rkdance@rkdc.org
Web Site: www.rkdc.org
Management:
   Artistic Director: Regina Klenjoski
Specialized Field: Modern Dance

50   RHAPSODY IN TAPS

4812 Matney Avenue
Long Beach, CA 90807
Phone: 714-838-3318
Fax: 714-838-4660
e-mail: davis7777@aol.com
Web Site: performingarts.net/Shafman/Rhapsody/
Management:
   Administrative Director: Kay L Davis
   Artistic Director: Linda Sohi-Donnell
   Development Consultant: Anne W Smith
Mission: To promote and perform the act of rhythm tap dance while exploring new choreographic directions.
Founded: 1981
Specialized Field: Rhythm Tap with Live Jazz
Status: Nonprofit
Budget: $40,000-$100,000
Organization Type: Performing; Touring

51   AEOLIAN BALLET THEATRE

914 Westwood Boulevard
Suite 250
Los Angeles, CA 90024
Phone: 310-367-6931
e-mail: info@aeolianballet.org
Web Site: www.aeolianballet.org
Officers:
   President: Stephen Penhoet
   Treasurer: Maria Serifica
Management:
   Executive Director: Maria Serafica
Mission: Dedicated to enriching people's lives through the experience of dance. The repertory includes classical to contemporary works from the great masterpieces of Fokine and Petipa to the choreographic experiments of promising unknowns.
Founded: 1996
Specialized Field: Professional Chamber Ballet Company
Status: Nonprofit
Volunteer Staff: 10
Paid Artists: 20

52   AISHA ALI DANCE COMPANY

3270 Kelton Avenue
Los Angeles, CA 90034-3002

Phone: 310-474-4867
Fax: 310-470-0342
e-mail: aisha@aisha-ali.com
Web Site: www.aisha-ali.com
Specialized Field: Dance & Music of the Middle East and North Africa

53 ALBERTO TOLEDANO & LOREEN ARBUS

8075 W Street
Suite 410
Los Angeles, CA 90048
Phone: 323-930-1244
Fax: 323-930-0186
e-mail: tanguero@tanguero.com
Web Site: www.tanguero.com

54 AMAN INTERNATIONAL MUSIC & DANCE ENSEMBLE

2333 Pontius Avenue
Los Angeles, CA 90064
Phone: 310-312-1648
Fax: 310-479-3388
e-mail: libermand@aol.com

55 AMAN INTERNATIONAL MUSIC AND DANCE COMPANY

400 S Main Street
Los Angeles, CA 92701
Phone: 213-626-8297
Fax: 213-620-8896
e-mail: amanex@aol.com
Management:
    Executive Director: RoseAnn Schoof
Mission: The preservation and presentation of America's multicultural heritage as expressed in its music, song and dance.
Founded: 1964
Specialized Field: Ethnic; Folk
Status: Professional; Nonprofit
Budget: $500,000-$1,000,000
Income Sources: Dance California; Dance USA
Organization Type: Performing; Touring; Educational

56 AVAZ INTERNATIONAL DANCE THEATRE

3756 Aloha Street
Los Angeles, CA 90027
Phone: 323-663-2829
Fax: 323-664-9041
e-mail: avazidt@aol.com
Web Site: www.avazinternationaldance.org
Management:
    Booking Agent: Gayle Hook
    Managing Director: Anthony Shay
Mission: Dedicated to preserving and performing the traditional dances and music of the Middle East, North Africa and Central Asia.
Founded: 1977
Specialized Field: Traditional; Contemporary
Status: Professional; Nonprofit
Paid Staff: 2
Paid Artists: 20

Budget: $250,000
Income Sources: Dance USA
Annual Attendance: 20,000
Type of Stage: Proscenium; Arch
Organization Type: Performing; Touring; Educational

57 BALLET FOLKLORICO DE MEXICO

10801 National Boulevard
Suite 220
Los Angeles, CA 90064
Phone: 310-474-4443
Fax: 310-446-9531
e-mail: afriedson@aol.com
Management:
    Chief Officer: Amalia Hernandez
    President: Adam Friedson
Mission: The Ballet Folklorico de Mexico is a reflection of the many kindred souls and spirits that make up the nation of Mexico. Brilliant and hauntingly meditative dances derived from long vanished Indian traditions.
Founded: 1952
Budget: $2,500,000+

58 BETHUNE THEATREDANSE

8033 Sunset Boulevard
Suite 221
Los Angeles, CA 90046
Phone: 323-874-0481
e-mail: ZBethune@aol.com
Web Site: www.bethunetheatredanse.org
Officers:
    President: Richard Sigler
    VP: Zita Rahbar
    Secretary/Treasurer: Jan Kalajian
Management:
    Artistic Director: Zina Bethune
    Administrative Director: Marcy Jacobs Hanigan
    Booking Contact: Rachel Cohen
    Producer: Paula Graber
    Production Associate: Paul Best
Mission: To combine multimedia and dramatic dance to create contemporary theatre art; to utilize stories drawn from screen plays, the literary world and television scripts, involving a broad range of multimedia art forms.
Founded: 1980
Specialized Field: Modern; Ballet; Theatrical Productions
Status: Professional; Nonprofit
Paid Staff: 8
Budget: $100,000-$200,000
Income Sources: Dance Resource Center; Chamber of Commerce
Organization Type: Performing; Touring; Resident; Educational

59 CADENCE ARTS NETWORK

10516 Clarkson Road
Los Angeles, CA 90064
Phone: 310-838-0849
Fax: 310-838-1922
e-mail: cadencearts@aol.com
Web Site: www.dance90210.com/Cadence.html
Management:
    Director: Rachel Cohen

Associate: Lori Perkovich
Mission: Cadence Arts Network is a development, booking, resource and referral network specializing in Dance, New Performance, World Music and Jazz.
Founded: 1989
Specialized Field: Dance; Cirque; World Music; Jazz

60 COLBURN KIDS TAP/L.A.
351 S Virgil Avenue
Los Angeles, CA 90020-1315
Phone: 213-621-2200
Fax: 213-621-2110
e-mail: louisehr@m.zar.use.edu
Web Site: www.usc.edu/dept/dance/p2_lacd.htnl
Management:
Artistic/Managing Director: Louise Reichlin
Artistic Director: Alfred Desio
Mission: To present the work of Louise Reichlin and Alfred Desio, to develop and educate a dance audience and to create performance opportunities in Los Angeles.
Income Sources: Dance Resource Center; Western Alliance of Arts Administrators
Performs At: Bing Theatre at USC; Japan America Theatre
Organization Type: Performing; Touring

61 COLLAGE DANCE THEATRE
2934-1/2 Beverly Glen Circle
Suite 25
Los Angeles, CA 90077
Phone: 818-784-8669
Fax: 818-981-4116
e-mail: duckler@earthlink.net
Web Site: www.collagedancetheatre.org
Officers:
Artistic Director: Heidi Duckler
Administrator: Linda Huggins
Mission: Founded by Artistic Director Heidi Duckler to take contemporary dance out of the studio, off the stage and directly into the community; to develop a new definition for the language of dance informed by environment. Committed to creating art in public, in nontraditional venues, fusing contemporary dance with visual art, theater and music; integrating community experiences with professional performance.
Budget: $100,000
Income Sources: Grants; Fundraising
Annual Attendance: 2,400

62 ELLE JOHNSON DANCE COMPANY
9628 Cresta Drive
Los Angeles, CA 90035-4004
Phone: 310-836-6396
Management:
Artistic Director: Elle Johnson
Specialized Field: Modern Dance
Notes: 6 dancers; music live and taped

63 JANIE GEISER
1938 Commonwealth Avenue
Los Angeles, CA 90027-2808
Phone: 323-906-1734

64 JAPAN AMERICAN COMMUNITY CENTER
244 S San Pedro Street
Los Angeles, CA 90012
Phone: 213-628-2727
Fax: 213-617-8576
e-mail: info@jacc.org
Web Site: www.jacc.org
Management:
Interim Officer: Cora Mirikitani
Director Administration: Victor Wong
Mission: Dedicated to presenting, perpetuating, transmitting and promoting Japanese and Japanese American art and culture to diverse audiences and to providing a center to enhance community programs.
Founded: 1980

65 JAZZ TAP ENSEMBLE
1416 Westwood Boulevard
Suite 207
Los Angeles, CA 90024
Phone: 310-475-4412
Fax: 310-475-4037
e-mail: jtensemble@aol.com
Web Site: www.jazztapensemble.com
Management:
Artistic Director: Lynn Dally
Managing Director: Gayle Hooks
Mission: Performing original tap choreography with live jazz music, the program introduces audiences to rhythm and improvisation and its development in American culture.
Founded: 1979
Specialized Field: Rhythm Tap Dance with live Jazz music
Status: Nonprofit
Paid Staff: 2
Paid Artists: 15
Budget: $200,000-$500,000
Income Sources: Grants; Ticket Sales

66 LORETTA LIVINGSTON AND DANCERS
1318 E Seventh Street
Suite 201
Los Angeles, CA 90021
Phone: 213-627-4684
Fax: 213-627-5875
e-mail: LLDances@aol.com
Web Site: www.LivingstonDance.com
Management:
Managing Director: David Plettner
Artistic Director: Loretta Livingston
Mission: Dedicated to the production of Loretta Livingston's choreography, the maintenance of a touring dance company and to providing educational and outreach programs.
Founded: 1984
Specialized Field: Modern
Status: Professional; Nonprofit
Budget: $200,000-$500,000
Income Sources: Dance/USA
Organization Type: Performing; Touring; Educational

67 LOS ANGELES BALLET
PO Box 712462
Los Angeles, CA 90071-7462
Phone: 213-833-3610
Fax: 714-991-8050
e-mail: aldeneau@netzero.net

68 LOUISE REICHLIN & DANCERS
351 S Virgil Avenue
Los Angeles, CA 90020-1315
Phone: 213-385-1171
Fax: 213-385-1171
e-mail: louisehr@mizar.usc.edu
Web Site: www.usc.edu/Dept/Dance/p2_lacd.html
Management:
    Artistic Director: Louise Reichlin
Mission: To create high quality concert work opportunities for LA artists, to enrich and enlarge an educated dance audience.
Founded: 1979
Specialized Field: Modern Dance
Budget: $40,000-$100,000

69 MAJIKINA HONRYU DANCE COMPANY
1738 Malcom Avenue
Suite 5
Los Angeles, CA 90024-5750
Phone: 310-475-7766
Fax: 310-475-7766
Management:
    Manager: Heather C Matsunaga
    Artistic Director: Aiko Majikina
Founded: 1977
Specialized Field: Classical; Folk; Traditional Dances of Okinaw.

70 NAOMI GOLDBERG/LOS ANGELES MODERN DANCE & BALLET
1110 Bates Avenue
Los Angeles, CA 90029
Phone: 323-663-9130
Fax: 323-663-5474
e-mail: maomigoldberg@msn.com
Management:
    Artistic Director/Choreographer: Naomi Goldberg

71 OBO ADDY'S OKROPONG
10516 Clarkson Road
Los Angeles, CA 90064
Phone: 310-838-1922
Fax: 310-838-1922
Web Site: www.dance90210.com/cadence.html
Management:
    Artistic Director: Obo Addy
Mission: World renowned master drummer of the GA people leads company of drummers and dancers based on the music of Ghana. A prominent member of the first generation of African musicians to bring their traditional and popular music worldwide.

72 RUDY PEREZ/DANCE COMPANY
1721 W Eight Street, Suite 409
PO Box 36614
Los Angeles, CA 90036
Phone: 213-931-3604
Management:
    Artistic Director: Rudy Perez
Mission: To present and produce experimental dance works.
Founded: 1970
Specialized Field: Modern
Status: Professional; Nonprofit
Organization Type: Performing; Touring
Notes: 5-7 dancers; taped music

73 SEN HEA HA
Cadence Arts Network
10516 Clarkson Road
Los Angeles, CA 90064
Phone: 310-838-0849
Fax: 310-838-1922
e-mail: cadencearts@aol.com

74 VALENTINA OUMANSKY DRAMATIC DANCE FOUNDATION
3433 Cahuenga Boulevard W
Los Angeles, CA 90068-1329
Phone: 323-850-9497
Fax: 323-876-9055
e-mail: valentina@dramaticdance.org
Web Site: www.dramaticdance.org
Officers:
    President: Tarumi Inouye
    Executive Treasurer: Karl Inouye
    VP: Susan Pintar
    Secretary: Marinell Dingman
Management:
    Artistic Director: Valentina Oumansky
Mission: To offer a literary based program of performing arts and video production that gives students another view of internalizing what they have already read.
Founded: 1973
Specialized Field: Dramatic dance
Status: Nonprofit
Volunteer Staff: 2
Paid Artists: 5
Budget: $250,000
Income Sources: Workshop; School Programs; Video Tape Productions
Affiliations: Los Angeles County Arts Commission
Facility Category: Studio Theatre
Seating Capacity: 50
Organization Type: Performing; Touring; Resident; Educational

75 VICTORIA MARKS PERFORMANCE COMPANY
11405 Biona Drive
Los Angeles, CA 90066
Phone: 310-636-2757
Fax: 310-636-2757
e-mail: vicmarks1@cs.com
Management:

Artistic Director: Victoria Marks
Mission: To provide a creative vehicle for the choreography of Victoria Marks; to bring the arts to diverse communities and educational situations.
Specialized Field: Modern
Status: Professional; Nonprofit
Budget: $40,000-$100,000
Organization Type: Performing; Touring; Resident; Educational

76 ZAPPED TAPS/ALFRED DESIO
Los Angeles Choreographers & Dancers
351 S Virgil Avenue
Los Angeles, CA 90020-1315
Phone: 213-385-1171
Fax: 213-385-1171
e-mail: louisehr@mizar.usc.edu
Web Site: www.usc.edu/dept/dance/p3_more.html#ZT
Management:
Artistic Director: Alfred Desio
Mission: To create high quality concert work opportunities for LA artists, to enrich and enlarge an educated dance audience.
Founded: 1979
Specialized Field: Tap
Status: Professional; Nonprofit
Income Sources: Dance Resource Center
Organization Type: Performing; Touring

77 CENTRAL WEST BALLET
3125 McHenry Avenue
Suite D
Modesto, CA 95350
Phone: 209-576-8957
Fax: 209-576-1308
e-mail: centralwestb@netscape.net
Web Site: wwww.centralwestballet.com
Management:
General Manager: Alyne Oppenheim
Mission: To offer performing and training opportunities to professionally minded dancers and to introduce balance as a viable art form to community.
Founded: 1987
Specialized Field: Dance
Volunteer Staff: 100
Paid Artists: 2
Non-paid Artists: 40
Budget: $250,000
Income Sources: Ads; Ticket Sales; Fund-Raising; Grants; Donations
Performs At: High school auditorium
Affiliations: Regional Dance America/Pacific
Annual Attendance: 10,000-14,000

78 INLAND PACIFIC BALLET
5050 Arrow Highway
Montclair, CA 91763
Phone: 909-482-1591
Fax: 909-482-1589
e-mail: ipballet@cyberg8t.com
Web Site: www.cyberg8t.cpm/ipballet
Officers:
President: Carl E Trinca
VP: Jim Morgan

Management:
Associate Director: Kevin Myers
Artistic Director: Victoria Koenig
Business Manager: Jerrad Roberts
Marketing Director: Tyrone Baker
Founded: 1994
Paid Staff: 7
Volunteer Staff: 20
Paid Artists: 3
Non-paid Artists: 11
Income Sources: Tickets Sales; Merchandise Contributed Income; Foundation; Corporate; Individual
Annual Attendance: 20,000
Facility Category: Opera House
Type of Stage: Proscenium
Seating Capacity: 2,500
Year Built: 1931
Year Remodeled: 1975
Cost: $600,000

79 LITTLE ANGELS
2029 Verdugo Boulevard
Suite 239
Montrose, CA 91020
Phone: 818-790-2393
Fax: 818-790-2544
e-mail: littleangersusa@aol.com
Management:
Booking Contact: Sunny Charla Asch
Specialized Field: Ethnic Korean Dance

80 UNIVERSAL BALLET
2029 Verdugo Boulevard
Suite 239
Montrose, CA 91020
Phone: 818-790-2393
Fax: 818-790-2544
e-mail: uballetusa@aol.com
Management:
Artistic Director: Oleg Vinogradov
Booking Contact/Associate Director: Sunny Charla Asch
Mission: To present the finest examples of the classical and contemporary ballet repertoire.
Specialized Field: Classical Ballet; Contemporary Ballet
Paid Staff: 50
Paid Artists: 60

81 TANCE DANZ
1512 Lilac Lane
Mountain View, CA 94043
Phone: 415-968-5959
Fax: 415-964-3264
Music Director: Carl Sitton
Public Relations: Cheryl Elliot
Mission: To extend the horizons of dance through arts interaction; to combine multimedia artists of many disciplines with dance.
Founded: 1980
Specialized Field: Modern; Ballet
Status: Professional; Nonprofit
Paid Staff: 5
Income Sources: Dance Action; Dance Bay Area
Performs At: Mt. View Theatre; McKenna Theatre

Organization Type: Performing; Touring
Notes: 8 dancers; taped music

82 AXIS DANCE COMPANY
1428 Alice Streetue
Suite 201
Oakland, CA 94612
Phone: 510-625-0110
Fax: 510-261-7050
e-mail: info@axisgdance
Web Site: www.axisdance.org
Management:
 Co-Director: Judith Smith
 Co-Director: Nicole Richter
Specialized Field: Modern Dance

83 CITICENTRE DANCE THEATRE
1428 Alice Street
Oakland, CA 94612
Phone: 510-451-1230
Fax: 510-451-1238
e-mail: cdftdance.sirius
Web Site: www.citicentredancetheatre.org
Management:
 Advancement Director: Elana Serrano
Mission: To foster heath and spiritual well-being in our community by increasing youth and family participation in African and African-American dance of the Diasporas.

84 DIMENSIONS DANCE THEATER
Alice Arts Center
1428 Alice Street, 3rd Floor
Oakland, CA 94612
Phone: 510-465-3363
Fax: 510-465-3364
e-mail: dimensionsdance@prodigy.net
Web Site: www.dimensionsdance.org
Mission: To create, perform, and teach dance that reflects the historical experiences and contemporary lives of African-Americans, and to promote the knowledge and appreciation of Africa and African dance forms.
Specialized Field: Modern Dance

85 NUBA DANCE THEATRE
1337 E 27th Street
Oakland, CA 94606
Phone: 510-532-4930
Fax: 510-532-4930
e-mail: nuba@earthlink.net
Management:
 Artistic Director: Evelyn Thomas
Founded: 1987
Specialized Field: Modern; Jazz; Ballet Dance Theatre
Paid Staff: 3
Volunteer Staff: 10
Paid Artists: 3
Non-paid Artists: 7
Performs At: Laney Theatre
Annual Attendance: 1050
Facility Category: Theatre; Studio; Mobile Stages
Organization Type: Performing; Touring: Educational
Notes: 11 dancers; multi-ethnic, multi-generational

86 OAKLAND BALLET
Alice Arts Center
1428 Alice Street
Oakland, CA 94612
Phone: 510-452-9288
Fax: 510-452-9557
Web Site: www.oaklandballet.org
Officers:
 President: H Lee Halterman
 VP: Steven Silberblatt
 Treasurer: Nancy Zastrow
 Secretary: Carol Cody
 CFO/COO: Tony Caparelli
Management:
 Marketing Director: Karen Kunzel
 Company Manager: Heidi Landgraf
Mission: Dedicated to the reconstruction, preservation and presentation of ballets from the Diaghilev era, as well as those by American and contemporary choreographers.
Founded: 1965
Specialized Field: Ballet
Status: Professional; Nonprofit
Paid Staff: 7
Volunteer Staff: 50
Paid Artists: 33
Budget: $1,000,000-$2,500,000
Annual Attendance: 42,000
Type of Stage: Proscenium
Seating Capacity: 3,000
Organization Type: Performing; Touring

87 ORCHES
Dancing, Teaching, Healing
530 E 8th Street
Suite 102
Oakland, CA 94606
Phone: 510-832-3835
Fax: 510-832-1102
e-mail: orches@earthlink.net
Web Site: www.guide.artsedeastbay.org
Management:
 Director: Peter Brown
Mission: Focus on dance, and its relationship to the richness of human life on earth.
Specialized Field: Modern Dance
Notes: 2 dancers; live and taped music

88 WING IT! PERFORMANCE ENSEMBLE
2273 Telegraph Avenue
Oakland, CA 94612
Phone: 510-814-9584
Fax: 510-836-3312
e-mail: bodywiz@aol.com
Web Site: www.bodywisdom.org
Founded: 1989
Specialized Field: Modern Improvisational dance; Theater; Song

89 WEST COAST CONSERVATORY BALLET
1014 W Collins
Orange, CA 92667-5537
Phone: 714-639-8525

Management:
    Director: Kristen Olsen Potts

90 DANCE PENINSULA BALLET
PO Box 154
Palos Verdes Estates, CA 90274
Phone: 310-524-4297
Fax: 310-326-7871
e-mail: ocean90710@aol.com
Management:
    Administrative Director: Pam Weiss
    Artistic Advisor: Patricia Stander

91 DON MCLEOD'S BUTOH THEATRE
Fremont Centre Theatre
1000 Fremont Avenue
Pasadena, CA 91030
Phone: 626-441-5977
Fax: 626-441-5976
e-mail: fct@fremontcentretheatre.com
Web Site: www.fremontcentretheatre.com
Management:
    Artistic Director: Don McLeod
Specialized Field: Modern Dance Theatre

92 PASADENA CIVIC BALLET
25 S Sierra Madre Boulevard
Pasadena, CA 91107
Phone: 626-792-0873
Fax: 626-356-0313
e-mail: info@pcballet.com
Web Site: www.pcballet.com
Management:
    Artistic Co-Director: Tania Grafos
    Artistic Co-Director: Diane DeFranco-Brown
    School Director: Zoe Pittokopitis
Mission: Committed to providing a semi-professional ballet experience, performance opportunities for young dancers, study abroad and assistance to those who dance as an avocation.
Founded: 1980
Specialized Field: Modern; Mime; Ballet; Jazz; Character; Hiphop
Status: Semi-Professional; Nonprofit
Paid Staff: 11
Income Sources: Pasadena Arts Council
Performs At: San Gabriel Civic Auditorium
Organization Type: Performing; Educational

93 PASADENA DANCE THEATRE
1985 E Locust Street
Pasadena, CA 91107
Phone: 626-683-3459
Fax: 626-683-3559
e-mail: cyoungpdt@aol.com
Web Site: www.pasadenadance.org
Officers:
    President: Larry Oviatt
    VP: Jean Simmervillo
    Treasurer: Ken Stroud
    Secretary: Abigail Lawerence
Management:
    Artistic Director: Cynthia Young
    Founding Director: Evelyn Lethone

    Music Director: Michael Roberts
    Associate Director: Laurence Blake
Mission: To advance dance through professional performance education and community outreach.
Founded: 1958
Specialized Field: Ballet
Status: Semi-Professional; Nonprofit
Paid Staff: 12
Volunteer Staff: 4
Paid Artists: 2
Non-paid Artists: 20
Income Sources: National Association for Regional Ballet
Organization Type: Performing; Touring; Resident

94 PETALUMA CITY BALLET
Petaluma School of Ballet
PO Box 4534
Petaluma, CA 94955
Phone: 707-762-3972
e-mail: petballet@aol.com
Web Site: www.sonic.net/~lblanc/pcb/
Management:
    Director: Ann Ringstad Derby
    Associate Director: Zoura Tompkins O'Neill

95 CAROLINA LUGO'S BRISAS DE ESPANA FLAMENCO DANCE COMPANY
1040 Pleasant Vally Drive
Pleasant Hill, CA 94523
Phone: 925-939-7850
Fax: 925-939-9773
e-mail: carolinalugo1@msn.com
Web Site: www.geocites.com/vienna/choir/5937

96 NADIA HAVA-ROBBINS
PO Box 990667
Redding, CA 96099
Phone: 530-229-7817
e-mail: turningpoint@snowcrest.net
Web Site: www.romabi.org/dance

97 TRAVELING BOHEMIANS/ROMANO KHELIBEN
PO Box 990667
Redding, CA 96099
Phone: 530-229-7817
e-mail: roma@romani.org
Web Site: www.romani.org/Dance

98 CALIFORNIA RIVERSIDE BALLET THEATRE
3840 Lemon Street
Riverside, CA 92501
Phone: 909-787-7850
Fax: 909-686-1240
e-mail: crballet@hotmail.com
Officers:
    Director: Glend Carhart-Hensly
    Administrator: Kathleen Riker
Management:

Chief Officer: Moira Kamgar
Office Manager: Fred Arens
Artistic Director: Glenda Carhart
Mission: To give young dancers the opportunity to perform in a professional atmosphere and provide high-calibre productions to the community.
Founded: 1968
Specialized Field: Modern; Ballet
Status: Professional; Nonprofit
Paid Staff: 75
Performs At: Landis Auditorium
Organization Type: Performing; Educational; Sponsoring

99 MAGIC CIRCLE REPERTORY THEATER

241 Vernon Street
Roseville, CA 95678
Phone: 916-782-1777
Fax: 916-782-1766
e-mail: bob@mcircle.org
Web Site: www.mcircle.org
Officers:
President: Dave Woolridge
VP: Cindy Nichols-Kitchell
Secretary: Harry Crabb
Treasurer: Ted Parker
Management:
Executive Producer: Robert C Gerould
Artistic Director: Rosemarie Gerould
Administrative Assistant: Teri Heitman
Education Outreach Director: Michelle Pabst
Marketing Director: Kris Hunt
Mission: To offer a high quality, full performing arts center for production and performance in the fields of dance, acting, and music. Additionally, we offer superior education and training of new talent in the areas of acting, dancing, technical support, production, and theatre management skills for all age groups. We will continue to invest in the future of our craft, to grow with the communities surrounding us, and to listen to our patrons.
Founded: 1987
Specialized Field: Live Theater
Budget: $500,000
Income Sources: Ads in the Program; Grants; Donations; Ticket Sales; Concessions; Sponsorships; Workshop Fees; Acting Class Fees
Performs At: Community Theatre
Affiliations: Roseville Theatre
Type of Stage: Proscenium
Seating Capacity: 500
Year Built: 1929
Year Remodeled: 2001
Rental Contact: Executive Director Robert Gerould

100 DALE SCHOLL DANCE/ART

801 41st Street
Sacramento, CA 95819
Phone: 916-451-3732
Fax: 916-451-1790
e-mail: pangeadesign@pacbell.net
Management:
Representative: Joan Liddicoat
Artistic Director: Dale Scholl

Mission: To provide an eclectic mix of theatre and dance.
Founded: 1982
Specialized Field: Modern; Ballet; Jazz; Theatre; Storytelling
Status: Professional; Nonprofit
Income Sources: Sacramento Area Dance Alliance
Organization Type: Performing; Resident

101 LAMBDA PLAYERS

1927 L Street
Sacramento, CA 95814
Phone: 916-442-0185
e-mail: lambdapl@pacbell.net
Web Site: www.lambdaplayers.org
Officers:
President: West Ramsey
Secretary: Maureen Gaynor
VP: Tom Swanner
Business Manager: Charles Peer
Management:
Production Manager: Stephen Abate
Secretary: Gregg Peterson
Business Manager: Charles Peer
Fund Development: West Ramesy
President: Marsha Swayze
VP: Greg Brooks
Affiliations: Sacramento Area Regional Theater Alliance and The League of Sacramento Theaters.

102 PHARES THEATRE BALLET OF SACRAMENTO

4430 Marconi Avenue
Sacramento, CA 95821
Phone: 916-484-1188
e-mail: pharesdance@webtv.net
Management:
Artistic Director: Marguerite Phares
Representative: Nancy Born
Co-Director: Stuart Carroll
Co-Director: Susan Carroll
Founded: 1967
Budget: $40,000-$100,000

103 SACRAMENTO BALLET

1631 K Street
Sacramento, CA 95814-4019
Phone: 916-552-5800
Fax: 916-552-5815
e-mail: info@sacballet.org
Web Site: www.sacballet.org
Officers:
President: John Webre
First VP: Bob Lucas
Second VP: Gina Pernetti
Management:
Arts Management Consultant: Carol Anne Muncaster
Artistic Director: Ron Cunningham
Development/Marketing: Becky Brover
Mission: To present professional performances in a wide range of standard and contemporary ballets in the classical mode to diverse audiences.
Founded: 1956
Specialized Field: Ballet
Status: Professional; Nonprofit

Paid Staff: 11
Volunteer Staff: 2
Paid Artists: 28
Non-paid Artists: 5
Budget: 2.1 million
Income Sources: Ticket Sales; Program Ads; Grants; Contributions
Performs At: Monclavi Center
Affiliations: Dance USA; NSFRE; Regional Dance Pacific America
Annual Attendance: 80,000
Facility Category: Community Center Theatre
Type of Stage: Proscenium
Seating Capacity: 2,426
Organization Type: Performing; Touring; Resident

---

104 CALIFORNIA BALLET COMPANY
4819 Ranson Court
San Diego, CA 92111
Phone: 858-560-6741
Fax: 858-560-0072
e-mail: jstubbs@earthlink.com
Web Site: www.californiaballet.org
Management:
   Director: Maxine Mahon
   Production Manager: Adrian Gonzalez
Mission: To perform, educate, and create new ballets.
Founded: 1967
Specialized Field: Ballet
Status: Semi-Professional; Nonprofit
Budget: $950,000
Income Sources: Membership; Tickets; CAC; San Diego City Commission for Arts and Culture; Sponsors
Performs At: Varies
Organization Type: Performing; Touring; Resident

---

105 CITY BALLET SAN DIEGO
941 Garnet Avenue
PO Box 99072
San Diego, CA 92169
Phone: 858-274-6058
Fax: 858-272-8375
e-mail: info@cityballet.org
Web Site: www.cityballet.org
Officers:
   President: Ann Hall
   VP: Ronald Cole
   Secretary: Susana Pregent
   Treasurer: Helen B Davis
Management:
   Artistic Director: Steven Wistrich
   Resident Choreographer: Elizabeth Wistrich
   Managing Director: JoAnne Emery
Mission: To produce high quality ballet performances as concerts, informal outreach presentations and educational programs.
Founded: 1993
Specialized Field: Ballet
Status: Nonprofit
Paid Staff: 2
Paid Artists: 10
Non-paid Artists: 9
Budget: $400,000
Income Sources: Ticket Sales; Donations
Performs At: Theatre

Annual Attendance: 16,000
Type of Stage: Fly Theatre; Proscenium Stage
Seating Capacity: 1,400

---

106 CIVIC DANCE COMPANY
2125 Park Boulevard
Metro Parks Administration Building
San Diego, CA 92101
Phone: 619-235-1195
Fax: 619-235-1112
Web Site: www.citydancearts.org
Management:
   Dance Specialist: Bonnie Ward
Mission: A performing outlet for the advanced dancers from 32 recreation centers - Rancho Bernardo to San Ysidro. The Civic Dance Company represents the Civic Dance Arts Program for the city of San Diego Park and Recreation Department, which has 2600 students throughout the county.
Founded: 1982
Specialized Field: Dance
Paid Staff: 18
Volunteer Staff: 120
Paid Artists: 4
Non-paid Artists: 40

---

107 MALASHOCK DANCE AND COMPANY
3103 Falcon Street
Suite J
San Diego, CA 92103
Phone: 619-260-1622
Fax: 619-260-1621
e-mail: lkincman@malashockdance.org
Web Site: www.malashockdance.org
Management:
   Artistic Director: John Malashock
   General Manager: Laurie Kincman
   Education/Outreach Director: Nina Malashock
Mission: The creation, production and performance of modern dance choreographed by John Malashock.
Founded: 1988
Specialized Field: Modern
Status: Professional
Paid Staff: 5
Paid Artists: 7-12
Budget: $200,000-$500,000
Income Sources: Government; Foundation; Corporate; Individuals
Affiliations: Dance/USA; SD Performing Arts League; TCG; CA Arts Council Touring Artists
Annual Attendance: 2000
Organization Type: Performing; Touring

---

108 SAN DIEGO DANCE ALLIANCE
625 Broadway
Suite 735
San Diego, CA 92101
Phone: 619-239-9255
Fax: 619-234-5853
e-mail: SDdanceALL@aol.com
Web Site: www.artmedia.com/organizations/sdada/
Officers:
   President: Danah Fayman
   VP: Jean Hellerich

Secretary: Bob Levy
Management:
    Executive Director: Fred Colby
    Development Director: Nadine Buchner
    Public Affairs Director: Albert Rodewald
    Project Director: William Conrow
Mission: To act as a catalyst in the development of dance appreciation in San Diego.
Founded: 1982
Specialized Field: Modern; Ballet; Ethnic
Status: Professional; Nonprofit
Paid Staff: 250
Income Sources: Association of Performing Arts Presenters: California Presenters; Western Alliance of Arts Administrators
Performs At: Spreduls Theatre; Civic Center
Organization Type: Educational; Presenter

109   SAN DIEGO DANCE THEATER

12246 Brickellia Street
San Diego, CA 92129
Phone: 858-484-7791
Fax: 858-822-3016
e-mail: jisaacs@cts.com
Web Site: www.sandiegodancetheater.org
Management:
    Artistic Director: Jean Isaacs
Mission: To create professional modern dance relevant to our geographical region and make it accessible to many people.
Founded: 1972
Specialized Field: Dance
Paid Staff: 3
Volunteer Staff: 10
Paid Artists: 12
Budget: $100,0000-$200,000
Income Sources: Public Grants; Foundations; Individual Donors; Ticket Sales
Annual Attendance: 4,000

110   SUSHI PERFORMANCE & VISUAL ART

320 Eleventh Avenue
San Diego, CA 92101
Phone: 619-235-8466
Fax: 619-235-8552
e-mail: vicki@sushiart.org
Web Site: www.sushiart.org
Management:
    Executive Director: Vicki Wolf
Mission: To present contemporary performance and dance by those artists working in experimental and meaningful form and content, and whose vision embodies the diversity of our rich cultural, ethnic, sexual and personal backgrounds.
Founded: 1980
Specialized Field: Contemporary Performance; Dance; Visual Art
Status: Professional; Nonprofit
Paid Staff: 1
Budget: $200,000
Income Sources: Grants; Individual Donations; Membership; Admissions
Annual Attendance: 4,000 - 6,000
Facility Category: Alternative Loft Space
Organization Type: Performing; Touring; Educational

111   ALONZO KINGS LINES BALLET

50 Oak Street
4th Floor
San Francisco, CA 94102
Phone: 415-863-3040
Fax: 415-863-1180
e-mail: info@linesballet.org
Web Site: www.linesballet.org
Management:
    Artistic Director: Alonzo King
Founded: 1982
Specialized Field: Dance
Paid Staff: 10
Volunteer Staff: 50
Paid Artists: 14
Budget: $1,000,000-$2,500,000

112   AMERICAN INDIAN DANCE THEATRE

2700 15 Avenue
San Francisco, CA 94127
Phone: 415-759-6410
Fax: 415-681-9801
e-mail: lindseyart@aol.com
Web Site: www.napama.org/lidsey.htm
Management:
    Producer: Barbara Schwei
    Artistic Director: Hanay Geiogamah

113   BALLET FOLCLORICO DO BRASIL

Gary Lindsey Artist Services
2700 15th Avenue
San Francisco, CA 94127
Phone: 415-759-6410
Fax: 415-681-9801
e-mail: lindseyart@aol.com
Web Site: www.napama.org/lindsey.htm
Management:
    Artistic Director: Amen Santo

114   BRENDA ANGIEL AERIAL DANCE

2700 15th Avenue
San Francisco, CA 94127
Phone: 415-759-6410
Fax: 415-681-8901
e-mail: lindseyart@aol.com
Web Site: www.napama.org/lindsey.htm
Management:
    Artistic Director: Brenda Angiel

115   CHINESE CULTURAL PRODUCTIONS - LILY CAI CHINESE DANCE COMPANY

Fort Mason Center
Building C-353
San Francisco, CA 94123
Phone: 415-474-4829
Fax: 415-474-1188
e-mail: info@ccpsf.org
Web Site: www.ccpsf.org
Management:
    Artistic Director: Lily Cai
    Executive Director: Gang Situ
    Education Director: Ann Lin

Mission: To promote greater public awareness of Chinese dance and music; to provide original contemporary work that is firmly rooted in Chinese cultural traditions; to challenge American conceptions of traditional Chinese and Chinese American culture; and to encourage our community artists to explore new expression.
Founded: 1989
Specialized Field: Dance
Status: Nonprofit Organization
Paid Staff: 4
Volunteer Staff: 10
Paid Artists: 7

116 CHITRESH DAS DANCE COMPANY
32 Saint Charles Avenue
San Francisco, CA 94132
Phone: 415-499-1601
Fax: 415-479-2724
e-mail: info@kathak.org
Web Site: www.kathak.org
Management:
   Artistic Director: Chitresh Das
Founded: 1980
Specialized Field: Dance
Paid Staff: 6
Volunteer Staff: 25
Paid Artists: 11
Budget: $285,000
Income Sources: Touring; Performances; Tuition

117 CORPUS ACROBATIC THEATRE
2700 15 Avenue
San Francisco, CA 94127
Phone: 415-759-6410
Fax: 415-681-9801
e-mail: lindseyart@aol.com
Web Site: www.napama.org/lindsey.htm

118 DANCE BRIGADE
3140 21st Street
Suite 107
San Francisco, CA 94110
Phone: 415-826-4441
Fax: 415-647-4588
e-mail: kkwickedwitch@yahoo.com
Web Site: www.dancemission.com/brigade/
Management:
   Managing Director: Raquel Lopez
   Artistic Director: Nina Finchter
   Artistic Director: Krissy Keefer
Mission: To expose the widest possible audience to socially-relevant dance.
Founded: 1986
Specialized Field: Modern; Ethnic
Status: Professional
Organization Type: Performing; Touring; Resident; Sponsoring

119 DANCE THROUGH TIME
2700 15 Avenue
San Francisco, CA 94127

Phone: 415-759-6410
Fax: 415-681-9801
e-mail: lindseyart@aol.com
Web Site: www.napama.org/lindsey.htm
Management:
   Executive Director: Lawrence Ewing

120 DANCERS' GROUP
1962 15th Street
San Francisco, CA 94114
Phone: 415-920-9181
Fax: 415-920-9173
Management:
   Director: Wayne Hazzard
Mission: To educate the community regarding dance in particular and the performing arts in general.
Founded: 1982
Specialized Field: Modern; Performance Art
Status: Professional; Semi-Professional; Nonprofessional; Nonprofit
Paid Staff: 2
Volunteer Staff: 5
Income Sources: Dance Bay Area
Organization Type: Performing; Educational; Sponsoring

121 DELLA DAVIDSON DANCE COMPANY
3153 17th Street
Box 328
San Francisco, CA 94110-1332
Phone: 415-553-7796
Fax: 415-553-7796
e-mail: delladance@earthlink.com
Management:
   Artistic Director: Della Davidson
   Executive Director: John Rush
Mission: To produce the original dance theatre work of Della Davidson.
Founded: 1976
Specialized Field: Modern
Status: Professional; Nonprofit
Income Sources: Theatre Artaud
Performs At: Theatre Artaud
Organization Type: Performing; Touring
Notes: 6 dancers; music live and taped

122 IRINA DVOROVENKO
2700 15th Avenue
San Francisco, CA 94127
Phone: 415-759-6410
Fax: 415-681-9801
Toll-free: 800-949-2745
e-mail: LindseyArt@aol.com
Web Site: www.napama.org/lindsey.htm

123 ISADORA DUNCAN DANCE CENTER
741 Lakeview Avenue
San Francisco, CA 94112
Phone: 415-587-0730
e-mail: RosarioVillasana@hotmail.com
Web Site: www.isadoraduncan.org
Management:
   Director: Rosario Villasana-Ruiz
Founded: 1989

Specialized Field: Modern; Historical
Status: Semi-Professional
Paid Staff: 4
Income Sources: Private
Performs At: Isadora Duncan Dance Center
Organization Type: Performing; Touring; Educational

124 JOE GOODE PERFORMANCE GROUP
3221 22nd Street
San Francisco, CA 94110
Phone: 415-648-4848
Fax: 415-648-5401
e-mail: joegoode@dnai.com
Web Site: www.joegoode.org
Management:
    Artistic Director: Joe Goode
Mission: To pierce the veil of toughness that we all have
in our lives and to uncover the vulnerable center, the
confused, flailing human part that we conceal and avoid.
Budget: $200,000-$500,000

125 JOSE GRECO II FLAMENCO DANCE COMPANY
2700 15th Avenue
San Francisco, CA 94127
Phone: 415-759-6410
Fax: 415-681-9801
Toll-free: 800-949-2745
e-mail: LindseyArt@aol.com
Web Site: www.napama.org/Lindsey.htm

126 KHADRA INTERNATIONAL DANCE THEATRE
5809 Mission Street
San Francisco, CA 94112
Phone: 415-337-2914
Fax: 415-337-2916
e-mail: khadrasf@aol.com
Officers:
    President: Deborah Zimmerman
Management:
    Artistic Director: Brooke Byrne
    Music Director: Jay Stebley
    Assistant Director: Lisa Taheosian
Mission: To make a unique artistic statement by drawing
on traditional folk music and dance; to capture the essence
of national character in theatrical presentations.
Founded: 1971
Specialized Field: Ethnic Dance
Status: Semi-Professional; Nonprofit
Paid Staff: 1
Volunteer Staff: 2
Paid Artists: 10
Non-paid Artists: 2
Budget: $40,000-$100,000
Income Sources: State; City; Corporate; Individual
Facility Category: Studio; Office
Type of Stage: Black Box
Stage Dimensions: 16x40
Rental Contact: Brooke Byrne
Organization Type: Performing; Touring; Resident;
Educational; Sponsoring

127 KULINTANG ARTS
474 Faxon Avenue
San Francisco, CA 94112
Phone: 415-239-0249
Fax: 415-239-0249
e-mail: info@kularts.org
Web Site: www.kularts.org
Officers:
    Board President: Francis Wong
    Board Secretary/Treasurer: Leslie Tyler
Management:
    Artistic Director: Alleluia Panis
    Administrator: Molly Barrons
    Graphic Designer: Tina Besa

128 LESLIE FRIEDMAN DANCE
Lively Foundation
2565 Washington Street
San Francisco, CA 94115
Phone: 415-346-8959
Fax: 650-964-6858
Management:
    Artistic Director: Leslie Friedman
Specialized Field: Modern Dance
Notes: 1-7 dancers; music live and taped

129 MARGARET JENKINS DANCE COMPANY
3973 25th Street #A
San Francisco, CA 94114-3812
Phone: 415-826-8399
Fax: 415-826-8392
e-mail: mjdcinc@aol.com
Management:
    Artistic Director: Margaret Jenkins
Mission: To perform the work of choreographer Margaret
Jenkins.
Founded: 1972
Specialized Field: Modern
Status: Professional; Nonprofit
Budget: $500,000-$1,000.000
Income Sources: California Confederation of the Arts;
American Arts Alliance; Dance USA; Dance California;
San Francisco Bay Area Dance Coalition
Performs At: Theatre Artaud; Yerba Buena Center for
the Arts
Organization Type: Performing; Touring; Resident;
Educational
Notes: 9 dancers; live and taped music

130 MASSENKOFF RUSSIAN FOLK FESTIVAL
357 Howth Street
San Francisco, CA 94117
Phone: 415-586-9654
Fax: 415-586-7987
e-mail: RussianFok@aol.com
Web Site:
www.members.aol.com/russianfok/music1/index.
Management:
    Singer/Director: Nikolai Massenkoff
    Artist Representative: Sandra Calvin

Mission: To provide entertainment and expand knowledge of Russian culture and people.
Founded: 1975
Specialized Field: Russian Music; Song; Dance
Facility Category: Flexible
Type of Stage: Flexible
Seating Capacity: 500-50,000

131 MAXIM BELOTSERKOVSKY
2700 15 Avenue
San Francisco, CA 94127
Phone: 415-759-6410
Fax: 415-681-9801
Toll-free: 800-949-2745
e-mail: LindseyArt@aol.com
Web Site: www.napama.org/Lindsey.htm

132 NANCY KARP AND DANCERS
4250 Horton Street, Studio 6
333 Valencia Street,Suite 302
San Francisco, CA 94103
Phone: 510-653-1195
Fax: 510-652-0898
e-mail: nkarp@dnai.com
Web Site: www.nancykarp.org
Management:
    Artistic Director: Nancy Karp
    President/Board of Directors: Lisa Clover
Founded: 1976
Specialized Field: Modern
Status: Professional; Nonprofit
Performs At: Cowell Theater; Theater Artaud
Type of Stage: Proscenium
Organization Type: Performing; Touring
Notes: 7 dancers, taped and live music

133 NATIONAL SONG AND DANCE COMPANY OF MOZAMBIQUE
2700 15 Avenue
San Francisco, CA 94127
Phone: 415-759-6410
Fax: 415-681-9801
Toll-free: 800-949-2745
e-mail: LindseyArt@aol.com
Web Site: www.napama.org/Lindsey.htm
Management:
    Artistic Director: David Abillio

134 NEVA RUSSIAN DANCE ENSEMBLE
2450 Sutter Street
San Francisco, CA 94115
Phone: 415-820-1405
Management:
    Artistic Director: Vladimir Riazantsev
    Business Manager: Michal Myers
Mission: Dedicated to the presentation and preservation of the ethnic character dances indigenous to Northern Russia, the Ukraine and Moldavia.
Founded: 1983
Specialized Field: Ethnic; Folk
Status: Professional; Nonprofit
Paid Staff: 2
Performs At: Russian Center of San Francisco

Organization Type: Performing; Touring; Resident; Educational

135 ODC THEATER
3153 17th Street
San Francisco, CA 94110
Phone: 415-626-6745
Fax: 415-863-9833
e-mail: theater@odcdance.org
Web Site: www.odctheatre.org
Management:
    Director: Andrew Wood
Mission: To develop informed, engaged and committed audiences and to advocate contemporary arts as an essential component to the economic and cultural development of our community.
Founded: 1980
Specialized Field: Dance; World/Ethnic Dance; World and New Music; Theatre; Opera; Poetry
Status: Professional; Nonprofit
Paid Staff: 6
Volunteer Staff: 2
Budget: $300,000
Annual Attendance: 18,000
Facility Category: Studio Theater
Type of Stage: Sprung Wood
Stage Dimensions: 48'x40'
Seating Capacity: 187
Year Built: 1920
Year Remodeled: 1980
Rental Contact: Director Andrew Wood
Organization Type: Performing; Touring; Resident; Educational

136 PURPLE MOON DANCE PROJECT
3543 18th Street #25
San Francisco, CA 94110
Phone: 415-552-1105
Fax: 415-552-0833
e-mail: purplemoondance@aol.com
Web Site: purplemoondance.org
Management:
    Artistic Director: Jill Toqawa
Specialized Field: Modern Dance

137 ROBERT FRIEDMAN PRESENTS
1353 4th Avenue
San Francisco, CA 94122
Phone: 415-759-1992
Fax: 415-759-6663
Toll-free: 800-706-2787
e-mail: info@rfpresents.com
Web Site: www.rfpresents.com
Officers:
    President: Robert Friedman
Founded: 1973

138 ROSA MONTOYA'S SCHOOL OF DANCE
3691 Mission Street
San Francisco, CA 94110-5817
Phone: 415-824-1960
Fax: 415-824-0934
e-mail: rosamonte@pacbell.net
Web Site: www.rosemontoya.com

Management:
  Artistic Director: Rosa Montoya

139 SAN DIEGO BALLET
2700 15th Avenue
San Francisco, CA 94127
Phone: 415-759-6410
Fax: 415-681-9801
Toll-free: 800-949-2745
e-mail: lindseyart@aol.com
Web Site: www.napama.org/lindsey.htm
Management:
  Artistic Director: Robin Morgan
  Associate Director: Thor Sutowski

140 SAN FRANCISCO BALLET
455 Franklin Street
San Francisco, CA 94102
Phone: 415-861-5600
Fax: 415-861-2684
e-mail: sfbmktg@sfballet.org
Web Site: www.sfballet.org
Officers:
  Chairman: Jim Herbert
  Chairman Emeritus: F Warren Hellman
  Vice Chairman: Stacey B Case
  Vice Chairman: James H Herbert, II
  Vice Chairman: Barbara L Rambo
  Secretary: Margaret G Gill
  Treasurer: James D Marver
Management:
  Artistic Director/Choreographer: Helgi Tomasson
  Executive Director: Glenn McCoy
  Development Director: Donna Blakemore
  Finance Director: J Mark Jenkins
  Marketing/Public Relations: Alvin A Henry
  Information Services Director: Steven Kaster
  Production Manager: Peter Butt
Founded: 1933
Specialized Field: Dance
Status: World Class Dance Company
Paid Artists: 69
Budget: 29,000,000
Annual Attendance: 100,000
Facility Category: War Memorial Opera House
Type of Stage: Dance; Opera
Seating Capacity: 3,200
Year Remodeled: 1996
Organization Type: Performing; Touring

141 SAN FRANCISCO ETHNIC DANCE FESTIVAL
Fort Mason
Building D
San Francisco, CA 94123-1382
Phone: 415-474-3914
Fax: 415-474-3922
e-mail: wawstaff@worldartswest.org
Web Site: www.worldartswest.org
Management:
  Executive Director: Sarah Shelley
Specialized Field: Dance; Ethnic
Budget: $60,000-$150,000
Season: June

Affiliations: Palace of Fine Arts
Seating Capacity: 1,000

142 SMUIN BALLET
300 Brannan Street
Suite 407
San Francisco, CA 94107
Phone: 415-495-2234
Fax: 415-495-2317
e-mail: info@smuinballet.org
Web Site: www.smuinballet.org
Management:
  Director: Michael Smuin
  Managing Director: James Kleinmann
  Marketing Director: Quintan Wikswo
Founded: 1994
Specialized Field: Ballet
Budget: $2.1 million
Income Sources: Ticket Sales; Donations

143 SWINGDANCE AMERICA
2700 15th Avenue
San Francisco, CA 94127
Phone: 415-759-6410
Fax: 415-681-9801
e-mail: lindseyart@aol.com
Web Site: www.napama.org/lindsey.htm

144 THEATER ARTAUD
450 Florida Street
499 Alabama Street,Suite 450
San Francisco, CA 94110
Phone: 415-437-2700
Fax: 415-437-2722
e-mail: info@theaterartaud.org
Web Site: www.theaterartaud.org
Officers:
  President: David Green
  Secretary/Treasurer: Sue Le Serere
  Executive Director: Kim Cook
Management:
  Artistic\Executive Director: Kim Cook
  Technical Director: Sean Riley
  Production Manager: David Szlaza
  Office Manager: Donnan Stone
  Technical Assistant: Lyndie Riemann
  House Manager: Kathleen O'Hara
  House Manager: Jennifer Ross
  Box Office: Michelle Mullholland
  Marketing/Publicity: Patrick Redington
Mission: To provide professional, technical and administrative services to performing arts companies; to present, produce and collaborate on productions and provide an expansive alternative performance space.
Specialized Field: Modern; Mime; Ballet; Jazz; Ethnic; Folk; Contemporary Work
Status: Professional
Income Sources: National Performance Network; California Presenters
Organization Type: Performing

145 WORLD ARTS WEST
Building D
Fort Mason Center
San Francisco, CA 94123
Phone: 415-474-3914
Fax: 415-474-3922
e-mail: wawstaff@worldartswest.org
Web Site: www.worldartswest.org
Officers:
  President: Herbert Rosenthal
Management:
  Acting Executive Director: Antigone Trimis
  Artistic Director: David Roche
  Executive Director: Sarah Shelly
Mission: To present and promote ethnic and cultural
diversity through the performance and teaching of world
dance traditions.
Founded: 1978
Specialized Field: Ethnic; Folk
Status: Nonprofit
Income Sources: Dance Bay Area; Association of
Performing Arts Presenters; Dance USA; California
Presenters
Performs At: Palace of Fine Arts; Cowell Theater; Other
Venues
Organization Type: Performing; Resident; Educational;
Sponsoring

146 YAELISA AND CAMINOS FLAMENCOS
Cadence Arts Network
50 Oak Street
4th Floor
San Francisco, CA 94610
Phone: 510-834-8272
Fax: 518-834-8146
e-mail: yaelisa@telocity.com
Web Site: www.caminosflamencos.com
Management:
  Artist Director: Yaelisa
Mission: Dedicated to creating and presenting flamenco
programs with a fresh, contemporary approach; to enrich
and educate the community by presenting innovative
contemporary works which reflect the nuevo flamenco
movement in Spain today.

147 ZACCHO DANCE THEATRE
1777 Yosemite Avenue 330
San Francisco, CA 94124
Phone: 415-822-6744
Fax: 415-822-6745
e-mail: zdt@sirius.com
Web Site: www.zaccho.org
Management:
  Artistic Director: Joanna Haigood
Specialized Field: Modern Dance
Notes: aerial choreography; site specific performance

148 ABHINAYA DANCE COMPANY OF SAN JOSE
476 Park Avenue
San Jose, CA 95110-2617

Phone: 408-993-9231
Fax: 408-277-3862
e-mail: Abhinaya_sj@yahoo.com
Web Site: www.abhinaya.com
Management:
  Artistic Director/Choreographer: Mythili Kumar
Mission: To present classical Indian dance.
Founded: 1981
Specialized Field: Ethnic; Indian
Organization Type: Performing

149 MARGARET WINGROVE DANCE COMPANY
1299 Del Mar Avenue
Suite 100
San Jose, CA 95110
Phone: 408-993-9233
Fax: 408-277-3862
Management:
  Artistic Director: Margaret Wingrove
Specialized Field: Modern Dance
Performs At: San Jose Stage Theater
Notes: 8-12 dancers; taped music

150 SAN JOSE CLEVELAND BALLET
42 Race Street
San Jose, CA 95109-1666
Phone: 408-288-2820
Fax: 408-993-9570
e-mail: ballet@sjcb.org
Web Site: www.sjcb.org
Management:
  Artistic Director: Dennis Nahat

151 SAN JOSE DANCE THEATRE
PO Box 612293
San Jose, CA 95161-2283
Phone: 408-286-9905
Fax: 408-293-0852
e-mail: sjdt@juno.com
Web Site: www.sjdt.org
Management:
  Executive Director: Pamela Stevens

152 PENINSULA BALLET THEATRE
126 Second Avenue, Suite 206
PO Box 1804
San Mateo, CA 94401
Phone: 650-340-9444
Fax: 650-340-9495
e-mail: Marketing@peninsulaballet.org
Web Site: www.peninsulaballet.org
Management:
  Artistic Director: Carlos Carvajal
  Operations Director: Sharon Torrano
  President: Christine Leslie
Mission: To provide the community with the educational
and cultural advantages of a resident ballet company and
to give the artist community roots not available in touring
companies.
Founded: 1967
Specialized Field: Ballet
Status: Professional; Nonprofit

Paid Staff: 3
Volunteer Staff: 75
Paid Artists: 26
Performs At: San Mateo Performing Arts Center
Organization Type: Performing; Resident

153 PERSPECTIVE DANCE THEATRE/RENO BALLET
Peninsula Ballet Theatre School
333 S B Street
PO Box 1804
San Mateo, CA 94401
Phone: 650-340-9444
Fax: 650-340-9495
e-mail: marketing@peninsulaballet.org
Officers:
   President: Christine Leslie
   VP: Carol Schwartz
   Secretary: William U Savage
   Treasurer: Keith Kaiser
Management:
   Artistic Director: Carlo Carvajal
   Music Director: Chris Christenson
Mission: To support and foster a vital arts community in the greater Bay Area through educational outreach and by engaging local art talent in the production and presentation of professional, live dance performances at affordable prices.
Specialized Field: Modern

154 JUNE WATANABE IN COMPANY
87 Mt. Rainier Drive
San Rafael, CA 94903
Phone: 415-499-1928
Fax: 415-499-1928
e-mail: jywaw@aol.com
Web Site: www.junewatanabeincompany.org
Management:
   Artistic Director: June Watanabe

155 MARIN BALLET/CENTER FOR DANCE
100 Elm Street
San Rafael, CA 94901
Phone: 415-453-6705
Fax: 415-453-5894
e-mail: mballet@pacbell.net
Web Site: www.marinballet.org
Management:
   Executive Director: Jane Greene
   Artistic Director: Cynthia Lucas
Mission: To provide excellent dance training and promote the art of dance in the community.
Founded: 1963
Specialized Field: Dance
Status: Nonprofit; Educational
Paid Staff: 6
Paid Artists: 15
Budget: $500,000-$1,000,000

156 AMAN FOLK ENSEMBLE
202 N Broadway
Santa Ana, CA 92701
Phone: 714-836-8006
e-mail: amanex@aol.com
Web Site: www.aman.net
Officers:
   President: Romalyn Tilghman
Management:
   Artistic Director: Barry Glass
   Director: Don Sparks
   Music Director: John Zeretzke
Mission: Features traditional dance and music from around the world in a fast-paced, energetic, contemporary program.
Founded: 1964

157 BETH SOLL & COMPANY
UC Santa Barbara
Dance Division
Santa Barbara, CA 93106
Phone: 805-971-1769
e-mail: soll@humanitas.ucsb.edu
Management:
   Dancer/Choreographer: Beth Soll

158 CHAMBER BALLET
PO Box 1046
Santa Barbara, CA 93102
Phone: 805-564-3568
Fax: 805-564-4282
Management:
   Director: Heidi Robitshek
   Artistic Director: Diane Knowles

159 SANTA BARBARA FESTIVAL BALLET
29 W Calle Laureles
PO Box 2327
Santa Barbara, CA 93105
Phone: 805-560-8883
Fax: 805-966-9521
Management:
   Artistic Director: Michele Rinaldi
   Co-Artistic Director: Denise Rinaldi
   Co-Artistic Director: Michele Anderson

160 STATE STREET BALLET
322-C State Street
Santa Barbara, CA 93101
Phone: 805-965-6066
Fax: 805-965-3590
e-mail: ssbdance@statetreeballet.com
Web Site: www.statestreetballet.com
Management:
   Artistic Director: Rodney Gustafson
Founded: 1994

161 SUMMERDANCE SANTA BARBARA
PO Box 91210
Santa Barbara, CA 93190-1210
Phone: 805-569-0706
Fax: 805-687-5153
e-mail: office@summerdance.com
Web Site: www.summerdance.com
Management:
   Executive Director: Dianne Vapnek

All listings are in alphabetical order by state, then city, then organization within the city.

162 SANTA CLARA BALLET

3086 El Camino Drive
Santa Clara, CA 95051
Phone: 408-247-9178
Fax: 408-248-3997
e-mail: scballet@bigfoot.com
Web Site: www.bigfoot.com/~scballet
Officers:
President: Dennis Mullen
VP: Jose Santos
Secretary: Nicholas Rendon, III
Treasurer: Josefa Villanueva
Management:
Artistic Director: Joesfa Villanueva
Mission: To stimulate and promote interest in ballet as an art form by providing high-quality ballet performances at a reasonable cost to the community. To provide opportunities to local dancers.
Founded: 1973
Specialized Field: Ballet; Jazz
Status: Semi-Professional; Nonprofit
Paid Staff: 3
Volunteer Staff: 5
Paid Artists: 8
Non-paid Artists: 15
Budget: $40,000-$100,000
Income Sources: Partially funded by the City of Santa Clara; memberships; donations; fund-raising
Performs At: Santa Clara Convention Center Theatre
Type of Stage: Wood
Seating Capacity: 607
Organization Type: Performing; Touring; Resident

163 DANCING CAT PRODUCTIONS

PO Box 639
Santa Cruz, CA 95061
Phone: 831-429-5085
Fax: 831-423-7057
e-mail: benc@dancingcat.com
Web Site: www.dancingcat.com
Management:
VP Marketing/Production: Ben Chruchill

164 DR. SCHAFFER AND MR. STERN DANCE ENSEMBLE

PO Box 8055
Santa Cruz, CA 95061-8055
Phone: 831-335-1861
Fax: 831-335-1876
e-mail: schafferkarl@fhda.edu
Web Site: www.schafferstern.org
Management:
Co-Artistic Director: Karl Schaffer
Co-Artistic Director: Erik Stern
Creative Collaborator: Gregg Lizenbery
Mission: Presents the artistic and educational work of Karl Schaffer and Erik Stern.
Founded: 1987
Specialized Field: Modern Dance
Paid Staff: 2
Paid Artists: 5
Income Sources: Grants fee for service; Touring; Donations
Notes: 2-5 dancers; math dance; taped music

165 JANLYN DANCE COMPANY
Great Dance for Kids

141 Shelter Lagoon Drive
Santa Cruz, CA 95060
Phone: 408-425-5951
Fax: 408-255-4114
e-mail: janlyndanc@aol.com
Management:
Artistic Director: Jayne King
Mission: To excite young minds about the world of modern dance.
Founded: 1979
Specialized Field: Modern Dance
Paid Artists: 4
Income Sources: Touring fees
Performs At: Schools
Affiliations: Young audiences of San Jose and Silicon Valley
Notes: Taped music; Great Dance in Space: The Solar Adventure

166 TANDY BEAL AND COMPANY

470 Front Street
Santa Cruz, CA 95060-4535
Phone: 831-429-1324
Fax: 831-429-1352
e-mail: foosbeal@aol.com
Management:
Artistic Director: Tandy Beal
Business Director: Shelly D'amour
Administrative Director: Nancy Matheson
Mission: The performance and production of the choreography of Tandy Beal.
Founded: 1974
Specialized Field: Modern
Status: Professional; Nonprofit
Budget: $500,000-$1,000,000
Income Sources: Dance USA; American Council for the Arts
Performs At: Cabrillo College
Organization Type: Performing; Touring
Notes: 1-12 dancers; taped music

167 ALLAN HANCOCK COLLEGE DANCE DEPARTMENT

800 S College Drive
Santa Maria, CA 93454
Phone: 805-922-6966
Fax: 805-928-7905
Toll-free: 866-354-5242
e-mail: ahcdance@hancock.cc.ca.us
Web Site: hancockcollege.org
Management:
Chairman: Linda Maxwell
Founded: 1967
Paid Staff: 50
Volunteer Staff: 200
Paid Artists: 10
Budget: $40,000-$100,000
Income Sources: Community College Budget; Box Office Receipts
Facility Category: Theater
Type of Stage: Thrust stage
Stage Dimensions: 40' x 40'

Year Built: 1967

---

168 DONNA STERNBERG & DANCERS
911 9th Street
Suite 206
Santa Monica, CA 90403
Phone: 310-260-1198
Fax: 310-260-1198
e-mail: dsdancers@earthlink.net
Web Site: www.dsdancers.com
Officers:
   President: Lynwood Davis
   VP: Michelle Tatum
   Secretary: Chris Bradford
Management:
   Artistic Director: Donna Sternberg
Mission: To develop an appreciation of dance by presenting compelling live performances and educational programs to audiences that are diverse in cultural outlook, economic class, age, ethnic background and gender.
Founded: 1985
Specialized Field: Modern Dance
Paid Staff: 1
Volunteer Staff: 2
Paid Artists: 6
Income Sources: Government Grants; Foundations; Business; Individuals; Ticket Sales; Contracted Performances and Teaching Programs
Notes: 5-6 dancers; music live and taped

---

169 KESHET CHAIM DANCE ENSEMBLE
4155 Dixie Canyon Avenue
Sherman Oaks, CA 91423
Phone: 818-784-0344
Fax: 818-896-1496
e-mail: general_info@kcdancers.org
Web Site: www.kcdancers.org
Management:
   Managing Director: Genie Benson
   Artistic Director: Eytan Avisar

---

170 SANTA CRUZ BALLET THEATRE
2800 S Rodeo Gulch Road
Soquel, CA 95073
Phone: 831-479-1600
Fax: 831-477-1606
e-mail: mclarty@jps.net
Management:
   Co-Artistic Director: Diane McLarty
   Co-Artistic Director: Robert Kelley

---

171 FRANCISCO MARTINEZ DANCE THEATRE
6723 Matilija Avenue
Valley Glen, CA 91405-4818
Phone: 818-988-2192
Fax: 818-988-2192
e-mail: fmdt@flash.net
Web Site: www.flash.net/~daj/fmdt
Management:
   Executive Director: David Allen Jones
   Artistic Director/Booking Manager: Francisco Martinez

Specialized Field: Modern Dance
Budget: $40,000-$100,000
Notes: 7 dancers; taped music

---

172 NESTING DOLLS
805 Venice Boulevard #4
Venice, CA 90291
Phone: 310-822-4836
Fax: 310-822-4836
e-mail: nestingdolls@candydarling.com
Web Site: www.candydarling.com/Nestingdolls
Management:
   Artistic Director/Choreographer: Cid Pearlman
   Theatre/Film Designer: Ron Davis
Specialized Field: Modern Dance

---

173 DIABLO BALLET
PO Box 4700
Walnut Creek, CA 94596
Phone: 925-943-1775
Fax: 925-943-1115
e-mail: diablo@diabloballet.org
Web Site: www.diabloballet.org
Management:
   Artistic Director: Lauren Jonas
   Executive Co-Director: Penelope Siiq
   Executive Co-Director: Carol Streeter
   Marketing Director: Victoria Montes

---

174 DANZA FLORICANTO/USA
4032 S Overcrest Drive
Whittier, CA 90601-1786
Phone: 562-695-3546
Fax: 562-695-3546
e-mail: floricanto@earthlink.net
Web Site: www.ocpac.org/fromthecenter/dance/danza_fl
Management:
   Artistic Director: Gema Sandoval
Founded: 1975

---

175 NAMAH ENSEMBLE
5756 Wallis Lane
PO Box 506
Woodland Hills, CA 91365
Phone: 310-592-7348
Fax: 818-887-7878
e-mail: bayaad@hotmail.com
Web Site: www.namah.net
Management:
   Manager: Maryann Brennen
   Artistic Director: Banafsheh Sayyad
   Composer/Performer: Pejman Hadadi
Mission: To express the ancient within a contemporary form by employing a style between ritual and performance, order and ecstasy, tradition and innovation.
Founded: 1994
Specialized Field: Contemporary Mystical Persian Dance and Music
Paid Staff: 1
Volunteer Staff: 1
Paid Artists: 6

Colorado

176 COLORADO DANCE FESTIVAL
2590 Walnut
Boulder, CO 80302
Mailing Address: PO Box 356, Boulder, CO. 80306
Phone: 303-442-7666
Fax: 303-449-7732
e-mail: colodancefest@earthlink.net
Web Site: www.cdf-dance.org
Officers:
    President: Noel Hefty
Management:
    Artistic Director: Dr. Michelle Hayes
    Program Coordinator: Susie Herman
    Executive Director: Katherine MacDiarmid
Mission: To develop new ideas in the arts through innovative dance and arts presentations, research, and education; to be an incubator for the research and development of new work in the area; to present programming of the highest quality that is inspiring and provocative; to respond to the changing needs of emerging artists.
Founded: 1979
Specialized Field: Multi-Media
Status: Professional; Nonprofit
Budget: $60,000-$150,000
Income Sources: University of Colorado
Season: July - August
Performs At: Boulder Festival Site
Facility Category: Various venues
Seating Capacity: 240 - 2,000
Organization Type: Performing; Touring; Resident; Educational; Sponsoring

177 HELANDER DANCE THEATER
PO Box 18685
Boulder, CO 80308
Phone: 303-473-9438
Fax: 303-449-4614
e-mail: chrissyln@yahoo.com
Management:
    Artistic Director: Danelle Helander
    Administrative Assistant: Chrissy Nelson
Mission: To make a vital contribution to the community through dance as a vehicle for greater understanding, sharing and healing for our local and global communities.
Specialized Field: Modern Dance Theater
Paid Staff: 1
Volunteer Staff: 15
Paid Artists: 10
Non-paid Artists: 3

178 LE CENTRE DU SILENCE MIME SCHOOL
PO Box 1015
Boulder, CO 80306-1015
Phone: 303-661-9271
Fax: 303-604-6046
e-mail: savital@concentric.net
Web Site: www.indranet.com/leds/html
Management:
    Founder/Director: Samuel Avital

Mission: To surpass the normal means of communication offered by the entertainment industry, and society's abuse of the spoken word; to perpetuate and educate in the Art of Silence - MIME.
Founded: 1971
Specialized Field: Mime; Movement Theatre; Masks; Acting

179 COLORADO SPRINGS DANCE THEATRE
7 E Bijou Street
Suite 209
Colorado Springs, CO 80903-1301
Phone: 719-630-7434
Fax: 719-442-2095
e-mail: csdance@sdance.org
Web Site: www.csdance.org
Officers:
    President: Debby Levinson
Management:
    Executive Director: John McLaughlin
Mission: To provide education and cultural enrichment for the region through sponsorship of world class dance companies.
Founded: 1977
Specialized Field: Modern; Ballet; Jazz; Ethnic; Folk; Other Types
Status: Nonprofit
Paid Staff: 3
Income Sources: Donations; Grants; Sponsorships
Annual Attendance: 12,000
Facility Category: Pikes Peak Center
Seating Capacity: 2,000
Year Built: 1977
Rental Contact: Cindy Ballard
Organization Type: Sponsoring

180 BALLET ARTS THEATRE
816 Acoma Street
Denver, CO 80204-4022
Phone: 303-825-7570
Fax: 303-456-1410
e-mail: balletartstheatre@yahoo.com
Management:
    Artistic Director: Paul Noel Fiorino

181 CLEO PARKER ROBINSON DANCE
119 Park Avenue W
Corner of 20th & Washington
Denver, CO 80205
Phone: 303-295-1759
Fax: 303-295-1328
e-mail: info@cleoparkerdance.org
Web Site: www.cleoparkerdance.org
Officers:
    President: Cleo Parker Robinson
    VP: Perry Hooks
    Secretary: Buddy Noel
Management:
    Executive Artistic Director/Founder: Cleo Parker Robinson
    Business Manager: Thomas E Robinson
    Marketing/Communications Director: Alexis Weltman

Booking/Development Manager: Malik Robinson
Lighting/Technical Director: Keith W Rice
Development Director: Erica Robertson
Operations Director: Terrie Bertley
Mission: To provide performances and programs for students, artists, and audiences worldwide, thereby fostering appreciation, access, and the development of new audiences for dance.
Founded: 1970
Specialized Field: Modern
Status: Professional; Nonprofit
Paid Staff: 7
Volunteer Staff: 1
Paid Artists: 18
Non-paid Artists: 0
Budget: $1,000,000-$2,500,000
Income Sources: Ensemble Performances; School; Government; Grants
Performs At: Theatre; 3 Studios
Affiliations: Denver Center for the Performing Arts
Facility Category: Concert Hall; Performance Center
Type of Stage: Proscenium
Seating Capacity: 300
Year Built: 1886
Rental Contact: Operations Director Mary Hart
Organization Type: Performing; Touring; Resident; Educational
Resident Groups: Cleo Parker Robinson Dance Ensemble

182   COLORADO BALLET

1278 Lincoln Street
Denver, CO 80203
Phone: 303-837-8888
Fax: 303-861-7174
e-mail: lindsay@coloradoballet.org
Web Site: www.coloradoballet.com
Management:
   Executive Director: Charles Gardenhire
   CEO/Artistic Director: Martin Fredmann
   Public Relations/Marketing Director: Michael Porto
   Group Sales Manager: Pedro Bernal
   Production Stage Manager: Arthur Espinoza
   Executive Director: Rita Sommers
   PR/Marketing Director: Keri Benell
Mission: To perform, present, tour and educate through classical and contemporary ballet.
Founded: 1951
Opened: 1961
Specialized Field: Ballet
Status: Professional; Nonprofit
Performs At: Denver Auditorium Theatre; Temple Hoyne Buell Theatre
Organization Type: Performing; Touring; Resident; Sponsoring

183   DANCE IN FLIGHT

816 Acoma Street
Denver, CO 80204
Phone: 303-825-7570
Fax: 303-422-1659
Specialized Field: Modern Dance

184   DEAFINITE MOTION

Ballet Arts Theatre
816 Acoma Street
Denver, CO 80204
Phone: 303-825-7570
Fax: 303-422-1659
e-mail: balletartstheat@sprintmail.com
Specialized Field: Modern dance
Notes: Deaf performance company

185   KIM ROBARDS DANCE

821 Acoma Street
Suite A-1
Denver, CO 80204
Phone: 303-825-4847
Fax: 303-825-4846
e-mail: krd@kimrobardsdance.org
Web Site: www.kimrobardsdance.org
Management:
   Artistic Director/CEO: Kim Robards
   Assistant to Director: LaRana Skalicky
   Dir/Promotions/Public Relations: David Sckolnik
Mission: To further inter-cultural understanding and to culturally enrich the lives of people of diverse ages and backgrounds through educating, creating, performing, and broadening the availability of modern dance as a performing art.
Founded: 1987
Specialized Field: Modern Dance
Paid Staff: 6
Volunteer Staff: 30
Paid Artists: 15
Budget: $100,000-$200,000

186   PREMIERE DANCE ARTS COMPANY

714 S Pearl Street
Denver, CO 80209-4213
Phone: 303-722-1206
Management:
   Artistic Director: Gwen Bowen
   Board Chairman: Patricia Sarmir
   Representative: Phyllis Thornburg

187   DAVID TAYLOR DANCE THEATRE

3435 S Inca Street
Suite C
Englewood, CO 80110
Phone: 303-789-2030
Fax: 303-789-2165
e-mail: david@dtdt.org
Web Site: www.dtdt.org
Officers:
   President: Cynthia Vigil
   VP: Jacques Berier
   Secretary: Carl Mack
   Treasurer: Spencer Meier
Management:
   Artistic Director: David Taylor
   Director Operations: Cynthia Vigil
   School Director: Michelle O'Bryan
   Administrative Director: Jackie Nagashina

Mission: To provide and present the highest standards in contemporary ballet performance, technical instruction and educational programs to the state of Colorado and throughout the Rocky Mountain region.
Founded: 1979
Specialized Field: Modern Ballet
Status: Professional; Nonprofit
Paid Staff: 25
Volunteer Staff: 6
Paid Artists: 11
Non-paid Artists: 8
Budget: $600,000
Income Sources: Box Office; Grants; Individual Contributions
Performs At: Lakewood Cultural Center; Town Hall Arts Center; Auditorium Theatre
Annual Attendance: 100,000
Facility Category: Performance
Type of Stage: Proscenium
Stage Dimensions: 44' x 32'
Organization Type: Performing; Educational
Comments: Artist Management: Gary Lindsey Artist Services

188 HANNAH KAHN DANCE COMPANY

4685 S Ogden Street
Englewood, CO 80110
Phone: 303-789-4181
Fax: 303-781-2292
e-mail: kahnhannah@yahoo.com
Web Site: www.youngaudiencescolorado.org/performances/
Officers:
    VP: Hannah Kahn
    President: Virginia Kontnik
Management:
    Artistic Director: Hannah Kahn
Mission: To produce the unique choreography of master teacher and choreographer Hannah Kahn. To educate the public about modern dance.
Founded: 1991
Specialized Field: Modern Dance
Status: Professional
Volunteer Staff: 1
Paid Artists: 10
Non-paid Artists: 1
Budget: $50,000
Income Sources: Grants; Contributions; Box Office; Performance & Teaching Fees; Classes
Annual Attendance: 7,000
Organization Type: Performing; Touring

189 CANYON CONCERT BALLET

1031 Conifer Street #3
Fort Collins, CO 80524-5313
Phone: 970-472-4156
Fax: 970-472-4158
e-mail: info@ccballet.org
Web Site: www.ccballet.org
Officers:
    Administrative Director: Marlys Schlei
Management:
    Artistic Director: Scott Ranagan

Connecticut

190 DANCE CONNECTICUT

224 Farmington Avenue
Hartford, CT 06105
Phone: 860-525-9396
Fax: 860-249-8116
Web Site: www.dancect.com
Officers:
    President: Greg Hughes
    Secretary: Lindsay Bauer
    Treasurer: Shirley Baskett
Management:
    Artistic Co-Director: Perry Lyman
    Artistic Co-Director/School Dir: Enid Lynn
    General Director: Margaret Wood
Mission: To maintain a full-time resident professional dance company and a school for the training of dance teachers and performers.
Founded: 1978
Specialized Field: Modern; Ballet
Status: Professional; Nonprofit
Paid Staff: 12
Income Sources: School of the Hartford Ballet
Performs At: The Bushnell Hall
Organization Type: Performing; Touring; Resident; Educational; Sponsoring

191 WORKS

233 Pearl Street
Hartford, CT 06103
Phone: 860-527-0226
Fax: 860-278-5461
e-mail: wmsdf@dancebase.com
Web Site: www.dancebase.com
Management:
    Artistic Director: Laura Glenn
Mission: To perform and teach via residencies throughout the United States and Europe.

192 DANCES FOR 2

6 Glynn Avenue
Middletown, CT 06457
Phone: 860-346-2210
Fax: 203-782-3596
e-mail: wfeuer@wesleyan.edu
Management:
    Co-Artistic Director: Willie Feuer
    Co-Artistic Director: Susan Matheke
Mission: The performance of duet concerts of modern and ballroom choreography using American composers and master teachers of modern technique, composition and ballroom dance.
Founded: 1979
Specialized Field: Modern; Ballroom; Ragtime
Status: Professional
Income Sources: Educational Center for the Arts; Wesleyan University
Performs At: Arts Hall; Wesleyan University
Organization Type: Performing; Touring; Educational

193 SACRED DANCE GUILD

305 Townsend Avenue
New Haven, CT 06512

Phone: 203-469-4277
Fax: 203-348-7981
e-mail: karen98jos@aol.com
Web Site: www.sacreddanceguild.org
Management:
    Executive Director: Karen Josephson

194 CONSERVATORY OF THE PERFORMING ARTS
79 W Street
New Milford, CT 06776
Phone: 860-354-2978
Fax: 860-350-0221
e-mail: arts@ctconservatory.com
Web Site: www.ctconservatory.com
Officers:
    President: Sarah Jane Chelminski
    VP: Clay Andres
    Treasurer: Jean Howard
    Secretary: Louise Read
Management:
    Executive Director: Kristin Marks
    Music Director: John Shackelford
    Dance Department Chairman: Robert Maiorano
    Theatre Department Chair: Heather McNeil
    Dance Department Co-Chair: Barbara Bravermau
Mission: Offers professional training in dance, music, theatre, and voice with an academic program for grades 7-12.
Founded: 1980
Specialized Field: Dance; Theatre; Music
Paid Staff: 1
Paid Artists: 30
Budget: $400,000
Income Sources: Tuition; Fundraising
Affiliations: Network of Performing Arts Schools
Annual Attendance: 420
Facility Category: Small; Informal
Type of Stage: Black Box
Seating Capacity: 75
Year Built: 1975
Resident Groups: Conservatory School

195 CONNECTICUT BALLET THEATRE
20 Acosta Street
Stamford, CT 06902
Phone: 203-964-1211
Fax: 203-961-1928
Web Site: www.hartnet.org/artsinct/MT_CT_Ballet.html
Management:
    Artistic Director: Brett Raphael
Mission: To offer quality classical and contemporary ballet to Connecticut and New England.
Founded: 1981
Specialized Field: Modern; Ballet
Status: Professional
Performs At: Palace Theatre of the Arts
Organization Type: Performing; Touring; Educational

196 ZIG ZAG BALLET
20 Acosta Street
Stamford, CT 06902

Phone: 203-964-1211
Fax: 203-961-1928
e-mail: zigzagballet@hotmail.com
Web Site: www.connecticutballet.com
Management:
    Director: Brett Raphael
Founded: 1999
Specialized Field: Dance
Paid Staff: 2
Paid Artists: 10
Budget: $250,000
Annual Attendance: 50,000

197 NUTMEG CONSERVATORY FOR THE ARTS
Nutmeg Ballet
58 Main Street
Torrington, CT 06790
Phone: 860-482-4413
Fax: 860-482-7614
e-mail: info@nutmegconservatory.org
Web Site: www.nutmegconservatory.org
Management:
    Artistic Director: Sharon E Dante
    Director/Student Services: Rose Ponte
Mission: To train and provide students with performance opportunities leading to professional careers in dance, music, and related disciplines.
Founded: 1971
Specialized Field: Ballet; Music
Status: Semi-Professional; Nonprofit
Paid Staff: 40
Paid Artists: 15
Budget: $500,000-$1,000,000
Facility Category: Dance/Music Instruction
Year Built: 2001
Organization Type: Performing; Touring; Resident; Educational; Sponsoring

198 MASK MESSENGERS
48 Hardscrabble Road
Warren, CT 06754
Phone: 416-534-8153
Fax: 416-534-1046
e-mail: faustwork@aol.com
Web Site: www.faustwork.com

199 MOMIX
35 Bell Hill Road
Washington Depot, CT 06793
Phone: 860-868-7454
Fax: 860-868-2317
e-mail: momix@snet.net
Web Site: www.momix.com
Management:
    Artistic Director: Moses Pendleton
    Company Manager: Jody Rutherford
Mission: Dance theatre.
Founded: 1980
Specialized Field: Modern; Dancer Illusionists
Status: Professional; Commercial
Budget: $500,000-$1,000,000
Organization Type: Performing; Touring
Notes: 5-8 dancers

200 PILOBOLUS DANCE THEATRE
PO Box 388
Washington Depot, CT 06794
Phone: 860-868-0538
Fax: 860-868-0530
e-mail: info@pilobolus.com
Web Site: www.pilobolus.com/pl.htm
Management:
   Manager: Susan Mandler
   Artistic Co-Director: Robby Barnett
   Artistic Co-Director: Alison Chase
   Artistic Co-Director: Jonathan Wolken
   Artistic Co-Director: Michael Tracy
Founded: 1971
Specialized Field: Modern
Status: Professional; Nonprofit
Performs At: Schubert Performing Arts Center
Organization Type: Performing; Touring; Resident

201 HARTT SCHOOL
University of Hartford
200 Bloomfield Avenue
West Hartford, CT 06117-1599
Phone: 860-768-4465
Fax: 860-768-4441
e-mail: harttadm@hartford.edu du
Web Site: www.hartford.edu/hartt/about/admin.asp
Officers:
   Executive Director: Micheal Yaffe
Management:
   Director of Admissions: Amy Becher
   Assistant Director Admissions: Leila Hawken
Mission: To offer internationally acclaimed conservatory training for musicians, dancers and actors, innovative programs for music and dance educators, and unique studies in Performance Management.
Founded: 1920
Specialized Field: Music; Dance; Theatre

Delaware

202 DELAWARE DANCE COMPANY
211 Newark Shopping Center
Newark, DE 19711
Phone: 302-738-2023
Web Site: www.delawaredance.org/
Officers:
   Administrative Director: Priscilla R Payson
   Secretary: Janan Crouse
   Treasurer: Jennifer Reynolds
Management:
   Artistic Director: Sunshine Webster Latshaw
   Ballet Mistress: Anne Horgan
   Ballet Mistress: Catherine Samardza
   General Manager: Rick Webster
   Artistic Advisor: Camille Izard
Mission: To provide quality dance performances throughout Delaware, Maryland and Pennsylvania while providing a venue for emerging dancers, choreographers and musicians to hone their professional skills.
Founded: 1978
Specialized Field: Modern; Ballet
Status: Professional; Nonprofit

Paid Staff: 30
Performs At: Dickinson Theatre; Delaware Theatre Company
Organization Type: Performing; Touring; Educational

203 MID-ATLANTIC BALLET
201 E Delaware Avenue
PO Box 161
Newark, DE 19715-0161
Phone: 302-266-6362
Fax: 302-661-0666
e-mail: kathleen@artsadcetera
Web Site: www.midatlanticballet.org
Management:
   Artistic Director: Sara T Warner
Founded: 1997

204 RUSSIAN BALLET CENTRE
641 W Newport Pike
Wilmington, DE 19732
Phone: 302-633-1577
Fax: 302-633-1577
Web Site: www.firststateballet.com
Management:
   Director: Kristina Dipple
Founded: 1999
Paid Staff: 3
Volunteer Staff: 12
Paid Artists: 6
Non-paid Artists: 45

District of Columbia

205 AFRICAN HERITAGE DANCERS & DRUMMERS
4018 Minnesota Avenue NE
Washington, DC 20019
Phone: 202-399-5252
Fax: 202-399-5252
e-mail: africanhdd@aol.com
Web Site: www.ahdd.org
Management:
   Managing Director: Melvin Deal

206 ARKA BALLET
PO Box 2098
Washington, DC 20013-2098
Phone: 301-587-6225
Fax: 301-587-6225
Web Site: www.arkaballet.org
Officers:
   President: Roudolf Kharatian
   Treasurer/Program Officer: Tania Chichmanian
   Secretary: Carolyn Wilks
Management:
   Artistic Director: Roudolf Kharatian
Mission: To make dance and the arts of the highest quality accessible to broad and diverse audiences; to nurture, develop and showcase international-level dance talent through inspiring and challenging choreography; to contribute to the continued development of the art of ballet as a form of expression.

Specialized Field: Ballet

207 CAPITOL BALLET COMPANY
1200 Delafield Place NW
Washington, DC 20011
Phone: 202-882-4039
Officers:
    President: Audrey Dickerson
    VP: Shirley Massengale
Founded: 1961
Specialized Field: Ballet
Status: Professional; Nonprofit
Paid Staff: 12
Organization Type: Resident

208 DANA TAI SOON BURGESS & COMPANY
1825 T Street NW
Washington, DC 20009
Phone: 202-588-1884
Fax: 202-588-1884
e-mail: movingforwarddanceco@compuserve.com
Web Site: www.movingforwarddance.com
Management:
    Manager: Jann Darsie
    Director/Founder: Dana Tai Soon Burgess
Specialized Field: Modern Dance

209 DANCE PLACE
3225 Eighth Street NE
Washington, DC 20017
Phone: 202-269-1600
Fax: 202-269-4103
Web Site: www.danceplace.org
Officers:
    Chairman: Kevin McQueen
    Vice Chairman: Rich Bernardi
    President: Alicia Luchowski
Management:
    Executive/Artistic Director: Carla Perlo
    Associate Artistic Director: Deborah Riley
    Public Relations: Sharon Witting
    Box Office: Nicole Pouliot
    Technical Director: Jessica Monchant
    Membership: Amanda Smith
Mission: To improve the quality of life in the Greater
Metropolitan area through the presentation of educational
and cultural programs.
Founded: 1980
Specialized Field: Modern; Ethnic
Status: Professional; Nonprofit
Budget: $800,000
Income Sources: Theater; Studio
Facility Category: Studio/Theatre/Community Center
Type of Stage: Black Box
Seating Capacity: 165
Year Built: 1936
Year Remodeled: 2000
Organization Type: Performing; Touring; Resident;
Educational; Sponsoring

210 DEBORAH RILEY DANCE PROJECTS
3255 8th Street NE
Washington, DC 20017-3502
Phone: 202-269-1600
Fax: 202-269-4103
Management:
    Artistic Director: Deborah Riley
Specialized Field: Modern Dance
Performs At: The Dance Place
Notes: 6 dancers; taped music

211 GALLAUDET DANCE COMPANY
Gallaudet University
800 Florida Avenue NE
Washington, DC 20002
Phone: 202-651-5591
Fax: 202-651-5861
e-mail: sue.gill@gallaudet.edu
Web Site: www.depts.gallaudet.edu/Dance
Management:
    Director: Diane Hottendorf
    Assistant Director: Sue Gill-Doleac
Mission: The Gallaudet Dance Company is a performing
arts group of approximately 15-20 deaf and hard of
hearing dancers. All members of the company are
undergraduate or graduate students at Gallaudet
University. They perform a variety of dance forms such as
jazz, hip-hop, tap, modern dance, and signs combined
with dance. The company has given performances
throughout the United States and abroad.
Specialized Field: Modern Dance and Signs combined
with Dance.
Organization Type: Educational; Performing
Notes: Company includes 15-20 dancers who are deaf or
hard-of-hearing

212 MAIDA WITHERS DANCE CONSTRUCTION COMPANY
800 21st Street NW
Washington, DC 20052
Phone: 202-994-0739
Fax: 202-994-9403
e-mail: withers@gwu.edu
Web Site: http://www.maidadance.com
Management:
    Artistic Director: Maida Withers
Mission: To create original dance works using technology
international collaborations; science/dance/technology.
Most dance works include visual art aspect.
Founded: 1974
Specialized Field: Post Modern Dance; New Media;
Multimedia
Paid Staff: 2
Volunteer Staff: 15
Paid Artists: 10
Budget: $89,000
Income Sources: Box Office; Foundation/Corporation
Support; Individual
Annual Attendance: 2500
Type of Stage: Proscenium & Thrust
Stage Dimensions: 60'x 50'

213 ST. MARK'S DANCE STUDIO
301 A Street SE
Washington, DC 20003-3805
Phone: 202-543-0054
Fax: 202-546-3695
Management:
   Director: Rosetta Brooks
Specialized Field: Modern Dance
Budget: $40,000-$100,000
Performs At: St. Mark's Church
Notes: 8 dancers; taped music

214 WASHINGTON BALLET
3515 Wisconsin Avenue NW
Washington, DC 20016
Phone: 202-362-3606
Fax: 202-362-1311
e-mail: wballet@washingtonballet.org
Web Site: www.washingtonballet.org
Officers:
   President: Kay Kendall
Management:
   Founder: Mary Day
   Executive Director: George Thompson
   Artistic Director: Septime Webre
Mission: To present a unique blend of classical and
contemporary ballet.
Founded: 1976
Specialized Field: Ballet
Status: Professional
Budget: $6 million
Income Sources: Earned; Donations
Performs At: John F Kennedy Center for the Performing
Arts; Warner Theatre
Organization Type: Performing; Touring

Florida

**215 CLASSICAL BALLET SCHOOL OF
VLADIMIR ISSAEV**
2646 Northeast 189th Terrace
Aventura, FL 33180
Phone: 305-935-3232
Fax: 305-935-1035
e-mail: info@classicalballetschool.com
Web Site: www.classicalballetschool.com
Management:
   Director: Vladimir Issaev
   School Manager: Ruby Issaev
Mission: Provide ballet training in the Vaganova Method.
Founded: 1997
Specialized Field: Ballet
Affiliations: Arts Ballet Theatre of Florida
Facility Category: 2,200 Square Feet/2 Studios/Marley
Covered Spring Floors

216 BOCA BALLET THEATRE
5620-B N Federal Highway
Boca Raton, FL 33487

Phone: 561-955-0709
Fax: 561-995-8356
e-mail: mail@bocaballet.org
Web Site: www.bocaballet.org
Management:
   Artistic Co-Director: Dan Guin
   Artistic Co-Director: Jane Tyree
Mission: To provide pre-professional training and
performing experience for local dancers and
choreographers.

217 MOMENTUM DANCE COMPANY
PO Box 331973
Coconut Grove, FL 33233-1973
Phone: 305-858-7002
Fax: 305-577-4521
e-mail: mdanceco@bellsouth.net
Web Site: www.momentumdance.com
Management:
   Artistic Director: Delma Iles
   Assistant Artistic Director: Jonah DelValle
   Rehearsal Mistress: Danella Bedford
Mission: To focus on producing new works, as well as
reconstructing works of historical significance; to act as a
modern dance resource for the community through
educational programs.
Founded: 1982
Specialized Field: Modern; Ballet; Jazz
Status: Professional; Nonprofit
Paid Staff: 2
Paid Artists: 12
Budget: $100,000-$200,000
Income Sources: Dance Umbrella; State Dance
Association of Florida
Organization Type: Performing; Touring; Resident;
Educational

218 GULFCOAST DANCE
2265 Peck Street
Fort Myers, FL 33902-1593
Phone: 941-334-3274
Fax: 941-334-8084
e-mail: picnichut@dr.com
Management:
   Director: Jeanne Bochette
Mission: To serve Southwestern Florida with dance
education and entertainment.
Founded: 1976
Specialized Field: Modern Dance; Ballet; Jazz Dance
Status: Nonprofit
Income Sources: Memberships; Grants; Events
Performs At: Mann Hall; Anderson Theater
Affiliations: Florida Dance Association
Facility Category: Studio Space
Type of Stage: Wood Sprung
Stage Dimensions: 25'x50'
Year Built: 1951
Year Remodeled: 2002
Organization Type: Performing

219 NORTHWEST FLORIDA BALLET
101 Chicago Avenue
PO Box 964
Fort Walton Beach, FL 32549

Phone: 850-664-7787
Fax: 850-664-7787
e-mail: NWFBallet@nwfl.net
Web Site: www.nwfl.net/nwfb
Officers:
   President: Barbara Beck Lord
   President Elect: Robert J Saxer
   Secretary: Judy Williams
   Treasurer: Carrie Wurdeman
Management:
   Artistic Director: Todd Eric Allen
   Assistant Director: Sharon Allen
   Founder: Bernadette Clements
Mission: To perform; to educate the public, as well as dancers; to enrich the cultural environment.
Founded: 1969
Specialized Field: Modern; Ballet; Jazz
Status: Professional; Semi-Professional; Nonprofit
Paid Staff: 12
Budget: $200,000-$500,000
Income Sources: Florida Dance Association
Organization Type: Performing; Touring; Resident; Educational; Sponsoring

220   MORCA DANCE THEATER

1206 NE 3rd Street
Gainsville, FL 98225
Phone: 352-271-8799
Fax: 352-271-0120
e-mail: morca@morca.com
Web Site: www.morca.com

221   BALLET ETUDES

415 W 51st Place
Hialeah, FL 33012
Phone: 305-827-1345
Fax: 305-828-9461
Web Site: aztec.asu.edu/ballet/
Management:
   Artistic Director: Susana Prieto
Mission: To realistically duplicate the experiences of a professional ballet company for serious young dancers. Under the guidance of its professional staff, Ballet Etudes is dedicated to providing the highest quality in dance education.
Founded: 1981
Specialized Field: Ballet
Status: Semi-Professional; Nonprofit
Income Sources: Dance Educators of America
Performs At: Jackie Gleason Theater
Organization Type: Performing; Touring; Educational

222   SCOTT EVANS PRODUCTIONS

PO Box 814028
Hollywood, FL 33081-4028
Phone: 954-963-4449
Fax: 954-967-8890
e-mail: evansprod@aol.com
Web Site: www.theentertainmentmall.com

223   FLORIDA BALLET AT JACKSONVILLE

123 E Forsyth Street
PO Box 4903
Jacksonville, FL 32202

Phone: 904-353-7518
Fax: 904-353-7709
Web Site: www.FloridaBallet.org
Officers:
   President: Leslie H Krieger PhD
   VP: Laurie Picinich-Byrd
   Treasurer: Micheal Kenney
   Secretary: Susan H Adams
Management:
   Artistic Director: Laurie Picinich-Byrd
Mission: To take a contemporary approach to performance of classical guest choreographers' ballet.
Founded: 1978
Specialized Field: Ballet
Status: Professional; Nonprofit
Budget: $40,000-$100,000
Organization Type: Performing; Touring; Resident

224   JACKSONVILLE BALLET THEATRE

10651 Atlantic Circle
Jacksonville, FL 32246
Fax: 904-721-0301
Management:
   Artistic Director: Dulce Anaya
Mission: To develop talent in the community through performance and enhancement of technique, acting ability and audience awareness.
Founded: 1970
Specialized Field: Modern; Ballet; Jazz
Status: Semi-Professional; Nonprofit
Performs At: Civic Auditorium
Organization Type: Performing; Educational

225   DEMETRIUS KLEIN DANCE COMPANY

811 Lake Avenue
Lake Worth, FL 33460
Phone: 561-586-1889
Fax: 561-586-1890
e-mail: klndnc@cs.com
Web Site: www.klein.bigstep.com
Management:
   Artistic Director: Demetrius Klein
   Executive Director: Kathleen Johnson Klein
Mission: To perform the works of Demetrius Klein with a maximum of a nine member performing company and to present modern dance on a local, regional, national and international level.
Founded: 1987
Specialized Field: Dance
Paid Staff: 4
Volunteer Staff: 10
Paid Artists: 10
Budget: $200,000-$500,000
Income Sources: Grants; Earned Income; Donations
Affiliations: Dans USA; Florida Dance Association
Annual Attendance: 10,000
Type of Stage: Sprung
Stage Dimensions: 30'x 40'
Seating Capacity: 500-700

226   FREDDICK BRATCHER & COMPANY

2263 SW 37th Avenue
Penthouse 1
Miami, FL 33145

Phone: 305-448-2021
Fax: 305-445-1412
Web Site: www.cdhfl.org
Officers:
  President: Jolie Cummings
  Chief Administrative Officer: Aaron Morris
  Artistic Director/Choreographer: Freddick Bratcher
Management:
  Managing Director: Maria Lemus
  Artistic Director: Freddick Bratcher
  Choreographer/Co-Dance Master: Gerard Ebitz
Mission: To provide South Florida with high-quality and innovative contemporary dance theater.
Founded: 1980
Specialized Field: Modern; Jazz
Status: Professional; Nonprofit
Performs At: Gusman Center for the Performing Arts
Organization Type: Performing; Touring; Educational

227 MAXIMUM DANCE COMPANY

9220 SW 158th Lane
Miami, FL 33157
Phone: 305-259-9775
Fax: 305-259-3160
Toll-free: 866-629-3262
e-mail: maxdance@att.net
Web Site: www.maximumdancecompany.com
Officers:
  President: Dennis Edwards
  Treasurer: Mark Steinberg
Management:
  Managing Director: Paul Wrong
  Artistic Co-Director: Yanis Pikieris
  Artistic Co-Director: David Palmer
Mission: To create and perform contemporary ballets of high energy passion and drama.
Founded: 1996
Specialized Field: Contemporary ballet
Paid Staff: 3
Paid Artists: 10
Budget: $1,000,000
Income Sources: Grants; Individual Donations; Touring; Ticket Sales

228 MIAMI DANCE THEATRE

10782 SW 133rd Court
SW 24th Street
Miami, FL 33165
Phone: 305-223-0370
Management:
  Co-Artistic Director: Judith Newman
  Co-Artistic Director: Mariana Alvarez-Brake
Mission: Dedicated to maintaining a classical ballet company for serious students ages 9 through 18.
Founded: 1980
Specialized Field: Ballet
Status: Nonprofit
Paid Staff: 27
Income Sources: Southeast Regional Ballet Alliance; Dance Umbrella
Organization Type: Performing

229 FLORIDA DANCE ASSOCIATION

500 71st Street
Suite 3
Miami Beach, FL 33141
Phone: 305-867-7111
Fax: 305-867-7121
Toll-free: 800-252-0808
e-mail: fldance@fldance.org
Web Site: www.fldance.org
Officers:
  President: Libby Patenaude
  President Elect: Patty Phillips
  Treasurer: Roberta Kjelgaard
  Secretary: Ellie Barrett
Management:
  Executive Director: Tom Thielen
  Operations Manager: Bill Doolin
Mission: To encourage excellence, support artistic and cultural diversity in dance, and increase opportunities for all people to experience dance and the arts.
Founded: 1974
Specialized Field: Modern; Ballet; Jazz; Ethnic; Folk
Status: Professional; Nonprofit
Paid Staff: 2
Volunteer Staff: 10
Paid Artists: 40
Budget: $400,000
Affiliations: Dance/USA; National Performance Network; Florida Cultural Alliance; Association of Performing Arts Presenters
Organization Type: Educational; Sponsoring; Service

230 MIAMI CITY BALLET

2200 Liberty Avenue
Miami Beach, FL 33139
Phone: 305-929-7000
Fax: 305-929-7002
e-mail: admin@miamicityballet.org
Web Site: www.miamicityballet.org
Management:
  Executive Director: Edward Villeua
  General Co-Manager: Pam Gardinel
  General Co-Manager: Mark Rosenblum
Mission: Dedicated to maintaining Florida's first fully-professional, major, resident ballet company and providing a variety of performances and outreach services statewide.
Founded: 1985
Specialized Field: Ballet
Status: Professional; Nonprofit
Budget: $8.5 million
Performs At: Dance Studios
Organization Type: Performing; Touring; Resident

231 ORLANDO BALLET

1111 N Orange Avenue
Suite 4
Orlando, FL 32804-6407
Phone: 407-426-1733
Fax: 407-426-1734
Web Site: www.orlandoballet.org
Officers:
  President: Tricia Earl
  Executive VP: Marty Hartley

Management:
    Executive Director: Laraine Frahm
    Marketing Director: Maria De La Roza
    Artistic Director: Fernando Bujones
    School Director: Peter Stark
    Executive Director: David Tompkins
Mission: To deliver dance to every corner of the community, from the schools to the theatres; to share the power and the joy of dance.
Founded: 1974
Specialized Field: Modern; Ballet; Jazz
Status: Professional; Nonprofit
Paid Staff: 53
Paid Artists: 28
Budget: $500,000-$1,000,000
Income Sources: State Dance Association of Florida
Organization Type: Performing; Touring; Sponsoring

---

232   KALEIDOSCOPE AND BALLET THEATRE
400 S Jefferson Street
Pensacola, FL 32501
Phone: 850-432-9546
Management:
    Artistic Co-Director: Judy Gomez
    Artistic Co-Director: Debbie Parrish
    Associate Co-Director: Patsy Hill
    Associate Co-Director: Nannette Whidby
Mission: To offer quality training and performing opportunities in classical ballet and modern dance for students in elementary through high school.
Founded: 1978
Specialized Field: Modern; Ballet
Status: Non-Professional; Nonprofit
Income Sources: Pensacola Dance Alliance
Organization Type: Performing; Resident; Educational

---

233   SARASOTA BALLET OF FLORIDA
5555 S Tamiami Trail
Sarasota, FL 34243-2141
Phone: 941-359-0099
Fax: 941-358-1504
Toll-free: 800-361-8388
e-mail: sarasotaballet@asolo.org
Web Site: www.sarasotaballet.org
Officers:
    President: Charles Knowles
    First VP: Daniel Kane
    Secretary: Diane L Muir
    Treasurer: C William Myers
Management:
    Artistic Director/CEO: Robert de Warren
    Operations Director: Jaime Roque
    Principal Ballet Master: Pavel Fomin
    Marketing Manager: Mary Elle Hunterov
Mission: To be committed to artistic excellence through the presentation of the highest quality of classical and contemporary dance, through the encouragement of choreographic talent, through the ongoing expansion of education programs and opportunities for community outreach and service, and through the participation in joint ventures with other regional arts organizations and dance companies.
Founded: 1990

Specialized Field: Professional Ballet
Paid Staff: 24
Volunteer Staff: 10
Paid Artists: 28
Budget: $2,500,000
Income Sources: Ticket Sales; Foundation and Corporate Grants; Individual Donations
Performs At: Van Wezel Performing Arts Hall; FSU Center for the Performing Arts
Affiliations: Sarasota Ballet Association
Annual Attendance: 35,000
Seating Capacity: 1700 and 500

---

234   THOMAS ARMOUR YOUTH BALLET
5818 SW 73rd Street
South Miami, FL 33143
Phone: 305-667-5985
Fax: 305-667-1024
e-mail: taballet@aol
Management:
    Artistic Co-Director: Thomas Armour
    Artistic Co-Director: Ruth Wiesen
Mission: To help young people enjoy and learn ballet prior to professional experience.
Founded: 1951
Specialized Field: Ballet
Status: Non-Professional; Nonprofit
Paid Staff: 30
Budget: $119,000
Income Sources: Private; Foundations; Corporate and Government
Performs At: Dade County Auditorium and Public Schools
Annual Attendance: 9,000
Organization Type: Performing; Resident

---

235   ST PETERSBURG CONCERT BALLET
2914 First Avenue N
St Petersburg, FL 33707
Phone: 727-327-4401
e-mail: nikolai@gte.net
Web Site: www.academyof balletarts.org
Management:
    Artistic Director: Suzanne Pomerantzeff
    Ballet Master: Sean Musselman
Mission: Provides serious dancers with an opportunity to perform professional level repertoire.
Founded: 1967
Specialized Field: Dance
Paid Staff: 3
Volunteer Staff: 6
Non-paid Artists: 15

---

236   LYNDA DAVIS
1716 Silverwood Court
Tallahassee, FL 32301
Phone: 850-877-4404
Fax: 850-644-1273
e-mail: idavis@garnet.acns.fsu.edu

---

237   TALLAHASSEE BALLET COMPANY
218 E Third Avenue
PO Box 772
Tallahassee, FL 32302

Phone: 850-222-1287
Fax: 850-224-7681
e-mail: tballet@unr.net
Web Site: www.tallaballet.com
Management:
   Artistic Director: Joyce Straub
   Associate Director: Kathryn Cashin
Mission: Nonprofit dance company which provides an outstanding training ground for emerging professionals while stimulating appreciation of the dance arts through quality productions of classical and contemporary works.
Founded: 1972
Specialized Field: Ballet
Status: Nonprofit
Paid Staff: 4
Volunteer Staff: 5
Non-paid Artists: 55
Budget: $200,000-$500,000
Affiliations: Florida Dance Association
Annual Attendance: 7,000-10,000
Organization Type: Performing; Resident; Educational

238   ACANTHUS DANCE

3524 W Paul Avenue
Tampa, FL 33611-3626
Phone: 813-835-1066
Fax: 813-253-7775
Management:
   Artistic Director: Richard Allan Ploch

239   FIRETHORN

10630 N 56th Street
Suite 211
Temple Terrace, FL 33617
Phone: 813-985-2555
Fax: 813-985-2555
Management:
   Director: Lucia Corsiglia Hatcher
Specialized Field: Modern Dance
Notes: 10 dancers; taped music

240   BALLET FLORIDA

500 Fern Street
West Palm Beach, FL 33401-5726
Phone: 561-659-1212
Fax: 561-659-2222
e-mail: admin@BalletFlorida.com
Web Site: WWW.BalletFlorida.com
Management:
   Artistic Director: Marie Hale
   Executive Director: A Harrison Cromer, Jr
Mission: The attainment of a dynamic synthesis of the aspiration of dancers, choreographers, and audiences through challenging all three of these components.
Founded: 1973
Specialized Field: Ballet
Status: Professional; Nonprofit
Budget: $2,500,000
Income Sources: Dance/USA
Organization Type: Performing; Touring; Resident; Educational

Georgia

241   ATHENS BALLET THEATRE
Athens School of Ballet
126 Barrington Drive
Athens, GA 30605
Phone: 706-353-2082
Web Site: www.itown.com/athens/abt/index.html
Officers:
   President: Ted Baumgartner
   VP: Randy Kemphouse
   Treasurer: Kathy Whitaker
Management:
   Artistic Director: Mary Ann Hale
Mission: To offer serious dance students an opportunity to further their training in a professional atmosphere.
Founded: 1973
Specialized Field: Ballet
Status: Nonprofit
Paid Staff: 23
Income Sources: Georgia Council of the Arts
Performs At: Athens School of Ballet
Facility Category: Civic center
Organization Type: Performing

242   CORE CONCERT DANCE COMPANY
Department of Dance
University of Georgia
Athens, GA 30602
Phone: 706-542-4415
Fax: 706-542-4084
e-mail: dance@coe.uga.edu
Web Site: www.coe.uga.edu/Dance//Companies/Core
Management:
   Artistic Director: Bala Sarasvati
Founded: 1991
Specialized Field: Modern Dance

243   UGA BALLET ENSEMBLE
University of Georgia
Department of Dance, Dance Building
Athens, GA 30602
Phone: 404-762-1416
Fax: 706-542-4084
e-mail: bsarasva@coe.uga.edu
Web Site: http://www.franklin.uga.edu
Management:
   Artistic Co-Director: Joan Buttram
   Artistic Co-Director: Bala Saravati
Founded: 1993
Income Sources: UGA Foundation; Student Activities; Grant Support

244   ATLANTA BALLET
1400 W Peachtree Street NW
Atlanta, GA 30309
Phone: 404-873-5811
Fax: 404-874-7905
e-mail: tckholm@atlantaballet.com
Web Site: www.atlantaballet.com
Officers:
   Chairman: Sam Moss
Management:
   Executive Director: Terrie Rouse

Artistic Director: John McFall
General Manager: Mark Komdat
Marketing Director: Tricia Ekholm
Mission: To provide professional ballet performances for the people of metropolitan Atlanta and the surrounding area.
Founded: 1929
Specialized Field: Ballet
Status: Professional; Nonprofit
Paid Staff: 27
Paid Artists: 45
Budget: $6,659,609
Income Sources: Dance USA; National Association for Regional Ballet
Performs At: Fabulous Fox Theatre
Annual Attendance: 75,000
Facility Category: Theatre
Seating Capacity: 4,500
Year Built: 1929
Year Remodeled: 1996
Rental Contact: Gene Conroy
Organization Type: Performing; Touring; Resident

245 BADU DANCE/HAKPOLOG DANCE INITIATIVE

PO Box 18504
Atlanta, GA 31126
Phone: 404-388-1271
Fax: 404-816-5556
e-mail: yawakwesi@aol.com, orhakpoloo1@aol.com
Officers:
  President: Menilyn T Herrick
  Secretary: Maria Garcia
Management:
  Artistic Director: Zelma Badu-Younge
Specialized Field: Modern Dance
Volunteer Staff: 3
Non-paid Artists: 3
Income Sources: Fund Raisers

246 BALLETHNIC DANCE COMPANY

2587 Cheney Street
PO Box 7749
Atlanta, GA 30344-3118
Phone: 404-765-1416
Fax: 404-762-6319
e-mail: ballethnic@mindspring.com
Web Site: www.ballethnic.org
Management:
  Co-Director: Nena Gilreath
  Co-Director: Waverly Lucas
Mission: To involve the community, especially youth and those who are financially less advantaged, in an appreciation of our unique art form.
Founded: 1990
Paid Staff: 4
Volunteer Staff: 8
Paid Artists: 9
Non-paid Artists: 7

247 BEACON DANCE COMPANY

410 W Trinity Place
Atlanta, GA 30030
Phone: 404-377-2929
Fax: 404-377-2929
Web Site: www.beacondance.org
Management:
  Artistic Director: D Patton White
Founded: 1952
Specialized Field: Modern; Ballet; Jazz
Status: Semi-Professional; Nonprofit
Paid Staff: 14
Organization Type: Performing; Educational

248 DANCERS COLLECTIVE OF ATLANTA

931 Monroe Drive
Suite 102
Atlanta, GA 30308
Phone: 404-233-7600
Fax: 404-873-3128
Web Site: www.dancerscollective.org

249 DANCING ON COMMON GROUND

PO Box 88674
Atlanta, GA 30338
Phone: 770-454-9654
Fax: 770-457-1825
e-mail: top@america.net
Web Site: www.topentertainment.com
Management:
  Managing Partner: Lorraine Rennie

250 FULL RADIUS DANCE

PO Box 54453
Atlanta, GA 30308
Phone: 404-724-9663
Fax: 404-724-9663
e-mail: dsdance@aol.com
Web Site: www.fullradiusdance.org
Officers:
  Chairman: Joffrey Scott Suprina
  Secretary: Rife Hughey
  Treasurer: Betty Bates
Management:
  Artistic/Executive Director: Douglas Scott
Specialized Field: Modern Dance

251 CHARNE FURCRON
Beacon Dance

PO Box 1553
Decatur, GA 30031-1553
Phone: 404-377-2929
Fax: 404-377-2929
e-mail: patton@beacondance.org
Web Site: www.beacondance.org

252 SEVERAL DANCERS CORE

PO Box 2045
Decatur, GA 30031-2045
Phone: 404-373-4154
Fax: 404-377-1815
e-mail: sdcinfo@mindspring.com
Web Site: www.severaldancerscore.org
Management:
  Artistic and Executive Director: Sue Schroeder

Mission: To create, present and produce contemporary dance.
Founded: 1980
Specialized Field: Dance
Paid Staff: 3
Volunteer Staff: 2
Paid Artists: 8
Non-paid Artists: 0
Budget: $270,000
Affiliations: The Field
Facility Category: Studio Theater

253 ROSALEE SHORTER
Baecon Dance
PO Box 1553
Devatur, GA 30031-1533
Phone: 404-377-2929
Fax: 404-377-2929
e-mail: patton@beacondance.org
Web Site: www.beacondance.org

254 GAINESVILLE BALLET
PO Box 1663
Gainesville, GA 30503
Phone: 770-532-4241
Fax: 770-534-8995
Web Site: www.gainesvilleballettheatre.org
Officers:
   President: Anne Gress
Management:
   Artistic Director: Judy Benton
   Managing Director: Victoria Burke
Mission: To further the cause of dance artistry in Northeast Georgia through productions of classical, neoclassical, jazz and modern dance.
Founded: 1974
Specialized Field: Modern; Ballet; Jazz
Status: Non-Professional; Nonprofit
Paid Staff: 35
Income Sources: Dance Coalition of Metro Atlanta; Southeast Regional Ballet Association
Performs At: Pearce Auditorium
Organization Type: Performing; Educational; Sponsoring

255 LAGRANGE BALLET
Music In Motion
241 Creek Ridge Drive
LaGrange, GA 30240-7726
Phone: 706-882-9085
e-mail: nanzdanz@charter.com
Management:
   Artistic Director: Nancy Theusen Gell
Mission: To enrich young lives through the art of dance.
Specialized Field: Contemporary Ballet, Jazz, Modern Dance, Musical Theater, Opera
Season: Georgia Summer Dance Conservatory - 3 weeks in July

256 THEATRE PLUS
Music in Motion Dance Company
241 Creek Ridge Drive Road
Lagrange, GA 30240

Phone: 706-882-9085
Fax: 607-257-9196
Toll-free: 877-646-3262
e-mail: nanzdanz@charter.net
Web Site: www.musicinmotion.com
Officers:
   President: Mary Ellis
   Director: Beth Hudson
Management:
   Artistic Director: Nancy Thuesen Gell
Mission: Music in Motion offers all types of dance presentation services including choreography, production staging, and instruction for classical and contemporary ballet, jazz, modern dance, musical theater and opera.

257 GEORGIA BALLET
31 Atlanta Street
3rd Floor
Marietta, GA 30060
Phone: 770-425-0258
Fax: 770-499-2144
e-mail: info@georgiaballet.org
Web Site: www.georgiaballet.simplenet.com
Officers:
   Business Director: Susan Laubacher
   School Director: Michele Ziemann-DeVos
   Development Director: Jennifer Truitt
   Administrative Assistant: Hollie Hittinger
Management:
   Artistic Director: Iris Hensley
   Ballet Master: Janusz Mazon
   Ballet Mistress: Gina Hyatt Mazon
Mission: Dedicated to promoting excellence in ballet performance and training, fostering an increased public awareness and appreciation for dance, and providing dedicated and talented dacers with the opportunity for advanced training and professional preforming venues.
Status: Nonprofit

258 PEGALOMANIA MOLLOY
2991 Black Bear Drive SE
PO Box 550151
Marietta, GA 30067-5789
Phone: 770-937-0187
Fax: 707-988-8983
e-mail: pegalomania@webmailbesssouth.net
Management:
   Artistic Director: Peggy Molloy

259 RUTH MITCHELL DANCE COMPANY
81 Church Street
Marietta, GA 30060
Phone: 770-426-0007
e-mail: thetoups@ix.netcom.com
Web Site: www.ruthmitchelldance.com
Officers:
   President: Sandra Ratchford
   VP: Courtney Kennedy
   Treasurer: Carmen Dillard
   President of the Guild: Judy Freeman
Management:
   Artistic Director: Ruth Mitchell
   Production Manager: Courtney Kennedy

Mission: To provide the community with a small, eclectic company to perform in places not suited for large ballet companies.
Founded: 1956
Specialized Field: Modern; Ballet; Jazz
Status: Professional; Nonprofit
Income Sources: National Association for Regional Ballet; Dance Coalition of Atlanta; Young Audiences of Atlanta
Organization Type: Performing; Touring

260   FESTIVAL BALLET COMPANY
416 Eagle's Landing Parkway
Stockbridge, GA 30281
Phone: 770-507-2775
Fax: 770-507-9182
e-mail: fbcatl@aol.com
Web Site: www.festivalballetatlanta.com
Management:
    Artistic Co-Director: Gregory Aaron
    Artistic Co-Director: Nicolas Pacana
    Company Manager: Allison Hannay
Mission: To thrill and move our audience, dancers, choreographers, students, supporters and staff with art and discipline; to enrich and inspire lives.
Founded: 1989
Paid Staff: 12
Volunteer Staff: 12
Paid Artists: 19
Non-paid Artists: 12
Budget: $ 300,000
Income Sources: Partners in Education; Grants; Donations; Ticket Sales
Affiliations: Clayton County Schools; Henry County Schools
Annual Attendance: 20,000

261   MYSTICAL ARTS OF TIBET
2092 Vista Center
Tucker, GA 30324
Phone: 404-716-5635
e-mail: mystical@drepung.org
Web Site: www.mysticalartsoftibet.org
Management:
    Director: Lobsang Tenzin
    Assistant Director: Irene S Lee
Mission: Program brings the ancient sacred visual and performing arts of Tibet of the West through the creation of Mandala Sand Painting exhibition and Sacred Music Sacred Dance Performance for world healing.
Founded: 1991

262   JAZZ DANCE THEATRE SOUTH
715 Parkside Drive
Woodstock, GA 30188-6057
Phone: 770-516-7229
Fax: 770-516-7229
Management:
    Artistic Director: Marcus R Alford
Mission: To provide performances, classes and lecture demonstrations that educate regarding jazz dance.
Founded: 1986
Specialized Field: Jazz
Status: Professional

Paid Staff: 4
Non-paid Artists: 12
Income Sources: Box Office; Tuition
Performs At: Cobb County Civic Center, Southern Polytechnic University
Organization Type: Performing; Touring; Resident; Educational

Hawaii

263   HAWAII STATE BALLET
1418 Kapiolani Boulevard
Honolulu, HI 96814
Phone: 808-947-2755
Web Site: www.hawaiistateballet.com
Officers:
    Assistant Director: Georgina Surles
    Director: John Landovsky
Management:
    Artistic Director: John Landovsky
Mission: The School's curriculum is designed to provide the highest standard of excellence in classical training.
Founded: 1983
Specialized Field: Ballet
Status: Professional; Nonprofit
Budget: $100,000
Income Sources: Ticket Sales
Performs At: Mamiya Theater
Type of Stage: Proscenium
Seating Capacity: 500
Organization Type: Touring; Resident

264   MEN DANCING-GREGG LIZENBERY DANCE PIONEERS
2101 Nuuanu
Suite 904
Honolulu, HI 96817
Phone: 808-533-2185
Fax: 808-942-9440
e-mail: lgreg@hawaii.edu
Management:
    Artist Representative: Marilyn Cristofori
Budget: $40,000-$100,000

Idaho

265   BALLET IDAHO
Esther Simplot Performing Arts Academy
501 S 8th Street, Suite A
Boise, ID 83702
Phone: 208-343-0556
Fax: 208-424-3129
e-mail: info@balletidaho.org
Web Site: www.balletidaho.org
Officers:
    Executive Director: Jack R Lemmon
    Director Marketing: Sonja Carter
    Director Development: Christine Jarski
    Director Academy: Jeff Giese
    President Board of Directors: Marilyn Beck
Management:

Marketing Director: Sonta Carter
Artistic Director: Toni Pimble
Mission: To promote the value of classical and contemporary dance in Idaho through excellence in performance and education.
Founded: 1971
Specialized Field: Modern; Ballet
Status: Professional
Paid Staff: 8
Paid Artists: 23
Budget: 1,150,000
Performs At: Morrison Center for the Performing Arts
Affiliations: Eugene Ballet Company
Annual Attendance: 14000
Seating Capacity: 2090
Organization Type: Performing; Touring; Resident; Educational; Sponsoring

266 OINKARI BASQUE DANCERS

1224 Rose Park Circle
Boise, ID 83702
Mailing Address: PO Box 1011 Boise, ID 83701
Phone: 208-336-8219
e-mail: yanci@msn.com
Officers:
Business Manager: Miren Artiach
Management:
Business Manager: John Kirtland
Boys Dance Director: Dan Ansotegui
Girls Dance Director: Toni Ansotegui
Historian: Julie Achabal
Sergeant-at-Arms: Ron Lemmon
Communicator: Ricardo Yancy
Mission: The promotion and enhancement of our culture through dance, song, language and education.
Specialized Field: Ethnic; Folk
Status: Nonprofit
Paid Staff: 70
Income Sources: Euskaldunak
Performs At: Boise Basque Center
Organization Type: Performing; Touring; Educational

267 FESTIVAL DANCE AND PERFORMING ARTS

University of Idaho
Building 203
Moscow, ID 83844-2403
Mailing Address: PO Box 442403 Moscow, ID 83844
Phone: 208-883-3267
Fax: 541-687-5745
e-mail: festdance@uidaho.edu
Officers:
Executive Director: Micki Panttaja
Mission: To offer the Inland Northwest the finest in performing arts; to provide performances as well as education and outreach.
Founded: 1989
Specialized Field: Dance; Musical Theatre
Status: Professional; Nonprofit
Paid Staff: 3
Income Sources: Pacific Northwest Arts Performers; Idaho Commission of the Arts; Washington State Arts Commission; Western Arts Foundation; Tickets; Contribution

Performs At: Beasly Performing Arts Coliseum; Washington State University
Type of Stage: Proscenium
Seating Capacity: 2,500
Organization Type: Performing; Educational; Sponsoring

Illinois

268 BALLET CHICAGO

218 S Wabash Avenue
Suite 2300
Chicago, IL 60604
Phone: 312-251-8838
Fax: 312-251-8840
e-mail: info@balletchicago.org
Web Site: www.balletchicago.org
Management:
Artistic Director: Daniel Duell
School Director: Patricia Blair
Development Director: Bridget Fraser
Mission: To develop future career classical dancers for Chicago and the dance world at large through the study and performance of the aesthetic and repertory of George Balanchine, this century's most influential and widely performed choreographer.
Founded: 1987
Specialized Field: Ballet
Status: Professional; Nonprofit
Organization Type: Performing; Touring; Educational

269 BREATRIZ RODRIGUEZ

70 E Lake Street
Suite 1300
Chicago, IL 60601-5917
Phone: 312-739-0120
Fax: 312-739-0119
e-mail: thejoffery@aol.com
Web Site: www.joffrey.com

270 CHICAGO DANCE AND MUSIC ALLIANCE

410 S Michigan Avenue
Suite 819
Chicago, IL 60605
Phone: 312-987-9296
Fax: 312-987-1127
e-mail: cmanet@voyager.net
Web Site: www.chicagoperformances.org
Officers:
Executive Director: Matthew Brockmeier
President: Jack Zimmerman
Mission: Provides direct services to members engaged in all genres of dance and music in the Chicago area, acts as an advocate on their behalf and disseminates information about their activities to the general public.
Founded: 1984
Specialized Field: Dance and Music; Arts Service
Status: Professional; Nonprofit
Paid Staff: 2
Budget: 250,000+

Income Sources: Earned Incme; Government and Foundation Grants; Individual Contributions
Organization Type: Service organization serving not-for-profit organizations and individual dance professionals

271 CHICAGO MOVING COMPANY

3035 N Hoyne
Chicago, IL 60618
Phone: 773-334-6019
Fax: 773-384-4292
Web Site: www.chicagomovingcompany.org
Management:
   Artistic Co-Director: Nana Shineflug
   Artistic Co-Director: Cindy Brandle
   Managing Director: Dennis Wise
Mission: To perform art that speaks to life; to touch the spirit of the audience, and engage them in feeling and reflections.
Founded: 1972
Specialized Field: Modern
Status: Professional; Nonprofit
Performs At: Columbia Dance Center
Organization Type: Performing; Touring; Educational

272 DANCE CENTER OF COLUMBIA COLLEGE

1306 S Michigan
Chicago, IL 60605
Phone: 312-344-8300
Fax: 312-344-8036
e-mail: info@dancecenter.org
Web Site: www.dancecenter.org
Officers:
   Chairman: Bonnie Brooks
Management:
   Executive Director: Phil Reynolds
   Outreach Coordinator: Sabrina Little
   Marketing Director: Heather Hartley
Mission: To provide dance instruction to a variety of people from culturally diverse backgrounds.
Founded: 1969
Specialized Field: Modern; Ballet; Jazz; Ethnic; Choreography; Improvisation
Status: Professional; Nonprofit
Paid Staff: 7
Paid Artists: 14
Budget: $2,100,000
Income Sources: Earned and Contributed Income
Performs At: Dance Center; Medina Temple; Harold Washington
Affiliations: APAP; IPN; MADTC
Annual Attendance: 10,000
Facility Category: Black Box
Type of Stage: Dance
Seating Capacity: 272
Year Built: 2000
Cost: $3,500,000
Rental Contact: Shannon Epplett
Organization Type: Performing; Educational

273 HUBBARD STREET DANCE CHICAGO

1147 W Jackson Boulevard
Chicago, IL 60607-2905
Phone: 312-850-9744
Fax: 312-455-8240
e-mail: gkalver@hubbardstreetdance.com
Web Site: www.hubbardstreetdance.com
Management:
   Executive Director: Gail Kalver
   Artistic Director: Jim Vincent
Founded: 1977
Paid Staff: 28
Paid Artists: 20
Budget: $2,500,000
Income Sources: Ticket Sales; Donations; Grants; Sponsorships
Affiliations: Lou Conte Dance Studio
Annual Attendance: 130,000
Facility Category: Dance Studio
Year Remodeled: 1998
Rental Contact: Julie Nakagowa Boettcher
Organization Type: Performing; Touring; Educational

274 JOEL HALL DANCERS & CENTER

1511 W Berwyn Street
Chicago, IL 60640
Phone: 773-293-0900
Fax: 773-293-1130
e-mail: joelhalldance@hotmail.com
Web Site: www.joelhall.org
Management:
   Artistic Director: Joel Hall
   Managing Director: Susan Dickson
   Associate Director: Vanessa Truvillion
   Associate Artistic Director: Nancy Teinowitz
Mission: To build and serve a constituency that is racially, ethnically, culturally and socially diverse; to promote a philosophy of inclusiveness; to enrich the lives of community members through dance education and performance
Founded: 1974
Specialized Field: Jazz; Ballet; Modern; Hip Hop; Tap; Egyptian. Children and Adults - Advanced Beginning Levels
Status: Professional; Nonprofit
Facility Category: Dance Studio
Organization Type: Performing; Touring; Resident; Educational

275 JOFFREY BALLET OF CHICAGO

70 E Lake Street
Suite 1300
Chicago, IL 60601
Phone: 312-739-0120
Fax: 312-739-0119
e-mail: information@joffrey.com
Web Site: www.joffrey.com
Officers:
   Chairman: Steve McMillan
   President: Gary E Holden
   Vice Chairman: Linda Chaplik Harris
   Vice Chairman: Pamela Stroebel
   Secretary: Carol Prins
   Assistant Secretary: Grace Barry
Management:
   Artistic Director: Gerald Arpino
   Executive Director: Laura D Gates

Mission: To preserve, recreate and present historical masterpieces of the twentieth century; to nurture, commission and present works of young artists, particularly Americans, to audiences worldwide; to present productions of its founders.
Budget: $2,500,000+
Income Sources: Tickets Sales; Touring; Contributions
Performs At: Auditorium Theatre

276 LIRA DANCERS OF THE LIRA ENSEMBLE

6525 N Sheridan Road
SKY905
Chicago, IL 60626
Phone: 773-539-4900
Fax: 773-508-7043
e-mail: lira@liraensemble.com
Web Site: www.liraensemble.com
Management:
   Artistic Director/General Manager: Lucyna Migala
   Choreographer: Anthony Dobrzynski
Mission: To perform historic and folk dance of Poland.
Non-paid Artists: 30
Budget: $200,000-$500,000
Organization Type: Performing

277 MORDINE AND COMPANY DANCE THEATRE

1016 N Dearborn Parkway
Chicago, IL 60640
Phone: 312-654-9540
Fax: 312-654-9542
e-mail: smordine@aol.com
Management:
   Artistic Director: Shirley Mordine
   General Manager: Lisa-Marie Smith
   Producing Director: Allen Doederlein
Mission: To create innovative dance works; to collaborate with outstanding artists; to conduct educational programs for high school students and young choreographers.
Founded: 1969
Specialized Field: Modern
Status: Professional; Nonprofit
Paid Staff: 3
Income Sources: Association for Performing Arts Presenters; Dance USA; Chicago Dance Coalition
Performs At: The Dance Center of Columbia College
Organization Type: Performing; Resident; Educational

278 MUNTU DANCE THEATRE

6800 S Wentworth
Room 396-E
Chicago, IL 60621
Phone: 773-602-1135
Fax: 773-602-1134
e-mail: muntudance@aol.com
Web Site: www.muntu.com
Officers:
   President: John Gray
Management:
   Company Manager: Carolyn Denne
Mission: The performance of traditional and contemporary African and African-American dance, music and folklore.

Specialized Field: Ethnic
Status: Professional; Nonprofit
Budget: $500,000-$1,000,000
Organization Type: Performing; Touring; Resident

279 NAJWA DANCE CORPS

1900 W Van Buren
Room 0505
Chicago, IL 60612
Phone: 312-850-7224
Fax: 773-929-9976
e-mail: zdoktor@aol.com
Management:
   Business Manager: Celeste Harrell
   Artistic Director: Najwa I
Mission: To perserve dance styles and techniques; to dance and entertain with dances of different areas in a historical context.
Founded: 1975
Specialized Field: Modern; Jazz; Ethnic
Status: Professional; Nonprofit
Budget: $40,000-$100,000
Income Sources: Chicago Dance Art Coalition; African-American Arts Alliance
Organization Type: Performing; Touring; Educational

280 RIVER NORTH CHICAGO DANCE COMPANY

1016 N Dearborn
Chicago, IL 60610
Phone: 312-944-2888
Fax: 312-944-2581
e-mail: info@rivernorthchicago.com
Web Site: www.rivernorthchicago.com
Management:
   Executive Director: Ann Marie Beyers
   Artistic Director: Frank Chaves
Mission: Established for the purpose of cultivating and promoting Chicago's wealth of jazz dance talent.
Founded: 1989
Specialized Field: Jazz; Contemporary Dance
Paid Staff: 3
Volunteer Staff: 1
Paid Artists: 15
Budget: $1,100,000
Income Sources: Performance Fees; Corporate, Foundation, and Government Contributions; Individual Contributions
Seating Capacity: 7,800
Year Built: 1979

281 TRINITY IRISH DANCE COMPANY

2936 N Southport
3rd Floor
Chicago, IL 60657
Phone: 773-549-6135
Fax: 773-549-6325
e-mail: trinitydancecompany@hotmail.com
Web Site: www.trinity-dancers.com
Management:
   Artistic Director: Mark Howard
   Company Manager: Michael Carr
Founded: 1990
Budget: $1,000,000-$2,500,000

Income Sources: Touring Revenue; Individual Grants; Corporation Grants

282 ZEPHYR DANCE
1627 N Oakley Avenue
Chicago, IL 60647-5318
Phone: 773-989-8225
Fax: 773-489-9930
Management:
Artistic Director: Michaelle Kranicke

283 JUDITH SVALANDER DANCE THEATRE
83 E Woodstock Street
Crystal Lake, IL 60014-4363
Phone: 815-455-2055
Fax: 815-477-0313

284 GUS GIORDANO JAZZ DANCE CHICAGO
614 Davis Street
Evanston, IL 60201
Phone: 847-866-6779
Fax: 847-866-9228
e-mail: ggjdc@giordanojazzdance.com
Web Site: www.giordanojazzdance.com
Officers:
President: Larry Adelson
VP: Lloyd Culbertson
VP: Randy Mehrberg
Treasurer: A. Steven Crown
Secretary: Ira Bodenstein
Management:
Artistic Director: Nan Giordano
Executive Director: Ben Hodge
Mission: To excite audiences about dance in general, specifically jazz dance.
Founded: 1962
Specialized Field: Jazz Dance; Contemporary
Status: Professional
Paid Staff: 3
Paid Artists: 16
Budget: $200,000-$500,000
Income Sources: Illinois Arts Council; Foundations; Ticket Sales; Performing Fees
Affiliations: Jazz Dance World Congress
Annual Attendance: 56,000
Organization Type: Performing; Touring; Educational

285 BALLET ENTRE NOUS
1237 Ridgewood Drive
Highland Park, IL 60035
Phone: 847-432-1510
e-mail: b.entrenous@att.net
Management:
Artistic Director: E. Marc Nevins

286 VON HEIDECKE'S CHICAGO FESTIVAL BALLET
1239 S Naper Boulevard
Naperville, IL 60540
Phone: 630-527-1052
Fax: 630-527-8427
Web Site: www.chicagofestivalballet.org

Officers:
Chairman: Christopher Rosean
Secretary: Sue Doser
Tresurer: Ron Pavlacka
Management:
Founder/Director: Kenneth von Heidecke
Artistic Honorary Advisor: Maria Tallchief
Artistic Advisor: Nathalie Krassovska
Studio Manager: Timothy Cremeens
Mission: To maintain the highest artistic standards and uncompromising quality of spirted performances through the traditions of classical ballet.
Status: Nonprofit

287 NATYAKALALAYAM DANCE COMPANY
620 Ridgewood Court
Oak Brook, IL 60523
Phone: 630-323-7835
Fax: 630-323-9752
e-mail: natyadc@aol.com
Web Site: www.natya.com
Management:
Artistic Director: Hema Rajagopalan
Mission: To promote the classical dance of India in today's contemporary world.
Founded: 1975
Specialized Field: Classical Dance of India, Performance and Teaching
Paid Staff: 3
Volunteer Staff: 8
Paid Artists: 2
Non-paid Artists: 25

288 MOMENTA
Academy of Movement and Music
605 Lake Street
Oak Park, IL 60302
Phone: 708-848-2329
Fax: 708-848-2391
e-mail: stephanieclemens@hotmail.com
Web Site: www.momenta-dance.org
Management:
Press Representative/Artistic Dir: Stephanie Clemens
Artistic Co-Director: Larry Ippel
Artistic Co-Director: James C Tenuta
Mission: To produce and present dance concerts.
Founded: 1983
Specialized Field: Dance - Historical Modern / Contemporary Choreography
Volunteer Staff: 3
Paid Artists: 15
Non-paid Artists: 50
Budget: $100,000
Income Sources: Tickets; Memberships; Fundraising
Performs At: Studio Theatre
Facility Category: Black Box Theatre
Type of Stage: Proscenium
Stage Dimensions: 45'x 30'x 125'
Year Built: 1983

289 PEORIA BALLET
8800 N Industrial Road
Peoria, IL 61615

Phone: 309-690-7990
Fax: 309-690-7991
e-mail: peoriaballet@juno.com
Web Site: www.peoriaballet.com
Officers:
   Chairman: Jim Maloof
   President Elect: Jim Roecker
   VP: Suzie Pschirrer
   Secretary: Linda Waldschmidt
Management:
   Artistic Director: Erich Yetter
   General Manager: Jamie Sanders
Mission: To further the participation, education and appreciation of all disciplines of dance as a cultural art form with a particular emphasis in ballet.
Founded: 1965
Specialized Field: Ballet
Status: Semi-Professional; Nonprofit
Paid Staff: 11
Paid Artists: 1
Budget: $400,000
Income Sources: Corporate and Private Donations; Grants; Fundraising Events; Tuition
Performs At: Peoria Civic Center
Organization Type: Performing; Touring; Resident

290 ROCKFORD DANCE COMPANY

711 N Main Street
Rockford, IL 61103
Phone: 815-963-3341
Fax: 815-963-3541
Web Site: www.rockforddancecompany.com
Management:
   Executive Director: Melissa Teske
   Artistic Director: Joy Xu
Mission: Committed to serving as an arts resource in dance through its presentations, performances and education.
Founded: 1972
Specialized Field: Modern; Ballet; Jazz
Status: Semi-Professional; Nonprofit
Paid Staff: 15
Organization Type: Performing; Resident; Educational; Sponsoring

291 PASCUAL OLIVERA AND ANGELA DEL MORAL AND COMPANY

7017 Lorel
Skokie, IL 60077
Phone: 847-675-7456
Fax: 847-675-7456
Officers:
   Director: Pascal Olivera
Mission: Dedicated to a romantic celebration of Spanish dance from the classical, to the folk, to the Flamenco.
Founded: 1977
Specialized Field: Ethnic
Status: Professional
Budget: $200,000-$500,000
Organization Type: Performing; Touring; Resident; Educational

292 SPRINGFIELD BALLET COMPANY

2820 S MacArthur
Springfield, IL 62704
Phone: 217-544-1967
Fax: 217-544-1968
e-mail: sbc@springnet1.com
Web Site: www.springnet1.com/sbc
Management:
   Artistic Director: Julie Guttas
   Company Manager: Merle E Shiffman
   Ballet Mistress/Marketing: Alica Wester
Mission: To use beauty, energy, and diversity of dance to speak to the community; to foster dance as the common language that encourages freedom of expression, bridges generations and cultures, and adds to the richness of life in Central Illinois.
Founded: 1975
Specialized Field: Modern; Ballet; Jazz; Folk
Status: Non-Professional; Nonprofit
Paid Staff: 30
Budget: $100,000-$200,000
Organization Type: Performing; Touring; Educational; Sponsoring

293 SALT CREEK BALLET

98 E Naperville Road
Westmont, IL 60559-1559
Phone: 630-769-1199
Fax: 630-769-0052
e-mail: saltcreekballet@aol.com
Web Site: www.saltcreekballet.org
Management:
   Co-Director: Sergey Kozadayev
   Co-Director: Zhanna Dubrovskaya
   Executive Director: Corinne M Pievog
Founded: 1985
Specialized Field: Dance
Paid Staff: 6
Volunteer Staff: 20
Paid Artists: 22
Non-paid Artists: 60
Budget: $750,000
Income Sources: Grants; Contributions; Ticket Sales
Annual Attendance: 10,000
Organization Type: Touring Company

294 TERESA Y LOS PREFERIDOS SPANISH DANCE COMPANY

729 Lake
Wilmette, IL 60091
Phone: 847-256-6614
Fax: 847-256-5318
e-mail: preferidos@aol.com
Management:
   Chief Officer: Teresa Cullen
Mission: To bring audiences the mystery and excitement of Spain with dazzling performances of regional, classical and Flamenco dances.
Specialized Field: Spanish Dance Repertory Company
Budget: $40,000-$100,000
Organization Type: Performing; Touring; Educational

295 INVENTIONS
1047 Gage Street
Winnetka, IL 60093
Phone: 847-446-0183
Fax: 847-446-0183
e-mail: inventions4@earthlink.net
Web Site: http://home.earthlink.net/~inventions4
Management:
    Co-Founder: T Daniel
    Co-Founder: Laurie Willets
    Co-Founder: John Bruce Yeh
    Co-Founder: Teresa Reilly
Mission: An innovative foursome that strikes out in a new direction! A visual slant to cleverly interpret Classical Music and Mime for the new Century.
Founded: 2000
Specialized Field: Music Ensemble
Status: Professional
Paid Staff: 2
Volunteer Staff: 2
Organization Type: Performing; Touring

296 T. DANIEL PRODUCTIONS
1047 Gage Street
Winnetka, IL 60093
Phone: 847-446-0183
Fax: 847-446-0183
e-mail: tdaniel@tdanielcreations.com
Web Site: tdanielcreations.com
Management:
    Artistic Co-Director/Co-Founder: T Daniel
    Artistic Co-Director/Co-Founder: Laurie Willets
Mission: To create, educate and tour theatrical productions, shows and concert programs dynamically based upon the Art of Mime for audiences of all ages.
Founded: 1971
Specialized Field: Visual Theatre Company
Status: Professional
Paid Staff: 2
Paid Artists: 2

Indiana

297 ANDERSON YOUNG BALLET THEATRE
29 E Dillon Street
PO Box 631
Anderson, IN 46016-1805
Phone: 765-643-2184
Management:
    Artistic Director: LouAnn Young

298 EVANSVILLE DANCE THEATRE
333 Plaza East Boulevard
Suite E
Evansville, IN 47715
Phone: 812-473-8937
Fax: 812-473-0392
e-mail: edt@danse.com
Web Site: www.edtdance.org
Officers:
    President: Mary Mably
Management:

School Director: Eckhard Heidrich
Director of Operations: Donna Bye
Administrative Assistant: Cari Dyke
Artistic Director: Donald Tolj
Ballet Mistress: Heather Ferranti Ferguson
Founded: 1981
Specialized Field: Ballet; Dance
Status: Professional; Nonprofit
Paid Staff: 12
Paid Artists: 7
Organization Type: Performing; Touring; Resident; Educational

299 FORT WAYNE BALLET
324 Penn Avenue
Fort Wayne, IN 46805
Phone: 219-484-9646
Fax: 219-484-9647
e-mail: carla@fortwayneballet.org
Web Site: www.fortwayneballet.com
Officers:
    President: Tom Swihart
    Treasurer: Sarah Strimennos
Management:
    Artistic/Executive Director: Karen Gibbons-Brown
    School Administrator: Carla Escosa
Mission: To stimulate interest in the art of dance by providing the community with an academy that encourages excellence and artistic achievement, and by producing quality dance productions and education outreach programs performed by established professionals and emerging local talent.
Founded: 1956
Specialized Field: Ballet; Jazz; Contemporary; Character
Status: Semi-Professional; Nonprofit
Paid Staff: 17
Volunteer Staff: 250
Budget: $500,000-$1,000,000
Income Sources: Fine Arts Foundation; Arts United of Greater Ft. Wayne
Performs At: Performing Arts Center
Affiliations: Arts United of Greater Ft. Wayne
Organization Type: Performing; Educational

300 FORT WAYNE DANCE COLLECTIVE
437 E Berry Street
Suite 203
Fort Wayne, IN 46802
Phone: 219-424-6574
Fax: 219-424-2789
e-mail: liz@fwdc.org
Web Site: www.fwdc.org
Officers:
    President: JJ Lane Carroll
    VP: Leslieen Reuymer
    Secretary: Cassandra Writz
    Treasurer: Joan Daley Uebelhoer
Management:
    Artistic Director: Liz Monnier
Mission: To promote and expand the development of human creativity and expression through movement, as well as to sustain and develop the Fort Wayne Dance Collective's traditions by presenting dance, inter- and

multi-disciplinary arts, and educational programs of the highest quality to diverse audiences and student populations.
Founded: 1979
Specialized Field: Modern Dance with a Multi Arts Focus
Status: Professional; Nonprofit
Paid Staff: 3
Paid Artists: 16
Budget: $300,000
Income Sources: Earned Income; Local Foundations; State and National Grants
Affiliations: Arts United
Annual Attendance: 10,000
Organization Type: Performing; Educational; Sponsoring; Video Producer for Public Access

301 BALLET INTERNATIONALE

502 N Capitol Avenue
Suite B
Indianapolis, IN 46204
Phone: 317-637-8979
Fax: 317-637-1637
e-mail: mail@balletinternationale.org
Web Site: www.balletinternationale.org
Management:
   CEO/Artistic Director: Eldar Aliev
   Executive Director: Pat Hanfor
   Company/Booking Manager: Nichole Waymire
   Public Relations/Marketing Director: Judy Donner
Mission: To stimulate the evolution of our community in those ways only possible with world class ballet.
Founded: 1973
Specialized Field: Modern; Ballet; Jazz
Status: Professional
Paid Staff: 23
Paid Artists: 26
Non-paid Artists: 1
Budget: $2,400,000
Affiliations: Association of Performing Arts Presenters; Arts Midwest; American Symphony Orchestra League; IPN; IAPAA; Indiana Advocates for the Arts
Facility Category: Murat Centre
Seating Capacity: 2,500
Organization Type: Performing; Touring; Resident; Educational; Sponsoring

302 DANCE KALEIDOSCOPE

4600 Sunset Avenue
Indianapolis, IN 46208-3485
Phone: 317-940-6555
Fax: 317-940-6557
e-mail: dancekal@netdirect.net
Web Site: www.dancekal.org
Officers:
   President Board of Trustees: Wayne Kreuscher
Management:
   Managing Director: Jan Virgin
   Artistic Director: David Hochoy
   Director Touring/Education: Tim Hubbard
   Director Development: Molly A Shane
Mission: The mission is to inspire, educate and entertain through the experience of outstanding contemporary dance.
Founded: 1972

Specialized Field: Modern Dance; Contemporary Dance
Status: Professional; Nonprofit
Paid Staff: 5
Paid Artists: 12
Budget: $1,032,000
Income Sources: Earned; Developed; Special Events
Performs At: Pike Performing Arts Center
Annual Attendance: 170,000
Organization Type: Performing; Touring; Resident

Iowa

303 CO' MOTION DANCE THEATER

129 E Seventh Street
Ames, IA 50010
Phone: 515-232-7374
Fax: 515-233-9290
e-mail: dance@comotion.org
Web Site: www.comotion.org
Officers:
   President: Gerald Sheble
   VP: Beth Clarke
   Secretary: Ron Jackson
   Treasurer: Larry Gleason
Management:
   Director: Valerie Williams
   General Manager: Susan Jackson
Mission: To bring high-caliber professional dance to Midwestern sponsors at affordable prices and to offer the highest quality in dance education to its students.
Founded: 1978
Specialized Field: Modern Dance
Status: Professional; Nonprofit
Paid Staff: 1
Paid Artists: 3
Non-paid Artists: 3
Performs At: The Ames City Auditorium
Organization Type: Performing; Touring; Resident; Educational

304 CO-MOTION DANCE

129 E 7th Street
Ames, IA 98102
Phone: 515-232-7374
Fax: 515-233-9290
e-mail: dance@comotion.org
Web Site: www.comotion.org
Officers:
   President: Paula Swenson
   VP: Jesse Jaramillo
   Treasurer: Barron Aoyama
   Secretary: Mary Lou McCollum
   Executive Director: Jane Hyde Walsh
Management:
   Artistic Director: Gail Heilbron
Mission: To cultivate a diverse and informed audience for professional modern dance.
Founded: 1979
Specialized Field: Modern
Status: Professional; Nonprofit
Organization Type: Performing; Touring; Educational; Sponsoring

305 IOWA DANCE THEATRE

6720 Hickman Road
Des Moines, IA 50322
Phone: 515-276-2694
Fax: 515-276-2694
Web Site: www.iowadancetheatre.com
Officers:
   Treasurer: Linda Snoddy
Management:
   Executive Director: Mary Joyce Lind
   Project Director: Janice Baker-Haines
   Co-Director: Lisa Hamilton
   Co-Director: Cathy Bergman
   Co-Director: Lana Lyddon-Hattan
   Head Chamber Dances: Kathleen Hurley
Mission: Dedicated to supporting a company of dancers who will perform and promote the art form of dance.
Founded: 1983
Specialized Field: Modern; Ballet; Jazz
Status: Semi-Professional; Nonprofit
Volunteer Staff: 15
Paid Artists: 12
Non-paid Artists: 15
Income Sources: Grants; Fundraisers
Performs At: Civic Center of Greater Des Moines
Annual Attendance: 5,000
Seating Capacity: 2,750
Year Built: 1979
Year Remodeled: 2000
Organization Type: Performing; Touring; Educational

Kansas

306 COHAN/SUZEAU DANCE COMPANY

University of Kansas
Murphy Hall-Department of Music
Lawrence, KS 66045
Phone: 785-841-6394
Fax: 785-864-5089
e-mail: suzeau@ku.edu
Web Site: www.cohansuzeau.com
Management:
   Co-Artistic Director: Patrick Suzeau
   Co-Artistic Director: Muriel Cohan
   Manager: Suan Whitfield

307 KANSAS REGIONAL BALLET

11728 Quivira Road
Overland Park, KS 66210
Phone: 913-451-9292
Fax: 913-498-2222
e-mail: krbdance@mindsping.com
Web Site: krb.ontheweb.nu
Officers:
   VP: Dennis Landsman
   President: Kathy Landsman
   Secretary: Linda Smith
   Treasurer: Dennis Landsman
Management:
   Artistic Co-Director: Kathy Landsman
   Artistic Co-Director: Dennis Landsman

Mission: To establish an outlet for aspiring young dancers to learn, practice, and perform all forms of dance in a professional atmosphere; to acquaint, educate, and enrich audiences of all ages.
Founded: 1979
Specialized Field: Ballet; Modern
Status: Pre-Professional; Nonprofit
Paid Staff: 2
Volunteer Staff: 27
Paid Artists: 4
Non-paid Artists: 27
Budget: $50,000
Income Sources: Fund Raisers; Grants; Ticket Sales
Performs At: Johnson Community College; Yardley Hall; The Carlson Center
Affiliations: Midstates Regional Dance America
Annual Attendance: 5,000
Facility Category: Community College
Type of Stage: Proscenium
Stage Dimensions: 55'x 45'
Seating Capacity: 1,300
Year Built: 1988
Rental Contact: Johnson County Community College
Organization Type: Performing; Touring; Educational

308 WICHITA CONTEMPORARY DANCE THEATRE

Witchita State University
1845 N Fairmount
Box 101
Wichita, KS 67260-0101
Phone: 316-978-3530
Fax: 316-978-3951
e-mail: renea.goforth@wichita.edu
Management:
   Director Dance: C Nicholas Johnson
   Assistant Director Dance: Renea Goforth
Mission: To provide high quality entertaining dance performances; to foster understanding and appreciation for dance through educational programs; to provide a venue for artists to live and work.

Kentucky

309 KENTUCKY BALLET THEATRE

736 National Avenue
Lexington, KY 40502
Phone: 859-252-5245
Fax: 859-252-7925
e-mail: info@kyballet.com
Web Site: www.kyballet.com
Officers:
   President: Jan Foody
   VP: Cynthia Bearley
   Treasurer: Danby Carter
   Secretary: Paul Evans Holbrook
   Public Relations: Larry Neuzel
Management:
   Artistic Director: Norbe Risco
   Public Relations: Sandy Robinson
Mission: To establish, through performance and education, a professional company and academy committed to the art of dance; to promote this fine art in

the Central Kentucky region and once established, broaden our service area to include regions where a need or interest exists.
Founded: 1998
Specialized Field: Dance Company/Academy

310   LEXINGTON BALLET

161 N Mill Street
Lexington, KY 40507
Phone: 859-233-3925
Fax: 859-255-2787
Web Site: www.lexingtonballet.org
Management:
  School Director: Lucia Montero
  Artistic Director: Frank Galvez
  Executive Director: Allen Porter
Mission: Committed to offering a variety of performances in contemporary and classical dance and to education, with a strong emphasis on classical ballet.
Founded: 1974
Specialized Field: Ballet
Status: Semi-Professional; Nonprofit
Paid Staff: 16
Budget: $200,000-$500,000
Organization Type: Performing; Resident

311   LOUISVILLE BALLET

315 E Main Street
Louisville, KY 40202-1215
Phone: 502-583-3150
Fax: 502-583-0006
e-mail: louballet3@ka.net
Web Site: www.louisvilleballet.org
Management:
  Artistic Director: Alun Jones
  Associate Artistic Director: Helen Starr
  Ballet Master: Vincent Falardo
  Ballet Master: Clark Reid
  Stage Manager/Lighting Designer: Michael T Ford
  Assistant Stage Manager: Jennyk Sabie
  Technical Director: Ted McQueen
  Costume Manager: Dan Fedie
Mission: To bring to the broadest audience high-quality professional dance.
Founded: 1952
Specialized Field: Modern; Ballet; Jazz
Status: Professional; Nonprofit
Paid Staff: 120
Budget: $1,000,000-$2,500,000
Income Sources: Dance USA; Southeast Regional Ballet Association
Affiliations: Dance USA; Southeast Regional Ballet Association
Organization Type: Performing; Touring; Resident; Educational; Sponsoring

Louisiana

312   BATON ROUGE BALLET THEATER

11017 Perkins Road
PO Box 82288
Baton Rouge, LA 70884

Phone: 225-766-8379
Fax: 225-766-8230
e-mail: brballet@entel.net
Web Site: www.brballet.org
Management:
  Artistic Co-Director: Sharon Mathews
  Artistic Co-Director: Molly Buchmann
  Director Development: Sonya Blanchard
Mission: To promote, aid and assist, in any manner whatsoever, the development, improvement and advancement of ballet by maintaining a performing dance company.
Founded: 1963
Specialized Field: Dance; Ballet and Modern
Status: Professional; Nonprofit
Budget: $200,000-$500,000
Income Sources: Ticket Sales; Grants; Donations
Organization Type: Performing; Touring; Resident

313   DELTA FESTIVAL BALLET OF NEW ORLEANS

3850 N Causeway Boulevard
Suite 119
Metairie, LA 70002
Phone: 504-836-7166
Fax: 504-836-7167
e-mail: dfballet@accesscom.net
Management:
  Artistic Director: Joseph Giacobbe
  Artistic Diector: Maria Giacobbe
  Administrative Director: Christines Hodgins
Mission: Advancing the art of dance through professional performance, education, cultural outreach and community involvement. Delta Festival Ballet is committed to arts-in-education.
Founded: 1969
Specialized Field: Ballet
Status: Professional; Nonprofit
Paid Staff: 15
Income Sources: National Association for Regional Ballet
Organization Type: Performing; Touring; Resident; Educational

314   NEW ORLEANS BALLET ASSOCIATION

305 Baronne Street
Suite 700
New Orleans, LA 70112
Phone: 504-522-0996
Fax: 504-595-8454
e-mail: jhamilton@nobadance.com
Web Site: www.nobadance.com
Officers:
  President: Cecile Gibson
  VP: Cynthia LeBreton
  Secretary: Conny Willems
  Treasurer: Guy Brierre
Management:
  Executive Director: Jenny R Hamilton
Mission: To cultivate an appreciation, understanding, and enjoyment of dance through presentation, education, and community service.
Founded: 1969
Specialized Field: Dance

Status: Nonprofit
Paid Staff: 7
Volunteer Staff: 520
Paid Artists: 15
Budget: $1,200,000
Income Sources: Box Office; Grants: Donations
Performs At: Mahalia Jackson Theater of the Performing Arts
Affiliations: Dance/USA; Association of Arts Presenters; Louisiana Presenters Network; Southwest Presenters
Annual Attendance: 15,000
Facility Category: Concert Hall
Type of Stage: Proscenium
Seating Capacity: 2,317
Organization Type: Sponsoring; Presenting; Educational

315 NEWCOMB DANCE COMPNAY

Department of Theatre and Dance
215 McWilliams Hall
New Orleans, LA 70118
Mailing Address: Tulane University
Phone: 504-865-5798
Fax: 504-865-6737
e-mail: dance@tulane.edu
Web Site: www.tulane.edu/~theatre
Management:
    Associate Professor: Alice Pascal Escher
Founded: 1984
Performs At: Dixon Hall
Type of Stage: Black Box; Proscenium
Seating Capacity: Proscenium theatre seats 1,000

316 SHREVEPORT METROPOLITAN BALLET

509 Marshall Avenue
Suite 1015
Shreveport, LA 71101
Phone: 318-459-1457
Fax: 318-459-1457
Web Site: www.shreveportmetroballet.org
Management:
    Director: Adrienne Brooks Williamson
    Director: Kendra Meiki
Mission: An educational vehicle for area young people to learn and perform ballet.
Founded: 1973
Specialized Field: Ballet
Status: Semi-Professional; Nonprofit
Paid Staff: 30
Performs At: The Shreveport Civic Theatre
Organization Type: Performing; Resident; Educational

Maine

317 BATES DANCE FESTIVAL

163 Wood Street
Lewiston, ME 04240-6016
Phone: 207-786-6381
Fax: 207-786-8282
e-mail: dancefest@bates.edu
Web Site: www.bates.edu/dancefest
Management:

Director: Laura Faure
    Associate Director/Registrar: Alison Hart
Mission: The Bates Dance Festival fosters a cooperative community in which choreographers, performers, educators, and students come together to study, perform, and create new work.
Founded: 1982
Specialized Field: Dance
Status: Professional
Paid Staff: 5
Volunteer Staff: 24
Paid Artists: 20
Budget: over $500,000
Income Sources: Public; Private; and Earned Income
Performs At: Schaeffer Theatre
Affiliations: Bates College
Annual Attendance: 4,000
Type of Stage: Sprung
Stage Dimensions: 28'x35'
Seating Capacity: 300
Year Built: 1952
Organization Type: Resident; Educational; Sponsoring

Maryland

318 BALLET THEATRE OF ANNAPOLIS

801 Chase Street
Annapolis, MD 21401
Phone: 410-263-8285
Fax: 410-626-1835
e-mail: btaballet@aol.com
Web Site: www.btaballet.org
Management:
    Executive Director: Lorraine Commeret
    Artistic Director: Edward Stewart
Founded: 1978
Specialized Field: Ballet
Status: Professional; Nonprofit
Paid Staff: 27
Budget: $200,000-$500,000
Organization Type: Touring; Resident

319 DOUG HAMBY DANCE

University of Maryland
Department of Dance, UMBC
1000 Hilltop Circle
Baltimore, MD 21250
Phone: 410-455-2950
Fax: 410-455-1046
e-mail: hamby@umbc.edu
Web Site: www.umbc.edu/newsevents/arts/dhd/
Management:
    Artistic Director: Doug Hamby
    Office of Arts/Culture: Thomas Moore
Budget: $40,000-$100,000

320 EVA ANDERSON DANCERS

5452 High Tor Hill
Columbia, MD 21048
Phone: 410-997-3899
Fax: 410-730-7411
Officers:

All listings are in alphabetical order by state, then city, then organization within the city.

President: Doris Williams
VP: Ernest Miller
Secretary: Yvette Shipley
Treasurer: Troy Burman
Management:
   Artistic Director: Eva Anderson
   Assistant Artistic Director: Yvette Shipley
Mission: To create dance based on the American experience with special emphasis on African-American experiences.
Founded: 1974
Specialized Field: Modern; Ethnic
Status: Professional
Budget: $40,000-$100,000
Organization Type: Performing; Touring; Educational

321 DANCE MATRIX

135 E Main Street
2nd Floor
Elkton, MD 21921
Phone: 410-620-5501
Fax: 410-392-5392
e-mail: janaea@crosslink.net
Web Site: www.dancematrix.org
Management:
   Artistic Director: Janaea Rose Lyn
Mission: To develop and present contemporary concert dance using musicians and composers on a project basis.
Founded: 1989
Specialized Field: Modern
Status: Professional
Paid Staff: 1
Volunteer Staff: 5
Paid Artists: 10
Budget: $50,000
Income Sources: Non Profit Organization
Performs At: Cecil Community College
Affiliations: Convergence Dance Centre
Type of Stage: Proscenium
Organization Type: Performing; Touring; Educational

322 FROSTBURG STATE UNIVERSITY: UNIVERSITY DANCE COMPANY

Dance Department, Division of Performing Arts
Frostburg State University
Frostburg, MD 21532
Phone: 301-687-4730
Fax: 301-687-7961
e-mail: bfischer@fsu.edu
Management:
   Artistic Director: Barry Fischer

323 NATIONAL TAP ENSEMBLE

PO Box 2439
Hagerstown, MD 21741-2439
Phone: 301-790-1180
Fax: 775-703-5519
Toll-free: 888-683-8277
e-mail: pr1@usatap.org
Web Site: www.usatap.org
Management:
   Public Relations Director: Miles Johnson
Mission: Over 2,000 programs performed worldwide.
Founded: 1988

Specialized Field: Performing Arts; Tap Dance; Jazz Music; American Vernacular Dance
Paid Staff: 3
Paid Artists: 12
Budget: $200,000-$500,000
Annual Attendance: 250,000

324 METROPOLITAN BALLET THEATRE AND ACADEMY

10076 Darnestown Road
Suite 202
Rockville, MD 20850
Phone: 301-762-1757
Fax: 301-762-1757
e-mail: mbta@erols.com
Web Site: www.metropolitanballettheatre.com
Management:
   Director: Suzanne Erlon
   Administrator: Gail Minning
Mission: Teaching dancers to be the best they can be.
Founded: 1989
Specialized Field: Dance; Ballet; Jazz
Status: Nonprofit
Paid Staff: 4

325 LIZ LERMAN DANCE EXCHANGE

7117 Maple Avenue
Takoma Park, MD 20912
Phone: 301-270-6700
Fax: 301-270-2626
e-mail: mail@danceexchange.org
Web Site: www.danceexchange.org
Officers:
   Chairman: Ronald Eichner
Management:
   Director Development: John Borstel
   Producing Director: Jane Hirshberg
Mission: To promote the belief that skills, discipline, expression, and beauty of dance can be a part of everyone's life; to perform at a wide variety of locations in the United States and Europe.
Founded: 1976
Specialized Field: Modern
Status: Professional; Nonprofit
Paid Staff: 8
Volunteer Staff: 4
Paid Artists: 9
Non-paid Artists: 6
Budget: $500,000-$1,000,000
Income Sources: Dance USA; Cultural Alliance of Greater Washington
Organization Type: Performing; Touring; Resident; Educational

Massachusetts

326 AMHERST BALLET

29 Strong Street
Amherst, MA 01002
Phone: 413-549-1555
e-mail: amhballet@the-spa.com
Web Site: www.the-spa.com/amherstballet/home.htm

Officers:
  President: Jerry Schoen
  VP: Edward Woodbridge
  Treasurer: Nancy Huntley
  Secretary: Andrea Leibson
Management:
  School Administrator: Therese Brady Donohue
  Artistic Director: Catherine Dahlinger Fair
Mission: The training of young people to perform for their peers, bringing an awareness of diversity and art through dance.
Founded: 1971
Specialized Field: Modern; Ballet; Jazz; Ethnic
Status: Non-Professional; Nonprofit
Paid Staff: 16
Budget: $100,000
Organization Type: Performing; Educational; Training

---

327   JACOB'S PILLOW DANCE FESTIVAL: SCHOOL/ARCHIVES/COMMUNITY PROGRAMS
358 George Carter Road
Becket, MA 01223
Mailing Address: PO Box 287, Lee, MA 01238
Phone: 413-637-1322
Fax: 413-243-4744
e-mail: info@jacobspillow.org
Web Site: www.jacobspillow.org
Management:
  Executive Director: Ella Baff
  General Manager: Charlotte Wooldridge
Mission: To support dance creation, presentation, education and preservation; and to engage and deepen public appreciation and support for dance.
Founded: 1933
Specialized Field: Ballet; Jazz; Modern; and Culturally Specific Dance
Status: Professional; Nonprofit
Budget: $3,800,000
Performs At: Doris Duke Studio Theatre; Ted Shawn Theatre
Annual Attendance: 70,000
Organization Type: Performing; Resident; Educational; Sponsoring

---

328   BOSTON BALLET
19 Clarendon Street
Boston, MA 02116-6107
Phone: 617-695-6950
Fax: 617-695-6995
Toll-free: 800-447-7400
Web Site: www.bostonballet.org
Officers:
  Chairman: John Humphrey
Management:
  Artistic Director: Mikko Nissien
  Public Relations Manager: Beth Olsen
Mission: To educate audiences and young professional dancers through community outreach and children's programming.
Founded: 1963
Specialized Field: Ballet
Status: Professional; Nonprofit
Performs At: Wang Theatre

Facility Category: Professional Repertory Ballet Company
Organization Type: Performing; Touring; Educational

---

329   DANCE UMBRELLA
515 Washington Street
5th Floor
Boston, MA 02111
Phone: 617-482-7570
Fax: 617-482-7571
e-mail: porganisak@danceumbrella.org
Web Site: www.danceumbrella.org
Management:
  Artistic Director: Paul Organisak
Performs At: Emerson Majestic Theatre

---

330   IMPULSE DANCE COMPANY
181 Mass Avenue
3rd Floor
Boston, MA 02115
Phone: 617-536-6989
Fax: 617-536-7696
e-mail: impdance@aol.com
Web Site: www.impulsedance.com
Management:
  Studio Manager: Lisa Paki
  Artistic Director: Adrienne T Hawkins
  Company Manager: Jeff Polster
Mission: To engender a universal appreciation of the art form of concert jazz dance.
Founded: 1972
Paid Staff: 3
Volunteer Staff: 10
Budget: $40,000-$100,000

---

331   MARCUS SCHULKIND DANCE COMPANY
252 W Newton Street
Suite 3
Boston, MA 02116-6482
Phone: 617-536-2962
Management:
  Artistic Director: Marcus Schulkind

---

332   TOPF CENTER FOR DANCE EDUCATION
551 Tremont Street
PO Box 180587
Boston, MA 02118
Phone: 617-482-0351
Fax: 617-542-9334
e-mail: info@topfcenter.org
Web Site: www.topfcenter.org
Officers:
  Chairman: Myran Parker-Brass
Management:
  Artistic Director: Suet May Ho
  Executive Director: Jari Poulin
Mission: To foster self esteem, cooperation and interracial understanding among diverse communities through dance instruction and performance opportunities.
Founded: 1974
Specialized Field: Dance; Education

Status: Professional; Nonprofit
Paid Staff: 20
Volunteer Staff: 150
Income Sources: Grants; Donations; Ticket Sales
Organization Type: Performing; Touring; Educational

333 INCA SON: MUSIC AND DANCE OF THE ANDES

Cambridge, MA 02238-1899
Mailing Address: PO Box 381899
Phone: 617-864-7041
Fax: 617-491-7098
e-mail: CIncaSonV@aol.com
Web Site: www.incason.com
Management:
    Founder/Creative Director: Cesar Villalobos
Founded: 1998
Specialized Field: Andean Music and Dance

334 JOSE MATEO'S BALLET THEATRE

400 Harvard Street
Harvard Square
Cambridge, MA 02138
Phone: 617-354-7467
Fax: 617-354-7856
Web Site: www.btb.org
Mission: To further the development of ballet as an art form through new works that make ballet relevant for today's diverse audiences; to offer programs of the highest quality and professional standards; to expand the role that dance plays in the cultural education and enrichment of our community.
Founded: 1986
Status: Nonprofit; Professional

335 MANDALA FOLK DANCE ENSEMBLE

PO Box 390642
Cambridge, MA 02139
Phone: 617-868-3641
e-mail: mandalafde@aol.com
Web Site: http://users.rcn.com/mandala.ma.ultranet/mand
Mission: The researching, preservation and performance of traditional folk dance and music from around the world; the broadening of cross-cultural awareness; the introduction of accessible dance to a broad audience.
Founded: 1965
Specialized Field: Ethnic; Folk
Status: Professional; Semi-Professional; Nonprofit
Paid Staff: 35
Income Sources: Massachusetts Council on the Arts; New England Foundation Tour Program; National Endowment for the Arts Dance Program
Performs At: John Hancock Hall
Organization Type: Performing; Touring; Resident; Educational

336 ST. PAUL'S SCHOOL BALLET COMPANY

St. Paul's School
325 Pleasant Street
Concord, MA 03301

Phone: 603-229-4689
Fax: 603-229-4679
e-mail: rwright@sps.edu
Web Site: www.sps.edu
Management:
    Dance Program Director: Rebecca Wright
Mission: To train young dancers in the art and technique of classical ballet while attaining a rigorous academic education.
Specialized Field: Dance
Performs At: Memorial Hall
Annual Attendance: 50
Facility Category: State of the Art Dance Studio
Type of Stage: Black Box

337 WALNUT HILL SCHOOL-BALLET

12 Highland Street
Natick, MA 01760
Phone: 508-650-5020
Fax: 508-653-9593
e-mail: admission@walnuthillarts.org
Management:
    Head of Ballet: Michael Owen
    Dean Admission: Matthew Derr
    Director Ballet Admission: Lorie Komlyn
Founded: 1893
Performs At: Keiter Performing Arts Center

338 ALBANY BERKSHIRE BALLET

51 N Street
Pittsfield, MA 01201
Phone: 413-445-5382
Fax: 413-445-5382
e-mail: webmaster@berkshireballet.org
Web Site: www.rpi.edu/~ruberd/nbb1
Management:
    Artistic Director: Madeline Cantarella Culpo
    Company Manager/Director: Marian Mendoz
    Ballet Master: William Cooley
    Music Director: John Culpo
    Administrative Assistant: Noreenor Reynolds
Founded: 1960
Specialized Field: Ballet
Affiliations: Koussevitsky Arts Centre; Centarella School of Dance

339 ART OF BLACK DANCE AND MUSIC

32 Cameron Avenue
Somerville, MA 02144
Phone: 617-666-1859
Fax: 617-776-8971
e-mail: abdm@aol.com
Officers:
    Board Member: William Taylor
    Board Member: Roberta Jackson
    Chief Operation: Richard Baarsvick
Management:
    Founder Director: De Ama Battle
Mission: To teach the history of mankind through dance, music and folklore; to educate and entertain using the culturally diverse expressions of our African heritage.
Founded: 1975
Specialized Field: Folklore
Status: Professional; Nonprofit

Paid Staff: 1
Volunteer Staff: 2
Paid Artists: 7
Non-paid Artists: 3
Income Sources: Massachusetts Cultural Council; Boston Cultural Council
Performs At: Various facilities
Annual Attendance: 30,000 - 50,000
Organization Type: Performing; Touring; Resident; Educational

Michigan

340 ANN ARBOR DANCE WORKS
1310 N University Court
University of Michigan Dance Department
Ann Arbor, MI 48109-2217
Phone: 734-763-5460
Fax: 734-763-5962
e-mail: delanghe@umich.edu
Web Site: www.music.umich.edu/departments/dance
Management:
  Co-Director/Choreographer: Gay Delanghe
  Co-Director/Choreographer: Bill De Young
  Co-Director/Choreographer: Jessica Fofel
  Co-Director/Choreographer: Sandra Torijan
  Co-Director/Choreographer: Ruth Leney-Midkiff
  Co-Director/Choreographer: Robin Wilson
  Co-Musical Director: Stephen Rush
  Technical Director: Mary Cole
Mission: Staging original and classic works of modern dance.
Founded: 1984
Specialized Field: Dance; Music
Status: Professional
Paid Artists: 9
Non-paid Artists: 10
Budget: $20,000
Income Sources: In-House Grants
Performs At: Betty Pease Studio Theater; University of Michigan Dance Building
Affiliations: University of Michigan; Department of Dance; School of Music
Annual Attendance: 800
Resident Groups: Dance Company of the University of Michigan.

341 DANCE GALLERY COMPANY
111 Third Street
Ann Arbor, MI 48103
Phone: 734-747-8885
Fax: 734-747-8885
e-mail: dancegallerystudio@ameritech.net
Management:
  Studio Manager: Noonie Anderson
  Rental Coordinator: Diane Black
Mission: To offer audiences quality modern dance and to promote and supply quality modern dance training.
Founded: 1981
Specialized Field: Modern Ballet Jazz
Status: Professional; Nonprofit
Income Sources: Michigan Council for Arts & Cultural Affairs; Washtenaw Council of Arts

Organization Type: Performing; Touring; Resident; Educational

342 UNIVERSITY OF MICHIGAN DANCE COMPANY
University of Michigan
Office of Major Events
530 S State Street, Box 554
Ann Arbor, MI 48109-1349
Phone: 734-936-9358
Fax: 734-936-9345
e-mail: kevgilman@umich.edu
Web Site: www.imich.edu/~mevents

343 MADAME CADILLAC DANCE THEATRE
15 E Kirby
Suite 903
Detroit, MI 48202
Phone: 313-875-6354
Fax: 313-875-2239
Web Site: www.artservemichigan.org/members/mdecadillac
Management:
  Artistic Director: Harriet Berg
  Business Manager: Matt Stockard
  Booking Agent: Callt Kypros
Mission: To tell the story of the American-French Colonial Period through performing 18th-century dance and music of the court and country.
Founded: 1982
Specialized Field: Ethnic; Folk; Historical
Status: Semi-Professional; Nonprofit
Organization Type: Performing; Touring; Educational

344 GRAND RAPIDS BALLET COMPANY
341 Ellsworth SW
Grand Rapids, MI 49503
Phone: 616-454-4771
Fax: 616-454-0672
e-mail: info@grballet.org
Web Site: www.grballet.org
Management:
  Artistic Director: Gordon P Schmidt
  Associate Artistic Director: Laura Berman
  Managing Director: Bob Bonolow
Budget: $1,000,000-$2,500,000

345 INTERLOCHEN DANCE ENSEMBLE
Interlochen Center for the Arts
PO Box 199
Interlochen, MI 49643-0199
Phone: 231-276-7200
Fax: 231-276-7885
e-mail: admissions@interlochen.org
Web Site: www.interlochen.org
Management:
  Dance Division Chair: Sharon Randolph
  Director Admissions: Thomas Bewley

346 KALAMAZOO BALLET COMPANY
326 W Kalamazoo Avenue
Kalamazoo, MI 49007

Phone: 616-343-3027
Fax: 616-342-8788
Web Site: www.kalamazoomi.com/ballet.htm
Management:
  Business Manager: Birgitte Scheele
  Artistic Director: Therese Bullard
Mission: To give dancers the opportunity to experience professional rehearsals and performances; to serve as a stepping stone to professional companies.
Founded: 1969
Specialized Field: Modern; Ballet; Ethnic; Folk
Status: Semi-Professional; Nonprofessional; Nonprofit
Paid Staff: 50
Income Sources: National Association for Regional Ballet; Mid-State Regional Dance America
Performs At: Civic Auditorium; Miller Auditorium
Organization Type: Performing; Touring; Educational

---

347 WELLSPRING/CORI TERRY & DANCERS

359 S Burdick Street
Kalamazoo, MI 49007
Phone: 616-342-4354
Fax: 616-342-4245
e-mail: wellspring@wellspringdance.com
Web Site: wellspringdance.com
Management:
  Artistic Director: Cori Terry
  Executive Director: Carol Snapp
  Touring/Facilities Coordinator: Heather Jach
Founded: 1981
Paid Staff: 9
Volunteer Staff: 13
Income Sources: Grants, Donations, Tickets Sales, Rentals
Performs At: State-of-the-art dance theatre and studio
Facility Category: Theatre/Studio
Type of Stage: Suspended Maple Floor
Seating Capacity: 120
Year Built: 2000
Rental Contact: Heather Jach

---

348 MINNESOTA DANCE ALLIANCE

528 Hennepin Avenue
Suite 510
Minneapolis, MI 55403
Phone: 612-340-1900
Fax: 612-340-9919
Management:
  Executive Director: June Wilson

---

349 EISENHOWER DANCE ENSEMBLE

1541 W Hamlin Road
Rochester Hills, MI 48309
Phone: 248-852-5850
Fax: 248-852-5875
e-mail: ederoche@juno.com
Web Site: www.ede-dance.org
Management:
  Artistic Director: Laurie Eisenhower
  Executive Director: Maury Okeru
  Company Manager: Anne Bak
  EDE Center for Dance Director: Francesca Pileci

Mission: To educate and inform the public about the art of dance through concert performances, educational residencies and workshops.
Founded: 1991
Specialized Field: Contemporary dance
Paid Staff: 5
Volunteer Staff: 15
Paid Artists: 9
Non-paid Artists: 2

Minnesota

---

350 MINNESOTA BALLET

301 W First Street
Suite 800
Duluth, MN 55802-1613
Phone: 218-529-3742
Fax: 218-529-3744
e-mail: info@minnesotaballet.org
Web Site: www.minnesotaballet.org
Officers:
  President: Liz Holt
Management:
  Executive/Artistic Director: Allen Fields
  Business/Accounting Manager: Willy McManus
  Associate Artistic Director: Robert Gardner
  Production: Kenneth Pogin
Mission: To maintain a high-quality school of ballet and a company of professional dancers; to present a regular series of performances.
Founded: 1965
Specialized Field: Ballet; Jazz
Status: Professional; Nonprofit
Paid Staff: 4
Volunteer Staff: 30
Paid Artists: 12
Budget: $200,000-$500,000
Income Sources: National Association for Regional Ballet
Performs At: Duluth Entertainment & Convention Center
Facility Category: Auditorium
Type of Stage: Proscenium
Stage Dimensions: 60'x45'
Seating Capacity: 2,400
Organization Type: Performing; Touring; Resident; Educational; Sponsoring

---

351 ETHNIC DANCE THEATRE

314 Clifton
Suite 105
Minneapolis, MN 55403
Phone: 612-870-8831
e-mail: info@ethnicdancetheatre.com
Web Site: www.ethnicdancetheatre.com
Officers:
  Chairman: Graham Thatcher
  Vice Chairman: Cindy Geiger
  Secretary: Jeanette Anderson
  Treasurer: Richard Van Puyvelde
  Company Manager: Sara Oxton
Management:
  Artistic Director/Co-Founder: Donald LaCourse
  Co-Founder: Jonathan Frey

Orchestra Director: Dee Langley
Vocal Director: Natalie Nowytski
Mission: Dedicated to the artistic and dynamic traditions of ethnic dance and music. Performs concerts and conducts residencies and public workshops.
Founded: 1974
Organization Type: Performing; Touring; Resident; Educational

352 HAUSER DANCE COMPANY AND SCHOOL

1940 Hennepin Avenue
Minneapolis, MN 55403
Phone: 612-871-9077
Fax: 612-870-0764
e-mail: nhdc@tcinternet.net
Web Site: tcfreenet.org/org/hauser
Officers:
   Chairman: Russ Christensen
   Treasurer: Heidi Jasmin
Management:
   Artistic Director: Heidi Hauser Jasmin
Mission: To promote and sustain the living language of modern dance. Accomplished by performing, fostering and teaching the constantly evolving Hauser Aesthetic. The goals of the organization are 1) artistic excellence and 2) access for all people to its programs.
Founded: 1961
Specialized Field: Modern Dance
Status: Professional; Nonprofit
Paid Staff: 2
Volunteer Staff: 15
Paid Artists: 6
Non-paid Artists: 10
Budget: $85,000
Income Sources: Foundations; Corporations; Individuals
Performs At: Nancy Hauser Memorial Theatre
Affiliations: Minnesota Dance Alliace
Annual Attendance: 1,500
Facility Category: Dance studio; Small black box theater
Stage Dimensions: 25'x35'
Seating Capacity: 100
Year Built: 1925
Year Remodeled: 1989
Organization Type: Performing; Touring; Educational; Sponsoring

353 MINNESOTA DANCE THEATRE

528 Hennepin Avenue
6th Floor
Minneapolis, MN 55403
Phone: 612-338-0627
Fax: 612-338-5160
e-mail: info@mndance.org
Web Site: www.mndance.org
Officers:
   President: David Lilly, Jr
Management:
   Artistic Director/Founder: Lise Houlton
   Development Director: Amy Braford Whitteg
Mission: Our legacy is a virtual library of dance repertoire from classical ballet to our own unique contemporary voice.
Founded: 1962

Specialized Field: Classical; Contemporary; Cutting Edge Choreography
Status: Professional; Nonprofit
Paid Staff: 14
Paid Artists: 35
Income Sources: Ticket Revenue; Donations; State Funding; Grants
Performs At: State Theatre; Illusion Theater; Fitzgerald Theater
Annual Attendance: 30,000
Organization Type: Performing; Touring; Resident; Educational

354 NORTHROP DANCE SEASON

84 Church Street SE
Minneapolis, MN 55455
Phone: 612-624-2345
Fax: 612-626-1750
Web Site: www.northrop.umn.edu
Management:
   Director: Dale Schatzlein
Mission: To offer an annual season featuring six to eight of the finest national and international dance companies.
Founded: 1919
Specialized Field: Dance
Status: Professional
Income Sources: Association of Performing Arts Presenters; International Society of Performing Arts Administrators
Performs At: Northrop Memorial Auditorium
Organization Type: Sponsoring

355 ZENON DANCE COMPANY AND SCHOOL

528 Hennepin Avenue
Suite 400
Minneapolis, MN 55403
Phone: 612-338-1101
Fax: 612-338-2479
e-mail: info@zenondance.org
Web Site: www.zenondance.org
Management:
   Artistic Director: Linda Z Andrews
   Managing Director: Ann Willemssen
   Business Manager: Sara Stevenson
   Scholarship Coordinator: Megan Flood
Mission: To sustain an artistically excellent, professional dance company in the Twin Cities.
Founded: 1983
Specialized Field: Modern; Ballet; Jazz
Status: Professional; Nonprofit
Paid Artists: 8
Facility Category: 2 Dance Studios
Stage Dimensions: 54'x46'; 56'x27'
Rental Contact: Managing Director Ann Willemssen
Organization Type: Performing; Touring; Resident; Educational

Mississippi

356 BALLET MISSISSIPPI
Mississippi Arts Center, Suite 106
PO Box 1787
Jackson, MS 39215-1787
Phone: 601-960-1560
Fax: 601-960-2135
e-mail: dkeary@netdoor.com
Management:
   Artistic Director: David Keary
   Executive Director: Joanna Hunt
Mission: To advance the study, understanding and
appreciation of ballet and other forms of dance.
Founded: 1982
Specialized Field: Ballet
Status: Professional; Nonprofit
Budget: $100,000-$200,000
Organization Type: Performing; Touring; Resident;
Educational

**357 USA INTERNATIONAL BALLET
COMPETITION**
PO Box 3696
Jackson, MS 39207-3696
Phone: 601-355-9853
Fax: 601-355-5253
e-mail: usaibc@netdoor.com
Web Site: www.usaibc.com
Management:
   Executive Director: Sue Lobrano
   Artistic Director: Peter Merz
   Public Relations/Marketing Director: Kathryn
   Stewart
   General Manager: Kathy Lyell
Mission: To provide an opportunity for dancers to test
themselves against recognized international standards of
dance excellence; to showcase their technical skills and
artistic talent; to provide a forum for communication and
intercultural exchange; and to educate, enlighten, and
develop future audience support for the art of dance.
Founded: 1979
Specialized Field: Dance
Status: Semi-Professional; Nonprofit
Performs At: Thalia Mara Hall
Annual Attendance: 36,000
Organization Type: Performing

Missouri

358 ALEXANDRA BALLET
68 E Four Seasons Center
Chesterfield, MO 63017
Phone: 314-469-6222
Fax: 314-469-6222
e-mail: amy@alexandraballet.org
Web Site: www.alexandraballet.org
Officers:
   President: Hillary Zimmerman
Management:
   Artistic Director: Alexandra Zaharias
   Ballet Mistress: Norma Gabriel
   Ballet Mistress: Laura Karmi

Ballet Mistress: Amy Scheers
Mission: Repertoire ranges from classic to contemporary.
Performance showcases original works through the
restaging of classics by locally and internationally known
choreographers and the collaboration of professional guest
artists.
Specialized Field: Regional Ballet Company

359 ST. LOUIS BALLET
218 THF Boulevard
Chesterfield, MO 63005
Phone: 636-537-1950
Fax: 636-537-2578
e-mail: info@stlouisballet.org
Web Site: www.stlouisballet.org
Management:
   Artistic Director: Gen Horiuchi
   Ballet Mistress: Ellen Costanza
   Resident Choreographer: Francis Patrelle

360 BALLET NORTH
6308 N Prospect Avenue
Gladstone, MO 64119-1825
Phone: 816-454-4859
Fax: 816-436-5788
e-mail: email@balletnorth.com
Web Site: www.balletnorth.com
Officers:
   Secretary: Alicia Nolte
   Treasurer: Heidi Luebbert
Management:
   Artistic Director: Laura Reinschmidt
   Production Designer: Matthew Reinschmidt
   Technical Director: Dan Fenger
Mission: To perform classic and modern ballets to all
ages and backgrounds in all areas.
Founded: 1976
Specialized Field: Classical and modern ballet
Status: Nonprofit
Paid Staff: 4
Volunteer Staff: 12
Paid Artists: 8
Non-paid Artists: 20
Budget: $55,000
Income Sources: Performance revenue; Fund raisers;
Grants
Affiliations: Independent
Facility Category: Professional theater

361 KANSAS CITY BALLET
1601 Broadway Boulevard
Kansas City, MO 64108-1207
Phone: 816-931-2232
Fax: 816-931-1172
Toll-free: 888-968-2538
e-mail: kcbinfo@kcballet.org
Web Site: www.kcballet.org
Management:
   Artistic Director: William Whitener
   General Manager: Kevin Amey
Mission: Founded and dedicated to the tradition of
classical ballet, Kansas City Ballet offers our community
region and dance profession dance experiences of the
highest quality.

Founded: 1957
Specialized Field: Dance; Ballet
Performs At: Lyric and Midland Theatre
Affiliations: MAC, National Endowment for the Arts
Annual Attendance: 48,000

362 STATE BALLET OF MISSOURI

1601 Broadway Street
Kansas City, MO 64108-1207
Phone: 816-931-2232
Fax: 816-931-1172
e-mail: jbentley@coop.crn.org
Web Site: www.stateballetofmissouri.org
Management:
 Artistic Director: William Whitener
 Executive Director: Jeffrey J Bentley
Mission: Committed to becoming the leading producer of world class ballet in the Midwest.
Founded: 1980
Specialized Field: Ballet
Status: Professional
Budget: $2,500,000
Organization Type: Performing; Touring

363 WYLLIAMS/HENRY DANCE THEATRE

209 S Olive Street
Kansas City, MO 64124
Phone: 816-235-2938
Fax: 816-531-4884
e-mail: henrym@umkc.edu
Management:
 Artistic Director: Mary Pat Henry

364 DANCE SAINT LOUIS

634 N Grand Boulevard
Suite 1102
Saint Louis, MO 63103
Phone: 314-534-5000
Fax: 314-534-5001
Web Site: www.dancestlouis.org
Management:
 General Manager: Laura Burkhart
 Executive Director: Sally A Bliss
Mission: Dedicated to enhancing the cultural well-being of greater St. Louis by creating and perpetuating interest, awareness and appreciation of dance as a major art form through concert presentations and educational activities.
Founded: 1966
Specialized Field: Modern; Mime; Ballet; Jazz; Ethnic; Folk
Status: Nonprofit
Paid Staff: 12
Income Sources: Dance USA
Performs At: Kiel Opera House; Edison Theatre; Washington University
Organization Type: Resident; Educational; Sponsoring

365 MID-AMERICA DANCE COMPANY

502 Mistletoe Lane
Saint Louis, MO 63108
Phone: 314-821-0660
e-mail: midamericadance@aol.com
Web Site: www.midamericadance.com
Officers:

Treasurer: Steve Butler
President: Cristin Viebranz
Development Director: Kate Meacham
Management:
 Artistic Director: Stacy West
 Booking Agent: Kate Meahcam
Mission: To provide high quality entertaining dance performances; to foster understanding and appreciation for dance through education programs; to provide a venue for artists to live and work; and to act as a preservation mechanism for valuable dances that may not otherwise survive.
Founded: 1976
Specialized Field: Modern
Status: Professional; Nonprofit
Paid Staff: 2
Non-paid Artists: 6
Income Sources: Regional Arts Comission; Missouri Arts Council; Arts & Education Council of St Louis; Private Foundations; Corporations; Individuals
Annual Attendance: 20,000
Organization Type: Performing; Touring; Educational

366 SAINT LOUIS BALLET

10 Kimler Drive, Suite C & D
PO Box 2101
Saint Louis, MO 63043
Phone: 314-567-4299
Fax: 314-567-4299
Web Site: www.stlouisballet.org
Management:
 Assistant to the General Director: Cynthia S Peak
 Artistic Director: Antoni Zalewski
Mission: To provide St. Louis and surrounding areas with a permanent, professional resident ballet company that performs both classical and contemporary works in the Ballet Russe tradition.
Founded: 1985
Specialized Field: Ballet
Status: Professional; Nonprofit
Budget: $200,000-$500,000
Income Sources: Grand Center
Organization Type: Performing; Touring; Resident; Educational

367 SAINT LOUIS CULTURAL FLAMENCO SOCIETY

PO Box 21818
Saint Louis, MO 63109
Phone: 314-781-1537
Fax: 314-781-6263
e-mail: marisel@saintlouisflamenco.com
Web Site: www.saitnlouisflamenco.com
Officers:
 Manager: Alvaro Molano
Management:
 Artistic Director: Marisel Salascruz
Mission: To promote and preserve the culture of Spain as expressed in dance, music, and song. To emphasize this, we use the carnation, the national flower of Spain, in our logo.
Founded: 1983
Specialized Field: Ballet
Status: Nonprofit

Paid Staff: 7
Income Sources: Dance St. Louis
Organization Type: Performing

368 SPRINGFIELD BALLET

400 S Avenue
Springfield, MO 65806
Phone: 417-864-1343
Fax: 417-864-6577
e-mail: spballet@mindspring.com
Web Site: www.springfieldballet.org
Officers:
   President: Russell Aldredge
   VP: Jennifer Penny
   Treasurer: Wayne Havarek
   Recording Secretary: Ann Hicks
Management:
   Executive Director: Phillip D McGuire
   School Director: Marsha Warnke
Mission: The education of students and the public in techniques of dance; performance at the highest possible level; presentation of guest dance companies.
Founded: 1976
Specialized Field: Modern; Ballet; Jazz; Tap
Status: Non-Professional; Nonprofit
Paid Staff: 10
Budget: $200,000-$500,000
Performs At: Landers Theatre; Vandivort Center; Coger Theater
Organization Type: Performing; Educational; Sponsoring

Montana

369 MONTANA BALLET COMPANY

221 E Main Street
Bozeman, MT 59715
Phone: 406-582-8702
Fax: 406-587-0595
e-mail: mtballet@gomotana.com
Web Site: www.montanaballet.com
Officers:
   President: Dianne Lorang
   VP: Susan Ledbetter
   Secretary: Leslee Finck
   Executive Director: Sandra Bellingham
Management:
   Artistic Director/Founder: Ann Bates
Mission: To train high school level professionally bound dancers; to present visiting dance companies; to outreach rural schools.
Founded: 1983
Specialized Field: Modern; Ballet; Jazz
Status: Professional; Nonprofit
Paid Staff: 3
Budget: $170,000
Performs At: Willson Auditorium
Facility Category: School
Stage Dimensions: 32'x 26'
Seating Capacity: 1,000
Organization Type: Performing; Touring; Educational; Sponsoring

Nebraska

370 NEBRASKA THEATRE CARAVAN

6915 Cass Street
Omaha, NE 68132
Phone: 402-553-4890
Fax: 402-553-6288
e-mail: info@omahaplayhouse.com
Web Site: omahaplayhouse.com
Management:
   Director Outreach/Touring: Richard L Scott
Mission: To provide quality theatrical experiences and educational opportunities to communities in which they would not otherwise be available. The caravan is the professional touring wing of the Omaha Community Playhouse.
Founded: 1976
Specialized Field: Local and National Tourtug

Nevada

371 NEVADA BALLET THEATRE

1651 Inner Circle
Las Vegas, NV 89134
Phone: 702-243-2623
Fax: 702-804-0365
e-mail: VAbrahm@nevadaballet.com
Web Site: www.nevadaballet.com
Management:
   Company Manager: Valerie Abraham
   Executive Director: Harry Ferris
Budget: $1,000,000-$2,500,000

372 NEVADA FESTIVAL BALLET

1790 W Fourth Street
Suite B
Reno, NV 89503
Phone: 775-785-7915
Fax: 775-785-7918
e-mail: leann@gbis.com
Officers:
   President: Michael McKeno
Management:
   Business Manager: Leann Pinguelo
Founded: 1984
Specialized Field: Dance

New Hampshire

373 BALLET NEW ENGLAND

PO Box 4501
Portsmouth, NH 03802-4501
Phone: 603-430-9309
Fax: 603-436-5396
e-mail: balletewengland@juno.com
Web Site: www.balletnewengland.org
Officers:
   Executive Director: Patsy L Lorentzen
   President: Jacinthe Grote
   VP: Mimi Gredy
   Secretary: Cathleen Marshall

Director: John S Cavanaugh
Director: Maureen Dwyer-Heinrichs
Director: Kathleen Murray
Director: Jennifer Ramsey
Management:
Co-School Director: Angela V Carter
Co-School Director: Martha M Soucy
Executive Director: Patsy L Lorentzen
Mission: Goal is to provide the finest in dance education with an emphasis in clinical ballet and to develop poise, self awareness and confidence through achievement.
Budget: $200,000-$500,000

New Jersey

374 ATLANTIC CONTEMPORARY BALLET

612 E Pine View Drive
Absecon, NJ 08205
Phone: 609-748-6625
Fax: 609-748-1068
e-mail: acbt@iname.com
Web Site: www.acbt.org
Founding Director: Phyllis Papa
Budget: $40,000-$100,000

375 NAI-NI CHEN DANCE COMPANY

PO Box 1121
Fort Lee, NJ 07024
Fax: 201-947-6380
Toll-free: 800-650-0246
e-mail: info@nainichen.org
Web Site: www.nainichen.org
Management:
Executive Director: Andrew Chiang
General Manager: Bonnie Hyslop
Mission: Bring the rich and elegant Asian dance tradition into the world of American choreography.
Founded: 1988
Specialized Field: Dance
Paid Staff: 3
Paid Artists: 10
Budget: $10,100,000
Income Sources: Tickets; Donations

376 RANDY JAMES DANCE WORKS

PO Box 4452
Highland Park, NJ 08904
Phone: 732-247-2653
Fax: 732-247-5353
e-mail: RJ4452@aol.com
Web Site: www.rjdw.org
Officers:
President: Bart Feller
VP: Philip Levy
Secretary: Susan Litt
Treasurer: Marvin Auerbach
Management:
Artistic Director: Randy James
National Booking Manager: Allison Schaeffer
Assistant Booking Manager: Sara Ketrow
Mission: Guided by the dynamic vision of Artistic Director Randy James who has built the company reflective of his personal dedication to ethnic and cultural diversity. The company is deeply committed to dance education and providing a forum for nurturing creative thoughts and ideas, and exposing the public to physical, emotional, mental and spiritual benefits of dance through the production of dance performances and workshops.
Founded: 1993
Paid Staff: 7
Volunteer Staff: 20
Paid Artists: 10
Budget: $100,000-$200,000
Income Sources: State Government; Foundations; Individual Supporters; Earned Income
Affiliations: Member of Dance USA, Dance NJ, DTW

377 ATTIC ENSEMBLE

83 Wayne Street
Jersey City, NJ 07302
Phone: 201-413-9200
Fax: 201-434-0568
Web Site: www.atticensemble.org
Founded: 1970
Income Sources: Donors; New Jersey Stage Council on the Arts; Hudson County Department of Cultural & Heritage Affairs

378 AVODAH DANCE ENSEMBLE

243 Fifth Street
Suite 9
Jersey City, NJ 07302
Mailing Address: HUC-JIR, One W 4th Street, New York, NY. 10012
Phone: 201-659-7072
Fax: 201-659-7072
e-mail: avodah@worldnet.att.net
Web Site: www.avodahdance.org
Officers:
President: Jesse Berger
VP: Renee Cook
Treasurer: Marianne Mendelson
Executive VP: JoAnne Tucker
Management:
Artistic Director: JoAnne Tucker
Mission: Avodah is a modern dance company that uses ancient sacred texts to connect and reconnect our spiritual selves to God and community. Reaching deep within the Jewish tradition, using dance, music and movement, Avodah strives to strengthen and further define Jewish idenity. Reaches out through cross-cultural collaborations. Avodah in Hebrew, connotes service or worship.
Founded: 1974
Specialized Field: Modern dance
Status: Professional
Paid Staff: 2
Paid Artists: 6
Budget: $75,000
Income Sources: Bookings; Grants; Individual Contributions
Organization Type: Performing; Touring; Resident; Educational

379 NEW JERSEY BALLET COMPANY

15 Microlab Road
Livingston, NJ 07039

Phone: 973-597-9600
Fax: 973-597-9442
e-mail: njballet@aol.com
Web Site: www.newjerseyballet.org
Officers:
  President: Michael K Furey Esq
  Executive VP: Carolyn Clark
  VP: Richard Meade Esq
  VP: Scott Morrison
  VP: Donald A Robinson
  Secretary: Peter Maloff
  Treasurer: Janice Colby
Management:
  Executive/Artistic Director: Carolyn Clark
  Artistic Co-Advisor: Eleanor D'Antuono
  Artistic Co-Advisor: Leonid Kozlov
  Artistic Co-Advisor: Edward Villella
  Assistant Artistic Director: Paul McRae
Mission: Makes the excitement of dance accessible to 150,000 New Jerseyans (live and through media) every year and maintains a repertory of exceptional breadth and quality including classical and contemporary works and ballets for children.
Founded: 1958
Specialized Field: Ballet; Dance
Status: Professional; Nonprofit
Budget: $1,000,000-$2,500,000
Organization Type: Performing; Touring; Educational

380   NEW JERSEY DANCE CENTER

202 Maplewood Avenue
Maplewood, NJ 07040
Phone: 973-762-3033
e-mail: info@newjerseydancecenter.com
Web Site: www.newjerseydancecenter.com
Management:
  Artistic Director: Anne Krohley
  Business Manager: Brian Gestring
Mission: To acquaint the community with dance.
Founded: 1982
Specialized Field: Ballet
Status: Semi-Professional; Commercial
Performs At: New Jersey Dance Theatre
Organization Type: Resident

381   RENATE BOUE DANCE COMPANY

239 Midland Avenue
Montclair, NJ 07042
Phone: 973-783-9845
Fax: 973-783-0001
e-mail: yass@bellatlantic.net
Officers:
  Chairperson: Barbara Francett
Management:
  Assistant Director: Muriel Daino
  Artistic Director: Renate Boue
Founded: 1972
Specialized Field: Modern
Status: Professional; Semi-Professional
Paid Staff: 4
Volunteer Staff: 15
Rental Contact: Julie Thompson
Organization Type: Performing; Educational

382   ST. JOHN'S RENAISSANCE DANCERS

239 Midland Avenue
Montclair, NJ 07042
Phone: 201-783-9845
Fax: 201-783-0001
Mission: The presentation of high quality dance and music of the Renaissance and the recreation of the splendor of 15th and 16th-century Europe.
Founded: 1979
Specialized Field: Historic Dance
Status: Professional
Organization Type: Performing; Touring; Educational

383   NATIONAL BALLET OF NEW JERSEY

5113 Church Road
Mount Laurel, NJ 08054
Phone: 856-235-5342
Fax: 856-235-6343
e-mail: balletnj@aol.com
Web Site: www.nationalballetnj.com
Management:
  Artistic Director: Kenna McAdams-Connor
  Co-Administrator: Gayle Gardiner
  Founder: Lorraine McAdams
Mission: To provide training and special coaching to young artists through a trainee and apprentice program, thereby providing exposure and professional appearances, performance opportunities and an introduction to dance as a profession.
Budget: $500,000-$1,000,000

384   AMERICAN REPERTORY BALLET

80 Albany Street
2nd Floor
New Brunswick, NJ 08901
Phone: 732-249-1254
Fax: 732-249-8475
e-mail: arbobragg@aol.com
Web Site: www.arballet.org
Management:
  Acting Executive Director: Oceola Bragg
  Artistic Director: Graham Lustig
Founded: 1978
Specialized Field: Ballet
Status: Professional; Nonprofit
Budget: $2,500,000+
Income Sources: George Street Playhouse, The State Theatre
Performs At: McCarter Theatre; Princeton State Theater
Organization Type: Performing; Resident; Touring; Educational

385   LKB DANCE

2 Chapel Drive
New Brunswick, NJ 08901
Phone: 732-742-1523
e-mail: leahkreutzer@hotmail.com
Management:
  Artistic Director: Leah Kreutzer
Mission: Modern dance repertory that deconstructs traditional forms to refelct contemporary issues such as women and gender, politics, and human relationships, presented in both concert and educational workshop settings.

Founded: 1999
Specialized Field: Modern Dance Company
Volunteer Staff: 3
Paid Artists: 8

386   IRINE FOKINE BALLET COMPANY
33 Chestnut Street
Ridgewood, NJ 07450-3803
Phone: 201-652-9653
Fax: 201-652-9286
Web Site: www.folkineballet.com
Management:
    Director: Irine Fokine
    Business Manager: Margaret Dunworth
Mission: To provide training for young dancers and bring ballet to young people in suburban communities.
Founded: 1956
Specialized Field: Ballet
Status: Semi-Professional
Budget: $100,000-$200,000
Organization Type: Performing; Touring; Educational

387   BROADWAY CENTER STAGE
South Orange, NJ
Mailing Address: PO Box 68 South Orange, NJ 07079
Phone: 973-378-3244
Fax: 973-378-3242
Toll-free: 888-447-8243
e-mail: squaredusa@comcast.net
Web Site: www.broadwaycenterstage.com
Management:
    Producer: Suzanne Ishee
    Business Manager: Lucy Bowers
    Marketing Director: Jean Kerley
Mission: Presenting the finest, most affordable Broadway programming available, the duo of Broadway stars captures the most memoriable moments of Broadway.
Founded: 1995
Specialized Field: Symphony; Performing Arts Series; Festivals; Corporate; Master Classes
Paid Staff: 3
Volunteer Staff: 1
Paid Artists: 6

388   CAROLYN DORFMAN DANCE COMPANY
2780 Morris Avenue
Suite 1-A
Union, NJ 07083
Phone: 908-687-8855
Fax: 908-686-5245
Toll-free: 800-887-9322
e-mail: cddc@infi.net
Web Site: www.CarolynDorfmanDanceCo.org
Officers:
    Board President: Jay Allen Berez
Management:
    Artistic Director: Carolyn Dorfman
    Executive Director: Tom Werder
    Company Manager: Andria Angelico
    Stage Manager: Wendy Thomas

Mission: To produce and perform the work of Artistic Director Carolyn Dorfman and guest artists, and to expand the understanding of dance as an art form by audiences of all ages.
Founded: 1982
Specialized Field: Modern Dance
Budget: $435,000

New Mexico

389   KESHET DANCE COMPANY
214 Coal Avenue SW
Albuquerque, NM 87102
Phone: 505-224-9808
Fax: 505-842-0309
e-mail: info@keshetdance.org
Web Site: www.keshetdance.org
Officers:
    President: Janet Mettard
Management:
    Artistic Director: Shira Greenberg
    Technical Director: Marla Wood
Mission: To inspire passion and open unlimited possibilities through the experience of dance by uniting professional dancers with the community.
Founded: 1996
Specialized Field: Dance, Modern
Paid Staff: 3
Volunteer Staff: 8
Paid Artists: 10
Non-paid Artists: 20
Budget: 250,000

390   NEW MEXICO BALLET COMPANY
4200 Wyoming Boulevard NE
Albuquerque, NM 87111
Mailing Address: PO Box 21518 Alburquerque, NM 87154
Phone: 505-292-4245
e-mail: nmballet@mandala.net
Web Site: www.nmballet.org
Officers:
    Chairman: June Leonard
    Executive Director: Mildred Ness
    Chair: Renee Mathews
    Secretary: Patty Soukup
    Treasurer: Beth Brown
    Historian: Donna Shiplet
Management:
    Artistic Director: Patricia Dickinson
    Guest Artist Liasion: Pamela Trent
Mission: To create and produce unique, innovative ballet and classical ballet performances for the people of New Mexico through dance education, ticket sales, major contributors, grants, and a strong volunteer Board and Guild.
Founded: 1972
Specialized Field: Ballet
Status: Nonprofessional; Nonprofit
Paid Staff: 40
Budget: $100,000-$200,000
Income Sources: Ticket Sales; Major Contributors; Grants

Organization Type: Performing; Touring

391 BILL EVANS DANCE COMPANY
PO Box 1126
Sandia Park, NM 87047
Phone: 505-286-0195
Fax: 505-277-9625
e-mail: billevansdance@hotmail.com
Web Site: billevansdance.org
Management:
Artistic Director: Bill Evans
Manager: Don Halquist
Mission: To support the creation and performance of
contemporary dance and rhythm tap dance work. To
support intensive workshops for teachers and students of
contemporary dance and rhythm tap dance.
Founded: 1975
Specialized Field: Dance
Status: Nonprofit; Tax Exempt
Paid Staff: 2
Volunteer Staff: 2
Paid Artists: 12
Non-paid Artists: 1
Budget: $100,000-$200,000
Income Sources: Ticket sales; grants
Annual Attendance: 7,000
Facility Category: Theatre
Type of Stage: Proscenium
Stage Dimensions: 40'x 35'
Seating Capacity: 420
Year Built: 1969
Year Remodeled: 1996
Resident Groups: Bill Evans Dance Company

392 ASPEN SANTA FE BALLET
550-B Saint Michaels Drive
Santa Fe, NM 87505
Phone: 505-983-5591
Fax: 505-992-1027
e-mail: jp@aspensantafeballet.com
Web Site: www.aspenballet.com
Management:
Executive Director: Jean-Philippe Malaty
Artistic Director: Tom Mossbrucker
Marketing Director: Brigitte Center
General Manager: Kerri Segell
Controller: Berry Roper
Office/Box Office Manager: Stacy Simon
Technical Director: Steve Myers
Mission: A company of twelve classically trained dancers
who perform an eclectic repertoire by some of the world's
foremost choreographers. Performs year-round at home in
Aspen and Santa Fe, and on tour throughout the United
States.
Founded: 1996

393 MARIA BENITEZ TEATRO FLAMENCO
PO Box 8418
Santa Fe, NM 87504-8418
Phone: 505-955-8582
Fax: 505-955-1726
e-mail: flamenco@mariabenitez.com
Web Site: www.mariabenitez.com
Management:

Artistic Director: Maria Benitez
Technical Director: Cecilio Benitez
Mission: To preserve, strengthen, and disseminate the
rich and diverse artistic heritage of Spain and Hispanic
people, enriching the lives not only of people of Spanish
ancestry, but all Americans.
Founded: 1971
Specialized Field: Professional Dance
Paid Staff: 6
Paid Artists: 18
Income Sources: Ticket Sales; Contributed Income
Performs At: Santa Fe: Maria Benitez Theatre
Annual Attendance: 30,000
Facility Category: Cabaret-Style
Type of Stage: Sprung Wood Floor
Stage Dimensions: 22x14
Seating Capacity: 200
Resident Groups: Maria Benitez Teatro Flamenco

394 SANTA FE FESTIVAL BALLET
PO Box 1595
Santa Fe, NM 87504-1595
Phone: 505-983-3362
Fax: 505-982-6718
e-mail: info@santafeballet.org
Web Site: www.aspeuballet.com
Management:
General Director: Henry Holth
Executive Director: Jean-Philippe Malaty
Artistic Director: Tom Mossbrucker
Director Development: Robin Cole
Development Associate/Aspen: Andrea Sprick
Mission: Company of eleven classically trained dancers
who perform an eclectic repertoire by some of the world's
foremost choreographers.
Budget: $200,000-$500,000

New York

**395 MAUDE BAUM & COMPANY: EBA
DANCE THEATRE**
351 Hudson Avenue
Albany, NY 12210
Phone: 518-465-9916
Fax: 518-465-9916
e-mail: ebadance@aol.com
Web Site: www.eba-arts.org
Officers:
Board President: Joel Rosenberg
Board Treasurer: Andrea Celli
Board Secretary: Laurence Wilson
Management:
Artistic Director: Maude Baum
Company Manager: Jennifer Newman
Mission: To create, perform and teach the art of Dance
Theatre; to educate through movement and drama; to
advance the art form in the community and throughout the
world.
Founded: 1962
Budget: $200,000-$500,000

396 COURANTE DANCE FOUNDATION
10 S Water Street
Athens, NY 12015
Phone: 518-945-1830
Fax: 518-945-1830
e-mail: courante@juno.com
Management:
    Director: Janis Pforisch
Mission: Dance and Theatre, specializing in historical
reconstruction.
Founded: 1981
Paid Staff: 1

397 BALLET LONG ISLAND
390 Central Avenue
Suite C
Bohemia, NY 11716
Phone: 631-567-4403
Fax: 631-567-3079
Web Site: www.expage.com/longislandballet
Management:
    Artistic Director: Debra Punzi
    Administrative Director: Donna Havranek
    Registrar: Sara Havranek
Mission: Our mission is to make dance available and
affordable to everyone. We have three main goals: to
support a professional ballet touring company; to maintain
a dance school with a Scholarship Program; to offer an
Apprentice Program for aspiring young dancers.
Founded: 1986
Specialized Field: Ballet Performance
Paid Staff: 3
Volunteer Staff: 25
Paid Artists: 14
Non-paid Artists: 20
Budget: $200,000-$500,000
Performs At: Islip Town Hall West; Long Island Ballet
Center Performance Space
Affiliations: Official School - Long Island Ballet Center
Annual Attendance: 40,000
Seating Capacity: 500

398 LES GUIRIVOIRES DANCE COMPANY
2195 Grand Concourse 6B
Bronx, NY 10453
Phone: 718-562-8656
Fax: 718-561-2761
e-mail: guiraudrm@aol.com
Web Site: www.geocities.com/Guiraud_1999
Management:
    Founder/Director: Rose Marie Guiraud
    Music Director: Emmett O McDonald
Mission: The promotion and preservation of African arts
and cultural exchange.
Founded: 1973
Specialized Field: African Dance Theatre
Paid Staff: 10
Volunteer Staff: 4
Paid Artists: 24

**399 MERIAN SOTO DANCE &
PERFORMANCE**
1001 Grand Concourse #10F
Bronx, NY 10452
Phone: 718-588-1936
Fax: 718-537-3973
e-mail: pepatian@aol.com
Management:
    Artistic Director: Merian Soto
    Associate Director: Jane Gabriels
Founded: 1983
Specialized Field: Dance
Paid Staff: 2
Paid Artists: 10

400 BRIGHTON BALLET THEATRE
3300 Coney Island Avenue
Brooklyn, NY 11235
Phone: 718-769-9161
Fax: 718-646-0376
e-mail: bb718@hotmail.com
Web Site: www.brooklynx.org
Officers:
    President: Irina Roizin
    Coordinator: Vladimir Lepisko
Mission: The Brighton Ballet Theatre, Russian Dance
Center is situated at the beautiful seashore of Coney
Island at the heart of the Russian cultural district.
Founded: 1988
Status: Not-for-Profit

401 BROOKLYN ARTS EXCHANGE
421 Fifth Avenue
Brooklyn, NY 11215
Phone: 718-832-0018
Fax: 718-832-9189
e-mail: info@bax.org
Web Site: www.bax.org
Management:
    Executive Director: Marya Warshaw
    General Manager: Vanessa Andato
Founded: 1991
Paid Staff: 5
Budget: $200,000-$500,000
Facility Category: Theatre and rehearsal studios
Stage Dimensions: 25'X 30'
Seating Capacity: 75

**402 CHARLES MOORE DANCE THEATRE:
DANCES AND DRUMS OF AFRICA**
397 Bridge Street
2nd Floor
Brooklyn, NY 11201
Phone: 718-467-7127
Fax: 718-624-7873
e-mail: CMDT397@aol.com
Management:
    Artistic Director: Ella Thompson-Moore
    Executive Director: Faryce Moore
    Company Director: Karen Bennett
Mission: The Dance Theater performs African, Caribbean
and African American works reconstructed and
choreographed by Charles Moore, Artistic Director, and
guest choreographers. Extensive research goes into each
work.
Founded: 1974
Specialized Field: Modern; Jazz; Ethnic; African
Diaspora

Status: Professional; Nonprofit
Paid Staff: 2
Volunteer Staff: 15
Paid Artists: 12
Income Sources: New York State Council Dance Arts; Department of Cultural Affairs; New York Division of the Humanities Education Department
Performs At: Charles Moore Center for Ethnic Studies
Organization Type: Performing; Touring; Educational

403 DANCEWAVE

72 7th Avenue
Brooklyn, NY 11217
Phone: 718-622-1810
Fax: 718-398-5539
e-mail: dwave@brainlink.com
Management:
   Executive/Artistic Director: Diane Jacobowitz
Founded: 1979
Specialized Field: Modern
Status: Professional
Paid Staff: 3
Paid Artists: 10
Performs At: Brooklyn Music School & Playhouse, other NYC theaters
Organization Type: Performing; Touring; Resident; Educational; Sponsoring

404 ISHANGI FAMILY AFRICAN DANCERS/SANKOTA

PO Box 400396
Brooklyn, NY 11240-0396
Phone: 718-919-2278
Fax: 718-919-7883
e-mail: ishangi1@aol.com
Web Site: members.aol.com/ishangi1/index.html
Mission: The objectives of the program are to introduce the student to the culture, dance, music, and history of West Africa, dispelling commonly held myths.
Budget: $40,000-$100,000

405 MARK MORRIS DANCE GROUP

3 Lafayette Avenue
Brooklyn, NY 11217-1415
Phone: 718-624-8400
Fax: 718-624-8900
e-mail: info@mmdg.org
Web Site: www.mmdg.org
Management:
   Artistic Director: Mark Morris
   General Director: Barry Alterman
   Managing Director: Nancy Umanoff
Mission: Dedicated to creating and performing the works of Mark Morris.
Founded: 1980
Specialized Field: Modern
Status: Professional; Nonprofit
Budget: $2,500,000
Organization Type: Performing; Touring

406 MARTHA BOWERS DANCE/THEATRE/ETCETERA

62 Midwood Street
Brooklyn, NY 11225
Phone: 718-287-2224
Fax: 718-875-4264
e-mail: MBOWERS3@aol.com
Management:
   Artistic Director: Martha Bowers
Mission: To create innovative performance works that involve diverse populations both within and beyond the confines of conventional theaters.
Founded: 1981
Budget: $40,000-$100,000

407 AFRICAN-AMERICAN CULTURAL CENTER'S AFRICAN DANCE & DRUM PERFORMING TROUPE

350 Masten Avenue
Buffalo, NY 14209
Phone: 716-884-2013
Fax: 716-885-2590
e-mail: aacc@pcom.net
Management:
   Dance Director: Naima O Robinson
   Drum Director: Theresa Mingo
   Executive Director: Agnes M Bain
Mission: By presenting traditional African dance and drum, the repertory Company provides art and entertainment, enlightening audiences in the breadth and scope of African culture.
Status: Semi-Professional; Nonprofit

408 PICK OF THE CROP DANCE

2495 Main Street
Suite 332
Buffalo, NY 14214
Phone: 716-837-6217
Fax: 716-837-6217
e-mail: curtstei@poc.org
Web Site: www.poc.org
Management:
   Artistic Director: Elaine Gardner
   Music/Executive Director: Curt Steinzor
   Company Manager: Laurie Lachiusa
Specialized Field: Dance
Budget: $100,000-$200,000

409 CHAUTAUQUA BALLET COMPANY

Chautauqua Institution
PO Box 28
Chautauqua, NY 14722
Phone: 716-357-6200
Fax: 716-357-9014
e-mail: info@chautauqua-inst.org
Web Site: www.ciweb.org
Officers:
   President: Scott McVay
   VP: Richard R Redington
Management:
   Programming Director: Marty Merkley
   Music Director/Symphony Orchestra: Uriel Segal
   General Manager, Chautauqua Opera: Jay Lesenger

Artistic Director Dance: Jean-Pierre Bonnefoux
Artistic Director, Theater: Rebecca Guy
Mission: To be a center for the arts, education, religion and recreation.
Founded: 1874
Specialized Field: Dance; Vocal Music; Instrumental Music; Theater; Grand Opera; Chamber Music
Status: Professional; Semi-Professional; Nonprofessional; Nonprofit
Paid Staff: 120
Paid Artists: 1500
Budget: $15,000,000
Income Sources: Box Office; Grants; Private Donations
Performs At: Amphitheater; Norton Hall; Lenna Hall
Affiliations: Opera America; Chamber Music America
Annual Attendance: 150,000
Organization Type: Performing; Religious; Educational; Recreational

410 EURYTHMY SPRING VALLEY ENSEMBLE
260 Hungry Hollow Road
Chestnut Ridge, NY 10977
Phone: 845-352-5020
Fax: 845-352-5071
e-mail: info@eurythmy.org
Web Site: www.eurythmy.org
Management:
   Artistic Director: Dorothea Mier
   Tour Coordinator: Marcia Rulfs
Mission: Bringing performances into hospitals and special care facilities.
Budget: $200,000-$500,000

411 MID-HUDSON BALLET COMPANY
4 Old Route 9
Fishkill, NY 12524
Phone: 845-897-2667
Fax: 845-897-7052
e-mail: www.estelleandalfonso.com
Officers:
   President: Gary Nagelhout
   Secretary: Beverly Smith
   Treasurer: Pat Maine
Management:
   Company Manager: Shirley Sedore
   Artistic Director: Estelle Alfonso
Mission: To promote interest in the art of dance, including but not limited to ballet; to organize, establish, produce, direct, and/or stage ballet and other classic and semi-classical performances and to foster and promote all activities and movements for the social, educational, and recreational benefits of its members and the public.
Founded: 1959
Specialized Field: Ballet
Status: Nonprofit
Income Sources: Northeast Regional Ballet; Dutchess County Arts Council
Performs At: Mid-Hudson Civic Center
Affiliations: Eisenhower Hall Theatre
Organization Type: Performing; Educational

412 ITHACA BALLET
105 Sheldon Road
Ithaca, NY 14850
Phone: 607-277-1967
Fax: 607-274-3672
e-mail: lbrantley@clarityconnect.com
Web Site: www.ithacaballet.org
Officers:
   President: Elisabeth Thorn
   VP: Charlotte Fogel
   Secretary: Elizabeth Schermerhorn
   Treasurer: Helene Wilmarth
Management:
   Co-Artistic Director: Alice Reid
   Co-Artistic Director: Cindy Ried
Mission: To bring classical and contemporary ballet to areas of upstate New York and Pennsylvania.
Founded: 1959
Specialized Field: Modern; Ballet
Status: Semi-Professional; Nonprofit
Budget: $40,000-$100,000
Organization Type: Performing; Touring

413 MUSIC IN MOTION DANCE COMPANY
National Headquarters
201 Hampton Road
Ithaca, NY 14850-1427
Phone: 607-257-6196
Fax: 607-257-6196
Toll-free: 877-646-3262
e-mail: MUSICNMOTI@aol.com
Web Site: www.musicinmotion.com
Officers:
   President/CEO: Barbara W Thuesen RDE
   VP/Georgia: Nancy Thuesen Gell
Management:
   RDE National Director/Founder NY: Barbara W Thuesen
   Artistic Director/Virginia: Darlene Stephens
   Artistic Director/Georgia: Nancy Thuesen Gell
   Coordinator/Spencer, New York: Grace Miller
Mission: To establish and present quality dance training centers and performances, license affiliates, train and certify teachers and choreographers.
Founded: 1966
Specialized Field: Dance; Ballet; Modern Jazz; Musical Theater; Certified Teacher & Choreographic Training
Paid Staff: 15
Volunteer Staff: 80
Paid Artists: 10
Non-paid Artists: 60
Budget: $50,000-$300,000
Income Sources: Classes; Worshops; Performances; Grants
Performs At: 4 Dance Centers with 3 Studios Each
Affiliations: Music in Motion Company and Academy; La Grange Ballet; Music in Motion Ensemble; Spencer Ballet Club; Georgia Summer Performing Arts Conservatory
Annual Attendance: 10000+
Facility Category: Arena
Type of Stage: Proscenium theatre

414 DINIZULU AFRICAN DANCERS, DRUMMERS AND SINGERS
Aims of Modzawe Cultural Center
11562 Sutphin Boulevard
Jamaica, NY 11434
Phone: 718-843-6213
e-mail: dance@dinizulu.com
Web Site: www.dinizulu.com/dance/
Officers:
   Executive Director: Alice Dinizulu
Management:
   Artistic Director: Esi-Ayisi Dinizulu
Mission: Dedicated to presenting the beauty and majesty of African culture through dance.
Founded: 1947
Specialized Field: Ethnic
Status: Professional; Nonprofit
Organization Type: Performing; Touring; Resident; Educational; Sponsoring

415 DEL-SE-NANGO OLDE TYME FIDDLERS ASSOCIATION
RD #3
PO Box 233
New Berlin, NY 13411
Phone: 607-843-6745
Mission: Dedicated to the preservation, promotion and perpetuation of the art of olde tyme fiddling, its music and dances.
Founded: 1978
Specialized Field: Folk
Status: Nonprofit
Paid Staff: 40
Organization Type: Performing; Educational; Sponsoring

416 EGLEVSKY BALLET
999 Herricks Road
New Hyde Park, NY 11040
Phone: 516-746-1115
Fax: 516-746-1117
Web Site: www.eglevskyballet.com
Management:
   Artistic Director: Ali Pourfarrokh
   Company Manager: Fleur Israel
Mission: To bring professional caliber ballet to Long Island audiences with mixed repertory.
Founded: 1961
Specialized Field: Ballet Company- Dance

417 AJKUN BALLET THEATRE
20 Chelsea Road
New Rochelle, NY 10805
Phone: 914-235-2265
Fax: 914-636-0534
e-mail: AJKUN@aol.com
Web Site: hometown.aol.com/maltak777/AjkunBallet
Management:
   Artistic Director: Leonard Ajkun
   Artistic Director: Chiara Ajkun

Mission: To share the experience of this art form with diverse audiences through showcases, residencies and performing arts-education, venues and programs. Seeks to introduce young talents to the professional world of dance.
Specialized Field: Ballet
Status: Non-Profit Corporation

418 AILEY II
211 W 61st Street
3rd Floor
New York, NY 10023
Phone: 212-767-0590
Fax: 212-767-0625
Web Site: www.alvinailey.org
Management:
   Artistic Director: Sylvia Waters
   Artistc Advisor: Judith Jamison
   Business Manager: Patrick Ayoung
Founded: 1974
Specialized Field: Modern DAnce

419 ALLNATIONS DANCE COMPANY
Performing Arts Foundation
500 Riverside Drive
New York, NY 10027
Phone: 212-316-8431
Fax: 212-316-8485
e-mail: alnatdanco@aol.com
Web Site: www.allnationsdance.com
Management:
   Artistic Director: Chuck Golden
   Founder/Executive Director: Herman Rottenberg
   Associate Director: Sophia Pachecano
Mission: The troupe is composed of dynamic ethnic dancers, who present their own cultures through music and dance, and unite with each other to perform dances from around the world.
Founded: 1967
Specialized Field: Ethnic
Status: Professional; Nonprofit
Budget: $100,000
Performs At: International House
Organization Type: Performing; Touring; Educational

420 ALPHA-OMEGA THEATRICAL DANCE COMPANY
711 Amsterdam Avenue
Suite 4E
New York, NY 10025
Phone: 212-749-0095
Fax: 212-749-0095
e-mail: alphaomegadance@aol.com
Management:
   Executive Director: Dolores Vanison-Blakely
   Artistic Director: Enrique Cruz De Jeses
   Assistant Director: Donna Clark
Mission: Committed to promoting knowledge and appreciation of artistic activities related to dance through schools, repertory ensembles and a professional company.
Founded: 1972
Specialized Field: Modern; Jazz
Status: Professional; Nonprofit
Paid Staff: 3

Volunteer Staff: 5
Paid Artists: 12
Budget: $69,000
Income Sources: Individual, NYSCA
Organization Type: Performing

421 ALVIN AILEY AMERICAN DANCE THEATER

211 W 61st Street
3rd Floor
New York, NY 10023
Phone: 212-767-0590
Fax: 212-767-0625
Web Site: www.alvinailey.org
Management:
Executive Director: Sharon Gersten Luckman
Artistic Director: Judith Jamison
Associate Artistic Director: Masazumi Chaya
General Manager/Production Director: James King
Director Marketing/Public Relations: Jodi Pam Krizer
Director Development: Bennett Rink
Mission: Alvin Ailey American Dance Theater is dedicated to the preservation of unique Black cultural expression and the enrichment of the American modern dance heritage.
Founded: 1958
Specialized Field: Modern; Ballet; Jazz; Ethnic
Status: Professional; Nonprofit
Budget: $14,000,000
Income Sources: Earned Revenue; Corporations; Foundations; Individuals
Performs At: City Center
Organization Type: Performing; Touring; Educational

422 AMANDA MCKERROW
Dube Zakin Management

67 Riverside Drive
New York, NY 10024
Phone: 212-877-3388
Fax: 212-799-8420

423 AMERICAN BALLET THEATRE

3890 Broadway
3rd Floor
New York, NY 10003-1278
Phone: 212-477-3030
Fax: 212-254-5938
e-mail: wchappell@abt.org
Web Site: www.abt.org
Officers:
Chairman: Gedalio Grinberg
President/Chair Nominating Comm: Edward A Fox
Vice Chairman: Mildred C Brinn
Vice Chairman: David Koch
Vice Chairman: Cindy L Sites
Secretary: Robin Neustein
VP/Chair Development Co: Elizabeth Harpel Kehler
VP/Treasurer: Brian J Heidtke
Management:
Artistic Director: Kevin McKenzie
Studio Company Manager: Dana Ball
Executive Director: Wallace Chappell
Director Finance: Nancy Fleeter

Assistant General Manager: Kristen Leonard
Dierctor Education: Mary Jo Ziesel
Mission: To develop a repertoire of the best ballets from the past and to encourage the creation of new works by gifted young choreographers, wherever they might be found.
Founded: 1940
Specialized Field: Ballet
Status: Professional
Budget: $2,500,000
Performs At: Metropolitan Opera House
Organization Type: Performing; Touring

424 AMERICAN BOLERO DANCE COMPANY: CARNEGIE HALL

881 7th Avenue
Suite 1204
New York, NY 10019
Phone: 212-315-2840
Fax: 212-315-2817
e-mail: ambolero@earthlink.com
Web Site: www.ambolero.com
Management:
President: Gabriela Granados

425 AMERICAN TAP DANCE ORCHESTRA

170 Mercer Street
New York, NY 10012
Phone: 212-243-6438
Fax: 212-243-6438
Web Site: nyctapfestival.com/ATDO/
Management:
Siegel Artist Management: Liz Silverstein
Siegel Artist Management: Ethel Siegel
Siegel Artist Management: Jane Lawrence Curtiss
Mission: Dedicated to celebrating, preserving and perpetuating one of America's few indigenous art forms, tap dance.
Founded: 1986
Specialized Field: Rhythm; Jazz; Tap Dance
Status: Professional; Nonprofit
Performs At: Woodpeckers Tap Dance Center
Organization Type: Performing; Touring; Educational

426 AMERICAN-INTERNATIONAL DANCE THEATRE

322 Duke Ellington Boulevard
New York, NY 100253471
Phone: 212-662-3468
Fax: 212-678-0571
e-mail: Ppress322@aol.com
Management:
Managing Director: Paulette Singer
Specialized Field: World Wide
Budget: $500,000

427 AMY HOROWITZ SOLO DANCE
Perspectives Communications

163 3rd Avenue, Suite 400
New York, NY 10003
Phone: 212-777-6206
Fax: 212-505-9963
e-mail: perspectivesusa@earthlink.net

Management:
Administrative Director: Paul Mitchell
Mission: Amy Horowitz seeks, through national and international performances of solo dance concerts, to magnify and illuminate aspects of the human condition and natural world, in hopes that rediscovery of timeless bonds will forge connections among diverse peoples.

428 AMY PIVAR PROJECTS

2440 Broadway
Suite 65
New York, NY 10024
Phone: 212-580-4445
Fax: 212-580-9031
e-mail: Pivardance@aol.com
Management:
Artistic Director: Amy Pivar
Artistic Director: Freda Rosen
Founded: 1991
Specialized Field: Dance/Theater
Budget: $100,000-$200,000

429 ANDREA DEL CONTE DANZA ESPANA

144 E 24th Street
New York, NY 10010-3730
Phone: 212-674-6725
Fax: 212-674-6725
e-mail: adelconte@aol.com
Web Site: www.delconte-danza.com
Management:
Artistic Director: Andrea Del Conte
Mission: The company is dedicated to interpreting and preserving the Spanish dance tradition for a wide range of audiences through performances and educational programming.

430 ANGLO-AMERICAN BALLET

250 W 54th Street
4th Floor
New York, NY 10019
Phone: 212-307-6909
Fax: 212-307-5412
e-mail: aabballet@aol.com
Web Site: www.anglo0american-ballet.org
Officers:
Founder/Chairman: Robert Kingsley
President: Catherine Kingsley
Secretary: Keith Nolan
Executive Committee: Larry Crabtree
Management:
Artistic Director: Catherine Kinglsey
Studio/Company Manager: Larry Crabtree
Mission: To present classical ballet and its relations to people of all ages, especially through educational and outreach specialty.
Founded: 1980
Specialized Field: Dance
Status: Nonprofit
Paid Staff: 2
Paid Artists: 9
Budget: $40,000-$100,000
Income Sources: Performance Fees; Donations; Training
Organization Type: Performing; Educational

431 ANIK BISSONNETTE

67 Riverside Drive
New York, NY 10024
Phone: 212-877-3388
Fax: 212-799-8420

432 ANNABELLA GONZALEZ DANCE THEATER

4 E 89th Street
P-C
New York, NY 10128-0645
Phone: 212-722-4128
Fax: 212-722-4128
e-mail: agdt@mindspring.com
Web Site: www.agdt.org
Officers:
Chairman of the Board: Richard E Grimmlez
Management:
Art/Executive Director: Annabella Gonzalez
Associate Director: Andrea Chait
Mission: To create excellent and original dances; to educate individuals of all ages and circumstances on modern dance, Mexican dance, jazz and creative improvisations.
Founded: 1976
Specialized Field: Modern; Ethnic
Status: Nonprofit
Paid Staff: 2
Volunteer Staff: 2
Paid Artists: 7
Budget: $40,000-$100,000
Income Sources: Government Foundations, Corporate Support; Individual Contributions
Affiliations: Dance Theater Worshop; ART/New York; The Association of Hispanic Arts
Annual Attendance: 5,000
Facility Category: Rental theatres, school theatres, libraries, etc.
Organization Type: Performing; Touring; Educational

433 APOLLO'S BANQUET

Grand Central Station
PO Box 523
New York, NY 10163
Phone: 203-838-1904
Fax: 203-838-1904
e-mail: louixiv203@aol.com
Management:
Artistic Director: Thomas Baird
Co-Director: Hugh Murphy
Mission: To present baroque dance and music of the highest quality possible in concert venues.
Founded: 1995
Specialized Field: Baroque Dance; Music

434 ASIAN AMERICAN DANCE THEATRE

26 Bowery
3rd Floor
New York, NY 10013
Phone: 212-233-2154
Fax: 212-766-1287
Management:
Artistic Director: Eleanor Yung
Manager: Ananya Chatterjea

Executive Director: Robert Lee
Mission: To advance traditional Asian dance and its synthesis with traditional dance through performing and visual art programs, concerts, exhibitions, a research center and a forum for critical exchange.
Founded: 1974
Specialized Field: Modern; Ethnic; Folk
Status: Professional; Nonprofit
Organization Type: Performing; Touring; Educational

435 BALLET GALAXIE

67 Riverside Drive
New York, NY 10024
Phone: 212-877-3388
Fax: 212-799-8420

436 BALLET HISPANICO OF NEW YORK

167 W 89th Street
New York, NY 10024
Phone: 212-662-6710
Fax: 212-362-7809
e-mail: info@ballethispanico.org
Web Site: www.ballethispanico.org
Officers:
  Chairman: Jody Gottfried Arnhold
  President: Thomas W Ostrander
  Secretary: Christopher Smeall
Management:
  Artistic Director: Tina Ramirez
  School Director: Zelma Bustillo
  Education Program Director: Josephine Irvine
Mission: Providing performances and training in traditional and contemporary Hispanic-American dance.
Founded: 1970
Specialized Field: Modern; Ballet; Ethnic
Status: Professional; Nonprofit
Paid Staff: 23
Paid Artists: 39
Budget: $3,000,000
Income Sources: Earned Revenue; Public and Private Sector Contributions
Affiliations: Dance/USA; Association of Performing Arts Presenters
Organization Type: Performing

437 BALLET MANHATTAN

61 W 62nd Street
Suite 17M
New York, NY 10023
Phone: 212-586-2699
Fax: 212-664-0743
Officers:
  VP: Charla Genn
Management:
  Executive Director: Paul Croitoroo
  Artistic Director: Charla Genn
  Development Director: Carollyn Philip
Mission: To perform eclectic works by contemporary choreographers to a wide audience throughout the world.
Founded: 1985
Specialized Field: Modern; Ballet
Status: Nonprofit
Budget: $100,000-$200,000
Organization Type: Performing; Touring

438 BALLET TECH

Lawrence A Wein Center for Dance and Theatre

890 Broadway
8th Floor
New York, NY 10003
Phone: 212-777-7710
Fax: 212-353-0936
e-mail: staff@ballettech.org
Officers:
  President: Eliot Feld
  VP: Geraldine Kunstadter
  Treasurer: Robert Freedman
  Secretary: Yvette Neier
Management:
  Choreographer Director: Eliot Field
  Operations/Finance Director: Maggie Christ
  Company Manager: Tiana Peterson
Mission: To provide tuition-free professional ballet training to gifted New York City public school children and to operate a professional ballet company.
Founded: 1974
Specialized Field: Ballet
Status: Professional; Nonprofit
Budget: $2,500,000
Performs At: Joyce Theater
Affiliations: The Ballet Tech School

439 BATTERY DANCE COMPANY

380 Broadway
Fifth Floor
New York, NY 10013
Phone: 212-219-3910
Fax: 212-219-3911
e-mail: battery@bway.net
Web Site: www.batterydanceco.com
Management:
  Artistic Director: Jonathan Hollander
  Manager: Medb McGearty
  International Cultural Exchange: Sven Van Damme
  Technical Director: Barry Steele
Mission: Performs on the world's stages, teaches, presents and advocates for the field of dance.
Founded: 1976
Specialized Field: Modern/comtemporary
Status: Professional
Paid Staff: 3
Volunteer Staff: 7
Paid Artists: 12
Budget: $200,000-$500,000
Income Sources: Pace University
Annual Attendance: 100,000
Facility Category: Mainstage Theaters; Outdoor Amphitheaters; Gallery Spaces
Organization Type: Performing; Touring; Resident; Educational; Sponsoring

440 BEBE MILLER COMPANY

140 2nd Avenue
Suite 404
New York, NY 10003
Phone: 212-777-1340
Fax: 212-777-1337
e-mail: bebemiller@aol.com

Management:
  Artistic Director: Bebe Miller
Mission: Dedicated to performing the works of Bebe Miller throughout the United States and abroad.
Founded: 1985
Specialized Field: Modern
Status: Professional; Nonprofit
Paid Staff: 2
Paid Artists: 6
Budget: $200,000-$500,000
Organization Type: Performing; Touring; Resident

441 BEVERLY BLOSSOM AND COMPANY

45 Tudor City Place
Suite 404
New York, NY 10017
Phone: 212-953-0651
Web Site: www.beverlyblossom.com
Management:
  Choreographer/Director: Beverly Blossom
Founded: 1981
Specialized Field: Modern; Theater Dance
Status: Professional
Income Sources: Circum-Arts
Organization Type: Performing; Touring

442 BILL T. JONES/ARNIE ZANE AND COMPANY

853 Broadway
Suite 1706
New York, NY 10003
Phone: 212-477-1850
Fax: 212-777-5263
e-mail: info@billtjones.org
Web Site: www.geocities.com/Broadway/Balconey/3252
Management:
  Executive Director: Jodi Bialburn
Mission: Promoting the works of choreographers Bill T. Jones and Amie Zane.
Founded: 1979
Specialized Field: Modern
Status: Professional; Nonprofit
Budget: $1,000,000-$2,500,000
Organization Type: Performing

443 BILL YOUNG & DANCERS

100 Grand Street
2nd Floor
New York, NY 10013
Phone: 212-925-6573
Fax: 212-925-6573
e-mail: wgy@panix.com
Web Site: www.pentacle.org
Management:
  Artistic Director: Bill Young

444 BLANCO & BLANCO

Old Chelsea Station
PO Box 985
New York, NY 10011

Phone: 212-362-6061
Fax: 212-877-0814
e-mail: blancoarts@aol.com
Web Site: www.blancopaf.org
Management:
  Co-Artistic Director: Carol Blanco
  Co-Artistic Director: R Michael Blanco
Mission: Blanco & Blanco, under the direction of Carol Blanco and R. Michael Blanco, is a collaborative company founded in 1992 which produces innovative cross-media performances in dance, theater, music and radio.
Founded: 1992
Status: Nonprofit 501(c)(3)

445 CAMI

165 West 57th Street
New York, NY 10019-2276
Phone: 212-841-9564
Fax: 212-841-9552
e-mail: info@cami.com
Web Site: www.cami.com
Founded: 1930
Specialized Field: Dance

446 CARLOTA SANTANA SPANISH DANCE COMPANY

154 Christopher Street
Suite 3D
New York, NY 10014
Phone: 212-229-9754
Fax: 212-229-1085
e-mail: santana@flamenco-vivo.org
Web Site: www.flamenco-vivo.org
Officers:
  Trustee: Donna Torres
  Trustee: Belen Fernandez
  Trustee: Deborah Freedman
  Trustee: Barbara B. Friedman
  Trustee: Janice P. Haggerty
  Trustee: Deborah Harper
  Trustee: Katherine Pacuba
  Trustee: Gilda Riccardi
  Trustee: Susan R.S. Schofield
Management:
  Artistic Director: Carlota Santana
  General Manager: Ann Stuart
Mission: To use flamenco to break down cultural barriers and to teach Spanish history and culture using flamenco as the focal point. Developing original flamenco works and unknown artists.
Founded: 1983
Specialized Field: Ethnic
Status: Professional; Nonprofit
Budget: $200,000-$500,000
Organization Type: Performing; Touring; Resident; Educational

447 CAROL FONDA AND COMPANY

20 E 17th Street
New York, NY 10003

Phone: 212-633-7202
Fax: 212-633-7204
e-mail: cfonda@dancenewyork.org
Web Site: www.dancenewyork.org
Officers:
  President: Lilly Chan
  VP: Robin Pell
  VP/Artistic Director: Carol Fonda
  Secretary: Maria Gordon Shydko
Management:
  Artistic Director: Carol Fonda
  Marketing Director: David Reynolds
  Development Director: Jillian Sweeney
  Public Relations Director: Maria Gordon Shydlo
  Director: Robin Pell
Mission: To support Arts-in-Education projects; to promote health and wellness projects.
Founded: 1978
Specialized Field: Modern
Status: Professional; Nonprofit
Paid Staff: 2
Volunteer Staff: 3
Paid Artists: 4
Budget: $40,000-$100,000
Income Sources: Professional training programs; Rental; Ticket sales
Facility Category: Studio/performance space
Type of Stage: Black Box
Stage Dimensions: 45 x 26
Seating Capacity: 65
Year Built: 2000
Rental Contact: Programs David Reynolds
Organization Type: Performing; Touring; Resident; Educational

448 CAROLYN LORD AND COMPANY

10 E 18th Street
Suite 3
New York, NY 10003
Phone: 212-924-7882
Fax: 212-989-6112
e-mail: carolyn@nais.com
Management:
  Artistic Director: Carolyn Lord

449 CELEBRATION TEAM OF NATIONAL DANCE INSTITUTE

594 Broadway
Room 805
New York, NY 10012
Phone: 212-226-0083
Fax: 212-226-0761
Web Site: www.nationaldance.org
Officers:
  Founder: Jacques d'Amboise
  Executive Director: Lesli Kapell
Management:
  Artistic Director: Ellen Weinstein
Mission: NDI's semi professional performing group is comprised of the 9-15 years olds drawn from the thousands of public school children that participate in NDI's in-school and Saturday programs. Each year, the programs of NDI inspire thousands of children, reaching across social, ethnic, and economic boundaries and including children facing physical and emotional challenges.

450 CHEN AND DANCERS

70 Mulberry Street
2nd Floor
New York, NY 10013
Phone: 212-349-0126
Fax: 212-349-0494
e-mail: info@htchendance.org
Web Site: www.htchendance.org
Officers:
  President: Thomas Lim
  Chairperson: Shirley Ubell
Management:
  Artistic Director: HT Chen
  Associate Director: Dian Dong
Mission: To perform contemporary works rooted in an Asian-American heritage.
Founded: 1978
Specialized Field: Modern
Status: Professional; Nonprofit
Paid Staff: 6
Volunteer Staff: 3
Non-paid Artists: 27
Income Sources: Association for Performing Arts Presenters
Affiliations: Dance/USA
Annual Attendance: 20,000
Facility Category: Black Box
Type of Stage: Marley floor for Modern Dance
Seating Capacity: 70
Year Built: 1892
Year Remodeled: 1988
Rental Contact: Artistic Director H. T. Chen
Organization Type: Performing; Touring; Resident; Educational

451 CHINESE FOLK DANCE COMPANY

NY Chinese Cultural Center
390 Broadway, 2nd Floor
New York, NY 10013
Phone: 212-334-3764
Fax: 212-334-3768
e-mail: nyccc390@aol.com
Web Site: www.chinesedance.org
Management:
  Executive Director: Amy Chin
  Artistic Director: Xiaoliang Yang
Mission: The performance, presentation and commission of traditional and contemporary dances in the Chinese idiom.
Founded: 1973
Specialized Field: Ethnic; Folk
Status: Professional; Nonprofit
Paid Staff: 5
Volunteer Staff: 2
Paid Artists: 20
Budget: $500,000
Annual Attendance: 150,000
Facility Category: Dance Studio
Rental Contact: Belle Lam
Organization Type: Performing; Touring; Educational

452 CHRISTINE CAMILLO
67 Riverside Drive
New York, NY 10024
Phone: 212-877-3388
Fax: 212-799-8420

453 CIA VINCENTE SAEZ
Bernard Schmidt Productions
461 W 49th Street, East Office
New York, NY 10019
Phone: 212-307-5046
Fax: 212-397-2459
e-mail: bschmidtpd@aol.com
Web Site: www.bernardschmidtproductions.com
Management:
    Artists Representative: Bernard Schmidt
Mission: Performers from around the world at the crossroads of innovation and tradition.
Specialized Field: Contemporary Dance With Moorish Inspiration from Spain.
Paid Staff: 2
Paid Artists: 8

454 COMPANY APPELS
420 W 24th Street
Suite 9E
New York, NY 10011
Phone: 212-242-1664
Fax: 212-242-1948
Management:
    Artistic Director: Jonathon Appels
Founded: 1979
Specialized Field: Modern Ballet; Modern Dance

455 CORTEZ & COMPANY - CONTEMPORARY BALLET
320 W 89th Street
Suite 1D
New York, NY 10024
Phone: 212-799-8682
Fax: 212-799-1561
e-mail: CorteznCo@aol.com
Web Site: www.cortezandcompany.com
Management:
    Artistic Director: Hernando Cortez
    Executive Director: Matthew Bruffee

456 CREACH/COMPANY
238 W 20th Street
Suite 1D
New York, NY 10011-5805
Phone: 212-924-5443
Fax: 212-924-5443
e-mail: TLCreach@aol.com
Web Site: www.pentacle.org
Management:
    Director: Terry Creach
Founded: 1980
Income Sources: New York Council for the Arts; Harkness Foundation for Dance; Meet the Composer; Joyce Mertz-Gilmore Foundations

457 CROSS PERFORMANCE
PO Box 143
New York, NY 10011
Phone: 646-602-9390
Fax: 646-602-9395
e-mail: mapp@multiartsprojects.com
Management:
    Artistic Director: Ralph Lemon
    Producing Director: Ann Rosenthal
Founded: 1995
Specialized Field: Dance; Theater

458 DANCE COLLECTIVE
463 W Street
953H
New York, NY 10014
Phone: 212-627-4275
Fax: 212-627-4275
e-mail: cnolte2344@aol.com
Web Site: www.nydancecollective.com
Management:
    Artistic Director: Carol Nolte
    Assistant Director: Renouard Gee
Mission: A professional modern dance company with 25 year artistic impetus to collaborate and communicate with diverse communities. Comprised of dancers from a variety of ethnic and cultural backgrounds, creative artists their own right, the company is committed to both community involvment and the expansion of creative potential.
Founded: 1974
Specialized Field: Modern
Status: Professional; Nonprofit
Paid Staff: 1
Volunteer Staff: 4
Paid Artists: 6
Affiliations: Dance Theatre Workshop; The Field
Organization Type: Performing; Touring

459 DANCE HK/NY
124 Chambers Street
New York, NY 10007
Phone: 212-962-2667
Fax: 212-962-2667
Management:
    Artistic Director: Rosalind Newman
    Executive Director: Thomas Borek
Mission: To present choreography of Artistic Director Rosalind Newman.
Founded: 1998
Specialized Field: Contemporary Music
Facility Category: Theater

460 DANCE JUNE LEWIS AND COMPANY
PO Box 2025
New York, NY 10159
Phone: 212-741-3044
Fax: 718-996-1433
Management:
    Publicity Manager: Mel Leifer
    Artistic Director: June Lewis
    Associate Artistic Director: Claudio Assante
Founded: 1968
Specialized Field: Modern/Contemporary

Status: Professional
Organization Type: Performing; Touring; Resident; Educational

461 DANCE THEATRE OF HARLEM

466 W 152nd Street
New York, NY 10031
Phone: 212-690-2800
Fax: 212-690-5762
Web Site: www.dancetheatreofharlem.org
Officers:
    CEO: Ernest M Littles
Management:
    Artistic Director: Arthur Mitchell
Mission: To maintain a professional dance company which provides creative and educational opportunities for young people.
Founded: 1969
Specialized Field: Ballet
Status: Professional; Nonprofit
Organization Type: Performing; Touring; Educational

462 DANCEBRAZIL

Capoeira Foundation
104 Franklin Street
New York, NY 10013
Phone: 212-382-0555
Fax: 212-278-8555
e-mail: sergygordeev@hotmail.com
Web Site: www.dancebrazil.org
Management:
    Artistic Director: Jelon Viera
    Associate Artistic Director: Nem Brite
Mission: To produce, perform and preserve traditional and contemporary Brazilian and Afro-Brazilian dance and music.
Specialized Field: Modern; Ethnic; Folk
Status: Professional; Nonprofit
Organization Type: Performing; Touring; Resident; Educational; Sponsoring

463 DANCEGALAXY

165 W 66th Street
Suite 15j
New York, NY 10023
Phone: 212-874-1061
Fax: 212-874-1061
e-mail: mbahiri@aol.com
Web Site: www.dancegalaxy.org
Management:
    Co-Artistic Director: Medhi Bahiri
    Agent: Harold Norris II
    Co-Artistic Director: Judith Fugate
Mission: Present high quality ballet at an affordable price.
Founded: 1997
Specialized Field: Dance (Ballet)

464 DANCES PATRELLE

PO Box 6802
New York, NY 10128
Phone: 212-722-7933
Fax: 212-722-7933
e-mail: info@dancepatrelle.org
Web Site: www.dancespatrelle.org
Management:
    Artistic Director: Frances Patrelle
Founded: 1988
Specialized Field: Ballet

465 DANCING IN THE STREETS

55 Avenue of the Americas
Suite 310
New York, NY 10013
Phone: 212-625-3505
Fax: 212-625-3510
e-mail: info@dancinginthestreets.org
Web Site: www.dancinginthestreets.org
Officers:
    President: Anthony Russell
Management:
    Executive Director/Producer: Aviva Davidson
    General Manager: Sarah Johnson
    Education Director: Rebecca Ashley
    Founder/Consulting Producer: Elise Bernhardt
Mission: Dancing in the streets transforms the experience of art in the community, by commissioning, producing and presenting site specific performance, nurturing its development, and promoting it as a public art form.
Founded: 1983
Specialized Field: Site specific performance
Status: Professional; Non Profit
Organization Type: Producing

466 DANSPACE PROJECT

St. Mark's Church
2nd Avenue and 10th Street
New York, NY 10003
Phone: 212-674-8112
Fax: 212-529-2318
e-mail: info@danspaceproject.org
Web Site: www.danspaceproject.org
Management:
    Executive Director: Laurie Uprichard
Mission: To offer innovative dance artists opportunities for growth and development through the support and presentation of their work.
Founded: 1974
Specialized Field: Modern; Experimental; Postmodern
Status: Professional; Nonprofit
Paid Staff: 5
Volunteer Staff: 15
Paid Artists: 30
Budget: $1,000,000
Performs At: Sanctuary Performace Space at St. Mark's Church
Annual Attendance: 15,000
Stage Dimensions: 36'x48'
Seating Capacity: 200
Year Built: 1799
Year Remodeled: 1980
Organization Type: Performing; Artists Services

467 DAVID GORDON/PICK UP PERFORMANCE COMPANY
47 Great Jones Street
New York, NY 10012
Phone: 212-529-1557
Fax: 212-529-1703
e-mail: pickupperformance@earthlink.net
Management:
  Director: David Gordon
  Associate Director: Ain Gordon
  Managing Director: Bruce Allardice
Mission: Dedicated to producing and promoting the work of David Gordon and Ain Gordon.
Founded: 1978
Specialized Field: Modern; Theater, Dance
Status: Professional; Nonprofit
Paid Staff: 2
Volunteer Staff: 122
Paid Artists: 20
Income Sources: Dance USA; Association for Performing Arts Presenters; Western Alliance of Arts Administrators
Organization Type: Performing; Touring; Resident

468 DOMINIC WALSH
252 W 76th Street
Suite 6E
New York, NY 10023
Phone: 212-724-3889
Fax: 212-874-5039
e-mail: markapl1@aol.com

469 DONALD WILLIAMS
Dube Zakin Management
67 Riverside Drive
New York, NY 10024
Phone: 212-877-3388
Fax: 212-799-8420

470 DOUG ELKINS DANCE COMPANY
PO Box 951
New York, NY 10011
Phone: 212-228-2071
Fax: 212-785-6739
e-mail: plam5678@aol.com
Management:
  Artistic Director: Doug Elkins
  Company Manager: Jane Weiner
  Financial Director: Lisa Nicks
  Booking: Cathy Zimmerman
Mission: Established to create and present the work of Doug Elkins and to provide dance education for all levels and ages.
Founded: 1987
Specialized Field: Modern; Street Styles; House Styles
Status: Professional; Nonprofit
Organization Type: Performing; Educational

471 DOUGLAS DUNN AND DANCERS
541 Broadway
New York, NY 10012

Phone: 212-966-6999
Fax: 212-274-1804
e-mail: ddunn@aol.com
Management:
  Artistic Director: Douglas Dunn
Mission: Dedicated to producing and promoting the works of contemporary choreographer Douglas Dunn.
Founded: 1976
Specialized Field: Modern
Status: Professional; Nonprofit
Income Sources: Pentacle/Danceworks
Organization Type: Performing; Touring; Educational

472 EIKO AND KOMA
246 W 38th
Floor 8
New York, NY 10018-5805
Phone: 212-278-8111
Fax: 212-278-8555
e-mail: info@pentacle.com
Web Site: www.pentacle.org
Management:
  Artistic Director/Choreographer: Eiko Otake
  Artistic Director/Choreographer: Koma Otake
Mission: Established to perform the theater choreography of Eiko and Koma.
Specialized Field: Contemporary
Status: Professional; Nonprofit
Organization Type: Performing; Touring; Resident; Educational

473 ELINOR COLEMAN DANCE ENSEMBLE
208 W 23rd Street
Suite 1600
New York, NY 10012-3239
Phone: 212-242-7660
Fax: 212-242-7640
e-mail: danse@nyct.net
Management:
  Artistic Director: Elinor Coleman
  Managing Director: Helena McDonagh
Founded: 1978
Specialized Field: Dance

474 ELISA MONTE DANCE COMPANY
1170 Broadway
Suite 912
New York, NY 10001
Phone: 212-251-0789
Fax: 212-251-0743
e-mail: E.MonteD@aol.com
Web Site: www.montebrowndance.org
Management:
  Artistic Director: Elisa Monte
  Artistic Director: David Brown
  Chairman: Nancy Perlman
  Managing Director: Amy Blackman
Budget: $200,000-$500,000

475 ERICA ESSNER PERFORMANCE CO-OP
13 W 82nd Street
Suite 3B
New York, NY 10024

e-mail: essner@eecop.org
Web Site: www.dancenet.org
Management:
　Director/Choreographer: Erica Essner
Mission: Striving for the essence of individuality, the cooperative process is revealed in the merging of unique and idiosyncratic movement styles based on each member of the company.
Specialized Field: Modern Dance

476　ERNESTA CORVINO'S DANCE CIRCLE COMPANY
451 W 50th Street
New York, NY 10019
Phone: 212-582-0571
Fax: 212-247-2564
Management:
　Director: Ernesta Corvino
　Ballet Mistress: Andra Corvino
　Manager: Gail S Block
Mission: To provide the public with high quality and affordable dance performances, as well as workshops and lecture demonstrations.
Founded: 1981
Specialized Field: Ballet
Status: Professional; Nonprofit
Performs At: Marymount Manhattan Theatre
Organization Type: Performing

477　ETHAN BROWN
67 Riverside Drive
New York, NY 10024
Phone: 212-877-3388
Fax: 212-799-8420

478　EUGENE JAMES DANCE COMPANY
PO Box 2504
New York, NY 10116
Phone: 212-564-1026
Fax: 212-564-1026
Management:
　Manager: Richard Williams
　Artistic Director: Eugene James
Mission: Dedicated to extending the contributions of Afro-American rhythms to dance.
Founded: 1967
Specialized Field: Modern; Ethnic
Status: Professional; Nonprofit
Volunteer Staff: 3
Organization Type: Performing; Touring; Resident

479　FELICE LESSER DANCE THEATER
484 W 43rd Street
Suite 9T
New York, NY 10036
Phone: 212-594-3388
Fax: 215-594-3388
e-mail: dance200faol.com
Web Site: www.fldt.org
Management:
　Artistic Director: Felice Lesser
Mission: To engage in the creation of new dance works; to perform, teach and tour.

Founded: 1975
Specialized Field: Modern; Ballet
Status: Professional; Nonprofit
Organization Type: Performing; Touring; Resident; Educational

480　GILMA BUSTILLO
67 Riverside Drive
New York, NY 10024
Phone: 212-877-3388
Fax: 212-799-8420

481　GINA GIBNEY DANCE
890 Broadway
Studio 5-2
New York, NY 10003
Phone: 212-677-8560
Fax: 212-677-8560
e-mail: ggdance@compuserve.com
Web Site: www.geocities.com/~gibneydance
Management:
　Artistic Director: Gina Gibney

482　ICE THEATRE OF NEW YORK
Pier 62
Room 312
New York, NY 10011
Phone: 212-929-5811
Fax: 212-929-0105
e-mail: itny@icetheatre.org
Web Site: www.icetheatre.org
Officers:
　Chairman: William Candee III
　Vice Chairman: R Palmer Baker
　President: Moira North
Management:
　Artistic Director: Moira North
　Associate Artistic Director: Douglas Webster
　Ensemble Director: Judy Blumberg
　General Manager: Michiko Simanjuntak
Mission: To build an artistic repertory of ice skating performance pieces; to allow professional skaters from various backgrounds to collaborate with choreographers, musicians and visual artists.
Founded: 1984
Specialized Field: Modern
Status: Professional; Nonprofit
Performs At: The Rink at Rockefeller Plaza
Organization Type: Performing; Touring; Educational

483　IMAGO
163 Amsterdam Avenue
Suite 121
New York, NY 10023
Phone: 212-799-4814
Fax: 212-874-3613
e-mail: AShafman@aol.com
Web Site: www.Arthur Shafman.com

484　JANIS BRENNER AND DANCERS
356 E 89th Street
Suite 5A
New York, NY 10128

Phone: 212-864-3874
Fax: 212-534-3227
e-mail: biles@circum.org
Web Site: www.circum.org
Management:
   Dancer/Choreographer/Singer: Janis Brenner
Mission: Established to perform the work of Janis Brenner and to conduct teaching workshops in technique, improvisation, composition, repertory and voice.
Founded: 1987
Specialized Field: Modern
Status: Professional; Nonprofit
Organization Type: Performing; Touring; Educational

485 ## JENNIFER MULLER: THE WORKS
131 W 24th Street
4th Floor
New York, NY 10011
Phone: 212-691-3803
Fax: 212-206-6630
e-mail: jennifermullertheworks.org
Management:
   Artistic Director: Jennifer Muller
   Executive Associate: Stephanie Tack
Mission: The Works is first and foremost devoted to creating dance that is ground-breaking both in form and content, expressive of contemporary society's concerns and performed with artistic integrity and excellence.
Founded: 1974
Specialized Field: Contemporary Dance
Status: Professional; Nonprofit
Paid Staff: 4
Volunteer Staff: 2
Paid Artists: 12
Budget: $200,000-$500,000
Organization Type: Performing; Touring; Resident

486 ## JOAN MILLER DANCE PLAYERS
1380 Riverside Drive
Suite 10B
New York, NY 10033
Phone: 212-568-8854
Fax: 212-795-5212
Management:
   Artistic Director/Choreographer: Joan Miller
   Company Manager: Sandra Bell
Mission: A unique, multi-ethnic, street smart, mixed media company with a zany sense of humor, a slightly off-beat point of view and an eclectic sense of dance theater.
Founded: 1969
Specialized Field: Modern; Ballet; Jazz; Ethnic
Status: Professional
Paid Staff: 5
Budget: $40,000-$100,000
Income Sources: Dance Theatre Workshop
Organization Type: Performing; Touring

487 ## JODY OBERFELDER DANCE PROJECTS
234 E 4th Street
Suite 16
New York, NY 10009

Phone: 212-777-6227
Fax: 212-995-0364
e-mail: jodyober@inch.com
Web Site: www.danceonline.com/d/jodyoberfelder
Management:
   Artistic Director: Jody Oberfelder

488 ## JOHN GARDNER
67 Riverside Drive
New York, NY 10024
Phone: 212-877-3388
Fax: 212-799-8420

489 ## JOLINDA MENENDEZ
67 Riverside Drive
New York, NY 10024
Phone: 212-877-3388
Fax: 212-799-8420

490 ## JOSE LIMON DANCE FOUNDATION
611 Broadway
Suite 905
New York, NY 10012
Phone: 212-777-3353
Fax: 212-777-4764
e-mail: info@limon.org
Web Site: www.limon.org
Management:
   Executive Director: Mark W Jones
   Artistic Director: Carla Maxwell
   Company Manager: Daniel Finney
Mission: This company presents modern classics, jazz works and other contemporary works through performances and residencies throughout the United States and abroad.
Founded: 1946
Specialized Field: Modern Dance
Status: Nonprofit
Paid Staff: 10
Paid Artists: 14
Budget: $1.5 Million
Income Sources: Corporate; Foundation; Government Grants; Individual Donations; Performance Fees; Liscensing Fees

491 ## JOSE MOLINA BAILES ESPANOLES
163 Amsterdam Avenue
Suite 121
New York, NY 10023
Phone: 212-799-4814
Fax: 630-563-1859
Management:
   International Limited: Arthur Shafman
   Artistic Director: Jose Molina
Mission: Committed to presenting American audiences with the best of all styles of Spanish dance.
Founded: 1962
Specialized Field: Ethnic
Status: Professional; Commercial
Organization Type: Performing; Touring

492 JOYCE TRISLER DANSCOMPANY

333 E 13th Street
#12
New York, NY 10003
Phone: 212-677-4351
Fax: 212-260-8491
e-mail: regina@danscompnay.com
Web Site: www.danscompany.com
Officers:
    President: Regina Larkin
    VP: Bettina May
    Secretary: Carmen De Lavallade
    Treasurer: Nicholas Petron
Management:
    Manager: Nicholas Petron
    Artistic Director: Regina Larkin
Mission: The Joyce Trisler Danscompany mission is to continue to bring American modern dance to contemporary prominence through our history and creativity, in performance and education.
Founded: 1975
Specialized Field: Modern/Lester Horton Technique
Paid Staff: 2
Volunteer Staff: 7
Paid Artists: 6
Budget: $10,000-20,000
Performs At: Olmstead Theatre; Adelphi University; Peridance Center
Facility Category: Studios; Theatre

493 JUILLIARD SCHOOL

The Juilliard School, Dance Division
60 Lincoln Center Plaza
New York, NY 10023
Phone: 212-799-5000
Fax: 212-724-0263
e-mail: news@juilliard.edu
Web Site: www.juilliard.edu
Management:
    Director Dance Division: Lawrence Rhodes
Mission: To provide dance training through performance.
Founded: 1951
Specialized Field: Contemporary; Ballet; Jazz; Ethnic; Tap
Status: Non-professional; Nonprofit
Paid Staff: 30
Budget: $500,000-$1,000,000
Organization Type: Performing; Resident

494 KAREN SCALZITTI-KENNEDY

252 W 76th Street
Suite 6E
New York, NY 10023
Phone: 212-724-3889
Fax: 212-874-5039
e-mail: markkapl1@aol.com

495 KATHAK ENSEMBLE & FRIENDS/CARAVAN

141 E 3rd Street
Apartment 12H
New York, NY 10009
Phone: 212-673-1282
Fax: 212-673-1282

Management:
    Artistic/Administrative Director: Janaki Patrik
Mission: To teach and perform classical Northern Indian Kathak dance with live musical accompaniment; to create new repertoire inspired by classical and modern Indian music, dance, poetry and mythology, but also informed by modern theatre techniques and by the need to communicate with a Western audience largely unfamiliar with the Indian aesthetic; to teach about Indian culture.
Founded: 1978
Specialized Field: Classical East Indian Dance

496 KATHY ROSE

10 Stuyvsant Oval
New York, NY 10009-2421
Phone: 212-353-9891
Fax: 212-353-9891
e-mail: kleo@bway.com
Web Site: www.krose.com
Management:
    Artistic Director: Kathy Rose
Specialized Field: Performance, Video, Installation

497 KEI TAKEI'S MOVING EARTH

28 Vesey Street
#2200
New York, NY 10007
Phone: 212-459-4383
Fax: 212-732-3926
Web Site: www2.gol.com/users/keitakei
Officers:
    Chairperson: Kei Takei
    President: Louise Roberts
    VP: Maldwyn Pate
    Secretary/Treasurer: Lawrence Brezer
Management:
    Executive Director: Laz Brezer
Mission: To perform the internationally acclaimed, award-winning choreography of Kei Takei.
Founded: 1969
Specialized Field: Modern
Status: Professional
Paid Staff: 8
Organization Type: Performing; Touring

498 KITCHEN

512 W 19th Street
New York, NY 10011
Phone: 212-255-5793
Fax: 212-645-4258
e-mail: info@thekitchen.org
Web Site: www.thekitchen.org
Officers:
    Co-Chairman: Philip Glass
    Co-Chairman: Robert Soros
    President: Molly Davies
    VP: John Parkinson, III
    VP: Elizabeth Kahn
    Vice Chairman: Frances Kazan
    Vice Chairman: Arthur Fleischer, Jr
    Treasurer: Oliver G. Gayley
    Secretary: Franny Heller Zorn
Management:
    Executive Director: Elise Bernhardt

Dance Curator: Dean Moss
New Media Director: Christine Young
Education/Outreach Curator: Treva Offut
Music Curator: John King
Director Press/Marketing: Isabell
Mission: The Kitchen is an interdisciplinary laboratory for visionary emerging and established artists. It has been a powerful force in shaping the cultural landscape of this country for almost three decades, and is internationally renowned for its early support of artists who have gone on to receive world-wide stature.
Founded: 1977
Specialized Field: Modern
Status: Professional; Nonprofit
Paid Staff: 20
Volunteer Staff: 10
Performs At: Black Box
Facility Category: Center for Music, Dance, Literature and Film.
Type of Stage: Black Box
Stage Dimensions: 44'x33'
Seating Capacity: 125
Year Built: 1985
Rental Contact: Sacina Yanow
Organization Type: Performing; Resident; Educational; Sponsoring

499 LABAN INSTITUTE OF MOVEMENT STUDIES

520 8th Avenue
3rd Floor
New York, NY 10018
Phone: 212-213-1162
Fax: 212-213-1225
e-mail: limssnyc@aol.com
Web Site: www.limsonline.org
Officers:
    Chair: Karen Bradley
    President: Virgina Reed
Management:
    Executive Director: Regina Miranda
    Certificate Director: Kristina Lindahl
    Financial Manager: Bernice Sobel
Mission: To teach Laban movement analysis, Bartenieff fundamentals on the introductory and professional level.
Founded: 1978
Specialized Field: Movement Analysis, Bartenieff Fundamentals Anatomy & Kinesiology
Status: Professional; Non-Professional; Nonprofit
Income Sources: National Association of Schools of Dance; Emergency Fund for Student Dancers; Dance Theatre Workshop: American Dinner Theatre Association; International Movement Therapists
Organization Type: Performing; Educational; Sponsoring

500 LAR LUBOVITCH DANCE COMPANY

229 W 42nd Street
8th Floor
New York, NY 10036-7201
Phone: 212-221-7909
Fax: 212-221-7938
e-mail: lubovitch@aol.com
Officers:

President: Katherine Bristor
Management:
    Executive Director: Richard J Caples
    Artistic Director: Lar Lubovitch
    Development Director: Farrall Dyhe
Mission: To create, perform and teach contemporary dance throughout the United States and the world.
Founded: 1968
Specialized Field: Modern
Status: Professional; Nonprofit
Paid Staff: 4
Volunteer Staff: 20
Paid Artists: 20
Budget: $1,000,000-$2,500,000
Affiliations: Dance USA; Association of Performing Arts Presenters
Annual Attendance: 15,000
Facility Category: Theater
Type of Stage: Proscenium
Rental Contact: Micheal Ranscht
Organization Type: Performing; Touring; Educational

501 LAURA (PER)FOREMAN(CE) ART THEATRE

94 Chambers Street
New York, NY 10003
Phone: 212-227-9067
Fax: 212-227-5895
Management:
    Choreographer/Director: Laura Foreman
    Representative: Hank O'Neal

502 LES BALLETS TROCKADERO DE MONTE CARLO

Box 46
Cathedral Station
New York, NY 10025
Phone: 212-865-7925
Fax: 212-865-7925
e-mail: info@trockadero.org
Web Site: www.trockadero.org
Officers:
    President: Eugene McDougle
    VP: Lucille Lewis Johnson
    Secretary/Treasurer: Troy Dorbin
Management:
    Director: Eugene McDougle
    Artistic Director: Tory Dobrin
Mission: To perform ballet parody.
Founded: 1973
Specialized Field: Ballet
Status: Professional; Nonprofit
Budget: $500,000-$1,000,000
Organization Type: Performing; Touring

503 LES GRANDS BALLETS DE LOONY

484 W 43rd Street
#32H
New York, NY 10036
Phone: 212-279-5169
Fax: 212-279-5169
e-mail: nephties@eathlink.net
Management:
    Artistic Director/Choreographer: Marco Galante

Mission: Marco Galantes goal is to present a show in which the work is solid, clever and very funny, a show which is diverse in its programming and is audience friendly.
Founded: 1992

---

504 LORI BELILOVE & COMPANY
141 W 26th Street
Isadora Duncan Dance Foundation
New York, NY 10001-6800
Phone: 212-691-5040
Fax: 212-627-0774
e-mail: info@isadoraduncan.org
Web Site: www.isadoraduncan.com
Officers:
   Chairman: Jim Belilove
   Treasurer: Martha Ferry
Management:
   Artistic Director: Lori Belilove
   General Manager: Fran Kirhser
   Associate Artistic Director: Cherlyn Smith
Mission: Expands public awareness and understanding of Isadora Duncan as a world famous performer and choreographer, innovator, feminist, educator, author and philosopher.
Founded: 1989
Specialized Field: Dance
Paid Staff: 6
Volunteer Staff: 20
Paid Artists: 12
Non-paid Artists: 5
Budget: $200,000
Income Sources: Grants; Individual & Corporate Contributions

---

505 LOTUS MUSIC & DANCE
109 W 27th Street
8th Floor
New York, NY 10001-6208
Phone: 212-627-1076
Fax: 212-675-7191
e-mail: info@lotusarts.com
Web Site: www.lotusarts.com
Management:
   Artistic Director: Kamala Cesar
   Administrative Director: Danon Alderson
Founded: 1989
Specialized Field: Multicultural Music & Dance

---

506 LOUIS ROBITAILLE
67 Riverside Drive
New York, NY 10024
Phone: 212-877-3388
Fax: 212-799-8420

---

507 LUCINDA CHILDS DANCE COMPANY
541 Broadway
New York, NY 10012
Phone: 212-431-7599
Fax: 212-431-7599
Officers:
   President: Lucinda Childs
Management:
   Artistic Director: Lucinda Childs

   General Manager: Amy Santos
Mission: Established to create and perform works by Lucinda Childs.
Founded: 1973
Specialized Field: Modern
Status: Professional; Nonprofit
Budget: $225,000
Organization Type: Performing; Touring; Resident; Educational

---

508 MANHATTAN TAP
PO Box 794
Grand Central Station
New York, NY 10163
Phone: 212-268-3731
Fax: 212-268-3718
e-mail: hcornell@manhattantap.org
Web Site: www.manhattantap.org
Management:
   Artistic Director: Heather Cornell
Founded: 1986
Paid Staff: 3
Paid Artists: 15
Budget: $100,000 - $250,000
Facility Category: Theater
Seating Capacity: 5,000

---

509 MARJORIE LIEBERT
New York, NY 10025
Mailing Address: PO Box 20456, Parkwest Station
Phone: 212-724-3238
Fax: 212-724-3238
Mission: To nurture and develop artistry and help healthy artists develop proper alignment. Rehabilitates injuries. Prevents future injuries. Reduces stress and develops muscles without stress.
Founded: 1980
Specialized Field: Ballet Classes, Coaching and Choreography

---

510 MARK DEGARMO AND DANCERS
Dynamic Forms
179 E Third Street
Suite 24
New York, NY 10009-7754
Phone: 212-353-1351
Fax: 212-267-8723
e-mail: pamarj@aol.com
Web Site: www.pamar.org
Management:
   Manager: Jan Michael Hanvik
Mission: Established to develop and perform the original choreography of Mark DeGarmo.
Founded: 1982
Specialized Field: Modern
Status: Professional
Income Sources: Dance USA
Organization Type: Performing; Touring; Resident; Educational

---

511 MARTHA GRAHAM DANCE COMPANY
153 E 53rd Street
Suite 5101
New York, NY 10022
Phone: 212-838-5886
Fax: 646-424-0341
e-mail: graham@aol.com
Officers:
   Chairman: Francis Mason
Management:
   Executive Director: Marvin Preston
   Finance Director: Nancy Lou Bright
   Administrative Director: Amy Harrison
Mission: Established to perform the original works of
Martha Graham.
Founded: 1926
Specialized Field: Modern
Status: Professional; Nonprofit
Organization Type: Performing; Touring; Educational

512 MARY ANTHONY DANCE THEATRE
736 Broadway
New York, NY 10003
Phone: 212-674-8191
Fax: 212-674-8191
Web Site: www.madt.org
Officers:
   President: Mary Anthony
Management:
   Artistic Director/Choreographer: Mary Anthony
   Associate Artistic Choreographer: Kun-Yang Lin
   Choreographer: Bertam Ross
Mission: To present modern dance through performances,
lecture-demonstrations and technique classes.
Founded: 1956
Specialized Field: Modern
Status: Professional; Nonprofit
Organization Type: Performing; Touring; Educational

513 MAURIZIO BELLEZZA
67 Riverside Drive
New York, NY 10024
Phone: 212-877-3388
Fax: 212-799-8420

**514 MERCE CUNNINGHAM DANCE
COMPANY**
55 Bethune Street
New York, NY 10014
Phone: 212-255-8240
Fax: 212-633-2453
e-mail: info@merce.org
Web Site: www.merce.org
Officers:
   Co-Chairman: Alvin Chereskin
   Co-Chairman: Sage F Cowles
   Vice Chairman: Suzanne Weil
   Treasurer: Anthony B. Creamer, III
Management:
   Artistic Director: Merce Cunningham
   Executive Director: Jeffrey James
   General Manager: Trevor Carlson

Mission: Committed to developing, understanding and
public interest in dance through performances, dance
instruction and videotapes.
Founded: 1964
Specialized Field: Modern
Status: Professional; Nonprofit
Income Sources: American Guild of Musical Artists;
National Association of Schools of Dance; Dance USA
Performs At: Merce Cunningham Studio
Organization Type: Performing; Touring; Educational

515 MICHAEL MAO DANCE
1841 Broadway
Suite 1008
New York, NY 10023
Phone: 212-757-9669
Fax: 212-757-4198
e-mail: admin@michaelmaodance.org
Web Site: www.michaelmaodance.org
Management:
   Marketing Director: Vadim Ghin
Mission: Dance Performance; Touring; Community
Outreach; Arts-in-Education; WSL Dance
Status: 501c3
Paid Staff: 3
Paid Artists: 15
Budget: $200,000-$500,000
Income Sources: NEA; NYSCA; DCA; Foundations;
Corporations; Fees; Tickets
Affiliations: ISPA; DTN; APAP

516 MIGUEL POVEDA
Bernard Schmidt Productions
461 W 49th Street, E Office
New York, NY 10019
Phone: 212-307-5046
Fax: 212-397-2459
e-mail: bschmidtpd@aol.com
Web Site: www.bernardschmidtproductions.com
Management:
   Artists Representative: Bernard Schmidt
Mission: Performers from around the world at the
crossroads of innovation and tradition.
Specialized Field: New Expression of Flamenco Singing
from Spain.
Paid Staff: 2
Paid Artists: 5

517 MIMI GARRARD DANCE COMPANY
155 Wooster Street
New York, NY 10012
Phone: 212-674-6868
Fax: 212-473-4710
e-mail: mimimgdc@aol.com
Web Site: www.seawright.net
Management:
   Artistic Director: Mimi Garrard
   Booking Manager: Liz Rodgers
Mission: Established to present original, professional
dance theatre productions to the public and offer classes
and workshops for individuals of all ages.
Founded: 1972
Specialized Field: Modern
Status: Professional; Nonprofit

Budget: $40,000-$100,000
Income Sources: Dance Theatre Workshop
Performs At: Mimi Garrard Dance Company
Organization Type: Performing; Touring; Resident

518 MOLISSA FENLEY
246 W 38th
Floor 8
New York, NY 10018-5805
Phone: 212-278-8111
Fax: 212-278-8555
e-mail: info@pentacle.org
Web Site: www.pentacle.org
Management:
 Artistic Director: Molissa Fenley
 Contact: Rosemary Quinn
Founded: 1985
Budget: $100,000-$200,000

519 MONTE BROWN DANCE COMPANY
39 Great Jones Street
New York, NY 10012
Phone: 212-251-0789
Fax: 212-251-0743
Web Site: www.montebrowndance.org
Officers:
 President: Elisa Monte
 Treasurer: David Brown
 Chairperson: Nathalie Berliet
Management:
 Managing Director: Bernard G Schmidt
Mission: To advance and enrich the art of dance through the presentation of the innovative choreography and outreach activities of Elisa Monte.
Founded: 1981
Specialized Field: Modern
Status: Professional; Nonprofit
Income Sources: Dance USA
Performs At: The Joyce Theater
Organization Type: Performing; Touring; Educational

520 MONTE/BROWN DANCE INTERNATIONAL TOURING
Bernard Schmidt Productions
461 W 49th Street, E Office
New York, NY 10019
Phone: 212-307-5046
Fax: 212-397-2459
e-mail: bschmidtpd@aol.com
Web Site: www.bernardschmidtproductions.com
Management:
 Artists Representative: Bernard Schmidt
Mission: Performers from around the world at the crossroads of innovation and tradition.
Specialized Field: Intense, Sensual Synthesis of Contempoary Dance, Music and Visuals.
Paid Staff: 3
Paid Artists: 15

521 MUNA TSENG DANCE PROJECTS
115 Christopher Street
4th Floor
New York, NY 10014

Phone: 212-627-5638
Fax: 212-645-5319
e-mail: MunaTseng@aol.com
Management:
 Artistic Director: Muna Tseng
Mission: Collaborative projects in cutting-edge East meets west contemporary dance theatre and photography, in New York City and on tour to the USA and internationally.
Founded: 1988
Specialized Field: Dance; Performance Art; Photography
Budget: $100,000

522 NATIONAL DANCE INSTITUTE
594 Broadway
Room 805
New York, NY 10012
Phone: 212-226-0083
Fax: 212-226-0761
e-mail: ndi@waterstreet.com
Web Site: www.nationaldance.org
Officers:
 Acting Chairman: Robert D Krinsky
Management:
 Founder: Jacques d'Amboise
 Executive Director: Lesli Kapell
 Artistic Director/Choreographer: Ellen Weinstein
Mission: To make the arts a foundation of children's education through the medium of dance; to reach children who would otherwise not have the opportunity to become involved in the arts.
Founded: 1976
Specialized Field: Modern; Jazz; Tap
Status: Nonprofit
Paid Staff: 50
Volunteer Staff: 100
Income Sources: Grants
Performs At: LaGuardia High School
Seating Capacity: 1,000
Organization Type: Performing; Educational

523 NEO LABOS DANCE THEATER
332 Bleecker Street
#G9
New York, NY 10014
Phone: 212-775-7091
Fax: 212-691-8661
e-mail: neolabos@worldnet.att.net
Web Site:
www.artswire.org/elsieman/neolabos/index.html
Management:
 Artistic Director: Michele Elliman
Budget: $40,000-$100,000

524 NETA PULVERMACHER AND DANCERS
39 Claremont Avenue
Apartment 41
New York, NY 10027
Phone: 212-316-3888
Fax: 212-316-9355
e-mail: npso@columbia.edu
Web Site: www.netacompany.org
Management:
 Artistic Director: Neta Pulvermacher

Mission: To present contemporary performance arts to the public.
Founded: 1987
Specialized Field: Modern; Ballet
Status: Professional
Paid Staff: 2
Budget: $40,0000-$200,000
Income Sources: Dance Theatre Workshop; Circum Arts
Organization Type: Performing; Touring; Resident; Educational; Sponsoring

525 NEUER TANZ

Bernard Schmidt Productions
461 W 49th Street, E Office
New York, NY 10019
Phone: 212-307-5046
Fax: 212-397-2459
e-mail: bschmidtpd@aol.com
Web Site: www.bernardschmidtproductions.com
Management:
   Artists Representative: Bernard Schmidt
Mission: Performers from around the world at the crossroads of innovation and tradition.
Specialized Field: Sophisticated Visual Imagery in Modern Dance from Germany.
Paid Artists: 10

526 NEW AMSTERDAM BALLET

290 Riverside Drive
New York, NY 10025
Fax: 212-678-0320
Management:
   Artistic Director: Martine van Hamel
Mission: To create new works on a project to project basis.
Founded: 1985
Specialized Field: Ballet Company
Volunteer Staff: 1
Paid Artists: 12

527 NEW DANCE GROUP STUDIO

254 W 47th Street
New York, NY 10036
Phone: 212-719-2733
Fax: 212-719-0457
e-mail: nadgac@aol.com
Web Site: www.ndg.org
Management:
   Artistic Director: Rick Schussel
   Business Manager: Sandy Lee
   Music Director: George Quincey
   General Manager: Kenneth Martin
Mission: To foster the art of dance through a wide range of classes, scholarships, rehearsal space and performance.
Founded: 1932
Specialized Field: Modern; Ballet; Jazz; Ethnic
Status: Professional; Nonprofit
Paid Staff: 10
Income Sources: Studio rental
Facility Category: Rehearsal/Casting Facility
Type of Stage: Studio
Seating Capacity: 80-100
Organization Type: Performing; Educational

528 NEW YORK CITY BALLET

New York State Theatre
20 Lincon Center
New York, NY 10023-6966
Phone: 212-870-5500
Fax: 212-870-7791
Web Site: www.nycballet.com
Officers:
   Chairman: Howard Solomon
   President: Robert I Lipp
   Treasurer: John L Vogelstein
   Secretary: Marilyn Laurie
Management:
   Founder: George Balanchine
   Founder: Lincoln Kirstein
   Founding Choreographer: Jerome Robbins
   Ballet Mistress: Rosemary Dunleavy
   Principal Conductor: Hugo Fiorrato
   Ballet-Master-in-Chief: Peter Martins
   External Affairs Director: Chris Ramsey
   General Manager: Anne Parsons
   Company Manager: Michele Lisi
Founded: 1948
Specialized Field: Ballet
Status: Professional; Nonprofit
Budget: $2,500,000
Performs At: New York State Theater
Facility Category: Proscenium
Seating Capacity: 2,779
Organization Type: Performing; Touring; Resident; Educational

529 NEW YORK THEATRE BALLET

30 East 31st Street
New York, NY 10016
Phone: 212-679-0401
Fax: 212-679-8171
e-mail: cami@cami.com
Web Site: www.members.aol.com/nytb
Management:
   Artistic Director: Diana Byer
   Executive Director: Gail Spangenberg
Founded: 1978
Specialized Field: Ballet; Dance
Paid Staff: 12
Paid Artists: 14
Budget: $500,000-$1,000,000

530 NICHOL HLINKA

Dube Zakin Management
67 Riverside Drive
New York, NY 10024
Phone: 212-877-3388
Fax: 212-799-8420

531 NILAS MARRTINS

252 W 76th Street
Suite 6E
New York, NY 10023
Phone: 212-724-3889
Fax: 212-874-5039
e-mail: markkapl1@aol.com

532 PABLO SAVOYE
Dube Zakin Management
67 Riverside Drive
New York, NY 10024
Phone: 212-877-3388
Fax: 212-799-8420

533 PARSONS DANCE COMPANY
229 W 42nd Street
Suite 800
New York, NY 10036
Phone: 212-247-3203
Fax: 212-247-3324
e-mail: parsonsnyc@aol.com
Web Site: www.parsonsdance.org
Management:
   Executive Director: Frank Sonntag
   Artistic Director: David Parsons
   Executive Director: Gray Montague
Mission: To create and perform modern dance; to educate and experiment.
Founded: 1985
Specialized Field: Modern; Ballet
Status: Professional
Budget: $1,000,000-$2,500,000
Organization Type: Performing; Touring; Resident; Educational

534 PASCAL RIOULT DANCE THEATRE
246 W 38th
Floor 8
New York, NY 10018-5805
Phone: 212-278-8111
Fax: 212-278-8555
e-mail: info@pentacle.org
Web Site: www.pentacle.org
Management:
   Artistic Director: Pascal Rioult
   Executive Director: Dan LaMorte
Budget: $200,000-$500,000

535 PAUL TAYLOR DANCE COMPANY
552 Broadway
2nd Floor
New York, NY 10012-3947
Phone: 212-431-5562
Fax: 212-966-5673
e-mail: jt@ptdc.org
Web Site: www.paultaylor.org
Officers:
   President: Norton Belknap
   Executive VP: Walter Scheuer
   VP: Carole K Newman
   VP/Treasurer: Elise Jaffe
   VP: Robert E Aberlin
   Secretary: Hazel Kandall
Management:
   Artistic Director and Founder: Paul Taylor
   Executive Director: Ross Kramberg
   Development: Emily Regas
   General Manager: John Tomlinson
   Director Marketing: Alan Olshan

Mission: The Paul Taylor Dance Foundation generates the resources Mr. Taylor needs to create new works; maintains the Paul Taylor Dance Company as one of the finest ensembles in the world; ensures that Mr. Taylor's work is seen by the largest possible audience; promotes the Taylor style through education initiatives; and preserves Mr. Taylor's dances for future generations. Sixteen member main Company.
Founded: 1966
Specialized Field: Modern
Status: Professional; Nonprofit
Paid Staff: 15
Volunteer Staff: 8
Paid Artists: 25
Budget: $4,700,000
Income Sources: Grants; Individual Donations; Ticket Sales; Matching Gifts; In Kind Donations; Touring Fees
Facility Category: Dance Studio/Dance School/Offices
Organization Type: Performing; Touring; Resident

536 PEARL LANG DANCE COMPANY AND FOUNDATION
382 Central Park W
New York, NY 10025
Phone: 212-866-2680
Fax: 212-866-2680
Management:
   Artistic Director: Pearl Lang
   Business Manager: Lois Schaffer
Founded: 1954
Specialized Field: Modern; Ethnic
Status: Professional; Nonprofit
Organization Type: Performing; Touring; Educational

537 PETRA
67 Riverside Drive
New York, NY 10024
Phone: 212-877-3388
Fax: 212-799-8420

538 PHYLLIS LAMHUT DANCE COMPANY
225 W 71st Street
#31
New York, NY 10023
Phone: 212-799-9048
Fax: 212-799-9048
e-mail: plamhut@msn.com
Management:
   Artistic Director: Phyllis Lamhut
Mission: To present the work of choreographer Phyllis Lamhut.
Founded: 1970
Specialized Field: Modern
Status: Professional
Organization Type: Performing; Touring; Resident; Educational

539 PHYLLIS ROSE DANCE COMPANY
Dance Vectors
102-00 Shore Front Parkway
Suite 10P
New York, NY 11694

Phone: 718-474-1672
Fax: 718-634-0348
e-mail: dancevectorsaol.com
Officers:
  President: Phyllis Rose
  Secretary: Ivy Rosen
  Treasurer: Susan Cherniak
Management:
  Company Director: Phyllis Rose
  Engagement Coordinator: Morgayne West
Mission: To provide arts-in-education experiences in the areas of dance, music, and folklore to young audiences, via performances, workshops and residency programs special focus on young audiences.
Founded: 1969
Specialized Field: Modern; Jazz; Ethnic; Folk; Novelty; Theatre
Status: Professional; Nonprofit
Paid Staff: 3
Volunteer Staff: 1
Paid Artists: 25
Budget: 100,000-200,000
Income Sources: Earned; Donations
Performs At: Touring
Organization Type: Performing; Resident; Educational; Sponsoring

540 POLISH AMERICAN FOLK DANCE COMPANY
58 W 58th Street
New York, NY 10019
Phone: 718-256-1423
Fax: 212-935-3706
Web Site: www.pafdc.org/main.htm
Management:
  Artistic Director: Stanley Pelc
Mission: Established to preserve and present the culture of Poland.
Founded: 1948
Specialized Field: Folk
Status: Nonprofessional; Nonprofit
Organization Type: Performing; Touring

541 POPPO & THE GOGO BOYS
165 W 26th Street
6th Floor
New York, NY 10001
Phone: 212-989-4819
Fax: 212-989-4819
e-mail: mikopop@gis.net
Management:
  Artistic Director: Poppo Shiraishi
  Manager: Miko Otake

542 REBECCA KELLY BALLET
151 W 50th Street
Suite 200
New York, NY 10001
Phone: 212-904-1422
Fax: 212-904-1426
e-mail: biles@circum.org
Web Site: www.circum.org
Management:
  Administrative Director: Craig Brashear

Artistic Director: Rebecca Kelly
Budget: $100,000-$200,000

543 RISA JAROSLOW AND DANCERS
250 8th Avenue
Suite 329
New York, NY 10018
Phone: 212-244-8962
e-mail: risajar@aol.com
Web Site: www.hightidedance.com
Management:
  Artistic Director: Risa Jaroslow
  Managing Director: Fran Smyth
Mission: Committed to bringing new dance and music to as wide an audience as possible and to expressing the essence of human relationships through dance.
Founded: 1985
Specialized Field: Modern
Status: Professional; Nonprofit
Paid Staff: 3
Volunteer Staff: 1
Paid Artists: 6
Budget: $170,000-180,000
Income Sources: Foundations; Government; Private Donors; Earned Income
Affiliations: Dance Theater Workshop
Annual Attendance: 2,000-3,000
Organization Type: Performing; Touring; Resident; Educational

544 ROD RODGERS DANCE COMPANY & STUDIOS
62 E 4th Street
New York, NY 10003
Phone: 212-674-9066
Fax: 212-674-9068
e-mail: rodgersstudio@aol.com
Web Site: rodrogersdance.com
Management:
  Artistic Director/Founder: Rod Rodgers
  General Manager: Rachel Lubell
  Coordinator Training Program: Kim Grier
Mission: In addition to touring, offering dance concerts and workshops. The Rodgers Company maintains a year round studio/school where training is offered in Afro-Haitian, several styles of jazz and modern dance techniques.
Founded: 1974
Specialized Field: Dance Concerts, Arts and Education Events, Training Studio Space Rental
Budget: $100,000-$200,000

545 SAEKO ICHINOHE DANCE COMPANY
159 W 53rd Street
Suite 22H
New York, NY 10019-6050
Phone: 212-757-2531
Fax: 212-757-3614
Web Site: www.instantmedia.com/saeko
Officers:
  President: Saeko Ichinohe
Management:
  Administrator: George Horishiga

Mission: To employ dance as an interpretive medium inspiring understanding between peoples and cultures; to offer indispensable nourishment for the heart, mind and soul through high quality programs which bring joy of movement to all ages, cultures and socio-economic groups; to contribute to the aesthetic development of dance by incorporating cultural heritages, strongly especially the Japanese tradition, into a framework of contemporary dance.
Founded: 1970
Specialized Field: Dance Performances; Lecture Demonstration; Master Class/Workshops; Mini-Performances for Children and Families
Paid Staff: 1
Volunteer Staff: 3
Paid Artists: 10
Budget: $40,000-$100,000

546 SALIA NI SEYDOU
Bernard Schmidt Productions
461 W 49th Street, E Office
New York, NY 10019
Phone: 212-307-5046
Fax: 212-397-2459
e-mail: bschmidtpd@aol.com
Web Site: www.bernardschmidtproductions.com
Management:
Executive Director: John Hassle
Mission: Performers from around the world at the crossroads of innovation and tradition.
Specialized Field: Combining African Rituals and Contemporary Dance from Burkina Faso, West Africa.
Paid Staff: 3
Volunteer Staff: 5

547 SCHOOL OF HARD KNOCKS
201 E 4th Street
New York, NY 10009
Phone: 212-533-9473
Fax: 212-260-5382
e-mail: info@yoshikochuma.org
Web Site: www.yoshikochuma.org
Management:
Artistic Director: Yoshiko Chuma
Manager: Bonnie Stein
Mission: The production of the works of Yoshiko Chuma and other members of the School of Hard Knocks.
Founded: 1979
Specialized Field: Post-Modern
Status: Nonprofit
Organization Type: Performing; Touring

548 SCOTT JOVOVICH
Dube Zakin Management
67 Riverside Drive
New York, NY 10024
Phone: 212-877-3388
Fax: 212-799-8420

549 SENSEDANCE
1425 3rd Avenue
#3C
New York, NY 10028

Phone: 212-717-6869
Fax: 212-717-6869
e-mail: rubsam@bceja.org
Web Site: www.sensedance.org
Management:
Artistic Director: Henning Rubsam
Music Director: Beata Moon
Mission: Contemporary/modern dance company - live and/or taped music.
Founded: 1991
Paid Staff: 2
Volunteer Staff: 2
Paid Artists: 9
Budget: $40,000-$100,000

550 SERGE CAMPARDON
67 Riverside Drive
New York, NY 10024
Phone: 212-877-3388
Fax: 212-799-8420

551 SOLARIS DANCE THEATRE & VIDEO
264 W 19th Street
Room 53
New York, NY 10011
Phone: 212-741-0778
Fax: 212-242-2201
e-mail: solaris@libertynet.org
Management:
Artistic Director: Henry Smith
Mission: To create experimental dance theatre through the workshop process and through cross-cultural performance; to create bonds with people otherwise unrecognized in our society.
Founded: 1976
Specialized Field: Modern; Ethnic; Folk; Martial Arts
Status: Professional; Nonprofit
Paid Staff: 4
Volunteer Staff: 6
Paid Artists: 12
Budget: $165,000
Income Sources: Grants; Performances
Performs At: Studio
Affiliations: Arts; Business Council
Organization Type: Performing; Touring; Resident; Educational

552 STEPHEN BEAGLEY
67 Riverside Drive
New York, NY 10024
Phone: 212-887-7338
Fax: 212-799-8420

553 STEPHEN PETRONIO DANCE COMPANY
140 2nd Avenue
Suite 504
New York, NY 10003
Phone: 212-473-1660
Fax: 212-477-3471
e-mail: spcdance@aol.com
Web Site: www.shaganarts.com
Management:

Artistic Director/Choreographer: Stephen Petronio
Managing Director: Tricia Pierson
Founded: 1984
Specialized Field: Modern
Status: Professional; Nonprofit
Organization Type: Performing; Touring

554 SUSAN MARSHALL & COMPANY

16A W 88th Street
New York, NY 10024
Phone: 212-873-9700
Fax: 212-873-1708
e-mail: rena@shaganarts.com
Web Site: wwwshaganarts.com
Management:
   Artistic Director/Choreographer: Susan Marshall
   Managing Director: Tia Levinson
   Booking Agent: Rena Shagan
Mission: Marshall's choreography illuminates the contemporary condition by interweaving movement, structure, imagery, and drama.
Founded: 1983
Specialized Field: Modern
Status: Professional; Nonprofit
Paid Staff: 4
Volunteer Staff: 3
Paid Artists: 8
Budget: $450,000
Income Sources: Dance USA
Organization Type: Performing; Touring

555 TAMARA HADLEY

67 Riverside Drive
New York, NY 10024
Phone: 212-877-3388
Fax: 212-799-8420

556 TRISHA BROWN COMPANY

625 W 55th Street
2nd Floor
New York, NY 10019
Phone: 212-582-0040
Fax: 212-582-9619
Web Site: www.trishabrowncompany.org
Officers:
   Chairman: Robert Raushchenberg
   President: Klaus Kertess
   VP: Jewella Brickford
Management:
   Artistic Director: Trisha Brown
   Executive Director: LaRue Allen
   Company Manager: Jodi White
Mission: To perform the contemporary dance of Trisha Brown.
Founded: 1964
Specialized Field: Modern
Status: Professional; Nonprofit
Paid Staff: 6
Paid Artists: 17
Budget: $1,000,000-$2,500,000
Organization Type: Performing; Touring; Resident; Educational

557 URBAN BUSH WOMEN

208 W 30th Street
#1105
New York, NY 10001
Phone: 212-695-2819
Fax: 212-695-3705
e-mail: Rcerritelli@ubwinc.org
Web Site:
www.fsu.edu/~svad/dance_pages/ubwhome.html
Officers:
   Chairman: Jawole Willa Jo Zollar
Management:
   Managing Director: Laurie Uprichard
   Artistic Director: Jawole Willa Jo Zollar
   Administative Director: Rhoda Cerritelli
Mission: To realize a creative vision continuously enriched by the folklore and religious traditions of Africans through movement, live music, a cappella vocalizations, and the drama and wit of the spoken word.
Specialized Field: Modern; Ethnic
Status: Non-Professional
Budget: $60,000-$150,000
Organization Type: Performing; Touring

558 VINCENT HANTAM

67 Riverside Drive
New York, NY 10024
Phone: 212-877-3388
Fax: 212-799-8420

559 WILLIAM DE GREGORY

67 Riverside Drive
New York, NY 10024
Phone: 212-877-3388
Fax: 212-799-8420

560 WOFA! PERCUSSION AND DANCE FROM GUINEA, WEST AFRICA

Bernard Schmidt Productions
461 W 49th Street, E Office
New York, NY 10019
Phone: 212-307-5046
Fax: 212-397-2459
e-mail: bschmidtpd@aol.com
Web Site: www.bernardschmidtproductions.com
Management:
   Artists Representative: Bernard Schmidt
Mission: Performers from around the world at the crossroads of innovation and tradition.
Specialized Field: Percussion and Dance-Rich Authentic African Tradion meets Contemporary Innovation.
Paid Artists: 10

561 WORLD MUSIC INSTITUTE

49 W 27th Street
Suite 930
New York, NY 10001
Phone: 212-545-7536
Fax: 212-889-2771
e-mail: wmi@worldmusicinstitute.org
Web Site: www.worldmusicinstitute.org
Officers:
   Chairperson: Zeyba Rahman

Management:
    Executive/Artistic Director: Robert H Browning
    Director Publicity: Helene Browning
    Associate Director: Isable Soffer
    Tour Coordinator: Leslie Malmed
Mission: World Music Institute is a not-for-profit organization dedicated to the research and presentation of the finest in traditional and contemporary music and dance from around the world. WMI supports and encourages musicians from immigrant communities and collaborates with universities, cultural organizations, and other presenting organizations that have similar goals.
Founded: 1985
Specialized Field: Ethnic; Folk; World Music; New Music
Status: Nonprofit
Paid Staff: 8
Performs At: Symphony Space; Town Hall; Merkin Hall
Annual Attendance: 35,000
Organization Type: Touring

562 POSEY DANCE COMPANY

PO Box 254
Northport, NY 11768-0254
Phone: 631-757-2700
Fax: 631-757-2107
e-mail: 74534.1660@compuserve.com
Management:
    Artistic Director: Elsa Posey
    Managing Director: Donna Brady
Mission: Education.
Founded: 1953
Specialized Field: Modern; Ballet; Jazz
Status: Professional; Nonprofit
Income Sources: American Dance Guild
Organization Type: Performing; Touring; Educational

563 DEBRA WEISS DANCE COMPANY

51 Summit Street
Nyack, NY 10960
Phone: 845-353-3860
Fax: 845-353-3860
e-mail: dnweiss@aol.com
Web Site: www.debraweissdance.org
Officers:
    Treasurer: Eric Bender
Management:
    Artistic Director/President: Debra Weiss
Mission: We use dance as a medium for storytelling and living history programs for children, teens, and adults. Much of our work is in schools and museums, where we supplement and enrich existing cirricula and exhibits with our programming.
Founded: 1983
Specialized Field: Storytelling history through dance; Arts-In-Education
Status: Professional; Nonprofit
Paid Staff: 1
Paid Artists: 6
Budget: $60,000
Affiliations: Arts Council of Rockland
Annual Attendance: 12,000
Organization Type: Performing; Touring; Resident; Educational

564 WESTCHESTER BALLET COMPANY

95 Croton Avenue
PO Box 694
Ossining, NY 10562
Phone: 914-941-4532
Fax: 941-923-7693
e-mail: info@westchesterballet.org
Web Site: www.westchesterballet.org
Officers:
    President: Kristina Lindbergh
    VP: Debbie Bassett
    Treasurer: Jeanette Sanders
    Secretary: Mary Levine
Management:
    Artistic Director: Jean Logrea
    Executive Director: Beth Fritz-Logrea
    Executive Director: Rosella Ranno
Mission: To promote the awareness and appreciation of dance through all the communitites of Westchester County NY.
Founded: 1950
Specialized Field: Ballet
Status: Professional; Semi-Professional; Non-Professional; Nonprofit
Paid Staff: 70
Performs At: Marymount College; Tarrytown
Organization Type: Performing; Educational

565 ANITA FELDMAN TAP/TAPPING MUSIC

34 Bogart Avenue
Port Washington, NY 11050
Phone: 516-944-6673
Fax: 516-944-6673
Mission: The company tours nationally and internationally including an annual NYC season.
Budget: $40,000-$100,000

566 ON QUEUE PERFORMING ARTISTS

517 County Highway 27
Richfield Springs, NY 13439
Phone: 315-858-1434
Fax: 315-858-1434
e-mail: info@onqueueartists.com
Web Site: www.onqueueartists.com
Management:
    Founder: Sandra P Bernegger
    Administrative Assistant: Frances Breslin
Mission: To promote the traditional performing arts of the world, including onnovations and hybridizations.
Founded: 1997
Specialized Field: World Music and Dance
Performs At: Association of Performing Arts Presenters; North American Folk Enthusists and Dance Alliance; Society Ethnicmusicology
Seating Capacity: 50-350

567 GARTH FAGAN DANCE

50 Chestnut Street
Rochester, NY 14604
Phone: 716-454-3260
Fax: 716-454-6191
Web Site: www.garthfagandance.org
Management:
    Founder/Artistic Director: Garth Fagan

General Manager: Grady S Bailey
Mission: To perform modern dance and compete on a national level, with original choreography by Garth Fagan.
Founded: 1970
Specialized Field: Modern; Ethnic
Status: Professional; Nonprofit
Budget: $1,000,000-$2,500,000
Organization Type: Performing; Touring; Resident; Educational

568 VANAVER CARAVAN

298 Mountain Road
Rosendale, NY 12472
Phone: 845-658-9748
Fax: 845-658-7332
e-mail: vanaverc@aol.com
Web Site: www.vanavercaravan.org
Officers:
  President: Livia Vanaver
  Officer: Julien Studley
  Officer: Paul Ellis
  Officer: Elizabeth Murphy
Management:
  Booking Manager: Barbara Mermell
  Artistic Director/President: Livia Vanaver
Mission: Over the past 26 years the Vanaver Caravan Dancers and musicians have been dedicated to performing.
Founded: 1972
Specialized Field: Modern; Ethnic; Folk; Live Music
Status: Professional; Nonprofit
Paid Staff: 4
Volunteer Staff: 10
Paid Artists: 25
Non-paid Artists: 12
Budget: $50,000
Organization Type: Performing; Touring; Educational

569 PAT CANNON'S FOOT & FIDDLE DANCE COMPANY

115 Johnsontown Road
Sloatsburg, NY 10974
Phone: 845-753-6950
Fax: 845-753-6949
e-mail: info@footandfiddle.com
Web Site: www.footandfiddle.com
Officers:
  President: Pat Cannon
Management:
  Artistic Director: Pat Cannon
  Music Director: Dave Keyes
  Office Manager: Carol Stout
Mission: To present a blend of clogging, square dance, tap dance, Irish step dancing, country music, bluegrass, swing, Cajun and rock and roll; to perform folk material with tap technique.
Founded: 1981
Specialized Field: Tap; Clogging; Swing; Irish Step
Status: Professional; Nonprofit
Paid Staff: 2
Paid Artists: 12
Budget: $180,000
Income Sources: Concert venues

Organization Type: Performing; Touring; Resident; Educational

570 MOWHAWK VALLEY BALLET

261 Genesee Street
Utica, NY 13501
Phone: 315-738-7646
Fax: 775-535-7110
e-mail: ballet@dreamscape.com
Web Site: www.mvballet.org
Officers:
  Administrative Director: Dominic Passalacqua
  Company Stage Manager: Steve Mackintosh
Management:
  Artistic Director: Delia Foley
  Technical Director: Joseph Rusnock
Founded: 1973
Year Built: 1920

571 TOMOV FOLKDANCE ENSEMBLE

66-12 48th Avenue
Woodside, NY 11377
Phone: 718-639-3465
Fax: 718-639-3465
e-mail: albkayassc@aol.com
Officers:
  VP: Albert Kay
Management:
  Director/Founder/Choreographer: George Tomov
Mission: TOMOV brings a rich, timeless tradition to the stage and transports the audience to a folk world of flashing color, lively movement and hauntingly beautiful melodies.
Founded: 1974
Specialized Field: Folk Dance and Songs
Volunteer Staff: 12
Non-paid Artists: 30
Budget: $40,000-$100,000

North Carolina

572 NORTH CAROLINA DANCE THEATRE

800 N College Street
Charlotte, NC 28206
Phone: 704-372-0101
Fax: 704-375-0260
e-mail: shannon@ncdance.org
Web Site: www.ncdance.org
Officers:
  Chair: Amy Blumenthal
  Chair-Elect: Robert G Beaven
  Founder: Robert Lindgren
  Secretary: Sandra McMullen
Management:
  Artistic Director/President: Jean-Pierre Bonnefoux
  Associate Artistic Director: Patricia McBride
  Associate Artistic Director: Jerri Kumery
Mission: To present the art of dance and dancers.
Founded: 1970
Specialized Field: Modern; Ballet
Status: Professional; Nonprofit
Budget: 4,200,000
Income Sources: Arts and Science Council of Charlotte

Performs At: North Carolina Blumenthal Performing Arts Center
Type of Stage: Proscenium
Stage Dimensions: 44'x34'
Seating Capacity: 1920
Year Built: 1992
Organization Type: Performing; Touring

573 AFRICAN-AMERICAN DANCE ENSEMBLE

120 Morris Street
Durham, NC 27701
Phone: 919-560-2729
Fax: 919-560-2743
e-mail: aade@vnet.net
Web Site: Africanamericandanceensemble.org
Officers:
   President: Willie Burt
   VP: Tamra Starck
   Secretary: Brandon Patterson
Management:
   Executive Director: James C Newlin
   Artistic Director: Chuck Davis
   Associate Artistic Director: Stafford C Berry, Jr
   Program Director: Normadien Woolbright
   Office Manager: Jean M Whitaker
Mission: The African-American Dance Ensemble seeks to preserve and share the finest traditions of African and African-American dance and music through research, education and entertainment. We celebrate traditional African culture, aesthetics and values as resources for all people and utilize these resources to encourage interracial cooperation.
Founded: 1984
Specialized Field: Dance
Paid Staff: 12
Volunteer Staff: 10
Paid Artists: 9
Budget: $500,000
Income Sources: Federal, State and Private Funding; Earned Income from Performances
Annual Attendance: 150,000

574 GREENSBORO BALLET

200 N Davie Street
Greensboro, NC 27401
Phone: 336-333-7480
Fax: 336-333-7482
Web Site: www.greensboroballet.org
Management:
   Artistic Director: Maryhelen Mayfield
   Marketing Director: Barry B Stoneking
Mission: To offer the highest caliber classical and contemporary ballet performances for our audiences.
Specialized Field: Dance
Paid Staff: 5
Paid Artists: 6
Non-paid Artists: 6

575 JAN VAN DYKE DANCE GROUP

306 Aberdeen Terrace
Greensboro, NC 27403-1817

Phone: 336-334-3043
Fax: 336-334-3238
e-mail: jevandyk@uncg.edu
Web Site: www.uncg.edu
Officers:
   President: Chas Hicks
   Secretary: Laura McDuffee
   Treasurer/Artistic Director: Jan Van Dyke
Management:
   Artistic Director: Jan Van Dyke
   Administrator: Kelley Mills
Mission: To present the work of Jan Van Dyke through a variety of professional performances and educational programs to all ages.
Founded: 1989
Specialized Field: Modern
Status: Professional; Nonprofit
Paid Staff: 1
Paid Artists: 9
Budget: $25,700,000
Income Sources: Grants; Fundraising; Donations; Ticket Sales
Affiliations: North Carolina Dance Project; UNC Greensboro Department of Dance; United Arts Council of Greensboro
Organization Type: Performing; Touring
Resident Groups: University of North Carolina at Greensboro

576 JOHN GAMBLE DANCE THEATER

490 Kallam Mill Road
Madison, NC 27025
Phone: 336-334-3042
Fax: 336-334-3238
e-mail: jjgamble@uncg.edu
Management:
   Artistic Director: John Gamble
   Associate Director: Virginia Ray Freeman
   Associate Director: Sherone Price
   Assistant Director: Emily E Daughtridge
   Assistant Director: Nikki Cox
Mission: Comprised of a multigenerational, multiracial company of 30 dancers, actors, and musicians. The JGDT addresses political and social issues through a blend of theater, dance, visual art, and music for the purpose of creating performances intended to stimulate thought and change.
Founded: 1989
Specialized Field: Dance; Theater
Income Sources: Public and Private Grants; Ticket Sales; Fundraisers
Affiliations: The University of North Carolina at Greensboro Center for Arts and Public Discourse

Ohio

577 OHIO BALLET

354 E Market Street
Akron, OH 44325
Phone: 330-972-7900
Fax: 330-972-7902
Web Site: www.ohioballet.com
Management:

General Manager: Lisa Winstel
Artistic Director: Heinz Poll
Associate Director: Barbara S Schubert
Artistic Administrator: Jane Starzman
Artistic Director: Jeffrey Graham Hughes
Mission: Delivering the magic of dance. To be a driving force creating a passion for dance.
Founded: 1968
Specialized Field: Ballet
Status: Professional; Nonprofit
Budget: $1,000,000-$2,500,000
Income Sources: Dance USA
Organization Type: Performing; Touring

578   CANTON BALLET

1001 N Market Avenue
Canton, OH 44702
Phone: 330-455-7220
Fax: 330-455-6977
e-mail: cantonballet@cantonballet.com
Web Site: www.cantonballet.com/ballet1.htm
Management:
    Artistic Director: Cassandra Crowley
    Managing Director: Lou Ann Gotch
    Office Manager: Deborah Sherrod
Mission: Committed to offering progressive levels of dance training of the highest quality and providing performance opportunities for dancers.
Founded: 1965
Specialized Field: Ballet
Status: Non-professional; Nonprofit
Paid Staff: 17
Budget: $600,000
Income Sources: Tuition; Performance Admissions; Memberships; Foundations; Funds for the Arts; Ohio Arts Council
Performs At: Palace Theatre
Affiliations: Regional Dance America; Ohio Citizens for the Arts; Ohio Dance
Organization Type: Performing; Touring; Resident; Educational

579   CINCINNATI BALLET

1555 Central Parkway
PO Box 14463
Cincinnati, OH 45214
Phone: 513-621-5219
Fax: 513-621-4844
e-mail: cballet@cincinnatiballet.com
Web Site: www.cincinnatiballet.com
Management:
    Artistic Director: Victoria Morgan
    Music Director: Carmon DeLeone
    Executive Director: John Zurick
    Public Relations Manager: Susan Eiswerth
    Marketing/Sales Director: Vanessa Torbeck
Mission: Committed to performing an extensive ballet repertoire in both Cincinnati and Knoxville.
Founded: 1958
Specialized Field: Ballet
Status: Professional
Income Sources: Dance USA; Ohio Dance
Performs At: Music Hall
Organization Type: Performing; Touring; Resident; Educational

580   CONTEMPORARY DANCE THEATER

1805 Larch Avenue
Cincinnati, OH 45224
Phone: 513-591-2557
Fax: 513-591-1222
e-mail: jfrsonj@aol.com
Web Site: www.cdt-dance.org
Officers:
    Board President: Elizabeth Collins
Management:
    Artistic Director: Jefferson James
    Assistant to the Director: Rachel James
    Technical Director: Dennis Reed
Mission: To promote the art of dance; to provide educational demonstrations and performances for the community and provide dance instruction; to present and produce dance.
Founded: 1972
Specialized Field: Modern; Jazz; Ethnic; Ballet; Tap; Improvisation; Hip Hop
Status: Professional; Nonprofit
Paid Staff: 2
Paid Artists: 7
Non-paid Artists: 12
Income Sources: Ohio Dance; Cincinnati Commission of the Arts; Dance Action
Performs At: The Dance Hall
Organization Type: Performing; Touring; Resident; Educational; Sponsoring

581   CLEVELAND STATE UNIVERSITY DANCE COMPANY

1983 Euclid Avenue
Dance Program
Cleveland, OH
Phone: 216-687-4883
Fax: 216-687-5410
e-mail: l.deering@csuohio.edu
Web Site: www.csuohio.edu/dance/main.htm
Management:
    Director: Lynn H Deering

582   DANCE CLEVELAND

1148 Euclid Avenue
Suite 311
Cleveland, OH 44115
Phone: 216-861-2213
Fax: 216-687-0022
e-mail: tward@dancecleveland.org
Web Site: www.dancecleveland.org
Officers:
    President: Jeffrey S Glazer
    VP Programing: Lucinda Lavelli
    VP Contributed Revenue: Ann Sethness
    VP Earned Revenues: Jeffrey Linton
    Secretary/Treasurer: Tom Leib
    VP/Trustees: Sheila Fox
Management:
    Executive Director: Stephanie Brown
    Marketing Director: Craig Rich
    Executive Director: Thomas P Ward

Mission: To foster an appreciation of and interest in dance in the Greater Cleveland Area through education and concert programming, the presentation of an annual concert series, dance education and dance/movement therapy programs.
Founded: 1956
Specialized Field: Modern; Mime; Ballet; Jazz; Folk
Status: Nonprofit
Income Sources: National Endowment for the Arts; Association for Performing Arts Presenters; International Society of Performing Arts Administrators; Arts Midwest; Dance USA; Arts Presenters
Performs At: Ohio Theatre; Playhouse Square Center
Organization Type: Educational; Sponsoring

583 REPERTORY PROJECT

2140 Lee Road
Suite 206
Cleveland, OH 44118
Phone: 216-397-3757
Fax: 216-397-7872
e-mail: info@repertoryproject.org
Web Site: www.repertoryproject.org
Officers:
    President Board of Trustees: Mark Walton
Management:
    Managing Director: Margaret Carlson
    Artistic Director: Hernando Cortez
Mission: To promote and develop interest in and appreciation for modern dance through performance, programs that promote learning and nurture wellness, audience and community dialogue and advocacy efforts to support the art form.
Founded: 1987
Specialized Field: Modern Dance
Paid Staff: 4
Volunteer Staff: 10
Paid Artists: 9

584 MORRISONDANCE

PO Box 18496
Cleveland Heights, OH 44118-0496
Phone: 216-241-9363
e-mail: sarah@morrisondance.com
Web Site: www.morrisondance.com
Management:
    Choreographer/Director: Sarah Morrison
    Artist/Designer: Scott Radke

585 BALLET METROPOLITAN

322 Mount Vernon Avenue
Columbus, OH 43215
Phone: 614-229-4860
Fax: 614-229-4858
e-mail: dance@balletmet.org
Web Site: www.balletmet.org
Officers:
    Chairman: Nancy Strause
    Executive Officer: Jeff Rich
Management:
    Artistic Director: David Nixon
    Dance Academy Administrator: Xandra Auderhalt
    Executive Director: Mary K Bailey

Mission: To maintain a resident professional ballet company; to develop a repertoire encompassing a range of classical and contemporary work; to provide educational audience development services to the community; to build a dance academy which provides professional training and vocational instruction.
Founded: 1980
Specialized Field: Ballet
Status: Professional; Nonprofit
Income Sources: National Association for Regional Ballet; Dance USA
Performs At: Ohio Theatre
Organization Type: Performing; Touring; Resident; Educational; Sponsoring

586 BALLETMET

322 Mount Vernon Avenue
Columbus, OH 43215-3841
Phone: 614-229-4860
Fax: 614-229-4858
e-mail: dance@balletmet.org
Web Site: www.balletmet.org
Management:
    Artistic Director: Gerard Charles
    Dance Academy: Chris Rogersurn
    Executive Director: Cheri Mitchell
    Company Manager: Carter Martin
Mission: To maintain a resident professional ballet company; to develop a repertoire encompassing a range of classical and contemporary work; to provide educational audience development services.
Founded: 1978
Specialized Field: Ballet
Status: Professional
Paid Staff: 110
Paid Artists: 27
Budget: $5,300,000
Income Sources: National Association for Regional Ballet; Dance USA; National Endowment for the Arts; Greater Columbus Arts Council; Ohio Arts Council
Performs At: Capitol Theatre
Organization Type: Performing; Resident; Touring; Educational

587 OHIO STATE UNIVERSITY DANCERS IN THE SCHOOLS

1813 N High Street
Columbus, OH 43210
Phone: 614-292-7935
Fax: 614-292-0939
e-mail: kennedy.74@osu.edu
Web Site: www.dance.ohio-state.edu
Management:
    Director: Margert Kennedy
Mission: Student performances for educational settings.
Specialized Field: Dance/dance education

588 CUYAHOGA VALLEY YOUTH BALLET

2315 State Road
Cuyahoga Falls, OH 44223
Phone: 330-928-6479
Fax: 330-928-4966
Web Site: www.cvyb.org
Officers:

President: Tom Hardy
VP: Andrea Kok
Recording Secretary: Gail Noble
Corresponding Secretary: Bernadette Harris
Treasurer: David Sarver
Management:
  Artistic Director: Nan Klinger
  Artistic Director: Mia Welch
  Assistant Artistic Director: Lori Klinger
Mission: To provide performing experience for talented young dancers, educating them in the realities of professional ballet; to educate area children and families in the appreciation of ballet as an art form at affordable prices.
Founded: 1975
Specialized Field: Modern; Ballet
Status: Pre-Professional; Nonprofit
Paid Staff: 33
Performs At: Akron Civic Theatre; EJ Thomas Hall
Organization Type: Performing; Resident; Educational

589 **DAYTON BALLET**
140 N Main Street
Dayton, OH 45402
Phone: 937-449-5060
Fax: 937-461-8353
e-mail: info@daytonballet.org
Web Site: www.daytonballet.org
Officers:
  President: Gregory McCann
  Chairman: Douglas Franklin
Management:
  Executive Director/Artistic Dir: Dermot Burke
  Artistic Associate: Gregory Robinson
  Financial Director: Lilia Shoemaker
Mission: To educate, enlighten, and entertain the widest audience possible. With the Miami Valley as a base, Dayton Ballet Association will maintain and further develop its artistic, managerial and technical resources.
Founded: 1937
Specialized Field: Ballet; Contemporary
Status: Nonprofit
Paid Staff: 25
Paid Artists: 20
Budget: $2,000,000
Income Sources: Ticket Revenue; Community Support; State and Local Government
Performs At: The Victoria Theatre; Schuster Performing Arts Center
Annual Attendance: 30,000
Seating Capacity: 1,100
Year Built: 1866
Year Remodeled: 1989
Organization Type: Performing

590 **DAYTON CONTEMPORARY DANCE COMPANY**
126 N Main Street
Suite 240
Dayton, OH 45402-1710
Phone: 937-228-3232
Fax: 937-223-6156
e-mail: office@dcdc.org
Web Site: www.dcdc.org

Management:
  Executive Director: Phyllis Brozozowska
  Artistic Director: Kevin Ward
Mission: The purpose of Dayton Contemporary Dance Company, a modern American dance company rooted in the African-American expirence, is to deliver contemporary dance of the highest quality to the broadest possible audience.
Founded: 1968
Specialized Field: Contemporary; Jazz; Modern
Status: Professional; Nonprofit
Paid Staff: 72
Paid Artists: 20
Non-paid Artists: 15
Budget: $1,600,000
Income Sources: Government; Corporate; Foundations; Individuals
Type of Stage: Proscenium
Organization Type: Performing; Touring; Resident

591 **RHYTHM IN SHOES**
126 N Main Street
Suite 420
Dayton, OH 45402
Phone: 937-226-7463
Fax: 937-910-1048
e-mail: rhythmshoe@aol.com
Web Site: www.rhythminshoes.org
Management:
  Artistic Director: Sharon Leahy
Paid Staff: 2
Paid Artists: 15
Budget: $200,000-$500,000

592 **SINCLAIR DANCE ENSEMBLE**
Blair Hall Theatre
444 W 3rd Street
Dayton, OH 45402
Phone: 937-512-2751
Fax: 937-512-2054
Toll-free: 800-315-3000
e-mail: pfox@sinclair.edu
Web Site: www.sinclair.edu
Management:
  Artistic Director: Patricia Fox
  Artistic Director: Dawn Quigley
  Artistic Director: Neil Vanderpool
Founded: 1978

593 **TOM AND SUSANA EVERT DANCE COMPANY**
Shore Cultural Centre
Euclid, OH 44123
Phone: 216-289-4144
Fax: 216-731-8354
e-mail: tomevert@aol.com
Officers:
  Chairman: Dennis Sutcliff
  President: Timothy Evert
  Treasurer: Thomas R Hawn
  Secretary: Hugh McKay
Management:
  Artistic Director: Tom Evert
  Administrative Assistant: Marcia Unger

Marketing Director: Susana Evert
Bookings: Lawrence L Evert Jr
Mission: To share the innate vitality of movement as a form of expression and the body as an instrument connected with the mind and spirit.
Founded: 1986
Specialized Field: Modern
Status: Professional; Nonprofit
Paid Staff: 1
Income Sources: Association for Performing Arts Presenters; Arts Midwest; Arts Presenters Network; Ohio Dance; Ohio Citizens Committee for the Arts
Performs At: Cleveland Play House
Organization Type: Performing; Touring; Resident; Educational; Special Events

594 ZIVILI: DANCES & MUSIC OF SOUTHERN SLAVIC COUNTRIES

1753 Loudon Street
Granville, OH 43023
Phone: 614-855-7805
Fax: 614-855-7805
e-mail: obenaufm@alink.com
Web Site: www.zivili.org -or- www.zivili.com
Officers:
Treasurer Director: Consatnce Leal
President Elect: Diane M Lease
Management:
Executive Director: Melissa Pintar Obenauf
Mission: To preserve the dance, music and song of the Croations, Slovenians, Serbs, Bosnians and Montenegrins.
Founded: 1973
Specialized Field: Ethnic
Status: Professional; Nonprofit
Performs At: Palace Theatre
Organization Type: Performing; Touring; Educational

595 LEAVEN DANCE COMPANY

Newman Center, Kent State University
1424 Horning Road
Kent, OH 44240
Mailing Address: 2292 Lynnwood Drive Stow OH, 44224
Phone: 330-688-8806
Fax: 330-686-6103
e-mail: leaven.km@juno.com
Web Site: www.leavendance.org
Management:
Artistic Director: Kathryn Mikelick
Mission: Leaven Dance Company is a professional dance ensemble whose work explores issues of spirituality, social concerns, peace, justice, and wellness through performances and worship and workshop venues.
Founded: 1992
Specialized Field: Dance
Paid Staff: 1
Volunteer Staff: 8
Paid Artists: 6

596 STUART PIMSLER DANCE & THEATER

1937 Glenwood Parkway
Minneapolis, OH 55422

Phone: 763-521-7738
e-mail: spdanth@aol.com
Web Site: innerart.com/spdt/
Management:
Artistic Director: Stuart Pimsler
Artistic Director: Suzanne Costello
Development: Robin Brooks
Mission: Committed to presenting performance work that comments on contemporary issues.
Founded: 1978
Specialized Field: Modern
Status: Professional
Paid Staff: 3
Paid Artists: 6
Budget: $200,000-$500,000
Income Sources: Ohio Dance; Association for Performing Arts Presenters; Alliance for Dance & Movement Arts
Organization Type: Performing

597 OBERLIN DANCE COMPANY

Oberlin College
30 N Professor Street
Oberlin, OH 44074
Phone: 440-775-8152
Fax: 440-775-8340
e-mail: paul.moser@berlin.edu
Web Site: www.oberlin.edu/~thedance/
Management:
Chair: Paul Moser
Associate Professor of Dance: Ann Cooper Albright
Mission: To provide a critical understanding and enhanced appreciation for theater, dance, and film arts and their relationship to others areas of liberal arts learning.
Performs At: Finney Chapel; Hall Auditorium; Warner Center

598 MIAMI UNIVERSITY DANCE THEATRE

106 E Phillips Hall
Oxford, OH 45056
Phone: 513-529-2730
Fax: 513-529-5006
e-mail: rosenblk@muohio.edu
Web Site: www.muohio.edu/dancetheatre
Management:
Artistic Director/General Manager: Lana Kay Rosenberg
Founded: 1933
Specialized Field: Dance
Performs At: Auditorium
Affiliations: OHW Dance; ACDFA
Annual Attendance: 1,100
Type of Stage: Proscenium
Seating Capacity: 730

599 CHILDREN'S BALLET THEATRE

PO Box 2255
Stow, OH 98801
Phone: 330-688-6065
Fax: 330-688-7781
e-mail: info@childrensballettheatre.org
Web Site: www.childrensballettheatre.org
Management:
Director: Joan Shelton-Mason

Artistic Director: Christine Meneer
Mission: To bring finest professional artists to
North-Central Washington.
Founded: 1985
Specialized Field: Ballet; Multi-Media Productions
Status: Semi-Professional; Nonprofit
Organization Type: Performing; Touring; Resident

600 TOLEDO BALLET ASSOCIATION
Westfield Shoppingtown Franklin Park
5001 Monroe Street
Toledo, OH 43623
Phone: 419-471-0049
Fax: 419-471-9005
e-mail: jjarrett@toledoballet.net
Web Site: www.toledoballet.net
Officers:
President: John Adams
Treasurer: Donna Dawson CPA
Secretary: Yolando Nora Calderon
Management:
Artistic Director: Nigel Burgoine
Business Director: Jennifer Jarrett
Mission: To provide performing opportunities for area
dancers, quality dance to the community, dance
scholarships and dance education.
Founded: 1958
Specialized Field: Ballet; Jazz
Status: Professional; Semi-Professional;
Nonprofessional; Nonprofit
Paid Staff: 23
Budget: $633,000
Income Sources: Various
Performs At: Stranahan Theater; Valentine Theater
Organization Type: Performing; Touring; Resident;
Educational; Sponsoring

601 BALLET WESTERN RESERVE
1361 5th Avenue
Youngstown, OH 44504
Phone: 330-744-1937
Fax: 330-744-2031
Management:
Director: Anita Lin O'Donnell
Office Manager: Kathy DuBois
Mission: Dedicated to promoting interest in ballet,
modern dance and jazz, arranging performances and
preparing students for performance and professional
dance careers.
Founded: 1979
Specialized Field: Modern; Ballet; Jazz
Status: Nonprofessional; Nonprofit
Performs At: Youngstown State University; Powers
Auditorium
Organization Type: Performing; Educational

Oklahoma

**602 WESTERN OKLAHOMA BALLET
THEATRE
Performing Company**
512 Frisco
PO Box 1593
Clinton, OK 73601
Phone: 508-323-3735
Management:
Artistic Director: Penny Askew
Mission: Dedicated to nurturing and promoting dance in
Western Oklahoma.
Founded: 1977
Specialized Field: Modern; Ballet
Status: Nonprofessional; Nonprofit
Paid Staff: 9
Income Sources: Regional Dance America; Southwestern
Regional Ballet Association
Performs At: Southwestern Oklahoma State University
Fine Arts
Organization Type: Performing; Educational

603 DUNCAN LAWTON CITY BALLET
1006 SW E Avenue
Lawton, OK 73501
Mailing Address: PO Box 3714 Lawton OK, 73502
Phone: 580-357-2700
Fax: 580-353-3527
e-mail: dlcballet@hotmail.com
Officers:
Chair: Dr. Lloyd A Dawe
Management:
Artistic Director/Founder: Margaret Gray
Managing Director: Roger Gray
Mission: Dedicated to the presentation of ballet.
Founded: 1994
Specialized Field: Ballet
Status: Nonprofit
Volunteer Staff: 3
Non-paid Artists: 16
Income Sources: Local Foundations
Performs At: Simon Center Theatre
Annual Attendance: 7,200

**604 OKLAHOMA FESTIVAL BALLET
School of Dance**
601 Elm Avenue
Room 429
Norman, OK 73019
Phone: 405-325-4051
Fax: 405-325-7024
e-mail: kyoung@ou.edu
Web Site: www.ou.edu/finearts/dance/index.htm
Management:
Director: Mary Margaret Holt
Artistic Advisor: Miquel Terekhov
Admistrative Assistant: Kathy Yuoung
Ballet Master: Donn Edwards
Mission: To present an eclectic repertoire through a
classical ballet company of young dancers.
Founded: 1984
Specialized Field: Ballet
Status: Semi-Professional

Paid Staff: 4
Non-paid Artists: 50
Budget: $200,000-$500,000
Income Sources: University of Oklahoma; Tours
Performs At: 5 Dance Studios
Annual Attendance: 5,500
Type of Stage: Proscenium arch stage
Stage Dimensions: 47 x 105
Seating Capacity: 643
Year Built: 1965
Year Remodeled: 2002
Organization Type: Performing; Touring; Resident; Educational

605 BALLET OKLAHOMA

7421 N Classen Boulvard
Oklahoma City, OK 73116
Phone: 405-843-9898
Fax: 405-843-9894
Web Site: www.balletoklahoma.com
Management:
Artistic Director: Bryan Pitts
Assistant to the Artistic Director: Laura Flagg-Pitts
Mission: To promote a professional resident ballet company and ballet school.
Founded: 1972
Specialized Field: Ballet; Jazz
Status: Professional
Paid Staff: 7
Volunteer Staff: 5
Paid Artists: 18
Budget: $1,000,000-$2,500,000
Organization Type: Performing; Touring; Resident; Educational; Sponsoring

606 OKLAHOMA CITY UNIVERSITY: SCHOOL OF AMERICAN DANCE & ART MANAGEMENT

2501 N Blackwelder
Oklahoma City, OK 73107
Phone: 405-521-5322
Fax: 405-521-5373
e-mail: jhs1017@aol.com
Management:
Dean: John Bedford

607 PRAIRIE DANCE THEATRE

2100 NE 52nd
Kirkpatrick Center
Oklahoma City, OK 73111
Phone: 405-424-2249
Fax: 405-475-9366
e-mail: co-mgr@prairiedance.org
Web Site: www.prairiedance.org
Management:
Executive Director: Beth Shumway
Mission: Prairie Dance Theatre offers full concerts of contemporary dance and is known for original works based on Southwestern and Native American themes.
Founded: 1978
Specialized Field: Modern; Ethnic; Folk
Status: Professional; Nonprofit
Budget: $100,000-$200,000

Income Sources: Kirpatrick Center Museum; MidAmerica Dance Network
Organization Type: Performing; Touring; Resident; Educational

608 TULSA BALLET

4512 S Peoria
Tulsa, OK 74105-4563
Phone: 918-749-6030
Fax: 918-749-0532
e-mail: admin@tulsaballet.org
Web Site: www.tulsaballet.org
Officers:
President: Cheryl Forrest
Chairman: Skipp Teel
Executive VP: Candace Trombka
VP/Strategic Range Planning: Kay Nixon
VP Finance/Budget: Donna Bost
Management:
Artistic Director: Marcello Angelini
Executive Director: Marc S Engel
Marketing Manager: Katy Hall
Mission: Tulsa Ballet Theatre is a professional ballet company whose purpose is to preserve the tradition of classical ballet; to promote the appreciation of contemporary dance; to create works of superior and enduring quality; and to educate through performances and outreach programs
Founded: 1956
Specialized Field: Ballet
Status: Professional; Nonprofit
Paid Staff: 24
Paid Artists: 30
Budget: $3,000,000
Income Sources: National Association for Regional Ballet; Dance USA
Affiliations: AACT; CCTC
Annual Attendance: 60,000
Seating Capacity: 2300
Organization Type: Performing; Touring

Oregon

609 DANCE AFRICA

University of Oregon, Department of Dance
1214 Unversity of Oregon
Eugene, OR 97403-1214
Phone: 541-346-3386
Fax: 541-346-3380
e-mail: mmoser@oregon.uoregon.edu
Management:
Director: Rita Honka
Founded: 1993
Specialized Field: Dance

610 DANCE THEATRE OF OREGON

8015 Dorris Street
Eugene, OR 97404
Phone: 541-689-9701
Fax: 541-688-9235
e-mail: dto@efn.org
Web Site: www.efn.org/~dto
Management:

Artistic Director: Marc Siegel
Artistic Director: Pamela Lehan-Siegel
Status: Nonprofit; Professional

611 EUGENE BALLET COMPANY
PO Box 11200
Eugene, OR 97440
Phone: 541-485-3992
Fax: 541-687-5745
e-mail: eballet@eugeneballet.org
Web Site: www.eugeneballet.org
Officers:
President: Susan Jones
VP: Kent Anderson
Secretary: Susan Kauble
Treasurer: Christine Allen
Marketing Director: Kelcey Boyce
Financial Manager: Sandy Naishtat
Management:
Artistic Director: Toni Pimble
Managing Director: Riley Grannan
Ballet Mistress/Regisseur: Lisa Moon
Ballet Master: Mark Lanham
Marketing Assistant: Sarah Bailen
Education Director: Sibyl Barnum
Computer Operations: Ray Brown
Mission: To provide quality professional dance productions and innovative educational services to a broad-based audience throughout the US.
Founded: 1978
Specialized Field: Ballet
Status: Professional; Nonprofit
Paid Staff: 5
Volunteer Staff: 2
Paid Artists: 20
Budget: $1,500,000
Income Sources: Individuals; Corporations; Foundations
Performs At: Hult Center for the Performing Arts
Annual Attendance: 25,000
Facility Category: Performing Arts Center
Type of Stage: Proscenium
Stage Dimensions: 52'x48'
Seating Capacity: 2,460
Year Built: 1982
Cost: $23 million
Organization Type: Performing; Touring; Resident; Sponsoring

612 BRITT FESTIVALS
PO Box 1124
Medford, OR 97501
Phone: 541-779-0847
Fax: 541-776-3712
e-mail: info@brittfest.org
Web Site: www.brittfest.org
Management:
Executive Director: Ron McUne
Music Director: Peter Bay
Marketing/Public Relations Director: Kelly Gonzales
Development Director: Ed Foss
Booking/Production Director: Mike Sturgill
Education Director: David MacKenzie
Mission: To present and sponsor, in Southern Oregon, performing arts of the highest quality for the education, enrichment and enjoyment of all.

Founded: 1963
Specialized Field: Classical; Jazz; Blues; Pop/Rock; Country; Folk; Bluegrass; World Music; Dance; Musical Theater; Comedy
Status: Professional; Nonprofit
Paid Staff: 12
Volunteer Staff: 600
Performs At: The Britt Gardens
Annual Attendance: 70,000
Facility Category: Outdoor Amphitheatre
Seating Capacity: 2200
Year Built: 1963
Year Remodeled: 1992
Organization Type: Performing; Touring; Resident; Educational; Sponsoring

613 BODYVOX
1300 NW Northrup Street
Portland, OR 972093
Phone: 503-229-0627
Fax: 503-229-0627
e-mail: info@bodyvox.com
Web Site: www.bodyvox.com
Officers:
President: Jamey Hampton
VP: Ashley Roland
Management:
Artistic Director: Jamey Hampton
General Manager: Una Loughran
Artistic Director: Ashley Roland
Mission: Bodyvox contemporary dance company performs and creates innovative multidisciplinary dance works.
Founded: 1998
Specialized Field: Contemporary Dance
Paid Staff: 4
Volunteer Staff: 20
Paid Artists: 13
Budget: $300,000
Income Sources: Artistic Fees; Private & Foundation Support

614 KATJA BIESANZ DANCE THEATER
3410 SW Water Avenue
Portland, OR 97201
Phone: 503-248-2207
Fax: 503-227-8481
e-mail: katja@teleport.com
Web Site: www.dance.org
Management:
Artistic Director: Katja Biesanz
Status: Nonprofit
Organization Type: Performing; Touring

615 METRO DANCERS
9933 SE Pine Street
Portland, OR 97216
Phone: 503-408-0604
Fax: 503-408-0495
e-mail: pdxmetarts@aol.com
Web Site: www.PDXMetroArts.org
Management:
Artistic Director: Nancy Yeamans
Mission: To make the arts accessible to everyone.

Founded: 1979
Specialized Field: Theatre; Music; Visual Arts
Status: Nonprofessional; Nonprofit
Paid Staff: 20
Volunteer Staff: 30
Income Sources: Regional Dance Association/Pacific
Type of Stage: Sprung Floor
Stage Dimensions: 40'x50'
Seating Capacity: 150
Year Built: 2000
Organization Type: Performing

616 OREGON BALLET THEATRE

818 SE 6th Avenue
Portland, OR 97214
Phone: 503-227-0977
Fax: 503-227-4186
e-mail: obt@obt.org
Web Site: www.obt.org
Officers:
 President: Scott Thomason
 VP: Fred Granum
 VP: Brad Miller
 Secretary: Michele O'Hara
 Treasurer: Barney Hyde
Management:
 Artistic Director: James Canfield
 Managing Director: Beth Barbre
 Music Director: Niel De Ponte
Mission: To offer the highest quality professional ballet to the people of Oregon, the Pacific Northwest and the US; to entertain and educate audiences, and to encourage the creative talents of dancers, choreographers, composers and musicians.
Founded: 1989
Specialized Field: Modern; Ballet; Jazz
Status: Professional; Nonprofit
Paid Artists: 18
Budget: $4.5 Million
Income Sources: Public and private funding organizations; Individual donations; Ticket sales gift; Boutique
Season: October - June
Performs At: Keller Auditorium, Newmark Theatre, Portland Center
Organization Type: Performing; Touring; Resident; Educational; Sponsoring

617 PIONEER COURTHOUSE SQUARE

701 SW 6th Avenue
Portland, OR 97204
Mailing Address: 715 SW Morrison, Portland, OR. 97205
Phone: 503-223-1613
Fax: 503-222-7425
Web Site: www.pioneersquare.citysearch.com
Management:
 General Manager: Jennifer Polver
 Events Management Coordinator: Stephanie Leeper
Budget: $400,000-1,000,000
Annual Attendance: 7.6 million
Facility Category: Public Space
Seating Capacity: 3,000

618 LITTLE BALLET THEATRE

PO Box 129
Warrenton, OR 97141
Phone: 503-860-1086
e-mail: lbt@clatsop.com
Web Site: www.clatsop.com
Management:
 Artistic Director: Jeanne Maddox Fastabend
Mission: To offer exposure to ballet to all people in Oregon's North Coast area.
Founded: 1978
Specialized Field: Ballet
Status: Non-Professional; Nonprofit
Paid Staff: 100
Performs At: Astoria High School Auditorium
Organization Type: Performing; Educational

Pennsylvania

619 ALLEGHENY BALLET COMPANY

1231 27th Avenue
Altoona, PA 16603
Phone: 814-943-6081
Fax: 814-337-0988
e-mail: BALLETALL@aol.com
Officers:
 Business Manager: Marjorie Lantz
Management:
 Artistic Director: Deborah Anthony
Specialized Field: Ballet
Status: Semi-Professional; Nonprofit
Performs At: Mishler Theatre
Organization Type: Performing; Resident

620 PITTSBURGH YOUTH BALLET

1033 Paxton Drive & Route 88
Bethel Park, PA 15102
Phone: 412-835-1250
Fax: 412-835-7969
e-mail: pybco@aol.com
Web Site: www.pybco.org
Management:
 Artistic Director: Jean Gedeon
Mission: To nurture and enhance the lives of children, establish a professional classic and contemporary Youth Company, and encourage new choreographers.
Founded: 1990
Specialized Field: Extension of the Pittsburgh Youth Ballet School
Status: Nonprofit

621 BALLET GUILD OF LEHIGH VALLEY
Pennsylvania Youth Ballet

556 Main Street
Bethlehem, PA 18018
Phone: 610-865-0353
Fax: 610-865-2698
e-mail: ythballet@aol.com
Web Site: www.bglv.org
Officers:
 President: Carol Dimopoulos
 VP: Barry Pell

All listings are in alphabetical order by state, then city, then organization within the city.

Secretary: Andrew Swantak
Treasurer: Harry Dimopoulos
Management:
    Production Manager: Garry Kasten
    Artistic Director: Oleg Briansky
    Artistic Director: Mireille Briane
Mission: Ballet Guild of Lehigh Valley, Inc. is a nonprofit organization dedicated to fostering the art of theatre dance, primarily classical ballet, through education and performances.
Founded: 1958
Specialized Field: Ballet
Status: Semi-Professional; Nonprofit
Paid Staff: 6
Budget: $200,000 - $250,000
Performs At: Zoellner Arts Center, Lehigh University
Organization Type: Performing; Educational

622 CENTRAL PENNSYLVANIA YOUTH BALLET

5 N Orange Street, Suite 3
PO Box 1773
Carlise, PA 17013
Phone: 717-245-1190
Fax: 717-245-1189
e-mail: info@cpyb.org
Web Site: www.cpyb.org
Officers:
    President: Tama M Carey
Management:
    Artistic Director: Marca Dale Weary
    Executive Director: Maurinda C Wingard
Mission: Dedicated to: the training of students in the art of classical ballet to the highest artistic standards; the performance of ballet as a component of student education; and the promotion of interest in the art form as a contribution to the cultural life of the extended community.
Founded: 1955
Specialized Field: Ballet
Status: Nonprofit
Affiliations: Resident Ball Company

623 CHINA DANCE THEATRE

Noble Plaza, Suite 212
801 Old York Road
Jenkintown, PA 19046-1611
Phone: 215-885-6400
Fax: 215-885-9929
e-mail: artists@rilearts.com
Web Site: www.rilearts.com

624 VOLOSHKY UKRAINIAN DANCE ENSEMBLES

856 Hamilton Drive
Jenkintown, PA 19046
Phone: 215-663-0294
Fax: 215-763-8503
e-mail: voloshky@mindspring.com
Web Site: www.voloshky.com
Management:
    Artistic Director: Taras Lewyckyi
    Assistant Artistic Director: Oleg Goudimiak
Founded: 1972

Specialized Field: Classical Ballet combined with traditional Ukrainian dance

625 STEVE LOVE'S NEW YORK EXPRESS ROLLER DANCE COMPANY

856 Hamilton Drive
Lafayette Hill, PA 19444
Phone: 610-828-7537
Fax: 610-940-0253
e-mail: brittonmgt@aol.com
Founded: 1985

626 NEW CASTLE REGIONAL BALLET

1807 Moravia Street
New Castle, PA 16101
Phone: 724-652-1822
Web Site: www.angelfire.com/pa4/ncrballet
Management:
    Director: Debbie Parou
    Artistic Director: Debbie Menichino Parou
Mission: To offer a program of proper ballet training to young dancers, an outlet to share their talent with the community, and a vehicle to educate the public in the art of ballet.
Founded: 1987
Specialized Field: Ballet; Jazz; Tap

627 DANCE AFFILIATES/AMERICAN BALLET COMPETITION

2000 Hamilton Street C-200
Philadelphia, PA 19130
Phone: 215-636-9000
Fax: 215-564-4206
e-mail: randy@dancecelebration.org
Web Site: www.dancecelebration.org
Officers:
    President: Ira Lefton, Esquire
    VP: Robert Fryling
    Secretary: James Goodwill
    Treasurer: Ed Hurd
Management:
    Artistic Director: F Randolph Swartz
    Director Development: Jane Bensignor
    Project Director/Ed. Coordinator: Anne-Marie Mulgrew
    Development Associate: Julianne Benstein
Mission: To advance the growth, development, and well being of the art of dance. As dance curators, we nurture the development of dance artists; serve as an intermediary between the touring artist and the audience, present new talent and new work.
Founded: 1972
Specialized Field: Modern; Ballet; Jazz; Ethnic; Folk
Status: Nonprofit
Paid Staff: 4
Volunteer Staff: 20
Budget: $1,000,000
Income Sources: Ticket Sales; Public & Private Funding
Performs At: Annenberg Center for the Performing Arts; Univ. of the Arts
Annual Attendance: 30,000
Facility Category: Theatre
Stage Dimensions: 48'x31'
Seating Capacity: 911

Year Built: 1972
Organization Type: Sponsoring

628 KORESH DANCE COMPANY

104 S 20th Street
PO Box 15815
Philadelphia, PA 19103
Phone: 215-751-0959
Fax: 215-665-0805
e-mail: info@koreshdance.org
Web Site: www.koreshdance.org
Management:
   Executive Director: Alon Koresh
Founded: 1991
Specialized Field: Dance

629 PENNSYLVANIA BALLET

1101 S Broad Street
Philadelphia, PA 19147
Phone: 215-551-7000
Fax: 215-551-7224
e-mail: paballet2@aol.com
Web Site: www.paballet.org
Officers:
   Chairman: Louise Reed
Management:
   Executive Director: Michael Scolamiero
   Artistic Director: Roy Kaiser
   Director Development: Jane Moses
   Director Marketing: Shawn Stone
   Music Director: Beatrice Jona Affron
   Education/Outreach Director: Phillip Juska
   Production Director: John Hoey
   Production Manager: Cheryl Harrison
Founded: 1963
Opened: 1962
Specialized Field: Ballet
Status: Professional; Nonprofit; Semi-Volunteer
Paid Staff: 55
Paid Artists: 40
Budget: $8,000,000
Income Sources: Earned; Unearned
Organization Type: Performing; Touring; Resident

630 PHILADELPHIA DANCE ALLIANCE

1429 Walnut Street
16th Floor
Philadelphia, PA 19102
Phone: 215-564-5270
Fax: 215-564-0497
e-mail: dance@libertynet.org
Web Site: www.libertynet.org/dance/
Management:
   Executive Director: Nancy J Dengler
Mission: An organization that provides the means to affect, enhance, and ensure the future health, stability and growth of the dance field.
Founded: 1971
Specialized Field: Dance

631 PHILDANCO/PHILADELPHIA DANCE COMPANY

9 N Preston Street
Philadanco Way
Philadelphia, PA 191042210
Phone: 215-387-8200
Fax: 215-387-8203
e-mail: phildanco@aol.com
Web Site: www.philadanco.org
Officers:
   Chairman: Spencer Werthemier, Esquire
Management:
   Artistic/Executive Director: Joan Myers Brown
   Managing Director: Vanessa Thomas
   Adminstrative Assistant: Reho Satchell
   Tour Representative: Baylin Artists
   Development/Research: Charlotte Sistron
   Fiscal Management: Donna Still
   Resident Choreographer: Milton Myers
   Managing Director: Venessa Thomas
   President: H Hetherington Smith
Mission: To perform instruct and train, offering tuition-free instruction and performing opportunities to young dancers.
Founded: 1970
Specialized Field: Modern; Ballet; Jazz
Status: Professional; Nonprofit
Paid Staff: 6
Volunteer Staff: 4
Paid Artists: 19
Budget: $1,000,000-$2,500,000
Income Sources: Dance USA; International Association for Blacks in Dance; American Dance Guild; Greater Philadelphia Cultural Alliance; PDA; Philadelphia C.C.
Affiliations: IABD; GRCA; Dance/USA; PDA; American Dance Guild
Annual Attendance: 60,000
Facility Category: Performing Arts Center
Type of Stage: Proscenium
Seating Capacity: 990
Organization Type: Performing; Touring; Resident; Educational

632 DANCE ALLOY

5530 Penn Avenue
Pittsburgh, PA 15206-3525
Phone: 412-363-4321
Fax: 412-363-4320
e-mail: info@dancealloy.org
Web Site: www.dancealloy.org
Officers:
   President: Jay Douglass
   VP: Mary K Austin
   Secretary: Larry Leahy
   Treasurer: Jaon Rigg S
Management:
   Artistic Director: Mark Taylor
   Company Manager: Barbara Thompson
   Executive Director: Cheryl Difatta
   Office Manager: Danieele Scherer
Mission: To create and perform new works of contemporary dance of high artistic merit and to teach dance by interacting with diverse communities in the Pittsburgh region, nationally and internationally.
Founded: 1976

Specialized Field: Contemporary Dance
Status: Professional; Nonprofit
Paid Staff: 6
Paid Artists: 5
Budget: $700,000
Income Sources: Foundations; Corporations; Government
Affiliations: Carnegie Museums of Pittsburgh; LABCO Dance; Pittsburgh Public Schools
Annual Attendance: 4,500
Facility Category: Dance Studio
Type of Stage: Studio
Seating Capacity: 100
Year Built: 1996
Rental Contact: Barbara Thompson
Organization Type: Performing; Touring; Educational

633 LABCO DANCE

1113 E Carson Street
3rd Floor
Pittsburgh, PA 15203
Phone: 412-481-6377
Fax: 412-481-5922
Toll-free: 800-607-0857
e-mail: labcodance@penn..com
Web Site: www.labcodance.com
Management:
   Co-Artistic Director: Evelyn Palleja-Vissicchio
Founded: 1996
Specialized Field: Dance
Paid Staff: 1
Volunteer Staff: 50
Paid Artists: 6
Non-paid Artists: 20

634 MARY MILLER DANCE COMPANY

601 Wood Street
Suite 12
Pittsburgh, PA 15222
Phone: 412-434-1169
Fax: 412-232-3262
e-mail: MaryMillerDance@aol.com
Web Site: www.marymillerdanceco.org
Management:
   Artistic Director: Mary Miller

635 PITTSBURGH BALLET THEATRE

2900 Liberty Avenue
Pittsburgh, PA 15201-1500
Phone: 412-454-9138
Fax: 412-281-9901
e-mail: pbt@uno.com
Web Site: www.pbt.org
Officers:
   Chairman: F James McCarl
   Vice Chair: Kears Pollock
   VP Finance/Treasurer: David J Lancia
   Secretary: Becky Torbin
Management:
   Artistic Director: Terrence S Orr
   Music Director/Principal Conductor: Akira Endo
   Ballet Mistress: Dana Arey
   Ballet Mistress: Mariannaen Tcherkassky
   Ballet Master: Roberto Munoz

Managing Director: Stephen B Libman
Assistant Pianist/Conductor: Michael Moricz
Company Pianist: Steven V Mitchell
Production Manager: David Holcomb
Mission: The presentation of quality professional ballet performances in Pittsburgh, regionally and nationally.
Founded: 1969
Specialized Field: Ballet
Status: Professional; Nonprofit
Budget: $2,500,000
Income Sources: National Endowment for the Arts; Dance USA
Organization Type: Performing; Touring; Resident; Educational

636 PITTSBURGH DANCE COUNCIL

910 Century Building
130 7th Street
Pittsburgh, PA 15222
Phone: 412-355-0330
Fax: 412-355-0413
e-mail: rspringer@dancecouncil.org
Web Site: www.dancecouncil.org
Officers:
   President: Victoria Eisenreich
Management:
   Executive Director: Paul Organisak
Mission: To incorporate diversity, balance and a high level of quality in all presentations and related activities. Committed to expanding the visibility, appreciation, and presentation of dance as an artform in the Pittsburgh area while nurturing the field of dance on local national and international levels.
Founded: 1969
Specialized Field: Modern; Ballet; Ethnic; Folk
Status: Nonprofit
Income Sources: Ticket Sales; Grants
Performs At: Benedum Center; Byham Theater
Organization Type: Sponsoring; Presenting

637 PENNSYLVANIA DANCE THEATRE

140 Kelly Alley
State College, PA 16801
Phone: 814-237-2188
Fax: 814-865-3039
e-mail: pdt@pdtdance.org
Web Site: www.pdtdance.org/home.html
Management:
   Artistic Director: Robert Steele
   Company Manager: Emma Gricar
Mission: To provide audiences with an overview of the mainstream as well as the cutting edge in modern dance.
Founded: 1979
Specialized Field: Modern
Status: Professional; Nonprofit
Paid Staff: 1
Budget: $100,000-$200,000
Organization Type: Performing; Touring; Educational

638 NOTARA DANCE THEATRE

700 Phillips Street
PO Box 1204
Stroudsburg, PA 18360

Phone: 570-421-1718
Fax: 570-422-1199
Officers:
   President: Sally Notara
   VP: Darrell Notara
Management:
   Co-Director: Sally Notara
   Co-Director: Darrell Notara

---

639   GREATER YORK YOUTH BALLET
Greater York Center for Dance Education
3524 E Market Street
York, PA 17402
Phone: 717-755-6683
Fax: 717-755-6688
e-mail: info@gycde.com
Web Site: www.gycde.com
Management:
   Artistic Director: Lori Pergament
Founded: 1971

Rhode Island

---

640   KELLI WICKE DAVIS/SHODA MOVING THEATRE
110 Highland Avenue
Barrington, RI 02806-4748
Phone: 401-245-6956
Fax: 401-245-6956
e-mail: kwickedavis@earthlink.net
Management:
   Artistic Director: Kelli Wicke Davis
Mission: Performances in theatre, movement design and performance art.
Founded: 1974
Specialized Field: Movement; Theatre; Dance
Paid Artists: 3
Affiliations: Director- SSDC

---

641   STATE BALLET OF RHODE ISLAND
52 Sherman Avenue
Lincoln, RI 02865
Phone: 401-334-2560
Fax: 401-334-0412
e-mail: himarsden@worldnet.att.net
Web Site: www.stateballet.com
Officers:
   Chairperson: Herci Marsden
   Vice Chairperson/Treasurer: Ana Mardsen Fox
   Recording Secretary: Barbara Ann Marsden
Management:
   Artistic Director: Herci Marsden
   General Manager: Ana Marsden Fox
   Rehearsal Assistant: Mia Nocera
   Rehearsal Assistant: Kari Ann Lavallee
Mission: To promote and maintain the highest standards of dance education and performance as Rhode Island's first established ballet company in residence.
Founded: 1960
Specialized Field: Ballet
Status: Semi-Professional; Nonprofit
Paid Staff: 4

Paid Artists: 8
Non-paid Artists: 60
Budget: $100,000
Income Sources: Admission; Benefactors; Members Contributor; Fund Raisers
Performs At: Roberts Hall Rhode Island College in Providence Auditorium
Affiliations: Braecrest School of Ballet
Annual Attendance: 10,000
Facility Category: Theatre
Stage Dimensions: 60'x80'
Seating Capacity: 1,000
Organization Type: Performing; Touring; Resident; Educational

---

642   ISLAND MOVING COMPANY
3 Charles Street
Newport, RI 02840
Mailing Address: PO Box 746, Newport, RI. 02840
Phone: 401-847-4470
Fax: 401-846-2902
e-mail: imcdance@yahoo.com
Web Site: www.newportarts.org
Officers:
   President: Sal DeRuggiero
   VP: Rachel Balaban
   Treasurer: Marc Tanguay
   Secretary: Pro Lyon
Management:
   Program Director: Cheryl Burns
   Artistic Director: Miki Ohlsen
   Director Development: Dominique Alfandre
Mission: The presentation of new choreography; the education of a dance audience; the training of young dancers.
Founded: 1982
Specialized Field: Modern; Ballet
Status: Professional; Nonprofit
Paid Staff: 6
Paid Artists: 15
Budget: $250,000
Income Sources: Admissions; Foundations; Grants; Membership; Residencies
Affiliations: Newport Academy of Ballet
Organization Type: Performing; Touring; Resident; Educational

---

643   EVERETT DANCE THEATRE
349 Hope Street
Providence, RI 02906
Phone: 401-831-9479
Fax: 401-455-0581
e-mail: info@everettdancetheatre.org
Web Site: www.everettdancetheatre.org
Management:
   Marketing Director: Therese Jungels
   Assistant Artistic Director: Aaron Jungels
Founded: 1985
Specialized Field: Theatre; Dance
Paid Staff: 3
Paid Artists: 15
Income Sources: Performances, Foundations
Annual Attendance: 15,000

644 FESTIVAL BALLET PROVIDENCE

825 Hope Street
Providence, RI 02906
Phone: 401-353-1129
Fax: 401-353-8853
e-mail: info@festivalballet.com
Web Site: www.festivalballet.com
Officers:
President: Don Wineburg
VP: Laura Love Rose
Treasurer: David Von Hemat
Secretary: Stacy Nakasians
Management:
Artistic Director: Milhailo Djuric
Managing Director: Lisa LaDew
Company Manager: Mark Fleisher
Mission: To thrill and move students, audiences, dancers, choreographers, supporters and staff, with art and discipline. We dance to enrich and inspire lives.
Founded: 1977
Specialized Field: Ballet
Status: Professional; Nonprofit
Paid Staff: 20
Paid Artists: 12
Non-paid Artists: 3
Budget: $1,500,000
Income Sources: Ticket Sales; School Tuition; Donations; Grants
Performs At: Providence Performing Arts Center; Veterans Memorial Aud.
Affiliations: The Festival Ballet Center for Dance Education
Annual Attendance: 35,000
Facility Category: Dance School; Performing Company
Type of Stage: Rent Providence Area Stages
Organization Type: Performing; Touring; Resident

645 GROUNDWERX MOVEMENT CENTER

95 Empire Street
PO Box 1346
Providence, RI 02903
Phone: 401-454-4564
Fax: 401-454-4564
e-mail: groundwerx@as220.org
Web Site: www.as220.org/Groundwerx

South Carolina

646 BYRNE MILLER DANCE THEATRE

PO Box 1667
Beaufort, SC 29901
Phone: 843-524-1117
Fax: 843-524-1117
e-mail: bmdt@gosiggy.com
Web Site: www.signature-is.net/~bmdt
Officers:
President: Jo Ann Graham
Management:
Artistic Director: Lesley Hendricks
Mission: A nonprofit organization founded by former dance instructor Byrne Miller and dedicated to bring world-class dance companies to Beaufort, organizing school workshops, artists' residencies and special student demonstrations.
Founded: 1971
Status: Nonprofit
Volunteer Staff: 20
Budget: $35,000-60,000
Performs At: John J. McVey Performing Arts Center

647 CHARLESTON BALLET THEATRE

477 King Street
PO Box 262
Charleston, SC 29401
Phone: 803-723-7334
Fax: 803-723-7334
e-mail: cbrpdc@aol.com
Web Site: www.charlestonballet.com
Officers:
President: Courtney Quattlebaum
VP: Linda Helmly
Treasurer: Andrea Crappa-Hurley
Secretary: Bradford Marshall
Management:
Artistic Director: Don Cantwell
Artistic Director: Patricia Cantwell
Resident Choreographer: Jill Eathorne Bahr
Company Manager: Kim Brantingham
Mission: To present dance of the highest quality to the Charleston Area and to provide training and performance opportunities for talented area dancers.
Founded: 1959
Specialized Field: Modern; Ballet; Jazz
Status: Professional; Nonprofit
Paid Staff: 10
Income Sources: National Association for Regional Ballet; Southeast Regional Ballet Association
Performs At: Gaillard Municipal Auditorium
Organization Type: Performing; Touring; Educational; Sponsoring

648 ROBERT IVEY BALLET

College of Charleston School of the Arts
1910 Savannah Highway
Charleston, SC 29407-9679
Phone: 843-556-1343
Fax: 843-757-0960
e-mail: ribart@mindspring.com
Web Site: www.home.mindspring.com
Officers:
President: Sandra Cook
Management:
Artistic Director: Robert Ivey
Mission: To promote and educate in the art of Dance.
Founded: 1977
Specialized Field: Modern; Ballet; Jazz; Guest Choreographers
Status: Semi-Professional; Nonprofit
Paid Staff: 50
Volunteer Staff: 3
Paid Artists: 3
Non-paid Artists: 30

Income Sources: Grants; Fundraiser; Donations; Addmission Sales
Performs At: Sottioe Theatre
Annual Attendance: 7,000
Facility Category: Rental Theatre
Type of Stage: Proscenium
Stage Dimensions: 48' x 32'
Seating Capacity: 785
Organization Type: Resident

---

649   SPOLETO FESTIVAL USA
478 E Bay Street
Suite 200
Charleston, SC 29403
Mailing Address: PO Box 157 Charleston, SC 29402
Phone: 843-579-3100
Fax: 843-723-6383
e-mail: receptionist@spoletousa.org
Web Site: www.spoletousa.org
Officers:
    Director Finance: Tasha Gandy
    Chairman of the Board: William B Hewitt
    President: Eric G Friberg
Management:
    Artistic Director: Joesph Flummerfrlt
    Music Director: Emmanuel Villaume
    General Director: Nigel Redden
    Producer: Nunally Kersh
Mission: To present opera, dance, theater, symphonic, choral and chamber music, jazz and visual arts exhibits of the highest quality; to serve as an educational environment for young artists and audiences alike.
Founded: 1977
Specialized Field: Opera; Chamber; Choral & Symphonic Music; Jazz; Theater; Dance
Status: Professional; Semi-Professional; Nonprofit
Paid Staff: 21
Income Sources: Opera America; Dance USA; Theatre Communications Group; National Institute for Music Theater; American Arts Alliance
Performs At: Gaillard Municipal Auditorium; Dock Street Theater
Organization Type: Performing; Educational; Sponsoring

---

650   CAROLINA BALLET
914 Pulaski Street
Columbia, SC 29201
Phone: 803-771-6303
Fax: 803-771-2625
e-mail: cmfu5678@aol.com
Web Site: www.carolinaballet.com
Officers:
    President: Jeff McKeeven
Management:
    Artistic Director: John Whitehead
    Director of Junior: Mimi Worrell
Paid Staff: 6
Volunteer Staff: 22
Paid Artists: 8
Non-paid Artists: 45

651   COLUMBIA CITY BALLET
PO Box 11898
Columbia, SC 29211
Phone: 803-799-7605
Fax: 803-799-7928
Toll-free: 800-899-7409
e-mail: ccballet@bellsouth.net
Web Site: www.columbiacityballet.com
Officers:
    President: Kara Sproles Mock
    Secretary: Susan Davis Gibson
    Treasurer: Derrick Stark
Management:
    Executive Artistic Director: William Starrett
    General Manager: Sydney Miller
Mission: Dedicated to presenting the art of dance to Columbia and its surrounding communities and contributing to the cultural and educational lives of audiences, dancers, and students.
Founded: 1961
Specialized Field: Ballet
Status: Professional; Nonprofit
Paid Staff: 8
Paid Artists: 30
Non-paid Artists: 6
Budget: $1,000,000
Income Sources: Box office; Grants; Corporate support
Performs At: Koger Center for the Arts
Annual Attendance: 125,000
Facility Category: opera
Type of Stage: Proscenium
Seating Capacity: 2,100
Year Built: 1989
Rental Contact: Michael Taylor
Organization Type: Performing; Touring; Resident; Educational

---

652   CAROLINA SCHOOL OF BALLET
872 Woodruff Road
Greenville, SC 29607
Phone: 864-349-2020
Fax: 864-297-7288
e-mail: AABALLET@aol.com
Management:
    Founder/Director: Barbara Selvey
    Art Director: Hannah Justo
    General Manager: Dolly Spigner
    Office Maknager: Emily Chester
    Ballet Mistress: Anita Pacylowski
Founded: 1974
Specialized Field: Ballet
Status: Non-Professional; Nonprofit
Paid Staff: 20
Volunteer Staff: 50
Paid Artists: 10
Non-paid Artists: 15
Performs At: Peace Center
Facility Category: Arts Facility
Seating Capacity: 200
Organization Type: Performing

---

653   GREENVILLE BALLET
9 Le Grande Boulevard
Greenville, SC 29607

Mailing Address: PO Box 8702
Phone: 864-238-6456
Fax: 864-841-3502
Management:
    Artistic Director: Andrew Kuharsky
    Associate Director: Merry Kuharksy
    General Mangager: Donna Wyman

Tennessee

654   BALLET TENNESSEE
John A. Patten Arts Center
3202 Kelly's Ferry Road
Chattanooga, TN 37419
Phone: 423-821-2055
Fax: 423-821-2456
e-mail: ballettenn@aol.com
Management:
    Artistic Director: Anna Baker
    Executive Director: Barry Van Cura
Mission: To make a positive impact on people of all ages, races, religions and economic backgrounds through the art of ballet by providing high quality performance and instruction.
Budget: $200,000-$500,000

655   CHATTANOOGA BALLET
PO Box 6175
Chattanooga, TN 37401
Phone: 423-870-1518
Fax: 423-892-1054
Web Site: www.chattanoogaballet.org
Officers:
    President: Meg Beene
    VP: James Fields
    Secretary: Diane Tingey
    Treasurer: J. Pat Williams
Management:
    General Director: Robert Willie
    School Director: Karen Smith
    Ballet Master: Frank Hay
Mission: To stimulate artistic growth and to increase public awareness and participation in the art of dance in our community and region through the following activities: The development and expression of a performing company with the emphasis on the continuing education and support of local students and professionals; the support and encouragement of choreographers through the commissioning of new works.
Founded: 1973
Specialized Field: Modern; Ballet; Jazz
Status: Nonprofit
Paid Staff: 11
Volunteer Staff: 100
Paid Artists: 9
Non-paid Artists: 40
Income Sources: William L. Montague Foundation; Allied Arts of Greater Chattanooga; Tennessee Arts Commission
Performs At: Fine Arts Center; University of Tennessee-Chattanooga
Affiliations: Tennessee Association of Dance; University of Tennessee

Organization Type: Performing; Touring; Resident; Educational; Sponsoring

656   BALLET MEMPHIS
7950 Trinity Road
Cordova, TN 38018
Phone: 901-737-7322
Fax: 901-737-7037
e-mail: wgriffin@balletmemphis.org
Web Site: www.balletmemphis.org
Management:
    Company/Touring Manager: Kathleen Shaffer
Founded: 1985
Specialized Field: Ballet; Classical; Contemporary
Status: Professional
Paid Artists: 24
Budget: $3,100,000
Performs At: Orpheum Theatre
Organization Type: Performing; Resident; Touring; Educational

657   TENNESSEE ASSOCIATION OF DANCE
PO Box 2432
Johnson City, TN 37605
Phone: 423-929-1129
Fax: 423-929-1129
e-mail: tndance@mounet.com
Web Site: www.tennesseedance.org
Officers:
    Executive Director: Judith Woodruf
Mission: To provide opportunities for education and the enhanced accessibility to dance; to serve the needs and represent the interests of dance artists and organizations; to provide leadership and advocacy; to promote cultural, social, and ethnic diversity within the dance field; to stimulate and nurture new ideas in dance; to promote the highest standards of excellence and integrity in all aspects.
Founded: 1971
Specialized Field: Modern; Ballet; Jazz; Tap
Status: Professional; Non-Professional; Nonprofit
Performs At: Middle Tennessee State University
Organization Type: Educational

658   CITY BALLET
PO Box 1664
Knoxville, TN 37901
Phone: 865-544-0495
Fax: 865-522-3043
e-mail: cityballet@nxs.net
Web Site: www.knoxballet.org
Officers:
    President: Mindy Coulter
Management:
    Executive Director: Ginger O Cook
Mission: To raise the calibre of dance in this area through public performances; to build technically proficient dancers through the use of professional teachers, choreographers, and performers brought in by the company.
Founded: 1988
Specialized Field: Modern; Ballet; Jazz
Status: Semi-Professional; Nonprofit
Paid Staff: 2

Budget: $550,000
Income Sources: Grants; Donations
Organization Type: Educational; Sponsoring

659 **TENNESSEE CHILDREN'S DANCE ENSEMBLE**

4216 Sutherland Avenue
Knoxville, TN 37919
Phone: 865-588-8842
Fax: 865-766-0345
e-mail: tcde@nxs.net
Web Site: www.korrnet.org/tcde
Management:
  Managing Director: Judy Robinson
  Artistic Director: Irena Linn
Mission: To function as a professional modern dance company, setting a high standard of excellence in dance using artists 8-17 years of age; to do all of the above in a positive atmosphere that teaches children to become future leaders.
Founded: 1981
Specialized Field: Modern Dance
Status: Professional; Nonprofit
Paid Staff: 5
Paid Artists: 22
Budget: $200,000-$500,000
Type of Stage: 7
Organization Type: Performing; Touring; Resident; Educational

660 **APPALACHIAN BALLET COMPANY**

215 W Broadway
Maryville, TN 37801
Phone: 865-982-8463
Fax: 865-982-9463
e-mail: kdorner@chartertn.net
Management:
  Artistic Director: Cheryl Van Metre
  Business Manager: Katharine Dorner
Mission: Providing high-quality dance performances for the greater Knoxville area since 1972. An Honor Company in the Southeast Regional Ballet Association, each year the company presents an opening performance at Pellissippi State.
Founded: 1972
Specialized Field: Ballet
Status: Semi-Professional; Nonprofit
Paid Staff: 32
Performs At: Knoxville Civic Auditorium; Tennessee Theater; Pellissippi State; Bijou Theater
Affiliations: Southeast Regional Ballet Association
Organization Type: Performing; Touring; Resident; Educational

661 **NASHVILLE BALLET**

3630 Redman Street
Nashville, TN 37209
Phone: 615-297-2966
Fax: 615-297-9972
e-mail: nashville.ballet@nashville.com
Web Site: www.nashvilleballet.org
Officers:
  President: Irwin Kuhn
  VP: Pat Emery

Treasurer: Claire Tucker
Secretary: Nancy Cheadle
Management:
  Executive Director: Paul Kaine
  Artistic Director: Paul Vasterling
  Director Marketing: Sarah Wnautson
  Music Director: Karen Lynne Deal
Mission: To develop a love and appreciation of ballet in our socially diverse community through high quality professional ballet performances, the School of Nashville Ballet, and educational outreach programs.
Founded: 1986
Specialized Field: Ballet
Status: Professional; Nonprofit
Paid Staff: 15
Paid Artists: 15
Budget: $1,000,000-$2,500,000
Organization Type: Performing; Touring; Educational

662 **TENNESSEE DANCE THEATRE**

615 5th Avenue S
Nashville, TN 37203
Phone: 615-248-3262
Fax: 615-248-3576
e-mail: tdt@artsynergy.org
Management:
  Artistic Director: Andrew Krichels
  Artistic Director: Donna Rizzo
  Executive Director: Edgardo Cora
  Marketing/Media Relations: Amanda Roche
  Dancer Development Director: Sonje Mayo
Mission: To nurture, develop and sustain the love, understanding and appreciation of the art of dance in Tennessee.
Founded: 1983
Specialized Field: Modern
Status: Professional; Nonprofit
Budget: $200,000-$500,000
Income Sources: Metro Division of Parks & Recreation
Organization Type: Performing; Touring; Resident

Texas

663 **LONE STAR BALLET**

1000 S Polk Street
Amarillo, TX 79101
Phone: 806-372-2463
Fax: 806-372-3131
e-mail: lonestarballet@yahoo.com
Web Site: www.handipages.com/lonestarballet
Officers:
  President: Dr. Robert Hansen
  VP: Leslie Richardson
  VP: Brian Smith
  Secretary: Jay Osborne
  Treasurer: Glenna Henderson
  Guild President: Angela Knapp
Management:
  Costume Mistress: Kathy McAfee
  Director Development: Jussen Smith
  General Manager: Cloris Thurston
  Founding Director: Neil Hess

Mission: To produce and promote the art of dance; present the traditional annual production of The Nutcracker; and award dance scholarships to students at West Texas A&M University.
Founded: 1976
Specialized Field: Ballet
Status: Nonprofit
Paid Staff: 5
Paid Artists: 30
Budget: $475,000
Income Sources: Mid-America Arts Alliance; Theatre Communications Group; Grants
Annual Attendance: 16,000
Facility Category: Civic Center
Seating Capacity: 2,300
Organization Type: Performing; Touring; Resident; Educational; Sponsoring

664 BALLET AUSTIN
Ballet Austin Academy
3002 Guadalupe
Austin, TX 78705
Phone: 512-476-9051
Fax: 512-472-3073
Web Site: www.balletaustin.org
Management:
  Artistic Director: Stephen Mills
  Executive Director: Cookie Ruiz
Mission: To involve and enrich Austin and surrounding communities through excellent and innovative performances and education; to achieve national recognition as one of the top classical ballet companies in the US.
Founded: 1956
Specialized Field: Ballet
Status: Professional; Nonprofit
Paid Staff: 16
Paid Artists: 47
Performs At: Performing Arts Center; University of Texas at Austin
Organization Type: Performing; Touring; Educational

665 DEBORAH HAY DANCE COMPANY
1783 Alta Vista Avenue
Austin, TX 78704
Phone: 512-472-0763
e-mail: deborahhay@aol.com
Web Site: www.deborahhay.com
Mission: To foster a discerning appreciation for the human body within the cultural construct of contemporary society, through dance as experienced by audience, student, and/or performer.
Founded: 1980
Specialized Field: Modern; New Dance
Status: Professional; Nonprofit
Organization Type: Performing; Touring

666 JOHNSON/LONG DANCE COMPANY
PO Box 516
Austin, TX 78757
Phone: 512-467-0704
Fax: 512-477-3908
e-mail: mh4arts@aol.com
Web Site: activemm.com/universe/about.htm

667 SHARIR DANCE COMPANY
3724 Jefferson Street
Austin, TX 78767
Phone: 512-458-8158
Officers:
  President: Margaret Perry
  VP: Beverly Reeve
  Secretary: Kim Weidman
  Treasurer: Chris Adams
Management:
  Artistic Co-Director: Jose Luis Bustamante
  Production Manager/Lighting: Amarante L Lucero
  Founder/Artistic Director: Yacov Sharir
  Managing Director: Cindy Goldberger
Mission: To promote the choreography of Yaco Sharir and Jose Luis Bustamante, foster experimentation and creativity of the highest artistic level, and to educate diverse audiences with outreach programs and a wide range of performance experiences of new dance, art, music and interactive technologies.
Founded: 1982
Specialized Field: Modern; Post-Modern
Status: Professional
Income Sources: University of Texas
Organization Type: Performing; Touring; Resident; Sponsoring

668 STILLPOINT DANCE
1112 N Lamar Blouevard
Austin, TX 78703
Mailing Address: PO Box 50432 Austin, TX 78763-0482
Phone: 512-474-2639
e-mail: stillpt@texas.net
Web Site: www.stillpointdance.com
Management:
  Composer: Jane Kaufmann
Mission: Stillpoint Dance work is deeply rooted in traditional modern dance, respecting the foundation from which modern dance evolved; acknowledging and revering history, and evolving and transcending in the present.
Founded: 1994

669 TAPESTRY DANCE COMPANY
507 B Pressler Street
Austin, TX 78703
Phone: 512-474-9846
Fax: 512-474-9212
e-mail: dance@tapestry.org
Web Site: www.tapestry.org
Officers:
  Academy Director: Sharon Marroguin
Management:
  Artistic Director: Acia Gray
Mission: Created with the goal of cross discipline choreography and training, the company supports the artistic development in the mixture of rhythm tap and percussion with contemporary ballet, jazz and modern creating new works.
Paid Staff: 3
Volunteer Staff: 10
Paid Artists: 6

670 DISCOVERY DANCE GROUP

PO Box 1953
Bellaire, TX 77402
Phone: 713-667-3416
Fax: 713-667-4717
e-mail: info@discoverydancegroup.org
Web Site: www.discoverydancegroup.org
Officers:
    President: Gretchen Irion
    Board VP: Elizabeth Celeste Humphries
    Secretary: Carol Andrews
    Treasurer: Christian Steed
Management:
    Executive/Artistic Director: Pamela
    Ybarguen-Stockman
    Managing Director: Jacqpea Frano Stockman
Mission: Dedicated to providing an outlet for talented dancers and further educating them in performance techniques and to perpetuating the unique Camille Long Hill technique and method.
Founded: 1965
Specialized Field: Modern; Ballet; Jazz; Ethnic
Status: Professional; Nonprofit
Paid Staff: 6
Budget: $150,000
Income Sources: Grants; Donations; Company Performance Income and Tution Income from Institute oF the Dance Arts
Affiliations: Cultural Arts Council of Houston
Organization Type: Performing; Touring; Educational

671 CORPUS CHRISTI BALLET

1621 N Mesquite
Corpus Christi, TX 78401
Phone: 361-882-4588
Fax: 361-881-9291
e-mail: ccballet@aol.com
Web Site: www.tamu.edu/ccballet
Management:
    Artistic Director: Cristina Stirling Munro
Founded: 1972
Specialized Field: Ballet
Status: Non-Professional; Nonprofit
Income Sources: Munro Ballet Studios
Performs At: Bayfront Plaza Auditorium
Organization Type: Performing; Touring; Resident; Educational; Sponsoring

672 DALLAS BLACK DANCE THEATRE

2627 Flora Street
PO Box 131290
Dallas, TX 75313-1290
Phone: 214-871-2376
Fax: 214-871-2842
e-mail: dbdt@verizon.net
Web Site: www.dbdt.com
Officers:
    Chairman: Marvin Robinson
Management:
    Founder/Artistic Director: Ann M Williams
    Executive Director: Zenetta Drew
    Operations Manager: Felicia White
Mission: To present ethnic dance as a meaningful art form.

Founded: 1976
Specialized Field: Modern; Jazz; Ethnic
Status: Nonprofit
Paid Staff: 6
Volunteer Staff: 3
Paid Artists: 10
Budget: $1,025,067
Income Sources: Corporate Sponsorship; City of Dallas; Individuals Donations, ticket sales/touring
Performs At: Majestic Theater; Meyerson Symphony Center; DMA
Affiliations: City of Dallas OCA; TCA; National Endowment for the Arts; IABA
Annual Attendance: 125,000
Facility Category: Majestic Theatre
Seating Capacity: 1,568
Year Built: 1921
Year Remodeled: 1984
Organization Type: Performing; Touring; Educational

673 DALLAS METROPOLITAN BALLET

6815 Hillcrest Avenue
Dallas, TX 75205
Phone: 214-361-0278
Fax: 509-692-2678
Management:
    Artistic Director: Ann Etgen
    Artistic Director: Bill Atkinson
Mission: Committed to building an audience for dance and to developing dancers in the Dallas area and the Southwest.
Founded: 1964
Specialized Field: Ballet
Status: Semi-Professional; Nonprofit
Paid Staff: 48
Volunteer Staff: 10
Paid Artists: 8
Non-paid Artists: 14
Income Sources: Ticket Sales; Donations; Grants; Fund Raisers
Performs At: McFarlin Auditorium; Southern Methodist University
Affiliations: Regional Dance America/Southwest
Organization Type: Performing; Touring; Resident; Educational

674 BALLET CONCERTO

3803 Camp Bowie Boulevard
Fort Worth, TX 761047-335
Phone: 817-989-7168
Fax: 817-989-7168
e-mail: mayra@mayraworthenballet.com
Web Site: www.balletconcerto.org
Management:
    Artistic Director: Margo Dean
Mission: Texas Ballet Concerto is a classically trained ballet company that is devoted to creating and presenting professional quality performances as it carries on the Ballet Russe tradition of exuberance in performing.
Founded: 1969
Specialized Field: Ballet
Status: Nonprofit
Paid Staff: 10
Income Sources: Southwest Regional Ballet Association
Organization Type: Performing

675 CONTEMPORARY DANCE/FORT WORTH

PO Box 11652
Fort Worth, TX 76110
Phone: 817-922-0944
Fax: 817-922-0944
e-mail: cdfw@cdfw.org
Web Site: www.cdfw.org
Management:
Co-Artistic Director/Executive Dir: Kerry L Kreiman
Co-Artistic Director: Susan Douglas Roberts

676 FORT WORTH DALLAS BALLET

6845 Green Oaks Road
Fort Worth, TX 76116
Phone: 817-763-0207
Fax: 817-763-0624
e-mail: Ballet@startext.net
Web Site: www.fwdballet.com
Management:
Artistic Director: Benjamin Houk
Executive Director: David Mallette
Company Manager: Mary Lynn Sloan
Budget: $2,500,000+

677 ALLEGRO BALLET OF HOUSTON

1570 S Dairy Ashford
Suite 200
Houston, TX 77077
Phone: 281-496-4670
Fax: 281-496-4670
e-mail: glendabrown@allegroballet.com
Web Site: www.allegroballet.com
Management:
Co-Artistic Director: Peggy Girouard
Co-Artistic Director: Glenda Brown
Ballet Mistress/Mgr/Associate Dir.: Vanessa Brown
Mission: Dedicated to offering a performing outlet for gifted dancers by presenting them in performances both at home and abroad in both classical and contemporary repertoire.
Founded: 1951
Specialized Field: Modern; Ballet; Jazz; Tap
Status: Semi-Professional; Nonprofit
Volunteer Staff: 6
Non-paid Artists: 15
Income Sources: Compaq; The Houston Chronicle; Houston Endowment; Radiant Engergy
Performs At: Jones Hall in Wortham; Mitchell Pavillion in Woodland
Affiliations: Regional Dance America
Annual Attendance: 10,000
Organization Type: Performing; Resident; Educational

678 CHRYSALIS REPERTORY DANCE COMPANY

PO Box 980398
Houston, TX 77098-0398
Phone: 713-661-9855
Fax: 713-664-0643
e-mail: drjsbak@gateway.net
Web Site: www.chrysalisdance.org
Officers:

President: Gay Ann Gustafson
VP: Jose Solis Jr, Esquire
Secretary: Harold Eisenman, Esquire
Treasurer: Ellin Grossman, PhD
Management:
Artistic Associate: Christine Lidvall
Director: Linda Phenix
Mission: To present innovative, quality dance to enhance Houston and other communities.
Founded: 1983
Specialized Field: Modern; Post-Modern; Community Residencies
Status: Professional; Nonprofit
Paid Staff: 3
Paid Artists: 7+
Budget: $100,0000
Income Sources: Individuals; Foundations; Corporations; Performances
Performs At: Heinen Theatre; Houston Community College
Facility Category: Proscenium and black box theaters
Organization Type: Performing; Touring; Resident; Educational; Sponsoring

679 CITY BALLET OF HOUSTON

9902 Long Point
Houston, TX 77055
Phone: 713-468-3670
Fax: 713-468-8708
Officers:
President-CBN: Jennifer Novoil
Management:
Co-Artistic Director: Margo Marshall
Co-Artistic Director: Dennis Marshall
Co-Artistic Director: Mary Arrington
Artistic Advisor: Frederic Franklin
Stage Director: Jennifer Mettar
Mission: To offer a training ground for young dancers and a showcase for choreographers, both local and well-established; to offer performances of high-quality at low ticket cost.
Founded: 1958
Specialized Field: Ballet
Status: Nonprofit
Volunteer Staff: 10
Paid Artists: 4
Non-paid Artists: 20
Income Sources: National Association for Regional Ballet; Southwest Regional Ballet Association
Performs At: Galveston Grand Opera House; Music Hall
Organization Type: Performing

680 HOUSTON BALLET

1921 W Bell
PO Box 130487
Houston, TX 77019
Phone: 713-523-6300
Fax: 713-523-4038
Toll-free: 800-828-2787
e-mail: adman@houstonballet.org
Web Site: www.houstonballet.org
Management:
Artistic Director: Ben Stevenson
Managing Director: CC Conner
Music Director: Ermanno Florio

Specialized Field: Ballet
Status: Professional; Nonprofit
Income Sources: Dance USA; National Corporate Fund for Dance
Performs At: Wortham Center for the Performing Arts
Organization Type: Performing; Touring; Resident; Educational

681   HOUSTON METROPOLITAN DANCE COMPANY AND CENTER

1202 Calumet @ San Jacinto
PO Box 980457
Houston, TX 77098
Phone: 713-522-6375
Fax: 713-849-9214
e-mail: houstonmet@aol.com
Web Site: www.houstonmet.com
Management:
    Executive Director: Michelle Smith
    Artistic Director: Dorrell Martin
    Educational Director: Kristie Kiser
Mission: To enhance the quality of life for individuals and society through instruction in, and the performance of dance. Committed to the development of dance using movement as a learning tool.
Founded: 1995
Specialized Field: Contemporary Dance
Status: Professional; Nonprofit
Paid Staff: 25
Volunteer Staff: 50
Paid Artists: 15
Non-paid Artists: 15
Income Sources: Grants; Foundation
Performs At: The Wortham Center
Annual Attendance: 10,000
Organization Type: Performing; Touring; Resident; Educational

682   TEXAS TAP ENSEMBLE

1763 W 34th Street
Houston, TX 77018
Phone: 713-686-9184
Fax: 713-664-2980
e-mail: texastap@yahoo.com
Officers:
    President: Cherie Krienitz
    Secretary: Jose Solis
    Treasurer: Elaine Frick
Management:
    Director: John F Truax
    Artistic Director: Paula Sloan
Mission: To produce not only good dancers and performers, but to nurture confidence and character in our future adults.
Founded: 1987
Specialized Field: Dance
Status: Nonprofit
Paid Staff: 5
Volunteer Staff: 10
Non-paid Artists: 50
Budget: $225,000
Income Sources: Grants; Corporate; Foundations
Performs At: 3 dance studios
Annual Attendance: 30,000

Facility Category: Dance studios

683   IRVING BALLET COMPANY

3333 N McArthur Boulevard
Irving, TX 75062
Phone: 972-252-2787
Fax: 972-254-0802
Management:
    Artistic Director: Dale Riley
Mission: Dedicated to expanding ballet audiences in the Irving area and establishing a permanent base for future dance audiences.
Founded: 1982
Specialized Field: Ballet; Jazz
Status: Semi-Professional
Paid Staff: 25
Income Sources: Irving Symphony; Cultural Affairs Council
Performs At: Irving Arts Center
Organization Type: Performing

684   KERRVILLE PERFORMING ARTS SOCIETY

PO Box 1884
Kerrville, TX 78029-1884
Phone: 830-896-5724
Fax: 830-257-8559
e-mail: dunnahoo@ktc.com
Officers:
    President: Eleanor Baldwin
    President/Guild: Martha Hensley
    President: Verna Benham
    President Elect, Guild: Lane Colvig
    Secretary: Jane Clint
Mission: Presents 6 national and international music and dance groups every season. Sponsors Hill County Youth Orchestra.
Founded: 1983
Specialized Field: Classical music
Status: Nonprofit
Income Sources: Tickets; Donations; Ad Campaign; Gala
Performs At: Trinity Baptist Church
Annual Attendance: 1,800
Facility Category: Municipal Auditorium
Seating Capacity: 1300
Organization Type: Performing

685   RIO GRANDE VALLEY BALLET

205 Pecan Boulevard
McAllen, TX 78501
Phone: 956-682-2721
Fax: 956-686-7175
e-mail: rgvb@earthlink.net
Management:
    Director: Deborah Case
Mission: Along with the finest in classical dance, Rio Grande Valley Ballet studies Mexican folklorico and flamenco with equal eye to studied authority. Working with professors of folk dances from as far away as Veracruz Mexico, the school and ballet seek authentic and moving expression in the dance forms native to South Texas. They have been chosen to travel throughout the state on numerous tours.
Founded: 1972

All listings are in alphabetical order by state, then city, then organization within the city.

Specialized Field: Ballet; Jazz; Ethnic; Folk
Status: Semi-Professional; Nonprofit
Paid Staff: 10
Volunteer Staff: 30
Paid Artists: 15
Non-paid Artists: 50
Budget: $40,000-$100,000
Organization Type: Performing; Touring; Resident; Educational; Sponsoring

686 PAMPA CIVIC BALLET

315 N Nelson
Pampa, TX 79065
Phone: 806-669-6361
Fax: 806-669-7293
Officers:
President: Mary Wilson
VP: Iris Day
Secretary: Linda Holt
Treasurer: Michael Epps
Company Representative: Ruth Riehart
Management:
Artistic Director: Jeanne M Willingham
Mission: To provide encouragement and performance opportunities to the more gifted and dedicated dancers in the area.
Founded: 1972
Specialized Field: Ballet
Status: Non-Professional; Nonprofit
Paid Staff: 20
Income Sources: Lesson Payments; Tickets
Performs At: M.K. Brown Auditorium
Facility Category: Civic Auditorium
Type of Stage: Proscenium
Stage Dimensions: 51x22
Seating Capacity: 1,200
Organization Type: Performing; Resident; Educational; Sponsoring

687 GUADALUPE FOLK DANCE COMPANY
Guadalupe Cultural Arts Center

1300 Guadalupe Street
San Antonio, TX 78207
Phone: 210-271-3151
Fax: 210-271-3480
e-mail: webmaster@guadalupeculturalarts.org
Web Site: guadalupeculturalarts.org
Officers:
Chairman: Hector Frousto
Management:
Executive Director: Maria Elenz Torralva Alonso
Mission: To preserve, promote, and develop the arts and culture of the Chicano/Latino/Native American peoples.
Founded: 1980
Specialized Field: Traditional Mexican Folklorico and Flamenco; Aztec Dance; Mambo; Salsa
Status: Nonprofit
Paid Staff: 23
Budget: $1,700,000
Income Sources: Federal; State; Local; Private
Performs At: Guadalupe Theater
Annual Attendance: 190,000
Type of Stage: Proscenium; Thrust
Seating Capacity: 379

Year Built: 1940
Year Remodeled: 1984
Cost: $1,000,000
Organization Type: Resident

688 SAN ANTONIO BALLET COMPANY

2800 NE Loop 410
Suite 307
San Antonio, TX 78212
Phone: 210-408-6970
Fax: 210-212-7775
Officers:
Administrative Director: Nancy Smith
Management:
Artistic Director: Vladimir Marek
Budget: $40,000-$100,000

689 SAN ANTONIO METROPOLITAN BALLET

2800 NE Loop 410
Suite 307
San Antonio, TX 78218
Phone: 210-656-1334
Fax: 210-656-1256
e-mail: dance@connallydance.com
Web Site: sametballet.org
Officers:
Board President: Freda Faley
VP: Maggie Rad
Treasurer: Daniel Lux
Secretary: Shannon Wickel
Management:
Artistic Director: Susan Beil Connally
Associate Director: Judith Clement Ghni
Mission: To provide high quality, low cost performances while developing local dance and choreographic talent.
Founded: 1983
Specialized Field: Dance
Paid Staff: 3
Volunteer Staff: 54
Paid Artists: 1
Non-paid Artists: 27
Budget: $100,000
Income Sources: Ticket Sales; Grants, Donations; Fund Raisers
Affiliations: Regional Dance America/Southwest
Facility Category: College Auditorium; City-Owned Theater
Seating Capacity: 600; 2500

690 CLEAR LAKE METROPOLITAN BALLET & REPERTORY THEATRE

17170 Mill Forest Road
Webster, TX 77598
Phone: 281-480-1466
Fax: 281-480-1622
e-mail: LMason4409@AOL.COM
Web Site: www.clmb.org
Management:
Executive/Artistic Director: Lynette Mason Gregg
Founded: 1976
Specialized Field: Dance, Theater
Status: Semi-Professional; Nonprofit
Paid Staff: 20

Volunteer Staff: 200
Paid Artists: 20
Non-paid Artists: 75
Budget: $800,000
Income Sources: Grants; Patrons; Government; Cities; Foundations
Performs At: University of Houston at Clear Lake
Annual Attendance: 11,000
Facility Category: University
Type of Stage: Proscenium
Stage Dimensions: 50'x60'
Seating Capacity: 500
Year Built: 1975
Rental Contact: Tyler Gavin
Organization Type: Performing

691 WICHITA FALLS BALLET THEATRE

3412 Buchanan
Wichita Falls, TX 76308
Phone: 940-322-2552
Fax: 940-322-2552
Web Site: www.wf.net/~wfbt/intro.html
Officers:
 President: Gari Boehm
 Secretary: Edith Huntington
 Treasurer: Patricia Thornton
Management:
 Co-Artistic Director: Patricia Thornton
 Co-Artistic Director: Gari Boehm
 Maintenance/Membership: Marie Lankford
 Ways and Means, Publicity: Judie Fager
 Hospitality: Cynthia Brock
 Marketing: Armando San Diego
 Tickets: Lynn Bassett
 Greek Night: Eleni Moshtaghi
Mission: Dedicated to nurturing the art of dance through ballet.
Founded: 1963
Specialized Field: Modern; Ballet
Status: Semi-Professional; Nonprofit
Paid Staff: 18
Income Sources: Southwest Regional Ballet Association
Performs At: Memorial Auditorium
Seating Capacity: 2,717
Organization Type: Performing; Touring; Resident

Utah

692 UTAH REGIONAL BALLET

PO Box 321
88 N 350 W
American Fork, UT 84003
Phone: 801-756-8091
Fax: 801-756-6545
e-mail: urbjacquel@mindspring.com
Officers:
 Treasurer: Stephen Shelley
Management:
 Artistic Director/Founder: Jacqueline Colledge
 URB Board President: Laura Bridgewater
 Board Member: Shauna Peterson
Mission: To provide enthusiastic audiences with quality programming.

Founded: 1980
Specialized Field: Ballet
Status: Professional; Nonprofit
Volunteer Staff: 50
Paid Artists: 11
Non-paid Artists: 19
Performs At: De Jong Concert Hall; Bringham Young University
Annual Attendance: Over 8,000 children
Organization Type: Performing; Touring

693 ODYSSEY DANCE UTAH

781 W 14600 S
Suite 1
Bluffdale, UT 84065
Phone: 801-495-3262
Fax: 801-495-3262
e-mail: Derryl@odysseydance.com
Web Site: www.ucdt.com
Officers:
 President: John Starrs
 VP: Kim DelGrosso
 Chairman: Ralph Hansen
 Board of Trustee: Greg Parrish
 Board of Trustee: Phyllis Parrish
 Associate Director: Bonnie Storey
 Public Relations: Melanie Doskocil
Management:
 Artistic Director: Derryl Yeager
Mission: To provide a home for some of Utah's great dancers, develop an enthusiastic and supportive audience, and remain financially stable and responsible.
Specialized Field: Classical and Jazz Dance
Income Sources: Ticket Sales
Performs At: Classical; Jazz
Stage Dimensions: 36'x24'

694 BALLET WEST

50 W 200 S
Salt Lake City, UT 84101-1642
Phone: 801-323-6883
Fax: 801-359-3504
e-mail: rlane@balletwest.org
Web Site: www.balletwest.org
Management:
 Executive Director: Johann Jacobs
 Artistic Director: Jonas Koge
 Company/Tour Manager: Richard Lane
Mission: Dedicated to presenting high quality ballet performances.
Founded: 1963
Specialized Field: Ballet
Status: Professional
Paid Staff: 30
Paid Artists: 46
Income Sources: Dance USA; Western Alliance of Arts Administrators; Association of Performing Arts Presenters
Organization Type: Performing; Touring; Resident; Educational

695 CLOG AMERICA

6645 Castleview Drive
Salt Lake City, UT 84128

Phone: 801-968-2411
Fax: 801-250-9491
e-mail: IAE123@aol.com
Web Site:
www.worldmusicevents.com/gallery/clogamerica
Officers:
    Director: Dennis H Cobia
    Co-Director: D Bryan Steele
Mission: The promotion of clogging workshops, festivals,
tours and performances throughout the USA and abroad.
Founded: 1970
Specialized Field: Folk
Status: Semi-Professional; Commercial
Paid Staff: 150
Income Sources: Utah Arts Council; National Clogging
Leaders Organization
Performs At: Scera Shell Amphitheatre
Organization Type: Performing; Touring; Educational

696   EASTERN ARTS INTERNATIONAL DANCE THEATER

PO Box 526362
Salt Lake City, UT 84152
Phone: 801-485-5824
e-mail: kstjohn@burgoyne.com
Web Site: www.easternartists.com
Officers:
    Dance Director: Katherine St John
    Music Director: Lloyd Miller
Management:
    Director: Katherine St. John
Mission: To promote time-honored traditions by offering
concerts, lectures, and workshops of cultures from Asia
and Eastern Europe.
Founded: 1960
Specialized Field: Ethnic
Status: Professional; Nonprofit
Paid Staff: 10
Income Sources: Western Alliance of Arts
Administrators; Society for Ethno-Musicology; Middle
East Studies Association; Society for Dance Ethnology
Organization Type: Performing; Educational;
Sponsoring

697   REPERTORY DANCE THEATRE

PO Box 510427
Salt Lake City, UT 84151-0427
Phone: 801-534-1000
Fax: 801-534-1110
e-mail: rdt@rdutah.org
Web Site: www.rdtutah.org
Officers:
    President: Francis Hanson
    Secretary: Tony Wolff
    Secretary: Margaret Landesmann
Management:
    Executive/Artistic Director: Linda C Smith
    Director Development: Susan Sandack
    Director Public Relations: Elaine Clark
    Booking Director: Lisa Dupaul Moran
    Stage Manager: Jeff Sturgis
    Lighting Designer: Nicholas Cavallaro
    Photographer: Scott Peterson

Mission: Repertory Dance Theatre is dedicated to the
creation, performance, perpetuation, and appreciation of
modern dance.
Founded: 1966
Specialized Field: Modern
Status: Professional
Paid Staff: 4
Paid Artists: 9
Budget: $500,000-$1,000,000
Organization Type: Performing; Touring; Resident;
Educational; Sponsoring

698   RIRIE WOODBURY DANCE COMPANY

138 W Broadway
Salt Lake City, UT 84101
Phone: 801-297-4241
Fax: 801-297-4237
e-mail: rwdance@aol.com
Web Site: www.ririewoodbury.com
Officers:
    Office Manager/Chairman: Kathy Black
    Vice Chairman: Amy Pahnke
    Secretary: Shirley Bliss
Management:
    Marketing/Public Relations: Jill Barnes
    Booking Manager: Jena Thompson
    Development: Daniel Morgan
    Associate Artistic Director: Charlotte Boye Christense
    Summer Workshop Coordinator: Kathy Black
Mission: Furthers contemporary dance as an accessible
and valued art form though performance and dance
education that raises the standards, deepens the
understanding and promotes personal connections with
contemporary dance.
Founded: 1964
Specialized Field: Modern
Status: Professional; Nonprofit
Budget: $500,000-$1,000,000
Organization Type: Performing; Touring; Resident;
Educational; Sponsoring

Vermont

699   BURKLYN BALLET THEATRE

Burlington, VT 05402
Mailing Address: PO Box 907, Island Heights, NJ 08732
Phone: 802-635-1390
Fax: 732-288-2663
e-mail: burklyn@aol.com
Web Site: www.burklynballettheatre.com
Officers:
    President: Angela Whitehill
Management:
    Artistic Director: Angela Whitehill
    Executive Director: James Whitehill
    Director Public Relations: Sandra Halbstein
    Director Operations: Arthur Leeth
Mission: A company of 20 professional, and 55
pre-professional dancers performing classical and
contemporary repertory in weekly performances
throughout the summer.
Founded: 1976
Specialized Field: Ballet

Status: Professional; Pre-Professional
Paid Staff: 12
Paid Artists: 20
Non-paid Artists: 55
Budget: $500,000
Income Sources: Box Office; Tuition
Performs At: Dibden Center for the Arts
Affiliations: Burklyn Youth Ballet
Annual Attendance: 2-5000
Facility Category: College Theatre
Type of Stage: Proscenium
Stage Dimensions: 42'x 39'
Seating Capacity: 600
Year Built: 1968
Year Remodeled: 1992
Organization Type: Performing; Touring; Educational

Virginia

700   REV. J. BRUCE STEWART

4327 Ravensworth Road
Suite 210
Annandale, VA 22003
Phone: 703-941-9422
Fax: 703-941-9422
e-mail: artwithyou@aol.com
Management:
  Artistic/Executive Director: Rev. Stewart
Mission: Teaching, performing and consulting services on the use of arts in worship, community building and personal spiritual development.
Founded: 1981
Specialized Field: Music; Drama; Dance; Clowning: Juggling: Storytelling; Mime; Poetry; Visual arts with all ages.

701   ARLINGTON DANCE THEATRE

PO Box 3091
Arlington, VA 22203
Phone: 703-524-4750
Fax: 703-524-4750
e-mail: adt1@erols.com
Web Site: www.arlingtonarts.org/adt/
Officers:
  President: Andrew Rylyk
  VP: Susan Tyson
  Secretary/Treasurer: Cheryl Scannell
Management:
  Youth Ballet Company Director: Martha Rutter
  Administrative Director: Amanda Smith
  School Director: Ann Kelly
Mission: To promote excellence in the performance and teaching of dance.
Founded: 1956
Specialized Field: Ballet; Jazz; Tap
Status: Semi-Professional; Nonprofit
Paid Staff: 16
Income Sources: Arlington County Cultural Affairs Office
Performs At: Thomas Jefferson Community Theatre
Organization Type: Performing; Educational

702   JANE FRANKLIN DANCE

3700 S Four Mile Run Drive
Arlington, VA 22206
Phone: 703-212-7680
Fax: 703-212-7680
e-mail: info@janefranklin.com
Web Site: www.janefranklin.com
Officers:
  Administrative Assistant: Carol Coteus
Management:
  Artistic Director: Jane Franklin
  Web Master: Michael Levy
Mission: Jane Franklin Dance is committed to the philosophy that dance can be a natural expression of ordinary experience. Emphasizing that dance arises from us all, Jane Franklin Dance aims to celebrate movement and make dance accessible to a wide range of audiences through community-based projects, educational outreach, collaborations with artists from other disciplines, and performance events.
Founded: 1995
Specialized Field: Dance
Status: Professional; Nonprofit
Paid Staff: 3
Organization Type: Performing; Touring; Educational

703   CONCERT BALLET OF VIRGINIA

11028 Leadbetter Road
Asheland, VA 23005
Phone: 804-798-0945
Officers:
  President: James St Germain
  VP: Pat Morris
  Public Relations: Jill Melichar
  Director: Robert Watkins
  Associate Director: Scott Boyer
  Executive Assistant: Thomas Rennie
  Technical Director: Deveaux Riddick
Mission: To provide a regular season of classical and contemporary innovative dance programming for the Richmond area along with statewide performances for the public as well as civic, educational and social organizations.
Founded: 1976
Specialized Field: Modern; Ballet; Jazz
Status: Non-Professional; Nonprofit; Commercial
Paid Staff: 15
Income Sources: Sacred Dance Guild
Performs At: The Woman's Club Auditorium; Blackwell Auditorium
Organization Type: Performing; Touring; Educational

704   BRISTOL BALLET COMPANY

628 Cumberland Street
Bristol, VA 24201
Phone: 276-669-6051
Fax: 276-669-9390
e-mail: bristoballet@hotmail.com
Management:
  Artistic Director: Mary Anne Snyder-Sowers
  Production Director: Nancy Peoples

Mission: To nurture, encourage and sustain community interest in the art of ballet; to make a contribution to the cultural progress and entertainment of the community and the larger Tri-cities Area.
Founded: 1959
Specialized Field: Ballet
Status: Nonprofit
Paid Staff: 15
Income Sources: Southeast Regional Ballet Association; Tennessee Arts Commission; Virginia Commission for the Arts
Performs At: Paramount Center
Organization Type: Performing

705 HAMPTON ROADS CIVIC BALLET

4607 Victoria Boulevard
Hampton, VA 23669
Phone: 757-722-8216
Officers:
   Director: Muriel Shelley Evans
Management:
   Ballet Mistress: Lisa Schultz
Mission: To provide live ballet performances at family prices; to provide performing experience for young dancers; to encourage young people to freely contribute to their community.
Founded: 1959
Specialized Field: Ballet
Status: Private; Nonprofit; Volunteer
Organization Type: Performing; Resident; Educational

706 COMMUNITY DANCE PROGRAM OF OLD DOMINION UNIVERSITY

Old Dominion University
Norfolk, VA 23529-0220
Phone: 757-683-5455
Fax: 757-683-4249
Management:
   Artistic Director: Istvan Ament

707 MALINI'S DANCES OF INDIA

1510 Bordeaux Place
Norfolk, VA 23509
Phone: 757-533-5594
Fax: 757-533-4616
e-mail: malinidance@hotmail.com
Web Site: www.arts.state.va.us
Officers:
   Artistic Director: Malini Srirama
   President: Vijaya Sarathy
Management:
   Artistic Director: Malini Sirama
Mission: To promote East Indian classical and folk dances through performances, lecture demonstrations, workshops and residencies.
Specialized Field: Ethnic
Status: Nonprofit
Paid Staff: 140
Organization Type: Performing; Touring; Resident; Educational; Sponsoring

708 VIRGINIA BALLET THEATRE

134 W Olney Road
Norfolk, VA 23510
Phone: 757-622-4822
Fax: 757-622-7904
e-mail: teric@virginiaballettheatre.com
Web Site: www.virginiaballettheatre.com
Management:
   Artistic Director: Frank Bove
   Artistic Director: Janina Bove
   Corporate Development: Teri Commander
Mission: Professional ballet dance theatre bringing dance and dance education to Hampton Roads and beyond.
Founded: 1961
Specialized Field: Ballet
Status: Non-Professional; Nonprofit
Paid Staff: 40
Volunteer Staff: 20
Organization Type: Performing; Resident

709 EZIBU MUNTU AFRICAN DANCE COMPANY

418 E Main Street
Richmond, VA 23201
Phone: 804-225-9209
e-mail: olaketu@aol.com
Officers:
   General Manager: Janine Bell
   Business Manager: C Rene Taylor
Management:
   Artistic Director: Faye Walker
   Drum Captain: Kurtne Patterson
Mission: A non-profit organization of educators, dancers, drummers, and other individuals dedicated to the promotion of knowledge and appreciation of African cultural values and artistic traditions.
Founded: 1973
Specialized Field: Ethnic; Folk
Status: Professional; Nonprofit
Organization Type: Performing; Touring; Educational

710 RICHMOND BALLET

407 E Canal Street
Richmond, VA 23219
Phone: 804-344-0906
Fax: 804-344-0901
e-mail: info@richmondballet.com
Web Site: www.richmondballet.com/main.asp
Officers:
   Chairman Faculty: Judy Jacob
Management:
   Artistic Director: Stoner Winslett
   Managing Director: Craig Margolis
   Managing Director: Ed Toch
   Media Relations Manager: Jennifer MacKenzie
Mission: To build an institution of integrity that addresses its community's needs, as well as its responsibilities to the art form; to provide the finest training to its dancers and students; and enhance the communty by providing significant education and outreach programs.
Founded: 1957
Specialized Field: Ballet
Status: Professional; Nonprofit
Budget: $2,500,000+

Organization Type: Performing; Touring; Resident; Educational

711 VIRGINIA COMMONWEALTH UNIVERSITY-DEPARTMENT OF DANCE & CHOREOGRAPHY

1315 Floyd Avenue
PO Box 843007
Richmond, VA 23284-7356
Phone: 804-828-1711
Fax: 804-828-7356
e-mail: mmcurtis@saturn.vcu.edu
Web Site: www.vcu.edu/artsweb/dance
Management:
   Chair: Martha Curtis
   Assistant Professor: Katrina South Clemans
Mission: VCU dance offers a vibrant, stimulating atmosphere where students are prepared for careers in the field of dance. VCU Dance also presents 3-6 professional companies each season.
Founded: 1981
Specialized Field: Dance, Choreography, Performance
Paid Staff: 6
Paid Artists: 24
Affiliations: NASD; CODA
Annual Attendance: 9,167
Facility Category: Theater
Seating Capacity: 225
Year Built: 1934
Year Remodeled: 1996
Rental Contact: Grace Street Theater House Manager Cynthia Theakston

712 MUSIC IN MOTION ACADEMY OF DANCE

629 N Lynnhaven Road
Virginia Beach, VA 23452-5831
Phone: 757-340-1534
Fax: 757-467-3045
e-mail: dasdance@aol.com
Web Site: www.musicinmotion.com
Management:
   Artistic Director: Darlene Stephens

Washington

713 PENINSULA DANCE THEATRE

515 Chester Avenue
Bremerton, WA 98310
Phone: 360-377-6214
Web Site: www.orgsites.com/wa/pdt
Management:
   Artistic Director: Lawan Morrison
Mission: Peninsula Dance Theatre is a non-profit volunteer organization dedicated to bringing all dance forms to the Kitsap Peninsula. Company members have professional instruction opportunities and scholarship opportunites to advance in their art. We accomplish this by providing guest instructors/choreographers and performance opportunites with three shows a year.
Specialized Field: Ballet
Status: Professional; Nonprofit

Performs At: Win Graulund Performing Arts Center
Organization Type: Performing; Resident

714 OLYMPIC BALLET THEATRE
Olympic Ballet School

700 Main Street
Anderson Cultural Center
Edmonds, WA 98020
Phone: 425-774-7570
Fax: 425-672-1152
e-mail: obt@eskimo.com
Web Site: www.olyballet.com/Theatre.htm
Management:
   Artistic Director: John Wilkins
   Artistic Director: Helen Wilkins
Mission: Dedicated to creating high-quality dance and providing training and performance opportunities for pre-professional dancers.
Founded: 1981
Specialized Field: Ballet
Status: Semi-Professional; Nonprofit
Paid Staff: 21
Budget: $200,000-$500,000
Income Sources: Pacific Regional Ballet Association
Organization Type: Resident

715 ARIA DANCE COMPANY

33631 9th Avenue S
Federal Way, WA
Phone: 253-924-0621
e-mail: info@intodance.com
Web Site: www.lassair.com
Officers:
   Executive Director: Ludwig Suju
Management:
   Artistic Director: Christina Vandenberg-Suju
   Event Coordinator: Cindy Mazzeo
Mission: Dedicated to helping dancers achieve self-discipline and artistic expression through dance. Also explores Modern, Jazz, Folk and Character dancing.
Specialized Field: Ballet
Status: Nonprofit

716 MEANY THEATRE

University of Washington
4001 University Way NE, Box 351150
Seattle, WA 98195
Phone: 206-543-4882
Fax: 206-685-2759
Web Site: www.meany.org
Officers:
   Chairman: Dr Buster Alvord
Management:
   Director: Matthew Krashan
   Director Business/Finance: Gayle Williams
   Director Development: John Idstrom
   Director Marketing: Jan Steadman
Specialized Field: Ballet; World Music & Dance; Classical Music
Status: Nonprofit
Paid Artists: 30
Income Sources: University of Washington
Performs At: Meany Hall
Organization Type: Sponsoring; Presenting

717 OCHEAMI
PO Box 31635
Seattle, WA 98103-1635
Phone: 206-329-8876
e-mail: ocheami@earthlink.net
Officers:
   Manager: Amma Anang
Management:
   Artistic Director: Kofi Anang
Mission: OCHEAMI is a group of artists whose common goal is the expression of the culture of West Africa through music and dance. The individuals represent a broad and diverse background: the diaspora, or growth and expansion, of Africa's influence in the realm of music and dance throughout the world; as well as the European, Caribbean, West Indian, South American and North American influence on music.
Founded: 1978
Specialized Field: Arts; Dance; Heritage/Historica; Multi-Discipline; Music
Status: Professional; Nonprofit
Organization Type: Performing; Touring; Educational

718 PACIFIC NORTHWEST BALLET
301 Mercer Street
Seattle, WA 98109
Phone: 206-441-9411
Fax: 206-441-2440
e-mail: marketing@pnb.org
Web Site: www.pnb.org
Officers:
   Executive Director: D David Brown
   Company Manager: Dwight Huttonn
Management:
   Artistic Director: Kent Stowell
   Artistic Director: Francia Russell
   Music Director/Conductor: Stewart Kershaw
   Associate Conductor/Company Pianist: Allan Dameron
Mission: Dedicated to maintaining a professional ballet company and school.
Founded: 1972
Specialized Field: Ballet
Status: Professional; Nonprofit
Budget: $12,000,000
Income Sources: Dance USA; American Arts Alliance; Washington State Arts Alliance
Organization Type: Performing; Touring; Resident

719 PAT GRANEY COMPANY
PO Box 20009
Seattle, WA 98102-1009
Phone: 206-329-3705
Fax: 206-329-3730
e-mail: biggirls@patgraney.org
Web Site: www.patgraney.org
Management:
   Artistic Director: Pat Graney
   Managing Director: Erin Nestor
Mission: To create, perform, and produce new dance and performance works. Pat Graney's work is distinctive in its diversity of style and character by integrating contemporary dance with other American movement forms.

Founded: 1990
Specialized Field: Dance
Status: Nonprofit
Paid Staff: 4
Volunteer Staff: 30
Paid Artists: 10
Budget: $200,000-$500,000
Income Sources: Individual Donors; Foundations; Corporate Grants

720 RADOST FOLK ENSEMBLE
PO Box 31295
Seattle, WA 98103
Phone: 206-860-5251
e-mail: admin@radost.org
Web Site: www.radost.org
Officers:
   Board President: Linda Folkers
Management:
   Artistic Director: Sidney Deering
   Artistic Director: Sarah Nofziger
Mission: To preserve the dance, music, and folklore of Eastern Europe through outstanding concert performances, development of authentic repertoire and stage choregoraphies, regular dance classes for children, and educational residencies in local s
Founded: 1976
Specialized Field: Ethnic Eastern Europe Dance and Music
Status: Semi-Professional; Nonprofit
Paid Staff: 1
Volunteer Staff: 4
Paid Artists: 8
Non-paid Artists: 12
Budget: $20,000
Income Sources: Touring Concerts; Teaching; Grants; Private Donations
Organization Type: Performing; Touring; Educational; Sponsoring

721 WORLD SERIES
University of Washington
Meany Hall
Seattle, WA 98195
Mailing Address: PO Box 351150
Phone: 206-543-4882
Fax: 206-685-2759
Web Site: meany.org
Management:
   Director: Matt Krashan
   Director Marketing/Public Relations: Jan Steadman
Mission: Committed to bringing world-class performers to the Seattle community via the University of Washington.
Specialized Field: Modern; Ballet; Jazz; Ethnic; World Music, Piano Recital, Chamber Music.
Status: Professional; Nonprofit
Paid Staff: 6
Paid Artists: 25
Performs At: Meany Theater
Organization Type: Performing; Touring; Educational

722 PERFORMING COMPANY OF PIONEER DANCE ARTS
172 Bell Meadow Lane
Sequim, WA 98382
Phone: 360-683-3693
Officers:
Director: Kathleen H Moore
Secretary: Gloria Price
Treasurer: Judy Lynn
Mission: Committed to raising dance-art awareness in the North Olympic Peninsula.
Founded: 1976
Specialized Field: Modern; Ballet; Jazz; Ethnic; Tap
Status: Non-Professional; Nonprofit
Paid Staff: 100
Performs At: Port Angeles High School Auditorium
Organization Type: Performing; Resident; Educational; Sponsoring

723 FILIPINIANA ARTS AND CULTURAL CENTER
569 N 166th Street
Shoreline, WA 98133
Phone: 206-542-7245
e-mail: rogerdelrosario@hotmail.com
Web Site: www.homestead.com/FDC_WA
Officers:
Director: Roger R DelRosario
Management:
Director: Roger R DelRosario
Mission: The Filipiniana Dance Company presents rich pageantry, elegant costumes, energetic music and graceful dances in a tapestry of Filipino folklore. Students will learn of the various cultural influences in this small country, and learn to apply this to their own communities.
Founded: 1970
Specialized Field: Ethnic
Status: Semi-Professional; Nonprofit
Volunteer Staff: 50
Non-paid Artists: 50
Budget: $25,000
Income Sources: Exhibits
Annual Attendance: 10,000
Organization Type: Performing; Touring; Resident; Educational; Sponsoring

724 TACOMA CITY BALLET
508 6th Avenue
Tacoma, WA 98402
Phone: 253-272-4219
Fax: 253-272-4219
Officers:
Chairman: John Hodder
Management:
Executive Director: Nikki Smith
Mission: To provide quality, fully-staged classical ballets for the Southern Puget Sound area.
Founded: 1955
Specialized Field: Ballet
Status: Semi-Professional
Paid Staff: 20
Income Sources: National Association for Regional Ballet; Pacific Regional Ballet Association
Performs At: Pantages Theater

Organization Type: Performing

725 TACOMA PERFORMING DANCE COMPANY
2315 6th Avenue
Tacoma, WA 98403
Phone: 253-627-8272
Officers:
Director: Jo Emery
Founded: 1967
Specialized Field: Modern; Ballet; Jazz
Status: Semi-Professional; Nonprofit
Performs At: Pantages Centre
Organization Type: Performing; Touring; Resident

West Virginia

726 CHARLESTON BALLET
822 Virginia Street E
Charleston, WV 25301
Phone: 304-342-6541
Fax: 304-345-1134
e-mail: chballet@newwave.net
Web Site: www.thecharlestonballet.com
Officers:
President: Michael Tassos
VP: Jennifer Goddard
Secretary: Milton Koslow
Treasurer: Colleen Reed
Management:
Artistic Director: Kim R Pauley
Office Manager: Elaine Baldwin
Mission: To present ballet concerts for professional and talented young dancers.
Founded: 1956
Specialized Field: Modern; Ballet; Folk
Status: Semi-Professional; Nonprofit
Paid Staff: 3
Volunteer Staff: 20
Paid Artists: 20
Non-paid Artists: 20
Organization Type: Performing; Touring

727 MID OHIO VALLEY BALLET COMPANY
PO Box 4204
1311 Ann Street
Parkersburg, WV 26104
Phone: 304-422-5538
Fax: 304-422-6730
e-mail: info@artswindow.org
Web Site: www.artswindow.org/movbal/movbmain.htm
Management:
Artistic Director: Norma Gunter
Budget: $1,000,000-$2,500,000

728 PARKERSBURG WHEELING BALLET COMPANY
PO Box 4204
Parkersburg, WV 26104
Phone: 304-422-5538
Toll-free: 800-882-1148
e-mail: info@artswindow.org

Officers:
President: Tom Wiseman
VP: D Dix
Secretary: S LeMasters
Treasurer: S. Stout
Management:
Artistic Director: N Gunter
Director: Suzy Gunter
Marketing Director: D Dix
Development Director: T Forster
Founded: 1981
Specialized Field: Ballet
Status: Professional; Nonprofit
Paid Staff: 40
Organization Type: Performing; Touring; Educational; Sponsoring

729 APPALACHIAN YOUTH JAZZ-BALLET COMPANY
605 D Street
South Charleston, WV 25303
Phone: 304-343-1076
Toll-free: 800-409-4646
Officers:
President: Ricklin Brown
VP: John Breed
Secretary: Catherine Halloran
Treasurer: Carol Velasquez
Management:
Artistic Director: Nina Denton
Mission: To provide talented aspiring dancers liaisons between the classroom and the professional stage; to enrich the community through concerts and lecture demonstrations; to provide inspiration to youngsters in the audience.
Founded: 1982
Specialized Field: Ballet; Jazz
Status: Nonprofit
Paid Staff: 2
Income Sources: Washington Community Education
Performs At: Charleston Civic Center; Municipal Auditorium
Organization Type: Performing; Touring; Educational

Wisconsin

730 LYNN DANCE COMPANY
W 8555 Deertail Road
Ladysmith, WI 54848
Phone: 715-532-6863
e-mail: taralynn@taralynnsdanceco.8m.com
Web Site: www.taralynnsdanceco.8m.com
Mission: To maintain the Chalicestream Dance Center for dance performance and teaching.
Founded: 1976
Specialized Field: Modern
Status: Professional
Performs At: Chalicestream Dance Center
Organization Type: Performing; Resident; Educational

731 KANOPY DANCE THEATRE
133 W Johnson Street
Madison, WI 53703
Phone: 608-255-2211
Officers:
President: Deirdre Wilson Garton
Secretary: David Egger
Treasurer: Colin Jefcoate
Management:
Associate Director: Robert E Cleary
Artistic Director: Lisa Andrea Thurell
General Clerical: Mary Beth Heydt
Mission: To maintain a full-time dance company and teaching studio, present concerts, conduct residencies and teach classes.
Founded: 1978
Specialized Field: Modern; Jazz
Status: Professional
Income Sources: Wisconsin Dance Council
Performs At: Kanopy Studio; Wisconsin Union Theatre
Organization Type: Performing; Touring; Resident; Educational; Sponsoring

732 MADISON SCOTTISH COUNTRY DANCERS
4206 Doncaster Drive
Madison, WI 53711
Phone: 608-274-0127
e-mail: crbuelow@facstaff.wisc.edu
Web Site: www.sprott.physics.wisc.edu/mscd/home.htm
Officers:
Chairperson: Priscilla Arsove
Chair: Nancy McClements
Treasurer: Scott Weiss
Secretary: Carol Buelow
Management:
Teacher: Norma Briggs
Teacher: Chuck Snowdon
Mission: To perform, teach, and promote Scottish country dancing and its music.
Founded: 1977
Specialized Field: Ethnic
Status: Non-Professional; Nonprofit
Paid Staff: 60
Income Sources: Royal Scottish Country Dance Society (Scotland)
Performs At: University of Wisconsin; Memorial Union
Organization Type: Performing; Educational

733 MELROSE MOTION COMPANY
1050 University Avenue
Madison, WI 53706
Phone: 608-262-1641
Fax: 608-265-3841
Management:
Director: Claudia Melrose
Assistant: Tim Glenn
Mission: To present works by Claudia Melrose and selected guest artists; to create and maintain high standards for dance in the Midwest; to educate and build audiences; to create a strong reputation for dance in the Midwest; to bring quality modern dance to the largest public eye possible.
Founded: 1985

Specialized Field: Modern
Status: Professional; Nonprofit
Paid Staff: 1
Income Sources: University of Wisconsin-Madison
Organization Type: Performing; Touring

734 MM COLBERT
1321 E Johnson Street
Madison, WI 53703
Phone: 608-257-9807
Officers:
   Chairperson: Nancy Idaka Sheran
Management:
   Director/Choreographer: MM Colbert
Mission: To present original modern ballets in collaboration with other living artists.
Founded: 1980
Specialized Field: Modern; Ballet; Jazz
Status: Nonprofit
Organization Type: Performing

735 TAPIT/NEW WORKS
1957 Winnebago Street
Madison, WI 53704
Phone: 608-244-2938
Fax: 608-244-9114
e-mail: tapit@mailbag.com
Web Site: www.tapitnewworks.org
Officers:
   VP: Bobbie Toney
   President: Mary Beth Gaffney
   Treasurer: Larry Lundy
   Secretary: Paul Neary
Management:
   Business Manager: Etta Gasport
   Associate Artistic Director: Danielle Dresden
   Associate Artistic Director: Donna Peckett
Mission: TAPIT/new works creates and produces original performance works and develops and promotes the art of tap dance. Through performances and educational activities, TAPIT speaks to people of all ages and socio-economic backgrounds.
Founded: 1985
Paid Staff: 2
Budget: $50,000-$120,000
Income Sources: Public; private; fees; tickets

736 WILLOW: A DANCE CONCERN
122 State Street
Lower Level
Madison, WI 251-5233
Phone: 608-280-9601
Management:
   Director: Phyllis Sanfilippo
Mission: To promote dance as a performing art and form of personal expression.
Founded: 1975
Specialized Field: Modern
Status: Nonprofit
Paid Staff: 5
Organization Type: Performing

737 MESOGHIOS DANCE TROUP
3813 S Meadow Drive
Middleton, WI 53562
Phone: 608-831-4485
Officers:
   President: Craig Schreiner
   President: Vicky Knoedler
   Secretary/Treasurer: William Knoedler
Management:
   Artistic Director: Vicky Knoedler
Mission: To perform Greek, Turkish and Russian ethnic and folk dances; to present and describe Greek and Turkish ethnic dress, decoration and custom.
Founded: 1978
Specialized Field: Ethnic; Folk
Status: Semi-Professional; Nonprofit
Paid Staff: 15
Organization Type: Performing; Educational

738 BETTY SALAMUN'S DANCECIRCUS
PO Box 1642
Milwaukee, WI 532011642
Phone: 414-277-8151
Fax: 414-277-8152
e-mail: dancecir@execpc.com
Web Site: www.dancecircus.org
Management:
   Artistic Director: Betty Salamun
   Financial Manager: David HB Drake
Mission: To create original dance, music and collaborative performances.
Founded: 1975
Specialized Field: Modern; Dance Environment; Collaborations
Status: Professional; Nonprofit
Paid Staff: 2
Volunteer Staff: 10
Paid Artists: 5
Budget: $95,000
Income Sources: Fees; Foundations
Affiliations: Dance USA
Annual Attendance: 45,000-50,000
Organization Type: Performing; Touring; Educational

739 KO-THI DANCE COMPANY
342 N Water, 7th Floor
PO Box 1093
Milwaukee, WI 53201-1093
Phone: 414-273-0676
Fax: 414-273-0727
e-mail: kkothi@aol.com
Web Site: www.ko-thi.org
Management:
   Chief Officer: Ferne Caulker
   Managing Director: Lydia LaGue
Mission: To promulgate and preserve the African, African-American, and Caribbean art forms.
Founded: 1969
Budget: $500,000-$1,000,000

740 MILWAUKEE BALLET
504 W National Avenue
Milwaukee, WI 53204

Phone: 414-643-7677
Fax: 414-649-4066
e-mail: 2thepointe@milwaukeeballet.org
Web Site: www.milwaukeeballet.org
Officers:
    CEO: Christine Harris
Management:
    Artistic Director: Simon Dow
    Ballet Mistress: Fiona Fuerstner
    Resident Conductor: Jamin Hoffman
Mission: To reveal this secret to those who will be entertained, moved and inspired by the beauty of the art form.
Founded: 1970
Specialized Field: Ballet
Status: Professional; Nonprofit
Budget: $4,800,000
Income Sources: Corporate/individual donation
Performs At: Uihlein Hall; Milwaukee Performing Arts Center
Organization Type: Performing; Touring; Resident; Educational

741   WILD SPACE DANCE COMPANY

PO Box 511665
820 E Knapp Street
Milwaukee, WI 53203
Phone: 414-271-0307
Fax: 414-271-6087
Management:
    Artistic Director: Debra Loewen
    Managing Director: Sheri Urban
Mission: Emphasizing the development of new movement styles, improvisation, original choreography, and highly theatrical dance events.
Founded: 1986
Specialized Field: Contemporary Dance
Status: Nonprofit
Paid Staff: 2
Paid Artists: 7

742   DANCE WISCONSIN

6332 Monona Drive
Monona, WI 53716
Phone: 608-221-4535
Fax: 608-221-9632
e-mail: DanceWI@mail.com
Web Site: www.dancewisconsin.com
Management:
    Artistic Director: Jo Jean Retrum
Mission: To promote and foster dance in Wisconsin and develop appreciation of the arts including dance, music and theatre by creating productions of the highest caliber geared towards entertaining, educating and enriching our diversified audience; to reach out to the community through demonstrations, special discounted shows and Dance in the Schools programs.
Founded: 1977
Specialized Field: Ballet
Status: Semi-Professional; Nonprofit
Volunteer Staff: 6
Paid Artists: 4
Non-paid Artists: 20
Budget: $100,000
Income Sources: Regional Dance America

Performs At: Madison Civic Center; Wisconsin Union Theatre; Milby Theatre
Seating Capacity: 2,000
Organization Type: Performing; Resident; Educational

743   LI CHIAO-PING DANCE

5973 Purcell Road
Oregon, WI 53575
Phone: 608-835-6590
Fax: 608-835-6592
e-mail: chiao-ping@education.wisc.edu
Web Site: www.lichinopingdance.org
Management:
    Projects Assistant: Dave Pansch
    Artistic Director: Li Chiao-Ping
Founded: 1990
Specialized Field: Dance
Paid Staff: 1
Volunteer Staff: 9
Paid Artists: 10
Budget: $80 k
Income Sources: Grants; Fees; Ticket Revenue

Alabama

744 ALABAMA SYMPHONY ORCHESTRA
3621 6th Avenue S
Birmingham, AL 35222
Phone: 205-251-6929
Fax: 205-251-6840
e-mail: orchestra@alabamasymphony.com
Web Site: www.alabamasymphony.org
Officers:
   President: Gloria N Moody
   Vice Chairman: H Corbin Day
Management:
   Executive Director: Kathy Yarbrough
   Music Director: Richard Westerfield
   Associate Conductor: Chris Confessore
   General Manager: Tim P Young
   Director Development: Nancy Caremichael
   Director Marketing/Public Relations: Pamela
   Satterfield
   Director Finance: Susan Trachtman
Mission: The Alabama Symphony Orchestra exists to
serve the citizens of Alabama by performing great music
and enriching lives through music. Strives to be a fine
regional orchestra that produces symphonic music of the
highest quality and provides outstanding outreach and
educational programs while maintaining its fiscal
strength.
Founded: 1933
Specialized Field: Symphony; Orchestra
Status: Nonprofit
Paid Staff: 20
Volunteer Staff: 610
Paid Artists: 54
Budget: $6 million
Income Sources: Box Office; Grants; Corporate and
Private Donations; Sponsorshipsans
Performs At: Alys Stephens Center; Performing Arts
Center
Affiliations: American Symphony Orchestra League;
American Federation of Musicians
Annual Attendance: 100,000+
Type of Stage: Proscenium
Stage Dimensions: 60x50
Seating Capacity: 1,300
Year Built: 1996
Rental Contact: Dan Gaincy
Organization Type: Performing

**745 RED MOUNTAIN CHAMBER
ORCHESTRA**
868 6th Street W
Birmingham, AL 35204
Phone: 205-714-8300
Fax: 205-251-9541
e-mail: sbeaudry@asfa.k12.al.us
Web Site: www.bham.net//rmco
Management:
   Manager/President: Suzanne Beaudry
   Artistic Consultant: Leslie Fillmer
   Consultant: Oliver Roosevelt
Mission: To educate and give pleasure to the public by
performing music not otherwise heard in Birmingham and
provide a musical outlet for players, conductors, and
soloists in the community.

Founded: 1981
Specialized Field: Instrumental Music; Classical
Orchestra Repertore
Budget: $35,000
Income Sources: State and Local Grants; Private Donors
Performs At: Colleges; Churches; Birmingham Museum
of Art
Affiliations: Birmingham Southern College
Annual Attendance: 1,200
Facility Category: Concert Hall
Type of Stage: Small Performance Space
Seating Capacity: 300

746 GADSDEN SYMPHONY ORCHESTRA
PO Box 13
Gadsden, AL 35902
Phone: 256-442-1208
Fax: 256-442-5460
e-mail: crabby@tds.net
Management:
   General Manager & Artistic Dir: Claudia Shelton
Founded: 1991
Specialized Field: Northeast Alabama
Volunteer Staff: 20
Budget: $35,000-$45,000
Income Sources: Local Contributions; Grants
Affiliations: American Symphony Orchestra League
Annual Attendance: 1,100
Facility Category: Concert Hall; Outdoor Ampitheatre
Seating Capacity: 800
Year Built: 1960
Year Remodeled: 1999

747 HUNTSVILLE CHAMBER MUSIC GUILD
UAH Library 333
301 Sparkman Drive NW
Huntsville, AL 35899
Phone: 256-824-6540
Fax: 256-824-6083
Web Site: www.hcmgeoncerts.uah.edu
Officers:
   President: Dr. Wilson Luquire
   VP: Chris McGraw
   Secretary: Ron Roberts
   Treasurer: David Brown
Mission: Dedicated to presenting established and rising
talents in chamber music.
Founded: 1953
Performs At: Roberts Recital Hall-University of
Alabama

**748 HUNTSVILLE SYMPHONY
ORCHESTRA**
PO Box 2400
Huntsville, AL 35804
Phone: 205-539-4818
Fax: 205-539-4819
e-mail: hso@ro.com
Web Site: www.hso.org
Management:
   Executive Director: David Todd
   Music Director: Taavo Virkhaus
   Symphony School Director: Evelyn Loehrlein

Mission: To serve the community as an aid to industrial development. The type industries for which Huntsville is known has brought an influx of people who are accustomed to the best in terms of their leisure time activities, and the Huntsville Symphony provides the quality of performances that these individuals demand.
Founded: 1954
Specialized Field: Symphony
Status: Non-Professional; Nonprofit; Commercial
Paid Staff: 75
Budget: $1,050,000-$3,600,000
Income Sources: American Symphony Orchestra League
Performs At: Von Braun Civic Center - Concert Hall
Organization Type: Performing; Educational; Sponsoring

749 HUNTSVILLE YOUTH ORCHESTRA

6806 Whitesburg Drive S
Huntsville, AL 35802
Phone: 256-880-0622
e-mail: hyo@traveller.com
Web Site: http://home.hiwaay.net
Officers:
 Administrative Director: Johnny Brewer
 Administrative Assistant: Kay Jones
Management:
 Music Director/Conductor: Gary Parks
Mission: To provide a rewarding and challenging experience for its members through performing good music; to awaken interest in symphonic literature in young people; to train those young people having outstanding talent.
Founded: 1962
Specialized Field: Orchestra; Chamber; Ensemble
Status: Non-Professional; Nonprofit
Paid Staff: 270
Income Sources: American Symphony Orchestra League (Youth Orchestra Division); Alabama Federation of Music; Alabama Arts Council
Performs At: Von Braun Civic Center
Organization Type: Performing; Touring; Educational; Sponsoring

750 MOBILE CHAMBER MUSIC SOCIETY

University of South Alabama Music Department
Laidlaw Performing Arts Center 1072
Mobile, AL 36688-0002
Phone: 251-460-6236
Fax: 334-460-7328
e-mail: music@mobilechambermusic.org
Web Site: www2.acan.net/~chambmus/
Management:
 Executive Director: Dr. Robert Wermuth
 Past President: Dan Silver
Mission: Present a six concert series
Founded: 1960
Volunteer Staff: 4

751 MOBILE SYMPHONY

257 Dauphin Street
Mobile, AL 36602

Phone: 251-432-2010
Fax: 251-432-6618
e-mail: mail@mobilesymphonyu.org
Web Site: www.mobilesymphony.org
Management:
 Executive Director: Christina Littlejohn
 Education Director: Sarah Wright
 Development Director: Amy Oliver
 Operations/Marketing Manager: David Hughes
 Administrative Assistant: Wanda Drews
Mission: Produce live symphonic music.
Founded: 1970
Paid Staff: 10
Paid Artists: 65
Budget: $260,000-1,050,000
Seating Capacity: 1,800

752 MONTGOMERY SYMPHONY ORCHESTRA

PO Box 1864
Montgomery, AL 36102
Phone: 334-240-4004
Fax: 334-240-4034
Management:
 Artistic Director: Thomas Hinds
 Manager: Helen Steineker
Mission: Dedicated to providing a symphony orchestra to the capital city.
Founded: 1976
Specialized Field: Symphony; Orchestra
Status: Semi-Professional; Volunteer
Non-paid Artists: 75
Income Sources: American Symphony Orchestra League
Performs At: Davis Theater for the Performing Arts
Seating Capacity: 1250
Organization Type: Performing; Educational

753 TUSCALOOSA SYMPHONY ORCHESTRA

614 Greensboro Avenue
Tuscaloosa, AL 35401
Mailing Address: PO Box 20001
Phone: 205-752-5515
Fax: 205-345-2787
Web Site: www.tsoonline.org
Management:
 Music Director & Conductor: Shinik Hahm
 Office Administrator: Kevin Hand
 Executive Director: Leslie Poss
Mission: To maintain an orchestra dedicated to superior performance and artistic innovation. The goal of the TSO is to expose the widest possible and most culturally diverse audiences to musical programs of the highest quality.
Founded: 1981
Paid Staff: 4
Volunteer Staff: 75
Paid Artists: 70
Budget: $260,000-1,050,000
Performs At: Moody Music Building; Concert Hall

Alaska

754 ANCHORAGE SYMPHONY ORCHESTRA

400 D Street
Suite 230
Anchorage, AK 99501
Phone: 907-274-8668
Fax: 907-272-7916
e-mail: aso@corecom.net
Web Site: www.anchoragesymphony.org
Officers:
  President: Robert Dickson
  President: Denis LeBlanc
  Secretary: AS Micky Becker
  Treasurer: Randy Pugh
  Legal Counsel: David Ruskin
  League President: Cheryll Boren Heinze
  ASOPA President: Martin Hoffer
Management:
  Executive Director: Sherri Reddick
  Music Director/Conductor: Randall Craig Fleischer
Mission: To enhance the quality of life by providing high-caliber orchestral music to an expanding audience.
Founded: 1946
Specialized Field: Symphony; Orchestra; Chamber; Ensemble
Status: Nonprofit
Budget: $900,000
Performs At: Alaska Center for the Performing Arts
Annual Attendance: 20,000
Seating Capacity: 200
Year Built: 1988
Organization Type: Performing; Educational

755 ANCHORAGE YOUTH SYMPHONY

PO Box 240541
Anchorage, AK 99524
Phone: 907-566-7297
Fax: 907-333-0576
e-mail: ancys@juno.com
Web Site: www.anchorageyouthsymphony.org
Officers:
  President: Terry Reeve
  Secretary: Gunnar Knapp
  Treasurer: Carolyn Smithhister
Management:
  Music Director/Conductor: Linn Weeda
  General Manager: Ron Flugum
Mission: Rehearsing and performing symphonic music of the masters; touring.
Founded: 1965
Specialized Field: Symphony; Orchestra
Status: Non-Professional; Nonprofit
Paid Staff: 2
Income Sources: American Symphony Orchestra League (Youth Orchestra Division)
Performs At: Alaska Center for the Performing Arts (three theatres)
Facility Category: Theatre
Seating Capacity: 750; 2,000; 300
Year Built: 1988
Cost: $87,000,000
Organization Type: Performing; Touring; Educational

756 FAIRBANKS SYMPHONY ASSOCIATION

PO Box 82104
Fairbanks, AK 99708
Phone: 907-479-3407
Fax: 907-474-6420
e-mail: fysymph2@uaf.edu
Web Site: www.fairbankssymphony.org
Officers:
  President: Mary Ann Borchert
  VP: Charles Davis, III
  Secretary: Ted Fathauer
  Treasurer: William Strauss
Management:
  Executive Director: Philip Koslow
  Librarian/Stage Manager: Lucas Clooten
  Operations Director: Rhonda Gilbertson
Mission: Supporting an active and vital symphony orchestra; promoting instrumental music in the schools, a youth orchestra program, orchestra village tours and other related events.
Founded: 1969
Specialized Field: Symphony; Orchestra; Chamber
Status: Nonprofit
Paid Staff: 4
Volunteer Staff: 100
Income Sources: American Symphony Orchestra League; Alaska Alliance on the Arts
Performs At: Charles W. Davis Concert Hall
Annual Attendance: 12,000
Seating Capacity: 1,000
Organization Type: Performing; Touting; Resident; Educational; Sponsoring
Resident Groups: Fairbanks Symphony Orchestra; Arctic Chamber Orchestra

757 RED HACKLE PIPE BAND

PO Box 82782
Fairbanks, AK 99708-2782
Phone: 907-479-5826
Fax: 907-474-6841
e-mail: fbrhb@mosquitonet.com
Web Site: www.mosquitonet.com/~fbrbh/
Management:
  Pipe Master: Bob White
  Assistant Pipe Master: Dennis Stephens
  Lead Drummer: Arthur L Robson
Mission: To present Scottish music (bagpipe) and Highland dance performances and instruction.
Founded: 1974
Specialized Field: Ethnic; Band
Status: Nonprofit
Paid Staff: 20
Organization Type: Performing; Educational

758 JOCELYN CLARK

1109 C Street
Juneau, AK 99801
Phone: 907-586-9601
e-mail: iiiz@jocelynclark.com
Web Site: jocelynclark.com
Management:
  USA Manager: Jocelyn Clark
  Dutch Manager: Makiko Goto
  German Manager: Il-Ryun Chung

Mission: Performance of new works for zheng, koto, kayagum, changgu, and quest artists.
Founded: 2001
Specialized Field: Chamber Music Ensemble

759 JUNEAU JAZZ AND CLASSICS

PO Box 22152
Juneau, AK 99802
Phone: 907-463-3378
Fax: 907-463-3378
e-mail: music@juneau.com
Web Site: www.jazzandclassics.org
Management:
  Music Director: Linda Rosenthal
  Executive Director: Pam Johansen
Mission: The presentation of an annual music festival in Juneau which features world-class jazz as well as classical artists.
Founded: 1987
Specialized Field: Instrumental; Jazz; Folk; Educational
Status: Professional; Nonprofit
Budget: $30,000-45,000
Season: May
Performs At: Juneau (Festival Site)
Seating Capacity: 1,000; 250; 250
Organization Type: Educational; Sponsoring

760 JUNEAU SYMPHONY

PO Box 21236
Juneau, AK 99802
Phone: 907-586-4676
Fax: 907-586-4676
e-mail: symphony@juneau.com
Web Site: www.juneau.com/symphony
Officers:
  President: Susan Burke
  VP: Lucy Merell
  Treasurer: Sharon Denton
  Secretary: Mary Ann Dlugosch
Management:
  Administrator: Jetta Whittaker
  Music Director: Kyle Wiley Pickett
  Concertmaster: Steve Tada
Budget: $35,000-100,000

Arizona

761 FLAGSTAFF SYMPHONY ORCHESTRA

PO Box 122
113-A E Aspen Avenue
Flagstaff, AZ 86002-0122
Phone: 928-774-5107
Fax: 928-774-5109
e-mail: symphony@flagstaff.az.us
Web Site: www.flagstaffsymphony.org
Management:
  Artistic Director: Randall Craig Fleischer
  Executive Director: Kathryn Joyce
  Marketing: Kathleen Seekatz
  Operations Manager: Karl Kein
Founded: 1949
Specialized Field: Symphony Orchestra
Paid Staff: 3

Volunteer Staff: 65
Paid Artists: 65
Budget: $260,000-1,050,000
Performs At: Ardrey Auditorium

762 MESA SYMPHONY ORCHESTRA

P0 Box 1308
Mesa, AZ 85211
Phone: 480-827-2143
Fax: 480-827-2070
e-mail: mesasymphony@earthlink.net
Web Site:
www.mesasymphonyorchestra.org/mesasymphony/
Management:
  Music Director/Conductor: Gordon J Johnson
  Executive Director: Kathryn Fellows
  Executive Assistant: Sandra Wallace
Paid Staff: 3
Volunteer Staff: 20
Paid Artists: 70
Budget: $150,000-260,000
Performs At: Chandler Central Arts
Annual Attendance: 60,000
Facility Category: 2 Halls, 1 Amphitheatre

763 PHOENIX CHAMBER MUSIC SOCIETY

Scottsdale Center for the Arts
PO Box 34235
Phoenix, AZ 85067
Phone: 602-252-0095
Management:
  Executive Director: Carol Olsen
Mission: To bring the world's finest chamber music ensembles to the Phoenix area.
Founded: 1959
Specialized Field: Chamber
Status: Nonprofit
Performs At: Scottsdale Center for the Arts
Organization Type: Sponsoring

764 PHOENIX SYMPHONY

455 N Third Street
Suite 390
Phoenix, AZ 85004
Phone: 602-495-1117
Fax: 602-253-1772
e-mail: info@phoenixsymphony.org
Web Site: www.phoenixsymphony.org
Officers:
  President: Willaim C Roche
  General Manager: Kendra Whitlock
  VP Development: Dale Hedding
  Marketing/Public Relations: Cyndi Suttle
  Chairman: Thomas MacGillivary
  Secretary: David Lindner
Management:
  Associate Conductor: Robert Moodyes
  Music Director: Hermann Michael
  Principal Pops Conductor: Doc Severinson
Mission: Establishing, maintaining and operating a symphonic performing group in the Phoenix metropolitan area; nurturing and promoting the knowledge and appreciation of music.
Founded: 1947

Specialized Field: Symphony; Orchestra; Chamber; Ensemble
Status: Professional; Nonprofit
Paid Artists: 75
Budget: $7,500,000
Performs At: Phoenix Symphony Hall; Orpheum Theatre; Sedona Cultural Park
Annual Attendance: 140,000
Facility Category: Symphony Hall
Seating Capacity: 2,500
Organization Type: Performing; Touring; Educational

765 YAVAPI SYMPHONY ASSOCIATION

288 N Alarcon Street
Prescott, AZ 86301
Phone: 928-776-4255
Officers:
CEO: Joan H Squires
Management:
Music Director: Hermann Michael
Mission: To offer an annual series featuring six to eight of the finest dance companies. Collaborates with Ballet Arizona, Arizona Opera, Arizona Theatre Company, Phoenix Bach Choir, Phoenix Boys Choir, Heard Museum and Arizona State University.
Founded: 1966
Specialized Field: Classics; Pops, Chamber Orchestra
Status: Nonprofit; Professional
Paid Artists: 75
Season: September-May
Performs At: Symphony Hall
Organization Type: Sponsoring; Performing; Touring

766 SCOTTSDALE SYMPHONY ORCHESTRA ASSOCIATION

3817 North Brown Avenue
PO Box 460
Scottsdale, AZ 85252
Phone: 480-945-8071
Fax: 480-946-8770
e-mail: sso@scotsymph.org
Web Site: www.scotsymph.org
Management:
Music Director: Irving A Fleming
Executive Director: Judith A Vagis
Founded: 1972
Budget: $150,000-260,000
Season: year round
Seating Capacity: 790

767 CHAMBER MUSIC SEDONA

PO Box 153
Sedona, AZ 86339-0153
Phone: 928-204-2415
Fax: 928-282-0893
e-mail: sedonacms@aol.com
Web Site: www.chambermusicsedona.org
Officers:
President: Jim Pease
Management:
Executive Director: Albert Harclerode
Founded: 1982
Budget: $200,000

Performs At: St. John Vianney Church; Museum of Northern Arizona
Affiliations: CMA, ACA
Annual Attendance: 4000
Seating Capacity: 250; 200

768 SEDONA JAZZ ON THE ROCKS

PO Box 889
Sedona, AZ 86339
Phone: 520-282-1985
Fax: 520-282-0590
Web Site: www.sedonajazz.com
Officers:
President: Gina Lohrey
Management:
Executive Director: Chris Irish
Mission: To preserve and promote jazz for the next generation.
Founded: 1982
Specialized Field: Jazz
Status: Nonprofit
Paid Staff: 3
Volunteer Staff: 200
Paid Artists: 50
Non-paid Artists: 4
Budget: $400,000
Income Sources: Box Office; Corporate Sponsors; Grants
Season: September
Performs At: Sedona Cultural Park (Festival Site)
Annual Attendance: 6,000
Facility Category: Various Venues
Seating Capacity: 200-4,500
Organization Type: Performing; Sponsoring

769 SUN CITIES CHAMBER MUSIC SOCIETY

10451 W Palmeras Drive
Suite 126-A
Sun City, AZ 85373-2044
Phone: 623-972-0478
Fax: 623-972-8815
e-mail: SCChmbrMusSoc@aol.com
Officers:
Artistic Adv Comittee Chair/2nd VP: Elsie Sterrenberg
Management:
Executive Director: Mona L Myhre
Mission: To present internationally acclaimed chamber music to the greater Phoenix area, providing a balance of established and emerging performers who are culturally diverse and, through school concerts and residencies, to foster lifelong appreciation of fine music.
Founded: 1976
Specialized Field: Chamber; Ensemble
Status: Nonprofit
Paid Staff: 1
Volunteer Staff: 12
Paid Artists: 6
Income Sources: NEA; Ariziona Commission on the Arts; WAA; Donors
Performs At: Bellevue Heights Church
Affiliations: CMA; WAA; Arizona Presenters Alliance
Annual Attendance: 3,500
Facility Category: Church

Stage Dimensions: 14'x75'
Seating Capacity: 575
Organization Type: Sponsoring

770 SYMPHONY OF THE WEST VALLEY
10451 Palemras Drive, Suite 210-N
Sun City, AZ pO box 14,
Phone: 623-972-4484
Fax: 623-972-4495
e-mail: symphonywestvalley@earthlink.net
Web Site: www.members.aol.com/scsywu/6.html
Officers:
   President: James Lapslay
Management:
   Music Director/Conductor: James Yestadt
   Executive Director: Richard Shelton
   Director of Development: Lisa Caldarella
Founded: 1968
Paid Staff: 4
Budget: $260,000-1,050,000
Income Sources: Individual Contributions; Corporate
Contributions; Grants
Performs At: Sundome Center for the Performing Arts;
Arizona State University West

771 ARIZONA STATE UNIVERSITY SYMPHONY ORCHESTRA & CHAMBER ORCHESTRA
Arizona State Unviersity
School of Music
Tempe, AZ 85287-0405
Phone: 480-965-3430
Fax: 480-965-2659
e-mail: Timothy.Russell@asu.edu
Web Site: www.music.asu.edu
Management:
   Manager/Conductor: Timothy Russell
Budget: $100,000-150,000
Performs At: Grady Gammage Auditorium
Annual Attendance: 15,000
Facility Category: Auditorium
Seating Capacity: 3000
Year Built: 1963

772 EASTERN ARIZONA COLLEGE-COMMUNITY ORCHESTRA
600 Church Street
Thatcher, AZ 85552
Phone: 520-428-8467
Fax: 520-428-8462
Management:
   Manager/Music Director: Trish Jordahl
Budget: $35,000

773 ARIZONA EARLY MUSIC SOCIETY
2937 E Beverly Drive
Tucson, AZ 85716
Phone: 520-889-4310
Fax: 520-722-8738
e-mail: aems@azearlymusic.org
Web Site: www.azearlymusic.org
Officers:
   Co-President: Jeffri Sanders

Co-President: Marth Salzman
Mission: Dedicated to the enrichment of contemporary
life with the music of the past.
Founded: 1982
Specialized Field: Medieval, Renaissance and Baroque
music
Budget: $10,000-20,000
Performs At: St. Philip's in the Hills Episcopal Church
Seating Capacity: 500

774 ARIZONA FRIENDS OF CHAMBER MUSIC
PO Box 40802
Tucson, AZ 85717
Phone: 520-577-3769
Fax: 520-881-2009
e-mail: friends@arizonachambermusic.org
Web Site: www.arizonachambermusic.org
Officers:
   President: Dr. Jean-Paul Bierny
Mission: Presenters of chamber music concerts.
Founded: 1947
Specialized Field: Chamber music
Paid Staff: 1/2
Volunteer Staff: 15
Paid Artists: 50
Budget: $200,000
Income Sources: Audience, Businesses, ACA, Pima
County
Performs At: Auditorium
Annual Attendance: 8,400
Facility Category: Theatre; Concert Hall
Type of Stage: thrust
Stage Dimensions: 9'x 24'
Seating Capacity: 550
Year Built: 1970

775 CATALINA CHAMBER ORCHESTRA
3924 W Ina Road, Suite 306
PO Box 64831
Tucson, AZ 85741
Phone: 520-624-0170
Fax: 520-624-0170
e-mail: info@catalinachamber.org
Web Site: www.catalinachamber.org
Management:
   Music Director: Enrique Lasansky
   Marketing: Ed Gabel
Mission: Dedicated to performing the rich and varied
repertoire for small orchestras which spans more than four
centuries.
Founded: 1991
Budget: $35,000-$100,000
Performs At: Berger Performing Arts Center

776 CIVIC ORCHESTRA OF TUCSON
PO Box 42764
Tucson, AZ 85733-2764
Phone: 612-798-0062
e-mail: civicorchestra@att.net
Web Site: www.civicorchestrampls.org
Officers:
   Co-President: Amy Crockett
   Co-President: Elizabeth Glidden

VP: Laurie Olmstead
Secretary: Faye Propsom
Treasurer: Barb Niles
President: Mary Crippen
Management:
Artistic Director: Dr. Hersel Kreloff
General Manager: Lee Oler
Music Director: Cary John Franklin
Budget: $35,000

777 PHILHARMONIA ORCHESTRA OF TUCSON
PO Box 41882
Tucson, AZ 85717-1882
Phone: 520-326-2793
Fax: 520-623-1500
e-mail: info@tpyo.org
Management:
Music Director: Suzette Battan
Mission: To provide the finest quality symphonic training and performance opportunities for young musicians in a professional environment that promotes advanced musical education, performance competition and responsibility through the presentation of high-quality symphonic concerts to the general public.
Specialized Field: Youth Symphony

778 SOUTHERN ARIZONA SYMPHONY ORCHESTRA
PO Box 43131
Tucson, AZ 85733
Phone: 520-323-7166
Web Site: www.zerogee.com/saso/home.html
Officers:
President/General Manager: Samuel R Kreiling
Management:
Music Director: Warren Cohen
Budget: $35,000
Seating Capacity: 60

779 TUCSON JAZZ SOCIETY
PO Box 1069
Tucson, AZ 85702-1069
Phone: 520-903-1265
Fax: 520-903-1266
e-mail: tjsmail@tucsonjazz.org
Web Site: www.tucsonjazz.org/
Officers:
Executive Director: Sandra Schuldmann
Management:
Volunterr Corrdinator: Gloria Butler
Teachnical Director: Ben Nead
Mission: To promote and present jazz.
Founded: 1977
Status: Professional; Nonprofit
Income Sources: National Jazz Service Organization; International Association of Jazz Educators
Organization Type: Sponsoring

780 TUCSON PHILHARMONIA YOUTH ORCHESTRA
PO Box 41882
Tucson, AZ 85717

Phone: 520-623-1500
e-mail: info@tpyo.org
Web Site: www.tpyo.org
Status: Nonprofit

781 TUCSON SYMPHONY ORCHESTRA
2175 N 6th Avenue
Tucson, AZ 85705
Phone: 520-792-9155
Fax: 520-792-9314
e-mail: admin@tucsonsymphony.org
Web Site: www.tucsonsymphony.org
Management:
Music Director/Conductor: George Hanson
Executive Director: Susan Franano
Founded: 1929
Paid Staff: 30
Paid Artists: 85
Budget: $4,098,500
Performs At: Tucson Convention Center Music Hall
Affiliations: ASOL, BMI, ASCAP
Facility Category: Music hall
Seating Capacity: 2,217

782 TUCSON WINTER CHAMBER MUSIC FESTIVAL
6429 E Calle de San Alberto
Tucson, AZ 85710-2115
Phone: 520-577-3769
Fax: 520-881-2009
e-mail: friends@arizonachambermusic.org
Web Site: www.arizonachambermusic.org/
Management:
Artistic Director: Peter Rejto
Executive Director: Dr. Jean Paul Bierny
Founded: 1948
Specialized Field: Instrumental
Volunteer Staff: 15
Paid Artists: 20
Budget: $60,000-$150,000
Season: February - March
Affiliations: Leo Rich Theatre; Tucson Convention Center
Seating Capacity: 550

Arkansas

783 ARKANSAS STATE UNIVERSITY AT BEEBE
ASU-Beebe
PO Box 1000
Beebe, AR 72012
Phone: 501-882-8324
Fax: 501-882-8324
Toll-free: 800-632-9985
e-mail: tdavis@asub.arknet.edu
Web Site: www.asub.edu
Officers:
Chair of Concert/Lecture Committee: Teddy Davis
Mission: The purpose of this institution is to provide high quality, affordable instruction and service programs.

784 SOUTH ARKANSAS SYMPHONY
315 E Oak
Suite 206
El Dorado, AR 71730
Phone: 870-862-0521
Fax: 870-862-0521
Toll-free: 800-792-0521
e-mail: sasomail@cox-internet.com
Management:
 Music/Executive Director: Kermit Poling
 Manager: Virginia Matthews
Mission: To promote symphonic music to the area and to introduce this music to children.
Founded: 1956
Specialized Field: El Dorado. Magnolic and Camden
Paid Staff: 2
Volunteer Staff: 23
Paid Artists: 50
Budget: $100,000-$150,000
Performs At: Municipal Auditorium; Harton Theatre

785 SYMPHONY SOCIETY OF NORTH ARKANSAS
123 A N Block
PO Box 1243
Fayetteville, AR 72701
Phone: 501-521-4166
Fax: 501-582-4252
Management:
 Executive Director: Alan Burdick
Mission: To provide four communities in Northwest Arkansas with classical, pops and educational concerts.
Founded: 1954
Specialized Field: Symphony; Orchestra
Status: Semi-Professional; Nonprofit
Paid Staff: 6
Income Sources: University of Arkansas
Performs At: Walton Arts Center
Organization Type: Performing; Educational

786 FORT SMITH SYMPHONY
405 Central Mall
PO Box 3151
Fort Smith, AR 72913
Phone: 501-452-7575
Fax: 501-452-8985
e-mail: FSSSymphony@aol.com
Web Site: www.fssymphony.org
Officers:
 President: Mark Rumsey
Management:
 Director: John Jeter
 Executive Director: Jerry Huff
 Director Finance/Administrative: Teri Ihrig
 Marketing Coordinator: Becky Yates
Mission: Dedicated to providing our community with excellent orchestral programs which entertain, educate and enhance the quality of life.
Founded: 1923
Paid Staff: 5
Volunteer Staff: 60
Paid Artists: 70
Budget: $260,000-$1,050,000
Performs At: Fort Smith Civic Center

Facility Category: Performing Arts Center
Seating Capacity: 1,400
Year Remodeled: 2000
Organization Type: Performing

787 HOT SPRINGS MUSIC FESTIVAL SYMPHONY ORCHESTRA
634 Prospect Avenue
Hot Springs, AR 71901-3918
Phone: 501-623-4763
Fax: 501-624-6440
e-mail: hsmusfest@prodig.com
Web Site: www.hotmusic.org
Management:
 Artistic Director: Richard Rosenberg
 Executive Director: Laura S Rosenberg

788 FOUNDATION OF ARTS
115 W Monroe
PO Box 310
Jonesboro, AR 72403-0310
Phone: 870-935-2726
Fax: 870-933-9505
e-mail: foa@insolwwb.net
Web Site: www.insolwwb.net/-foa
Officers:
 Executive Director: Sherri Greuel
 Marketing Director/Box Office: Danita Martin
 Education Director: Lara Shelton
 Technical Director: Brett Kellett
Management:
 Music Director: Dr. Neale King Bartee
 Executive Director: Margaret Peacock
 Education Director: Lara Shelton
 Marketing/Box Office: Danita Martin-Wilkins
Mission: Education, Community Theatre Workshops, Guest Directors, etc. to conduct workshops. Emphasis on youth, but offered to all ages.
Founded: 1978
Paid Staff: 5
Budget: $35,000-$100,000
Income Sources: Box Office, Grants, Private Donation, Class Tuition
Annual Attendance: 25,000
Facility Category: Theatre
Type of Stage: Proscenium
Seating Capacity: 670
Year Built: 1940
Year Remodeled: 2000
Rental Contact: Executive Director Sherri Greuel
Resident Groups: Nea Symphony, Theatre on the Ridge, Act Experience, Jonesboro City Ballet

789 ARKANSAS SYMPHONY ORCHESTRA
2417 N Tyler
PO Box 7328
Little Rock, AR 72207
Phone: 501-666-1761
Fax: 501-666-3193
e-mail: asoinfo@alitel.net
Web Site: www.arkansassymphony.org
Management:
 Music Director: David Itkin
 Executive Director: William Vickery

Budget: $1,050,000-$3,600,000
Performs At: Robinson Center Music Hall
Seating Capacity: 2,609

790   PINE BLUFF SYMPHONY ORCHESTRA
512 Pine Street
Suite 205
Pine Bluff, AR 71601
Mailing Address: PO Box 1594, Pine Bluff, AR.
71613-1594
Phone: 870-536-7666
Fax: 870-536-8355
Management:
   Music Director: Charles Jones Evans
   Executive Director: William H Fox, Jr
Mission: To give students an opportunity to improve and
continue their skills and to raise their sights in life; to
expose our community to a quality of music we would
rarely hear otherwise.
Founded: 1987
Budget: $150,000-$260,000
Seating Capacity: 1,900

California

791   BAKERSFIELD SYMPHONY ORCHESTRA
1328 34th Street
Suite A
Bakersfield, CA 93301
Phone: 661-323-7928
Fax: 661-323-7331
e-mail: jfarrere@bakersfieldsymphony.org
Web Site: www.bakersfieldsymphony.org/
Management:
   Music Director: John Farrer
Budget: $260,000-$1,050,000
Performs At: Bakersfield Convention Center

792   BERKELEY SYMPHONY ORCHESTRA
2322 Shattuck Avenue
Berkeley, CA 94704
Phone: 510-841-2800
Fax: 510-841-5422
e-mail: mail@berkeleysymphony.org
Web Site: www.berkeleysymphony.org
Management:
   Executive Director: Catherine Barker-Henwood
   Music Director: Kent Nagano
   Bookeeper/Data Manager: Shohei Sawada
   Administrative Assistant: Recardo Antoni
   Personnel Manager: Elizabeth Gibson
Mission: To present traditional and contemporary
symphony literature.
Founded: 1969
Specialized Field: Symphony; Orchestra
Status: Semi-Professional
Paid Staff: 37
Performs At: Zellerbach Hall; University of California at
Berkeley
Organization Type: Performing

793   BERKELEY YOUTH ORCHESTRA
Laney College Music Department
PO Box 1294
Berkeley, CA 94701
Phone: 510-540-0812
Fax: 510-464-3264
e-mail: info@berkeley-youth-orchestra.org
Web Site: www.berkeley-youth-orchestra.org
Officers:
   President: Linda Kay
   Manager: Penny Boys
Management:
   Music Director: Ann Krinitsky
   Woodwind And Brass Coach: Jay Lehmann
   Assistant: Josh Walden

**794   CALIFORNIA CHAMBER ORCHESTRA
& CHAMBER OPERA**
907 Keeler Avenue
Berkeley, CA 94708-1419
Phone: 510-524-3682
Fax: 510-524-3683
e-mail: edida@earthlink.net
Management:
   Artistic Director: Edgar J Braun
   Manager: Janet Mitchell
Budget: $260,000-$1,050,000

795   CONCERTO AMABILE
San Francisco Early Music Society
PO Box 10151
Berkeley, CA 94709
Phone: 510-528-1725
Fax: 510-528-1725
Management:
   Artistic Director: Kathleen Kraft
Mission: To present the finest in baroque repertoires, with
particular emphasis on lesser-known composers.
Specialized Field: Chamber; Ensemble; Instrumental
Group
Status: Professional; Nonprofit
Organization Type: Performing; Touring

796   SAN FRANCISCO CHAMBER ORCHESTRA
907 Keeler Avenue
Berkeley, CA 94708-1419
Phone: 510-524-3682
Fax: 510-524-3683
Web Site: www.sdco.org/sdco.html
Management:
   Music Director: Edgar Braun
   Manager: Janet Mitchell
Budget: $260,000-$1,050,000

797   SAN FRANCISCO EARLY MUSIC SOCIETY
PO Box 10151
Berkeley, CA 94709

Phone: 510-528-1725
Fax: 510-528-1725
e-mail: sfems@sfems.org
Web Site: www.sfems.org
Officers:
   Administrative Assistant: Susan Hedges
Mission: Dedicated to serving as an umbrella organization in Northern California for early music activities and to creating an appreciative and supportive environment for the study and performance of medieval, renaissance and baroque music by both amateurs and professionals in Northern California.
Founded: 1975
Specialized Field: Early European Music
Status: Nonprofit
Seating Capacity: 150
Organization Type: Educational; Sponsoring

798   YOUNG PEOPLE'S SYMPHONY ORCHESTRA

PO Box 5539
Berkeley, CA 94705
Phone: 510-849-9776
Fax: 510-849-9777
e-mail: ypsomanager@hotmail.com
Web Site: www.ypsomusic.org
Officers:
   President: Edward Levitch
   VP/Executive Director Emeritus: Ljuba Davis
Management:
   Operations Director: David E Davis
   Music Director/Conductor: David Ramadanoff
Mission: To provide young musicians between the ages of 13 and 21 an opportunity to expand their musical experience under the guidance of professionals through the rehearsal and performance of a wide range of symphonic and chamber music repertoire.
Founded: 1935
Paid Staff: 2
Paid Artists: 10
Budget: $100,000
Performs At: Dean Lesher Regional Center for the Arts
Rental Contact: Operations Manager David Davis

799   LOS ANGELES PERFORMING ARTS ORCHESTRA

2250 Gloaming Way
Beverly Hills, CA 90210
Phone: 310-276-2731
Fax: 310-275-8245
Management:
   Acting Director: Nedra Zachary
   Contractor: Jenice Rosen
Founded: 1981
Specialized Field: Official orchestra for the Loren I. Zachary Society National Vocal Competition for Young Opera Singers; Grand Finals Concert
Volunteer Staff: 3
Paid Artists: 25
Budget: $15,000
Performs At: Wilshire Ebell Theatre
Annual Attendance: 1270
Facility Category: Theatre
Type of Stage: Proscenium

Seating Capacity: 1170
Year Built: 1927
Year Remodeled: 1989

800   PLAYBOY JAZZ FESTIVAL

9320 Wilshire Boulevard
#302
Beverly Hills, CA 90212
Phone: 310-786-7400
Fax: 310-786-7440
Web Site: www.playboy.com
Management:
   Communications Director: Bill Farley
   Festival Manager: Jonne-Marie Switzler
Mission: Providing a community service; enabling the residents of Los Angeles to enjoy jazz.
Founded: 1979
Specialized Field: Jazz
Status: Professional
Budget: $1.5-2 Million
Season: June Weekend
Performs At: Hollywood Bowl (Festival Site)
Seating Capacity: 17,900
Organization Type: Sponsoring

801   YOUNG MUSICIANS FOUNDATION DEBUT ORCHESTRA

195 S Beverly Drive
Suite 414
Beverly Hills, CA 90212
Phone: 310-859-7668
Fax: 310-859-1365
e-mail: YMFmusic@aol.com
Web Site: www.YMF.org
Management:
   Music Director: Wilson Hermanto
   Executive Director: Edith Rugolo
Budget: $260,000-$1,050,000
Performs At: Wilshire Ebell Theatre

802   ASIA AMERICA SYMPHONY ORCHESTRA

608 Silver Spur Road #320
Bolling Hills Estates, CA 90274
Phone: 310-377-8977
Fax: 310-377-8949
e-mail: AASA608@aol.com
Web Site: www.commasoft.com/aaso
Management:
   Music Director: David Benoit
   Manager: Ted T Tanaka
Mission: To promote music and cultural exchange by offering a broad variety of activities designed to educate and enrich the diverse communities of Southern California.
Budget: $150,000-$260,000
Performs At: Torrance Cultural Arts Center

803   SOUTHEAST SYMPHONY

PO Box 3576
Burbank, CA 91508

Phone: 818-504-0600
Fax: 818-504-9291
e-mail: sesaschol@hotmail.com
Officers:
   President: Rosemarie Cook-Glover
   VP: Myrtle Moore
   VP: Lorraine Julian
Management:
   Music Director: John Dennison
   Artistic Director: Jacqueline Broussard
Mission: Free concerts, apprenticeships, scholarships and educational programs.
Founded: 1948
Specialized Field: Symphony Concerts
Paid Staff: 14
Volunteer Staff: 30
Paid Artists: 60
Budget: $100,000-$150,000
Income Sources: Grants; Memberships; Donations
Affiliations: Association of California Symphony Orchestras
Seating Capacity: 1,100

---

804   SAN FERNANDO VALLEY SYMPHONY
20210 Haynes Street
Canoga Park, CA 91306
Phone: 818-347-4807
Fax: 818-883-3148
Officers:
   President: Jonathan Laurie
   VP: Leon Wood
Management:
   Music Director: James Elza Domine
   Associate Conductor: Nancy Ross
Mission: To present classical concerts.
Founded: 1980
Specialized Field: Symphonic; Classical
Status: Professional; Semi-Professional; Nonprofit
Income Sources: Association of California Symphony Orchestras; San Fernando Valley Arts Council
Performs At: Main Stage Theater; Pierce College-Soka Campus
Organization Type: Performing; Touting; Resident; Educational; Sponsoring

---

805   CARMEL BACH FESTIVAL
PO Box 575
Carmel, CA 93921
Phone: 831-624-1521
Fax: 831-624-2788
e-mail: info@bachfestival.org
Web Site: www.bachfestival.org
Officers:
   President: Natalie Stewart
Management:
   Music Director: Bruno Weil
   Artistic Director: Nana Faridany
   Executive Managing Director/VP: William Witnbergen
Mission: Performing the works of Johann Sebastian Bach, as well as other classical compositions.
Founded: 1935
Specialized Field: Instrumental; Opera; Choral; Childrens'; Educational
Status: Professional; Nonprofit

Paid Staff: 35
Paid Artists: 100
Non-paid Artists: 30
Budget: $2,300,000
Income Sources: Private Donations
Season: July - August
Performs At: Carmel (Festival Site)
Affiliations: Various Sites in the vicinity of Carmel-by-the-Sea
Annual Attendance: 17,000
Facility Category: Community Auditorium
Type of Stage: Proscenium
Seating Capacity: 733; 400; 250; 200
Year Built: 1928
Organization Type: Performing; Educational

---

806   CHAMBER MUSIC MONTEREY BAY
PO Box 221458
Carmel, CA 93922-1458
Phone: 831-625-2212
Fax: 831-625-2212
Web Site: www.chambermusicmontereybay.org/
Officers:
   President: Amy Anderson
   VP: Bob Haltrop
   Secretary: Laura Burian
   Treasurer: Judith Midgley
   Second VP: Renate Wunsch
Mission: To present high-quality chamber music at a minimum cost; to sponsor an annual competition for young musicians.
Founded: 1967
Specialized Field: Chamber
Status: Nonprofit
Paid Staff: 2
Volunteer Staff: 14
Paid Artists: 5
Budget: $105,000
Income Sources: Donations; Ticket Sales; Grants
Annual Attendance: 3,000
Facility Category: Theatre and Community Center
Type of Stage: Proscenium
Seating Capacity: 700
Year Built: 1940
Year Remodeled: 2002
Organization Type: Sponsoring

---

807   MONTEREY BAY SYMPHONY
PO Box 146
Carmel, CA 93921-0146
Phone: 831-372-6276
Fax: 831-373-8450
Officers:
   President: Ron A Weitzman
   VP: Morley Brown
   VP: Bert Saunders
   Secretary: Edie Karas
   Secretary: Donna Jett
   Treasurer: Charles R. Glick
Management:
   Music Director: Jack Bayes
   Music Director: Sharon Jones
   Music Director: Carol Christensen
Mission: To present free concerts, currently five per year.
Founded: 1985

Specialized Field: Music
Volunteer Staff: 20
Paid Artists: 56
Budget: $35,000-$100,000
Performs At: Naval Postgraduate School

808 MONTEREY COUNTY SYMPHONY ASSOCIATION
10th Street Between Mission and San Carlos
PO Box 3965
Carmel, CA 93921
Phone: 831-624-8511
Fax: 831-624-3837
Toll-free: 800-697-1138
e-mail: info@montereysymphony.org
Web Site: www.montereysymphony.org
Officers:
   President: Alycs M Nunes
   VP/Long Range Planning: Thomas Ruth
   VP Development: Joann Taylor Johnson
   VP Marketing: Mollie Hedges
Management:
   Executive Director: Joseph Truskot
   Director of Operations: Joan DeVisser
   Music Director: Kate Tamarkin
   Chorus Director: Leroy Kromm
Mission: To produce high-quality classical music for the people of Monterey Bay, Salinas Valley, San Benito County and Big Sur.
Founded: 1946
Specialized Field: Symphony; Orchestra; Chamber; Ensemble
Status: Professional; Nonprofit
Paid Staff: 6
Paid Artists: 80
Budget: $1,500,000
Income Sources: Association of California Symphony Orchestras; American Symphony Orchestra League
Performs At: Sunset Theatre; Sherwood Hall; Pacific Grove Middle School
Affiliations: ACSO; American Symphony Orchestra League
Annual Attendance: 20,000
Seating Capacity: 733; 1511
Year Remodeled: 2002
Organization Type: Performing

809 CALIFORNIA WIND ORCHESTRA
PO Box 1503
Carmichael, CA 95609
Phone: 916-489-2576
e-mail: lehr@gotnet.net
Web Site: www.cawinds.com
Officers:
   Board President: Ken McCollum
Management:
   Music Director: Dr Lester E Lehr
Mission: To bring the joy of live professional wind music to the Greater Sacramento Valley and beyond.
Founded: 1995
Specialized Field: Wind Ensemble
Status: Professional; Tax Exempt
Performs At: The Crest Theater

810 CARSON-DOMINQUEZ HILLS SYMPHONY
PO Box 5425
Carson, CA 90749-5425
Phone: 310-243-3543
Fax: 310-243-3947
e-mail: bbccandy@earthlink.net
Web Site: www.bbccandy.com
Management:
   Music Director: Dr. Frances Steiner
   Executive Director: Alyce Bledsoe
Mission: To offer a wide range of repertoire: works by Mozart, Beethoven, Stravinsky, and contemporary music such as the West Coast premiere of the 1996 Pulitzer Prize winning composition in music by George Walker, as well as more popular music, such as Tchaikovsky's 1812 Overture, music from West Side Story, and highlights of Showboat.

811 CALIFORNIA E.A.R. UNIT FOUNDATION
29654 Driver Avenue
Castaic, CA 91384
Phone: 661-775-9975
Fax: 661-775-3855
e-mail: amy@earunit.org
Web Site: earunit.org
Management:
   Executive Director: Amy Knoles
   Director: Dorothy Stone
Mission: Dedicated to the performance, promotion, and creation of some of the most exciting music of our time.
Founded: 1982
Specialized Field: Chamber; Electronic & Live Electronic, Contemporary Chamber Music
Status: Professional; Nonprofit
Paid Staff: 2
Volunteer Staff: 2
Paid Artists: 6
Performs At: Los Angeles County Museum of Art
Organization Type: Performing; Touring; Resident; Educational
Resident Groups: New Chamber Music

812 BESSIE BARTLETT FRANKEL FESTIVAL OF CHAMBER MUSIC
Scripps College, Music Department
1030 Columbia
Claremont, CA 91711
Phone: 909-607-3266
Fax: 909-621-8323
e-mail: kkosakow@scrippscol.edu
Web Site: www.scrippscol.edu/~dept/Music/music.html
Management:
   Music Department: Jane O'Donnell
Specialized Field: Instrumental
Season: September - March
Performs At: Balch Auditorium; Scripps College; Claremont (Festival Site)
Affiliations: Balch Auditorium; Humanities Auditorium
Facility Category: Auditorium
Seating Capacity: 300

813 CLAREMONT SYMPHONY ORCHESTRA

840 North Indian Hill Boulevard
Claremont, CA 91711
Phone: 909-626-4868
Fax: 626-798-3890
Web Site: www.csz.com/cso/
Officers:
   President: Barbara Bonzo
Management:
   Conductor: James Fahringer
Budget: $35,000
Performs At: Bridges Hall of Music

814 POMONA COLLEGE ORCHESTRA

Pomona College, Music Department
340 N College Avenue
Claremont, CA 91711
Phone: 909-621-8155
Fax: 909-621-8645
Web Site: www.music.pomona.edu/orchestra
Management:
   Music Director: Eric Lindholm
Budget: $35,000
Performs At: Bridges Hall of Music
Annual Attendance: 2500-3000
Seating Capacity: 600
Year Built: 1915
Year Remodeled: 2001

815 CULVER CITY-MARINA DEL REY-WESTCHESTER SYMPHONY

PO Box 4846
Culver City, CA 90231
Phone: 310-839-5537
Fax: 323-255-1998
Management:
   Music Director/Conductor: Frank Fetta
   Manager: Helene Mirich-Spear
Budget: $35,000-$100,000
Performs At: Veterans Memorial Auditorium

816 HENRY MANCINI INSTITUTE

10811 Washington Boulevard
Suite 300
Culver City, CA 90232
Phone: 310-845-1900
Fax: 310-845-1909
e-mail: hmi@manciniistitute.org
Web Site: www.manciniinstitute.org
Management:
   Managing Director: Kelly Connaughton
   Program Administrator: Jill Packard

817 CYPRESS POPS ORCHESTRA

PO Box 434
Cypress, CA 90630
Phone: 714-826-8872
Fax: 714-828-4276
e-mail: Dallen8075@aol.com
Web Site: www.cypresspops.com
Officers:
   President: Darlene Allen

VP: Joanne Harrison
   Treasurer: Marcia Durbin
   Secretary: Jean Harries
Management:
   Music Director: John E Hall III
Status: Nonprofit
Budget: $75,000-$125,000
Seating Capacity: 1,000

818 CAPISTRANO VALLEY SYMPHONY

24582 Del Prado
Suite F
Dana Point, CA 92629
Phone: 949-240-8584
Fax: 949-240-0467
e-mail: info@sjc.net
Web Site: www.cvsymphony.com
Management:
   Music Director: Carlos Spiga
   Administrator: Tracy Nishimuta
Mission: To bring the highest quality symphonic music and educational programs.
Founded: 1984
Budget: $150,000-$260,000

819 TASSAJARA SYMPHONY ORCHESTRA

696 San Ramon Valley Boulevard
Danville, CA 94526
Phone: 925-820-2494
e-mail: greatmusic@tassajarasymphony.org
Web Site: www.tassajarasymphony.org
Officers:
   President: David Summers
   Secretary: John Carr
   Treasurer: Melanie Prole
Management:
   Founding Musical Director: Sara Jobin
   Artistic Director: Dawn Wade
   Public Relations: Cheryl Williamson
Mission: Aims to provide an exciting and enjoyable playing environment that encourages camraderie and emphasizes fine ensemble playing.
Founded: 1998
Specialized Field: Music Performance
Paid Staff: 2
Volunteer Staff: 10
Paid Artists: 45
Budget: $140,000
Income Sources: Donors; Grants
Performs At: Community Church and Regional Center for the Arts
Annual Attendance: 1500

820 DOWNEY SYMPHONY ORCHESTRA

PO Box 763
Downey, CA 90241-0763
Phone: 818-884-6301
Fax: 818-884-4677
e-mail: upbow3@aol.com
Officers:
   Preident: William Hare
Management:
   Music Director: Thomas Osborn

All listings are in alphabetical order by state, then city, then organization within the city.

Mission: Provide Symphonic music to Southeast Los Angeles and also through our Music in the School program to elementary schools in Downey.
Founded: 1956
Specialized Field: Symphonic music
Status: Professional; Nonprofit
Paid Staff: 20
Volunteer Staff: 10
Paid Artists: 60
Performs At: Downey Civic Center
Organization Type: Performing

821   IMPERIAL VALLEY SYMPHONY

1904 Johnson Lane
PO Box 713
El Centro, CA 92243-0713
Phone: 760-355-6287
Fax: 760-355-6398
e-mail: joel@imperial.cc.ca.us
Web Site: http://faculty.imperial.cc.ca.us
Management:
  Music Director/Conductor: Joel Jacklich
Founded: 1974
Specialized Field: Music; Symphony Orchestra
Paid Staff: 1
Volunteer Staff: 4
Paid Artists: 25
Non-paid Artists: 35
Budget: $20,000
Affiliations: American Symphony Orchestra League
Annual Attendance: 1950
Seating Capacity: 1050
Year Built: 1996

822   SAN DIEGO CHAMBER ORCHESTRA

2210 Encinitas Boulevard
Suite M
Encinitas, CA 92024-4378
Phone: 760-753-6402
Fax: 760-753-2089
Toll-free: 888-848-7326
e-mail: levenson@sdco.org
Web Site: www.sdco.org
Officers:
  President: Bill Weber
  VP: Elsie Weston
  Secretary: Susan Snow
  CFO: Leslie Ross
Management:
  Artistic Director: Donald Barra
  Executive Director: Jeffrey Levenson
  Marketing/PR Director: Sharon Fendrich
  President: Bill Weber
  VP: Elsie V Weston
  CFO: Leslie Ross
  Secretary: Susan H Snow
Mission: To provide a resident small orchestra of the highest professional caliber for the greater San Diego area.
Founded: 1984
Specialized Field: Symphony; Orchestra; Chamber
Status: Professional; Nonprofit
Paid Staff: 5
Volunteer Staff: 1
Paid Artists: 150

Budget: $1.3 million
Income Sources: Ticket Sales; Donations; Sponsors
Performs At: Performance Halls and Public Areas
Affiliations: American Symphony Orchestra League; Association of California Symphony Orchestras
Annual Attendance: 40,000
Seating Capacity: 100-3,000
Organization Type: Performing
Resident Groups: Chamber Orchestra

823   LOS ANGELES MOZART ORCHESTRA

3330 Barham Boulevard #207
Encino, CA 91416
Mailing Address: PO Box 17643, Encino, CA. 91416
Phone: 323-874-6316
Fax: 323-874-2684
e-mail: info@lamozart.org
Web Site: www.lamozart.com
Officers:
  President: Virginia Van Osdel, DDS
  VP: Nancy MacLachlan
  Treasurer: Cheryl Jordan
  Secretary: Larry Kurens
  President Emeritus: Patricia Oliansky
  President Emeritus: Neil Bennett
Management:
  Music Director: Lucinda Carver
  Executive Director/Asst Conductor: Debra Cheverino
  Music Director Emeritus/Conductor: David Keith
Mission: As the premiere organization in Southern California specializing in the work of Mozart and his contemporaries, the LAMO presents distinctive, world-class performances of its repertoire to the multi-cultural population of its region. Through its concerts and innovative educational programming, LAMO strives to make the high artistic quality embodied in its work accessible to its diverse community.
Specialized Field: Chamber orchestra specializing in Mozart and his contemporaries
Budget: $260,000-$1,050,000
Performs At: Zipper Hall; Colburn School for the Performing Arts

824   FREMONT SYMPHONY ORCHESTRA

PO Box 104
Fremont, CA 94537
Phone: 510-794-1652
Fax: 510-794-1658
e-mail: info@fremontsymphony.org
Web Site: www.fremonsymphony.org
Officers:
  Executive Director: Abastasia Herold
Management:
  Music Director: David Sloss
  Personnel Manager: Carole Klein
Mission: To provide and develop, for the greater Fremont area, a professional symphony orchestra. The orchestra will fulfill the community's needs and wants by offering a balanced program of established symphonic repertoire.
Founded: 1964
Specialized Field: Symphony; Orchestra; Ensemble; Music; Music Education
Status: Professional; Semi-Professional
Paid Staff: 5
Volunteer Staff: 45

Paid Artists: 100
Budget: $350,000
Income Sources: Ticket Sales; Government; Corporate &
Foundation Grants; Individual Contributions;
Fund-raising Events
Performs At: Smith Center at Ohlone College
Affiliations: American Symphony Orchestra League;
ACSO; Fremong Chamber; American Society of
Composers, Authors and Publishers
Annual Attendance: 2,500-6,000
Facility Category: Theatre
Type of Stage: Proscenium
Stage Dimensions: 30x30
Seating Capacity: 405
Year Built: 1995
Rental Contact: Susan Wodiska
Organization Type: Performing; Educational

825 FRESNO PHILHARMONIC

2610 West Shaw Lane
Suite 103
Fresno, CA 93711-3332
Phone: 559-261-0600
Fax: 559-261-0700
Web Site: www.fresnophil.org
Officers:
    President: Rick Docker
    First VP: Larry Hagoplan
    Secreatry: Kay Whitten
    Treasurer: JD Northway
Management:
    Music Director: Theodore Kuchar
    Executive Director: Robert Lippert
Founded: 1954
Specialized Field: Symphony; Orchestra
Status: Professional; Nonprofit
Paid Artists: 80
Budget: $ 1.8 Million
Income Sources: Association of California Symphony
Orchestras
Performs At: Saroyan Theatre
Organization Type: Performing; Touring; Resident

826 PHILIP LORENZ MEMORIAL
KEYBOARD CONCERTS

PO Box 14162
Fresno, CA 93650
Phone: 559-278-2337
Fax: 559-278-6800
e-mail: andreasw@csufresno.edu
Web Site: www.keyboardconcerts.com
Management:
    Artistic Director: Andreas Werz
Founded: 1971
Specialized Field: Music; Piano Recitals
Status: Nonprofit
Paid Staff: 5
Volunteer Staff: 4
Paid Artists: 3
Performs At: The Concert Hall, Callifornia State
University, Fresno
Seating Capacity: 450

827 SOUTH VALLEY SYMPHONY

PO Box 1347
Gilroy, CA 95021-1347
Phone: 408-842-3934
Fax: 408-842-0672
e-mail: pvklogck@garlic.com
Officers:
    President: Al Navaroli
    Treasurer: Paul V Kloecker
Management:
    Music Director/Conductor: Henry Mollicone
Founded: 1974
Specialized Field: Symphony Music
Paid Staff: 2
Volunteer Staff: 10
Non-paid Artists: 40
Budget: $35,000-$100,000

828 GLENDALE SYMPHONY

PO Box 4626
Glendale, CA 91203
Phone: 818-500-8720
Fax: 818-500-8014
e-mail: info@glendalesymphony.org
Web Site: www.glendalesymphony.org
Officers:
    President: Robert Bornhoeft
Management:
    Office Manager: Jamie Bornhoeft
Mission: To bring the world of fine music to the broadest
possible community. We present annual seasons of
scheduled concerts of the familiar classical repertoire-
works that, over the years, have become accepted
masterpieces. In doing so, we advance the cause of fine
music and help stimulate an active cultural life in our
community, and the fellowship that goes with it, year
round.
Founded: 1924
Specialized Field: Symphony; Orchestra
Status: Professional; Nonprofit
Income Sources: American Symphony Orchestra League
Performs At: Alex Theater
Organization Type: Performing; Educational

829 GLENDALE YOUTH ORCHESTRA

PO Box 4401
Glendale, CA 91222-0401
Phone: 818-321-3083
Fax: 818-403-0180
Web Site: www.glendale-online.com/gyo
Officers:
    President: Eitan Sadeh
    VP: Elinor Lloyd
    Treasurer: Alan Kleinsasser
    Secretary: Sue Kelly
Management:
    Music Director: Brad Keimach
    Orchestra Manager: Vonnie Banerdt
Mission: To provide qualified young musicians an
environment in which to explore, comprehend, appreciate
and develop a lasting interest in music in a quality
orchestral setting. As orchestra members, to perform

concerts of standard symphonic music; to learn the value of achievement, teamwork, and discipline; to work with top teaching professionals as coaches.
Founded: 1989
Status: Nonprofit
Budget: $35,000-$100,000
Performs At: Alex Theatre

830 RUSSIAN RIVER JAZZ FESTIVAL

3rd Street
PO Box 1913
Guerneville, CA 95446
Phone: 707-869-3940
Fax: 707-869-0147
Management:
 Office Manager: Kathryn Marceau
Mission: Bringing top name jazz and related performers to perform in an outdoor venue while benefitting local programs for the community and its youth.
Founded: 1976
Specialized Field: Vocal Music; Instrumental Music; Festivals
Status: Nonprofit
Paid Staff: 5
Organization Type: Performing

831 RUSSIAN RIVER CHAMBER MUSIC

1803 Vine Street
#136
Healdsburg, CA 95448
Phone: 707-524-8700
Fax: 707-431-7622
e-mail: info@russianrivermusic.org
Web Site: www.russianrivermusic.org
Officers:
 President: Jay M Behmke
 VP: Al Merck
 Treasurer: Chris Baldenhofer
Management:
 Artistic Director: Gary McLaughlin
Mission: To present live concerts of the highest quality in the heart of Sonoma County's wine country.
Founded: 1992
Performs At: Healdsburg Federated Church
Seating Capacity: 300

832 HOLLYWOOD BOWL ORCHESTRA

The Hollywood Bowl
2301 N Highland Avenue
Hollywood, CA 90078
Phone: 323-850-2095
Fax: 323-512-2966
e-mail: slinder@laphil.org
Web Site: www.hollywoodbowl.org
Officers:
 President: Robert I Weingarten
 VP: Anthon Cannon
 VP: Donald De Brier
 Treasurer: Dennis Kent
 Secretary: Alan Wayte
Management:
 Manager: Steve Linder
 Principal Conductor: John Mauceri
 Operations Manager: Christi Brockway

 COO: Patricia Mitchell
 Generl Manager: Gail Samuel
 Concert Master: Bruce Dukov
Founded: 1991
Seating Capacity: 17,695

833 INDIAN WELLS DESERT SYMPHONY

74-935 Highway 111
Suite 115
Indian Wells, CA 92210
Phone: 760-773-5988
Fax: 760-772-5083
e-mail: cashinmktg@aol.com
Officers:
 Business Manager: Marilyn Benachowski
Management:
 Music Director: Edwin R Benachowski

834 PHILHARMONIC SOCIETY OF ORANGE COUNTY

2082 Business Center Drive
Suite 100
Irvine, CA 92612
Phone: 949-553-2422
Fax: 949-553-2421
e-mail: contactus@philharmonicsociety.org
Web Site: www.philharmonicsociety.org
Management:
 Executive Director: Dean Corey
Mission: To foster, promote and increase the knowledge and appreciation of the arts through the presentation of performances by musical artists of national and international stature.
Performs At: Orange County Performing Arts Center
Seating Capacity: 2900

835 MARIN COMMUNITY COLLEGE SYMPHONY

835 College Avenue
Kentfield, CA 94904
Phone: 415-457-8811
Fax: 415-485-0135
Management:
 Music Director/Conductor: Norman Masonson
Mission: To foster cultural advancement in the community.
Founded: 1960
Specialized Field: Symphony; Orchestra; Chamber; Instrumental Group
Status: Non-Professional; Nonprofit
Paid Staff: 2
Performs At: Fine Arts Theatre
Organization Type: Performing; Educational

836 LA JOLLA CHAMBER MUSIC SOCIETY

7946 Ivanhoe Street, Suite 309
PO Box 2168
La Jolla, CA 92037
Phone: 858-459-3724
Fax: 858-459-3727
e-mail: ljcms@ljcms.org
Web Site: www.ljcms.org
Officers:

Chairman: Sue Hodges
VP: Paul Jacobs
VP: Dr. K Chung Hesselink
VP: Howard Robin
Secretary: Sue Hodges
Treasurer: Javade Chaudhri
Management:
  Executive Director: Mary Lou Aleskie
  Managing Director: Kathryn Martin
  Production/Education Director: Hannes Kling
  Artistic Operations Manager: Dan Bourla
Mission: To present the world's finest muscians and ensembles.
Founded: 1968
Specialized Field: Symphony; Chamber; Ensemble; Recitals; Summerfest
Status: Professional; Nonprofit
Paid Staff: 15
Budget: $3,000,000
Income Sources: Ticket Sales; Contributions
Performs At: Sherwood Auditorium; Civic Theatre; Copley Symphony Hall
Annual Attendance: 35,000
Organization Type: Performing; Presenting

---

837 LA JOLLA SYMPHONY & CHORUS ASSOCIATION
9500 Gilman Drive
UCSD Box 0361
La Jolla, CA 92093-0361
Phone: 858-534-4637
Fax: 858-534-9947
e-mail: cycollins@ucsd.edu
Web Site: www.lajollasymphony.com
Management:
  Executive Director: Sylvia Grace
  Operations Manager: Cindy Collins
Mission: The LaJolla Symphony & Chorus is a musical performing group dedicated to inspiring San Diego with the joy of music. Our orchestra and chorus perform ground-breaking orchestral and choral music along with traditional favorites from the classical repertoire. We are also dedicated to bringing music education to the public schools of San Diego.
Status: Nonprofit
Budget: $150,000-$260,000
Performs At: Mandeville Center for the Performing Arts

---

838 MOZART CLASSICAL ORCHESTRA
23251 Peralta
Suite N
Laguna Hills, CA 92653
Phone: 949-830-2950
Fax: 949-581-3066
e-mail: info@mozartorchestra.org
Web Site: www.mozartorchestra.org
Management:
  Music Director/Conductor: Ami Porat
Founded: 1980
Budget: $150,000-$260,000
Performs At: St. Andrews Presbyterian Church; Irvine Barclay Theatre

---

839 LAGUNA CHAMBER MUSIC SOCIETY
13 Doheny
Laguna Niguel, CA 92677
Phone: 949-249-2404
Fax: 949-249-8370
e-mail: Lagunachmu@earthlink.net
Management:
  Artistic Director: Glenda Van Der Zaag
Mission: To present a series of chamber music concerts for the public and to present music education programs in schools.
Founded: 1959
Specialized Field: Chamber Music
Paid Staff: 1
Performs At: Irvine Barclay Theatre; Artist's Theatre
Seating Capacity: 750; 450

---

840 CONCERT IN THE VINEYARDS
5050 Arroyo Road
Livermore, CA 94550
Phone: 925-456-2406
Fax: 925-456-2401
Management:
  Program Director: Geirgine Woodward

---

841 LIVERMORE-AMADOR SYMPHONY
PO Box 1049
Livermore, CA 94551-1049
Phone: 925-447-3672
Fax: 810-283-0188
e-mail: info@livamsymph.org
Web Site: www.livamsymph.org
Officers:
  Secretary Board of Directors: Richard Hatfield
Management:
  Music Director: Dr. Arthur Barnes
Founded: 1963
Specialized Field: Music
Budget: $35,000-$100,000
Performs At: First Presbyterian Church
Seating Capacity: 450

---

842 LONG BEACH SYMPHONY ORCHESTRA
555 E Ocean Boulevard
Suite 106
Long Beach, CA 90802
Phone: 562-436-3203
Fax: 562-491-3599
e-mail: ibso@ibso.org
Web Site: www.lbso.org
Management:
  Executive Director: Jack Fishman
  Music Director: Enrique Arturo Diemecke
Mission: To offer quality symphonic music.
Founded: 1935
Specialized Field: Symphony; Orchestra
Status: Nonprofit
Paid Staff: 13
Volunteer Staff: 300
Paid Artists: 83
Performs At: Terrace Theater
Seating Capacity: 3,000
Organization Type: Performing

---

843 PENINSULA SYMPHONY ORCHESTRA

146 Main Street
Suite 207
Los Altos, CA 94402
Phone: 650-941-5291
Fax: 650-941-5292
e-mail: music@peninsulasym.org
Web Site: www.peninsulasym.org
Management:
   Music Director/Conductor: Mitchell Sardou Klein
   Executive Director: Margarit Rinderknecht
Founded: 1949
Budget: $150,000-260,000
Performs At: San Mateo Performing Arts Center; Flint Center

844 AMERICAN YOUTH SYMPHONY

2376 Westwood Boulevard
2nd Floor
Los Angeles, CA 90064
Phone: 310-234-8355
Fax: 310-234-9785
e-mail: music@aysymphony.org
Web Site: www.aysymphony.org
Officers:
   Chairman: Elise Rips
Management:
   Executive Director: Anne E Gimbel
Mission: To provide free concerts for the Los Angeles community and to educate the professional musicians of tomorrow.
Founded: 1964
Specialized Field: Symphony; Orchestra
Status: Non-Professional; Nonprofit
Paid Staff: 6
Volunteer Staff: 60
Paid Artists: 110
Budget: $620,000
Income Sources: American Symphony Orchestra League (Youth Orchestra Division)
Performs At: Royce Hall; UCLA
Annual Attendance: 12,000
Organization Type: Performing; Educational

845 INTERNATIONAL ASSOCIATION OF JAZZ APPRECIATION

PO Box 48146
Los Angeles, CA 90048
Phone: 325-295-0644
Fax: 323-295-3786
Officers:
   Founder/President: William J MD
Mission: To preserve jazz music through education and presentation.
Founded: 1982
Specialized Field: Orchestra; Ensemble; Band
Status: Nonprofit
Organization Type: Performing; Educational

846 LOS ANGELES BACH FESTIVAL

First Congregational Church
540 S Commonwealth Avenue
Los Angeles, CA 90020-1298
Phone: 213-385-1345
Fax: 213-487-0461
e-mail: musicinfo@fccla.org
Web Site: www.fccla.org
Management:
   Music Director: Thomas Summerville
Specialized Field: Instrumental; Choral; Folk
Budget: $20,000-$35,000
Affiliations: First Congregational Church of Los Angeles
Seating Capacity: 150; 1,000

847 LOS ANGELES CHAMBER ORCHESTRA

707 Wolshire Boulevard
Suite 1850
Los Angeles, CA 90017
Phone: 213-622-7001
Fax: 213-955-2071
e-mail: laco@laco.org
Web Site: www.laco.org
Officers:
   President: Lois Evans
   Chairman: Edward J Nowaker, Jr
   VP: Scott Bottles
   Treasurer: Gregory Soukup
   Treasurer: Simon H Clark
   Assistant Treasurer: Martin Recchuite
Management:
   Executive Director: Ruth L Eliel
   General Manager: Andrea Laguni
   Director Finance: Thomas Mallen
   Director Marketing: Nicolette Atkins
   Music Director: Jeffrey Kahane
   Concertmaster: Margaret Batjer
Mission: To perform high-quality concerts of the chamber orchestra repertoire, from Baroque and early Classical works to the compositions of the 19th and 20th century specifically written for small orchestra, including works by living composers.
Founded: 1968
Specialized Field: Orchestra; Chamber
Status: Professional; Nonprofit
Paid Staff: 12
Paid Artists: 43
Budget: $2.2 million
Income Sources: Ticket Sales; Contributed income from foundations; Corporations; Government agenies; Individual donations
Performs At: Alex Theatre Glandale
Affiliations: American Symphony Orchestra League; Association of California Symphony Orchestras; Western Arts Alliance; International Society of Performing Art
Organization Type: Performing; Touring; Resident

848 LOS ANGELES DOCTORS SYMPHONY ORCHESTRA

PO Box 27353
Los Angeles, CA 90027-0353
Phone: 323-662-1045
Fax: 323-857-3307
e-mail: maestro@ladso.org/ethelred2@aol.com
Web Site: www.ladso.org
Officers:
   President/Orchestra Council: Bernard Bagish
   VP: Ethel McClatchey

Secretary: Nora Graham
Treasurer: Ken Alexander
Management:
   Music Director: Ivan Shulman
Mission: To provide for the comradeship of music for its musicians, to contribute culturally to the community, to help raise funds for medical and other charities and provide concerts at low cost to the public.
Founded: 1953
Specialized Field: Orchestra
Volunteer Staff: 10
Non-paid Artists: 3
Budget: $15,000
Income Sources: Dues; Grants; Donations
Performs At: No Official Base
Annual Attendance: 4,000

849 LOS ANGELES PHILHARMONIC ORCHESTRA

135 N Grand Avenue
Los Angeles, CA 90012
Phone: 213-972-7300
Fax: 213-617-3065
Web Site: www.laphil.org
Officers:
   Chairman: Barry A Sanders
   President: Robert I Weingarten
   VP: Dr. Hansonia Caldwell
   Treasurer: Dennis M. Kent
   Secretary: Alan Wayte
Management:
   Music Director: Esa-Pekka Salonen
   General Manager: Gail Samuel
   Managing Director: Deborah Borda
Budget: $50,000,000+
Performs At: Dorothy Chandler Pavilion; Hollywood Bowl (summer)

850 SANTA CECILIA ORCHESTRA

2759 W Broadway
Los Angeles, CA 90041
Phone: 323-259-3011
Fax: 323-257-0889
e-mail: Santaceciliao@aol.com
Web Site: scorchestra.org
Management:
   Music Director/Conductor: Sonia Marie De Leon De Vega
Founded: 1992
Paid Staff: 2
Volunteer Staff: 3
Paid Artists: 64
Performs At: Greystone Mansion

851 UNIVERSITY OF SOUTHERN CALIFORNIA THORNTON SYMPHONY

USC, Thornton School of Music
Music Faculty Building, Room 409
Los Angeles, CA 90089-0851
Phone: 213-740-3132
Fax: 213-740-3217
Management:
   Assistant: Barrie Duffus-Tucker
Budget: $35,000

Performs At: Bovard Auditorium

852 COMMUNITY SYMPHONY PEPPERDINE
Music Department

24255 Pacific Coast Highway
#4462
Malibu, CA 90263
Phone: 310-456-4462
Fax: 310-456-4077
Web Site: www.pepperdine.edu
Management:
   Music Director/Conductor: Thomas Osborn
Mission: To provide training for musicians and symphonic experience for diverse audiences.
Founded: 1983
Specialized Field: Symphony
Status: Semi-Professional
Paid Staff: 38
Performs At: Smothers Theatre; Pepperdine University
Organization Type: Performing

853 MILL VALLEY CHAMBER MUSIC SOCIETY

PO Box 5121
Mill Valley, CA 94942
Phone: 415-381-1056
Fax: 415-381-2039
e-mail: lsnyder@microweb.com
Officers:
   President: Larry Snyder
Mission: The presentation of an annual subscription series of five concerts per season.
Founded: 1974
Specialized Field: Chamber; Ensemble; Instrumental Group
Status: Nonprofit
Organization Type: Educational; Sponsoring

854 SADDLEBACK CHAMBER PLAYERS
Saddleback College

28000 Marguerite Parkway
Mission Viejo, CA 92692-3635
Phone: 949-582-4763
Fax: 949-347-8653
e-mail: genglish@saddleback.cc.ca.us
Web Site: www.saddleback.cc.ca.us
Management:
   Director Performing Arts: Geofrey L English
Budget: $35,000
Seating Capacity: 400

855 MODESTO SYMPHONY

3509 Coffee Road
Suite D-1
Modesto, CA 95355
Phone: 209-523-4156
Fax: 209-523-0201
e-mail: mso@modestosymphony.org
Web Site: www.modestosymphony.org
Officers:
   President: Carl Boyett
   First VP: Sylvester Aguilar

Management:
   Executive Director: Camille Reed
   Music Director: Darryl One
Mission: To serve the region as a professional orchestra constantly striving for the highest quality attainable.
Founded: 1931
Specialized Field: Symphony
Status: Professional; Nonprofit
Paid Staff: 10
Volunteer Staff: 3
Budget: $1.7 Million
Income Sources: Association of California Symphony Orchestras; American Symphony Orchestra League
Performs At: Modesto Junior College Auditorium
Seating Capacity: 940
Organization Type: Performing; Educational

856 LOS ANGELES CLASSICAL CHINESE ORCHESTRA

876 N Garfield Avenue
Montebello, CA 90640
Phone: 626-282-7940
Fax: 626-282-7086
e-mail: lacco@chinamusic.org
Web Site: www.chinamusic.org
Officers:
   President: Sally Ho
Management:
   Music Director: Christopher Fu
   Manager: Willy Fong
Mission: To introduce classic Chinese music to American audiences.
Founded: 1989
Specialized Field: Classical Music
Paid Staff: 12
Volunteer Staff: 24
Paid Artists: 20
Non-paid Artists: 40
Budget: $260,000-$1,050,000
Income Sources: Fund raising; Ticket sales; Selling CD's and books.
Seating Capacity: 1,490

857 MUSIC IN THE VINEYARDS NAPA VALLEY CHAMBER MUSIC FESTIVAL

PO Box 432
Mt. Helena, CA 94574
Phone: 707-578-5656
Fax: 707-578-5699
e-mail: gadams@sonic.net
Web Site: www.napavalleymusic.org
Officers:
   President: David Marsten
   VP: Robilee F Deane
Management:
   Executive Director: Gail V Adams
   Artistic Director: Michael Adams
   Music Director: Daria Adams
   Development Director: Melinda Mendelson

Mission: Dedicated to bringing together outstanding artists to perform in the vineyard settings of the Napa Valley so that performers and audience alike can experience the intimacy of chamber music as it was intended to be performed.
Founded: 1995
Specialized Field: Instrumental
Budget: $140,000
Season: August
Performs At: Napa Valley (Festival Site)
Affiliations: Various vineyards and related venues
Seating Capacity: 150 - 250

858 NAPA VALLEY SYMPHONY

2407 California Boulevard
Napa, CA 94558
Phone: 707-226-6872
Fax: 707-226-3046
e-mail: info@napaval;leysymphony.org
Web Site: www.napavalleysymphony.org
Officers:
   President: Scott Mathes
   VP: Lonne Carr
   VP: Jeff Omodt
   Treasurer: Winnie St.John
   Secretary: Tom Illgen
Management:
   Executive Director: Tom Illgen
   Development Director: Steve Gallion
   Operations Manager: Theresa Gabel
   Patrons Service Assistant: Karen Pearson
   Music Director/Conductor: Asher Raboy
Mission: To provide the Napa Valley with Symphonic music performances of high standards; to offer music education programs for youth.
Founded: 1933
Specialized Field: Symphony
Status: Nonprofit
Paid Staff: 10
Paid Artists: 55
Budget: $1 Million
Performs At: Lincoln Theatre; Yountville
Annual Attendance: 15,000
Organization Type: Performing; Educational

859 CSUN YOUTH ORCHESTRAS

California State University Northridge
18111 Nordhoff Street
MUSC 149
Northridge, CA 91330-8314
Phone: 818-677-3074
Fax: 818-677-3164
Management:
   Music Director/Conductor: Jerry D Luedders
   General Manager: Melanie Dimmick
   Executive Director: Dave Pier
Paid Staff: 1
Volunteer Staff: 20
Paid Artists: 3
Budget: $100,000
Performs At: Performing Arts Community Center
Annual Attendance: 5,000-6,000
Type of Stage: Proscenium
Year Built: 1994

860 MUSIC HUB
PO Box 437
Novato, CA 94948
Phone: 415-898-8381
Fax: 415-898-8381
e-mail: ctingle@earthlink.net
Web Site: www.MusicHubAgency.com

861 OAKLAND EAST BAY SYMPHONY
400-27th Street
Suite 501
Oakland, CA 94609
Phone: 510-444-0801
Fax: 510-444-0863
e-mail: admin@oebs.org
Web Site: www.oebs.org
Officers:
    President: Mike Sanford
    Executive VP: Jim Hasler
    VP: Robert Keenan
    VP: Meckila Pierce
    Treasurer: Christopher Toohey
    Secretary: Dawn Uribe
Management:
    Music Director: Michael Morgan
    Executive Director: Jennifer Duston
Mission: To present live professional symphonic and collaborative artistic performances to diverse audiences in Oakland and neighboring communities. To serve as a community resource, offering educational outreach and community services to schools, businesses and other organizations.
Founded: 1988
Specialized Field: Instrumental Music
Paid Staff: 7
Paid Artists: 85
Budget: $260,000-1,050,000
Performs At: Paramount Theatre

862 OAKLAND JAZZ ALLIANCE
1330 Broadway #1030
Oakland, CA 94612
Phone: 510-839-2440
Fax: 510-268-9065
Officers:
    President: Buddy Montgomery
    VP: David Montgomery
    Secretary: Majors Harrison
    Treasurer: Dr. Alan Werblin
Management:
    Executive Director: Charla Montgomery
Mission: To preserve, develop and express jazz music; to develop serious young artists.
Founded: 1987
Specialized Field: Vocal Music; Instrumental Music; Festivals
Status: Nonprofit
Paid Staff: 1
Organization Type: Performing; Educational

863 OAKLAND YOUTH ORCHESTRA
1428 Alice Street
Room 202M
Oakland, CA 94612

Phone: 510-832-7710
Fax: 510-832-2571
e-mail: stack@oyo.org
Web Site: www.oyo.org
Management:
    Music Director: Michael Morgan
    Executive Director: Barbara Stack
Mission: Education and performance.
Founded: 1964
Budget: $150,000

864 OJAI CAMERATA
PO Box 733
Ojai, CA 93024
Phone: 805-289-4890
Fax: 805-488-3374
Web Site: www.camerata.thacher.org/
Officers:
    President: Christine Beirne
Management:
    Music Director: Miguel del Aguila
Budget: $35,000
Performs At: Ventura City Hall; Los Angeles County Museum of Art

865 CHAPMAN UNIVERSITY SYMPHONY ORCHESTRA & CHAMBER ORCHESTRA
Chapman University
One University Drive
Orange, CA 92866
Phone: 714-997-6914
Fax: 714-744-7671
Management:
    Music Director/Conductor: John Koshak
    Manager: Samuel Nordcum
    Assistant Manager: David Whitehill
Budget: $100,000-150,000
Facility Category: Concert Hall
Seating Capacity: 999

866 ORANGE COUNTY YOUTH SYMPHONY ORCHESTRA
Chapman University
Orange, CA 92866
Phone: 714-997-6914
Fax: 714-744-7671
Web Site: www.ocyso.org
Management:
    Music Director/Conductor: John Koshak
Budget: $35,000-100,000
Seating Capacity: 999

867 CALIFORNIA YOUTH SYMPHONY
441 California Avenue, #5
Palo Alto, CA 94306
Phone: 650-325-6666
Fax: 650-325-1243
e-mail: info@cys.org
Web Site: www.cys.org
Management:
    Executive Director: James Hogan
    Executive Assistant: Ching Ying Pang

Music Director and Conductor: Leo Eylar
Mission: Offering young musicians the opportunity to perform in a high quality symphony orchestra.
Founded: 1952
Specialized Field: Symphony
Status: Non-Professional; Nonprofit
Paid Staff: 3
Volunteer Staff: 25
Paid Artists: 5
Non-paid Artists: 480
Performs At: Flint Center in Cupertino
Affiliations: American Symphony Orchestra League (Youth Orchestra Division); Association of California Symphony Orchestras
Annual Attendance: 8,000
Organization Type: Performing; Educational

---

868   EL CAMINO YOUTH SYMPHONY

2439 Birch Street
Suite 3
Palo Alto, CA 94306
Phone: 650-327-2611
Fax: 650-327-0338
e-mail: ecys@earthlink.net
Web Site: www.ecys.org
Officers:
    President: Wendy Littman
    VP: Stella Chen
    Secretary: Jean Mach
    Treasurer: Bob Adler
Management:
    Music Director: Dr. Camilla Kolchinsky
    Executive Director: Cathy Spieth
Mission: The El Camino Symphony is dedicated to music education by providing a nurturing environment for the training and development of young musicians from our culturally diverse community and by encouraging a lasting appreciation of music; and music excellence by providing quality performance opportunities for our muscians and presenting outstanding musical events for the community.
Budget: $260,000-1,050,000
Performs At: Spangenburg Theatre

---

869   CHAMBER ORCHESTRA OF THE SOUTH BAY

PO Box 2095
Palos Verdes Peninsula, CA 90274
Phone: 310-373-3151
Fax: 310-373-3151
e-mail: rmiller675@aol.com
Web Site: www.palosverdes.com/chamberorchestra
Officers:
    President: Robert Miller
Management:
    Music Director: Dr. Frances Steiner
Mission: To serve as the only fully-professional classical orchestra resident in a South Bay venue of Los Angeles.
Founded: 1983
Volunteer Staff: 7
Paid Artists: 36
Budget: $130,000-150,000
Income Sources: Ticket Sales; Contributions
Performs At: Norris Theatre for the Performing Arts

Affiliations: American Symphony Orchestra League; Association of California Symphony Orchestra
Annual Attendance: 2,200
Facility Category: Theatre
Type of Stage: Proscenium
Seating Capacity: 450
Year Built: 1983

---

870   COLEMAN CHAMBER CONCERTS

202 S Lake Avenue
Suite 201
Pasadena, CA 91101
Phone: 626-793-4191
Fax: 818-787-1294
e-mail: krfccma@aol.com
Web Site: www.coleman.caltech.edu
Management:
    Executive Director: Kathy R Freedland
Mission: To present international chamber ensembles, both established and emerging.
Founded: 1904
Specialized Field: Chamber
Status: Nonprofit
Paid Staff: 1
Income Sources: Western Alliance of Arts Administrators; Chamber Music America; California Presenters.
Performs At: Beckman Auditorium
Seating Capacity: 1,150
Organization Type: Sponsoring

---

871   PASADENA POPS

20 S Altadena Drive
Pasadena, CA 91107
Phone: 626-792-7677
Fax: 626-792-3410
e-mail: pasadenapops@earthlink.net
Web Site: www.pasadenapops.com
Officers:
    President: Thomas Leddy
    Treasurer: Philip Miles
    Secretary: Gail Belansky
Management:
    Executive Director: Janet Skinner Wells
Status: Professional; Nonprofit

---

872   PASADENA SYMPHONY

2500 E Colorado Boulevard
#260
Pasadena, CA 91107
Phone: 626-793-7172
Fax: 626-793-7180
e-mail: contact@pasadenasymphony.org
Web Site: www.pasadenasymphony.org
Management:
    Music Director: Jorge Mester
    Executive Director: Karine Beesley
Founded: 1928
Specialized Field: Symphony; Orchestra
Status: Professional
Budget: $1,050,000-3,600,000
Performs At: Pasadena Civic Auditorium
Seating Capacity: 2,965
Organization Type: Performing

873 SOUTHWEST CHAMBER MUSIC
595 E Colorado Boulevard
Suite 211
Pasadena, CA 91101
Phone: 626-685-4455
Fax: 626-685-4458
Toll-free: 800-726-7141
e-mail: mail@swmusic.org
Web Site: www.swmusic.org
Management:
  Executive Director: Jan Karlin
  Artistic Director: Jeff von der Schmidt
Mission: Southwest Chamber Music provides Southern California with programs designed to energize and renew the standard repertory of chamber music by intergrating the best of contemporary, world and early music in concerts of wide appeal to the general public.
Performs At: Norton Simon Museum; Colburn School of Performing Arts, Huntington Library
Seating Capacity: 300; 400; 250

874 CALIFORNIA SYMPHONY ORCHESTRA
1603 Oak Park Boulevard
Pleasant Hill, CA 94523
Phone: 925-280-2490
Fax: 925-280-2494
e-mail: info@californiasymphony.org
Web Site: www.californiasymphony.org
Management:
  Music Director: Barry Jekowsky
  Executive Director: Stacey Street
Founded: 1986
Specialized Field: Instrumental music
Paid Staff: 9
Volunteer Staff: 62
Paid Artists: 5
Budget: $1,050,000-3,600,000
Performs At: Hofmann Theatre; Concord Pavilion; Todos Santos Plaza
Annual Attendance: 15,850

875 SHASTA SYMPHONY ORCHESTRA
PO Box 496006
Redding, CA 96049
Phone: 530-225-4761
Fax: 530-225-4830
e-mail: rfiske@shastacollege.edu
Web Site: www.library.shastacollege.edu/music/
Management:
  Music Director: Dr. Richard Allen Fiske
  General Manager: William Justice
Budget: $150,000-260,000
Seating Capacity: 474

876 REDLANDS SYMPHONY ASSOCIATION
1200 E Colton
PO Box 3080
Redlands, CA 92373-0999
Phone: 909-335-5202
Fax: 909-335-5213
e-mail: symphony@redlands.edu
Web Site: www.RedlandsSymphony.com
Officers:
  President: Bob Clark

  VP: Helen Nics
  Secretary: Mary Briccetti
  Treasurer: Phillip Doolittle
Management:
  Executive Director: Walter Collins
  Personnel Contractor: John Gates
  Music Director/Conductor: Jon Robertson
  Office Manager: Denise Derda
Mission: Developing and maintaining an excellent symphony orchestra which offers an annual series of concerts; coordinating outreach programs.
Founded: 1958
Specialized Field: Vocal Music; Instrumental Music
Status: Professional; Nonprofit
Income Sources: American Symphony Orchestra League; Association of California Symphony Orchestras
Performs At: Memorial Chapel; University of Redlands
Organization Type: Performing; Educational

877 BEACH CITIES SYMPHONY
PO Box 248
Redondo Beach, CA 90277
Phone: 310-379-9725
Fax: 310-798-2834
Web Site: www.geocities.com/Athens/Thebes/2642/
Officers:
  Board Chairman: Martin Klood
  President: Robert Peterson
Management:
  Orchestra Manager: Rebecca Rutkowski
  Librarian: John Wisniewski
  Music Director/Conductor: Barry Brisk
Mission: To present an annual season of free masterworks for orchestra in the South Bay.
Founded: 1951
Specialized Field: Symphony
Status: Semi-Professional; Nonprofit
Income Sources: American Symphony Orchestra League; Symphony League of Los Angeles County
Performs At: Darsee Auditorium; El Camino College
Organization Type: Performing

878 REDWOOD SYMPHONY
1031 16th Avenue
Redwood City, CA 94063
Phone: 650-366-6872
Fax: 650-366-6872
e-mail: RedwoodSym@aol.com
Web Site: www.redwoodsymphony.org
Officers:
  Chairman: Kristin Link
Management:
  Music Director/Conductor: Dr. Eric Kujawsky
  Executive Director: Eric Kujawsky
  Public Relations: Griff Derryberry
Founded: 1985
Budget: $35,000
Performs At: Canada College Theater

879 RIVERSIDE COUNTY PHILHARMONIC
PO Box 1601
Riverside, CA 92502
Phone: 909-787-0251
Fax: 909-787-8933

All listings are in alphabetical order by state, then city, then organization within the city.

Management:
   Music Director: Patrick Flynn
   Executive Director: Patricia Korzec
Mission: To provide the Inland area with symphonic music for the general public and provide music education to local schools.
Founded: 1958
Specialized Field: Symphony; Orchestra
Status: Professional; Nonprofit
Paid Staff: 4
Volunteer Staff: 10
Non-paid Artists: 70
Budget: $260,000-1,050,000
Income Sources: Ticket Sales; Contributions; Grants
Performs At: Municipal Auditorium; Gardiner W. Spring Auditorium
Annual Attendance: 1,200
Seating Capacity: 1,600
Organization Type: Performing

880 ORCHESTRA SONOMA

5409 Synder Lane
Rohnert Park, CA 94928
Phone: 707-569-9169
Fax: 707-569-9169
Web Site: www.members.aol.com/orchsonoma/
Management:
   Conductor: Nan Washburn
   Manager: Karen Zimmerman
Budget: $100,000-150,000
Performs At: Spreckels Performing Arts Center

881 CAMELLIA SYMPHONY ASSOCIATION

PO Box 19786
Sacramento, CA 95819
Phone: 916-929-6655
Fax: 916-929-4292
e-mail: camelliaorch@aol.com
Web Site: camelliasymphony.org
Management:
   General Manager: Roberta McCellain
   Music Director/Conductor: Eugene F Castillo
Mission: To expand the growth of music in the Sacramento area by presenting unique repertoire; to provide opportunities for area musicians and composers; to offer performances at reasonable prices.
Founded: 1963
Specialized Field: Orchestra
Status: Semi-Professional; Nonprofit
Paid Staff: 73
Income Sources: American Symphony Orchestra League; Association of California Symphony Orchestras
Performs At: Memorial Auditorium
Annual Attendance: 8,000
Facility Category: Church + Community Center Theater
Seating Capacity: 2400
Organization Type: Performing

882 SACRAMENTO PHILHARMONIC ORCHESTRA

Esquire Plaza Building
1215 K Street, Suite 920
Sacramento, CA 95814
Phone: 916-329-9310
Fax: 916-564-9872
e-mail: sacphil@hotmail.com
Web Site: www.sacramentophiharmonic.org
Officers:
   President: Frank Radoslovich
   Secretary: David G Simon
   Treasurer: Brooks H Erickson
Management:
   Music Director/Conductor: Michael Morgan
   Execuitve Director: Lana Rossi
Budget: $260,000-1,050,000
Performs At: Community Center Theater

883 SACRAMENTO YOUTH SYMPHONY & ACADEMY OF MUSIC

3443 Ramona Avenue
Suite 22
Sacramento, CA 95826
Phone: 916-731-5777
Fax: 916-736-3874
e-mail: office@sacys.org
Web Site: www.sacys.org
   President: Kurt Mathews
   Second VP: Eugene Borack
   Secretary: Pennie Nixon
   Treasurer: Darryl Nixon
Management:
   Music Director: Michael Neumann
   Manager: Jennifer Smart
Budget: $100,000-150,000

884 CHAMBER MUSIC IN NAPA VALLEY

4050 Spring Mounttain Road
Saint Helens, CA 94574
Phone: 707-963-1391
Fax: 707-963-4512
Web Site: www.chambermusicnapa.org
Management:
   Director: John Kongsgaard
Performs At: United Methodist Church
Seating Capacity: 320

885 SAN BERNARDINO SYMPHONY ORCHESTRA

362 W Court Street
San Bernardino, CA 92401
Phone: 909-381-5388
Fax: 909-381-5380
e-mail: sbsymphony@aol.com
Web Site: sanbernardinosymphony.org
Officers:
   President: Mark Edwards
   First VP: Mary Schnepp
   Secretary: Bobbie Terrell
   Treasurer: Lucia Powell
Management:
   Artistic Director: Carlo Pointi Jr
   Director Operations: Judy Brewer
   Administrative Assistant: Jodee Ballard
   Personal Manager: John Gates
Mission: To present regular series of symphonic concerts; to present the best of the musical culture, both popular and classical, of our neighboring country, Mexico. The

San Bernardino Symphony Orchestra is committed to a broadly based program of community musical education through pre-concert lectures and talks from the podium, through docent programs and in-schools instrumental demonstrations.

Founded: 1929
Paid Staff: 2
Volunteer Staff: 25
Paid Artists: 5
Budget: $347,000
Income Sources: Box Office; Donations; Special Events; Fundraising
Performs At: California Theatre for the Arts
Affiliations: American Symphony Council Orchestra; Broadcast Music, Inc.
Facility Category: Theatre
Type of Stage: Wood
Stage Dimensions: 28'x56'
Seating Capacity: 1,728
Year Built: 1928

886 MAINLY MOZART FESTIVAL

121 Broadway
Suite 374
San Diego, CA 921013
Mailing Address: PO Box 124705 San Diego, CA 92112-4705
Phone: 619-239-0100
Fax: 619-233-4292
e-mail: admin@mainlymozart.org
Web Site: www.mainlymozart.org
Officers:
  Chairman: Edward Richards
  President: Christopher Weil
  Treasurer: Jim Rosenfield
  Secretary: Linda Satz
Management:
  Artistic Director: David Atherton
  Executive Director: Nancy S Laturno
  Development Director: Alexandra Pearson
  Director Administration: Dalouge Smith
Founded: 1989
Specialized Field: Classical Music; Jazz; Education
Status: Nonprofit
Paid Staff: 7
Paid Artists: 80
Budget: $700,000 - 800,000
Income Sources: Box Office; Grants; Donations
Affiliations: Spreckels Theatre; Neurosciences Institution
Annual Attendance: 5,000
Seating Capacity: 1,500

887 SAN DIEGO EARLY MUSIC SOCIETY

3510 Dove Court
San Diego, CA 92103-3904
Phone: 619-291-8246
Fax: 619-688-1684
e-mail: sdems@sdems.org
Web Site: www.sdems.org
Officers:
  President: Evelyn Lakoff
  VP: Penelope Hawkins
  Treasurer: Laurent Planchon
  Secretary: Angela Quinn
Management:

  Concert Manager: Vera Kalmijn
Mission: To encourage the appreciation of medieval, renaissance, and baroque music; to present two series of six concerts each, outreach programs, and annual workshop for instrumentalists and vocalists.
Founded: 1981
Specialized Field: Early Music (Classical)
Paid Staff: 1
Budget: $65,000
Income Sources: Box Office; Members; Ads; Grants
Performs At: St. James-by-the-Sea; Sherwood Auditorium At S.D. Museum of Contemporary Art, La Jolla; S.D. Museum of Art
Affiliations: Early Music America; SDPAL
Annual Attendance: 2,500
Seating Capacity: 400; 500; 100

888 SAN DIEGO SYMPHONY ORCHESTRA

1245 7th Avenue
San Diego, CA 92101
Phone: 619-235-0800
Fax: 619-235-0005
e-mail: sandiegosymphony@sandiegosymphony.
Web Site: www.sandiegosymphony.com
Officers:
  President: Ben G Clay
  VP: Harold B Dokmo, Jr
  Treasurer: James Lewis Bowers, PhD
  Secretary: Marilyn Allen Sawyer
Management:
  Executive Director: Douglas Gerhart
  Artistic Director: Jung-Ho Pak
  Office Manager: LeAnna Zevely
  Receptionist: Trivian Lewis
  General Manager/Director Orchestra: Drew Cady
  Controller/Director Finance: Julie Hecker
  Director Marketing: Yvonne Dows
  Development Director: John De Michele
  Production Stage Manager: Elizabeth Stephens
Mission: To present the highest quality performances of classical music to the San Diego community.
Founded: 1910
Specialized Field: Symphony; Orchestra
Status: Professional; Nonprofit
Income Sources: American Symphony Orchestra League; Association of California Symphony Orchestras
Performs At: Copley Symphony Hall
Organization Type: Performing; Educational; Sponsoring

889 SAN DIEGO YOUTH SYMPHONY

PO Box 124670
1650 El Prado, #207A
San Diego, CA 92101
Phone: 619-233-3232
Fax: 619-233-3236
e-mail: sdys@sdys.org
Web Site: www.sdys.org
Management:
  Artistic Director: Jeff Edmons
  Executive Director: Susan Rumley
Mission: Dedicated to the development and enhancement of the musical experience through the teaching and performances of classical repertoire. As the most comprehensive orchestral training program for the youth

of San Diego, we strive to provide each student with outstanding training and performance opportunities through classical music.
Founded: 1945
Specialized Field: Music Education
Paid Staff: 2
Paid Artists: 3
Budget: $150,000-260,000
Performs At: Concert Hall
Seating Capacity: 2,400

890 TIFERETH ISRAEL COMMUNITY ORCHESTRA
6660 Cowles Mountain Boulevard
San Diego, CA 92119-1899
Phone: 619-697-6001
Fax: 619-265-2550
Management:
   Music Director: David Amos
   Manager: Steven Foster
Founded: 1974
Specialized Field: Orchestra in San Diego County
Paid Staff: 3
Volunteer Staff: 70
Paid Artists: 2
Non-paid Artists: 12
Budget: $15,000
Income Sources: Tickets, donations
Annual Attendance: 4000
Facility Category: Social Hall
Seating Capacity: 400-1500

891 CHAMBER MUSIC WEST FESTIVAL
San Francisco Conservatory of Music
1201 Ortega Street
San Francisco, CA 94122
Phone: 415-564-8086
Fax: 415-759-3499
Management:
   Festival Corrdinator: Timothy Bach
Mission: Offering advanced students and faculty the opportunity to perform with outstanding guest artists and providing Bay Area audiences with concerts featuring highly imaginative programming.
Specialized Field: Chamber
Status: Professional; Nonprofit
Performs At: Hellman Hall
Organization Type: Performing; Educational

892 KRONOS QUARTET
1235 A 9th Avenue
PO Box 225340
San Francisco, CA 94122
Phone: 415-731-3533
Fax: 415-664-7590
e-mail: kronos@kronosarts.com
Web Site: www.kronosquartet.org
Officers:
   Chairman: Donlyn Lyndon
   President: David Harrington
   VP: John Sherba
   Treasurer: Hank Dutt
   Secretary: Jennifer Culp
Management:

   Managing Director: Janet Cowperthwaite
   Associate Director: Laird Rodet
   Production Director: Larry Neff
   Office Manager: Leslie Dean Mainer
Mission: To develop, perform, and record new work for the string quartet.
Founded: 1973
Specialized Field: Chamber; Ensemble
Status: Professional; Nonprofit
Paid Staff: 6
Paid Artists: 4
Budget: $1.5 Million
Income Sources: Earned; Contributions
Affiliations: Association of Performing Arts Presenters; Western Arts Alliance; Chamber Music America; National Academy of Recording Arts Sciences
Annual Attendance: 1,000,000
Organization Type: Performing; Touring; Sponsoring

893 MIDSUMMER MOZART FESTIVAL
World Trade Center
#250G
San Francisco, CA 94111
Phone: 415-292-9620
Fax: 415-954-0852
e-mail: wolfgang@midsummermozart.org
Web Site: www.midsummermozart.org
Officers:
   Chairman: James M Rockett
   President: Wendell Rider
   Treasurer: Richard Heath
Management:
   Music Director/Conductor: George Cleve
   Executive Director: Helena Zaludova
   Librarian: Marta Tobey
   Public Relations Manager: Alexandra Ivanoff
   Associate Advisory Administrator: Clark Griffith
Mission: To present the music of Wolfgang Amadeus Mozart to expanding Bay Area audiences through performances of unparalleled excellence.
Founded: 1975
Specialized Field: Instrumental
Status: Professional; Nonprofit
Budget: $10,000
Income Sources: American Symphony Orchestra League; California Confederation of the Arts; Association of California Symphony Orchestras
Season: July
Affiliations: Various venues throughout California
Seating Capacity: 928; 700; 315; 600; 300
Organization Type: Performing

894 NEW CENTURY CHAMBER ORCHESTRA
580 Washington Street
Suite 311
San Francisco, CA 94111
Phone: 415-433-6226
Fax: 415-433-6227
e-mail: nshapiro@ncco.org
Web Site: www.ncco.org
Management:
   Music Director: Krista Bennion Feeney
   Executive Director: Parker E Monroe

Marketing/Audience Coordinator: Nina Shapiro
Mission: The misson of the New Century Chamber Orchestra is to be a virtuoso, conductorless ensemble, which creates - through performance, education, and accessibility, a persons connection with its audience, conveying the passion and joy of the music directly to its listeners.
Founded: 1992
Specialized Field: Music
Paid Staff: 6
Volunteer Staff: 25
Paid Artists: 17

895 PAUL DRESHER ENSEMBLE ELECTRO-ACOUSTIC BAND
Musical Traditions
333 Valencia Street
Suite 301
San Francisco, CA 94103-3552
Phone: 415-558-9540
Fax: 510-843-4057
e-mail: pauld@dresherensemble.org
Web Site: www.dresherensemble.org
Officers:
    President: Paul Dresher
    VP: Robin Kirck
Management:
    Business Manager: Carrie Boram
    Artistic Director: Paul Dresher
    Executive Director: Robin Kirck
Mission: To integrate traditional acoustic instrumentation with the recent advances in musical technology; to create diverse new repertory using the resources of this integration; to break down boundries between different styles.
Founded: 1984
Status: Professional; Nonprofit
Organization Type: Performing; Touring; Educational

896 PHILHARMONIA BAROQUE ORCHESTRA
180 Redwood Street
Suite 200
San Francisco, CA 94102-3281
Phone: 415-252-1288
Fax: 415-252-1488
e-mail: info@philharmonia.org
Web Site: www.philharmonia.org
Management:
    Music Director: Nicholas McGegan
    Executive Director: Robert Birman
    Artistic Director: Jeff Phillips
Mission: The performance of 17th and 18th century music using instruments of the period.
Founded: 1981
Specialized Field: Orchestra; Historical Performance
Status: Professional; Nonprofit
Performs At: Herbst Theatre
Organization Type: Performing; Touring

897 ROVA SAXAPHONE QUARTET
333 12th Street
San Francisco, CA 94103
Phone: 415-487-1701
Fax: 415-487-1501
e-mail: info@rova.org
Web Site: www.rova.org
Management:
    Administrator: David Cook
Mission: An ensemble of musicians from Europe, the US and Canada performing music inspired by jazz and world music.
Founded: 1977
Specialized Field: Jazz Ensemble; New Music Ensemble
Status: Professional; Nonprofit
Paid Staff: 2
Paid Artists: 4
Organization Type: Performing; Touring

898 SAN FRANCISCO COMMUNITY MUSIC CENTER ORCHESTRA
544 Capp Street
San Francisco, CA 94110
Phone: 415-647-6015
Fax: 415-647-3890
e-mail: info@sfmusic.org
Web Site: www.sfmusci.org
Management:
    Conductor/Musical Director: Urs Leonhardt Steiner
    General Manager: Linda Hitchcock
Budget: $100,000-150,000
Performs At: First Congregational Church

899 SAN FRANCISCO CONTEMPORARY MUSIC PLAYERS
44 Page Street
Suite 604A
San Francisco, CA 94102
Phone: 415-252-6235
Fax: 415-621-2533
e-mail: info@sfcmp.org
Web Site: www.sfcmp.org
Officers:
    President: Anne Baldwin
    VP: Didier de Fontaine
    Secretary: Patti Deuter
    Treasurer: Margot Golding
Management:
    Executive Director: Adam L Frey
Mission: To professionally perform contemporary chamber music using a mixed ensemble.
Founded: 1971
Specialized Field: Chamber; Ensemble
Status: Professional; Nonprofit
Paid Staff: 3
Paid Artists: 14
Budget: 300,000
Income Sources: Government and foundation grants; Individual donations; Ticket sales
Performs At: Yerba Buena Center for the Arts
Annual Attendance: 2,000
Facility Category: Arts Center
Seating Capacity: 350-740
Organization Type: Performing; Touring

900 SAN FRANCISCO CONSERVATORY OF MUSIC
1201 Ortega Street
San Francisco, CA 94122
Phone: 415-564-8086
Fax: 415-759-3499
Web Site: www.sfcm.edu
Management:
   President: Colin Murdoch
   Acting Dean: Timothy Bach
   Director Administration: Patricia Berkowitz
Mission: The training of classical musicians for professional careers in performing, composing, conducting and teaching.
Founded: 1917
Specialized Field: Orchestra; Chamber; Ensemble; Electronic & Live Electronic
Status: Nonprofit
Performs At: Hellman Hall
Organization Type: Performing; Educational

901 SAN FRANCISCO JAZZ SPRING SEASON
SF Jazz
3 Embarcadero Center, Lobby Level
San Francisco, CA 94111
Phone: 415-398-5655
Fax: 415-398-5569
Toll-free: 800-850-7353
e-mail: sfjazz@sfjazz.org
Web Site: www.sfjazz.org
Officers:
   Chairman: Fred Brown
   President: Randall Kline
   Treasurer: Michael Lazarus
   Secretary: Corinne Beauvais
Management:
   Publicist: Audrey Faine
   Development Director: Dave Barrett
   Executive Director: Randell Kline
Mission: Offering the finest Bay Area and national jazz performers in San Francisco venues.
Founded: 1983
Specialized Field: Dance; Vocal Music; Instrumental Music; Festivals; Jazz
Status: Professional; Nonprofit
Paid Staff: 22
Volunteer Staff: 300
Paid Artists: 40
Non-paid Artists: 25
Budget: $4 million
Annual Attendance: 30,000
Organization Type: Performing; Resident; Educational

902 SAN FRANCISCO SYMPHONY
Louise M. Davies Symphony Hall
201 Van Ness Avenue
San Francisco, CA 94102
Phone: 415-552-8000
Fax: 415-431-6857
Toll-free: 800-696-9689
e-mail: gleasner@sfsymhpony.org
Web Site: www.sfsymphony.org
Officers:

President: Nancy H Bechtle
Management:
   Executive Director: Brent Assink
   Music Director: Michael Tilson Thomas
   Chorus Administrator: Gregory Boals
   Director Artistic Planning: Gregg Gleasner
   Artistic Administrator: Michael Bartlett
   Director Communications: Karen Ames
   Director Marketing/Sales: Michele L Prisk
   Director: John Kieser
   Technical Director: Timothy Carless
Mission: To achieve recognition as a great orchestra; to serve the community; to attain the appropriate balances of financial and organizational strength.
Founded: 1911
Specialized Field: Symphony; Orchestra
Status: Professional; Nonprofit
Budget: $150,000-400,000
Performs At: Louise M. Davies Symphony Hall; Flint Center
Affiliations: American Symphony Orchestra League; Association of California Symphony Orchestras
Organization Type: Performing; Touring; Resident; Educational

903 SAN FRANCISCO SYMPHONY YOUTH ORCHESTRA
Louise M. Davies Symphony Hall
San Francisco, CA 94102
Phone: 415-552-8000
Fax: 415-431-6857
Management:
   Director Education Programs: Ronald Gallman
   Music Director/Conductor: Alasdair Neale
   Director Youth Orchestra: Ronald Gallman
Mission: To present the best pre-professional, performance training program for Bay Area, young musicians.
Founded: 1981
Specialized Field: Symphony; Orchestra
Status: Non-Professional; Nonprofit
Income Sources: American Symphony Orchestra League (Youth Orchestra Division)
Performs At: Louise M. Davies Symphony Hall
Organization Type: Performing; Touring; Resident; Educational; Sponsoring

904 WOMEN'S PHILHARMONIC
44 Page Street
Suite 604-D
San Francisco, CA 94102
Phone: 415-437-0123
Fax: 415-437-0121
e-mail: info@womensphil.org
Web Site: www.womensphil.org/
Officers:
   President: Robyn Bramhall
   VP: Terrie Baune
   Secretary: Mu'afrida Bell
   Acting Treasurer: Judy Patrick
   Voting Member: Mary Stiles
Management:
   President Board of Directors: Robyn Bramhall
   Executive Director: Kristina Kohler

Program/Development Coordinator: Paul Volstad
Mission: Increase public relations and public awareness of women in classical music, both historical and contemporary, and to advance the careers of women composers, conductors and performers.
Founded: 1981
Specialized Field: Orchestra; Chamber; Ensemble, Advocacy
Status: Professional; Nonprofit
Paid Staff: 2
Volunteer Staff: 20
Paid Artists: 60
Income Sources: American Symphony Orchestra League; Association of California Symphony Orchestras; American Music Conference; American Society of Composers, Authors and Publishers
Performs At: First Congregational Church
Organization Type: Performing; Touring; Resident; Educational

905 HEWLETT-PACKARD SYMPHONY ORCHESTRA

436 River Rock Court
San Jose, CA 95136
Phone: 408-447-3166
Fax: 408-447-2697
e-mail: hpso@hpisrhi.cup.hp.com
Web Site: www.hpl.hp.com/hpsymphony
Management:
Principal Conductor: George Yefchak
Manager: Herb Gellis
Assistant Conductor: Dan Dickerman
Budget: $35,000

906 SAN JOSE CHAMBER MUSIC SOCIETY

PO Box 108
San Jose, CA 95103-0108
Phone: 408-286-5111
Fax: 408-868-0131
e-mail: sjcmsmusik@aol.com
Web Site: www.sjliving.com
Management:
Artistic Director: Ted Lorraine
Founded: 1986
Status: Nonprofit
Income Sources: Donations
Seating Capacity: 340

907 SAN JOSE JAZZ SOCIETY

60 S Market Street
Suite 1150
San Jose, CA 95113
Mailing Address: PO Box 1170 San Jose, CA. 95109
Phone: 408-288-7557
Fax: 408-288-7598
e-mail: jazzmaster@sanjosejazz.org
Web Site: www.sanjosejazz.org
Management:
Associate Director Education: Rob Roman
General Director: Henry A Schiro
Mission: To bring jazz to the Silicon Valley community through performance and education. The San Jose Jazz Society presents jazz to the public in myriad ways including free concerts, festivals, hands-on workshops,

clinics, master classes, commissions for new works, and education and outreach initiatives. SJJS's goal is to enhance the community's awareness of this indigenous music.
Founded: 1986
Specialized Field: Music
Status: Nonprofit
Income Sources: Grants; Donations; Sponsors; Members
Annual Attendance: 150,000

908 SAN JOSE SYMPHONY

100 N Almaden Avenue
San Jose, CA 95110
Phone: 408-287-7383
Fax: 408-286-6391
e-mail: info@sanjosesymphony.org
Web Site: www.sanjosesymphony.org
Officers:
Chairperson: Marie R Bianco
President: Richard S Gourley
Secretary/Treasurer: Michael D McSweeney
Management:
Interim CEO: Richard S Courely
Founded: 1879
Specialized Field: Symphony; Orchestra; Ensemble
Status: Professional; Nonprofit
Paid Staff: 30
Volunteer Staff: 12
Paid Artists: 80
Budget: $6,500,000
Income Sources: Ticket Sales; Donations; Grants
Performs At: Center for Performing Arts; Flint Center
Affiliations: American Symphony Orchestra League, Association of California Symphony Orchestras
Annual Attendance: 200,000
Seating Capacity: 2,600
Organization Type: Performing; Educational

909 SAN JOSE TAIKO GROUP

PO Box 26895
San Jose, CA 95159
Phone: 408-293-9344
Fax: 408-293-9366
e-mail: sjtaiko@taiko.org
Web Site: www.taiko.org
Management:
Managing Director: Roy Hirabayashi
Creative Director: PJ Hirabayashi
Mission: To feature the taiko (Japanese drum) as the principle instrument in a contemporary performing arts form.
Founded: 1973
Specialized Field: Ethnic; Instrumental Group
Status: Professional; Nonprofit
Paid Staff: 1
Paid Artists: 5
Non-paid Artists: 12
Organization Type: Performing; Touring; Educational

910 SOUTH BAY GUITAR SOCIETY

19 N Second Street
Suite 102
San Jose, CA 95113

Phone: 408-292-0704
Fax: 408-280-0407
e-mail: sbgs@sbgs.org
Web Site: www.sbgs.org
Officers:
  President: Jerry Snyder
  VP: Tom Ingalz
  Treasurer: Karel Vystrcil
Management:
  Artistic Director: Daniel Roest
  Director: Stanley Lee
  Director: Rick Rodriguez
  Director: Vern Glick
Mission: To make classical guitar music accessible to people of diverse cultures, ages, abilities and economic means by offering performance opportunities to professional and amateur muscians, providing classical guitar music education, and by presenting the music of many cultures to the public.
Founded: 1986

911 PACIFIC CHAMBER SYMPHONY

1155 East 14th Street
Suite 215
San Leandro, CA 94577
Phone: 510-352-3945
Fax: 510-352-3947
e-mail: cponca@aol.com
Web Site: www.classicalphi.org
Management:
  Music/Executive Director: Lawrence Kohl
  Marketing/Development: Laura Bajuk
Budget: $260,000-1,050,000
Performs At: Neighborhood Theater; Valley Community Theater

912 SAN LUIS OBISPO MOZART FESTIVAL

PO Box 311
San Luis Obispo, CA 93406
Phone: 805-781-3008
Fax: 805-781-3011
e-mail: info@mozartfestival.com
Web Site: www.mozartfestival.com
Officers:
  Associate Conductor: Jeffrey Kahane
Management:
  Music Director: Clifton Swanson
  Executive Director: Curtis Pendleton
Mission: To present a classical music festival highlighting Mozart and other classical and contemporary composers.
Founded: 1970
Specialized Field: Instrumental; Opera; Choral; Jazz; Childrens'; Ethnic; Educational
Status: Professional; Nonprofit
Budget: $150,000-$400,000
Season: July - August
Performs At: Throughout San Luis Obispo County (Festival Sites)
Affiliations: San Luis Performing Arts Center; Wineries; Chapels
Seating Capacity: 1,300
Organization Type: Performing; Educational

913 SAN LUIS OBISPO SYMPHONY

PO Box 658
San Luis Obispo, CA 93406
Phone: 805-543-3533
Fax: 805-781-3534
e-mail: staff@slosymphony.com
Web Site: www.slosymphony.com
Management:
  Music Director: Michael Nowak
  Executive Director: Sandi Sigurdson
Paid Staff: 6
Volunteer Staff: 1
Paid Artists: 75
Budget: $260,000-1,050,000
Income Sources: Ticket Sales; Donations; Grants
Seating Capacity: 1,100

914 CALIFORNIA PHILHARMONIC ORCHESTRA

1120 Huntington Drive
San Marino, CA 91108
Phone: 626-300-8200
Fax: 626-300-8010
e-mail: info@calphil.org
Web Site: www.calphil.org
Officers:
  Chairman: Robert W Miller
  President: Lynn Caffrey Gabriel
  VP: S Robert Zeilstra
  Secretary: Leslie C. Green
  Treasurer: Linda Lowr
Management:
  Music Director: Victor Vener
  Executive Director: Andre C Vener
Mission: To bring excellent professional performances of great music to the widest possible audience.
Founded: 1997
Paid Staff: 10
Volunteer Staff: 500
Paid Artists: 70

915 MARIN SYMPHONY ORCHESTRA

4340 Redwood Highway
Suite 409C
San Rafael, CA 94903-2104
Phone: 415-479-8100
Fax: 415-479-8110
e-mail: greatmusic@marinsymphony.org
Web Site: www.marinsymphony.org
Officers:
  President: Louis Bartolini
  VP: Steve Borden
  Secretary: Abe Froman
  Treasurer: David Bott
Management:
  Artistic Director: Alasdair Neale
  Executive Director: Noralee Monestere
Mission: To bring classical music to the people of Marin County.
Founded: 1952
Paid Staff: 3
Volunteer Staff: 30
Paid Artists: 84
Budget: $260,000-1,050,000

Performs At: Marin Veterans' Auditorium in San Rafael
Seating Capacity: 2,000
Architect: Frank Lloyd Wright

916 MARIN SYMPHONY YOUTH ORCHESTRA

4340 Redwood Highway
Suite 409
San Rafael, CA 94903
Phone: 415-479-8100
Fax: 415-479-8110
Management:
  Conductor/Director MSY Programs: Leslie Stewart
  Conductor: George Thompson
Mission: To provide quality musical training, education and scholarship opportunities for young people in the community.
Founded: 1955
Specialized Field: Symphony Youth Orchestra
Status: Non-Professional; Nonprofit
Paid Staff: 40
Income Sources: American Symphony Orchestra League (Youth Orchestra Division)
Performs At: San Rafael High School Auditorium
Organization Type: Performing; Touring; Educational; Sponsoring

917 PACIFIC SYMPHONY ORCHESTRA

1231 E Dyer Road
Suite 200
Santa Ana, CA 92705-5606
Phone: 714-755-5788
Fax: 714-755-5789
e-mail: pso@pso.org
Web Site: www.pacificsymphony.org
Officers:
  President: John E Forsyte
  Chairman: Michael S Gordon
Management:
  Music Director: Carl St. Clair
  VP: James T Medvitz
Mission: To shape and build a cultural awareness of lasting impact and value.
Budget: $3,600,000-10,000,000
Performs At: Orange County Performing Arts Center

918 MUSIC ACADEMY OF THE WEST SUMMER FESTIVAL

1070 Fairway Road
Santa Barbara, CA 93108
Phone: 805-969-4726
Fax: 805-969-0686
e-mail: festival@musicacademy.org
Web Site: www.musicacademy.org
Officers:
  President: David L Kuehn
Management:
  Artistic Operations Manager: Mirna Gofuken
  Director of Communications: Diane Eagle Kataoka
Mission: To provide the best possible instruction and inspiration for gifted young musicians, instrumental and vocal, through its summer schools and festival.
Founded: 1947
Specialized Field: Summer classical music training

Budget: $1,050,000-3,600,000
Income Sources: Individual Contributions; Foundations; Corporations
Performs At: Lobero Theatre
Annual Attendance: 25,000
Facility Category: 3 Halls
Seating Capacity: 680; 382; 195
Year Built: 1970

919 SANTA BARBARA CHAMBER ORCHESTRA

PO Box 90903
Santa Barbara, CA 93190
Phone: 805-687-7820
Fax: 805-687-8850
e-mail: info@sbco.org
Web Site: www.sbco.org
Officers:
  President: Joe Campanelli
  Chairman: Wendy Edmunds
  CFO: Donald Lafler
  Secretary: Jack Catlett
Management:
  Music Director: Heiichiro Ohyama
  Executive Director: Catherine Richardson
Founded: 1978
Specialized Field: Chamber Orchestra
Paid Staff: 6
Paid Artists: 70
Budget: $430,000
Performs At: Lobero Theatre
Annual Attendance: 11,000

920 SANTA BARBARA SYMPHONY ASSOCIATION

1900 State Street
Suite G
Santa Barbara, CA 93101-2429
Phone: 805-898-9626
Fax: 805-898-9326
e-mail: mail@thesymphony.org
Web Site: www.thesymphony.org
Officers:
  Board President: Linda Hedgepeth
Management:
  Music Director: Gisele Ben-Dor
  Executive Director: John Robinson
Mission: To impel interest in performance, composition, and the lifetime adventure of knowledgeable listening.
Founded: 1953
Paid Staff: 8
Volunteer Staff: 3
Budget: $1,050,000-3,600,000
Performs At: Arlington Theatre
Annual Attendance: 40,000

921 WEST COAST CHAMBER ORCHESTRA

1812 La Coronilla Drive
Santa Barbara, CA 93109
Phone: 805-962-6609
Fax: 805-962-6609
e-mail: info@westcoastsymphony.com
Web Site: www.westcoastsymphony.com

All listings are in alphabetical order by state, then city, then organization within the city.

Mission: To present the finest music at the best possible price and to employ the finest local musicians available.
Founded: 1966
Specialized Field: Symphony; Orchestra; Chamber
Status: Professional; Nonprofit
Paid Staff: 20
Income Sources: Old Spanish Days Fiesta
Performs At: Courthouse; Sunken Gardens; Lobero Theater
Organization Type: Performing

922 SANTA CRUZ BAROQUE FESTIVAL

PO Box 482
Santa Cruz, CA 95061
Phone: 831-457-9693
Fax: 831-425-1260
e-mail: info@scbarique.org
Web Site: www.scbaroque.org
Officers:
  President: William Visscher
  VP: Micheal McKay
  Screetary/Treasurer: Frank Kaehler
Management:
  General Manager: Linda K Fawcett
  Artistic Director: Linda Burman-Hall
Mission: Offering a series of early music concerts each spring.
Founded: 1974
Specialized Field: Instrumental
Status: Professional; Nonprofit
Budget: $10,000-$20,000
Season: February - May
Facility Category: Various auditoriums
Seating Capacity: 400
Organization Type: Performing; Sponsoring

923 SANTA CRUZ COUNTY SYMPHONY

200 7th Avenue
Suite 225
Santa Cruz, CA 95062
Phone: 831-462-0553
Fax: 831-462-0598
e-mail: sccs@santacruzsymphony.com
Web Site: www.santacruzsymphony.com
Management:
  Music Director: John Larry Granger
  Interim Executive Director: Barry Bouifas
Founded: 1957
Paid Staff: 4
Paid Artists: 80
Budget: $260,000-1,050,000
Annual Attendance: 15,000
Facility Category: Civic Auditorium
Seating Capacity: 1,300
Year Built: 1930

924 SCOTT HARRIS BIG BAND

216 Alhambra Avenue
Suite C
Santa Cruz, CA 95062
Phone: 408-248-7999
Fax: 408-248-7900
e-mail: scott@scottharris.com
Management:

Director: Scott Harris
Mission: To present Big Band music of the 1920's-40's purely for audience entertainment.
Founded: 1980
Specialized Field: Instrumental Group; Band; Swing
Status: Professional; Commercial
Paid Staff: 14
Organization Type: Performing; Touring

925 BRENTWOOD-WESTWOOD SYMPHONY ORCHESTRA

1010 19th Street
Suite 8
Santa Monica, CA 90403
Phone: 310-829-3149
Fax: 310-829-3149
Management:
  Founder/Conductor: Alvin Mills
  Executive Secretary: Grusha Paterson Mills
Budget: $100,000-150,000
Performs At: Los Angeles County Museum Broadcast Auditorium

926 LOS ANGELES BAROQUE ORCHESTRA

1007 Montant Avenue
#304
Santa Monica, CA 90403
Phone: 323-664-2535
Fax: 310-393-6423
e-mail: music@labaroque.org
Web Site: www.labaroque.org
Management:
  Music Director: Gregory Maldonado
  Managing Director: Annette Simons
Budget: $260,000-1,050,000
Performs At: Water Garden; Zipper Concert Hall; Miles Memorial Playhouse

927 SANTA MONICA SYMPHONY ORCHESTRA

PO Box 3101
Santa Monica, CA 90403
Phone: 310-841-4152
Fax: 310-838-7411
Web Site: www.smsymphony.org
Officers:
  President: David Bendett
  VP: Nathaniel Trives
  Treasurer: Sonia Luna
  Secretary: Susan McKellar
Management:
  Music Director: Allen Robert Gross
  Executive Director: David Bendett
  Director: Maynard Ostrow
  Director: Innis Richards
  Director: Elizabeth Sheffield
  Director: William Worcester
  Director: Steve Fletcher
  Director: John Dunkelberger
Budget: $35,000-100,000
Seating Capacity: 3,000

928 SANTA ROSA JUNIOR COLLEGE CHAMBER MUSIC SERIES
1501 Mendocino Avenue
Santa Rosa, CA 95401
Phone: 707-527-4372
Fax: 707-527-4870
e-mail: rdunham@santarosa.edu
Management:
   Community Education Director: Roberta Dunham
Performs At: Randolph Newman Auditorium
Seating Capacity: 200

929 SANTA ROSA SYMPHONY
50 Mark W Springs Road
Suite 405
Santa Rosa, CA 95403
Phone: 707-546-8742
Fax: 707-546-0460
e-mail: info@santarosasymphony.com
Web Site: www.santarosasymphony.com
Officers:
   President: Pam Chanter
Management:
   Executive Director: Alan Silow
   Marketing Director: Sara Obuchowski
   Director Finance/Administration: Jed Coffin IV
   Director Development: Connie Wolfe
   Administrative Assistant: Patricia Gingelli
   Education Director: Cindy Weichei
Mission: To inspire and engage people with the highest quality musical performances and educational programs.
Founded: 1927
Specialized Field: Symphony; Orchestra; Chamber; Ensemble
Status: Nonprofit
Paid Staff: 18
Volunteer Staff: 100
Paid Artists: 80
Budget: $2.2 Million
Income Sources: Underwriters, Grants, Donations, Endowments, Ticket Sales
Performs At: Luther Burbank Center for the Arts
Annual Attendance: 50,000
Organization Type: Performing; Resident; Educational

930 NEW VALLEY SYMPHONY ORCHESTRA
PO Box 57018
Sherman Oaks, CA 91413-2018
Phone: 818-773-1095
Fax: 818-789-5402
e-mail: nvso2@aol.com
Officers:
   President: Sarah Fisk
   Treasurer: Chuck Denet
Management:
   Music Director: James A Swift
   Assistant Music Director: Myk Price
Founded: 1970
Paid Staff: 3
Volunteer Staff: 25
Paid Artists: 65
Non-paid Artists: 10
Budget: $35,000-100,000

Income Sources: Donations and Union Trust fund
Performs At: Hall of Liberty
Annual Attendance: 3000
Facility Category: 1500 Seat Auditorium
Type of Stage: very shallow
Stage Dimensions: depth- 30ft

931 STANFORD SYMPHONY ORCHESTRA
Stanford University
Braun Music Center Room 121
Stanford, CA 94305-3076
Phone: 650-723-4304
Fax: 650-725-2686
e-mail: music.dept@forsythe.stanford.edu
Web Site: www.stanford.edu/group/Music
Officers:
   President: Shannon Delaney
   Treasurer: Benjamin Ko
Management:
   Music Director: Ann Krinitsky
   Administrative Director: Mario Champagne
Founded: 1891
Specialized Field: Music
Status: Nonprofit
Paid Staff: 2
Volunteer Staff: 5
Budget: $35,000-100,000
Performs At: Dinkelspiel Auditorium

932 FRIENDS OF CHAMBER MUSIC OF STOCKTON
PO Box 4874
Stockton, CA 95204
Phone: 209-572-7127
Fax: 209-572-7218
e-mail: spencem@sutterhealth.org
Officers:
   President: Michael Spencer
   Secretary: Janet Bonner
   VP: Carole Gilbertson
Management:
   President: Dr. Michael Spencer
   Secrtary: Janet Bonner
   VP: Carole Gilbertson
Mission: Presentation of chamber music.
Founded: 1955
Specialized Field: Chamber Music
Status: Nonprofit
Volunteer Staff: 8
Paid Artists: 19
Income Sources: Ticket Sales
Performs At: Conservatory of Music
Seating Capacity: 900

933 STOCKTON SYMPHONY ASSOCIATION
1151 W Robinhood Drive
Suite C-4
Stockton, CA 95207
Phone: 209-951-0196
Fax: 209-951-1050
e-mail: admin@stocktonsymphony.org
Web Site: www.stocktonsymphony.org
Officers:
   President: Douglas B Wied

VP Finance: Teresa Mandella
VP Board Development: John Vera
VP Fund Development: Leslie Sherman
VP Marketing: Robert A. Penezic
VP Education: Janet Bonner
Treasurer: Sara Cortes
Secretary: Ned Hopkins
Management:
   Music Director/Conductor: Peter Jaffe
   Executive Director: Franklin M Fine
Founded: 1926
Specialized Field: Symphony; Orchestra
Status: Professional; Nonprofit
Income Sources: American Symphony Orchestra League; Association of California Symphony Orchestras
Performs At: San Joaquin Delta College
Organization Type: Performing; Educational

934 UNIVERSITY SYMPHONY ORCHESTRA

University of the Pacific
Stockton, CA 95211
Phone: 209-946-2415
Fax: 209-946-2770
Management:
   Music Director: Dr. Michael A Allard
Budget: $35,000
Performs At: Faye Spanos Concert Hall

935 NOVA VISTA SYMPHONY

PO Box 60312
Sunnyvale, CA 94088
Phone: 408-245-3116
Fax: 408-925-2042
e-mail: novavista@juno.com
Web Site: www.novavista.org
Officers:
   President: Gerald Brady
Management:
   Music Director: Navroj Mehta
Budget: $35,000
Performs At: Foothill College Auditorium

936 CONEJO POPS ORCHESTRA

3648 Mountclef Boulevard
Thousand Oaks, CA 91358
Phone: 805-492-2764
Fax: 805-498-7092
Management:
   Music Director: Elmer Ramsey
Mission: Dedicated to maintaining a non-profit corporation for the education and enhancement of the musical, cultural and social interests of the community, through the medium of a symphony orchestra.
Founded: 1961
Specialized Field: Symphony; Chamber
Status: Semi-Professional; Nonprofit
Paid Staff: 37
Income Sources: American Symphony Orchestra League
Performs At: Preus-Brandt Forum; California Lutheran University
Organization Type: Performing

937 NEW WEST SYMPHONY ASSOCIATION

2100 E Thousand Oaks Boulevard
Suite D
Thousand Oaks, CA 91362
Phone: 805-497-5800
Fax: 805-497-5839
e-mail: info@newwestsymphony.org
Web Site: www.newwestsymphony.org
Officers:
   President: Judy Linton
   Secretary: Shary Carr
   Treasurer/Chair Finance Committee: S Douglas Smith, Jr
Management:
   General Manager: Jim Reeves
   Music Director: Boris Brott
Mission: To present concerts of classical music for the community; to foster and promote an increased public knowledge and appreciation of concert music.
Founded: 1995
Specialized Field: Symphony; Chamber; Ensemble
Status: Professional; Nonprofit
Paid Staff: 8
Budget: $1,500,000
Performs At: Oxnard Civic Auditorium
Annual Attendance: 30,000
Facility Category: Multi-Purpose Theatre
Type of Stage: Proscenium
Organization Type: Performing

938 EL CAMINO COLLEGE - COMMUNITY ORCHESTRA

16007 S Crenshaw Boulevard
Torrance, CA 90506
Phone: 310-660-3732
Fax: 310-660-3792
e-mail: DTETER@elcammo.cc.aa.us
Management:
   Music Director/Conductor: Dane Teter
Mission: To train college musicians; to provide community musicians with an opportunity to read and perform a greater variety of music than in other local groups.
Founded: 1949
Specialized Field: Orchestra
Status: Non-Professional; Nonprofit
Paid Staff: 2
Performs At: Marsee Auditorium
Organization Type: Performing; Educational

939 NEW CENTURY PLAYERS

California Institute of the Arts
24700 McBean Parkway
Valencia, CA 91355
Phone: 661-253-7817
Fax: 661-255-0938
Toll-free: 800-545-2787
e-mail: info@music.calarts.edu
Web Site: www.music.calarts.edu
Officers:
   Secretary: Roxanne Chenault
Management:
   Artistic Director: David Rosenboom

Mission: The ensemble is comprised of accomplished and versatile musicians who merge high-quality performance with skillfull teaching methods and present concerts in traditional chamber music combining performance with commentary.
Founded: 1970
Specialized Field: Symphony; Orchestra; Chamber; Ensemble; Ethnic; Folk; Instrumental Group; Electronic & Live Electronic; Band
Status: Professional; Nonprofit
Performs At: Roy O. Disney Music Hall
Seating Capacity: 75
Year Built: 1970
Year Remodeled: 1994
Organization Type: Resident

940 VALLEJO SYMPHONY ASSOCIATION

3467 Sonoma Boulevard, Suite 10
PO Box 568
Vallejo, CA 94590
Phone: 707-643-4441
Fax: 707-643-5746
e-mail: info@VallejoSymphony.org
Web Site: www.VallejoSymphony.org
Officers:
   President: Karen Clare
   VP: Dan Federick
   Secretary: Mary Eichbauer
   Treasurer: Nanacy Fuller Lett
Management:
   Music Director: David Ramadanoff
   Personnel Manager: Craig McAmis
   Operations Manager: Paul Coddington
   Librarian: Marta Tubey
Founded: 1931
Specialized Field: Symphony Orchestra
Paid Staff: 42
Volunteer Staff: 18
Paid Artists: 85
Budget: $100,000-150,000

941 VICTOR VALLEY SYMPHONY ORCHESTRA

PO Box 160
Victor Valley College
Victorville, CA 92393
Phone: 760-245-4271
Fax: 760-245-9745
Management:
   Music Director/Conductor: KC Manji
   Manager: Art Baker
Budget: $35,000-100,000
Seating Capacity: 493

942 TULARE COUNTY SYMPHONY

200 W Oak Street, PO Box 1201
Tulare County Library Building 2nd Floor
Visalia, CA 93279
Phone: 559-732-8600
Fax: 559-737-4586
e-mail: tcsymph@mindinfo.com
Web Site: www.tcsymphony.org
Officers:
   President: Phil Bourdette

VP: Steve Post
Secretary: Roger Hall
Treasurer: Walter Deissler
Management:
   Music Director/Conductor: David Andre
   General Manager: Brooke Mack
Mission: To promote and foster the appreciation of all music; to further adult participation in creative musical activity; to promote the education and development of young musicians.
Founded: 1960
Specialized Field: Symphony; Orchestra
Status: Professional; Nonprofit
Paid Staff: 2
Volunteer Staff: 20
Paid Artists: 75
Income Sources: Association of California Symphony Orchestras
Performs At: L.J. Williams Theatre
Organization Type: Performing; Resident; Educational

943 DIABLO SYMPHONY ORCHESTRA

1601 Civic Drive
PO Box 2222
Walnut Creek, CA 94595
Phone: 925-295-1401
Fax: 925-685-4143
e-mail: patshirl@infi.net
Web Site: www.cyberfair.gsn.org/woodside/diabsym.htm
Management:
   Music Director/Conductor: Joyce Johnson-Hamilton
   President: Patrick J Campbell
Mission: To provide a community orchestra in which professionally trained classical musicians, with careers other than music, can play quality classical music in a regional arts theater. To make avaliable quality classical music to the community citizens at reasonable ticket prices. To provide a platform for education of young generation performers in classical music to insure continuation of the music.
Founded: 1962
Specialized Field: Symphony; Orchestra
Status: Professional; Nonprofit
Paid Staff: 7
Volunteer Staff: 15
Paid Artists: 12
Budget: 125,000
Income Sources: Tickets; Sponsors; Members; American Symphony Orchestra League; Association of California Symphony Orchestras
Performs At: Regional Arts Center
Affiliations: Yen Liang Annual Youth Artist Competition
Annual Attendance: 7,000
Facility Category: Art Center Music Hall
Type of Stage: 3 Stage Music Hall
Stage Dimensions: 40x50
Seating Capacity: 100; 300; 800
Year Built: 1989
Organization Type: Performing; Sponsoring

944 SACRAMENTO JAZZ JUBILEE

2787 Del Monte Boulevard
West Sacramento, CA 95691

Phone: 916-372-5277
Fax: 916-372-3479
e-mail: stjs@earthlink.net
Web Site: www.sacjazz.com
Management:
 Executive Director: Roger Krum
 Business Manager: Vivan Abraham
Mission: To preserve and promote traditional jazz music.
Founded: 1974
Specialized Field: Jazz
Paid Staff: 5
Budget: $2 million
Income Sources: Admissions; Sponsorships; Grants; Food concession sales; Souvenir sales
Season: May
Affiliations: 40 Sacramento Area Venues (Indoor & Outdoor)
Annual Attendance: 100,000
Seating Capacity: 250-2,500

945 RIO HONDO SYMPHONY ASSOCIATION
PO Box 495
Whittier, CA 90608
Phone: 562-947-5907
e-mail: rhsymphony@gtemail.net
Web Site: www.whittierbiz.com/rhsymphony
Officers:
 President: Louis Galindo
Management:
 Conductor: Wayne Rienecke
Mission: To provide free concerts of symphonic music to all residents of Whittier and surrounding cities known as the Rio Hondo Area; to encourage young talented musicians through Young Artist Auditions.
Founded: 1933
Specialized Field: Symphony; Orchestra
Status: Nonprofit
Paid Staff: 25
Income Sources: Rio Hondo Symphony Guild
Performs At: Whittier Union High School Auditorium
Organization Type: Performing; Resident

946 WHITTIER COLLEGE BACH FESTIVAL
PO Box 634
13406 East Philadelphia Street
Whittier, CA 90608
Phone: 562-907-4237
Fax: 562-907-4237
e-mail: dlozano@whittier.edu
Management:
 Director: Danilo Lozano
Specialized Field: Instrumental
Budget: $10,000
Season: March
Performs At: Whittier College Campus (Festival Site)
Facility Category: Whittier College Memorial Chapel & other venues
Seating Capacity: 300

947 SAN FERNANDO VALLEY SYMPHONY ORCHESTRA
20210 Haynes Street
Winnetka, CA 91306
Phone: 818-347-4807
Fax: 818-883-3148
e-mail: JDomine@aol.com
Web Site: www.sfvsymphony.com/home.htm
Management:
 Music Director: James Domine
Budget: $35,000-100,000

948 WEST VALLEY CHAMBER ORCHESTRA
Pierce College Music Department
6201 Winnetka Avenue
Woodland Hills, CA 91371
Phone: 818-347-0551
Fax: 810-710-2943
Management:
 Conductor: Rowan Taylor
 Assistant Director: Timothy J Durand
Mission: To offer free concerts to the community year-round.
Founded: 1972
Specialized Field: Orchestra
Status: Non-Professional; Nonprofit
Paid Staff: 15
Organization Type: Performing; Resident; Educational

949 HARMONIA BAROQUE PLAYERS
19795 Villager Circle
Yorba Linda, CA 92886-4452
Phone: 714-970-8545
Fax: 714-970-8439
e-mail: gmfrankl@earthlink.net
Web Site: www.ocartsnet.org/harmonia/
Management:
 Director: Marika Frankl
Mission: Harmonia Baroque has been established to perform rich and plentiful repertoire written for small ensembles in the Renaissance and Baroque period. The ensemble is committed to perform not only the popular works, but also the lesser-known masterpieces of these times. The groups is also deeply committed to providing affordable and high quality performances.
Founded: 1984
Specialized Field: Baroque Chamber Music
Volunteer Staff: 15
Non-paid Artists: 6
Income Sources: Box Office; Private Donations
Season: 9 concerts annually
Performs At: Three Southern California Churches
Affiliations: Arts Orange County
Annual Attendance: 700

Colorado

950 BOULDER BACH FESTIVAL
PO Box 1896
Boulder, CO 80306
Phone: 303-494-3159
Fax: 303-494-4940
e-mail: BolderBach@aol.com
Web Site: www.boulderbachfest.org
Management:

Music Director: Robert Spillman
Executive Director: Cheryl Staats
Specialized Field: Instrumental; Choral
Paid Staff: 1
Volunteer Staff: 200
Paid Artists: 40+
Budget: $100,000
Income Sources: Admissions; donations; grants
Season: January
Performs At: Boulder (Festival Site)
Affiliations: First Prebyterian Church
Annual Attendance: 2,500
Seating Capacity: 800

951 BOULDER PHILHARMONIC ORCHESTRA

Dairy Center for the Arts
250 Walnut Street, Suite 6
Boulder, CO 80302-5700
Phone: 303-449-1343
Fax: 303-443-9203
e-mail: info@peakarts.org
Web Site: www.peakarts.org
Management:
   Executive Director: William Lightfoot
   Conductor/Music Director: Oswald Lehnert
Mission: To enhance lives through the experience of arts, by providing access, creating connections and preserving creativity.
Founded: 1956
Specialized Field: Symphony; Orchestra
Status: Non-Professional; Nonprofit
Paid Staff: 60
Income Sources: American Symphony Orchestra League; Western Alliance of Arts Administrators
Performs At: Macky Auditorium Concert Hall
Organization Type: Performing; Sponsoring

952 SINFONIA OF COLORADO
Dairy Center for the Arts

2590 Walnut Street
Suite 6
Boulder, CO 80302
Phone: 303-449-1343
Fax: 303-443-9203
e-mail: info@peakarts.com
Web Site: www.peakarts.com
Management:
   Music Director: Theodore Kuchar
   Executive Director: William C Lightfoot
Founded: 1997
Budget: $150,000-260,000
Performs At: First Presbyterian Church; Trinity Church

953 BRECKENRIDGE MUSIC INSTITUTE ORCHESTRA

PO Box 1254
217 S Ridge Street
Breckenridge, CO 80424
Phone: 970-453-9142
Fax: 970-453-9143
e-mail: bmynro@breckenridgemusicfestival.net
Web Site: www.breckenridgemusicfestival.net

Management:
   Music Director: Gerhardt Zimmermenn
   Executive Director: Jeff D Braum
   Administrator/Marketing/Programs: Sara Anton
Mission: Provide musicians the experience necessary to enhance their skills through an intense repertory performance experience.
Specialized Field: Instrumental; Multi-media; Opera; Choral; Jazz; Folk; Theatre; Educational
Paid Staff: 16
Volunteer Staff: 35
Budget: $260,000-1,050,000
Performs At: Riverwalk Center
Facility Category: Amphitheater
Seating Capacity: 750

954 NATIONAL REPERTORY ORCHESTRA

PO Box 6336
217 S Ridge Street
Breckenridge, CO 80424
Phone: 970-453-9142
Fax: 970-453-9143
e-mail: bmi@sni.net
Web Site: www.sni.net/bmi-nro
Management:
   Conductor: Carl Topilow
   Executive Director: Jeff Baum
   Administrator/Marketing/Programs: Kaye E Mers
Mission: Education and performance.
Paid Staff: 16
Volunteer Staff: 35
Budget: $260,000-1,050,000
Performs At: Riverwalk Center at Breckenridge
Facility Category: Amphitheater
Seating Capacity: 750

955 COLORADO SPRINGS SYMPHONY ORCHESTRA

619 N Cascade
PO Box 1692
Colorado Springs, CO 80901
Phone: 719-633-4611
Fax: 719-633-6699
e-mail: lori@cssymphony.org
Web Site: www.cssymphony.org
Officers:
   President: Shawn Raintree
   VP: Denny Weber
   VP: Nora Courier
   Treasurer: Ann Fetsch
   Secretary: Dr. Pam Shockley
   Past President: Mary Ellen McNally
   President-Elect: Penny Whitney
Management:
   Executive Director: Daniel J Hart
   Conductor/Music Director: Christopher Wilkins
   Director Marketing/Development: Douglas Ismail
   Music Director: Lawrence Smith
Mission: To offer symphonic music; to sponsor other performing-arts productions and music education programs in the schools.
Founded: 1922
Specialized Field: Symphony; Orchestra; Chamber
Status: Professional; Nonprofit

Income Sources: National Endowment for the Arts; American Symphony Orchestra League
Performs At: Pikes Peak Center
Organization Type: Performing; Educational; Sponsoring

---

956 **CRESTED BUTTE CHAMBER MUSIC FESTIVAL**
PO Box 992
Crested Butte, CO 81224
Phone: 970-349-5864
Fax: 970-349-5864
Management:
  Artistic Director: Claire Jolivet
  Administrative Director: Karrie Tenley
Specialized Field: Instrumental; Choral; Folk; Ethnic
Budget: $20,000-$35,000
Season: July - August
Performs At: Crested Butte, CO (Festival Site)
Facility Category: Crested Butte Chamber Music Festival
Seating Capacity: 250

---

957 **COLORADO SYMPHONY ORCHESTRA**
999 18th Street
Suite 2055
Denver, CO 80202
Phone: 303-292-5566
Fax: 303-293-2649
e-mail: admin@coloradosymphony.org
Web Site: www.coloradosymphony.org
Officers:
  President/CEO: Del Hock
  Chairman Board of Trustees: Jerome Kern
  Vice Chair: Cy Harvey
Management:
  Associate Conductor: Adam Flatt
  Executive Assistant/ Office Manager: Kristina Morise
Mission: To be recognized as Colorado's premier full-time professional symphonic music resource.
Founded: 1922
Specialized Field: Symphony; Orchestra
Status: Professional; Nonprofit
Paid Staff: 23
Paid Artists: 134
Non-paid Artists: 250
Budget: $2.4 Million
Income Sources: Ticket Revenue; Donations From Individuals; Foundations; Businesses; Public Agencies
Performs At: Boettcher Concert Hall
Annual Attendance: 150,000
Facility Category: Concert hall, performance center
Type of Stage: In the round
Stage Dimensions: 35 x 80
Orchestra Pit: 1
Seating Capacity: 2,684
Year Built: 1974
Organization Type: Performing; Touring; Resident; Educational; Sponsoring
Resident Groups: Colorado Symphony Orchestra

---

958 **DENVER MUNICIPAL BAND**
2253 Bellaire Street
Denver, CO 80207
Phone: 303-388-0183
Fax: 303-322-8608
Web Site: www.dmamusic.org/dmb/
Management:
  Conductor: Ed Lenicheck
  Manager: Gerald Endsley
Mission: Presenting free summer concerts in Denver parks.
Founded: 1891
Specialized Field: Band
Status: Professional
Income Sources: Association of Concert Bands
Organization Type: Performing

---

959 **DENVER YOUNG ARTISTS ORCHESTRA**
2828 Speer Boulevard
Suite 230
Denver, CO 80211
Phone: 303-433-2420
Fax: 303-433-2428
e-mail: info@dyao.org
Web Site: www.dyao.org
Management:
  Music Director: Adam Flatt
Paid Staff: 2
Volunteer Staff: 10
Paid Artists: 2
Non-paid Artists: 85
Budget: $150,000
Income Sources: Grants; Ticket sales; Member fees
Performs At: Boettcher Concert Hall
Affiliations: Colorado Chamber Players
Annual Attendance: 5,000

---

960 **SAN JUAN SYMPHONY**
PO Box 1073
Durango, CO 81302
Phone: 970-259-2342
Fax: 970-247-7520
e-mail: navarro@sanjuansymphony.com
Web Site: www.sanjuansymphony.com
Officers:
  President: Diane Van Berg
Management:
  Executive Director: Marge Navarro
  Music Director: Arthur Post
Founded: 1973
Specialized Field: Symphony Orchestra
Budget: $35,000- $100,000
Income Sources: Foundation Grants
Affiliations: ASOL
Annual Attendance: 4000
Seating Capacity: 800/ 600

---

961 **ARAPAHOE PHILHARMONIC**
4301 S Broadway
Suite 103
Englewood, CO 80110-5786
Phone: 303-781-1892
Fax: 303-781-4918
e-mail: apo@qadas.com
Web Site: www.arapahoe.phil.org
Management:

Music Director/Conductor: Vincent C LaGuardia, Jr
Orchestra Administrator: Suzi Piegols
Mission: Dedicated to providing quality live orchestra performances for the community's enjoyment, appreciation and education.
Founded: 1953
Specialized Field: Symphony (Volunteer)
Budget: $35,000-100,000
Income Sources: Box Office; Donations; Grants
Performs At: Orchard Road Christian Church
Annual Attendance: 5,000

962 COLORADO STATE UNIVERSITY ORCHESTRA
Colorado State University
Music Department
Fort Collins, CO 80523-1778
Phone: 970-491-5529
Fax: 970-491-7541
Management:
　Manager/Conductor: Dr. William Runyan
Budget: $35,000
Seating Capacity: 700

963 FORT COLLINS SYMPHONY ORCHESTRA
PO Box 1963
Fort Collins, CO 80522
Phone: 970-482-4823
Fax: 970-482-4858
e-mail: note@fcsymphony.org
Web Site: www.fcsymphony.org
Officers:
　President: Jody Johnson
　VP: Steve Hogan
　Secretary: Sharyn Salmen
　Treasurer: Rex Wells
Management:
　Executive Director: Donna Visocky
Mission: To educate, entertain, and enhance the cultural environment.
Founded: 1949
Paid Staff: 4
Volunteer Staff: 100
Paid Artists: 100
Budget: $391,000
Income Sources: Individual and corporate donations; Foundations
Performs At: Lincoln Center Auditorium
Affiliations: American Symphony Orchestra League
Annual Attendance: 10,000
Facility Category: City Auditorium Concert Hall
Type of Stage: Proscenium
Seating Capacity: 1,180
Year Remodeled: 1979
Rental Contact: David Siever

964 JEFFERSON SYMPHONY ORCHESTRA
1806 Jackson Avenue
PO Box 546
Golden, CO 80401

Phone: 303-278-4237
Fax: 303-278-1205
e-mail: jsomusic@juno.com
Web Site: www.jeffersonsymphony.com
Officers:
　President: Jack Galland
　VP Finance: Larry Lucero
　VP Activities: Helen Leith
　VP Performance: Joan Havercroft
　Secretary: John Bluner
　Treasurer: Jellymmeison Nichols
　VP Marketing: Doris McGowan
Management:
　Office Manager: Monika Taylor
　Bookkeeper: Dawn Reitmair
　Fundraiser: Bob Kliner
　Music Director/Conductor: T Gordon Parks
Mission: To provide performing opportunities for serious musicians; to provide good symphonic music; to maintain a position which educates the public of all ages to the pleasure of classical and light classical music.
Founded: 1953
Specialized Field: Symphony; Orchestra; Ensemble
Status: Semi-Professional; Nonprofit
Paid Staff: 2
Volunteer Staff: 150
Budget: $275,000
Income Sources: Chamber of Commerces
Performs At: Green Centre; Colorado School of Mines
Annual Attendance: 5000
Facility Category: auditorium
Seating Capacity: 1,100
Year Built: 1973
Organization Type: Performing

965 GRAND JUNCTION MUSICAL ARTS ASSOCIATION
225 N 5th #120
Grand Junction, CO 81501
Phone: 970-243-6787
Fax: 970-243-6792
e-mail: info@gjsymphony.org
Web Site: www.gjsymphony.org
Management:
　Manager: Cynthia Rhodes
　Music Director: Kirk Gustafson
Mission: To provide Western Colorado with high quality classical music.
Founded: 1977
Specialized Field: Symphony; Orchestra; Band; Chorus; Children's Choir
Status: Nonprofit
Performs At: Grand Junction High School Auditorium
Organization Type: Performing; Touring; Educational; Sponsoring

966 GREELEY PHILHARMONIC ORCHESTRA
801 8th Street
Suite 220F
Greeley, CO 80631-3900

Mailing Address: PO Box 1535, Greeley CO. 80632-1535
Phone: 970-356-6406
Fax: 970-352-8761
e-mail: greeley.phil@juno.com
Officers:
   President: John T Coppom
   VP: Bill Kehl
   Treasurer: Brad Ewing
   Secretary: Dimitria Hurst
Management:
   Conductor: Howard Skinner
   Administrator: Merte Cunningham
Founded: 1911
Specialized Field: Symphonic Orchestra Performances
Paid Staff: 4
Paid Artists: 80
Budget: $260,000-1,050,000
Income Sources: Tickets; Grants; Fund Drives; Sponsors
Performs At: Union Colony Civic Auditorium
Annual Attendance: 12,000
Facility Category: Performance Hall
Seating Capacity: 1,665
Year Built: 1984
Rental Contact: Jill Dominghez

967 SYMPHONY, OPERA & CHAMBER ORCHESTRA

University Orchestras
Fraiser 18, 401 20th Street
Greeley, CO 80639
Mailing Address: Box 28 Greeley, CO 80639
Phone: 970-351-2273
Fax: 970-351-2639
e-mail: rguyver@arts.unco.edu
Web Site: www.arts.unco.edu/music/orchestras.html
Management:
   Director Orchestras: Dr. Russell Guyver
   Administrative Assistant: Liz Mares
Budget: $35,000
Income Sources: Fees
Performs At: Union Colony Civic Center; Foundation Hall

968 UNIVERSITY OF NORTHERN COLORADO SYMPHONY ORCHESTRA

University Orchestras
Fraiser 18
Greeley, CO 80639
Phone: 970-351-2385
Fax: 970-351-1923
e-mail: artsinfo@arts.unco.edu
Web Site: www.arts.unco.edu/music/orchestras.html
Management:
   Music Driector: Dr. Russell Guyver
   Program Assistant: Julie-Ann Jordan
Budget: $35,000
Performs At: Union Colony Civic Center; Foundation Hall

969 LONGMONT SYMPHONY ORCHESTRA

PO Box 74
Longmont, CO 80502
Phone: 303-772-5796
Fax: 303-678-0642
Web Site: www.longmont.com/lso
Management:
   Music Director: Dr. Robert Olson
   Executive Director: Natasha Tiff
Budget: $150,000-260,000
Performs At: Vance Brand Civic Auditorium

970 PUEBLO SYMPHONY ORCHESTRA

2200 Bonfort Boulevard
Pueblo, CO 81001
Phone: 719-549-2385
Fax: 719-549-2468
Management:
   Executive Director: Tom Christner
   Music Director/Conductor: Jacob Chi
Mission: The symphony presents eclectic programs appealing to many different tastes, and engages in a variety of educational and community outreach programs, and sponsors the Pueblo Youth Symphony.
Founded: 1928
Specialized Field: Orchestra
Status: Nonprofit
Income Sources: American Symphony Orchestra League
Performs At: Memorial Hall; Hoag Hall; University of Southern
Organization Type: Performing

971 STRINGS IN THE MOUNTAINS

1875 Ski Time Square Drive
PO Box 774627
Steamboat Springs, CO 80477
Phone: 970-879-5056
Fax: 970-879-7460
e-mail: strings@stringsinthemountains.org
Web Site: www.stringsinthemountains.org
Officers:
   President/CEO: Kay Clagett
   Financial Manager: Anne Degroff
Management:
   Music Director: Katherine Collier
   Music Director: Yizhak Schotten
   Artistic Director: Andres Cardenes
   Executive Director/Festival Manager: Betse Grassby
   Marketing/Development Director: Sheri Steiner
   Youth Program Dir/Facility Manager: Jessie Burns
Mission: Dedicated to presenting the highest possible quality chamber music in the inspiring atmosphere of Steamboat Springs.
Founded: 1988
Specialized Field: Instrumental; Opera; Jazz; Childrens' Chamber Music
Status: Professional; Nonprofit
Paid Staff: 5
Volunteer Staff: 125
Paid Artists: 170
Budget: $1,000,000
Income Sources: American Symphony Orchestra League; Chamber Music America; Western Arts Alliance; Private and Corporate Donations; Grants; Ticket Sales
Season: July - August
Performs At: Tensile Fabric Structure
Facility Category: Strings Music Tent
Stage Dimensions: 13'x30'

Seating Capacity: 540
Year Built: 1982
Rental Contact: Facility Manager Jessie Burns
Organization Type: Performing

972 TYER CHAMBER MUSIC FESTIVAL

PO Box 115
Telluride, CO 81435
Phone: 970-728-8686
Fax: 970-728-8686
Toll-free: 800-525-3455
e-mail: klangs@rmi.net
Web Site: www.telluride.com/chamber.html
Management:
   Director: Roy Malan
   Director: Robin Sutherford
   President: Kay Langstaff
Specialized Field: Instrumental
Budget: $10,000
Season: August
Performs At: Telluride [Festival Site]
Facility Category: Sheridan Opera House
Seating Capacity: 240

Connecticut

973 HARTFORD JAZZ SOCIETY

116 Cottage Grove Road
Room 204
Bloomfield, CT 06002
Phone: 860-242-6688
Fax: 830-242-6688
Management:
   President: Betty Ector
   Program Director: Bill Sullivan
Mission: Dedicated to presenting 7-11 concerts a year in
Hartford, promoting and keeping jazz music alive in the
area and offering community programs on jazz.
Founded: 1960
Specialized Field: Jazz
Status: Professional
Performs At: Hartford Holiday Inn
Organization Type: Sponsoring

974 GREATER BRIDGEPORT SYMPHONY ORCHESTRA

446 University Avenue
Bridgeport, CT 06604
Phone: 203-576-0263
Fax: 203-367-0064
Web Site: www.bridgeportsymphony.org
Officers:
   Chairman: Robert S Tellalian
   President: Richard Hiendlmayr
   VP: Thomas Trotta
   Treasurer: H. Michael Keden
   Assitant Treasurer: Humphrey T. Nichols, II
   Corporate Secretary: Barbara P. Bellinger
   Recording Secretary: Jena Maric
Management:
   Music Director/Conductor: Gustav Meier
   Executive Director: Jena Maric

Founded: 1945
Budget: $260,000-1,050,000
Performs At: Klein Memorial Auditorium
Facility Category: Auditorium
Seating Capacity: 1,468

975 ASTON MAGNA FOUNDATION FOR MUSIC AND THE HUMANITIES

PO Box 3167
Danbury, CT 06813
Phone: 203-792-4662
Fax: 203-744-7244
Toll-free: 800-875-7156
e-mail: info@astonmagna.org
Web Site: www.astonnmagna.org
Officers:
   Chairman: Robert B Strassler
Management:
   Executive Director: Ronnie Boriskin
   Artistic Director: Daniel Stepner
   Academy/Outreach Director: Raymond Erickson
   Festival Administrator: Joseph Oorchard
   Academy/Outreach Administrator: Constance
   Baldwin
   Business Manager: Florence Lynch
Mission: Presenting baroque and classical music on
period instruments; sponsoring educational programs
connecting the music with the society and culture in
which it was written.
Founded: 1972
Specialized Field: Chamber; Early Music
Status: Professional; Nonprofit
Paid Staff: 4
Volunteer Staff: 6
Performs At: St. James Church Festival in Great
Barrington, MA
Organization Type: Performing; Touring; Educational;
Sponsoring

976 DANBURY MUSIC CENTRE

256 Main Street
Danbury, CT 06810
Phone: 203-748-1716
Fax: 203-794-1308
e-mail: dmc1935@snet.net
Web Site: www.danbury.org/MusicCtr
Officers:
   President: Dennis Nazzaro
   Secretary: John W Cherry
   Treasurer: Dawn Ellen Whaley
Management:
   Executive Director: Nancy F Sudik
Mission: To sponsor musical organizations, instrumental
and vocal, in which persons of a wide variety of musical
backgrounds are encouraged to study and to perform
classical and modern compositions to improve their
ability and to share the joy of music with the people of
greater Danbury.
Founded: 1935
Specialized Field: Music, Primarily Classical
Status: Semi-Professional; Non-Professional; Nonprofit
Paid Staff: 15
Volunteer Staff: 35
Paid Artists: 20

Non-paid Artists: 800
Budget: $240,000
Income Sources: Private Support; Corporate & Businesses; City & State; Grants; Trustfunds; Tuition; Tickets
Performs At: Marian Anderson Recital Hall
Annual Attendance: 12,000
Seating Capacity: 175 - 1,200
Organization Type: Performing; Educational; Sponsoring

977 GREATER BRIDGEPORT SYMPHONY YOUTH ORCHESTRA
PO Box 645e
Fairfield, CT 06430-0645
Phone: 203-227-6695
e-mail: bupton2@aol.com
Web Site: www.gbyo.org
Management:
   Music Director: Robert Genualdi
   General Manager: Barb Upton
Mission: To offer young musicians in the Greater Bridgeport area a quality orchestral experience.
Founded: 1961
Specialized Field: Symphony; Orchestra
Status: Non-Professional
Performs At: Fairfield High School
Organization Type: Performing; Educational

978 CONNECTICUT PHILHARMONIC ORCHESTRA
1127 W Putnam Avenue
Room 207
Greenwich, CT 06230
Phone: 828-253-3315
Fax: 828-258-0357
e-mail: RHBAKER@prodigy.net
Management:
   Music Director: Robert Hart Baker
   General Manager: Alexander Kopple
Mission: To give orchestra concerts to the New York, New Jersey, Connecticut metro area.
Founded: 1976
Specialized Field: Symphony Orchestra
Budget: $35,000-100,000
Income Sources: Ticket Sales, Donations
Performs At: Various Auditoriums

979 GREENWICH SYMPHONY ORCHESTRA
PO Box 35
Greenwich, CT 06836
Phone: 203-869-2664
Fax: 203-622-3980
Web Site: www.greenwichsym.org
Officers:
   President: Richard W. Radcliffe
Management:
   Conductor/Musical Director: David Gilbert
Mission: To offer a subscription series, youth concert series and chamber players series.
Founded: 1958
Budget: $260,000-1,050,000
Facility Category: Greenwich High School Auditorium
Seating Capacity: 850

980 SYMPHONY ON THE SOUND
RD 1, 18 Zygmont Lane
Greenwich, CT 06830
Phone: 203-661-7413
Fax: 203-661-7413
Management:
   Music Director/Conductor: Joseph Leniado-Chira
   General Manager: PM Lewis
Budget: $35,000-100,000

981 CHAMBER MUSIC PLUS
PO Box 231463
Hartford, CT 06123
Phone: 860-278-7148
Fax: 860-278-7248
e-mail: cmp@chambermusicplus.org
Web Site: www.chambermusicplus.org
Management:
   Co-Founder/Artistic Director: Harry Clark
   Co-Founder/Pianist: Sanda Schuldmann
Founded: 1980
Paid Staff: 3
Paid Artists: 8
Budget: $400,000

982 CONNECTICUT CLASSICAL GUITAR SOCIETY
PO Box 1528
Hartford, CT 06114-1528
Phone: 860-249-7041
Fax: 860-693-2651
e-mail: info@ccgs.org
Web Site: www.ccgs.org
Officers:
   Executive Director: Beatrice Birdman
Management:
   Artistic Director: Daniel Salazar
Mission: To serve the general public and classical guitarists by providing a forum for listening, learning, performing and teaching.
Founded: 1985
Income Sources: Funded in part by the Connecticut Commission of the Arts; The Greater Hartford Arts Council; Takamine Guitar; The Roberts Foundation: The D'Addario Foundation

983 HARTFORD SYMPHONY ORCHESTRA
228 Farmington Avenue
Hartford, CT 06105-3596
Phone: 860-246-8742
Fax: 860-247-1720
e-mail: info@hartfordsymphony.com
Web Site: www.hartfordsymphony.org
Officers:
   President: Millard H Pryor, Jr.
   VP Finance: Thomas R Wildman, Esquire
   VP Marketing: Robinson A Grover
   VP Administration: John H. Beers
Management:
   Executive Director: Charles Owens
   Orchestra Manager: Keith Powell
Mission: To bring music and educational programs of the highest artistic standards to the widest possible audience.
Founded: 1934

Performs At: Bushnell
Annual Attendance: 142,000
Seating Capacity: 2,805

984 MANCHESTER SYMPHONY ORCHESTRA/CHORALE

PO Box 861
Manchester, CT 06045-0906
Phone: 860-659-8260
e-mail: musicsix@cox.net
Web Site: www.msoc.org
Officers:
    President: Sherrill Stott
    VP: Ann Benson Frost
    Treasurer: John Belbruno
Management:
    Chorale Artistic Director: Mark Bailey
    Orchestra Artistic Director: Per Brevig
Mission: To offer a performing outlet for talented volunteers and bring good classical music to the community.
Founded: 1960
Specialized Field: Symphony; Orchestra; Chorale
Status: Non-Professional; Nonprofit; Volunteer; Community
Paid Staff: 150
Income Sources: Artist-in-Residence Manchester High School
Performs At: Manchester High School
Organization Type: Performing; Resident

985 MERIDEN SYMPHONY ORCHESTRA

PO Box 124
Meriden, CT 06450
Phone: 203-238-3855
Fax: 203-686-0172
Officers:
    President: Dr. Daniel Schwartz
Management:
    Personnel Manager: Marta Boratgis
    Marketing Director: Brenda J Vumbaco
Mission: To perform 3-4 concerts per season and one free Independence Day concert.
Founded: 1948
Volunteer Staff: 10
Budget: $100,000-150,000
Income Sources: Grants; Donations; Box Office
Annual Attendance: 3,000

986 NEW BRITAIN SYMPHONY ORCHESTRA

PO Box 1253
New Britain, CT 06050-1253
Phone: 860-826-6344
Fax: 860-826-6344
e-mail: nbso@msn.com
Web Site: www.geocities.com/nbsymph2000
Management:
    Conductor: Jerome Laszloffy
    Executive Director: Gina Kahn
Mission: Performs annual four-concert seasons, additional outdoor concerts and varied music enrichment programs for school children. Comprised of more than 65 instrumentalists and engages selected guest artists.

Founded: 1950
Specialized Field: Symphony; Orchestra
Status: Nonprofit
Performs At: Vincent Sala Auditorium; New Britain High School
Organization Type: Performing

987 SILVERMINE GUILD CHAMBER MUSIC SERIES

1037 Silvermine Road
New Canaan, CT 06840
Phone: 203-996-9700
Fax: 203-996-2763
Management:
    Coordinator: Carol Nordgren
Performs At: Gillford Hall

988 CONNECTICUT CHAMBER ORCHESTRA

PO Box 3398
New Haven, CT 06515
Phone: 860-612-4371
Fax: 860-612-4371
Management:
    Music Director/Conductor: Sayard Stone
    Manager: Sheila Gardiner
Mission: Connecticut's first chamber orchestra has performed in several European cities and in Mexico. In addition to its regular performances in New Haven, the orchestra plays for elementary students, sponsors choral and band festivals for high school students and sponsors the Young Artists Concerts.
Budget: $35,000-100,000

989 NEW HAVEN SYMPHONY ORCHESTRA

70 Audubon Street
3rd Floor
New Haven, CT 06510
Phone: 203-865-0831
Fax: 203-789-8907
Toll-free: 800-292-6476
e-mail: newhavensymphony@cshore.com
Web Site: www.newhavensymphony.com
Officers:
    Officer: Charles A O'Malley III
    President: Robert Dannies
Management:
    Executive Director: Michael MacLeod
    Director Development: Jim Wright
    Box Officer Manager: Don Hackett
    Administrative Assistant: Dorian Trifiro
Mission: The New Haven Orchestra is one of the oldest orchestras in the United States. Concerts take place in Woolsey Hall on the Yale University Campus, and the symphony also performs at schools, public parks and community centers in pursuit of our mission to reach a diverse audience and promote excellence in the performing arts.
Founded: 1894
Specialized Field: Orchestral Music
Paid Staff: 13
Paid Artists: 70
Budget: $2 million

Income Sources: Box Office; Sponsorship; Individual Contribution
Performs At: Woolsey Hall
Annual Attendance: 100,000

---

990 PHILHARMONIA ORCHESTRA OF YALE
PO Box 208246
New Haven, CT 06520-8246
Phone: 203-432-1978
Fax: 203-432-7448
e-mail: glenn.mortimer@yale.edu
Web Site: www.yale.edu/schmus
Management:
   Artistic Director: Lawrence Leighton Smith
   Manager: Glenn Mortimer
Budget: $35,000
Performs At: Woolsey Hall

---

991 EASTERN CONNECTICUT SYMPHONY
289 State Street
New London, CT 06320
Phone: 860-443-2876
Fax: 860-444-7601
e-mail: ectsymphony@snet.net
Web Site: www.ectsymphony.com
Officers:
   President: Alan Proctor
   VP: Neil Ruenzel
   Secretary: Tom Castle
   Treasurer: David Zuckerbraun
Management:
   Executive Director: Isabelle G Singer
   Assistant to the Executive Director: Tina DuBosque
Mission: To offer the people of Eastern Connecticut high quality musical performances, with an emphasis on orchestral concerts.
Founded: 1946
Specialized Field: Symphony; Orchestra; Ensemble
Status: Professional
Paid Staff: 5
Volunteer Staff: 10
Paid Artists: 75
Budget: $750,000
Income Sources: Ticket Sales; Grants; Corporate Sponsorships; Individual Donations; Fundraising Events
Performs At: Garde Arts Center
Annual Attendance: 8,400
Facility Category: Restored theater at Garde Arts Center
Seating Capacity: 1440
Year Built: 1926
Year Remodeled: 1998
Organization Type: Performing; Educational

---

992 NORFOLK CHAMBER MUSIC FESTIVAL/YALE SUMMER SCHOOL OF MUSIC
Ellen Battell Stoeckel Estate
Route 44 & 272
Norfolk, CT 06058-0545
Phone: 860-542-3000
Fax: 860-542-3004
e-mail: norfolk@yale.edu
Web Site: www.yale.edu/norfolk
Management:
   Director: Joan Panetti
   Operations Manager: Deanne Chin
Mission: To provide chamber-music performances and professional training.
Founded: 1941
Specialized Field: Instrumental; Folk; Educational
Status: Professional; Nonprofit
Paid Staff: 12
Paid Artists: 70
Budget: $60,000 - 150,000
Season: Late June - late August
Performs At: The Music Shed
Annual Attendance: 17,500
Facility Category: Indoor
Seating Capacity: 1,000
Rental Contact: Elaine C. Carroll
Organization Type: Performing; Educational

---

993 AMERICAN CLASSICAL ORCHESTRA
50 Washington Street
Norwalk, CT 06854
Phone: 203-838-6995
Fax: 203-838-6998
e-mail: amerclassorch@juno.com
Web Site: www.Americanclassicalorchestra.com
Officers:
   Chairman: Ron Hahn
   President: Nancy Vick
   Treasurer: Peter Burmin
   VP: Allan Bernard
Management:
   Music Director: Thomas Crawford
   Artistic Administrator: Tim Fry
   Education Director: Mae Miller
   Executive Director: Senja Foster
Mission: To support period instrument performance and education at its subscription series at Norwalk Concert Hall. Repertoire spans the Baroque period through early Romantic.
Founded: 1985
Specialized Field: Performs on period instruments
Paid Staff: 6
Volunteer Staff: 25
Paid Artists: 45
Budget: $260,000-700,000
Seating Capacity: 1,062

---

994 NORWALK SYMPHONY ORCHESTRA
83 E Avenue
Suite 207
Norwalk, CT 06851
Phone: 203-847-8844
Fax: 203-866-2290
e-mail: norwalksym@mags.net
Web Site: www.norwalksymphony.org
Management:
   Conductor: Jesse Levine
   Executive Director: Larry Berger
Budget: $260,000-1,050,000
Seating Capacity: 1,063

995 NORWALK YOUTH SYMPHONY

PO Box 73
Norwalk, CT 06856-0073
Phone: 203-866-4100
Fax: 203-866-0012
e-mail: nwkysym@optonline.net
Web Site: www.norwalkyouthsymphony.org
Officers:
Chairman: John Harmon
Management:
Executive Director: Carolyn Phillips
Mission: To enrich the lives of young people within a musical community. We provide the finest possible training, practice and performance opportunities, enabling our students to learn, share and enjoy the power of music.
Founded: 1956
Specialized Field: Youth Symphony
Status: Nonprofit
Paid Staff: 1
Paid Artists: 3
Budget: $800,000
Income Sources: Tuition; Box Office; Donations; Grants
Performs At: Norwalk Concert Hall
Affiliations: ASOL; MCNC; ASCAP: BMI
Annual Attendance: 5,500
Seating Capacity: 1,000
Organization Type: Performing; Educational

996 RIDGEFIELD SYMPHONY ORCHESTRA

3 Big Shop Lane
PO Box 289
Ridgefield, CT 06877
Phone: 203-438-3889
Fax: 203-438-0222
e-mail: symphony@ridgefield-ct.com
Web Site: www.ridgefieldsymphony.org
Officers:
President: Sabina Slavin
VP: Joesph Kreitz
Treasurer: Leroy T Kling
Management:
Music Director: Sidney Rothstein
Mission: Present classical music programs of highest quality to Ridgefield and surroundings communities.
Founded: 1964
Specialized Field: Symphony
Status: Professional; Nonprofit
Paid Staff: 1
Volunteer Staff: 34
Paid Artists: 70+
Budget: $450,000
Income Sources: American Symphony Orchestra League; Broadcast Music Incorporated; American Society of Composers, Authors and Publishers
Performs At: High School Auditorium
Annual Attendance: 6,000
Type of Stage: Proscenium
Seating Capacity: 880
Organization Type: Performing

997 STAMFORD SYMPHONY ORCHESTRA

263 Tresser Boulevard
Stamford, CT 06901
Phone: 203-325-1407
Fax: 203-325-8762
e-mail: info@stamfordsymphony.org
Web Site: www.stamfordsymphony.org
Officers:
Acting President: James Marpe
Management:
Executive Director: Barbara J Soroca
Music Director: Roger Nierenberg
Mission: To provide the Fairfield County area with the finest in symphony music.
Founded: 1968
Specialized Field: Symphony; Orchestra; Ensemble
Status: Professional; Nonprofit
Paid Staff: 7
Budget: $1 million
Income Sources: Ticket sales; contributions; grants
Performs At: Palace Theatre of the Arts
Annual Attendance: 20,000
Organization Type: Performing; Resident; Educational

998 YOUNG ARTISTS PHILHARMONIC

Ridgeway Station
PO Box 3301
Stamford, CT 06905
Phone: 203-532-1278
Fax: 203-532-1278
Web Site: www.syap.org
Management:
Manager: Frances Lourie
Music Director: Salvatore Princiotti
Mission: To develop musical excellence among talented young artists in the area through membership in Young String Ensemble (Elementary), Young People's Orchestra (Middle School) and Young Artists Philharmonic (High School).
Founded: 1960
Specialized Field: Three Orchestras, two flue ensembles and two jazz ensembles.
Status: Non-Professional; Nonprofit
Paid Staff: 150
Performs At: Stamford High School
Organization Type: Performing; Educational

999 WILLIMANTIC ORCHESTRA

532 Browns Road
Storrs, CT 06268
Phone: 860-423-5807
Fax: 860-429-6863
Management:
Conductor: David Vaughan
Manager: Scott Lehmann
Budget: $35,000
Performs At: Shafer Auditorium; Eastern Connecticut State University

1000 WALLINGFORD SYMPHONY ORCHESTRA

333 Christian Street
PO Box 6023
Wallingford, CT 06492-0088
Phone: 203-697-2261
Fax: 203-697-2396
Web Site: www.iimsnet.com/wso.htm

All listings are in alphabetical order by state, then city, then organization within the city.

Officers:
President: Elizabeth Mitchell
Management:
Music Director/Conductor: Philip T Ventre
Founded: 1974
Paid Staff: 0
Paid Artists: 65
Budget: $35,000-100,000
Income Sources: Subscription; Individual Contribution; Corporate
Performs At: Paul Mellon Arts Center; Chiate Rosemary Hall
Facility Category: Theater
Seating Capacity: 780
Year Built: 1972

1001 WATERBURY SYMPHONY ORCHESTRA
83 Bank Street
PO Box 1762
Waterbury, CT 06721
Phone: 203-574-4283
Fax: 203-756-3507
e-mail: waterbury.symphony@snet.net
Web Site: www.waterburysymphony.org
Officers:
President: Gail McTaggart, Esquire
First VP: De Bare Saunders
Second VP: Jane Sendzimer
Treasurer: Jane Sabatini
Secretary: Nancy Grasing
Management:
Conductor: Leif Bjaland
Administrative Director: Jennifer Zembruski
Personnel Manager: Dante Galuppo
Specialized Field: Central CT including New Haven, Litchfield, and Fairfield Counties
Paid Staff: 3
Volunteer Staff: 75
Paid Artists: 70
Budget: $260,000-1,050,000
Income Sources: Annual Fund, Corporate Sponsors, Memberships, Grants
Performs At: College Stage and Warner Theatre
Facility Category: Community College
Type of Stage: Proscenium
Stage Dimensions: 38x34
Seating Capacity: 800

1002 CONNECTICUT YOUTH SYMPHONY
The Hartt School
200 Bloomfield Avenue
University of Hartford
West Hartford, CT 06117
Phone: 860-768-7768
Fax: 860-768-4777
e-mail: harttcomm@mail.hartford.edu
Web Site: www.hartford.edu/hartt.community
Management:
Music Director: Dan D'Addio
Director: Michael Yatfe
Founded: 1930
Specialized Field: Music
Budget: $35,000
Income Sources: Tuition; Fundraising

Performs At: Lincoln Theater
Affiliations: Hartt School
Annual Attendance: 1,500
Seating Capacity: 700

1003 ORCHESTRA NEW ENGLAND
1124 Campbell Avenue
West Haven, CT 06516
Phone: 203-934-8863
Fax: 203-934-8379
Web Site: www.orchestranewengland.org
Management:
Music Director/Conductor: James Sinclair
General Manager: Joseph Russo
Mission: To perform the highest quality of orchestral music for as many people as possible.
Founded: 1975
Specialized Field: Orchestra
Status: Professional; Nonprofit
Paid Staff: 3
Non-paid Artists: 25
Budget: $200,000
Income Sources: Fundraising
Performs At: Battell Chapel; Yale University
Annual Attendance: 3,000
Seating Capacity: 850

Delaware

1004 NEWARK SYMPHONY ORCHESTRA
PO Box 7775
Newark, DE 19714-7775
Phone: 302-366-8491
Fax: 302-366-8491
e-mail: webmaster@newarksymphony.org
Web Site: www.newarksymphony.org
Management:
Music Director: Roman Pawlowski
Personel Manager: Jennifer Hugh
Business Manager: Adrian Harding
Mission: To offer volunteer musicians the opportunity to play symphonic literature; to provide live performances for the community.
Founded: 1966
Specialized Field: Symphony
Status: Non-Professional; Nonprofit
Paid Staff: 80
Income Sources: University of Delaware
Performs At: University of Delaware
Organization Type: Performing

1005 BRANDYWINE BAROQUE
PO Box 730
Wilmington, DE 19899
Phone: 302-594-4544
Fax: 302-594-4538
e-mail: brandywinebaroq@mindspring.com
Management:
Artistic Director: Karen Flint
Administrative Director: Robert Munsell
Specialized Field: Chamber Music
Budget: $100,000-150,000

1006 DELAWARE SYMPHONY ASSOCIATION
PO Box 1870
Wilmington, DE 19899
Phone: 302-656-7374
Fax: 302-656-7754
Web Site: www.desymphony.org
Management:
 Executive Director: Curtis Long
Mission: To educate, inspire, challenge and entertain a diverse and expanding range of individuals with quality symphonic music.
Founded: 1929
Specialized Field: Symphony; Orchestra; Chamber; Ensemble; Instrumental Group
Status: Professional; Nonprofit
Income Sources: American Symphony Orchestra League
Performs At: Grand Opera House
Organization Type: Performing; Educational

1007 DICKINSON THEATRE ORGAN SOCIETY
PO Box 7263
Wilmington, DE 19803-0296
Phone: 302-995-2603
e-mail: redtos@voicenet.com
Web Site: www.geocities.com/dtoskimball
Management:
 Chairman Publicity: Connie Mead
Mission: The presentation of theatre organ concerts on the theatre pipe organ in the Dickinson High School Auditorium.
Founded: 1970
Status: Professional; Semi-Professional; Nonprofit
Performs At: Dickinson High School Auditorium
Organization Type: Sponsoring

1008 MID-ATLANTIC CHAMBER MUSIC SOCIETY
2314 Rideway Road
Wilmington, DE 19899
Phone: 302-654-7283
Fax: 302-654-7283
e-mail: info@midatmusic.org
Web Site: www.midatmusic.org
Management:
 Artistic Director: Diane Monroe

District of Columbia

1009 UNITED STATES AIR FORCE BAND
201 McChord Street
Bolling AFB
Bolling AFB, DC 20332-0202
Phone: 202-767-4224
Fax: 202-767-0686
Web Site: www.bolling.af.mil/band/
Management:
 Commander/Conductor: Col. Lowell E Graham
 Vice Commander/Associate Conductor: Major Frank Grzych
 The Singing Sergeants Director: 1st Lt. Chad Steffey
 The Air Force Strings Director: 1st Lt. Donald Schofield
 Ceremonial Brass Director: 1st Lt. Michael Mench
 Director Operations: CMSgt. Mark Williams
 Director Public Affairs: CMSgt. Daisy Jackson
Mission: The United States Air Force Band performs national and international concert tours to support Air Force and Department of Defense public awareness, community relations objectives and international understanding.
Founded: 1941
Specialized Field: Symphony; Orchestra; Chamber; Ensemble; Instrumental Group; Electronic & Live Electronic; Band
Status: Professional; Nonprofit
Paid Staff: 209
Volunteer Staff: 1
Budget: $1,800,000
Income Sources: American Symphony Orchestra League; Music Educators National Conference; National Bandmasters Association; American Bandmasters Association
Performs At: DAR Constitution Hall
Organization Type: Performing; Touring

1010 CHARLIN JAZZ SOCIETY
2025 I Street NW
Suite 501
Washington, DC 20006
Phone: 202-686-2816
Fax: 202-686-4870
Web Site: www.dcmdva-arts.org/sourdeth/newpage2.htm
Management:
 Director: Linda S Wernick-Cassell
Mission: Dedicated to nourishing jazz as a national treasure.
Founded: 1979
Specialized Field: Orchestra; Ensemble; Instrumental Group; Band
Status: Professional; Nonprofit
Income Sources: Washington Performing Arts Society; Ellington School of the Arts; George Washington University
Performs At: John F. Kennedy Center for the Performing Arts
Organization Type: Performing; Touring; Resident; Educational

1011 CONTEMPORARY MUSIC FORUM
2801 Upton Street NW
Washington, DC 20007
Phone: 202-333-4529
Web Site: www.contemporarymusic.org
Management:
 Personnel Director: Helmut Braunlich
 Program Director: Tony Stark
Mission: To provide the Greater Washington area with quality contemporary music performances.
Founded: 1973
Specialized Field: Chamber
Status: Nonprofit
Performs At: Armand Hammes Auditorium; Corcoran Gallery
Organization Type: Performing; Resident

1012 DC YOUTH ORCHESTRA PROGRAM

Brightwood Station
PO Box 56198
Washington, DC 20011
Phone: 202-723-1612
Fax: 202-726-1900
Web Site: www.dcyop.cpb.org
Management:
   Director: Lyn McLain
   Assistant Director Administration: Carol Rende
   Assistant Director of Music: Erika Schulte
   Director Development: Wing-Chi Chan
Mission: To provide children ages 5-19 with an instrumental music training center.
Founded: 1960
Specialized Field: Symphony; Orchestra; Chamber
Status: Nonprofit
Income Sources: American Symphony Orchestra League Youth Orchestra Division
Organization Type: Performing; Touring; Educational

1013 GEORGE WASHINGTON UNIVERSITY SYMPHONY ORCHESTRA

George Washington University
801 22nd Street NW, Suite B144
Washington, DC 20052
Phone: 202-994-6245
Fax: 202-994-9038
e-mail: gwmusic@gwu.edu
Web Site: www.gwu.edu/~music
Officers:
   Chairman: Roy J Guenther
Management:
   Manager/Conductor: Piotr Gajewslei
Mission: Performs 2 concerts per year of traditional orchestral repertoire, often featuring soloists from within the ensemble, the faculty and the professional community.
Founded: 1961
Budget: $35,000
Performs At: Lisner Auditorium

1014 KENNEDY CENTER OPERA HOUSE ORCHESTRA

John F. Kennedy Center
2700 F Street NW
Washington, DC 20566-0012
Phone: 202-416-8215
Fax: 202-416-8216
e-mail: lhhearn@kennedy-center.org
Management:
   Music Director: Heinz Fricke
   Orchestra Personnel/Operation Mgr: Laura Hutchason Hearn
Budget: $1,050,000-3,600,000
Performs At: Kennedy Center Opera House

1015 NATIONAL GALLERY ORCHESTRA

National Gallery of Art
Washington, DC 20565
Phone: 202-842-6075
Fax: 202-842-2407
e-mail: G-Manos@nga.gov
Web Site: www.nga.gov
Management:
   Music Director: George Manos
   Music Program Specialist: Stephen Ackert
Mission: To provide the public with free concerts at the National Gallery of Art.
Founded: 1941
Specialized Field: Symphony; Orchestra; Chamber; Ensemble
Status: Nonprofit
Paid Staff: 8
Performs At: Museum Garden Courts; National Gallery
Seating Capacity: 500
Organization Type: Performing

1016 NATIONAL MUSICAL ARTS

PO Box 39162
Washington, DC 20016
Phone: 301-946-0355
Fax: 336-855-8494
e-mail: pgraypiano@msn.com
Officers:
   Chairman: Jane Siena
   Secretary: Christopher Griner
   President Friends of NMA: Charles Cleland
Management:
   Artistic Director: Patricia Gray
Mission: To revolutionize the way audiences experience musically innovative live performances and outreach projects, and by exploring music's role throughout the biosphere via transdisciplinary projects.
Founded: 1980
Specialized Field: Chamber; Ensemble
Status: Professional; Nonprofit
Paid Staff: 2
Paid Artists: 20
Budget: $150,000
Income Sources: Grants; Corporations; Friends' donations
Annual Attendance: 3,000
Facility Category: Auditorium
Type of Stage: Speaker Stage
Seating Capacity: 650
Year Built: 1970
Organization Type: Performing; Touring; Resident
Resident Groups: National Music Arts

1017 NATIONAL SYMPHONY ORCHESTRA ASSOCIATION

Kennedy Center for the Performing Arts
2700 F Street Northwest
Washington, DC 20566
Phone: 202-467-4600
Fax: 202-416-8585
Toll-free: 800-444-1324
Web Site: www.kennedy-center.org
Management:
   Music Director: Leonard Slatkin
   Executive Assistant: Beverly Harris
   General Manager: Jean Hamilton
   Assistant Conductor: Anthony Aibel
   Assistant Conductor: Takao Kanayama
   President: Robert C Jones
   General Manager: Jean Hamilton
   Director Operations: Kate Gorecki

Artistic Administrator: C Ulrich Bader
Mission: To nurture, promote and expand the musical knowledge and appreciation of the public through performances of symphonic and other music.
Founded: 1930
Specialized Field: Symphony; Orchestra; Chamber
Status: Nonprofit
Income Sources: American Symphony Orchestra League; John F. Kennedy Center for the Performing Arts
Performs At: John F. Kennedy Center for the Performing Arts
Organization Type: Performing; Touring

1018 THEATER CHAMBER PLAYERS
JFK Center for the Performing Arts
4227 46th Street NW
Washington, DC 20016
Phone: 202-363-6700
Fax: 202-416-8585
e-mail: theaterplay@theaterchamberplayers.org
Web Site: www.theaterchamberplayers.org/
Management:
  Artistic Director: Leon Fleisher
  Artistic Director: Dina Koston
Mission: Committed to introducing its audience to works by contemporary American and European composers which are not heard on other series, along with standard chamber music repertoire. Over thirty distinguished musicians, many of whom have internationally acclaimed careers, perform regularly with Theater Chamber Players.
Founded: 1968
Specialized Field: Chamber
Status: Professional
Income Sources: Chamber Music America; Cultural Alliance of Greater Washington
Performs At: John F. Kennedy Center for the Performing Arts
Organization Type: Performing; Touring; Resident; Educational

1019 WASHINGTON BACH CONSORT
5125 MacArthur Boulevard NW
Suite 42
Washington, DC 20016-3300
Phone: 202-686-7500
Fax: 202-686-6200
e-mail: bachconsort@olg.com
Web Site: bachconsort.org
Officers:
  President: Walter H Lubsen, Jr
  VP: Charles Reifel
  Secretary: David H Ehrlich
  Treasurer: Robert S. Inglis
Management:
  Music Director: Dr. J Reilly Lewis
  Executive Director: Stephen B Barko
Mission: To perform to the highest artistic standards the music of JS Bach and his Baroque contemporaries; to expand our audience through concerts, collaborations with other performing ensembles, media appearances, marketable recordings, and tours; to promote current and future appreciation of Bach in our community through compelling music education programs presented by members of the Consort.

Founded: 1977
Specialized Field: Washington Metropolitan Area
Paid Staff: 5
Volunteer Staff: 20
Paid Artists: 50
Budget: $260,000-1,050,000

1020 WASHINGTON CHAMBER SYMPHONY
1099 22nd Street NW
#602
Washington, DC 20037-1822
Phone: 202-452-1321
Fax: 202-728-1134
e-mail: WCSymphony@aol.com
Web Site: www.WCSymphony.org
Officers:
  President: Elizabeth Loker
  VP: Lisa Heideman
  VP: Norman Sinel
  VP: Katherine Menz Werble
  Secretary: Eric Smith
Management:
  Executive Director: Rhonda L Halverson
  Maestro: Stephen Simon
  Concert Operations Director: Carmen J Stoll
  Development Manager: Kenneth A Oldham Jr
Mission: The Symphony presents classical music from all periods with a focus on music composed for chamber orchestras; provides performances by both established and emerging classical music professionals and composers; and develops interactive educational programs for children and adults.
Founded: 1976
Specialized Field: Symphony; Chamber
Status: Professional; Nonprofit
Paid Staff: 5
Budget: $1,000,000
Income Sources: Ticket Sales; Donors
Performs At: John F. Kennedy Center for the Performing Arts
Affiliations: American Symphony Orchestra League
Seating Capacity: 475
Organization Type: Performing; Touring; Resident; Educational; Sponsoring

1021 WASHINGTON SYMPHONY ORCHESTRA
2437 15th Street NW
Washington, DC 20009
Phone: 202-986-6030
Fax: 202-986-6968
Web Site: www.wsodc.org
Officers:
  President: Lucy M Duncan
  Treasurer: Frederick P Birks
  Secretary: Bettie J Graham
  VP Development: L/Col Robert J. Hawley
  President Emeritus: Douglas Metz
  President Emeritus: Milton Kotler
Management:
  Executive Director: Warren R Cecconi, Jr
  Development Coordinator: Cassie W Ross
  Executive Assistant: Cindy Dyrda
  VP Operations: Henry T Keegan

Music Director: Julius P Williams
Mission: To perform and promote symphonic music to build bridges among the culturally diverse communities of Washington, DC and the world in such a way that it will distinguish it from all others by the quality and innovation of its service, education and performance to both new and seasoned music lovers.
Founded: 1934
Annual Attendance: 3,500

1022 COMMODORES

617 Warrington Avenue SE
Washington Navy Yard, DC 20374-5054
Phone: 202-433-6093
Fax: 202-433-4108
e-mail: public.affairs@navyband.navy.mil
Web Site: www.navyband.navy.mil
Management:
  Master Chief Musician/Music Dir: Leland V Gause
Mission: To provide music for such ceremonies, functions and other occasions as may be directed by proper authority in order to best represent the Navy in a musical capacity at the seat of government and elsewhere as directed.
Founded: 1969
Specialized Field: Jazz
Organization Type: Performing; Touring; Educational

1023 COUNTRY CURRENT

617 Warrington Avenue SE
Washington Navy Yard, DC 20374-5054
Phone: 202-433-6093
Fax: 202-433-4108
e-mail: public.affairs@navyband.navy.mil
Web Site: www.navyband.navy.mil
Management:
  Senior Chief Musician: Wayne C Taylor
Mission: To provide music for such ceremonies, functions and other occasions as may be directed by proper authority in order to best represent the Navy in a musical capacity at the seat of government and elsewhere as directed.
Founded: 1973
Specialized Field: United States Navy Premier Country/Bluegrass Music Group
Organization Type: Performing; Touring

1024 CRUISERS

617 Warrington Avenue SE
Washington Navy Yard, DC 20374-5054
Phone: 202-433-6093
Fax: 202-433-4108
e-mail: public.affairs@navyband.navy.mil
Web Site: www.navyband.navy.mil
Management:
  Master Chief Musician: Gerard J Ascione
  Musician First Class: Kenneth H Carr
  Musician First Class: John L Fisher
  Musician First Class: Benjamin L Grant
  Musician First Class: John T Parsons

Mission: To provide music for such ceremonies, functions and other occasions as may be directed by proper authority in order to best represent the Navy in a musical capacity at the seat of government and elsewhere as directed.
Founded: 1999
Specialized Field: United States Navy Premier Rock Ensemble
Organization Type: Performing; Touring

1025 UNITED STATES NAVY BAND

617 Warrington Avenue SE
Washington Navy Yard, DC 20374-5054
Phone: 202-433-3676
Fax: 202-433-4108
e-mail: public.affairs@navyband.navy.mil
Web Site: www.navyband.navy.mil
Management:
  Operations Officer: Stuart B McLean
  Master Chief Musician/Pub Affairs: Jon T Youngdahl
  Commander/Officer in Charge: Ralph M Gambone
  Lieutenant/Assistant Leader: Melvin P Kessler
  Lieutenant/Third Officer: Isaac Daniel, Jr
Mission: To provide music for such ceremonies, functions and other occasions as may be directed by proper authority in order to best represent the Navy in a musical capacity at the seat of government and elsewhere as directed.
Founded: 1925
Specialized Field: Premier United States Navy Musical Organization; Also maintains a chorus as well as jazz, country, rock and chamber ensembles
Annual Attendance: 1,500,000
Organization Type: Performing; Touring; Educational

Florida

1026 MIAMI INTERNATIONAL PIANO FESTIVAL

20191 E Country Club Drive
Suite 709
Aventura, FL 33180
Phone: 305-935-5115
Fax: 305-935-9087
e-mail: giselle@miamipianofest.com
Web Site: www.miamipianofest.com
Officers:
  Chairman: Jack Brodsky
  Secretary: Karen Dornbusch
Management:
  Artistic Director: Giselle Brodsky
  Executive Director: Agnes Youngblood
Founded: 1997
Specialized Field: Music; Piano
Status: Nonprofit
Paid Staff: 2
Volunteer Staff: 10
Paid Artists: 15
Budget: $360,000
Income Sources: Private Donations; Grants; Ticket Sales; Merchandise
Season: February

Performs At: Lincoln Theatre
Annual Attendance: 5,000
Facility Category: Lincoln Theatre
Seating Capacity: 700

1027 BOCA POPS ORCHESTRA
100 NE First Avenue
Boca Raton, FL 33432-3987
Phone: 561-393-7677
Fax: 561-393-7364
e-mail: mlmcgrew@bellsouth.net
Web Site: www.bocapops.org
Officers:
  Chairman: Stuart Flaum
  Vice Chairman: Marvin Satisky
  Secretary: Daniel Cope
  Tresurer: Jay Galeota
Management:
  Music Director/Conductor: Crafton Beck
  President/CEO: Edward Cordick
  Director Marketing: Michele McGrew
Mission: To provide quality entertainment and educational programs within the community.
Founded: 1951
Specialized Field: Palm Beach and Broward Counties
Status: Nonprofit
Paid Staff: 12
Volunteer Staff: 15
Paid Artists: 100
Budget: $2,600,000
Income Sources: Individual and Corporate Donations; Grants; Ticket Sales
Performs At: Kravis Center; Spanish River Center; Bailey Concert Hall

---

1028 CHAMBER MUSIC SOUTH
22467 Ensenada Way
Boca Raton, FL 33433
Phone: 561-488-1037
Fax: 561-218-8676

1029 MIAMI BACH SOCIETY/TROPICAL BAROQUE MUSIC FESTIVAL
PO Box 4034
Coral Gables, FL 33114
Phone: 305-669-1376
Fax: 305-669-1376
e-mail: JGaubatz@msn.com
Web Site: miamibachsociety.org
Officers:
  President: Mark Hart
  VP: George Berberian
  Secretary: Claire Veater
  Treasurer: Myriam Ribenborm
Management:
  Artistic Director: Donald Oglesby
  Executive Director: Kathy Gaubatz
  Artistic Director: Robert Heath
Mission: To perform and present the music of Johann Sebastian Bach and his baroque composer contemporaries to the people and visitors of the sociable Florida community.
Founded: 1984
Paid Staff: 4

Budget: $300,000
Income Sources: Corporations; Government; Indivdual Donations; Ticket Sales
Annual Attendance: 5,000
Organization Type: Performing and Presenting Musical Organization
Resident Groups: MBS Chorus and Orchestra

1030 DAYTONA BEACH SYMPHONY SOCIETY
100 S Beach Street, Suite 200
PO Box 2
Daytona Beach, FL 32115
Phone: 904-253-2901
Fax: 904-253-5774
e-mail: dbss@bellsouth.net
Web Site: www.dbss.org
Management:
  President: Bobbi L Coleman
  VP: Lloyd Collins
  Managing Director: Rob Rothman
Mission: To bring people and music together.
Founded: 1952
Specialized Field: Symphony; Orchestra; Chamber
Status: Nonprofit
Performs At: Peabody Auditorium
Annual Attendance: 20,000
Organization Type: Sponsoring

1031 FLORIDA INTERNATIONAL FESTIVAL FEATURING THE LONDON SYMPHONY ORCHESTRA
901 6th Street
PO Box 1310
Daytona Beach, FL 32115-1310
Phone: 386-252-1511
Fax: 386-238-1663
e-mail: fifcfce@fif-lso.org
Web Site: www.fif-lso.org
Management:
  General Manager: Dewey Anderson
Founded: 1974
Specialized Field: Music
Paid Staff: 6
Volunteer Staff: 100
Paid Artists: 200
Budget: $400,000 - 1,000,000
Income Sources: Ticket Sales; Contributions; Grants
Season: July
Performs At: Daytona Beach area [Festival Site]; Various
Annual Attendance: 2,000-40,000
Facility Category: Peabody Aud; Ocean Cntr; Ormond Beach Cntr; etc.
Seating Capacity: 250 - 8,000

1032 PINELLAS YOUTH SYMPHONY
PO Box 2755
Dunedin, FL 34697-2755
Phone: 727-438-3149
Fax: 727-733-7901
e-mail: psymanager@yahoo.com
Web Site: http://pysmusic.org
Officers:

President: Kenneth Heffner
VP Operations: Wayne Raymond
Treasurer: J Gerrard Correa
Executive Director: Beth Romanov
Management:
  Music Director: Robert Romanski
  Artistic Director: Mark Sforzini
  Artistic Advisor: Thomas Wilkins

1033 FLORIDA PHILHARMONIC ORCHESTRA

3401 NW 9th Avenue
Fort Lauderdale, FL 33309-5903
Phone: 954-561-2997
Fax: 954-561-1390
Toll-free: 800-226-1812
Web Site: www.flaphil.com
Officers:
  Chairman: Robert E Levinson
  Boca Raton Vice Chairman: Morton Levy
  Dade Vice Chairman: Rose4 Green
Management:
  Executive Director: Connie F Linsler
  Music Director: James Judd
  Director Orchestra Operations: Neilnda Birnbaum
  Resident Conductor: Glen Cortese
  Associate Conductor: Igor Gruppman
  Development Director: Barbara Fead
  Public Relations: Bonnie Arnold
  Marketing: Ed Cambron
Mission: To maintain a symphony orchestra; to further the cultural and educational purposes of South Florida.
Founded: 1985
Specialized Field: Symphony
Status: Professional; Nonprofit
Paid Staff: 35
Volunteer Staff: 2
Paid Artists: 88
Non-paid Artists: 140
Performs At: War Memorial Auditorium; Florida Atlantic University
Organization Type: Performing; Touring; Resident; Educational

1034 SOUTHWEST FLORIDA SYMPHONY ORCHESTRA & CHORUS ASSOCIATION

8695 College Parkway
Suite 212-1
Fort Myers, FL 33919
Phone: 941-433-3040
Fax: 941-433-3089
e-mail: swflso@swflso.org
Web Site: swflso.org
Officers:
  President: Michael K Sheeley
  First VP: J Thomas Uhler
  Second VP: Michael Peceri
  Secretary: Dorothy Kollmar
  Treasurer: Morton Crane
Management:
  Music Director: Paul Nadler

Mission: Committed to sharing their passion for music with the entire Southwest Florida community through continuous improvement of the artistic quality, programmatic breath and cultural relevance of our concert programs and presentations.
Budget: $1,050,000-3,600,000
Performs At: Barbara B. Mann Performing Arts Hall

1035 GAINESVILLE SYMPHONY ORCHESTRA

PO Box 7011
Gainesville, FL 32605-7011
Phone: 352-336-5448
Fax: 352-336-4266
Web Site: www.afn.org/~gso
Officers:
  President: Karl Ashley
  VP: Lawrence Lokken
Management:
  Executive Director: Julia Diana
  Music Director/Conductor: Dr. Raymond Chobaz
Founded: 1983
Specialized Field: Baroque to 20th century music.
Annual Attendance: 10,000

1036 MELBOURNE CHAMBER MUSIC SOCIETY

501 S Sonora Circle
PO Box 033403
Indialantic, FL 32903
Phone: 321-725-6806
Fax: 321-725-6806
Web Site: www.melbournechambermusicsociety.com
Officers:
  President: Anneke Bertsch
Management:
  President: Anneke Bertsch
Mission: To bring in internationally known artists to the members and the community.
Founded: 1978
Specialized Field: Chamber Music for Brevard County

1037 JACKSONVILLE SYMPHONY ORCHESTRA

300 W Water Street
Suite 200
Jacksonville, FL 32202
Phone: 904-354-5479
Fax: 904-354-9238
Toll-free: 877-662-6731
e-mail: info@jaxsymphony.org
Web Site: www.jaxsymphony.org
Officers:
  Chairman: Ar Carpenter
  Chairman Elect: Steve Halverson
  Secretary: Isabelle Davis
  Treasurer: Gerald J Pollack
Management:
  Music Director: Fabio Mechetti
  Executive Director: Alan Hopper
  Artistic Administrator: Cecil S Cole
  Administrator/Finance Director: Jim Lynn
  Human Resources: Sally Pettegrew

Mission: To provide performances of high artistic quality designed to reach the broadest possible audience; to strive to not only inspire and challenge its audience with classical music, but also provide educational and public service programs.
Founded: 1949
Specialized Field: Symphony; Orchestra; Chamber
Status: Professional; Nonprofit
Paid Staff: 25
Paid Artists: 52
Budget: $6,600,000
Income Sources: Ticket sales; Private donations; Grants
Performs At: Robert E. Jacoby Symphony Hall; Times Union Center For The Performing Arts
Annual Attendance: 175,000
Type of Stage: Platform
Seating Capacity: 1800
Year Built: 1997
Year Remodeled: 1999
Rental Contact: Director Adina Alford
Organization Type: Performing; Touring; Educational

1038 KEY WEST SYMPHONY

1025 White Street
PO Box 744
Key West, FL 33041
Phone: 305-292-1774
Fax: 305-292-5623
e-mail: kwso@bellsouth.net
Web Site: www.keywestsymphony.com
Management:
    Music Director/Conductor: Sebrina Maria Alfonso
Founded: 1998
Specialized Field: Symphony/Music
Paid Staff: 3
Paid Artists: 80
Performs At: Tennessee Williams Fine Arts Center

1039 IMPERIAL SYMPHONY ORCHESTRA

1037 S Florida Avenue, Suite 125
PO Box 2623
Lakeland, FL 33803
Phone: 863-688-3743
Fax: 863-686-2881
e-mail: iso_lkld@yahoo.com
Web Site: www.imperialsymphony.org
Officers:
    President: Martha Linder
Management:
    Music Director/Conductor: Mark Thielen
    Executive Director: Colleen Burton
    Concertmaster: Arthur Pranno
    Music Manager: Ann Satterfield
Mission: The Imperial Symphony Orchestra is committed to the high quality performance of symphonic music in order to educate, entertain, and inspire audiences and enrich the lives of the people of Polk County and neighboring communities.
Budget: $260,000-1,050,000
Performs At: The Lakeland Center

1040 BREVARD SYMPHONY ORCHESTRA

1500 Highland Avenue
PO Box 361965
Melbourne, FL 32936-1965
Phone: 407-242-2024
Fax: 407-259-4716
Toll-free: 800-345-8591
e-mail: bso@iu.net
Web Site: www.geocities.com/Vienna/Strasse/2235
Status: Not-for-profit
Income Sources: North Central/South Guilds

1041 FRIENDS OF CHAMBER MUSIC OF MIAMI

du Pont Building, Suite 1619
169 E Flagler Street
Miami, FL 33131-1211
Phone: 305-373-3101
Fax: 305-381-8734
Officers:
    President: Julian H Kreeger
Performs At: Gusman Concert Hall, University of Miami

1042 MIAMI CHAMBER SYMPHONY

5690 N Kendall Drive
Miami, FL 33156
Phone: 305-858-3500
Fax: 305-857-5001
Management:
    Music Director/Manager: Burton Dines
    Office Manager: Jean Bailly
Mission: The symphony performs subscriptions series concerts at Gusman Hall on the University of Miami campus featuring world-class soloists.
Founded: 1981
Specialized Field: Symphony; Chamber
Status: Professional; Nonprofit
Budget: 150,000
Income Sources: American Symphony Orchestra League
Performs At: Gusman Concert Hall
Organization Type: Performing

1043 MIAMI CLASSIC GUITAR SOCIETY

PO Box 0725
Miami, FL 33265
Phone: 305-412-2494
Fax: 305-412-2494
e-mail: mcgs_guitar@hotmail.com
Officers:
    President: Carlos Molina
Management:
    President: Carlos Molina
Mission: Concert Series/Master Classes/Lectures
Founded: 1987
Specialized Field: Classical Guitar
Volunteer Staff: 4
Paid Artists: 6
Budget: $45,000
Income Sources: Grants; Sponsors; Members; Ticket Sales
Performs At: Theaters; Churches
Annual Attendance: 2,000
Seating Capacity: 300

1044 SOUTH FLORIDA YOUTH SYMPHONY

12645 SW 114 Avenue
Miami, FL 33176
Phone: 305-238-2729
Fax: 305-252-9876
e-mail: marj-@rocketmail.com
Web Site: www.sfys.net
Officers:
President: Emma Alvarez
First VP: Patricia Lefebvre
Second VP: Marcoantonio Real
Corresponding Secretary: Larry Howell
Secretary Recording: Vashti Laing
Treasurer: Terrie Garmendia
Assistant Treasurer: Hung Pham
Management:
Executive Musical Director: Marjorie Hahn
Mission: To broaden the horizons of young talented musicians in the area of symphonic music; to train them in the performance of this music, in conducting and for solos; to offer a junior string training program for beginning students.
Founded: 1964
Specialized Field: Orchestra; Chamber; Ensemble
Status: Nonprofit
Paid Staff: 8
Volunteer Staff: 5
Budget: $120,000
Income Sources: Donations; Grants; Admissions
Annual Attendance: 3,500
Organization Type: Performing; Educational
Resident Groups: All

1045 NEW WORLD SYMPHONY

541 Lincoln Road
Miami Beach, FL 33139
Phone: 305-673-3330
Fax: 305-673-6749
Toll-free: 800-597-3331
e-mail: admin@nws.org
Web Site: www.nws.org
Officers:
Chairman: Robert E Hoffman
Chairman: Howard Frank
Vice Chairman/Secretary: Laurie Wynne
Vice Chairman/Treasurer: William L. Morrison
Vice Chairman: Ronald W. Drucker
Vice Chairman: Ronald G. Stone
Management:
President/CEO: Howard Herring
Artistic Operations: Douglas Mericott
Artistic Director: Michael Tilson-Thomas
CFO: David Phillips
VP Development: Jonathan Peterson
Dean of Musicians: Patricia Nutt
Mission: To maintain a national advanced-training program that prepares gifted young orchestral musicians (ages 21-30) for full-time professional music careers and provides participants the opportunity to study and perform with distinguished conductors and solo artists.
Founded: 1987
Specialized Field: Symphony; Orchestra; Chamber; Education
Status: Professional; Nonprofit
Paid Staff: 48

Budget: $7.8 Million
Income Sources: Endowment; contributions; ticket sales
Annual Attendance: 22,000
Facility Category: Theatre
Type of Stage: Sprung Beech
Stage Dimensions: 49'32 x 42'4 x 25
Seating Capacity: 705
Year Built: 1936
Year Remodeled: 1988
Cost: $3,000,000
Organization Type: Performing; Touring

1046 NAPLES PHILHARMONIC ORCHESTRA

5833 Pelican Bay Boulevard
Naples, FL 34108
Phone: 941-597-1111
Fax: 941-597-8163
Toll-free: 800-597-1900
e-mail: orchestra@naplesphilcenter.org
Web Site: www.naplesphilcenter.org
Officers:
President/CEO: Myra Janco Daniels
VP Operations/Program: Naomi Buck
CFO: Pablo Veintimilla
Management:
Music Director: Christopher Seaman
Principal Pops Conductor: Erich Kunzel
Orchestra Manager: Chuck Gottschalk
Mission: To present for all ages the best that is affordable in visual as well as performing arts.
Founded: 1989
Specialized Field: Orchestra, Dance, Theatre, Comedy, Opera, Ballet
Paid Staff: 250
Paid Artists: 85
Budget: $3,600,000-10,000,000
Performs At: Philharmonic Center for the Arts

1047 CENTRAL FLORIDA SYMPHONY
Citrus County Committee

3001 SW College Road
Ocala, FL 34478
Phone: 352-873-5808
Fax: 352-237-8737
Web Site: www.nccentral.com/cfsymphony/symphony.htm
Officers:
Treasurer: George M Durgin Jr
President: Mona Wiegand
Management:
Music Director/Conductor: James Plondke
Founded: 1975
Budget: $35,000-100,000
Performs At: CFCC Fine Arts Auditorium; Lecanto Auditorium

1048 ORLANDO PHILHARMONIC ORCHESTRA

PO Box 540203
Orlando, FL 32854-0203
Phone: 407-896-6700
Fax: 407-896-5512
Web Site: www.orlandophil.org
Management:

Music Director: Hal France
Principal Guest Conductor: Alfred Savia
Acting Manager: Mark Fischer
Budget: $1,050,000-3,600,000
Seating Capacity: 2,500

1049 UNIVERSITY OF CENTRAL FLORIDA ORCHESTRA
University of Central Florida
Dept. of Music, 215 Student Union
PO Box 163245
Orlando, FL 32816-1354
Phone: 407-823-6471
Fax: 407-823-5244
e-mail: jholt@pegasus.cc.ucf.edu
Web Site: pegasus.cc.ucf.edu/~osa/
Management:
    Music Director/Conductor: John C Whitney
    Manager: Matt Boone
    Assistant Director: Jean Holt
Budget: $35,000
Seating Capacity: 500

1050 GREATER PALM BEACH SYMPHONY ASSOCIATION
235 Sunrise Avenue
Palm Beach, FL 33480
Phone: 561-655-2657
Fax: 561-655-9113
e-mail: jjtighe1@bellsouth.net
Web Site: www.expresspages.com/g/greaterpbsymphony/
Officers:
    Co-Chairwoman: Joan Tighe
    Co-Chairman: John Tighe
Management:
    Music Director: Naxim Gershunoff
Mission: To bring quality music programs to Palm Beach.
Founded: 1963
Volunteer Staff: 2
Paid Artists: 60
Budget: $200,000
Income Sources: contributions
Annual Attendance: 2,500
Facility Category: multi-venues
Seating Capacity: 1,000

1051 PALM BEACH POPS
231 Bradley Place
Palm Beach, FL 33480
Phone: 561-832-7677
Fax: 561-832-9686
e-mail: pbp@aol.com
Web Site: www.palmbeachpops.org
Officers:
    Chairman: Kenneth G Langone
    President: W Robert Lappin
    VP: Steven A Levin
    Secretary/Treasurer: James F. Fitzgerald
Management:
    Music Director: Bob Lappin
    Director of Operations: Cheryl Parker
    Marketing Director: Ryan Dorsche
    Director of Development: Alexa Radd

Mission: To preserve the heritage of America's great composers and lyricists, and to celebrate the great performers of the past and present.
Budget: $1,050,000-3,600,000
Performs At: Kravis Center for the Performing Arts; Broward Center

1052 PENSACOLA JAZZFEST
PO Box 18337
Pensacola, FL 32523-8337
Phone: 850-433-8382
Fax: 850-433-1969
e-mail: nvickers@cs.com
Web Site: www.artsnwfl.org/jazz
Management:
    Executive Director: F Norman Vickers
    Executive Secretary: Patricia Ashton

1053 PENSACOLA SYMPHONY ORCHESTRA
PO Box 1705
Pensacola, FL 32598
Phone: 850-435-2533
Fax: 850-444-9910
Web Site: www.pensacolasymphony.com/index2.html
Management:
    Music Director/Conductor: Peter Rubardt
    Executive Director: Innes Richards
Budget: $260,000-1,050,000
Performs At: Saenger Theatre

1054 SYMPHONY OF THE AMERICAS
199 N Ocean Boulevard
Suite 200
Pompano Beach, FL 33062
Phone: 954-545-0088
Fax: 954-545-9088
e-mail: sympamer@aol.com
Web Site: www.symphonyoftheamericas.org
Management:
    Music Director: James Brooks-Bruzzese
    Executive Director: Renee LaBonte
Founded: 1988
Specialized Field: South Florida
Paid Staff: 4
Paid Artists: 5
Budget: $260,000-1,050,000
Income Sources: Sponsers; Grants; Donations; Program Ads
Performs At: Broward Performing Arts Center
Affiliations: None

1055 GULF COAST SYMPHONY ORCHESTRA
PO Box 1759
Sanibel Island, FL 33957
Phone: 941-472-6197
Fax: 941-481-4620
e-mail: GCSymOrch@aol.com
Web Site: www.naples.net
Management:
    Music Director: Andrew M Kurtz
    Executive Director: Martha Cox
Founded: 1996
Volunteer Staff: 150
Budget: $35,000-100,000

Performs At: Barbara B. Mann Performing Arts Hall

1056 FLORIDA WEST COAST BRASS QUINTET

709 N Tamiami Trail
Sarasota, FL 34236
Phone: 941-953-4252
Fax: 941-953-3059
e-mail: symphony@fwcs.org
Web Site: www.fwcs.org
Management:
  Executive Director: Joseph McKenna
  General Manager: Trevor Cramer
  Marketing Director: Linda Joffe
  Development Director: Kristina Kelly
  Education Director: Elizabeth Power
Mission: To promote chamber music locally, statewide, and nationally both presenting and providing broad-based educational programs of the highest quality.
Founded: 1986
Specialized Field: Brass Ensemble
Status: Professional; Nonprofit
Performs At: Holley Hall
Facility Category: Performing; Resident; Touring

1057 FLORIDA WEST COAST NEW ARTISTS PIANO QUARTET

709 N Tamiami Trail
Sarasota, FL 34236
Phone: 941-953-4252
Fax: 941-953-3059
e-mail: symphony@fwcs.org
Web Site: www.fwcs.org
Management:
  Executive Director: Joseph McKenna
  General Manager: Trevor Cramer
  Business Manager: Susan Lagg-May
  Marketing Director: Linda Joffe
  Development Director: Kristina Kelly
  Education Director: Elizabeth Power
Mission: To promote chamber music locally, statewide, and nationally by both presenting and providing broad-based educational programs of the highest quality.
Founded: 1991
Specialized Field: String Ensemble
Status: Professional; Nonprofit
Paid Artists: 4
Income Sources: Ticket Sales
Performs At: Holley Hall
Organization Type: Performing; Resident; Touring

1058 FLORIDA WEST COAST SYMPHONY

709 N Tamiami Trail
Sarasota, FL 34236
Phone: 941-953-4252
Fax: 941-953-3059
e-mail: symphony@fwcs.org
Web Site: www.fwcs.org
Officers:
  President: Hope Luther
  VP: Bryan Langton
  VP: Beatrice Friedman
Management:
  Executive Director: Joseph McKenna

Artistic Director: Leif Bialand
  General Manager: Trevor Cramer
Mission: To present orchestral music and community education programs of the highest quality in a three-county area on Florida's Gulf Coast.
Founded: 1949
Specialized Field: Music
Status: Nonprofit
Budget: $4 million
Income Sources: Concert Tickets Sales; Donations; Grants
Performs At: Van Wezel Performing Arts Hall; Holley Hall
Organization Type: Performing; Resident

1059 FLORIDA WEST COAST WIND QUINTET

709 N Tamiami Trail
Sarasota, FL 34236
Phone: 941-953-4252
Fax: 941-953-3059
e-mail: symphony@fwcs.org
Web Site: www.fwcs.org
Management:
  Executive Director: Joseph McKenna
  General Manager: Trevor Cramer
  Business Manager: Susan Lagg-May
  Marketing Director: Linda Joffe
  Development Director: Kristina Kelly
  Education Director: Elizabeth Power
Mission: To promote chamber music locally, statewide, and nationally both presenting and providing broad-based educational programs of the highest quality.
Founded: 1984
Specialized Field: Wind Ensemble
Status: Professional; Nonprofit
Performs At: Holley Hall
Facility Category: Performing; Resident; Touring

1060 FLORIDA WEST COAST YOUTH ORCHESTRAS

709 N Tamiami Trail
Sarasota, FL 34236
Phone: 941-953-4252
Fax: 941-953-3059
e-mail: symphony@fwcs.org
Web Site: www.fwcs.org
Management:
  Executive Director: Joseph McKenna
  General Manager: Trevor Cramer
  Business Manager: Susan Lagg-May
  Marketing Director: Linda Joffe
  Development Director: Kristina Kelly
  Education Director: Elizabeth Power
  Assistant Education Director: Jim Cliff
Mission: The Florida West Coast Symphony Orchestra Program consists of six orchestras, affording students the opportunity to participate in an orchestra comparable to their skill level. Students audition each year to participate.
Founded: 1956
Specialized Field: Youth Philharmonic; Youth Symphony; Symphonic Winds; Symphonic Strings; String Orchestra One; String Orchestra Two
Status: Non-Professional; Nonprofit

Income Sources: Donations, Grants
Performs At: Van Wezel Performing Arts Hall; Holley Hall
Facility Category: Performing; Resident; Touring
Organization Type: Performing; Educational

1061 FLORIDA WIND QUINTET

709 N Tamiami Trail
Sarasota, FL 34236
Phone: 941-953-4252
Fax: 941-953-3059
e-mail: symphony@fwcs.org
Web Site: www.fwcs.org
Management:
   General Manager: Trevor Cramer
Mission: The resident wind quintet of the Florida West Coast Symphony; presents concerts to the community.
Founded: 1984
Specialized Field: Ensemble
Status: Professional; Nonprofit
Paid Artists: 5
Income Sources: Florida West Coast Music
Performs At: Holley Hall
Organization Type: Performing; Resident

1062 JAZZ CLUB OF SARASOTA

330 S Pineapple Avenue
#111
Sarasota, FL 34236
Phone: 941-366-1552
Fax: 941-366-1553
e-mail: mail@clubsarasota.com
Web Site: www.jazzclubsarasota.com
Officers:
   President: Jerry Roucher
Mission: To promote and preserve jazz.
Founded: 1980
Paid Staff: 1
Volunteer Staff: 60
Paid Artists: 100
Non-paid Artists: 10
Performs At: Auditorium

1063 NEW ARTISTS STRING QUARTET

709 N Tamiami Trail
Sarasota, FL 34236
Phone: 941-953-4252
Fax: 941-953-3059
e-mail: symphony@fwcs.org
Web Site: www.fwcs.org
Management:
   Executive Director: Joseph McKenna
   General Manager Florida West Coast: Trevor Cramer
Mission: To provide a showcase for new, young string players in the Florida West Coast Symphony.
Founded: 1967
Specialized Field: Ensemble
Status: Professional; Nonprofit
Paid Artists: 4
Income Sources: Florida West Coast Symphony
Performs At: Holley Hall
Organization Type: Performing; Touring; Resident

1064 BIG BEND COMMUNITY ORCHESTRA

3321 Dartmoor Drive
Tallahassee, FL 32312
Phone: 850-893-4567
Fax: 850-668-4870
Management:
   Conductor/Artistic Director: Waldie Anderson
   Manager: Ginny Densmore
Mission: Community Orchestra Provides area with The Artist Series
Founded: 1994
Specialized Field: Tallahasee, FL
Budget: $35,000-100,000
Seating Capacity: 1,200

1065 TALLAHASSEE SYMPHONY ORCHESTRA

1345 Thomasville Road
Tallahassee, FL 32303
Phone: 850-224-0461
Fax: 850-222-9092
e-mail: info@tsolive.org
Web Site: www.tsolive.org/index1.html
Officers:
   Founding Chairman: Ret Adm Philip Ashler
   Secretary: Tim Atkinson
   President: Segundo Fernandez
   Executive VP Fund Development: Bobby Bacon
Management:
   Executive Director: Lois D Griffin
   Manager TYSO: Debra Herman
   Artistic Advisor: Jon Piersol
Mission: Dedicated to maintaining a high-quality symphony orchestra in Tallahassee; committed to superior quality and to furthering cultural opportunities in the community.
Founded: 1981
Specialized Field: Symphony
Status: Professional; Nonprofit
Paid Staff: 3
Income Sources: American Symphony Orchestra League
Performs At: Ruby Diamond Auditorium
Organization Type: Performing; Resident

1066 FLORIDA ORCHESTRA

101 S Hoover Boulevard
#100
Tampa, FL 33609
Phone: 813-286-1170
Fax: 813-286-2316
e-mail: ticketing@floridaorchestra.org
Web Site: www.flordiaorchestra.org
Officers:
   Chairman: David Fischer
   Immediate Past Chair: Raymond Murray
   Secretary: Susan Betzer
   Treasurer: David Zimmerman
Management:
   Executive Director: Leonard Stone
   Music Director Designate: Stefan Sanderling
   Director Operations: Jeff Bram
   Financial Officer: Christine Stone
Mission: To serve the Tampa Bay Area and the state of Florida with high-quality symphonic music.

Founded: 1968
Specialized Field: Symphony; Orchestra
Status: Professional; Nonprofit
Paid Staff: 25
Paid Artists: 80
Budget: $8,400,000
Income Sources: Ticket Sales; Private & Corporate Donations; Fundraising Events
Performs At: Mahaffrey Theater
Annual Attendance: 150,000
Organization Type: Performing; Touring; Resident; Educational

1067 VENICE SYMPHONY

PO Box 1561
Venice, FL 34284
Phone: 941-488-1010
Fax: 941-488-7074
e-mail: venicesymphony@aol.com
Web Site: www.thevenicesymphony.org
Management:
  Music Director: Wesley John Schumacher
  Executive Director: Jean Peters
Mission: Perform concerts; cultivate; promote; and sponsor an appreciation of musical arts in the community; and secure the interests of patrons of these arts.
Founded: 1973
Specialized Field: Classical Music
Paid Staff: 5
Paid Artists: 100
Budget: $326,000
Income Sources: Tickets; Contributions; Grants
Performs At: Church of the Nazarene
Annual Attendance: 11,875
Facility Category: Church
Seating Capacity: 625
Organization Type: Performing

1068 FLORIDA SYMPHONY YOUTH ORCHESTRA

PO Box 2328
Winter Park, FL 32790
Phone: 407-999-7800
Fax: 407-898-5250
e-mail: fsyo@fsyo.org
Web Site: www.fsyo.org
Officers:
  President: Joseph Wise
  VP: Michael Muszynski
  Secretary: David Whitfield
  Treasurer: Toni Strollo Holbrook
Management:
  Music Director: Andrew Lane
  Executive Director: Beverly Hendricks
Mission: To provide an educationally sound musical experience that will motivate students to fulfill their potential and strive for excellence, building an appreciation of the performing arts and the audiences of the future.
Founded: 1957
Paid Staff: 3
Volunteer Staff: 120
Paid Artists: 3
Budget: $150,000-260,000

Income Sources: Box Office; Grants; Private Donations
Performs At: Performing Arts Centre
Annual Attendance: 16,000
Seating Capacity: 2,359
Organization Type: Performing Arts Center

Georgia

1069 ALBANY SYMPHONY ASSOCIATION

PO Box 70065
Albany, GA 31707
Phone: 229-430-6799
Fax: 229-430-6798
Web Site: www.albanysymphony.org
Officers:
  President: David Hardin
  Treasurer: John Stephenson
  Secretary: Wilhelmina Hall
Management:
  General Manager: Amy Spinosa
  Music Director: Claire Fox Hillard
  Assistant Marketing: Robert Drake
Mission: Dedicated to providing and promoting quality symphonic music for Southwest Georgia through the maintenance of a symphony orchestra and related educational activities.
Founded: 1964
Specialized Field: Symphony; Orchestra
Status: Professional
Paid Staff: 5
Volunteer Staff: 10
Budget: $275,000
Income Sources: American Symphony Orchestra League; Albany Arts Council
Performs At: Municipal Auditorium; Albany
Facility Category: Municipal Auditorium
Seating Capacity: 980
Year Built: 1915
Year Remodeled: 1993
Organization Type: Performing; Educational

1070 GEORGIA SOUTHWESTERN STATE UNIVERSITY CHAMBER CONCERT SERIES

800 Wheatley Street
Americus, GA 31709-4693
Phone: 229-931-2204
Fax: 229-931-2927
e-mail: jem@canes.gsw.edu
Officers:
  Fine Arts Department Chairman: Julie Megginson
Specialized Field: Music
Performs At: Fine Arts Theatre
Seating Capacity: 250

1071 ATLANTA CHAMBER PLAYERS

Peachtree Center Station
PO Box 56834
Atlanta, GA 30343

Phone: 404-872-4952
Fax: 404-875-8822
e-mail: paulapeace@atlmyg.org
Web Site: www.atlantachamberplayers.com
Management:
   Artistic Director: Paula Peace
   Business Manager: Ed Trafford
Mission: Atlanta Chamber Players is a professional ensemble of musicians committed to offering audiences world class traditional and contemporary masterpieces as well as commissioned new works.
Founded: 1976
Specialized Field: Chamber
Status: Professional; Nonprofit
Paid Staff: 3
Paid Artists: 7
Performs At: Georgia State University Recital Hall; Kennesaw State University
Organization Type: Performing; Touring; Resident; Educational

---

1072 **ATLANTA JAZZ FESTIVAL**
Atlantic Bureau of Cultural Affairs

675 Ponce De Leon
Atlanta, GA 30308
Phone: 404-817-6851
Fax: 404-658-6945
Management:
   Bureau Director: Barbara Bowser
   Festivals Manager: Jackie Davis
Mission: To offer a showcase for talented local and national performers; to provide Atlanta citizens with jazz music.
Specialized Field: Dance; Vocal Music; Instrumental Music
Status: Professional; Nonprofit
Performs At: Grant Park
Organization Type: Performing; Educational

1073 **ATLANTA SYMPHONY ORCHESTRA**

1293 Peachtree Street NE
Suite 300
Atlanta, GA 30309
Phone: 404-733-4900
Fax: 404-733-4901
e-mail: ASO@woodruffcenter.org
Web Site: www.atlantasymphony.org
Officers:
   President: Allison Vulgamore
   VP: John Sparrow
   Chairman: Jere Drummond
   VP Marketing: Charles Wade
Management:
   Music Director: Robert Spano
   Music Director Emeritus: Yoel Levi
   Principal Guest Conductor: Donald Runnicles
   Conductor Youth Orchestra: Jere Flint
   Concertmaster: Cecilia Arzewski
   President: Allison Vulgamore
   General Manager: John Sparrow
   Operations Manager: Sandra Schaffer
Mission: To provide Atlanta area audiences with quality symphonic concerts for their enjoyment.
Founded: 1945

Specialized Field: Symphony; Orchestra; Chamber
Status: Professional; Nonprofit
Paid Staff: 50
Paid Artists: 99
Income Sources: American Symphony Orchestra League
Performs At: Symphony Hall; Chastain Park Amphitheatre
Facility Category: Concert Hall
Type of Stage: Full Theater Facilities
Seating Capacity: 1749 / 82
Year Built: 1968
Rental Contact: Operations Manager Sandra Schaffer
Organization Type: Performing

1074 **ATLANTA SYMPHONY YOUTH ORCHESTRA**

1293 Peachtree Street NE
Suite 300
Atlanta, GA 30309
Phone: 404-733-4870
Fax: 404-733-4901
e-mail: melanie.darby@woodruffcenter.org
Web Site: www.atlantasymphony.org
Officers:
   Parents Association President: Lynda Martin
   President Elect: Beth Gibson
   Secretary: Ken Morris
   Treasurer: Diane Foust
Management:
   Conductor: Jere Flint
   Director Education: Susan Merritt
   Coordinator/Youth & Family Programs: Melanie Darby
Founded: 1974
Specialized Field: Performance; educational
Paid Staff: 60
Volunteer Staff: 22
Paid Artists: 100
Non-paid Artists: 120
Budget: $35,000-100,000
Performs At: Robert W Woodruff Arts Center
Seating Capacity: 1748
Rental Contact: Sandi Schaffer

1075 **CHASTIAN PARK AMPHITHEATRE ATLANTA SYMPHONY ORCHESTRA SUMMER POPS**

1293 Peachtree Street NE
Suite 300
Atlanta, GA 30309
Phone: 404-733-4886
Fax: 404-733-4999
e-mail: rschastian@aol.com
Web Site: www.classicchastian.org
Management:
   Director: Rudi Schlegel
   Program Coordinator: Peter Wasserman
   Production/ Stage Manager: Lee Freeman
Founded: 1973
Paid Staff: 30
Volunteer Staff: 200
Budget: $6 million
Income Sources: Tickets; sponsors
Season: June - August

Performs At: Chastian Park [Festival Site]
Affiliations: Atlanta Symphony Orchestra
Annual Attendance: 160,000
Facility Category: Chastian Park Amphitheatre
Type of Stage: Plywood/ Shell
Seating Capacity: 6,291
Year Built: 1933
Year Remodeled: 1989
Resident Groups: Atlanta Symphony Orchestra

1076 EMORY SYMPHONY ORCHESTRA

Emory University, Musical Department
1804 N Decatur
Atlanta, GA 30322
Phone: 404-727-6445
Fax: 404-727-0074
e-mail: music@emory.edu
Web Site: www.emory.edu/MUSIC
Management:
    Music Director/Conductor: Scott A Stewart

1077 SPELMAN COLLEGE FRESH IMAGES CHAMBER MUSIC SERIES

PO Box 246
350 Spelman Lane Southwest
Atlanta, GA 30314
Phone: 404-223-7680
Fax: 404-215-7771
e-mail: kjohns10@spelman.edu
Web Site: www.spelman.edu
Officers:
    Chairman Music Department: Kevin Johnson
Specialized Field: Music
Performs At: Sisters Chapel

1078 AUGUSTA SYMPHONY ORCHESTRA

1301 Greene Street, Suite 200
PO Box 579
Augusta, GA 30903-0579
Phone: 706-826-4705
Fax: 706-826-4735
e-mail: sandraself@augustasymphony.org
Web Site: www.augustasymphony.org
Officers:
    President: Elizabeth Rogers
    VP Development: Joseph Huff
    VP/Community Affairs: Dr. Charles Wolf
    Treasurer: Hugh McCutheon
Management:
    Music Director/Conductor: Donald Portnoy
    Executive Director: Sandra Sutton Self
    Ticket Manager/Communications: Adria Gunter
    Director Communications: Donna Branch
Mission: To be the premier provider of orchestra music for the greater Augusta region.
Founded: 1954
Paid Staff: 14
Volunteer Staff: 3
Paid Artists: 250
Budget: $1,000,700
Income Sources: Tickets; Contracts; Support Groups; Annual Fund Contributions (Corporate, Individual, Foundations)

Performs At: Performing Arts Theatre; Augusta State University; Ball Auditorium
Annual Attendance: 35,000
Facility Category: Performance Arts Theatre; Bell Auditorium
Seating Capacity: 800; 2,200
Year Built: 1950
Year Remodeled: 2000
Resident Groups: Augusta Symphony String Quartet; Augusta Symphony Woodwind Trio

1079 COLUMBUS SYMPHONY ORCHESTRA

101 13th Street
PO Box 1499
Columbus, GA 31902
Phone: 706-323-5059
Fax: 706-323-7051
e-mail: customerservice@columbussymphony.com
Web Site: www.csoga.org
Management:
    Executive Director: Terri Parodi
    Music Director/Conductor: George Del Gobbo
    Personnel Manager: Jeanette Ross
    Marketing Director: Becky Young
    Development Director: Patty Young
Mission: To provide quality music to area residents.
Founded: 1855
Specialized Field: Symphony
Status: Semi-Professional
Paid Staff: 8
Volunteer Staff: 3
Budget: $715,000
Income Sources: American Symphony Orchestra League
Performs At: Three Arts Theatre
Annual Attendance: 25,000
Facility Category: Theatre
Seating Capacity: 1,668
Organization Type: Performing; Touring; Resident; Educational; Sponsoring

1080 GAINESVILLE SYMPHONY ORCHESTRA

422 Brenau Avenue
PO Box 162
Gainesville, GA 30503
Phone: 770-532-5727
Fax: 770-535-0554
e-mail: gso-pam@mindspring.com
Management:
    Music Director: Larry Sims
    Executive Director: Pam Slaton
Founded: 1981
Paid Staff: 2
Volunteer Staff: 30
Non-paid Artists: 80
Budget: $35,000-100,000
Performs At: Pearce Auditorium
Annual Attendance: 5,000
Rental Contact: Laura Nagel

1081 MACON SYMPHONY ORCHESTRA

400 Poplar Street
Macon, GA 31201

Phone: 478-301-5300
Fax: 478-301-5505
e-mail: mso@maconsymphony.com
Web Site: www.maconsymphony.com
Officers:
   President - Elect: Katherine B Vitale
   VP Development: Detra J Wright
   VP Audience Development: Suzanne F Newman
   Treasurer: James C Banks
   Recording Secretary: Nancy Brown Cornett
   Cooresponding Secretary: Susan M Morton
Management:
   President: Kim T Schnell
   General Manager: Doris Wood
   Music Director/Conductor: Adrian Gnam
   Marketing/Development Director: John E Sweat
Mission: To offer live quality classical music performances for the enjoyment of the community; to foster the appreciation of music through educational programs.
Specialized Field: Orchestra
Status: Professional; Nonprofit
Paid Staff: 6
Volunteer Staff: 1
Paid Artists: 75
Budget: $650,000
Income Sources: Ticket Sales, Donations, Grants
Performs At: Grand Opera House
Annual Attendance: 12,000+
Seating Capacity: 1,025
Year Built: 1887
Year Remodeled: 2000
Organization Type: Performing; Resident; Educational

1082   COBB SYMPHONY ORCHESTRA

PO Box 452
Marietta, GA 30061
Phone: 770-499-3488
Fax: 770-424-5541
e-mail: webmaster@cobbsymphony.org
Web Site: www.cobbsymphony.org
Management:
   Music Director: Steven Byess
   Executive Director: Hillary Wagy
   Music Director: Lynne Webster
Budget: $150,000-260,000
Performs At: Stillwell Theatre

1083   ROME SYMPHONY ORCHESTRA

540 Broad Street
PO Box 553
Rome, GA 30161
Phone: 706-291-7967
Fax: 706-291-3840
e-mail: symphony@romesymphony.org
Web Site: www.romesymphony.org
Officers:
   President: Barbara L Beninato
   VP: Katie Dempsey
   Treasurer: Ira Levy
   Secretary: Suzanne Smith
Management:
   Executive Director: Mary Ann K Bray
   Music Director/Conductor: Philip O Rice

Mission: The vision of the RSO, within the context of available resources, is to promote, educate, and entertain. Presents performances of the highest artistic level, performs a diverse repertoire; provides opportunities for area musicians to use their talents and training, cultivate and expands musical appreciation, offers educational musical appreciation, and offers educational musical experiences.
Founded: 1921
Specialized Field: Music
Paid Staff: 2
Volunteer Staff: 5
Paid Artists: 65
Budget: $35,000-100,000
Income Sources: Donations; Ticket Sales; Program Sales; Fund Raisers
Performs At: City Hall
Seating Capacity: 1,094

1084   ORCHESTRA ATLANTA

1000 Holcomb Woods Parkway
Suite 112
Roswell, GA 30076
Phone: 770-992-2559
Fax: 770-998-6877
e-mail: orchatl@aol.com
Web Site: www.orchestraatlanta.com
Management:
   Manager: Charles Little
Founded: 1984
Paid Staff: 1
Volunteer Staff: 10
Paid Artists: 15
Non-paid Artists: 8
Budget: $100,000-150,000
Performs At: Roswell Cultural Arts Center

1085   DEKALB SYMPHONY ORCHESTRA

PO Box 1313
Tucker, GA 30085
Phone: 404-299-4341
Fax: 404-299-4271
e-mail: dso@dekalbsymphony.com
Web Site: www.dekalbsymphony.com
Officers:
   Chairman: Paul Tylor
Management:
   Artistic Director: Thomas Anderson
   Manager: Richard Rogers
Founded: 1964
Budget: $140,000
Performs At: Marvin Cole Auditorium
Annual Attendance: 8,000
Facility Category: College Auditorium
Seating Capacity: 500

1086   VALDOSTA SYMPHONY ORCHESTRA

Valdosta State University
Valdosta, GA 31698
Phone: 229-333-5804
Fax: 229-259-5578
e-mail: jploendue@valdosta.edu
Web Site: www.valdosta.edu/music
Management:

Music Director: Samuel Wong
Interior Executive Director: John Graham
Orchestra Director: Dr. J Ploendue

Hawaii

1087 CHAMBER MUSIC HAWAII
1466 Akeakamaie Street
Honolulu, HI 96816
Phone: 808-738-0202
Fax: 808-738-0202
Management:
Executive Director: Susan Haas
Mission: To provide the people of Hawaii with chamber music through support of resident chamber music ensembles.
Specialized Field: Chamber; Ensemble
Status: Professional; Nonprofit
Organization Type: Presenting

1088 HAWAII CHAMBER ORCHESTRA SOCIETY
3810 Maunaloa Avenue
Honolulu, HI 96816
Phone: 808-734-0397
Fax: 808-926-8004
Management:
Music Director: Herbert Ward
General Manager/Opera Director: Jacqueline Ward
Mission: To increase interest in and appreciation of classical music.
Founded: 1967
Specialized Field: Chamber; Ensemble; Opera
Status: Professional; Nonprofit
Organization Type: Performing; Educational

1089 HAWAII YOUTH SYMPHONY ASSOCIATION
1110 University Avenue
Suite 201
Honolulu, HI 96826-1508
Phone: 808-941-9706
Fax: 808-941-4995
e-mail: admin@hiyouthsymphony.org
Web Site: www.hiyouthsymphony.org
Management:
Music Director: Henry Miyamura
Executive Director: Bonnie Hilton
Mission: Dedicated to nurturing the educational and artistic development of student musicians.
Founded: 1964
Specialized Field: Symphony; Orchestra-Youth
Status: Nonprofit
Paid Staff: 20
Volunteer Staff: 50
Paid Artists: 6
Budget: $600,000
Income Sources: Registration; Grants; Donations; Sponsorships; Tickets
Performs At: Neal S. Blaisdell Center Concert Hall
Affiliations: ASOL, HAAE
Organization Type: Performing; Educational

1090 HONOLULU CHAMBER MUSIC SERIES
Box 2233
Honolulu, HI 96804
Phone: 808-528-8226
Fax: 808-956-9422
e-mail: tslaught@outreach.hawaii.edu
Officers:
President: Andrew Bunn
Performs At: Orvis Auditorium

1091 HONOLULU SYMPHONY ORCHESTRA
650 Iwilei Road
Suite 202
Honolulu, HI 96817
Phone: 808-524-0815
Fax: 808-524-1507
e-mail: jmancuso@honolulusymphony.com
Web Site: www.honolulusymphony.com
Management:
Music Director: Samuel Wong
Executive Director: Steve Bloom
Orchestra Manager: Jim Mancuso
Stage Coordinator: Kenji Stevens
Artist Coordinator: Kristin McEntee
Director Marketing: Alan Rakov
Founded: 1900
Budget: $3,600,000-10,000,000
Performs At: Neal Blaisdell Concert Hall

1092 UNIVERSITY OF HAWAII AT MANOA
2530 Dole Street
Honolulu, HI 96822
Phone: 808-956-2042
Fax: 808-956-9657
Web Site: www.hawaii.edu
Management:
Director: Barbara Furstenberg
Marketing/Production Coordinator: Cheryl Kohashi
Program Specialist: Suzanne Shoemaker
Secretary: Susan Yokouchi
Mission: Dedicated to presenting quality musical, dance, theater and special attractions to Hawaii audiences, including the Honolulu Chamber Music Series.
Founded: 1907
Specialized Field: Chamber; Ensemble; Ethnic; Instrumental Group; Solo
Status: Professional
Income Sources: Western Alliance of Arts Administrators; Association for Performing Arts Presenters
Performs At: Blaisdell Concert Hall; Orvis Auditorium
Organization Type: Sponsoring

1093 MAUI PHILHARMONIC SOCIETY
95 Mahalani Street
Wailuku, HI 96793
Phone: 808-244-3771
Fax: 808-242-1857
Web Site: www.mauisymphony.com
Performs At: Various Auditoriums

1094 MAUI SYMPHONY ORCHESTRA
PO Box 1033
Wailuku, HI 96793
Phone: 808-986-8400
Fax: 808-242-6867
e-mail: info@mauisymphony.com
Web Site: www.mauisumphony.com
Officers:
    President: Frank Blackwell
Management:
    Music Director/Conductor: James French
Mission: To give native musicians an opportunity to
perform; to provide the Maui community with a
permanent resident orchestra; to provide an opportunity
for local performers and choreographers to display their
talents through association with the orchestra; to premiere
original works.
Founded: 1979
Specialized Field: Symphony; Orchestra; Ethnic
Status: Semi-Professional; Nonprofit
Paid Staff: 40
Income Sources: American Symphony Orchestra
League; Maui Community Arts Council
Performs At: Baldwin Auditorium; Wailuku
Organization Type: Performing

Idaho

1095 BOISE CHAMBER MUSIC SERIES
1910 University Drive
Boise, ID 83725-1560
Phone: 208-426-1216
Fax: 208-426-1771
e-mail: jbelfy@boisestate.edu
Management:
    Manager: Jeanne Belfy
Performs At: Morrison Center Recital Hall

1096 BOISE PHILHARMONIC ASSOCIATION
516 S 9th Street
Boise, ID 83702
Phone: 208-344-7849
Fax: 208-336-9078
Toll-free: 888-300-7849
e-mail: info@boisephilharmonic.org
Web Site: www.boisephilharmonic.org
Officers:
    Board President: Stephen S Trott
Management:
    Music Director: James Ogle
    Executive Director: Anthony C Boatman
    Marketing Director: Jennifer Brink
Founded: 1887
Paid Staff: 10
Volunteer Staff: 50
Paid Artists: 72
Budget: $1.3 million
Performs At: Morrison Center for the Performing Arts
Annual Attendance: 50,000

1097 IDAHO CLASSICAL GUITAR SOCIETY
550 W Fort Street
Room 667
Boise, ID 83724
Phone: 208-384-1518
Fax: 208-334-9715

1098 MAGIC PHILHARMONIC ORCHESTRA
428 E Highway 81
Burley, ID 83318
Phone: 208-678-9534
Fax: 208-678-9116
e-mail: jzd@pmt.org
Officers:
    President: Wayne Hurst
    Treasurer: Bob Daley
    Secretary: Sesan Neibaur
Management:
    Librarian: Jo Dayley
Founded: 1983
Volunteer Staff: 75
Paid Artists: 2
Non-paid Artists: 4
Budget: $35,000
Performs At: King Fine Arts Center

1099 IDAHO FALLS SYMPHONY
498 A Street
Suite A
Idaho Falls, ID 83402
Phone: 208-529-1080
Fax: 208-529-1097
e-mail: ifsymphsrv.net
Web Site: www.srv.net/~ifsymph/Home.html
Management:
    Conductor/Music Director: George Adams
    Business Manager: Linda Watts
Mission: Instrumental music.
Founded: 1955
Specialized Field: Symphony; Orchestra
Status: Semi-Professional; Nonprofit
Paid Staff: 4
Volunteer Staff: 21
Income Sources: American Symphony Orchestra League
Performs At: Civic Auditorium
Annual Attendance: 10,000+
Seating Capacity: 948
Organization Type: Performing; Resident; Educational

1100 AUDITORIUM CHAMBER MUSIC SERIES
University of Idaho
Moscow, ID 83844-4015
Phone: 208-885-7557
Fax: 208-885-7254
e-mail: chambermusic@uidaho.edu
Management:
    Director: Mary DuPree
    Administrative Assistant: Matthew Pilcher
Mission: Four concert series and residency activities.
Paid Staff: 2
Paid Artists: 20
Performs At: University Auditorium

1101 WASHINGTON IDAHO SYMPHONY
PO Box 9185
Moscow, ID 83843
Phone: 509-335-3581
Fax: 509-335-2220
Web Site: www.c-5.com/symphony/
Management:
    Executive Director: Cecilia Lund
Mission: To offer the enjoyment of music to people of all ages and provide area musicians an opportunity to participate in an orchestra or chorus.
Founded: 1972
Specialized Field: Symphony; Ensemble
Status: Non-Professional; Nonprofit
Paid Staff: 40
Income Sources: American Symphony Orchestra League
Organization Type: Performing; Resident; Educational

1102 IDAHO STATE CIVIC SYMPHONY
Campus Box 8099
Pocatello, ID 83209
Phone: 208-282-3479
Fax: 208-236-4884
e-mail: hurlangi@isu.edu
Management:
    Music Director/Conductor: Dr. Thom Ritter George
    Manager: Angela Hurley
Budget: $100,000-150,000
Performs At: Goranson Hall

1103 MAGIC VALLEY SYMPHONY
PO Box 1805
315 Falls Avenue
Twin Falls, ID 83303-1805
Phone: 208-734-6549
Fax: 208-733-6161
Officers:
    President: George Halsell
Management:
    Conductor: Theodore H Hadley
    Business Manager: H Richard Cook
    Librarian: Jan Olsen
Mission: Committed to enhancing the cultural life of the community and providing an outlet for performers.
Founded: 1959
Specialized Field: Symphony; Orchestra
Status: Non-Professional; Nonprofit
Paid Staff: 3
Budget: $25,500
Income Sources: Ticket Sales; Donations
Performs At: College of Southern Idaho Fine Arts Auditorium
Affiliations: American Society of Composers, Authors and Publishers
Annual Attendance: 2,000
Facility Category: Junior College
Seating Capacity: 900
Year Built: 1970
Organization Type: Performing

Illinois

1104 ALTON SYMPHONY ORCHESTRA
PO Box 1205
Alton, IL 62002
Phone: 618-467-2326
Fax: 618-465-7435
e-mail: info@altonsymphony.org
Web Site: www.altonsymphony.org
Officers:
    President: Mark Landon
    VP: Bud-Emmerson Shultz, Jr
    Secretary: Judy Roth
    Treasurer: Debbie Kelley
Management:
    Manager: Dr. Frank M Boals
Mission: To provide a training ground for the development of instrumental abilities of area musicians; to increase interest in orchestral music; to present concerts to the public.
Founded: 1946
Specialized Field: Symphony
Status: Non-Professional; Nonprofit
Income Sources: Illinois Council of Orchestras
Performs At: Hatheway Hall; Lewis & Clark Community College
Organization Type: Performing

1105 FOX VALLEY SYMPHONY
WCC-Aurora Campus
5 E Galena Boulevard
Aurora, IL 60506
Phone: 630-896-1133
Fax: 630-906-4127
Web Site: www.focol.org/~fvso/
Management:
    Music Director: Fusao Kajima
    General Manager: Bobbie Thornton
Founded: 1966
Paid Staff: 7
Volunteer Staff: 125
Paid Artists: 65
Budget: $35,000-100,000
Performs At: Paramount Arts Center

1106 SINFONIETTA AMERICANA
39432 N Avenue
Beach Park, IL 60099-3602
Phone: 847-872-3707
Fax: 847-872-6860
Management:
    Music Director: Samuel Korngold
    General Manager: David Tannenbaum
Budget: $150,000-260,000

1107 BELLEVILLE PHILHARMONIC
116 N Jackson Street
Belleville, IL 62220
Phone: 618-235-5600
Fax: 618-235-4975
Web Site: www.bellphil.com
Management:
    Administrator: Kathleen J AuBuchon
    Office Manager: Kathly Albers

Mission: Committed to serving the interests of music and musicians in the Greater Belleville area.
Founded: 1867
Specialized Field: Symphony; Orchestra; Instrumental Group
Status: Non-Professional; Nonprofit
Paid Staff: 100
Organization Type: Performing; Educational

1108 ILLINOIS CHAMBER ORCHESTRA

PO Box 3094
Bloomington, IL 61702
Phone: 309-661-2662
Fax: 309-827-2726
Web Site: ilsymphony.org
Management:
   Executive Director: Maureen Earley
   Orhcestra Manager: Eileen Johnson
   Conductor: Karen Deal
Budget: $100,000-150,000
Performs At: Sangamon State University Auditorium; Braden Auditorium

1109 CENTRALIA PHILHARMONIC ORCHESTRA

Centralia Cultural Society
1250 E Rexford Street
Centralia, IL 62801
Phone: 618-532-2951
Fax: 618-532-2964
e-mail: artcntr@msn.com
Web Site: www.centraliaarts.org
Management:
   Administrative Coordinator: Jane Pacey
Founded: 1961
Specialized Field: Orchestra; Choral; Theatre; Art; Dance
Status: Nonprofit
Paid Staff: 1
Budget: $150,000
Income Sources: Ticket Sales; Donations; Patrons; Trust Funds
Annual Attendance: 25,000
Seating Capacity: 300
Year Built: 1971
Year Remodeled: 1981

1110 CHAMPAIGN-URBANA SYMPHONY ORCHESTRA

701 Devonshire Drive, C-24
Champaign, IL 61820-7337
Phone: 217-351-9139
Fax: 217-351-1698
e-mail: music@cusymphony
Web Site: www.cusymphony.org
Officers:
   President: Bill Volk
   VP: Ernest Gullerud
   Secretary: George Perlstein
   Treasure: Peggy Schneider
Management:
   Music Director/Conductor: Steven Larsen
   General Manager: Sue Crawford
   Aministrative Assistant: Dori Johnson

Mission: To provide live, symphonic music performances of the highest quality and music education for our community's children.
Budget: $150,000-260,000
Performs At: Krannert Center for the Performing Arts

1111 EASTERN SYMPHONY ORCHESTRA

Eastern Illinois University
Department of Music
Charleston, IL 61920
Phone: 217-581-3111
Fax: 217-581-7137
e-mail: cfrrr@eiu.edu
Web Site: www.eiu.edu/~music
Management:
   Director Orchestral Activities: Richard Robert Rossi
Volunteer Staff: 20
Paid Artists: 15
Non-paid Artists: 60
Budget: $50,000
Performs At: Dvorak Hall

1112 AMERICAN FESTIVAL ORCHESTRA CHICAGO CHAMBER PLAYERS

1020 S Monitor Avenue
Chicago, IL 60644
Phone: 773-261-6922
Fax: 773-282-9404
Management:
   Music Director/Conductor: George William Kuhs
   Manager: Charles Matyas
Mission: To maintain a year round studio/school where training is offered in Afro-Haitian, Several styles of jazz and modern dance techniques.

1113 ANNUAL CHICAGO JAZZ FESTIVAL

Mayor's Office of Special Events
121 N LaSalle Street
Chicago, IL 60602
Phone: 312-744-3315
Fax: 312-744-0613
e-mail: specialevents@cityofchicago.org
Web Site: www.cityofchicago.org/specialevents
Management:
   Coordinator: Jennifer J Washington
Mission: To present a festival, free to the public featuring jazz in all of its forms.
Founded: 1979
Specialized Field: Vocal Music; Instrumental Music; Jazz
Status: Professional
Performs At: Symphony Music Shell; Petrillo Music Shell
Organization Type: Performing

1114 CHICAGO CHAMBER ORCHESTRA

332 S Michigan Avenue
Suite 1143
Chicago, IL 60604
Phone: 312-822-5570
Fax: 262-605-1148
e-mail: KoberDieter@aol.com
Web Site: www.geocities.com/fiala4825
Management:

Founder Musical Director/Conductor: Dieter Kober

1115 CHICAGO SINFONIETTA

188 West Randolphi Street
Suite 1601
Chicago, IL 60601
Phone: 312-236-3681
Fax: 312-235-5429
Officers:
    Chairperson: Michelle Collins
    President: Roger G Wilson
    VP: Weldon Rougeau
    Secretary: Robert Wootton
Management:
    Music Director: Paul Freeman
    General Manager: Thomas De Walle
    Development Administrator: Maria Mowbray
    Director Marketing: Ferris O'Shaughnessy
Mission: Offering classical music in original orchestration and promoting ethnic diversity in the concert hall.
Founded: 1986
Specialized Field: Classical, Jazz, World
Status: Nonprofit
Paid Staff: 16
Volunteer Staff: 120
Paid Artists: 65
Non-paid Artists: 1
Income Sources: Chicago Music Alliance
Performs At: Lund Auditorium; Rosary College
Organization Type: Performing; Touring; Educational

1116 CHICAGO SYMPHONY ORCHESTRA

220 S Michigan Avenue
Chicago, IL 60604
Phone: 312-294-3000
Fax: 312-294-3329
Toll-free: 800-223-7114
e-mail: info@chicagosymphony.org
Web Site: www.chicagosymphony.org
Officers:
    President: Henry Fogel
    Assistant to President: Margaret Smith
    Administrative Assistant: Julie Taylor
    Secretary of the Board: Kim Briggs
    Director Martketing: Joyce Idema
    Director Finance: Tom Hallett
Management:
    Executive Director: Henry Fogel
    Music Director: Daniel Barenboim
    Artistic Administrator: Martha Gilmer
    Principal Guest Conductor: Pierre Boulez
    Music Director Laureate: Sie George Solti
    Chorus Director: Duain Wolfe
    Composer in Residence: Augusta Read Thomas
    Manager: Vanessa Moss
Founded: 1890
Specialized Field: Symphony; Orchestra
Status: Nonprofit
Income Sources: American Symphony Orchestra League
Organization Type: Performing

1117 CHICAGO YOUTH SYMPHONY ORCHESTRA

410 S Michigan Avenue
Suite 833
Chicago, IL 60605
Phone: 312-939-2207
Fax: 312-939-2015
e-mail: cyso@cyso.org
Web Site: www.cyso.org
Officers:
    President: Toby J Bishop
    VP: Elaine Felder
    VP: Rose Ann Grundman
    VP: Ernest Haberli
    VP: Fred Morrison
    VP: Wendy W. Reynes
    VP: John Schaldweiler
    VP: Debra Yates
    Secretary: John Roberts
Management:
    Executive Director: Jeannette Kreston
    Music Director: Allen Tikham
    Director Of Operations: Pam Baker
    Marketing And Program Manager: Erin Fusco
Mission: To provide the finest quality orchestral training and performance opportunities for Chicagoland musicians 8 - 18
Founded: 1946
Specialized Field: Instramental music
Status: Nonprofit
Paid Staff: 12
Budget: $848,450
Income Sources: Government; Foundations/Corporations; Benefit; Individuals
Performs At: Orchestra Hall
Facility Category: Large Rehearsal/Performance Hall
Organization Type: Performing; Touring; Sponsoring

1118 CLASSICAL SYMPHONY ORCHESTRA & THE PROTEGE PHILHARMONIC

333 S State Street
Chicago, IL 60604
Phone: 312-341-1521
Fax: 312-341-1835
e-mail: clasorch@interaccess.com
Web Site: homepage.interaccess.com/~clasorch
Management:
    Music Director: Joseph Glymph
Budget: $150,000-260,000
Performs At: Preston Bradley Hall

1119 CSO PRESENTS

220 S Michigan Avenue
Chicago, IL 60604
Phone: 312-294-3333
Fax: 312-294-3329
Web Site: www.chicagosymphony.org
Officers:
    President: Henery Fogel
Management:
    Music Director: Daniel Barenboim
Budget: $400,000-$1,000,000
Performs At: Orchestra Hall at Symphony Center

1120 NEW BLACK MUSIC REPERTORY ENSEMBLE
Center for Black Music Research
Columbia College, 600 S Michigan
Chicago, IL 60605
Phone: 312-344-7559
Fax: 312-344-8029
Web Site: www.cbmr.org
Officers:
   Director: Resita M Sands, Jr
Management:
   Coordinator of Perf. Activities: Coleridge Parkinson
Mission: To perform works by black composers from 1700 to the present.
Founded: 1988
Specialized Field: Chamber; Ensemble; Ethnic
Status: Professional; Nonprofit
Paid Staff: 13
Paid Artists: 40
Income Sources: Columbia College, Federal and State Grants, Foundation and Corporate Grants
Organization Type: Performing; Touring

1121 PERFORMING ARTS CHICAGO
410 S Michigan Avenue
#911
Chicago, IL 60605
Phone: 312-663-1628
Fax: 312-663-1043
e-mail: mail@pachicago.org
Web Site: www.pachicago.org
Officers:
   Chair: Helyn Goldenberg
   President Director: Maya Polsky
   President: Judy Neisser
   Treasurer: David Ellis
Management:
   Executive Director: Susan Lipman
   Programs Manager: CJ Mitchell
   Director: Christy Uchida
   Operations Manager: Laurell Zahrobsky
   Development Assistant: Brigid Flynn
Mission: Performing Arts Chicago is dedicated to the presentation of new work by local, national, and international artists from a wide cultural spectrum, and in doing so, reaching out in collaboration with the Chicago arts and education communities to challenge our diverse urban audience.
Founded: 1959
Specialized Field: Chamber; Theater; Dance; Puppetry
Status: Professional; Nonprofit
Paid Staff: 6
Budget: $1,000,000
Performs At: The Civic Theater
Organization Type: Performing; Resident; Educational; Sponsoring

1122 ROOSEVELT UNIVERSITY ORCHESTRA: CHICAGO COLLEGE OF PERFORMING ARTS
430 S Michigan Avenue
Chicago, IL 60605
Phone: 312-341-3780
Fax: 312-341-6358
Web Site: www.roosevelt.edu
Management:
   Chief Resident Conductor: Steven Squires
Specialized Field: Theatre Conservatory, Music Conservatory Community Academy
Performs At: Rudolph Ganz Memorial Hall

1123 UNIVERSITY OF CHICAGO PROFESSIONAL INSTRUMENTAL MUSIC SERIES
The PRISM Series
1212 E 59 Street
Chicago, IL 60637-1604
Phone: 773-955-9339
Fax: 773-702-1195
e-mail: epstein@cs.uchicago.edu
Management:
   Artistic Advisor: Charles Pikler
Performs At: Mandel Hall

1124 UNIVERSITY OF CHICAGO SYMPHONY ORCHESTRA
1010 E 59th Street
Chicago, IL 60637
Phone: 773-702-3427
Fax: 773-753-0558
e-mail: KKohlerh@midway.uchicago.edu
Web Site: http://music.uchicago.edu
Officers:
   President: Gilberto Zaldivar
   VP: Rene Buch
   Secretary/Treasurer: Robert Weber Federico
Management:
   Music Director/Conductor: Barbara Schubert
   Director Public Relations: Kristine Kohler-Hall
Budget: $100,000
Performs At: Leon Mandel Hall
Affiliations: University of Chicago

1125 DANVILLE SYMPHONY ORCHESTRA
2917 N Vermillion Street
Danville, IL 61832
Phone: 217-443-5300
Fax: 217-443-5313
e-mail: dso@soltec.org
Web Site: www.danvillesymphony.org
Management:
   Executive Director: Janet Picllo
   Music Director: Jeremy A Swerling
   Administrative Director: Linda Pollert
Mission: To serve our community and to inspire it to achievement and excellence by presenting music at the highest possible levels of artistic excellence.
Founded: 1967
Specialized Field: Symphony; Orchestra; Chamber
Status: Semi-Professional; Nonprofit
Paid Staff: 2
Paid Artists: 80
Budget: $190,000
Income Sources: Illinois Council of Orchestras; Illinois Presenters Network

Performs At: High School Auditorium; David Palmer Civic Center
Seating Capacity: 1,700
Organization Type: Performing; Educational

1126 MILLIKIN-DECATUR SYMPHONY ORCHESTRA
Millikin University
1184 W Main
Decatur, IL 62522
Phone: 217-424-6300
Fax: 217-420-6652
e-mail: mluxner@mail.millikin.edu
Web Site: www.millikin.edu
Management:
    Music Director/Conductor: Michael Luxner
    Artistic Administrator: Lois Sanner
Budget: $150,000-260,000
Performs At: Kirkland Center Theatre

1127 NORTHWEST SYMPHONY ORCHESTRA
PO Box 1491
Des Plaines, IL 60016
Phone: 847-317-9343
Web Site: www.northwestsymphonyorchestra.org
Officers:
    President: Diane Macewicz
Management:
    Music Director: Anthony Spain PhD
Founded: 1987
Budget: $35,000
Performs At: Highline Performing Arts Center
Seating Capacity: 900

1128 ELGIN SYMPHONY ORCHESTRA
20 Du Paga Court
Elgin, IL 60120
Phone: 847-888-4000
Fax: 847-888-0400
e-mail: boxoffice@elignsymphony.org
Officers:
    President: John Totten
    Secretary: Sue Ollman
    Treasure: Daniel Westrope
    VP Marketing: Elizabeth Erotas-Rouzer
Management:
    Music Director: Robert Hanson
    Executive Director: Michael Pastreich
Founded: 1950
Specialized Field: Symphony Orchestra

1129 ELMHURST SYMPHONY ORCHESTRA
PO Box 345
Elmhurst, IL 60126
Phone: 630-941-0202
Fax: 630-941-0627
e-mail: elmso@aol.com
Management:
    Music Director: Stephen Alltop
    Symphony Manager: Charlene Campbell
    Executive Director: Susan Fuller
Founded: 1959

Specialized Field: Symphony Orchestra
Paid Staff: 3
Volunteer Staff: 35
Paid Artists: 27
Non-paid Artists: 53
Budget: $250,000
Performs At: Hammerschmidt Memorial Chapel at Elmhurst College
Annual Attendance: 4,500
Facility Category: Chapel
Type of Stage: Closed Proscenium
Seating Capacity: 853

1130 BACH WEEK FESTIVAL IN EVANSTON
PO Box 6133
Evanston, IL 60204-6133
Phone: 847-945-7929
Fax: 847-945-1106
e-mail: bachwk@aol.com
Web Site: www.bachweek.org
Management:
    Music Director: Richard R Webster
    General Manager: Anne Harris
Season: May
Facility Category: Saint Luke's Episcopal Church, Evanston
Seating Capacity: 450

1131 SYMPHONY II
1123 Emerson Street
Suite 207
Evanston, IL 60201
Phone: 847-866-6888
Fax: 847-866-0966
e-mail: symphonyII@yahoo.com
Web Site: www.symphony-II.org
Officers:
    President: Dr. James Berkenstock
Management:
    Music Director: Larry Rachleff
    Artistic Administrator: Barbara Haffner
Mission: The ensemble is dedicated to building new audiences for serious music by offering moderately priced concerts, at the highest professional level, in convenient venues. Its presentations of the full range symphonic works embody the excitement of live performances and exemplify a special relationship between performers and audiences.
Budget: $260,000-1,050,000
Performs At: Pick - Staiger Concert Hall

1132 DUPAGE SYMPHONY
PO Box 488
Glen Ellyn, IL 60137
Phone: 630-690-8644
Fax: 630-690-8644
Web Site: www.dupagesymphony.org
Management:
    Music Director/Conductor: Barbara Schubert
    Business Manager: Doris Purdie
Mission: To provide area citizens an opportunity to hear live music; to offer a performance outlet for musicians.
Founded: 1954

Specialized Field: Symphony; Orchestra; Chamber; Ensemble
Status: Non-Professional; Nonprofit
Paid Staff: 65
Income Sources: Illinois Council of Orchestras
Performs At: Dupage County Auditorium
Organization Type: Performing; Touring

1133 NEW PHILHARMONIC
College of DuPage
425 22 Street
Glen Ellyn, IL 60137
Phone: 630-942-3005
Fax: 630-790-9806
e-mail: bauerH@CDnet.cod.edu
Management:
  Music Director: Harold Bauer
Budget: $150,000-260,000
Seating Capacity: 800

1134 WHEATON SYMPHONY ORCHESTRA
344 Spring Avenue
Glen Ellyn, IL 60137
Phone: 630-790-1430
Fax: 630-790-9703
Management:
  General Manager: Donald C Mattison
  Music Director: Peter Lipari
Mission: Dedicated to performing the music of 19th and 20th-century composers which was composed for large orchestras.
Founded: 1959
Specialized Field: Symphony
Status: Non-Professional
Volunteer Staff: 2
Income Sources: American Symphony Orchestra League
Performs At: Hubble Middle School Main Auditorium
Affiliations: Hubble Middle School
Seating Capacity: 550
Year Built: 1930
Year Remodeled: 1985
Organization Type: Performing

1135 CHAMBER MUSIC SOCIETY OF THE NORTH SHORE
PO Box 470
Glencoe, IL 60022
Phone: 847-835-5084
e-mail: iris@interaccess.com
Web Site: www.cmsns.org
Officers:
  President: Iris Cosnow
  Administrator: Sandra Weiss
Founded: 1984
Specialized Field: Chamber Music
Performs At: Pick-Staiger Concert Hall
Seating Capacity: 900

1136 MIDWEST YOUNG ARTISTS
878 Lyster Road
Highwood, IL 60201

Phone: 847-926-9898
Fax: 847-926-4787
e-mail: mya@mya.org
Web Site: www.mya.org
Officers:
  President: Richard Sugar
  VP: John Chipman
  Secretary: Tom Sharp
  Treasurer: Tom Drake
Management:
  Director: Dr. Allan Dennis
  Director Administration: Karen Dennis
  Director Development: Richard Gage
Founded: 1993
Paid Staff: 6
Paid Artists: 18
Budget: $260,000-1,050,000
Income Sources: Tuition; Ticket Sales; Program Ad Revenues
Performs At: Pick - Staiger Concert Hall
Affiliations: Illinois Council of Orchestras

1137 LAKE FOREST SYMPHONY
50 E Old Mill Road
Lake Forest, IL 60045-3844
Phone: 847-295-2135
Fax: 847-295-2747
e-mail: lfsymphony@aol.com
Web Site: www.lakeforestsymphony.com
Officers:
  Treasurer: Donald R Smith
Management:
  Music Director: Alan Heatherington
  President: Charles Fry
  Controller: Gayle Heatherington
  Director Marketing: Jaon Meigs
Mission: Present five classical concerts during the regular season.
Founded: 1956
Specialized Field: Symphony Orchestra
Paid Staff: 5
Volunteer Staff: 1
Budget: $260,000-1,050,000
Income Sources: Donations; Ticket Sales
Performs At: Drake Theater; Barat College
Annual Attendance: 1,200
Type of Stage: Thrust
Seating Capacity: 640
Year Built: 1960

1138 CEDARHURST CHAMBER MUSIC
PO Box 923
Mount Vernon, IL 62864
Phone: 618-242-1236
Fax: 618-242-9530
e-mail: Shar@midwest.net
Web Site: www.cedarhurst.org
Management:
  Executive Director: Sharon Bradham
Mission: Presenting a series of chamber music concerts for the broad Southern Illinois audience; featuring performers from Illinois as well as the rest of the United States and overseas.
Founded: 1979

Specialized Field: Orchestra; Chamber; Ensemble; Ethnic
Status: Professional; Nonprofit
Income Sources: Chamber Music America; Illinois Presenters Network
Performs At: Main Gallery; Mitchell Art Museum
Type of Stage: Portable
Stage Dimensions: 16' x 24'
Seating Capacity: 200
Year Built: 1973
Year Remodeled: 1991
Organization Type: Sponsoring

1139 NORTHBROOK SYMPHONY ORCHESTRA

899 Skokie Boulevard
#LL12
Northbrook, IL 60062
Phone: 847-272-0755
Fax: 847-272-0787
e-mail: nso@theramp.net
Web Site: www.northbrooksymphony.org
Officers:
    President: Susan Laing
    Treasurer: Joseph Kitzes
    VP Administration: John Amrein
    VP Marketing: James Kahan
    Secretary: Linda Wachtel
Management:
    Music Director: Lawrence Rapchak
    General Manager: JC Wacholz
    VP Development: Judith Gelleerd
Mission: To offer classical music concerts at an affordable price as well as outreach programs.
Founded: 1980
Specialized Field: Classical Symphony Orchestra; Education Outreach
Paid Staff: 2
Volunteer Staff: 30
Paid Artists: 75
Non-paid Artists: 25
Budget: $260,000-1,050,000
Income Sources: Ticket Sales; Foundations; Corporate & Individual Donations; Special Events
Performs At: Sheely Center for the Performing Arts
Affiliations: CHG Music Alliance; Illinois Council of Orchestra; American Symphony Orchestra League
Annual Attendance: 10,000
Seating Capacity: 1,484

1140 SYMPHONY OF OAK PARK & RIVER FOREST

PO Box 3564
Oak Park, IL 60303
Phone: 708-524-1892
Fax: 708-524-9892
e-mail: KCM908@aol.com
Web Site: www.symphonyoprf.com
Management:
    Music Director: Jay Friedman
Budget: $35,000-100,000

1141 ILLINOIS PHILHARMONIC ORCHESTRA

377 Artists Walk
Park Forest, IL 60466
Phone: 708-481-7774
Fax: 708-481-7998
Web Site: www.ipomusic.org
Management:
    Music Director: Carmon DeLeone
    Executive Director: Thomas Vitek
Budget: $260,000-1,050,000

1142 PEORIA SYMPHONY ORCHESTRA

203 Harrison
Peoria, IL 61602
Phone: 309-637-2787
Fax: 309-637-7388
e-mail: execdir@peoriasymphony.org
Web Site: www.peoriasymphony.org
Officers:
    President: Sidney Banwart
    VP: Walter Kuppman
    Treasurer: Bill O'Malley
    Secretary: Winsley Durand, Jr
Management:
    Music Director: David Commanday
    Executive Director: Judy Furniss
Mission: We provide excellent performances of fine music to a large and diverse audience in a variety of settings. Through a team effort of musicians, volunteers, staff and boards, we develop aggressive programs of education, marketing, and development. Cooperative efforts with local organizations enable us to enrich the mind, life, and culture which is the soul of our community.
Budget: $950,000
Performs At: Peoria Civic Center

1143 QUINCY SYMPHONY ORCHESTRA

428 Main Street
Suite 270
Quincy, IL 62301
Phone: 217-222-2856
Fax: 217-222-2869
e-mail: qsoa@adams.net
Web Site: www.adams.net/~qsoa
Officers:
    President: Anda Zirnitis
Management:
    General Manager: Stacy Taylor
    Managerial Assistant: Pam Snider
Mission: To provide the area with fine orchestral music; to offer local musicians the opportunity to perform; to provide educational programs.
Founded: 1947
Specialized Field: Symphony; Orchestra; Chamber
Status: Non-Professional; Nonprofit
Paid Staff: 45
Volunteer Staff: 40
Budget: $130,000
Income Sources: Grants; Donations; Tickets
Performs At: Quincy Junior High School Auditorium
Organization Type: Performing; Resident; Educational

1144 AUGUSTANA SYMPHONY ORCHESTRA
Augustana College
639 38 Street
Rock Island, IL 61201
Phone: 309-794-7307
Fax: 309-794-7678
e-mail: acedu@augustana.edu
Management:
   Music Director: Daniel Culver
   Cultural Events Director: Dan Urton
Budget: $35,000
Performs At: Centennial Hall

1145 MENDELSSOHN CLUB
415 N Church Street
Rockford, IL 61103-6881
Phone: 815-964-9713
Fax: 815-964-9929
e-mail: info@mendelssohnclub.org
Web Site: www.mendelssohnclub.org
Management:
   Executive Director: Lynn Andreini
Mission: To promote, support and present quality music
for all.
Founded: 1884
Specialized Field: Music
Paid Staff: 5
Volunteer Staff: 45
Paid Artists: 41
Non-paid Artists: 406
Affiliations: Rockford Area Arts Council; Illinois Arts
Council
Facility Category: Auditorium with Stage
Stage Dimensions: 18'x 40'
Seating Capacity: 220
Year Built: 1952
Year Remodeled: 2002

1146 ROCKFORD AREA YOUTH SYMPHONY ORCHESTRA
Riverfront Museum Park
711 N Main Street
Rockford, IL 61103-6903
Phone: 815-965-0049
Fax: 815-965-0642
e-mail: info@rockfordsymphony.com
Web Site: www.rockfordsymphony.com
Officers:
   President: DeWayne Fellows
Management:
   RSO Musical Director/Conductor: Steven Larsen
   RSO Executive Director: Scott Provancher
   RAYSO Conductor: Hsien-Liang Lien
Founded: 1965
Specialized Field: Youth instruction/Performance
Paid Staff: 1
Paid Artists: 6
Non-paid Artists: 65
Budget: $260,000-1,050,000
Income Sources: Grants; Ticket sales; Individual gifts;
Sponsorshipos
Performs At: Coronado Theatre

1147 ILLINOIS CHAMBER SYMPHONY
12 S 1st Avenue
Saint Charles, IL 60174
Phone: 630-377-6423
Fax: 630-377-3105
Officers:
   President: Charles Brown
   VP: Jeffrey Hunt
   Secretary/Treasurer: William Simmons
Management:
   Music Director: Stephen Squires
   Marketing Director: Robert Murphy
   Executive Director: Catherine Squires
   Librarian: Tim Juergensen
   Personnel Manager: Amy Scarlato
Mission: Promoting live classical music of the highest
artistic caliber and furthering cultural growth in the state
of Illinois.
Founded: 1983
Specialized Field: Orchestra; Chamber
Status: Professional; Nonprofit
Income Sources: Indiana Orchestra Consortium; Kane
County Tourism Association; American Symphony
Orchestra League; Fox Valley Arts Council
Performs At: Norris Cultural Arts Center; Baker
Methodist Church
Organization Type: Performing

1148 SKOKIE VALLEY SYMPHONY ORCHESTRA
9501 Skokie Boulevard
Skokie, IL 60077
Phone: 847-679-9501
Fax: 847-679-1879
Web Site: www.skokievalleysymphony.org
Management:
   Music Director: Dr. Donald Chen
   General Manager: Laura Gunderson
Mission: Our community symphony, the Skokie Valley
Symphony Orchestra, was founded in 1962 by musicians
who wanted to enrich the lives of others through music.
Founded: 1962
Specialized Field: Symphony
Budget: $35,000-100,000
Income Sources: Ticket sales; Donations; Grants
Affiliations: Illinois Council of Orchestra's
Facility Category: Concert Hall
Type of Stage: Proscenium
Seating Capacity: 839
Year Built: 1996

1149 ILLINOIS SYMPHONY ORCHESTRA
PO Box 5191
Springfield, IL 62705-5191
Phone: 217-522-2838
Fax: 217-522-7374
e-mail: info@ilsymphony.org
Web Site: ilsymphony.org
Management:
   Executive Director: Mauren Early
Budget: $260,000-1,050,000

1150 SPRINGFIELD SYMPHONY ORCHESTRA
Capitol Avenue
Springfield, IL 62701
Phone: 413-733-2291
Fax: 413-781-4129
e-mail: info@springfieldsym.org
Web Site: www.masslive.com
Management:
    General Manager: Linda G Moore
    Music Director/Conductor: Kenneth Kiesler
    Orchestra Manager: Judith Lampert
Mission: To sponsor, promote and assist in the presentation of symphonic concerts; encourage and develop a desire for symphonic music; instruct, assist and develop musical abilities; assist in training and education; provide concerts, musical programs and other entertainment.
Founded: 1921
Specialized Field: Symphony; Orchestra; Chamber; Ensemble
Status: Professional; Nonprofit
Income Sources: American Symphony Orchestra League; Chamber Music America; Illinois Arts Alliance
Performs At: Braden Auditorium at Illinois State University
Organization Type: Performing; Touring; Resident; Educational

1151 SINFONIA DA CAMERA
909 W Oregon
Urbana, IL 61801
Phone: 217-244-4350
Fax: 217-244-4350
e-mail: sinfonia@uiuc.edu
Web Site: www.sinfonia.uiuc.edu/sinfonia
Management:
    Music Director: Ian Hobson
    General Manager: Rebecca Hill Riley
    Director Development: Susan Kingston
Budget: $150,000-260,000
Performs At: Foellinger Great Hall

1152 WAUKEGAN SYMPHONY ORCHESTRA & CONCERT CHORUS
39 Jack Benny Drive
Waukegan, IL 60085
Phone: 847-244-1660
Fax: 847-662-0592
e-mail: wkarts@waukeganparks.org
Web Site: www.waukeganparks.org/jbc
Management:
    Music Director: Stephen Blackweldor
    Performance Supervisor: Rik Covalinski
Paid Staff: 2
Paid Artists: 6
Non-paid Artists: 60
Budget: $100,000-150,000
Income Sources: Waukegan Park District Corporation, grants
Performs At: Orlin D. Trapp Auditorium
Annual Attendance: 1500
Facility Category: Auditorium
Type of Stage: Proscenium

Seating Capacity: 1500

1153 CHINESE CLASSICAL ORCHESTRA AND EDUCATIONAL PROGRAM
PO Box 5275
Woodridge, IL 60517-0275
Phone: 630-910-1551
Fax: 630-910-1561
Web Site: www.chinesemusic.net
Officers:
    President: Dr. Sin-yan Shen
    VP: Kok-Koon Ng
Management:
    Director Concert Lecture Department: Dr. Yuan-Yuan Lee
Mission: The music society is the largest Chinese music educational service institution in North America; publishes the Chinese Music Monograph Series, the international journal of Chinese Music, and educational material on music and acoustics.
Founded: 1976
Specialized Field: Symphony; Orchestra; Chamber; Ensemble; Ethnic; Folk; Instrumental Group; Electronic & Live Electronic
Status: Professional; Nonprofit
Budget: $260,000 - $1,050,000
Organization Type: Performing; Touring; Resident; Educational; Sponsoring

1154 SILK AND BAMBOO ENSEMBLE
Chinese Music Society of North America
PO Box 5275
Woodridge, IL 60517-0275
Phone: 630-910-1551
Fax: 630-910-1561
Web Site: www.chinesemusic.net
Management:
    Music Director/Conductor: Dr. Sin-yan Shen
    Manager: Johson Hsu
Mission: To create chamber music of the 21st century; to perform works utilizing silk and bamboo instrumentation and just intervals; to tour internationally and in the US year round.
Founded: 1981
Specialized Field: Chamber; Ensemble; Ethnic; Instrumental Group
Status: Professional; Nonprofit
Budget: $260,000 - 1,050,000
Organization Type: Performing; Touring; Educational

1155 WOODSTOCK MOZART FESTIVAL
PO Box 734
Woodstock, IL 60098
Phone: 630-983-7072
Fax: 630-717-7782
e-mail: mozartfest@aol.com
Web Site: www.mozartfest.org
Officers:
    President: Louis La Coque
Management:
    General Director: Anita Whelan
    Artistic Advisor: Mark Peskanov
Founded: 1987
Paid Staff: 3

Paid Artists: 40
Budget: $130,000
Income Sources: Individuals, Corporations, Foundations
Facility Category: Woodstock Opera House (121 Van Buren Street)
Seating Capacity: 412
Year Built: 1889
Year Remodeled: 1977

Indiana

1156   ANDERSON SYMPHONY ORCHESTRA ASSOCIATION

1124 Meridian Street
Suite C
Anderson, IN 14016
Phone: 317-644-2111
Fax: 317-642-1477
Officers:
   President: Marion Hovermale
   Treasurer: John Kane
Management:
   Music Director: Richard Sowers
   Exeutive Director: Pamela Coletti
Founded: 1978
Paid Staff: 74
Budget: $150,000-260,000
Performs At: Paramount Theatre Centre

1157   BLOOMINGTON SYMPHONY ORCHESTRA

PO Box 1823
Bloomington, IN 47402
Phone: 812-331-2320
Fax: 812-331-2320
e-mail: bso@bloomington.in.us
Web Site: www.bloomington.in.us/bso
Management:
   General Manager: Anne Marie Dix
Mission: Strives to provide serious music to the community; to encourage interest in hearing and participating in serious music; and to offer a professional environment for performing that music for both amateurs and professionals.

1158   CARMEL SYMPHONY ORCHESTRA

11 First Avenue NE
PO Box 761
Carmel, IN 46032
Phone: 317-844-9717
Fax: 317-844-9916
e-mail: office@carmelsymphony.com
Management:
   Executive Director: Alan Davis
   Office Manager: Denise Ryan
Mission: To educate children of all ages with music.
Founded: 1975
Status: Nonprofit
Paid Staff: 3
Paid Artists: 13
Non-paid Artists: 60
Budget: $150,000-175,000

Income Sources: Box Office; Grants; Donations
Affiliations: American Symphony Orchestra League
Annual Attendance: 15,000
Organization Type: Performing; Educational

1159   COLUMBUS INDIANA PHILHARMONIC

393 Commons Mall
Columbus, IN 47201
Phone: 812-376-2638
Fax: 812-376-2567
e-mail: info@columbus-in-phil.org
Web Site: www.columbus-in-phil.org
Officers:
   President: Kaye Ellen Conner
   VP: Ronald F Sewell
   Treasurer: Robert Williamson
   Secretary: Bruce Pollert
   Immediate Past President: Jane B. Hoffmeister
Management:
   Manager: Alice O. Curry
   Administrative Assistant: Elizabeth Mullich
   Music Director: David Bowden
Mission: To enhance the quality of life in our community so that all citizens have the opportunity to be touched by live, classical music in a manner and style meaningful to them.
Founded: 1986
Specialized Field: Symphony
Status: Semi-Professional; Nonprofit
Budget: $260,000-$1,050,000
Income Sources: American Symphony Orchestra League; Indiana Orchestra Consort; Indiana Arts Commission; Columbus Area Arts Council
Performs At: Columbus North Erne Auditorium
Facility Category: Orchestra Professional
Organization Type: Performing; Educational; Sponsoring

1160   BETHANY-ELKHART COUNTY SYMPHONY ASSOCIATION

410 S Main Street, Suite 3
PO Box 144
Elkhart, IN 46515
Phone: 219-293-1087
Fax: 219-522-2270
e-mail: symphonyoftheheart@juno.com
Management:
   Conductor: Dr. Kenley Inglefield
   Executive Director: Bethany J Schaubert
Budget: $100,000-150,000
Performs At: Elco Performing Arts Center

1161   EVANSVILLE PHILHARMONIC ORCHESTRA

530 Main Street
PO Box 84
Evansville, IN 47708
Phone: 812-425-5050
Fax: 812-426-7008
e-mail: euphil@evansvillephilharmonic.org
Web Site: www.evansvillephilharmonic.org
Officers:
   President: Philip Fisher
   VP: James Dodd

Secretary: Thomas F Clayton
Treasurer: Ken Robinson
Board of Director: Danny Bateman
Management:
  Executive Director: Ken Krantz
  Administrative Assistant: Sandy Oldham
  Director Marketing: Lynette McClusky
Mission: To provide the Tri-State Area of Southern Indiana, Illinois and Kentucky with symphonic music of the highest quality; to present programs for adult audiences and students in the school systems.
Founded: 1934
Specialized Field: Symphony; Orchestra; Chamber; Ensemble
Status: Professional
Paid Staff: 18
Budget: $2,000,000
Income Sources: American Symphony Orchestra League; Indiana Orchestra Consortium; Evansville Arts & Education Council
Performs At: Victory Theatre
Seating Capacity: 1,800
Year Remodeled: 1998
Organization Type: Performing; Educational

1162 FORT WAYNE PHILHARMONIC ORCHESTRA

2340 Fairfield Avenue
Fort Wayne, IN 46807
Phone: 219-744-1700
Fax: 219-456-8555
Web Site: www.FortWaynePhilharmonic.com
Officers:
  Chairman: Michael McCollum
  Secretary: Nancy Stewart
  Treasurer: John Shoaff
Management:
  Music Director: Edvard Tchivzhel
  Assistant Conductor: David Borsnold
  Director Concert Operations: Laura Bordner
  President: Christopher Guerin
Founded: 1946
Specialized Field: Performing, educational
Paid Staff: 22
Paid Artists: 88
Budget: $4,100,000
Income Sources: Box office, grants, private donations
Performs At: Embassy Theatre
Affiliations: America Symphony Orchestra League, Indiana Orchestra Consortium
Annual Attendance: 220,000
Type of Stage: Proscenium
Seating Capacity: 2434
Year Built: 1928

1163 NEW WORLD YOUTH SYMPHONY ORCHESTRA

10815 Brenda Court
Fortville, IN 46040
Phone: 317-877-1155
Fax: 317-485-5247
Management:
  Music Director: Susan Kitterman
  Business Manager: Susan Bever

Budget: $100,000-150,000
Performs At: Circle Theater

1164 DEPAUW UNIVERSITY CHAMBER SYMPHONY

DePauw University
600 S Locust Street
Greencastle, IN 46135
Phone: 765-658-4388
Fax: 765-658-4401 .
Web Site: osmith@depauw.edu
Management:
  Conductor: Orcenith Smith
Budget: $6,000
Performs At: Kresge Auditorium
Type of Stage: Concert Stage
Stage Dimensions: 60'x 40'
Year Built: 1976
Rental Contact: 765-658-4828 Byron Craft

1165 DEPAUW UNIVERSITY SYMPHONY ORCHESTRA

DePauw University
600 S Locust Street
Greencastle, IN 46135
Phone: 765-658-4388
Fax: 765-658-4401
e-mail: osmith@depauw.edu
Management:
  Conductor: Orcenith Smith
Mission: Teaching our repertoire and concert touring.
Founded: 1974
Budget: $8,000
Performs At: Kresge Auditorium
Affiliations: American Symphony Orchestra League
Type of Stage: Concert Stage
Stage Dimensions: 60'x 40'
Seating Capacity: 1500
Year Built: 1976
Rental Contact: 765-658-4828 Byron Craft
Organization Type: Touring

1166 AMERICAN CONSERVATORY OF MUSIC

252 Wildwood Road
Hammond, IN 46324
Phone: 219-931-6000
Fax: 219-931-6089
e-mail: registrar@americanconservatory.edu
Web Site: www.americanconservatory.edu
Officers:
  Registrar: Dr. Mary Ellen Newson
  President: Theodora Schulze
  Dean: Dr. Marvin Zaporyn
  Chairman Emeritus: Dr. Richard Schulze
  Chairman: Dr. Otto Schulze
Founded: 1886

1167 INDIANAPOLIS CHAMBER ORCHESTRA

Clowes Memorial Hall
4600 Sunset Avenue
Indianapolis, IN 46208-3443

Phone: 317-940-9607
Fax: 317-940-6551
e-mail: ico@butler.edu
Web Site: www.icomusic.org
Management:
   Music Director: Kirk Trevor
   Executive Director: Chad Miller
Budget: $260,000-1,050,000
Seating Capacity: 2,200

1168 INDIANAPOLIS SYMPHONY ORCHESTRA

45 Monument Circle
Indianapolis, IN 46204
Phone: 317-262-1100
Fax: 317-262-1159
e-mail: iso@indyorch.org
Web Site: www.indyorch.org
Officers:
   President/CEO: Richard R Hoffert
   Chairman: James B Steichen, MD
Management:
   VP/General Manager: Thomas R Ramsey
   VP Finance/Administration: Susan L Prenatt
   VP Marketing: Ellen Schantz
   VP Development: Kevin Garvey
   Director Public Relations: Thomas N Akins
Mission: To perform live symphonic music at the highest artistic level; to promote, support and sustain interest in symphonic music in Indiana; to present programs that enrich, entertain and challenge all audiences.
Founded: 1930
Specialized Field: Symphony; Orchestra; Chamber; Ensemble
Status: Professional; Nonprofit
Paid Staff: 60
Paid Artists: 90
Budget: $23 Million
Income Sources: Ticket Sales; Contributions; Endowment
Performs At: Hilbert Circle Theatre
Affiliations: ASOL
Annual Attendance: 500,000+
Type of Stage: Proscenium
Stage Dimensions: 50x40
Seating Capacity: 1786
Year Built: 1916
Year Remodeled: 2002
Organization Type: Performing; Touring; Resident; Educational

1169 INTERNATIONAL VIOLIN COMPETITION OF INDIANAPOLIS

32 E Washington Street
Suite 1320
Indianapolis, IN 46204
Phone: 317-637-4574
Fax: 317-637-1302
e-mail: kwok@violin.org
Web Site: www.violin.org
Management:
   Executive Director: Glen Kwok
   Director Public Relations: Cathleen Partlon Strauss
   Director Operations: Mindy Miller

Director Development: JoEllen Bendall
Mission: To enhance the tradition of classical music and to heighten the cultural profile of Indiana and its capital city.
Founded: 1979
Specialized Field: Chamber Music
Paid Staff: 4

1170 PHILHARMONIC ORCHESTRA OF INDIANAPOLIS

17 W Market
Suite 910
Indianapolis, IN 46204
Phone: 317-916-0178
Fax: 317-656-8754
Web Site: www.philharmonicindy.org
Officers:
   President: Deana Slater
   VP: Craig Parmerlee
   Treasurer: Joyce Boxman
   Secretary: Rolanda Haycox
Management:
   General Manager: Jeff Maess
   Artistic Director: Orcenith Smith
Mission: We provide educational opportunities to the community and enhance the musical growth of volunteer membership.
Founded: 1940
Specialized Field: Symphony; Orchestra; Chamber
Status: Non-Professional; Nonprofit
Paid Staff: 3
Paid Artists: 7
Non-paid Artists: 80
Budget: $100,000-150,000
Performs At: Caleb Mills Hall
Organization Type: Performing; Resident; Educational

1171 SYMPHONY ON THE PRAIRIE
Indianapolis Symphony Orchestra

45 Monument Circle
Indianapolis, IN 46204-2919
Phone: 317-262-1100
Fax: 317-262-1159
Toll-free: 800-366-8457
e-mail: ttolokan@indyorch.org
Web Site: www.indyorch.org
Officers:
   President/CEO: Richard R Hoffert
   VP/General Manager: Thomas R Ramsey
Management:
   Artistic Director: Toby Tolokan
   Media Relations Manager: Tim Northcutt
Founded: 1982
Paid Staff: 50
Paid Artists: 150
Budget: $21,000,000
Income Sources: Box Office; Fees; Sponsorship; Contributions
Season: June - September
Performs At: Conner Prairie, Fishers [Festival Site]
Affiliations: Indianapolis Symphony Orchestra
Annual Attendance: 100,000
Facility Category: Conner Prairie Fishers, In.
Type of Stage: Concrete with Risers, Shell

Seating Capacity: 14,000
Year Built: 1982
Year Remodeled: 1991
Resident Groups: Indianapolis Symphony Orchestra

1172 BUTLER UNIVERSITY SYMPHONY ORCHESTRA

4600 Sunset Avenue
Indianpolis, IN 46208
Phone: 317-940-9346
Fax: 317-940-9930
Toll-free: 800-368-6852
e-mail: info@butler
Web Site: www.butler.edu
Management:
    Conductor: Jackson Wiley
Performs At: Clowes Memorial Hall

1173 KOKOMO SYMPHONY

2601 S Webster Street
PO Box 6115
Kokomo, IN 46904-1659
Phone: 765-455-1659
Fax: 765-453-0048
e-mail: ksoexec@kokomosymphony.org
Web Site: www.kokomosymphony.org
Management:
    Executive Director: Paul L Wood
Mission: To maintain a local orchestra, chorus and youth orchestra; to provide the highest quality of music under the direction of a capable conductor; to provide musical education programs in underserved areas.
Founded: 1971
Specialized Field: Symphony; Orchestra; Chamber
Status: Nonprofit
Paid Staff: 2
Volunteer Staff: 460
Paid Artists: 65
Budget: $239,000
Income Sources: American Symphony Orchestra League; Indiana Orchestra Consortium; Indiana Advocates for the Arts
Performs At: Havens Auditorium
Affiliations: ASOL
Annual Attendance: 5400
Facility Category: Auditorium
Seating Capacity: 905
Organization Type: Performing; Touring; Resident; Educational; Sponsoring

1174 LAFAYETTE SYMPHONY

111 N 6th
PO Box 52
Lafayette, IN 47902
Phone: 765-742-6463
Fax: 765-742-2375
Web Site: www.dcwi.com/~lso
Officers:
    President: Doug Gutridge
    VP: Sandy Bollenbacher
    Treasurer: Chuck Wolpat
    Secretary: Mary Beth Buescher
Management:
    General Manager: Cecily Dresser

Music Director/Conductor: Anne Harrigan
Office Administrator: Sue Ebert
Marketing Coordinator: Beverly Reid
Mission: To offer symphonic literature for the education and enjoyment of residents of the Greater Lafayette Area.
Founded: 1951
Specialized Field: Symphony; Orchestra
Status: Semi-Professional; Nonprofit
Budget: $260,000-$1,050,000
Income Sources: American Symphony Orchestra League; Indiana Orchestra Consortium
Performs At: Long Center for the Performing Arts
Organization Type: Performing; Educational

1175 TIPPECANOE CHAMBER MUSIC SOCIETY

638 N Street
Lafayette, IN 47901
Phone: 765-497-6440
Fax: 765-583-2386
Management:
    Artistic Director: Verna Aloe
Mission: Fosters and promotes the appreciation of chamber music. Promotes the pursuit of musical excellence in the area's youth through diverse educational programs, including master classes, coaching and special school programs.
Founded: 1997
Specialized Field: Music
Status: Nonprofit

1176 MARION PHILHARMONIC ORCHESTRA

PO Box 272
Marion, IN 46952
Phone: 765-662-0012
Fax: 765-662-2667
e-mail: mpo@comteck.com
Web Site: www.qws.com/mpo
Officers:
    President: Jerry Albrecht
    VP: Jim Fordham
    Secretary: Susan Munn
    Treasurer: Bob Hogan
Management:
    Music Director: Diane Persson
    Business Manager: Marion Philharmonic
Founded: 1969
Paid Staff: 80
Budget: $150,000-260,000
Performs At: Marion High School Auditorium

1177 MUNCIE SYMPHONY ORCHESTRA

2000 University Avenue
Bail State University
Muncie, IN 47306
Phone: 765-285-5531
Fax: 765-285-9128
e-mail: manager@munciesymphony.com
Web Site: www.munciesymphony.com
Officers:
    President: Jerome J Gassen
    VP: Don Whitaker
    Past President: Paul C Powers

Secretary: Charles Hetrick
Management:
    Executive Director: Judy A Kirkwood
Mission: To stimulate, educate, and entertain audiences in East Central Indiana, and to provide meaningful musical experience for professional, community, and student musicians, through the performance of fine music and other activities.
Founded: 1948
Specialized Field: Symphony
Status: Semi-Professional; Nonprofit
Paid Staff: 11
Paid Artists: 80
Income Sources: American Symphony Orchestra League; American Society of Composers, Authors and Publishers; Broadcast Music Incorporated; Indiana Orchestra Consortium
Performs At: Emens Auditorium
Affiliations: Ball State University
Organization Type: Performing; Educational

1178 NORTHWEST INDIANA SYMPHONY ORCHESTRA AND SOCIETY

1040 Ridge Road
Munster, IN 46321
Phone: 219-836-0525
Fax: 219-836-0690
e-mail: info@nwisymphony.org
Web Site: www.nwisymphony.org
Officers:
    President: Tom Katsahnias
    VP: Marie Hibbs
    Treasurer: David LeBar
    Secretary: Alicia Tassaro
Management:
    Music Director/Conductor: Kirk Muspratt
    Executive Director: Judith Walker
    Marketing Director: Kim Radu
    Development Director: Daniel Root
Mission: Dedicated to presenting subscription, special, and children's concerts and maintaining the Youth Orchestra and Chorus.
Founded: 1941
Specialized Field: Symphony; Orchestra; Chamber; Ensemble
Status: Professional; Nonprofit
Budget: $1,000,000
Income Sources: Grants; Donations; Ticket Sales
Performs At: Star Plaza Theatre; Merrillville
Organization Type: Performing; Resident; Educational

1179 CHANTICLEER STRING QUARTET

944 Woods Road
Richmond, IN 47374
Phone: 765-966-6214
Fax: 765-973-4570
Management:
    Founder/Violinist/Agent: Caroline Klempe Green
Mission: Sharing in creative ways with people in all walks of life and of all ages the beauty of chamber music.
Founded: 1977
Specialized Field: Chamber
Status: Professional; Nonprofit
Organization Type: Performing; Touring; Educational

1180 RICHMOND SYMPHONY ORCHESTRA

380 Hub Etchison Parkway
PO Box 982
Richmond, IN 47374
Phone: 765-966-5181
Fax: 765-973-3346
e-mail: rso@infocom.com
Web Site: www.richmondsymphony.org
Officers:
    President: Terri Logan
    First VP: Jeff Jackson
    VP: Diana Pappin
    Secretary: Bobbi Whitlock
    Treasurer: Carol Smyth
Management:
    Music Director/Conductor: Guy Victor Bordo
    Executive Director: Laura Hinkley
Founded: 1957
Budget: $260,000-1,050,000
Performs At: Civic Hall Performing Arts Center

1181 SOUTH BEND SYMPHONY ORCHESTRA

120 W LaSalle
Suite 404
South Bend, IN 46601-1305
Phone: 219-232-6343
Fax: 219-232-6627
e-mail: managingdirector@sbsymphony.com
Web Site: sbsymphony.org
Management:
    Music Director/Conductor: Tsung Yeh
    Managing Director/Executive VP: W Mack Richardson
Mission: To perform classical, pops, chamber orchestra, and educational programs.
Founded: 1932
Specialized Field: Symphony Orchestra
Paid Staff: 11
Paid Artists: 95
Budget: $1,050,000-3,600,000
Income Sources: Sales; Contributions; Investments
Performs At: Morris Performing Arts Center
Affiliations: ASOL
Annual Attendance: 150,000
Type of Stage: Proscenium
Seating Capacity: 2,500
Year Built: 1920
Year Remodeled: 2000
Cost: 16,000,000
Rental Contact: Dennis Andres

1182 TERRE HAUTE SYMPHONY ORCHESTRA

25 N 6th Street
Terre Haute, IN 47807
Phone: 812-242-8476
Fax: 812-232-2781
Toll-free: 800-878-8476
e-mail: thso@juno.com
Web Site: www.terrehautesymphony.org
Officers:
    President: Dr. Wieke Van der Weiden Bejamin
    Secretary: Richard Layton

Treasurer: Lowell Bourne
Management:
  Executive Director: Jean Elliott Williams
  Music Director: David Bowden
  Librarian/Resident Composer: Daniel Powers
  Personnel Manager: Laura Q Savage
  Personnel Manager: Chad Roseland
  Bloomington Contractor: Gesa Kordes
  Stage Manager: Alice Yuritic
  House Manager: Emily L Fisher
  Box Office Assitant: Julliane Brandt
Mission: To increase the enjoyment and cultural enrichment of audiences in the Wabash Valley area by maintaining an orchestra dedicated to excellent performances of symphonic literature.
Founded: 1926
Specialized Field: Symphony
Status: Professional
Paid Staff: 8
Paid Artists: 80
Budget: $345,000
Income Sources: Private; Corporate; State
Performs At: Tilson Auditorium; Indiana State University
Annual Attendance: 7,500
Facility Category: Music hall
Seating Capacity: 1478
Year Remodeled: 2002
Rental Contact: 812-237-3737 Hulman Center
Organization Type: Performing; Educational; Run-Outs

1183 VALPARAISO UNIVERSITY SYMPHONY ORCHESTRA

VU Center for the Arts
Valparaiso, IN 46383
Phone: 219-464-5455
Fax: 219-464-5244
e-mail: sarah.rothaar@valpo.edu
Web Site: www.valpo.edu
Management:
  Conductor: Dennis Friesen-Carper
  Arts Development Director: Sarah C Rothaar
Budget: $35,000

Iowa

1184 AMES TOWN AND GOWN CHAMBER MUSIC ASSOCIATION

3222 Oaklnad Street
Ames, IA 50014-3518
Phone: 515-292-3891
e-mail: ForrestPS@aol.com
Web Site: www.amestownandgown.org
Officers:
  President: Karl Gwiasda
  VP: Linda Hagge
  Secretary: Sherry Dragula
Management:
  Artistic Director: Paula Forrest Helmuth
Mission: The presentation of four to six chamber music concerts annually.
Founded: 1950

Specialized Field: Chamber; Ensemble; Instrumental Group
Status: Nonprofit
Income Sources: Iowa State University Music Department
Performs At: Iowa State University Music Hall Recital Hall
Organization Type: Sponsoring

1185 CENTRAL IOWA SYMPHONY

PO Box C
Ames, IA 50014-1018
Phone: 515-292-4466
Fax: 515-292-4115
e-mail: wholger@msn.com
Web Site: www.cisymphony.org
Officers:
  President: Willa Holger
  Secretary: Sue Proescholdt
  Treasurer: Tom Jackson
Management:
  Music Director/Conductor: Mark A Laycock
Mission: To foster quality performance of orchestral music for the people of the Central Iowa communities; to offer satisfying musical experience for its musicians; and to provide leadership in the arts community.
Budget: $35,000-100,000
Performs At: Ames City Hall Auditorium

1186 WATERLOO-CEDAR FALLS SYMPHONY ORCHESTRA

Gallagher-Bluedorn Center
Cedar Falls, IA 50614-0803
Phone: 319-273-3373
Fax: 319-273-3363
e-mail: information@wcfsymphony.org
Web Site: www.wcfsymphony.org
Officers:
  President: Kathleen Wernimont
  President-Elect/VP: Richard Congdon
  Secretary: Charles Wheeland
  Treasure: Louis Fettkether
Management:
  Executive Director: Rachel Falland
Mission: To educate, entertain, and enrich listeners of all ages through community outreach by presenting performances of the highest quality, representing the full range of orchestral repertoire.
Founded: 1930
Specialized Field: Symphony; Orchestra; Chamber; Ensemble
Status: Nonprofit
Paid Staff: 7
Income Sources: American Symphony Orchestra League; American Society of Composers, Authors and Publishers; Broadcast Music Incorporated
Performs At: Kersenbrock Auditorium
Annual Attendance: 15,000
Facility Category: Performing Arts Center
Seating Capacity: 1,500
Year Built: 2000
Organization Type: Performing

1187 CEDAR RAPIDS SYMPHONY ORCHESTRA
205 2nd Avenue SE
Cedar Rapids, IA 52401
Phone: 319-366-8206
Fax: 319-366-5206
Web Site: www.crsymphony.org
Management:
 Executive Director: Marc D Levy
 Music Director/Conductor: Christian Tiemeyer
Founded: 1922
Specialized Field: Symphony; Orchestra; Chamber; Ensemble
Status: Professional; Nonprofit
Budget: $1,050,000-$3,600,000
Income Sources: American Symphony Orchestra League
Performs At: Paramount Theatre
Organization Type: Performing; Educational

1188 CLINTON SYMPHONY ORCHESTRA
PO Box 116
Clinton, IA 52733-0116
Phone: 319-243-2049
Officers:
 President: Richard J Phelan
Management:
 Music Director: Steven Martyn Zike
Budget: $35,000-100,000

1189 QUAD CITY SYMPHONY ORCHESTRA ASSOCIATION
327 Brady Street
PO Box 1144
Davenport, IA 52805-1144
Phone: 563-322-0931
Fax: 563-322-6864
e-mail: info@qcsymphony.com
Web Site: www.qcsymphony.com
Officers:
 President: Patricia E Duffy
 Executive VP: Dan Churchill
 Secretary: Beth Dietz
 Treasurer: Sue Hansey
 Honorary Chairman: Elsie von Maur
Management:
 Executive Director: Lance O Willett
 Orchestra Manager: Dennis Loftin
 Music Director/Conductor: Donald Schleicher
 Marketing Director: Karen Brooke
Mission: Dedicated to supporting symphonic performances; committed to fostering, stimulating and encouraging orchestral ensemble and other music through developmental programs and scholarships.
Founded: 1915
Specialized Field: Symphony; Orchestra
Status: Professional; Nonprofit
Paid Staff: 6
Volunteer Staff: 375
Paid Artists: 90
Budget: $1,600,000
Income Sources: Ticket Sales; Contributions; Fund-raising
Performs At: Centennial Hall; Rock Island; Adler Theater; Davenport

Affiliations: American Symphony Orchestra League; Illinois Council of Orchestra
Annual Attendance: 40,000
Facility Category: Theatres
Type of Stage: Proscenium
Seating Capacity: 2,350; 1,620
Year Built: 1931
Year Remodeled: 1984
Organization Type: Performing; Educational

1190 QUAD CITY YOUTH STRING ENSEMBLE
327 Brady Street
Davenport, IA 52801
Mailing Address: PO Box 1144, Davenport, IA. 52805
Phone: 319-322-0931
Fax: 319-322-6864
e-mail: LWillett@qcsymphony.com
Web Site: www.qcsymphony.com
Management:
 Director: Dortha Dewit
 Executive Director: Lance Willett
Paid Staff: 1
Budget: $5,000
Performs At: Adler Theatre; Centennial Hall
Annual Attendance: 500
Facility Category: Recital Hall

1191 QUAD CITY YOUTH SYMPHONY ORCHESTRA
327 Brady Street
Davenport, IA 52801
Mailing Address: PO Box 1144, Davenport, IA. 52805
Phone: 319-322-0931
Fax: 319-322-6864
e-mail: lwillett@qcsymphony.com
Web Site: www.qcsymphony.com
Management:
 Music Director/Conductor: Thomas Hageman
 Executive Director: Lance Willett
Mission: Nonprofit
Founded: 1915
Paid Staff: 2
Budget: $35,000
Performs At: Adler Theatre; Centennial Hall
Annual Attendance: 8,000
Seating Capacity: 1620

1192 LUTHER COLLEGE SYMPHONY ORCHESTRA
Luther College
700 College Drive
Decorah, IA 52101
Phone: 319-387-8206
Fax: 319-387-1076
Toll-free: 800-369-8863
e-mail: boxoffice@crsymphony.org
Web Site: www.luthercollege.edu
Management:
 Music Director: Daniel Baldwin
 Manager: Marlene Runyon
Budget: $35,000
Performs At: Center for Faith & Life

1193 DES MOINES SYMPHONY

221 Walnut Street
Des Moines, IA 50309
Phone: 515-280-4000
Fax: 515-280-4005
e-mail: info@dmsymphony.org
Web Site: www.dmsymphony.org
Management:
   Music Director/Conductor: Joseph Giunta
Founded: 1937
Specialized Field: Symphony; Orchestra; Chamber; Ensemble
Status: Professional; Nonprofit
Paid Staff: 9
Budget: $1,700,000
Income Sources: Ticket Sales; Grants; Private Donations
Performs At: Civic Center of Greater Des Moines
Affiliations: American Symphony Orchestra League
Annual Attendance: 80,000
Facility Category: Civic Center
Type of Stage: Proscenium
Stage Dimensions: 61'x30'
Seating Capacity: 2,653
Year Built: 1979
Organization Type: Performing; Educational

1194 DRAKE SYMPHONY ORCHESTRA

Drake University
Music Department
Des Moines, IA 50311
Phone: 515-271-2108
Fax: 515-271-2558
e-mail: john.canarina@drake.edu
Web Site: www.drake.edu/artci/Music_Dept/
Management:
   Orchestral Studies Director: John Canarina
Budget: $35,000
Performs At: Sheslow Auditorium

1195 DUBUQUE SYMPHONY ORCHESTRA

PO Box 881
Dubuque, IA 52004
Phone: 319-557-1677
Fax: 319-557-9841
e-mail: dbqsymhpony@mwci.net
Management:
   General Manager: Robert A Birman
   Operations Manager: Mary Ellen Rogers
   Librarian: Tracey Rush
Mission: To provide quality performances; to offer educational programs in the field of classical music.
Founded: 1959
Specialized Field: Symphony; Orchestra; Chamber; Ensemble
Status: Semi-Professional; Nonprofit
Income Sources: Symphony League
Performs At: Five Flags Center Theatre
Organization Type: Performing; Resident; Educational; Sponsoring

1196 DES MOINES COMMUNITY ORCHESTRA

PO Box 1796
Johnston, IA 50306
Phone: 515-964-4562
Web Site: www.desmoinescommunityorchestra.org
Officers:
   President: Rich Gordley
   VP: Kathy Scott
   Treasurer: Laura Valle
   Secretary: Kendall Childs
   Social: Deb Gordley
   Music Acquisition: Rich Gordley
   Fund Raising: George Mosley
Management:
   Music Director/Conductor: Carl Johnson
Budget: $35,000
Performs At: Hoyt Sherman Place

1197 SOUTHEAST IOWA SYMPHONY ORCHESTRA

601 N Main
Mount Pleasant, IA 52641
Phone: 319-385-8021
Fax: 319-385-6352
Web Site: www.geocities.com/Broadway/Orchestra/1844
Management:
   Conductor/Music Director: Robert McConnell
   Manager: Joy Rayman Anderson
Mission: Dedicated to educating, encouraging and performing orchestral music in Southeast Iowa.
Founded: 1950
Specialized Field: Symphony; Orchestra
Status: Non-Professional; Nonprofit
Paid Staff: 40
Income Sources: American Symphony Orchestra League; Broadcast Music Incorporated; American Society of Composers, Authors and Publishers
Performs At: James Madison Auditorium; Iowa Wesleyan Chapel Auditorium
Organization Type: Performing

1198 OTTUMWA SYMPHONY ORCHESTRA

PO Box 173
Ottumwa, IA 52501
Phone: 515-684-4294
Fax: 515-682-8255
Officers:
   President: John Cobler
Management:
   Music Director: Tony Chang
Budget: $35,000-100,000
Performs At: St. John Auditorium

1199 CENTRAL COLLEGE COMMUNITY ORCHESTRA

Central College, Music Department
812 University
Pella, IA 50219
Phone: 641-628-5295
Fax: 641-628-5316
e-mail: lawsone@central.edu
Web Site: www.central.edu
Management:
   Conductor: Eric Lawson
Budget: $35,000
Performs At: Douwstra Performing Arts Center
Facility Category: Auditorium

Seating Capacity: 650
Rental Contact: Lowell Olivier

1200 NORTHWEST IOWA SYMPHONY ORCHESTRA

498 4th Avenue NW
Sioux Center, IA 51250
Phone: 712-722-6230
Fax: 712-722-4496
e-mail: niso@dordt.edu
Web Site: www.dordt.edu/niso
Management:
    Music Director: Henry Duitman
    Manager: James Koldenhoven
Budget: $35,000
Seating Capacity: 1,200

1201 SIOUX CITY SYMPHONY ORCHESTRA

520 Pierce Street, Suite 273
PO Box 754
Sioux City, IA 51102
Phone: 712-277-2111
Fax: 712-252-0224
e-mail: SiouxCitySymOrch@aol.com
Web Site: www.siouxcitysymphony.com
Management:
    Executive Director: Teresa Sumpter
    Operations Manager/Office Manager: Trinette
    Patterson
    Marketing Assistant: Siri Caltvedt
    Education Director: Kevin Engel-Cartie
    Music Director/Conductor: Stephen R Radcliffe
Mission: To perform at concerts and to educate.
Founded: 1915
Specialized Field: Symphony; Orchestra; Ensemble
Status: Professional; Nonprofit
Paid Staff: 5
Paid Artists: 100
Budget: $800,000
Income Sources: Sponsors; Grants; Individual Giving;
Ticket Sales
Performs At: Eppley Auditorium
Seating Capacity: 2500
Year Built: 1927
Year Remodeled: 2001
Cost: $9,200,000
Organization Type: Performing; Resident; Educational

1202 SIOUXLAND YOUTH SYMPHONY ORCHESTRA

520 Pierce Street, Suite 273
PO Box 754
Sioux City, IA 51101
Phone: 712-277-2111
Fax: 712-252-0224
Management:
    Chairman: Richard Bogenriof

1203 WARTBURG COMMUNITY SYMPHONY ORCHESTRA

Wartburg College
222 9th Street NW
Waverly, IA 50677

Phone: 319-352-8370
Fax: 319-352-8501
Web Site: www.wartburg.edu/symphony
Management:
    Music Director/Conductor: Dr. Janice E Wade
Founded: 1952
Specialized Field: Symphony Orchestra
Volunteer Staff: 20
Paid Artists: 5

Kansas

1204 EMPORIA SYMPHONY ORCHESTRA

Box 4029
Emporia, KS 66801-5087
Phone: 316-341-5431
Fax: 316-341-5073
Management:
    Music Director: Allan Comstock
    Chairman: Marie Miller

1205 HAYS SYMPHONY ORCHESTRA

Fort Hays State University
Hays, KS 67601
Phone: 913-628-5360
Fax: 913-628-4096
Web Site: www.ellisco.org/symphony.htm
Management:
    Conductor/Music Director: Christine Webber
Mission: Offering Western Kansas musical and cultural
activities and providing music students with artistic and
educational opportunities.
Founded: 1920
Specialized Field: Symphony; Orchestra
Status: Nonprofit
Paid Staff: 2
Income Sources: American Society of Composers,
Authors and Publishers; American Symphony Orchestra
League
Performs At: Beach/Schmidt Performing Arts Center
Organization Type: Performing; Educational

1206 HUTCHINSON SYMPHONY ASSOCIATION

PO Box 1241
Hutchinson, KS 67504-1241
Phone: 620-728-0246
Fax: 620-728-8157
Web Site: http://hutchsymphony.org
Management:
    Conductor/Musical Director: Daniel Delisi
Budget: 100,000

1207 NEWTON MID-KANSAS SYMPHONY ORCHESTRA

300 E 27th Street
PO Box 245
North Newton, KS 67117
Phone: 316-283-0814
Fax: 316-284-5286
Web Site: www2.southwind.net/~newtorch
Officers:

Manager: Jill Gatz
Management:
  Music Director: Daniel Hege
Founded: 1956
Paid Staff: 1
Volunteer Staff: 20
Paid Artists: 2

1208 YOUTH SYMPHONY ASSOCIATION OF KANSAS

7301 Mission Road
Suite 143
Shawnee Mission, KS 66208
Phone: 913-722-6810
Fax: 913-722-6806
e-mail: ysymph@crn.org
Web Site: www.crn.org/kcys
Management:
  Music Director/Conductor: Dr. Glenn Block
Mission: To provide educational opportunities for young musicians by performing before community-wide audiences and by inspiring excellence in performance.
Budget: $260,000-1,050,000

1209 TOPEKA SYMPHONY

PO Box 2206
Topeka, KS 66601-2206
Phone: 785-232-2032
Fax: 785-232-6204
e-mail: tso@TopekaSymphony.org
Web Site: www.TopekaSymphony.org
Management:
  Music Director/Conductor: John Strickler

1210 COLUMBIAN THEATRE: MUSEUM & ART CENTER

PO Box 72
521 Lincoln Avenue
Wamego, KS 66547-0072
Phone: 785-456-2029
Fax: 785-456-9498
Toll-free: 800-899-1893
e-mail: ctheatre@wamego.net
Web Site: www.wamego.com/to/columbian/default.html
Management:
  Artistic Director: Scott Kickhaefer
Performs At: Peddicord Playhouse

1211 WICHITA SYMPHONY

Century II Concert Hall
225 W Douglas
Wichita, KS 67202
Phone: 316-267-5259
Fax: 316-267-1937
e-mail: symphony@wso.org
Web Site: www.wso.org
Management:
  General Manager: Mitchell Berman
  Music Director/Conductor: Andrew Sewell
Mission: To rpovide Southcentral Kansas with the highest quality of cultural, educational and entertainment presentations through the maintencance of a symphony orchestra and related activities.

Founded: 1944
Specialized Field: Symphony; Orchestra; Chamber
Status: Professional; Nonprofit
Paid Staff: 6
Volunteer Staff: 350
Paid Artists: 95
Budget: $2.15 million
Income Sources: Ticket Sales; Donations; Program Advertising; Performance Fees; Investment Income
Performs At: Century II Concert Hall
Facility Category: Convention Center
Stage Dimensions: 49'x60'x29'
Seating Capacity: 2,250
Year Built: 1969
Organization Type: Performing; Touring; Educational; Sponsoring

Kentucky

1212 BOWLING GREEN-WESTERN SYMPHONY ORCHESTRA

416 E Main Street
Bowling Green, KY 42101
Phone: 270-782-2787
Fax: 270-782-2894
Web Site: www.wku.edu/Dept/Academic/AHSS/Music/
Management:
  Music Director/Conductor: Jooyong Ahn
Mission: Offering the people of Southern Kentucky classical music.
Founded: 1982
Specialized Field: Symphony; Orchestra; Chamber
Status: Semi-Professional; Nonprofit
Paid Staff: 35
Income Sources: American Symphony Orchestra League
Performs At: Van Meter Auditorium
Organization Type: Performing; Resident; Educational

1213 CENTRAL KENTUCKY YOUTH ORCHESTRAS

161 N Mill Street
Lexington, KY 40507-1125
Phone: 859-254-0796
Fax: 859-254-9644
e-mail: ckyo@ckyo.org
Web Site: www.ckyo.org
Officers:
  President: Linda Helm
  Seceretery: Sharon Melchior
  Tresurer: Jeff Garstka
Management:
  Music Director: William Briggs
Mission: Dedicated to the musical education and growth of its student members. Provides performance opportunities, motivational workshops, small group instruction, travel, mentoring and social interaction.

1214 CHAMBER MUSIC SOCIETY OF CENTRAL KENTUCKY

Box 12032
Lexington, KY 40579

Phone: 859-224-7003
e-mail: mlfrey00@uky.edu
Web Site: www.uky.edu/OtherOrgs/CMSCK
Mission: The purpose of this society is to foster and promote chamber music in Central Kentucky and the organization remains the only one in the area devoted exclusively to the presentation of music written for small ensembles.
Founded: 1950
Status: Nonprofit

1215 LEXINGTON PHILHARMONIC SOCIETY

161 N Mill Street
Lexington, KY 40507
Phone: 859-233-4226
Fax: 859-233-7896
Web Site: www.lexingtonphilharmonic.org
Officers:
  President: Dr. Michael J Morrill
  President Elect: Larry Deener
  Foundation Chairman: John Burrus
  Secretary: Sharon C. Reed
  Guild President: Doris King Shepherd
  Guild President Elect: Cindy Leveridge
  Chamber of Commerce: Barbara Wagner
Management:
  Music Director/Conductor: George Zack
  Executive Director: Peter Kucirko
  Orchestra Representative: Elaine Cook
Mission: To offer entertainment and enjoyment to the local community.
Founded: 1961
Specialized Field: Symphony; Chamber; Ensemble
Status: Nonprofit
Income Sources: Lexington Arts & Cultural Council; Kentucky Arts Council
Performs At: Singletary Center for the Arts
Organization Type: Performing; Educational
Comments: Special Seating and Facilities; Program in Large Type: Assistive Listening Devices

1216 LOUISVILLE BACH SOCIETY

4607 Hanford Lane
Louisville, KY 40207
Phone: 502-585-2224
Fax: 502-893-7954
Web Site: www.louisvillebachsociety.org
Management:
  Music Director: Melvin Dickinson
Mission: To perform the choral and orchestral music of Bach, as well as other baroque, modern, classical and romantic composers.
Founded: 1964
Specialized Field: Orchestra; Choral
Status: Nonprofit
Paid Staff: 80
Income Sources: Kentucky Arts Council; Greater Louisville Fund for the Arts; American Federation of Musicians
Performs At: University of Louisville
Organization Type: Performing; Touring; Resident; Educational

1217 LOUISVILLE CHAMBER MUSIC SOCIETY

University of Louisville
School of Music
Louisville, KY 40292
Phone: 502-852-0978
Fax: 502-852-0520
e-mail: Ostling@louisville.edu
Officers:
  Artist/Program Committee Chairman: Dr. Acton Ostling, Jr
Performs At: Recital Hall

1218 LOUISVILLE ORCHESTRA

300 W Main Street
Louisville, KY 40202
Phone: 502-587-8681
Fax: 502-589-7870
Web Site: www.louisvilleorchestra.org
Management:
  Executive Director: Tim King
  Director of Operations: Michael Beattie
  Music Director: Uriel Segal
  Principal Pops Conductor: Robert Bernhardt
  Associate Conductor: Robert Franz
  Development Manager: Goma Cpsbu
  Director Marketing: Diana Dinicola
  Production Coordinator: Adrienne Hinkebein
  Director Finance: Tonya McSorley
Mission: To bring the finest orchestral music to our region; to provide an educational resource; to maintain our own recording company that commissions, performs and records new music for our time.
Founded: 1937
Specialized Field: Symphony; Orchestra; Chamber
Status: Professional; Nonprofit
Paid Staff: 18
Paid Artists: 70
Budget: $6,000,000
Income Sources: American Symphony Orchestra League; American Arts Alliance; Greater Louisville Fund for the Arts
Performs At: Whitney Hall; Macauley Auditorium
Annual Attendance: 205,000
Organization Type: Performing; Touring; Educational; Sponsoring

1219 LOUISVILLE YOUTH ORCHESTRA

623 W Main
Louisville, KY 40208
Phone: 502-582-0135
Fax: 502-582-0149
Management:
  Music Director: Daniel Spurlock
  Executive Director: Melody Welsh
Mission: To provide high quality musical experiences and the opportunity of performing for the benefit of the community and its young musicians regardless of race, creed, or economic circumstances.
Founded: 1958
Specialized Field: Orchestra
Status: Nonprofit
Income Sources: Greater Louisville Fund for the Arts; Youth Performing Arts Council

Performs At: Youth Performing Arts Center
Organization Type: Performing; Educational

1220 KENTUCKY SYMPHONY

PO Box 72810
Newport, KY 41072
Phone: 859-431-6216
Fax: 859-431-3097
e-mail: info@kyso.org
Web Site: www.kysc.org
Management:
   Music/Executive Director: James R Cassidy
   General Manager: Angela Williamson
Mission: To culturally enrich, educate and entertain the residents of Northern Kentucky and Greater Cincinnati through unique and innovative presentations designed to make symphonic music and the concert experience, accessible and affordable.
Founded: 1992
Paid Staff: 2
Volunteer Staff: 45
Paid Artists: 90
Non-paid Artists: 4
Budget: $550,000
Income Sources: Event Entertainment
Annual Attendance: 45,000
Seating Capacity: 637-10,000

1221 OWENSBORO SYMPHONY ORCHESTRA

122 E 18th Street
Owensboro, KY 42303-3751
Phone: 270-684-0661
Fax: 270-683-0740
e-mail: info@owensborosymphony.org
Web Site: www.owensborosymphony.org
Officers:
   President: Robert G Reed
   President Elect: Leslie Hines
   Secretary: Sandy Wood
   Treasurer: Joe Hancock
Management:
   Executive Director: M Wade Kelly
   Music Director/Conductor: Nicholas Palmer
   General Manager: Paula Knott
Mission: To enhance the cultural environment of Western Kentucky through performances of symphonic music.
Founded: 1966
Specialized Field: Symphony; Orchestra
Status: Professional; Nonprofit
Paid Staff: 5
Volunteer Staff: 3
Paid Artists: 75
Budget: $759,000
Income Sources: American Symphony Orchestra League
Performs At: River Park Center
Annual Attendance: 7,400
Facility Category: Performing Arts Center
Seating Capacity: 1,482
Year Built: 1991
Rental Contact: Assistant Director Roxi Witt
Organization Type: Performing; Touring; Resident; Educational; Recording

1222 PADUCAH SYMPHONY ORCHESTRA

2101 Broadway
Paducah, KY 42002-1763
Mailing Address: PO Box 1763
Phone: 270-444-0065
Fax: 270-444-0065
Toll-free: 800-738-3727
e-mail: symphony@apex.net
Web Site: www.paducahsymphony.com
Management:
   General Manager: Leslie Rude
   Music Director/Conductor: Dr. Jordan Tang
Paid Staff: 12
Volunteer Staff: 75
Paid Artists: 100
Budget: $400,000+

Louisiana

1223 RAPIDES SYMPHONY ORCHESTRA

PO Box 12093
Alexandria, LA 71315-2093
Phone: 318-442-9709
Fax: 318-442-9755
Management:
   Conductor: William Kushner
Founded: 1967
Specialized Field: Community Based Orchestra
Paid Staff: 1
Volunteer Staff: 30
Non-paid Artists: 50

1224 BATON ROUGE SYMPHONY ORCHESTRA

9623 Brookline Avenue
Baton Rouge, LA 70809
Phone: 225-927-2776
Fax: 225-923-2772
e-mail: info@brso.org
Web Site: www.brso.org
Officers:
   President: Robert Harvill
   President Elect: Dan Ahem
   Treasurer: Bob Abbott
   Secretary: Ziad Alem
Management:
   Executive Director: JL Nave
   Director Operations: Craig Hahn
Mission: To offer professional quality orchestral performances in symphony and related arts.
Founded: 1947
Specialized Field: Symphony; Orchestra; Chamber; Ensemble
Status: Nonprofit
Paid Staff: 13
Paid Artists: 84
Performs At: Riverside/Centroplex Theatre for Performing Arts
Annual Attendance: 36,000
Seating Capacity: 1,897
Organization Type: Performing

1225 ACADIANA SYMPHONY ORCHESTRA
412 Travis Street
PO Box 53632
Lafayette, LA 70505
Phone: 337-232-4277
Fax: 337-237-4712
e-mail: info@acadianasymphony.org
Web Site: www.acadianasymphony.org
Management:
 Music Director: Xiao-Lu Li
 Executive Director: Marie Orgeron
Mission: To promote music and music education with focus on the youth throughout the entire region of Acadiana.
Founded: 1984
Paid Staff: 5
Paid Artists: 9

1226 LAKE CHARLES SYMPHONY
PO Box 3102
Lake Charles, LA 70602
Phone: 337-433-1611
Fax: 337-433-1615
e-mail: lclasym@aol.com
Web Site: www.lcymphony.org
Officers:
 President: Lucie Earhart
Management:
 Executive Director: Debbie Reed
Founded: 1958
Specialized Field: Symphony Orchestra
Status: Nonprofit
Paid Staff: 2
Volunteer Staff: 50
Paid Artists: 70
Affiliations: Southwest Regional Ballet Association

1227 JEFFERSON SYMPHONY ORCHESTRA
1118 Clearview Parkway
Metairie, LA 70001
Phone: 504-885-2000
Fax: 504-885-3437
e-mail: jpasinfo@jpas.org
Web Site: www.jpas.org
Management:
 Music Director/Conductor: Dennis G Assaf

1228 MONROE SYMPHONY ORCHESTRA
PO Box 4353
Monroe, LA 71211-4353
Phone: 318-435-0029
Fax: 318-435-6761
e-mail: symphony@bayou.com
Web Site: www.bayou.com/symphony
Management:
 Music Director: Dr. Roger Jones
 Executive Director: Naomi Cordill
Mission: To provide the region with live symphonic music of quality and to educate the public about its music.
Founded: 1971
Specialized Field: Northeast Louisiana and South Arkansas

1229 LOUISIANA PHILHARMONIC ORCHESTRA
305 Baronne Street
Suite 600
New Orleans, LA 70112
Phone: 504-523-6530
Fax: 504-595-8468
e-mail: dohara@lpomusic.com
Web Site: www.lpomusic.com
Officers:
 Orchestra President: Ann Cohen
 President: Hugh W Long
Management:
 Executive Director: Sharon Litwin
 Artistic Administrator: Kenneth K Kussmann
 Conductor/Music Director: Klauspeter Seibel
 Director Marketing/Public Relations: Dennis O'Hara
 Controller: Joe Toups
 Manager Box Office: Tamara R Clement
 Assistant Manager/Box Office: Jewdeia L Williams
 Operations Manager: K Kussmann
 Orchestra Personnel Manager: Jack Gardner
Mission: Strives to continue its artistic growth, continue its financial success, provide cultural enrichment to the community, and have many more sell out performances in the future.
Founded: 1991
Specialized Field: LPO makes music history by being the only full-time, player-managed symphony orchestra in the United States.
Paid Staff: 15
Volunteer Staff: 100
Paid Artists: 70
Budget: 4 Million
Income Sources: Ticket Sales, Contributions, Grants
Season: September-May
Performs At: Orpheum Theater
Annual Attendance: 50,000
Facility Category: Theatre
Type of Stage: Orchestra
Seating Capacity: 1800
Year Built: 1921
Rental Contact: Jeff Montalbaro

1230 NEW ORLEANS CONCERT BAND
UNO Box 522
New Orleans, LA 70148-0522
Phone: 504-455-9380
e-mail: nocb@email.com
Web Site: www.gnofn.org/~nocb
Officers:
 President: John Risey
 VP: Norman Robinson
 Secretary: Jackie Gillane
 Treasurer: Donna Thompson
 Board Member: Keith Buccola
 Board Member: Steve Carter
 Board Member: Henry Lowentritt
 Board Member: Ed Mulderick
 Board Member: Charlene Strain
Management:
 Conductor: Dr. Richard Dugser
Mission: An adult community band providing quality music at free concerts.
Founded: 1915

Specialized Field: Music - wind ensemble
Status: Professional; Non-Professional
Paid Artists: 80
Budget: $5,000
Income Sources: Dues, grants
Performs At: University of New Orleans Recital Hall
Affiliations: Association of Concert Bands
Annual Attendance: 10,000
Facility Category: University owned
Seating Capacity: 85
Year Built: 1965
Organization Type: Resident

1231 NEW ORLEANS JAZZ AND HERITAGE FOUNDATION

1205 N Rampart Street
New Orleans, LA 70116
Phone: 504-522-4786
Fax: 504-522-5456
Toll-free: 800-854-4714
Web Site: www.nojhf.org
Officers:
   Executive Director: Wali Abdel-Ra'oof
Management:
   Program Director: Sharon Martin
Mission: The presentation and preservation of Louisiana's culture and music.
Founded: 1970
Specialized Field: Festivals
Status: Nonprofit
Paid Staff: 12
Organization Type: Performing

1232 SHREVEPORT SYMPHONY ORCHESTRA

619 Louisiana Avenue
Suite 400
Shreveport, LA 71101
Mailing Address: PO Box 205
Phone: 318-222-7496
Fax: 318-222-7490
e-mail: office@shreveportsymphony.com
Web Site: www.shreveportsymphony.com
Officers:
   President: Dr. David Lilien
   Treasurer: Sidney E Kent
   Secretary: Anna Epling
   Chairman: Virginia Shehee
   President Board Development: Gene Eddy
   VP Education/Outreach: Janie Samuels
   VP Development: Donald A Webb
   Member-At-Large: Debbie Rathburn
Management:
   Music Director/Conductor: Dennis Simons
   Marketing Director: Melissa Baldwin
Mission: Dedicated to providing the three-state area with the highest possible quality musical performances.
Founded: 1947
Specialized Field: Symphony; Orchestra; Chamber; Ensemble
Status: Professional; Nonprofit
Paid Staff: 12
Budget: 1.2 million

Income Sources: American Symphony Orchestra League, Annual Fund, Ticket Sales
Performs At: Civic Theatre
Affiliations: American Symphony Orchestra League; Chamber of Commerce
Type of Stage: Proscenium
Seating Capacity: 1,737
Year Built: 1963
Organization Type: Performing; Touring; Educational

Maine

1233 MAINE MUSIC SOCIETY

PO Box 711
Auburn, ME 04240
Phone: 207-782-1403
Fax: 207-783-1851
e-mail: mms@gwi.net
Web Site: www.mainemusicsociety.org
Officers:
   President: Judith W Andrucki
   VP: Charles W Scheib
   Treasurer: Jeffrey R Gosselin
Management:
   Artistic Director: Peter Frewen
Mission: The Maine Music Society supports the artistic and educational activities of the professional Maine Chamber Ensemble and the auditioned, mixed-voice Androscoggin Chorale.
Founded: 1991
Status: Nonprofit
Income Sources: Maine Community Foundation; Davis Family Foundation; Helen & George Ladd Charitable Foundation; Maine Arts Commision; Maine Humanities Commission
Performs At: Orchestral; Chamber and Coral Music; Educational Programs
Affiliations: American Symphony Orchestra League; Maine Arts Sponsors Association; Androscoggin County Chamber of Commerce; Maine Association of Non-Profits

1234 BANGOR SYMPHONY ORCHESTRA

PO Box 1441
Bangor, ME 4402-1441
Phone: 207-942-5555
Fax: 207-990-1272
Toll-free: 800-639-3221
e-mail: symphony@bangorsymphony.com
Web Site: www.bangorsymphony.com
Management:
   Executive Director: Susan Jonason
Mission: The Bangor Symphony Orchestra performs locally as well as on tour.
Founded: 1896
Specialized Field: Symphony; Orchestra; Chamber; Ensemble
Status: Professional; Nonprofit
Paid Staff: 7
Paid Artists: 90
Income Sources: American Symphony Orchestra League; Greater Bangor Arts Council
Performs At: Bangor Opera House

Annual Attendance: 12,000
Organization Type: Performing; Touring; Resident; Sponsoring

1235 ARCADY MUSIC SOCIETY
PO Box 780
Bar Harbor, ME 04609
Phone: 207-288-3151
Fax: 207-288-3151
e-mail: arcady@arcady.org
Web Site: www.arcady.org
Management:
Artistic Director: Masanobu Ikemiya
Mission: To offer the finest contemporary and classical music to Maine residents, particularly chamber music and presentations for youth.
Founded: 1981
Specialized Field: Vocal Music; Instrumental Music; Festivals
Status: Professional; Nonprofit
Paid Staff: 2
Volunteer Staff: 30
Paid Artists: 70
Budget: $307,000
Income Sources: Chamber Music America
Organization Type: Performing; Educational; Sponsoring

1236 BOWDOIN SUMMER MUSIC FESTIVAL
6300 College Station
Bowdoin College
Brunswick, ME 04011
Phone: 207-373-1400
Fax: 207-373-1441
e-mail: bsmf@blazenetme.net
Web Site: www.summermusic.org
Officers:
Chairman of the Board: Hugh Phelps
Vice Chair: William A Rogers
Treasurer: Lester Hodgdon
Secretary: Nancy R Connery
Management:
Artistic Director: Lewis Kaplan
Executive Director: Peter Simmons
Admissions Director: Jen Means
Business Manager: Chris Murray
Mission: To provide the most promising music students from around the world with opportunities to further their musical development, and to present chamber music performed to the highest standards by distinguished professional musicians.
Founded: 1964
Specialized Field: Chamber
Status: Nonprofit
Budget: $1,100,000
Income Sources: Contributions; Ticket Sales; Tution
Performs At: Crooker Theater, Brunswick High School
Affiliations: Chamber Music America; Major Conservatories; Maine Performing Arts Network
Annual Attendance: 10,000
Seating Capacity: 600
Year Built: 1995
Organization Type: Educational; Presenting

1237 PIERRE MONTEUX SCHOOL
PO Box 157
Hancock, ME 04640
Phone: 207-422-3931
Fax: 207-422-9122
e-mail: www.monteuxschool.org
Web Site: pmonteux@aol.com
Officers:
Chamber Music Instructor: Claude Monteux
Management:
Administrative President: Nancie Monteux-Barendse
Music Director: Michael Jinbo
Mission: To acquaint young conductors and future orchestra musicians with the full symphonic repertoire.
Founded: 1943
Specialized Field: Instrumental Music; Symphony
Status: Professional; Nonprofit
Organization Type: Performing; Educational

1238 ATLANTIC CHAMBER ORCHESTRA
PO Box 4866
Portland, ME 04112-4866
Phone: 207-797-4011
Fax: 207-780-9697
Web Site: www.acopresents.com
Founded: 1999
Income Sources: Grants; Donors

1239 LARK SOCIETY FOR CHAMBER MUSIC
PO Box 11
Portland, ME 04112
Phone: 207-761-1522
Fax: 207-780-6554
e-mail: larksq@ctel.net
Mission: Committed to supporting and presenting a Portland concert series and educational presentations by the Portland String Quartet. Presenters of the Portland Concert Series, and supporters of the PSQ's outreach activities, we promote chamber music and music education in the state of Maine.
Specialized Field: Chamber; Ensemble
Status: Professional
Income Sources: Chamber Music America
Organization Type: Performing; Touring; Resident; Educational

1240 PORTLAND SYMPHONY ORCHESTRA
477 Congress Street
PO Box 3573
Portland, ME 04104
Phone: 207-773-6128
Fax: 207-773-6089
e-mail: psobox@portlandsymphony.com
Web Site: www.portlandsymphony.com
Officers:
President: Peter Haynes
Management:
Executive Director: Jane E Hunter
Director of Marketing: Camille Cook
Director/Finance & Office Operation: Sharon W Berry
Music Director/Conductor: Toshiyuki Shimada
Orchestra Manager: Andrew Kipe

Mission: The PSO is a professional orchestra aspiring to the highest artistic quality; serving its city, state, and Northern New England. Its mission is to engage diverse audiences in the enjoyment of live orchestral music.
Founded: 1924
Specialized Field: Symphony; Orchestra
Status: Nonprofit
Paid Staff: 9
Budget: $2.5 Million
Performs At: Merrill Auditorium
Organization Type: Performing

1241 BAY CHAMBER CONCERTS

10 Summer Street
PO Box 228
Rockport, ME 04856
Phone: 207-236-2823
Fax: 207-230-0454
Toll-free: 888-707-2770
e-mail: info@baychamberconcerts.org
Web Site: www.baychamberconcerts.org
Officers:
   President: Martha Rogers
   Secretary: Monica Kelly
   Treasurer: Frank Beane
Management:
   Artistic Director: Thomas Wolf
   Director Marketing/Communications: Kathy Maloney
   Administrative Coordinator: Anne Tani
Mission: To nurture music appreciation, with emphasis on chamber music, among residents of Maine.
Founded: 1960
Specialized Field: Instrumental and Vocal Music
Status: Professional
Paid Staff: 4
Budget: $500,000
Performs At: Rockport Opera House
Facility Category: Opera House; Strom Auditorium
Type of Stage: Proscenium; Auditorium
Seating Capacity: 400; 800
Organization Type: Performing

Maryland

1242 ANNAPOLIS CHAMBER ORCHESTRA
Maryland Hall for the Creative Arts

801 Chase Street
Annapolis, MD 21401
Phone: 410-263-1906
Fax: 410-263-5989
e-mail: annapolischorale@erols.com
Web Site: www.annapolischorale.org
Officers:
   President: John Vickerman
   VP: Jim Harle
   Treasurer: Marilyn Rhodovi
   Secretary: Katherine Hilton
Management:
   Music Director: J Ernest Green
   General Manager: Pamela Godfrey
Founded: 1973
Annual Attendance: 12,000

1243 BALTIMORE CLASSIC GUITAR SOCIETY

4607 Maple Avenue
Baltimore, MD 21227
Phone: 410-247-5320
e-mail: president@bcgs.org
Web Site: www.bcgs.org
Officers:
   President: David Hepple
Mission: To promote awareness of the classical as an art form.

1244 BALTIMORE SYMPHONY ORCHESTRA

Joseph Meyerhoff Symphony Hall
1212 Cathedral Street
Baltimore, MD 21201-5545
Phone: 410-783-8000
Fax: 410-783-8077
e-mail: tweber@baltimoresymphony.org
Web Site: www.baltimoresymphony.org
Management:
   President: John Gidwitz
   VP Artistic/Education Programming: Lucinda Williamsch
   Music Director: Yuri Temirkanov
Founded: 1916
Specialized Field: Symphony
Status: Professional
Income Sources: American Symphony Orchestra League; American Arts Alliance
Performs At: Joseph Meyerhoff Symphony Hall
Organization Type: Performing
Notes: Low vision, hearing assistance, wheelchair access

1245 CONCERT ARTISTS OF BALTIMORE

1114 St. Paul Street
Baltimore, MD 21202-2615
Phone: 410-625-3525
Fax: 410-625-9343
e-mail: cab@cabalto.org
Web Site: www.cobalto.org
Management:
   Director: Edward Polochick
   Managing Director: Felice Homann
Mission: To present varied classical music programs, featuring an all professional orchestra and vocal ensemble.
Founded: 1987
Paid Staff: 4
Volunteer Staff: 10
Paid Artists: 70
Budget: $ 300,000
Income Sources: Grants; Ticket Sales; Corporate Foundations; Individual Giving
Annual Attendance: 7,500-10,000

1246 PEABODY CONSERVATORY OF MUSIC

1 E Mount Vernon Place
Baltimore, MD 21202-2397
Phone: 410-659-8140
Fax: 410-659-8140
e-mail: lpollack@peabody.jhu.edu
Management:
   Concert Manager: Elizabeth Pollack

Performs At: Miriam A. Friedberg Concert Hall

1247 UNIVERSITY OF MARYLAND BALTIMORE COUNTY SYMPHONY
Fa 509, 1000 Hilltop Circle
Baltimore, MD 21250
Phone: 410-455-2942
Fax: 410-455-1181
e-mail: benton@umbc.edu
Web Site: research.umbc.edu/~morin/colleg.htm
Management:
 Music Department Chair: Dr. Linda Dusman
Performs At: Fine Arts Building

1248 MONTGOMERY COUNTY YOUTH ORCHESTRA
PO Box 30036
Bethesda, MD 20824-0036
Phone: 301-654-2018
e-mail: info@mcyo.org
Web Site: www.mcyo.org
Officers:
 First VP: Joan Maps Ducore
 Second VP: Deborah Johnson
 Tresurer: Ginny Jacoby
 Secretary: Georganne Larsen
Management:
 Senior Youth Orchestra Conductor: Olivia W Gutoff
Mission: Mission of the orchestras is to nurture, develop, and advance young, talented musicians in a quality orchestral program.
Founded: 1946

1249 MARYLAND PRESENTS
Clarice Smith Performing Arts Center
University of Maryland
College Park, MD 20742-5611
Phone: 301-405-7846
Fax: 301-405-5977
e-mail: rclevela@deans.umd.edu
Web Site: www.claricesmithcenter.umd.edu
Management:
 Executive Director: Susan Farr
 Associate Director Communications: Amy Harrison
 Director of Cultural Participation: Ruth Waalkes
Founded: 2001
Paid Staff: 50
Performs At: The Inn and Conference Center
Annual Attendance: 250,000
Facility Category: Performing Arts Center with 6 stages
Year Built: 2001
Rental Contact: Claudia Telliho

1250 UNIVERSITY OF MARYLAND: INTERNATIONAL WILLIAM KAPELL PIANO COMPETITION & FESTIVAL
Clarice Smith Performing Arts Center
University of Maryland
College Park, MD 20742
Phone: 301-405-8174
Fax: 301-405-5977
Web Site: www.claricesmithcenter.umd.edu
Founded: 1971

Specialized Field: Piano Competition
Status: Nonprofit
Income Sources: University of Maryland
Season: 2003
Performs At: Clarice Smith Performing Arts Center
Organization Type: Educational; Sponsoring

1251 CANDLELIGHT CONCERT SOCIETY
8970-A Route 108
Columbia, MD 21045
Phone: 410-715-0034
Fax: 410-715-0034
Management:
 Executive Director: Bonita J Bush
Mission: To offer Central Maryland audiences professional chamber music.
Founded: 1974
Specialized Field: Instrumental Music; Chamber Music; Children
Status: Professional; Nonprofit
Paid Staff: 1
Volunteer Staff: 75
Budget: $178,000
Income Sources: Columbia Foundations; MSAC; HCAC; Chamber Music America; Contributions
Season: October - May
Performs At: Smith Theatre; Howard Community College
Annual Attendance: 16,000
Type of Stage: Proscenium
Seating Capacity: 417
Organization Type: Performing; Sponsoring

1252 SUSQUEHANNA SYMPHONY ORCHESTRA
Forest Hill, MD 21050
Mailing Address: PO Box 485
Phone: 410-838-6465
Fax: 410-515-4438
e-mail: sbzbari@erols.com
Management:
 Music Director: Sheldon Bair
Mission: The Susquehanna Symphony Orchestra is a non profit community orchestra, providing education and entertainment for Harford County, Maryland.

1253 MARYLAND YOUTH SYMPHONY ORCHESTRA
PO Box 27
Glenwood, MD 21738
Phone: 410-442-5645
Fax: 410-489-7268
e-mail: mgattomyso@aol.com
Web Site: member.aol.com/mgattomyso/orchestra.htm
Management:
 Music Director: Angelo Gatto
 General Manager: Marharet Gatto
Mission: The symphony provides the opportunity for talented young musicians to learn and perform major symphonic repertoire at a high professional level, thus providing cultural enrichment for both performer and audience
Founded: 1964
Specialized Field: Symphonic Music

Paid Staff: 3
Paid Artists: 6

1254 MUSIC AT PENN ALPS
177 Casselman Road
PO Box 309
Grantsville, MD 21536
Phone: 301-895-5881
Fax: 301-895-5881
e-mail: fbolton@gcnet.net
Web Site: www.musicatpennalps.net
Management:
    Program Director: Fred C Bolton
Mission: Chamber Music Concerts.
Founded: 1992
Specialized Field: Chamber Music
Volunteer Staff: 14
Paid Artists: 35

1255 MARYLAND SYMPHONY ORCHESTRA
13 E Potomac Street
Hagerstown, MD 21740
Phone: 301-797-4000
Fax: 301-797-2314
e-mail: info@mdsymphony.com
Web Site: www.mdsymphony.com
Management:
    Executive Director: Marc D Lavy
    Operations Manager: Elaine Braun
    Marketing Director: Brenda Bush
    Box Office Manager: Beth Ann Deodorff
    Administrative Assistant: Carolyn Reed
Founded: 1982
Specialized Field: Symphony
Status: Professional
Paid Staff: 5
Budget: $1,000,000
Income Sources: Donors; Grants
Performs At: Maryland Theatre
Annual Attendance: 20,000
Seating Capacity: 1377
Organization Type: Performing

1256 PRINCE GEORGE'S PHILHARMONIC
6611 Kenilworth Avenue
Riverdale, MD 20738
Mailing Address: PO Box 1111
Phone: 301-454-1462
Fax: 301-454-1454
Mission: The Philharmonic's partnership with Prince George's County schools helps cultivate a new generation of musicians and audiences. With a focus on helping children develop to their fullest potential, the schools and orchestra together clarify the best role for each to play.
Organization Type: Performing; Educational

1257 JEWISH COMMUNITY CENTER SYMPHONY
6125 Montrose Road
Rockville, MD 20852
Phone: 301-881-0100
Fax: 301-881-5512
Web Site: www.jccso.org

Management:
    Music Director: Joel Lazar

1258 NATIONAL CHAMBER ORCHESTRA SOCIETY
850 Avery Road
Rockville, MD 20851
Phone: 301-762-8580
Fax: 301-762-8581
e-mail: natchorch@aol.com
Web Site: www.nationalchamberorch.org
Officers:
    President: Dieneke Johnson
    VP: Ruth Berman
    VP: Nathan Kuniners
    Treasurer: Katherine Reeves
    Secretary: Joel Alper
Management:
    Administrator: Cara Hupprich
    Music Director/Conductor: Piotr Gajewski
Mission: To provide concerts and programs that foster an appreciation for great classical music.
Specialized Field: Orchestra; Chamber
Status: Professional; Nonprofit
Paid Staff: 3
Volunteer Staff: 5
Paid Artists: 32
Budget: $350,000
Performs At: Duke Ellington School of the Arts; F. Scott Theatre
Annual Attendance: 8,000
Facility Category: Theatre
Organization Type: Resident

1259 BALTIMORE CHAMBER ORCHESTRA
1818 Potspring Road
Suite 202
Timonium, MD 21093
Phone: 410-308-0402
Fax: 410-308-0403
e-mail: jpelton@baltchamberorch.org
Web Site: www.baltchamberorch.org
Management:
    Music Director: Anne Harrigan
    Executive Director: Penelope Swenson
Founded: 1984
Income Sources: Legg Mason; Lockheed Martin; The Rouse Company
Annual Attendance: 8,000

Massachusetts

1260 NORTH SHORE PHILHARMONIC ORCHESTRA
PO Box 95
Beverly, MA 01915-0095
Phone: 617-631-6513
Fax: 617-247-3087
e-mail: nsphil@hotmail.com
Web Site: www.nspo.org
Officers:
    President: Robert A Marra, Jr

VP: Mary Miller
Treasurer: William Justin Shahan
Secretary: Thad Coverdale
Management:
  Manager: Herbert A Cohen
  Music Director: Max Hobart
Mission: Committed to providing access to quality music at an affordable price to communities on Boston's North shore; to developing, training and providing opportunities for young muscians; and to providing a large range of programs.
Founded: 1948
Specialized Field: Symphony; Orchestra
Status: Semi-Professional; Nonprofit
Paid Staff: 35
Organization Type: Performing; Resident

1261 ALEA III

855 Commonwealth Avenue
Boston, MA 02215
Phone: 617-353-3340
Fax: 781-793-8902
e-mail: kalogeras@earthlink.net
Officers:
  Chairman: John Doverio
  President: George Demeter
  Co-President: Ellen Demeter
  Treasurer: Samuel Headrick
Management:
  Executive Administrator: Alexandros Kalogeras
  Music Director: Theodore Antoniou
Mission: Dedicated to performing and promoting twentieth century classical music and supporting the work of contemporary composers.
Founded: 1979
Specialized Field: Chamber; Ensemble; Electronic & Live Electronic
Status: Professional; Nonprofit
Income Sources: Boston University
Performs At: Tsai Performance Center
Organization Type: Performing; Resident

1262 BOSTON POPS ORCHESTRA

Symphony Hall
301 Massachusetts Avenue
Boston, MA 02115
Phone: 617-266-1492
Fax: 617-638-9493
Web Site: www.bso.org
Management:
  Conductor: Keith Lockhart
  Manager: Tony Beadle
  Artistic Administrator: Dennis Alves
  Sales & Marketing Director: Kim Noltemy
  Director Finance: Thomas D May
  Operations Manager: Christopher W Ruigomez
  Chorus Manager: Felicia A Burrey
  Production Coordinator: Jana Gimenez
Opened: 1885
Specialized Field: Orchestra; Pops; Popular Selections
Status: Professional; Nonprofit
Income Sources: Memberships
Performs At: Symphony Hall
Organization Type: Performing; Touring

1263 BOSTON SYMPHONY CHAMBER PLAYERS

Symphony Hall
301 Massachusetts Avenue
Boston, MA 02115
Phone: 617-266-1492
Fax: 617-638-9367
Web Site: www.bso.org
Management:
  Orchestra Manager: Ray F Wellbaum
  Artistic Administrator: Anthony Fogg
Mission: The Chamber Players comprise the 12 first-chair players of the Boston Symphony Orchestra. They present programs of standard and contemporary literature not only in Boston and at Tanglewood, but on tour throughout this country and abroad, especially to audiences in locations which would not ordinarily be able to hear the Boston Symphony Orchestra in person.
Founded: 1964
Specialized Field: Chamber; Ensemble
Status: Professional; Commercial
Income Sources: Boston Symphony Orchestra
Performs At: Jordan Hall; Tanglewood
Organization Type: Performing; Touring

1264 BOSTON SYMPHONY ORCHESTRA

Symphony Hall
301 Massachusetts Avenue
Boston, MA 02115
Phone: 617-638-9270
Fax: 617-638-9367
e-mail: pkramer@bso.org
Web Site: www.bso.org
Officers:
  Chairman Emeritus: Nelson J Darling, Jr
  Chairman: JP Barger
  Vice Chairman: Lewis S Dabney
  Vice Chairman: John H. Fitzpatrick
  President: George H. Kidder
  Vice Chairman: Archie C. Epps
  Vice Chairman/Treasurer: William J. Poorvu
Management:
  Managing Director: Mark Volpe
  Assistant Managing Director: Daniel R Gustin
  Finance & Business Director: Michael G McDonough
  Artistic Administrator: Evans Mirageas
  Director Public Relations: Caroline Smedvig
  Director Development: Josiah Stevenson
  Orchestra Manager: Ray F Wellbaum
  Music Director: Seiji Ozawa
Mission: To bring great music to the widest possible audience; the Boston Symphony Orchestra, Inc. is the parent organization of the Boston Symphony Orchestra, the Boston Pops, the Boston Symphony Chamber Players, Tanglewood and the Tanglewood Music Center. To foster and maintain an organization dedicated to the making of music consonant with the highest aspirations of musical art.
Founded: 1881
Specialized Field: Symphony; Orchestra; Chamber; Ensemble
Status: Professional; Nonprofit
Performs At: Symphony Hall Tanglewood
Organization Type: Performing; Touring; Resident; Educational

1265 DINOSAUR ANNEX MUSIC ENSEMBLE
PO Box 5824
Boston, MA 02114
Phone: 617-482-3852
Fax: 617-482-4972
e-mail: manager@dinosaurannex.org
Web Site: www.dinosaurannex.org
Management:
　Artistic Director: Scott Wheeler
　Manager: Michael J Veloso
Mission: Presenting the best in contemporary music for chamber ensemble.
Founded: 1975
Specialized Field: Orchestra; Chamber; Ensemble; Instrumental Group; Electronic & Live Electronic
Status: Professional; Nonprofit
Paid Staff: 1
Paid Artists: 22
Performs At: First and Second Church; Boston
Organization Type: Performing

1266 GREATER BOSTON YOUTH SYMPHONY ORCHESTRAS
855 Commonwealth Avenue
Boston, MA 02215
Phone: 617-353-3348
Fax: 617-353-5205
Web Site: www.gbyso.org
Officers:
　President: David M Welch
　VP: Pamela Petri Humphrey
　Secretary: Anne Cademenos
　Treasurer: Doris Fritz Welch
Management:
　Executive Director: Catherine Weiskel
　Music Director: Federico Cortese
　Orchestra Manager: Ed Feingold
　Director Public Relations/Marketing: Jessica Tanner
　Director of Development: Ryan Losey
Mission: To organize and promote a youth orchestra program that provides the highest quality musical education, training and performance opportunities for young people.
Founded: 1958
Specialized Field: Symphony; Orchestra; Chamber
Status: Non-Professional; Nonprofit
Paid Staff: 5
Volunteer Staff: 25
Budget: $800,000
Income Sources: Boston University; Public/Private Grants; Tuition
Affiliations: Boston University
Organization Type: Performing; Touring; Resident; Educational

1267 HANDEL AND HAYDN SOCIETY
300 Massachusetts Avenue
Boston, MA 02115
Phone: 617-262-1815
Fax: 617-266-4217
e-mail: info@handelandhaydn.org
Web Site: www.handelandhaydn.org
Management:
　Music Director: Grant Llewellyn
　Conductor Laureate: Christopher Hogwood
　Executive Director: Mary Deissler
Mission: Dedicated to promoting the performance, study, composition and appreciation of music.
Founded: 1815
Specialized Field: Chamber; Ensemble; Choral
Status: Professional; Nonprofit
Paid Staff: 16
Budget: $2,600,000
Performs At: Symphony Hall; Jordan Hall
Annual Attendance: 40,000
Organization Type: Performing; Touring; Educational; Sponsoring

1268 MASSACHUSETTS YOUTH WIND ENSEMBLE
290 Huntington Avenue
Boston, MA 02115
Phone: 617-585-1130
Fax: 617-585-1135
e-mail: prep@newenglandconservatory.edu
Management:
　Music Director/Conductor: Michael Mucci
　Extension Division Dean, NE: Mark Churchill
Mission: Providing exceptionally talented high school musicians with an opportunity to study and perform the quality literature written for wind, brass, and percussion instruments.
Founded: 1970
Specialized Field: Chamber; Ensemble; Instrumental Group; Band
Status: Nonprofit
Income Sources: New England Conservatory
Performs At: Jordon Hall
Organization Type: Performing; Touring; Educational

1269 NEW ENGLAND PHILHARMONIC
6 Hemenway Street
Boston, MA 02140
Phone: 617-868-1222
Fax: 617-868-1222
Web Site: www.nephilharmonic.org
Officers:
　President: Kathleen Cragin Brittan
　VP: Jennifer Snodgrass
　Secretary/Director of Development: Jeff Bigler
　Treasurer: John Guthrie
Management:
　General Manager: Brian Ritter
　Music Director: Richard Pittman
　Personnel Manager: Elizabeth Dinwiddie
Mission: To nurture and encourage the enjoyment and appreciation of new and unusual orchestral music and perform standard orchestral literature in community locations.
Founded: 1976
Specialized Field: Orchestra
Status: Non-Professional
Paid Staff: 65
Income Sources: American Symphony Orchestra League
Performs At: Sanders Theatre; Cambridge; Dwight Hall
Organization Type: Performing; Resident

212　　*All listings are in alphabetical order by state, then city, then organization within the city.*

1270   BROCKTON SYMPHONY ORCHESTRA
PO Box 143
Brockton, MA 02303
Phone: 508-588-3841
Fax: 419-818-5426
e-mail: exec.dir@brocktonsymphony.org
Web Site: www.brockstonsymphony.org
Management:
   Music Director/Conductor: Jonathan Cohler
   Executive Director: Andrea Bates
Founded: 1948

1271   BOSTON BAROQUE
PO Box 380190
Cambridge, MA 02238
Phone: 617-484-9200
Fax: 617-489-9713
e-mail: info@bostonbaroque.org
Web Site: www.bostonbaroque.org
Management:
   Founder/Music Director: Martin Pearlman
   Executive Director: Carole Friedman
   Administrative Assistant: Amanda Chace
   Operations Manager: Laurie R Szablewski
Mission: To present performances of Baroque and
classical music on period instruments with a chorus.
Founded: 1973
Specialized Field: Orchestra; Chorus
Status: Professional; Nonprofit
Income Sources: Memberships
Performs At: Jordan Hall
Organization Type: Performing; Touring; Resident

1272   BOSTON CHAMBER MUSIC SOCIETY
10 Concord Avenue
Cambridge, MA 02138-2322
Phone: 617-349-0086
Fax: 617-349-0080
e-mail: bcms1@shore.net
Web Site: www.bostonchambermusic.org
Officers:
   Chairman: James Marten
   President: Gary Seligson
   Clerk: Winthrop Minst
   Treasurer: Donald Robbins
Management:
   Artistic Director: Ronald Thomas
   Executive Director: Mary S Jaffee
   Concert Manager: Wen Huang
Mission: To provide Boston's concert-going public with
exceptional performance of the great chamber music
repertoire of the 18th, 19th, and 20th centuries while
fostering understanding and appreciation of the artform.
Founded: 1982
Specialized Field: Chamber Music
Paid Staff: 4
Budget: $480,000
Income Sources: Box Office; Grants; Contributions
Performs At: Concert Hall

1273   BOSTON MUSICA VIVA
114 Auburn Street
4th Floor
Cambridge, MA 02138

Phone: 617-354-6910
Fax: 617-354-8513
e-mail: bmv@pobox.com
Web Site: www.bmv.org
Officers:
   President: Micheline de Bievre
   Treasurer: Grant Anderson
   Clerk: Robert Soorian
Management:
   General Manager: Miguel A Rodriguez
   Music Director: Richard Pittman
Mission: To promote the work of living American
composers as well as comtemporary classics.
Founded: 1969
Specialized Field: Chamber; New Music
Status: Professional
Paid Staff: 2
Volunteer Staff: 4
Paid Artists: 10
Budget: $450,000
Income Sources: Box Office; Grants; Donations
Performs At: Edward Pickman Hall; Blackman
Auditorium; Tsai Performance Center
Affiliations: Chamber Music America
Organization Type: Performing; Touring; Educational

**1274   BOSTON PHILHARMONIC
ORCHESTRA**
295 Huntington Avenue
Suite 210
Cambridge, MA 02115
Phone: 617-236-0999
Fax: 617-236-8613
e-mail: office@bostonphil.oeg
Web Site: www.bostonphil.org
Management:
   General Manager: Rod Birtles
Mission: Committed to reaching and educating a wide
audience in fine arts.
Founded: 1979
Specialized Field: Symphony; Orchestra
Status: Professional; Semi-Professional; Nonprofit
Paid Staff: 4
Paid Artists: 60
Non-paid Artists: 25
Budget: $1,000,000
Income Sources: Arts Boston
Performs At: Jordan Hall; Sanders Theater; Symphony
Hall
Annual Attendance: 7,000
Organization Type: Performing; Touring

**1275   CAMBRIDGE SOCIETY FOR EARLY
MUSIC: CHAMBER MUSIC SERIES**
Box 336
Cambridge, MA 02238-0336
Phone: 617-489-2062
Fax: 617-489-0686
e-mail: csem@csem.org
Web Site: www.csem.org
Management:
   Music Director: Bernard Brauchli

Mission: To entertain, enlighten, educate, and in general promote the rich musical culture of five centuries of Western music occuring up to the early nineteenth century.
Performs At: Fogg Art Museum

1276 HARVARD-RADCLIFFE ORCHESTRA
Harvard University
Music Building
Cambridge, MA 02138
Phone: 617-496-6276
Fax: 617-496-8081
e-mail: hro@hcs.harvard.edu
Web Site: hcs.harvard.edu/~hro/home.html
Management:
Conductor: Dr. James Yannatos

1277 KLEZMER CONSERVATORY BAND
83 Inman Street
Cambridge, MA 02139
Phone: 617-354-2884
Fax: 617-776-0955
Web Site: www.klezmerconservatory.com
Management:
Business Manager Aaron Concert Man: James Guttmann
Mission: To offer Yiddish instrumental and vocal music with many influences (Jazz, Dixieland, Ragtime, Latin and Broadway).
Founded: 1980
Specialized Field: Ethnic; Folk; Band
Status: Professional
Organization Type: Performing; Touring

1278 MUSICAMADOR
199 Pemberton Street
Cambridge, MA 02140
Phone: 617-492-1515
Fax: 617-492-1515
e-mail: mail@musicamador.com
Web Site: www.musicamador.com
Management:
Director: Rosi Amador
Managing Director: Nina Korican
Mission: Agent
Specialized Field: Music

1279 PRO ARTE CHAMBER ORCHESTRA
99 Bishop Allen Drive
Cambridge, MA 02139
Phone: 617-661-7067
Fax: 617-492-6596
Web Site: www.proarte.org
Management:
Executive Director: Ryan Fleur
Music Director: Isaiah Jackson
Chair: W. Easley Hamner
President: Barbara Englesberg
Mission: Seeks to make classical music accessible to the entire community. Through our Access to the Best Music program, low income, at-risk, disabled, and elderly individuals experience fine music.
Founded: 1978

Specialized Field: Orchestra; Chamber
Status: Professional; Nonprofit
Paid Staff: 9
Volunteer Staff: 510
Paid Artists: 40
Budget: $550,000
Income Sources: Ticket Sales; Contributed Sources
Performs At: Sanders Theater
Annual Attendance: 6,500
Seating Capacity: 1,200
Year Built: 1870
Year Remodeled: 1994
Organization Type: Performing

1280 CONCORD BAND
Box 302
Concord, MA 01742
Phone: 978-897-9969
Fax: 978-369-1367
Web Site: www.concordband.org
Officers:
President: BP Troup
Treasurer: J Grace
Management:
Music Director: Dr. William G McManus
Manager/Librarian: J Kemson
Fundraising: L Matson
Founded: 1959
Specialized Field: Band
Status: Non-Professional; Nonprofit
Paid Staff: 70
Income Sources: Association of Concert Bands
Organization Type: Performing

1281 CONCORD ORCHESTRA
PO Box 381
Concord, MA 01742
Phone: 978-369-4967
e-mail: jlbo@rcn.com
Management:
Conductor: Richard Pittman
Mission: Dedicated to providing our amateur musicians the enjoyment of playing music and offering good music to the community.
Founded: 1952
Specialized Field: Symphony; Orchestra
Status: Non-Professional; Nonprofit
Paid Staff: 70
Income Sources: American Symphony Orchestra League
Organization Type: Performing

1282 INTERNATIONAL MUSIC NETWORK
278 Main Street
Gloucester, MA 01930
Phone: 978-283-2883
Fax: 978-283-2330
Web Site: www.imnworld.com
Management:
Co-Director/Co-Owner: AnneMarie Southard
Co-Director/Co-Owner: Scott Southard
International Agent: Scott Southard
European Agent: Katherine McVicker
International Coordinator: Kristen Teixeria
Accountant: Pat Lefebvre

Contract Administrator: Laurie Zylicz
Mission: Booking agency
Founded: 1989
Specialized Field: Jazz & World Music

1283 PIONEER VALLEY SYMPHONY

7 Franklin Street
Greenfield, MA 01301
Phone: 413-773-3664
Fax: 413-772-6800
e-mail: pvsc@javanet.com
Web Site: www.pvso.org
Management:
Music Director: Paul Phillips
Mission: To serve the Pioneer Valley.

1284 SYMPHONY PRO MUSICA

Main Street, Suite 3A
PO Box 332
Hudson, MA 01749
Phone: 978-562-0939
Fax: 978-562-0939
e-mail: spm@symphonypromusical.org
Web Site: www.symphonypromusica.org
Management:
Music Director: Mark Churchill
Mission: Symphony Pro Musica have enriched the cultural life of our communities with live performances of the best symphonic music from the eighteenth, nineteenth, and twentieth centuries.
Founded: 1983
Specialized Field: Classical Music
Paid Staff: 2
Volunteer Staff: 15
Paid Artists: 6
Non-paid Artists: 65

1285 BERKSHIRE CHAMBER MUSIC SOCIETY

PO Box 155
Lenox, MA 01240-0155
Phone: 413-637-3636
Fax: 413-637-4599
e-mail: Quartets@bcn.net
Management:
Artistic Director: Edgar Feldman

1286 THAYER SYMPHONY ORCHESTRA

14 Monument Square
Suite 406
Leominster, MA 01453
Phone: 978-466-1800
Fax: 978-466-1000
e-mail: info@thayersymphony.org
Web Site: www.thayersymphony.org
Management:
General Manager: Francis Wada
Conductor/ Artistic Director: Toshimasa Francis Wada
Executive Director: Kathleen Corcoran

Mission: To sustain and develop a symphony orchestra of the highest quality for the education, enrichment, and pleasure of the citizens and musicians of Central Massachusetts.
Founded: 1973
Specialized Field: Symphony
Status: Semi-Professional; Nonprofit
Paid Staff: 20
Income Sources: American Symphony Orchestra League; North Central Massachusetts Chamber of Commerce
Organization Type: Performing; Educational

1287 INDIAN HILL SYMPHONY

PO Box 1484
Littleton, MA 01460
Phone: 978-486-9524
Fax: 978-486-9844
e-mail: susan@indianhillmusic.org
Web Site: www.indianhillmusic.org
Management:
Music Director: Bruce Hangen
Executive Director: Susan Randazzo
Founded: 1974
Paid Staff: 75
Annual Attendance: 7,000
Facility Category: various venues

1288 TUFTS UNIVERSITY: MUSIC DEPARTMENT

20 Professor Row
Medford, MA 02155
Phone: 617-627-3350
Fax: 617-627-3712
e-mail: rblackman@infonet.tufts.edu

1289 MELROSE SYMPHONY ORCHESTRA

PO Box 175
Melrose, MA 02176
Phone: 781-662-0641
Fax: 781-662-0641
e-mail: millierich@aol.com
Web Site: melrosesymphony.org
Officers:
President: Millie Rich
First VP: Anne Fremont-Smith
Second VP: Katherine Radley
Secretary: Rita Moore
Treasurer: Albert J Traveis
Management:
Executive Director: Millie Rich
Mission: To give the citizens of Melrose and surrounding area an opportunity to participate in the joy of music.
Founded: 1918
Specialized Field: Symphony; Orchestra
Status: Nonprofit
Volunteer Staff: 17
Paid Artists: 1
Non-paid Artists: 72
Performs At: Memorial Building (590 Main Street, Melrose)
Annual Attendance: 5,000
Facility Category: Auditorium Performance Center
Type of Stage: Performance Stage

Stage Dimensions: 30x40
Seating Capacity: 900
Year Built: 1912
Rental Contact: 7189794185 Millie Rich
Organization Type: Performing

1290 BOSTON CLASSICAL ORCHESTRA

Box 152
Newton, MA 02468
Phone: 617-423-3883
Fax: 617-527-4764
Web Site: www.bostonclassicalorchestra.org
Officers:
   President: Wendy Spector
   VP: Cristina Fernandaz-Haegg
   Secretary: Stephen J Gaal
Management:
   Executive Secretary: Robert Brink
   Manager: Quindara Dodge
   Music Director: Harry Ellis Dickson
Mission: To offer outstanding performances of the chamber orchestra repertoire in an intimate setting, concentrating on music of the Classical period. Through imaginatively presented live concerts in a relaxed atmosphere, the BCO seeks to foster a sense of connection between audience and performers and to strengthen its appeal to a growing and varied public.
Founded: 1980
Specialized Field: Symphony; Orchestra; Chamber
Status: Professional; Nonprofit
Performs At: Faneuil Hall
Organization Type: Performing

1291 NEWTON SYMPHONY ORCHESTRA

61 Washington Park
Newton, MA 02460
Phone: 617-965-2555
Fax: 617-965-0450
e-mail: newtonsymphony@compuserve.com
Web Site: www.newtonsymphony.org
Officers:
   President: Walter F Carter
   VP: Andris Vizolis
   Secretary: Nancy O'Brien
   Treasurer: Joel Corman
Management:
   Administrative Coordinator: Arks Smith
   Music Director/Conductor: Jeffrey Rink
   Personnel Manager: Mark Perreovlt
Mission: To provide area volunteer musicians the opportunity to maintain and develop their skills, and to enhance music appreciation, promote cross-cultural understanding, and build community through outreach programs for students and seniors.
Founded: 1965
Specialized Field: Symphony Orchestra
Status: Nonprofit; Volunteer
Paid Staff: 3
Volunteer Staff: 7
Paid Artists: 10
Non-paid Artists: 60
Budget: $100,000
Income Sources: Box office; grants; private donations
Performs At: Rashi Auditorium
Annual Attendance: 3,000 - 4,000

Seating Capacity: 852
Organization Type: Performing

1292 CAPE COD CHAMBER MUSIC FESTIVAL

Formerly Cap & Islands Chamber Music Festival
216C Orleans Road
Nickerson Corners
North Chatham, MA 02650
Phone: 508-945-8060
Fax: 508-945-8059
Toll-free: 800-229-5739
e-mail: contact@capecodchambermusic.org
Web Site: www.capecodchambermusic.org
Officers:
   President: Lawrence M Handley
   Treasurer: Laura S Emmons
   Secretary: George Dillion
Management:
   Artistic Director: Nicholas Kitchen
   Executive Directoror: Pamela Patrick
   Director Development: Lynne Pleffner
Mission: To present the finest classical and contemporary chamber music by both world-class ensembles and exceptional young emerging artists to Cape Cod audiences; to develop new and younger audiences for chamber music; to commission new chamber works whenever possible; and to provide educational activities and programs which encourage, broaden and deepen appreciation of the chamber music art form.
Founded: 1979
Specialized Field: Festivals
Status: Professional; Nonprofit
Paid Staff: 3
Paid Artists: 30
Facility Category: Usually churches
Seating Capacity: 250 - 300
Organization Type: Performing; Educational

1293 SMITH COLLEGE ORCHESTRA

Smith College Musical Department
Sage Hall, Smith College
Northampton, MA 01063
Phone: 413-585-3150
Fax: 413-585-3180
e-mail: jhirsh@smith.edu
Management:
   Conductor: Jonathan Hirsh
Performs At: Concert Halls

1294 STOCKBRIDGE CHAMBER CONCERTS AT SEARLES CASTLE

68 Kenilworth Street
Pittsfield, MA 01201
Phone: 413-442-7711
Fax: 413-442-7711
Toll-free: 888-528-7728
e-mail: elizabethhagenah@altavista.com
Officers:
   President: Elizabeth A Hagenah
   VP: Dr. David Anderegg
   Treasurer: Dr. Norma Thompson

Management:
   Artistic Director/Founder: Elizabeth A Hagenah
   Clerk: Eunice Agar
Mission: To promote cultural activities and help outstanding young talents by giving them scholarship performances with mature artists.
Founded: 1975
Specialized Field: Vocal Music; Instrumental Music; Festivals
Status: Professional; Nonprofit
Paid Artists: 15
Budget: $16,000 - $22,000
Income Sources: Ticket sales, contributions
Performs At: Searles Castle
Affiliations: Chamber Music America (member)
Annual Attendance: 175
Facility Category: Concert hall and reception atrium
Type of Stage: Small elevated
Seating Capacity: 175, 250 childrens programs
Year Built: 1886
Rental Contact: At John Dewey Academy Dr. Thomas Bratter
Organization Type: Performing; Touring; Resident; Educational; Sponsoring
Resident Groups: Stockbridge Chamber Concerts (summer)

1295 PLYMOUTH PHILHARMONIC ORCHESTRA

16 Court Street
Plymouth, MA 02361
Mailing Address: PO Box 3174, Plymouth, MA 12361
Phone: 508-746-8008
Fax: 508-746-0115
e-mail: thephil@adelphia.com
Web Site: www.plymouthphilharmonic.com
Officers:
   President: Louise Woodruff
   VP: Thomas Hurley
   VP: Michael Coleman
   Secretary/Clerk: Donna Frugoli
   Treasurer: Paul Kiley
   VP: N. Thompson Bosanquet
Management:
   Executive Director: Roberta J Otto
   Office Manager: Linda Hurley
   Development Manager: Christine Wells
   Marketing Specialist: Judith Ingram
   Music Director/Conductor: Steven Karidoyanes
Mission: To present excellent, professional symphonic music to the broadest possible audience and to encourage a life-long love of music through a variety of educational programs.
Founded: 1913
Specialized Field: Symphony; Orchestra; Chamber; Ensemble
Status: Professional; Semi-Professional; Nonprofit
Paid Staff: 8
Paid Artists: 75
Budget: $519,468
Income Sources: Ticket Sales; Grants; Contributions
Performs At: Memorial Hall - Plymouth, Massachusetts
Affiliations: American Symphony Orchestra League; Plymouth County Development Council; Plymouth Area Chamber of Commerce

Annual Attendance: 15,500
Facility Category: Municipal Auditorium
Seating Capacity: 1285
Year Built: 1926
Year Remodeled: 2002
Organization Type: Performing; Educational; Sponsoring

1296 ROCKPORT CHAMBER MUSIC FESTIVAL

PO Box 312
Rockport, MA 01966
Phone: 978-546-7138
e-mail: rcmf@shore.net
Web Site: www.rcmf.org
Officers:
   President: Phillip D Cutter MD
   VP: Dianne Anderson
   VP: Barbara Sparks
   Treasurer: William Hausman
   Clerk/Secretary: Mollie Byrnes
Management:
   Artistic Director: David Deveau
Mission: The presentation of a 16-concert series in June, featuring chamber ensembles performing alone and in collaboration.
Specialized Field: Chamber
Status: Professional; Nonprofit
Performs At: Rockport Art Association
Organization Type: Presenting

1297 MUSICORDA FESTIVAL & SUMMER STRING PROGRAM

PO Box 557
South Hadley, MA 01075
Phone: 413-538-2590
Fax: 413-538-3021
e-mail: musicorda@aol.com
Web Site: www.musicorda.org
Management:
   Artistic Director: Leopold Teraspulsky
   Executive Director: Jacqueline Melnick
Mission: To forge an international community of artists and students dedicated to sharing their joy in making music and to enriching the lives of diverse audiences through excellence in performance and education.
Founded: 1987
Specialized Field: Instrumental Music
Status: Professional; Nonprofit
Paid Staff: 4
Volunteer Staff: 4
Performs At: Chapin Auditorium; Mount Holyoke College
Facility Category: Concert Hall
Seating Capacity: 800
Organization Type: Performing; Touring; Resident; Educational

1298 SPRINGFIELD ORCHESTRA ASSOCIATION

75 Market Place
1ST Floor
Springfield, MA 01103

Phone: 413-733-0636
Fax: 413-781-4129
Management:
   Music Director: Kevin Rhodes
   Executive Director: Michael Jonnes
Mission: To provide symphonic music and other musical entertainment to the residents of Western Massachusetts; to nurture music appreciation.
Specialized Field: Symphony
Status: Professional; Nonprofit
Performs At: Springfield Symphony Hall
Organization Type: Performing; Touring; Educational

1299 MARTHA'S VINEYARD CHAMBER MUSIC SOCIETY

PO Box 4189
Vineyard Haven, MA 02568
Phone: 508-696-8055
Fax: 508-696-8055
e-mail: mvcms@vineyard.net
Web Site: mvcms.vineyard.net/
Officers:
   President: Daniel J Culkin
   VP: Dr. Sofia Anthony
   Treasurer: Marilyn Hollinshea
   Secretary: Susan Phelps
Management:
   Executive Director: Nancy Rogers
   Artistic Director: Delores Stevens
Mission: To produce chamber music concerts, promote and support classical music learning opportunities and create awareness of the value and significance of fine music on the island.
Founded: 1971
Specialized Field: Chamber Music
Status: Professional; Nonprofit
Paid Staff: 1
Paid Artists: 30
Budget: $100,000
Income Sources: Box Office; Grants; Private Donations
Performs At: Old Wharling Church; Chilmark Community Center
Annual Attendance: 2,800
Facility Category: Historic Church; Peformance & community Center
Type of Stage: Proscenium
Seating Capacity: 500; 200

1300 NEW ENGLAND STRING ENSEMBLE

599 N Avenue, Suite 8
PO Box 2012
Wakefield, MA 01880
Phone: 781-224-1117
Fax: 781-224-3547
e-mail: info@nese.net
Web Site: www.nese.net
Officers:
   President: Gordon Conrad
   VPresident: James Wisdom
   Tresurer: Bob Sanferrare
   Clerk: John Wall
Management:
   Music Director: Susan Davenny Wyner
   Executive Director: Peter Stickel

   Orchestra Manager: John Bumstedd
Mission: The New England String Ensemble was founded to bring string music both to the concertgoing public and to those who might not overwise have the opportunity to hear a professional string orchestra.
Founded: 1994
Specialized Field: Classical Music
Paid Staff: 3
Volunteer Staff: 2
Paid Artists: 30
Annual Attendance: 390,000
Facility Category: Concet Hall
Seating Capacity: 1,000

1301 BRANDEIS UNIVERSITY DEPARTMENT OF MUSIC

PO Box 5491110
South Street
Waltham, MA 02454-9110
Phone: 781-736-3310
Fax: 781-736-3320
e-mail: music@brandies.edu
Web Site: www.brandeis.edu/departments/music
Mission: Pesenting a university concert series including Professional Series, Concerts at Noon and student performances.
Founded: 1940
Specialized Field: Orchestra; Chamber; Ensemble; Instrumental Group; Electronic & Live Electronic
Status: Professional; Non-Professional; Nonprofit
Performs At: Slosberg Recital Hall
Organization Type: Performing; Resident

1302 BOSTON CIVIC SYMPHONY ORCHESTRA OF BOSTON

PO Box 859
Westwood, MA 02090
Phone: 617-923-6333
Fax: 781-329-7293
e-mail: csoboston@aol.com
Web Site: www.csob.org
Management:
   Music Director/Conductor: Max Hobart

1303 WILLIAMS CHAMBER PLAYERS

Williams College Department of Music
54 Chaplin Hall Drive
Williamstown, MA 01267
Phone: 413-597-2736
Fax: 413-597-3100
Management:
   Chair/Department Music: Douglas B Moore
   Concert Manager: Ernest Clark
Mission: To bring high-quality performance of chamber music repertoire to Williams students and the community-at-large.
Founded: 1999
Specialized Field: Chamber
Status: Professional; Nonprofit
Performs At: Brooks-Rogers Recital Hall; Bernhard Music Center
Organization Type: Performing; Touring; Resident

1304 QUINCY SYMPHONY ORCHESTRA
PO Box 2
Wollaston, MA 02170
Phone: 781-961-3790
Fax: 617-376-1297
e-mail: deneb@gis.net
Web Site: http://quincysymphony.org
Officers:
President: Barbara Clement
First VP: Lee Salerno
Second VP: Roberta Kopelman
Secretary: Eleanor Nelson
Treasurer: David Levy
Management:
Music Director: Yoichi Udagawa
Founded: 1954

1305 CAPE ANN SYMPHONY ORCHESTRA
712A Main Street
Yarmouth Port, MA 02675
Phone: 508-326-1111
Fax: 508-362-7916
e-mail: casadvbe@shore.net
Management:
Music Director: Yoichi Udagawa

1306 CAPE SYMPHONY ORCHESTRA
712A Main Street
Yarmouth Port, MA 02675-2000
Phone: 508-362-1111
Fax: 508-326-7916
e-mail: csoadmin@capesymphony.org
Web Site: www.capesymphony.org
Officers:
President: Daniel Sepico
VP: Kenneth Brock
Management:
Music Director/Conductor: Royston Nash
Executive Director: Eric Borenstein
Director Development: Pamela Morrill
Mission: The program is designed to encourage appreciation and to futher develop the students understanding of classical music.

Michigan

1307 ADRIAN SYMPHONY ORCHESTRA
110 S Madison Street
Adrian, MI 49221
Phone: 517-264-3121
Fax: 517-264-3833
e-mail: aso@adrian.edu
Web Site: www.aso.org
Management:
Executive Director: Susan Hoffman
Music Director: John Dodson
Mission: To remain Lenawee County's premiere musical ensemble and Adrian College's professional orchestra-in-residence; to perform classical, family, holiday, pops, chamber and young peoples' concerts.
Founded: 1981

Specialized Field: Symphony; Orchestra; Chamber; Ensemble
Status: Professional; Nonprofit
Paid Staff: 5
Budget: $350,000
Income Sources: American Symphony Orchestra League; Michigan Orchestra Association
Performs At: Dawson Auditorium
Affiliations: Adrian College
Organization Type: Performing; Touring; Resident; Educational

1308 ALMA SYMPHONY ORCHESTRA
614 W Superior Street
Alma, MI 48801
Phone: 517-463-7167
Fax: 517-463-7277
Toll-free: 800-321-2562
e-mail: Scripps@alma.edu
Management:
Music Director: Douglas Scripps

1309 ANN ARBOR SYMPHONY ORCHESTRA
527 E Liberty
Suite 208B
Ann Arbor, MI 48104
Phone: 734-994-4801
Fax: 734-994-3949
e-mail: a2so@a2so.com
Web Site: a2so.com
Officers:
President: Martha A Darling
VP: J. Robert Gates
Secretary: Jane Wilkinson
Treasurer: Gerard H. Spencer
Past President: Walter G. Byers
Management:
Executive Director: Mary Steffek Blaske
Personnel Manager: Gregg Emerson Powell
Librarian: Kathleen Grimes
Operations Manager: Daniel Getty
Music Director: Arie Lipsky
Founded: 1928
Specialized Field: Symphony; Orchestra
Status: Professional
Paid Staff: 9
Paid Artists: 100
Budget: $850,000
Income Sources: Tickets; Contributions; Special Events
Performs At: Michigan Theater
Annual Attendance: 18,000
Organization Type: Performing; Educational

1310 UNIVERSITY OF MICHIGAN SCHOOL OF MUSIC: MICHIGAN YOUTH PROGRAMS
1100 Baits Drive
Ann Arbor, MI 48109-2085
Phone: 734-763-1279
Fax: 734-647-0140
e-mail: sumgraro@umich.edu
Web Site: www.music.umich.edu/resources/myo/index.html
Management:

Director: Donald Sinta

**1311 UNIVERSITY OF MICHIGAN
SYMPHONY ORCHESTRAS**
1100 Baits Drive
Ann Arbor, MI 48109-2085
Phone: 734-764-5575
Fax: 734-763-5097
e-mail: aderente@umich.edu
Web Site: www.music.umich.edu
Management:
   Music Director: Kenneth Kiesler
   Managing Director: David R Aderente
Budget: $35,000
Performs At: Hill Auditorium

**1312 BATTLE CREEK SYMPHONY
ORCHESTRA**
PO Box 1613
Battle Creek, MI 49016
Phone: 269-963-1911
Fax: 269-966-2547
e-mail: bcso@musiccenterscmi.com
Officers:
   President: Penny DeGarmo
Management:
   Music Director/Conductor: Matthew Hazelwood
   General Manager: Glenn Klassen
Mission: The performance of classical and pops concerts.
Founded: 1899
Specialized Field: Symphony; Orchestra; Chamber
Status: Professional; Nonprofit
Paid Staff: 6
Paid Artists: 80
Budget: $500,000
Income Sources: American Symphony Orchestra
League; Michigan Council for Arts and Cultural Affairs;
United Arts Council
Performs At: WK Kellogg Auditorium
Organization Type: Performing; Educational

**1313 BIRMINGHAM-BLOOMFIELD
SYMPHONY**
1592 Buckingham
Birmingham, MI 48009
Phone: 248-645-2276
Fax: 248-645-2276
Web Site: www.bbso.org
Management:
   Executive Director: Carla Lamphere
   Personnel Manager: Jon Boyd
   Librarian: Eldonna May
   Administrative Assistant: Joe Labuta
Mission: To foster an appreciation of the musical arts.
Founded: 1975
Specialized Field: Symphony; Orchestra; Ensemble
Status: Professional; Nonprofit
Income Sources: American Society of Composers,
Authors and Publishers; Michigan Orchestra Association;
Michigan Orchestra Volunteer Association
Performs At: Temple Beth El
Organization Type: Performing; Educational

1314 CADILLAC SYMPHONY ORCHESTRA
PO Box 435
Cadillac, MI 49601
Phone: 231-779-0701
Fax: 231-876-1180
Web Site: www.cadillacmichigan.com/symphony
Officers:
   President 'CSO' Orchestra: Carol Buckholz
   VP: Laurie Melstrom
Management:
   Music Director: William J Donahue
Founded: 1973
Paid Staff: 1
Volunteer Staff: 18
Non-paid Artists: 75
Budget: $40,000
Income Sources: Ticket Sales, Patrons Drive
Performs At: High School Auditorium
Annual Attendance: 3500
Facility Category: Auditorium
Seating Capacity: 734
Year Built: 1984

1315 MACOMB SYMPHONY ORCHESTRA
PO Box 381062
4-4575 Garfield
Clinton Township, MI 48038
Phone: 810-286-2045
Fax: 810-286-2068
e-mail: CookT@Macomb.cc.mi.us
Web Site: www.macombsymphony.org
Management:
   Music Director: Thomas Cook
Founded: 1974
Specialized Field: Orchestra
Paid Staff: 2
Volunteer Staff: 28
Paid Artists: 82
Non-paid Artists: 6
Budget: $35,000-100,000
Seating Capacity: 1,230
Year Built: 1981
Year Remodeled: 2002

**1316 DEARBORN ORCHESTRAL SOCIETY /
DEARBORN SYMPHONY**
PO Box 2063
Dearborn, MI 48123
Phone: 313-565-2424
Fax: 313-565-2411
Web Site: www.dearbornsymphony.com
Officers:
   President: Sandra Butler
   VP: Carolyn Carr
   Treasurer: John Carr
Management:
   Music Director: Kypros Markou
   Office Manager: Debora Brazakis
Paid Staff: 3
Income Sources: Donations; Corporate Support
Annual Attendance: 5,000
Facility Category: Ford Community and Performing Arts
Center
Seating Capacity: 1,201

Year Built: 2001

1317 DETROIT SYMPHONY ORCHESTRA

3663 Woodward Avenue
Suite 100
Detroit, MI 48201
Phone: 313-576-5100
Fax: 313-576-5101
e-mail: info@detroitsymphony.com
Web Site: www.detroitsymphony.com
Officers:
   President: Emil Kang
   VP: Susan Burns
Management:
   Music Director: Neeme Jarvi
   Executive Director: Emil Kang
Mission: Today the Orchestra offers a variety of educational programs and resources, including the Detroit Symphony Civic and Sinfonia Orchestras and free educational concerts.
Founded: 1914
Specialized Field: Symphony; Orchestra
Status: Professional; Nonprofit
Performs At: Orchestra Hall; Meadow Brook Music Festival
Organization Type: Performing; Touring; Resident; Educational; Sponsoring

1318 CHAMBER MUSIC SOCIETY OF DETROIT

31731 Northwestern Highway
Suite 168W
Farmington Hills, MI 48334-1654
Phone: 248-737-9980
Fax: 248-737-9981
e-mail: chambermusicsocietyofdetroit@algxmail.com
Web Site: www.ComeHearCMSD.org
Officers:
   President: Lois R Beznos
Management:
   Administrative Director: Karen T Isble
Founded: 1944
Performs At: Seligman Performing Arts Center; Orchestra Hall
Affiliations: Chamber Music America
Seating Capacity: 715; 2,035

1319 FLINT SCHOOL OF PERFORMING ARTS: YOUTH ENSEMBLES

1025 E Kearsley
Flint, MI 48503
Phone: 810-238-1350
Fax: 810-238-6385
e-mail: fim@thefim.com
Web Site: www.thefim.com
Management:
   Music Director: Davin Pierson Torre
   Marketing Director: Chris Ferris
Annual Attendance: 3500

1320 FLINT SYMPHONY ORCHESTRA

Flint Institute of Music
1025 E Kearsley Street
Flint, MI 48503
Phone: 810-238-1350
Fax: 810-238-6385
Web Site: www.thefim.com/fso
Management:
   Manager: Tom Glasscock
Founded: 1917
Specialized Field: Symphony; Orchestra
Status: Professional; Nonprofit
Budget: $260,000-1,50,000
Performs At: James H. Whiting Auditorium
Organization Type: Performing; Resident; Educational

1321 GRAND RAPIDS SYMPHONY

169 Louis Campau Promenade NW
Suite One
Grand Rapids, MI 49503
Phone: 616-454-9451
Fax: 616-454-7477
e-mail: grsinfo@grsymphony.org
Web Site: www.grsymphony.org
Officers:
   Chairperson: Thomas Hilliker
Management:
   President: William A Ryberg
   VP Marketing/Public Relations: Karen Mueller
   Public Relations Manager: Carol Tanis
   VP Development: Jan McKinnon
Mission: The purpose of the Grand Rapids Symphony Society is to provide concerts of orchestral and chamber music and educational programs of the highest quality to the widest possible audience.
Founded: 1929
Specialized Field: Symphony; Orchestra; Chamber; Ensemble
Status: Nonprofit
Paid Staff: 25
Paid Artists: 75
Budget: $6.2 million
Income Sources: Concert and Event Income; Grants; Private Donations
Annual Attendance: 200,000
Organization Type: Performing; Touring; Resident; Educational

1322 GRAND RAPIDS YOUTH SYMPHONY

220 Lyon Street NW
Suite 415
Grand Rapids, MI 49503
Phone: 616-454-9451
Fax: 616-454-7477
Management:
   Conductor: John Varineau
   Outreach Director: Pam French
Mission: The Grand Rapids Youth Symphony affords the area's finest young musicians the opportunity to perform orchestal compositions ats a high standard.
Founded: 1959
Specialized Field: Symphony; Orchestra
Status: Non-Professional; Nonprofit
Paid Staff: 80

Income Sources: American Symphony Orchestra League (Youth Orchestra Division); Grand Rapids Symphony
Performs At: Forest Hills Northern High School Auditorium
Organization Type: Performing; Educational

1323 ST. CECILIA MUSIC SOCIETY
24 Ransom Avenue NE
Grand Rapids, MI 49503
Phone: 616-459-2224
Fax: 616-459-2997
e-mail: scms_pwp@iserv.net
Web Site: www.scmsonline.org
Management:
   Executive Director: Sharon Mack
   Music Director: Philip Pletcher
Mission: To promote and support chamber music performance in Western Michigan, specifically Grand Rapids.
Specialized Field: Music Education and Performance
Status: Nonprofit
Paid Staff: 20
Volunteer Staff: 300
Paid Artists: 50
Non-paid Artists: 100
Budget: $700,000
Income Sources: Membership, Grants, Corporate funding
Performs At: Royce Auditorium
Annual Attendance: 35,000
Facility Category: Historic Landmark Building
Type of Stage: Proscenium
Seating Capacity: 650
Year Built: 1894
Year Remodeled: 1998
Organization Type: Sponsoring

1324 PRO MUSICA OF DETROIT
181 Beaupre Avenue
Grosse Pointe Farms, MI 48236-3448
Phone: 313-885-0793
Fax: 313-885-6685
e-mail: alex@suczek.com
Web Site: www.promusicadetroit.com
Officers:
   First VP: Alice Haidostian
   Second VP: Dr. Hershel Sandberg
   Secretary: Ann Kondak
   Treasurer: James Diamond
   President: Alexander Suczek
Mission: To present world-class emerging performers in debut recitals; to offer performances of composers.
Founded: 1927
Specialized Field: Vocal Music; Instrumental Music; Composers' New Works; World Class Musical Artist Debuts
Status: Professional; Nonprofit
Volunteer Staff: 40
Paid Artists: 3-30
Budget: $60,000
Income Sources: Ticket Sales; Membership; Endowment; Corporate Sponsors
Performs At: Recital Hall of the Detroit Institute of the Arts
Annual Attendance: 3,000
Facility Category: Auditorium; Concert Hall

Seating Capacity: 1,100
Year Built: 1927
Organization Type: Performing

1325 HILLSDALE COLLEGE COMMUNITY ORCHESTRA
Hillsdale College
Hillsdale, MI 49242
Phone: 517-437-7341
Fax: 517-437-3923
Management:
   Music Director/Manager: James A Holleman
Budget: $35,000
Performs At: Markel Auditorium; Sage Center for the Arts

1326 HOLLAND CHAMBER ORCHESTRA
583 Riley
Holland, MI 49424
Mailing Address: PO Box 8084, Holland, MI. 49422-8084
Phone: 616-786-3172
Fax: 616-393-7616
e-mail: hco@macatawa.org
Management:
   Music Director: Mihai Craioveanu
   Orchestra Director: Thomas Working
Mission: Belongs to the community and allows adult musicians to share their love of music and further develop their talents; provides enjoyable and informative programs to promote classical music and inspire our listeners.
Budget: $35,000

1327 HOLLAND SYMPHONY ORCHESTRA
294 W Lakewood
PO Box 8054
Holland, MI 49422-8084
Phone: 616-494-0256
Fax: 616-392-7871
e-mail: hso@hollandsymphony.org
Web Site: www.hollandsymphony.org
Management:
   Executive Director: Kay Walvoord
Founded: 1990
Specialized Field: Orchestra
Paid Staff: 4
Volunteer Staff: 30
Paid Artists: 1
Non-paid Artists: 80
Budget: $100,000
Income Sources: Donations; Ticket Sales; Grants; Corporate Sponsorships
Performs At: High School Performing Arts Centers
Annual Attendance: 4000
Facility Category: Performing Arts Center
Seating Capacity: 942

1328 HOPE COLLEGE ORCHESTRA
Hope College, Music Department
127 E 12th Street
Holland, MI 49423

Phone: 616-394-7652
Fax: 616-395-7182
e-mail: ritsema@hope.edu
Management:
   Conductor: Robert Ritsema
Mission: The presentation of concerts on campus as well as in other cities.
Founded: 1949
Specialized Field: Orchestra; Chamber
Status: Non-Professional; Nonprofit
Paid Staff: 60
Budget: $35,000
Income Sources: American Symphony Orchestra League; Michigan Orchestra Association
Performs At: Dimnent Chapel
Organization Type: Performing; Touring; Resident; Educational

---

1329   KEWEENAW SYMPHONY ORCHESTRA OF MICHIGAN TECHNOLOGICAL UNIVERSITY

Michigan Technological University
1400 Townsend Drive, Fine Arts, 209 WAHC
Houghton, MI 49931
Phone: 906-487-2067
Fax: 906-487-3347
e-mail: jbhanson@mtu.edu
Web Site: www.fa.mtu.edu
Management:
   Music Director: Jeffery Bell-Hanson
   Arts Director: Dr. Milton Olsson
Founded: 1971
Budget: $35,000-100,000
Performs At: Rozsa Center for the Performing Arts
Affiliations: ASOL

1330   CHAMBER MUSIC SOCIETY OF KALAMAZOO

The Epic Center
359 S Burdick, Suite 200B
Kalamazoo, MI 49007
Phone: 616-382-0882
Fax: 616-349-9229
e-mail: Billmaxey@cs.com
Officers:
   President: William Maxey
Performs At: Civic Auditorium

1331   FONTANA CONCERT SOCIETY

359 S Burdick
Suite 200
Kalamazoo, MI 49007
Phone: 616-382-7774
Fax: 616-382-0812
e-mail: fontana@iserv.net
Web Site: www.fontanafestival.org
Officers:
   Administrative Assistant: Janlee Rothman
   Administrative Assistant: Ann Meade Sanders
Management:
   Director: Anders Dahlberg
   Assistand Director: Cori Sommers
   Financial Advisor: Wendy Biddle

Mission: Offering diverse high quality chamber music programs in a relaxed rural setting.
Founded: 1980
Specialized Field: Vocal Music; Instrumental Music; Festivals
Status: Professional; Nonprofit
Performs At: The Art Emporium
Organization Type: Performing; Sponsoring

1332   KALAMAZOO SYMPHONY ORCHESTRA

359 S Burdick Street
Suite 100
Kalamazoo, MI 49007
Phone: 616-349-7759
Fax: 616-349-9229
e-mail: symphony@iserv.net
Web Site: www.kalamazoosymphony.com
Officers:
   President: Kathie Vander Ploeg
   President Elect: Ken Miller
Management:
   Music Director/Conductor: Raymond Harvey
   Executive Director: Stacy Ridenour
   Director Marketing/Promotion: Holly J Kellar
   Development Director: Joan Thomas
   Education Director: Jane Rooks Ross
Mission: To support a professional symphony orchestra and staff; to present concerts of symphonic music and related programs of the highest possible artistic level; to support effective regional music education; to serve and involve the people of the greater Kalamazoo area in the Symphony Society.
Founded: 1921
Specialized Field: Symphony; Orchestra; Chamber; Ensemble
Status: Professional; Nonprofit
Paid Staff: 12
Paid Artists: 85
Budget: $2,000,000
Income Sources: Individual & Corporate Sponsors; Local; State & National Grants
Performs At: Miller Auditorium
Annual Attendance: 25,000
Seating Capacity: 3,496
Organization Type: Performing; Educational

1333   GREATER LANSING SYMPHONY ORCHESTRA

230 N Washington Square
Suite 100
Lansing, MI 48933
Phone: 517-487-5001
Fax: 517-487-0210
e-mail: info@ lansingsymphony.org
Web Site: www.lansingsymphony.org
Officers:
   President: James Sauage
   Treasurer: Roy Pentilla
   Secretary: David Nussdorfer
Management:
   General Manager: Judith Moore
   Operations Manager: Kara McGillicuddy
   Director Education/Outreach: Gretchen Morse

Administrative Assistant: Kristy Brown
Mission: To provide the finest possible quality symphonic music and educational service to residents of the Greater Lansing area.
Founded: 1930
Specialized Field: Symphony; Orchestra; Chamber; Ensemble
Status: Professional; Nonprofit
Performs At: Wharton Center for Performing Arts
Affiliations: American Symphony Orchestra League
Organization Type: Performing; Educational

1334 LIVONIA SYMPHONY ORCHESTRA

30499 Plymouth Road
Livonia, MI 48150
Phone: 734-421-1111
Fax: 734-464-8713
e-mail: promoman@kelseypromo.com
Officers:
President: Robert Bennett
Management:
Music Director/Conductor: Volodymyr Schesiuk
Budget: $100,000-150,000

1335 MIDLAND SYMPHONY ORCHESTRA

1801 W St. Andrews Road
Midland, MI 48640
Phone: 989-631-4234
Fax: 989-631-7890
e-mail: peterson@mcfta.org
Management:
General Manager: Judyth L. Peterson
Mission: Encouraging and supporting the Midland Symphony Orchestra in its pursuit of artistic excellence.
Founded: 1936
Specialized Field: Symphony; Orchestra; Chamber; Ensemble; Instrumental Group
Status: Professional; Semi-Professional; Non-Professional; Nonprofit
Income Sources: Michigan Orchestra Association; American Symphony Orchestra League
Performs At: Midland Center for the Arts
Organization Type: Performing; Touring; Educational; Sponsoring

1336 MUSIC SOCIETY: MIDLAND CENTER FOR THE ARTS

1801 W St. Andrews
Midland, MI 48640
Phone: 517-631-1072
Fax: 517-631-7890
Web Site: www.mcfta.org/main.html
Management:
Artistic Director: Dr. Victor A Klimash
Mission: Committed to providing performing and educational opportunities that would not otherwise exist.
Founded: 1943
Specialized Field: Orchestra; Chamber; Ensemble; Folk; Instrumental Group; Band
Status: Nonprofit
Performs At: Midland Center for the Arts
Organization Type: Performing; Educational; Sponsoring

1337 WEST SHORE YOUTH SYMPHONY ORCHESTRA

425 W Western Avenue
Suite 409
Muskegon, MI 49440
Phone: 231-726-3231
Fax: 231-722-6913
e-mail: info@wsso.org
Web Site: www.wsso.org
Officers:
Executive Director: Gretchen Cheney Rhoades
President: A Sawyer
Mission: To bring fine live music to the West Michigan area.
Founded: 1940
Specialized Field: Symphony; Orchestra; Chamber
Status: Professional; Nonprofit
Paid Staff: 5
Budget: 12,500
Type of Stage: thrust
Stage Dimensions: 30' x 50'
Seating Capacity: 1,700
Year Remodeled: 1999
Organization Type: Performing

1338 PLYMOUTH SYMPHONY

470 Forest Place, Suite 18
PO Box 6349
Plymouth, MI 48170-0379
Phone: 734-451-2112
Fax: 734-451-3458
e-mail: plymouthsymphony@aol.com
Web Site: www.plymouthsymphony.com
Officers:
President: Linda Alvarado
VP: John Lewis
Secretary: Robert Pray
Treasurer: Michelle Burger
Management:
Executive Director: Darlene A Dreyer
Music Director/Conductor: Nan Washburn
Office Manager: Pat Derderian
Mission: To provide high quality orchestral and music education experiences for the surrounding community.
Founded: 1945
Specialized Field: Southeast Michigan Orchestra
Paid Staff: 8
Volunteer Staff: 50
Paid Artists: 80
Budget: $271,000
Income Sources: Ticket sales; Grants; Donations; Auction; Raffle
Performs At: Variety of public venues
Affiliations: ASOL
Facility Category: Churches, auditoriums, banquet halls

1339 SAGINAW BAY ORCHESTRA

310 Johnson Street
PO Box 415
Saginaw, MI 48606

Phone: 989-755-6471
Fax: 989-755-1420
Toll-free: 877-755-7276
e-mail: sbso@msn.com
Web Site: www.saginabayorchestra.com
Management:
   Music Director/Conductor: Leo Najar
   Executive Director: Tamara Grefe
Founded: 1935
Paid Staff: 3

1340 SOUTHWEST MICHIGAN SYMPHONY ORCHESTRA

513 Ship Street
Saint Joseph, MI 49085
Phone: 269-982-4030
Fax: 269-982-4181
e-mail: info@smso.org
Web Site: www.smso.org
Management:
   General Manager: Jeffrey G White
   Music Director: Robert Vodnoy
Mission: To present concerts and sponsor an orchestra; to provide music educational activities.
Founded: 1950
Specialized Field: Symphony; Orchestra
Status: Professional
Performs At: Mendel Center; Lake Michigan College
Organization Type: Performing; Educational

1341 DETROIT CHAMBER WINDS

17348 W 12 Mile Road
Suite 192
Southfield, MI 48076
Phone: 248-559-2095
Fax: 248-559-2098
e-mail: chambermusic@juno.com
Web Site: www.detroitchamberwinds.org
Management:
   Artistic Advisor: H. Robert Reynolds
   Executive Director: Maury Okun
Mission: To offer performances of works featuring between 6 and 20 winds.
Specialized Field: Chamber
Status: Professional; Nonprofit
Organization Type: Performing

1342 METROPOLITAN YOUTH SYMPHONY

PO Box 244
Southfield, MI 48037
Phone: 503-239-4566
Toll-free: 888-752-9697
e-mail: mysgm@teleport.com
Management:
   President: Philip Lanzisera
   Music Director: Lajos Baloghn
   Conductor: Dr. John Richards
   Conductor: Bill Hunt

1343 LAKE ST. CLAIR SYMPHONY ORCHESTRA

21120 Benjamin
PO Box 806249
St. Clair Shores, MI 48080
Phone: 586-775-8138
Fax: 810-776-1012
e-mail: tulrich@home.com
Web Site: www.lscso.com
Officers:
   President: Tom Ulrich
   VP: Walter Lewis
Management:
   Music Director: Charles Burke
Mission: To promote and provide a symphony orchestra for the residents of the communities adjacent to Lake St. Clair; to provide a continuing educational program in symphonic music for students of the various school districts in the communities served by the Orchestra; and to provide a community-based organization for the expression and enjoyment of the music.
Founded: 1962
Specialized Field: Symphony; Orchestra
Status: Semi-Professional; Nonprofit
Budget: $35,000-100,000
Income Sources: American Symphony Orchestra League; Michigan Orchestra Association
Performs At: Schaublin Auditorium
Organization Type: Performing

1344 TRAVERSE SYMPHONY ORCHESTRA

123 1/2 E Front Street
PO Box 1247
Traverse City, MI 49685
Phone: 231-947-7120
Fax: 231-947-8118
e-mail: tso@tso-online.org
Web Site: www.tso-online.org
Management:
   Executive Director: Andy Burlow
Founded: 1951
Specialized Field: Symphony; Orchestra; Chamber
Status: Professional
Budget: $500,000
Income Sources: Ticket Sales; Grants; Donations; Sponserships
Annual Attendance: 7,000
Organization Type: Performing; Touring; Sponsoring

Minnesota

1345 BEMIDJI SYMPHONY ORCHESTRA

Bemidji State University
1500 Birchmont Drive
Bemidji, MN 56601-2699
Phone: 218-755-3364
Fax: 218-755-4369
e-mail: mmatalamaki@nmptv.org
Management:
   Music Director: Dr. Thomas L Swanson

Mission: Dedicated to communicating the richness of a variety of African cultures and customs through dance, rythm, and song in an exciting, energetic and colorful manner.
Budget: $35,000
Performs At: Bangsberg Fine Arts Complex Theatre & Recital Hall

1346 DULUTH-SUPERIOR SYMPHONY ORCHESTRA

506 W Michigan Street
Duluth, MN 55802
Phone: 218-733-7575
Fax: 218-733-7537
Web Site: www.dsso.com
Management:
    Executive Director: Andrew Berryhill
    Music Director: Markand Thakar
Mission: To generate the required financial and artistic resources to maintain the finest possible symphony orchestra as well as related programs and services; to develop future musicians and audiences.
Founded: 1932
Specialized Field: Symphony; Orchestra; Chamber; Ensemble
Status: Professional; Nonprofit
Budget: $1,000,000
Income Sources: American Symphony Orchestra League; Saint Louis County Heritage & Arts Center
Performs At: Duluth Auditorium
Annual Attendance: 40,000
Facility Category: DECC Auditorium
Type of Stage: Normal Stage
Seating Capacity: 2,400
Year Built: 1966
Organization Type: Performing; Educational

1347 DULUTH-SUPERIOR YOUTH ORCHESTRAS & SINFONIA

506 W Michigan Street
Duluth, MN 55802
Phone: 218-733-7575
Fax: 218-733-7537
Mission: To offer a learning and performing experience for students in the Youth Orchestra (high school) and Sinfonia (junior and senior high school).
Founded: 1940
Specialized Field: Symphony; Orchestra; Chamber; Ensemble
Status: Non-Professional; Nonprofit
Paid Staff: 100
Income Sources: American Symphony Orchestra League (Youth Orchestra Division); Duluth-Superior Symphony Orchestra
Organization Type: Performing; Educational

1348 HEARTLAND SYMPHONY ORCHESTRA

PO Box 241
Little Falls, MN 56345
Phone: 320-632-0960
Fax: 320-632-9025
Toll-free: 800-826-1997
Management:
    Music Director: Richard Haglund

Business Manager: William Adkins
Mission: To bring orchestral music to concert-goers in our area, to aquaint young people with the beauty of classical music, and to provide an opportunity for trained musicians to play together.
Founded: 1977
Status: Nonprofit
Budget: $35,000-100,000
Performs At: Tornstrom Auditorium; Charles Martin Auditorium

1349 MANKATO SYMPHONY ORCHESTRA

120 South Broad Street
Mankato, MN 56001
Mailing Address: PO Box 645 Mankato MN, 56002
Phone: 507-625-8880
Fax: 507-625-5792
e-mail: mso@mnic.net
Web Site: www.symphony.mankato.com
Officers:
    Executive Director: Jane Stetta
    President: Lisa Haman
    VP: Lorin Ruthenbeck
    Secretary: Sally Trask
    Treasurer: Ann Coleman
Mission: The orchestra plays five subscription concerts each year plus three Youth Concerts, and provides many educational and artistic opportunities to area students, including the Young artist and Young Composer contests. The orchestra also plays one free outdoor concert in June.
Founded: 1952
Specialized Field: Symphony; Orchestra
Status: Non-Professional; Nonprofit
Paid Staff: 1
Volunteer Staff: 65
Paid Artists: 90
Budget: $190,000
Income Sources: Grants; Sponsors; Contributions
Performs At: Mankato West High School Auditorium
Facility Category: High school auditorium
Organization Type: Performing; Resident; Educational

1350 CIVIC ORCHESTRA OF MINNEAPOLIS

PO Box 50604
Minneapolis, MN 55405-0604
Phone: 612-332-4842
Fax: 612-649-1288
e-mail: peltier@winternet.com
Management:
    Music Director: Cary John Franklin
Budget: $35,000

1351 GREATER TWIN CITIES YOUTH SYMPHONIES

528 Hennepin Avenue
Suite 404
Minneapolis, MN 55403
Phone: 612-870-7611
Fax: 612-870-7613
e-mail: mail@gtcys.org
Web Site: www.gtcys.org
Officers:
    President: Loisd Hesselroth
    Treasurer: Kerry Spaven

VP: Nancye Rystrom
Secretary: Kristin Schoephoerster
Management:
Interim Artistic Director: Marlene Pauley
Operations Manager: Devin Thomas
Office Manager: Denise Culshaw
Executive Director: Christine Corcoran
Mission: In the conviction that music nourishes the mind, body, and spirit of the individual and enriches the community, the Greater Twin Cities Youth Symphonies provides a rigorous and inspiring orchestral experience for qualifying young muscians.
Founded: 1972
Specialized Field: Symphony; Chamber; Ensemble
Status: Non-Professional; Nonprofit
Paid Staff: 6
Paid Artists: 8
Non-paid Artists: 5
Budget: $645,000
Performs At: Orchestra Hall; Landmark Center
Organization Type: Performing; Touring; Educational

1352 METROPOLITAN SYMPHONY ORCHESTRA

PO Box 581213
Minneapolis, MN 55458-1213
Phone: 651-645-4283
e-mail: info@msoa.net
Officers:
President: William Schrickel
VP: Terry Wilson
Treasurer: Scott Simmons
Secretary: Scott Simmons
Management:
Music Director: William Intriligator
General Manager: Mark Warhol
Budget: $35,000

1353 MINNESOTA ORCHESTRA

Orchestra Hall
1111 Nicollet Mall
Minneapolis, MN 55403
Phone: 612-371-5600
Fax: 612-371-0838
Toll-free: 800-292-4141
e-mail: info@mnorch.org
Web Site: www.minnesotaorchestra.org
Officers:
President: David J Hyslop
VP/General Manager: Robert R Neu
VP/CFO: E Benton Gill
VP Marketing: Stephen Baker
Management:
Music Director: Osmo Vanska
VP Development: Mary Ellen Kuhi
Director of Public Affairs: Gwen Pappas
Director Educational Activities: Jim Bartsch
Manager Outreach: Mele Willis
Mission: The Minnesota Orchestra is one of the nations leading symphony orchestras presenting more than 200 concerts a year, including classical programs, pop concerts, family concerts and a summer festival.
Founded: 1903

Specialized Field: Vocal Music; Instrumental Music; Festivals; Grand Opera
Status: Professional; Nonprofit
Paid Artists: 95
Income Sources: Concert Performances
Performs At: Orchestra Hall
Annual Attendance: 400,000
Type of Stage: Permanent acoustic shell
Seating Capacity: 2,450
Year Built: 1974
Year Remodeled: 1997
Rental Contact: Mark Georgesen
Organization Type: Performing; Touring; Resident; Educational; Sponsoring

1354 MINNESOTA SINFONIA

901 N 3rd Street
Suite 112
Minneapolis, MN 55403
Phone: 612-871-1701
Fax: 612-871-1701
e-mail: mnsinfonia@aol.com
Web Site: www.mnsinfonia.org
Officers:
Chair Emeritus: David Zimmerman
Treasurer: Chad Bailey

1355 WALKER ART CENTER

725 Vineland Place
Minneapolis, MN 55403
Phone: 612-375-7624
Fax: 612-375-7618
e-mail: information@walkerart.org
Web Site: www.walkerart.org
Management:
Director: Kathy Halbreich
Performing Arts Curator: Philip Bither
Mission: Serving as a regional and international catalyst for emerging forms of expression; engaging audiences in the issues which are shaping contemporary arts.
Specialized Field: Visual, performing and media arts
Status: Professional; Nonprofit
Paid Staff: 150
Performs At: Walker Art Center Auditorium
Facility Category: Multidiscliplinary Arts Center
Seating Capacity: 350
Organization Type: Performing; Touring; Resident; Educational; Sponsoring; Exhibition

1356 FARGO-MOORHEAD SYMPHONY ORCHESTRA AND ASSOCIATION

810 Fourth Avenue S
Suite 250
Moorhead, MN 56560
Phone: 218-233-8397
Fax: 218-236-1845
e-mail: fmsymphony@i29.net
Web Site: www.fmsymphony.org
Management:
Executive Director: Bill Law

Mission: To provide our region with the opportunity to experience live orchestral music, including performances by local, regional, national, and international guest artists; to provide musicians in the community with the opportunity to perform.
Founded: 1931
Paid Staff: 8
Paid Artists: 75
Budget: $260,000-1,050,000
Income Sources: Individual; Corporate; Foundations
Performs At: Reineke Fine Arts Center
Annual Attendance: 15,000
Facility Category: Concert hall- University
Stage Dimensions: 987
Seating Capacity: 1,000
Year Built: 1990
Rental Contact: 7012817932 Division of Fine Arts

1357 SAINT OLAF COLLEGE ORCHESTRA

Saint Olaf College
1520 St Olaf Avenue
Northfield, MN 55057
Phone: 507-646-3179
Fax: 507-646-3527
e-mail: ericksor@stolaf.edu
Web Site: www.stolaf.edu/depts/music/stolaf_orch
Management:
   Conductor: Steven Amundson
   Manager: Richard Erickson
Budget: $35,000-100,000
Performs At: Skoglund Center Auditorium
Seating Capacity: 4,000

1358 ROCHESTER CIVIC MUSIC

201 4th Street SE
Suite 170
Rochester, MN 55904
Phone: 507-285-8076
Fax: 507-281-6055
Web Site: www.ci.rochester.mn.us/music
Management:
   General Manager: Steven J Schmidt
Mission: To offer a comprehensive and coordinated music program for area residents.
Founded: 1933
Specialized Field: Presenter; Producer
Status: Professional; Government Agency
Performs At: Mayo Civic Center
Organization Type: Performing; Touring; Resident; Educational; Sponsoring

1359 ST. CLOUD SYMPHONY ORCHESTRA

PO Box 234
Saint Cloud, MN 56302-0234
Phone: 320-257-3114
e-mail: stcloudsymphony@paramountarts.org
Web Site: www.stcloudsymphony.com
Management:
   Music Director: Lawrence Eckerling
   Executive Director: Dian Gray

Mission: To present high quality performance of orchestral music and educational outreach activities to the St. Could area, encourage participation by local and area musicians and to further the understanding and appreciation of orchestral music.
Founded: 1975
Budget: $100,000-150,000
Performs At: Benedicta Arts Center; Ritchse Auditorium

1360 451ST ARMY BAND

Fort Snelling
Building 506
Saint Paul, MN 55111
Phone: 612-713-3339
Fax: 612-713-3519
Management:
   Commander/Band Master: CW4 Bruce J Hedblom
   Assistant Conductor: SSG Robert A Lake
Mission: Representing the 88th United States Army Reserve Command to the military and to the general public as well as promoting and encouraging the performing arts.
Founded: 1923
Specialized Field: Ensemble; Ethnic; Folk; Band
Status: Professional; Nonprofit
Organization Type: Performing; Touring; Educational

1361 MINNESOTA STATE BAND

651 Mackubin Street N
Saint Paul, MN 55103-1624
Phone: 651-282-4077
Web Site: www.mnband.org
Management:
   Music Director/Conductor: Joseph Komro
   Public Relations: Neil Danielson
   Stage Manager: Adam Torres
   Concert Coordinator: Helmut Kahlert
Mission: Dedicated to furthering the musical development and appreciation of America's concert band and wind ensemble movement.
Founded: 1898
Specialized Field: Ensemble; Ethnic; Instrumental Group; Band
Status: Professional; Nonprofit
Paid Staff: 70
Income Sources: Association of Concert Bands
Organization Type: Performing; Touring; Educational

1362 SAINT PAUL CHAMBER ORCHESTRA

Hamm Building, 408 St. Peter Street
Suite 500
Saint Paul, MN 55102-1497
Phone: 651-292-3248
Fax: 651-292-3281
e-mail: info@spcomail.org
Web Site: www.thespco.org
Officers:
   President/Managing Director: Bruce Coppock
   Immediate Post Chairman: AJ Huss, Jr
   Chairman: Lowell J Noteboom
   Treasurer: Sallie Lilienthal
   Secretary: Terry T. Saario
Management:
   Baroque Serires Director: Nicholas McGegan

Music Director: Andreas Delfs
Director Finance: Beth Villaume
Mission: To present a world-class professional chamber orchestra in the Twin Cities, dedicated to superior performance and artistic innovation, for the enrichment of community life and world audiences.
Founded: 1959
Specialized Field: Orchestra; Chamber; Ensemble
Status: Professional; Nonprofit
Paid Artists: 33
Budget: $9,200,000
Income Sources: Government & Corporate Donors; Sales
Season: 38 weeks
Performs At: Ordway Center for the Performing Arts
Affiliations: American Symphony Orchestra League; Association of Performing Arts Presenters
Organization Type: Performing; Touring; Resident; Educational; Recording

Mississippi

1363 GULF COAST SYMPHONY

PO Box 542
Biloxi, MS 39533-0542
Phone: 228-435-9800
Fax: 228-435-9807
e-mail: gcso@worldnet.att.net
Web Site: www.gulfcoastsymphony.net
Officers:
    President: Harold Roberts
    VP: Jim Wooten
    Secretary: Peggy Schloegel
    Music Director/Conductor: John Wesley Strickler
Management:
    Executive Director: Natalie Robohm
    Development Director: Signe Cutrone
Mission: The presentation of symphonic music to Gulf Coast residents.
Founded: 1963
Specialized Field: Symphony
Status: Professional; Nonprofit
Paid Staff: 3
Volunteer Staff: 150
Paid Artists: 4
Budget: $460,000
Performs At: Saenger Theatre; Biloxi
Annual Attendance: 20,000
Facility Category: Theater
Seating Capacity: 1,050
Rental Contact: Lee Hood
Organization Type: Performing; Touring; Educational

1364 UNIVERSITY OF SOUTHERN MISSISSIPPI SYMPHONY

PO Box 5081
Hattiesburg, MS 39406-5081
Phone: 601-261-1305
Fax: 601-261-1308
Management:
    Music Director/Conductor: Jay Dean
Budget: $100,000-150,000
Performs At: Bennett Auditoirum
Seating Capacity: 1,000

1365 MISSISSIPPI SYMPHONY ORCHESTRA

201 E Pascagoula Street
PO Box 2052
Jackson, MS 39225-2052
Phone: 601-960-1565
Fax: 601-960-1564
Toll-free: 800-898-5050
e-mail: development@msorchestra.com
Web Site: www.msorchestra.com
Officers:
    Chairman: Alan Leach
Management:
    President/CEO: Robert A Reed
    Director Finance: Sarajean Babin
    Director Operations: Richard Hudson
    Director Education: Patrick Johnson
    Music Director & Conductor: Crafton Beck
Founded: 1944
Specialized Field: Symphony; Orchestra; Chamber; Pops/ Popular Selections
Paid Staff: 7
Volunteer Staff: 1
Budget: $1,300,000
Performs At: Brianwood Presbyterian; Thalia Mara Hall; Galloway United Methodist Church
Seating Capacity: 2430

1366 MISSISSIPPI YOUTH SYMPHONY ORCHESTRA

PO Box 2052
Jackson, MS 39225-2052
Phone: 601-960-1565
Fax: 601-960-1564
Toll-free: 800-898-5050
e-mail: jerryo@msorchestra.com
Web Site: www.msorchestra.com
Officers:
    Director Public Relations: Heather Clancy
Management:
    Executive Director: Robert Reed
    Education Director: Jacqueline Perry
    Conductor MS Youth Symphony Orc.: Tim Li
    MS Youth Symphony Orchestra: Stephine Garrett
    MS Youth Cadet Orchestra: Melane Franklin
Mission: To promote education and appreciation of classical music through participation in the junior or senior youth orchestras.
Specialized Field: Symphony; Orchestra
Status: Non-Professional; Nonprofit
Income Sources: American Symphony Orchestra League(Youth Orchestra Division)
Performs At: Chastain Junior High School
Organization Type: Performing; Touring; Educational

1367 MERIDIAN SYMPHONY ORCHESTRA

910 Highway 19 N
PO Box 2171
Meridian, MS 39307
Phone: 601-693-2224
Fax: 601-482-8824
e-mail: mso@netdoor.com
Web Site: www.msnnetdoor.com
Management:
    Music Director: Claire Fox Hillard

General Manager: Carolyn Abdella
Budget: $260,000-1,050,000
Performs At: Meridian Community College Auditorium
Seating Capacity: 600

1368 TUPELO SYMPHONY ORCHESTRA ASSOCIATION

PO Box 474
Tupelo, MS 38802
Phone: 662-842-8433
Fax: 662-842-9565
e-mail: tupelo symphony@netdoor.com
Web Site: www.tupelo symphony.com
Officers:
   President: Robert Mark Ledbetter
   Executive VP: Nancy Diffee
   Secretary: Sandy Morris
   Development: Bob Schreiner
Management:
   Music Director: Louis Lane
   Executive Director: WF Sparks
   Executive Administrator: Margaret Anne Murphey
   Orchestra Manager: David East
Mission: To offer high quality performances of symphonic works.
Founded: 1971
Specialized Field: Symhpony; Orchestra
Status: Professional
Volunteer Staff: 3
Budget: $150,000-260,000
Income Sources: Contributors/Corporate/Ticket sales/Grants
Performs At: Tupedo Civic Auditorium
Affiliations: American Symphony Orchestra League
Facility Category: Civic Auditorium
Seating Capacity: 1,100
Year Built: 1965
Year Remodeled: 2000
Organization Type: Performing; Touring

Missouri

1369 MISSOURI SYMPHONY SOCIETY

203 S 9th Street
Columbia, MO 65201
Phone: 573-875-0600
Fax: 573-449-4214
e-mail: motheatre@socket.net
Web Site: www.missouritheatre.com
Mission: The enhancement of the cultural environment through fine music, education and the nurturing of young musicians.
Founded: 1971
Specialized Field: Symphony; Orchestra; Chamber
Status: Professional; Nonprofit
Paid Staff: 40
Budget: $375,000
Income Sources: Pops Orchestra; Chamber Orchestra Festival Symphony
Performs At: Missouri Theatre
Type of Stage: Proscenium
Seating Capacity: 1,220
Year Built: 1928

Rental Contact: Executive Director David A White
Organization Type: Performing; Touring; Educational; Sponsoring

1370 INDEPENDENCE SYMPHONY ORCHESTRA

3408 Trail Ridge Dirive
Independence, MO 64055
Phone: 816-373-8151
Fax: 816-220-6511
e-mail: LynnP12@juno.com
Web Site: www.indepsymphony.org
Officers:
   President: Rick Henks
   VP: Chelle Farrand
   Treasurer: Helen Newlin
   Secretary: Betty Liston
Management:
   Music Director: Jack Ergo
   Executive Director: Alan Tyree
Budget: $35,000
Seating Capacity: 1500-5000

1371 FRIENDS OF CHAMBER MUSIC

4643 Wyandotte Street
Suite 201
Kansas City, MO 64112-1542
Phone: 816-561-9999
Fax: 816-561-8810
Toll-free: 877-697-3287
e-mail: marketing@chambermusic.org
Web Site: www.chambermusic.org
Officers:
   Chairman of the Board: Steve Karbank
Management:
   Executive Director: Cynthia Siebert
   Marketing Director: Marcy Chiasson Medler
Status: Not-for-profit

1372 KANSAS CITY CHAMBER ORCHESTRA

11 East 40th Street
Kansas City, MO 64111
Phone: 816-960-1324
Fax: 816-960-1325
e-mail: kcco@earthlink.net
Management:
   Music Director/Conductor: Bruce Sorrell
Founded: 1987
Specialized Field: Instrumental Music
Budget: $150,000-200,000
Income Sources: Donations, Grants, Ticket sales

1373 KANSAS CITY SYMPHONY

1020 Central
Suite 300
Kansas City, MO 64105-1672
Phone: 816-471-1100
Fax: 816-471-0976
e-mail: tkutey@kcsymphony.org
Web Site: www.kcsymphony.org
Officers:
   President: Shirley Bush Helzberg
   VP: Robert A Kipp

VP: Michael D Fields
VP: Arthur B. Krause
Secretary/Treasurer: William B. Taylor
Management:
Music Director: Anne Manson
Executive Director: Roland E Valliere
Assistant to the Executive Director: Mary Allen
Director Marketing/Public Relations: Rose Sinn

1374 NORTHLAND SYMPHONY ORCHESTRA
PO Box 12255
Kansas City, MO 64152
Phone: 816-759-1260
Fax: 816-759-9084
e-mail: northlandsymphonyorchestra@yahoo.com
Web Site: www.geocities.com/vienna/8988/
Management:
Music Director/Conductor: James Murray III
Mission: To offer professional, amateur and student musicians an opportunity to preform fin orchestral music and free public concerts fir diverse audiences.
Budget: $35,000
Performs At: Park Hill South School Auditorium
Seating Capacity: 950

1375 UNIVERSITY OF MISSOURI-KANSAS CITY CONSERVATORY SYMPHONY ORCHESTRA
4949 Cherry Street
Kansas City, MO 641110
Phone: 816-235-2731
Fax: 816-235-5265
e-mail: olsonrh@umkc.edu
Web Site: www.umck.edu
Management:
Music Director: Robert Olson
Seating Capacity: 612

1376 LIBERTY SYMPHONY ORCHESTRA
PO Box 30
Liberty, MO 64068
Phone: 816-781-7700
Fax: 816-415-5012
e-mail: tickets@libertysymphony.com
Web Site: www.libertysymphony.com
Officers:
President: Bill Matteson
Secretary: Ruth Ann Rooney
Treasurer: David Noyes
Management:
Conductor: Dr. Phillip C Posey
Manager: Laurie Spence
Mission: To help satisfy the growing need for a musical outlet in the northern metropolitan area in general and the Liberty community in particular; to complement and enhance the already-rich cultural environment of the community by bringing people and music together; to provide a further dimension for the quality of life in our community.
Founded: 1970
Paid Staff: 3
Volunteer Staff: 30
Paid Artists: 22

Non-paid Artists: 58
Budget: $50,000
Income Sources: Sponsors; Patrons; Donors; Grants; Box Office
Performs At: Liberty Performing Arts Theatre; Liberty Community Center
Affiliations: Missouri Citizens for the Arts; American Symphony Orchestra League; Missouri Arts Council; Liberty Chamber of Commerce
Annual Attendance: 4,200
Facility Category: Performing Arts Theatre
Seating Capacity: 700
Year Built: 1991
Organization Type: Performing; Educational

1377 SAINT JOSEPH SYMPHONY SOCIETY
120 S Eighth Street
Saint Joseph, MO 64501
Phone: 816-233-7701
Fax: 816-233-6704
e-mail: stjosymphony@aol.com
Officers:
President: Jane Hausman
VP: Dr. Richard Bell
Treasurer: Mark Matthews
Secretary: Diane Nicholas
Management:
Executive Director: Allison E Stewart
Mission: To present symphonic concerts and educational activities for the citizens of Northwest Missouri and Eastern Kansas.
Founded: 1959
Specialized Field: Symphony
Status: Professional; Nonprofit
Paid Staff: 5
Paid Artists: 60
Performs At: Missouri Theatre
Organization Type: Performing; Educational

1378 NEW MUSIC CIRCLE
142 Willow Brook Road
Saint Louis, MO 63146
Phone: 314-432-6073
Fax: 314-567-5384
e-mail: alumrod@aol.com
Management:
Music Director: Rich O'Donnell
Mission: To advocate for new music; to commission new works; to promote promising composers and ensembles.
Specialized Field: Electronic & Live Electronic; New Music; Avant Garde
Status: Professional; Nonprofit
Organization Type: Presenting

1379 SAINT LOUIS CLASSICAL GUITAR SOCIETY
PO Box 11425
Saint Louis, MO 63105
Phone: 314-567-5566
e-mail: guitarsl@inlink.com
Web Site: www.guitarstlouis.org
Officers:
President: William Ash

Mission: To promote and foster an understanding and appreciation of the guitar, to encourage a high standard in instruction and performance, to encourage the creation and preservation of music for the guitar to sponsor the society.
Status: Nonprofit
Budget: $10,000-$20,000
Performs At: The Ethical Society

1380 SAINT LOUIS PHILHARMONIC ORCHESTRA

PO Box 220437
Saint Louis, MO 63122
Phone: 314-421-3600
Web Site: www.stlphilharmonic.org
Officers:
  President: Marilyn K Humiston
  VP: Stephen Larmore
  Secretary: Doug Kenner
  Treasurer: David Lyon
Mission: To offer musicians an opportunity to play good music under the direction of an able conductor.
Founded: 1860
Specialized Field: Symphony
Status: Non-Professional; Nonprofit
Performs At: Scottish Rite Cathedral
Organization Type: Performing

1381 SAINT LOUIS SYMPHONY ORCHESTRA

Powell Symphony Hall
718 N Grand Boulevard
Saint Louis, MO 63103
Phone: 314-533-2500
Fax: 314-286-4142
Toll-free: 800-232-1880
e-mail: carlaj@slso.org
Web Site: www.slso.org
Officers:
  Chairman: Virginia Weldon
  President/Executive Director: Don Roth
  Secretary: Richard Duesenberg
  Treasurer: Dr. Wilfred R. Konneker
  CFO: John Fraser
Management:
  General Manager: Carla Johnson
  Chorus Director: Amy Kaiser
  Director Artistic Administration: Kathleen Van Bergen
  Acting Stage Manager: Mike Lynch
  Director Marketing: Stephen Duncan
  Concertmaster: David Halen
Founded: 1879
Specialized Field: Symphony
Status: Professional; Nonprofit
Budget: $27,000,000
Performs At: Powell Symphony Hall at Grand Center
Seating Capacity: 2,700
Organization Type: Performing; Touring; Educational

1382 SAINT LOUIS SYMPHONY YOUTH ORCHESTRA

Powell Symphony Hall
718 N Grand Boulevard
Saint Louis, MO 63103
Phone: 314-533-2500
Fax: 314-286-4142
Web Site: www.slso.org/performers/yo.htm
Management:
  Manager: Margaret Neilson
  Music Director: David Amado
  Founder: Leonard Slatkin
Mission: The Saint Louis Symphony Youth Orchestra was founded in 1970 by Leonard Slatkin to acquaint young instrumentalists with the atmosphere of a professional orchestra, to introduce them to the environment of the Saint Louis Symphony and to provide them with the opportunity of investigating and performing a wide spectrum of symphonic music.
Founded: 1970
Specialized Field: Symphony; Orchestra; Chamber
Status: Non-Professional; Nonprofit
Paid Staff: 100
Income Sources: American Symphony Orchestra League (Youth Orchestra Division)
Performs At: Powell Symphony Hall at Grand Center
Organization Type: Performing; Touring; Educational; Sponsoring

1383 KANSAS CITY YOUTH SYMPHONY ASSOCIATION OF KANSAS

7301 Mission Road
Suite 143
Shawnee Mission, MO 66208
Phone: 913-722-6810
Fax: 913-722-6806
e-mail: ysymph@crn.org
Web Site: www.crn.org/kcys
Management:
  Music Director/Conductor: Glenn Block
Mission: To provide educational opportunities for young muscians by performing before community-wide audiences and by inspiring excellence in performance.

1384 SPRINGFIELD SYMPHONY ASSOCIATION

1536 E Division
Springfield, MO 65803
Phone: 417-864-6683
Fax: 417-864-8967
Web Site: www.orion.org/~symphony/history.html
Officers:
  President: Randal L Saul
  VP: Jason Hemingway
  Treasurer: Lisa C Officer
  Secretary: Sheryl Wachter
  Guild President: Libby Falk
Management:
  Executive Director: Dana C Randall
  Conductor: Charles Bontrager
Mission: To provide the highest level of symphonic music and music education to all of Southwest Missouri, commensurate with sound fiscal policies.
Founded: 1934
Specialized Field: Symphony
Status: Semi-Professional
Income Sources: American Symphony Orchestra League; Missouri Arts Council

Performs At: Juanita K. Hammons Hall for the Performing Arts
Organization Type: Performing

1385 KIRKWOOD SYMPHONY ORCHESTRA

PO Box 410053
St Louis, MO 63141
Phone: 314-569-3220
Fax: 314-569-3220
Web Site: www.claytonsymphony.org
Officers:
    President: Rusell A Willis
Management:
    Conductor: James E Richards
Budget: $35,000
Performs At: St. John's Lutheran Church
Seating Capacity: 500

1386 CENTRAL MISSOURI STATE UNIVERSITY SYMPHONY ORCHESTRA

Music Department
Utt 109
Warrensburg, MO 64093
Phone: 660-543-4330
Fax: 660-543-8271
e-mail: rutland@cmsu1.cmsu.edu
Web Site: www.cmsu.edu/music
Officers:
    Chairman Music Department: Charles McAdams
Management:
    Music Director/Conductor: John Rutland
Mission: To give university students and community members exposure to the standard orchestral repertoire and serve as a cultural force within the greater Warrensburg area.
Founded: 1871
Specialized Field: Kansas City
Paid Staff: 2
Paid Artists: 1
Non-paid Artists: 55
Budget: $35,000
Performs At: Hart Recital Hall
Seating Capacity: 350

Montana

1387 BILLINGS SYMPHONY SOCIETY

201 N Broadway
Suite 350
Billings, MT 59103
Phone: 406-252-3610
Fax: 406-252-3353
e-mail: symphony@billingssymphon.org
Web Site: www.billingssymphony.org/
Management:
    Music Director: Dr. Uri Barnea
    Chorale Director: David Barnet
    General Manager: Maxine Pihlaja
Mission: To offer the community and the region live symphonic music.
Founded: 1951
Specialized Field: Symphony; Orchestra

Status: Semi-Professional; Nonprofit
Budget: $260,000-1,050,000
Income Sources: American Symphony Orchestra League; Montana Association of Symphony Orchestras
Performs At: The Alberta Bair Theater for the Performing Arts
Seating Capacity: 1,200
Organization Type: Performing

1388 YELLOWSTONE CHAMBER PLAYERS

1204 Rimhaven Way
Billings, MT 59102
Phone: 406-248-2832
Fax: 406-248-2832
e-mail: mclamonaca@hotmail.com
Officers:
    Board Member: Mary LaMonaca
    VP: Delores Vigessa
    Secretary: Lisa Lombardy
    Treasurer: Ramona Turnbull
Management:
    President: Elizabeth Adcock
    Ticket Manager: Caron Schultz
Mission: The performance of a wide variety of chamber music, from string quartets and piano quintets, to small ensembles employing clarinet, flute and guitar.
Founded: 1980
Specialized Field: Chamber; Ensemble; Instrumental Group
Status: Professional; Nonprofit
Volunteer Staff: 20
Paid Artists: 15
Income Sources: Friends of YCP; Donations; Business Sponsors
Performs At: Churches; Small Recital Halls
Annual Attendance: 1,000
Organization Type: Performing; Touring; Resident

1389 GREAT FALLS SYMPHONY ASSOCIATION

Civic Center Building
PO Box 1078
Great Falls, MT 59403
Phone: 406-453-4102
Fax: 406-453-9779
e-mail: info@gfsymphony.org
Web Site: www.gfsymphony.org
Management:
    Executive Director: Carolyn Valacich
    Music Director/Conductor: Gordon J Johnson
    Choir Director: Kathy McIntosh
Mission: To serve as the primary source of cultural and educational service to North Central Montana. Performances include the symphony orchestra with guest artists, choir, musical theatre, ballet, opera and resident string quartet recitals as well as public school demonstrations.
Founded: 1959
Specialized Field: Symphony; Orchestra; Symphonic Choir; Chamber Ensemble; Youth Orchestra
Status: Professional; Nonprofit
Paid Staff: 8
Paid Artists: 65
Non-paid Artists: 80

Budget: $450,000-$500,000
Income Sources: American Symphony Orchestra League; Montana Association of Symphony Orchestras; Tickets
Performs At: Great Falls Civic Center
Annual Attendance: 35,000
Seating Capacity: 1,776
Organization Type: Performing; Touring; Resident; Educational; Sponsoring

1390 HELENA SYMPHONY SOCIETY

15 N Ewing Street
PO Box 1073
Helena, MT 59624
Phone: 406-442-1860
Fax: 406-443-6620
e-mail: helenasymphony@hotmail.com
Web Site: www.helenasymphony.org
Officers:
   President: John Mundinger
   VP: Frank Graham
   Secretary: Ross Common
Management:
   Executive Director: Leslie Gilkey
   Music Director: Eric Funk
   Chorale Director: Gary Funk
Mission: The presentation of classical and popular symphony concerts, including choral and chamber concerts.
Founded: 1955
Specialized Field: Symphony; Orchestra; Chamber; Ethnic
Status: Nonprofit
Paid Staff: 4
Volunteer Staff: 20
Non-paid Artists: 140
Budget: $175,000
Income Sources: American Society of Composers; Authors and Publishers; Broadcast Music Incorporated; Donations; Tickets
Performs At: Helena Civic Center
Affiliations: American Symphony Orchestra League; Montana Association of Symphony Orchestra
Organization Type: Performing; Educational

1391 MISSOULA SYMPHONY ASSOCIATION

111 N Higgins Avenue
Suite 208
Missoula, MT 59802
Phone: 406-721-3194
Fax: 406-721-7985
e-mail: mslasymphony@hotmail.com
Officers:
   President: David Nelson
Management:
   Executive Director: John Driscoll
Mission: To present artistic programs of excellence to Missoula and the surrounding areas, provide an opportunity for young persons and develop an interest in the arts through concerts and master classes.
Founded: 1954
Specialized Field: Symphony
Status: Nonprofit
Paid Staff: 4
Paid Artists: 10

Non-paid Artists: 60
Budget: $200,000
Income Sources: American Symphony Orchestra League
Performs At: University Theatre
Annual Attendance: 7,500
Facility Category: University Theatre
Stage Dimensions: 37'x 36'
Seating Capacity: 1,040
Year Built: 30's
Year Remodeled: 1997
Organization Type: Performing; Sponsoring

Nebraska

1392 HASTINGS SYMPHONY ORCHESTRA

Fuhr Hall
9th and Ash
Hastings, NE 68901
Phone: 402-461-7361
Fax: 402-461-7428
e-mail: jjohnson@hastings.edu
Web Site: www.hastingsnet.com/symphony
Management:
   Music Director/Conductor: Dr. James Johnson
   Executive Secretary: Joyce Grothen
Mission: To enrich the cultural environment for people of all ages by providing quality, live performances of music in a symphonic setting, music education, and performance opportunities for talented musicians.
Founded: 1926
Specialized Field: Symphony; Orchestra; Chamber
Status: Non-Professional; Nonprofit
Paid Staff: 2
Volunteer Staff: 20
Paid Artists: 25
Non-paid Artists: 50
Budget: $60,000
Income Sources: Tickets; Contributions; Grants
Performs At: Hastings Masonic Temple
Annual Attendance: 6000
Facility Category: City Auditorium
Organization Type: Performing; Touring; Resident; Educational
Resident Groups: American Symphony Orchestra League

1393 KEARNEY AREA SYMPHONY ORCHESTRA

University of Nebraska at Kearney
Music Department, 2506 12th Avenue
Kearney, NE 68849
Phone: 308-865-8618
Fax: 308-865-8806
e-mail: crockerr@unk.edu
Officers:
   President: Dick Hock
Management:
   Interim Conductor: Dr. Ron Crocker
Budget: $35,000
Income Sources: Donations; Ads
Performs At: Auditorium
Annual Attendance: 350
Seating Capacity: 500

1394 LINCOLN CIVIC ORCHESTRA

216 N 11 Street
Suite 202
Lincoln, NE 68508-1401
Phone: 402-477-8446
Fax: 402-477-8222
e-mail: lco@artsincorparated.org
Management:
Music Director: Dr. Pat Fortney
Executive Director: Dean W Haist
Mission: Offering community members an opportunity to perform serious music.
Specialized Field: Orchestra
Status: Nonprofit
Paid Staff: 130
Budget: $35,000
Performs At: O'Donnell Aud.; Rogers Arts Center; Nebraska Wesleyan Univ.
Organization Type: Resident

1395 LINCOLN FRIENDS OF CHAMBER MUSIC

5211 W Chadderton Circle
Lincoln, NE 68521
Phone: 402-472-5121
Fax: 402-472-8962
e-mail: jkraus1@unl.edu
Web Site: www.lfem.org
Officers:
President: Joe Kraus
Head Artists Subcommittee: Anne Chang-Barnea
Mission: Presenting chamber music; promoting community appreciation of chamber music; aiding talented local chamber music artists.
Founded: 1965
Specialized Field: Instrumental Music
Status: Nonprofit
Volunteer Staff: 15
Budget: $25,000
Income Sources: Ticket Sales; Donations; Grants
Performs At: Sheldon Art Gallery Auditorium
Annual Attendance: 1250
Facility Category: Art Gallery Auditorium
Stage Dimensions: 25'W x 10'D
Seating Capacity: 300
Year Built: 1963
Rental Contact: P.J. Jacobs
Organization Type: Sponsoring

1396 LINCOLN SYMPHONY ORCHESTRA

233 S 13th Street
Suite B102
Lincoln, NE 68508
Phone: 402-476-2211
Fax: 402-476-2236
e-mail: info@lincolnsymphony.com
Web Site: lincolnsymphony.com
Officers:
President: James Strasheim
Management:
Music Director: Edward Polochick
Executive Director: Edward Williams
Founded: 1925
Specialized Field: Symphony; Orchestra

Status: Professional; Nonprofit
Paid Staff: 5
Volunteer Staff: 4
Paid Artists: 78
Budget: $260,000- $ 1,050,000
Performs At: Lied Center for the Performing Arts; Kimball Recital Hall
Affiliations: American Symhpony Orchestra League
Seating Capacity: 2285/ 850
Organization Type: Performing; Sponsoring

1397 LINCOLN YOUTH SYMPHONY

7201 Woody Creek Lane
Lincoln, NE 68501
Phone: 402-423-5343
Fax: 435-797-3150
Officers:
President: Joyce Glaesemann
Secretary: Linda Maack
Treasurer: Carl Olson
Administrator: Richard Scott
Business Manager: Micheal Swartz
Management:
Music Director/Conductor: Dr Brain Moore
Mission: The Lincoln Youth Symphony Orchestra was organized to perform symphonic literature unable to be played within regular school instruction through participation in the Youth Orchestra or the Junior Youth Orchestra.
Founded: 1953
Specialized Field: Symphony; Orchestra
Status: Non-Professional; Nonprofit
Paid Staff: 76
Income Sources: American Symphony Orchestra League (Youth Orchestra Division); Lincoln Public Schools
Performs At: Kimball Recital Hall; University of Nebraska
Organization Type: Performing; Touring; Educational; Sponsoring

1398 NEBRASKA JAZZ ORCHESTRA

216 N 11 Street
Suite 202
Lincoln, NE 68508-1401
Phone: 402-477-8446
Fax: 402-477-8222
e-mail: njo@artsincorporated.org
Management:
Music Director: Ed Love
Executive Director: Dean Haist
Founded: 1975
Budget: $35,000- $100,000
Performs At: Ramada Hotel & Conference Center; Joslyn Art Museum, Omaha
Seating Capacity: 450/ 1500

1399 OMAHA AREA YOUTH ORCHESTRAS

PO Box 34518
Omaha, NE 68134-0518
Phone: 402-238-2044
Fax: 402-238-2310
e-mail: oayo@radiks.net
Web Site: www.oayo.org
Officers:

President: Kathleen Vance
Secretary: Dara Spivack
Treasurer: Craig Vance
President-Elect: Ron Mimick
Management:
   Music Director: Aviva Segall
   General Manager: Jan Braden
   Associate Conductor: Jennifer L Bloomgarden
Mission: To enhance the musical education of aspiring and talented young musicians through the medium of orchestral performance; to help them become appreciative listeners; and to build discipline, cooperation, and other skills necessary for a group accomplishment.
Founded: 1958
Specialized Field: Symphony; Orchestra; Chamber; Ensemble
Status: Non-Professional; Nonprofit
Paid Staff: 6
Volunteer Staff: 250
Budget: $200,000
Income Sources: American Symphony Orchestra League; Omaha Symphony Guild; ASTA; Music Educators National Conference; Nebraska Arts Council
Performs At: University Recital Hall
Annual Attendance: 7,000-8,000
Organization Type: Performing; Educational; Sponsoring

1400 OMAHA SYMPHONY

1605 Howard Street
Omaha, NE 68102
Phone: 402-342-3836
Fax: 402-342-3819
e-mail: bravo@omahasymphony.org
Web Site: www.omahasymphony.org
Officers:
   President/CEO: Fred Bronstein
Management:
   General Manager: Sara A Pflueger
   Operations Manager: Sherrie Goeden
   Operations Assitant: Tara M Cowherd
   Personnel Manager: Jay Wise
Founded: 1921
Specialized Field: Symphony; Orchestra; Chamber; Ensemble
Status: Professional; Nonprofit
Paid Staff: 27
Paid Artists: 70
Budget: $4,500,000
Income Sources: American Symphony Orchestra League; National Endowment for the Arts; Nebraska Arts Council
Organization Type: Performing; Touring; Resident; Educational; Sponsoring

1401 OMAHA SYMPHONY CHAMBER ORCHESTRA

1605 Howard Street
Omaha, NE 68102
Phone: 402-342-3836
Fax: 402-342-3819
e-mail: bravo@omahasymphony.org
Web Site: www.omahasymphony.org
Management:

CEO: Fred Bronstein
   General Manager: Sara Pflueger
Budget: $1,050,000- $3,600,000
Performs At: Orpheum Theatre; Joslyn Art Museum; Witherspoon Concert Hall
Seating Capacity: 2750/ 1174

Nevada

1402 CARSON CITY SYMPHONY

PO Box 2001
Carson City, NV 89702-2001
Phone: 775-883-4154
Fax: 775-883-4371
e-mail: ehbugli@aol.com
Web Site: www.members.aol.com/CCSymphony
Officers:
   President: Elinor Bugli
   VP: Grant Mills
   Treasurer: Charlotte Tucker
   Secretary: Edith Isidoro-Mills
Management:
   Music Director/Conductor: David Bugli
   Director Chamber Singers: Judy Monson
Mission: To provide amateur and volunteer professional musicians with opportunity to learn and perform various musical styles to entertain and educate the community.
Founded: 1984
Specialized Field: Educational performances
Status: Nonprofit
Paid Artists: 3
Non-paid Artists: 55
Budget: $25,000
Income Sources: Memberships; Ticket sales; Grants; Donations
Performs At: Concert Hall at Carson City Community Center
Affiliations: Carson Chamber Singers, Brewery Arts Center
Annual Attendance: 2,000
Facility Category: Concert hall in community center
Type of Stage: Proscenium
Seating Capacity: 800

1403 CHAMBER MUSIC SOUTHWEST

UNLV Department of Music
4505 Maryland Parkway
Las Vegas, NV 89154-5025
Phone: 702-895-3332
Fax: 702-895-4239
e-mail: pkreider@ccmail.nevada.edu
Management:
   Chair: Dr. Paul Kreider
Mission: Promoting the cause of high quality chamber music in Southern Nevada; nurturing appreciation of great music in Las Vegas.
Founded: 1987
Specialized Field: Chamber; Ensemble; Instrumental Group
Status: Professional; Nonprofit
Paid Staff: 8
Income Sources: University of Nevada-Las Vegas; KNPR-FM

Performs At: Artemus W. Ham Hall; Judy Bayley Theatre
Organization Type: Performing; Touring; Educational

1404 LAS VEGAS CIVIC SYMPHONY

821 Las Vegas Boulevard N
Las Vegas, NV 89101
Phone: 702-229-6211
Fax: 702-382-5199
Web Site: www.ci.las-vegas.nv.us
Management:
   Cultural Supervisor: Patricia L Harris
   Cultural Center Coordinator: Ellis Rice
   Cultural Publicist: Stephanie Fosse
Mission: Provide culturally enriched performances and classes to the Greater Las Vegas area.
Specialized Field: Music, Theatre, Dance and Visual arts.
Paid Staff: 20
Paid Artists: 50
Non-paid Artists: 200
Budget: $260,000- $1,050,000
Performs At: Reed Whipple Cultural Arts Center
Seating Capacity: 300

1405 LAS VEGAS PHILHARMONIC

1289 S Torrey Pines Drive
Las Vegas, NV 89146
Phone: 702-258-5438
e-mail: lvphil@anv.net
Web Site: www.lasvegasphilharmonic.com
Officers:
   Chairman: Richard Plaster
   President: Susan Tompkins
   Treasurer/Secretary: Carolyn Kenton
   Administrative Manager: Anita Meyer
   Executive Director: William Marion
   First VP: Lou Emmert
   Second VP: Lynn Wiender
Management:
   Music Director/Conductor: Harold L Weller
   Associate Conductor: Richard McGee
Founded: 1998

1406 NEVADA SYMPHONY ORCHESTRA

4505 Maryland Parkway
VNLV Department of Music
Las Vegas, NV 89154
Phone: 702-895-3332
Fax: 702-895-4239
Web Site: www.nevadasymphony.org
Officers:
   President: M Rex Baird
   VP: Bruce B Borgelt
   Secretary: Collen Schoeder
   Treasurer/ President Elect: B. Michl Lloyd
Management:
   Artistic Director: Virko Baley
   Executive Dorector: Judith Markham
   Director Operations: Timothy Bonenfant
   Chairman: Paul Kreider
Mission: To offer symphonic performances, services and educational opportunities to the Las Vegas community.
Founded: 1980
Specialized Field: Vocal Music; Instrumental Music

Status: Professional; Nonprofit
Organization Type: Performing; Educational; Sponsoring

1407 RENO CHAMBER ORCHESTRA

PO Box 547
Reno, NV 89504
Phone: 775-323-6393
Fax: 775-323-6711
e-mail: info@renochamberorchestra.org
Web Site: www.renochamberorchestra.org
Officers:
   President: V Robert Payant
Management:
   Music Director: Vahe Khochayan
   Executive Director: Scott Faulkner
   Operations Manager: Chris Morrison
Mission: To provide the highest quality performance of repertoire written for the smaller orchestra and educate and promote the appreciation of the music among diverse audiences.
Paid Staff: 4
Volunteer Staff: 45
Paid Artists: 40 +
Budget: $300,000- $350,000
Income Sources: Individual contributions; Tickets sales; Foundations; Grants; Corparate solicitions
Performs At: Nightingale Concert Hall
Facility Category: Concert Hall
Seating Capacity: 615

1408 RENO PHILHARMONIC

925 Riverside Drive
Suite 3
Reno, NV 89503
Phone: 775-348-9413
Fax: 775-348-0643
e-mail: rponv@aol.com
Web Site: www.renophilharmonic.com
Management:
   Music Director: Barry Jekowsky
Mission: To bring the best of symphonic music to the Truckee Meadows and surrounding communities; to ensure a high quality musical experience; to bring that musical experience to the youth of our community; to foster strong individual and corporate support for the Reno Philharmonic; to engage in sound business and fiscal planning and execution; to work in cooperation with the other local arts groups.

New Hampshire

1409 NEVERS' 2ND REGIMENT BAND

PO Box 2352
Concord, NH 03819
Phone: 603-642-6623
e-mail: info@neversband.org
Web Site: www.neversband.org
Officers:
   Treasurer: Doug Osborne
   Secretary: Deborah Lincoln
   Member-at-Large: Peter Clark
   Business Manager: George West

Management:
Conductor: Jiffi Rainie
Interim Conductor: Douglas Osborne
Mission: To perpetuate its tradition of live, high quality performances of music for the benefit and enjoyment of all people; to promote and demonstrate the continuing relevance of modern and traditional concert band music and to preserve the history of the Band's regimental origins.
Founded: 1861
Specialized Field: Band
Status: Semi-Professional; Nonprofit
Paid Staff: 6
Paid Artists: 30
Income Sources: City of Concord
Affiliations: American Federation of Musicians
Facility Category: Outdoors; Wagner Bandwagon
Seating Capacity: unlimited
Year Built: 1968
Organization Type: Performing

1410 APPLE HILL CENTER FOR CHAMBER MUSIC

Apple Hill Road
PO Box 217
East Sullivan, NH 03445
Phone: 603-847-3371
Fax: 603-847-9734
e-mail: info@applehill.org
Web Site: www.applehill.org
Officers:
President: John Hoffman
VP: Julian Bergeron
Secretary: Carl Helmers
Board Treasurer: Drew Landry
Management:
Executive Director/Pianist: Eric Stumacher
Administrative Associate: April Weed
Fiscal Manager: Claudia Jacobs
Summer School Administrator: Lisa Tatesian
Mission: To further the performing and teaching of chamber music at the highest standard and in so doing to play for peace. It pursues these goals through the internationally celebrated performance and coaching of its Artists-in-Residence, the Apple Hill Chamber Players.
Founded: 1971
Specialized Field: Chamber; Ensemble Music
Status: Professional; Semi-Professional; Non-Professional; Nonprofit
Paid Staff: 6
Paid Artists: 5
Performs At: Louise Shonk Kelly Concert Barn
Organization Type: Performing; Resident; Educational; Sponsoring

1411 NEW HAMPSHIRE PHILHARMONIC ORCHESTRA

83 Hanover Street
4th Floor
Manchester, NH 03101
Phone: 603-647-6476
Fax: 603-647-4130
e-mail: info@nhpo.com
Officers:

President: Walter Zanchuk
VP: Adele Baker
Secretary: George Jobel
Treasurer: John Gunther
Management:
Executive Director: Steven A Olans
Mission: To offer classical concerts; to enhance music education; to provide opportunities for nonprofessionals to work with music professionals.
Founded: 1905
Specialized Field: Symphony; Orchestra
Status: Professional; Non-Professional; Nonprofit
Paid Staff: 2
Volunteer Staff: 2
Paid Artists: 2
Non-paid Artists: 65
Budget: $100,000
Income Sources: Box office; donations; foundations
Performs At: Palace Theatre
Annual Attendance: 10,000
Facility Category: Concert Hall
Type of Stage: Proscenium
Seating Capacity: 850
Year Built: 1920
Year Remodeled: 1975
Organization Type: Performing; Resident; Educational

1412 NEW HAMPSHIRE SYMPHONY ORCHESTRA

1087 Elm Street #306
Manchester, NH 03105-1298
Phone: 603-669-3559
Fax: 603-623-1195
Toll-free: 800-639-9320
e-mail: info@nhso.org
Web Site: www.nhso.org
Management:
Music Director: Kenneth Kiester
Director Marketing: Jennifer Marble
Office Manager: Holly Foster
Founded: 1974
Specialized Field: Symphony; Orchestra
Status: Professional; Nonprofit
Season: July - August
Performs At: Palace Theatre and Music Hall in Portsmouth, NH
Affiliations: American Symphony Orchestra League
Organization Type: Performing; Touring; Educational

New Jersey

1413 MONMOUTH SYMPHONY ORCHESTRA

Seaview Square Mall
Suite 263
Asberry Park, NJ 07712
Phone: 732-775-7008
Fax: 732-758-6420
e-mail: maestro@monmouthsymphony.com
Web Site: www.monmouthsymphony.com
Management:
Conductor: Roy D Gussman
Manager: ET Hunter
Budget: $35,000- $100,000

Performs At: Paramount Theatre, Asbuty Park
Seating Capacity: 1,700

1414 COLONIAL SYMPHONY
246 B Madisonville Road
Basking Ridge, NJ 07920
Phone: 908-766-7555
Fax: 908-953-9799
e-mail: CCSeries@aol.com
Web Site: www.colonialsymphony.org
Officers:
  President: Mark C Rosenblum
  VP: Carol Wead
  VP: Daniel H Olmsted
  Vice-President: Ross Longfield
  Treasurer: Thomas P. Bintinger
  Secretary: Lawrence J. Hunt
Management:
  Music Director/Conductor: Yehuda Gilad
  Executive Director: Suzanne Samson
Mission: Dedicated to nurturing and sustaining a superior orchestra performing a balance of classical and contemporary music and enhancing the understanding of music through education.
Founded: 1950
Specialized Field: Symphony
Status: Professional; Nonprofit
Paid Staff: 2.5
Volunteer Staff: 12
Paid Artists: 50
Budget: $500,000
Income Sources: Corporate donations; Individual donations; Government endowments; Foundations
Performs At: Community Theatre in Morristown, N.J.
Affiliations: American Symphony Orchestra League
Annual Attendance: 5,000
Facility Category: Community Theatre of Morristown
Organization Type: Performing; Educational

1415 ORCHESTRA OF ST. PETER BY THE SEA
PO Box 215
Bay Head, NJ 08742
Phone: 732-920-4444
Fax: 732-477-6277
Web Site: www.franj.org
Management:
  Music Director/Manager: Alphonse Stephenson
  Music Director/Conductor: Maestro Alphonsestephenson
Performs At: Touring orchestra

1416 BLOOMFIELD MANDOLIN ORCHESTRA
PO Box 1776
Bloomfield, NJ 07003
Phone: 973-748-0081
e-mail: nj.mandolins@worldnet.att.net
Web Site: www.geocites.com/nashville/7090/
Officers:
  President: Arthur Coppola
  VP/Manager: Peter Longo
  Secretary: Ella Theting
  Treasurer: Robert Elsinger

Management:
  Conductor: Gabriel Nevola
Mission: The Bloomfield Federation of Music sponsors our non-profit community orchestra.
Founded: 1932
Specialized Field: Symphony
Status: Nonprofit
Paid Staff: 2
Volunteer Staff: 44
Income Sources: New Jersey Orchestra Association
Performs At: North Junior High School
Organization Type: Performing

1417 BAY ATLANTIC SYMPHONY
PO Box 872
Bridgeton, NJ 08302
Phone: 856-451-1169
Fax: 856-451-4380
Web Site: www.bayatlanticsymphony.org
Management:
  Music Director: Jed Gaylin
Founded: 1983
Budget: $260,000-1,050,000
Income Sources: Bell Atlantic Foundation; Woodruff Energy; Pine Street Web Works

1418 SOLID BRASS
5 Sunset Drive
Chatham, NJ 07928-1141
Phone: 201-701-0674
Fax: 201-701-0674
e-mail: haislip@solidbrass.com
Web Site: www.solidbrass.com/menu.html
Management:
  Co-Management: Paul Goldberg
Mission: Preserving and perpetuating brass chamber music through performance, recording, composing and related activities.
Founded: 1982
Specialized Field: Chamber; Ensemble
Status: Professional
Non-paid Artists: Yes
Organization Type: Performing; Touring; Educational

1419 PHILHARMONIC OF SOUTHERN NEW JERSEY
PO Box 1750
Cherry Hill, NJ 08034
Phone: 856-779-2600
Fax: 609-654-8792
e-mail: raineyo@geocities.com
Web Site: www.psnj.org
Officers:
  President: Yole Patterson
  VP: Jack Paolin
  Secretary: Barbara Travaline
  Treasurer: Madelyn Niessner
Management:
  Music Director: Philip Travaline
Mission: To provide quality classical music for the community and to offer rehearsal/performance opportunities for the talented musician.
Budget: $35,000- $100,000
Performs At: Forrest Rowland Auditorium

Seating Capacity: 1,300

1420 NEW JERSEY INTERGENERATIONAL ORCHESTRA

PO Box 432
Cranford, NJ 07016
Phone: 908-709-0084
Fax: 908-709-6724
e-mail: njiorch@aol.com
Web Site: www.bobdevlin.com/njio.html
Management:
    Conductor/Executive: Lorraine Marks
Mission: To nurture the belief that senior citizens can share their wisdom and become vital resources for children by bringing youth and the elderly together to share experiences that promote mutual growth and understanding between generations.
Founded: 1994
Status: Non-Professional
Paid Staff: 3
Volunteer Staff: 10
Paid Artists: 30
Non-paid Artists: 100

1421 HADDONFIELD SYMPHONY

41 S Haddon Avenue
Suite 7
Haddonfield, NJ 08033
Phone: 856-429-1880
Fax: 856-428-5634
e-mail: symphony@haddonfield-symphony.org
Web Site: www.haddonfield-symphony.org
Officers:
    President: Trevor Orthmann
Management:
    Music Director: Rossen Milanov
Mission: Dedicated to enriching the musical lives of the residents of the state of New Jersey.
Founded: 1952
Specialized Field: Symphony; Orchestra
Status: Professional; Nonprofit
Paid Staff: 6
Organization Type: Performing; Educational

1422 LYRIC THEATRE

PO Box 3128
Hoboken, NJ 07030
Phone: 201-217-2628
Fax: 201-795-4757
Web Site: www.thelyrictheatre.org
Management:
    Artistic Director/Conductor: Franco Bertacci
    Manager Director: Ronald J Asher
Mission: To present a broad range of music from classical to contemporary, true to the vision of the composer; to provide performing venues for the professionals of tomorrow; to develop synergism between seasoned performers and young artists.
Paid Staff: 4
Paid Artists: 45
Performs At: Hoboken H.S. Auditorium/ other venues
Seating Capacity: 850

1423 NEW JERSEY CITY UNIVERSITY ORCHESTRA

2039 Kennedy Boulevard
New Jersey University/Music Department
Jersey City, NJ 07305
Phone: 201-200-2017
Fax: 201-200-3130
e-mail: eraditz@njcu.edu
Management:
    Music Director: Edward Raditz
Paid Staff: 2
Volunteer Staff: 10
Paid Artists: 3
Budget: $35,000
Performs At: Margaret William Auditorium, New Jersey City University
Annual Attendance: 3000
Facility Category: Theatre\Auditorium
Seating Capacity: 1,000
Year Built: 1960
Year Remodeled: 1975

1424 NEW JERSEY MUSIC SOCIETY

311 Claremont Avenue
Montclair, NJ 07042
Phone: 973-746-6068
Fax: 973-746-0685
e-mail: njchambermusicsociety@att.net
Web Site: njcms.org
Management:
    Executive Director: Michael Lawson
    Assistant Executive Director: Marie Figueredo
    Artist in Residence: Paquito D'Rivera
Mission: To create, produce and maintain a repertoire of outstanding musical performances in classical, jazz and world music with core artists-in-residence and frequent nationally prominent guest artists. To provide new opportunities to a wider audience through innovative and stimulating children's programs, family concerts and workshops in area school system.
Founded: 1974
Specialized Field: Chamber
Status: Professional; Nonprofit
Performs At: Montclair Art Museum; Union Congregatinal Church
Organization Type: Performing; Touring; Resident; Educational

1425 WEST JERSEY CHAMBER MUSIC SYMPHONY & SOCIETY

101 Bridgeboro Road
Moorestown, NJ 08057
Phone: 856-778-1899
Fax: 856-234-3666
Management:
    Music Director: Joel Krott
    Executive Assistant: Cindi Schneider
Founded: 1980
Specialized Field: Orchestra; Chamber; Choral
Status: Professional; Nonprofit
Paid Staff: 2
Volunteer Staff: 15
Paid Artists: 40
Budget: $35,000 - $100,000

Performs At: Various churches and schools
Organization Type: Performing; Touring

1426 NEW JERSEY YOUTH SYMPHONY

570 Central Avenue
Murray Hill, NJ 07974
Phone: 908-771-5544
Fax: 908-771-9839
e-mail: office@njys.org
Web Site: www.njys.org
Management:
 Executive Director: Linda Abrams
 Artistic Director: Barbara Barstow
Mission: To provide talented young musicians with orchestral and related music education experiences that will enable them to reach their highest potential as performers and listeners.
Founded: 1979
Specialized Field: Instrumental Music
Status: Non-Professional; Nonprofit
Non-paid Artists: 95
Budget: $500,000
Organization Type: Performing; Touring; Educational

1427 PARADISE CHAMBER ORCHESTRA

PO Box 427
Neptum, NJ 07753
Phone: 732-774-0028
Fax: 732-988-9635
e-mail: P.L.Paradise@aol.com
Management:
 Manager/Musical Director: Paul Paradise
Budget: $35,000- $100.000
Performs At: Sanders Theater
Seating Capacity: 1,000

1428 CATHEDRAL BASILICA OF THE SACRED HEART CONCERT SERIES

89 Ridge Street
Newark, NJ 07104
Phone: 973-484-2400
Fax: 973-497-9336
e-mail: jmiller@cathedralbasilica.org
Web Site: www.cathedralbasilica.org/concert/
Management:
 Director Music Ministry: John J Miller
Mission: Offering quality musical programs to Newark area residents.
Founded: 1983
Specialized Field: Symphony; Orchestra; Chamber; Ensemble

1429 GREATER NEWARK ORCHESTRA

2 Central Avenue
Newark, NJ 07102
Phone: 973-624-3713
Fax: 973-624-2115
e-mail: info@njsymphony.org
Web Site: www.njusymphony.org
Management:
 Music Director: Gabriel Gordon
 Education Director: Maria Araujo
 Chamber Orchestra Director: Henry Kao

Specialized Field: Music Performance
Budget: $35,000- $100,000
Performs At: New Jersey Performing Arts Center
Seating Capacity: 2,700

1430 NEW JERSEY SYMPHONY ORCHESTRA

2 Central Avenue
Newark, NJ 07102
Phone: 973-624-3713
Fax: 973-624-2115
e-mail: information@njsymphony.org
Web Site: www.njsymphony.org
Officers:
 President: Lawrence J Tamburrit
 General Operation: Susan Stucker
 Chairman: Victor Parsonnet
 Executive Vice Chairman/Treasurer: Victor Bauer
Management:
 Music Director: Zdenek Macal
Mission: To engage the people of New Jersey by performing the full syphonic repertoire at the highest caliber in a variety of settings for diverse audiences.
Founded: 1922
Specialized Field: Symphony; Orchestra; Chamber; Ensemble
Status: Professional; Nonprofit
Paid Staff: 43
Volunteer Staff: 76
Budget: $14.5 Million
Performs At: New Jersry Performing Arts Center; John Harms Center for the Arts/Englewood; Community Theatre/Morristown; State Theatre
Affiliations: War Memorail Trenton
Seating Capacity: 2,600/1,900
Organization Type: Performing

1431 OCEAN CITY POPS

901 Asbury Avenue
Ocean City, NJ 08226
Phone: 609-398-9585
Fax: 609-339-0374
Web Site: www.oceancitypops.org
Management:
 Music Director: William Scheible
 Executive Director: Michael Dattilo
Budget: $250,000- $1,050,000
Performs At: auditorium
Seating Capacity: 930

1432 PLAINFIELD SYMPHONY ORCHESTRA

PO Box 5093
Plainfield, NJ 07061
Phone: 908-561-5140
Fax: 732-932-1768
e-mail: psonj@aol.com
Web Site:
www.members.tripod.com/Plainfield_Symphony/
Officers:
 President: Keith McCoy
Management:
 Music Director/Conductor: Sabin Pautza
 Executive Director: Tim Espar

All listings are in alphabetical order by state, then city, then organization within the city.

Mission: To prepare and present musical programs of a symphonic type; to stimulate interest in symphonic music in the Central New Jersey area; to provide educational opportunities through youth and family concerts; and to provide a medium of performance for talented nonprofessional musicians.
Founded: 1919
Specialized Field: Instrumental Music
Paid Staff: 2
Paid Artists: 30
Non-paid Artists: 20
Budget: $35,000- $100,000
Performs At: Crescent Avenue Presbyterian Church
Seating Capacity: 750

1433 GREATER PRINCETON YOUTH ORCHESTRA

PO Box 3037
Princeton, NJ 08540
Phone: 609-936-8700
Fax: 609-936-8771
e-mail: mws8487@aol.com
Web Site: www.gpyo.org
Officers:
  President: Richard Bilotti
  VP: Stuart Barudin
  Treasurer: Peter Cahill
  Secretary: Noreen Coutin
Management:
  Music Director: Fernando Rucciay
  Manager Co-ord: Evelyn Krosnck
  Operations Manager: Melinda Strauss
Mission: To provide exciting and unique educational opportunites for many of our community's young people. Through their involvement in the Orchestra, gifted young musicians from across Central New Jersey and Pennsylvania hone their skills as performers in a large orchestra and in chamber music groups, and learn to work with others in pursuing common goals.
Founded: 1961
Budget: $35,000- $100,000
Performs At: Richard Auditorium, Princeton University
Seating Capacity: 868

1434 PRINCETON SYMPHONY ORCHESTRA

PO Box 250
Princeton, NJ 08542
Phone: 609-497-0020
Fax: 609-497-0904
e-mail: pcs7@ix.netcom.com
Web Site: princetonsymphony.org
Officers:
  President: John J Hamel III
Management:
  Music Director/Conductor: Mark Laycock
  Executive Director: Joshua Worby
Mission: To present the finest classical compositions from the widest range, including unusual and seldom heard works; to enhance audience appreciation of the often unfamiliar works through lectures and presentations; to create an outstanding performance opportunity for the many excellent musicians in the Central New Jersey region; and to reach out to new audiences both geographically and demographically.

Founded: 1986
Paid Artists: 55
Budget: $250,000- $1,050,000
Performs At: Richardson Auditorium
Seating Capacity: 870

1435 RIDGEWOOD SYMPHONY ORCHESTRA

PO Box 176
Ridgewood, NJ 07451-0176
Phone: 201-612-0118
Fax: 201-445-2762
Web Site: www.ridgewoodsymphony.org
Officers:
  President: E Sosinsky
  Secretaryident: Ellen Hill
  Treasurer: Richard A Marri
Management:
  General Manager: Karin A Todd
  House Manager: John Pinsl
  Personnel Manager: Sylvia Rubin
  Personnel Manager: Louise Butler
Founded: 1940
Specialized Field: Symphony Orchestra
Paid Staff: 4
Volunteer Staff: 10
Non-paid Artists: 90
Budget: $90,000
Income Sources: Box Office; Grants; Private Donations; Fundraising
Performs At: Benjamin Franklin Middle School Auditorium
Annual Attendance: 3,700
Seating Capacity: 775

1436 SUMMIT SYMPHONY

100 Morris Avenue
Summit, NJ 07901
Phone: 908-277-2932
Fax: 908-277-2978
Management:
  Music Director: James Sadewhite
  Manager Orchestra Personnel: Barry Davidson
Mission: To offer orchestra music to Summit and surrounding communities and provide an opportunity for nonprofessionals to perform major works.
Founded: 1937
Specialized Field: Symphony
Status: Non-Professional; Nonprofit
Income Sources: Summit Board of Recreation; New Jersey Council on the Arts
Performs At: Summit Senior High School; Summit Middle School
Organization Type: Performing

1437 BERGEN PHILHARMONIC ORCHESTRA

PO Box 174
Teaneck, NJ 07666
Phone: 201-837-1980
Management:
  Music Director: David Gilbert
  Chairman: Lois Marshall

1438 GARDEN STATE PHILHARMONIC SYMPHONY ORCHESTRA
7 Hadley Avenue
Toms River, NJ 08753
Phone: 732-349-6277
Fax: 732-349-2401
e-mail: garden1idt.net
Web Site: www.islandhts.com/garden.htm
Management:
Music Director/Conductor: Anthony LaGruth
Mission: Dedicated to maintaining a professional orchestra in Ocean County and surrounding NJ counties, that will give concerts of the highest cultural and educational value for the community and to providing both educational and training programs as well as fostering activities to encourage appreciation of music.
Founded: 1956
Specialized Field: Symphony; Orchestra
Status: Professional; Nonprofit
Paid Staff: 30
Volunteer Staff: 2
Paid Artists: 70
Income Sources: Grants
Performs At: Toms River High School North; The Strand Theatre
Seating Capacity: 1200
Organization Type: Performing

1439 GARDEN STATE PHILHARMONIC SYMPHONY YOUTH ORCHESTRA
7 Hadley Avenue
Toms River, NJ 08753
Phone: 732-349-6277
Fax: 732-349-2401
e-mail: garden@idt.net
Web Site: www.islandhts.com/garden.htm
Management:
Conductor: Les Hollander
Executive Director: Alan G Moore
Budget: $250,000- $1,050,000
Performs At: Toms River H.S. Auditorium/ Ocean County College Arts Center
Seating Capacity: 1,266/ 604

1440 GREATER TRENTON SYMPHONY ORCHESTRA
28 W State Street
Suite 202
Trenton, NJ 08608
Phone: 609-394-1338
Fax: 609-394-1394
e-mail: info@trentonsymphony.org
Web Site: www.trentonsymphony.org
Management:
Executive Director/Conductor: John Peter Holly
Mission: To offer residents of the greater Trenton area high-quality performances of classical music for orchestra.
Founded: 1921
Specialized Field: Symphony; Orchestra
Status: Professional; Nonprofit
Performs At: War Memorial Theater
Organization Type: Performing; Educational

1441 UNITY CONCERTS OF NEW JERSEY
Montclair State University
Life Hall 134
Upper Montclair, NJ 07043
Phone: 973-655-4086
Fax: 973-655-5366
e-mail: unitycon@aol.com
Web Site: www.unityconcerts.org
Management:
Administrator: Lindsay Gambini
Mission: To provide the finest classical music concerts to Northern New Jersey.
Founded: 1920
Specialized Field: Instrumental Music; Classical
Status: Nonprofit
Budget: $150,000-400,000
Income Sources: Private Foundations/Grants; Business/Corporate Donations; Box Office; Government Grants; Individual Donations
Performs At: Montclair Community Auditorium; Mt. Hebron School Auditorium
Organization Type: Sponsoring

1442 PHILHARMONIC ORCHESTRA OF NEW JERSEY
PO Box 4064
Warren, NJ 07059
Phone: 908-226-7300
Fax: 908-226-7337
e-mail: info@ponj.org
Web Site: www.ponj.org
Management:
Music Director/Conductor: George Marriner Maull
Manager Director: Virgina Johnson
Executive Director: Hewitt V Johnson
Mission: To perform concerts and to increase the apperciation of classical music through educational offerings.
Founded: 1987
Specialized Field: Central & Northern New Jersey & New York City
Paid Staff: 95
Budget: $250,000- $1,050,000
Performs At: New Jersey Performing Arts Center
Seating Capacity: 2,800/785

1443 ORCHESTRA AT WILLIAM PATERSON COLLEGE
William Paterson College
300 Pompton Road
Wayne, NJ 07470
Phone: 973-720-2694
Fax: 973-720-2408
e-mail: orchestra@wpunj.edu
Web Site: www.wpunj.edu/arts_culture/orchestra/
Management:
Music Director/Conductor: Murry Colosimo
Executive Director: William Huston
Orchestra Manager: Nancy Clancy
Business Manager: Sheri Newberger
Mission: To increase arts offerings and education within New Jersey's tri-county area; to present dynamic performances of great orchestral music played by outstanding musicians.

Founded: 1986
Specialized Field: Orchestra
Status: Professional
Paid Staff: 8
Performs At: Shea Center for the Performing Arts
Seating Capacity: 960
Organization Type: Performing

1444 ARBOR CHAMBER MUSIC SOCIETY

PO Box 2901
Westfield, NJ 07090
Phone: 908-232-1116
Fax: 908-232-2423
e-mail: arbormusic@comcast.net
Web Site: www.westfieldnj.com/arbormusic
Management:
   Director: Lenore Fishman Davis
Mission: To bring the highest artistic standards of chamber music performance to New Jersey's audiences, to educate audiences and to develop the next generation of listeners and musicians.
Founded: 1991
Status: Professional
Income Sources: Private Foundations; Business/Corporate Donations; Box Office; Individual Donations
Performs At: Union City Arts Center; St. Paul's Episcopal Church-Westfield
Organization Type: Performing; Touring; Educational

1445 WESTFIELD SYMPHONY ORCHESTRA

224 E Broad Street
Suite 5
Westfield, NJ 07090
Phone: 908-232-9400
Fax: 908-232-2446
e-mail: wso@westfieldnj.com
Web Site: www.westfieldsymphony.com
Officers:
   President: Louis Franez
   Treasurer: Alan Smith
   First VP: Norman Luka, MD
   Second VP: Mark Fleder
Management:
   Executive Director: Nicole E DeNigro
   Music Director: David Wroe
Mission: To bring the highest quality professional music to the central New Jersey area; to provide education programs for grades 1-12 in the area.
Founded: 1983
Specialized Field: Symphony
Status: Professional; Nonprofit
Paid Staff: 5
Volunteer Staff: 5
Paid Artists: 106
Budget: $500,000
Income Sources: Government Grants; Box Office; Corporate Donations; Foundation Contributions; Individual Donations
Performs At: Union County Arts Center; The Presbyterian Church, Westfield
Affiliations: American Symphony Orchestra League; Westfield Area Chamber of Commerce; Center for Nonprofits

Organization Type: Performing; Resident; Touring; Educational
Comments: For information concerning accessibility for special needs, call (908) 232-9400

New Mexico

1446 CHAMBER ORCHESTRA OF ALBUQUERQUE

PO Box 35081
Albuquerque, NM 87176-5081
Phone: 505-881-2078
Fax: 505-881-2634
e-mail: coaoch@aol.com
Web Site: coa.aosys.com
Management:
   Music Director/Conductor: David Oberg
   Operations Manager: Diane Bonnell
Mission: To provide a broad range of listening and participatory musical opportunities to the State of New Mexico; to maintain a professional orchestra whose work enriches the quality of community life.
Founded: 1976
Specialized Field: Orchestra
Status: Professional; Nonprofit
Paid Staff: 3
Paid Artists: 1
Performs At: St. John's United Methodist Church
Organization Type: Performing

1447 NEW MEXICO SYMPHONY ORCHESTRA

3301 Menaul Boulevard NE
Suite 4
Albuquerque, NM 87107
Mailing Address: PO Box 30208, Albuquerque, NM. 87190-0208
Phone: 505-881-9590
Fax: 505-881-9456
e-mail: postmaster@nmso.org
Web Site: www.nmso.org/
Officers:
   Marketing/Public Relations: Mark Amo
   Development Director: Joan Allen
   Ticket Office Manager: Betsy Ball
   Administration Assistant: Laura Merritt
   Orchestra Personnel Manager: Kurt Civilette
   Librarian: Lisa DiCarlo
   Box Office Assistant: Irene Garcia
   Executive Director: Kevin Hagen
   Production Manager: Robin Rupe
Management:
   Principal Pops Conductor: Michael Krajewski
   Resident Conductor/Choral Director: Roger Melone
   Music Director: Guillermo Figueroa
Mission: To present live concerts of music for small ensembles through full orchestra in both educational and concert settings.
Founded: 1932
Specialized Field: Symphony; Orchestra
Status: Professional; Nonprofit
Paid Staff: 22
Paid Artists: 80

Income Sources: American Symphony Orchestra
League; American Arts Alliance
Performs At: Popejoy Hall
Organization Type: Performing; Educational

1448 SOUTHWEST SYMPHONY

PO Box 101
Hobbs, NM 88240
Phone: 505-738-1041
Fax: 505-392-5980
e-mail: swshobbs@hotmail.com
Officers:
   President: Mark T Sanchez
Management:
   Music Director: Dr. Mark Jelinek
   Executive Director: Bill Razo
Founded: 1983
Paid Staff: 2
Volunteer Staff: 120
Budget: $100,000- $150,000
Income Sources: Fund Drives: Season Tickets, Grants,
Donations
Performs At: Auditorium
Seating Capacity: 2,000

1449 LAS CRUCES SYMPHONY ORCHESTRA

PO Box 1622
Las Cruces, NM 88004
Phone: 505-646-3709
Fax: 505-646-1086
e-mail: lcsymphony@mailcity.com
Web Site: www.lascrucessymophony.com
Officers:
   President: Marianna Burden
   VP: Herb Adams
   Treasurer: Tom Tate
   Secretary: Nancy Carlson
   VP: Nita Swartz
Management:
   Music Director/Conductor: Dr. Lonnie D Klein
   Manager: Erica Zenzer
Paid Staff: 1
Volunteer Staff: 70
Paid Artists: 8
Non-paid Artists: 1
Budget: $100,000- $150,000
Income Sources: Box Office; Grants; Private Donations
Performs At: NMSU Performance Center
Affiliations: American Symphony Orchestra League
Annual Attendance: 8,000
Facility Category: Music Hall
Type of Stage: Thrust
Seating Capacity: 540
Year Built: 1985

1450 ROSWELL SYMPHONY ORCHESTRA

W Office Plaza
1717 W Second, Suite 112
Roswell, NM 88201
Phone: 505-623-5882
Fax: 505-623-5882
Toll-free: 800-300-9822
e-mail: rso@dfn.com
Web Site: www.harrosdev.com/rso

Officers:
   President: James Monteith
Management:
   Music Director: John Farrer
   Manager: Shirley Ann Munroe
   Director/Financial & Office: Melynda Roberson
Founded: 1960
Specialized Field: Symphony Orchestra
Paid Staff: 3
Paid Artists: 84
Budget: $150,000- $260,000
Income Sources: Tickets; Grants; Gifts; Fund Raising
Performs At: Pearson Auditorium
Affiliations: American Symphony Orchestra League
Annual Attendance: 11,000
Facility Category: Auditoriums
Seating Capacity: 930

1451 MUSIC FROM ANGEL FIRE

130 Grant Avenue
#201
Santa Fe, NM 87501
Mailing Address: PO Box 502, Angel Fire, NM. 87710
Phone: 505-377-3233
Fax: 505-989-4773
Toll-free: 888-377-3300
e-mail: info@musicfromangelfire.org
Web Site: www.musicfromangelfire.org
Management:
   General Director: John W Giovando
   Artistic Director: Ida Kavafian
   Executive Administrator: Nancy Ondov
   Associate Director: Lynne S Mazza
Mission: To bring world-class chamber music performed
by international artists to the Northern New Mexico
communities of Angel Fire and Taos, and to Las Vegas.
Founded: 1984
Specialized Field: Chamber Music
Status: Professional; Nonprofit
Paid Staff: 2
Volunteer Staff: 30
Paid Artists: 38
Budget: $600,000
Affiliations: Chamber Music America; America
Symphony Orchestra League
Annual Attendance: 15,000
Facility Category: Concert Hall; Venues in Taos, Angel
Fire and Las Vegas
Organization Type: Performing

1452 SANTA FE PRO MUSICA

1405 Luisa Street
PO Box 2091
Santa Fe, NM 87504
Phone: 505-988-4640
Fax: 505-984-2501
Toll-free: 800-960-6680
e-mail: info@santafepromusica.com
Web Site: www.santafepromusica.com
Officers:
   President: Poykon Kohr
Management:
   Executive Director: David Provost
   Artistic Director: Tom O'Connor
   Operations Manager: Tallie Tolen

All listings are in alphabetical order by state, then city, then organization within the city.

Mission: To provide the highest quality chamber music possible and make youth programs available to the public.
Founded: 1980
Specialized Field: Symphony; Orchestra; Chamber
Status: Professional; Nonprofit
Paid Staff: 7
Budget: $900,000
Performs At: Lensic Theatre
Annual Attendance: 14,000
Organization Type: Performing; Touring; Educational

1453 SANTA FE SYMPHONY

551 W Cordova Road, Suite D
PO Box 9692
Santa Fe, NM 87504
Phone: 505-983-3530
Fax: 505-982-3888
e-mail: symphony@rt66.com
Web Site: www.sf-symphony.org
Management:
  Founder/General Director: Gregory Heltman
  Operations Manager: Diane Stengle
  Music Director: Steven Smith
  Chorus Director: Linda Raney
Founded: 1984
Specialized Field: Symphony; Orchestra; Chamber; Chorus
Status: Professional; Nonprofit
Paid Staff: 5
Volunteer Staff: 40
Paid Artists: 100
Non-paid Artists: 80
Budget: $650,000
Income Sources: Ticket Sales; Grants; Contributions
Performs At: Lensic Performing Arts Center
Affiliations: Santa Fe Performing Arts Association
Annual Attendance: 11,000
Facility Category: Theatre
Type of Stage: Proscenium
Stage Dimensions: 40' x 50'
Seating Capacity: 791
Year Built: 1977
Organization Type: Performing; Resident; Educational; Sponsoring

New York

1454 ALBANY SYMPHONY ORCHESTRA

19 Clinton Avenue
Albany, NY 12207
Phone: 518-465-4755
Fax: 518-465-3711
e-mail: ASO@GLOBAL2000.NET
Web Site: www.albanysymphony.com
Officers:
  Chairman: Alan P Goldberg
  VP: John L Riley
Management:
  Music Director/Conductor: David Alan Miller
  General Manager: Sharon Walsh

Mission: To give quality performances of classical music, with an emphasis on the establishment of an American symphonic repertoire, at the same time developing programs which bring a new audience.
Founded: 1931
Specialized Field: Instrumental music
Status: Professional; Nonprofit
Paid Staff: 6
Volunteer Staff: 250
Paid Artists: 68
Budget: $1.1 million
Income Sources: American Symphony Orchestra League
Performs At: Palace Theatre; Troy Savings Bank Music Hall
Annual Attendance: 16,000
Seating Capacity: 2,800; 1,250
Organization Type: Performing

1455 CAPITOL CHAMBER ARTISTS

263 Manning Boulevard
Albany, NY 12206
Mailing Address: 263 Manning Boulevard, Albany, NY. 12206
Phone: 518-458-9231
Fax: 518-458-9231
e-mail: ccartist@crisny.org
Web Site: www.capitolchamber.qpg.com/
Management:
  Director: Mary Lou Saetta
Mission: Performing the highest quality chamber music and educating a new audience.
Founded: 1969
Specialized Field: Chamber
Status: Professional; Nonprofit
Annual Attendance: 15,000
Organization Type: Performing; Touring; Resident; Educational

1456 GOLIARD CHAMBER SOLOISTS

Goliard Concerts
21-65 41st Street
Astoria, NY 11105
Phone: 718-728-8927
Fax: 718-728-8927
e-mail: goliardcts@aol.com
Management:
  Artistic Director: Patricia Handy
  Executive Director: Limor Tomer
  General Director: James Blanton
  Development Associate: Gregg Lauterbach
Mission: Performing eclectic chamber music in various vocal and instrumental combinations.
Founded: 1983
Specialized Field: Chamber
Status: Professional; Nonprofit
Paid Staff: 3
Volunteer Staff: 1
Paid Artists: 40
Performs At: Merkin Concert Hall at the Abrahman Goodman House
Organization Type: Performing; Touring; Presenting

1457 AUBURN CHAMBER ORCHESTRA
17 Nelson Street
Auburn, NY 13021-2649
Phone: 315-252-0065
Officers:
President: Ramon Cornwall
Management:
Conductor: Robert Connell
President: Karen Deming
Budget: $35,000
Performs At: auditorium
Seating Capacity: 1,000

1458 GENESSE SYMPHONY
PO Box 391
Batavia, NY 14021
Phone: 585-343-0350
e-mail: deward@frontiernet.net
Web Site: www.iinc.com/nonprof/gso
Officers:
President: Joan Ward
VP: Melinda Hay
Secretary: Ann Reid
Treasurer: Henry Emmans
Management:
Music Director: Raffaele Ponti
Board President: Joan Ward
Orchestra Manager: Jeanette Partis

1459 BINGHAMTON PHILHARMONIC ORCHESTRA
31 Front Street
Binghamton, NY 13905
Phone: 607-622-6717
Fax: 607-722-6526
e-mail: info@binhamtonphilharmonic.org
Web Site: www.binghamtonphilharmonic.org
Officers:
President: Linda Biemot
VP: Robert Pausher
Treasure: Matt Schaefer
Secretary: Leslie Levene
Management:
Executive Director: Stephan Raube-Wilson
Conductor/Artistic Director: John Covelli
Marketing Director: Cynthia K Kelly
Stage Manager: Alan Mica
Development Associate: Sandra J Griffiths
Accounts Manager: Lucille A Bush
Office Manager: June M Christensen
Mission: Presentation of classical and pops concerts.
Founded: 1996
Specialized Field: Orchestra; Pops/Popular Selections
Status: Professional; Nonprofit
Paid Staff: 6
Paid Artists: 76
Budget: $260,000-1,050,000
Income Sources: Ticket sales; grants
Performs At: Forum Theatre; Anderson Center at Bingham University
Annual Attendance: 17,000
Seating Capacity: 1,188; 1,590
Organization Type: Performing

1460 BRONX ARTS ENSEMBLE ORCHESTRA
Golf House
Van Cortlandt Park
Bronx, NY 10471
Phone: 718-601-7399
Fax: 718-549-4008
e-mail: baeconcert@aol.com
Web Site: www.bronxartsensemble.org
Management:
Executive/Artistic Director: William Scribner
Mission: Offering chamber music programs and chamber orchestras at a variety of locations in the Bronx at affordable prices.
Founded: 1972
Specialized Field: Symphony; Chamber
Status: Professional; Nonprofit
Paid Staff: 5
Volunteer Staff: 10
Budget: $260,000-1,050,000
Income Sources: Various
Performs At: Fordham University
Organization Type: Performing; Resident; Educational
Resident Groups: Fordham University

1461 BARGEMUSIC
Fulton Ferry Landing
Brooklyn, NY 11201
Phone: 718-624-2083
Fax: 718-624-1155
e-mail: Laurengrn@aol.com
Web Site: www.bargemusic.org
Management:
Artistic Director: Ik-Hwan Bae
Executive Director: Margaret Barclay
Program Coordinator: Cheryl Schiele
President: Olga Bloom
Business Manager: Keith O'Brien
Administrative Assistant: Caroline Hansen
Mission: Presenting year-round chamber music concerts on a permanently moored barge in New York Harbor.
Founded: 1977
Specialized Field: Instrumental Music
Status: Nonprofit
Budget: $150,000-400,000
Income Sources: Chamber Music America
Organization Type: Performing

1462 BROOKLYN FRIENDS OF CHAMBER MUSIC
Lafayette Avenue Presbyterian Chruch
85 S Oxford Street
Brooklyn, NY 11217
Phone: 212-825-1221
Fax: 718-951-5412
e-mail: wflecknaf@aol.com
Management:
Manager: Wanda Fleck
Mission: Six chamber music concerts, commissioning of new work.
Founded: 1988
Specialized Field: Chamber Music
Volunteer Staff: 10
Paid Artists: 50

1463 BROOKLYN PHILHARMONIC ORCHESTRA

30 Lafayette Avenue
Brooklyn, NY 11217
Phone: 718-636-4137
Fax: 718-622-3777
Web Site: www.brooklynphil.org
Officers:
  Chairman: Stanley H Kaplan
  President: Robert C Rosenberg
  Honorary Chairman: I Stanley Kriegel
  Treasurer: Richard Kane
  Executive VP: Craig Matthews
  Executive VP: John Tamberlane
Management:
  Executive Director: Joseph Horowitz
  Artistic Director: Maurice Edwards
  Director Development: Jana Strauss
  Operations Manager: Eri Klein
  Music Director: Robert Spano
Mission: To bring the best in standard and modern repertoire at the lowest possible prices and best performance level to the borough of Brooklyn and Greater New York, as well as free concerts to the general public in the parks and in the schools.
Founded: 1954
Specialized Field: Symphony; Orchestra; Chamber; Ensemble; Ethni
Status: Professional; Nonprofit
Paid Staff: 80
Income Sources: Opera House
Performs At: Brooklyn Academy of Music
Organization Type: Performing; Educational

1464 BROOKLYN SYMPHONY ORCHESTRA

PO Box 334
Brooklyn, NY 11202
Phone: 718-852-0677
Fax: 718-951-5412
Web Site: www.artanwords.com/BHMS.html
Officers:
  President: Jaye Zuckerman
Management:
  Music Director: Nicholas Armstrong
Budget: $35,000
Performs At: Church of Saint Ann and The Holy Trinity
Seating Capacity: 500

1465 SEM ENSEMBLE

25 Columbia Place
Brooklyn, NY 11201
Phone: 718-488-7659
Fax: 718-243-0964
e-mail: pusem@aol.com
Officers:
  President: Jerald Ordover
  Secretary: Paula Cooper
Management:
  Artistic director: Peter Kotik
  Managing Director: Martina Perry
Mission: To offer performances of and education in new music.
Specialized Field: Orchestra; Chamber
Status: Professional

Performs At: Willow Place Auditorium
Organization Type: Performing; Touring; Resident; Educational

1466 ARS NOVA MUSICIANS CHAMBER ORCHESTRA

136 Goethe Street
Buffalo, NY 14206
Phone: 716-894-2456
Fax: 716-894-2456
e-mail: arsnovamusicians@aol.com
Management:
  Music Director/Conductor: Marylouise Nanna
  Manager Director: Susan Willet
Founded: 1974
Specialized Field: West New York
Budget: $35,000- $100,000
Performs At: various locations

1467 BUFFALO CHAMBER MUSIC SOCIETY

67 Covington Road
Buffalo, NY 14216
Phone: 716-838-2383
Fax: 716-838-2383
e-mail: bcms@earthlink.net
Web Site: www.bflochambermusic.org
Management:
  Executive Director: Clementina Fleshler
Mission: Present world renowned chamber ensembles in Western New York.
Founded: 1924
Specialized Field: Chamber Music
Budget: $60,000-150,000
Income Sources: Subscriptions
Performs At: Kleinhans Music Hall
Annual Attendance: 7000
Seating Capacity: 700

1468 CHAUTAUQUA SYMPHONY ORCHESTRA

Chautauqua Institution
PO Box 28
Chautauqua, NY 14722
Phone: 716-357-6217
Fax: 716-357-9014
Toll-free: 800-836-2787
e-mail: cso@ciweb.org
Web Site: www.CIWEB.org
Management:
  Music Director: Uriel Segal
  VP/Program Director: Marty Merkley
  Personnel Manager: Jason Weintraub
Founded: 1929
Specialized Field: Symphony; Orchestra
Status: Professional; Nonprofit
Budget: $1,300,000
Income Sources: American Symphony Orchestra League
Performs At: Amphitheater; Chautauqua Institution
Organization Type: Performing; Resident; Educational

1469 PHILHARMONIA VIRTUOSI CORPORATION
145 Palisade Street
Dobbs Ferry, NY 10522
Phone: 914-973-7729
Fax: 914-693-7040
Toll-free: 800-475-7220
e-mail: info@pvmusic.org
Web Site: www.pVmusic.org
Officers:
    Chairman: Marvia Liftson
    President: Lucille Werlinich
    VP/Treasurer: Denny P Jacobson
    Secretary: Deborah Senft
Management:
    Music Director: Richard Kapp
Mission: To perform an exceptionally broad spectrum of music from the 1600s to the present; to remain a flexible ensemble that performs orchestra concerts with up to 45 players and chamber music programs with as few as three.
Founded: 1968
Specialized Field: Orchestra; Chamber
Status: Professional; Nonprofit
Paid Staff: 5
Volunteer Staff: 60
Paid Artists: 100
Budget: $650,000
Organization Type: Performing; Touring; Educational; Recording

1470 ISLIP ARTS COUNCIL CHAMBER MUSIC SERIES
50 Irish Lane
East Islip, NY 11730
Phone: 631-224-5420
Fax: 631-224-5440
e-mail: iacouncil@aol.com
Web Site: www.isliparts.org
Officers:
    President: Helene Katz
    VP: Nicholas Wartella
    Secreaty: Jean Lipshie
    Treasurer: Edward E. Wankel
Management:
    Executive Director: Lillian Barbash
    Co-Directror: Jodi Gianni
    Artist Administrator: Dorothy Kalson
    Clerk Typist: Angela Wallace
Mission: To present a variety of disciplines ranging from fine classical music to young persons' programs to avant garde performance art; to enable and emerging art organizations to gain information and assistance from the Arts Council library and staff in applying for not-for-profit status, funding, computer services, publicity, mailing lists, etc.
Founded: 1974
Specialized Field: Vocal Music; Instrumental Music
Status: Professional; Nonprofit
Budget: $250,000
Income Sources: Town of Islip; Suffolk County
Performs At: Sayville Schools; Dowling College
Type of Stage: Semi-Thurst
Organization Type: Performing

1471 FOREST HILLS SYMPHONY ORCHESTRA OF QUEENS
160-08 25th Drive
Flushing, NY 11358
Phone: 516-785-2532
Fax: 516-785-8027
e-mail: Fhso44@aol.com
Management:
    Music Director: Franklin Verbsky
    Manaer: Marilyn Verbsky

1472 JULIUS GROSSMAN ORCHESTRA
PO Box 26
Oakland Gardens Station
Flushing, NY 11364
Phone: 718-776-5914
Management:
    Music Director: Julius Grossman
    Manager: Arthur Serating

1473 WESTERN NEW YORK CHAMBER ORCHESTRA
Mason Hall
State University College
Fredonia, NY 14063
Phone: 716-673-3463
Fax: 716-673-3154
Officers:
    President: James Merrins
    VP: Lydia Evans
    Secretary: Ruth Mohoney
    Treasurer: John Wrigley
Management:
    Executive Director: James East
    Artistic Director: Joel Revzen
    Business/Orchestra Manager: Signe Rominger
Mission: To present concerts throughout Western New York, Pennsylvania and on tour; to sponsor a chamber orchestra and chamber music series; to sponsor an ensemble-in-residence at the State University of New York, Fredonia School of Music.
Founded: 1981
Specialized Field: Orchestra; Chamber
Status: Professional; Nonprofit
Paid Staff: 3
Volunteer Staff: 1
Paid Artists: 55
Income Sources: Arts Council for Chautauqua County; Fund for the Arts in Chautauqua County
Performs At: King Concert Hall; State University of New York
Organization Type: Performing; Touring; Resident; Educational; Sponsoring

1474 FRIENDS OF MUSIC ORCHESTRA
Brodie Fine Arts Building
State University of New York - Geneseo
Geneseo, NY 14454
Phone: 716-243-2958
Fax: 716-245-5826
Management:
    Music Director: James Walker

Mission: To provide to the Geneseo Valley region a wide range of repertoire on a professional level, with emphasis on new music for chamber orchestra.
Founded: 1970
Specialized Field: Orchestra
Status: Professional; Profit
Volunteer Staff: 12
Paid Artists: 38
Non-paid Artists: 1
Performs At: Saint Michael's Church
Organization Type: Performing; Educational; Sponsoring

1475 GENESEO CHAMBER SYMPHONY

Brodie Fine Arts Building
State University of New York-Geneseo
Geneseo, NY 14454
Phone: 716-245-5824
Fax: 716-245-5826
Management:
　Music Director: James Walker
Mission: Committed to providing younger performers an opportunity to interact with respected, established artists in performance as well as educational environments.
Founded: 1970
Specialized Field: Chamber
Status: Semi-Professional; Nonprofit
Paid Staff: 39
Performs At: Wadsworth Auditorium
Organization Type: Performing; Educational; Sponsoring

1476 TREMONT STRING QUARTET

PO Box 396
Geneseo, NY 14454
Phone: 716-243-4429
Fax: 716-245-5005
Management:
　Artistic Director: Richard Balkin
　Executive Director: James Kirkwood
Mission: Performing the best contemporary and standard chamber music repertory in venues throughout the world.
Specialized Field: Chamber
Status: Professional; Nonprofit
Organization Type: Performing; Touring; Resident; Educational; Sponsoring

1477 QUEENS SYMPHONY ORCHESTRA

80-00 Copper Avenue
Building 22
Glendale, NY 11385
Phone: 718-326-4455
Fax: 718-326-4499
e-mail: qso@queenssymphony.org
Web Site: www.queenssymphony.org
Officers:
　President: Harry Chain
　Executive VP: Elsi Levy
　Executive VP: Nick Webster
　VP: David Stein
　Treasurer: Wingson Wong
Management:
　Executive Director: Sophia Foglia
　General Manager: Lynda Herndon

President: Dr. Harry Heinemann
Executive VP: Nick Webster
Executive VP: Elsi Levy
VP: David Stein
Treasurer: Wingson Wong
Founded: 1953
Specialized Field: Symphony
Status: Professional; Nonprofit
Income Sources: American Symphony Orchestra League
Performs At: Colden Center for the Arts; Queens College
Organization Type: Performing

1478 GLENS FALLS SYMPHONY ORCHESTRA

7 Lapham Place
PO Box 2036
Glens Falls, NY 12801
Phone: 518-793-1348
Fax: 518-793-9122
e-mail: gfso.off@netheaven.com
Management:
　Music Director: Charles Peltz
　Executive Director: Robert B Rosoff

1479 GREAT NECK PHILHARMONIC

38 Hicks Lane
Great Neck, NY 11024
Phone: 516-482-4225
Management:
　Music Director: Mark Russell Amsterdam
　Executive Director: Susan Amsterdam

1480 FOUNDATION FOR BAROQUE MUSIC

165 Wilton Road
Greenfield Center, NY 12833
Phone: 518-893-7527
Fax: 518-893-2351
e-mail: rconant@baroquefestival.org
Web Site: www.baroquefestival.org
Officers:
　President: Robert Conant
　VP: Nancy Conant
　Secretary/Treasurer: James P Ketterer
Management:
　Artistic Director: Robert Conant
Mission: Promoting 17th and 18th century music by performing with historically accurate techniques on period instruments.
Founded: 1959
Specialized Field: Dance; Vocal Music; Instrumental Music; Festivals
Status: Professional; Nonprofit
Paid Staff: 1
Volunteer Staff: 2
Paid Artists: 28
Budget: $32,000
Income Sources: New York State Council on Arts; Private & Business Donations
Performs At: Baroque Festival Studio
Affiliations: ALA; SCAC; Early Music America; Chamber Music America; Greater Saratoga Chamber of Commerce
Annual Attendance: 800
Facility Category: Chamber music hall - all wood

Stage Dimensions: 25'x40'
Seating Capacity: 110
Year Built: 1973
Year Remodeled: 1996
Rental Contact: President Robert Conant
Organization Type: Performing; Resident; Educational

1481 WESTCHESTER PHILHARMONIC

111 N Central Avenue
Suite 425
Hartsdale, NY 10530
Phone: 914-682-3707
Fax: 914-682-3716
e-mail: office@Westchesterphil.org
Web Site: www.westchesterphil.org
Officers:
   President: Tony Riotto
   VP: Cris Ansnes
   Secretary: Ruth Toff
   Treasurer: Barbara Merson
Management:
   Executive Director: Elaine C Carroll
   Music Director: Paul Lustig Dunkel
   Personnel Manager: Jonathan Taylor
   Box Office Manager: Andrew Drew
Mission: The New Orchestra of Westchester is committed
to bringing the highest quality music to the Westchester
area with a goal of featuring music by living American
composers as part of annual programming.
Founded: 1983
Specialized Field: Symphony Orchestra
Status: Professional; Nonprofit
Paid Staff: 10
Volunteer Staff: 50
Paid Artists: 100
Budget: $1,450,000
Income Sources: Westchester Council for Arts; New
York State Coucil on Arts; National Endowment for the
Arts
Performs At: Performing Arts Center; State University of
New York
Annual Attendance: 27,650
Organization Type: Performing; Educational

1482 COLUMBIA FESTIVAL ORCHESTRA

PO Box 416
Hudson, NY 12534
Phone: 518-392-7198
Fax: 519-392-7198
Web Site: www.columbiafestivalorchestra.org
Management:
   Art Director: Gwen Gould
   Manager: Benjamin Harms

1483 CAYUGA CHAMBER ORCHESTRA

116 N Cayuga Street
Ford Hall, Ithaca College
Ithaca, NY 14850
Phone: 607-273-8981
Fax: 607-273-4816
Management:
   General Manager: Danielle Farnbaugh

1484 NEW DIRECTIONS CELLO FESTIVAL

501 Linn Street
Ithaca, NY 14850
Phone: 607-277-1686
Fax: 607-277-1686
Toll-free: 877-665-5815
e-mail: info@newdirectionscello.com
Web Site: www.newdirectionscello.com
Management:
   Director: Chris White
   Education Director: Sera Surslen
Mission: To bring together cellists and others interested in
nonclassical uses of cello (jazz, blues, folk, rock, etc.).
Workshops, jams, concerts.
Founded: 1995
Specialized Field: Music
Paid Staff: 2
Volunteer Staff: 10
Paid Artists: 12
Budget: Under $10,000
Income Sources: Sponsors, Participants, Donations
Season: July 11 - 13, 1999
Performs At: University of Connecticut, Storrs [Festival
Site]
Annual Attendance: 100
Facility Category: Mehden Auditorium/Recital Hall
Stage Dimensions: 50x25
Seating Capacity: 500
Year Built: 1985
Cost: $150 - 3 day

1485 JAMESTOWN CONCERT ASSOCIATION

315 N Main Street
Suite 200
Jamestown, NY 14701-5124
Phone: 716-487-1522
Fax: 716-483-5051
e-mail: icamusic@excite.com
Officers:
   President: R Richard Corbin
   VP: Sally Ulrich
   Treasurer: F John Fuchs
   Secretary: Mary Weeden
Management:
   Programming: Sally Ulrich
Mission: Purpose of presenting live classical
performances in the Jamestown area.
Founded: 1934
Volunteer Staff: 16
Income Sources: Arts Association Chautauqua County
Performs At: Civic Center
Organization Type: Educational; Sponsoring

1486 LAKE GEORGE JAZZ WEEKEND
Lake George Arts Project

Canada Street
Lake George, NY 12845
Phone: 518-668-2616
Fax: 518-668-3050
Officers:
   President: Ed Ostberg
Management:
   Executive Director: John Strong
   Music Director: Paul Pines

Mission: Sponsoring a two-day jazz festival every September featuring nationally acclaimed as well as emerging jazz artists.
Specialized Field: Instrumental Music; Jazz
Status: Professional; Nonprofit
Performs At: Shepard Park Bandstand
Organization Type: Performing; Touring

1487 BEETHOVEN FESTIVAL

Friends of the Arts
Locust Valley, NY 11560
Mailing Address: PO Box 702
Phone: 516-922-0061
Fax: 516-922-0770
e-mail: info@friendsofthearts.com
Web Site: www.friendsofthearts.com
Management:
   Executive Director: Theodora Bookman
Mission: Presenting Beethoven's lifetime body of work during one spectacular weekend.
Founded: 1981
Specialized Field: Instrumental Music
Status: Professional; Nonprofit
Performs At: Planting Fields Arboretum
Organization Type: Performing

1488 LONG ISLAND BAROQUE ENSEMBLE

PO Box 7
Locust Valley, NY 11560
Phone: 631-724-7386
Fax: 631-864-4426
e-mail: pkbarts@aol.comm
Officers:
   President: Edward Pressman
   Treasurer: Alfred Zoller
   Secretary: Viein Barathan
   VP: Alice Ross
Management:
   Artistic Director: Sonia Grib
   Administator: Patricia Berman
Mission: Performing early music on period instruments in conjunction with vocal specialists.
Founded: 1970
Specialized Field: Chamber; Ensemble
Status: Professional; Nonprofit
Paid Staff: 2
Volunteer Staff: 10
Budget: $40,000
Income Sources: Government; Counties; Private; Ticket Sales
Performs At: St. Andrews Lutheran Church
Annual Attendance: 2,000
Organization Type: Performing; Touring; Educational

1489 LONG ISLAND PHILHARMONIC

One Huntington Quadrangle
Suite LL-09
Melville, NY 11747
Phone: 631-293-2223
Fax: 631-293-2655
e-mail: liphil@fnol.net
Web Site: www.liphilharmonic.com
Officers:
   President: Larry Austin
   Chairman: David H Peirez
   Chairman Emeritus: Barry R Shapiro
   Secretary and Counsel: Rocco S Barrese
   Treasurer: Joesph F Purcell
Management:
   Executive Director: Karen L Barnes
   Marketing/Project Manager: Shari M Levitz
   Orchestra/Production Manager: Matthew E Flood
Founded: 1979
Specialized Field: Symphony; Orchestra; Chamber
Status: Professional
Budget: $2,000,000
Performs At: Tilles Center; Staller Center
Organization Type: Performing; Resident; Educational

1490 NOMADICS

PO Box 1073
Millbrook, NY 12545
Phone: 845-677-3319
Fax: 845-677-3319
e-mail: flautist107@yahoo.com
Web Site: www.thenomadics.com
Officers:
   Public Relations: Lynnette Benner
Mission: To expose people, children in particular, to ethnic music from countries other than our own. We perform Ethnic Folk Music, discuss its history, performance practices and traditional instruments. Some of the countries we touch on are Sweden, Austria, The British Isles, Turkey, Argentina and many others. Our concerts are interactive and informative.
Founded: 2001
Specialized Field: World Folk, Celtic, Classical, Colonial
Paid Staff: 2
Paid Artists: 2
Performs At: Various Venues
Affiliations: American Federation of Musicians

1491 DEL-SE-NANGO OLDE TYME FIDDLERS ASSOCIATION

RD #3
PO Box 233
New Berlin, NY 13411
Phone: 607-843-6745
Mission: Dedicated to the preservation, promotion and perpetuation of the art of olde tyme fiddling, its music and dances.
Founded: 1978
Specialized Field: Folk
Status: Nonprofit
Paid Staff: 40
Organization Type: Performing; Educational; Sponsoring

1492 TANNERY POND CONCERTS

PO Box 446
New Lebanon, NY 12125
Phone: 413-442-7813
Toll-free: 888-820-1696
Web Site: www.regionnet.com
Officers:
   President: Brenda Archer Adams
   VP: Lois E Dickson
   Treasurer: Brian Baker

Secretary: Cindy Puccio
President Emeritus: Christina Wirth
Management:
  Artistic Director: Christian Steiner
  Administrative Director: Linda McGinley Papas
Performs At: Tannery Pond

1493 AEOLIAN CHAMBER PLAYERS
173 Riverside Drive
New York, NY 10024
Phone: 212-595-4688
Fax: 212-595-8431
e-mail: Lewiskap@aol.com
Management:
  Director: Lewis Kaplan
Mission: Committed to performing a broad repertoire of music from the classical to the contemporary.
Founded: 1961
Specialized Field: Chamber
Status: Professional
Income Sources: National Endowment for the Arts; New York State Council on Arts; Bowdoin Summer Music Festival
Organization Type: Performing; Touring; Resident

1494 AFFILIATE ARTISTS
37 W 65th Street
New York, NY 10023
Phone: 212-580-2000
Management:
  President/Artistic Director: Richard C Clark
  Director Programs/Development: Joseph Chart
Mission: To help develop the careers of the nation's most promising young performing artists; to help develop audiences for the arts throughout the country; to develop corporate and foundational support for the arts.
Specialized Field: Soloists
Status: Professional; Nonprofit
Organization Type: Resident; Educational; Sponsoring

1495 AMERICAN COMPOSERS ORCHESTRA
1775 Broadway
Suite 525
New York, NY 10019
Phone: 212-977-8495
Fax: 212-977-8995
e-mail: aco@americancomposers.org
Web Site: www.americancomposers.org
Officers:
  President: Francis Thorne
Management:
  Executive Director: Michael Geller
  Music Director: Steven Sloane
  Artistic Director: Robert Beaser
  Conductor Laureate: Dennis Russell Davies
Mission: The ACO's purpose is to discover, produce and present the widest possible spectrum of American repertoire, past and present, in performances of the highest quality, thereby focusing national awareness and support of American composers and their music.
Founded: 1976
Specialized Field: Symphony; Orchestra
Status: Professional; Nonprofit
Paid Staff: 7

Paid Artists: 84
Budget: $1,900,000
Income Sources: American Symphony Orchestra League
Performs At: Carnegie Hall
Annual Attendance: 20,000
Organization Type: Performing

1496 AMERICAN SYMPHONY ORCHESTRA
850 7th Avenue
Suite 503
New York, NY 10019-5230
Phone: 212-581-1365
Fax: 212-489-7188
e-mail: executivedirector@americansymphony.org
Web Site: www.americansymphony.org
Management:
  Executive Director: Lynne Meloccaro
  Music Director: Leon Botstein
  Composer in Residence: Richard Wilson
  Resident Conductor: Eckart Preu
  Assistant Conductor: Thomas Carling
  Director Operations: Alex Johnston
  Director Development: Suzanne Konowitz
  Assoc. Director of Marketing: Tobin Fowler
  Personnel Manager: Ronald Seil
Mission: American Symphony Orchestra is the only self-governing orchestra in the United States with a subscription series at Carnegie Hall. It is also a resource organization providing musical service to communities nurturing young artists.
Founded: 1962
Specialized Field: Symphony; Orchestra; Ensemble
Status: Professional; Nonprofit
Paid Staff: 8
Performs At: Carnegie Hall
Organization Type: Performing

1497 AMERICAN TAP DANCE ORCHESTRA
170 Mercer Street
New York, NY 10012
Phone: 212-243-6438
Fax: 212-243-6438
Web Site: nyctapfestival.com/ATDO/
Management:
  Siegel Artist Management: Liz Silverstein
  Siegel Artist Management: Ethel Siegel
  Siegel Artist Management: Jane Lawrence Curtiss
Mission: Dedicated to celebrating, preserving and perpetuating one of America's few indigenous art forms, tap dance.
Founded: 1986
Specialized Field: Rhythm; Jazz; Tap Dance
Status: Professional; Nonprofit
Performs At: Woodpeckers Tap Dance Center
Organization Type: Performing; Touring; Educational

1498 ASSOCIATION FOR THE ADVANCEMENT OF CREATIVE ARTS
PO Box 187
Times Square Station
New York, NY 10108
Phone: 212-594-7149
Fax: 212-594-7149

Mission: To provide a forum for composers and performers to perform their own original music.
Specialized Field: Ensemble
Status: Professional; Nonprofit
Organization Type: Performing

1499 BACHANALIA CHAMBER ORCHESTRA

400 W 43rd Street
Suite 7D
New York, NY 10036
Phone: 212-239-5906
Fax: 212-239-5906
Management:
    Artistic Director: Nina Beilina

1500 BLOOMINGDALE SCHOOL OF MUSIC

323 W 108th Street
New York, NY 10025
Phone: 212-663-6021
Fax: 212-932-9429
Web Site: www.bloomingdalemusic.org
Management:
    Executive Director: Lawrence Davis
Mission: To promote, foster and develop the love of and interest for the musical arts.
Founded: 1964
Specialized Field: Orchestra; Chamber; Ensemble; Ethnic; Folk; Electronic & Live Electronic
Status: Professional; Nonprofit
Income Sources: National Guild of Community Schools of the Arts
Organization Type: Performing; Educational; Sponsoring

1501 CARNEGIE CHAMBER PLAYERS

514 W 110th Street
Suite 41
New York, NY 10025
Phone: 212-645-7424
Management:
    Artistic Director: Richard Goldsmith
    Artistic Director: Yari Bond
Mission: The promotion of chamber music in a mixed string and woodwind ensemble; the commissioning of new works; the performing of a traditional chamber music repertoire.
Specialized Field: Chamber; Ensemble
Status: Professional; Nonprofit
Performs At: Montshire Science Museum; Norwich VT
Organization Type: Performing; Touring; Resident; Educational

1502 CHAMBER MUSIC AMERICA

545 8th Avenue
New York, NY 10018
Phone: 212-875-5784
Fax: 212-875-5779
Web Site: www.chamber-music.org
Management:
    Executive Director: Dean K Stein
    Chairman: Robert L Bogomolny
    President: Robert Martin
    VP: Lucy Miller
    VP: Phillip Ying

    Secretary: Barbara Barcly
    Treasurer: Thomas Van Straaten
    CEO: Margaret M Mioi
Mission: To make chamber music a vital part of American cultural life through promoting professional chamber music.
Founded: 1977
Specialized Field: Chamber
Status: Professional; Nonprofit
Organization Type: Educational; Service Organization

1503 CHAMBER MUSIC SOCIETY OF LINCOLN CENTER

70 Lincoln Center Plaza
10th Floor
New York, NY 10023
Phone: 212-875-5775
Fax: 212-875-5799
Web Site: www.chambermusicsociety.org
Management:
    Executive Director: Norma Hurlburt
    Director Artistic Planninf/Tour: Martha Bonta
    Director Development: Edward Harsh
    Manager Touring: Kate Sobel
Mission: To present chamber music concerts.
Founded: 1969
Specialized Field: Chamber; Ensemble; Instrumental Group
Status: Professional; Nonprofit
Performs At: Alice Tully Hall
Organization Type: Performing; Touring; Resident; Educational

1504 CHINESE MUSIC ENSEMBLE OF NEW YORK

149 Canal Street
New York, NY 10002
Phone: 212-925-6110
e-mail: info@chinesemusic.org
Web Site: www.geocities.com
Officers:
    Director: Yu-chiung Teng
    Associate Director: Terence Yeh
    Associate Director: Oiman Chan
Management:
    Director: Tsuan-Nien Chang
Mission: To introduce the music of China to Western audiences.
Founded: 1961
Specialized Field: Ensemble; Ethnic; Folk
Status: Semi-Professional; Nonprofit
Organization Type: Performing; Touring; Educational

1505 CITY SYMPHONY ORCHESTRA OF NEW YORK

311 W 34th Street
New York, NY 10001
Phone: 212-947-3362
Fax: 212-465-2367
Management:
    Artistic Director: David Eaton
    Personnel Contractor: Leonid Fleishaker

Mission: The presentation of young performers at the major concert halls in New York City; the presentation of performances and music by artists of different ethnic backgrounds.
Specialized Field: Symphony; Chamber
Status: Professional; Nonprofit
Performs At: Carnegie Hall; Alice Tully Hall
Organization Type: Performing

1506 CLASSICAL QUARTET

225 W 99th Street
New York, NY 10025
Phone: 212-222-2700
Web Site: saturdaybrass.org
Officers:
  President: Nancy Wilson
  Treasurer: David Miller
Management:
  Artist Representative: Beverly Simmons
Mission: The Classical Quartet was founded to present masterpieces of the Classic Era, string quartets of Haydn, Mozart, Beethoven and their contemporaries, on period instruments.
Founded: 1979
Specialized Field: Chamber; Ensemble
Status: Professional
Performs At: Saint Michael's Church
Organization Type: Performing; Touring; Resident; Educational

1507 COLUMBIA UNIVERSITY ORCHESTRA

Music Department
806 Dodge Hall, Columbia University
New York, NY 10027
Phone: 212-854-5409
Fax: 212-854-8191
Management:
  Music Director/Conducter: Jeffrey F Milarsky
  Conductor: George Rothman

1508 CONCORDIA

330 7th Avenue
21st Floor
New York, NY 10001
Phone: 212-967-1290
Fax: 212-629-0508
Officers:
  President: Joel Hirschtritt
  Chairman: Tomio Taki
  Executive Director: Leslie Stilfeman
Management:
  Artistic Director: Mafia Alsop
Mission: Unique and adventurous fifty piece orchestra dedicated to breaking down the barriers between jazz and classical music by presenting innovative concerts combining American Symphonic masterpieces, orchestral jazz and commissioned premieres.
Founded: 1984
Specialized Field: Orchestra; Chamber
Status: Professional; Nonprofit

1509 CONCORDIA ORCHESTRA

850 7th Avenue
Suite 1206
New York, NY 10025
Phone: 212-581-2392
Fax: 212-262-9165
e-mail: cordiaorch@aol.com
Web Site: www.concordiaorchestra.org
Management:
  Art Director: Marin Alsop
  Co-Director: Gabriella Blanco
  Co-Director: Lorna Dolci

1510 COSMOPOLITAN SYMPHONY ORCHESTRA

PO Box 231045
New York, NY 10023-1045
Phone: 212-873-7784
Fax: 212-873-7784
Management:
  Artistic Director Chamber Players: Eric Grossman
  Managing Director: Rita Asen
Mission: To present live symphonic music and/or chamber music to a diverse audience at low to moderate prices.
Volunteer Staff: 20
Paid Artists: 35

1511 EARLY MUSIC FOUNDATION

1047 Amsterdam Avenue
New York, NY 10025
Phone: 212-749-6600
Fax: 212-932-7348
e-mail: info@earlymusicny.org
Web Site: www.earlymusicny.org
Officers:
  President: Janice Haggerty
Management:
  General Manager: Gene Murrow
  Artistic Director: Frederick Renz
  Development Manager: Chris Tokar
Mission: Fosters public knowledge, understanding and appreciation of music of the medieval, Renaissance and baroque eras through performances and recording of the highest artistic quality by its two performing ensembles.
Founded: 1974
Specialized Field: Early Music
Status: Professional; Nonprofit
Paid Staff: 2
Paid Artists: 7
Budget: $350,000
Income Sources: Early Music America
Performs At: Cathedral of Saint John the Divine
Organization Type: Performing; Touring; Resident

1512 EOS ORCHESTRA

161 6th Avenue
Suite 902
New York, NY 10013
Phone: 212-691-6415
Fax: 212-691-6648
Web Site: www.eosorchestra.com
Management:
  Artistic Director/Conductor: Jonathan Sheffer

Executive Director: Stephen Vann
Director Operations/Education: Lee Ellen Hreem
Director Development: Johanna Burlingham
Specialized Field: Performing Series/Music

1513 JAZZ AT LINCOLN CENTER'S ESSENTIALLY ELLINGTON JAZZ FESTIVAL
33 W 60th Street
11th Floor
New York, NY 10023-7999
Phone: 212-258-9800
Fax: 212-258-9900
e-mail: info@jazzatlincolncenter.org
Web Site: www.jazzatlincolncenter.org
Officers:
President/CEO: Hughlyn F Fierce
Management:
Artistic Director: Wynton Marsalis
Mission: To promoting the appreciation and understanding of jazz through performance, education and preservation.
Founded: 1991
Specialized Field: Jazz
Status: Not-for-Profit
Performs At: Lincoln Center of Performing Arts
Organization Type: Performing; Touring; Education; Residence

1514 LITTLE ORCHESTRA SOCIETY OF NEW YORK
330 W 42nd Street
12th Floor
New York, NY 10036-6902
Phone: 212-971-9500
Fax: 212-971-9501
Management:
Music Director: Dino Anagnost
Managing Director: John Kordel
General Manager: Hugo Hoogenboom
Director Development: Judith Inglis
Director Marketing Development: Amand Ramaswamy
Founded: 1947
Specialized Field: Scripted Classical Music Concerts for Children and Adults
Paid Staff: 13
Volunteer Staff: 12
Paid Artists: 60

1515 LYRIC CHAMBER MUSIC SOCIETY OF NEW YORK
20 W 64th Street
Suite 27H
New York, NY 10023
Phone: 212-875-4230
Fax: 212-496-9928
e-mail: LyricCMS@aol.com
Web Site: www.lyricny.org
Management:
Artistic Director: Dr. Joan Thomson Kretschmer
Executive Director: Peggy Flaum

Mission: To provide exceptionally gifted musicians an opportunity to perform chamber music.
Founded: 1997
Specialized Field: Chamber Music
Paid Staff: 1
Volunteer Staff: 1

1516 MARGOT ASTRACHAN MUSIC
1050 5th Avenue
New York, NY 10028
Phone: 212-722-6394
Fax: 212-828-9026
Management:
Owner: Margot Astrachan
Founded: 1994
Specialized Field: Theatre, Cabaret

1517 MUSIC BEFORE 1800
Corpus Christi Church
529 W 121st Street
New York, NY 10027
Phone: 212-666-0675
Fax: 212-666-9266
e-mail: mb1800@aol.com
Web Site: http://members.aol.com/mb1800
Mission: Offering performances of vocal and instrumental chamber music from before 1800.
Founded: 1975
Specialized Field: Chamber
Status: Professional
Income Sources: Chamber Music America; Early Music America
Performs At: Corpus Christi Church
Organization Type: Performing; Sponsoring

1518 NATIONAL ORCHESTRAL ASSOCIATION
475 Riverside Drive
Suite 249
New York, NY 10115
Phone: 212-870-2009
Fax: 212-870-2129
Specialized Field: Orchestra; Chamber
Status: Nonprofit
Performs At: Carnegie Hall
Organization Type: Educational

1519 NEW YORK CHAMBER SYMPHONY
130 W 56th Street
Suite 710
New York, NY 10019
Phone: 212-262-6927
Fax: 212-246-3204
e-mail: elaine@nycs.org
Web Site: www.nycs.org
Management:
VP Managing Director: Sharon Griffin
Director Operations: Cymthia Baker
Administrative Assistant: Claresa Fisher
Director Finance: Dale Hirschman
Director Marketing/Public Relations: Abbe Krieger
Development Associate: Dr. Roberta Zlokower

1520 NEW YORK CONSORT OF VIOLS

201 W 86th Street
New York, NY 10024
Phone: 212-580-9787
Fax: 212-496-8014
e-mail: jdavidoff@nyconsortofviols.org
Web Site: www.consortofviols.org
Management:
   Artistic Director: Judith Davidoff
Mission: Performing the vast repertoire of music for
violas from the Renaissance and Baroque periods;
encouraging the composition of new works for the viola.
Founded: 1972
Specialized Field: Chamber
Status: Professional; Nonprofit
Paid Staff: 1
Paid Artists: 4
Organization Type: Performing; Touring; Educational

1521 NEW YORK HARP ENSEMBLE

140 W End Avenue
Suite 3K
New York, NY 10023
Phone: 212-799-5989
Fax: 212-799-5989
Management:
   Music Director: Dr. Aristid von Wurtzler
   Metropolitan Artists Management:
Mission: To perform concerts worldwide; to offer new
contemporary compositions for four harps; to provide
master classes; to produce recordings and appear in
television performances.
Founded: 1970
Specialized Field: Chamber
Status: Professional; Nonprofit
Organization Type: Performing; Touring; Resident;
Educational

1522 NEW YORK PHILHARMONIC

65th Street at Broadway
New York, NY 10023
Phone: 212-875-5000
Fax: 212-875-5717
Web Site: www.newyorkphilharmonic.org
Management:
   Music Director: Kurt Masur
   Principal Guest Conductor: Sir Colin Davis
   Laureate Conductor, 1943-1990: Leonard Bernstein
   Acting Executive Director: Bill Thomas
   Assistant/Executive Director: Susan O'Dell
   Administrative Assistant: Luisa Enriquez
   Artistic Coordinator: Monica Parks
   Controller: Pamela Katz
   Office Services Administrator: Eddie Duffy
Founded: 1842
Specialized Field: Symphony; Orchestra; Chamber
Status: Professional
Income Sources: American Symphony Orchestra League
Performs At: Avery Fisher Hall
Organization Type: Performing; Touring; Resident;
Educational

1523 NEW YORK PHILOMUSICA CHAMBER ENSEMBLE

105 W 73rd Street
#4C
New York, NY 10023
Phone: 212-580-9933
Fax: 212-580-3902
e-mail: staff@nyphilomusica.org
Web Site: www.nyphilomusia.org
Management:
   Artistic Director: Robert Johnson
   General Manager: Lori Diffendaffer
Mission: Performing and recording the music written
from 1750 to the present for wind, strings and piano, with
guest soloists.
Founded: 1971
Specialized Field: Chamber; Ensemble
Status: Professional; Nonprofit
Performs At: American Concert Hall; Merkin Concert
Hall
Organization Type: Performing; Recording

1524 NEW YORK POPS

881 7th Avenue
Suite 903
New York, NY 10019
Phone: 212-765-7677
Fax: 212-315-3199
e-mail: info@newyorkpops.org
Web Site: www./newyorkpops.org
Management:
   Founder/Musical Director: Skitch Henderson
   Executive Director: James M Johnson
Mission: Publicly-supported, not-for-profit corporation
dedicated to broadening public awareness and enjoyment
of America's rich popular music heritage through
presentation of orchestral concerts of the highest quality
in traditional and non-traditional settings.
Founded: 1983
Specialized Field: Symphony
Status: Professional; Nonprofit
Paid Staff: 5
Paid Artists: 79
Budget: 2.1 million
Income Sources: Concert Fees, Ticket Sales, and
Institutional Support From Individuals, Corporations,
Foundations, and Government Sources.
Performs At: Carnegie Hall
Affiliations: American Syphony Orchestra League, NYC
& Company
Facility Category: Concert Hall
Organization Type: Performing; Touring

1525 NEW YORK YOUTH SYMPHONY

850 7th Avenue
Suite 505
New York, NY 10019-5230
Phone: 212-581-5933
Fax: 212-582-6927
e-mail: info@nyyouthsymphony.org
Web Site: www.nyyouthsymphony.org
Officers:
   Chairperson: Leslie J Garfield
   President: Edward S Cohen

Vice Chairman: Robert L Poster
Treasurer: Benson J. Chapman
Management:
   Executive Director: Barry Goldberg
   Music Director: Paul Haas
Mission: New York Youth Symphony is established as the premier orchestra in metropolitan New York offering a unique learning experience and musical showcase for the gifted, young musician, conductor, soloist and composer.
Founded: 1963
Specialized Field: Symphony; Chamber Music Program; Jazz Band
Status: Non-Professional; Nonprofit
Paid Staff: 5
Volunteer Staff: 60
Budget: $1,000,000
Income Sources: Contributions; Ticket Sales
Performs At: Carnegie Hall
Affiliations: American Symphony Orchestra League; Chamber Music America
Annual Attendance: 14,000
Seating Capacity: 2,800
Organization Type: Performing; Educational; Sponsoring

1526   NORTH/SOUTH CONSONANCE

Cathedral Station
PO Box 698
New York, NY 10025-0698
Phone: 212-663-7566
Fax: 212-663-7566
e-mail: info@northsouthmusic.org
Web Site: www.nsmusic.com
Mission: Performing and furthering the music of living composers with particular emphasis on music from the Americas.
Founded: 1980
Specialized Field: Chamber; Ensemble; Instrumental Group; Electronic & Live Electronic; New Music
Status: Professional; Nonprofit
Income Sources: Chamber Music America
Performs At: Merkin Hall; Weil Recital Hall
Organization Type: Performing; Touring; Resident; Educational

1527   ORCHESTRA OF ST. LUKE'S

330 W 42nd Street
9th Floor
New York, NY 10036
Phone: 212-594-6100
Fax: 212-594-3291
e-mail: nlhayashi@orchestraofstlukes.org
Web Site: www.orchestraofstlukes.org
Management:
   Director Artistic Planning: Elizabeth Ostrow
   Executive Director/President: Marianne C Lockwood
   Director Operations: Valerie Broderick
   Director Marketing: Noel Hayashi
   Director Education: Rosalyn Bindman
   Director Development: Keith Wiggs
Mission: St. Lukes is a gathering of outstanding musicians whose purpose is to bring the beauty of music and the enlightened communication that is unique to music to as broad an audience as possible.
Founded: 1974

Specialized Field: Orchestra
Status: Professional; Nonprofit
Paid Staff: 15
Income Sources: St. Luke's Chamber Ensemble
Performs At: Merkin Concert Hall; Carnegie Hall
Organization Type: Performing

1528   ORPHEUS CHAMBER ORCHESTRA

490 Riverside Drive
New York, NY 10027
Phone: 212-896-1700
Fax: 212-896-1717
Web Site: www.orpheusnyc.com
Management:
   Executive Director: Harvey Seipter
Mission: To provide members an opportunity to work in collaboration on the selection and interpretation of pieces.
Founded: 1972
Specialized Field: Orchestra; Chamber
Status: Professional; Nonprofit
Performs At: Carnegie Hall
Organization Type: Performing; Touring

1529   PEOPLES' SYMPHONY CONCERTS

201 W 54th Street
New York, NY 10019
Phone: 212-586-4680
Fax: 212-581-4029
e-mail: psc@franksalomon.com
Management:
   Manager: Frank E Salomon

1530   PRO PIANO NEW YORK RECITAL SERIES

Pro Piano
85 Jane Street
New York, NY 10014
Phone: 212-206-8794
Fax: 212-633-1207
e-mail: ricard@propiano.com
Web Site: www.propiano.com
Management:
   Founder/Executive Director: Ricard de La Rosa
   Artistic Director: Chitose Okashiro
Mission: Present pianists to perform at Weill Hall NYC annually.
Budget: $60,000-150,000
Performs At: Weill Recital Hall at Carnegie Hall

1531   QUINTET OF THE AMERICAS

134 Bowery
New York, NY 10013
Phone: 718-230-5189
Fax: 718-398-2737
e-mail: quintet@aol.com
Web Site: www.quintet.org
Management:
   Director: Barbara Oldham
Mission: The presentation of chamber music and contemporary music, with an emphasis on North and South America.
Founded: 1976
Specialized Field: Chamber; Ethnic

Status: Professional; Nonprofit
Paid Staff: 3
Paid Artists: 5
Performs At: Center for Inter-American Relations
Organization Type: Performing; Touring; Resident; Educational

1532 RIVERSIDE SYMPHONY

225 W 99th Street
New York, NY 10025
Phone: 212-864-4197
Fax: 212-864-9795
e-mail: riverside@riversidesymphony.org
Web Site: www.riversidesymphony.org
Management:
Artistic Director: Anthony Korf
Conductor/Music Director: George Rothman
Production Manager: Johnathan Salter
Mission: To present new and less-familiar work; to present emerging artists; to produce American music.
Specialized Field: Symphony; Orchestra
Status: Professional; Nonprofit
Budget: $500,000
Performs At: Alice Tully Hall Lincoln Center
Organization Type: Performing; Resident; Educational

1533 ROULETTE INTERMEDIUM

228 W Broadway
New York, NY 10013
Phone: 212-219-8242
Fax: 212-219-8773
e-mail: info@roulette.org
Web Site: www.roulette.org
Officers:
President: Jim Staley
Management:
Program Director: Jim Staley
Projects Director: David Weinstein
Managing Director: Suzanne Youngerman
Mission: To be a presenting organization and facility for innovative composers and musicians through its concert series, commissions and recording distribution services; to support a broad range of new music by young established artists.
Specialized Field: Chamber; Ensemble; Ethnic; Folk; Instrumental Group; Electronic & Live Electronic; Band
Status: Nonprofit
Performs At: Roul
Organization Type: Presenting

1534 SAINT LUKES CHAMBER ENSEMBLE

130 W 42nd Street
Suite 804
New York, NY 10036
Phone: 212-594-6100
Fax: 212-594-6100
Web Site: www.orchestraofstlukes.org/chamber.htm
Management:
Artistic Director: Michael Feldman
Executive Director: Marriane C Lockwood
Mission: Encompasses St. Luke's Chamber Ensemble, Orchestra of St. Luke's, Children's Free Opera and Dance of New York.
Specialized Field: Orchestra; Chamber

Status: Nonprofit
Performs At: Avery Fisher Hall; Merkin Concert Hall; Brooklyn
Organization Type: Performing; Touring; Educational; Sponsoring

1535 SATURDAY BRASS QUINTET

St. Michael's Episcopal Church
225 W 99th Street
New York, NY 10025
Phone: 212-222-2700
Fax: 212-678-5916
Mission: Presenting classics of the brass chamber genre; soliciting and performing new selections for brass.
Specialized Field: Chamber
Status: Professional; Nonprofit
Organization Type: Performing; Touring; Resident; Educational

1536 SHEILA-NA-GIG MUSIC

513 E 13th Street
#3
New York, NY 10009
Phone: 212-260-2302
Fax: 212-260-9645
e-mail: sngmusic@earthlink.net
Web Site: www.sheilanagig.com
Management:
Director: Brendan Jamieson
Mission: To represent artists from Ireland, Scotland and the US in world and acoustic music.
Founded: 1998
Specialized Field: Tazent Agency

1537 ST. PATRICK'S CATHEDRAL CHAMBER MUSIC SERIES

St. Patrick's Cathedral
460 Madison Avenue
New York, NY 10022
Phone: 212-753-2261
Fax: 212-753-3925
e-mail: mlchamber@aol.com
Management:
Manager: Monica Avitsur
Budget: $10,000

1538 TISCH CENTER FOR THE ARTS

1395 Lexington Avenue
New York, NY 10128
Phone: 212-415-5740
Fax: 212-415-5738
Director: Hanna Gaifman
Managing Director: Anna Lisa Browns
Specialized Field: Orchestra; Chamber; Ensemble; Pops; Theatre; Jazz
Status: Nonprofit
Performs At: Kaufmann Concert Hall
Organization Type: Performing; Educational

1539 ONONDAGA CIVIC SYMPHONY ORCHESTRA
Ed Brennan
4870 Coventry Road
North Syracuse, NY 13215
Phone: 315-488-5133
e-mail: ejbrennan@aol.com
Management:
   President: Ed Brennan
   VP: Fred Wenthen

1540 CATSKILL SYMPHONY ORCHESTRA
PO Box 14
Oneonta, NY 13820
Phone: 607-436-2670
Fax: 607-436-2718
Management:
   General Manager: Deborah Wolfanger
   Personnel Manager: Charles England
Mission: Bringing quality music to the immediate and outlying areas of Central New York State.
Founded: 1972
Specialized Field: Symphony; Orchestra
Status: Professional; Nonprofit
Paid Staff: 7
Performs At: Hunt Union; State University of New York-Oneonta
Organization Type: Performing; Educational

1541 WAVERLY CONSORT
Patterson, NY 12563
Mailing Address: PO Box 286
Phone: 845-878-3723
Fax: 845-878-3817
Management:
   Artistic Director: Michael Jaffee
Mission: The presentation of early music to audiences in NY and across the country.
Founded: 1964
Specialized Field: Ensemble
Status: Professional; Nonprofit
Organization Type: Performing; Touring

1542 HUDSON VALLEY PHILHARMONIC
35 Market Street
Poughkeepsie, NY 12601
Phone: 845-473-5288
Fax: 845-473-2074
e-mail: SLAMARCA@bardavon.org
Web Site: WWW.BARDAVON.ORG
Management:
   Music Director: Randall Craig Fleischer
   Executive Director: Chris Silva
   Managing Director: Stephen LaMarca
Mission: Dedicated to sponsoring and supporting a professional symphony orchestra which will present performances of the highest artistic quality and further the musical growth of the region.
Founded: 1959
Specialized Field: Symphony; Orchestra; Chamber
Status: Professional

Income Sources: American Symphony Orchestra League; American Society of Composers, Authors and Publishers; Broadcast Music Incorporated
Performs At: Ulster Performing Arts Center; Bardavon 1869 Opera House
Organization Type: Performing; Resident; Sponsoring

1543 CHAMBER MUSIC AT RODEF SHALOM WITH STEPHEN STARKMAN & FRIENDS
51 Ackerthook Road
Rhinebeck, NY 12572
Phone: 845-876-2742
Management:
   Artistic Director: Stephen Starkman
Budget: $10,000-20,000
Seating Capacity: 500+

1544 RHINEBECK CHAMBER MUSIC SOCIETY
PO Box 465
Rhinebeck, NY 12572
Phone: 845-876-2870
Web Site: www.geocities.com/rhinebeckcms/
Management:
   Artistic Director: Kurt Grishman
Budget: $10,000-20,000
Performs At: Church of Messiah

1545 MAMADOU DIABATE
517 County Highway 27
Richfield Springs, NY 13439
Phone: 315-858-1434
Fax: 315-858-1434
e-mail: info@onqueuartists.com
Web Site: www.onqueuartists.com
Management:
   Founder/Agent: Sandra Bernegger
   Administrative Assistant: Linda Van Slyke
   Administrative Assistant: Frances Breslin
Mission: To perform music from Mali, touring with balafon, ngoni, guitar, players and singer, Abdoulaye Diabate.
Founded: 1997
Specialized Field: World Music: Mali
Paid Staff: 4

1546 MATAPAT
517 County Highway 27
Richfield Springs, NY 13439
Phone: 315-858-1434
Fax: 315-858-1434
e-mail: info@onqueuartists.com
Web Site: www.onqueuartists.com
Management:
   Founder/Agent: Sandra Bernegger
   Administrative Assistant: Linda Van Slyke
   Administrative Assistant: Frnaces Breslin
Mission: To perform the traditional music, song and dance of Quebec with contempoary and world music influences.
Founded: 1997
Specialized Field: Music and Dance of Quebec

Paid Staff: 3
Paid Artists: 3

1547 EASTMAN PHILHARMONIA

26 Gibbs Street
Eastman School of Music
Rochester, NY 14604-2599
Phone: 716-274-1110
Fax: 716-274-1110
Management:
  Music Director: Mendi Rodan
  Concert Manager: Andrew Green

1548 GREECE SYMPHONY ORCHESTRA

950 E Avenue
Rochester, NY 14607
Phone: 716-663-4693
Fax: 716-581-1015
Management:
  Director: David Fetler
Mission: Committed to enhancing the cultural life of
Greece and the surrounding area through free concerts and
other performances and to sponsoring young artists
competitions in local schools.
Founded: 1968
Specialized Field: Orchestra
Status: Semi-Professional; Nonprofit
Paid Staff: 65
Income Sources: Greece (NY) Performing Arts Society
Organization Type: Performing; Sponsoring

1549 QUARTET PROGRAM

1163 E Avenue
#4
Rochester, NY 14607
Phone: 585-274-1592
Fax: 585-442-4282
e-mail: ccastleman@aol.com
Web Site: www.quartetprogram.com
Officers:
  Chairman: Joesph Cuningham
Management:
  Director: Charles Castleman
Mission: Develop individual and ensemble skills and
explore group dynamics for the finest preprofessional
musicians.
Founded: 1970
Specialized Field: Instrumental Music
Status: Professional; Nonprofit
Paid Staff: 15
Paid Artists: 8
Non-paid Artists: 40
Performs At: Bucknell Hall
Organization Type: Performing; Resident; Educational;
Sponsoring

1550 ROCHESTER CHAMBER ORCHESTRA

950 E Avenue
Rochester, NY 14607
Phone: 716-473-6711
Fax: 716-271-8879
Web Site: www.rochester.edu/College/MUR/ursourco/
Management:
  Director: David Fetler

Mission: Offering the Rochester community an
outstanding chamber orchestra repertoire from the 17th
century to the present; presenting newly commissioned
works.
Founded: 1964
Specialized Field: Orchestra
Status: Professional; Nonprofit
Performs At: Asbury First Methodist Church
Organization Type: Performing; Sponsoring

1551 SOCIETY FOR CHAMBER MUSIC IN ROCHESTER

PO Box 20715
Rochester, NY 14602
Phone: 716-359-1000
Fax: 716-359-1132
e-mail: hai@eznet.net
Management:
  Manager: Deborah Dunham
Budget: $35,000-60,000
Performs At: Memorial Art Gallery Auditorium; Roberts
Wesleyan Auditorium

1552 SARATOGA PERFORMING ARTS CENTER

Saratoga Spa State Park
Saratoga Springs, NY 12866
Phone: 518-587-9330
Fax: 518-587-3330
e-mail: info@spar.org
Web Site: www.spac.org
Officers:
  Honorary Chairman: Cornelius Whitney
  Chairman: Charles V Wait
  President: Herbert A Chesbrough
  Secretary: Walter M. Jeffords, Jr
  Treasurer: Harold N. Langlitz
Mission: To host performing arts events.
Founded: 1966
Specialized Field: Dance; Vocal Music; Instrumental
Music; Theater; Grand Opera
Status: Professional; Nonprofit
Budget: $11 Million
Income Sources: International Association of Auditorium
Managers; New York Performing Arts Association;
Membership ticket sales
Affiliations: Summer home of New York City Ballet,
Philadelphia Orchestra and Saratoga Chamber Music
Festival
Annual Attendance: 350,000
Facility Category: Ampitheatre
Type of Stage: Proscenium
Stage Dimensions: 80 W x 60 D
Seating Capacity: 5100
Year Built: 1966
Organization Type: Performing; Educational;
Sponsoring

1553 EMPIRE STATE POPS: SYMPHONY AND CHAMBER ORCHESTRA

130 Garth Road
Suite 123
Scarsdale, NY 10583

Phone: 914-723-2694
Fax: 914-723-3460
Management:
    Music Director: Earl Groner
    Executive Director: L Gerald Marshall

1554 STATEN ISLAND SYMPHONY

1 Campus Road
Staten Island, NY 10301
Phone: 718-390-3426
Fax: 718-420-4145
e-mail: sisymphony@aol.com
Officers:
    President: Sandra Sperry
Management:
    Office Manager: Marie Penza
    Executive Director: Elizabeth LaCause
Founded: 1980
Specialized Field: Classical Music
Paid Staff: 3
Volunteer Staff: 20
Paid Artists: 10
Non-paid Artists: 40

1555 ROSEWOOD CHAMBER ENSEMBLE

43-31 39th Street
Sunnyside, NY 11104
Phone: 718-784-6160
Mission: Providing the community with quality classical music and offering musical education to young people.
Founded: 1980
Specialized Field: Chamber; Ensemble
Status: Professional; Nonprofit
Organization Type: Performing; Educational

1556 SYRACUSE FRIENDS OF CHAMBER MUSIC

35 Drumlins Terrace
Syracuse, NY 13224
Phone: 315-446-0994
Fax: 315-446-0994
Web Site: www.syr.edu/arts/chambermusic/
Management:
    Music Director: Henry Palocz
Mission: To provide high quality chamber music concerts to Central New York audiences.
Founded: 1950
Specialized Field: Chamber Music
Volunteer Staff: 10
Budget: $20,000-35,000
Performs At: High School Auditorium

1557 SYRACUSE SYMPHONY ORCHESTRA

411 Montgomery Street
Syracuse, NY 13202
Phone: 315-424-8222
Fax: 315-424-1131
Toll-free: 800-724-3810
e-mail: webmaster@syracusesymphony.org
Web Site: www.syracusesymphony.org
Management:
    Music Director: Daniel Hege
    Resident Conductor: Grant Cooper

Conductor Emeritus: Kazuyoshi Akiyama
Mission: To maintain and further develop a resident, professional symphony orchestra; to produce musical performances of the highest artistic quality; to fulfill the cultural, educational and entertainment needs of the Central and Northern New York communities we serve.
Founded: 1960
Specialized Field: Symphony; Orchestra; Chamber
Status: Professional; Nonprofit
Income Sources: American Symphony Orchestra League; Association of Performing Arts Presenters
Performs At: John H. Mulroy Civic Center
Organization Type: Performing; Touring; Resident; Educational

1558 SYRACUSE SYMPHONY YOUTH ORCHESTRA

411 Montgomery Street
Syracuse, NY 13202
Phone: 315-424-8222
Fax: 315-424-1131
Web Site: www.syracusesymphony.org
Officers:
    Chairman: Dr. Arthur Rosenbaum
Management:
    Conductor: Kenneth Andrews
    Orchestra Manager: Cornelia Brewster
    Education Manager: Cher Leszczewicz
    Youth String/Orchestra Conductor: Muriel Bodley
Founded: 1961
Specialized Field: Symphony; Orchestra
Status: Non-Professional; Nonprofit
Paid Staff: 80
Income Sources: American Symphony Orchestra League (Youth Orchestra Division); Syracuse Symphony Orchestra
Performs At: H.W. Smith Elementary School
Organization Type: Performing; Touring; Resident; Educational

1559 ROCKLAND SUMMER INSTITUTE - ORCHESTRAL & CHAMBER MUSIC STUDIES

PO Box 161
Tallman, NY 10982
Phone: 845-357-7011
Fax: 845-357-7011
e-mail: RSImusic@aol.com
Web Site: www.RSImusic.org
Management:
    Founder/Associate Artistic Director: Dr. Edward Michael Gold

1560 FRIENDS OF CHAMBER MUSIC OF TROY

45 Maple Avenue
Troy, NY 12180-5129
Phone: 518-266-0044
Fax: 518-276-2649
e-mail: herroi@rpi.edu
Web Site: www.friendsofchambermusic.org
Officers:
    President: Isom Herron

Management:
   Programming: Susan Blandy
Founded: 1949
Specialized Field: Calssic Music
Budget: $10,000-20,000
Performs At: Kiggins Hall; Emma Willard School

1561 TROY CHROMATICS CONCERTS
PO Box 1574
Troy, NY 12181
Phone: 518-273-0038
Fax: 518-273-1564
Mission: Providing world class artists and programs to New York State's capital region.
Founded: 1895
Specialized Field: Symphony; Chamber; Ensemble; Soloists
Status: Nonprofit
Performs At: Troy Savings Bank Music Hall
Organization Type: Sponsoring

1562 NASSAU SYMPHONY SOCIETY
185 California Avenue
Uniondale, NY 11553
Phone: 516-565-0646
Fax: 516-481-3382
Management:
   Executive Director: Sherry Smolev
Mission: The performance of the highest quality symphonic music for residents of all ages on Long Island.
Specialized Field: Symphony
Status: Professional; Nonprofit
Performs At: John Cranford Adams Playhouse; Hofstra University
Organization Type: Performing; Educational

1563 CHAMBER MUSIC SOCIETY OF UTICA
310 Genesee Street
Utica, NY 13502
Phone: 315-822-4392
e-mail: jimit@borg.com
Web Site: www.uticachambermusic.org
Management:
   Trustee: James Taylor
   Head Music Selection: Dr. Jon Magendanz
Mission: The presentation of an annual series of high-quality chamber music concerts.
Specialized Field: Chamber music
Status: Nonprofit
Budget: $10,000-$20,000
Performs At: Munson-Williams-Proctor Museum of Art Auditorium
Annual Attendance: 1,200
Facility Category: Arts Museum
Type of Stage: Open
Stage Dimensions: 15x30
Seating Capacity: 271
Year Remodeled: 1992
Organization Type: Presenting

1564 AMHERST SYMPHONY ORCHESTRA
67 Blossom Heath
PO Box 1083
Williamsville, NY 14221
Phone: 716-633-4606
Fax: 716-836-4972
e-mail: SLT@adelphia.net
Web Site: www.amherts.com/AmherstSymphony
Management:
   Music Director: Steven Thomas
   General Manager: Joan E Fishburn
Budget: $35,000- $100,000
Performs At: Amherst Middle School
Seating Capacity: 1475

1565 CHAMBER PLAYERS INTERNATIONAL
45 Crossways Park Boulevard
Woodbury\, NY 11797
Fax: 212-481-7690
Toll-free: 877-444-4488
Performs At: Poway Center for the Performing Arts
Seating Capacity: 850

1566 MAVERICK CONCERTS
PO Box 102
Woodstock, NY 12498
Phone: 845-679-8217
Web Site: www.maverickconcerts.org
Mission: To provide Sunday afternoon chamber music concerts in summer.
Specialized Field: Chamber
Status: Professional; Nonprofit
Performs At: Maverick Concert Hall
Organization Type: Performing

North Carolina

1567 ASHEVILLE CHAMBER MUSIC SERIES
25 Brook Forest Drive
Arden, NC 28704
Mailing Address: PO Box 1003 Arden, NC 28802
Phone: 828-298-5085
e-mail: marybarth@aol.com
Web Site: http://www.main.nc.us
Officers:
   President: Dr. Harold Rotman
   VP: Philip Walker
   Secretary: Perien Gray
   Treasurer: JH Wynn
Management:
   Program Director: Bill van der Hoeven
Mission: To provide chamber music concerts.
Founded: 1952
Specialized Field: Instrumental Music
Status: Non-Professional; Nonprofit
Budget: $10,000-20,000
Income Sources: Chamber Music America
Organization Type: Performing

1568 HOWARD HANGER JAZZ FANTASY
31 Park Avenue N
Asheville, NC 28801

All listings are in alphabetical order by state, then city, then organization within the city.

Phone: 828-254-1174
Fax: 828-254-1174
Toll-free: 800-345-1174
e-mail: info@howardhanger.com
Web Site: www.howardhanger.com
Management:
   Music Director: Howard Hanger
Mission: Performing new age as well as traditional jazz; introducing children aged 6-12 to jazz.
Founded: 1966
Specialized Field: Ensemble; Electronic & Live Electronic
Status: Professional
Paid Artists: 4
Organization Type: Performing; Touring; Educational

1569 MOORE COMMUNITY BAND
Route 1
PO Box 98
Cameron, NC 28326
Phone: 919-245-7267
Management:
   Director: David Sieberling
Mission: Offering the opportunity to perform quality band literature; supporting community programs.
Founded: 1984
Specialized Field: Band
Status: Nonprofit
Paid Staff: 35
Income Sources: Sandhills Arts Council
Performs At: Performing Arts Center
Organization Type: Performing; Resident

1570 CAROLINA PRO MUSICA
PO Box 32022
Charlotte, NC 28232
Phone: 704-334-3468
Fax: 704-333-5239
e-mail: kjacob@vnet.net
Web Site: www.carolinapromusica.org
Officers:
   Executive Director: Karen Hite Jacob
   Education Director: Holly Wright Maurer
   Outreach: Rebecca Miller Saunders
Management:
   Artistic Director: Karen Hite Jacob
   Research: Edward Ferrell
Mission: The performance of music primarily written before 1800 in an historically-correct style, on period instruments.
Founded: 1977
Specialized Field: Early Music ensemble; Medieval trough Baroque; Concerts; Educational Programs.
Status: Professional; Nonprofit
Paid Artists: 4
Budget: $15,000- $20,000
Income Sources: Ticket sales; Education grants; Promoters
Performs At: St. Mary's; St. Martin's
Affiliations: Early Music America
Annual Attendance: 750
Facility Category: Churches. St. Mary's; St. Martin's
Seating Capacity: 125/175
Year Built: 1925
Year Remodeled: 1975

Organization Type: Performing; Touring; Educational; Sponsoring
Resident Groups: Belmont Abbey College, Belmont NC

1571 CHAMBER MUSIC OF CHARLOTTE
2114 Amboy Court
Charlotte, NC 28205
Phone: 704-535-3024
Mission: To foster the composition, performance and enjoyment of chamber music.
Founded: 1977
Specialized Field: Chamber
Status: Professional; Semi-Professional; Nonprofit
Paid Staff: 15
Organization Type: Performing; Educational

1572 CHARLOTTE PHILHARMONIC ORCHESTRA AND CHORUS
PO Box 470987
Charlotte, NC 28247-0987
Phone: 704-846-2788
Fax: 704-847-6043
e-mail: info@charlottephilharmonic.org
Web Site: www.charlottephilharmonic.org
Officers:
   Chairman: Dr. J Arlen Smith
   President: Albert E Moehring
   Treasurer: C Chandler
Management:
   Maestro: Albert E Moehring
   Orchestra Manager: Patricia Moehring
   Choral Director: Marc Setzer
   Administrative Assistant: Barbara Guenzi
Mission: Perform a variety of musical entertainment, classical/popular. Provide educational programming for all ages.
Founded: 1990
Specialized Field: Orchestra; Chorus
Status: Not-for-profit; Professional Symphonic Orchestra; Amateur Volunteer Chorus
Paid Staff: 4
Volunteer Staff: 100
Paid Artists: 125
Budget: $705,000
Income Sources: Box Office, Private Donations, Grants/Gifts
Affiliations: American Symphony Orchestra League, Association of Symphony Orchestras of North Carolina, Chamber of Commerce, Charlotte Convention Center
Annual Attendance: 15-20,000
Facility Category: Performing Arts Center/Concert Hall
Type of Stage: Proscenium
Stage Dimensions: 60 x 30
Seating Capacity: 2,100
Year Built: 1993

1573 CHARLOTTE SYMPHONY
201 S College Street
Suite 110 - College Street Level
Charlotte, NC 28244
Phone: 704-972-2003
Fax: 704-972-2012
e-mail: scottb@charlottesymphony.org
Web Site: www.charlottesymphony.org

Officers:
   Chairperson: Elizabeth J McLughlin
Management:
   Executive Director: Richard L Early
   Music Director: Christof Perick
Founded: 1932
Specialized Field: Symphony; Orchestra; Ensemble
Paid Staff: 25
Budget: $7.1 Million
Income Sources: American Symphony Orchestra
League; Association of Symphony Orchestras of North
Carolina; Arts Advocates of North Carolina
Performs At: North Carolina Blumenthal Performing
Arts Center
Facility Category: Multi-purpose performing arts center
Type of Stage: Proscenium
Stage Dimensions: 55 W x 50 D
Seating Capacity: 2097
Year Built: 1992
Cost: $65 Million
Rental Contact: Booking Manager NC Blumenthal

1574 QUEENS UNIVERSITY: QUEENS FRIENDS OF MUSIC CHAMBER SERIES

1900 Selwyn Avenue
Charlotte, NC 28274
Phone: 704-337-2204
Fax: 704-337-2356
e-mail: deanjm@queens.edu
Web Site: www.queens.edu
Management:
   Artistic Director: Paul Nitsch
Founded: 1983
Specialized Field: Chamber Music
Paid Staff: 1
Volunteer Staff: 28
Paid Artists: 6
Budget: $10,000-20,000
Income Sources: Donations; Ticket Sales
Performs At: Dana Auditorium
Annual Attendance: 1,200
Year Built: 1961
Year Remodeled: 1995

1575 CHAMBER ARTS SOCIETY

PO Box 90685
Duke University
Durham, NC 27708
Phone: 919-660-3356
Fax: 919-660-3381
Management:
   Director: Robert Bryant
   Director Institute of Art, Duke Uni: Kathy Silbiger
Mission: Committed to providing five or six chamber
music concerts of the highest possible quality annually,
with an emphasis on string quartet.
Founded: 1945
Specialized Field: Chamber
Status: Nonprofit
Paid Staff: 2
Volunteer Staff: 6
Budget: $60,000
Income Sources: Tickets Sales; Contributions Institute of
the Arts

Performs At: Bryan Center
Annual Attendance: 3,000
Seating Capacity: 600
Organization Type: Sponsoring

1576 MALLARME CHAMBER PLAYERS

Durham Arts Council
120 Morris Street
Durham, NC 27701
Phone: 919-560-2788
Fax: 919-560-2743
e-mail: mallarme@mindspring.com
Web Site: www.marllarmemusic.org
Officers:
   President: Jimmy Gibbs
   VP: Shelly Green
Management:
   Artistic Director: Anna Ludwig Wilson
   Office Manager: Robin Vail
Mission: To perform concerts that enhance that intamacy
of communication that is the special province of chamber
music, with professional artists featuring all of the
orchestral instruments.
Founded: 1984
Specialized Field: Chamber Music
Paid Staff: 2
Paid Artists: 30
Budget: $150,000
Income Sources: Earned Revenue; Corporate;
Foundations Grants; Individual Donors; Merchandise
Performs At: People Security Insurance Theatre
Affiliations: North Carolina Arts Council
Annual Attendance: 10,000

1577 CUMBERLAND COUNTY FRIENDS OF THE ORCHESTRA

1624 Ireland Drive
Fayetteville, NC 28304
Phone: 910-484-8121
Fax: 910-323-4127
Officers:
   President: David J Phleeger
   Secretary: Rita Warren
   Treasurer: Lynn Gloyeski
Management:
   Orchestra Coordinator: Janice Swoope
Mission: To maintain a community support group for the
Cumberland County School Orchestra Program, lending
volunteer hours and financial aid where needed to
maintain excellence in the program.
Founded: 1980
Specialized Field: Orchestra
Status: Nonprofit
Organization Type: Educational; Sponsoring

1578 HIGHLAND BRITISH BRASS BAND ASSOCIATION

2405 Morganton Road
Fayetteville, NC 28303
Phone: 910-484-0281
Officers:
   Chairman: Robert Downing

Mission: To provide suitable outlet for musically talented adults who are interested in promoting good band music in the British Brass Band format for the instruction and edification of the general public.
Founded: 1980
Specialized Field: Band
Status: Semi-Professional; Nonprofit
Income Sources: Arts Council of Fayetteville & Cumberland County
Performs At: Methodist College
Organization Type: Performing

1579 GREENSBORO SYMPHONY ORCHESTRA

200 N Davie Street, Suite 328
PO Box 20303
Greensboro, NC 27420
Phone: 336-335-5456
Fax: 336-335-5580
e-mail: gsoadmin@mindspring.com
Web Site: www.greensborosymphony.org/home.html
Officers:
President: Robert Lavietas
Librarian: Erik Salzwedel
Management:
Music Director: Barry Auman
Music Director: Stuart Malina
Executive Director: Lisa Crawford
Mission: To strive seriously for the highest quality of performance, with the ultimate goal of attaining a truly professional sound, the love of playing orchestral literature remaining the prime factor for participation.
Founded: 1977
Specialized Field: Orchestra
Status: Professional
Income Sources: City of Greensboro
Performs At: War Memorial Auditorium
Organization Type: Performing

1580 PHILHARMONIA OF GREENSBORO

200 N Davie Street, Box 2
The Music Center, City Arts
Greensboro, NC 27401
Phone: 336-373-2549
Fax: 336-373-2659
Management:
Music Director: Robert Gutter
Executive Director: Lynn H Donovan

1581 SUMMER STRINGS ON THE MEHERRIN

303 S Elm Street
Greenville, NC 27858
Phone: 919-752-2542
Officers:
President: John R Kernodle, Jr
Secretary: Angela Seawell
Management:
Music Director: Paul Topper
Chowan College Officer: James Chamblee
Mission: Summer Strings on the Meherrin offers a three-week program for 12 to 18-year-old bowed string players to improve their musicianship and techniques and to present chamber music concerts.
Founded: 1972

Specialized Field: Chamber; Ensemble
Status: Nonprofit
Income Sources: Chowan College
Performs At: Daniels Hall; Chowan College
Organization Type: Performing; Resident; Educational

1582 HENDERSONVILLE SYMPHONY ORCHESTRA

HS Auditorium 800
PO Box 1811
Hendersonville, NC 28793
Phone: 828-697-5884
Fax: 828-697-5765
e-mail: hso@brinet.com
Web Site: www.hendersonvillesymphony.org
Officers:
President: Lynn Kitts
VP: Tom Sauter
Management:
Music Director: Dr. Thomas Joiner
Manager: Sandie Salvaggio-Walker
Orchestra: Candace Norton
Founded: 1971
Paid Staff: 4
Paid Artists: 65
Budget: $211,000

1583 WESTERN PIEDMONT SYMPHONY

243 3rd Avenue NE
Suite 1-N
Hickory, NC 28601
Phone: 828-324-8603
Fax: 828-324-1301
e-mail: wpsymphony@charles.net
Web Site: www.wpsymphony.org
Officers:
President: Adam Neilly
Treasurer: Lynn Loehr
Secretary: Nancy Rockett
Management:
Music Director/Conductor: John G Ross
Executive Director: Frances Balcher
Business Manager: Rochelle Hull
Founded: 1964
Income Sources: Unifour; Fund-raisers
Performs At: P.E. Monroe Auditorium

1584 SMOKY MOUNTAIN BRITISH BRASS

PO Box 1467
Lake Juanaluska, NC 28745
Phone: 828-253-6842
e-mail: smbrass@asapgroup.com
Web Site: http://www.smbrass.com
Management:
General Manager: Bert Wiley
Artistic Director: Dr. William Bryant
Mission: Offering quality music for brass band covering all artists and eras.
Founded: 1981
Specialized Field: Chamber; Band
Status: Semi-Professional
Organization Type: Performing; Touring; Educational

1585 TRINKLE BRASS WORKS

803 W 24th Street
Lumberton, NC 28358
Phone: 919-671-4556
Officers:
President: Steven Trinkle
VP: Genie Burkett
Secretary: Dr. Alan Kalkor
Treasurer: Joel Gordon
Mission: Established in 1977 to provide art centers, universities and schools with concerts and lecture-recitals in brass and percussion chamber music. Concerts include performances on Renaissance, Baroque and modern instruments.
Founded: 1977
Specialized Field: Chamber; Ensemble; Instrumental Group
Status: Professional; Nonprofit
Income Sources: Wisconsin Arts Board
Organization Type: Performing; Touring; Resident; Educational

1586 NORTH CAROLINA SYMPHONY

2 E South Street
Raleigh, NC 27601
Phone: 919-733-2750
Fax: 919-733-9920
e-mail: tickets@ncsymphony.org
Web Site: www.ncsymphony.org
Officers:
Chairman: William P Furr
Vice Chairman: Henry Mitchell
Secretary: Carolyn Turner
Treasurer: Wade Reece
Management:
Music Director/Conductor: Gerhardt Zimmermann
Artistic VP: Scott Freck
Assistant Conductor: Jeffrey. Pollock
Stage Manager: Granville H Spry, III
Assistant Stage Manager: Prentis Lambert
Mission: Presenting live orchestral music for residents of North Carolina; providing music education programs in the schools.
Founded: 1932
Specialized Field: Symphony; Orchestra; Chamber; Ensemble
Status: Professional; Nonprofit
Budget: $8.4 Million
Income Sources: American Symphony Orchestra League
Organization Type: Performing; Touring; Resident; Educational; Sponsoring

1587 RALEIGH RINGERS

8516 Sleepy Creek Drive
Raleigh, NC 27613
Phone: 919-847-7574
Fax: 919-847-7574
Web Site: www.rr.org
Management:
Director: David M Harris
Honorary Associate Director: Fred Gramann
Artistic Consultant: Dr. William A Payn
Status: Nonprofit

1588 RALEIGH SYMPHONY ORCHESTRA

Long View Center
119 S Pason Street, PO Box 25878
Raleigh, NC 27611-5878
Phone: 919-546-9755
Fax: 919-546-0251
Web Site: raleighsymphony.com
Management:
Music Director: Alan Neilson
Executive Director: Rachel M Parnell
Founded: 1979
Specialized Field: Music

1589 TAR RIVER CHORAL & ORCHESTRAL SOCIETY

The Dunn Center 1200
PO Box 8255
Rocky Mount, NC 27804
Phone: 252-985-3055
Web Site: www.abouttroc.org
Management:
Music Director/Conductor: Lorenzo Muti
General Manager: Beth Kupsco

1590 SALISBURY SYMPHONY ORCHESTRA

PO Box 4264
Salisbury, NC 28145
Phone: 704-637-4314
Fax: 704-637-4268
e-mail: mshives@catawba.edu
Web Site: www.ci.salisbury.nc.us/symphony
Officers:
President: Martha West
VP: Jean Owen
Secretary: Judy Robinson
Management:
Music Director/Conductor: David Hagyes
Mission: Performing symphonic music and increasing musical appreciation in the area; offering four full concerts annually, including one free concert for youth.
Founded: 1966
Specialized Field: Symphony; Orchestra
Status: Professional; Nonprofit
Paid Staff: 3
Paid Artists: 70
Budget: $241,900
Income Sources: Ticket Sales; Program Ads; Sponsorships; Contributions
Performs At: Varick Auditorium; Livingstone College
Seating Capacity: 1,500
Year Built: 1964
Organization Type: Performing; Educational

1591 PADDYWHACK

Route 2
PO Box 60
Tryon, NC 28782
Phone: 704-894-8091
Mission: Playing and promoting 16th-19th century popular music.
Founded: 1978
Specialized Field: Ensemble; Ethnic; Folk; Band
Status: Semi-Professional
Income Sources: Schiele Museum

Organization Type: Performing; Touring; Educational

1592 WILMINGTON SYMPHONY ORCHESTRA

4608 Cedar Avenue
Suite 105
Wilmington, NC 28403
Phone: 910-791-9262
Fax: 910-791-8970
Web Site: www.wilmingtonsymphony.org
Officers:
President: John R Stike
Treasurer: Ralph Godwin
Management:
Executive Director: Reed M Wallace
Mission: To provide music of the highest integrity and performance quality to the community.
Founded: 1971
Specialized Field: Symphony
Status: Non-Professional; Nonprofit
Paid Staff: 3
Budget: $250,000
Income Sources: Box office; Private donations; Grants
Performs At: Kenan Auditorium
Annual Attendance: 6,000
Seating Capacity: 987
Organization Type: Performing; Educational

1593 NORTH CAROLINA SCHOOL OF THE ARTS SYMPHONY ORCHESTRA

North Carolina School of the Arts
School of Music, 15335 Main Street
Winston-Salem, NC 27127
Phone: 336-770-3255
Fax: 336-770-3248
e-mail: suemiller@ncarts.com
Web Site: www.ncarts.edu/
Management:
Conductor: Serge Zehnacker
Dean: Robert Yekovich
Founded: 1963

1594 WAKE FOREST UNIVERSITY SYMPHONY ORCHESTRA

Reynolda Station
Box 7345
Winston-Salem, NC 27109
Phone: 336-758-5100
Fax: 336-758-4935
e-mail: dhagy@wfu.edu
Management:
Conductor: Dr. David Hagy

1595 WINSTON-SALEM PIEDMONT TRIAD SYMPHONY ASSOCIATION

610 Coliseum Drive
Winston-Salem, NC 27106
Phone: 336-725-1035
Fax: 336-725-3924
e-mail: mvale@wssymphony.org
Web Site: www.wssymphony.org
Officers:
Operations/Stage Manager: Beverley Naiditch

Financial Manager: Selina Carter
Management:
Executive Director: E Merritt Vale
Music Director: Peter Perret
Director Marketing Development: William Cole
Box Office Manager: Tinay Jeffers
Mission: Presenting the finest symphonic as well as choral literature; providing high quality music education for Winston-Salem and Forsythe County children.
Founded: 1947
Specialized Field: Symphony; Orchestra; Chamber; Ensemble
Status: Professional; Nonprofit
Paid Staff: 9
Paid Artists: 80
Budget: $1.4 million
Income Sources: American Symphony Orchestra League; Broadcast Music Incorporated; American Society of Composers, Authors and Publishers; Association of Symphony Orchestras of North Carolina
Performs At: E. Stevens Center for the Performing Arts
Annual Attendance: 100,000
Seating Capacity: 1,380
Year Remodeled: 1985
Organization Type: Performing; Resident; Educational

North Dakota

1596 BISMARCK-MANDAN ORCHESTRAL ASSOCIATION

215 N 6th Street
Bismarck, ND 58501
Phone: 701-258-8345
Fax: 701-258-8345
e-mail: lundberg@tic.bisman.com
Web Site: www.bmso.net
Officers:
President: William Pearce
Treasurer: Al Wolf
Treasurer: Richard Weber
Management:
Executive Director: Susan Lundberg
Music Director: Thomas Wellin
Mission: To share orchestral music and educational programs of all kinds with the public in many venues.
Founded: 1975
Specialized Field: Symphony; Orchestra; Instrumental Group
Status: Nonprofit
Paid Staff: 3
Volunteer Staff: 200
Paid Artists: 70
Budget: $300,000
Income Sources: Private; Corporate; Grants
Performs At: Belle Mehus City Auditorium
Annual Attendance: 4,000
Facility Category: Auditorium
Type of Stage: Conventional
Stage Dimensions: 40 x 60
Seating Capacity: 836
Year Built: 1914
Year Remodeled: 1997
Cost: 32.5 Million

Organization Type: Performing

1597 GREATER GRAND FORKS SYMPHONY ORCHESTRA

PO Box 7084
Grand Forks, ND 58202-7084
Phone: 701-777-3359
Fax: 701-777-3320
e-mail: ggfso@und.nodake.edu
Management:
   Music Director: Timm Rolek
   Executive Director: Jennifer Elting
   Theatre Symphony Music Director: James Popejoy
Mission: The greater Grand Forks Symphony Association is a regional center for classical music performance and education.
Paid Staff: 3
Paid Artists: 50
Non-paid Artists: 10

1598 INTERNATIONAL MUSIC CAMP

1725 11th Street SW
Minot, ND 58701
Phone: 701-838-8472
Fax: 701-838-8472
e-mail: info@internationalmusiccamp.com
Web Site: www.internationalmusiccamp.com
Officers:
   President: Vern Gerig
   VP: Clifford Grubb
   Secretary: Roy Johnson
   Treasurer: Randy Hall
Management:
   Camp Director: Joseph T Alme
Mission: To develop a greater appreciation among students of all nations through their mutual interest in the arts.
Founded: 1956
Specialized Field: Band choral, Piano, Jazz (vocal and instrumental), Dance, Chamber Music, Orchestra (Full and Strings only) and visual Arts.
Status: Professional; Semi-Professional; Non-Professional; Nonprofit
Paid Staff: 250
Volunteer Staff: 25
Paid Artists: 150
Budget: $600,000
Income Sources: Camp Fees
Performs At: International Music Camp
Annual Attendance: 3,000
Facility Category: Open Auditorium; Performing Arts Center
Stage Dimensions: 60' x 100'
Seating Capacity: 2000; 500
Year Built: 1982
Year Remodeled: 1999
Cost: $1,500,000
Rental Contact: Joseph T Alme
Organization Type: Performing; Resident; Educational

1599 MINOT SYMPHONY ASSOCIATION

500 University Avenue W
Minot, ND 58707
Phone: 701-858-4228
Fax: 701-858-3823
Web Site: warp6.cs.misu.nodak.edu/music/mso/
Officers:
   President: Lou Whitmer
   Treasurer: David Herzig
   Conductor: Dr. Daniel Hornstein
Mission: To foster and perpetuate the Minot Symphony Orchestra, a college-community orchestra.
Founded: 1965
Specialized Field: Symphony; Orchestra
Status: Professional; Nonprofit
Paid Staff: 70
Income Sources: North Dakota Council of Arts; Minot Area Council of Arts; North Dakota Arts Alliance; American Symphony Orchestra League; National Endowment for the Arts
Performs At: McFarland Auditorium
Organization Type: Performing; Resident

Ohio

1600 AKRON SYMPHONY ORCHESTRA

17 N Broadway
Akron, OH 44308
Phone: 330-535-8131
Fax: 330-535-7302
e-mail: generalinformation@arkonsymphony.org
Web Site: www.akronsymphony.org
Officers:
   President: Richard Kemph
Management:
   Executive Director: Jeffrey K Sperry
   Director Marketing/Public Relations: Wendy Turrell
Mission: To provide the community with the finest quality symphonic and choral music; to educate the local public with respect to classical and contemporary music; and to extend special support to worthy local individual artists and projects.
Founded: 1949
Specialized Field: Instrumental Music; Vocal Music
Status: Professional; Nonprofit
Paid Staff: 8
Volunteer Staff: 2
Paid Artists: 83
Budget: $1.2 million
Income Sources: American Symphony Orchestra League; Ohio Arts Council; Private/Corporate Donations; Grants; Funding
Performs At: E.J. Thomas Performing Arts Hall
Facility Category: University Performing Arts Hall
Seating Capacity: 3,000
Organization Type: Performing; Educational

1601 AKRON YOUTH SYMPHONY ORCHESTRA

17 N Broadway
Akron, OH 44308-1946
Phone: 330-535-8131
Fax: 330-535-7302
e-mail: WTurrell@akronsymphony.org
Web Site: www.akronsymphony.org
Management:

Music Director/Conductor: Ya-Hui Wang
Executive Director: Jeffrey K Sperry
Director Marketing: Wendy A Turrell
Founded: 1949
Specialized Field: Symphony; Orchestra; Youth Symphony; Chorus
Status: Professional; Nonprofit
Paid Staff: 75
Income Sources: Akron Symphony Orchestra; American Symphony Orchestra League (Youth Orchestra Division)
Performs At: E.J. Thomas Performing Arts Hall
Organization Type: Performing; Educational; Sponsoring

1602 ASHLAND SYMPHONY ORCHESTRA
PO Box 13
Ashland, OH 44805
Phone: 419-289-5115
Fax: 419-289-5329
e-mail: symphony@ashland.edu
Officers:
President: Annette Shaw
VP: Julia Wright
Secretary: Ann Gutherie
Treasurer: Don Eiserling
Management:
General Manager: Lawrence Hiner
Music Director/Conductor: Arie Lipsky
Office Manager: Linda Workman
Personnel/Production Manager: Ron Marenchin
Mission: Offering symphonic orchestra programs to all residents of Ashland as well as the surrounding area.
Founded: 1970
Specialized Field: Symphony; Orchestra
Status: Semi-Professional; Nonprofit
Volunteer Staff: 35
Paid Artists: 7
Budget: $155,000
Income Sources: Box Office; Private Donations; Business Donations
Performs At: Hugo Young Theatre
Affiliations: American Symphony Orchestra League
Annual Attendance: 3,500-6,000
Organization Type: Performing; Educational

1603 ASHTABULA CHAMBER ORCHESTRA
3325 W 13th Street
Ashtabula, OH 44004
Mailing Address: PO Box 415 Ashtabula, OH 44005
Phone: 440-964-3322
e-mail: hdra!alltel.net
Web Site: www.ashtabulaareaorchestra.com
Officers:
President: Joesph Petros
VP: May Lou Jaskela
Treasurer: Betty Heitikko
Secretary: Dianne Lahti
Management:
Music Director: Michael Gelfand
Mission: To educate the people of the area in all types of stringed music; to provide string ensemble music for public enjoyment; to encourage young people on strings.
Founded: 1982
Specialized Field: Orchestra; Chamber
Status: Non-Professional; Nonprofit

Paid Staff: 35
Income Sources: Kent State University; Ashtabula Campus
Performs At: Kent State University Auditorium; Ashtabula Campus
Organization Type: Performing; Resident

1604 CLEVELAND POPS ORCHESTRA
24000 Mercantile Road
Unit 10
Beachwood, OH 44122
Phone: 216-765-7677
Fax: 216-765-1931
e-mail: morgenstern@clevelandpops.com
Web Site: www.clevelandpops.com
Management:
Music Director: Carl Topilow
Executive Director: Shirley Morganstern
Marketing Director: Gordon Petitt
Mission: To present pops music of the highest artistic quality that is entertaining and exciting to a wide and diverse audience.
Founded: 1994

1605 OHIO CHAMBER ORCHESTRA
3659 Green Road #118
Beachwood, OH 44122
Phone: 216-464-1755
Fax: 216-464-8628
e-mail: oco@ix.netcom.com
Officers:
President: Paul R Bunker
Chairman Executive Committee: William Steffee MD
Executive Vice Chairman: Robert H Jackson
Treasurer: James E. Wilcosky
Secretary: Martha Vail
President Ohio Chamber Orchestra: Norma Glazer
Management:
Executive Director: Eugenia L Epperson
Mission: To perform at the highest artistic level possible programs specializing in works written specifically for chamber orchestra in appropriate (intimate) settings, featuring soloists of local and international standing.
Founded: 1972
Specialized Field: Symphony; Orchestra; Chamber; Ensemble
Status: Professional
Performs At: The Cleveland Play House
Organization Type: Performing; Touring; Resident

1606 SUBURBAN SYMPHONY ORCHESTRA
PO Box 22653
Beachwood, OH 44122
Phone: 216-449-2389
Management:
Music Director: Martin Kessler
General Manager: Paul Pride
Mission: To offer accomplished professionals and nonprofessionals an opportunity to be part of a symphony orchestra; to present five free concerts each season.
Founded: 1954
Specialized Field: Symphony; Orchestra

Status: Professional; Semi-Professional; Non-Professional; Nonprofit
Paid Staff: 70
Performs At: Beachwood High School Auditorium
Organization Type: Performing

1607 BALDWIN-WALLACE COLLEGE SYMPHONY ORCHESTRA

275 Eastland Road
Fanny Nast Gamble Auditorium 650
Berea, OH 44017
Phone: 440-826-2362
Fax: 440-826-3239
Web Site: www.bw.edu
Management:
   Conductor: Dwight Ottman
   Conservatory of Music Director: Dr. Catherine Jarjisian

1608 VENTI DA CAMERA

Bowling Green State University
Bowling Green, OH 43403
Phone: 419-372-2955
Fax: 419-372-2938
Management:
   Oboe/College Musical Arts: John Bentley
   Flute/College Musical Arts: Christina Jennings
   Clarinet; College of Musical Arts: Kevin Schempf
   Bassoon College of Musical Arts: Winston Collier
   Horn; College of Musical Arts: Rosemary Williams
Mission: Presenting works composed for wind quintet as well as other ensembles and offering a wide-ranging repertoire to a broad audience.
Founded: 1965
Specialized Field: Chamber; Woodwind Quintet
Status: Professional
Income Sources: Bowling Green State University College of Music
Performs At: Bryan Recital Hall
Annual Attendance: 800
Facility Category: Recital Hall
Stage Dimensions: 50'x30'
Seating Capacity: 250
Year Built: 1976
Organization Type: Performing; Touring; Resident; Educational

1609 CANTON SYMPHONY ORCHESTRA

1001 Market Avenue N
Canton, OH 44702-1024
Phone: 330-452-3434
Fax: 330-452-4429
e-mail: lmoorhouse@cantonsymphony.org
Web Site: www.cantonsymphony.org
Officers:
   President: Robert L Leibeusperger
Management:
   Executive Director: Linda V Moorhouse
   Music Director: Gerhardt Zimmerman
Mission: To maintain an orchestra of the highest quality as a cultural and educational resource and to bring the enjoyment and enrichment of great music to increasing numbers of citizens in Northeastern Ohio.
Founded: 1937

Specialized Field: Symphony; Orchestra; Chamber; Ensemble
Status: Professional; Nonprofit
Paid Staff: 5
Paid Artists: 17
Income Sources: American Symphony Orchestra League
Performs At: William E. Umstattd Performing Arts Hall
Seating Capacity: 1490
Year Built: 1976
Organization Type: Performing

1610 CANTON YOUTH SYMPHONY

1001 North Market Avenue
Canton, OH 44702
Phone: 330-452-3434
Fax: 330-452-4429
Management:
   Manager: Linda V Moorhouse
   Conductor: John Russo
Founded: 1962
Specialized Field: Symphony; Orchestra
Status: Non-Professional; Nonprofit
Income Sources: American Symphony Orchestra League (Youth Orchestra Division); Canton Symphony Orchestra
Performs At: Fine and Professional Arts Building
Organization Type: Performing; Educational; Sponsoring

1611 DAYTON CLASSICAL GUITAR SOCIETY

8530 Cherrycreek Drive
Centerville, OH 45458
Phone: 937-435-1858
e-mail: music@mccutcheon.com
Officers:
   President: Jim McCutcheon
Founded: 1975
Budget: $1,000
Annual Attendance: 500-700
Seating Capacity: 175

1612 CCM PHILHARMONIA & CONCERT ORCHESTRA

College-Conservatory of Music
PO Box 210003
Cincinnati, OH 45221-0003
Phone: 513-556-9420
Fax: 513-556-2698
e-mail: gibsonmi@email.uc.edu
Management:
   Music Director: Mark Gibson
   Assistant Dean Performance Mgmt: Katherine Mohylsky

1613 CINCINNATI CHAMBER ORCHESTRA

1406 Elm Street
Cincinnati, OH 45202-7517
Phone: 513-723-1182
Fax: 513-723-1057
e-mail: cco@one.net
Web Site: w3.one.net/~cco
Officers:
   President/CEO: Robert Chavez
   VP: Larry Olivier

Secretary: Florence Koetters
Treasurer: Bill Riggs
Management:
    Executive Director: David Steele]
    Operations Manager: Berton Herrlinger
    Music Director: Mischa Santora
Mission: To bring to the stage repertoire ranging from legendary masterpieces to exhilarating premieres.
Founded: 1974
Paid Staff: 3
Paid Artists: 32
Budget: $325,000
Organization Type: Performing; Touring; Educational

1614 CINCINNATI ORCHESTRA

1621 Laval Drive
Cincinnati, OH 45255
Phone: 513-474-1584
Fax: 513-474-1584
e-mail: pstanbery@rml.net
Web Site: www.hfso.org
Management:
    Music Director: Paul Stanbery
Mission: Presentation of symphonic concerts, educational activities and pops.
Paid Staff: 4
Volunteer Staff: 16
Paid Artists: 75

1615 CINCINNATI SYMPHONY AND POPS ORCHESTRA

1241 Elm Street
Cincinnati, OH 45210
Phone: 513-621-1919
Fax: 513-744-3535
Web Site: www.cincinnatisymphony.org
Officers:
    Chairman: Daniel J Hoffheimer
    Vice Chair: James B Reynolds
    President: Steven Monder
    Secretary: J Marvin Quin II
    Treasurer: Marilyn J Osborn
    Immediate Past Chairman: Peter S Strange
Management:
    General Manager: Janell Weinstock
    Orchestra Manager: David A Crane
    Marketing Director: Dianne L Cooper
    Public Relations Director: Rosemary Weathers
    Finance Director: Donald C Auberger Jr
    Development Director: Kenneth A Goode
Mission: To establish life-long relationships with the community, promoting active participation in music; and to encourage participants to listen, appreciate, advocate, perform, volunteer and contribute.
Founded: 1895
Specialized Field: Vocal Music; Instrumental Music
Status: Professional; Nonprofit
Performs At: Music Halland
Organization Type: Sponsoring

1616 CINCINNATI SYMPHONY YOUTH ORCHESTRA

1241 Elm Street
Music Hall
Cincinnati, OH 45210
Phone: 513-621-1919
Fax: 513-744-3535
Management:
    Educational Activities Manager: Anne Cushing-Reid

1617 CLASSICAL PIANO SERIES

Xavier University
3800 Victoria Parkway
Cincinnati, OH 45207-2717
Phone: 513-745-3161
Fax: 513-745-2083
e-mail: heim@admin.xu.edu
Web Site: www.xu.edu
Management:
    Director: Father Jack Heim
Budget: $20,000-35,000
Performs At: University Center Theatre
Seating Capacity: 395

1618 CLERMONT PHILHARMONIC

1621 Laval Drive
Cincinnati, OH 45255
Phone: 513-732-2561
Fax: 513-474-1584
e-mail: pstanbery@rml.net
Management:
    Music Director: Paul Stanbery
    General Manager: Angelo Santoro

1619 JAZZ GUITAR SERIES

Xavier University
3800 Victoria Parkway
Cincinnati, OH 45207-2717
Phone: 513-745-3161
Fax: 513-745-2083
e-mail: heim@admin.xu.edu
Web Site: www.xu.edu
Management:
    Director: Father Jack Heim
Budget: $20,000-35,000
Performs At: University Center Theatre
Seating Capacity: 395

1620 JAZZ PIANO SERIES

Xavier University
3800 Victoria Parkway
Cincinnati, OH 45207-2717
Phone: 513-745-3161
Fax: 513-745-2083
e-mail: heim@admin.xu.edu
Web Site: www.xu.edu
Management:
    Director: Father Jack Heim
Budget: $20,000-35,000
Performs At: University Center Theatre
Seating Capacity: 395

1621 LINTON CHAMBER MUSIC SERIES/ENCORE!
1223 Central Parkway
Cincinnati, OH 45214
Phone: 513-381-6868
Fax: 513-381-6888
e-mail: lintoninc@aol.com
Web Site: www.wguc.org/linton
Management:
    Artistic Director: Richard Waller
    Executive Director: Anne Black
Budget: $20,000-35,000
Performs At: First Unitarian Church; Cinicinnati City Council Chambers

1622 CLEVELAND CHAMBER SYMPHONY
2001 Euclid Avenue
Cleveland, OH 44115
Phone: 216-687-9243
Fax: 216-687-9279
e-mail: ccscsu@csuohio.edu
Web Site: www.csuohio.edu/ccs
Officers:
    Managing Director: Stephen Olans
    Administrative Coordinator: Jeff Zdanowicz
    Personnel Manager: James Taylor
Management:
    Artistic Director/Founder: Dr. Edwin London
    Associate Conductor: Andrew Rindfleisch
    Program Annotator: Robert Finn
Mission: Works to commission, perform, record and promote the dissemination of musical works exclusively by composters of our time.
Founded: 1980
Paid Staff: 3
Paid Artists: 37
Budget: $400,000 - 500,000
Income Sources: Individuals; Government & Distinguished Private Foundations; Ohio Arts Council
Performs At: Drinko Recital Hall
Affiliations: National Endowment for the Arts; The Ohio Arts Council; The Ohio Board of Regents; The Cleveland Foundation; The George Gund Foundation
Annual Attendance: 2,700 - 3,300
Facility Category: Recital Hall
Type of Stage: Proscenium
Seating Capacity: 300
Year Built: 1990
Rental Contact: Facilities Coordinator Toni Lovejoy

1623 CLEVELAND INSTITUTE OF MUSIC
11021 E Boulevard
Cleveland, OH 44106
Phone: 216-791-5000
Fax: 216-791-3063
e-mail: cimmktg@po.cwro.edu
Web Site: www.cim.edu
Officers:
    President: David Cerone
Management:
    Director Marketing/Communications: Susan M Schwartz
Mission: To provide talented students with a professional, world-class education in the art of music.

Founded: 1920
Specialized Field: Music
Paid Staff: 65
Paid Artists: 180
Budget: $13,175,000
Affiliations: Cleveland International Piano Competition; Art Song Festival; Western Reserve University
Annual Attendance: 47,000
Facility Category: Music
Seating Capacity: 550
Year Built: 1961
Rental Contact: Lori Wright
Resident Groups: Faculty and Student Performers

1624 CLEVELAND JAZZ ORCHESTRA
PO Box 31666
Cleveland, OH 44131
Phone: 216-524-2263
Fax: 216-524-8349
Web Site: www.clevelandjazz.org
Officers:
    President: Jill Brotman
    VP: Jim Remond
Management:
    Managing Director: Larry Patch Paciorek
    Music Director: Jack Schantz
Mission: To establish Cleveland Jazz Orchestra in Northeast Ohio; to enhance availability and quality of jazz; to assist in educating young musicians; to encourage involvement and training of minority musicians.
Founded: 1985
Specialized Field: Ensemble; Instrumental Group; Band
Status: Professional; Nonprofit
Paid Staff: 2
Volunteer Staff: 6
Paid Artists: 80
Income Sources: Cuyahoga Community College; Northeast Ohio Jazz Society; Cleveland Playhouse
Annual Attendance: 5,000
Organization Type: Performing; Resident; Educational; Sponsoring

1625 CLEVELAND OCTET
1510 Crest Road
Cleveland, OH 44121
Phone: 216-381-9031
Fax: 216-291-0502
Officers:
    Founder/Director: Erich Eichhorn
Management:
    Columbia Artist Management, NY:
Mission: To present and perform rarely performed masterpieces for ensembles of six to eight players.
Founded: 1977
Specialized Field: Chamber; Ensemble
Status: Professional; Nonprofit
Income Sources: Cleveland Museum of Art; Cleveland Orchestra
Performs At: Cleveland Museum of Art
Organization Type: Performing; Touring

1626 CLEVELAND ORCHESTRA
11001 Euclid Avenue
Severance Hall
Cleveland, OH 44106
Phone: 216-231-7372
Fax: 216-231-0202
e-mail: info@clevelandorchestra.com
Web Site: www.clevelandorch.org
Officers:
   Chairman: Larry Milder
Management:
   Executive Director: Reobert Porco
   Music Director: Christoph Von Dohnanyi
   Manager: Nancy Bell Cue
   Director Choruses: Robert Porco
   Concert Master: William Preucil
Founded: 1918
Specialized Field: Symphony; Orchestra; Ensemble
Status: Professional; Nonprofit; Semi-Volunteer
Paid Staff: 6
Volunteer Staff: 168
Income Sources: American Symphony Orchestra League
Performs At: Severence Hall; Blossom Music Center
Organization Type: Performing; Touring; Resident;
Educational; Sponsoring

1627 CLEVELAND ORCHESTRA YOUTH ORCHESTRA
11001 Euclid Avenue
Severance Hall
Cleveland, OH 44106-1796
Phone: 216-231-7352
Fax: 216-231-4077
e-mail: chaff@clevelandorchestra.com
Web Site: www.clevelandorch.com
Management:
   Music Director: Steven Smith
   Manager: Christine Haff-Paluck
Founded: 1985
Specialized Field: Northern Ohio
Paid Staff: 1
Paid Artists: 1

1628 CLEVELAND PHILHARMONIC ORCHESTRA
8702 Bessemer Avenue
PO Box 16251
Cleveland, OH 44116
Phone: 216-556-1800
Management:
   General Manager: Martha Hamilton
   Music Director/Conductor: William B Slocum
Mission: Providing performances of quality at reasonable
ticket prices; to train aspiring musicians; to offer
musicians a technical education.
Founded: 1938
Specialized Field: Symphony; Orchestra
Status: Semi-Professional; Nonprofit
Paid Staff: 60
Income Sources: American Symphony Orchestra
League; Saint Vincent Quadrangle Association
Performs At: Cuyahoga Community College
Organization Type: Performing; Resident; Sponsoring

1629 NORTHEAST OHIO JAZZ SOCIETY
4614 Prospect Avenue
#533
Cleveland, OH 44103-4393
Phone: 216-426-9900
Fax: 216-426-9906
Web Site: www.nojs.org
Budget: $60,000-150,000

1630 SHAKER SYMPHONY ORCHESTRA
27090 Cedar Road
Stone Gardens
Cleveland, OH 44122
Phone: 216-378-1801
Management:
   Conductor: Dr. J Layne

1631 TRINITY CHAMBER ORCHESTRA
2021 E 22nd Street
Cleveland, OH 44115-2489
Phone: 216-579-9745
Fax: 216-771-3657
e-mail: mpainc@aol.com
Management:
   Personal Manager: Sandra Baxter
Performs At: Trinity Cathedral

1632 UNIVERSITY CIRCLE CHAMBER ORCHESTRA
Music Department
Case Western Reserve University
Cleveland, OH 44106
Phone: 216-368-2400
Fax: 216-368-6557
Web Site:
www.cwru.edu/artsci/musc/ensembles/orchestra.
Management:
   Music Department Case Western Rese:
Mission: Offering an opportunity to university students as
well as interested amateurs, to perform stimulating
repertoire in a pleasant but serious atmosphere.
Specialized Field: Symphony; Orchestra; Chamber;
Ensemble; Instrumental Group
Status: Non-Professional; Nonprofit
Paid Staff: 18
Income Sources: Case Western Reserve University
Performs At: Harkness Chapel
Organization Type: Performing; Resident; Educational

1633 CLEVELAND CHAMBER MUSIC SOCIETY
1991 Lee Road
Suite 205
Cleveland Heights, OH 44118
Phone: 216-371-3071
Fax: 216-371-5415
Web Site: www.clevelandchambermusic.org
Founded: 1949
Paid Staff: 1
Budget: $60,000-150,000
Income Sources: Ticket Sales; Endowment
Performs At: Fairmount Temple Auditorium; Church of
the Convenant

Annual Attendance: 2,800
Facility Category: Rent
Seating Capacity: 736

1634 HEIGHTS CHAMBER ORCHESTRA

PO Box 18413
Cleveland Heights, OH 44118
Phone: 216-921-4339
Fax: 440-775-8886
e-mail: susanblackwell@hotmail.com
Web Site: http://members.core.com/15/CA/gh461/hco
Officers:
  President: Susan Blackwell
  VP: Sue Schieman
  Treasurer: Marlene Englander
  Secretary: Carl Boyd
Management:
  Concert Master: Gino Raffaeli
  Conductor: John Fioritto
Mission: To provide the community with an orchestra and the schools with music education.
Founded: 1983
Specialized Field: Symphony; Orchestra
Status: Nonprofit
Paid Staff: 52
Income Sources: Cleveland Heights Board of Education; Cleveland Heights Parks & Recreation Department
Performs At: Performing Arts Center; Cleveland Heights High School
Organization Type: Performing

1635 COLUMBUS CHAMBER MUSIC SOCIETY

PO Box 14445
Columbus, OH 43214
Phone: 614-267-2267
e-mail: info@columbuschambermusic.org
Web Site: www.columbuschambermusic.org
Officers:
  President: Ivan Mueller
  VP: Robert Wilhelm
  Secretary: Sally Cleary Griffiths
  Treasurer: John Dickinson
Status: Non Profit
Budget: $35,000-60,000
Seating Capacity: 500

1636 COLUMBUS SYMPHONY ORCHESTRA

55 East State Street
Columbus, OH 43215
Phone: 614-228-8600
Fax: 614-224-7273
Web Site: www.columbussymphony.com
Officers:
  Chairman: Linda Kass
Management:
  Executive Director/President: Daniel Hart
  General Manager: Susan L Rosenstock
  Music Director: Alessandro Siciliani
  Public Relations Manager: Linda Brill
Mission: To nurture and further the public's musical knowledge through educational activities and musical performances.
Founded: 1950

Specialized Field: Symphony; Orchestra; Chamber; Ensemble
Status: Professional
Budget: $10.8 million
Income Sources: American Symphony Orchestra League
Performs At: Ohio Theatre; Mershon Auditorium
Annual Attendance: 205,000
Organization Type: Performing; Educational; Sponsoring

1637 COLUMBUS SYMPHONY YOUTH ORCHESTRAS

55 East State Street
Columbus, OH 43215
Phone: 614-228-9600
Fax: 614-224-7273
e-mail: eberman@columbysymphony.org
Web Site: csyoa.org
Management:
  Music Director/Conductor: Peter Stafford Wilson
  Education Director: Jane Hahn
  Youth Orchestra Manager: Erica C Berman
Mission: To provide the highest quality educational and performance experiences for Central Ohio's most gifted instrumentalists.
Founded: 1955
Specialized Field: Symphony; Orchestra; Chamber
Status: Non-Professional; Nonprofit
Paid Staff: 7
Income Sources: American Symphony Orchestra League (Youth Orchestra Division); Columbus Symphony Orchestra; donations; tuiton
Performs At: Mess Hall, Capital University; Capitol Theatre; Verne Ritte Center; Hughes Auditorium; Ohio State University
Organization Type: Performing; Touring; Educational

1638 JAZZ ARTS GROUP OF COLUMBUS

709 College Avenue
Columbus, OH 43209
Phone: 614-235-3999
Fax: 614-235-9744
Officers:
  President: Jim Brock
  VP: Bob Ackerman
  Treasurer: Mark Shary
  Secretary: Ethel Shapiro
Management:
  General Manager/Artistic Director: Ray Eubanks
  Operations: Margaret Barr
  Marketing/Development: Mitch Swain
  Box Office: Andy Houser
Mission: To present and perform America's only indigenous art form.
Founded: 1972
Specialized Field: Orchestra; Jazz
Status: Professional; Nonprofit
Income Sources: City of Columbus Music in the Air
Performs At: Batelle Auditorium; Palace Theatre
Organization Type: Performing; Touring; Resident; Educational

1639 PRO MUSICA CHAMBER ORCHESTRA OF COLUMBUS
243 N 5th Street
Columbus, OH 43215
Phone: 614-464-0066
Fax: 614-464-4141
Web Site: www.promusicacolumbus.org
Management:
   Executive Director: Alan Silon
   Music Director/Conductor: Dr. Timothy Russell
Mission: To establish a partnership with the audience in order to understand and fulfill audience needs for a variety of entertaining and enlightening musical performances as well as educational experiences.
Founded: 1978
Specialized Field: Symphony; Orchestra; Chamber
Status: Professional; Nonprofit
Paid Staff: 7
Budget: $800,000
Performs At: Southern Theatre
Seating Capacity: 939
Year Built: 1896
Year Remodeled: 1999
Organization Type: Performing; Touring

1640 DAYTON PHILHARMONIC ORCHESTRA ASSOCIATION
Memorial Hall
125 E 1st Street
Dayton, OH 45402
Phone: 937-224-3521
Fax: 937-223-9189
e-mail: info@daytonphilharmonic.com
Web Site: www.daytonphilharmonic.com
Management:
   Executive Director: Curtis Long
   Music Director: Neal Gittleman
   Public Relations Coordinator: Allyson Crawford
Mission: Maintaining and nurturing the highest quality professional symphonic orchestra; offering live concerts that promote cultural enhancement.
Founded: 1933
Specialized Field: Symphony; Orchestra; Chamber
Status: Professional; Nonprofit
Paid Staff: 21
Volunteer Staff: 3
Paid Artists: 90
Non-paid Artists: 350
Income Sources: American Symphony Orchestra League; American Arts Alliance; American Council for the Arts
Performs At: Montgomery County's Memorial Hall; Dayton Convention Center
Organization Type: Performing; Resident; Educational; Sponsoring

1641 DAYTON PHILHARMONIC YOUTH ORCHESTRA
Memorial Hall
125 E 1st Street
Dayton, OH 45402
Phone: 937-224-3521
Fax: 937-223-9189
e-mail: info@daytonphilharmonic.com
Web Site: www.daytonphilharmonic.com
Management:
   Conductor: Patrick Reynolds
   Director Education: Gloria Pugh
   Conductor Junior String Orchestra: Karen Jones
Mission: To give aspiring young musicians of the Dayton area an opportunity to work together studying challenging orchestral music; to attempt to strengthen and expand the musical skills, knowledge, talent and experience through the study of the symphonic orchestral literature.
Founded: 1982
Specialized Field: Symphony; Orchestra
Status: Professional; Nonprofit
Paid Staff: 15
Volunteer Staff: 3
Non-paid Artists: 90
Income Sources: American Symphony Orchestra League (Youth Orchestra Division); Ohio Music Club; Dayton Philharmonic Orchestra
Performs At: Concert Hall; Wright State University
Organization Type: Performing; Educational

1642 SOIREES MUSICALES PIANO SERIES
834 Riverview Terrace
Dayton, OH 45407-2433
Phone: 937-228-5802
Fax: 937-228-2380
e-mail: hagpia@interaxs.net
Web Site: www.soireesmusicales.com
Management:
   Series Director: Donald C Hageman
Founded: 1969
Specialized Field: Solo Recitals-Piano
Volunteer Staff: 7
Budget: $10,000-20,000
Performs At: Shiloh Church

1643 CENTRAL OHIO SYMPHONY ORCHESTRA
PO Box 619
Delaware, OH 43015
Phone: 740-362-1799
Fax: 740-362-1733
Toll-free: 888-999-2676
e-mail: mail@coso-orchestra.org
Web Site: www.COSO-Orchestra.oeg
Management:
   Executive Director: Warren W Hyer
   Interim Conductor: Jamie Morales Matos
Founded: 1978
Specialized Field: Symphony Orchestra
Paid Staff: 4
Paid Artists: 65
Non-paid Artists: 10
Budget: $120,000
Annual Attendance: 20,000
Facility Category: Concert Hall
Seating Capacity: 1,079
Year Built: 1893
Year Remodeled: 1980

1644 HAMILTON-FAIRFIELD SYMPHONY & CHORALE

101 S Monument Street
Fairfield Auditorium 950
Hamilton, OH 45011
Phone: 513-895-5151
Fax: 513-474-1584
e-mail: pstanbery@rml.net
Web Site: www.hfso.org
Management:
    Music Director/Conductor: Paul Stanbery
    General Manager: Rita Line

1645 MUSIC FROM THE WESTERN RESERVE

Western Reserve Academy
116 College Street
Hudson, OH 44236
Phone: 330-650-9714
Fax: 330-688-4839
Officers:
    President: Bruce F Rothmann, MD
    VP: Walter Watson
    Treasurer: Robert L Henke
    Secretary: David Hunter, Esquire
    Recording Secretary: Diana Truyell
Management:
    Concert Manager: Lola Rothmann
Mission: Showcasing the abundant musical talent of Northeast Ohio.
Founded: 1982
Specialized Field: Chamber Music
Status: Nonprofit
Volunteer Staff: 6
Budget: $10,000
Performs At: The Chapel, Western Reserve Academy
Annual Attendance: 600-700
Seating Capacity: 450
Year Built: 1836
Organization Type: Sponsoring

1646 LAKELAND CIVIC ORCHESTRA

Lakeland Community College
Lakeland Performing Arts Center 430
Kirtland, OH 44094-5198
Phone: 440-953-7091
Fax: 440-975-4738
Management:
    Orchestra Director: Kathryn Harsta
    General Manager: Lawrence Aulderheide

1647 LAKESIDE SYMPHONY

236 Walnut Avenue
Lakeside, OH 43440
Phone: 419-798-4461
Fax: 419-798-5033
e-mail: schedule@lakesideohio.com
Web Site: www.lakesideohio.com
Management:
    Executive Director: Bud Cox
    Music Director: Robert L Conquist
    Program Director: G Keith Addy

Mission: To maintain a professional resident orchestra for part of the summer season at Lakeside.
Founded: 1925
Specialized Field: Symphony; Orchestra; Chamber
Status: Professional; Nonprofit
Paid Staff: 75
Volunteer Staff: 60
Paid Artists: 10
Performs At: Hoover Auditorium
Organization Type: Performing; Resident; Educational

1648 LIMA SYMPHONY ORCHESTRA

PO Box 1651
67 Town Square
Lima, OH 45802
Phone: 419-222-5701
Fax: 419-222-6587
e-mail: staff@limasymphony.org
Web Site: www.limasymphony.com
Officers:
    Symphony Board President: Linda Burkhalter
    VP: Tom Leininger
    Secretary: Scott Shafer
    Friends of the Symphony, President: Kim Shanahan
Management:
    Music Director/Conductor: Crafton Beck
    Executive Director: Paul Assenheimer
    Personnel Manager: Anita Sims Skinner
Mission: Promoting the public's musical appreciation and knowledge through live musical performances, including chamber, opera and symphonic.
Founded: 1953
Specialized Field: Symphony; Orchestra; Chamber
Status: Semi-Professional; Nonprofit
Paid Staff: 8
Volunteer Staff: 1
Paid Artists: 85
Budget: $350,000- $400,000
Income Sources: American Symphony Orchestra League
Performs At: Veterans Memorial Civic and Convention Center
Seating Capacity: 1,670
Organization Type: Performing; Educational; Sponsoring

1649 MANSFIELD SYMPHONY ORCHESTRA

PO Box 789
Mansfield, OH 44901-0789
Phone: 419-522-2726
Fax: 419-524-7005
e-mail: tomc@rparts.org
Web Site: www.rparts.org
Management:
    President/CEO: Dr. Thomas J Carlo
Facility Category: Theater
Type of Stage: Proscenium
Seating Capacity: 1406
Year Built: 1928
Year Remodeled: 1982

1650 RICHLAND PERFORMING ARTS

138 Park Avenue W
Mansfield, OH 44902

Phone: 419-524-5927
Fax: 419-524-7098
Officers:
   President: William McIntyre
   VP: Jeanne Alexander
   Secretary: J Brad Preston
   Treasurer: Dan Scurci
Management:
   General Manager: Dr. Thomas J Carto
   Music Director/Conductor: Jeff Holland Cook
   Development Director: Janet E Keeler
Mission: To present symphony concerts mainly from symphony repertoire including educational and pops programming.
Founded: 1930
Specialized Field: Symphony; Orchestra; Ensemble
Status: Professional; Nonprofit
Income Sources: American Symphony Orchestra League; ORACLE; OCCA
Performs At: Renaissance Theatre
Organization Type: Performing; Touring; Educational

1651 MIDDLETOWN SYMPHONY ORCHESTRA

130 N Verity Parkway
PO Box 411
Middletown, OH 45042
Phone: 513-424-2426
e-mail: mso@middletownsymphony.com
Web Site: http://www.middletownsymphony.com
Officers:
   President: John Ritan
Management:
   Music Director: Carmon DeLeone
Founded: 1941

1652 SOUTHEASTERN OHIO SYMPHONY ORCHESTRA

PO Box 42
New Concord, OH 43762
Phone: 740-826-8197
Fax: 740-826-8404
e-mail: PgeMaker@aol.com
Management:
   Music Director: Laura E Schumann
   Executive Director: Elizabeth E Broschart

1653 TUSCARAWAS PHILHARMONIC

PO Box 406
New Philadelphia, OH 44663
Phone: 330-364-1843
Fax: 330-364-1843
Officers:
   President: Steve Jenkins
   VP: Sheila Snead
   Secretary: Patricia Karnosh
   Treasurer: Patricia Tolloti
Management:
   Music Director/Conductor: Eric Benjamin
   General Manager: Melanie Winn
   Finance Manager: Robert L Henke
Mission: To offer musical enjoyment to all ages and enhance the cultural development of the community.
Founded: 1935

Specialized Field: Symphony; Orchestra
Status: Semi-Professional; Nonprofit
Paid Staff: 35
Performs At: Dover High School
Annual Attendance: 4,000 - 6,000
Facility Category: Auditorium
Type of Stage: Proscenium
Seating Capacity: 1,084
Organization Type: Performing

1654 NORTHERN OHIO YOUTH ORCHESTRAS

39 S Main
Suite 244
Oberlin, OH 44074
Phone: 440-775-3059
Fax: 440-774-6160
e-mail: noyo@apk.net
Management:
   Music Dirrector: Dr. Joanne Erwin
   General Manager: Gretchen Faro

1655 OBERLIN BAROQUE ENSEMBLE

Conservatory of Music
Oberlin College
Oberlin, OH 44074
Phone: 440-775-8121
Fax: 440-775-8886
Mission: The ensemble performs 17th and 18th-century compositions on period instruments.
Founded: 1973
Specialized Field: Chamber; Ensemble; Instrumental Group
Status: Professional
Income Sources: Oberlin College Conservatory of Music
Performs At: Oberlin Conservatory
Organization Type: Performing; Touring; Resident; Educational

1656 MIAMI UNIVERSITY SYMPHONY ORCHESTRA

209 A Presser
Hall Auditorium 730
Oxford, OH 45056
Phone: 513-529-1966
Fax: 513-529-3027
e-mail: muso@muohio.edu
Web Site: www.fna.muohio.edu/muso/
Management:
   Music Director: Jamie Morales-Matos

1657 MIAMI WIND QUINTET

Department of Music
Miami University
Oxford, OH 45056
Phone: 513-529-1809
Fax: 513-529-3841
Management:
   Director Audience Development: Jeanne Conners
Mission: Offering chamber music composed for winds; assisting young wind players.
Founded: 1985
Specialized Field: Chamber; Instrumental Group

Status: Professional
Income Sources: Miami University
Performs At: Souers Recital Hall; Miami University
Organization Type: Performing; Touring; Resident; Educational

1658 SPRINGFIELD SYMPHONY ORCHESTRA
PO Box 1374
300 S Fountain Avenue
Springfield, OH 45501
Phone: 937-325-8100
Fax: 937-325-2299
e-mail: info@springfieldsym.org
Web Site: www.springfieldsym.org
Officers:
　President: Melinda Marsh
　VP: Baird Tipson
Management:
　Executive Director: A. Diane Schoeffler
　Music Director/Conductor: Peter Stafford Wilson
Mission: Providing the best symphonic music for the community; offering music education to youth.
Founded: 1944
Specialized Field: Symphony; Chamber
Status: Professional; Nonprofit
Paid Staff: 60
Paid Artists: 80
Budget: $850,000
Income Sources: American Symphony Orchestra League
Performs At: Kuss Auditorium; Clark State Performing Arts Center
Affiliations: Clark State College
Annual Attendance: 1,200
Seating Capacity: 1,200
Organization Type: Performing; Sponsoring

1659 TOLEDO JAZZ SOCIETY
425 N St Claire Street
Toledo, OH 43604
Phone: 419-241-5299
Fax: 419-241-4777
e-mail: toledo@toledojazzsociety.org
Web Site: www.toledojazzsociety.org
Officers:
　President: Jon Richardson
　VP: Jeff Jaffe
　Secretary: AC Alrey
　Executive Director: Jori Lynch Jex
Mission: Promoting the performance of jazz and its preservation as an art form; providing concerts, educational programs and lectures.
Founded: 1980
Specialized Field: Orchestra; Ensemble; Band
Status: Professional; Nonprofit
Paid Staff: 4
Volunteer Staff: 10
Paid Artists: 100
Income Sources: Association of Performing Arts Presenters; Arts Midwest
Performs At: The Embers
Organization Type: Performing; Resident; Educational; Sponsoring

1660 TOLEDO SYMPHONY
1838 Parkwood
Suite 310
Toledo, OH 43604
Phone: 419-241-1272
Fax: 419-321-6890
Toll-free: 800-348-1253
e-mail: music@toledosymphony.com
Web Site: www.toledosymphony.com
Officers:
　Chairman: Joe Maghiochetti
Management:
　President/CEO: Robert Bell
　Production Manager: Ray Clark
　Orchestra Manager: Keith McWatters
Mission: To furnish performances of the highest artistic caliber to the widest possible audience; to conduct public service and education functions.
Founded: 1943
Specialized Field: Symphony; Orchestra; Chamber; Ensemble; Instrumental Group
Status: Professional; Nonprofit
Performs At: Toledo Museum of Art Peristyle
Organization Type: Performing; Touring; Educational

1661 WESTERVILLE SYMPHONY
28 S State Street
PO Box 478
Westerville, OH 43081
Phone: 614-890-5523
Fax: 614-882-2085
e-mail: wsymphony@otterbein.edu
Web Site: www.westervillesymphony.org
Officers:
　President: Donna Kerr
　VP: John Gale
　Secretary: Lyle Barkhymer
　Treasurer: Michael Howard
　Executive Director: Jeanne Browne
Management:
　Music Director: Peter Stafford Wilson
Mission: A non-profit, charitable corporation functioning as an aesthetic, educational and cultural resource, presenting performances primarily of symphonic music; an artistic outlet for amateur and semi-professional musicians.
Founded: 1982
Specialized Field: Symphony; Orchestra; Ensemble
Status: Non-Professional; Nonprofit
Paid Staff: 50
Performs At: Cowan Hall; Otterbein College
Organization Type: Performing; Educational

1662 WOOSTER SYMPHONY ORCHESTRA
College of Wooster
217 Scheide Music Center
Wooster, OH 44691
Phone: 330-263-2047
Fax: 330-263-2051
e-mail: jlindberg@acs.wooster.edu
Management:
　Contact: Jeffrey Lindberg
Mission: Bringing the community live orchestral repertoire.

Founded: 1915
Specialized Field: Symphony; Orchestra
Status: Non-Professional
Paid Staff: 1
Volunteer Staff: 5
Paid Artists: 18
Non-paid Artists: 55
Budget: $20,000
Income Sources: Women's Committee; ticket sales
Performs At: McGaw Chapel
Affiliations: Colllege of Wooster
Annual Attendance: 6,000 per concert
Organization Type: Performing; Resident

1663 CHAMBER MUSIC YELLOW SPRINGS

Box 448
Yellow Springs, OH 45387
Phone: 937-767-2912
Fax: 937-767-9350
e-mail: mary.t.white@wright.edu
Officers:
    President: Mary T White
Mission: Performing professional chamber music of high quality.
Founded: 1983
Specialized Field: Chamber Music
Status: Professional; Nonprofit
Budget: 25-30,000
Income Sources: Donations: Grants; Tickets
Performs At: First Presbyterian Church
Seating Capacity: 240
Organization Type: Sponsoring

1664 YOUNGSTOWN SYMPHONY ORCHESTRA

260 Federal Plaza W
Youngstown, OH 44503
Phone: 330-744-4269
Fax: 330-744-1441
e-mail: symphony@cboss.com
Web Site: www.youngstownsymphony.com
Management:
    Executive Director: Patricia C Syak
    Theatre Coordinator: Leslie A Brown
Founded: 1931
Specialized Field: Performing, educational
Status: Professional; Nonprofit
Paid Staff: 7
Paid Artists: 500
Budget: $200,000
Income Sources: American Symphony Orchestra League
Performs At: Youngstown Symphony Center; Edward W. Powers Auditorium
Annual Attendance: 131,347
Facility Category: Auditorium
Type of Stage: Proscenium
Stage Dimensions: 60 x 40
Seating Capacity: 2310
Year Built: 1931
Year Remodeled: 1968
Cost: 1.5 Million
Rental Contact: Theatre Coordinator Leslie A. Brown
Organization Type: Performing; Resident; Educational
Resident Groups: Youngstown Symphony Orchestra

Oklahoma

1665 BARTLESVILLE SYMPHONY ORCHESTRA

Bartlesville Community Center
300 E Adams Boulevard
Bartlesville, OK 74005
Phone: 918-333-7989
Fax: 918-333-7989
e-mail: lauren@bartlesvillesymphony.org
Web Site: www.bartlesvillesymphony.org
Management:
    Music Director/Conductor/Manager: Lauren Green
Mission: Offering community musicians and audiences an opportunity to experience symphonic professional quality symphonic musical expirences and world-class quest soloists.
Founded: 1957
Specialized Field: Symphony; Orchestra
Status: Non-Professional; Nonprofit
Paid Staff: 1
Volunteer Staff: 2
Paid Artists: 20
Non-paid Artists: 45
Budget: $200,000
Income Sources: Tickets; Donations; Fundraising Products
Performs At: Bartlesville Community Center
Annual Attendance: 4,000
Facility Category: Auditoriuam
Type of Stage: Proscenium
Seating Capacity: 1700
Year Built: 1982
Cost: $ 13 Million
Organization Type: Resident

1666 OKLAHOMA MOZART INTERNATIONAL FESTIVAL

500 SE Dewey, Suite A
PO Box 2344
Bartlesville, OK 74005
Phone: 918-333-9900
Fax: 918-336-9525
e-mail: jmswindell@okmozart.com
Web Site: www.okmozart.com
Management:
    Executive Director: Peggy Ball
    Artistic Director: Ransom Wilson
    Development Director: Linda Cubbage
    Public Relations Director: Jeanette Swindell
Founded: 1985
Specialized Field: Dance; Vocal Music; Instrumental Music; Festivals; Grand Opera
Status: Professional; Nonprofit
Paid Staff: 8
Volunteer Staff: 800
Paid Artists: 50
Non-paid Artists: 0
Budget: $890,000
Income Sources: Oklahoma State Arts Council; National Endowment for the Arts; Individuals; Businesses
Performs At: Bartlesville Community Center
Annual Attendance: 30,000
Facility Category: Concert Hall, Community Center

Seating Capacity: 1700
Year Built: 1982
Organization Type: Sponsoring
Resident Groups: New York Orchestra

1667 ENID-PHILLIPS SYMPHONY ORCHESTRA

300 W Cherokee
Suite 109
Enid, OK 73701
Phone: 405-237-9646
Fax: 405-237-7646
Management:
    Artistic Director: Douglas Newell
    Administrative Associate: Eleanor Hornbaker
Founded: 1906
Specialized Field: Symphony; Orchestra
Status: Professional; Nonprofit
Income Sources: American Symphony Orchestra League
Performs At: Eugene S. Briggs Auditorium
Organization Type: Performing; Educational

1668 LAWTON PHILHARMONIC ORCHESTRA

PO Box 1473
Lawton, OK 73502
Phone: 580-248-2001
Fax: 580-248-2200
e-mail: lawphil@sirinet.net
Web Site: www.lawton-philharmonic.org
Management:
    Executive Director: Laura Doser
    Music Director/Conductor: Miriam Burns
Mission: To provide high quality cultural experiences to Southwest Oklahoma.
Founded: 1962
Specialized Field: Symphony Orchestra
Status: Professional
Paid Staff: 3
Volunteer Staff: 40
Paid Artists: 62
Budget: $260,000
Income Sources: Box office; Grants; Private donations
Performs At: McMahon Memorial Auditorium
Affiliations: American Symphony Orchestra League
Annual Attendance: 10,000
Facility Category: Concert Hall
Seating Capacity: 1,560
Year Built: 1962
Year Remodeled: 2000
Organization Type: Performing; Touring; Resident; Educational; Sponsoring

1669 JAZZ IN JUNE

PO Box 2405
Norman, OK 73070
Phone: 405-325-3388
e-mail: dkritten@swbell.net
Web Site: www.jazzinjune.org
Management:
    Executive Director: Phoebe Morales
Mission: To offer Oklahoma residents a jazz festival.
Founded: 1985
Specialized Field: Vocal Music; Instrumental Music

Status: Professional; Semi-Professional
Income Sources: American Federation of Musicians
Organization Type: Performing

1670 UNIVERSITY OF OKLAHOMA SYMPHONY ORCHESTRA

Catlett Music Center University of Oklahoma
500 W Boyd
Norman, OK 73019
Phone: 405-325-7731
Fax: 405-325-7574
e-mail: duilio@ou.edu
Web Site: www.ou.eduou.edu
Management:
    Artistic Director/Conductor: Duilio Dobrin
    Assistant Conductor: Yiannis Hadjiloizou
    Personnel Director: Shara Long
    Operations Director: Timothy Verville
Founded: 1920
Paid Staff: 6
Performs At: Catlett Music Center

1671 CHAMBER MUSIC IN OKLAHOMA

PO Box 54624
Oklahoma City, OK 73154-1624
Phone: 405-974-3333
Fax: 405-974-3844
Web Site: www.cmok.org
Officers:
    Vice President & Treasurer: Brad Ferguson
    Vice President & Special Projects: Mary J Rutherford
    Secretary: Martha Blaine
Management:
    Artists & Bookings: Dr Mark A Everett
    Publicity & Webmaster: Dr. H Dean Everett
Founded: 1960
Specialized Field: Chamber
Status: Nonprofit
Budget: $20,000-35,000
Performs At: Christ the King Church

1672 GO FOR BAROQUE

PO Box 20178
Oklahoma City, OK 73120
Phone: 405-840-0278
Mission: To offer formal baroque concerts and young people's concerts.
Founded: 1982
Specialized Field: Chamber; Ensemble
Status: Professional
Organization Type: Performing; Touring; Educational

1673 OKLAHOMA CITY PHILHARMONIC ORCHESTRA

428 W California
Suite 210
Oklahoma City, OK 73102
Phone: 405-232-7575
Fax: 405-232-4353
e-mail: info@okcphilharmonic.org
Web Site: www.okcphilharmonic.org
Officers:
    President: John P McMillin

President Elect: Michael Joseph
VP: Grace Ryan
Treasurer: Doug Stussi
Management:
Music Director/Conductor: Joel Levine
Executive Director: Edward Walker
General Manager: Joe Ragan
Finance Director: Vanessa Etheridge
Mission: Performing classical, orchestral, and popular music; entertaining and educating; enhancing the cultural environment of Oklahoma City as well as the state.
Founded: 1988
Specialized Field: Symphony; Orchestra
Status: Professional; Nonprofit
Performs At: Rose State Performing Arts Theatre
Affiliations: American Symphony Orchestra League; Allied Arts of Oklahoma City
Organization Type: Performing; Resident

1674 CONCERTIME

11317 E 4th Street
Tulsa, OK 74128-2006
Phone: 918-438-2582
Fax: 918-437-1848
e-mail: organist@mciworld.com
Web Site: www.webtek.com/concertime
Management:
Manager: Alta Selvey
Mission: To continue cultivating audiences to enjoy chamber music.
Founded: 1954
Specialized Field: Chamber
Status: Professional; Nonprofit
Income Sources: Chamber Music America
Performs At: John H. Williams Theater; Tulsa Performing Arts Center
Organization Type: Performing; Educational

1675 SINFONIA

PO Box 35956
Tulsa, OK 74153-5956
Phone: 918-488-0398
Fax: 918-488-0396
Management:
Director: Dana Rushin
Performs At: Tulsa Community College Performing Arts Center for Education

1676 TULSA PHILHARMONIC

2901 S Harvard Avenue
Suite A
Tulsa, OK 74114
Phone: 918-747-7473
Fax: 918-747-7496
e-mail: info@tulsaphilharmonic.org
Web Site: www.tulsaphilharmonic.org
Officers:
President: Dr. Gordon D Lantz
VP: Larry E Lee
VP: Richard B Williamson
Secretary: Robert K. Gardnine
Treasurer: Ronald R. Glass
Management:
CEO: Thomas Greedom

Director Operations: Wendy Jones
Stage Manager: Tomnt Cortwright
Librarian: Marc Facci
Personnel Manager: Phillip Wachowski
Mission: To offer live performances of symphony music.
Founded: 1947
Specialized Field: Symphony; Orchestra; Chamber; Ensemble
Status: Professional; Nonprofit
Performs At: Tulsa Performing Arts Center; Brady Theater
Affiliations: Walter Arts Center at Holland Hall School
Organization Type: Performing; Touring; Resident; Educational; Sponsoring

1677 TULSA YOUTH SYMPHONY ORCHESTRA

2901 S Harvard Avenue
Tulsa, OK 74114
Phone: 918-747-7473
Fax: 918-747-7496
e-mail: tulsaphil@mail.webtek.com
Web Site: www.webtek.com/tulsaphil
Management:
Conductor/Administrator: Ronald Wheeler
Administrative Assistant: Michelle Olson
Mission: Tulsa Youth Symphony Orchestra aims to encourage and develop students' musical abilities through rehearsal, concert performance and regular contact with professional musicians, offering training and performance opportunities.
Founded: 1963
Specialized Field: Symphony; Orchestra; Chamber
Status: Non-Professional; Nonprofit
Paid Staff: 85
Income Sources: American Symphony Orchestra League (Youth Orchestra Division); Tulsa Philharmonic
Performs At: Union High School Performing Arts Center
Seating Capacity: 1,900
Organization Type: Performing; Touring; Educational
Resident Groups: Philharmonic Society; Tulsa Area Youth Association

Oregon

1678 CHAMBER MUSIC CONCERTS

SOSC
1250 Siskiyou Boulevard
Ashland, OR 97520
Phone: 541-552-6419
Fax: 541-552-6380
e-mail: chamber-music@sou.edu
Web Site: www.sou.edu/cmc
Management:
Founder/Director: Dr Gregory Fowler
Assistant: Lesley Pohl
Mission: To offer Southern Oregon residents the highest possible quality of chamber music.
Founded: 1984
Specialized Field: Chamber
Status: Professional; Nonprofit
Performs At: SOSC Music Building Recital Hall
Organization Type: Performing

1679   ROGUE VALLEY SYMPHONY
SOU Music Hall
1250 Siskiyou Boulevard
Ashland, OR 97520
Phone: 541-552-6354
Fax: 541-552-6353
e-mail: office@rvsymphony.org
Web Site: www.rvsymphony.org
Officers:
   President: Julia Lester
   Past President: Gary Lorre
   Secretary: Mary Jo Bergstrom
   Treasurer: Barbara Johnson
Management:
   Executive Director: Francis Van Ausdal
   Music Director/Conductor: Arthur Shaw
Founded: 1966
Paid Staff: 6
Paid Artists: 73
Budget: $449,150
Performs At: SOU Music Recital Hall
Annual Attendance: 20,000
Facility Category: 3 Facilities

1680   CHAMBER MUSIC CORVALLIS
3904 NW Clarence Circle
Corvallis, OR 97330
Phone: 541-757-0086
Fax: 541-757-2520
e-mail: orloffc@proaxis.com
Web Site: www.violins.org
Officers:
   Chairman: Carole Orloff
Budget: $35,000-60,000
Performs At: LaSells Stewart Center

1681   OSU-CORVALLIS SYMPHONY ORCHESTRA
Oregon State University
Benton Hall 101
Corvallis, OR 97331-2502
Phone: 541-737-4061
Fax: 541-737-4268
e-mail: mcarlson@orst.edu
Management:
   Music Director/Conductor: Marian Carlson

1682   EMERALD CHAMBER PLAYERS
3080 Potter
Eugene, OR 97405
Phone: 541-344-0483
e-mail: ORVALETTER@netscape.net
Management:
   Convener: Orval Etter
Mission: To provide amateurs with opportunities to play and perform chamber music.
Founded: 1962
Specialized Field: Orchestra; Chamber; Ensemble; Instrumental Group
Status: Non-Professional; Nonprofit
Organization Type: Performing

1683   EUGENE SYMPHONY
115 W 8th Avenue
Eugene, OR 97401
Phone: 541-687-9487
Fax: 541-687-0527
e-mail: info@eugenesymphony.org
Web Site: www.eugenesymphony.org
Management:
   Executive Director: Rebekah Lambert
   Personal Manager: Deanna McGlothin
Mission: Offering professional excellence in musical performances for the enrichment of a broad audience.
Founded: 1966
Specialized Field: Symphony; Orchestra
Status: Professional; Nonprofit
Paid Staff: 7
Volunteer Staff: 2
Paid Artists: 80
Non-paid Artists: 0
Budget: $1.4 million
Income Sources: American Society of Composers, Authors and Publishers; American Symphony Orchestra League
Performs At: Hult Center for the Performing Arts
Facility Category: Hult Center for the Performing Arts
Seating Capacity: 2400
Year Built: 1982
Organization Type: Performing; Resident

1684   OREGON BACH FESTIVAL
1257 University of Oregon
Eugene, OR 97403
Phone: 541-346-5666
Fax: 541-346-5669
Toll-free: 800-457-1486
e-mail: saltzman@oregon.ugregon.edu
Web Site: www.bachfest.uoregon.edu
Management:
   Artistic Director: Helmuth Rilling
   Executive Director: H Royce Saltzman
   Marketing Director: George Evano
Mission: To offer high quality performances that elevate the spirits of both performers and audiences.
Founded: 1970
Specialized Field: Choral-Orchestral
Status: Professional; Nonprofit
Paid Staff: 8
Budget: 1.3 Million
Income Sources: Box office, grants, private donqtions
Performs At: University of Oregon School of Music; Beall Concert
Affiliations: University of Oregon School of Music
Annual Attendance: 33,000
Facility Category: Concert Hall
Type of Stage: Proscenium
Seating Capacity: 2500/550
Organization Type: Performing; Resident; Educational

1685   OREGON MOZART PLAYERS
541 Willametta Street
Suite 308
Eugene, OR 97401

Phone: 541-345-6648
Fax: 541-345-7849
e-mail: omp@pacwest.net
Web Site: www.oregonmozart.org/
Management:
   Music Director: Andrew Massey
Mission: To offer chamber orchestra music; to provide talented, local musicians with opportunities to perform as orchestra members and soloists as well as in chamber ensembles.
Founded: 1982
Specialized Field: Orchestra; Chamber
Status: Professional; Nonprofit
Performs At: Hult Center For The Performing Arts; Beall Concert
Organization Type: Performing; Touring; Resident; Educational

1686 PACIFIC UNIVERSITY COMMUNITY WIND ENSEMBLE

Pacific University
Music Department
Forest Grove, OR 97116
Phone: 503-357-6151
Fax: 503-359-2910
Management:
   Conductor: Michael Burch-Pesses
Mission: To provide music students with educational training; to offer community members a performing outlet.
Founded: 1849
Specialized Field: Orchestra; Chamber
Status: Non-Professional; Nonprofit
Performs At: University Center
Organization Type: Performing; Resident; Educational

1687 MT HOOD POPS ORCHESTRA

PO Box 1641
Gresham, OR 97030
Phone: 503-669-1937
Fax: 503-667-2848
e-mail: pierikm@teleport.com
Management:
   Music Director: Ben Brooks
   Orchestra Manager: Dmarilyn Pierik
Mission: To provide for the performance of contemporary and classical music and to help promote the fine arts in the Eastern part of Multnoman, Clackamps and Clark counties.
Specialized Field: Music
Paid Artists: 65
Performs At: Auditorium

1688 GRANDE RONDE SYMPHONY ORCHESTRA

PO Box 824
La Grande, OR 97850
Phone: 541-962-3352
Fax: 541-962-3596
Management:
   Music Director: Steven Ward
Performs At: Loso Hall

1689 BRITT FESTIVALS

PO Box 1124
Medford, OR 97501
Phone: 541-779-0847
Fax: 541-776-3712
Toll-free: 800-882-7488
e-mail: info@brittfest.org
Web Site: www.brittfest.org
Officers:
   Board President: Tim Gerking
Management:
   Executive Director: Ron McUne
   Music Director: Peter Bay
   Marketing/Public Relations Director: Kelly Gonzales
   Development Director: Ed Foss
   Booking/Production Director: Mike Sturgill
   Education Director: David MacKenzie
Mission: To present and sponsor, in Southern Oregon, performing arts of the highest quality for the education, enrichment and enjoyment of all.
Founded: 1963
Specialized Field: Classical; Jazz; Blues; Pop/Rock; Country; Folk; Bluegrass; World Music; Dance; Musical Theater; Comedy
Paid Staff: 12
Volunteer Staff: 600
Performs At: Outdoor Auditorium
Annual Attendance: 70,000
Facility Category: Outdoor Amphitheatre
Seating Capacity: 2200
Year Built: 1963
Year Remodeled: 1992

1690 OREGON EAST SYMPHONY

424 S Main
Pendleton, OR 97801
Phone: 541-276-0320
Fax: 541-278-6114
e-mail: oes@ucinet.com
Management:
   Executive Director: Cheryl Marier
Founded: 1976
Specialized Field: Symphony
Paid Staff: 2
Volunteer Staff: 10
Paid Artists: 70
Non-paid Artists: 30
Budget: $125,000
Income Sources: Sales; Grants; Sponsorship
Performs At: Vert Auditorium
Annual Attendance: 4,000
Facility Category: Hall
Type of Stage: Wooden
Stage Dimensions: 40 x 30
Seating Capacity: 750
Year Built: 1925
Year Remodeled: 1995

1691 CHAMBER MUSIC NORTHWEST

522 SW Fifth Avenue
Suite 725
Portland, OR 97204

Phone: 503-223-3202
Fax: 503-294-1690
e-mail: info@cmnw.org
Web Site: www.cmnw.org
Officers:
 Educations & Communications Manager: Adrienne Leverette
Management:
 Executive Director: Linda Magee
 Artistic Director: David Shifrin
 Operations Director: Franck Avril
 Finance Director: Katherine King
 Marketing Manager: Garen Horgend
Mission: To present an annual summer music festival (five weeks/25 concerts) with world renowned performers in residence; to present concerts and educational activities on a year-round basis.
Founded: 1971
Specialized Field: Chamber; Ensemble; Classical Music
Status: Professional; Nonprofit
Paid Staff: 6
Volunteer Staff: 50
Paid Artists: 75
Budget: One Million
Affiliations: Kaul Auditorium at Reed College; Cabell Theatre at Catlin Gabel School
Annual Attendance: 19,000
Facility Category: Small Concert Hall (private college)
Seating Capacity: 550
Year Built: 1998
Organization Type: Performing
Notes: Wheelchair seating available

1692 CHAMBER MUSIC SOCIETY OF OREGON
1935 NE 59th Avenue
Portland, OR 97213-4117
Phone: 503-287-2175
e-mail: delorenzoh@earthlink.net
Web Site: www.oregonchambermusic.org
Officers:
 President: Patricia Ann Haim
 VP: Dr. Floyd Grant Jackson
 Secretary: Beatrice Matin
 Treasurer: John B. Gould
 Executive Director: Hazel M. DeLorenzo
Mission: To promote music in our schools for its value in teaching children how to learn.
Founded: 1973
Specialized Field: Orchestra; Chamber; Ensemble; Instrumental Group
Status: Non-Professional; Nonprofit
Performs At: St. Philip Neri Church; Hood River Middle School
Organization Type: Performing; Resident; Educational

1693 COLUMBIA SYMPHONY ORCHESTRA
PO Box 6559
Portland, OR 97228
Phone: 503-234-4017
Fax: 503-234-4017
e-mail: cso@pacifier.com
Web Site: www.columbiasymphony.org
Officers:

President: Susan Charon
Management:
 Executive Director: Betsy Hatton
 Director Development: Kathryn Oliver
 Music Director/Conductor: Huw Edwards
Founded: 1982
Paid Staff: 2
Volunteer Staff: 20
Paid Artists: 65
Non-paid Artists: 8
Performs At: Auditorium
Facility Category: Church
Seating Capacity: 600

1694 FRIENDS OF CHAMBER MUSIC
PO Box 397
Portland, OR 97207
Phone: 503-224-9842
Fax: 503-725-8215
Mission: To present a season of five chamber-music concerts annually; to sponsor outreach activities, including workshops and master classes.
Specialized Field: Chamber
Status: Nonprofit
Organization Type: Presenting

1695 FRIENDS OF CHAMBER MUSIC
PO Box 397
Portland, OR 97207
Phone: 503-224-9842
Fax: 503-725-8215
e-mail: info@focm.org
Web Site: focm.org
Management:
 Executive Director: Pat Zagelow
Budget: $200,000
Income Sources: Tickets; Contributors
Performs At: Lincoln Hall Auditorium; Portland State University
Annual Attendance: 7,000
Type of Stage: Proscenium
Seating Capacity: 476

1696 METROPOLITAN YOUTH SYMPHONY
PO Box 5254
Portland, OR 97208
Phone: 503-239-4566
Toll-free: 888-752-9697
e-mail: mysgm@teleport.com
Web Site: www.metroyouthsymphony.org
Management:
 Music Director/Conductor: Lajos Balogh
 Conductor Symphonic Band: Dr. John K Richards
 Conductor Concert Orchestra: Bill Hunt
 Associate Conductor: Mike Ott
 Associate Conductor: Nita Van Pelt
 Conductor Preparatory Band: Larry Wells
 Conductor Overture Orchestra: Kathie Reed
Specialized Field: The Metropolitan Youth Symphony (MYS) is a non-profit educational organization, with over 400 talented young musicians.
Performs At: Arlene Schnitzer Concert Hall; Intermediate Theater

1697 OREGON SYMPHONY
921 SW Washington
Suite 200
Portland, OR 97205
Phone: 503-228-4294
Fax: 503-228-4150
e-mail: symphony@orsymphony.org
Web Site: www.orsymphony.org
Management:
  Conductor: James DePreist
  Associate Conductor: Norman Leyden

1698 PORTLAND BAROQUE ORCHESTRA
1020 SW Taylor Street
Suite 275
Portland, OR 97205
Phone: 503-222-6000
Fax: 503-226-6635
e-mail: admin@pbo.org
Web Site: www.pbo.org/
Officers:
  President: Jon Kruse
  VP: John Hammerstad
  Secretary: Gretchen Boehmer
  Treasurer: Roy Abramowitz
Management:
  Artistic Director: Monica Huggett
  Operations Manager: W Kellogg Thorsell
  Box Office Manager: Carol Cartier
Founded: 1984
Specialized Field: Baroque music performed on period instruments.
Status: Tax-exempt

1699 PORTLAND CHAMBER ORCHESTRA ASSOCIATION
PO Box 9024
Portland, OR 97205
Phone: 503-227-7902
Fax: 503-227-7066
Officers:
  President: Ellwood Miller
  VP: Mildred Berthelsdorf
  Treasurer: Margaret Sutherland
  Recording Secretary: Jane Perkins
Management:
  Director: Mildred Berthelsdorf, MD
  Conductor: Anthony Armore
Mission: To present free and/or low fee concerts of fine chamber music by outstanding local talent.
Founded: 1946
Specialized Field: Classical Orchestra
Paid Artists: 30
Budget: $44,948
Income Sources: Private; Foundations; Grants; Endowments; Business/corporate donations; Individual donations
Performs At: Scottish Rite Center
Annual Attendance: 255/concert
Facility Category: Performing Arts Center
Type of Stage: Raised
Seating Capacity: 400

1700 PORTLAND STATE UNIVERSITY PIANO RECITAL SERIES
PO Box 751
Portland, OR 97207
Phone: 503-725-5400
Fax: 503-725-8215
e-mail: zagelop@mail.pdx.edu
Web Site: www.fpa.pdx.edu/prs/
Management:
  Executive Director: Pat Zagelow
  Artistic Director: Harold Gray
Mission: The piano recital series is dedicated to presenting the finest pianists in the world in recital settings and outreach activities for the purpose of enriching and educating our community.
Founded: 1978
Paid Staff: 2
Paid Artists: 10
Budget: $200,000
Income Sources: Tickets; Contributions
Performs At: Lincoln Hall Auditorium
Annual Attendance: 6,000
Type of Stage: Proscenium
Seating Capacity: 476

1701 PORTLAND STRING QUARTET WORKSHOP AT COLBY COLLEGE
PO Box 6782
Colby College
Portland, OR 04101
Phone: 207-774-5144
Fax: 207-761-2406
e-mail: arpeggio@worldnet.att.net

1702 PORTLAND YOUTH PHILHARMONIC ASSOCIATION
1119 SW Park Avenue
Portland, OR 97205
Phone: 503-223-5939
Fax: 503-223-5003
e-mail: information@portlandyouthphil.org
Web Site: www.portlandyouthphil.org
Officers:
  President: Bruce Samson
  VP: George C Reinmiller
  Corporate Secretary: Wayne Landeverk
  Treasurer: Robert M. Nibley
Management:
  Music Director/Conductor: Mei-Ann Chen
  Executive Director: Paul Barthelemy
Mission: It is the purpose of the Portland Youth Philharmonic to maintain the finest possible resident youth orchestra in order to inspire, train and educate young people in the performance and appreciation of symphonic music and to provide a cultural asset to the community.
Founded: 1924
Specialized Field: Symphony; Orchestra; Ensemble
Status: Non-Professional; Nonprofit
Paid Staff: 7
Non-paid Artists: 206
Budget: $500,000
Income Sources: American Symphony Orchestra League (Youth Orchestra Division)

Performs At: Arlene Schnitzer Concert Hall; Civic Auditorium
Organization Type: Performing; Touring; Resident; Educational

1703 ROSE CITY CHAMBER ORCHESTRA

PO Box 6652
Portland, OR 97228-6652
Phone: 503-921-2785
e-mail: info@rosecity.org
Web Site: www.rosecity.org
Mission: The Rose City Chamber Orchestra was formed in Portland, Oregon by a group of dedicated musicians with the goal to achieve the highest quality musical experience, enjoyed by both performers and the community.
Founded: 1998
Specialized Field: Community chamber orchestra

1704 SINFONIA CONCERTANTE ORCHESTRA

1640 SE Holly Street
Portland, OR 97214
Phone: 503-231-1421
Fax: 503-236-1655
e-mail: sueminde@aol.com
Management:
    Artistic Director & Conductor: Stefan Minde
Mission: To provide the community of the greater metropolitan area with outstanding performances that preserve the classical music tradition. To support mentoring and educational programs for students.
Founded: 1990
Specialized Field: Chamber Orchestra
Volunteer Staff: 20
Performs At: Lewis & Clark College; Evans Hall; St. Mary's Cathedral

1705 UMPQUA SYMPHONY ASSOCIATION

PO Box 241
Roseburg, OR 97470
Phone: 503-672-4320
Web Site: members.nbci.com/UmpquaSymphony/
Management:
    Production Director: Bob Robbins
    President: Loren Hinkle
    VP: Virginia Roth
    Secretary: Barbara Dugas
    Treasurer: Deborah Dixon
Mission: To offer the local community classical music.
Founded: 1955
Specialized Field: Symphony; Orchestra; Chamber; Ensemble; Instrumental Group
Status: Nonprofit
Performs At: Umpqua Community College Auditorium
Organization Type: Sponsoring

1706 CAMERATA MUSICA

PO Box 2782
Salem, OR 97302
Phone: 503-364-8263
Fax: 503-362-3290
e-mail: gstubble@willamette.edu
Web Site: www.open.org
Officers:
    President: George Struble
Mission: To present free chamber music concerts by local professional musicians. Concerts presented on Sunday afternoons, seven Sundays a year.
Founded: 1976
Specialized Field: Chamber music
Status: Professional; Non-Professional; Nonprofit
Volunteer Staff: 3
Paid Artists: 30
Budget: $5,000
Income Sources: Patrons; Grants; Memorial Gifts; Donations at concerts
Performs At: Salem Public Library Lecture Hall
Affiliations: Mid-Valley Arts Council, Salem
Annual Attendance: 1,600
Seating Capacity: 300
Year Built: 1990
Rental Contact: Camerata Musica (free)
Organization Type: Performing; Sponsoring

1707 SALEM CHAMBER ORCHESTRA

PO Box 768
Salem, OR 97308
Phone: 503-378-5483
e-mail: kkenaston@willamette.edu
Web Site: www.open.org/~scomusic/
Management:
    Executive Director: Kimberly Kenaston
Mission: The Salem Chamber Orchestra, through a partnership between Willamette University and the Salem-Keizer community, enriches the Willamette Valley by promoting classical music that entertains, educates, and provides performance opportunities for Willamette students and area musicians.
Founded: 1984
Specialized Field: Classical Music
Paid Staff: 2
Volunteer Staff: 4
Paid Artists: 15
Non-paid Artists: 35
Performs At: Smith Auditorium Willamette university

1708 SUNRIVER MUSIC FESTIVAL CHAMBER ORCHESTRA

PO Box 4308
Sunriver, OR 97707
Phone: 541-593-1084
Fax: 541-593-6959
e-mail: srmusic@coinet.com
Web Site: www.sunrivermusic.org
Officers:
    President: Bergen Bull
Management:
    Executive Director: Lori Noack
    Office Manager: Joan Fields
Mission: Present quality performances of classical music and educational programs for the youth of Central Oregon.
Founded: 1971

Specialized Field: Central Oregon
Paid Staff: 3
Volunteer Staff: 200
Budget: $250,000
Income Sources: Private; Business; Grants
Performs At: Great Hall
Annual Attendance: 3,500

Pennsylvania

1709 ALLENTOWN SYMPHONY ASSOCIATION

Symphony Hall
23 N 6th Street
Allentown, PA 18101
Phone: 610-432-6715
Fax: 610-871-0142
e-mail: info@allentownsymphony.org
Web Site: www.allentownsymphony.org
Officers:
President: John Berseth
Management:
Music Director/Conductor: Diane M Whittry
Executive Director: Robert Ditmars
Mission: To promote cultural values by providing high quality symphonic music and performing arts events, with broad community appeal, and education concerning them, in Allentown's historic Symphony Hall.
Founded: 1950
Specialized Field: Symphony; Orchestra; Performing Arts; Comedians
Status: Nonprofit
Income Sources: American Symphony Orchestra League; Association of Pennsylvania Orchestras; Lehigh Valley Arts Council; American Society of Composers, Authors and Publishers
Performs At: Symphony Hall
Annual Attendance: 20,000
Seating Capacity: 1246
Year Built: 1899
Year Remodeled: 1998
Rental Contact: John Ebert
Organization Type: Performing; Educational

1710 ALTOONA SYMPHONY ORCHESTRA

1331 12th Avenue, Suite 107
PO Box 483
Altoona, PA 16603
Phone: 814-943-2500
Fax: 814-943-7115
Web Site: www.altoona.net/symphony/home
Officers:
President: Al Massod
VP: Karen Shauf
Second VP: Phil Sukenik
Secretary: Edith Isacke
Assistant Secretary: Judy Halbritter
Treasurer: Heidi Rexford
Assistant Treasurer: Robert Lamort
Management:
Music Director: Nicolas Palmer
Executive Director: A Diane Schoeffler
Accounts Manager: Bruce Brower

Personnel Manager/Librarian: Sandy Woodward
Office Manager: Nancy Bickel
Mission: To provide the highest quality fine arts performances to everyone in our community.
Specialized Field: Orchestra

1711 NORTHEASTERN PENNSYLVANIA PHILHARMONIC

957 Broadcast Center
Avoca, PA 18641-1654
Phone: 570-457-8301
Fax: 570-457-5901
e-mail: info@nepaphil.org
Web Site: www.nepaphil.org
Officers:
President: Susan S Belin
VP Administration: Nicholas H Niles
VP Development: Anna Cervenak
VP Marketing/Public Relations: Mark Thomas
Treasurer: Thomas Robinson
Assistant Treasurer: Richard I. Rosenthal
Management:
Executive Director: Glenn T Roberts
Music Director/Conductor: Clyde Mitchell
Operations Manager: Jamie Kurtz
Director Development: Karen Kelly Mears
Marketing/Public Relations: Lisa Philips
Executive Assistant: Jean Spindler
Education Manager: Laura Craig
Mission: To produce the highest quality symphony orchestra and chamber ensemble performances possible; to provide musical services; to maintain an organizational environment in which local and national talent serve as a cultural resource.
Founded: 1972
Specialized Field: Symphony; Orchestra
Status: Professional; Nonprofit
Paid Staff: 11
Paid Artists: 64
Income Sources: American Symphony Orchestra League; Citizens for the Arts in Pennsylvania
Performs At: Masonic Temple; Kirby Center for the Performing Arts
Organization Type: Performing; Touring; Educational

1712 ERIE PHILHARMONIC

1006 State Street
Erie, PA 16501
Phone: 814-455-1375
Fax: 814-455-1377
e-mail: eriephil@ncinter.net
Web Site: www.eriephil.org
Management:
Music Director: Hugh Keelan
Executive Director: William F Faust
Mission: To offer symphonic, youth orchestra and pops concerts; to provide quality music educational experiences; to exhibit leadership in cultural affairs of the tri-state area.
Founded: 1913
Specialized Field: Symphony; Orchestra
Status: Nonprofit; Professional
Paid Staff: 12
Volunteer Staff: 120

Income Sources: Individual; Foundation; Grants
Performs At: Warner Theatre
Seating Capacity: 2500
Organization Type: Performing

1713 WESTMORELAND SYMPHONY ORCHESTRA

105 N Pennsylvania Avenue
Greensburg, PA 15601
Phone: 724-837-1850
Fax: 724-837-1342
e-mail: info@westmorelandsymphony.org
Web Site: www.westmorelandsymphony.org
Officers:
  President: JoAnn R Lightcap
  Treaurer: William Friedlander
Management:
  Music Director: Kypros Markov
  Executive Director: Morris A Brand
Mission: Expanding accessibility to the cultural enrichment provided by music; offering enjoyment, inspiration and motivation.
Founded: 1969
Specialized Field: Symphony; Orchestra; Ensemble
Status: Semi-Professional; Nonprofit
Paid Staff: 4
Budget: $450,000
Performs At: Palace Theatre
Seating Capacity: 1,300
Organization Type: Performing; Educational

1714 GREENVILLE SYMPHONY SOCIETY

PO Box 364
Greenville, PA 16125
Phone: 724-588-2911
Web Site: www.geocites.com/Vienna/Strasse/2224
Management:
  Manager: John H Evans
  Personnel Director: Vicki Poe
  Personnel Director: Jamie Scott
  Librarian: Jean Sankey
  Music Director/Conductor: Paul Chenevey
Mission: To provide music education through performances.
Founded: 1927
Specialized Field: Symphony; Orchestra
Status: Nonprofit
Income Sources: Pennsylvania Council on the Arts
Performs At: Passavant Memorial Center; Thiel College
Organization Type: Performing

1715 CENTRAL PENNSYLVANIA FRIENDS OF JAZZ

PO Box 10738
Harrisburg, PA 17105
Phone: 717-540-1010
Fax: 717-540-7735
e-mail: pajazz@epix.net
Web Site: www.pajazz.org
Officers:
  President: Ray Bogardus
  First VP: Frank Paul
  Second VP: Keith Thomas
  Third VP: Karen Sheaffer

  Treasurer: Fred Guion
  Secretary: Bunny Hottenstein
Management:
  Executive Director: Dave Lazorcik
Mission: To present, promote and preserve America's unique art form, jazz.
Founded: 1980
Specialized Field: Instrumental Music; Festivals
Status: Nonprofit
Paid Staff: 30
Budget: $76,000
Income Sources: Allied Arts Fund; Metro Arts of Central Pennsylvania; Mellon Bank; PA Council on the Arts
Facility Category: Hotel Ballroom
Organization Type: Performing; Educational; Sponsoring

1716 HARRISBURG SYMPHONY ASSOCIATION

800 Corporate Circle
Suite 101
Harrisburg, PA 17110
Phone: 717-545-5527
Fax: 717-545-6501
Web Site: www.harrisburgsymphony.org/
Management:
  Music Director: Stuart Malina
Mission: To offer Central Pennsylvania quality symphonic music.
Founded: 1930
Specialized Field: Symphony; Orchestra
Status: Professional; Nonprofit
Paid Staff: 15
Volunteer Staff: 300
Income Sources: Grants; Ticket Sales; Fundraising; Corporate and Individual Donations
Performs At: The Forum
Annual Attendance: 140,000
Facility Category: The Forum, State-owned Hall
Seating Capacity: 1,763
Year Built: 1931
Organization Type: Performing

1717 HARRISBURG YOUTH SYMPHONY ORCHESTRA

128 Locust Street
Harrisburg, PA 17101
Phone: 717-545-5527
Fax: 717-545-6501
Web Site: www.angelfire.com/pa3/hyso/
Management:
  Music Director/Conductor: Dr. Ronald E Schafer
Mission: To provide young people with an opportunity to participate in an orchestra.
Specialized Field: Symphony; Orchestra
Status: Non-Professional; Nonprofit
Paid Staff: 70
Income Sources: American Symphony Orchestra League (Youth Orchestra Division)
Performs At: Susquehanna Township Middle School
Organization Type: Performing; Touring; Educational; Sponsoring

1718 HERSHEY SYMPHONY ORCHESTRA

PO Box 93
Hershey, PA 17033
Phone: 717-533-8449
Fax: 717-520-9227
e-mail: hsogm@itech.net
Web Site: www.hersheysymphony.org
Management:
  Music Director: Dr. Sandra Dackow
  Assistant Coordinator: Robert Sproul
  Concertmistress: MaryLee Yerger
  General Manager: Diane Cook
  Personnel Manager: KellyLee Yerger
  Librarian: Kim Elicker
  Archivist: Annette Kilpatrick
Founded: 1969
Paid Staff: 7
Non-paid Artists: 15

1719 BALTIMORE CONSORT

801 Old York Road 1206
Jenkinstown, PA 19046
Phone: 215-885-6400
Fax: 215-885-9929
e-mail: artists@rilearts.com
Web Site: www.file.com
Management:
  Artist Management: Joanne Rile
Mission: To perform popular music of the fifteen and sixteen hundreds from England, France and Scotland.
Founded: 1980
Specialized Field: Chamber; Ensemble; Folk; Instrumental Group
Status: Professional; Nonprofit
Income Sources: Walters Art Gallery
Organization Type: Performing; Touring; Resident; Educational

1720 JOHNSTOWN SYMPHONY ORCHESTRA

227 Franklin Street
Suite 302
Johnstown, PA 15901
Phone: 814-535-6738
Fax: 814-535-6739
e-mail: info@johnstownsymphony.org
Web Site: www.johnstownsymphony.org
Officers:
  President: Karen Azer
  Past President: Edward Sheenan, Jr
  President Elect: David Mordan
  Secretary: Adelle Pickling
  Treasurer: Gordon Smith
  VP: Terry Stevens
Management:
  Executive Director: Amy Baldonieri
  Business Manager: Lawrence R Samay
  Administrative Assistant: Helen Chilcot
  Music Director: Istvan Jaray
Mission: To provide classical music for greater Johnstown area residents.
Founded: 1929
Specialized Field: Symphony; Orchestra; Chamber
Status: Professional
Paid Staff: 7

Paid Artists: 160
Non-paid Artists: 80
Budget: $616,000
Income Sources: Individuals; Corporations; Grants; Sponsors
Annual Attendance: 16,680
Facility Category: Auditorium
Seating Capacity: 1,000
Year Built: 1990
Rental Contact: Patricia Carnivali
Organization Type: Performing

1721 KENNETT SYMPHONY

105 S Broad Street
PO Box 72
Kennett Square, PA 19438
Phone: 215-444-6363
Fax: 610-925-1599
e-mail: symphony@kennett.net
Web Site: www.symphony@kennett.net
Management:
  Office Manager: Kathy Douglas
Founded: 1940
Volunteer Staff: 3

1722 LEHIGH VALLEY CHAMBER ORCHESTRA

PO Box 20641
Lehigh Valley, PA 18002
Phone: 610-266-8555
Fax: 610-266-8525
e-mail: lvco@fast.net
Web Site: www.lvco.org
Management:
  Executive Director: Llyena Boylan
  Music Director: Donald Spieth
  Office Manager: Holly Stackhouse
Mission: To support and appreciate classical music through performances of the highest standard of excellence; to enhance the quality of life in our community by fostering musical heritage and promoting contemporary American music, providing educational programming and presenting virtuoso performers of international stature; to create and seek opportunities to enhance our reputation.
Founded: 1979
Specialized Field: Orchestra
Status: Professional; Nonprofit
Paid Staff: 3
Volunteer Staff: 100
Paid Artists: 100
Income Sources: Individual; Government; Business
Performs At: Dorothy & Dexter Baker Center for the Arts
Annual Attendance: 8,000-10,000
Seating Capacity: 500
Organization Type: Performing; Touring; Educational; Recording

1723 MCKEESPORT SYMPHONY ORCHESTRA

PO Box 354
McKeesport, PA 15134-0354

Phone: 412-672-1168
Fax: 412-460-1415
e-mail: mso@trfn.clpgh.org
Web Site: www.trfn.clpgh.org
Management:
   Concertmaster: Warren Davidson
   Assistant Conductor & Choral Dir: Yugo Sava Ikach
Mission: To present orchestra concerts and other musical events of professional quality for the benefit of the public.

1724 ALLEGHENY CIVIC SYMPHONY

Music Department
Allegheny College
Meadville, PA 16335
Phone: 814-332-3356
e-mail: rbond@allegro.edu
Management:
   Conductor: Robert Bond
Mission: To provide student artists with an opportunity to perform with experienced musicians; to offer high quality performances.
Founded: 1957
Specialized Field: Symphony
Status: Semi-Professional; Nonprofit
Paid Staff: 60
Income Sources: Allegheny College
Performs At: Raymond P. Shafer Auditorium
Organization Type: Performing; Educational

1725 RIVERSIDE SYMPHONIA

136 Buckmanville Road
New Hope, PA 08530
Phone: 215-862-3300
Web Site: www.riverside-symphonia.org
Management:
   Music Director: Mariusz Simolij
   Executive Director: Benita Ryan
Founded: 1990
Budget: $150,000- $260,000
Performs At: auditorium
Seating Capacity: 450

1726 CHAMBER MUSIC SOCIETY OF BETHLEHEM

PO Box 447
Old Zionsville, PA 18068-0447
Phone: 610-435-7611
Fax: 610-967-6569
Web Site: www.cmsob.org
Officers:
   President: Jennifer H Scavuzzo
   VP: Philip Metzger
   Treasurer: Edward Walakovits
   Secretary: Margery Metzger
Mission: To offer chamber music; to promote educational activities.
Founded: 1951
Specialized Field: Chamber
Status: Nonprofit
Budget: $50,000
Income Sources: Subscriptions; Donations; Tickets Sales
Annual Attendance: 1,500
Seating Capacity: 425
Organization Type: Performing; Sponsoring

1727 BACH FESTIVAL OF PHILADELPHIA

8419 Germantown Avenue
Philadelphia, PA 19118
Phone: 215-247-2224
Fax: 215-247-4070
e-mail: bach@bach-fest.org
Web Site: www.bach-fest.org
Officers:
   President: Toni Carey
   Treasurer: Emilio Bonelli
   VP: Samuel Swansen
   Secretary: Jeanette Cord
Management:
   Executive Director: Sharon R Derstine
Mission: The Bach Festival of Philadelphia is dedicated to enriching the community through concerts and educational programs presented by some of the best Baroque interpreters in the world.
Founded: 1976
Specialized Field: Vocal Music; Instrumental Music; Festivals
Status: Professional; Nonprofit
Paid Staff: 2
Volunteer Staff: 8
Income Sources: Government; Corporate and private foundations; Donations; Ticketsales; Advertising books
Performs At: Churches, Performance halls
Annual Attendance: 2,000-3,000
Organization Type: Educational; Presenting

1728 CHESTNUT BRASS COMPANY

PO Box 30165
Philadelphia, PA 19103
Phone: 215-204-6792
Fax: 215-204-9792
Web Site: www.chestnutbrass.com/
Mission: Offering a historical perspective on brass instruments to the public.
Founded: 1977
Specialized Field: Chamber; Ensemble; Instrumental Group; Jazz
Status: Professional; Nonprofit
Income Sources: Greater Philadelphia Cultural Alliance; Temple University; Esther Boyle School
Organization Type: Performing; Touring; Resident; Educational

1729 CONCERTO SOLOISTS

Walnut Street Theatre Building
9th and Walnut Streets
Philadelphia, PA 19107
Phone: 215-574-3550
Fax: 215-574-3598
Web Site: www.wstonline.org
Management:
   Artistic/Music Director: Marc Mostovoy
   General Manager: Ken Wesler
   Artistic Administrator: Kelli Marshall
Mission: To belong to the Philadelphia community as one of its cultural institutions.
Founded: 1964
Specialized Field: Orchestra; Chamber; Ensemble; Instrumental Group
Status: Nonprofit

Income Sources: Greater Philadelphia Arts Council; Performing Arts League of Philadelphia; American Symphony Orchestra League
Performs At: Walnut Street Theatre; Church of the Holy Trinity
Organization Type: Performing; Touring; Resident; Educational; Sponsor Produced

1730 MARLBORO SCHOOL OF MUSIC
135 South 18th Street
Philadelphia, PA 19103
Phone: 215-569-4690
Fax: 215-569-9497
e-mail: marlboro@dplus.net
Web Site: www.marlboromusic.org
Management:
   General Manager: Anthony P Checchia
Mission: Professional school providing advanced training for chamber musicians.
Founded: 1951
Specialized Field: Chamber Music
Status: Professional; Nonprofit
Income Sources: Grants; Ticket Sales; Endowments; Patron Gifts
Performs At: Marlboro College Concert Hall
Annual Attendance: 8,000+
Seating Capacity: 670
Organization Type: Performing; Educational

1731 PHILADELPHIA CHAMBER MUSIC SOCIETY
135 S 18th Street
Philadelphia, PA 19103
Phone: 215-569-8587
Fax: 215-569-9497
e-mail: mail@philadelphiachambermusic.org
Web Site: www.pcmsnet.org
Officers:
   Chairman: Jerry G Rubenstein
   Vice-Chairman: M Todd Cooke
   President: Elizabeth P Glendinning
   VP: Horace W Schwarz
   Treasurer: Park B Dilks
   Secretary: Sandor S Shapiro MD
Management:
   Artistic Director: Anthony Checchia
   Executive Director: Philip Maneval
   Administrator/Concert Manager: Miles Cohen
   Development Director: Derek Delaney
   Marketing Director: Susan Grody
Mission: The Philadelphia Chamber Music Society (PCMS) is one of the largest, most accessible music presenting forums in the United States.
Founded: 1986
Performs At: Perelman Theater; Pennsylvania Convention Center

1732 PHILADELPHIA CLASSICAL GUITAR SOCIETY
2038 Sansom Street
Philadelphia, PA 19103
Phone: 215-567-2972
Fax: 215-963-9950
e-mail: membership@phillyguitar.org
Web Site: www.phillyguitar.com
Officers:
   Acting President: Joseph Mayes
   Secretary: Arnold Gessel
   Treasurer: George Thomas
Management:
   Artistic Director: Joseph Mayes
   Marketing Director: Michael Simmons
Mission: To present and foster classical guitar-related activities throughout the Greater Philadelphia area; to provide a forum for informal performance, lectures, outreach, and communication between fellow classical guitar enthusiasts.
Specialized Field: Chamber Music
Status: Professional; Nonprofit
Paid Staff: 40
Budget: $10,000-20,000
Income Sources: Ticket Sales; Patron Gifts; Grants
Performs At: Pennsylvania Convention Auditorium
Seating Capacity: 610

1733 PHILADELPHIA ORCHESTRA ASSOCIATION
260 S Broad Street
16th Floor
Philadelphia, PA 19102
Phone: 215-893-1900
Fax: 215-875-7649
e-mail: philadelphia_orchestra@philorch.org
Web Site: www.philorch.org
Officers:
   Vice Chairman (Rpac Oversight): Robert J Butera
   Vice Chairman (Artistic): John G Christy
   Vice Chairman (Planning): Peter G Ernster
   Vice Chairman (Education): Carole Haas Gravagno
   Vice Chairman Marketing: Beverly A Harper
   Vice Chairman (Human Resources): Martin A Heckscher
   Vice Chairman (Development): John N Park, Jr
   (Nominating & Governance): Robert H Rock
   Vice Chairman (Investments): Ellen C Wolf
Management:
   President/CEO: Joseph H Kluger
   Music Director/Conductor: Wolfgang Sawallisch
   Director Finance: Ben Hayllar
   Executive VP: Shel Thompson
   Chairman: Richard L Smoot
   Vice Chairman/Audit: Roland K Bullard II
   Director Public Relations: Judith Kurnick
   Director Development: Maria T Giliotto
   Director Ecucation: Gary Alan Wood
Mission: Maintaining the Philadelphia Orchestra's preeminence as one of the city's outstanding cultural assets.
Founded: 1900
Specialized Field: Symphony; Orchestra
Status: Professional; Nonprofit
Income Sources: American Symphony Orchestra League
Performs At: Academy of Music
Seating Capacity: 2,897
Organization Type: Performing

1734 PHILADELPHIA YOUTH ORCHESTRA

PO Box 41810
Philadelphia, PA 19101-1810
Phone: 215-563-7308
Fax: 215-545-7399
e-mail: info@pyos.org
Web Site: www.pyos.org
Officers:
   President: James Goodchild
Management:
   Music Director/Conductor: Joseph Primavera
   Executive Director: Louis Scaglione
Mission: To promote, encourage and foster the study and practice of music by making available to deserving and talented youth opportunities for orchestra instruction and supervision of their work and to provide concerts for promoting musical art and its appreciation.
Founded: 1939
Specialized Field: Symphony; Orchestra; Chamber; Ensemble
Status: Non-Professional; Nonprofit
Paid Staff: 2
Volunteer Staff: 200
Non-paid Artists: 190
Income Sources: American Symphony Orchestra League (Youth Orchestra Division); Greater Philadelphia Cultural Alliance
Performs At: Academy of Music
Facility Category: Theatres; Schools
Organization Type: Performing; Touring; Educational

1735 PIFFARO: THE RENAISSANCE BAND

739 N 25th Street
Philadelphia, PA 19130
Phone: 215-235-8469
Fax: 215-235-8469
e-mail: piffaro1@aol.com
Web Site: www.piffaro.com
Officers:
   Chairman: William Gross
Management:
   Director: Robert Wiemken
   Director: Joan7 Kimball
Mission: Performing early Baroque and Renaissance music using period instruments.
Founded: 1980
Specialized Field: Chamber; Ensemble; Early Music
Status: Professional; Nonprofit
Paid Staff: 3
Volunteer Staff: 10
Paid Artists: 7
Budget: $170,000
Income Sources: Government; Pennsylvania Council Art Foundation; Ticket sales; Concert fees
Organization Type: Performing; Touring; Educational

1736 PRESIDENTIAL JAZZ WEEKEND

African-American History Museum
701 Arch Street
Philadelphia, PA 19106
Phone: 215-574-0380
Fax: 215-574-3110
Management:
   Jazz Live Director: Rhoda Blount

Museum Director: Dr. Rowena Stewart
Mission: To celebrate the classical music of African-Americans.
Founded: 1989
Specialized Field: Vocal Music; Instrumental Music; Festivals; Ethnic
Status: Professional; Semi-Professional; Nonprofit
Income Sources: Greater Philadelphia Cultural Alliance; American Association of Museums; Coalition of Afro-American Organizations
Organization Type: Performing; Educational; Sponsoring

1737 RELACHE ENSEMBLE

715 S Third Street
Philadelphia, PA 19147
Phone: 215-574-8246
Fax: 215-574-0253
e-mail: relache@att.net
Web Site: www.relache.org/indexWin.htm
Management:
   Executive Artistic Director: Joseph Franklin
   Director Planning/Development: Arthur Stidfole
   Director Educational Projects: Laurel Wyckoff
Mission: Developing, producing and presenting the works of living composers.
Specialized Field: Chamber; Ensemble; Instrumental Group; Electronic & Live Electronic; Contemporary Music
Status: Professional; Nonprofit
Performs At: Mandell Theater
Organization Type: Performing; Touring; Resident; Educational; Sponsoring

1738 PITTSBURGH CHAMBER MUSIC SOCIETY

PO Box 81066
Pittsburgh, PA 15217-0566
Phone: 412-624-4129
Fax: 412-624-6461
e-mail: pcahmber@pitt.edu
Web Site: www.trfn.clpgh.org/pcms
Management:
   Executive Director: Natalie Forbes
Mission: Presenting chamber music; commissioning new works; providing educational outreach.
Founded: 1961
Specialized Field: Chamber
Status: Professional; Nonprofit
Paid Staff: 2
Income Sources: Chamber Music America; PA Presenters
Performs At: The Carnegie Music Hall
Organization Type: Sponsoring

1739 PITTSBURGH NEW MUSIC ENSEMBLE
Duquesne University School of Music

Pittsburgh, PA 15282
Mailing Address: PO Box 99476
Phone: 412-682-2955
Fax: 412-682-2955
e-mail: prime@pnme.org
Officers:
   President: Bruce Wilder

VP: Liza Weis
Secretary: Roger Dannenberg
Treasurer: Bonnie Hellman
Management:
Executive Director: Michelle Greenlaw
Artistic Director: Kevin Noe
Mission: To encourage the creation, performance, dissemination and appreciation of contemporary music, with special emphasis on American Music and living composers.
Founded: 1976
Specialized Field: Chamber; Instrumental Group; Contemporary Chamber Ensemble
Status: Professional; Nonprofit
Paid Staff: 2
Paid Artists: 50
Income Sources: Chamber Music America
Performs At: Levy Hall at The Fulton Theatres
Organization Type: Performing; Touring; Resident; Educational; Sponsoring

1740 PITTSBURGH SYMPHONY ORCHESTRA

Heinz Hall
600 Penn Avenue
Pittsburgh, PA 15222
Phone: 412-392-4900
Fax: 412-392-4909
e-mail: PSO_inquiries@pittsburghsymphony.or
Web Site: www.pittsburghsymphony.org
Officers:
President: Tom Todd
Executive VP: Gideon Toeplitz
Management:
Music Director: Mariss Jansons
Mission: Striving for and attaining excellence in artistic achievement.
Founded: 1895
Specialized Field: Symphony; Orchestra; Chamber
Status: Nonprofit
Income Sources: Pittsburgh Symphony Society
Performs At: Heinz Hall for the Performing Arts
Seating Capacity: 2,661
Organization Type: Performing; Touring; Educational; Presenting

1741 PITTSBURGH YOUTH SYMPHONY ORCHESTRA ASSOCIATION

Heinz Hall
600 Penn Avenue
Pittsburgh, PA 15222-3259
Phone: 412-392-4872
Fax: 412-392-3326
e-mail: info@pittsburghyouthsymphony.org
Web Site: www.pittsburghsymphony.org
Officers:
President: Jerry Gindrele
VP: Suzanne Cafferty Ross
Secretary: Bethne Cheberenchic
Treasurer: Roberts Milspaw
Management:
Music Director: Edward Cumming
Managing Director: Craig Johnson
Personnel Manager/Librarian: Mara Coffman

Special Projects Coordinator: Eve Goodman
Mission: To provide the best possible musical training to members of the orchestra and to develop new audiences for symphonic music among youth.
Founded: 1946
Specialized Field: Symphony; Orchestra; Chamber; Ensemble
Status: Non-Professional; Nonprofit
Income Sources: Grants; Foundations; Corporate/Individual Contribution
Performs At: Pittsburgh Symphony Heinz Hall
Annual Attendance: 5,000
Seating Capacity: 2663
Organization Type: Performing; Touring; Resident; Educational; Sponsoring

1742 RENAISSANCE AND BAROQUE SOCIETY OF PITTSBURGH

303 S Craig Street
PO Box 10156
Pittsburgh, PA 15213
Phone: 412-682-7262
Fax: 412-682-5253
e-mail: director@rbsp.org
Web Site: www.rbsp.org
Management:
Executive Director: Ann F Mason
President: Rosemary Hogan
VP: Laura Haibeck
Secretary: Susan Godfrey
Treasurer: Margaret M Barth
Mission: Sponsoring national and international touring ensembles who use period instruments to perform early music.
Founded: 1969
Specialized Field: Orchestra; Chamber; Early Music Presenter
Status: Professional
Performs At: Synod Hall; Sacred Heart Cathedral
Organization Type: Sponsoring
Comments: Special parking/entry for handicap access; Large print programs

1743 RIVER CITY BRASS BAND

PO Box 6436
Pittsburgh, PA 15212
Phone: 412-322-7222
Fax: 412-322-6821
Toll-free: 800-292-7222
e-mail: kshaffer@rcbb.com
Web Site: www.rcbb.com
Officers:
Chairman: Michael C Barbarita
Management:
Conductor: Denis Colwell
Executive Director: Marilyn Thomas
Contracted Performances Rep.: Milton Orkin
General Manager: Joseph Zuback
Mission: The mision of the River City Brass Band is to propagate and perpetuate musical culture, primarily American musical culture, across a broad spectrum of the public through the presentation of brass band

All listings are in alphabetical order by state, then city, then organization within the city.

performances, educational programs and the production of recordings. The River City Brass Band has as its central obligation service to the people of Western Pennsylvania.
Founded: 1981
Specialized Field: Band
Status: Professional; Nonprofit
Paid Staff: 8
Paid Artists: 28
Budget: $2 million
Income Sources: Association of Performing Arts Presenters; American Concert Band; National Endowment for the Arts
Performs At: Carnegie Music Hall
Annual Attendance: 140,000
Organization Type: Performing; Touring; Resident; Educational; Recording

1744 TAMBURITZANS FOLK ENSEMBLE

1801 Boulevard of the Allies
Pittsburgh, PA 15219
Phone: 412-396-5185
Fax: 412-396-5583
e-mail: stafura@duq2.cc.duq.edu
Web Site: www.duq.edu/Tamburitzans
Management:
Managing Director: Paul G Stafura
Mission: The Duquesne University Tamburitzans is dedicated to preserving and perpetuating the cultural heritages of Eastern Europe and its neighbors through performance, while awarding scholarships to talented and deserving student performers.
Founded: 1937
Specialized Field: Ensemble; Ethnic; Folk
Status: Non-Professional; Nonprofit
Paid Staff: 40
Income Sources: Duquesne University
Organization Type: Performing; Touring

1745 READING SYMPHONY ORCHESTRA

136 N 6th Street
Reading, PA 19601-3502
Phone: 610-373-7557
Fax: 610-373-5446
e-mail: readingsym@aol.com
Web Site: www.readingsymphony.com
Management:
Executive Director: Charles Weiser
Music Director/Conductor: Sidney Rothstein
Mission: Providing the city of Reading and Berks County with high quality orchestral concerts.
Founded: 1912
Specialized Field: Symphony
Status: Professional; Nonprofit
Paid Staff: 10
Non-paid Artists: 80
Income Sources: Grants; Ticket Sales; Fundraisers
Performs At: Rajah Theatre
Annual Attendance: 10,000+
Seating Capacity: 2,150
Organization Type: Performing; Educational; Sponsoring

1746 NITTANY VALLEY SYMPHONY

PO Box 1375
State College, PA 16804-1375
Phone: 814-231-8224
Fax: 814-231-0140
e-mail: info@nvs.org
Web Site: www.nvs.org
Management:
Music Director: Michael Jinbo
Mission: Pledging to program the best in orchestral music, it presents six concerts a year, including one specially designed for families.
Founded: 1967
Specialized Field: Orchestra
Status: Nonprofit
Income Sources: Ticket Revenue; Grants; Foundation Earnings; Donor Contributions

1747 VILLANOVA UNIVERSITY CHAMBER SERIES

Office of Musical Activities
Villanova University
Villanova, PA 19085
Phone: 610-519-7214
Fax: 610-519-7596
Management:
Manager: Peter Marino
Budget: $20,000-35,000
Performs At: St. Mary's Hall

1748 WILLIAMSPORT SYMPHONY ORCHESTRA

360 Market Street
Room 3
Williamsport, PA 17701-6315
Phone: 570-322-0227
Fax: 570-327-7662
e-mail: symphony@uplink.net
Web Site: www.williamsportsymphony.org
Management:
Music Director: Robin Fountain
Mission: To be a cultural asset to the community by providing quality orchestral music, education and performance opportunities for regional talent to an ever-expanding audience.

Rhode Island

1749 KINGSTON CHAMBER MUSIC FESTIVAL AT URI

PO Box 1733
Kingston, RI 02881
Phone: 401-874-2060
Fax: 401-874-2380
e-mail: sadd@egr.uri.edu
Web Site: www.mce.uri.edu
Management:
Artistic Director/Violin: David Kim
Mission: To provide outstanding classical music programs in New England. Offers both summer and winter concerts, and also outreach programs at local area schools.

Founded: 1989
Specialized Field: Classical music
Volunteer Staff: 15
Paid Artists: 1045
Budget: $60,000
Income Sources: Donations; Ticket sales
Affiliations: University of Rhode Island
Annual Attendance: 2800

1750 UNIVERSITY OF RHODE ISLAND SYMPHONY ORCHESTRA

Music Department
University of Rhode Island
Kingston, RI 02881
Phone: 401-874-2764
Fax: 401-874-2772
e-mail: music@etal.uri.edu
Web Site: www.uri.edu/artsci/mus
Management:
   Conductor: Ann Danis
Performs At: Recital Hall, Fine Arts Center

1751 BROWN UNIVERSITY ORCHESTRA

Brown University
Box 1924
Providence, RI 02912
Phone: 401-863-1472
Fax: 401-863-1256
e-mail: orchestra@brown.edu
Web Site: www/brown.edu/Orchestra
Management:
   Music Director: Paul Phillips
Founded: 1918
Specialized Field: Instrumental Music
Performs At: Sayles Hall

1752 RHODE ISLAND CHAMBER MUSIC CONCERTS

Brown University
Box 1903
Providence, RI 02912
Phone: 401-863-2416
e-mail: BROWNVM.edu
Management:
   Executive Assistant: Jeanne D Fonda
Budget: $10,000-20,000
Performs At: Alumni Hall

1753 RHODE ISLAND CIVIC CHORALE & ORCHESTRA

33 Chestnut Street
Providence, RI 02903
Phone: 401-521-5670
Fax: 401-521-5276
e-mail: ricco@ids.net
Web Site: www.ricco.org
Management:
   Music Director: Dr. Edward Markward
Performs At: Veterans Memorial Auditorium

1754 RHODE ISLAND COLLEGE SYMPHONY ORCHESTRA

Roberts Hall 215
Rhode Island College
Providence, RI 02908
Phone: 401-874-2431
Fax: 401-874-2772
Web Site: www.uri.edu/artsci/mus
Management:
   Music Director: Dr. Edward Markward
Performs At: Roberts Auditorium

1755 RHODE ISLAND PHILHARMONIC ORCHESTRA AND MUSIC SCHOOL

222 Richmond Street
Providence, RI 02903
Phone: 401-831-3123
Fax: 401-831-4577
e-mail: information@ri-philharmonic.org
Web Site: www.ri-philharmonic.org
Officers:
   Executive Director: David M Wax
   Operations Director: David W Gasper
Founded: 1945
Specialized Field: Symphony
Status: Professional; Nonprofit
Paid Staff: 10
Paid Artists: 72
Income Sources: Individual; Corporate; Foundation Grants
Performs At: VMA Arts and Cultural Center
Seating Capacity: 2,100
Organization Type: Performing; Resident; Educational

South Carolina

1756 ANDERSON SYMPHONY ORCHESTRA

126 Foxcroft Way
Anderson, SC 29621
Phone: 864-224-5508
Officers:
   President: Marion Hovermale
   Treasurer: John Kane
Management:
   Music Director: Richard Sowers
   Exeutive Director: Pamela Coletti
Founded: 1978
Specialized Field: Affiiate of the Anderson Symphony Orchestra Association.
Paid Staff: 74
Budget: $150,000-260,000
Performs At: Paramount Theatre Centre

1757 CHARLESTON SYMPHONY ORCHESTRA

77 Calhoun Street
Charleston, SC 29403
Phone: 843-723-7528
Fax: 843-722-3463
e-mail: darrell@charlestonsymphony.com
Web Site: www.charlestonsymphony.com
Officers:

President: Bronwyn Lester
Management:
    Executive Director: Darrell G Edwards
    Music Director/Conductor: David Stahl
    Associate Conductor: Bundit Ungrangsee
    Assistant Manager: Cynthia Branch
Mission: Offering South Carolina residents quality musical performances; educating children through the use of smaller orchestras and ensembles.
Founded: 1936
Specialized Field: Symphony; Orchestra; Chamber; Ensemble
Status: Professional; Nonprofit
Paid Staff: 11
Volunteer Staff: 1
Budget: $2.5 Million
Income Sources: Ticket Sales; Business; Individual Contributions; Grants
Performs At: Gaillard Municipal Auditorium
Facility Category: Multipurpose
Seating Capacity: 2730
Organization Type: Performing; Touring; Resident; Educational

1758 SPOLETO FESTIVAL USA

478 E Bay Street
Suite 200
Charleston, SC 29403
Mailing Address: PO Box 157 Charleston, SC 29402
Phone: 843-579-3100
Fax: 843-723-6383
e-mail: receptionist@spoletousa.org
Web Site: www.spoletousa.org
Officers:
    Director Finance: Tasha Gandy
    Chairman of the Board: William B Hewitt
    President: Eric G Friberg
Management:
    Artistic Director: Joesph Flummerfrlt
    Music Director: Emmanuel Villaume
    General Director: Nigel Redden
    Producer: Nunally Kersh
Mission: To present opera, dance, theater, symphonic, choral and chamber music, jazz and visual arts exhibits of the highest quality; to serve as an educational environment for young artists and audiences alike.
Founded: 1977
Specialized Field: Opera; Chamber; Choral & Symphonic Music; Jazz; Theater; Dance
Status: Professional; Semi-Professional; Nonprofit
Paid Staff: 21
Income Sources: Opera America; Dance USA; Theatre Communications Group; National Institute for Music Theater; American Arts Alliance
Performs At: Gaillard Municipal Auditorium; Dock Street Theater
Organization Type: Performing; Educational; Sponsoring

1759 CAROLINA YOUTH SYMPHONY

PO Box 534
Greenville, SC 29602
Phone: 864-232-3963
e-mail: gordon@carolinayouthsymphony.com
Web Site: www.carolinayouthsymphony.com

Management:
    Executive Director: Lee Elmore
    Conductor/Repertory Orchestra: James Kilgus
    Director: Leslie W Hicken

1760 GREENVILLE SYMPHONY ORCHESTRA

The Symphony Center
S Main Street
Greenville, SC 29601
Phone: 803-232-0344
Fax: 803-240-3113
Web Site: www.greenvillesymphony.org
Management:
    Office Manager: Patricia G Quarles
    Operations Manager: Julie Greer
    Music Director/Conductor: Edvard Tchivzhel
    General Manager: Joel E Keller
    Ticket Manager: Edith K Diver
    Librarian: Susan Bocook
Mission: Providing our community with the highest quality musical entertainment and education.
Founded: 1948
Specialized Field: Symphony; Chamber; Ensemble; Pops
Status: Professional
Income Sources: American Symphony Orchestra League; American Society of Composers, Authors and Publishers; Broadcast Music Incorporated
Performs At: Peace Center for the Performing Arts
Organization Type: Performing; Resident; Educational

1761 CONVERSE COLLEGE SINFONIETTA

Converse College
580 E Main Street
Spartanburg, SC 29302-0006
Phone: 864-596-9021
Fax: 864-596-9167
e-mail: paul.davis@converse.edu
Web Site: www.converse.edu
Management:
    Conductor: Paul Davis
Mission: College student orchestra.
Founded: 1899
Paid Staff: 2

South Dakota

1762 BROOKINGS CHAMBER MUSIC SOCIETY

Music Department
S Dakota State University, Brookings
Brookings, SD 57007
Phone: 605-688-5187
Fax: 605-688-4307
Web Site: web.sdstate.edu/sites/bcms
Officers:
    President: Dan Kemp
Management:
    Program Coordinator: John F Colson
Mission: Offering the South Dakota State University community and the Brookings area the highest quality artists and ensembles.

Founded: 1982
Specialized Field: Orchestra; Chamber; Ensemble; Instrumental Group
Status: Nonprofit
Volunteer Staff: 16
Paid Artists: 20
Budget: $18,000
Income Sources: Season tickets; Gate; Donations; Endowments; Grants
Performs At: Peterson Recital Hall
Affiliations: SDSU
Annual Attendance: 1,800
Facility Category: Recital Hall
Type of Stage: Open
Stage Dimensions: 40' x 25'
Seating Capacity: 350
Year Built: 1980
Year Remodeled: 1995
Organization Type: Performing; Educational; Sponsoring

1763 SOUTH DAKOTA STATE UNIVERSITY CIVIC SYMPHONY

Music Department
S Dakota State University
Brookings, SD 57007
Phone: 605-688-5187
Fax: 605-688-4307
e-mail: john_brawand@sdstate.edu
Management:
   Music Director/Conductor: John Browand
Mission: Performing symphonic literature from Baroque through contemporary and highlighting outstanding soloists.
Founded: 1966
Specialized Field: Symphony; Orchestra
Status: Non-Professional; Nonprofit
Paid Staff: 3
Paid Artists: 10
Non-paid Artists: 40
Budget: $10,000
Income Sources: South Dakota State University; South Dakota Arts Council; Corporate Sponsors; Local Businesses
Performs At: Peterson Recital Hall
Facility Category: Performing Arts Center
Type of Stage: Concert Hall
Stage Dimensions: 96'x63'
Seating Capacity: 1000
Year Built: 2001
Cost: $6.4 million
Organization Type: Performing; Educational

1764 BLACK HILLS SYMPHONY ORCHESTRA

Rapid City, SD
Mailing Address: PO Box 2246, Rapid City SD 57709
Phone: 605-348-4676
Web Site: www.rapidnet.com/~ecorwin/symphony
Management:
   Conductor: Jack Knowles
   Concertmaster: Coral White

Mission: To promote music appreciation and knowledge in the area; to offer opportunities for local musicians to grow through performance and education.
Founded: 1931
Specialized Field: Symphony; Orchestra
Status: Nonprofit
Paid Staff: 10
Performs At: Rushmore Plaza Civic Center Theater
Organization Type: Performing; Resident; Educational

1765 SOUTH DAKOTA SYMPHONY

300 N Dakota
Suite 116
Sioux Falls, SD 57104
Phone: 605-335-7933
Fax: 605-335-1958
e-mail: sdsymphony@sdsymphony.org
Web Site: www.sdsymphony.org
Officers:
   Executive Director: Tom Bennett
   Administrative Assistant: Linda Clement
   Marketing Coordinator: Heidi Sehr
   President: Fene Uher
Management:
   Music Director: Susan Haig
Mission: Providing the highest quality orchestral music to the people of the Northern Plains, the South Dakota Symphony takes leadership in enhancing the cultural environment of the region, developing an understanding and interest in the people of the state for fine artistic expression.
Founded: 1922
Specialized Field: Symphony; Orchestra; Chamber; Ensemble
Status: Professional; Nonprofit
Paid Staff: 8
Paid Artists: 10
Budget: $1,500,000
Income Sources: Ticket Sales, Donations, grants, fundraising events
Performs At: Washington Pavilion of Arts and Science
Facility Category: Performing arts center
Type of Stage: Multi-purpose
Stage Dimensions: 50'x60'
Seating Capacity: 1,850
Year Remodeled: 1998
Rental Contact: Jeff Venekamp
Organization Type: Performing; Touring; Resident; Educational

Tennessee

1766 CHATTANOOGA SYMPHONY AND OPERA

630 Chestnut Street
Chattanooga, TN 37402
Phone: 423-267-8583
Fax: 423-265-6520
e-mail: info@chattanoogasymphony.org
Web Site: www.chattanoogasymphony.org
Management:
   Executive Director: John Wehrle
   Music Director: Robert Bernhardt

Specialized Field: Grand Opera; Lyric Opera; Light Opera; Operetta; Symphony
Status: Professional; Nonprofit
Paid Staff: 40
Budget: $1.2 Million
Income Sources: Tennesseans for the Arts; Opera America; American Symphony Orchestra League
Performs At: Tivoli Theatre
Annual Attendance: 50,000 - 75,000
Facility Category: Theatre and Outdoor
Seating Capacity: 1700
Organization Type: Performing; Touring; Educational

1767   JACKSON SYMPHONY ASSOCIATION

1903 N Highland, Suite 6
PO Box 3429
Jackson, TN 38303
Phone: 901-427-6440
Fax: 901-427-6417
Toll-free: 800-951-6440
e-mail: jso@aeneas.net
Web Site: www.jso.tn.org
Officers:
  Executive Director: Fran Goldman
  President: Michele T Jackson
  Development Director: Jessica Barnes
  Education Coordinator: Lynn White
  Secretary: Jan Boud
  String Specialist: Adam Crane
  VP: Dave Moore
  Chairman Finance Committee: Bill Snipes
  President Symphony League: Nancy McMahon
Management:
  Music Director: Dr. Jordan Tang
  Executive Director: Fran Goldman
Mission: To support a performing orchestra of increasing quality for Jackson and its surrounding area; to promote the preservation of our musical heritage and audience exposure to the finer aspects of that heritage by providing programs that are attractive and entertaining.
Founded: 1961
Specialized Field: Symphony; Orchestra
Status: Semi-Professional
Paid Staff: 6
Volunteer Staff: 1
Budget: $600,000
Performs At: The Jackson Civic Center
Affiliations: American Symphony Orchestra League
Annual Attendance: 30,000
Organization Type: Performing; Touring; Resident; Educational

1768   JOHNSON CITY SYMPHONY ORCHESTRA

3201 Bristol Highway
Suite 2, PO Box 533
Johnson City, TN 37605
Phone: 423-926-8742
Fax: 423-926-8979
e-mail: jcsymphony@juno.com
Web Site: www.jcsymphony.com
Officers:
  Chairman: Sharon Green
Management:

  Conductor: Lewis Dalvit
  General Manager: Joel Phillips
Mission: To be a vital regional force providing orchestral music for all ages through education, entertainment, and cultural enrichment.
Founded: 1969
Specialized Field: Symphony Orchestra
Paid Staff: 4
Volunteer Staff: 1
Paid Artists: 70
Non-paid Artists: 5
Budget: $ 191,900
Income Sources: Tennessee Arts Commission Grant; Johnson City Area Arts Council Grant; Corporate and Individual Sponsorships and Contributions; Foundation Grants
Performs At: College Chapel; City Auditorium; Bristol Motor Speedway
Affiliations: ASOL; BMI
Annual Attendance: 20,000
Seating Capacity: 1194

1769   KINGSPORT SYMPHONY ORCHESTRA

1200 E Center Street
Kingsport, TN 37660
Phone: 423-392-8423
Fax: 423-392-8428
e-mail: ksorch@aol.com
Web Site: www.kso.bigstep.com
Management:
  Music Director: Cyrus Ginwala
  Executive Director: Ann Meyers
  Personnel Mgr./Education Director: Elaine Barker
  Office Manager: Judy Branfield
Mission: To offer the public orchestral concerts as well as educational programs.
Founded: 1947
Specialized Field: Symphony; Orchestra; Chamber; Ensemble; Instrumental Group
Status: Semi-Professional; Non-Professional; Nonprofit
Paid Staff: 4
Volunteer Staff: 1
Paid Artists: 75
Budget: $285,000
Income Sources: Tickets sales, TN Arts, Commission grants, private contribution,corp. contributions
Performs At: Tom F Reid Employee Center
Affiliations: ASOL
Facility Category: Auditorium
Seating Capacity: 1,700 +
Organization Type: Performing; Resident; Educational; Sponsoring

1770   KNOXVILLE SYMPHONY ORCHESTRA

708 Gay Street
Knoxville, TN 37902
Phone: 865-523-1178
Fax: 865-546-3766
Web Site: www.ksoknox.org/
Management:
  Executive Director: Constance Harrison
  Director Development: Martha Weaver
Mission: To offer the region of East Tennessee a symphony orchestra for its enjoyment and education.
Founded: 1935

Specialized Field: Symphony; Orchestra
Status: Professional; Nonprofit
Performs At: Tennessee Theater
Organization Type: Performing; Touring; Educational

1771 MEMPHIS SYMPHONY ORCHESTRA AND YOUTH SYMPHONY ORCHESTRA

3100 Walnut Grove Road
Suite 501
Memphis, TN 38111-3598
Phone: 901-324-3627
Fax: 901-324-3698
e-mail: opsdir@memphissymphony.org
Web Site: www.memphissymphony.org
Officers:
   Chairman: David Ferraro
   Chairman Elect: George E Cates
   President/Executive Director: Martha Ellen Maxwell
Management:
   Music Director/Conductor: David Loebel
   Resident Conductor: Vincent L Danner
   Director Operations: Amylou Porter
   Personnel Manager: Doug Mayes
Founded: 1952
Specialized Field: Symphony; Orchestra; Chamber
Status: Professional; Nonprofit
Paid Artists: 75
Performs At: Eudora Auditorium
Affiliations: American Symphony Orchestra League; Memphis Arts Council
Organization Type: Performing; Educational; Sponsoring

1772 NASHVILLE SYMPHONY

2000 Glen Echo Road
Suite 204
Nashville, TN 37215
Phone: 615-783-1200
Fax: 615-783-1575
Web Site: www.nashvillesymphony.org
Officers:
   Chairman: Martha R Ingram
   Secretary: Pamela K Pfeffer
   Treasurer: David Williams II
   Vice-Chairman: Joseph K Presley
   Vice-Chairman: Lou Todd
   Vice-Chairman: Anne Russell
Management:
   Music Director: Kenneth Schermerhorn
   Associate Conductor: Byung-Hyun Rhee
   Executive Director: Alan D Valentine
   Executive Assistant: Laura Faust
Mission: Dedicated to enhancing the quality of life in Nashville and the surrounding communities by providing opportunities for all citizens to enjoy live performances of symphonic music in its various forms.
Founded: 1946
Specialized Field: Symphony; Orchestra; Chamber
Status: Professional
Income Sources: American Symphony Orchestra League; American Arts Alliance; American Society of Composers, Authors and Publishers; Broadcast Music Incorporated

Performs At: Tennessee Performing Arts Center; War Memorial Auditorium
Organization Type: Performing; Resident; Touring; Educational

1773 OAK RIDGE SYMPHONY ORCHESTRA

205 Badger Road
PO Box 4271
Oak Ridge, TN 37831-4271
Phone: 423-483-5569
Fax: 423-483-3960
e-mail: orcma@kornet.org
Web Site: www.kornet.org/Orcma
Management:
   Artistic Director/Conductor: John D Welsh
   Choral Director: Rosemary Ahmad
   Office Administrator: C Anne Brackins
   Operations Manager: Robert Adamcik
Mission: Offering the community quality music; providing gifted performers with an outlet.
Founded: 1942
Specialized Field: Symphony; Orchestra
Status: Semi-Professional; Nonprofit
Paid Staff: 35
Income Sources: American Symphony Orchestra League; Tennesseans for the Arts
Performs At: Oak Ridge High School Auditorium
Organization Type: Performing; Educational

1774 SEWANEE FESTIVAL ORCHESTRAS / SEWANEE MUSIC FESTIVAL

University of the South
735 University Avenue
Sewanee, TN 37383-1000
Phone: 931-598-1225
Fax: 931-598-1706
e-mail: ssmf@sewanee.edu
Web Site: sewaneetoday.sewanee.edu/ssmf/
Management:
   Artistic Director: Dr. Steven Shrader
   Associate Director: Frank Shaffer
   Director Admission: Katherine Lehman
   Festival Coordinator: Kory Vrieze
Founded: 1957

Texas

1775 ABILENE PHILHARMONIC ASSOCIATION

402 Cypress
Suite 130
Abilene, TX 79601
Phone: 915-677-6710
Fax: 915-676-6343
Web Site: www.abilene.com/philharmonic/home.html
Management:
   Music Director/Conductor: George Yaeger
   Manager/Librarian: Ed Allcorn
   Executive Secretary: Susan Saver
Mission: Offering the finest in symphonic literature to Abilene area residents.
Founded: 1950

Specialized Field: Symphony; Orchestra
Status: Professional; Nonprofit
Income Sources: American Symphony Orchestra League
Performs At: Abilene Civic Center
Organization Type: Performing; Educational

1776 AMARILLO SYMPHONY

PO Box 2586
1000 Polk Street
Amarillo, TX 79105-2586
Phone: 806-376-8782
Fax: 806-376-7127
e-mail: symphony@arn.net
Web Site: www.amarillosymphony.org
Management:
   Executive Director: Jason S Wright
   Music Director: James Setapen
Mission: Providing symphonic music to residents of the Texas Panhandle; expanding musical appreciation and knowledge in the area.
Founded: 1924
Specialized Field: Symphony; Orchestra; Chamber; Ensemble
Status: Professional; Nonprofit
Paid Staff: 6
Budget: $1,300,000
Income Sources: Tickets; Donations
Performs At: Amarillo Civic Center
Affiliations: American Symphony Orchestra League
Annual Attendance: 80,000
Facility Category: Auditorium; Outdoor
Seating Capacity: 2,300
Year Built: 1960
Organization Type: Performing; Educational

1777 AUSTIN CHAMBER MUSIC CENTER

4930 Burnet Road
Suite 203
Austin, TX 78756
Phone: 512-454-7562
Fax: 512-454-0029
e-mail: info@austinchambermusic.org
Web Site: www.austinchambermusic.org
Management:
   Director: Felicity Coltman
   Business Manager: Ora Shay
   Education Coordinator: Lisa Link
   Arts Management Apprentice: Erin Hill
Mission: To improve the quality of community life by nurturing and expanding the knowledge, understanding, and appreciation of chamber music through education and performance.
Founded: 1981
Specialized Field: Chamber
Status: Professional; Nonprofit
Paid Staff: 4
Budget: $275,000
Income Sources: Grants from government; Foundations and corporations; Underwriting; Individuals and corporations; Ticket sales
Annual Attendance: 13,000
Facility Category: Various locations
Organization Type: Performing; Educational; Sponsoring

1778 AUSTIN CLASSICAL GUITAR SOCIETY

PO Box 49704
Austin, TX 78765
Phone: 512-832-1789
Web Site: www.main.org/acgs
Officers:
   President: Mike Harris
Management:
   Executive Director: Walter Laich
Budget: $10,000

1779 AUSTIN SYMPHONY ORCHESTRA SOCIETY

1101 Red River
Austin, TX 78701
Phone: 512-476-6064
Fax: 512-476-6242
e-mail: tickets@austinsymphony.org
Web Site: www.austinsymphony.org
Officers:
   President: Joe Long
Management:
   Executive Director: Jim Reagan
   Music Director: Peter Bay
   Director Educational Programs: Diana Eblen
   Assistant to Executive Director: Barbara Uhlaender
Mission: To enhance the cultural quality of life for the adults and young people of Austin and Central Texas by providing excellence in music performance and educational programs.
Founded: 1911
Specialized Field: Symphony; Orchestra; Chamber; Ensemble; Ethnic; Folk; Band
Status: Professional
Paid Staff: 15
Budget: $3.8 million
Season: September-April
Performs At: University of Texas Theater for the Performing Arts
Affiliations: ASOL
Annual Attendance: 400,000
Organization Type: Performing; Touring; Resident; Educational; Sponsoring

1780 SYMPHONY OF SOUTHEAST TEXAS

4345 Phelan
Suite 105
Beaumont, TX 77707
Phone: 409-892-2257
Fax: 409-892-0117
e-mail: sost@aol.com
Web Site: www.arts.state.tx.us/caltca/calregions.cfm
Management:
   Interm Executive Director: Joseph Carlucci
Mission: Offering residents of Southeast Texas high quality musical performances of all types.
Founded: 1953
Specialized Field: Symphony; Orchestra
Status: Semi-Professional; Nonprofit
Paid Staff: 5
Income Sources: American Symphony Orchestra League; American Society of Composers, Authors and Publishers; Broadcast Music Incorporated
Performs At: Julie Rogers Theatre

Organization Type: Performing; Resident

1781 BRAZOS VALLEY SYMPHONY ORCHESTRA

800 S Coulter
PO Box 3524
Bryan, TX 77802
Phone: 979-779-6100
e-mail: office@bvso.org
Web Site: www.bvso.org
Officers:
President: Keith Brooks
First VP: Douglas Menarchik
Second VP: Jim Singleton
Secretary: Jennifer de Jong
Treasurer: Kay Dobbins
Management:
Music Director/Conductor: Marcelo Bussiki
Concermaster: Javier Chaparro
Mission: To bring fine orchestral music to the Brazos Valley, home of Bryan/College Station and Texas A&M University. Each year, with generous support from our patrons, the BVSO puts on a full season of performances that delight young and old alike
Founded: 1981
Specialized Field: Symphony; Orchestra; Chamber
Status: Non-Professional
Organization Type: Performing

1782 CORPUS CHRISTI CHAMBER MUSIC SOCIETY

4709 Curtis Clark
Corpus Christi, TX 78411
Mailing Address: PO Box 60124 Corpus Christi, TX 78466-0124
Phone: 361-855-0264
Fax: 361-698-1620
e-mail: jallison@the-1.net
Management:
Program Director: Joan Allison
President: Stephen Hilmy
Mission: To prmote the appreciation and enjoyment of chamber music by bringing the world's finest ensembles.
Founded: 1984
Specialized Field: Music
Volunteer Staff: 25
Paid Artists: 15
Budget: $20,000-35,000
Income Sources: Private Donors; foundations; ticket sales
Performs At: Wolfe Recital Hall; Richardson Auditorium
Affiliations: Chamber Music America
Annual Attendance: 1,600
Facility Category: Recital Hall; Auditorium
Seating Capacity: 300; 1,800

1783 TEXAS JAZZ FESTIVAL SOCIETY

403 N Shoreline Boulevard
Corpus Christi, TX 78403
Phone: 361-883-4500
Fax: 361-883-4500
e-mail: james@microtek-sales.com
Web Site: www.texasjazz-fest.org/
Management:

Festival Originator: Al Beto Garcia
Mission: Producing the Texas Jazz Festival to the public annually, free of charge; promoting and preserving American jazz.
Founded: 1969
Specialized Field: Vocal Music; Instrumental Music; Festivals
Status: Professional; Nonprofit
Performs At: Bayfront Plaza Convention Center
Organization Type: Performing

1784 CHAMBER MUSIC INTERNATIONAL

PO Box 140092
Dallas, TX 75214
Phone: 972-385-7267
Fax: 214-324-1868
e-mail: cmi1998@yahoo.com
Web Site: community.dallasnews.com
Management:
General Manager: Anita Schmidt
Paid Staff: 1
Paid Artists: 26
Budget: $100,000
Performs At: St. Barnabas Presbyterian Church

1785 DALLAS BACH SOCIETY

PO Box 140201
Dallas, TX 75214-0201
Phone: 214-320-8700
e-mail: DBachSoc@cs.com
Web Site: www.dallasbach.org
Management:
Artistic Director: James Richman
General Manager: Angeline Churchill
Mission: Uniting the finest vocalist and instrumentalists specializing in Baroque and Classical period music, brings lively and informed performances of Handel, Bach, Vivaldi, Mozart and friends to the Dallas-Fort Worth area, featuring outstanding performers from around the Metroplex, New York, the United States and abroad, to assure the highest professional standards of performance practice and technical virtuosity.
Founded: 1982
Specialized Field: Orchestra; Chamber; Choral
Status: Professional; Semi-Professional; Nonprofit
Paid Staff: 20
Income Sources: Chorus America; International Bach Society
Performs At: Dallas Museum of Art; Saint Thomas Aquinas Church
Organization Type: Performing; Sponsoring

1786 DALLAS CHAMBER MUSIC SOCIETY

4808 Drexel Drive
Dallas, TX 75205
Phone: 214-526-7301
e-mail: dcms@netscape.net
Web Site: dcms.us
Officers:
President: George Lee, Jr
VP Development/Financial: Bill Barstow
VP Membership/Accommodations: Arend-Julius Koch
Secretary: Pat Baldwin

Management:
  Manager: Don Ort
  Artistic Director: Dorothea Kelley
Mission: To offer Dallas audiences low cost chamber music concerts of the highest professional quality.
Founded: 1954
Specialized Field: Instrumental Music
Status: Professional; Nonprofit
Performs At: Caruth Auditorium; Southern Methodist University
Organization Type: Performing; Sponsoring

1787 DALLAS CLASSIC GUITAR SOCIETY

PO Box 190823
Dallas, TX 75219
Phone: 214-528-3733
Fax: 214-528-4842
e-mail: dcgs@dallasguitar.org
Web Site: www.dallasguitar.org
Management:
  General Manager: Donna Ward
Mission: The purpose of the Dallas Classic Guitar Society is to promote the appreciation and understanding of the classical guitar and its music, from historical derivatives and related instruments to contemporary counterparts. We do this through the presentation of the best guitar artists in Classical music (Renaissance through Contemporary), Flamenco, South American, Folk, Jazz, Blues, and beyond.
Founded: 1979
Specialized Field: Guitar - classical
Status: Nonprofit
Paid Staff: 1
Income Sources: Grants; Donations
Performs At: Meyerson Symphony Center, Mesquite Arts Center
Annual Attendance: 3000 - 5000
Facility Category: Concert Halls
Seating Capacity: 500 and 1500
Organization Type: Performing; Resident; Educational; Sponsoring

1788 GREATER DALLAS YOUTH ORCHESTRA ASSOCIATION

Sammons Center for the Ars
3630 Harry Hines Boulevard
Dallas, TX 75219
Phone: 214-528-7747
Fax: 214-522-9174
e-mail: info@gdyo.org
Web Site: www.gdyo.org
Management:
  Executive Director: Charles R Moore
  Artistic Director: Richard Giangiulio
Mission: To provide serious Dallas area student musicians with ensemble training performance opportunities.
Founded: 1972
Specialized Field: Symphony; Orchestra; Ensemble
Status: Non-Professional; Nonprofit
Income Sources: Tuition; Diversified Grants
Performs At: Morton H Meyerson Symphony Center
Affiliations: American Symphony Orchestra League
Annual Attendance: 15,000

Organization Type: Performing; Resident; Educational

1789 VOICES OF CHANGE

8609 NW Plaza Drive
#438
Dallas, TX 75225
Phone: 214-378-8670
Fax: 214-378-5043
e-mail: voicesofchange@mail.com
Web Site: www.voicesofchange.org
Officers:
  Office Administrator: Donna Mendro
  President: Helen Tieber
  VP/Treasurer: Russell Horn
  Secretary: Jani Leuschel
Management:
  Artistic Director: Jo Boatright
  Co-Artistic Director: Sheilds-Collins Bray
Mission: To present the works of living composers and classics of the 20th & 21st centuries; to offer a seasonal series, tours, monthly radio broadcasts, recordings, special-event concerts and commissions.
Founded: 1975
Specialized Field: Chamber; Ensemble
Status: Professional; Nonprofit
Paid Staff: 2
Budget: $115,000
Income Sources: Tickets, Gifts, Grants
Performs At: Caruth Auditorium; Southern Methodist University
Affiliations: Chamber Music America; Southern Methodist University; American Music Center; Meet the Composers; Texas Commission on the Arts
Annual Attendance: 5,000
Organization Type: Performing; Touring; Resident; Educational

1790 WALDEN PIANO QUARTET/WALDEN CHAMBER MUSIC SOCIETY

PMB 729
PO Box 29081
Dallas, TX 75372
Phone: 214-750-1561
Fax: 214-369-4711
e-mail: laucl@excite.com
Management:
  Management Consultant: Clara Lau
Founded: 1981
Specialized Field: Chamber Music
Status: Professional
Paid Staff: 1
Volunteer Staff: 1
Paid Artists: 5
Budget: $20,000-35,000
Income Sources: Private; City; Foundations
Performs At: Sanctuary, First Unitarian Church
Annual Attendance: 1,200
Stage Dimensions: 15 x 20
Year Built: 1965

1791 SOUTH TEXAS SYMPHONY ASSOCIATION

1201 W University
Edinburg, TX 78539

Mailing Address: PO Box 2832 McAllen, TX 78501
Phone: 956-393-2293
Fax: 956-393-2290
e-mail: southtexassymphony@prodigy.net
Web Site: www.southtexassymphony.com
Officers:
   President: Suzie McDonald
   VP: Bill Buerns
   Secretary: Matt Weber
   Treasurer: Cecilio Rodriguez
Management:
   Administrator: Glynda Boykin
   Administrative Secretary: Velma Ranirez
   Clerk: Rolando Gonzalez
Mission: Promoting, nurturing and supporting symphonic music performances in South Texas.
Founded: 1976
Specialized Field: Symphony; Chamber
Status: Semi-Professional; Nonprofit
Paid Staff: 78
Volunteer Staff: 40
Budget: $529,000
Income Sources: American Symphony Orchestra League; Pan American University
Performs At: Pan American University Fine Arts Auditorium
Annual Attendance: 6,500
Facility Category: Fine Arts Center
Seating Capacity: 1,055
Organization Type: Performing; Resident; Educational

1792 EL PASO PRO-MUSICA

3557 N Mesa
PO Box 13328
El Paso, TX 79913-3328
Phone: 915-833-9400
Fax: 915-833-9425
e-mail: info@elpasopromusica.org
Web Site: www.elpasopromusic.org
Officers:
   Chairman/President: Ellen Lacy
   President Elect: Jaime Lowensberg
Management:
   Executive Director: Karen Paul
   Office Manager: Nancy Ellis
Mission: Promoting musical and cultural growth in the El Paso area; presenting chamber music and a chamber music festival.
Founded: 1977
Specialized Field: Chamber Music
Status: Professional; Nonprofit
Organization Type: Performing; Educational; Presenter

1793 EL PASO SYMPHONY ORCHESTRA

PO Box 180
El Paso, TX 79942
Phone: 915-532-3776
Fax: 915-533-8162
e-mail: epsoorg@htp.net
Web Site: www.epso.org
Officers:
   Chairman: William V Ballew, III
Management:
   Executive Manager: Ruth Ellen Jacobson
   Music Director/Conductor: Gurer Aykal

Mission: Fostering appreciation of symphonic music in the El Paso area.
Founded: 1930
Specialized Field: Symphony; Orchestra
Status: Professional; Nonprofit
Paid Staff: 100
Budget: $1,000,000
Income Sources: Ticket sales, contributions
Performs At: El Paso Civic Center Theatre
Annual Attendance: 35,000
Facility Category: Theatre
Seating Capacity: 2,400
Organization Type: Performing; Educational; Sponsoring

1794 CLIBURN CONCERTS

Van Cliburn Foundation
2525 Ridgmar Boulevard, Suite 307
Fort Worth, TX 76116
Phone: 817-738-6536
Fax: 817-738-6534
e-mail: clistaff@cliburn.org
Web Site: www.cliburn.org
Officers:
   President: Richard Rodzinski
Management:
   General Manager: Maria Guralnik
Mission: To produce the Cilburn Piano Series.
Founded: 1962
Status: Professional; Nonprofit
Budget: $150,000-400,000
Performs At: Nancy Lee & Perry R. Bass Performance Hall

1795 FORT WORTH SYMPHONY ORCHESTRA

330 E 4th Street
Suite 200
Fort Worth, TX 76102
Phone: 817-665-6500
Fax: 817-665-6600
e-mail: admin@fwsymphony.org
Web Site: www.fwsymphony.org
Officers:
   Executive Director: Ann Koonsman
Management:
   Music Director: Miguel Harth-Bedoya
   General Manager: John Toohey
   Production Manager: Jim Brady
   Marketing Manager: Stacey Newman
Mission: To provide the leadership and financial support required to maintain a symphony orchestra of first rank and to build an internationally-recognized chamber orchestra, dedicated to artistic development and performances of superior quality.
Founded: 1925
Specialized Field: Symphony; Orchestra; Chamber
Status: Professional; Nonprofit
Paid Staff: 25
Volunteer Staff: 400
Paid Artists: 80
Budget: $9,900,000
Income Sources: Ticket Sales; Grants; Individual & Corporate Donors

Performs At: Tarrant County Convention Center; Ed Landreth Auditorium
Affiliations: American Symphony Orchestra League
Annual Attendance: 290,000
Rental Contact: Rental Contact Carl Davis
Organization Type: Performing; Touring

1796 YOUTH ORCHESTRA OF GREATER FORT WORTH

4401 Trail Lake Drive
Orchestra Hall
Fort Worth, TX 76109
Phone: 817-923-3121
Fax: 817-924-0007
e-mail: yofwex@yahoo.com
Web Site: www.geocites.com/Vienna/Strasse/7287/
Management:
   General Manager: David Goudy
Mission: Educating young musicians from the ages of 3 to 22.
Founded: 1965
Specialized Field: Orchestra
Status: Nonprofit
Paid Staff: 1
Volunteer Staff: 100
Paid Artists: 6
Budget: $200,000
Income Sources: Grants; tuitions; concerts
Performs At: Orchestra Hall
Annual Attendance: 4,000
Type of Stage: Proscenium
Stage Dimensions: 70x40
Seating Capacity: 384
Year Built: 1940
Year Remodeled: 1980
Rental Contact: 817-921-6222 Mike Haley
Organization Type: Performing; Touring; Educational

1797 DALLAS BRASS

4321 Clemson Drive
Garland, TX 75042
Phone: 972-276-7114
Web Site: www.dallasbrass.com/
Management:
   Director: Michael Levin
   Booking Coordinator: Wiss Rudd
Mission: Striving to bridge musical gaps from classical to pop.
Founded: 1982
Specialized Field: Ensemble; Instrumental Group
Status: Professional; Commercial
Organization Type: Performing; Touring; Resident; Educational

1798 GARLAND SYMPHONY ORCHESTRA

1721 Reserve
Garland, TX 75042
Phone: 972-926-0611
Fax: 972-926-0811
Web Site: www.garlandsymphony.org/
Officers:
   President: Dick Sutton
   VP: Mike Lancaster
   Secretary: Celia Swiger

Treasurer: Rick Trimble
Management:
   Music Director: Robert Carter Austin
   Assistant General Manager: Richard Stieber
Mission: Presenting the finest possible concerts.
Founded: 1978
Specialized Field: Symphony; Orchestra
Status: Professional; Nonprofit
Performs At: Garland Performing Arts Center
Organization Type: Performing; Educational

1799 CLEAR LAKE SYMPHONY

PO Box 890582
Houston, TX 77289-0582
Phone: 713-639-0702
e-mail: arthurs@blkbox.com
Web Site: www.serve.com/Violin
Management:
   General Manager: Betty Wall
   Music Director: Charles Johnson
Mission: To present classical music for the residents of the Bay area and to provide opportunities to qualified musicians both to perform with a classical orchestra and to participate in the music education of the area.
Founded: 1976
Specialized Field: Symphony; Orchestra
Status: Non-Professional; Nonprofit
Paid Staff: 34
Income Sources: National Symphony Orchestra League
Performs At: Clear Lake Theatre; Gloria Dei Lutheran Church Auditorium
Organization Type: Performing

1800 HOUSTON CIVIC SYMPHONY ORCHESTRA

4378 Harrest Lane
Houston, TX 77004-6606
Phone: 713-747-0018
e-mail: harris@bcm.tmc.edu
Web Site: www.civicsymphony.org
Officers:
   President: Mark Andrews
   VP: John Snyder
   Secretary: Susan Weaver
   Treasurer: Betty Thompson
Management:
   Music Director: Clifton Evans
   Assistant Conductor: Richard Spitz
Mission: To provide a playing and performance opportunity for professional and nonprofessional musicians who earn the major portion of their livelihood outside full-time, professional music performances.
Founded: 1967
Specialized Field: Symphony; Orchestra; Chamber
Status: Semi-Professional; Nonprofit
Paid Staff: 65
Income Sources: University of Houston
Performs At: Cullen Hall; University of Houston
Organization Type: Performing

1801 HOUSTON EARLY MUSIC

PO Box 271193
Houston, TX 77277

Phone: 713-432-1744
e-mail: info@HoustonEarlyMusci.org
Web Site: www.HoustonEarlyMusic.org
Officers:
President: Rodney Koenig
Secretary: Bettie Anderson
Treasurer: Terece McGovern
Management:
Executive Director: Helga Aurisch
Artistic Director: Nancy Ellis
Mission: Houston Early Music is a chartered, non-profit, organization whose purpose is to present historically-informed performances of early music from the European traditions and other world cultures in concerts featuring internationally renowned vocal, instrumental and chamber musicians. In addition, we reach out to new and diverse audiences through a cross-disciplinary educational program.
Founded: 1968
Specialized Field: Chamber; Ensemble; Ethnic; Folk; Dance
Status: Professional; Nonprofit
Paid Staff: 8
Organization Type: Educational; Sponsoring

1802 HOUSTON FRIENDS OF MUSIC

Shepperd School of Music, Rice University
PO Box 1892
Houston, TX 77251
Phone: 713-348-5400
Fax: 713-348-5405
e-mail: friends@rice.edu
Web Site: www.ruf.rice.edu/friends
Management:
Administrative Director: Alicia D Less
Mission: Presenting chamber ensembles of national and international reputation; developing new audiences.
Founded: 1959
Specialized Field: Chamber; Ensemble; Instrumental Group
Status: Professional; Nonprofit
Income Sources: Shepherd School of Music
Performs At: Seude Concert Hall
Organization Type: Performing; Sponsoring

1803 IRVING SYMPHONY ORCHESTRA ASSOCIATION

225 E John Carpenter Freeway
Suite 120
Irving, TX 75062
Phone: 972-831-8818
Fax: 972-831-8817
e-mail: irvingsymphony@irvingsymphony.com
Web Site: www.irvingsymphony.com
Officers:
President: Rene Castilla
President Elect: Beverly Adams
Secretary: Nancie Rissing
Treasurer: Carol Little
Management:
Music Director/Conductor: Hector Guzman
Executive Director: Marguerite Korkmas
Mission: Offering Irving and its surrounding communities outstanding music.

Founded: 1962
Specialized Field: Symphony; Orchestra
Status: Nonprofit
Paid Staff: 1
Volunteer Staff: 220
Paid Artists: 85
Performs At: Carpenter Performance Hall
Affiliations: ASOL; TASO
Organization Type: Performing

1804 LAREDO PHILHARMONIC ORCHESTRA

PO Box 1399
Laredo, TX 78042
Phone: 956-727-8886
e-mail: lpo@laredophilharmonic.org
Web Site: www.laredophilharmonic.org
Management:
Music Director/Conductor: Terence Frazor
Co-President: Consuelo Lopez
Co-President: Elmo Lopez
Executive VP: Teresa Nimcham
Mission: Contributing to the cultural enrichment of Laredo and the surrounding area.
Founded: 1980
Specialized Field: Symphony; Orchestra; Chamber
Status: Professional; Nonprofit
Performs At: Laredo Civic Center
Organization Type: Performing; Touring; Resident; Educational

1805 LONGVIEW SYMPHONY ORCHESTRA

PO Box 1825
Longview, TX 75606
Phone: 903-236-9739
Web Site: www.longviewtx.com
Management:
Music Director/Conductor: Tonu Kalam
Business Manager: Gary Bruns
Mission: Presenting the highest calibre orchestral music to Texas citizens.
Founded: 1968
Specialized Field: Symphony; Orchestra
Status: Semi-Professional; Nonprofit
Volunteer Staff: 36
Paid Artists: 75
Budget: $260,000
Income Sources: Ticket sales; Grants; Contributions
Performs At: T.G. Field Auditorium
Annual Attendance: 5,000
Organization Type: Performing; Resident; Educational

1806 LUBBOCK SYMPHONY ORCHESTRA

1313 Broadway
Suite 2
Lubbock, TX 79401
Phone: 806-762-1688
Fax: 806-762-1824
e-mail: iso@door.net
Web Site: www.lubbocksymphony.org
Management:
Executive Director: Pam Parkman
Music Director/Conductor: Andrews Sill

Mission: Offering the Lubbock Area symphonic music and an enhanced quality of life.
Founded: 1942
Specialized Field: Symphony; Orchestra; Chamber; Ensemble
Status: Professional; Nonprofit
Paid Staff: 8
Volunteer Staff: 450
Paid Artists: 84
Budget: $900k
Income Sources: American Symphony Orchestra League; American Society of Composers, Authors and Publishers
Performs At: Lubbock Memorial Civic Center
Annual Attendance: 12,000
Seating Capacity: 1,400
Organization Type: Performing; Educational

1807 MARSHALL SYMPHONY ORCHESTRA
Marshall, TX 75671
Mailing Address: PO Box 421
Phone: 903-935-5266
Fax: 903-938-3531
Management:
   Artistic Director/Conductor: Leonard Kacenjar
   Management Consultant: Fran Hurley
Mission: To provide local musicians with an opportunity to perform along with professional musicians; to provide symphonic music for area audiences.
Founded: 1952
Specialized Field: Symphony; Orchestra
Status: Semi-Professional; Nonprofit
Paid Staff: 45
Income Sources: Marshall Regional Arts Council; Texas Association of Symphony Orchestras
Performs At: Marshall Civic Center Theatre
Organization Type: Performing

1808 MIDLAND-ODESSA SYMPHONY AND CHORALE
3100 LaForce Boulevard
PO Box 60658
Midland, TX 79711
Phone: 915-563-0921
Fax: 915-498-9251
e-mail: symphony@mosc.org
Web Site: www.mosc.org
Management:
   Executive Director: Jeannine Donnelly
   Music Director/Conductor: Nyela Basney
Mission: To offer residents of the Permian Basin symphonic, chamber and choral music.
Founded: 1962
Specialized Field: Symphony; Orchestra; Chamber; Ensemble
Status: Nonprofit
Paid Staff: 6
Volunteer Staff: 100
Paid Artists: 65
Budget: $670,000
Income Sources: Tickets; Grants; Donations
Affiliations: ASOL
Annual Attendance: 10,000
Organization Type: Performing; Educational

1809 SAN ANGELO SYMPHONY ORCHESTRA AND CHORALE
PO Box 5922
San Angelo, TX 76902
Phone: 915-658-5877
Fax: 915-653-1045
e-mail: mercyla@sanangelosymphony.org
Web Site: www.sanangelosyphony.org
Officers:
   President: Fred Key
   VP: Doris Rousselot
   Secretary: Johnell Vincent
   Treasurer: Bill McKinney
   Past President: Teady George
Management:
   Music Director/Conductor: Hector Guzman
   Executive Director: Mercyla Sheiburne
Mission: To further cultural advancement and enjoyment of symphonic music in the San Angelo area.
Founded: 1948
Specialized Field: Symphony
Status: Professional; Non-Professional; Nonprofit
Paid Staff: 140
Income Sources: Broadcast Music Incorporated; American Society of Composers, Authors and Publishers; American Symphony Orchestra League
Performs At: City Auditorium
Annual Attendance: 50,000
Seating Capacity: 1,590
Organization Type: Performing

1810 SAN ANTONIO CHAMBER MUSIC SOCIETY
PO Box 12702
San Antonio, TX 78212
Phone: 210-408-1558
Fax: 210-408-1558
e-mail: bat@ccsi.com
Web Site: www.ccsi.comg
Officers:
   President: Dale Bennett
   VP Administration: Diane Stevens
   VP Membership: Daavid Shapiro
   Financial Secretary: Mary K Vaughan
   Treasurer: William Montville
   Secretary: George M Vaughan
Management:
   Artist Committee: Ruth J Guriuitz
   Artist Committee: Marilyn Cockburn
Mission: Chamber music series featuring world chamber music artists.
Founded: 1943
Specialized Field: Chamber music ensembles
Volunteer Staff: 25
Paid Artists: 5
Budget: $35,000-60,000
Performs At: Incarnate Word College Auditorium

1811 SAN ANTONIO SYMPHONY
222 E Houston Street
Suite 200
San Antonio, TX 78205

Phone: 210-554-1000
Fax: 210-554-1008
Web Site: www.sasymphony.org
Management:
   Music Advisor: Christopher Wilkins
   Executive Director: Steven R Brosvik
   Gen. Manager/Artistic Administrator: Lawrence J
   Fried
   Public Relations: Nancy Diehl
Mission: Providing an outstanding professional symphony; meeting cultural, entertainment and educational needs of the community.
Founded: 1939
Specialized Field: Symphony; Orchestra
Status: Professional; Nonprofit
Paid Staff: 21
Paid Artists: 77
Budget: $7,500,000
Income Sources: American Symphony Orchestra League
Performs At: Majestic Theatre
Seating Capacity: 2400
Organization Type: Performing; Educational

1812 YOUTH ORCHESTRAS OF SAN ANTONIO
Department of Parks & Recreation
950 E Hildebrand Avenue
PO Box 120396
San Antonio, TX 78212
Phone: 210-737-0097
Fax: 210-732-7233
e-mail: musicdir@stic.net
Web Site: www.yosa.org
Management:
   Music Director: Brendon Townsend

1813 MID-TEXAS SYMPHONY ORCHESTRA
Texas Lutheran University
1000 W Court Street
PO Box 3216-TLU
Seguin, TX 78155
Phone: 830-372-8089
Fax: 830-372-8112
e-mail: mts@tlu.edu
Web Site: www.segurn.net/orgimtsymphony
Officers:
   President: Bill Dean
Management:
   Stage Manager: Kappa Kappa Psi
Founded: 1978
Specialized Field: Symphony Orchestra
Paid Staff: 1

1814 SHERMAN SYMPHONY ORCHESTRA
900 N Grand Avenue
Suite 61567
Sherman, TX 75090
Phone: 903-813-2251
Fax: 903-813-2273
e-mail: ddominick@austinc.edu
Web Site: shermansymphony.com
Management:
   Conductor: Daniel Dominick

Mission: To offer concert performances featuring standard orchestral repertoire to area audiences; to provide guest appearances by nationally-known soloists.
Founded: 1966
Specialized Field: Symphony; Orchestra
Status: Non-Professional; Nonprofit
Paid Staff: 2
Volunteer Staff: 40
Paid Artists: 30
Budget: $50,000
Performs At: Wynne Chapel
Annual Attendance: 3,200
Facility Category: College Chapel; City Concert Hall
Seating Capacity: 300; 1,300
Year Built: 1930
Year Remodeled: 2000
Organization Type: Performing; Educational; Sponsoring

1815 EAST TEXAS SYMPHONY ORCHESTRA
305 S Broadway
Suite 603
Tyler, TX 75702
Phone: 903-592-1427
Fax: 903-592-7649
Web Site: www.etso.org/
Officers:
   VP Operations: Jean Davoust
   President/CEO: Les Talbert
   President Elect: LaVerne Gollop
   VP Administration: Nancy Wrenn
Mission: To bring excellent orchestral music to East Texas.
Founded: 1936
Specialized Field: Symphony; Orchestra
Status: Professional; Semi-Professional
Paid Staff: 7
Paid Artists: 70
Performs At: Cowan Performing Arts Center; UT-Tyler
Affiliations: American Symphony Orchestra League
Seating Capacity: 2,073
Organization Type: Performing

1816 WACO SYMPHONY ORCHESTRA
600 Austin Avenue, Suite 22
PO Box 1201
Waco, TX 76703
Phone: 254-754-0851
Fax: 254-752-8611
e-mail: exdir@wacosymphony.com
Web Site: www.wacosymphony.com
Management:
   Executive Director: Susan Taylor
Founded: 1962

1817 WICHITA FALLS SYMPHONY ORCHESTRA
30005 Garnett
Parker Square
Wichita Falls, TX 76308
Phone: 940-723-6202
Fax: 817-322-4480
Web Site: members.aol.com/WFSO/WFSO.htm
Management:

Manager: Alex Rouggieri
Music Director/Conductor: Theodore Plute
Mission: Offering the community the highest quality of symphonic music; educating area youth.
Founded: 1946
Specialized Field: Symphony; Orchestra
Status: Nonprofit
Performs At: Memorial Auditorium
Organization Type: Performing

Utah

1818 UTAH CLASSICAL GUITAR SOCIETY
1466 E 920 S
Provo, UT 84606

Management:
President: James Mahood
Program Director: David Norton
Secretary: Stephen Hanka
Mission: Furthering performance and study of classical guitar repertoire in Utah.
Founded: 1984
Specialized Field: Chamber
Status: Nonprofit
Paid Staff: 5
Performs At: First Presbyterian Church; Salt Lake City
Organization Type: Performing

1819 CHAMBER MUSIC SOCIETY OF SALT LAKE CITY
807 N Juniperpoint Drive
Salt Lake City, UT 84103
Phone: 801-364-1322
Fax: 801-581-4148
e-mail: wwallcomp@aol.com
Officers:
President: Edward Epstein
VP: Naomi Feigel
Treasurer: Paul Griffin
Secretary: Linda Schweikand
Management:
Program Chair: Fran Wilcox
Transportation Chair: David George
President: Edward Epstein
Mission: To entertain and enlighten.
Founded: 1966
Specialized Field: Chamber Music
Budget: $40,000-45,000
Income Sources: Ticket Sales; Contributions
Performs At: Libby Gardner Auditorium - David Gardner Hall
Facility Category: Auditorium
Seating Capacity: 650
Year Remodeled: 1999

1820 EASTERN ARTS INTERNATIONAL DANCE THEATER
PO Box 526362
Salt Lake City, UT 84152

Phone: 801-485-5824
e-mail: kstjohn@burgoyne.com
Web Site: www.easternartists.com
Officers:
Dance Director: Katherine St John
Music Director: Lloyd Miller
Management:
Director: Katherine St. John
Mission: To promote time-honored traditions by offering concerts, lectures, and workshops of cultures from Asia and Eastern Europe.
Founded: 1960
Specialized Field: Ethnic
Status: Professional; Nonprofit
Paid Staff: 10
Income Sources: Western Alliance of Arts Administrators; Society for Ethno-Musicology; Middle East Studies Association; Society for Dance Ethnology
Organization Type: Performing; Educational; Sponsoring

1821 GINA BACHAUER INTERNATIONAL PIANO FOUNDATION
Salt Lake City, UT 84147
Mailing Address: PO Box 11664
Phone: 801-521-9200
Fax: 801-521-9202
e-mail: gina@bachauer.com
Web Site: www.bachauer.com
Officers:
Chairman: Linda M Babcock
Vice Chairman: Jeffrey T Simmons
Secretary/Treasurer: Taylor Vriens
Management:
Artistic Director/Founder: Dr. Paul C Pollei
Associate Artistic Director: Massimiliano Frani
Executive Director: Kimberly Garnn
Marketing/PR Director: Tracey Turner
Mission: To further the pianistic art by holding international piano competitions, solo recitals and educational sessions; to enrich the community and build an artistic and educational environment for musicians and nonmusicians alike.
Founded: 1976
Specialized Field: Classical Piano
Status: Nonprofit
Paid Staff: 8
Performs At: Symphony Hall; Salt Lake City Assembly Hall
Organization Type: Performing; Educational; Sponsoring

1822 GRANITE YOUTH SYMPHONY
340 E 3545 S
Salt Lake City, UT 84115
Phone: 801-268-8542
Fax: 801-263-6128
Management:
PhD Staff Assoc., Music Education: Ellis C Worthen
Mission: Dedicated to studying and performing standard symphonic literature.
Founded: 1957
Specialized Field: Symphony; Orchestra; Instrumental Group

Status: Nonprofit
Income Sources: Granite School District
Organization Type: Performing; Touring; Educational

1823 ORCHESTRA AT TEMPLE SQUARE

50 E North Temple Street
20th Floor
Salt Lake City, UT 84150
Phone: 801-240-4150
Fax: 801-240-4886
e-mail: Bradfordbd@ldschurch.org
Officers:
  President: Mac Christensen
  Manager: Brent R Peterson
Management:
  Director: Barlow D Bradford
Founded: 1999
Paid Staff: 2
Volunteer Staff: 6
Non-paid Artists: 110
Performs At: Tabernacle on Temple Square
Affiliations: The Church of Jesus Christ of Latter-day Saints
Annual Attendance: 10,000
Facility Category: Church

1824 SALT LAKE SYMPHONY

220 Morris Avenue
Suite 200
Salt Lake City, UT 84115
Phone: 801-463-2440
e-mail: contact@saltlakesymphony.com
Web Site: www.saltlakesymphony.org
Management:
  Music Director/Conductor: James Michael Caswell
Founded: 1976
Income Sources: Individuals; Corporations
Performs At: Abravanel Hall; Jeanne Wagner Concert Hall; Temple Square

---

1825 UNIVERSITY OF UTAH: DEPARTMENT OF MUSIC

1395 E President's Circle
Room 204
Salt Lake City, UT 84112-0030
Phone: 801-581-6762
Fax: 801-581-5683
e-mail: robertwalzel@music.utah.edu
Web Site: www.music.utah.edu
Officers:
  Chairman: Edgar J Thompson
Performs At: David P. Gardner Hall; Libby Gardner Concert Hall; Chamber Music Hall; Dumke Recital Hall; Mckay Music Library

---

1826 UTAH SYMPHONY

123 W S Temple
Salt Lake City, UT 84101
Phone: 801-533-5626
Fax: 801-521-6634
e-mail: info@utahsymphony.org
Web Site: www.utahsymphony.org
Officers:

Chairman: Scott Parker
Management:
  Music Director: Keith Lockhart
  Principal Guest Conductor: Pavel Koganrson
  Assistant Conductor: Scott O'Neill
  Assistant Conductor: Kory Katseanes
  Assistant Stage Manager: Rick Cave
  Assistant Stage Manager: Joielle Adams
Mission: To maintain a symphony orchestra capable of providing performances of the highest possible quality; to provide performance opportunities for skilled professional musicians; to foster musical education for persons of all ages.
Founded: 1940
Specialized Field: Symphony
Status: Professional; Nonprofit
Budget: $12,000,000
Income Sources: American Symphony Orchestra League; American Arts Alliance
Performs At: Symphony Hall
Annual Attendance: 200,000
Facility Category: Concert Hall
Seating Capacity: 2,800
Year Built: 1979
Architect: $12,000,000
Organization Type: Performing; Educational

Vermont

1827 BURLINGTON DISCOVER JAZZ FESTIVAL

230 College Street
Burlington, VT 05401
Phone: 802-863-7992
Fax: 802-864-3927
e-mail: info@discoverjazz.com
Web Site: www.discoverjazz.com
Officers:
  Director for the Performing Arts: Andrea Rogers
Management:
  Director: Michael Bandelato
  Director Marketing/Development: Tara Perkins
  Chief Programming Officer: Arnie Malina
Mission: Offering the widest possible range of jazz and music educational programs; ticketed and free events.
Founded: 1984
Specialized Field: Vocal Music; Instrumental Music; Festivals
Status: Nonprofit
Paid Staff: 2
Volunteer Staff: 350
Budget: $300,000
Income Sources: Burlington City Arts; Flynn Center
Performs At: Multi-disciplinary
Annual Attendance: 45,000
Facility Category: city-wide (Burlington)
Organization Type: Performing; Educational; Sponsoring

1828 VERMONT MOZART FESTIVAL

110 Main Street
Burlington, VT 05401

Phone: 802-862-7352
Fax: 802-862-2201
Toll-free: 800-639-9097
Web Site: www.vtmozart.com/
Management:
   Executive Director: Laura Cole
   Associate Director: Regina Gonzales
Mission: To create opportunities for young people to appreciate and pursue excellence in music.
Founded: 1973
Specialized Field: Vocal Music; Instrumental Music; Festivals
Status: Professional; Nonprofit
Income Sources: Ticket sales, sponsorship, membership
Organization Type: Performing

1829 VERMONT SYMPHONY ORCHESTRA
2 Church Street
Suite 19
Burlington, VT 05401-4457
Phone: 802-864-5741
Fax: 802-864-5109
Toll-free: 800-876-9293
e-mail: info@vso.org
Web Site: www.vso.org
Officers:
   Chairman: John Dinse
   Vice Chairman: Ken Singer
   Treasure: Jesse F Sammis, III
   Secretary: Patricia Mandeville
Management:
   Executive Director: Alan Jordan
   Orchestra Manager: Eleanor Long
   Music Director: Jaime Laredo
Founded: 1934
Specialized Field: Symphony; Ensemble
Status: Professional; Nonprofit
Paid Staff: 14
Paid Artists: 54
Budget: $1,400,000
Performs At: Flynn Theatre
Affiliations: American Symphony Orchestra League
Annual Attendance: 65,100
Organization Type: Performing; Touring; Educational

1830 VERMONT YOUTH ORCHESTRA
PO Box 905
Burlington, VT 05402
Phone: 802-658-4708
Fax: 802-658-4810
e-mail: info@vyo.org
Web Site: www.vyo.org
Management:
   Manager: Carolyn Long
   Music Director/Conductor: Troy Peters
   Executive Director: Caroline W Widdon
Mission: Exposing young people to music, with an emphasis on classical.
Founded: 1964
Specialized Field: Symphony; Orchestra
Status: Non-Professional; Nonprofit
Paid Staff: 85
Budget: $400,000
Income Sources: American Symphony Orchestra League (Youth Orchestra Division)

Performs At: Flynn Theatre, local schools
Organization Type: Performing; Educational

1831 BANJO DAN AND THE MID-NITE PLOWBOYS
25 Kent Street
Montpelier, VT 05602
Phone: 802-229-5733
e-mail: banjodan@pshift.com
Management:
   Band Leader/Booking Agent: Dan Lindner
Mission: A professional 4 or 5 piece band available to play bluegrass music at concerts, schools and festivals.
Founded: 1972
Specialized Field: Folk
Status: Professional
Organization Type: Performing

Virginia

1832 FAIRFAX SYMPHONY ORCHESTRA
4024 Hummer Road
Annandale, VA 22003
Phone: 703-642-7200
Fax: 703-642-7205
e-mail: info@fairfaxsymphony.org
Web Site: www.fairfaxsymphony.org
Officers:
   President: R Dennis McArver
Management:
   Executive Director: Rachel Garrity
Mission: To provide high quality orchestra performances as well as music appreciation and education programs to enhance the quality of life in the metropolitan Washington area.
Founded: 1957
Specialized Field: Symphony; Orchestra; Chamber; Ensemble; Instrumental Group
Status: Professional; Nonprofit
Budget: $1,200,000
Performs At: George Masson University
Affiliations: American Symphony Orchestra League; SOI
Organization Type: Performing; Touring; Resident; Educational

1833 HESPERUS
3706 N 17th Street
Arlington, VA 22207
Phone: 703-525-7550
Fax: 703-908-9207
Management:
   Artistic Director: Scott Reiss
   Producing Director: Tina Chancey
Mission: To trace, through music, the cultural parallels existing between the Old and New Worlds.
Specialized Field: Chamber; Folk; Early Music; Classical
Status: Professional; Nonprofit
Performs At: Smithsonian Institute; National Museum of America
Organization Type: Touring; Resident

1834 CHARLOTTESVILLE CLASSICAL GUITAR SOCIETY

4685 Pelham Drive
Earlysville, VA 22936
Phone: 434-973-0115
Fax: 434-975-3935
e-mail: dave@rediscov.com
Web Site: www.avenue.org/ccgs
Officers:
   President: David Edwards
   VP: Keith Stevens
Management:
   President: David L Edwards
   VP: Keith Stevens
Mission: Develop interest in the Classical Guitar, educate and perform community service.
Founded: 1993
Specialized Field: classical guitar
Status: active
Volunteer Staff: 4
Paid Artists: 2
Non-paid Artists: 6
Budget: $3,000
Income Sources: Donations; Ticket Sales
Facility Category: Church
Type of Stage: Elevated
Seating Capacity: 250
Year Built: 1900

1835 WASHINGTON AND LEE UNIVERSITY CONCERT GUILD

Washington and Lee University
201 DuPont Hall, Department of Music
Lexington, VA 24450
Phone: 703-463-8855
Fax: 540-463-8104
e-mail: gaylardt@wlu.edu
Web Site: http://music.wlu.edu/guild.htm
Management:
   Music Department: Timothy Gaylard
Mission: To bring nationally and internationally recognized classical artists to the campus.
Specialized Field: Chamber; Soloist; Opera
Status: Professional; Nonprofit
Paid Artists: 4
Performs At: Lenfest Centre
Organization Type: Educational; Sponsoring

1836 TIDEWATER CLASSICAL GUITAR SOCIETY

PO Box 1171
Norfolk, VA 23501
Phone: 757-627-6229
Web Site: www.ptcs.cx

1837 RICHMOND SYMPHONY ORCHESTRA

300 West Franklin Street
Richmond, VA 23220
Phone: 804-788-4717
Fax: 804-788-1541
Web Site: www.richmondsymphony.com/
Management:
   Music Director: Mark Russell Smith
   Executive Director: Michele Walter
   Assistant Executive Director: Felicia Pompa
   Office Manager: Nancy Wyatt
   Accounting Manager: Celia Powell
   Associate Conductor: Gerard Edeistein
   Orchestra Manager: Patricia Vorhis
   Operations Assistant: Jennifer Green
   Manager Chorous: Barbie Baker
Mission: To perpetuate the orchestral tradition, develop audience enthusiasm, educate future generations of concert goers, and contribute to the enjoyment of the art of symphonic music. We invite you and encourage you to join with us in carrying out the Richmond Symphony's mission.
Founded: 1908
Specialized Field: Symphony; Orchestra; Chamber; Ensemble
Status: Professional; Nonprofit
Income Sources: American Symphony Orchestra League; Indiana Orchestra Consortium
Performs At: Civic Auditorium
Organization Type: Performing; Resident; Educational

1838 ROANOKE SYMPHONY ORCHESTRA

541 Luck Avenue
Suite 200
Roanoke, VA 24016
Phone: 540-343-9127
Fax: 540-343-0065
Toll-free: 866-277-9127
e-mail: music@rso.com
Web Site: www.rso.com
Officers:
   President: W Tucker Lemon
   VP: Rita Bishop
   VP: Melissa Giles
   VP: R Jay Irons
Management:
   Music Director: David Wiley
   Executive Director: Jane Kenworthy
   Director/Public Relations: Joe Cobb
Mission: To enrich lives, educate, and entertain audiences in Western Virginia with the highest quality instrumental and choral concerts, and to enhance traditional performances with innovative programming in a welcoming acoustical environment.
Founded: 1953
Status: Nonprofit; Education
Paid Staff: 10
Paid Artists: 1
Budget: $1.7 million
Income Sources: Gifts and ticket sales
Facility Category: Civic Center/Auditorium
Seating Capacity: 2,400/848

1839 VIRGINIA BEACH SYMPHONY ORCHESTRA

PO Box 2544
Virginia Beach, VA 23450
Phone: 757-671-8611
Fax: 757-671-8704
e-mail: VBSOED@aol.com
Web Site: www.vbso.org
Officers:

President: L Jean Stewart
VP: Harvey Stokes
Secretary: Anna Stewart
Treasurer: Lee Edmondson
Management:
  Music Director/Conductor: David S Kunkel
  Executive Director: Wendy T Young
  Concertmaster: Dora M Mullins
Mission: The Virginia Beach Symphony provides a high quality music for everyone, affords an opportunity for players, and young musicians. We perform over 18 concerts a year for the citizens of Virginia Beach and the Hampton Roads area.
Founded: 1981
Specialized Field: Symphony Orchestra
Paid Staff: 8
Volunteer Staff: 150
Paid Artists: 2
Non-paid Artists: 100
Performs At: Pavilion Theater, Virginia Beach
Affiliations: ASCAP; BMI; American Symphony Orchestra; Virginians for the Arts; Central Business District; Cultural Alliance of Greater Hampton Roads Chamber
Annual Attendance: 55,000
Facility Category: Theater; Convention
Type of Stage: Proscenium
Seating Capacity: 1000
Year Built: 1981
Rental Contact: Mary Collins

Washington

1840 BELLEVUE PHILHARMONIC ORCHESTRA

924 Bellevue Eay NE, 2nd Floor
PO Box 1582
Bellevue, WA 98009
Phone: 425-455-4171
Fax: 425-455-9170
e-mail: kate.neville@bellphil.org
Web Site: www.bellevuephilharmonic.org
Management:
  Executive Director: Andrea Singleton Schmidt

1841 BREMERTON SYMPHONY ORCHESTRA

PO Box 996
535B 6th Street
Bremerton, WA 98337
Phone: 206-373-1722
Fax: 360-405-1158
e-mail: symphony@symphonic.org
Web Site: www.symphonic.org
Officers:
  President: Anita Williams
  First VP: Caron Cromwell
  Second VP: Mahlon Christensen
  Secretary: Nancyen Reid
Management:
  Music Director/Conductor: John Welsh
  Executive Director: Laurie Strange
  General Manager: Laurie Strange

Mission: To bring high quality classical instrumental and vocal music to our diverse communities; to serve the skilled amateur musicians of the region by providing performance opportunities; and develop enthusiasm and love of music for the enrichment of the cultural environment of the West Sound.
Founded: 1942
Specialized Field: Symphony; Orchestra; Ensemble
Status: Non-Professional; Nonprofit
Paid Staff: 60
Paid Artists: 10
Budget: $200,000
Income Sources: American Symphony Orchestra League
Performs At: Bremerston High School; Admiral Theatre
Organization Type: Performing; Resident; Educational

1842 CASCADE SYMPHONY ORCHESTRA

PO Box 550
Edmonds, WA 98026
Phone: 425-778-4688
Fax: 425-672-3951
Management:
  Conductor: Ropen Shakarian
  Executive Director: Ruby Fusaro
Mission: Performing symphonic literature which ranges from the baroque to the contemporary.
Founded: 1962
Specialized Field: Symphony; Orchestra; Chamber; Ensemble
Status: Semi-Professional; Non-Professional
Income Sources: American Symphony Orchestra League; Broadcast Music Incorporated; American Society of Composers, Authors and Publishers; American Federation of Musicians
Performs At: Puget Sound Christian College
Organization Type: Performing; Resident; Sponsoring

1843 OLYMPIA SYMPHONY ORCHESTRA

3400 Capitol Boulevard S
Suite 203
Olympia, WA 98501-3351
Phone: 360-753-0074
Fax: 360-753-4735
e-mail: ladams@olympiasymphony.com
Web Site: www.olympiasymphony.com
Officers:
  President: Renee C Ries
  First Vice President: Owen G Reese Jr, MD
  Second Vice President: Cheryl Helpenstell
  Secretary: Diane Jenkins
  Treasurer: Phil Jones
  Executive Director: Catherine Von Bechtolsheim
  Olympia Symphony Guild President: Joyce Allen
Management:
  General Manager: Cynthia Morrison
  Music Director/Conductor: Ian Edlund
Mission: To encourage the growth and development of the symphony orchestra and maintain the orchestra; to promote musical and cultural entertainment in diverse forms; to provide the musicians of Thurston County and its surrounding areas with the opportunity to play in a symphony.
Founded: 1970
Specialized Field: Symphony; Orchestra
Status: Professional; Nonprofit

Income Sources: American Symphony Orchestra League
Performs At: Washington Center for the Performing Arts
Organization Type: Performing; Educational

1844 MID-COLUMBIA SYMPHONY
716 Jadwin
PO Box 65
Richland, WA 99352
Phone: 509-943-6602
Fax: 509-946-7917
e-mail: email@midcolumbiasymphony.org
Web Site: www.midcolumbiasymphony.org
Officers:
Executive Director: Ken Pointer
Management:
Concert Manager: Carma Kimball
Music Director/Conductor: Dr Robert Bode
Mission: The Mid-Columbia Symphony is committed to implementing an inclusive strategy that embraces everyone in the region, creating a cultural entity that is a source of regional pride, creating and implementing a strong educational program.
Founded: 1945
Specialized Field: Symphony; Orchestra
Status: Non-Professional; Nonprofit
Income Sources: American Symphony Orchestra League
Performs At: Richland High School Auditorium
Organization Type: Performing; Resident; Educational

1845 EARLY MUSIC GUILD OF SEATTLE
2366 Eastlake Avenue E
Suite 335
Seattle, WA 98102
Phone: 206-325-7066
Fax: 206-860-9151
e-mail: emg@earlymusicguild.org
Web Site: www.earlymusicguild.org
Management:
Executive Director: August Denhard
Mission: Presenting an annual international six concert series featuring touring ensembles.
Founded: 1977
Specialized Field: Chamber; Early Music
Status: Professional; Nonprofit
Budget: $250,000
Organization Type: Educational; Sponsoring

1846 NORTHWEST CHAMBER ORCHESTRA
1305 4th Avenue
#522
Seattle, WA 98101
Phone: 206-343-0445
Fax: 206-343-3955
e-mail: boxoffice@nwco.org
Web Site: www.nwco.org
Officers:
President: Mark Charles Paben
VP: James Simpkins
VP: Bruce King
Secretary: Katie Matison
Treasurer: Maureen Swanson
Management:
Executive Director: Deborah K Daoust
Artistic Director: Marjorie Kransberg-Talvi

Music Director/Principal Conductor: Ralf Gothoni
Mission: To present pre-baroque through contemporary repertoire for chamber orchestra and ensembles. NWCO accomplishes this through concerts, tours, educational outreach programs, broadcasts, free public concerts and recordings. Includes a core of twenty string players with adjunct musicians added based on the repertoire.
Founded: 1973
Specialized Field: Orchestra; Chamber
Status: Professional; Nonprofit
Paid Staff: 3
Volunteer Staff: 2
Paid Artists: 25
Budget: $600,000
Income Sources: American Federation of Musicians
Performs At: Nordstrom Recital Hall; Benarova Hall
Annual Attendance: 11,000
Facility Category: Concert Hall
Seating Capacity: 532
Year Built: 1999
Organization Type: Performing; Touring; Resident; Educational

1847 PHILADELPHIA STRING QUARTET
PO Box 45776
Seattle, WA 98145
Phone: 206-527-8839
Fax: 206-526-8621
Web Site: www.musicfest.net/
Management:
Executive Director: Alan Iglitzin
Mission: Performing string quartets; producing the Olympic Music Festival.
Founded: 1960
Specialized Field: Chamber
Status: Professional; Nonprofit
Organization Type: Performing; Touring; Educational; Sponsoring

1848 PUGET SOUND CHAMBER MUSIC SOCIETY
93 Pike Street
#315
Seattle, WA 98101
Phone: 253-383-2674
Fax: 253-383-1709
Officers:
President: Stuart Rolfe
Management:
Executive Director: Kyle Siebrecht
Mission: To offer the highest quality chamber music festival.
Specialized Field: Chamber
Status: Nonprofit
Organization Type: Presenting

1849 SEATTLE BAROQUE
2366 Eastlake Avenue E
Suite 428
Seattle, WA 98102
Phone: 206-322-3118
Fax: 206-322-3119
e-mail: info@seattlebaroque.org
Web Site: www.seattlebaroque.org/

All listings are in alphabetical order by state, then city, then organization within the city.

Management:
    Music Director: Ingrid Matthews
    Artistic Director: Bryon Schenkman
    Executive Director: Joann Mendelsohn
    Marketing/Development Coordinator: Karen Nestvold
Mission: To awaken contemporary audiences to the vitality of 17th and 18th century music through historically informed performance of both familiar and unknown works.
Founded: 1993
Specialized Field: Classical Music
Paid Staff: 6
Volunteer Staff: 6
Paid Artists: 35

1850 SEATTLE SYMPHONY ORCHESTRA

200 University Street
PO Box 21906
Seattle, WA 98111-3906
Phone: 206-215-4700
Fax: 206-215-4701
e-mail: info@seattlesymphony.org
Web Site: www.seattlesymphony.org
Officers:
    Co-Chairman: Alexandra A Brookshire
    Co-Chairman: Cyrus R Vance, Jr
    Vice Chair: Alexander W Clouts
    Vice Chair: Robert L Collett
    Vice Chair: David Friedenberg
Management:
    Executive Director: Deborah R Card
Mission: To present symphonic music of the highest quality in a distinctive way for the enjoyment, enrichment and education of the people of the Pacific Northwest.
Founded: 1903
Specialized Field: Symphony; Orchestra; Chamber; Ensemble; Instrumental Group
Status: Professional; Nonprofit
Paid Staff: 63
Volunteer Staff: 270
Paid Artists: 90
Budget: $20,000,000
Income Sources: Ticket Sales; Donations
Performs At: Benaroya Hall, Seattle
Annual Attendance: 338,000
Facility Category: Symphony Hall
Seating Capacity: 2500; 540
Year Built: 1998
Cost: $11.8 Million
Rental Contact: Troy Skubitz
Organization Type: Performing; Resident; Educational

1851 SEATTLE YOUTH SYMPHONY ORCHESTRA

11065 5th NE
Suite A
Seattle, WA 98125
Phone: 206-362-2300
Fax: 206-361-9254
e-mail: info@syso.org
Web Site: www.syso.org/
Management:
    Executive Director: Daniel Petersen

    Box Office Manager: John Empey
    Community Relations Director: Stuart Wolferman
Mission: To offer performances that promote music appreciation.
Founded: 1942
Specialized Field: Symphony; Orchestra
Status: Nonprofit
Paid Staff: 7
Volunteer Staff: 100
Paid Artists: 100
Non-paid Artists: 999
Income Sources: American Society of Composers, Authors and Publishers; Broadcast Music Incorporated
Performs At: Seattle Center Opera House
Organization Type: Performing; Educational

1852 SPOKANE SYMPHONY ORCHESTRA

929 W Sprage
Spokane, WA 99201
Phone: 509-326-3136
Fax: 509-326-3921
e-mail: info@spokanesymphony.org
Web Site: www.spokanesymphony.org/
Officers:
    President: Elizabeth Cowles
Management:
    Executive Director: John Hancock
    Music Director: Fabio Mechetti
    Director Marketing: Annie Matton
    Director Marketing: Amanda Livingston
Mission: The Spokane Symphony Society believes that orchestral music nurtures the human spirit and is integral to the presentation and development of our American culture. We are committed to providing performances of the symphonic and chamber orchestra repertoire and to promoting educational and cultural activities which will enhance the knowledge and appreciation of that music for people of all ages.
Founded: 1945
Specialized Field: Symphony; Orchestra; Chamber
Status: Professional; Nonprofit
Paid Staff: 17
Volunteer Staff: 20
Paid Artists: 65
Budget: $3.4 million
Income Sources: Ticket Sales; Contributions; Endorsement
Performs At: Spokane Opera House
Affiliations: ASOL
Annual Attendance: 150,000
Organization Type: Performing; Touring; Resident; Educational; Sponsoring

1853 TACOMA PHILHARMONIC

901 Broadway
Tacoma, WA 98402
Phone: 253-272-0809
Fax: 253-591-0537
e-mail: info@TacomaPhilharmonic.org
Web Site: www.tacomaphilharmonic.org
Management:
    Executive Director: Andrew Wood
Founded: 1936
Specialized Field: Classical Music
Paid Staff: 2

Volunteer Staff: 24
Budget: $150,000-400,000
Income Sources: Grants; Donations; Ticket Sales
Performs At: Pantages Theater
Annual Attendance: 7,600+
Seating Capacity: 1,186

1854 TACOMA SYMPHONY ORCHESTRA
738 Broadway, Suite 301
PO Box 19
Tacoma, WA 98401
Phone: 253-272-7264
Fax: 253-274-8187
e-mail: tacomasymphonyorchstra@hotmail.com
Management:
 Executive Director: Mitchell Owens
 Music Director: Harvey Felder
 Administrative Assistant: Karen Pickett
Mission: To offer the community affordable classical music.
Founded: 1959
Specialized Field: Symphony; Orchestra
Status: Professional; Nonprofit
Paid Staff: 10
Performs At: Pantages Theatre
Organization Type: Performing

1855 TACOMA YOUTH SYMPHONY
901 Broadway Plaza
Suite 500
Tacoma, WA 98402
Phone: 253-627-2792
Fax: 253-627-1682
e-mail: tacomayouthsymphony@msn.com
Web Site: www.tacomayouthsymphony.org/
Management:
 Executive Director: Dr. Loma L Mosley
 Artistic Director: Dr. Paul-Elliot Cobbs
Mission: Committed to the development of the Tacoma Youth Symphony Association as a quality music education organization that attracts and sustains the highest level of musical excellence for training and performance in the Puget Sound area. The TYSA challenges young musicians to pursue musical excellence, to seek intellectual stimulation, and to experience the love and joy of music making.
Founded: 1962
Specialized Field: Symphony; Orchestra; Chamber; Ensemble
Status: Non-Professional; Nonprofit
Paid Staff: 9
Volunteer Staff: 120
Paid Artists: 8
Non-paid Artists: 15
Income Sources: American Symphony Orchestra League (Youth Orchestra Division)
Performs At: Pantages Centre
Organization Type: Performing; Educational

1856 WALLA WALLA SYMPHONY
PO Box 92
Walla Walla, WA 99362

Phone: 509-529-8020
Fax: 509-529-1353
e-mail: wwsorch@wwics.com
Web Site: www.symphony.com
Officers:
 President: Martin Thorson
 VP: Barbara Stubblefield
 Secretary: Gretchen de Grasse
 Treasurer: Dudley Joyce
Management:
 Executive Director: Russ Martin
 Production Assistant: Trudy Ostby
Mission: Continuing the tradition of outstanding symphonic music; bringing high-quality performances to the entire community, including children.
Founded: 1906
Specialized Field: Symphony; Orchestra
Status: Non-Professional; Nonprofit
Paid Staff: 7
Paid Artists: 80
Budget: $300,000
Performs At: Cordinet Hall
Annual Attendance: 10,000
Seating Capacity: 1,384
Organization Type: Performing

1857 YAKIMA SYMPHONY ORCHESTRA
32 N 3rd Street
Yakima, WA 98901
Phone: 509-248-1414
Fax: 509-457-0980
e-mail: yaksymarch@aol.com
Web Site: symphony.artsyakima.org/lobby.html
Management:
 General Manager: Brooke Creswell
 Director Development: Noel Moxley
 Administrative Assistant: Sue Chirco-Coontz
Mission: Performing and promoting symphonic music.
Founded: 1971
Specialized Field: Symphony; Orchestra
Status: Professional; Nonprofit
Paid Staff: 6
Paid Artists: 65
Income Sources: American Symphony Orchestra League
Performs At: Capitol Theatre
Seating Capacity: 1,500
Year Built: 1971
Organization Type: Performing; Educational

1858 YAKIMA YOUTH ORCHESTRA
PO Box 307
Yakima, WA 98907
Phone: 509-966-3394
Fax: 509-457-0980
Management:
 Conductor: Dennis Clauss
Specialized Field: Symphony; Orchestra; Chamber
Status: Non-Professional; Nonprofit
Paid Staff: 20
Income Sources: Yakima Symphony Orchestra
Organization Type: Performing; Educational

West Virginia

1859 CHARLESTON CHAMBER MUSIC SOCIETY
PO Box 641
Charleston, WV 25323
Phone: 304-344-5389
Fax: 304-344-5389
e-mail: ndavids@aol.com
Management:
Executive Director: N David Stem
Mission: To bring outstanding chamber-music ensembles to Charleston.
Founded: 1941
Specialized Field: Chamber; Ensemble
Status: Nonprofit
Paid Staff: 1
Volunteer Staff: 7
Budget: $40,000
Income Sources: Association of Performing Arts Presenters; Chamber Music America
Performs At: Christ Church United Methodist
Affiliations: Association od Performing Arts Presenters; Chamber Music America
Annual Attendance: 1500
Facility Category: Church Sanctuary
Type of Stage: 3/4 Round
Seating Capacity: 400+
Organization Type: Performing; Sponsoring

1860 MONTCLAIRE STRING QUARTET
1205 Oakmont Road
Charleston, WV 25314
Phone: 304-345-5743
Fax: 304-342-0152
Web Site: www.wvsymphony.org/montclaire_string_quartet.
Officers:
President: John L McClaugherty
Management:
Executive Director: Paul Helfrich
Mission: To present the highest quality string quartet repertoire throughout the state of West Virginia; to provide leadership in the West Virginia Symphony Orchestra; to present educational programs in West Virginia schools.
Founded: 1982
Specialized Field: Symphony; Chamber; Ensemble; Instrumental Group
Status: Professional
Paid Artists: 4
Performs At: Kanawha United Presbyterian Csrch
Organization Type: Performing; Touring; Resident; Educational; Sponsoring

1861 HUNTINGTON CHAMBER ORCHESTRA
800 5th Avenue
PO Box 2434
Huntington, WV 25701
Phone: 304-525-0670
Fax: 304-525-0670
e-mail: symphony@ezxv.com
Officers:
President: Jim Morgan

Secretary: Sue Woods
Treasurer: Gray Hampton
Management:
Manager: Asley Orr
Music Director: Kimo Furumoto
Personnel Manager: Sandy White
Mission: To perform the finest music written for chamber orchestras.
Founded: 1970
Specialized Field: Orchestra; Chamber
Status: Professional; Nonprofit
Paid Staff: 3
Income Sources: American Symphony Orchestra League
Performs At: Huntington Galleries
Organization Type: Performing; Resident

1862 WHEELING SYMPHONY
1025 Main Street
Suite 307
Wheeling, WV 26003
Phone: 304-232-6191
Fax: 304-232-6192
e-mail: wso@wheelingsymphony.com
Web Site: www.wheelingsymphony.org
Officers:
President Board of Directors: Betty H Mullen
Management:
Executive Director: Susan C Hogan
Mission: To provide balanced and diversified musical programs which broaden audience appreciation and improve the quality of life in our area.
Founded: 1926
Specialized Field: Symphony; Orchestra
Status: Professional; Nonprofit
Paid Staff: 10
Income Sources: Grants; Donations; Ticket Sales
Performs At: Capitol Music Hall
Organization Type: Performing; Touring; Resident; Educational

Wisconsin

1863 BELOIT JANESVILLE SYMPHONY ORCHESTRA
PO Box 185
Beloit, WI 53512
Phone: 608-363-2554
Fax: 608-363-2718
e-mail: bjso@www.beloit.edu
Web Site: www.beloit.edu/~bjso
Officers:
President: Leslie Brunsell
VP: Bonnie Welter
Management:
Music Director: Robert Tomaro
Executive Director: Nancy Sonntag
Founded: 1953
Specialized Field: Instrumental Music
Paid Staff: 5
Volunteer Staff: 130
Paid Artists: 80

INSTRUMENTAL MUSIC / Wisconsin

1864 FOND DU LAC SYMPHONIC BAND
536 E Tenth Street
PO Box 1779
Fond du Lac, WI 54916
Phone: 920-907-7678
e-mail: marthur@fdlsymphonicband.org
Officers:
   President: Kathy Nachtwey
   VP: James Neujahr
   Secretary: Tess Flaherty
Management:
   Music Director: Raymond C Wifler
   Manager: Mary A Arthur
   Treasurer: Mary Liz Julka
   Equipment Manager: Bruce Zabel
   Librarian: Joan Perry
Mission: To provide quality musical entertainment for our area and beyond; to enhance the image of the concert band as a performing medium; to provide a sophisticated performing opportunity for adult instrumentalists.
Founded: 1898
Specialized Field: Band
Status: Semi-Professional; Nonprofit
Paid Staff: 20
Income Sources: Association of Concert Bands; American Federation of Musicians
Organization Type: Performing; Touring

1865 GREEN BAY SYMPHONY ORCHESTRA
115 S Jefferson Street
PO Box 222
Green Bay, WI 54305
Phone: 920-435-3465
Fax: 920-435-1427
Web Site: www.gbsymphony.org/
Officers:
   President: Kent Ciak
   VP: Jim Bowley
   Treasurer: Jean Vande Hey
Management:
   Executive Director: John Kelley
   Business Manager: Pete Schmeling
   Education Driector: Jill Quigley
   Administrative Assistant: Dana Blodgett
Mission: To promote orchestras and performances of the highest quality for the enjoyment of ever-widening audiences and pursue educational experiences for youth and adults through musical collaborations.
Founded: 1914
Specialized Field: Symphony; Orchestra; Chamber
Status: Nonprofit
Paid Staff: 7
Volunteer Staff: 135
Paid Artists: 71
Income Sources: American Symphony Orchestra League; Association of Wisconsin Symphony Orchestra
Performs At: Weidner Center for The Performing Arts
Organization Type: Performing; Educational

1866 CARTHAGE CHAMBER MUSIC SERIES
2001 Alford Drive
Kenosha, WI 53140-1994
Phone: 262-551-8500
Fax: 262-551-6208
e-mail: sjoerd1@carthage.edu
Web Site: www.carthage.edu/departments/music/chamser.ht
Officers:
   Chairman Music Department: Dr. RD Sjoerdsma
Budget: $20,000-35,000
Performs At: Siebert Chapel

1867 KENOSHA SYMPHONY ASSOCIATION
4917 68th Street
Kenosha, WI 53142
Phone: 262-654-9080
Fax: 262-654-4445
e-mail: ddr3@ocronet.net
Web Site: www.kenosksymphony.org
Officers:
   President: Joseph Mayne
   First VP: Donnalee Bain
   Second VP: Dr. Greg Lyne
   Secretary: Ksthleen Braun
   Treasurer: Donald Michie
Management:
   General Manager: Deborah Dunlap Ruffolo
Mission: To provide a symphony orchestra in a community setting.
Founded: 1941
Specialized Field: Symphony; Orchestra; Chamber
Status: Professional; Semi-Professional; Non-Professional; Nonprofit
Paid Staff: 1
Volunteer Staff: 50
Paid Artists: 70
Income Sources: Kenosha Unified Schools
Performs At: Reuther Auditorium
Organization Type: Performing; Educational

1868 MADISON SYMPHONY ORCHESTRA
6314 Odana Road
Madison, WI 53719
Phone: 608-257-3734
Fax: 608-280-6192
e-mail: info@madisonsymphony.org
Web Site: www.madisonsymphony.org
Officers:
   President: Doug Reuhl
Management:
   Executive Director: Richard Mackie
Founded: 1926
Specialized Field: Symphony
Status: Professional
Paid Staff: 9
Paid Artists: 90
Budget: $2,000,000
Performs At: Oscar Meyer Theatre
Affiliations: Civic Center Box Office
Annual Attendance: 40,000+
Facility Category: Multi Purpose Performance Hall
Seating Capacity: 2,110
Organization Type: Performing; Educational

1869 WISCONSIN CHAMBER ORCHESTRA

22 N Carroll Street, Suite 104
PO Box 171
Madison, WI 53701-0171
Phone: 608-257-0638
Fax: 608-257-0611
e-mail: wco@chorus.net
Web Site: www.wcoconcerts.com
Officers:
   President: Richard Leeping
   VP: Jill Sommers
   Treasurer: Don Rahn
   Secretary: Chris Berry
Management:
   Executive Director: Robert Sorge
   Music Director: Andrew Sewell
Mission: To perform musical works.
Founded: 1962
Specialized Field: Orchestra; Chamber
Status: Professional; Nonprofit
Performs At: Capitol Square; First Congregational
Church; Wisconsin Union Theater
Seating Capacity: 1,200
Organization Type: Performing

1870 WISCONSIN YOUTH SYMPHONY ORCHESTRAS

1625 Humanities Building
455 N Park Street
Madison, WI 53706
Phone: 608-263-3320
Fax: 608-265-3751
Web Site: www.wyso.music.wisc.edu/
Officers:
   President: Liz Quilliam
   Treasurer: Evan Richards
   Secretary: David Lovell
Management:
   Music Director: James R Smith
   Executive Director: Shelia Dunn Joneleit
   Operations Coordinator: Amy Wregand
   Development Director: Sarah Seres
   Administrative Assistant: Elizabeth Allman
   Associate Music Director: Tom Buchhauser
Mission: To meet the symphonic needs of the
musically-talented youth of Southern Wisconsin.
Founded: 1966
Specialized Field: Orchestra
Status: Nonprofit
Paid Staff: 25
Volunteer Staff: 50
Performs At: Mills Concert Hall; University of
Wisconsin
Annual Attendance: 2,500
Facility Category: music hall
Stage Dimensions: 40x40
Seating Capacity: 750
Organization Type: Performing; Touring; Educational

1871 MARSHFIELD-WOOD COMMUNITY SYMPHONY

2000 W 5th Street
Marshfield, WI 54449
Phone: 715-387-1147
Fax: 715-389-6517
Officers:
   President: Sarah Hanson
Management:
   Conductor: Timothy McCollum
Mission: To present the best music possible for the least
possible cost.
Founded: 1965
Specialized Field: Symphony; Orchestra
Status: Nonprofit
Income Sources: American Symphony Orchestra League
Performs At: Fine Arts Building Theatre
Organization Type: Performing; Educational

1872 FOX VALLEY SYMPHONY

1477 Kenwood Center
Menasha, WI 54952
Phone: 920-729-5000
Fax: 920-729-5468
e-mail: info@foxvalleysymphony.com
Web Site: www.foxvalleysymphony.com/
Officers:
   President, Fox Valley Symphony: Tom Gottsacker
   President Symphony League: Priscilla Daniels
Management:
   Executive Director: Carley Miller
   Music Director: Brian Goner
Mission: To provide symphonic music for all; to sponsor
youth orchestras and to introduce school children to
orchestra music.
Founded: 1966
Specialized Field: Symphony
Status: Nonprofit
Paid Staff: 7
Volunteer Staff: 125
Paid Artists: 65
Budget: $424,000
Performs At: Pickard Auditorium; Lawrence University
Chapel
Annual Attendance: 6000
Organization Type: Performing; Resident; Educational;
Sponsoring

1873 MILWAUKEE SYMPHONY ORCHESTRA

700 N Water Street
Suite 700
Milwaukee, WI 53202
Phone: 414-291-6010
Fax: 414-291-7610
Toll-free: 800-291-7605
e-mail: info@milwaukeesymphony.org
Web Site: www.milwaukeesymphony.org
Officers:
   VP Marketing: Judith Keysevling
   Chairman: Judy Jorgensen
   Immediate Past-Chairman: Stephen E Richman
   Public Relations Associate: Tricia Zielinski
   Human Resources Manager: Diane Quinn
Management:
   Auditions Coordinator: Mary Novak
Founded: 1959
Specialized Field: Symphony; Orchestra
Status: Professional; Nonprofit
Paid Staff: 5

All listings are in alphabetical order by state, then city, then organization within the city.

Budget: $16M
Income Sources: Ticket Sales; Fees for Services; United Performing Arts Fund; Wisconsin Arts Board; Milwaukee County CAMPAC
Performs At: Performing Arts Center; Uihlein Hall
Annual Attendance: 270,000
Organization Type: Performing; Touring; Educational; Recording

1874 MILWAUKEE YOUTH SYMPHONY ORCHESTRA
929 N Water Street
Milwaukee, WI 53202
Phone: 414-272-8540
Fax: 414-272-8549
e-mail: general@myso.org
Web Site: www.myso.org
Officers:
    President: Angela Johnston
    VP: Patricia Anders
    VP: Margarete Harvey
    VP: JoAnne Krause
    Vice President: Travers Price
    Secretary: Sandra Ammon
    Treasurer: Jamshed Patel
Management:
    Executive Director: Frances S Richman
    Director Arts/Resident Conductor: Carter Simmons
    Music Director/Senior Symphony: Margery Deutsch
Mission: Provides training in the finest techniques of orchestral and ensemble musicianship to students ages 8-18 in the greater Milwaukee area, through our extensive schedule of rehersals and performances.
Founded: 1956
Specialized Field: Symphony; Orchestra; Chamber; Ensemble
Status: Non-Professional; Nonprofit; Youth Orchestra
Budget: $475,000
Performs At: Uihlein Hall
Annual Attendance: 10,000

1875 PRESENT MUSIC
1840 N Farwell Avenue
Suite 301
Milwaukee, WI 53202
Phone: 414-271-0711
Fax: 414-271-7998
e-mail: info@presentmusic.org
Web Site: www.presentmusic.org
Management:
    Artistic Director: Kevin Stalheim
    Managing Director: Daniel Petry
Mission: To enhance appreciation of music through small ensemble productions featuring contemporary concert music presented in a way that is provocative, engaging and fun.
Founded: 1982
Specialized Field: Chamber; Ensemble; Instrumental Group
Status: Professional; Nonprofit
Paid Artists: 16
Budget: $425,000

Income Sources: Private Foundations; Business/Corporate Donations; Government Grants; Individual Donations
Annual Attendance: 5,000
Facility Category: Art Museum
Seating Capacity: 750
Year Built: 2001
Organization Type: Performing; Touring; Resident; Educational; Recording

1876 OSHKOSH SYMPHONY ORCHESTRA
290 City Center
PO Box 522
Oshkosh, WI 54902
Phone: 920-233-7510
Fax: 620-233-5091
Officers:
    President: John Bermingham
    Executive VP: Sam Adams
    Secretary: Victoria Beltran
    Treasure: Stuart N. Tribbey
    Executive Director: Susan Traska
    Marketing Director: Mary Whitlock
Management:
    Business Manager: Rebecca Spurlock
Founded: 1940
Specialized Field: Symphony; Orchestra
Status: Semi-Professional
Income Sources: Association of Wisconsin Symphony Orchestra; American Symphony Orchestra League
Performs At: Osh Kosh Civic Auditorium
Organization Type: Performing

Wyoming

1877 WYOMING SYMPHONY ORCHESTRA
111 Westsecond Street
Suite 103
Casper, WY 82601
Mailing Address: PO Box 667 Casper, WY 82602
Phone: 307-266-1478
Fax: 307-266-4522
e-mail: wso@coffey.com
Web Site: www.wyomingsymphony.com
Officers:
    President: Bobbie Brown
Management:
    Executive Director: Jennifer Thompson
    Music Director: Jonathan Shames
    Librarian: Roger Hedlund
Mission: To enhance cultural life; to expand childrens' musical horizons; to offer area musicians a performance outlet.
Founded: 1950
Specialized Field: Symphony; Orchestra
Status: Professional; Nonprofit
Paid Staff: 4
Paid Artists: 75
Budget: $300,000
Income Sources: City of Casper; Wyoming Council on the Arts; National Endowment for the Arts; American Symphony Orchestra League; Private Foundations

Performs At: John F. Welsh Auditorium; Natrona County High School
Affiliations: American Symphony Orchestra League
Annual Attendance: 6,400
Facility Category: High School
Organization Type: Performing; Touring; Educational

1878 CHEYENNE SYMPHONY ORCHESTRA

PO Box 851
Cheyenne, WY 82003
Phone: 307-778-8561
Fax: 307-634-7512
Management:
    Executive Director: Christine De Poorter
    Music Director: Mark Russell
Mission: Presenting excellent professionally performed symphonic music to as wide as possible an audience, emphasizing educational outreach.
Founded: 1954
Specialized Field: Symphony; Orchestra; Chamber
Status: Professional; Nonprofit
Income Sources: American Symphony Orchestra League; Symphony & Choral Society of Cheyenne
Performs At: Cheyenne Civic Center
Organization Type: Performing; Educational

Alabama

1879 BIRMINGHAM MUSIC CLUB
2023 4th Avenue N
Birmingham, AL 35203
Phone: 205-252-7548
Fax: 205-328-7677
Web Site: www.bhammusic.org/about.html
Officers:
    Interim Executive Director: Kathleen West

1880 OPERA BIRMINGHAM
1817 3rd Avenue N
Birmingham, AL 35203
Phone: 205-322-6737
Fax: 205-322-6206
e-mail: operabham@wwisp.com
Web Site: www.operabirmingham.org
Officers:
    President: John T Natter
    Guild President: Summer Currier
Management:
    General Director: John D Jones
    Principal Conductor: Steven White
    Education/Outreach Manager: Mary K Jackson
    Office Manager: Yvonne Henderson
Mission: Opera Birmingham is committed to creating the finest opera productions, developing local and regional talent through competition and exposure to major artists, and preserving the operatic art form through community-wide education.
Performs At: Alabama Theater

1881 HUNTSVILLE OPERA THEATER
8802 Willow Hills Drive
Huntsville, AL 36660-1633
Phone: 334-476-7377
Fax: 334-476-7373
e-mail: mbeutjer@hiwaay.net
Web Site: www.huntsvilleopera.com/hot.html
Officers:
    President: Steve Russell
    Guild President: Sonja Bruek
Management:
    General Director/Princ Conductor: Jerome Shannoni
    Administrative Director: Merv White-Spunner
    Financial Secretary: Nancy Thomas
    Education Director: Charles Smoke
    Publications Manager: Sarah Wright
    Marketing Director: Larry Wooley
    Development Director: Paul Klotz
Mission: Nurturing the growth of young dancers, singers and technicians.
Founded: 1981
Specialized Field: Grand Opera
Status: Nonprofit
Performs At: Von Braun Civic Center - Playhouse
Organization Type: Performing

1882 MOBILE OPERA
2152 Airport Boulevard
PO Box 66633
Mobile, AL 36602
Phone: 251-432-6772
Fax: 251-431-7613
e-mail: GenDir@aol.com
Web Site: www.mobileopera.org
Officers:
    President: Laureen H Lynnell
    Executive VP: Duane Graham
    First VP: Earl G Jackson
    Treasurer: Celia Sapp
Management:
    General Director: Jerome Shannon
    Executive Assistant: Kathleen Garner
    Ticketing Services: Nancy Tomas
    Development Director: Darby McClintock
Mission: Present professional productions of opera and musical thatre and programs dedicated to in school arts education and community outreach while providing performance opportunities for national and regional artists.
Founded: 1946
Specialized Field: Grand Opera
Paid Staff: 4
Volunteer Staff: 10
Paid Artists: 150
Budget: $700,000
Income Sources: Opera America
Performs At: Mobile Saenger Theatre
Annual Attendance: 9,120
Type of Stage: Proscenium
Seating Capacity: 1,900
Year Built: 1963

Alaska

1883 ALASKA LIGHT OPERA THEATRE
639 W International Airport Road
#34
Anchorage, AK 99502
Fax: 907-345-2568
Officers:
    President: James Feeney
    VP: Duane Heyman
    Treasurer: Frank Danner
    Secretary: Jacquie Turpin
Management:
    General Director: Gloria Marinacc Allen
    Administrative Assistant: Judy O'Neal
Mission: To produce professional-quality musical theatre; to produce musical-theatre education programs for Alaska school children; to provide professional development to Alaskan musical-theatre performers through the Resident Artists Program.
Founded: 1984
Specialized Field: Light Opera
Status: Professional; Nonprofit
Performs At: Fourth Avenue Theatre
Organization Type: Performing; Resident; Educational

1884 ANCHORAGE CONCERT CHORUS
PO Box 103738
Anchorage, AK 99510

All listings are in alphabetical order by state, then city, then organization within the city.

Phone: 907-274-7464
Fax: 907-563-5980
e-mail: concertchorus@gci.net
Web Site: www.anchorageconcertchorus.org
Officers:
  President: Becky Oberrecht
Management:
  Executive Director: Jennifer Duford
  Conductor: Grant Cochran
Mission: To serve Anchorage and surrounding communities by fostering excellence in choral music through world-class vocal performance, community events, and music education.
Founded: 1947
Specialized Field: Choral
Status: Nonprofit
Paid Staff: 2
Volunteer Staff: 160
Budget: $170,000
Income Sources: Municipality of Anchorage; Alaska State Council on the Arts
Performs At: Alaska Center for the Performing Arts
Affiliations: Chorus America
Annual Attendance: 12,000-16,000
Organization Type: Performing
Resident Groups: Alaska Center for the Performing Arts

1885 ANCHORAGE OPERA COMPANY

1507 Spar Avenue
Anchorage, AK 99501-1812
Phone: 907-279-2557
Fax: 907-279-7798
e-mail: info@anchorageopera.org
Management:
  Artistic Director: Peter H Brown
  Executive Director: Edward Bourgeois
  Music Administrator: Kristin Quigley-Brye
  Director Development: Charlotte Fox
Performs At: Alaska Center for the Performing Arts

1886 FAIRBANKS CHORAL SOCIETY AND CHILDREN'S CHOIR

University of Alaska-Fairbanks
PO Box 900174
Fairbanks, AK 99775
Phone: 907-456-1144
Fax: 907-456-7464
Web Site: www.mosquitonet.com/~sing/
Management:
  Music Director: Dr. Suzanne Summerville
Mission: Sponsoring the Fairbanks Children's Choir, Sing-It-Yourself Messiah, and CHORUS!.
Founded: 1984
Specialized Field: Choral
Status: Non-Professional; Nonprofit
Performs At: University of Alaska; Fairbanks Concert Hall
Organization Type: Performing; Educational; Sponsoring

1887 FAIRBANKS LIGHT OPERA THEATRE

PO Box 72787
Fairbanks, AK 99707

Phone: 907-456-3568
Fax: 907-456-3662
Web Site: www.flot.org
Officers:
  President: Theresa Reed
  VP: Tami Holland
  Treasurer: Phyllis Church
  Secretary: Dorothea Moravec
Mission: To offer our community musical theatre and light opera.
Founded: 1969
Specialized Field: Light Opera
Status: Non-Professional; Nonprofit
Performs At: Hering Auditorium; Alaskaland Civic Center
Organization Type: Performing; Touring

1888 JUNEAU ORATORIO CHOIR

PO Box 32760
Juneau, AK 99803-2760
Phone: 907-789-0320
Fax: 907-586-6261
e-mail: mackinnon@gci.net
Officers:
  President: J Allan MacKinnon
Management:
  Artistic Director: J Allan MacKinnon

Arizona

1889 ARIZONA OPERA

4600 N 12th Street
Phoenix, AZ 85014
Phone: 602-266-7464
Fax: 602-266-5806
e-mail: contact@azopera.com
Web Site: www.azopera.com
Officers:
  CFO: Heather Davis
  Director Operations: Leilani M Rothrock
  Director Marketing: Laura Schairer
  Director Development: Julia L. Waterfall
  Director Education: Deanna Hoying
  Chief Accountant: Suzette Griffen
  Production Manager: Polly Monroe
  Development Associate: Andrea McSwain
Management:
  Director Artistic Operations: Tom Wright
  Principal Conductor: Cal Stewart Kellogg
  Box Office Manager - Tucson: Nancy Williams
  Box Office Manager-Phoenix: Michael Tomaszek
  Box Office Associate: Terri Staats
  Box Office Associate: Paloma Routh
  Administrative Associate: Melanie Booth
  Artistic Administrative Assistant: Shannon Whidden
  Chorus Director: John Massaro
Mission: To offer grand opera to Arizona, in both the Tucson and Phoenix areas.
Founded: 1972
Specialized Field: Grand Opera
Status: Professional; Nonprofit
Budget: $5,400,000

Income Sources: Contributed Income; Corporate; Government; Foundations; Individual Donations
Performs At: Tucson Community Center Music Hall; Phoenix Symphony Hall
Annual Attendance: 80,000
Organization Type: Performing

1890 ORPHEUS MALE CHORUS OF PHOENIX

PO Box 217
Phoenix, AZ 85001
Phone: 602-271-9396
e-mail: john@orpheus.org
Web Site: www.orpheus.org
Officers:
   President: Loyld Weberg
Management:
   Music Director: John Brown
Mission: Offering an outlet for men who love singing; employing music as a tool for furthering goodwill.
Founded: 1929
Specialized Field: Choral
Status: Non-Professional; Nonprofit
Paid Artists: 2
Non-paid Artists: 40+
Income Sources: Dues; CD Sales; Contract Concerts; Patron Contributions
Performs At: Trinity Cathedral, Camelback Bible Church, Dupherm Theatre
Organization Type: Performing; Touring

1891 PHOENIX BACH CHOIR

PO Box 16956
Phoenix, AZ 85011-6956
Phone: 602-253-2224
Fax: 602-253-5772
e-mail: office@bachchoir.org
Web Site: www.bachchoir.org
Management:
   Executive Director: Joel M Rinsema

1892 PHOENIX BOYS CHOIR

1131 E Missouri Avenue
Phoenix, AZ 85014
Phone: 602-264-5328
Fax: 602-264-6778
e-mail: lynn@boyschoir.org
Web Site: www.boyschoir.org
Management:
   Artistic Director: Georg Stangelberger
   Executive Director: Mary Ann Pulk
   General Manager: Lynn Tuttle
Mission: To educate boys in the art of singing.
Founded: 1948
Specialized Field: Choral, Children
Paid Staff: 6
Volunteer Staff: 100
Paid Artists: 6

1893 ARIZONA OPERA

3501 N Mountain Avenue
Tucson, AZ 85719

Phone: 520-293-4336
Fax: 520-293-5097
e-mail: contact@azopera.com
Web Site: www.azopera.com
Management:
   General Director: David Speers
Mission: To offer grand opera to Arizona, in both the Tucson and Phoenix areas.
Founded: 1972
Specialized Field: Grand Opera
Status: Professional; Nonprofit
Paid Staff: 30
Budget: $5,400,000
Income Sources: Contributed Income; Corporate; Government; Foundations; Individual Donations
Performs At: Tucson Community Center Music Hall; Phoenix Symphony Hall
Annual Attendance: 80,000
Organization Type: Performing

1894 DESERT VOICES

PO Box 270
Tucson, AZ 85702-0270
Phone: 520-791-9662
Fax: 520-624-3360
e-mail: office@desertvoices.org
Web Site: www.desertvoices.org
Officers:
   President: John Kissler
   VP: Mary Webber
   Secretary: Anne Levy
   Treasurer: Heath Howe
Mission: Arizona premiere GLBT chorus.
Founded: 1988
Status: Nonprofit
Income Sources: Arizona Commission on the Arts; National Endowment for the Arts; Tucson Pima Arts Council; Amazon Foundation; Southern Arizona Community Foundation

1895 TUCSON ARIZONA BOYS CHORUS

5770 E Pima Street
Tucson, AZ 85712
Phone: 520-296-6277
Fax: 520-296-6751
e-mail: tabc@boyschorus.org
Web Site: www.boyschorus.org
Officers:
   President: Bob Patrick
   VP: John Bradyck
   Treasurer: Larry Lamy
   Secretary: John Brayton
Management:
   Director: Dr. Julian M Ackerley
   General Manager: Carol M Williams
Mission: Presents a varied program including traditional boychoir repertoire, songs of the southwest with trick rodeo roping, a choreographed medley of popular tunes aaaaaaand stirring patriotic selections.
Founded: 1939
Specialized Field: Choral Performing Arts
Paid Staff: 4
Paid Artists: 5
Budget: $680,000

Income Sources: Performance Fees; Ticket Sales; Fundraising Programs; Corporate Partners; Foundation Support; Governmental Grants
Affiliations: International SocietyO Children's Choral and Performing Arts; Alliance For Arts and Understanding; American Choral Directors Association

1896 WASHINGTON CHORUS
1010 Wisconsin Avenue NW
Suite 310
Washington, AZ 20007
Phone: 202-342-6221
Fax: 202-342-8208
e-mail: staff@thewashingtonchorus.org
Web Site: www.thewashingtonchorus.org
Officers:
  Chair Board of Trustees: Nancy Ignatius
  Vice Chair Board of Trustees: Catherine French
  Vice Chair Board of Trustees: August Schumach
  Secretary: Katherine Roberts
Management:
  Music Director: Robert Shafer
  Executive Director: Dianne Peterson
  Director Finance/Administration: Alison Combes
  Direcror Development: Eric Stevenson
Mission: The Washington Chorus shares, preserves and advances the art of choral singing to help expirence the transforming power od choral music.
Founded: 1961
Paid Staff: 8
Non-paid Artists: 200
Budget: $807,000
Income Sources: Individual; Foundation; Corporate & Government Support; Ticket Sales
Performs At: Kennedy Center Concert Hall
Annual Attendance: 25,000
Facility Category: Concert Hall

Arkansas

1897 OPERA IN THE OZARKS AT INSPIRATION POINT
19 S Hills Loop
Holiday Island, AR 72631
Phone: 501-253-8595
Fax: 501-253-8595
e-mail: operintheozarks@ipa.net
Web Site: www.opera.org
Management:
  General Director: James Swiggart
  Artistic Director: Vern Sutton
Specialized Field: Instrumental; Opera; Childrens'; Educational
Budget: $60,000-$150,000
Season: May - July
Affiliations: South Central of National Federated Music Clubs
Facility Category: Amphitheater
Seating Capacity: 300

California

1898 BERKELEY OPERA
1678 Shattuck Svenue
Suite 312
Berkeley, CA 94709
Phone: 510-841-1903
e-mail: webmaster@berkeleyopera.com
Web Site: www.berkeleyopera.com/dsm/index.html
Management:
  General Director: Richard Goodman
  Audition Secretary: Jane Rateaver
  Orchestra Manager: Bonnie Lockett
  Artistic Director: Jonathan Khuner
Mission: The presentation of opera.
Founded: 1979
Specialized Field: Lyric Opera
Status: Semi-Professional
Paid Staff: 20
Income Sources: Theater Bay Area
Performs At: Julia Morgan Theater; Hillside Club Theater
Organization Type: Performing

1899 CALIFORNIA CHAMBER ORCHESTRA & CHAMBER OPERA
907 Keeler Avenue
Berkeley, CA 94708-1419
Phone: 510-524-3682
Fax: 510-524-3683
Management:
  Artistic Director: Edgar J Braun
  Manager: Janet Mitchell
Budget: $260,000-$1,050,000

1900 LOS ANGELES CONCERT OPERA ASSOCIATION
2250 Gloaming Way
Beverly Hills, CA 90210
Phone: 310-276-2731
Fax: 310-275-8245
Management:
  Acting Director: Nedra Zachary
Mission: To provide young opera singers with performance opportunities, and to provide lesser-known opera, and Viennese operetta.
Founded: 1987
Specialized Field: Opera and Operettas in concert version
Status: Nonprofit
Paid Artists: 30
Performs At: Wilshire Ebell Theatre
Organization Type: Performing

1901 ANGELES CHORALE
23501 Park Sorrento #106
Calabasas, CA 91302
Phone: 818-591-1735
Fax: 818-591-1738
e-mail: angeleschorale@sbcglobal.net
Web Site: www.angeleschorale.org
Officers:
  Chairman of the Board: Werner Keller
Management:

All listings are in alphabetical order by state, then city, then organization within the city.

Executive Director: Rae MacDonald
Artistic Director: Donald Neuon
Mission: To make a significant statement for choral excellence in Southern California; to enhance the cultural environment of the Los Angeles area through quality choral/orchestral concerts; to broaden musical interest in, and appreciation for, fine choral music for audiences representing the diverse spectrum of population in Southern California; and to perform a full range of musical styles.
Founded: 1975
Paid Staff: 1
Volunteer Staff: 1
Paid Artists: 20
Non-paid Artists: 125
Budget: $180,000
Income Sources: Tickets; Donations; Grants
Performs At: Concert hall
Annual Attendance: 4,000
Facility Category: Royce Hall, UCLA + Bel Air Presbyterian Church
Seating Capacity: 1,400
Year Remodeled: 1994
Cost: $5,000

1902 HIDDEN VALLEY OPERA ENSEMBLE
PO Box 116
Carmel Valley, CA 93924
Phone: 831-659-3115
Fax: 831-659-7442
e-mail: hvms@aol.com
Web Site: hiddenvalleymusic.org
Management:
   General Director: Peter Meckel
Mission: Arts training for pre-professional and early professional artists
Founded: 1963
Specialized Field: Vocal; Instrumental Ensembles
Paid Staff: 25
Volunteer Staff: 50
Paid Artists: 30
Non-paid Artists: 30

1903 CAPITOL OPERA SACRAMENTO
6219 Ross Avenue
Carmichael, CA 95608
Phone: 916-944-2149
Fax: 916-944-1282
e-mail: ljs@softcom.net
Web Site: www.capopera.com
Management:
   General Director: Kathleen Torchia-Sizemore
Mission: To keep opera alive and provide performing opportunities for developing artists.
Founded: 1990
Specialized Field: Opera; Music
Volunteer Staff: 10
Income Sources: Tickets; Donations; Seasonal Subscriptions
Affiliations: AACT; Opera America
Annual Attendance: 5,000
Facility Category: Small Theater
Type of Stage: Black Box
Seating Capacity: 50
Year Remodeled: 1993

1904 ALL AMERICAN BOYS CHORUS
PO Box 1527
Costa Mesa, CA 92628
Phone: 714-708-1670
Fax: 714-557-5447
e-mail: taabc@aol.com
Web Site: www.allamericanboyschorus.org
Management:
   Executive Director: Anthony S Manrique
   Music Director: David TR Albulario
   Production Manager: Jason Gannon
   Marketing Director: Juan Ayala
Mission: To provide each member with the training, motivation, and opportunity to develop and exercise qualities of leadership within an exceptional program of choral music conducted in an environment of high moral standards.
Founded: 1970

1905 MASTER CHORALE OF ORANGE COUNTY
660 W Baker
Suite 273
Costa Mesa, CA 92626
Mailing Address: PO Box 2156, Costa Mesa, CA. 92628
Phone: 714-997-6504
Fax: 714-556-6341
e-mail: info@whmc.org
Management:
   Music Director: Dr. William D Hall
   Associate Music Director: Dr. Thomas Sheets
   Administrative Director: Sheri Sheperd
   Administrative Assistant: Jean Updegraff
Founded: 1956
Specialized Field: Choral
Status: Nonprofit
Paid Staff: 140
Budget: $10,000
Performs At: Orange County Performing Arts Center
Organization Type: Performing

1906 WILLIAM HALL MASTER CHORALE
660 W Baker
Suite 273
Costa Mesa, CA 92626
Mailing Address: PO Box 2156, Costa Mesa, CA. 92628
Phone: 714-556-6262
Fax: 714-556-6341
e-mail: info@whmc.org
Web Site: www.chapman.edu/music/links/whmc.html
Management:
   Music Director: William Hall
   Administration Director: Jean Updegraff
   Public Relations Director: Vicki Heston

1907 FULLERTON CIVIC LIGHT OPERA
218 W Commonwealth Avenue
Fullerton, CA 92832
Phone: 714-526-3832
Fax: 714-992-1193
e-mail: marilyn@fclo.com
Web Site: www.fclo.com
Officers:
   President: Gordon Haag

Management:
General Manager: Griff Duncan
Artistic Director: Jan Duncan
Group Sales: Marilyn Gianotti
Mission: To present live stage musicals and nationwide costume and scenery rentals.
Founded: 1971
Specialized Field: Light Opera; Operetta; Musical Theatre
Status: Professional; Nonprofit
Paid Staff: 34
Volunteer Staff: 40
Paid Artists: 90
Non-paid Artists: 40
Budget: $1.6 million
Income Sources: Ticket Sales; Costume/Scenery Rentals; Contributions
Performs At: Plummer Auditorium
Affiliations: National Alliance of Musical Theatre Producers
Annual Attendance: 50,000
Facility Category: Stage Auditorium
Type of Stage: Proscenium
Stage Dimensions: 36x31
Seating Capacity: 1,314
Year Built: 1934
Year Remodeled: 1993
Cost: $2,700,000
Rental Contact: Fullerton Union High School District
Organization Type: Performing; Resident

1908 SACRAMENTO CHORAL SOCIETY AND ORCHESTRA

11230 Gold Express Drive
#310-217
Gold River, CA 95670
Phone: 916-492-7761
Fax: 916-965-0884
Web Site: www.sacramentochoral.com
Officers:
President: Jim McCormick
VP: James Jepson
Second VP/Conductor: Donald Kendrick
Secretary: Marya Kasch
Treasurer: Truman Rishard
Management:
Marketing/Public Relations: Leah Vande Berg
Mission: To continue the tradition of performing important choral orchestral masterworks for the community; to develop an appreciation of choral music in the community; to encourage choral music education and creativity through workshops, clinics and mentoring; to achieve professional standards of performance; to secure a lasting foundation as a symphonic music organization.
Founded: 1996
Status: Nonprofit

1909 ALBERT MCNEIL JUBILEE SINGERS OF LOS ANGELES

447 Herondo Street, #210
Hermosa Beach, CA 90254
Phone: 310-379-7807
Fax: 310-318-9240
e-mail: AlMcNeil@aol.com

Management:
Director: Albert McNeil
Personal Representative: Walter Gould
Founded: 1968
Paid Staff: 1

1910 CASA ITALIANA OPERA COMPANY

4911 Melrose Avenue
Hollywood, CA 90029
Phone: 323-463-2996
Fax: 310-411-9349
e-mail: murphy@econ/ucla.edu
Web Site: www.casaitaliana.org
Management:
General Director: Mario E Leonetti
Performs At: Casa Italiana Hall and Theater; Wilshire Ebell Theater

1911 LONG BEACH CIVIC LIGHT OPERA

PO Box 20280
Long Beach, CA 90801
Phone: 562-435-7605
Fax: 310-372-8685
Management:
Managing Director: Pegge Logefeil
Producer: Martin Wiviott
Mission: Maintaining artistic excellence in professional musical theatre; training young people and preprofessionals in musical theatre.
Founded: 1950
Specialized Field: Light Opera; Operetta
Status: Professional; Nonprofit
Performs At: Terrace Theater
Organization Type: Performing

1912 LONG BEACH OPERA

6372 Pacific Coast Highway
PO Box 14895
Long Beach, CA 90803
Phone: 562-985-8152
Fax: 310-596-8380
Web Site: www.lbopera.com/
Management:
General Director: Michael Milenski
Mission: Offering professional opera to Southern California; nurturing childrens' love of opera and performing arts.
Founded: 1978
Specialized Field: Grand Opera; Lyric Opera
Status: Professional; Nonprofit
Paid Staff: 25
Performs At: Center Theater; Terrace Theater
Organization Type: Performing; Educational

1913 CALIFORNIA FESTIVAL OPERA

6156 Buena Vista Terrace
Los Angeles, CA 90042
Phone: 323-255-7884
Fax: 323-255-1998
Management:
Artistic Director: Frank Fetta
Performs At: Redlands Bowl

1914 LOS ANGELES CHAMBER SINGERS & CAPPELLA
2055 Kelton Avenue
Los Angeles, CA 90025
Phone: 310-575-9790
Fax: 310-575-3405
e-mail: voices@lacs.org
Web Site: www.lacs.org
Management:
   Music Director: Peter Rutenberg
Mission: Los Angeles Chamber Singers excels in the art
and performance of choral chamber music; preserves and
promotes the art form; favors repertoire that is
accompanied, of historical or musical signifiance to any
era, aspecially contemporary; fa
Founded: 1990
Paid Staff: 1
Paid Artists: 25

1915 LOS ANGELES MASTER CHORALE
The Music Center
135 N Grand Avenue
Los Angeles, CA 90012
Phone: 213-626-0624
Fax: 213-626-0196
e-mail: lamc@lamc.org
Web Site: www.lamc.org
Officers:
   Chairman: Edward J McAniss
   President: Mark Foster
   Treasurer: V Charles Jackson
Management:
   Music Director: Paul Salamunovich
   Founder/Music Director Laureate: Roger Wagner
   General Manager: Marjorie Lindbeck
   Assistant General Manager: Mark Praigg
   Composer in Residence: Morten Lauridsen
   Rehearsal Accompanist: Dwayne Condon
   Director Chamber Singers: Nancy Sulahian
Mission: To educate the public in the art of choral singing
and to foster an appreciation of the art form.
Specialized Field: Choral
Status: Professional
Paid Staff: 37
Income Sources: Individual Contributions
Performs At: Dorothy Chandler Pavilion
Organization Type: Performing; Resident; Educational

1916 LOS ANGELES OPERA
135 N Grand Avenue
Suite 327
Los Angeles, CA 90012
Phone: 213-972-7219
Fax: 213-687-3490
e-mail: wehelpyou@laopera.com
Web Site: www.laopera.org
Officers:
   President: Marc I Stern
   Chairman Emeritus: Richard Seaver
   Chairman/CEO: Leonard I Green
   Secretary/Treasurer: Eugene P. Stein
   Chairman of the Executive Committee: Bernard A.
   Greenburg
   Vice Chairman: Roy L. Ash

   Vice Chairman: Audrey Skirball-Kenis
   Vice Chairman: Flora Thornton
   Director Finance/Administration: Jeb Bonner
Management:
   Executive Director: Ian White-Thomson
   Artistic Director: Placido Domingo
   Principal Conductor: Kent Nagano
   Artistic Administrator: Edgar Baitzel
   Director Finance/Administration: Jeb Bonner
   Director Human Resources: Pat Brady
   Costume Director: Kristine Haugan
   Director Public Relations: Gary Murphy
   Director Community Programs: Stacy Brigtman
Mission: To present opera at its highest professional
standard with international guest artists and a resident
company.
Founded: 1986
Specialized Field: Grand Opera
Status: Professional; Nonprofit
Income Sources: Ticket Revenue, Contributed Income
Performs At: Dorothy Chandler Pavilion
Annual Attendance: 160,000
Facility Category: Performing Arts Center
Type of Stage: Proscenium
Seating Capacity: 3,086
Year Built: 1964
Organization Type: Performing; Resident; Educational

1917 OPERA A LA CARTE
PO Box 39606
Los Angeles, CA 90039
Phone: 626-791-0844
Web Site: www.gilbertandsullivan.com
Management:
   Director: Richard Sheldon
Founded: 1970

1918 ROGER WAGNER CHORALE
1260 Devon Avenue
Los Angeles, CA 90024
Phone: 310-859-9259
Fax: 310-859-1927
e-mail: jwc94muse@aol.com
Management:
   Conductor: Jeannine Wagner

1919 UNIVERSITY OF SOUTHERN CALIFORNIA OPERA
Ramo Hall, #208B
University Park
Los Angeles, CA 90089
Phone: 213-740-3109
Fax: 213-740-3217
Management:
   Opera Manager/Professor: William Williams
   Resident Director/Conductor: William Vendice
   Stage Director: Frans Boerlage
Mission: Providing a performance outlet and training for
talented young singers in all aspects of performance;
presenting two full operas as well as various single
scenes.
Founded: 1940
Specialized Field: Grand Opera; Lyric Opera; Light
Opera; Operetta

Status: Semi-Professional; Nonprofit
Paid Staff: 25
Income Sources: University of Southern California
Performs At: Bing Theater
Organization Type: Performing; Touring; Educational

1920 TOWNSEND OPERA PLAYERS

605 H Street
Modesto, CA 95354
Mailing Address: PO Box 4519, Modesto, CA. 95352
Phone: 209-523-6426
Fax: 209-579-0532
e-mail: TOP@ainet.com
Web Site: townsendoperaplayers.com
Officers:
  President: Robert Fisk
  Secretary: Judy Schmidt
  Treasurer: Dale McKinney
Management:
  Founder/General Director: Erik Buck Townsend
  Operations Manager: Erika Townsend
  Production Coordinator: Barbara Wesley
  Membership/Production: Barbara Wesley
  Education Director: Charles Sheaffer
  Public Relations/Marketing: Martha Martin
Mission: Performing great opera as well as classics of American Musical Theatre for the enjoyment of San Joaquin Valley and surrounding area residents.
Founded: 1982
Specialized Field: Grand Opera; Lyric Opera; Light Opera; Operetta
Status: Professional; Nonprofit
Paid Staff: 4
Paid Artists: 100
Non-paid Artists: 150
Budget: $400,000
Income Sources: Membership, Grants, Donation and Ticket Sales
Annual Attendance: 10,000
Facility Category: High School Auditorium
Stage Dimensions: 44'x38'x16'
Seating Capacity: 1,100
Year Built: 1900
Organization Type: Performing; Touring; Educational

1921 SCHOLA CANTORUM

1605 W El Camino Real
Suite 200
Mountain View, CA 94040-2459
Phone: 650-254-1700
Fax: 650-254-1701
e-mail: info@scholacantorum.org
Web Site: www.scholacantorum.org
Officers:
  Chairman: Henry Lesser
Management:
  Music Director: Gregory Wait
  Executive Director: Nicola Rees
Mission: To celebrate the joy of singing with our community: by performing choral music of all styles, including masterpieces and commissioned works; by educating and inspiring our singers and our audiences.
Founded: 1964
Specialized Field: Choral Music
Status: Non-professional; Nonprofit

Paid Staff: 4
Volunteer Staff: 3
Paid Artists: 2
Budget: $218,000
Income Sources: Ticket Sales; Grants; Donations; Sponsorships;
Annual Attendance: 5,000

1922 BAROQUE CHORAL GUILD

688 W Dana Street
Mountian View, CA 94041
Phone: 650-969-4095
Web Site: www.bcg.org
Officers:
  President: Wendy Bartlett
  Vice-President/Treasurer: Carol Handelman
  Secretary: David Vossbrink
Management:
  Music Director: Sanford Dole
  Managing Director: Audrey Wong
Status: Nonprofit

1923 MUSICAL AMERICA

North Hollywood High School
5231 Colfax Avenue
North Hollywood, CA 91607
Phone: 818-980-3095
Management:
  Director: Cornelia Korney
Mission: Educating through the presentation of fine choral music; providing the community with entertainment.
Founded: 1969
Specialized Field: Choral
Status: Semi-Professional; Non-Professional
Income Sources: Los Angeles Unified School District
Performs At: North Hollywood High School
Organization Type: Performing; Touring; Educational

1924 KITKA WOMEN'S VOCAL ENSEMBLE

1201 Martin Luther King Jr Way
Suite 103
Oakland, CA 94612
Phone: 510-444-0323
Fax: 510-444-1013
e-mail: info@kitka.org
Web Site: www.kitka.org
Officers:
  President: Rodney Pasion
  Treasurer: Chitra Arunasalam
  VP: Norman Gelbart
Management:
  Director: Shira Cion
  Artistic Co-Director: Juliana Graffagna
  Artistic Co-Director: Janet Kutulas
  Office Manager: Leslie Bonnet
Mission: To build audiences for music rooted in Eastern European traditions through live performances, educational programs, recordings, and radio broadcasts.
Founded: 1979
Specialized Field: World Music; Chroal Music
Paid Staff: 3
Paid Artists: 10
Non-paid Artists: 9

Budget: $300,000
Income Sources: National Endowment for the Arts; California Arts Council; Alameda County Art Comission; City of Oakland; Hewlett Foundation; Rockefeller Foundation; Zellerbach Foundation
Affiliations: Folk Alliance; Chorus America; Western Arts Alliance
Annual Attendance: 12,000-24,000
Facility Category: Concert Halls, Festivals

1925 OAKLAND YOUTH CHORUS

2619 Broadway
Oakland, CA 94612
Phone: 510-287-9700
Fax: 510-832-2211
e-mail: mail@oaklandyouthchorus.org
Web Site: www.oaklandyouthchorus.org
Management:
  Managing Director: Bea Andrade
  Artistic Director: Trente Morant
Mission: Providing multicultural youth from ages 14-21 with quality professionally-directed training; to advance the choral art form.
Founded: 1974
Specialized Field: Choral
Status: Professional; Nonprofit
Paid Staff: 12
Non-paid Artists: 80
Budget: $6,000
Performs At: First Presbyterian Church; Calvin Simmons Theater
Organization Type: Performing; Touring; Sponsoring

1926 WILLIAM HALL CHORALE

333 N Glassell Avenue
Orange, CA 92866
Phone: 714-997-6891
Fax: 714-997-6504
Officers:
  Founder: Dr. William D Hall

1927 WEST BAY OPERA

221 Lambert Street
Palo Alto, CA 94306
Phone: 650-424-9999
Fax: 650-324-1215
e-mail: davidsloss@earthlink.net
Web Site: www.wbopera.org
Officers:
  Business Manager: Ben DeBolt
  Development Officer: Matthew Gilmartin
  Production Manager: Michele Sullivan
Management:
  General Director: Maria Holt
Mission: Dedicated to providing quality opera performances as well as expanding opportunities for participation; committed to providing training for opera performers.
Founded: 1955
Specialized Field: Grand Opera; Lyric Opera; Light Opera
Status: Semi-Professional; Nonprofit
Paid Staff: 40
Performs At: Lucie Stern Theatre

Organization Type: Performing; Educational

1928 LIGHT OPERA THEATRE OF SACRAMENTO

PO Box 188093
Sacramento, CA 95818-8093
Phone: 916-978-5800
e-mail: info@lightoperasac.org
Web Site: www.lightoperasac.org
Officers:
  Board President: Robin Henson
  Business Manager: Bill Bourne
Management:
  Artistic Director: Mike Baad
  Artistic Director: Debbie Baad

1929 SACRAMENTO MASTER SINGERS

PO Box 215501
Sacramento, CA 95821
Phone: 916-338-0300
Fax: 916-334-1808
e-mail: REHchoir@aol.com
Web Site: www.mastersingers.org
Officers:
  President: Chris Webster
Management:
  Music Director: Ralph Hughes
  Business Manager: Carol Barbieri

1930 SACRAMENTO MEN'S CHORUS

PO Box 188726
Sacramento, CA 95818
Phone: 916-484-5789
e-mail: info@sacmenschorus.org
Web Site: www.sacmenschorus.org
Management:
  Business Manager: Frank Lawler
Founded: 1985
Specialized Field: Choral
Status: Non-Professional; Nonprofit
Paid Staff: 30
Performs At: First United Methodist
Organization Type: Performing; Touring

1931 SACRAMENTO OPERA

3811 J Street
Sacramento, CA 95816
Mailing Address: PO Box 161027, Sacramento, CA. 95816
Phone: 916-737-1000
Fax: 916-737-1032
e-mail: sacopera@pacbell.net
Web Site: www.sacopera.org
Officers:
  President: Michael A Nelson
  Secretary/Treasurer: Joanne Bodine
  Board Chairman: Nina Ankele
Management:
  Executive Director: George Sinclair
  Artistic Director: Timm Rolek
Mission: To produce outstanding regional opera; to develop & cultivate public interst in opera & its allied arts; and to further music education.

Founded: 1947
Specialized Field: Opera
Status: Professional; Nonprofit
Paid Staff: 1
Paid Artists: 1
Income Sources: Opera America
Performs At: Sacramento Community Center Theatre
Organization Type: Performing; Educational

1932 SAN DIEGO CHILDREN'S CHOIR
PO Box 910411
San Diego, CA 92191
Phone: 760-632-5467
Fax: 760-632-8244
e-mail: sdcc@worldnet.att.net
Web Site: www.sdcchoir.org
Management:
    Administrator: James Campbell
Founded: 1990
Specialized Field: Music; Choral Music Education
Budget: $250,000
Affiliations: Chorus America; ACDA;
Annual Attendance: 10,000
Facility Category: Different Venues
Type of Stage: Traditional at all venues
Stage Dimensions: varies
Seating Capacity: 200-2100

1933 SAN DIEGO COMIC OPERA/LYRIC OPERA SAN DIEGO
610 A Street
Suite 101
San Diego, CA 92101
Phone: 619-239-8836
Fax: 619-231-0662
e-mail: comicoperapr@hotmail.com
Web Site: www.sdcomicopera.com
Officers:
    President: Roberto Cueva
    VP: Richard Brown
    Secretary: Kristin Schuler Hint
    Treasurer: William Mayleas
Management:
    General Director: Leon Nataker
    Artistic Director: J Sherwood Montgomery
    PR/Marketing Director: Kathleen Switzer
    Business Manager: Sue Boland
Mission: To offer quality musical theater; to provide creative employment for area professional artists; to train young artists as they move toward professional careers.
Founded: 1979
Specialized Field: Light Opera; Operetta; Musical Theater
Status: Professional; Nonprofit
Paid Staff: 6
Budget: $500,000
Income Sources: Ticket Sales; Membership Dues; Foundations; Grants
Performs At: Indoor Casa del Prado Theater
Affiliations: San Diego Performing Arts League; Opera America; San Diego Arts & Culture Coalition; Downtown Partnership
Annual Attendance: 15,000
Facility Category: Rental

Seating Capacity: 550
Organization Type: Performing; Touring; Resident; Educational

1934 SAN DIEGO MEN'S CHORUS
3749 Park Boulevard
PO Box 33825
San Diego, CA 92163
Phone: 619-296-7664
Fax: 619-296-3471
e-mail: sdchorus@pacbell.net
Web Site: www.sdmc.org
Officers:
    President: Jonathon N Myatttt
    VP: Todd D Ebert
    Treasurer: Jamie Royak
    Secretary: Tony Hammond
Management:
    Artistic Director: Dr. Robert Engle
Mission: To foster unity and a love of music through our performances.
Founded: 1985
Specialized Field: Choral
Status: Non-Professional; Nonprofit
Paid Staff: 2
Volunteer Staff: 130
Budget: $150,000
Income Sources: Membership Dues; Ticket Sales; Individual & Business Donations
Performs At: First Unitarian Universalist Church
Affiliations: GALA Choruses
Annual Attendance: 5,000
Seating Capacity: 541
Organization Type: Performing; Touring
Comments: Donates $4,000 annually to local HIV/AIDS organizations

1935 SAN DIEGO OPERA
1200 3rd Avenue
18th Floor, Civic Center Plaza
San Diego, CA 92101-4112
Phone: 619-232-7636
Fax: 619-231-6915
e-mail: sdostaff@sdopera.com
Web Site: www.sdopera.com
Officers:
    President: William R Stensrud
    Executive VP: Robert B Horsman
    VP Finance: L Renee Comeau
    VP Special Projects: James L. Fitzpatrick
    VP Marketing/Membership: Lisa Briggs
    VP Individual Gifts: Iris Lynn Strauss
    Secretary: James H. Amos Jr.
Management:
    General Director: Ian D Campbell
    Director Administration: Michael G Murphy
    Director Strategic Planning: Ann S Campbell
    Resident Conductor: Karen Keltner
    Director Education/Outreach: Nicolas M Reveles
    Director Marketing/Public Relations: Todd Schultz
    Director Production: Ronald G Allen
    Director Finance: John Sleeper
Performs At: Civic Theatre

All listings are in alphabetical order by state, then city, then organization within the city.

1936 STARLIGHT MUSICAL THEATRE
1549 El Padro - Balboa Park
PO Box 3519
San Diego, CA 92101
Phone: 619-544-7800
Fax: 619-544-0496
Management:
  Executive Director: CE Bud Farnks
  Producing Artistic Director: Don Ward
  Producing Artistic Director: Bonnie Ward
Mission: The preservation and promotion of the art form of musical theatre.
Founded: 1946
Specialized Field: Light Opera; Musical Theatre
Status: Professional; Nonprofit
Performs At: Starlight Bowl; Civic Theatre; Spreckles Theatre
Organization Type: Performing; Educational

1937 MEROLA OPERA PROGRAM
War Memorial Opera House
301 Van Ness Avenue
San Francisco, CA 94102
Phone: 415-565-6427
Fax: 415-255-6774
e-mail: rjones@sfopera.com
Web Site: www.sfopera.com/merola
Management:
  Administrator: Renata Jones
  President: Rusty Rolland
Mission: Discovering and developing professional opera singers; sponsoring the Merola Opera Program at the San Francisco Opera and the San Francisco Opera Center auditions.
Founded: 1954
Specialized Field: Grand Opera; Lyric Opera
Status: Nonprofit
Income Sources: Central Opera Service
Performs At: War Memorial Opera House
Rental Contact: Bill Bowles
Organization Type: Educational; Sponsoring

1938 OPERA CENTER SINGERS
War Memorial Opera House
301 Van Ness Avenue
San Francisco, CA 90039
Phone: 415-565-3239
Fax: 415-255-6774
e-mail: BBowles@SFOpera.com
Web Site: www.sfopera.com
Management:
  Director: Sheri Greenawald
  Sales Manager: Bill Bowles
Rental Contact: Bill Bowles

1939 POCKET OPERA
44 Page Street #200
San Francisco, CA 94102
Phone: 415-575-1100
Fax: 415-575-1104
e-mail: info@pocketopera.org
Web Site: www.pocketopera.org
Officers:
  President: Paula March Romanovsky
  Secretary: Robin Rodricks
  Treasurer: Mel Bricmmeier
Management:
  Artistic Director: Donald Pippin
Mission: Pocket Opera was created to address the need to preserve and promote accessibility of the broad range of operatic literature for English-speaking audiences at affordable ticket prices.
Founded: 1977
Specialized Field: Grand Opera; Lyric Opera; Light Opera; Operetta
Status: Professional; Nonprofit
Paid Staff: 4
Budget: $450,000
Income Sources: Central Opera Service
Organization Type: Performing; Touring; Resident

1940 SAN FRANCISCO BACH CHOIR
3145 Geary Boulevard, #210
San Francisco, CA 94118-3300
Phone: 415-922-6562
Fax: 415-922-2819
e-mail: singet@flash.net
Web Site: www.sfbach.org
Management:
  Artistic Director: David P Babbitt

1941 SAN FRANCISCO CHANTICLEER
1182 Market Street
Suite 216
San Francisco, CA 94102
Phone: 415-252-8589
Fax: 415-252-7941
Web Site: www.chanticleer.org
Officers:
  Founder: Louis Botto
  President & Secretary: Christine Bullin
  Chairman: Lynn DW Luckow
  Vice Chair: Barbara M. Barclay
  Treasurer: David S. Hugle
Management:
  General Director: Christine Bullin
  Business Manager: Jess Perry
  Music Director: Joseph Jennings
Mission: To present professional a cappella vocal music; to elevate choral music standards; to produce a unique ensemble sound which utilizes the entire male vocal range.
Founded: 1978
Specialized Field: Choral
Status: Professional; Nonprofit
Paid Staff: 9
Paid Artists: 12
Budget: $2,300,000
Income Sources: Contributed; Government; Foundation & Individual; Earned Income; Tour Fees; Ticket Sales; Recording Sales
Performs At: Bay Area Churches
Affiliations: Chorus America
Organization Type: Performing; Touring; Resident; Educational

1942 SAN FRANCISCO CHORAL ARTISTS
601 Van Ness Avenue
Suite E 3344
San Francisco, CA 94102
Phone: 415-979-5779
e-mail: info@sfca.org
Web Site: www.sfca.org
Officers:
  President: Maureen Stone
Management:
  Music Director: Claire Giovannetti
  Associate Conductor: Doug Wyatt
  Development Manager: Teresa Byrne
  Publicity: Audrey Wong
Mission: To develop and maintain an outstanding performing choral ensemble dedicated to the art of modern classical music.
Specialized Field: Choral
Status: Professional; Nonprofit
Performs At: Calvary Presbyterian Church; St. Mark's Episcopal
Organization Type: Performing

1943 SAN FRANCISCO GIRLS CHORUS AND ASSOCIATION
1337 Sutter
PO Box 15397
San Francisco, CA 94115-0397
Phone: 415-673-1511
Fax: 415-673-0639
e-mail: info@sfgc.org
Web Site: www.sfgirlschorus.org
Management:
  Artistic Director: Susan McMane
  Executive Director: Janet Garvin
  Director Marketing/Communication: Jay Krohnengold

1944 SAN FRANCISCO OPERA
War Memorial Opera House
301 Van Ness Avenue
San Francisco, CA 94102-4509
Phone: 415-861-4008
Fax: 415-621-7508
Web Site: www.sfopera.com
Officers:
  Chairman: Franklin P Johnson, Jr
  President of the Association: William W Godward
  VP: Francis W Chen
  VP: Howard H. Leach
  VP: Leslie P. Hume
  VP/Treasurer: Doreen Woo Ho
  Secretary: Robert E. Sullivan
  Chairman Emeritus: Reid W. Dennis
Management:
  General Director: Pamela Rosenberg
  Music Director: Donald Runnicles
  Artistic Administrator: Brad Trexell
Mission: To enhance cultural life; to present masterworks of opera with the San Fransico Opera Orchestra and outstanding casts; to offer training and outreach; to nurture new audiences and talent.
Founded: 1923
Specialized Field: Opera

Budget: 51 Million
Income Sources: Private and Corporate Donations; Instituional Gifts; Ticket Sales; Government Assistance
Performs At: War Memorial Opera House

1945 SAN FRANCISCO OPERA CENTER
War Memorial Opera House
301 Van Ness Avenue
San Francisco, CA 94102
Phone: 415-861-4008
Fax: 415-255-6774
e-mail: chancock@sfopera.com
Web Site: www.sfopera.com
Management:
  Director: Sheri Greenwald
  Administrative Director: Curt Hancock
Mission: To utilize the various affiliate components of the San Francisco Opera Association in a comprehensive and unique professional training program for artists.
Founded: 1982
Specialized Field: Grand Opera; Lyric Opera; Light Opera; Operetta
Status: Professional; Nonprofit
Performs At: Cowell Theater; Herbst Thater; Old First Chruch; Yerba Buena Theater; Stern Grove
Rental Contact: Bill Bowles
Organization Type: Performing; Touring; Resident; Educational; Sponsoring

1946 SAN FRANCISCO SYMPHONY CHORUS
San Francisco Symphony
Pouise M. Davies Symphony Hall
San Francisco, CA 94102
Phone: 415-552-8000
Fax: 415-431-6857
Web Site: www.sfsymphony.org
Officers:
  President: Nancy H Bechtle
  VP: John D Goldman
  VP: Robert D Glynn, Jr
  VP: Eff W. Martin
  Secretary: Robert R. Tufts
Management:
  Chorus Director: Vance George
  Chorus Administrator: Gregory Boals
Mission: Recognition as a world-class chorus; performance of a wide repertoire of fine music under leading conductors.
Founded: 1973
Specialized Field: Symphonic
Status: Professional; Nonprofit
Performs At: Louise M. Davies Symphony Hall
Organization Type: Performing

1947 WESTERN OPERA THEATER
War Memorial Opera House
301 Van Ness Avenue
San Francisco, CA 94102-4509
Phone: 415-565-3239
Fax: 415-255-6774
e-mail: BBowles@SFOpera.com
Web Site: www.sfopera.com/wot
Management:
  Director: Richard Harrell

Tour Manager: William Bowles
Rental Contact: Bill Bowles

1948 AMERICAN MUSICAL THEATER OF SAN JOSE

1717 Technology Drive
San Jose, CA 95110
Phone: 408-453-7100
Fax: 408-453-7123
Toll-free: 888-455-7469
e-mail: amtsj@amtsj.org
Web Site: www.amtsj.org
Officers:
    Chairman of the Board: John P Traub
    Vice Chairman: John Dennis
    Secretary: Chuck Berger
    Treasurer: John Kelm
Management:
    Artistic Director: Dianna Shuster
    President/Executive Producer: Stewart Slater
    Director Sales: Moorea Warren
Founded: 1934
Specialized Field: Performing Arts
Paid Staff: 55
Volunteer Staff: 80
Paid Artists: 40
Non-paid Artists: 10
Season: August - September
Performs At: San Jose Center for the Performing Arts
Annual Attendance: 150,000
Seating Capacity: 2,600

1949 OPERA SAN JOSE

2149 Paragon Drive
San Jose, CA 95131
Phone: 408-437-4450
Fax: 408-437-4455
e-mail: info@operasj.org
Web Site: www.operasj.org
Officers:
    President: Frank Veloz
    VP/Chair of Finance: Sharon McCorkle
    Secretary: Jack Schneider
Management:
    General/Artistic Director: Irene Dalis
    Music Director: David Rohrbaugh
    Business Manager: Michelle Shields
    Administrative Assistant: Valerie Peters
    Director/Marketing: Larry Hancock
    Director Communications: Christine Spielberger
    Corporate Relations Manager: Glen Won
Mission: To maintain and enhance a professional opera company of artistic excellence; to provide principally in opera of all periods and secondarily in operetta; to provide opera singers with professional development and performance opportunities; to develop, educate and entertain.
Founded: 1984
Specialized Field: Lyric Opera; Operetta
Status: Professional; Nonprofit
Paid Staff: 18
Volunteer Staff: 155
Paid Artists: 224
Budget: $2,765,000

Performs At: Montgomery Theater
Seating Capacity: 519
Organization Type: Performing; Touring; Educational; Sponsoring

1950 MASTERWORKS CHORALE

1700 W Hillsdale Boulevard
San Mateo, CA 94402
Phone: 650-574-6210
Fax: 650-574-6303
e-mail: chorale@masterworks.org
Web Site: www.masterworks.org
Management:
    Music Director: Richard Garrin
    Executive Director: J Peter Jensen
    Music Director Emeritus: Galen Marshall

1951 OPERA PACIFIC

600 W Warner Avenue
Santa Ana, CA 92707
Phone: 714-546-6000
Fax: 714-546-6077
e-mail: lrobinson@operapacific.org
Web Site: www.operapacific.org
Officers:
    Chairman: Patrick Seaver
Management:
    Artistic Director: John DeMain
    Executive Director: Martin G Hubbard
    Producing Director/Artistic Advisor: Mitchell Krieger
    Marketing/Development Director: Adrian Stevens
    Music Administrator/Chorusmaster: Henri Venanzi
    Director Finance: Bree Noble
Mission: To present a broad repertoire of opera and American musicals with the highest artistic standards; to provide opportunities for emerging opera talent; to reach out to area communities with educational and performance opportunities.
Founded: 1986
Specialized Field: Grand Opera
Status: Professional; Nonprofit
Performs At: Orange County Performing Arts Center
Affiliations: Opera America
Organization Type: Performing; Touring; Resident; Educational

1952 PACIFIC CHORALE

1221 E Dyer Road
Suite 230
Santa Ana, CA 92705
Phone: 714-662-2345
Fax: 714-662-2395
e-mail: contactus@pacificchorale.org
Web Site: www.pacificchorale.org
Management:
    Artistic Director/Conductor: John Alexander
    Executive Director: Julie Bussell
    Assistant Conductor: Dennis Houser
Mission: Committed to the highest quality performance and recording of existing choral masterworks, and to the creation, performance, and recording of future masterworks. We will enrich and educate our current audience as well as singers and audiences of the future.

Founded: 1968
Specialized Field: Choral
Status: Semi-Professional; Nonprofit
Paid Staff: 7
Paid Artists: 40
Non-paid Artists: 130
Budget: $1.2 million
Income Sources: Ticket revenue, Contributions
Performs At: Orange County Performing Arts Center
Affiliations: Chorus America, ACDA
Annual Attendance: 10,000+
Organization Type: Performing; Touring; Educational

1953 OPERA SANTA BARBARA

PO Box 4505
123 W Padre Street
Santa Barbara, CA 93140-4505
Phone: 805-898-3890
Fax: 805-898-3892
Toll-free: 800-563-7181
e-mail: opera@SBOpera.com
Web Site: www.operasb.com
Officers:
    President: Sandra L Urquhart
    VP: Frederick Sidon
    Secretary: Marilyn Crawford
    Treasurer: Mary Penny
Management:
    Artistic Director/Conductor: Valery Ryvkin
    Artistic Director: Joan Rutkowski
    Administrative Director: Christopher D Snell
    Production Coordinator: Nicolai Scott Jussila
Mission: To reintroduce this art form to our schools. The Education Department arranges for noontime performances in local high and junior high schools featuring arias from the current production; students then attend the full dress rehearsal.
Founded: 1994
Specialized Field: Opera
Status: Tax free nonprofit
Paid Staff: 4
Volunteer Staff: 75
Paid Artists: 100
Performs At: Lobero Theater

1954 LA MARCA AMERICAN VARIETY SINGERS

2655 W 230th Place
Torrance, CA 90505
Phone: 310-325-8708
Fax: 310-325-8708
e-mail: lamarcamusic@lycos.com
Web Site: www.lamarcamusic.tripod.com
Management:
    Director/Manager: Priscilla LaMarca
Mission: Entertaining, educating and promoting the arts as well as the American spirit.
Founded: 1974
Specialized Field: Lyric Opera; Light Opera; Choral; Folk; Show Choirs
Status: Professional; Nonprofit; Commercial
Paid Staff: 2
Income Sources: International Federation of Festival Organizations

Organization Type: Performing; Touring; Resident; Educational

1955 VENTURA COUNTY MASTER CHORALE & OPERA ASSOCIATION

Box 7388
Ventura, CA 93006
Phone: 805-653-7282
Fax: 805-653-7282
Management:
    Artistic/Musical Director: Dr. Burns Taft

1956 DIABLO LIGHT OPERA COMPANY

PO Box 5034
Walnut Creek, CA 94596
Phone: 925-939-6161
Fax: 925-944-1565
Web Site: www.dloc.org
Officers:
    President: Bobbi Bach
Management:
    Artistic Advisor: Rhoda Klitsner
    Producer: Grete Egan
Mission: Dedicated to enriching our community by producing quality musicals and light opera and by providing educational opportunities in the arts.
Founded: 1960
Specialized Field: Light Opera; Operetta; Musical Theatre
Status: Non-Professional; Nonprofit
Paid Staff: 50
Performs At: Regional Center for the Arts
Organization Type: Performing; Educational

1957 FESTIVAL OPERA ASSOCIATION

675 Ygnacio Vally
#B125
Walnut Creek, CA 94596
Phone: 925-944-9610
Fax: 310-441-9349
e-mail: festop@hotcocco.infi.net
Management:
    Artistic Director: Olivia Stapp
Performs At: Hofmann Theater; Regional Center for the Arts

Colorado

1958 ASPEN OPERA THEATER CENTER

2 Music School Road
Aspen, CO 81611
Phone: 970-925-3254
Fax: 970-925-3802
e-mail: festival@aspenmusic.org
Web Site: www.aspenmusicfestival.com
Officers:
    President/CEO: Don Roth
Management:
    General Manager: James Berdahl
    Music Director: David Zinman
    Artistic Administrator: NancyBell Coe
Founded: 1949

Performs At: Wheeler Opera House
Annual Attendance: 5000
Facility Category: Opera House
Type of Stage: Proscenium
Stage Dimensions: 27 x 24
Seating Capacity: 490
Year Built: 1889
Year Remodeled: 1984

1959 WHEELER OPERA HOUSE

320 E Hyman Avenue
Aspen, CO 81611
Phone: 970-920-5790
Fax: 970-920-5780
e-mail: nidat@ci.aspen.co.us
Web Site: www.wheeleroperahouse.com
Management:
Executive Director: Nida Tautvydas
Founded: 1985
Specialized Field: Dance; Vocal Music; Instrumental Music; Theatre
Status: Nonprofit
Income Sources: Association of Performing Arts Presenters
Performs At: Wheeler Opera House
Year Built: 1889
Year Remodeled: 1984
Organization Type: Sponsoring

1960 AURORA SINGERS

Fox Arts Center
PO Box 9
Aurora, CO 80040
Phone: 303-361-2910
Fax: 303-361-2952
Web Site: www.best.com/~gds/aurora.html
Management:
Music Director/Conductor: Ken Johnson
Cultural Arts Administrator: Alice Lee Main
Mission: Providing Aurora residents with a chance to perform before an audience.
Founded: 1977
Specialized Field: Choral
Status: Non-Professional
Paid Staff: 50
Income Sources: City of Aurora
Performs At: Aurora Fox Arts Center
Organization Type: Performing; Resident

1961 COLORADO SPRINGS CHORALE

16 E Platte
PO Box 2304
Colorado Springs, CO 80901
Phone: 719-634-3737
Fax: 719-473-0077
e-mail: csc@cschorale.org
Web Site: www.cschorale.org
Officers:
Chairman: Linda Madden
Vice Chairman: Kenneth Myers
Secretary: Marie Gardner
Treasurer: Sandra Damron
Management:
Artistic Director/Conductor: Doanld P Jenkins

Executive Director: Mark Dempsey
Mission: To contribute to the cultural richness of the Pikes Peak Region while providing an artistically rewarding choral experience for talented singers.
Founded: 1956
Specialized Field: Auditioned Chorus
Status: Professional; Nonprofit
Paid Staff: 4
Non-paid Artists: 150
Budget: $150,000
Income Sources: Grants; Donations; Ticket Sales
Performs At: Pikes Peak Center
Seating Capacity: 1885
Organization Type: Performing; Resident

1962 MOSAIC

27 S Tejon
PO Box 2304
Colorado Springs, CO 80903
Phone: 719-634-3737
Fax: 719-473-0077
Officers:
Chairman: Ken Myers
Vice Chairman: Sylvia Hutson
Secretary: Myrtis Thompson
Treasurer: James Price
Management:
Manager: Carolyn Schwartz
Mission: A representative ensemble of the Colorado Springs Chorale, performing a repertoire of diverse musical styles, performing in schools, service clubs, retirement homes and businesses, and private and public functions.
Founded: 1990
Specialized Field: Choral
Status: Non-Professional; Nonprofit
Paid Staff: 12
Organization Type: Performing; Resident; Educational

1963 CENTRAL CITY OPERA HOUSE ASSOCIATION

621 17th Street
Suite 1601
Denver, CO 80293
Phone: 303-292-6500
Fax: 303-292-4958
Toll-free: 800-851-8175
e-mail: admin@centralcityopera.org
Web Site: www.centralcityopera.org
Management:
Artistic Director Emeritus: John Moriarty
General Director: Pelham G Pearce
Director Marketing: Deb Hruby
Mission: Central City Opera is the nations fifth oldest opera comapany. The national summer opera festival draws patrons from 46 states, presenting works of artistic excellence from standard and 20th century repertoire.
Founded: 1932
Specialized Field: Opera
Paid Staff: 17
Paid Artists: 100
Budget: $2,500,000
Income Sources: Scientifrand Cultural Facilities District
Season: July - August

Performs At: Central City (Festival Site)
Affiliations: Opera America League of Historic-America Theatres
Annual Attendance: 27,000
Facility Category: Opera House
Type of Stage: Proscenium
Stage Dimensions: 25x34x171/2
Seating Capacity: 552
Year Built: 1878
Cost: $23,000 (built)

1964 COLORADO CHILDREN'S CHORALE

518 17 Street
Suite 760
Denver, CO 80202
Phone: 303-892-5600
Fax: 303-892-0828
e-mail: mail@childrenschorale.org
Web Site: www.childrenschorale.org
Officers:
  President: Jim Billings
  VP: Libby Kirkpatrick
  Secretary: Ruth Silver
  Treasurer: Susan Holmes
  Member at Large: Bryan Pulte
Management:
  Artistic Director: Deborah DeSantis
Mission: Providing the nation with a performing-arts group that features children and strives for excellence.
Founded: 1974
Specialized Field: Choral
Status: Professional; Nonprofit
Paid Staff: 45
Organization Type: Performing; Touring; Educational

1965 OPERA COLORADO

695 S Colorado Boulevard
Suite 20
Denver, CO 80246
Phone: 303-778-1500
Fax: 303-778-6533
e-mail: info@operacolorado.org
Web Site: www.operacolorado.org
Officers:
  Chairman: Jack Finlaw
Management:
  Artistic Director: James Robinson
  General Director: Peter Russell
  Director Marketing: Rex Fuller
  Development Director: Susan Evans
Mission: To develope a better appreciation and understanding of opera throughout the community; to produce the highest quality performances of grand operas in their original languages with projected English supertitles translation.
Founded: 1981
Specialized Field: Grand Opera
Status: Professional; Nonprofit
Paid Staff: 75
Budget: $2,000,000-5,000,000
Income Sources: Opera America
Rental Contact: Gordon Robertson
Organization Type: Performing; Resident; Educational

1966 DURANGO CHORAL SOCIETY

780 Main Avenue
Suite 214
Durango, CO 81301
Mailing Address: PO Box Durango, CO 81302
Phone: 970-247-7251
Fax: 970-382-6910
e-mail: mack_1@fortlewis.edu
Web Site: www.durangochoralsociety.com
Officers:
  President: Gene M Bradley
  Executive Vice-President: Bob Westerwick
  VP Development: Wynn Berven
  Treasurer: Bob Dolphin
  Assistant Treasurer: Sarah Jones
  Secretary: Trisha Burbach
Management:
  Executive Director/Musical Director: Diane Vandenberg
Mission: To provide fine choral and orchestral performances for the four-corners area.
Founded: 1961
Specialized Field: Choral
Status: Semi-Professional
Paid Staff: 45
Income Sources: American Choral Directors Association
Organization Type: Performing; Touring; Resident; Educational; Sponsoring

1967 LARIMER CHORALE

Box 884
Fort Collins, CO 80522
Phone: 970-491-1209
Fax: 970-491-4142
e-mail: paddy@colostate.edu
Web Site: www.fortnet.org/lc
Officers:
  VP: Jan Painter
  Secretary: Halli Freddy
  Treasurer: Andrew Hinds
Management:
  Production Manager: Paddy Shannon
Mission: To bring classical choral music to Northern Colorado by singing choral music of the masters.
Founded: 1977
Paid Staff: 5
Volunteer Staff: 30
Paid Artists: 8
Non-paid Artists: 105
Budget: $80,000+
Income Sources: Audiences, grants, fundraising
Performs At: Lincoln Center
Annual Attendance: 4,000+
Facility Category: Large community auditorium building, 2 stages
Type of Stage: Large for 200 singers/50 symphony
Seating Capacity: 1180, smaller stage 350
Year Built: 1978

1968 OPERA FORT COLLINS

PO Box 701
Fort Collins, CO 80524

Phone: 970-482-0220
e-mail: opera@fortnet.org
Web Site: www.Fortnet.org/opera
Management:
  Artistic Director: Elizabeth Elliott

Connecticut

1969 DANBURY MUSIC CENTRE
256 Main Street
Danbury, CT 06810
Phone: 203-748-1716
Fax: 203-794-1308
e-mail: dmc1935@snet.net
Web Site: www.danbury.org/MusicCtr
Officers:
  President: Dennis Nazzaro
  Secretary: John W Cherry
  Treasurer: Dawn Ellen Whaley
Management:
  Executive Director: Nancy F Sudik
Mission: To sponsor musical organizations, instrumental and vocal, in which persons of a wide variety of musical backgrounds are encouraged to study and to perform classical and modern compositions to improve their ability and to share the joy of music with the people of greater Danbury.
Founded: 1935
Specialized Field: Music, Primarily Classical
Status: Semi-Professional; Non-Professional; Nonprofit
Paid Staff: 15
Volunteer Staff: 35
Paid Artists: 20
Non-paid Artists: 800
Budget: $240,000
Income Sources: Private Support; Corporate & Businesses; City & State; Grants; Trustfunds; Tuition; Tickets
Performs At: Marian Anderson Recital Hall
Annual Attendance: 12,000
Seating Capacity: 175 - 1,200
Organization Type: Performing; Educational; Sponsoring

1970 NEW ENGLAND LYRIC OPERETTA
PO Box 1007
Darien, CT 06820
Phone: 203-655-0566
Fax: 203-655-8066
Officers:
  Chairman: Stephen Pierson
Management:
  Artistic Director: William H Edgerton
Mission: Performing the entire range of American and European operetta.
Founded: 1986
Status: Professional; Nonprofit
Performs At: Rich Forum; Stauford Center for the Arts
Organization Type: Performing; Resident

1971 FAIRFIELD COUNTY CHORALE
61 Unguowa Road
Fairfield, CT 06430

Phone: 203-254-1333
Fax: 203-319-8273
e-mail: fairfieldcountyc@aol.com
Web Site: www.fairfieldcountychorale.org
Officers:
  President: Lucinda Kuuth
Management:
  Music Director: Johannes Somary
  Executive Director: Evelyn Averill
Mission: To perform classical choral music with professional orchestra and soloists, in the manner in which the composer intended it. To present this to people living in Fairfield County, with the hope of enriching their musical lives.
Founded: 1965
Paid Staff: 3
Budget: $80,000
Income Sources: Tickets; Advertisement Sales; Donations; Fund Raising
Performs At: Norwalk Concert Hall
Annual Attendance: 2,000
Facility Category: Concert Hall
Seating Capacity: 1,064
Rental Contact: City of Norwalk

1972 GREENWICH CHORAL SOCIETY
PO Box 5
Greenwich, CT 06836
Phone: 203-622-5136
Fax: 203-325-8762
Management:
  Music Director/Conductor: Paul F Mueller
  Executive Director: Greg Wold
Mission: To offer audiences a wide variety of choral music for their enjoyment and education.
Founded: 1925
Specialized Field: Choral
Status: Nonprofit
Performs At: State University of New York at Purchase
Organization Type: Performing

1973 CONNECTICUT OPERA
226 Farmington Avenue
Hartford, CT 06105
Phone: 830-527-0713
Fax: 860-293-1715
Web Site: www.connecticutopera.org
Officers:
  Chairman: John G Ewen
  Vice Chairman: Thomas K Standish
  President: Calvin S Price
Management:
  Artistic/General Director: Willie Waters
  Managing Director: Maria L Levy
Mission: To preserve and advance the operatic art form; to make opera accessible to a diverse population; to educate, enlighten and entertain through the medium of opera; to assist young artists, directors, designers and technicians.
Founded: 1942
Specialized Field: Grand Opera; Light Opera; Operetta
Status: Professional
Paid Staff: 10
Income Sources: Opera America
Performs At: Horace Bushnell Memorial Hall

All listings are in alphabetical order by state, then city, then organization within the city.

Organization Type: Performing; Touring; Resident; Educational; Sponsoring

1974 CONNECTICUT CHORAL ARTISTS (CONCORA)

52 Main Street
New Britain, CT 06051
Phone: 860-224-7500
Fax: 860-827-8890
e-mail: concoramail@aol.com
Web Site: www.concora.org
Officers:
  President: John Coghill
Management:
  Executive Director: Jane Penfield
  Artistic Director: Richard Coffey
  Director Operations: Jane Penfield
  Administrative Assistant: Yvonne Cherry
Mission: To perform the finest choral music in a professional manner.
Founded: 1974
Specialized Field: Choral
Status: Professional; Nonprofit
Paid Staff: 5
Paid Artists: 60
Budget: $275,000
Income Sources: Government; Foundations; Individuals
Affiliations: Chorus America
Organization Type: Performing; Touring; Resident; Educational

1975 GREATER NEW BRITAIN OPERA ASSOCIATION

1615 Stanley Street
New Britain, CT 06051
Phone: 860-224-2466
Fax: 860-584-9687
Management:
  General Manager: Kenneth A Larson
Mission: To offer a showcase for young artists cast in principal roles; to expose Connecticut youth to opera through work-study programs and classes.
Founded: 1976
Specialized Field: Grand Opera
Status: Professional; Nonprofit
Organization Type: Performing; Resident

1976 YALE RUSSIAN CHORUS

Yale Station
PO Box 202032
New Haven, CT 06520
Phone: 203-432-4776
e-mail: yrc@yale.edu
Web Site: www.yale.edu/yrc
Officers:
  President: Ashley Lucas
  VP: Hsien Seow
Management:
  Music Director: Mark Bailey
  Conductor: Mark Bailey
  Assistant Conductor: Benjamin Warfield
Founded: 1953

1977 CONNECTICUT GRAND OPERA AND ORCHESTRA

15 Bank Street, Mezzenine Level
Stamford, CT 06901
Phone: 203-327-2867
Fax: 203-327-1417
e-mail: mail@ctgrandopera.org
Web Site: www.ctgrandopera.org
Officers:
  Chairman: Robert A Wilson
  Secretary: Robert Scrofani
  Treasurer: Philip Giordano
Management:
  General Director: Laurence Gilgore
  Administrative Director: Arlene Arend
Mission: Dedicated to presenting to area residents and visitors world-class operatic and orchestral performances featuring international music talent and innovative productions.
Founded: 1978
Specialized Field: Grand Opera
Status: Professional
Paid Staff: 6
Volunteer Staff: 40
Income Sources: American Guild of Musical Artists; International Association of Theatrical Stage Employees
Performs At: Palace Theatre of the Arts; Klein Auditorium
Organization Type: Performing; Resident

1978 PRO ARTE CHAMBER SINGERS OF CONNECTICUT

PO Box 4251
Stamford, CT 06905
Phone: 203-322-5970
Management:
  Managing Director: Cynthia King
Mission: Presenting the full depth of choral repertoire, ranging from medieval times to the contemporary.
Founded: 1974
Specialized Field: Choral
Status: Professional
Performs At: First Presbyterian Church
Organization Type: Performing; Touring

1979 CONNECTICUT CONCERT OPERA

PO Box 370341
West Hartford, CT 06137-0341
Phone: 860-722-2300
Fax: 860-726-1839
e-mail: ctconcert@aol.com
Management:
  Artistic Director: Wayne Rivera
  President: John Wadhams
  VP: Robert Merritt
Mission: To present less frequently heard operas in original language with supertitles in concert format to expand opera opportunites in Connecticut and Western Massachusetts.
Founded: 1991
Specialized Field: Concert Opera
Volunteer Staff: 25
Paid Artists: 30

Delaware

1980 DIAMOND STATE CHORUS OF SWEET ADELINES
42 Craig Road
Bear, DE 19701
Phone: 609-358-8995
Fax: 302-378-0935
Web Site: www.diamondstatechorus.org
Officers:
    President: Emily Pinder
    VP: Louisa Leipold
    Secretary: Sylvia Taggart
    Treasurer: Celia Renal
Management:
    Chores Manager: Becky Diamond
Mission: Entertaining and educating the public in barber shop harmony as an American art form.
Founded: 1978
Specialized Field: Choral
Status: Semi-Professional; Nonprofit
Paid Staff: 50
Organization Type: Performing; Educational

1981 MADRIGAL SINGERS OF WILMINGTON
Faith Presbyterian Church
PO Box 9241
Newark, DE 19714
Phone: 302-368-1407
Fax: 215-358-5789
Web Site: www.madrigal-singers.org
Officers:
    President: Barbara Tilton
    Secretary of Board: Carolyn Zoldos-Crowell
    Treasurer: Brian Hanson
Management:
    Director: Virginia Vaalburg
Mission: Presenting Renaissance as well as other chamber music, both a capella and accompanied, with performers in period costumes, for the community's enjoyment and enrichment.
Founded: 1959
Specialized Field: Choral
Status: Semi-Professional; Nonprofit
Paid Staff: 20
Organization Type: Performing; Touring; Educational

1982 GRAND OPERA HOUSE
818 Market Street Mall
Wilmington, DE 19801
Phone: 302-658-7897
Fax: 302-652-5346
e-mail: grandopera@grandopera.org
Web Site: www.grandopera.org
Management:
    Executive Director: Kenneth A Wesler
    Associate Director: Stephen Bailey
    Marketing Director: Mary K Davis
    Director Production: Rick Neidig
    Director Development: Jennifer Mackey
    Controller: Barbara Kelly
    Director Operations: Jamie Bowman
    Media Manager: Paige Wolf

Founded: 1871
Specialized Field: Dance; Classical; Jazz; Theater; Folk; Rock; Opera; Children's Shows; Comedy
Status: Professional; Nonprofit
Performs At: Grand Opera House
Affiliations: Association of Performing Arts Presenters; League of Historic American Theatres
Seating Capacity: 1190; 300
Year Built: 1871
Year Remodeled: 1973
Rental Contact: Jennifer Uro
Organization Type: Performing; Educational; Sponsoring

1983 OPERA DELAWARE
818 N Market Street, Suite 200
PO Box 432
Wilmington, DE 19899-0432
Phone: 302-658-8063
Fax: 302-659-4991
e-mail: opinfo@operadel.org
Web Site: www.operadel.org
Officers:
    President: John W Rollins III
    Treasurer: John Rollins
    VP: Charles Platznzie
    VP: Linda O'Conner
Management:
    General Director: Leland P Kimball III
    Managing Director: Julie W Van Blancom
    Marketing Director: Cindy Frankey
Mission: Mission is to enrich the cultural life of people in the Deleware Valley by producing opera, educational and outreach programs.
Founded: 1948
Specialized Field: Grand Opera
Status: Semi-Professional
Paid Staff: 90
Volunteer Staff: 30
Paid Artists: 80
Budget: $1.5 million
Income Sources: Opera America; Central Opera Service; American Arts Alliance
Performs At: Grand Opera House
Annual Attendance: 27,000
Type of Stage: Proscenium
Stage Dimensions: 38x30
Seating Capacity: 1,100
Year Built: 1876
Year Remodeled: 1976
Organization Type: Performing; Educational

District of Columbia

1984 CATHEDRAL CHORAL SOCIETY
Washington National Cathedral
Massachusetts & Wisconsin Avenues NW
Washington, DC 20016-5098
Phone: 202-537-8980
Fax: 202-537-5648
e-mail: choralsociety@cathedral.org
Web Site: www.cathedralchoralsociety.org
Officers:

All listings are in alphabetical order by state, then city, then organization within the city.

President: Roberta J Duffy
VP: Steven W Smith
Secretary: Neal Jackson
Treasurer: Gerald Padwe
Management:
  Music Director: J Reilly Lewis
  Executive Director: Mark W Ohnmacht
Founded: 1942
Specialized Field: Choral Music
Paid Staff: 7
Paid Artists: 3
Non-paid Artists: 220
Budget: $1,044,400
Performs At: Washington National Cathedral
Affiliations: Chorus America; Cultural Alliance of Greater Washington
Annual Attendance: 23,626
Facility Category: Cathedral
Seating Capacity: 1618
Year Built: 1907

1985 CHORAL ARTS SOCIETY OF WASHINGTON

5225 Wisconsin Avenue NW
2nd Floor, Suite 603
Washington, DC 20015
Phone: 202-244-3669
Fax: 202-244-4244
e-mail: choralarts@choralarts.org
Web Site: www.choralarts.org
Officers:
  Chairman: Eric Frauntelle
  Treasurer: Charles E Hoyt
  Vice Chairman: Patrica B Sagon
  Vice Chair: Elizabeth Holleman
  Secretary: Lorraine Wallace
  Immediate Past Chair: Anne Keiser
  General Counsel: David Brown
  Vice Chair: Cinnie Fehr
Management:
  Music Director: Norman Scribner
  Executive Director: Judith Brophy
  Director Development: John Chappell
  Director Public Relations: Carrie Halpert
  General Counsel: David N Brown
  Chorus President: Jim McHugh
  Associate Conductor: Joseph Holt
  Director Comm./Education Programs: Alicia Mills
Mission: Committed to the highest standards of excellence in its programming and performance.
Founded: 1965
Specialized Field: Choral
Status: Non-Professional; Nonprofit
Paid Staff: 10
Non-paid Artists: 190
Budget: $2,000,000
Income Sources: Individual Donors; Corporate; Government and Foundation Grants; Gifts
Performs At: John F. Kennedy Center for the Performing Arts
Affiliations: Kennedy Center; Chorus America
Annual Attendance: 17,500
Type of Stage: Concert Hall
Organization Type: Performing; Resident

1986 CHORUS AMERICA

1156 15th Street NW
Suite 310
Washington, DC 20005
Phone: 202-331-7577
Fax: 202-331-7599
e-mail: service@chorusamerica.org
Web Site: www.chorusamerica.org
Officers:
  President: John Alexander
Management:
  Office Manager: Adam Hall
  Executive Director: Ann Meier Baker
Mission: To promote the high quality and artistic growth of vocal ensembles; to stimulate further development of remuneration for singers; to encourage greater understanding, appreciation and enjoyment of choral music by all segments of society.
Founded: 1977
Specialized Field: Choral
Status: Nonprofit
Paid Staff: 7
Volunteer Staff: 2

1987 MASTER CHORALE OF WASHINGTON

1200 29th Street NW
Suite LL2
Washington, DC 20007
Phone: 202-471-4050
Fax: 202-471-4051
e-mail: singing@masterchorale.org
Web Site: www.masterchorale.org
Officers:
  Executive Director: Lea Joergenson
  Director Concert Operations: Dennis Martin
  Marketing/Box Office Manager: Ian Buckwalter
  Chairman: Barbara Esau
  First Vice Chairman: Jean Riddelll
  Treasurer: Eric Schweizer
  Secretary: Melissa Krause
Management:
  Music Director: Donald McCullough
Mission: To present choral music concerts.
Founded: 1967
Specialized Field: Choral
Status: Professional; Semi-Professional; Nonprofit
Paid Staff: 5
Volunteer Staff: 4
Paid Artists: 12
Non-paid Artists: 128
Budget: $951,911
Performs At: John F. Kennedy Center for the Performing Arts
Organization Type: Performing

1988 MASTER CHORALE CHAMBER SINGERS

1200 29th Street NW
LL 2
Washington, DC 20007
Phone: 202-471-4050
Fax: 202-471-4051
e-mail: singing@masterchorale.org
Web Site: www.masterchorale.org

Management:
    Music Director: Donald McCullough
    Concert Operations Director: Dennis Martin
    Executive Director: Lea Joergenson

1989 OPERA MUSIC THEATER INTERNATIONAL

1201 Pennsylvania Avanue
Suite 300
Washington, DC 20004
Phone: 202-661-4716
Fax: 202-661-4699
e-mail: mail@omti.org
Web Site: www.omti.org
Management:
    General Director: James McCully, Jr

1990 SUMMER OPERA THEATRE COMPANY

Music School- CUA
620 Michigan Avenue NE
Washington, DC 20064
Phone: 202-526-1669
Fax: 202-319-5433
e-mail: webmaster@summeropera.org
Web Site: www.summeropera.org
Officers:
    Chairman: Leilane G Mehler
    Vice Chairman and Dev. Chairman: Elizabeth C Sara
    Secretary: Jaqueline Havener
    Treasurer: Helen Toomey
    Membership Chairman: Mary Frances Lombard
    Board/Staff Liaison: F. Victoria Tresansky
Management:
    Founder/General Manager: Elaine R Walter, PhD
    Administrative Director: Deanne M Walter
Mission: To seek, promote and present young artists ready for work with major opera and musical theatre companies; to offer more established artists the opportunity to prepare and perform new roles.
Founded: 1978
Specialized Field: Grand Opera; Lyric Opera; Operetta
Status: Professional; Nonprofit
Paid Staff: 4
Volunteer Staff: 4
Paid Artists: 200
Budget: $750,000
Income Sources: Private Donations/ Grants/ Box Office
Performs At: The Hartke Theatre
Annual Attendance: 5,900
Facility Category: Theatre
Organization Type: Performing; Resident; Educational

1991 UNITED STATES AIR FORCE SINGING SERGEANTS

Bolling Air Force Base
201 McChord Street
Washington, DC 20332-0202
Phone: 202-767-5665
Fax: 202-767-0686
e-mail: bandpublicaffairs@bolling.af.mil
Web Site: www.bolling.af.mil\band
Management:
    Conductor: Lt. Daniel Price
    Manager: CMSgt. Julianne Turrentine

Founded: 1945
Paid Artists: 25
Affiliations: Chorus America; American Choral Directors Association

1992 VOCAL ARTS SOCIETY

1818 24th Street NW
Washington, DC 20008
Phone: 202-265-8177
Fax: 202-265-7164
e-mail: gperman@aol.com
Web Site: www.vocalartssociety.org
Officers:
    President: Gerald Perman
    Chair Board of Director: Martha Ellison
    Treasurer: Ernest Hamel
    Secretary: Mary Lynne McElroy
Management:
    Artistic Director: Gerald Perman
    Executive Director: Nancy E Petris
Mission: To promote the classical recital and bring to the Greater Washington area the finest vocals artists in programs of the great and largely underpreformed song literature.
Founded: 1990
Specialized Field: Metropolitan Washington, D.C.
Paid Staff: 1
Paid Artists: 22
Budget: $170,000
Income Sources: Board/Audience Contributions; Foundation Grants
Performs At: Terrace Theater of the Kennedy Center; French Embassy
Annual Attendance: 3,600
Facility Category: Recital Hall
Seating Capacity: 475; 800

1993 WASHINGTON BACH CONSORT

5125 MacArthur Boulevard
Suite 42
Washington, DC 20016-3300
Phone: 202-686-7500
Fax: 202-686-6200
e-mail: bachconsort@olg.com
Web Site: bachconsort.org
Officers:
    President: Ann Meier
    Treasurer: Robert Inglis
    Secretary: Craig Hosmer
Management:
    Music Director: J Reilly Lewis
Mission: Perform to the highest artistic standards the music of JS Bach and his Baroque contemporaries. Expand our audience through concerts, collaborations with other performing ensembles, media appearances, marketable recordings, and tours. Promote current and future appreciation of Bach in our community through compelling music education programs presented by members of the Consort.
Founded: 1977
Specialized Field: Choral; Orchestral
Status: Professional; Nonprofit
Organization Type: Performing; Touring; Educational

1994 WASHINGTON CONCERT OPERA

3509 Connecticut Avenue NW
PMB 730
Washington, DC 20037
Phone: 202-364-5826
Fax: 202-986-4530
e-mail: wcopera@erols.com
Web Site: www.wcopera.org
Management:
    General Director: Stephen Crout
Performs At: Kennedy Center Concert Hall

1995 WASHINGTON OPERA

2600 Virginia Avenue NW
Suite 104
Washington, DC 20037
Phone: 202-295-2420
Fax: 202-295-2479
Toll-free: 800-876-7372
e-mail: info@dc-opera.org
Web Site: www.dc-opera.org
Officers:
    President: Michael R Sonmenreich
    Board of Trustees, Life Chairperson: Mrs. Eugene B
    Casey
    Chairperson: James V Kimsey
    Chair of the Executive Committee: Mrs. Cristine F
    Hunter
Management:
    Director Develpoment: Richard Russell
    Artistic Director: Placido Domingo
    Marketing Director: Trish Taylor Schuman
Mission: To provide highest quality opera; to broaden
public awareness and understanding of opera through
education and community programming; to support
development of young American singers; to encourage
work of new composers to maintain opera as a living art
form.
Founded: 1956
Specialized Field: Grand Opera; Lyric Opera; Light
Opera; Operetta
Status: Professional; Nonprofit
Paid Staff: 60
Volunteer Staff: 150
Budget: $30,000,000
Income Sources: Box Office; Grants; Private Donations
Performs At: John F. Kennedy Center for the Performing
Arts
Affiliations: OPERA America; Washington Opera
Guild/Edcuational
Annual Attendance: 135,500
Type of Stage: Open Stage; Proscenium
Seating Capacity: 2,200
Organization Type: Performing; Resident; Educational
Notes: Access for persons with disabilities. To reserve
wheelchairs, call 202-426-8340 (TTY 416-8524).

1996 COUNTRY CURRENT

617 Warrington Avenue SE
Washington Navy Yard, DC 20374-5054
Phone: 202-433-6093
Fax: 202-433-4108
e-mail: public.affairs@navyband.navy.mil
Web Site: www.navyband.navy.mil
Management:
    Senior Chief Musician: Wayne C Taylor
Mission: To provide music for such ceremonies, functions
and other occasions as may be directed by proper
authority in order to best represent the Navy in a musical
capacity at the seat of government and elsewhere as
directed.
Founded: 1973
Specialized Field: United States Navy Premier
Country/Bluegrass Music Group
Organization Type: Performing; Touring

1997 CRUISERS

617 Warrington Avenue SE
Washington Navy Yard, DC 20374-5054
Phone: 202-433-6093
Fax: 202-433-4108
e-mail: public.affairs@navyband.navy.mil
Web Site: www.navyband.navy.mil
Management:
    Master Chief Musician: Gerard J Ascione
    Musician First Class: Kenneth H Carr
    Musician First Class: John L Fisher
    Musician First Class: Benjamin L Grant
    Musician First Class: John T Parsons
Mission: To provide music for such ceremonies, functions
and other occasions as may be directed by proper
authority in order to best represent the Navy in a musical
capacity at the seat of government and elsewhere as
directed.
Founded: 1999
Specialized Field: United States Navy Premier Rock
Ensemble
Organization Type: Performing; Touring

1998 SEA CHANTERS

617 Warrington Avenue SE
Washington Navy Yard, DC 20374-5054
Phone: 202-433-6093
Fax: 202-433-4108
e-mail: public.affairs@navyband.navy.mil
Web Site: www.navyband.navy.mil
Management:
    Master Chief Musician: John R Bury
    Chief Musician/Musical Director: Keith D Hinton
Mission: To provide music for such ceremonies, functions
and other occasions as may be directed by proper
authority in order to best represent the Navy in a musical
capacity at the seat of government and elsewhere as
directed.
Founded: 1956
Specialized Field: Traditional Choral Music; Sea
Chanteys; Broadway Musicals
Organization Type: Performing; Touring

Florida

1999 PICCOLO OPERA COMPANY

24 Del Rio Boulevard
Boca Raton, FL 33432-4734
Fax: 561-394-0520
Toll-free: 800-282-3161
Officers:

President: Marjorie Gordon
VP: Milton J Miller
Secretary: Merry Silber
Treasurer: M. Gordon
Management:
Executive Director: Marjorie Gordon
Mission: A travelling troupe of professional singers, available throughout the year. Opera in English for adults and youngsters.
Founded: 1963
Status: Nonprofit; Professional; Traveling Company
Budget: Varies
Income Sources: Performances; Grants to Sponsors
Affiliations: Free-Lance Traveling Company
Organization Type: Travelling troupe

2000 GOLD COAST OPERA

3501 SW Davie Road
Fort Lauderdale, FL 33314
Phone: 954-201-6578
Fax: 954-752-8449
Web Site: www.goldcoastopera.org
Management:
General Director: Thomas Cavendish
Principal Stage Director: Malcolm Srnold
Mission: To offer the Pompano Beach area top-quality, fully-staged musical works spanning musical theatre and comic opera as well as other operatic productions.
Founded: 1979
Specialized Field: Operetta; Muiscal Theatre
Status: Professional; Nonprofit
Paid Staff: 20
Income Sources: Opera America
Performs At: Omni Auditorium; Bailey Hall; Coral Springs Civic Center
Organization Type: Performing; Touring; Educational

2001 OPERA GUILD

333 SW Second Street
Fort Lauderdale, FL 33312
Phone: 954-728-9700
Fax: 954-728-9702
Management:
General Manager: William H Martin
Mission: Promoting opera and the newer performing arts.
Founded: 1944
Specialized Field: Grand Opera
Status: Nonprofit
Income Sources: Junior Opera Guild/Children's
Performs At: Broward Center for the Performing Arts
Organization Type: Touring

2002 FLORIDA GRAND OPERA

1200 Coral Way
Miami, FL 33145
Phone: 305-854-1643
Fax: 305-856-1042
e-mail: info@fgo.org
Web Site: www.fgo.org
Management:
General Director: Robert Heuer
Public Relations Director: Eveliny Bastos-Klein
Artistic Administation Director: Karl Hesser
Music Director: Stewart Robertson

Budget: 10,000,000

2003 ORLANDO OPERA

1111 N Orange Avenue
Orlando, FL 32804
Phone: 407-426-1717
Fax: 407-426-1705
Web Site: www.orlandoopera.org
Officers:
President: George Fender
Management:
General Manager: Robert Swedberg
Director Development: Joan Sberro
Director Marketing: Laura Knight
Director Education: Greg Ruffer
Founded: 1958
Specialized Field: Grand Opera
Status: Professional
Income Sources: Opera America
Performs At: Bob Carr Performing Arts Center
Organization Type: Performing

2004 CHORAL SOCIETY OF PENSACOLA

1000 College Boulevard
Room 803
Pensacola, FL 32504
Phone: 850-484-1806
Fax: 850-484-1835
Web Site: www.artsnwfl.org/choralsociety
Management:
Music Director/Conductor: William Clarke
Mission: The performance of choral literature.
Founded: 1935
Specialized Field: Choral
Status: Semi-Professional; Nonprofit
Paid Staff: 82
Income Sources: Arts Council of North West Florida; Chorus America; Florida Cultural Action Alliance
Performs At: Saenger Theatre; Cokesbury United Methodist Church
Organization Type: Performing; Resident

2005 PENSACOLA OPERA

PO Box 1790
Pensacola, FL 32598-1790
Phone: 850-433-6737
Fax: 850-433-1082
e-mail: pensacolaopera@att.net
Web Site: www.pensacolaopera.com
Officers:
Chairman: Jan Cavanaugh
Vice-Chairman: Ann Marie Boweyer
Treasurer: Michael Eiser
Secretary: Joanne Bujnoski
Management:
General Director: Philip M Dobard
Artistic Director: Kyle Marrero
Director Development/Unified Incom: Tracey E Mitchell
Educational Coordinator: Ann Ferguson
Administrative Assistant: Barbara Lake
Mission: To provide professional opera production and education.
Founded: 1983

Specialized Field: Opera
Paid Staff: 7
Volunteer Staff: 15
Paid Artists: 75
Non-paid Artists: 40
Budget: $350,000
Income Sources: Ticket Sales; Public and Private Contributions; Other Income
Performs At: Vaudeville Era Theater
Affiliations: OPERA America
Annual Attendance: 12,000
Facility Category: Performing
Type of Stage: Proscenium
Seating Capacity: 1,800

2006 SARASOTA OPERA ASSOCIATION

61 N Pineapple Avenue
Sarasota, FL 34236
Phone: 941-366-8450
Fax: 941-955-5571
Toll-free: 888-673-7212
e-mail: info@sarasotaopera.org
Web Site: www.sarasotaopera.org
Officers:
   Chairman: Joseph L Berner
   Vice Chairman: Edward C Bavaria
Management:
   Artistic Director: Victor De Renzi
   Executive Director: Susan J Danis
   Public Relations: Greg Parry
   House Manager: Chris Burtless
Mission: To continue to bring quality opera to our community and to showcase it in our own opera house; to educate the general community in an appreciation of opera and send our outreach programs into the schools of both Manatee and Sarasota counties; to offer statewide touring programs.
Founded: 1959
Specialized Field: Grand Opera
Status: Professional; Nonprofit
Paid Staff: 25
Paid Artists: 200
Income Sources: Opera America; Central Opera Service; American Guild of Musical Artists
Performs At: Sarasota Opera House
Organization Type: Performing; Educational; Sponsoring

2007 TAMPA BAY GAY MEN'S CHORUS

Tampa Bay Arts
3000 34th Street S
Suite C-206
St. Petersburg, FL 33711
Phone: 727-865-9004
Fax: 727-866-1006
e-mail: tbgmc@aol.com
Web Site: www.tampabayarts.com
Management:
   Interim Director: Randy Leonard

2008 FLORIDA STATE OPERA AT FLORIDA STATE UNIVERSITY

School of Music
002 HMU
Tallahassee, FL 32306-1180
Phone: 850-645-4903
Fax: 850-644-2566
e-mail: opera@cmr.fsu.edu
Officers:
   President, Florida State University: Sandy D'Alamberte
   Dean School of Music: Jon Piersol
Management:
   Director Opera Activities: Douglas Fisher
   Production Manager: June Dollar
   Technical Director: James Meade
   Stage Director/Professor Opera: Matthew Lata
Mission: Providing training for students at Florida State University; serving as a quality cultural resource.
Founded: 1963
Specialized Field: Grand Opera; Lyric Opera; Operetta; Music Theatres
Status: Semi-Professional; Nonprofit
Paid Staff: 10
Volunteer Staff: 200
Performs At: Ruby Diamond Auditorium; Opperman Music Hall
Affiliations: National Opera Association; Central Opera Service; TOG
Organization Type: Performing

2009 MASTER CHORALE OF TAMPA BAY

PO Box 20591
Tampa, FL 33622-0591
Phone: 813-258-9468
Fax: 813-258-0988
e-mail: MChorale@tampabay.rr.com
Web Site: www.masterchorale.com
Officers:
   Chairman: Robert B Hicks
   Operations Manager: Sandy Ray
Management:
   Music/Artistic Director: Richard Zielinski
Mission: To enrich the community by performing and sustaining high quality choral music.
Paid Staff: 3

2010 SPANISH LYRIC THEATER

2819 Safe Harbor Drive
Tampa, FL 33618
Phone: 813-936-0217
Fax: 813-936-0217
Management:
   Artistic Director: Rene Gonzalez
Performs At: Tampa Bay Performing Arts Center

2011 PALM BEACH OPERA

415 S Olive Avenue
West Palm Beach, FL 33401
Phone: 561-833-3709
Fax: 561-833-8294
e-mail: pbopera@pbopera.org
Web Site: www.pbopera.org
Management:

General Director: R Joseph Barnett
Director Marketing: Michele Eassa
Mission: Producing operas as well as allied musical performances.
Founded: 1961
Specialized Field: Grand Opera
Status: Professional; Nonprofit
Performs At: Kravis Center for the Performing Arts
Organization Type: Performing; Touring; Resident; Educational

2012 FLORIDA LYRIC OPERA

5111 Clarcona Ocoee Road
Winter Park, FL 33702
Phone: 407-292-2143
Fax: 407-523-4279
e-mail: administration@centralfloridalyricopera.com
Web Site: www.centralfloridalyricopera.com
Officers:
President: Millicent Barimo
VP: Marie Hillman
Secretary: Marcia Davis
Treasurer: Mary Collier
Management:
General Manager: Rosalia Maresca
Mission: To promote area talent; to discover, direct and train talented performers in every aspect of musical performance.
Founded: 1988
Specialized Field: Grand Opera; Lyric Opera; Light Opera; Operetta
Status: Professional
Organization Type: Performing; Educational

Georgia

2013 ATLANTA BOY CHOIR

1215 S Ponce de Leon Avenue
Atlanta, GA 30306
Phone: 404-378-0064
Fax: 404-378-4722
e-mail: abchoir@bellsouth.net
Web Site: www.atlantaboychoir.org
Officers:
Administrative/Business Manager: Roberta Kahne
Management:
Director: Fletcher Wolfe
Administrative/Business Manager: Roberta Kahne

2014 ATLANTA OPERA

728 West Peachtree NW
Atlanta, GA 30308-1139
Phone: 404-881-8801
Fax: 404-881-1711
Toll-free: 800-356-7372
e-mail: info@atlantaopera.org
Web Site: www.atlantaopera.org
Officers:
Chairman: Shepard B Ansley
President: Barbara D Stewart
VP: Jack Gillfillan
Treasurer: Ronald R. Antinori
Secretary: Kevin J. Saunders

Management:
Artistic Director: William Fred Scott
Executive Director: Alfred D Kennedy
Artistic Administrator: Sarah D Wikle
Education Coordinator: Brenda Pruitt
General Manager: Russel P Allen
Director Marketing: Amy Moudy
Mission: To present opera productions of the highest standards possible, while fostering education about the art form and encouraging growth with services and programs designed to fill the needs of the community
Founded: 1979
Specialized Field: Grand Opera; Lyric Opera
Status: Professional; Nonprofit
Paid Staff: 23
Volunteer Staff: 40
Paid Artists: 200
Non-paid Artists: 10
Budget: $5.4 Million
Income Sources: Ticketing, Foundations, Individuals, Coporate, Government
Performs At: Alliance Theatre; Symphony Hall
Annual Attendance: 50,000+
Seating Capacity: 4514
Year Built: 1920
Organization Type: Performing; Educational

2015 ATLANTA SYMPHONY ORCHESTRA CHORUS

Robert W. Woodruff Arts Center
1292 Peachtree Street NE
Atlanta, GA 30309
Phone: 404-733-4901
Fax: 404-733-4901
Web Site: www.atlantasymphony.org
Management:
Conductor: Robert Shaw
Choral Administrator: Nola Frank
Specialized Field: Grand Opera; Operetta; Arias
Status: Non-Professional; Nonprofit; Volunteer
Performs At: Robert W. Woodruff Arts Center Symphony Hall
Organization Type: Performing; Touring

2016 ATLANTA YOUNG SINGERS OF CALLANWOLDE

980 Briarcliff Road NE
Atlanta, GA 30306
Phone: 404-873-3365
Fax: 404-873-0756
e-mail: aysc@bellsouth.net
Web Site: www.aysc.org
Management:
Music Director: Paige Mathis
Executive Director: Sharon D Moore
Staff Accompanist: William E Krape
Founded: 1975
Specialized Field: Music-Childrens Choir
Paid Staff: 2
Volunteer Staff: 200
Paid Artists: 5
Budget: $300,000
Income Sources: Grants; Donations; Performances
Annual Attendance: 30,000-60,000

2017 CHORAL GUILD OF ATLANTA
PO Box 550772
Atlanta, GA 30355
Phone: 404-223-6362
Fax: 770-641-1385
e-mail: info@cgatl.org
Web Site: www.cgatl.org
Management:
    Conductor/Director: William Noll
Mission: Recognition as the foremost large civic chorus in the metro Atlanta area; performance of major works of nonstandard repertoire; increasing financial solvency.
Specialized Field: Choral
Status: Semi-Professional; Nonprofit
Organization Type: Performing; Touring

2018 TROIKA BALALAIKES
World Artists
3126 Bolero Drive
Atlanta, GA 30341
Phone: 770-939-4343
Fax: 770-908-1231
e-mail: lynnmc@mindspring.com
Web Site: www.lynnmcconnell.com
Specialized Field: Russian Folk and World Music
Affiliations: Cucanandy (Irish), Cowboy Envy, Deluxe Vaudeville Orchestra, Atlanta Brassworks, Hotlanta (Dixieland), Mariachi Vasqukez, Else Witt

2019 AUGUSTA OPERA ASSOCIATION
1301 Greene Street
Suite 100
Augusta, GA 30903
Phone: 706-826-4710
Fax: 706-826-4732
e-mail: KBopera@aol.com
Web Site: augustaopera.org
Officers:
    President: Sandra Blackwood
    Treasurer: Davenport Bruker
    Secretary: Doris Begley
    Executive VP: Gerald Chamber S
Management:
    Managing Director: Katherine DeLoach
    Artistic Director: Mark Flint
    Administrative Assistant: Donna Jannikrtner
    Marketing Associate: Mary Ann Woodworth
Mission: Strives to present opera music theater productions of the highest standards while encouraging growth of the art form through its programs and outreach services.
Founded: 1967
Specialized Field: Grand Opera; Lyric Opera; Light Opera; Operetta
Status: Professional
Paid Staff: 3
Volunteer Staff: 35
Paid Artists: 221
Non-paid Artists: 128
Budget: $500,000
Income Sources: Subscriptions; Single Ticket Sales; Iundividual Donations; Foundations; Corporations; Government Grants
Performs At: Imperial Theatre

Affiliations: Opera America
Annual Attendance: 9,000
Seating Capacity: 850
Organization Type: Performing; Resident; Educational

2020 GRAND OPERA HOUSE SEASON AT THE GRAND
651 Mulberry Street
Macon, GA 31201
Phone: 912-301-5460
Fax: 912-301-5469
e-mail: goss_km@mercer.edu
Web Site: www.mercer.edu/thegrand
Management:
    Managing Director: Karen Lambert
    Artistic Administration Director: Karen Goss
Performs At: Grand Opera House

Hawaii

2021 HAWAII ECUMENICAL CHORALE
3752 Old Pali Road
Honolulu, HI 96817
Phone: 808-595-3447
Fax: 808-521-4595
Management:
    Artistic Director: Eileen Lum
Mission: To provide an opportunity for local singers to participate in more challenging music than average choirs offer; to sponsor a local choral composition contest to encourage indigenous choral work.
Founded: 1979
Specialized Field: Grand Opera; Choral; Ethnic; Folk
Status: Semi-Professional; Nonprofit
Volunteer Staff: 4
Affiliations: State Foundation on Culture and the Arts
Organization Type: Performing; Resident; Educational

2022 HAWAII OPERA THEATRE
987 Waimanu Street
Honolulu, HI 96814
Phone: 808-596-7858
Fax: 808-596-0379
Toll-free: 800-836-7372
e-mail: hotopera@hawaii.rr.com
Web Site: www.hawaiiopera.org
Management:
    General Director: J Mario Ramos
    General/Artistic Director: Henry G Akina
Mission: To offer opera in Hawaii.
Founded: 1962
Specialized Field: Grand Opera
Status: Professional; Nonprofit
Income Sources: Opera America; Central Opera Service
Performs At: Neal S. Blaisdell Center-Concert Hall
Orchestra Pit: 1
Organization Type: Performing; Touring; Resident; Educational

2023 HONOLULU CHILDREN'S OPERA CHORUS
PO Box 22304
Honolulu, HI 96822
Phone: 808-521-2982
Fax: 808-521-4595
Officers:
  Business Manager: Malla Ka'ai
Management:
  Music Director: Nola A Nahulu
  Accompanist: Wendy Chang
Mission: Developing and nurturing the performing arts by means of choral music; providing educational and artistic resources for Hawaii.
Founded: 1961
Specialized Field: Grand Opera; Light Opera; Choral; Ethnic
Status: Nonprofit
Organization Type: Performing; Educational

2024 OAHU CHORAL SOCIETY
3215 Pali Highway
Honolulu, HI 96817-5202
Phone: 808-595-0327
Fax: 808-595-8616
e-mail: OahuChoral@aol.com
Web Site: www.oahuchoral.com
Management:
  Music Director: Timothy Carney
  President: Linda Fuller
  VP: Peter Tirbak
Founded: 1978
Status: Nonprofit

Idaho

2025 BIOTZETIK BASQUE CHOIR
PO Box 1011
Boise, ID 83701
Phone: 208-336-8219
Management:
  Business Manager: John Kirtland
  Business Manager: Miren Artiach
  Communicator: Ricardo Yanci
Mission: The promotion and enhancement of our culture through dance, song, language and education.
Specialized Field: Ethnic; Folk
Status: Nonprofit
Paid Staff: 70
Income Sources: Euskaldunak
Performs At: Boise Basque Center
Organization Type: Performing; Touring; Educational

2026 BOISE MASTER CHORALE
PO Box 2244
Boise, ID 83701
Phone: 208-344-7901
e-mail: info@boisemasterchorale.org
Web Site: www.boisemasterchorale.org
Officers:
  President: Alana Seacord
  Secretary: Cindy Geile

Treasurer: Bob Ball
Membership: Diane Campbell
Program Director: Leon Collins
Advertising: Barbara Myhre
Management:
  Conductor: Carson Wong
  Stage Manager: Randall Pierson
Mission: Offering the community fine choral music; enabling community members to participate in a high quality choral group.
Specialized Field: Choral
Status: Professional; Semi-Professional; Nonprofit
Paid Staff: 125
Performs At: Saint John's Cathedral; Morrison Center for the Arts
Organization Type: Performing

2027 OPERA IDAHO
516 S 9th Street
Suite B
Boise, ID 83702
Phone: 208-345-9116
Fax: 208-336-9078
e-mail: operaidaho@espaa.org
Web Site: www.operaidaho.org
Management:
  Executive Director: Peter Southwell-Sander
  Artistic Director: Timothy Lindberg
Performs At: Morrison Center; Esther Simplot Performing Arts Annex

Illinois

2028 BELLA VOCE
410 S Michigan
Suite 716
Chicago, IL 60605
Phone: 312-461-0723
Fax: 312-461-0487
e-mail: mail@bellavoce.org
Web Site: www.bellavoce.org
Management:
  General Manager: Caitlin Strokosch
Mission: Presenting historically-based performances of masterworks from the Renaissance and 19th-20th centuries.
Founded: 1982
Specialized Field: Choral
Status: Semi-Professional; Nonprofit
Paid Staff: 2
Volunteer Staff: 30
Paid Artists: 24
Budget: $125,000
Income Sources: Grants; Donations; Concert tickets; CD's
Annual Attendance: 2,500
Organization Type: Performing

2029 CHICAGO A CAPPELLA
2936 N Southport Avenue
Suite 210
Chicago, IL 60657

Phone: 773-296-0165
Fax: 773-296-0968
Toll-free: 800-746-4969
e-mail: info@chicagoacappella.org
Web Site: www.chicagoacappella.org
Management:
   Executive Director: Matthew Greenberg
   Artistic Director: Jonathan Miller
Mission: Nine professional vocal soloists committed to furthering the art of singing together without instruments. Chicago a cappella aims to speak directly to the human spirit, through repertoire from the ninth to the twenty-first centuries.
Founded: 1993
Specialized Field: Repertoire from ninth to twenty-first centuries.
Status: Professional
Performs At: Civic Center Music Hall

2030 CHICAGO CHILDREN'S CHOIR

78 E Washington
Chicago, IL 60602
Phone: 312-849-8300
Fax: 312-849-8309
e-mail: info@ccchoir.org
Web Site: www.ccchoir.org
Management:
   Artistic Director: Josephine Lee
   Development Director: Pam Sullivan
   Marketing Director: Pat Washington
Founded: 1956
Specialized Field: Choral; Folk
Status: Semi-Professional
Paid Staff: 31
Volunteer Staff: 100
Budget: $2,500,000
Income Sources: Performance Fees; Corporate; Civic and Private Sponsorships
Performs At: Concert halls, churches, etc.
Annual Attendance: 1500
Organization Type: Performing; Touring; Educational

2031 CHICAGO OPERA THEATER

70 E Lake Street
Suite 540
Chicago, IL 60601-5907
Phone: 312-704-3420
Fax: 312-704-8421
e-mail: BDickie@chicagooperatheater.org
Web Site: www.chicagooperatheater.org
Management:
   General Director: Brian Dickie
   Finance/Administrator Director: Jean Fox
   Operations Director: Deborah Oberschelp
   Box Office Manager: Alexis Klussner
   Artistic Administrator: Roger Weitz
   Controller: Michael Cunningham
   Production Manager: Brad Gonda
Mission: To present Classical, Baroque, and 20th century operas with a strong empasis on education for people young and old.
Founded: 1974
Specialized Field: Major Works of Classical; Baroque; 20th Century Operas
Status: Professional

Type of Stage: Athenaeum

2032 CHICAGO SYMPHONY CHORUS

Symphony Center
220 S Michigan Avenue
Chicago, IL 60604
Phone: 312-294-3430
Fax: 312-294-3450
e-mail: chorus@cso.org
Web Site: www.cso.org
Management:
   Executive Director: Karen Deschere
   Chorus Director: Duain Wolfe
Mission: Performance with a leading symphony orchestra.
Founded: 1957
Specialized Field: Choral
Status: Professional; Semi-Professional; Nonprofit
Paid Artists: 105
Non-paid Artists: 80
Budget: $1,000,000
Performs At: Orchestra Hall; Ravinia Festival
Organization Type: Performing; Touring; Educational

2033 CHORAL ENSEMBLE OF CHICAGO

2335 N Orchard Street
Chicago, IL 60614
Phone: 773-935-3800
Fax: 773-878-8605
Management:
   Music Director: Scott Arkenberg
   Music Director-Emeritus: George Estevez

2034 LIRA CHAMBER CHORUS

6525 N Sheridan Road
#SKY905
Chicago, IL 60626
Phone: 773-539-4900
Fax: 773-508-7043
e-mail: lira@liraensemble.com
Web Site: www.liraensemble.com
Management:
   Artistic Director/General Manager: Lucyna Migala
Mission: To bring back Polish Culture into American life.
Paid Staff: 5
Paid Artists: 50

2035 LIRA CHILDREN'S CHORUS (DZIECI)

6525 N Sheridan Road
#SKY905
Chicago, IL 60626
Phone: 773-539-4900
Fax: 773-508-7043
Management:
   Artistic Director/General Manager: Lucyna Migala

2036 LIRA SINGERS

6525 N Sheridan Road
#SKY905
Chicago, IL 60626

Phone: 773-539-4900
Fax: 773-508-7043
e-mail: lira@liraensemble.com
Web Site: www.liraensemble.com
Management:
   Artistic Director/General Manager: Lucyna Migala
   Assistant Manager: Susan Smentek
Mission: The Lira Ensemble is the nation's only professional performing arts company specializing in Polish music, song, and dance.
Organization Type: Performing

2037 LYRIC OPERA CENTER FOR AMERICAN ARTISTS

20 N Wacker Drive
Chicago, IL 60606
Phone: 312-332-2244
Fax: 312-345-8425
Web Site: www.lyricopera.org
Management:
   Director: Richard Pearlman
   Manager: Dan Novak
Founded: 1974
Specialized Field: Grand Opera; Lyric Opera; Light Opera
Status: Professional; Nonprofit
Income Sources: Lyric Opera of Chicago
Organization Type: Performing; Educational

2038 LYRIC OPERA OF CHICAGO

20 N Wacker Drive
Suite 840
Chicago, IL 60606
Phone: 312-332-2244
Fax: 312-419-8345
Web Site: 7ww.lyricopera.org
Management:
   Artistic Director: Matthew A Epstein
   General Director: William Mason
   Music Director Designate: Sir Andrew Davis
Mission: Offering quality opera to Chicago area residents.
Founded: 1954
Specialized Field: Grand Opera
Status: Professional; Nonprofit
Income Sources: Lyric Opera Center for American Artists
Performs At: Civic Opera House
Seating Capacity: 3,563
Organization Type: Performing; Sponsoring

2039 MUSIC OF THE BAROQUE CHORUS & ORCHESTRA

100 N LaSalle Street
Suite 1610
Chicago, IL 60602
Phone: 312-551-1415
Fax: 312-551-1444
e-mail: baroque@baroque.org
Web Site: www.baroque.org
Officers:
   Chairman: Elbert O Hand III
Management:
   Executive Director: Karen Fishman
   Music Director: Jane Glover

Director Marketing/Communications: Anne Penway
Mission: To perform and increase audience appreciation for choral and orchestral music of the 17th and 18th centuries.
Founded: 1972
Specialized Field: Repertorie Chorus & Orchestra
Paid Staff: 6
Paid Artists: 60
Budget: $1,500,000
Performs At: Church Venues
Annual Attendance: 13,000
Facility Category: Church venues
Type of Stage: Varies
Seating Capacity: 600-2,521

2040 WILLIAM FERRIS CHORALE

690 W Belmont Avenue
Chicago, IL 60657
Phone: 773-325-2000
Fax: 773-325-9293
e-mail: wfchorale@aol.com
Web Site: www.mt-carmel.org
Management:
   Executive Director: John Vorrasi
Founded: 1972

2041 WINDY CITY PERFORMING ARTS

3023 N Clark
#329
Chicago, IL 60657
Phone: 773-404-9242
Fax: 773-404-6815
e-mail: wcpa@windycitysings.org
Web Site: www.windycitysings.org
Management:
   Executive Director: Todd J Ruppenthal
   Music Director: Michael Querio
Founded: 1979
Specialized Field: musica/choral
Paid Staff: 2
Volunteer Staff: 20
Paid Artists: 6
Non-paid Artists: 100
Budget: $400,000
Annual Attendance: 5,000

2042 MILLIKIN UNIVERSITY OPERA THEATRE

1184 W Main Street
Decatur, IL 62522-2084
Phone: 217-424-6300
Fax: 217-420-6652
Toll-free: 800-373-7733
e-mail: trmorris@mail.millikin.edu
Web Site: www.millikin.edu
Management:
   Dean Fine Arts: Stephen Fiol
   Director School of Music: Mary Ellen Poole
   Director Opera Studies: Terry Morris
   Director/Departments/Theatre/Dance: Barry Pearson
Mission: To provide professional training and numerous performance opportunities for undergraduates in productions including scenes, chamber operas, fully produced operas and musical theatre.

Founded: 1955
Specialized Field: Grand Opera; Lyric Opera; Operetta
Status: Nonprofit
Paid Staff: 4
Budget: $15,000
Income Sources: Annual budget; ticket sales
Performs At: Kirkland Fine Arts Center, Albert Taylor Hall, Kaeuper Hall
Affiliations: Opera America, Musical America
Annual Attendance: 2,000
Type of Stage: Proscenium w/hydraulic pit
Organization Type: Educational

2043 DOWNERS GROVE CHORAL SOCIETY

PO Box 655
Downers Grove, IL 60515-0655
Phone: 630-515-0030
Fax: 630-910-8254
e-mail: rdunkman@aol.com
Management:
   Music Director/Conductor: Robert Holst
   Orchestra Manager: Patricia Smith

2044 L'OPERA PICCOLA

1840 Fox Run Drive
Unit D
Elk Grove, IL 60007
Phone: 312-560-1072
Fax: 847-823-3165
e-mail: sasha@loperapiccola.org
Web Site: www.loperapiccola.org
Officers:
   President: Jerry Lee Brown
   Treasurer: John Sasser
   Board Director: Edward C Reicin
Management:
   Executive Director/General Manager: Sasha Gerritson Brauer
   Artistic Director: Shifra Werch
   Music Director: David Richards
   Executive Producer: Madeline Nelson
Mission: To provide traditional Italian opera to the world by linking thye singers of today with the success of tomorrow.
Founded: 1996
Specialized Field: Opera
Status: Nonprofit
Paid Staff: 4
Volunteer Staff: 250
Budget: $250,000
Income Sources: Grants; Individual Donations; Ticket Sales
Performs At: Athenaeum Theatre
Annual Attendance: 6,000
Seating Capacity: 985

2045 LIGHT OPERA WORKS

927 Noyes Street
Evanston, IL 60201
Phone: 847-869-7930
Fax: 847-869-6388
e-mail: postmaster@light-opera-works.org
Web Site: www.light-opera-works.org
Management:

General Director: Bridget McDonough
Artistic Director: Lara Teeter
Business Manager: Mike Kotze
Production Manager: Julie Newland
Mission: Producing professional light opera.
Founded: 1980
Specialized Field: Light Opera; Operetta; Musical Comedy
Status: Professional; Nonprofit
Paid Staff: 5
Paid Artists: 35
Budget: $950,000
Income Sources: Box office; grants; donations
Performs At: Cahn Auditorium
Affiliations: National Opera Association, Opera America, League of Chicago Theatres, Chicago Music Alliance
Annual Attendance: 20,000
Type of Stage: Proscenium
Stage Dimensions: 45 x 35 x 22
Year Built: 1940
Year Remodeled: 1994
Organization Type: Performing

2046 DUPAGE OPERA THEATER

Arts Center,College of Dupage
Glen Ellyn, IL 60137
Phone: 630-942-3005
Fax: 630-790-9806
e-mail: bauerh@cdnet.cod.edu
Web Site: www.cod.edu
Management:
   Artistic Director: Harold Bauer
Performs At: Arts Center

2047 GLEN ELLYN CHILDREN'S CHORUS

799 Roosevelt Road
Building 6, Suite 100
Glen Ellyn, IL 60137
Phone: 630-858-2471
Fax: 630-858-2476
e-mail: info@gechildrenschorus.org
Web Site: www.gechildrenschorus.org
Management:
   Music Director: Emily Ellsworth
   Executive Director: Joana Welles
Mission: To provide any interested child, regardless of previous musical experience, with an outstanding performance-based music education program offered in a positive and nurturing environment which fosters self-esteem and personal growth.
Founded: 1964
Specialized Field: Choral; Children's
Status: Non-Professional; Nonprofit
Organization Type: Performing; Touring; Educational

2048 MOLINE BOYS CHOIR

3426 23rd Avenue
Moline, IL 61265
Phone: 309-764-3109
e-mail: mobocho@aol.com
Management:
   Director: Kermit Wells
   Manager: Margaret Mangelsdorf

Mission: To perform choral literature of a variety of styles; to provide vocal/choral training to boys of talent, interest and ability.
Founded: 1948
Specialized Field: Choral
Status: Nonprofit
Paid Staff: 2
Volunteer Staff: 1
Organization Type: Performing; Touring; Educational

2049 OPERA ILLINOIS

331 Fulton Street
Suite 309
Peoria, IL 61602
Phone: 309-673-7253
Fax: 309-673-7211
e-mail: Frontdesk@operaillinois.com
Web Site: www.operaillinois.com
Officers:
   President: Karl Kuppler
   Vice-President: Camille Gibson
   Treasurer: Mildred Arends
Management:
   Executive Director: Margaret Swain
   Artistic Director: Flora Contino
   General Manager: William Swain
   Production Manager: Richard Weil
Mission: The mission is to enhance the cultural, educational and economic life of Downstate Illinois by the promotion of opera and the production of professional opera performances
Founded: 1972
Specialized Field: Opera; Classical Music; Theater
Paid Staff: 5
Volunteer Staff: 25
Budget: $565,000
Income Sources: Ticket Revenue; Contributed Revenue
Performs At: Peoria Civic Center Theater
Affiliations: Opera America
Annual Attendance: 10,000+
Facility Category: Peorkia, Civic Center, Theatre
Type of Stage: Proscenium
Stage Dimensions: 45'x35'x45'
Seating Capacity: 2131
Year Built: 1981

2050 MUDDY RIVER OPERA COMPANY

428 Maine Street
Suite 270
Quincy, IL 62301-3930
Phone: 217-222-2856
Fax: 217-222-2869
Officers:
   President: Avril Marie Bernzen
Management:
   Artistic Director: Avril Marie Bernzen
   Music Conductor: Fr. Dennis Scharer
Founded: 1989
Volunteer Staff: 16
Annual Attendance: 2000
Facility Category: Several theatres
Seating Capacity: 500-650

2051 AUGUSTANA CHOIR

Office of Cultural Events, Augustana College
639 38th Street
Rock Island, IL 61201
Phone: 309-794-7307
Fax: 309-794-7678
e-mail: acedu@augustana.edu
Web Site: www.augustana.edu
Management:
   Conductor: John Hurty
   Manager: Dan Urton

2052 ARCH-OPERA HOUSE OF SANDWICH

140 E Railroad Street
Sandwich, IL 60548
Phone: 815-786-2555
Fax: 815-786-7012
e-mail: operahouse@sannauk.com
Web Site: www.sandwichoperahouse.com
Officers:
   President: Barbara Hoffman
Management:
   Executive Director: Sandra Black
Founded: 1878
Specialized Field: Performing Arts Center
Paid Staff: 2
Volunteer Staff: 200
Budget: $50,000-$100,000
Performs At: ARCH-Opera House of Sandwich
Affiliations: Rockford Arts Council, Illinois Presenters Newtork, Fox Valley Arts Council
Annual Attendance: 25,000
Facility Category: Restored 1878 Opera House
Type of Stage: Proscenium arch
Stage Dimensions: 20 x 20
Seating Capacity: 310
Year Built: 1878
Year Remodeled: 1986
Cost: $1.75 Million
Rental Contact: Executive Director Sandra Black

2053 WAUKEGAN CONCERT CHORUS

39 Jack Benny Drive
Waukegan, IL 60087
Phone: 847-360-4742
Fax: 847-662-0592
e-mail: wkarts@waukeganparks.org
Web Site: www.waukeganparks.org/jbc
Management:
   Director: Stephen Blackweider
   Performance Supervisor: Rik Covalinski
Non-paid Artists: 30

2054 WAUKEGAN SYMPHONY ORCHESTRA & CONCERT CHORUS

39 Jack Benny Drive
Waukegan, IL 60085
Phone: 847-244-1660
Fax: 847-662-0592
e-mail: wkarts@waukeganparks.org
Web Site: www.waukeganparks.org/jbc
Management:
   Music Director: Stephen Blackweldor
   Performance Supervisor: Rik Covalinski

Paid Staff: 2
Paid Artists: 6
Non-paid Artists: 60
Budget: $100,000-150,000
Income Sources: Waukegan Park District Corporation, grants
Performs At: Orlin D. Trapp Auditorium
Annual Attendance: 1500
Facility Category: Auditorium
Type of Stage: Proscenium
Seating Capacity: 1500

2055 WOODSTOCK OPERA HOUSE

121 Van Buren Street
Woodstock, IL 60098
Phone: 815-338-4212
Fax: 815-334-2284
e-mail: ophsedir@woodstock-il.com
Web Site: www.woodstock-il.com
Management:
    Executive Director: John Scharres
Mission: Providing McHenry County, Illinois with a cultural center; showcasing Illinois artists as well as American and international performers; working closely with the local Woodstock community.
Founded: 1890
Specialized Field: Dance; Vocal Music; Instrumental Music; Theater; Festivals
Status: Nonprofit
Paid Staff: 15
Volunteer Staff: 20
Income Sources: International Society of Performing Arts Administrators; Association of Performing Arts Presenters
Performs At: Woodstock Opera House
Annual Attendance: 55,000
Facility Category: theatre
Type of Stage: Proscenium
Stage Dimensions: 24'x26'
Seating Capacity: 420
Year Built: 1890
Year Remodeled: 1974
Organization Type: Performing; Resident; Educational; Sponsoring

Indiana

2056 INDIANAPOLIS OPERA

250 E 38th Street
Indianapolis, IN 46205
Phone: 317-283-3531
Fax: 317-923-5611
e-mail: ticket@indyopera.org
Web Site: www.indyopera.org
Officers:
    President: Norman Oman
Management:
    Executive Director: John Pickett
    Artistic Director: James Caraher
    Director Resource Development: Samuel J Smith
    Marketing/Customer Relations: Matthew Tippel
Mission: To produce and present opera in performances of the highest quality and to develop audiences for opera.

Founded: 1975
Specialized Field: Grand Opera; Lyric Opera; Light Opera; Operetta
Status: Professional; Nonprofit
Paid Staff: 10
Paid Artists: 130
Budget: $2,312,000
Performs At: Clowes Memorial Hall; Butler University
Affiliations: Opera America
Annual Attendance: 16,800
Facility Category: Multiple use, concert/ performance hall
Type of Stage: Proscenium
Stage Dimensions: 52'x 60'
Year Built: 1965
Organization Type: Performing; Touring; Resident; Educational; Sponsoring
Resident Groups: Indianapolis Opera Ensemble

2057 INDIANAPOLIS SYMPHONIC CHOIR

4600 Sunset Avenue
Indianapolis, IN 46208
Phone: 317-940-6461
Fax: 317-940-8461
e-mail: davel@iquest.net
Web Site: www.iquest.net/~ischoir
Management:
    Director: James Bagwell

2058 MACALLISTER

PO Box 1941
Indianapolis, IN 46206
Phone: 317-546-6387
Fax: 317-546-6399
e-mail: opera@iquest.net
Officers:
    President: PE MacAllister
    VP: Melvin Carroway
    Secreetary: Dede Commons
    Treasurer: Alan Thompson
Management:
    General Director: Elaine Bookwalter
    President/Board of Directors: PE MacAllister
Mission: To provide opera opportunities for young artists through opera productions and sponsorship of the MacAllister Awards, the largest sponsored, nonrestricted opera competition on the continent; to provide, through productions, training for young artists, both artistic and technical.
Founded: 1980
Specialized Field: Grand Opera; Lyric Opera; Light Opera; Operetta; Competition
Status: Professional; Nonprofit
Paid Staff: 2
Income Sources: Central Opera Service; Butler University Romantic Festival
Performs At: Frederic M. Ayers Auditorium
Organization Type: Performing; Touring; Sponsoring

2059 PELLA OPERA HOUSE

611 Franklin Street
PO Box 326
Pella, IN 50219

Phone: 641-628-8628
Fax: 641-628-8628
e-mail: pellaophouse@lisco.net
Web Site: www.pellaoperahouse.com
Management:
   General Manager: Barbara Filer
   Assistant Manager: Emily Riley
   Volunteer Coordinator: Vicki Meyers
Mission: Present a variety of performing arts throughout the year for entertainment and educational purposes. To enhance and support the arts community.
Founded: 1900
Specialized Field: Performing Arts
Paid Staff: 2
Volunteer Staff: 30
Budget: $260,000
Income Sources: Ticket Sales; Donations; Tours
Annual Attendance: 32,000
Type of Stage: Proscenium
Stage Dimensions: 22x22
Seating Capacity: 324
Year Built: 1900
Year Remodeled: 1990
Cost: $2,000,000
Rental Contact: Emily Riley

2060 WHITEWATER OPERA COMPANY

211 S 5th Street
Richmond, IN 47374
Phone: 765-962-7106
Fax: 765-962-7451
e-mail: wocop@infocom.com
Web Site: www.infocom.com/~wocop
Officers:
   President: Paul Hemker
   VP: Russ Peterson
   Secretary: Carolyn Blakey
   Treasurer: Jerry Planck
Management:
   Office Manager: Carolyn Jensen
   General Director: Curtis Tucker
Mission: A resident opera company which presents one-act and full-length operas. Provides schools and organizations with educational operatic programs.
Founded: 1972
Specialized Field: Grand Opera; Lyric Opera; Light Opera; Operetta
Status: Professional; Nonprofit
Budget: $200,000
Performs At: Civic Hall Performing Arts Center
Affiliations: Opera America
Organization Type: Performing; Touring; Educational

2061 VALPARAISO UNIVERSITY CHORALE

Valparaiso University Music Department
Valparaiso, IN 46383
Phone: 219-464-5455
Fax: 219-464-5244
Web Site: www.valpo.edu/music/chorale/flash
Management:
   Conductor: Christopher M Cock
   Tour Manager: Dot Neuchterlein

2062 DORIAN OPERA THEATRE

Decorah, IA 52101
Phone: 563-387-1089
Fax: 563-387-1076
e-mail: dorianop@luther.edu
Web Site: www.luther.edu/~dot
Officers:
   President: Robert Lillie
   VP: Justine Lionberger
   Secretary/Treasurer: Lynette Wilson
   Director Marketing: Vicki Bjerke
Management:
   Managing Director: David Judisch
   Artistic Director: Jessica Paul
Mission: Offering performance experience to young professionals as well as student artists.
Founded: 1985
Specialized Field: Lyric Opera; Light Opera; Operetta
Status: Semi-Professional; Nonprofit
Paid Staff: 25
Performs At: Luther College Center for Faith and Life
Organization Type: Touring; Resident; Educational

2063 DES MOINES CHORAL SOCIETY

8345 University Blouevard
Suite F-1
Des Moines, IA 50325
Phone: 515-273-5255
Fax: 515-225-6363
e-mail: DMCS@assoc-serv.com
Web Site: www.members.aol.com/dmchoral
Officers:
   President: Wayne Bauman
   VP/Community Relations: LuAnn White
   Treasurer: Carolyn Knittle
   Secretary: Lois O'Donnell
Management:
   Artistic Director/Conductor: Janet Davis
   Executive Director: Jan Gemar
Mission: To inform, educate and stimulate the public toward a better appreciation of choral music.
Specialized Field: Performing; Educational
Paid Staff: 1
Paid Artists: 6
Budget: $85,000
Income Sources: Tickets; Grants; Private Donations
Affiliations: Chorus America; Metro Alliance of Greater Des Moines
Annual Attendance: 2,000

2064 DES MOINES METRO OPERA

106 W Boston
Indianola, IA 50125-8175
Phone: 515-961-6221
Fax: 515-961-8175
e-mail: dmmopera@aol.com
Web Site: www.dmmo.org
Officers:
   President: Mary Kelly
   President Elect: Kimberly Shadur
   Secretary: Linda Kniep
   Treasurer: Tom McKlveen

Management:
Artistic Director: Robert L Larsen
Executive Director: Jerilee M Mace
Development/Community Rel. Director: Robert Montana
Artistic Administrator: Michael Egel
Mission: To provide a stage for young American artists, produce high quality performances and educate audiences to opera in the Midwest.
Founded: 1973
Specialized Field: Opera
Status: Professional; Nonprofit
Paid Staff: 71
Volunteer Staff: 115
Paid Artists: 105
Budget: 1.8 Million
Income Sources: Revenue and contributions
Season: June - July
Performs At: Indianola (Festival Site)
Affiliations: Opera America
Annual Attendance: 8,000
Facility Category: Blank Performing Arts Center
Type of Stage: Proscenium with thrust stage
Seating Capacity: 488
Year Built: 1972
Rental Contact: Jim Lile
Organization Type: Performing; Touring; Resident; Educational
Resident Groups: OPERA Iowa - 13 week tour

Kansas

2065 TOPEKA SYMPHONY CHORUS
PO Box 2206
Topeka, KS 66601-2206
Phone: 785-232-2032
Fax: 785-232-6204
e-mail: tso@topekasymphony.org
Management:
Director: Skip Ellis
Manager: Timothy Jones

Kentucky

2066 KENTUCKY OPERA
Kentucky Opera Building
101 S 8th Street
Louisville, KY 40202
Phone: 502-584-4500
Fax: 502-584-7484
Toll-free: 800-690-9236
Web Site: www.kyopera.org
Management:
Press/Media Releations Manager: Patrick Riedling
General Director: Deborah Sandler
Finance Director: Brett Landow
Development Director: Jeff Sodowsky
Marketing Director: Steve Kelley
Mission: To entertain and educate a broad, diverse audience by producing opera of the highest quality.
Founded: 1952

Specialized Field: Grand Opera; Lyric Opera; Light Opera; Operetta
Status: Professional; Nonprofit
Paid Staff: 20
Volunteer Staff: 200
Paid Artists: 80
Budget: $2,200,000
Income Sources: Fund for the Arts; mainstage performances, education programs, public/private philanthropy
Performs At: Kentucky Center for the Arts; Whitney Hall
Annual Attendance: 14,000/25,000 edu
Type of Stage: Proscenium
Stage Dimensions: 59'9"x52'6"x32'
Seating Capacity: 2,406
Year Built: 1983
Year Remodeled: 2002
Organization Type: Performing; Touring; Educational

2067 LOUISVILLE BACH SOCIETY
4607 Hanford Lane
Louisville, KY 40207
Phone: 502-585-2224
Fax: 502-893-7954
Web Site: www.louisvillebachsociety.org
Management:
Music Director: Melvin Dickinson
Mission: To perform the choral and orchestral music of Bach, as well as other baroque, modern, classical and romantic composers.
Founded: 1964
Specialized Field: Orchestra; Choral
Status: Nonprofit
Paid Staff: 80
Income Sources: Kentucky Arts Council; Greater Louisville Fund for the Arts; American Federation of Musicians
Performs At: University of Louisville
Organization Type: Performing; Touring; Resident; Educational

2068 LOUISVILLE CHORUS
6303 Fern Valley Pass
Louisville, KY 40228
Phone: 502-968-6300
Fax: 502-962-1094
e-mail: chorus@flyinghands.com
Web Site: fastzone.com/chorus/
Officers:
Treasurer: George Brown
Secretary Board of Directors: Sue Juetty
Management:
Music Director: Daniel Spurlock
Executive Director: Therese Davis
Mission: To foster the art of vocal music; to provide a high-quality musical experience, representing a wide variety of styles from the Renaissance to the present.
Founded: 1939
Specialized Field: Choral
Status: Semi-Professional; Nonprofit
Paid Staff: 4
Income Sources: Corporations
Organization Type: Performing; Touring; Educational; Sponsoring

Louisiana

2069 BATON ROUGE GILBERT AND SULLIVAN SOCIETY

746 Main Street
Baton Rouge, LA 70898
Phone: 225-343-0067
e-mail: brgns@aol.com
Web Site: www.members.aol.com/brgns
Mission: Performing excerpts from and full-length productions of Gilbert and Sullivan operettas.
Founded: 1975
Specialized Field: Operetta
Status: Non-Professional; Nonprofit
Paid Staff: 35
Performs At: Baton Rouge Little Theatre
Organization Type: Performing

2070 JPAS CHILDREN'S CHORUS/YOUTH CHORALE

Jefferson Performing Arts Society
1118 Clearview Parkway
Metairie, LA 70001
Phone: 504-885-2000
Fax: 504-885-3437
e-mail: jpasinfo@jpas.org
Web Site: www.jpas.org
Officers:
    Chairman: Hannah Cunningham
    President: Wayne Keating
    Past President: Dr. Bud Willis
    Secretary: Subhash Kulkarni
Management:
    Director: Andrea Babin
    Accompanist: William Prante
    Conductor: Joey Winters
    Conductor: Dr. Louise LaBruyere
Mission: To provide a complete music education experience for young people.
Founded: 1984
Specialized Field: Choral Music; Opera Music Theater
Paid Staff: 4
Volunteer Staff: 20
Paid Artists: 10
Non-paid Artists: 130
Budget: $150,000
Income Sources: JPAS; Tuitions

2071 WOMEN'S GUILD OF THE NEW ORLEANS OPERA

3512 Taft Park
Metairie, LA 70002-4558
Phone: 504-899-1945
Fax: 504-529-7668
Web Site: www.neworleansopera.org
Officers:
    President: Veronica Porteo Scheinuk
Mission: To support the New Orleans Opera Association through fund-raising; to educate.
Founded: 1942
Status: Professional; Nonprofit
Organization Type: Educational; Sponsoring

2072 NEW ORLEANS OPERA ASSOCIATION

305 Baronne
Suite 500
New Orleans, LA 70112-1618
Phone: 504-529-2278
Fax: 504-529-7668
Toll-free: 800-881-4459
Web Site: www.neworleansopera.org
Officers:
    President: Lois Hawkins
    Executive VP: Robert Monroe
    Treasurer: Ronald Dyer
    Secretary: Charles Dupin
Management:
    General Director: Robert Lyall
    Music Administrator/Chorus Master: Carol Rausch
    Scenic Studios Manager: G. Alan Rusnak
    Director Operations: Rebecca Hildabrant
Mission: Providing the highest quality grand opera for Louisiana and its surrounding area.
Founded: 1942
Specialized Field: Grand Opera
Status: Professional; Nonprofit
Budget: $2.5 Million
Income Sources: Individual; Corporate; Foundation; Ticket Sales
Season: October- April
Performs At: Mahalia Jackson Theater of the Performing Arts
Annual Attendance: 18,500
Facility Category: Theater
Year Built: 1975
Organization Type: Performing; Resident; Educational

2073 SYMPHONY CHORUS OF NEW ORLEANS

72 Neron Place
New Orleans, LA 70118
Phone: 504-861-4230
Fax: 504-866-2838
e-mail: SteveEdw@aol.com
Web Site: www.lpomusic.com/scno.htm
Management:
    Music Director: Steven Edwards

2074 SHREVEPORT OPERA

212 Texas Street
Suite 101
Shreveport, LA 71101
Phone: 318-227-9503
Fax: 318-227-9518
e-mail: edillners@shreveopera.org
Web Site: www.shreveopera.org
Officers:
    President: Dr. F Scott Kennedy
    VP: Ron Voss
    Treasurer: Robert Conway
    Secretary: Judy McColgan
Management:
    General Director: Eric T Dillner
    Development Director: Karen A Edwards
    Production Manager: Dawn Huertas
Mission: To provide professional opera and to tour children's opera to schools throughout the region.

Founded: 1949
Specialized Field: Opera
Status: Professional; Nonprofit
Paid Staff: 6
Volunteer Staff: 250
Paid Artists: 10
Non-paid Artists: 125
Income Sources: Opera Guild; Corporations; Grants; Foundations; Division of Arts
Performs At: Civic Theater
Affiliations: Opera America
Annual Attendance: 6000
Facility Category: Civic Theater
Seating Capacity: 1750
Organization Type: Performing; Touring; Resident; Educational

Maine

2075 MAINE MUSIC SOCIETY
PO Box 711
Auburn, ME 04240
Phone: 207-782-1403
Fax: 207-783-1851
e-mail: mms@gwi.net
Web Site: www.mainemusicsociety.org
Officers:
  President: Judith W Andrucki
  VP: Charles W Scheib
  Treasurer: Jeffrey R Gosselin
Management:
  Artistic Director: Peter Frewen
Mission: The Maine Music Society supports the artistic and educational activities of the professional Maine Chamber Ensemble and the auditioned, mixed-voice Androscoggin Chorale.
Founded: 1991
Status: Nonprofit
Income Sources: Maine Community Foundation; Davis Family Foundation; Helen & George Ladd Charitable Foundation; Maine Arts Commision; Maine Humanities Commission
Performs At: Orchestral; Chamber and Coral Music; Educational Programs
Affiliations: American Symphony Orchestra League; Maine Arts Sponsors Association; Androscoggin County Chamber of Commerce; Maine Association of Non-Profits

2076 PORTLAND OPERA REPERTORY THEATRE
437 Congress Street
PO Box 7733
Portland, ME 04112
Phone: 207-879-7678
Fax: 207-879-7681
e-mail: portopera@aol.com
Web Site: www.portopera.org
Officers:
  President: Jack Riddle
Management:
  Artistic/General Director: Bruce Hangen
  Administrative Assistant: Diane York

Production Manager: Joanne Greene
Founded: 1995
Paid Staff: 3
Volunteer Staff: 2
Budget: $500,000
Income Sources: Corporate; Individual Support
Annual Attendance: 6,000
Facility Category: Municipal Theatre
Type of Stage: Proscenium
Stage Dimensions: 52'x40'x35'
Seating Capacity: 1830
Year Built: 1912
Year Remodeled: 1997

2077 PORTLAND SYMPHONIC CHOIR
PO Box 1517
Portland, ME 04104
Phone: 503-223-1217
Fax: 503-223-1217
Web Site: www.pschoir.org
Management:
  Director: Dr. Bruce Browne
  Assistant Director: Debbie Glaze
Founded: 1946

2078 BAY CHAMBER CONCERTS
10 Summer Street
PO Box 228
Rockport, ME 04856
Phone: 207-236-2823
Fax: 207-230-0454
Toll-free: 888-707-2770
e-mail: info@baychamberconcerts.org
Web Site: www.baychamberconcerts.org
Officers:
  President: Martha Rogers
  Secretary: Monica Kelly
  Treasurer: Frank Beane
Management:
  Artistic Director: Thomas Wolf
  Director Marketing/Communications: Kathy Maloney
  Administrative Coordinator: Anne Tani
Mission: To nurture music appreciation, with emphasis on chamber music, among residents of Maine.
Founded: 1960
Specialized Field: Instrumental and Vocal Music
Status: Professional
Paid Staff: 4
Budget: $500,000
Performs At: Rockport Opera House
Facility Category: Opera House; Strom Auditorium
Type of Stage: Proscenium; Auditorium
Seating Capacity: 400; 800
Organization Type: Performing

2079 OPERA MAINE
Wind Rising, 99 Bay View
Steuben, ME 04680
Phone: 207-546-4495
Fax: 207-546-4495
e-mail: info@operamaine.org
Web Site: www.operamaine.org
Management:

Artistic Director: David Katz
Executive Director: Diane Kern

Maryland

2080 ANNAPOLIS OPERA
801 Chase Street
Room 304
Annapolis, MD 21401
Phone: 410-267-8135
Fax: 410-267-6440
e-mail: admin@annapolisopera.org
Web Site: www.annapolisopera.org
Management:
  President: Jean Jackson
Mission: To bring affordable opera to the residents of Maryland, educate audiences about opera as an art form, provide opportunities for local artists and technical personnel to involve themselves in all phases of opera production, and discover emerging talent among young Maryland vocal artists through an annual vocal competition.
Founded: 1973
Specialized Field: Grand Opera; Light Opera; Operetta
Status: Professional; Non-Professional; Nonprofit
Paid Staff: 3
Volunteer Staff: 30
Paid Artists: 70
Non-paid Artists: 125
Budget: $320,000
Income Sources: Tickets; Donations; Grants
Performs At: Maryland Hall for the Creative Arts
Annual Attendance: 6,500
Organization Type: Performing; Educational

2081 BALTIMORE CHORAL ARTS SOCIETY
1316 Park Avenue
Baltimore, MD 21217
Phone: 410-523-7070
Fax: 410-523-7097
Toll-free: 800-750-0875
e-mail: info@baltimorechoralarts.org
Web Site: www.baltimorechoralarts.org
Officers:
  President: Arnold Paskoff
  VP: Linda C Goldberg
  Treasurer: Jeffrey Austin
  Secretary: Andrea Bowman-Moore
Management:
  Music Director: Tom Hall
  Executive Director: Sandra N Smith
  Administrative Director: Laura Byrne
  Chorus Manager: Ellen Clayton
Founded: 1966
Specialized Field: Choral, Orchestral
Paid Staff: 4
Volunteer Staff: 1
Paid Artists: 65
Non-paid Artists: 75
Budget: $500,000

Income Sources: Ticket Sales; Contributions; Maryland State Arts Council; Baltimore County Commission on Arts & Science; Mayor's Advisory Committee on Art & Culture; Local Contributors
Performs At: Joseph Meyerhoff Symphony Hall; Krausbaar Auditorium
Affiliations: Member of Chorus America
Annual Attendance: 15,000

2082 BALTIMORE OPERA COMPANY
110 W Mount Royal Avenue
Suite 306
Baltimore, MD 21201
Phone: 410-625-1600
Fax: 410-625-6474
e-mail: JHarp@baltimoreopera.com
Web Site: www.baltimoreopera.com
Management:
  Music Director: James Harp
Founded: 1950
Specialized Field: Opera
Volunteer Staff: 50
Paid Artists: 300
Budget: $7 million
Annual Attendance: 60,000
Facility Category: Opera House
Type of Stage: Proscenium
Seating Capacity: 2460
Year Built: 1894
Year Remodeled: 1981

2083 BALTIMORE SYMPHONY CHORUS
1212 Cathedral Street
Baltimore, MD 21201
Phone: 410-783-8100
Fax: 410-783-8077
e-mail: tweber@baltimoresymphony.org
Web Site: www.baltimoresymphony.org
Management:
  Music Director: Yurird Temirkanov
  Manager:
Mission: The choir is the choral arm of the Baltimore Symphony and performs when the Symphony needs singers.
Specialized Field: Choral
Status: Nonprofit
Performs At: Joseph Meyerhoff Symphony Hall
Organization Type: Performing

2084 HANDEL CHOIR OF BALTIMORE
3600 Clipper Mill Road
Suite 240
Baltimore, MD 21218
Phone: 410-366-6544
e-mail: music@handelchoir.org
Web Site: www.charm.net/~hcob
Officers:
  President: Audrey Theis
  VP: Howard Kymptom
  Treasurer: John Keenan
Management:
  Music Director: Herbert Dimmock
Founded: 1934
Status: Nonprofit

Income Sources: Southwest Airlines; David Ashton & Associates

2085 OPERA VIVENTE
811 Cathedral Street
Baltimore, MD 21201
Phone: 410-547-7997
Fax: 847-557-2175
e-mail: info@operavivente.org
Web Site: www.operavivente.org
Management:
  General Director: John Bowen
  Music Director: Aaron Sherber

2086 MASTERWORKS CHORUS & ORCHESTRA
PO Box 34677
Bethesda, MD 20827-0677
Phone: 301-840-0008
Fax: 301-309-3691
e-mail: mwchorus@aol.com
Web Site: www.masterworkschorus.org/mc
Management:
  Artistic Director: Dr. Stanely Engebreston

2087 WASHINGTON SAVOYARDS
PO Box 34584
Bethesda, MD 20827
Phone: 202-965-7678
Web Site: www.savoyards.org
Officers:
  President: Nancy Weiss
  VP: Blair Eigss
  Treasurer: Robert Ritter
  Production: Scott Kennison
Founded: 1973
Performs At: Theater of the Duke Ellington School of the Arts

2088 CHILDREN'S OPERA THEATER
3203 Pickwick Lane
Chevy Chase, MD 20815
Phone: 301-656-2442
Fax: 301-656-2442
Management:
  Artistic Director: Michael Kaye
Mission: Introducing and involving youth in opera; providing employment for artists as they make the transition to a professional career.
Founded: 1976
Specialized Field: Light Opera; Choral
Status: Professional; Nonprofit
Organization Type: Touring; Educational

2089 COLUMBIA PRO CANTARE
5404 Iron Pen Place
Columbia, MD 21044
Phone: 410-465-5744
Fax: 419-730-8634
e-mail: cantare@concentric.net
Web Site: www.ns.connext.net/~columbiaprocantare
Founded: 1977

2090 INSTITUTE OF MUSICAL TRADITIONS
PO Box 629
Glen Echo, MD 20812
Phone: 301-587-4434
Fax: 301-263-0030
e-mail: imtfolk@imtfolk.org
Web Site: imtfolk.org
Management:
  Executive Director: Betsy Platt

2091 CHILDREN'S CHORUS OF MARYLAND
100 E Pennsylvania Avenue
Suite 202
Towson, MD 21286
Phone: 410-494-1480
Fax: 410-494-4673
e-mail: ccm@ccmsings.com
Web Site: www.ccmsings.org
Officers:
  President: Mary Weller
  VP: Micheal Marsh
  Secretary: Micheal Mauro
  Treasurer: Joanne Rubin
  Executive Director: Ramona Galey
Management:
  Atistic Director: Betty Bertaux
Mission: The Chorus of Maryland is dedicated to excellence in choral music education and performance for musical children through a program that offers graded music instruction based on child development curriculum, professional public performances and community outreach.

Massachusetts

2092 VALLEY LIGHT OPERA
PO Box 2143
Amherst, MA 01004-2143
Phone: 413-549-1098
e-mail: wcvenmen@attbi.com
Web Site: www.vlo.org
Management:
  General Manager: Bill Venman
Mission: Promotes broad participation and produces fine entertainment.
Founded: 1975
Specialized Field: Light Opera
Status: Non-Professional; Nonprofit
Performs At: Amherst Regional High School Auditorium
Organization Type: Performing

2093 BOSTON CAMERATA
140 Clarendon Street
Boston, MA 02116
Phone: 617-262-2092
e-mail: info@bostoncamerata.com
Web Site: www.hometown.aol.com/Boscam/index.html
Officers:
  Administrative Director: Richard Maloney
Management:
  Music Director: Joel Cohen
Founded: 1954

2094 BOSTON LYRIC OPERA COMPANY

45 Franklin Street
4th Floor
Boston, MA 02110-1300
Phone: 617-542-4912
Fax: 617-542-4913
Web Site: www.blo.org
Officers:
  Chairman: Sherif A Nada
  President: Horace H Irvine II
  Treasurer: Catherine Greir
  Clerk: Donald M. Robbins, Esquire
Management:
  General Director: Janice Del Sesto
  Artistic Director: Leon Major
  Music Director: Stephen Lord
  Communications Manager: Mara Littman
Mission: To present a varied repertoire of works accessible to a broad segment of the community, productions featuring both young American artists of promise and the most highly-regarded figures in the world of opera.
Founded: 1976
Specialized Field: Lyric Opera
Status: Professional
Paid Staff: 30
Volunteer Staff: 38
Budget: 8.5 Million
Income Sources: Opera America; Memberships; National Endowment for the Arts; Massachusetts Cultural Council
Performs At: Shubert Theatre
Annual Attendance: 60,000 - 70,000
Seating Capacity: 1550
Organization Type: Performing

2095 CANTATA SINGERS

PO Box 979
Boston, MA 02117
Phone: 617-267-6502
Fax: 617-267-9463
e-mail: bach@cantatasingers.org
Web Site: www.cantatasingers.org
Management:
  Music Director: David Hoose
  Executive Director: Lisa Stiller
  Public Relations: Barbara Raney
Founded: 1964
Specialized Field: Choral Music
Status: Nonprofit
Paid Staff: 3
Volunteer Staff: 5
Paid Artists: 20
Non-paid Artists: 44
Budget: $400,000
Income Sources: Ticket sales; contributions; government endowments
Performs At: Rented Hall
Affiliations: Chorus America
Annual Attendance: 7,000
Facility Category: Rented Concert Hall at New England Conservatory
Rental Contact: Jon Wulp

2096 HANDEL AND HAYDN SOCIETY

300 Massachusetts Avenue
Boston, MA 02115
Phone: 617-262-1815
Fax: 617-266-4217
e-mail: info@handelandhaydn.org
Web Site: www.handelandhaydn.org
Management:
  Music Director: Grant Llewellyn
  Conductor Laureate: Christopher Hogwood
  Executive Director: Mary Deissler
Mission: Dedicated to promoting the performance, study, composition and appreciation of music.
Founded: 1815
Specialized Field: Chamber; Ensemble; Choral
Status: Professional; Nonprofit
Paid Staff: 16
Budget: $2,600,000
Performs At: Symphony Hall; Jordan Hall
Annual Attendance: 40,000
Organization Type: Performing; Touring; Educational; Sponsoring

2097 OPERA NEW ENGLAND

45 Franklin Street
4th Floor
Boston, MA 02110-1300
Phone: 617-542-4912
Fax: 617-542-4913
Web Site: www.one.org
  Vice President: Barbara Barclay
  VP: Hagnette Cumitz
  VP: Norma Peterson
  VP: Sonya Sohopick
  Secretary: Anne Chemiavsky
  Treasurer: Robert W. Burmester
Management:
  Artistic Director: Linda C Black
Mission: To present seasons of opera for children and for general audiences. As the regional development program of The Opera Company of Boston, we present productions prepared by The Opera Company of Boston. Since 1983, our chapter has presented only productions for children.
Founded: 1973
Specialized Field: Lyric Opera; Light Opera
Status: Professional; Nonprofit
Income Sources: Opera Company of Boston
Organization Type: Educational; Sponsoring

2098 BRAINTREE CHORAL SOCIETY

346 Washington Street
PMB #154
Braintree, MA 02184
Phone: 508-583-5662
e-mail: braintreechoral@bigfoot.com
Web Site: www.neighborhoodlink.com/org/bcs
Management:
  Music Director: Deborah Smith
Mission: Promoting interest in choral music.
Founded: 1923
Specialized Field: Choral
Status: Non-Professional; Nonprofit
Paid Staff: 4
Organization Type: Performing

2099 KLEZMER CONSERVATORY BAND
83 Inman Street
Cambridge, MA 02139
Phone: 617-354-2884
Fax: 617-776-0955
Web Site: www.klezmerconservatory.com
Management:
    Business Manager Aaron Concert Man: James
    Guttmann
Mission: To offer Yiddish instrumental and vocal music
with many influences (Jazz, Dixieland, Ragtime, Latin
and Broadway).
Founded: 1980
Specialized Field: Ethnic; Folk; Band
Status: Professional
Organization Type: Performing; Touring

2100 RADCLIFFE CHORAL SOCIETY
Holden Chapel, Harvard University
Cambridge, MA 02138
Phone: 617-495-5730
Fax: 617-496-5166
e-mail: rcs@hcs.harvard.edu
Web Site: www.hcs.harvard.edu/~rcs/main.html
Officers:
    President: Jennifer Hoang
Management:
    Conductor: Jameson Marvin
    Manager: Michelle Schutz

**2101 COLLEGE LIGHT OPERA COMPANY
ON CAPE COD**
PO Box 906
Falmouth, MA 02541
Phone: 508-548-0668
Fax: 440-774-8485
e-mail: bob.haslun@oberlin.edu
Web Site: www.collegelightopera.com
Officers:
    President: DeWitt C Jones, III
    Treasurer: Robert A Haslun
    Secretary: Ursula R Haslun
Management:
    Producer/General Manager: Robert A Haslun
    Producer/Business Manager: Ursula R Haslun
Mission: Musical theatre training ground for
undergraduates.
Founded: 1969
Specialized Field: Light Opera; Operetta; Musical
Theatre
Status: Non-Professional; Nonprofit
Paid Staff: 15
Non-paid Artists: 32
Budget: $300,000
Income Sources: Box Office; Annual Fund
Performs At: Highfield Theatre
Annual Attendance: 16,200
Type of Stage: Proscenium
Seating Capacity: 300
Year Built: 1947
Year Remodeled: 1999
Cost: $450,000
Organization Type: Performing; Resident; Educational

2102 COMMONWEALTH OPERA
140 Pine Street
Florence, MA 01062
Phone: 413-586-5026
Fax: 413-587-0380
Toll-free: 866-733-6737
e-mail: commopr1@aol.com
Web Site: www.commonwealthopera.org
Officers:
    President: Gerry Katz
    VP: Richard Strongren
    Treasurer: Anita Regish
    Guild President: Katherine Willey
Management:
    Artistic Director: Richard R Rescia
    Executive Director: Dora Lewis
Mission: Enhancing professional opportunities in and
appreciation of grand opera and broadway musicals in the
region.
Founded: 1977
Specialized Field: Grand Opera; Lyric Opera
Status: Semi-Professional
Paid Staff: 3
Volunteer Staff: 40
Budget: 250,000
Income Sources: Tickets; Sponsors; Donations
Performs At: Calvin Theatre; Smith College
Organization Type: Performing; Touring

2103 BERKSHIRE OPERA COMPANY
40 Railroad Street
Great Barrington, MA 01230
Phone: 413-644-9000
Fax: 413-644-9030
e-mail: info@berkshireopera.org
Web Site: www.berkshireopera.org
Management:
    General Director: Linda Jackson
    Artistic Director: Joel Revzen
    Director Finance/Administration: Melissa Thomson
Mission: To produce and present the very finest in
professional opera. To provide and enhance educational
programming and community activities to people of all
ages in Berkshire County.
Founded: 1985
Specialized Field: Lyric Opera; Chamber Opera
Status: Professional; Nonprofit
Budget: $1.3 million
Income Sources: Berkshire Hills Visitors Bureau
Performs At: Mahaiwe Theater
Annual Attendance: 3,000
Seating Capacity: 700
Year Built: 1905
Rental Contact: Al Shwartz
Organization Type: Performing; Touring; Resident;
Educational

2104 PRISM OPERA
5 Linebrook Road
Ipswich, MA 02148
Phone: 978-356-1787
Toll-free: 888-236-8181
e-mail: prism@prismopera.org
Web Site: www.prismopera.org

Management:
Artistic Director: Thomas Stumpf
Executive Director: Arthur Rishi
Mission: Prism Opera is committed to producing effective and moving productions of operatic masterpieces, with a special emphasis on neglected works and on twentieth century repertoire.
Founded: 1995

2105 MASTER SINGERS

PO Box 172
Lexington, MA 02173
Phone: 781-862-6459
e-mail: msingers@themastersingers.org
Web Site: www.themastersingers.org
Officers:
President: Sarah Getty
Treasurer: Shaylor Lindsay
Secretary: Virginia Fitzgerald
Management:
Music Director: Adam Grossman
Accompanist: Eric Mazonson
Mission: To present the chamber chorus repertoire of all eras in an intimate setting aimed at maximum enjoyment for both singers and listeners.
Founded: 1967
Specialized Field: Choral
Status: Nonprofit
Paid Staff: 30
Income Sources: Massachusetts Cultural Alliance
Performs At: First Parish Church in Lexington
Organization Type: Performing; Touring

2106 LONGWOOD OPERA

42 Hawthorne Avenue
Needham, MA 02192
Phone: 781-455-0960
Fax: 781-455-0960
e-mail: Encore@LongwoodOpera.org
Web Site: www.home.earthlink.net/~brumit
Management:
General Director: J Scott Brumit

2107 ZAMIR CHORALE OF BOSTON

P0 Box 590126
Newton Centre, MA 02459
Phone: 617-731-0025
Toll-free: 866-926-4720
e-mail: manager@zamir.org
Web Site: www.zamir.org
Officers:
Chairman: Joyce Bohnen
Co-Treasurer: Marvin Mandelbaum
Clerk: Andrew M Greene
Management:
General Manager: Jan A Woiler
Music Director: Joshua Jacobson
Accompanist: Edwin Swanborn
Mission: To promote, develop and encourage the growth of Jewish choral music through scholarship, performances, recordings and educational programs.
Founded: 1969
Specialized Field: Choral; Ethnic
Status: Non-Professional; Nonprofit

Paid Staff: 5
Organization Type: Performing; Touring; Resident; Educational

2108 MASTERWORKS CHORALE

PO Box 620692
Newton Lower Falls, MA 02162
Phone: 781-235-6210
Fax: 617-738-0052
Management:
General Manager: Maria D Hagigeorges
Mission: The performance of major choral works.
Founded: 1940
Specialized Field: Choral
Status: Semi-Professional; Nonprofit
Paid Staff: 120
Performs At: Sanders Theatre; Harvard University
Organization Type: Performing; Touring

2109 SMITH COLLEGE GLEE CLUB & CHOIRS

Smith College, Music Department
Northhampton, MA 01063
Phone: 413-585-3150
Fax: 413-585-3180
Management:
Choir/Chorale: Pamela Getmick

2110 GLORIAE DEI ARTES FOUNDATION

PO Box 2831
Orleans, MA 02653
Phone: 508-255-3999
Fax: 508-240-1989
e-mail: gdc@gdaf.org
Web Site: www.gdaf.org
Officers:
President: Sarah R Kanaga
Management:
Director: Elizabeth C Patterson
Business Manager: Barbara B Manuel
Concert Manager: Karen E Moore
Mission: The persuit of excellence in the performing and visual arts and to the inspiration and education of others. The foundation encompasses twelve arts groups and soloist, including the world renowned choir Gloriae Dei Cantores, Spirit of America band, Stages Theatre Company, Tapestry Dance Company, Archangelus Brass Ensemble, Gloria Dei Ringers, Vox Caeli Sinfonia, Gloriae Dei Chamber Ensemble, Master Schola educational series.
Status: Nonprofit

2111 BERKSHIRE LYRIC THEATRE

PO Box 347
Pittsfield, MA 01202
Phone: 413-499-0258
e-mail: info@berkshirelyric.org
Web Site: www.berkshirelyric.org
Officers:
President: Donald Phipps
VP: Sharyl Noroian
VP: Tom Sherer
Secretary: Sue Burke

Treasurer: Kathleen Kelley
Management:
   Director: Robert P Blafield
Mission: To present choral concerts and light opera.
Founded: 1963
Specialized Field: Light Opera; Choral
Status: Nonprofit
Paid Staff: 40
Organization Type: Performing

2112 PAUL MADORE CHORALE

PO Box 992
Salem, MA 01970-6092
Phone: 781-639-8062
Fax: 781-639-8065
e-mail: djmurph@mediaone.net
Officers:
   President: Kathleen Snarry
   Vice President: Chris Lemoine
   Treasurer: Marcia Hunkins
   Recording Secertary: Eileen Mackey
   Corresponding Secretary: Elaine Shindle
   Librarian: Judy Pierce
Management:
   Director: Paul Madore
   Orchestra Manager: Alan Hawery
   Chorus Manager: Donna Murphy
Mission: Offering choral masterpieces for the enjoyment
and cultural advancement of the North Shore/Boston
areas.
Founded: 1966
Specialized Field: Oratoric
Status: Semi-Professional; Nonprofit
Volunteer Staff: 1
Paid Artists: 1
Budget: $50,000
Income Sources: Box Office; Private Donations
Performs At: Churches; Municipal Buildings
Affiliations: Salem Chamber of Commerce; Greater
Boston Choral Consortium
Organization Type: Performing

2113 FINE ARTS CHORALE

779 Main Street
South Weymouth, MA 02190
Phone: 617-337-3023
Toll-free: 800-230-7555
Officers:
   President: Deborah Kohl
   VP: Kate Lacatell
   Secretary: Eleanor MacDonald
   Treasurer: Louise Bacon
Management:
   Music Director/Founder: Peter L Edwards
Mission: The presentation of sacred choral masterworks
accompanied by a professional orchestra and soloists.
There are no dues required.
Founded: 1966
Specialized Field: Choral
Status: Non-Professional; Nonprofit
Paid Staff: 130
Organization Type: Performing

2114 REVELS

80 Mount Auburn Street
Watertown, MA 02472
Phone: 617-972-8300
e-mail: infor@revels.org
Web Site: www.revels.org
Officers:
   President: Michael E Kolowich
   VP: Brian O'Donovan
   Treasurer: J Patrick Kinney III
Management:
   Executive Director: Gayle Rich
   Artistic Director: Patrick Swanson
   Music Director: George Emlen
   Makerting And Public Relations: Alan Casso
   Development Director: Marissa Timmins
   Art Director: Sue Ladr
   Business Manager: Kimberly Luiggi
   Office Manager: Jennifer Sur
   Production Manager: Virginia D Morton
Mission: Offering performances and recordings that
promote the appreciation of traditional songs, music,
customs and rituals.
Founded: 1971
Specialized Field: Musical Theatre
Status: Nonprofit
Paid Staff: 60
Performs At: Sanders Theatre; Harvard University
Organization Type: Performing; Educational

2115 OPERA APERTA

PO Box 701
Weston, MA 02493
Phone: 781-899-3112
Fax: 781-893-4288
e-mail: robertalamb@opera-aperta.org
Web Site: www.opera-aperta.org
Management:
   Director: Roberta Pearle Lamb
Mission: To provide musically satisfying, dramatically
engaging artistic productions to Boston's growing
audience for the opera; to bring opera to the community,
expanding the audience beyond the already initiated.

2116 SALISBURY LYRIC OPERA

11 Chamberlain Parkway
Worcester, MA 01602
Phone: 508-799-3848
Fax: 508-792-3067
Management:
   Co-Director: Richard Monroe

Michigan

2117 OPERA! LEWANEE

110 S Madison Street
Cornelius House
Adrian, MI 49221
Phone: 517-264-3121
Fax: 517-264-3833
e-mail: aso@lni.net
Web Site: www.aso.org

Officers:
  Co-Chair: Robert Bell
  Co-Chair: Muriel Bell
Management:
  Artistic Director: David Katz
  Producer: Jimmy Hilburger
Mission: To create grand opera performances for the citizens of Lenawee County, Michigan; to sponsor the Friedrich Schorr Memorial Performance Prize in Voice; to collaborate between the Adrian Symphony and the Croswell Opera House.
Founded: 1989
Specialized Field: Grand Opera; Lyric Opera; Operetta
Status: Professional; Nonprofit
Income Sources: National Opera Association; Opera America
Performs At: Croswell Opera House
Organization Type: Performing; Resident; Educational

2118 BOYCHOIR OF ANN ARBOR
1100 N Main Street
Ann Arbor, MI 48104
Phone: 734-663-5377
Fax: 734-663-0001
e-mail: office@aaboychoir.org
Web Site: www.aaboychoir.org
Management:
  Director: Dr. Thomas Strode
Mission: To offer vocal and choral training, and performance opportunities, to musically gifted boys with unchanged voices.
Founded: 1986
Status: Nonprofit
Paid Staff: 3
Volunteer Staff: 60
Budget: $65,000
Income Sources: Tuition; Donations; Grants
Affiliations: Royal School of Church Music

2119 COMIC OPERA GUILD
PO Box 1922
Ann Arbor, MI 48106
Phone: 734-973-3264
Fax: 734-973-6281
e-mail: mgillett@umich.edu
Web Site:
www.personal.umich.edu/~mgillet/coghome.htm
Officers:
  President: Andy Stimpson
  Secretary: Shanna Kaminski
  Treasurer: George Valenta
Management:
  Managing Director: Thomas Petiet
Mission: The Comic Opera Guild was formed for the purpose of creating and developing interest in comic opera as a separate theatrical form. The touring approach is fundamental to this purpose because of the potential in reaching large numbers of people unacquainted with comic opera.
Founded: 1973
Specialized Field: Operetta
Status: Professional; Semi-Professional; Nonprofit
Paid Staff: 6
Volunteer Staff: 40
Paid Artists: 25

Non-paid Artists: 50
Performs At: Michigan Theater; Mendelssohn Theater
Organization Type: Performing; Touring; Resident

2120 UNIVERSITY MUSICAL SOCIETY CHORAL UNION
881 N University Avenue
Ann Arbor, MI 48109-1011
Phone: 734-763-8997
Fax: 734-647-1171
Toll-free: 800-221-1229
e-mail: choralunion@umich.edu
Web Site: www.ums.org
Officers:
  Chairperson: Beverly Geltner
  Vice Chair: Lester Monts
  Secretary: Prue Rosenthal
  Treasurer: David Featherman
Management:
  Director Programming: Michael Kondziolka
  Director Administration: John Kennard
  Director Development: Susan McClanahan
  Director Marketing: Sara Billmann
Mission: To provide professional theatre, dance and music for Southeastern Michigan students and residents.
Founded: 1879
Specialized Field: Music; Dance; Theater
Status: Non-Professional; Nonprofit
Paid Staff: 30
Budget: $8,000,000
Income Sources: Ticket Sales; Fundraising
Performs At: Hill Auditorium; University of Michigan
Affiliations: Association of Performing Arts Presenters; International Society of Performing Arts Administrators
Annual Attendance: 150,000
Organization Type: Performing; Touring; Resident; Educational

2121 UNIVERSITY OF MICHIGAN GILBERT AND SULLIVAN
The Michigan League Building
911 N University
Ann Arbor, MI 48109
Phone: 734-647-8436
e-mail: umgassexec@umich.edu
Web Site: www.umgass.org
Officers:
  President: Daniel Florip
  VP: Julia Head
  Secretary: Andriana Pachella
  Treasurer: Elizabeth Crabtree
Management:
  Company Promoter: Matthew D Grace
  Ticket Manager: Barbara Fleming
  Programme: James Allen
Founded: 1947
Specialized Field: Operetta
Status: Non-Professional; Nonprofit
Paid Artists: 30
Performs At: Mendelssohn Theatre; University of Michigan
Organization Type: Performing; Resident; Educational

2122 CHEBOYGAN AREA ARTS COUNCIL/OPERA HOUSE
403 N Huron Street
PO Box 95
Cheboygan, MI 49721
Phone: 231-627-5432
Fax: 231-627-2643
e-mail: jpl@nmo.net
Web Site: www.theoperahouse.org
Officers:
   President: Jeff Swadling
   VP: Ron Berg
   Treasurer: Alice Barron
   Secretary: Gussie Williams
Management:
   Executive Director: Joann P Leal
   Stage Technician: Jerry Bronson
Mission: To promote and encourage cultural and educational activities within the Straits Area of Northern Michigan, and to provide services that stimulate and encourage participation in and appreciation of the arts.
Founded: 1972
Specialized Field: Multi-disciplinary
Status: Nonprofit
Budget: $250,000
Income Sources: Membership; Ticket Sales; Fundraisers; Grants; Other Earned Income
Performs At: Opera House
Affiliations: Association of Performing Arts Presenters; MACAA; LHAT
Annual Attendance: 30,000
Facility Category: Historic Theatre
Type of Stage: Proscenium
Stage Dimensions: 34x20
Seating Capacity: 582
Year Built: 1877
Year Remodeled: 1984
Rental Contact: Joann P. Leal
Organization Type: Educational; Sponsoring

2123 TIBBITS OPERA FOUNDATION AND ARTS COUNCIL
14 S Hanchett Street
Coldwater, MI 49036
Phone: 517-278-6029
Fax: 517-279-7594
e-mail: boxoffice@tibbits.org
Web Site: www.tibbits.org
Officers:
   President: Molly VanStone
   Vice President of the Board: Connie Winbigler
Management:
   Executive Director: Christine Delaney
   Business Manager/Box Office Manager: Rose Goras
   Production Manager: Susan Merrill
   Artistic Director: harles Burr
Mission: To foster enrichment of life by preserving the historic Tibbits Opera House and supporting arts culture and education.
Founded: 1964
Specialized Field: Dance; Vocal Music; Instrumental Music; Theater; Children's Theatre; Festivals; Lyric Opera; Art Gallery

Status: Professional; Semi-Professional; Non-Professional; Nonprofit
Paid Staff: 5
Income Sources: Membership; Ticket Sales; Annual Auction; Grants - Michigan Council for Arts and Cultural Affairs; Michigan Humanities Council; Branch County Community Foundation; Corporate
Performs At: Tibbits Opera House
Facility Category: Theatre/Opera House
Type of Stage: Proscenium
Stage Dimensions: 25'x30'
Seating Capacity: 499
Year Built: 1882
Year Remodeled: 1965
Rental Contact: Carolyn Stewart
Organization Type: Performing; Touring; Resident; Educational; Sponsoring
Resident Groups: Tibbits Summer Theatre - Professional Repertory Company

2124 MICHIGAN OPERA THEATRE
1526 Broadway
Detroit, MI 48226
Phone: 313-961-3500
Fax: 313-237-3412
e-mail: webadministrator@motopera.org
Web Site: www.michiganopera.org
Management:
   General Director: Dr David DiChiera
   Facilities Director: Karen Tjaden
   COO: Brett Batterson
   Production Director: David Osborne
   Administration Director: John Eckstrom
   Marketing Director: Steve Haviaras
   Assistant Marketing Director: Susan Fazzini
Mission: To be one of the outstanding opera companies in the United States, serving as a major cultural resource.
Founded: 1971
Specialized Field: Grand Opera; Operetta; Dance; Musical Theatre
Status: Professional; Nonprofit
Paid Staff: 54
Volunteer Staff: 800
Paid Artists: 74
Budget: 12,000,000
Income Sources: Earned and Unearned
Performs At: Stage; Rehearsal Room
Affiliations: International Association of Auditorium Managers
Annual Attendance: 194,608
Facility Category: Performing Arts
Type of Stage: Proscenium
Stage Dimensions: 65x110
Seating Capacity: 2,800
Year Built: 1922
Year Remodeled: 1996
Rental Contact: Facilities Director Karen Tjaden
Organization Type: Performing; Touring

2125 RACKHAM SYMPHONY CHOIR
555 Brush Street
Number 2311
Detroit, MI 48226

Phone: 313-272-0333
Fax: 313-272-5111
e-mail: info@mail.rackhamchoir.org
Web Site: www.rackhamchoir.org
Management:
  Music Director: Suzanne Mallare Acton
  Assistant Director And Accompanist: Donald Kukier
  Managing Director: Anne Bak
Mission: To provide choral symphonic performances featuring the works of the classical masters to the Detroit metropolitan area.
Founded: 1949
Specialized Field: Choral
Status: Nonprofit
Paid Staff: 60
Organization Type: Performing; Educational

2126 OPERA LITE

PO Box 405
Dearborn
Farmington Hills, MI 48121
Phone: 248-888-7640
Management:
  Managing Director: David Pulice
  Assistant Director: Amy Kutt
Founded: 1986
Specialized Field: Light Opera
Organization Type: Performing; Touring; Resident

2127 OPERA GRAND RAPIDS

161 Ottawa NW
Suite 204
Grand Rapids, MI 49503
Phone: 616-451-2741
Fax: 616-451-4587
Web Site: www.operagr.com/
Management:
  Executive Director: John Peter Jeffries
  Artistic Director: Robert Lyall
  Public Relations/Marketing Director: Veronica Komar
Mission: To enhance the quality of life in the Grand Rapids area and Western Michigan by providing professional-quality operatic/musical theater productions; to raise the level of appreciation and understanding of opera in all residents.
Founded: 1967
Specialized Field: Grand Opera; Musical Theatre
Status: Professional; Nonprofit
Paid Staff: 6
Budget: $1.2 million
Performs At: DeVos Hall; Van Andel Arena
Annual Attendance: 17,000
Seating Capacity: 2,340
Year Built: 1979
Organization Type: Performing; Educational; Sponsoring

2128 HOLLAND CHORALE

PO Box 1513
Holland, MI 49422-1513

Phone: 616-494-0256
Fax: 616-395-2481
e-mail: hollandchorale@novagate.com
Web Site: www.hollandchorale.org/
Management:
  Music Director: Gary Bogle
  Assistant Director: Richard Cory
Volunteer Staff: 85

2129 FONTANA CONCERT SOCIETY

821 W South Street
Kalamazoo, MI 49007
Phone: 616-382-0826
Fax: 616-382-0812
Management:
  Interim Co-Director: I Fu Wang
  Interim Co-Director: Robert Humiston
  General Manager: Janet Karpus
Mission: To offer quality, diverse chamber music programs in a relaxed, rural setting.
Founded: 1980
Specialized Field: Vocal Music; Instrumental Music; Festivals
Status: Professional; Nonprofit
Performs At: The Art Emporium
Organization Type: Performing; Sponsoring

2130 SAGINAW CHORAL SOCIETY

326 S Jefferson Avenue
Saginaw, MI 48607-1270
Phone: 517-753-1812
Fax: 989-753-1043
e-mail: scsmusic@tm.net
Web Site: www.saginawchoralsociety.com/
Officers:
  President: Joan McGlaughlin
Management:
  Project Development Director: Marce Wiltse
  Business Manager: Lee Wright
Mission: To provide an opportunity for quality singers to join together in singing and performing fine choral music so as to contribute to the enjoyment, musical growth and education of the residents of Saginaw Valley. Regularly performs master works from the classical choral music literature, as a priority in maintaining the firm artistic integrity of the organization.
Founded: 1935
Specialized Field: Community Chorus

Minnesota

2131 AUGSBURG CHOIR

Augsburg College
2211 Riverside Avenue
Minneapolis, MN 55454
Phone: 612-330-1276
Fax: 612-330-1264
e-mail: hendricp@augsburg.edu
Web Site: www.augsburg.edu
Management:
  Choral Activities Director: Peter A Hendrickson

2132 MINNESOTA CHORALE

528 Hennepin Avenue
Suite 211
Minneapolis, MN 55408
Phone: 612-333-4866
Fax: 612-344-1504
Officers:
  President: Joyce Gordon
  Vice President: Chris Trost
  Secretary: Malcolm MacLean
  Treasurer: Ed Robinson
Management:
  Executive Director: Rebecca Scheele
  Operations/Management Assistant: Carolann Haley
Mission: The Minnesota Chorale is a nationally acclaimed symphonic chorus with a signature flexibility to perform masterfully in ensembles ranging from 20 to 200 voices. Celebrates the human voice in its ability to educate, enrich, and inspire.
Founded: 1972
Specialized Field: Choral
Status: Semi-Professional; Nonprofit
Paid Staff: 130
Income Sources: Chorus America
Performs At: Orchestra Hall; Ordway Music Theatre
Organization Type: Performing

2133 MINNESOTA OPERA

620 N First Street
Minneapolis, MN 55401
Phone: 612-333-2700
Fax: 612-333-0869
e-mail: staff@mnopera.org
Web Site: www.mnopera.org
Officers:
  President/CEO: Kevin Smith
  Artistic Director: Dale Johnson
Management:
  President: Kevin Smith
  Artistic Director: Dale Johnson
Mission: To produce opera and opera education programs at the highest artisic level that inspire and entertain our audiences and enrich the cultural life of our community.
Founded: 1963
Specialized Field: opera
Status: Professional; Nonprofit
Income Sources: Opera America
Performs At: Ordway Music Theatre
Annual Attendance: 55,000
Facility Category: Rent Ordway Center for the Performing Arts
Seating Capacity: 1764
Year Built: 1985
Organization Type: Performing; Touring; Resident; Educational; Recording

2134 NATIONAL LUTHERAN CHOIR

3355 Hiawatha Avenue S
PO Box 6450
Minneapolis, MN 55406
Phone: 612-722-2301
Fax: 612-722-0962
e-mail: info@nlca.com
Web Site: www.nlca.com

Management:
  Executive Director/General Manager: Chris Anderson
  Music Director: David Cherwien
Mission: The presentation of sacred choral music in a live settiong and on recorded mediums.
Founded: 1986
Specialized Field: Choral
Status: Professional
Paid Staff: 3
Volunteer Staff: 35
Non-paid Artists: 63
Budget: $250,000
Income Sources: Ticket Sales; General Donations; Corporate Donations
Affiliations: American Council for the Arts; American Lutheran Church Musicians; Chorus America
Annual Attendance: 25,000
Organization Type: Performing

2135 TWIN CITIES GAY MEN'S CHORUS

528 Hennepin Avenue
Suite 307
Minneapolis, MN 55403
Phone: 612-339-7664
Fax: 612-332-8141
e-mail: chorus@tcgmc.org
Web Site: www.tcgmc.org
Officers:
  Executive Director: Joann Usher
  Board Chair: Dwight Jogner
Management:
  Artistic Director: Stan Hill
Founded: 1981
Specialized Field: Choral
Status: Nonprofit; Professional
Paid Staff: 3
Non-paid Artists: 150
Budget: $684,000
Income Sources: Ticket sales; merchandise; contributions
Performs At: Ted Menn Concert Hall
Annual Attendance: 9,000
Facility Category: Concert hall
Seating Capacity: 1,100
Organization Type: Performing, Touring, Recording

2136 VOCALESSENCE

1900 Nicollet Avenue
Minneapolis, MN 55403
Phone: 612-547-1451
Fax: 612-547-1484
e-mail: info@vocalessence.org
Web Site: www.vocalessence.org
Management:
  Artistic Director: Philip Brunelle
Mission: Founded as The Plymouth Music Series, explores the interaction of voices and instruments through innovative programming of music, both newly-commissioned and rarely heard.
Founded: 1969
Specialized Field: Choral; Vocal Music
Paid Staff: 10
Volunteer Staff: 0
Paid Artists: 100
Non-paid Artists: 80

2137 MINNETONKA CHAMBER CHOIR
Music Association of Minnetonka
18285 Highway 7
Minnetonka, MN 55345
Phone: 952-401-5954
Fax: 952-401-5959
Web Site: www.musicassociation.org
Management:
  Director: Roger Satrang Hoel

2138 MINNETONKA SYMPHONY CHORUS
Music Association of Minnetonka
18285 Highway 7
Minnetonka, MN 55305
Phone: 952-401-5954
Fax: 952-401-5959
Web Site: www.musicassociation.org
Management:
  Director: Roger Satrang Hoel

2139 CONCORD SINGERS OF NEW ULM
PO Box 492
New Ulm, MN 56073
Phone: 507-354-8850
Fax: 507-354-8853
e-mail: concords@newulmtel.net
Web Site: concordsingers.com
Officers:
  President: Henk Exoo
  VP: Lenny Donahue
  Secretary: Dick Wilbrecht
  Treasurer: Joe Meyer
Management:
  Manager: Tom Paluch
  Director: Bob Beusmann
Mission: Good singing; fellowship and good will extended to the enjoyment and culture of the people and development of the musical art and promotion of community relations for the city of New Ulm; to keep alive the German language through song.
Founded: 1931
Specialized Field: Choral; Ethnic
Status: Non-Professional; Nonprofit
Organization Type: Performing; Sponsoring

2140 SAINT OLAF CHOIR
Saint Olaf College
1520 Saint Olaf Avenue
Northfield, MN 55057-1098
Phone: 507-646-3179
Fax: 507-646-3527
Management:
  Music Director/Conductor: Anton Armstrong
  Manager: BJ Johnson
Founded: 1912

2141 ROCHESTER ORCHESTRA & CHORALE
PO Box 302
Rochester, MN 55903-0302
Phone: 507-286-8742
Fax: 507-280-4136
Toll-free: 877-286-8742
e-mail: office@roandc.org
Web Site: www.roandc.org
Officers:
  President: Kathryn Karseu
  Past President: Carolyun Rorie
  Secretary: Dianna Horntvedt
Management:
  Executive Director: Elizabeth W Wall
  Music Director: Jere Lantz
  Business Administrator: Amy Lindstrom
Mission: Rochester Orchestra and Chorale seeks to serve our community and region by preserving, nurturing and advancing the art of music through education and high quality performances that seek to touch the soul.
Founded: 1919
Specialized Field: Symphony; Orchestra; Chamber; Ensemble; Chorale
Paid Staff: 3
Volunteer Staff: 80
Paid Artists: 75
Non-paid Artists: 80
Budget: $328,000
Income Sources: Ticket Sales; Contributions; Grants
Performs At: Mayo Civic Center; Rochester Assembly of God Church
Affiliations: ASOL
Annual Attendance: 7,000-8,000
Facility Category: Mayo Civic Center

2142 MINNESOTA CENTER CHORALE
PO Box 7833
Saint Cloud, MN 56302
Phone: 320-363-4467
Fax: 320-363-6097
e-mail: pwelter@csbsju.edu
Management:
  Music Director: Philip Welter
Paid Staff: 1
Budget: $60,000
Annual Attendance: 3,000
Facility Category: Auditorium
Year Built: 1965

2143 QUITE LIGHT OPERA COMPANY
PO Box 7374
Saint Cloud, MN 56302
Phone: 320-259-4515
Fax: 320-363-6097
Management:
  Managing/Music Director: Philip Welter
Budget: $20,000
Performs At: Technical High School Auditorium

2144 NORTH STAR OPERA
1863 Eleanor Avenue
Saint Paul, MN 55116
Phone: 651-224-1640
e-mail: steve@northstaropera.org
Web Site: www.northstaropera.com
Management:
  Artistic Director: Steve Stucki

All listings are in alphabetical order by state, then city, then organization within the city.

Artistic Director: Steven Stucki
Mission: Developing and showcasing highly-talented, well-qualified professional musicians, singers and related personnel of the local area and upper Midwest; sponsoring college internship programs.
Founded: 1980
Specialized Field: Lyric Opera; Light Opera; Operetta
Status: Professional; Nonprofit
Performs At: O'Shaughnessy Auditorium; Drew Fine Aris Theatre
Organization Type: Performing; Touring; Resident; Educational

2145 DALE WARLAND SINGERS

2300 Myrtle Avenue
Suite 120
St Paul, MN 55114
Phone: 651-632-5870
Fax: 651-632-5873
Web Site: www.dalewarlandsingers.org
Officers:
President: Robin M Keyworth
Vice President: Dan V Schmechel
Treasurer: James W Peter
Secretary: David Cooper
Management:
Music Director: Dale Warland
General Manager: Debra Harrer
Founded: 1972
Specialized Field: Choral Music
Paid Staff: 10
Volunteer Staff: 5
Paid Artists: 40

Mississippi

2146 GULF COAST OPERA THEATRE

PP Box 118
Biloxi, MS 39533-0118
Phone: 228-374-4200
Fax: 228-374-0152
Web Site: www.datasync.com/~micksch/gco.htm
Management:
General Director: David Daniels
Mission: Educating Mississippi Gulf Coast residents regarding musical theatre and opera.
Founded: 1973
Specialized Field: Grand Opera; Operetta; Musical Theatre
Status: Semi-Professional; Nonprofit
Paid Staff: 40
Performs At: Saenger Theatre for the Performing Arts
Organization Type: Performing; Resident

2147 CENTER FOR OPERA & MUSIC THEATRE

PO Box 5081
Hattiesburg, MS 39533-5081
Phone: 601-261-1305
Fax: 601-261-1308
e-mail: jcdean@netdoor.com
Management:

Director: Jay Dean
Performs At: Mannoni Performing Arts Auditorium

2148 SOUTHERN ARTS FESTIVAL OPERA

PO Box 5081
Hattiesburg, MS 39406-5081
Phone: 601-261-1310
Fax: 601-261-1308
e-mail: jcdean@netdoor.com
Management:
Director: Jay Dean
Performs At: Mannoni Performing Arts Auditorium

2149 MISSISSIPPI OPERA ASSOCIATION

PO Box 1551
Jackson, MS 39215
Phone: 601-960-1528
Fax: 601-960-1526
e-mail: info@msoperaa.org
Web Site: www.msopera.org
Management:
Artistic Director: Garold Whisler
Executive Director: Patton Rice
Mission: To promote and encourage the appreciation and study of opera; developing opera talent.
Founded: 1944
Specialized Field: Grand Opera; Lyric Opera; Light Opera; Operetta; Musical Theatre
Status: Professional; Nonprofit
Volunteer Staff: 3
Income Sources: Opera America
Performs At: Jackson Municipal Auditorium
Organization Type: Performing; Touring; Educational

Missouri

2150 SAINT LOUIS CHAMBER CHORUS

PO Box 11558
Clayton, MO 63105
Phone: 636-458-4343
Fax: 314-993-6458
e-mail: maltworm@inlink.com
Web Site: www.iwc.com/slcc
Management:
Assistant Conductor: Brian Reeves
Executive Director: Linda Ryder
Music/Artistic Director: Philip Barnes
Rehearsal Accompanist: Martha Shaffer
Mission: To educate and inspire by presenting in concert choral works of unusual rarely performed music by outstanding composers, usually a cappella.
Founded: 1957
Specialized Field: Choral
Status: Professional; Nonprofit
Paid Staff: 4
Volunteer Staff: 18
Paid Artists: 36
Income Sources: Arts & Education Council of Greater St. Louis; Regional Arts Commission of St. Louis; Missouri Arts Council; Gateway Foundation; Mercantile Bank
Affiliations: American Choral Directors Association; Chorus America

Organization Type: Performing; Educational

2151 HEARTLAND MEN'S CHORUS

PO Box 32374
Kansas City, MO 64171-5374
Phone: 816-931-3338
Fax: 816-531-1367
e-mail: hmc@hmckc.org
Web Site: hmckc.org
Management:
    Executive Director: Rick Fisher
    Music Director: Joseph P Nadeau
Mission: A not-for-profit, volunteer chorus of gay and
gay-sensitive people joining together to make a positive
cultural contribution to the entire community; advancing
men's choral music through excellence in performance.
Founded: 1986
Specialized Field: Choral Music
Status: Non-Professional; Nonprofit
Paid Staff: 3
Paid Artists: 20
Non-paid Artists: 120
Budget: 269,000
Income Sources: Program revenues; Donations
Performs At: The Folly Theater
Affiliations: Gay and Lesbian Association Choruses;
Chorus America
Annual Attendance: 5,000
Seating Capacity: 1,078
Year Built: 1900
Year Remodeled: 2000
Organization Type: Performing

2152 LYRIC OPERA OF KANSAS CITY

Lyric Theatre
1029 Central
Kansas City, MO 64105-1677
Phone: 816-471-4933
Fax: 816-471-0602
Web Site: www.kc-opera.org
Management:
    Artistic Director: Ward Holmquist
    General Director: Evan R Luskin
Mission: To present opera theatre with American artists
singing in English.
Founded: 1958
Specialized Field: Grand Opera; Lyric Opera; Operetta
Status: Professional; Nonprofit
Paid Staff: 21
Paid Artists: 120
Budget: $3.8 million
Income Sources: Ticket Sales; Contributions
Performs At: Lyric Theatre
Affiliations: Opera America
Annual Attendance: 20,000
Type of Stage: Proscenium
Stage Dimensions: 50'x36'
Seating Capacity: 1640
Year Built: 1926
Year Remodeled: 1974
Organization Type: Performing; Touring; Resident

2153 KANSAS CITY SYMPHONY CHORUS

William Jewell College
Music Department
Liberty, MO 64068
Mailing Address: 800 West 47 Street, Kansas City, MO.
64112
Phone: 816-781-7700
Fax: 816-415-5027
e-mail: epleya@william.jewell.edu
Web Site: www.jewell.edu
Management:
    Director: Arnold Epley

2154 BACH SOCIETY OF SAINT LOUIS

634 N Grand Boulevard
Saint Louis, MO 63103-1002
Phone: 314-652-2224
Fax: 314-652-0450
e-mail: bachsociety@worldnet.att.net
Web Site: www.bachsociety.org
Officers:
    Chairman: Dan Lesicko
    Vice Chairman: Sally M Williams
    Treasurer: Susan Thomson
    Secretary: Ellen Walters
Management:
    Music Director/Conductor: Dr. A Dennis Sparger
    Executive Director: Alayne D Smith
Mission: To educate, enrich and entertain the people of
the St. Louis region by performing the choral works of
Johann Sebastian Bach and other composers.
Founded: 1941
Paid Staff: 1
Paid Artists: 25
Non-paid Artists: 35
Budget: $250,000
Income Sources: Individual & Corporate Contributions;
Local; Regional & State Grants
Annual Attendance: 5,000

2155 OPERA THEATRE OF SAINT LOUIS

539 Garden Avenue
PO Box 191910
Saint Louis, MO 63119
Phone: 314-961-0171
Fax: 314-961-7463
e-mail: info@opera-stl.org
Web Site: www.opera-stl.org
Officers:
    Chairman: Janet McAfee Weakley
    Vice Chair: Arnold W hen Donaldver
    Vice Chair: Jo Ann Harmon
    Vice Chair: Donna M. Wilinson
    Treasurer: Terry Crow
Management:
    General Director: Charles R MacKay
    Artistic Director: Colin Graham
    Music Director: Stephen Lord
    Director Finance: Brenda Malottke
Mission: To offer opera in English; to provide career
advancement for young American singers; to offer the
direction of renowned conductors and directors.
Founded: 1976

Specialized Field: Grand Opera; Lyric Opera; Light
Opera; Operetta
Status: Nonprofit; Professional
Paid Staff: 20+
Paid Artists: 72
Budget: $6,500,000
Income Sources: 75% From Contributions
Performs At: Loretto-Hilton Center for the Performing
Arts
Affiliations: Missouri Arts Council; regional Arts
Commission; National Endowment for the Arts; Arts &
Education Council of Greater Saint Louis
Annual Attendance: 29,000
Facility Category: Theater
Type of Stage: Thrust
Seating Capacity: 987
Rental Contact: Stephen Ryan
Organization Type: Performing; Touring; Educational

2156 SAINT LOUIS SYMPHONY CHORUS
718 N Grand Boulevard
Saint Louis, MO 63103
Phone: 314-286-4110
Fax: 314-286-4142
e-mail: richarda@slso.org
Management:
  Manager: Richard Ashburner
  Chorus Director: Amy Kaiser
  Accompanist: Gail Hintz
Mission: Performing orchestral works with a chorus.
Founded: 1977
Specialized Field: Choral
Status: Professional; Non-Professional; Nonprofit
Paid Staff: 2
Paid Artists: 26
Non-paid Artists: 114
Income Sources: Chorus America
Performs At: Powell Symphony Hall
Organization Type: Performing; Touring; Educational

**2157 SAINT LOUIS SYMPHONY CHILDREN'S
CHOIRS**
2842 N Ballas
Saint Louis, MO 63131
Phone: 314-993-9626
Fax: 314-993-0264
Management:
  Artistic Director: Barbara Berner
  Program Administrator: Patricia J Niehaus

2158 SPRINGFIELD REGIONAL OPERA
1433 E Republic Road
Springfield, MO 65806
Phone: 417-881-0713
Fax: 417-881-1019
e-mail: opera@sropera.com
Web Site: www.sropera.com
Officers:
  President: Maggie Wilcox-Burton
Management:
  Executive Director: Marie Murphree
  Education Director: Susan Brummel
  Music Director: Robert Quebbeman

Mission: Providing Springfield and Southwest Missouri
with operatic experiences of the highest possible calibre
through performance and education.
Founded: 1979
Specialized Field: Grand Opera; Lyric Opera; Light
Opera; Operetta
Status: Professional; Nonprofit
Paid Staff: 4
Paid Artists: 45
Non-paid Artists: 30
Budget: $189,000
Income Sources: Box office, grants, private donations
Performs At: Landers Theatre; Hammons Hall
Affiliations: Opera America
Annual Attendance: 7,000
Seating Capacity: 2200
Organization Type: Performing

Montana

**2159 BILLINGS SYMPHONY ORCHESTRA &
CHORALE**
201 N Broadway
Suite 350
Billings, MT 59101
Phone: 406-252-3610
Fax: 406-252-3353
e-mail: symphony@billingssysymphony.org
Web Site: www.billingssymphony.org
Officers:
  President: Robert Griffin
  VP: Jon Phillips
  Secretary: John Green
  Treasurer: Nicki Larson
Management:
  Music Director/Conductor: Uri Barnea
  Executive Director: Rina Reynolds
Mission: To encourage artistic excellence and offer
symphonic performances and educational programs to the
region.
Founded: 1950
Specialized Field: Orchestra; Chorale
Status: Nonprofit
Paid Staff: 4
Paid Artists: 85
Budget: $260,000-1,050,000
Income Sources: Individual; Businesses; Foundations;
Government; Ticket Revenue
Performs At: Alberta Bair Theater for the Performing
Arts
Annual Attendance: 30,000

2160 MONTANA CHORALE
214 24th Street SW
Great Falls, MT 59406
Phone: 406-453-0248
Fax: 406-453-7248
e-mail: info@montana-chorale.org
Web Site: www.montana-chorale.org
Officers:
  President: Ann Cogswell
  VP: Lorrin Darby
  Treasurer: Sharon Knowles

Management:
Artistic Director: Kenyard Smith
Mission: To inspire and develop the choral arts in Montana, provide continuing education and employment for professional singers in Montana and develop an artistic climate with international reputation in Montana.
Founded: 1976
Specialized Field: Choral
Status: Professional; Nonprofit
Income Sources: Chorus America
Performs At: Great Falls Civic Center
Organization Type: Performing; Touring; Sponsoring

Nebraska

2161 CLARION CHAMBER CHORALE

PO Box 31366
Omaha, NE 68131
Phone: 402-597-1240
Fax: 402-597-1254
e-mail: stane@collegiumusa.com
Web Site: clarionchamberchorale.org
Management:
Artistic Director: Stanley Schmidt
Associate Director: Richard Palmer
Mission: Presenting concerts focusing on choral literature for chamber ensembles.
Founded: 1982
Specialized Field: Choral
Status: Semi-Professional; Nonprofit
Paid Staff: 3
Volunteer Staff: 33
Non-paid Artists: 33
Income Sources: Clarion Choral Foundations
Performs At: First United Methodist Church
Organization Type: Performing; Touring

2162 OPERA OMAHA

1625 Farnam
Omaha, NE 68102
Phone: 402-346-4398
Fax: 402-346-7323
Toll-free: 877-846-7872
Web Site: www.operaomaha.org
Officers:
President: George H Heider
President Elect: David Gardels
Management:
Executive Director: Joan Desens
Artistic Director: Hal France
Founded: 1958
Specialized Field: Opera
Status: Professional; Nonprofit
Paid Staff: 13
Budget: $2.4 million
Income Sources: Individuals; Foundations; Corporations; NEA; Nebraska Arts Council; Douglas County; NE Ticket Income
Performs At: Orpheum Theatre; Witherspoon Concert Hall
Annual Attendance: 9,000
Facility Category: Theater
Type of Stage: Proscenium

Stage Dimensions: 54'w x 30'h x 44'd
Seating Capacity: 2,500
Year Built: 1927
Year Remodeled: 2002
Organization Type: Performing; Touring; Resident; Educational; Sponsoring

Nevada

2163 NEVADA OPERA THEATRE

4080 Paradise Road
Suite 15
Las Vegas, NV 89109
Phone: 702-699-9775
Fax: 702-699-9831
Management:
General/Artistic Director: Eileen Hayes
Performs At: Artemus West Ham Concert Hall

2164 NEVADA OPERA ASSOCIATION

925 Riverside Drive
Suite 5
Reno, NV 89505
Mailing Address: PO Box 3256
Phone: 775-786-4046
Fax: 775-786-4063
e-mail: nevadaopera@aol.com
Web Site: www.nevadaopera.com
Management:
Managing Director: Karen L Haas
Artistic Director: Robin Stamper
Marketing Director: Zoe Rose
Mission: To produce quality professional opera for the broadest possible audience.
Founded: 1968
Specialized Field: Grand Opera; Lyric Opera; Light Opera; Operetta
Status: Professional; Nonprofit
Paid Staff: 6
Volunteer Staff: 10
Income Sources: Corporate & Donors
Performs At: Pioneer Center for the Performing Arts
Organization Type: Performing; Resident

New Hampshire

2165 CLAREMONT OPERA HOUSE

City Hall on Tremont Square
PO Box 664
Claremont, NH 03743
Phone: 603-542-0064
Fax: 603-542-7014
e-mail: twincloud@pobox.com
Web Site: www.claremontoperahouse.com
Management:
Executive Artistic Director: Thom Wolke
Mission: Multi-use performing arts center.
Opened: 1977
Specialized Field: Upper Connecticut Valley
Budget: $150,000
Income Sources: Tickets; Membership; Sponsers

Affiliations: APAP; APNNE
Annual Attendance: 15,000
Facility Category: Theatre
Type of Stage: Proscenium
Seating Capacity: 780
Year Built: 1897
Year Remodeled: 1975

2166 OPERA NORTH

40 N College Street
Hanover, NH 03755
Phone: 603-643-1946
Fax: 603-448-0999
e-mail: opera.north@valley.net
Web Site: www.operanorth.org
Officers:
  President: Virginia Rolett
  President Elect: Caroline Vaillant
  Treasurer: Timothy Wager
  Secretary: Carl Brandon
Management:
  Artistic Director: Louis Burkot
  Executive Director: Patricia Compton
  Producer: Florence Klausner
  Director Productions: Ron Luchsinger
Mission: To produce opera for Northern New England
with the highest musical and dramatic standards; to
recognize that opera is both entertaining and spiritually
enriching, we seek diversified audience through
educational and performance programs. Opera North is
also committed to the development of young artists
through performance opportunities and production
experience.
Founded: 1981
Specialized Field: Opera
Paid Staff: 3
Volunteer Staff: 350
Paid Artists: 150
Budget: $540,000
Income Sources: Ticket Sales, Grants, Contributions
Performs At: Lebanon Opera House
Affiliations: Opera America
Annual Attendance: 11,000
Facility Category: Auditorium
Type of Stage: Proscenium
Stage Dimensions: 30 x 30 x 27
Seating Capacity: 800
Year Built: 1920
Year Remodeled: 2001

2167 LEBANON OPERA HOUSE

51 N Park Street
PO Box 384
Lebanon, NH 03766
Phone: 603-448-0400
Fax: 603-448-0444
e-mail: lebanon.opera.house@valley.net
Web Site: www.lebanonoperahouse.org
Management:
  Executive Director: Partridge Boswell

2168 METRO LYRIC OPERA

PO Box 35
Allenhurst, NJ 07711
Phone: 732-531-2378
Fax: 732-531-2752
e-mail: metrolyricopera@yahoo.com
Web Site: www.metrolyricopera.org
Officers:
  President: John Mullins
  VP: John Plunkett
  Secretary: Joan Benoist
Management:
  Founder And Artistic Director: Era Tognoli
  Assistant Artistic Director: Luccio Zachary
  Conductor: Anton Coppola
Mission: To bring opera of a high standard to all people at
popular prices; to create a professional outlet for
deserving young artists as well as experienced
professionals; to bring opera in English to public schools.
Founded: 1959
Specialized Field: Grand Opera; Operetta
Status: Professional
Income Sources: Monmouth Opera Guild
Performs At: Paramount Theatre; Strand Theatre
Organization Type: Performing; Educational;
Community Service

2169 NORTH JERSEY CHORAL SOCIETY

St Matthews Evangelical Lutheran Church
173 N Washington Avenue
Bergenfield, NJ 07621
Phone: 201-387-9505
Fax: 201-387-0025
e-mail: njchoral@hotmail.com
Web Site: community.nj.com/cc/njchoral
Officers:
  President: John P Pieroni
Management:
  Artistic Director: Lawrence A Constance

2170 AUREUS QUARTET

22 Lois Avenue
Demarest, NJ 07627-2220
Phone: 201-767-8704
Fax: 201-767-8704
e-mail: AureusQuartet@aol.com
Management:
  Artistic Director: James J Seiler
  Manager: David Saybrook
Founded: 1982
Paid Staff: 2
Paid Artists: 4

2171 PHILOMUSICA CHOIR

PO Box 6032
East Brunswick, NJ 08816-6032
Phone: 732-545-8434
e-mail: info@philomusic.org
Web Site: www.philomusic.org/
Officers:
  President: Elizabeth Dixon
  VP: Jonathan Butler

All listings are in alphabetical order by state, then city, then organization within the city.

Treasurer: Phyllis Chudnick
Secretary: Jeffrey Aaron
Management:
Director: Dennis Boyle
Mission: Excellence in choral sound, performance and musicianship.
Founded: 1969
Specialized Field: Choral Works; Early Sacred Music; Madrigals; Folk Songs; Gospel
Status: Non-Professional
Non-paid Artists: 40+
Affiliations: Middlesex County Cultural/Heritage Commission
Organization Type: Performing; Touring

2172 VERISMO OPERA/NEW JERSEY ASSOCIATION OF VERISMO OPERA

PO Box 3024
Fort Lee, NJ 07024-9024
Phone: 201-342-1970
Fax: 201-224-6911
Web Site: www.njavo.org
Officers:
President: Giovanni Simone
VP: Lucine Amara
VP: Evelyn Quaife
VP: Stan Staniloff
Secretary: Fran Staniloff
Treasurer: Adora Crager
Management:
Artistic Director: Lucine Amara
Music Director: Anthony Morss
Director Marketing: Robert Caminiti
Box Office Manager: Mary Briggs
Mission: The New Jersey Association of Verismo Opera has been a part of the New Jersey music scene since 1989. It began by sponsoring a vocal competition and an opera workshop.
Founded: 1989
Specialized Field: Opera

2173 RARITAN VALLEY CHORUS

PO Box 6044
Hillsborough, NJ 08844
Phone: 908-281-8509
e-mail: rvchoralsociety@musician.org
Web Site: www.princetonol.com/groups/rvchorusociety/
Management:
Conductor: Mark Trautman
Mission: A community based ensemble of varying ages, backgrounds and careers. The choir is open to all residents of the region and offers a range of musical experiences unparalleled in Central New Jersey.
Founded: 1990

2174 NEW JERSEY STATE OPERA

50 Park Place
10th Floor
Newark, NJ 07102
Phone: 973-623-5757
Fax: 973-623-5761
e-mail: newjerseystateop@aol.com
Web Site: www.newjerseystateopera.org
Officers:

Secretary: Florence A Infante
Treasurer: CG Haagensen
President: Anthony V Boccabella
Management:
Artistic Director: Alfredo Silipigni
Artistic Director: Maestro Alfredo Silipigni
Assistant Artistic Director: Donna Lawrence
Founded: 1966
Specialized Field: Opera
Status: Professional
Paid Staff: 50
Income Sources: Essex County Arts Council; New Jersey State Arts Council
Performs At: New Jersey Performing Arts Center; Prudential Hall
Seating Capacity: 2,750
Organization Type: Performing

2175 ARS MUSICAL CHORALE & ORCHESTRA

PO Box 525
Paramus, NJ 07653
Phone: 201-358-6405
Fax: 201-358-6405
e-mail: arsmusica@hotmail.com
Web Site: www.arsmusica.org
Management:
Music Director: Italo Marchini

2176 PRO ARTE CHORALE

400 Paramus Road
Paramus, NJ 07652
Phone: 201-445-9052
Fax: 201-445-1421
Officers:
President: Howard Hanes
Management:
Music Director: David Crone
Managing Director: Wendy Dockray
Chorus Manager: Sharonian Sauer
Founded: 1964
Specialized Field: Performing chorus (volunteer)
Paid Staff: 2
Paid Artists: 4
Budget: $130,000
Income Sources: State grant, corporation foundation, private donations, ticket sales, fund raisers, membership dues
Performs At: Concert hall, church/temple
Affiliations: Chorus America

2177 AMERICAN BOYCHOIR

19 Lambert Drive
Princeton, NJ 08540
Phone: 609-924-5858
Fax: 609-924-5812
Web Site: www.americanboychoir.org
Officers:
Chairman: Chester W Douglass
President: John Ellis
Management:
Music Director: Vincent Metallo
General Manager: Janet Kaltenbach

Mission: The Boychoir includes choristers from throughout North America, who are students at the internationally-renowned boarding and day choir school (which offers a full academic program).
Founded: 1937
Specialized Field: Choral
Status: Professional; Nonprofit
Paid Staff: 42
Budget: $3,000,000
Organization Type: Performing; Touring; Educational

2178 PRINCETON PRO MUSICA CHORUS & ORCHESTRA

PO Box 1313
Princeton, NJ 08542
Phone: 609-683-5122
Fax: 609-683-9676
e-mail: prinpromusica@aol.com
Web Site: www.princetopromusic.org
Officers:
  President: Bernard McMullan
  Treasurer: Betsy Whittlsey
Management:
  Managing Director: Karen Peters
  Music Director: Frances Fowler Slade
Mission: To perform masterpieces of the choral repertoire with a professional orchestra and soloists.
Founded: 1979
Specialized Field: Choral
Status: Nonprofit
Paid Staff: 4
Volunteer Staff: 25
Paid Artists: 30
Non-paid Artists: 120
Income Sources: NJSCA; Individuals
Performs At: Richardson Auditorium; Princeton University
Affiliations: Chorus America; Art Pride
Organization Type: Performing

2179 WESTMINSTER CHOIR

101 Walnut Lane
Princeton, NJ 08540-3899
Phone: 609-921-7100
Fax: 609-921-3012
e-mail: wccinfo@rider.edu
Web Site: www.westminster.rider.edu
Management:
  Conductor: Joseph Flummerfelt
  Accompanist/Assistant Director: Nancianne Parrella
  Manager: Tricia Kersh
Founded: 1920
Specialized Field: Choral Music

2180 RIDGEWOOD GILBERT AND SULLIVAN OPERA COMPANY

975 E Ridgewood Avenue
Ridgewood, NJ 07450
Phone: 201-385-9314
Web Site: www.dancaster.com/RidgewoodGandS/
Officers:
  President: Unfilled
  VP: Joan Barker
  Treasurer: April Jacobs

Secretary: Phil Sternenberg
Business Manager: Judy Rosenthal
Member at Large: Mike Wiley
Member at Large: Eileen Karlson
Member-At-Large: Tim Schwartz
Management:
  Stage Director: Wilbur Watkin Lewis
  Music Director: Chester Wolfson
  Business Manager: Jack Strangfeld
Mission: Presenting Gilbert and Sullivan operas; fostering appreciation of Gilbert and Sullivan operas, music and drama.
Founded: 1937
Specialized Field: Light Opera
Status: Non-Professional; Nonprofit
Paid Staff: 50
Income Sources: American Association of Community Theatres
Performs At: Ben Franklin Middle School
Organization Type: Performing; Touring

2181 COMMUNITY OPERA

417 Morris Avenue # 22
Summit, NJ 07901
Phone: 908-277-1934
Mission: Showcasing opera singers as well as modern composers.
Founded: 1981
Specialized Field: Grand Opera; Operetta
Status: Professional
Income Sources: Orpheus Society
Performs At: Hudson Guild; South Street Seaport-Fulton Center

2182 SUMMIT CHORALE

PO Box 265
Summit, NJ 07902-0265
Phone: 908-464-0959
Fax: 908-464-0959
e-mail: robertgrubb@home.com
Web Site: www.summitchorale.org
Management:
  Music Director: Garyth Nair
  Trearsurer/Business Manager: Robert J Grubb
Mission: To promote and cultivate choral music by providing an opportunity for those who enjoy ensemble singing to explore the rich heritage of choral music while studying and singing under the best professional leadership obtainable; to foster public appreciation and enjoyment of choral music through performance as well as educational and community outreach endeavors.
Founded: 1909
Status: Non-professional
Volunteer Staff: 12
Paid Artists: 2-60
Budget: $70,000
Income Sources: Private; Public; Box Office; Grants; Fundraising
Performs At: University; Churches; Schools
Organization Type: Performing; Education

2183 CHORAL ARTS SOCIETY OF NEW JERSEY
PO Box 2036
Westfield, NJ 07091
Phone: 908-756-5154
Officers:
   President: James Zgoda
   VP: Ted Schirm
   Treasurer: Linda Jacobey
   Secretary: Suzanne Beeny
Management:
   Music Director: Evelyn Bleeke
Mission: To study, perform and promote choral works.
Founded: 1962
Specialized Field: Choral
Status: Non-Professional
Organization Type: Performing

New Mexico

2184 OPERA SOUTHWEST
515 15th Street NW
Albuquerque, NM 87104
Phone: 505-243-0591
e-mail: operaSW@aol.com
Web Site:
www.unm.edu/~shapiro/MUSIC/opera_southwest.ht
Officers:
   President: Sheila Johnson
Management:
   Production Manager/General Director: Justine
   Tate-Opel
   Artistic Director: Kyle Marrero
   Music Director: Michael Butterman
Mission: To present fully staged, costumed operas with
accomplished musicians at the highest artistic level.
Founded: 1972
Specialized Field: Grand Opera; Lyric Opera; Light
Opera; Operetta
Status: Professional; Nonprofit
Paid Staff: 30
Income Sources: Central Opera Service
Performs At: KiMo Theatre
Organization Type: Performing; Educational

2185 SANGRE DE CRISTO CHORALE
PO Box 4462
Santa Fe, NM 87502-4462
Phone: 505-662-9717
Fax: 505-665-4433
e-mail: busmgr@sdc-chorale.org
Web Site: www.sdc-chorale.org
Officers:
   Board President: Andrea Poole
   President Elect: Gary Buff
   Development Chair: Gary Bell
   Performanace Chair: Joan Ellis
Management:
   Director: Sheldon Kalberg
   Business Manager: Hastings Smith
Mission: Performance of choral music and educational
outreach.
Founded: 1978

Volunteer Staff: 10
Paid Artists: 35
Budget: $52,000
Income Sources: Admissions; Contributions;
Advertising; Grants
Performs At: Churches, Hotels
Annual Attendance: 1,800
Facility Category: Various venues: churches, hotels
Type of Stage: Choral Risers off Floor

2186 SANTA FE DESERT CHORALE
500 Montezuma
Suite 118-B
Santa Fe, NM 87501
Phone: 505-988-2282
Fax: 505-988-7522
Toll-free: 800-244-4011
e-mail: info@desertchorale.org
Web Site: www.desertchorale.org
Officers:
   President: Mary Ann Nelson
Mission: To perform music from the choral repertoire
within the last five centuries, especially Baroque and
modern.
Founded: 1982
Specialized Field: Choral
Status: Professional; Nonprofit
Income Sources: Chorus America
Performs At: Santuario de Guadalupe; Loretto Chapel
Organization Type: Performing; Educational

2187 SANTA FE SYMPHONY ORCHESTRA AND CHORUS
PO Box 9692
Santa Fe, NM 87504
Phone: 505-983-3530
Fax: 505-982-3888
Toll-free: 800-480-1319
Web Site: sf-symphony.org
Management:
   Founder/General Director: Gregory Heltman
   Operations Manager: Diane Stengle
   Development Director: Jennifer Schiffmacher
   Music Director: Steven Smith
Budget: $550,000
Income Sources: Contributions; Ticket Sales; Grants
Performs At: Lensic Performing Arts Center
Seating Capacity: 800

New York

2188 ALBANY PRO MUSICA
PO Box 3850
Albany, NY 12203-0850
Phone: 518-438-6548
e-mail: info@albanypromusica.org
Web Site: www.albanypromusica.org
Management:
   Artistic Director/Conductor: David Griggs-Janower
Mission: To be a mixed chorus of selected volunteers
who are dedicated to the enhancement of the cultural life
in upstate New York and their own musical growth.

Albany Pro Musica achieves these objectives through professional quality a cappella performance and accompanies choral repertoire drawn from diverse traditions and styles.
Founded: 1981
Performs At: Civic and community musical events
Affiliations: Albany Symphony Orchestra

2189 TRI-CITIES OPERA COMPANY

315 Clinton Street
Binghamton, NY 13905
Phone: 607-729-3444
Fax: 607-797-6344
e-mail: info@tricitiesopera.com
Web Site: www.tricitiesopera.com
Officers:
President: Grant Best
First VP: Dr. Fran Goldman
Second First President: Juames Thomas
Treasurer: Dirk Olds
Management:
Artistic Director: Duane Skrabalak
Associate Artistic Director: Peter Sicilian
Executive Diector: Reed Smith
Marketing/Development Director: Kim Eaton
Mission: Mission is to produce opera.
Founded: 1949
Specialized Field: Grand Opera
Status: Professional; Nonprofit
Paid Staff: 50
Budget: $1,000,000
Income Sources: American Guild of Musical Artists; American Federation of Musicians; International Association of Theatrical Stage Employees
Performs At: Broome County Forum
Affiliations: Binghamton University
Annual Attendance: 15,000
Seating Capacity: 1500
Year Built: 1920
Year Remodeled: 1975
Organization Type: Performing; Resident; Educational

2190 BRONX OPERA COMPANY

5 Minerva Place
Bronx, NY 10468
Phone: 718-365-4209
Fax: 718-563-8379
Web Site: www.bronxopera.org
Officers:
President: Eva Schulz
Treasurer: Manny Nadelman
Management:
Artistic Director: Michael Spierman
Assistant Artistic Director: Ben Spierman
Production Manager: Gayle Jeffries
Mission: Bronx Opera has established a record of continuous growth, excellence and community involvement.
Founded: 1967
Specialized Field: New York City
Status: Nonprofit

2191 PARKCHESTER CHORUS

Parkchester Station
PO Box 300
Bronx, NY 10462
Phone: 718-892-0178
Fax: 718-292-5607
e-mail: lnanko@cardinalhayes.org
Officers:
President: Mary Ellen Vicari
Management:
Director: Lorraine C Nanko
Founded: 1939
Specialized Field: Community Chorus
Paid Staff: 1
Volunteer Staff: 10
Budget: $5,000
Income Sources: Bronx Council on the Arts; Fund Raisers
Performs At: Church
Annual Attendance: 600

2192 AMERICAN OPERA PROJECTS

138 S Oxford Street
Brooklyn, NY 11217
Phone: 718-398-4024
Fax: 718-398-3489
e-mail: info@aopinc.org
Web Site: www.americanoperaprojects.org/
Management:
Artistic Director/Founder: Grethe Berrett Holby
Managing Director: Charles Jarden
Performs At: SoHo Center
Seating Capacity: 100

2193 REGINA OPERA COMPANY

1251 Tabor Court
Brooklyn, NY 11219
Phone: 718-232-3555
Fax: 718-232-3555
e-mail: linda@reginaopera.org
Web Site: www.reginaopera.org
Officers:
President: Marie Cantoni
Executive VP: Francine Garber-Cohen
VP/Legal Advisor: Linda Cantoni
Mission: Training young professionals and showcasing experienced directors and performers.
Founded: 1970
Specialized Field: Grand Opera; Broadway; Ethnic Music; Operetta
Status: Semi-Professional; Nonprofit
Volunteer Staff: 15
Non-paid Artists: 50
Budget: Under $100,000
Income Sources: Public & Private Funding; Ticket Sales
Performs At: Regina Hall
Annual Attendance: 5,000
Facility Category: School; Auditorium (revised)
Type of Stage: Proscenium
Stage Dimensions: 30'x18'
Seating Capacity: 325
Organization Type: Performing

2194 BUFFALO PHILHARMONIC CHORUS & CHAMBER SINGERS
PO Box 176
Buffalo, NY 14207-0176
Phone: 716-447-1927
Fax: 716-874-0486
e-mail: mcolquhoun@earthlink.net
Management:
    Business Manager: Michael Colquhoun
Founded: 1936
Paid Staff: 3
Volunteer Staff: 15
Paid Artists: 10
Non-paid Artists: 100

2195 CHAUTAUQUA OPERA
Chautauqua Institution
PO Box 28
Chautauqua, NY 14722
Phone: 716-357-6200
Fax: 716-357-9014
Toll-free: 800-836-2787
e-mail: info@chautauqua-inst.org
Web Site: www.chautauqua-inst.org
Management:
    Artistic/General Director: Jay Lesenger
Mission: Offering opera in English with young, emerging artists; training young singers.
Founded: 1929
Specialized Field: Grand Opera; Lyric Opera; Light Opera; Operetta
Status: Professional
Income Sources: Opera America
Performs At: Norton Hall
Organization Type: Performing; Resident; Educational

2196 BERKSHIRE-HUDSON VALLEY FESTIVAL OF OPERA
PO Box 454
Clavarack, NY 12513
Phone: 518-851-6778
Fax: 518-851-6778
e-mail: +coc@mhonline.com
Officers:
    President: Alberto Figols
    VP: Glenn Wilder
    Secretary/Treasurer: Anne de Figols
Management:
    Artist Representative: Ramon Alsina
Mission: To bring live professional opera and dance to people who would not normally have access to productions on a regular basis; primarily serving Massachusetts, the Southern Berkshires and the Hudson Valley.
Founded: 1971
Specialized Field: Dance; Vocal Music; Instrumental Music; Theater; Lyric Opera; Grand Opera
Status: Professional; Nonprofit
Volunteer Staff: 5
Budget: Varies
Income Sources: Tickets; Sponsors; Donations; Grants
Affiliations: Touring Concert Opera Comapny
Annual Attendance: 5,000 - 10,000
Organization Type: Performing; Touring

2197 GLIMMERGLASS OPERA
PO Box 191
Cooperstown, NY 13326
Phone: 607-547-5704
Fax: 607-547-6030
e-mail: glimmer@telenet.net
Web Site: www.glimmerglass.org/
Management:
    General Director: Esther Nelson
    Music Director: Stewart Robertson
Mission: To produce new, little known, and familiar operas and works of music theater in innovative productions which capitalize on the intimacy and natural setting of The Alice Busch Opera Theater; to promote an artistically challenging work environment for young American performers, and to engage important directors, designers and conductors who provide high standards of achievement.
Founded: 1975
Specialized Field: Vocal Music; Lyric Opera; Grand Opera
Status: Professional; Nonprofit
Paid Staff: 25
Income Sources: Opera America
Season: July - August
Performs At: Alice Busch Opera Theater
Facility Category: Theater
Seating Capacity: 900
Year Built: 1987
Organization Type: Performing

2198 1891 FREDONIA OPERA HOUSE
PO Box 384
Fredonia, NY 14063
Phone: 716-679-0891
Fax: 716-679-3175
e-mail: operahouse@netsync.net
Web Site: www.fredopera.org
Management:
    Executive Director: Elizabeth Booth
Mission: To present the best in music and theatre, including classical, jazz, and folk.
Founded: 1891
Paid Staff: 3
Volunteer Staff: 60

2199 ITHACA OPERA ASSOCIATION
116 N Cayuga Street
Ithaca, NY 14850
Phone: 607-272-0168
Fax: 607-273-4816
e-mail: bigd@starflinn.com
Web Site: hammer.prohosting.com/~ioa/
Management:
    Director: Dale Finn
Mission: Bringing the Finger Lakes area high quality entertainment; employing talented local and regional performers.
Founded: 1949
Specialized Field: Grand Opera; Lyric Opera; Light Opera; Operetta; Musical Theatre
Status: Professional; Nonprofit
Paid Staff: 20
Income Sources: New York State Coucil on Arts

Performs At: Barnes Hall; Cornell University
Organization Type: Performing; Touring; Educational

2200 DELAWARE VALLEY OPERA

PO Box 188
Narrowsburg, NY 12764
Phone: 845-252-3910
Web Site: www.libertynet.org/dvoc/
Management:
General Manager: Gloria Krause
Founded: 1986
Specialized Field: Light Opera; Operetta
Status: Semi-Professional; Nonprofit
Paid Staff: 40
Performs At: Tusten Theatre; Sullivan County
Community College
Organization Type: Performing; Educational

2201 NEW ROCHELLE OPERA

PO Box 112
New Rochelle, NY 10802
Phone: 914-576-0365
Fax: 914-235-1027
Toll-free: 800-576-0365
e-mail: frybody@aol.com
Web Site: www.angelfire.com/ny/nropera
Management:
Executive Director: Camille Coppola
Company Coordinator: Billie Tucker
Founded: 1985
Volunteer Staff: 15+
Budget: $65,000
Income Sources: Box Office; Grants; Contributions
Performs At: New Rochelle Library Theatre
Annual Attendance: 3000
Facility Category: Theatre
Type of Stage: Proscenium
Stage Dimensions: 18 x 30
Seating Capacity: 150
Year Built: 1979

2202 AMATO OPERA THEATRE

319 Bowery
New York, NY 10003
Phone: 212-228-8200
Fax: 646-654-6952
e-mail: info@amato.org
Web Site: www.amato.org
Officers:
President: Anthony Amato
Management:
Executive Director: Irene Frydel Kim
Artistic Director: Anthony Amato
Mission: The Amato Opera Theater, has survived on a
collective artistic desire to present grand opera that is
good theater and, at the same time, has created a platform
for aspiring young artists.
Founded: 1948
Specialized Field: Grand Opera; Light Opera
Status: Professional; Semi-Professional; Nonprofit
Paid Staff: 3
Volunteer Staff: 25
Non-paid Artists: 200
Budget: $160,000

Income Sources: Tickets; Donations
Seating Capacity: 107
Organization Type: Performing

2203 AMERICAN CHAMBER OPERA COMPANY

PO Box 909
Ansonia Station
New York, NY 10032
Phone: 212-781-0857
Fax: 718-596-2038
Management:
Executive Director: Doug Anderson
Stage Manager: George Zarr
Mission: Presenting full productions of chamber operas
with strong dramatic and musical values.
Founded: 1983
Specialized Field: Chamber Opera
Status: Professional; Nonprofit
Performs At: Riverside Church Theatre
Organization Type: Performing

2204 AMERICAN OPERA MUSIC THEATER

400 W 43rd Street
Suite 19-D
New York, NY 10036
Phone: 212-594-1839
Fax: 212-695-4350
e-mail: corto@mindspring.com
Management:
Artistic Director: Diana Corto
Administrator: C Miles
Stage Director: Theodore Mann
Mission: Promote emerging artists with major talent,
prsent new famililar music, with costumed and staged
quality productions.
Paid Staff: 3
Volunteer Staff: 3
Paid Artists: 50
Budget: $250,000
Income Sources: Corporate; Donations; Service
Revenues
Performs At: Theatres; Schools; Alternate spaces
Annual Attendance: 30,000
Facility Category: Theaters
Type of Stage: Proscenium, round
Stage Dimensions: 26 x 35 minimum
Seating Capacity: 500 - 3,000

2205 AMERICAN-INTERNATIONAL LYRIC THEATRE

322 Duke Ellington Boulevard
New York, NY 10025-3471
Phone: 212-662-3468
Fax: 212-678-0517
e-mail: Ppress322@aol.com
Web Site: members.aol.com/ppress322/music1/index.htm
Management:
Managing Director: Paulette Singer
Artistic Director: Russell Miller
Founded: 1985
Paid Staff: 3
Paid Artists: 50
Budget: $500,000

Season: Year round

2206 BOYS CHOIR OF HARLEM
2005 Madison Avenue
New York, NY 10035-1298
Phone: 212-289-1815
Fax: 212-289-4195
e-mail: BCH@mindspring.com
Web Site: www.boyschoirofharlem.org
Officers:
President: Dr. Walter J Turnbull
Management:
Executive VP: Horace Turnbull
Company Manager: Hilda Cabrera
Mission: The Boys Choir of Harlem program evolves directly from our mission and a vision of consistent, compassionate, communal strength in raising children.
Specialized Field: Choral music / Artistic Education
Paid Staff: 60
Paid Artists: 32
Non-paid Artists: 28
Season: One or two tours a year
Comments: Boys Choir age are 9 to 18 years.

2207 CANTERBURY CHORAL SOCIETY
2 E 90th Street
Church of the Heavenly Rest
New York, NY 10128
Phone: 212-222-9458
Fax: 212-222-9458
e-mail: dodlsey@aol.com
Management:
Conductor: Charles D Walker
Founded: 1952
Paid Staff: 1
Paid Artists: 12
Non-paid Artists: 100
Performs At: Church
Annual Attendance: 2,000
Facility Category: Church
Seating Capacity: 900
Year Built: 1929

2208 CHILDREN'S AID SOCIETY CHORUS
219 Sullivan Street
New York, NY 10012
Phone: 212-533-1675
Fax: 212-583-7519
e-mail: information@caschorus.org
Web Site: www.childrensaidsociety.org
Management:
Music Director: Elizabeth C Parker
Assistant Director: Rachel Gahan
Mission: Strives to provide every child, regardless of socioeconomic situation, the opportunity to study and perform quality choral music with other children from New York City.
Founded: 1997
Specialized Field: Choral

2209 COLLEGIATE CHORALE
881 7th Avenue
Carnegie Hall Studios #1201
New York, NY 10019

Phone: 212-664-1390
Fax: 212-568-5948
Web Site: collegiatechorale.org/
Management:
Music Director: Robert Bass
Manager: Lauren Scott

2210 DICAPO OPERA THEATRE
184 E 76th Street
New York, NY 10021
Phone: 212-288-9438
Fax: 212-744-1082
e-mail: medicapo@aol.com
Web Site: www.dicapo.com
Management:
General Director: Michael Capasso
Artistic Director: Diane Martindale
Season: September - June
Performs At: Dicapo Theatre
Facility Category: Theatre
Type of Stage: Proscenium
Stage Dimensions: 40'x 40'
Seating Capacity: 200
Rental Contact: General Director Michael Capasso

2211 EARLY MUSIC FOUNDATION
1047 Amsterdam Avenue
New York, NY 10025
Phone: 212-749-6600
e-mail: info@EarlyMusicNY.org
Web Site: www.earlymusicny.org
Management:
Artictic Director: Frederick Renz

2212 GRACE CHURCH CHORAL SOCIETY
802 Broadway
New York, NY 10003
Phone: 212-254-2000
Fax: 212-673-4938
e-mail: pallen@gracechnyc.org
Web Site: www.gracenyc.org
Management:
Organist/Master Choriters: Patrick Allen
Conductor: John Maclay
Founded: 1961
Paid Staff: 2
Volunteer Staff: 6
Paid Artists: 12
Non-paid Artists: 100
Performs At: Church
Affiliations: Grace Church in New York
Annual Attendance: 2,400

2213 HOLY TRINITY BACH CHOIR
3 W 65th Street
New York, NY 10023
Phone: 212-978-4321
Fax: 212-877-6816
e-mail: rde10023@aol.com
Web Site: www.holytrinitynyc.org
Officers:
President: Timothy Cage
Management:
Cantor: Richard Erickson

Office Manager: Tobin Schmuck
Mission: To bring the music of Bach to the community in context of worship.
Founded: 1968
Specialized Field: Choral/Sacred Music
Paid Staff: 2
Volunteer Staff: 3
Paid Artists: 25
Income Sources: Donations; Offerings; Endowment
Facility Category: Church
Seating Capacity: 550
Year Built: 1904
Resident Groups: Bach Choir; Period In

2214 I CANTORI DI NEW YORK
PO Box 1376
New York, NY 10185
Phone: 212-439-4758
e-mail: info@cantorinewyork.com
Web Site: www.cantorinewyork.com
Officers:
President: Tyler Cutforth
VP: Pamela M Reich
Treasurer: Ilse de Veer
Secretary: Brian Hopkins
Management:
Conductor: Bart Folse
General Manager: Paul Schleuse
Artistic Director: Mark Shapiro
Mission: Presenting a wide range of choral music, juxtaposing the classic with the contemporary.
Founded: 1984
Specialized Field: Choral
Status: Semi-Professional
Organization Type: Performing

2215 L'OPERA FRANCAIS DE NEW YORK
PO Box 3151
New York, NY 10008
Phone: 212-349-7009
Fax: 212-349-7009
e-mail: lofny@mindspring.com
Web Site: www.interlog.com/~abel/lofny.html
Management:
Artistic Director: Yves Abel
General Manager: Antonio Tessitore
Mission: Offering American audiences French lyric opera.
Founded: 1988
Specialized Field: Lyric Opera
Status: Professional
Income Sources: French Institute; Alliance Francaise
Performs At: Alice Tull Hall; Kaye Playhouse
Organization Type: Performing

2216 LA GRAN SCENA OPERA COMPANY
211 E 11th Street
Suite 9
New York, NY 10003
Phone: 212-460-9124
Fax: 212-460-9124
e-mail: irasiff@aol.com
Web Site: www.granscena.org
Management:

Artistic Director: Ira Siff
Managing Director: Antonio Tessitore
Founded: 1981
Specialized Field: Opera Parody
Paid Staff: 2
Volunteer Staff: 6
Paid Artists: 15
Non-paid Artists: 0
Budget: $150,000
Income Sources: Funding and Performances
Performs At: Various Auditoriums
Annual Attendance: varies
Facility Category: varies

2217 MASTERWORK CHORUS
310 W 55th Street
Suite 1K
New York, NY 10019
Phone: 212-246-7091
Fax: 212-262-8762
Management:
Executive Director: Robert A Buckley

2218 METROPOLITAN OPERA
Lincoln Center
New York, NY 10023
Phone: 212-362-6000
e-mail: metinfo@visionfoundry.com
Web Site: www.metopera.org
Mission: From its opening in 1883, the Metropolitan Opera has been one of the world's leading opera companies. Today, the Met's preeminent position rests on the elements that established its reputation: high quality performances with many of the world's most renowned artists, a superior company of orchestral and choral musicians, a large repertory of works, and the resources to make performances available to the public.
Founded: 1883
Specialized Field: Orchestra; Choral
Season: January-December

2219 MUSIC-THEATRE GROUP
30 W 26th Street
Suite 1001
New York, NY 10010-2011
Phone: 212-366-5260
Fax: 212-366-5265
Management:
Producing Director: Diane Wondisford
Mission: Commissioning, developing and producing innovative music theatre.
Founded: 1971
Specialized Field: Music Theatre
Status: Professional; Nonprofit
Paid Staff: 5
Paid Artists: 50
Income Sources: Opera America
Organization Type: Performing; Touring

2220 MUSICA SACRA
165 W 86th Street
New York, NY 10023
Phone: 212-721-6500
Officers:

President: Jonathan Prinz
VP: Robert F Langley
VP: Robert Brauer
Secretary: Barbara G. Landau
Treasurer: Gerald W. Richman
Management:
   General Manager: Elizabeth Bond
Mission: Performing choral works that span the ages.
Founded: 1973
Specialized Field: Choral
Status: Professional
Performs At: Lincoln Center; Carnegie Hall
Organization Type: Performing

2221 NEW AMSTERDAM SINGERS
PO Box 373
New York, NY 10025
Phone: 212-568-5948
e-mail: info@nasingers.org
Web Site: www.nasingers.org
Management:
   Executive Director: James Backmon
   Music Director: Clara Longstreth
Mission: The New Amsterdam Singers, directed by Clara Longstreth, is a mixed chorus of seventy skilled singers specializing in a cappella and double chorus repertoire.

2222 NEW YORK CHORAL SOCIETY
881 7th Avenue
Studio 1201
New York, NY 10019
Phone: 212-247-3878
Fax: 973-948-4878
e-mail: nychoral@yahoo.com
Web Site: www.nychoral.org
Officers:
   President: James Hagen
   Treasurer: Joanne Lawson
   Executive VP: Lisa Guida
   Secretary: Grace E Lee
Management:
   Executive Director: John Lawson
   Music Director: John Daly Goodwin
Mission: Presenting performances in Carnegie Hall of choral masterpieces as well as lesser-known works.
Founded: 1958
Specialized Field: Choral
Status: Non-Professional; Nonprofit
Paid Staff: 280
Volunteer Staff: 50
Paid Artists: 2
Performs At: Carnegie Hall; Lincoln Center
Organization Type: Performing; Touring

2223 NEW YORK CITY OPERA
20 Lincoln Center
New York State Theatre
New York, NY 10023
Phone: 212-870-5630
Fax: 212-724-1120
e-mail: webmaster@nycopera.com
Web Site: www.nycopera.org
Management:
   General/Artistic Director: Paul Kellogg

Executive Producer: Sherwin Goldman
Associate Artistic Director: Robin Thompson
Director Marketing: Claudia Kennan Hough
Mission: Producing grand opera; developing and presenting young American artists; presenting opera as theater.
Founded: 1944
Specialized Field: Grand Opera; Musical Theatre
Status: Professional
Budget: $ 34 Million
Income Sources: Opera America
Performs At: New York State Theatre; Lincoln Center
Annual Attendance: 275,000+
Seating Capacity: 2,763
Organization Type: Performing; Touring; Resident; Educational

2224 NEW YORK CONCERT SINGERS
75 E End Avenue
Suite 9L
New York, NY 10028
Phone: 212-879-4412
Fax: 212-879-4412
e-mail: jclurman@aol.com
Officers:
   Chairman: Judith Clurman
   Vice Chair/Treasurer: Marcia Klugman
   Vice Chair: Bruce Ruben
   Secretary: Paul Olsen
Management:
   Music Director/Conductor: Judith Clurman
Mission: To present choral programs, vocal chamber programs and symphony programs.
Founded: 1988
Specialized Field: Choral
Status: Professional
Paid Staff: 2
Paid Artists: 50
Performs At: Lincoln Center; European Tour; 92nd Street
Organization Type: Performing; Educational

2225 NEW YORK GILBERT AND SULLIVAN PLAYERS
251 West 91st Street
#4C
New York, NY 10024
Phone: 212-769-1000
Fax: 212-769-1002
e-mail: info@nygasp.org
Web Site: www.nygasp.org
Officers:
   President: Carol Davis
   Vice President: Albert Bergeret
   Treasurer: Derek Hughes
   Secretary: John Behonek
Management:
   Artistic Director: Albert Bergeret
Mission: Producing and promoting Gilbert and Sullivan's works, along with related works employing orchestras as well as small ensembles.
Founded: 1974
Specialized Field: Operetta; Musical Theatre
Status: Professional

Paid Staff: 2
Paid Artists: 80
Budget: $1,500,000
Income Sources: Sales; Individual Contributions; Fees for Performance; Government Endowments
Performs At: Symphony Space; City Center; Tour
Affiliations: Actors' Equity Association; American Federation of Musicians of the United States and Canada
Annual Attendance: 25,000
Facility Category: Performing Arts Theatre/Symphony
Type of Stage: Proscenium
Stage Dimensions: 48 x 30
Seating Capacity: 2500
Year Remodeled: 2001
Cost: $35,000
Rental Contact: Eugene Lowery
Organization Type: Performing; Touring; Resident; Educational

2226 NEW YORK OPERA PROJECT

461 Central Park W
Suite 4D
New York, NY 10025
Phone: 212-749-6603
Fax: 212-749-6603
e-mail: 110227.546@compuserve.com
Management:
  Artistic Director: Fredrick Martell
  Music Director: Paul Mueller
Founded: 1993
Paid Staff: 2
Volunteer Staff: 3

2227 NEW YORK TREBLE SINGERS

210 W 89th Street # 4L
#4L
New York, NY 10024-1811
Phone: 212-496-0094
Fax: 212-496-0094
e-mail: vsdavidson@nytreblesinger.org
Web Site: www.nytreblesingers.org
Management:
  Conductor: Virginia S Davidson
Mission: To perform works for womens voices and promote good will through music.
Founded: 1985
Specialized Field: Classical Vocal
Paid Staff: 1
Volunteer Staff: 3
Paid Artists: 13

2228 NOONDAY CONCERTS

74 Trinity Place
New York, NY 10006-2088
Phone: 212-602-0768
Fax: 212-602-9630
Web Site: www.trinitywallstreet.org
Management:
  Director Trinity Concerts: Earl Tucker
Founded: 1933
Specialized Field: New York, New Jersey, Connecticut
Paid Staff: 2
Budget: $300,000
Income Sources: Foundations; Corporations

Performs At: St. Paul's Chapel & Trinity Church
Affiliations: APAP, ISPA, CMA
Annual Attendance: 16,000
Facility Category: Church

2229 OPERA EBONY

2109 Broadway
New York, NY 10023
Phone: 212-874-7245
Fax: 212-877-2110
e-mail: infor@operaebony.org
Web Site: www.operaebony.org
Management:
  Music Director: Wayne Sanders
  Artistic Director: Benjamin Matthews
  Special Projects Director: Mohammed Hatim
Mission: Discovering and promoting singers, composers, directors, choreographers and technicians.
Founded: 1973
Specialized Field: Grand Opera; Ethnic; Folk; 20th Century Works
Status: Professional; Nonprofit
Income Sources: The American Music Center; Opera America
Performs At: Aaron Davis Hall
Organization Type: Performing; Touring; Educational

2230 OPERA NORTHEAST/CHILDREN'S OPERA THEATRE

PO Box 6700
New York, NY 10128
Phone: 212-472-2168
Fax: 212-472-6910
Web Site: www.operamgt.com
Management:
  Artistic Director: Donald Westwood
  Administrative Director: Tracy Throne
Mission: Build a first-class touring organization to produce and present authentic classical lyric theatre.
Founded: 1972
Specialized Field: Opera, Operetta, Young Audiences
Status: Professional; Nonprofit
Paid Staff: 6
Volunteer Staff: 10
Paid Artists: 30
Budget: $250,000
Organization Type: Performing; Touring; Educational

2231 OPERA ORCHESTRA OF NEW YORK

239 W 72nd Street
Suite 2R
New York, NY 10023
Phone: 212-799-1982
Fax: 212-721-9170
e-mail: info@oony.org
Web Site: www.oony.org/
Management:
  Music Director: Eve Queler
  Director Development: Yvonne Altmann
  General Manager: Alix Barthelmes
Mission: To offer the public an opportunity to enjoy operas which are little-known or rarely heard.
Founded: 1971
Specialized Field: Grand Opera; Lyric Opera

Status: Professional; Nonprofit
Budget: $1.5 million
Income Sources: Ticket sales and donations
Performs At: Carnegie Hall
Organization Type: Performing; Sponsoring

2232 ORATORIO SOCIETY OF NEW YORK

881 7th Avenue
Carnegie Hall, Suite 504
New York, NY 10019-3321
Phone: 212-247-4199
e-mail: webmaster@oratoriosocietyofny.org
Web Site: www.oratoriosocietyofny.org
Officers:
　　Chairperson: Ellen L Blair
　　President: Richard A Pace
　　VP: Evelyn R Arcudi
　　VP: Mary-Jo P. Noren-Iacovino
　　VP: Janet Plucknett
　　Treasurer/Archivist: Marie Gangemi
　　Secretary: Edwin D. Robertson
Management:
　　Music Director: Lyndon Woodside
Mission: Dedicated to the performance of classical choral music. Most performances are given at Carnegie Hall which was built for the Society by its president Andrew Carnegie.
Founded: 1873
Specialized Field: Choral
Status: Non-Professional; Nonprofit
Paid Staff: 200
Performs At: Carnegie Hall
Organization Type: Performing; Touring; Resident; Educational

2233 PALA OPERA ASSOCIATION

200 Riverside Boulevard
PHZA
New York, NY 100690917
Phone: 212-874-7866
Fax: 212-769-0563
e-mail: elizabethfalk@usa.net
Officers:
　　President: Elizabeth Falk
　　VP: Martin Piecuch
　　VP: Richard Woitach
　　VP: Timothy Lindberg
Management:
　　Producer/Artistic Director: Elizabeth Falk
　　Music Director: Timothy Lindberg
　　Chief Music Consultant: Richard Woitach
　　Conductor: Matrin Piecuch
Mission: To offer high-calibre, ascending artists with professionalism and elegance, accompanied by a chorus and full orchestra; providing them the opportunity to be heard by discerning, paying audiences as well as critics.
Founded: 1989
Specialized Field: Grand Opera; Opera/Theater Combinations
Status: Professional
Paid Staff: 2
Budget: 75,000-100,000
Income Sources: Contibutors
Performs At: Town Hall; Players
Organization Type: Performing

2234 SHEILS-NA-GIG MUSIC

New York, NY 10009
Mailing Address: PO Box 2349
Phone: 212-260-2302
Fax: 212-260-9645
e-mail: sngmusic@earthlink.net
Web Site: www.sheilanagig.com
Management:
　　Director: Brandan Jamieson

2235 MATAPAT

517 County Highway 27
Richfield Springs, NY 13439
Phone: 315-858-1434
Fax: 315-858-1434
e-mail: info@onqueuartists.com
Web Site: www.onqueuartists.com
Management:
　　Founder/Agent: Sandra Bernegger
　　Administrative Assistant: Linda Van Slyke
　　Administrative Assistant: Frnaces Breslin
Mission: To perform the traditional music, song and dance of Quebec with contempoary and world music influences.
Founded: 1997
Specialized Field: Music and Dance of Quebec
Paid Staff: 3
Paid Artists: 3

2236 LAKE GEORGE OPERA FESTIVAL

480 Broadway
Suite 336
Saratoga Springs, NY 12866
Phone: 518-584-6018
Fax: 518-584-6775
e-mail: lgopera@aol.com
Web Site: www.lakegeorgeopera.org
Officers:
　　President: Robert C Miller
　　Business Manager: Patty Finnerty
Management:
　　General Director: William Florescu
　　Director Development: Roberta Ricci
　　Director Education: Betty Ramsbacher
Mission: To rpoduce the highest quality professional opera' develop the next generation of srtists through our Apprentice program' and to bring students the riches of the arts through our opera in the schools program.
Founded: 1962
Specialized Field: Opera
Paid Staff: 5
Paid Artists: 95
Budget: $800,000
Income Sources: Endowment; Individual Contributions; Tickets; Private/Public Grants
Performs At: Spac Little Theater; Saratoga Springs State Park
Affiliations: Opera America Professional Company Member
Annual Attendance: 16,000
Type of Stage: Modified Proscenium
Seating Capacity: 500
Cost: $22-$54

2237 SCHENECTADY LIGHT OPERA COMPANY

PO Box 1006
Schenectady, NY 12301-1006
Phone: 518-393-5732
Web Site: www.sloctheater.com
Officers:
President: Mellissa Jacijan
Secretary: Melinda Zarnoch
Treasurer: Mary Zarnoch
Management:
Business Manager: Joseph Concra
Mission: To present Broadway Musicals.
Founded: 1926
Specialized Field: Broadway Musicals
Status: Nonprofit
Affiliations: NYSTA
Organization Type: Performing

2238 CANTICUM NOVUM SINGERS

2 Cove Road
South Salem, NY np590-1023
Phone: 914-763-3453
Fax: 914-763-1998
e-mail: hrconductor1@aol.com
Web Site: www.csis.pace.edu/wos/
Officers:
Chairman: Robert Havemeyer
Vice President: Edie Rosenbaum
Management:
Artistic Director/Conductor: Harold Rosenbuam
Executive Director: Richard Pickett
Founded: 1973
Specialized Field: Music; Performance; Choral; Music
Paid Staff: 1
Non-paid Artists: 24
Budget: $21,000
Income Sources: Individuals; Tickets; Merchandise; Contracted Services; Contributions; Fund Raisers
Affiliations: In Residence at Bloomingdale School of Music
Annual Attendance: 1,500

2239 NEW YORK VIRTUOSO SINGERS

2 Cove Road
South Salem, NY 10590
Phone: 914-763-3453
Fax: 914-763-1998
e-mail: hrconductor1@aol.com
Web Site: www.nyvirtuoso.org
Officers:
Chairman: Robert Havemeyer
Vice President: Edie Rosenbaur
Management:
Artistic Director/Conductor: Harold Rosenbaum
Executive Director: Richard Pickett
Mission: To perform chamber choral works from all periods with a special emphasis on 20th century repertoire; to commission, perform and record premieres.
Founded: 1988
Specialized Field: Music; Choral Music; Performance
Status: Professional; Nonprofit
Paid Staff: 1
Paid Artists: 16

Budget: $55,000
Income Sources: Foundations; Corporation; Individuals; Tickets; Merchandise; Contracted Services
Performs At: Merkin Concert Hall
Annual Attendance: 3,000
Facility Category: Concert Halls, Churches
Organization Type: Performing

2240 WESTCHESTER ORATORIO SOCIETY

Box 6
South Salem, NY 10590
Phone: 914-763-3453
Fax: 914-763-3453
e-mail: bobmcdon@cs.com
Web Site: csis.pace.edu/wos/
Management:
Music Director/Conductor: Harold Rosenbuam

2241 SYRACUSE OPERA

PO Box 1223
Syracuse, NY 13201-1223
Phone: 315-475-5915
Fax: 315-475-6319
e-mail: info@syracuseopera.com
Web Site: www.syracuseopera.com
Management:
General Director: Catherine Wolff
Artistic Director: Richard McKee
Mission: To produce for the community professional opera performances of the highest quality promoting young talent from across the country and cultivate a further appreciation of opera within the region, specifically Syracuse and the surrounding six county area by means of outreach and educational programs.
Founded: 1974
Specialized Field: Grand Opera; Lyric Opera; Light Opera; Operetta
Status: Professional; Nonprofit
Paid Staff: 10
Budget: $1M
Income Sources: New York State Coucil on Arts; County of Onandaga; Natural Heritage Trust; Corporations; Foundations; Individuals
Performs At: Crouse-Hinds Concert Theater
Seating Capacity: 2,042
Organization Type: Performing; Touring; Resident; Educational

2242 TAGHKANIC CHORALE

PO Box 144
Yorktown Heights, NY 10598-0144
Phone: 914-737-6707
Web Site: taghkanicchorale.ontimeonline.com/
Officers:
President: Peter Hauge
VP: Pat Miller
Secretary: Sandra Strubbe
Treasurer: Dale Sharp
Management:
Music Director: Johannes Somary
Music Director: Dennis Keene
Mission: Preparation and performance of choral works with emphasis on quality and authenticity.
Founded: 1967

Specialized Field: Choral
Status: Semi-Professional; Nonprofit
Paid Staff: 100
Income Sources: Chorus America
Organization Type: Performing; Educational

North Carolina

2243 CAROLINA VOICES

1900 Queens Road
Charlotte, NC 28207
Phone: 704-374-1564
Fax: 704-372-8733
Web Site: www.carolinas.org
Management:
  Music Director: Jocelyn Thompson
  Music Director: Bob Pritchard
  Music Director: Bonnie Brown
  Music Director: Scott McKenzie
  Director: Jacqueline Robinson
Mission: To enrich and educate our community by sharing our passion for quality choral music and uniting the voices of all people in celebration of music, the international language of the soul.
Founded: 1956
Specialized Field: Choral Arts
Paid Staff: 10
Volunteer Staff: 1
Non-paid Artists: 175
Annual Attendance: 30,000

2244 CHARLOTTE PHILHARMONIC CHORUS

PO Box 470987
Charlotte, NC 28247-0987
Phone: 704-846-2788
Fax: 704-847-6043
Web Site: www.charlottephilharmonic.org
Officers:
  President: Deborah L Gould
Management:
  Choral Director: Marc S Setzer
Founded: 1994
Performs At: The Carriage Club of Charlotte

2245 OPERA CAROLINA

345 N College Street
Suite 409
Charlotte, NC 28202
Phone: 704-332-7177
Fax: 704-332-6448
e-mail: elaine@operacarolina.org
Web Site: www.operacarolina.org
Officers:
  Chairman: Philip W Norwood
  Chair Elect: Fred Lawrence
  Secretary: Emmy Lou Burchet
  Treasurer: Gerald P Carroll
Management:
  General Director: James Meena
  Director Marketing: Elaine Spallone
  Director Production: Steve Dellinger

Artistic Administrator: Chad Calvert
Mission: To inspire the region's diverse population through the presentation of excellent professional opera, operetta, music, theatre, and education and outreach programs that elevate the quality of life in the Carolinas.
Founded: 1948
Specialized Field: Opera; operetta; music theater
Status: Professional; Nonprofit
Paid Staff: 13
Paid Artists: 150
Budget: $2,500,000
Income Sources: Private Foundations/Grants/Endowments; Business/Coporate Donation; Government Grants; Individual Donations
Performs At: North Carolina Performing Arts Center
Affiliations: Opera America
Annual Attendance: 12,000
Facility Category: Performing Arts Center
Type of Stage: Proscenium
Stage Dimensions: 60'x43'
Year Built: 1970
Year Remodeled: 1992
Rental Contact: NC Performing Arts Center
Organization Type: Performing; Touring; Resident; Educational

2246 DURHAM CIVIC CHORAL SOCIETY

120 Morris Street
Durham, NC 27701
Phone: 919-560-2733
Web Site: www.choral-society.org
Officers:
  President: Dan Gunselman
  VP: Florence Nash
  Secretary: Celia Grasty Lata
  Treasurer: Lynn Wilson
Management:
  Publicity Chair: Rick Johnston
  Membership Chair: Nancy Team
  Development Chair: Rachel Steelman
  Conductor: Rodney Wynkoop
Mission: Our mission is to bring together persons who share a common interest in high-quality performance of significant choral literature, both sacred and secular.
Founded: 1949
Specialized Field: Choral
Status: Non-Professional; Nonprofit
Paid Staff: 154
Performs At: Duke University Chapel; Baldwin Auditorium
Organization Type: Performing

2247 CHORAL SOCIETY OF GREENSBORO

200 N Davie Street
Box 2
Greensboro, NC 27401
Phone: 336-373-2549
Fax: 336-373-2659
Web Site: www.greensboro.com/choral/
Management:
  Conductor: William Carroll
  Executive Director: Lynn H Donovan
Mission: Sharing musical understanding, appreciation, accomplishment and musicianship with the public.
Founded: 1984

Specialized Field: Choral
Status: Non-Professional
Paid Staff: 200
Income Sources: City of Greensboro; The Music Center
Performs At: Dana Auditorium
Organization Type: Performing

2248 GREENSBORO OPERA COMPANY

1828 Banking Street
Greensboro, NC 27408
Phone: 336-273-9472
Fax: 336-273-9481
Web Site: www.people-places.com/youthchorus/
Management:
   Administrator: Mary C Eubanks
Mission: Enhancing cultural life in the Greensboro area through developing and promoting a quality program of operas and education.
Founded: 1981
Specialized Field: Grand Opera
Status: Professional; Nonprofit
Income Sources: Opera America; Central Opera Service
Performs At: War Memorial Auditorium; Carolina Theatre
Organization Type: Performing; Educational; Sponsoring

2249 RALEIGH BOYCHOIR

1329 Ridge Road
Raleigh, NC 27607
Mailing Address: PO Box 12481, Raleigh, NC. 27605
Phone: 919-881-9259
Fax: 919-881-0971
e-mail: rbc@ipass.net
Web Site: www.raleighboychoir.org
Management:
   Founder/Director: Thomas E Sibley
Mission: To educate and train boys in the art of singing; to perform the finest music in the boychoir tradition; to contribute to musical life in the greater Raleigh area; and to enhance North Carolina's cultural reputation. The Raleigh Boychoir experience develops character, discipline, leadership, and a strong commitment to excellence.
Founded: 1968
Specialized Field: Music, Vocal
Paid Staff: 3
Volunteer Staff: 5
Paid Artists: 2

2250 TAR RIVER CHORAL & ORCHESTRAL SOCIETY

The Dunn Center 1200
PO Box 8255
Rocky Mount, NC 27804
Phone: 252-985-3055
Web Site: www.abouttroc.org
Management:
   Music Director/Conductor: Lorenzo Muti
   General Manager: Beth Kupsco

2251 PIEDMONT CHAMBER SINGERS

PO Box 10269
Winston-Salem, NC 27108
Phone: 336-722-4022
e-mail: mlevigne@piedmontchambersingers.org
Web Site: www.piedmontchambersingers.org
Officers:
   President: Ed Carlson
   VP: Martha Claire Henzler
   Secretary: Joe Crocker
   Treasurer: Ken Carpenter
Management:
   Director-Emeritus: Donald L Armitage
   Music Director: James Allbritten
Mission: Over the past two decades, PCS has gained a loyal following of supporters and patrons.
Founded: 1977

2252 PIEDMONT OPERA THEATRE

900 W 1st Street
Winston-Salem, NC 27101
Phone: 336-725-7101
Fax: 336-725-7131
e-mail: info@piedmontopera.org
Web Site: www.piedmontopera.org/
Officers:
   President: Guy Rudsill
   Treasurer: Gerard R Gunzenhauser
   Secretary: Clyde Fitzgerald
   VP Education: Margaret Kolb
   VP Education: Margaret Kolb
Management:
   Interim Manager: Rhonda Ozerman
Mission: To create and support consistently superior opera theatre productions and programs that ensure recognition of the company as an important community asset for entertainment and education, a force in city development, and a magnet attraction for regional and national audiences.
Founded: 1978
Specialized Field: Grand Opera; Lyric Opera; Light Opera; Operetta
Status: Professional; Nonprofit
Income Sources: Opera America; Central Opera Service; National Opera Association; Arts Council; Winston-Salem
Performs At: Roger L. Stevens Center for the Performing Arts
Organization Type: Performing; Resident; Educational

2253 WINSTON-SALEM PIEDMONT TRIAD SYMPHONY ASSOCIATION

610 Coliseum Drive
Winston-Salem, NC 27106
Phone: 336-725-1035
Fax: 336-725-3924
e-mail: mvale@wssymphony.org
Web Site: www.wssymphony.org
Officers:
   Operations/Stage Manager: Beverley Naiditch
   Financial Manager: Selina Carter
Management:
   Executive Director: E Merritt Vale
   Music Director: Peter Perret

All listings are in alphabetical order by state, then city, then organization within the city.

Director Marketing Development: William Cole
Box Office Manager: Tinay Jeffers
Mission: Presenting the finest symphonic as well as choral literature; providing high quality music education for Winston-Salem and Forsythe County children.
Founded: 1947
Specialized Field: Symphony; Orchestra; Chamber; Ensemble
Status: Professional; Nonprofit
Paid Staff: 9
Paid Artists: 80
Budget: $1.4 million
Income Sources: American Symphony Orchestra League; Broadcast Music Incorporated; American Society of Composers, Authors and Publishers; Association of Symphony Orchestras of North Carolina
Performs At: E. Stevens Center for the Performing Arts
Annual Attendance: 100,000
Seating Capacity: 1,380
Year Remodeled: 1985
Organization Type: Performing; Resident; Educational

North Dakota

2254 FARGO-MOORHEAD OPERA COMPANY

1104 2nd Avenue S
Suite 316
Fargo, ND 58103
Phone: 701-239-4558
Fax: 701-476-1991
Toll-free: 877-687-7469
e-mail: director@fmopera.org
Web Site: www.fmopera.org
Officers:
   President: Glenda Haugen
   VP: Larry Dorn
   Treasurer: Ardis Furham
   Secretary: Marv Degerness
Management:
   Executive Director: Rebecca Sundel-Schoenwald
Mission: To produce two operas a year, performing each twice.
Founded: 1968
Specialized Field: Grand Opera; Lyric Opera; Light Opera; Operetta
Status: Professional; Nonprofit
Paid Staff: 3
Paid Artists: 12
Budget: $268,250
Income Sources: National Endowment for the Arts; Alex Stern Family Foundation; Daytons Project Imagine; Cities of Fargo; Bush Foundation; Midnight Foundation; Moorhead FM Area Foundation
Annual Attendance: 3,600
Facility Category: Concert Hall
Organization Type: Performing; Touring; Educational
Resident Groups: Minnesota Association of Community Theatres, Lake Agassiz Arts Council, US Assoc. Community Theatre

2255 INTERNATIONAL MUSIC CAMP

1725 11th Street SW
Minot, ND 58701
Phone: 701-838-8472
Fax: 701-838-8472
e-mail: info@internationalmusiccamp.com
Web Site: www.internationalmusiccamp.com
Officers:
   President: Vern Gerig
   VP: Clifford Grubb
   Secretary: Roy Johnson
   Treasurer: Randy Hall
Management:
   Camp Director: Joseph T Alme
Mission: To develop a greater appreciation among students of all nations through their mutual interest in the arts.
Founded: 1956
Specialized Field: Band choral, Piano, Jazz (vocal and instrumental), Dance, Chamber Music, Orchestra (Full and Strings only) and visual Arts.
Status: Professional; Semi-Professional; Non-Professional; Nonprofit
Paid Staff: 250
Volunteer Staff: 25
Paid Artists: 150
Budget: $600,000
Income Sources: Camp Fees
Performs At: International Music Camp
Annual Attendance: 3,000
Facility Category: Open Auditorium; Performing Arts Center
Stage Dimensions: 60' x 100'
Seating Capacity: 2000; 500
Year Built: 1982
Year Remodeled: 1999
Cost: $1,500,000
Rental Contact: Joseph T Alme
Organization Type: Performing; Resident; Educational

Ohio

2256 CINCINNATI BOYCHOIR

1926 Mills Avenue
Cincinnati, OH 45212
Phone: 513-396-7664
Fax: 513-396-7664
e-mail: cincyboychoir@junco.com
Management:
   Music Director: Randall Wolfe
   Office Manager: Karen Stimpert
Mission: To provide high quality music, education, and performance opportunities to boys with unchanged voices and choral music to greater Cincinnati and other regions.
Founded: 1965
Specialized Field: Choral
Status: Nonprofit
Paid Staff: 2
Volunteer Staff: 10
Paid Artists: 2
Non-paid Artists: 110
Facility Category: Rehearsal Hall
Year Built: 1896
Organization Type: Performing; Touring; Resident; Educational

2257 CINCINNATI OPERA

1241 Elm Street
Cincinnati, OH 45210
Phone: 513-621-1919
Fax: 513-744-3520
Web Site: www.cincinnatiopera.com/2001
Management:
   Artistic Director: Nicholas Munilasis
   Managing Director: Patricia K Beggs
Mission: To provide opera to the Cincinnati and Tri-State Area.
Founded: 1920
Specialized Field: Grand Opera; Lyric Opera; Operetta
Status: Professional; Nonprofit
Paid Staff: 28
Income Sources: Opera America
Performs At: Music Hall
Organization Type: Performing

2258 CLEVELAND ORCHESTRA CHORUS

11001 Euclid Avenue
Cleveland, OH 44106
Phone: 216-231-7300
Fax: 216-231-0202
Officers:
   Chairperson: Margaret B Robinson
   The Cleveland Orchestra Chorus Oper:
Management:
   Director Choruses: Gareth Morrell
   Coordinator Choruses: Nancy Gage
   Librarian: Eleanor Kushnick
   Accompanist/Soloist: Joela Jones
   Assitant Accompanist: Betty Meyers
   Assitant Accompanist: Donald Shelhorn
Mission: To assist the Cleveland Orchestra in performing choral-orchestral works.
Founded: 1952
Specialized Field: Choral; Concert Opera; Pops
Status: Non-Professional; Nonprofit
Paid Staff: 170
Performs At: Severence Hall; Blossom Music Center
Organization Type: Performing; Touring; Resident

2259 LYRIC OPERA CLEVELAND

11300 Juniper Road
PO Box 06198
Cleveland, OH 44106
Phone: 216-231-2484
Fax: 216-231-5502
e-mail: lyric@en.com
Web Site: www.lyricoperacleveland.org/
Officers:
   President: Don Scippione
   President Guild: Becky Elliot
Management:
   Artistic Director: Johnathan Field
   Managing Director: Michael Radice
   Operations Director: Cliff Wilson
   Business Manager: Andrew Hawkins
Mission: To utilize talented artists from the North in music theatre productions; to uncover new ideas, fresh concepts and illuminating perspectives in every work it produces; to emphasize training opportunities for professional development.

Founded: 1974
Specialized Field: Lyric Opera; Light Opera; Operetta; Musical Theatre
Status: Professional; Nonprofit
Paid Staff: 4
Paid Artists: 30
Non-paid Artists: 2
Budget: $500,000
Income Sources: Tickets, Cleveland Foundation, Gund & Kyles
Performs At: Cleveland Institute of Music
Annual Attendance: 4,800
Facility Category: Professional Theatre
Type of Stage: Proscenium
Stage Dimensions: 30 X 40
Seating Capacity: 500
Organization Type: Performing; Resident; Educational; Sponsoring

2260 SAINT SAVA FREE SERBIAN ORTHODOX CHURCH

2151 W Wallings
Cleveland, OH 44147
Phone: 216-741-3002
Management:
   Director: Dragica Zamiska
Mission: To encourage and perpetuate Serbian music, dance, language, culture and heritage.
Founded: 1982
Specialized Field: Ethnic; Folk
Status: Non-Professional; Nonprofit
Income Sources: Saint Sava Free Serbian Orthodox Church; School Congregation; Cleveland Area Arts Council
Organization Type: Performing; Touring; Resident; Educational

2261 COLUMBUS SYMPHONY CHORUS

55 E State Street
Columbus, OH 43215
Phone: 614-228-9600
Fax: 614-224-7273
Management:
   Conductor: Ronald J Jenkins
   Assistant to Conductor: Lois Zook
Mission: To expose the public to great music.
Founded: 1960
Specialized Field: Choral
Status: Non-Professional; Nonprofit
Income Sources: Columbus Symphony Orchestra
Performs At: Ohio Theatre
Organization Type: Performing; Resident; Educational

2262 DAYTON OPERA ASSOCIATION

138 N Main Street
Dayton, OH 45402
Phone: 937-228-0662
Fax: 937-228-9612
Web Site: www.daytonopera.org
Officers:
   President: Mark Light
   Executive Director: Diane Kennedy
Management:
   Artistic Director: Thomas Bankston

Mission: To increase appreciation for opera through education; to present and promote opera of high quality to the Dayton region in balanced programs; to utilize international artists; to encourage local and regional artistic development.
Founded: 1960
Specialized Field: Grand Opera; Operetta; Musical Theatre
Status: Professional; Nonprofit
Paid Staff: 30
Budget: 1.3 million
Income Sources: Box Office; Grants; Private Donations
Performs At: Memorial Hall
Affiliations: Opera America; American Arts Alliance; Dayton Performing Arts Fund
Facility Category: War Memorial Theater
Type of Stage: Proscenium
Stage Dimensions: 58 x 36 x 26
Seating Capacity: 2,501
Year Built: 1902
Year Remodeled: 1953
Organization Type: Performing; Resident; Educational

2263 HAMILTON-FAIRFIELD SYMPHONY & CHORALE

101 S Monument Street
Fairfield Auditorium 950
Hamilton, OH 45011
Phone: 513-895-5151
Fax: 513-474-1584
e-mail: pstanbery@rml.net
Web Site: www.hfso.org
Management:
Music Director/Conductor: Paul Stanbery
General Manager: Rita Line

2264 LANCASTER CHORALE

PO Box 251
Lancaster, OH 43130
Phone: 614-569-4306
Web Site: www.lancasterchorale.com/
Officers:
President: Cathy Tolbert
Mission: To perform the finest choral literature, encompassing a wide range of styles, idioms and periods. The Chorale is characterized by its unique versatility, control, precision and blend.
Founded: 1985
Specialized Field: Choral
Status: Professional
Income Sources: Chorus America
Organization Type: Performing; Touring

2265 SORG OPERA COMPANY

65 S Main Street
PO Box 906
Middletown, OH 45044
Phone: 513-425-0180
Fax: 513-425-0181
e-mail: sorgopera@core.com
Web Site: www.sorgopera.org
Officers:
President: William Teager
VP: William Hilsmier

Secretary: Charles Robertson
Treasure: Paul Dirkes
Management:
General Director: Curtis Tucker
Administrative Assistant: Nicki Finkelman-Gividen
Marketing/Development Director: Charles Wente
Mission: To enrich the quality of life in the Miami Opera Valley through the presentation of exceptional productions, the development of cultural awareness through opera education and the encouragment of community pride and participation.
Founded: 1990
Paid Staff: 3
Paid Artists: all
Budget: $339,000
Performs At: Sorg Opera House
Affiliations: Opera America
Seating Capacity: 700

2266 OHIO LIGHT OPERA

College of Wooster
329 E University Street
Wooster, OH 44691
Phone: 330-263-2345
Fax: 330-263-2272
e-mail: OH_LT_OPERA@acs.wooster.edu
Web Site: www.wooster.edu/OHIOLIGHTOPERA/
Management:
Artistic Director: Steven Daigle
Music Director: J. Lynn Thompson
Founded: 1979
Specialized Field: Lyric theatre
Budget: $800,000
Income Sources: Private Donations, Ticket Sales
Performs At: Freedlander Theatre
Annual Attendance: 22,000
Seating Capacity: 394

Oklahoma

2267 CIMARRON CIRCUIT OPERA COMPANY

PO Box 1085
Norman, OK 73070
Phone: 405-364-8962
Fax: 405-364-8962
e-mail: ccoc@telepath.com
Web Site: www.ccocopera.org/
Management:
Artistic Director: Thomas Carey
Music Director: Lisa Anderson
Technical Director: Alan Parker
Mission: Offering training and experience to young Oklahoma singers; bringing opera to areas in Oklahoma where residents normally wouldn't have access to performances.
Founded: 1975
Specialized Field: Grand Opera; Lyric Opera; Light Opera; Children's Opera
Status: Professional; Nonprofit
Paid Staff: 5
Income Sources: Central Opera Service; Mid-America Arts Alliance

Performs At: Sooner Theatre; Holmberg Hall
Organization Type: Performing; Touring; Sponsoring

2268 CANTERBURY CHORAL SOCIETY
428 W California
#100
Oklahoma City, OK 73102-2454
Phone: 405-232-7464
Fax: 405-232-7465
e-mail: sing@canterburychoralsociety.org
Management:
    Executive Director: James B Hughes
Founded: 1969
Specialized Field: choral music
Paid Staff: 10
Non-paid Artists: 475

2269 OKLAHOMA OPERA AND MUSIC THEATER COMPANY
Oklahoma City University
2501 N Blackwelder
Oklahoma City, OK 73106
Phone: 405-521-5316
Fax: 405-521-5971
Toll-free: 800-633-7242
Web Site: www.okcu.edu
Management:
    Dean: Mark Edward Parker
Mission: Offering the public high quality performances; providing students with a professional arena in which to develop their talents.
Founded: 1904
Specialized Field: Grand Opera; Lyric Opera; Light Opera; Operetta; Choral
Status: Non-Professional; Nonprofit
Income Sources: Oklahoma City University
Performs At: Kirkpatrick Theater
Organization Type: Performing; Educational

2270 LIGHT OPERA OKLAHOMA - LOOK
Harwelden
2210 S Main
Tulsa, OK 74114
Phone: 918-583-4267
Fax: 918-583-1780
e-mail: eric@lightoperaok.org
Web Site: www.lightoperaok.org
Management:
    Artistic Director: Eric Gibson
    Artistic Director Emeritus/Founder: John Everitt
Mission: To preserve and create awareness of the musical comedy/operetta art form by producing a festival of such every summer in Tulsa, OK.
Founded: 1984
Specialized Field: Music Comedy; Operetta; Plays
Paid Staff: 3
Volunteer Staff: 10
Paid Artists: 100
Non-paid Artists: 10
Budget: $300,000-350,000
Income Sources: Foundations; Corporations
Performs At: University of Tulsa School of Theatre
Annual Attendance: 6000-7500
Seating Capacity: 375

2271 TULSA OPERA
1610 S Boulder
Tulsa, OK 74119
Phone: 918-582-4035
Fax: 918-592-0380
Web Site: www.tulsaopera.com
Officers:
    President: Scott Filstrup
    Chairman: Jonathan Helmerich
Management:
    General Director: Carol I Crawford
    Director Finance/Planning: Elena Jackson-Forsyth
    Director Operations: Amanda Foust
Mission: To produce opera of artistic integrity and enrich the regional community through innovative education and outreach programs.
Founded: 1948
Specialized Field: Grand Opera
Status: Professional; Nonprofit
Paid Staff: 15
Volunteer Staff: 100
Income Sources: Opera America; American Arts Alliance; Arts & Humanities Council of Tulsa
Performs At: Chapman Music Hall
Organization Type: Performing; Sponsoring

Oregon

2272 EUGENE OPERA
PO Box 11200
Eugene, OR 97440
Phone: 541-485-3985
Fax: 541-683-3783
e-mail: mail@eugeneopera.com
Web Site: www.eugeneopera.com
Officers:
    President: Guendolyn Griffith Lienallen
Management:
    Artistic Director: Robert Ashens
    Managing Director: Peter Geddeis
    Marketing/Public Relations Director: Karen Bednaiz
Mission: The production of opera.
Founded: 1976
Specialized Field: Grand Opera; Lyric Opera; Light Opera; Operetta
Status: Professional; Nonprofit
Paid Staff: 6
Volunteer Staff: 20
Budget: $800,000
Income Sources: Ticket Sales, Grants, Fund Raising
Performs At: Huh Center for the Performing Arts
Seating Capacity: 2,400
Year Built: 1982
Organization Type: Performing; Educational

2273 PORTLAND OPERA
1515 SW Morrison
Portland, OR 97205
Phone: 503-241-1407
Fax: 503-241-4212
e-mail: admin@portlandopera.org
Web Site: www.portlandopera.org
Management:

General Director: Robert Bailey
Founded: 1964
Specialized Field: Grand Opera; Lyric Opera; Light Opera; Operetta
Status: Professional; Nonprofit
Paid Staff: 50
Budget: $6.7 Million
Performs At: Portland Keller Auditorium
Affiliations: Opera America
Annual Attendance: 48,000
Facility Category: Auditorium
Type of Stage: Proscenium
Stage Dimensions: 30 x 60 x 43
Seating Capacity: 3,000
Year Built: 1917
Year Remodeled: 1967
Rental Contact: Lori Leyba Kramer
Organization Type: Performing; Touring; Resident

Pennsylvania

2274 MARY GREEN SINGERS

990 Old Huntingdon Pike
Huntingdon Valley, PA 19006
Phone: 215-572-5063
Fax: 215-884-5432
Officers:
   Music Director/Conductor: Mary Woodmansee Green
Mission: Tax-exempt, non-profit cultural and educational institution.
Founded: 1986
Specialized Field: Choral
Status: Semi-Professional; Nonprofit
Paid Staff: 1
Volunteer Staff: 6
Non-paid Artists: 150
Organization Type: Performing; Touring; Educational

2275 FULTON OPERA HOUSE

12 N Prince Street
PO Box 1865
Lancaster, PA 17608
Phone: 717-394-7133
Fax: 717-397-3780
e-mail: admin@athenfulton.org
Web Site: www.athenfulton.org
Officers:
   President: Ellen Groff
   VP: Philip R Wenger
   Secretary: Liz Habecker
   Treasurer: Ellie Aurand
Management:
   Managing Director: Rod McCullough
   Artistic Director: Michael D Mitchell
   Theatre Advancement: Deidre Simmons
Founded: 1852
Specialized Field: Musical; Theatrical Group
Status: Professional; Nonprofit
Budget: $2,100,000
Income Sources: Earned and Contributed
Performs At: Fulton Opera House
Annual Attendance: 100,000+
Facility Category: Theatre

Type of Stage: Proscenium
Seating Capacity: 684
Year Built: 1852
Year Remodeled: 1995
Architect: $9,500,000
Rental Contact: Managing Director Rod McCullough
Organization Type: Performing; Touring; Educational

2276 LANCASTER OPERA COMPANY

PO Box 8382
Lancaster, PA 17604
Phone: 717-392-0885
Fax: 717-392-5650
e-mail: info@lancasteropera.com
Web Site: www.lancasteropera.com
Management:
   Executive Council: Kelly Knouse
   Artistic Director: Scott Drackley
   Board President: Paul Fulmer
   Marketing Manager: Dianne Fussaro
Founded: 1951
Specialized Field: Opera
Status: Nonprofit
Paid Staff: 1
Volunteer Staff: 25
Non-paid Artists: 120
Budget: $130,000
Income Sources: Tickets; Grants; Annual Appeal; Corporate Funding
Performs At: Fulton Opera House
Annual Attendance: 5,000+
Facility Category: 150 year-old theater
Type of Stage: Proscenium
Seating Capacity: 684
Year Built: 1852

2277 ACADEMY OF VOCAL ARTS OPERA THEATRE

1920 Spruce Street
Philadelphia, PA 19103
Phone: 215-735-1685
Fax: 215-732-2189
e-mail: info@avaopera.org
Web Site: www.avaopera.org
Officers:
   President: Albert W Mandia
   VP: John A Nyheim
   VP: Laren Pitcairn
   VP: James McKee Ridgway
   VP: Conant Scott Rogers
   Secretary: Martha R Hurt
Management:
   Executive Director: K James McDowell
   Music Director: Christofer Macatsoris
   Director Marketing/Public Relations: Maryann Devine
Mission: To train young singers for international careers in opera, and present in operas and recitals.
Founded: 1934
Specialized Field: Opera
Paid Staff: 33
Non-paid Artists: 25
Performs At: Helen Corning Warden Theater; Academy of Music

Affiliations: N.A.S.M.
Seating Capacity: 180

2278 CHORAL ARTS SOCIETY OF PHILADELPHIA
1616 Walnut Street
Suite 711
Philadelphia, PA 19103
Phone: 215-545-8634
Fax: 215-545-8637
e-mail: info@choralarts.com
Web Site: www.choralarts.com
Management:
 Artistic Director: David J Tang
 Executive Director: Kim Shiley
 Assistant Conductor: Elizabeth Braden
Mission: The presentation of a choral and symphonic repertoire spanning all musical periods.
Founded: 1982
Specialized Field: Choral
Status: Professional; Nonprofit
Paid Staff: 140
Performs At: Mann Music Center; Academy of Music; Kimmel Center; Churches; Cathedrals
Organization Type: Performing; Touring; Educational

2279 LYRIC OPERA THEATRE STREET
1608 S Broad
Philadelphia, PA 19145-1509
Phone: 215-755-1288
Fax: 215-551-1444
e-mail: llotop@aol.com
Web Site: surf.2/llotop.com
Officers:
 President: AC Pugliese
 VP/Secretary: Margaret Kastle
Mission: To provide repertoire experience for deserving amateur, professional and semi-professional singers.
Founded: 1987
Specialized Field: Grand Opera; Lyric Opera
Status: Nonprofit
Paid Staff: 2
Volunteer Staff: 10
Paid Artists: 10
Non-paid Artists: 50
Budget: $35,000-$60,000
Organization Type: Performing; Educational

2280 MENDELSSOHN CLUB OF PHILADELPHIA
1218 Locust Street
Philadelphia, PA 19107
Phone: 215-735-9922
Fax: 215-573-3786
e-mail: mcchorus@philadelphia.libertynet.or
Web Site: www.libertynet.org
Officers:
 President: James B Straw
 Chairman: C Christopher Cannon
 Vice Chairman: Dennis Alter
 Vice Chairman: Sara A Cerato
 Vice Chairman: Laurie Wagman
 VP: Benjamin Alexander
 VP: Jack R Bershad

VP: Richard A Doran
VP/Treasurer: Albert E Piscopo
Management:
 Executive Director: Jack Mulroney
 Producing Artistic Director: Robert B Driver
 Marketing/Communications: Gary Gansky
 Production: Susan Ashbaker
Mission: Mendelssohn's Club's mission has been to challenge, enrich, serve and fulfill its singing members, patrons and audiences through the excellence of its performances.
Founded: 1874
Specialized Field: Choral
Paid Staff: 1
Volunteer Staff: 5
Paid Artists: 12
Non-paid Artists: 160
Budget: $222,000
Income Sources: Ticket Sales; Government and Foundation Grants; Individual Contributions
Performs At: Various: Symphony Halls to churches

2281 OPERA COMPANY OF PHILADELPHIA
Graham Building, 20th Floor
One Penn Square West
Philadelphia, PA 19102
Phone: 215-981-1450
Fax: 215-981-1455
Web Site: www.operaphilly.com
Officers:
 President: John P Mulroney
 Chairman: H Douglas Paxson
Management:
 General Director: Robert B Driver
 Marketing/Communications Director: Craig Robert Hamilton
 President: C Christopher Cannon
 Competition Director: Grey Nemeth
 Executive Director: John P Mulroney
 Director Development: Lisa Ketcham
 Chorus Master: Donald Nally
Mission: To present original productions of classical opera literature featuring renowned artists and promising young singers. OCP also sponsors the world's largest voice competition—the Opera Company of Philadelphia/Luciano Pavarotti International Voice Competition.
Founded: 1975
Specialized Field: Grand Opera
Status: Professional; Nonprofit
Income Sources: Opera America; Greater Philadelphia Cultural Alliance
Performs At: Academy of Music
Organization Type: Performing

2282 PHILADELPHIA GAY MEN'S CHORUS
1315 Spruce Street
Philadelphia, PA 19107-5601
Phone: 215-731-9230
Toll-free: 877-462-7464
e-mail: pgmchorus@juno.com
Web Site: www.pgmc.org
Management:
 Artistic Director: Elliot Jones

Mission: The Philadelphia Gay Men's Chorus is a diverse group of gay men and their supporters dedicated to continuing a tradition of excellence in the choral arts. Through our music and our presence we seek to improve the lives of our members, to touch the gay community, and to reach out to all people in the tri-state area.
Founded: 1981

2283 PHILADELPHIA SINGERS

1211 Chestnut Street
Suite 610
Philadelphia, PA 19107
Phone: 215-751-9494
Fax: 215-751-9490
e-mail: onfo@philadelphiasingers.org
Web Site: www.philadelphiasingers.org
Officers:
   President: Doralene Davis
   VP: Robert E Mortensen
   VP: Chef Fritz Blank
   Secretary: Michael M. Mills
   Treasurer: James K. Abel
Management:
   Executive Director: David Baney
   Music Director: David Hayes
   General Manager: Robert E Mortensen
   Office Administration: Matthew Seneca
Mission: To produce high quality choral music and offer opportunities for professional singers.
Founded: 1972
Specialized Field: Choral
Status: Professional
Paid Staff: 8
Volunteer Staff: 2
Paid Artists: 60
Non-paid Artists: 60
Performs At: Academy of Music; Church of the Holy Trinity
Affiliations: Resident Chorus of the Philadelphia Orchestra
Organization Type: Performing

2284 SINGING CITY

123 S 17th Street
Philadelphia, PA 19103
Phone: 215-569-9067
Fax: 215-569-9088
e-mail: info@singingcity.org
Web Site: www.singingcity.org
Officers:
   President: Robert H Holmes, MD
Management:
   Music Director: Jeffery Brillhart
Mission: Present choral music concerts, educational and community outreach programs.
Founded: 1948
Specialized Field: Choral Music
Paid Staff: 4
Volunteer Staff: 3
Budget: $235,000
Income Sources: Charitable Donations; Contracted Musical Engagements

2285 BACH CHOIR OF PITTSBURGH

425 6th Avenue
Suite 1220
Pittsburgh, PA 15219
Phone: 412-454-0800
Fax: 412-394-4280
e-mail: BACHCHOIR@aol.com
Web Site: www.artswire.org/bachoir
Management:
   Artistic Director: Dr. Brady R Allred
   Managing Director: Ellen Sheppard

2286 MENDELSSOHN CHOIR OF PITTSBURGH

PO Box 334
Pittsburgh, PA 15230-0334
Phone: 412-281-3310
Fax: 412-381-0739
e-mail: themcp@bellatlantic.net
Web Site: www.mendelssohnchoir.org/
Management:
   Music Director/Conductor: Robert Page
   Executive Director: Suzanne M Vertosick

2287 OPERA THEATER OF PITTSBURGH

PO Box 110108
Pittsburgh, PA 15232
Phone: 412-624-3500
Fax: 412-624-3525
e-mail: OperaTheatrePgh@netscape.net
Management:
   Founder: Mildred Posvar
   Director of Operations: Cynthia Kroneberg
Mission: To offer professional opera to people outside of metropolitan centers; to introduce opera to children; to nurture emerging professionals.
Specialized Field: Grand Opera; Children's Opera; Chamber Opera
Status: Professional; Nonprofit
Budget: $35,000-$60,000
Performs At: Byham Theatre; Hazlett theatre
Affiliations: Carnegie Mellon University
Seating Capacity: 1,200
Organization Type: Performing; Touring; Educational

2288 PITTSBURGH CLO

719 Liberty Avenue
Pittsburgh, PA 15222
Phone: 412-281-3973
Fax: 412-281-5339
e-mail: mail@pittsburgclo.com
Web Site: www.pitsburgclo.org

2289 PITTSBURGH CAMERATA

PO Box 81546
Pittsburgh, PA 15217
Phone: 412-421-5884
e-mail: gmluley@pittsburghcamerata.org
Web Site: www.pittsburgcamerata.org
Officers:
   Business Manager: Gail Luley
Management:
   Artistic Director: Rebecca Rollett

All listings are in alphabetical order by state, then city, then organization within the city.

Business Manager: Gail Luley

2290 PITTSBURGH CIVIC LIGHT OPERA

719 Liberty Avenue
Benedum Center
Pittsburgh, PA 15222
Phone: 412-281-3973
Fax: 412-281-5339
e-mail: mail@pittsburghCLO.org
Web Site: www.pittsburghclo.org
Management:
   Director Education/Outreach: Meredith Adams
   Artistic Director Outreach: Buddy Thompson
Mission: To perpetuate, preserve and create musical, light opera and drama productions for the cultural and educational enrichment of our audiences, primarily in Western Pennsylvania and, secondarily, the United States.
Founded: 1946
Specialized Field: Light Opera; Operetta
Status: Professional; Nonprofit
Income Sources: Musical Theater Works; National Musical Theater Network
Season: June - August
Performs At: Benedum Center for the Performing Arts
Seating Capacity: 2,837
Organization Type: Performing; Educational

2291 PITTSBURGH OPERA

801 Penn Avenue
Pittsburgh, PA 15222-3681
Phone: 412-281-0912
Fax: 412-281-4324
e-mail: info@pittsburghopera.org
Web Site: www.pittsburghopera.org
Officers:
   President: H Woodruff Turner
   Secretary: Gracia Sheptak
   Treasurer: Kenneth Brand
Management:
   General Director/VP: Mark Weinstein
   Artistic Director: Christopher Hahn
   Music Director: John Mauceri
Mission: To culturally enrich Pittsburgh and the tri-state area and to draw national and international attention to the region.
Founded: 1939
Specialized Field: Grand Opera
Status: Professional; Nonprofit
Paid Staff: 30
Volunteer Staff: 300
Paid Artists: 300
Budget: $7.5 Million
Income Sources: Ticket Sales; Contributions; Grants
Performs At: Benedum Center for the Performing Arts
Affiliations: Opera America
Annual Attendance: 39,000
Facility Category: Opera House/Multi-purpose Theatre
Type of Stage: Proscenium
Seating Capacity: 2,770
Organization Type: Performing

2292 PITTSBURGH CONCERT CHORALE

PO Box 252
Warrendale, PA 15086

Phone: 412-635-7654
Fax: 412-635-0583
e-mail: pccsing@nauticom.net
Web Site: www.pghconcertchorale.org/about.html
Officers:
   President: Donald Maragon
   VP: Susan Mancuso
   VP: Charles Morrissey
   VP: Steve Radr
Management:
   Founder: Dr. Clark Bedford
   Executive Director: Betty Snyder
Mission: To share the joy of fine choral music with exceptional volunteer singers of the community.
Founded: 1985
Specialized Field: Ensemble chorale
Status: Volunteer; Not-for-Profit; Tax-Emept
Paid Staff: 1
Paid Artists: 2
Non-paid Artists: 85
Budget: $18,500
Income Sources: Ticket Sales, Grants, Government, Individuals
Performs At: Orchard Hill Church; Ingomar Methodist Church; Jewish Commuknity Center
Affiliations: Chorus America, Greater Pittsburgh Arts Alliance, Northern Allegheny County Chamber of Commerce
Annual Attendance: 3200

Rhode Island

2293 RHODE ISLAND CIVIC CHORALE AND ORCHESTRA

33 Chestnut Street
Providence, RI 02903
Phone: 401-521-5670
e-mail: info@ricco.org
Web Site: www.ricco.org
Officers:
   President: Chester S Labedz, Jr
   First VP: Roberta Padula
   Second VP: Margaret Gidley
   Third VP: Herman Eschentacher
   Secretary: David T. Riedel
   Treasurer: Walter Hope, Jr
   Assistant Treasurer: Joseph A. Goldkamp
Management:
   Director/Conductor: Edward Markward
Mission: To provide artistic enrichment to the public and the singers through presentation of at least three concerts of major choral works per year. These concerts feature the singers of the chorale, along with professional orchestra and soloists
Founded: 1957
Specialized Field: Choral; Chamber
Status: Nonprofit
Paid Staff: 70
Performs At: Veterans Memorial Auditorium; Grace Church
Organization Type: Performing

2294 CHORUS OF WESTERLY
119 High Street
Westerly, RI 02891
Phone: 401-586-8663
Fax: 401-586-1370
e-mail: notes@chorusofwesterly.org
Web Site: www.chorusofwesterly.org
Officers:
  President: Emily Rinnegan
  VP: Gail Lewis
  Treasurer: J Austin Murphy
  Recording Secretary: Olive Tamm
  Corresponding Secretary: Anne Utter
Management:
  Music Director: George Kent
  Manager: Aurea Davis
Mission: To perform, with artistic intergrity, both the major classic works of the choral literature and new or lesser-known pieces of merit; to educate children and adults of diverse backgrounds in the appreciation, understanding, and performance of great music; to grow and develop steadily as an organization important to the cultural experiences of the region.
Founded: 1959
Paid Staff: 6
Non-paid Artists: 200
Budget: $600,000
Income Sources: Tickets; Conferance Fees; Gifts; Grants
Performs At: The Chorus of Westerly Performance Hall
Affiliations: Chorus America
Annual Attendance: 30,000
Facility Category: Historic Church Building
Seating Capacity: 440
Year Built: 1886
Year Remodeled: 1991
Rental Contact: Aurea Davis

South Carolina

2295 NEWBERRY OPERA HOUSE
Box 357
Newberry, SC 29108-0221
Phone: 803-276-5179
Fax: 803-276-9993
e-mail: nbyopera@aol.com
Web Site: newberryoperahouse.com
Management:
  Executive Director: Deborah Smith
Budget: $400,000-1,000,000
Stage Dimensions: 29'x25'
Seating Capacity: 426
Year Built: 1881
Year Remodeled: 1996
Architect: $5,500,000

Tennessee

2296 CHATTANOOGA BOYS CHOIR
4315-B Brainerd Road
Chattanooga, TN 37411

Phone: 423-622-3033
Fax: 423-622-1182
e-mail: cbchoir@vei.net
Web Site: www.chattanoogaboyschoir.com/
Management:
  Administrative Assistant: Linda A Smith
  Music Director: Ron Starnes
Mission: To offer comprehensive training that inspires boys to love and appreciate good music.
Founded: 1954
Specialized Field: Choral
Status: Professional; Nonprofit
Paid Staff: 11
Organization Type: Performing; Touring

2297 CHATTANOOGA SYMPHONY AND OPERA ASSOCIATION
630 Chestnut Street
Chattanooga, TN 37402
Phone: 423-267-8583
Fax: 423-265-6520
e-mail: csoa@chattanooga.net
Web Site: www.chattanoogasymphony.org
Management:
  Executive Director: John Wehrle
  Music Director: Robert Bernhardt
Founded: Symp
Specialized Field: Grand Opera; Lyric Opera; Light Opera; Operetta; Symphony
Status: Professional; Nonprofit
Paid Staff: 40
Budget: $60,000-$150,000
Income Sources: Tennesseans for the Arts; Opera America; American Symphony Orchestra League
Performs At: Tivoli Theatre
Seating Capacity: 1,680
Organization Type: Performing; Touring; Educational

2298 KNOXVILLE OPERA COMPANY
602 S Gay Street, Suite 700
PO Box 16
Knoxville, TN 37901-0016
Phone: 865-524-0795
Fax: 865-524-7394
e-mail: info@knoxvilleopera.com
Web Site: www.knoxvilleopera.com/
Officers:
  President: Joseph De Leese
  President Elect: Sammie Lynn Puett
  Secretary: Fuad Mishu
  Treasurer: Ruth Love
Management:
  General Director: Robert Lyall
  Business Manager: Ann Broadhead
  Production Manager: Don Townsend
Mission: To produce opera and musical theatre performances at current standards; to provide performance opportunities for developing American artists; to develop an appreciation for the art form through a program of opera education.
Founded: 1976
Specialized Field: Grand Opera; Lyric Opera; Light Opera; Musical Theatre
Status: Professional; Nonprofit

Paid Staff: 160
Income Sources: Opera America
Performs At: Civic Auditorium
Organization Type: Performing; Sponsoring

2299 LINDENWOOD CONCERTS

2400 Union Avenue
Memphis, TN 38112
Phone: 901-458-1652
Fax: 901-458-0145
e-mail: Chris.Nemec@lindenwood.net
Web Site: www.lindenwood.net
Management:
   Director: Gary Beard
   Producer: Chris Nemec
Mission: To present the musical arts in a setting of a church, as in 17th and 18th century Europe; to provide high quality cultural events at an affordable price.
Founded: 1979
Paid Staff: 2
Volunteer Staff: 50
Paid Artists: 15
Non-paid Artists: 95
Income Sources: Box Office and Benefactors
Affiliations: AGO; ACDA; Choristers Guild; Disciples of Christ
Annual Attendance: 1,000
Facility Category: Church Sanctuary with Pipe Organ and Grand Piano
Seating Capacity: 1,000
Year Built: 1966
Year Remodeled: 1996
Rental Contact: Chris Nemec
Resident Groups: Gary Beard Chorale; Lindenwood Chancel Choir

2300 NASHVILLE OPERA ASSOCIATION

3628 Trousdale Drive
Suite D
Nashville, TN 37204
Phone: 615-832-5242
Fax: 615-832-5243
e-mail: nashopera@nashvilleopera.org
Web Site: www.nashvilleopera.org
Management:
   Executive Director: Carol Penterman
   Company Manager: Lynn Newcomb
Mission: To present operatic productions to middle Tennesseeans.
Founded: 1981
Specialized Field: Grand Opera; Lyric Opera; Light Opera
Status: Professional; Nonprofit
Paid Staff: 14
Paid Artists: 60
Budget: $1.6 million
Income Sources: Contributed and Earned Income
Season: September - April
Performs At: Andrew Jackson Hall; Polk Theatre
Affiliations: Opera America
Annual Attendance: 13,000
Organization Type: Performing; Educational

2301 NASHVILLE SYMPHONY CHORUS

209 10 Avenue South
#448
Nashville, TN 37203
Phone: 615-255-5600
Fax: 615-255-5656
Web Site: www.nashvillesymphony.com/history/chorus
Management:
   Chorus/Musical Director: George Mabry

Texas

2302 ABILENE OPERA ASSOCIATION

PO Box 6611
Abilene, TX 79608
Phone: 915-676-7372
Fax: 915-690-6660
e-mail: YouSeeJane@aol.com
Web Site: www.abileneopera.com/
Management:
   Producer: Jane Guitar
Mission: To promote opera appreciation in West Texas by locally producing professional caliber grand opera and to foster local talent utilizing professional means.
Founded: 1980
Budget: $35,000-$60,000
Performs At: Paramount Theatre
Seating Capacity: 1,200

2303 AUSTIN LYRIC OPERA

901 Barton Springs Road
PO Box 984
Austin, TX 78767
Phone: 512-472-5927
Fax: 512-472-4143
Toll-free: 800-316-7372
e-mail: frontdesk@austinlyricopera.org
Web Site: www.austinlyricopera.org
Officers:
   Chairman: Paul Burns
   President: Betty King
Management:
   General Director: Joseph McClain
   Business Manager: Jeanne Lynch
   Marketing: David Burger
   Development: Gregory Perrin
   Public Relations: Molly Browning
Mission: To promote and support opera; to foster public awareness of opera as a fine art.
Founded: 1985
Specialized Field: Grand Opera; Lyric Opera
Status: Professional; Nonprofit
Budget: $5,000,000
Income Sources: Central Opera Service
Season: November, January, March
Performs At: University of Texas Performing Arts Center
Annual Attendance: 48,000
Facility Category: Concert Hall
Type of Stage: Proscenium
Seating Capacity: 2,872
Organization Type: Performing; Educational

2304 CHORUS AUSTIN
PO Box 204361
Austin, TX 78720
Phone: 512-719-3300
Fax: 512-719-3339
e-mail: info@chorusaustin.org
Web Site: www.chorusaustin.org
Officers:
Treasur/Secretary: Stephen Falky
Vice Chairman: Jerry Goodrich
Chairman: David Marks
Management:
Executive Director: Vicki Buterbauch
Artistic Director: Dr. Kenneth Sheppard

2305 BEAUMONT CIVIC OPERA
4350 Thomas Glen
Beaumont, TX 77706
Phone: 409-892-5408
e-mail: blackda@lub002.lamar.edu
Management:
Conductor: L Randolph Babin
Business Manager: Delores Black
Mission: Presenting fine musical productions in Southwest Texas and giving young performers opportunities.
Founded: 1962
Specialized Field: Grand Opera; Light Opera; Operetta; Musical Comedy
Status: Nonprofit
Budget: $35,000-$60,000
Income Sources: Opera America
Performs At: Julie Rogers Theatre for the Performing Arts
Seating Capacity: 1,775
Organization Type: Resident

2306 TEXAS A&M UNIVERSITY OPERA & PERFORMING ARTS
PO Box J-1
College Station, TX 77844-9081
Phone: 979-845-1661
Fax: 979-845-8043
e-mail: anne-black@tamu.edu
Web Site: www.opas.tamu.edu
Management:
Executive Director: Anne Black
Budget: $400,000-1,000,000

2307 DALLAS OPERA
8350 N Central Expressway
Campbell Center 1, Suite 210, LB 1-11
Dallas, TX 75206
Phone: 214-443-1043
Fax: 214-443-1060
e-mail: suzannec@dallasopera.org
Web Site: www.dallasopera.org
Officers:
President: Martin J Weiland
Management:
Music Director: Graeme Jenkins
Director Artistic Administration: Jonathon Pell
Mission: The Dallas Opera is an opera company committed to the presentation of opera at the international level. It enriches the community through performances of grand and chamber opera, operatic concerts, recitals and attendant education and community service programs.
Founded: 1957
Specialized Field: Grand Opera
Status: Professional; Nonprofit
Paid Staff: 30
Budget: $10,298,000
Performs At: Music Hall at Fair Park
Affiliations: Opera America; American Arts Alliance; Texas Arts Alliance
Annual Attendance: 79,754
Seating Capacity: 3,420
Rental Contact: Director of Production John Gage
Organization Type: Performing; Educational; Sponsoring

2308 DALLAS SYMPHONY CHORUS
Dallas Symphony Association
Meyerson Symphony Center
2301 Flora Street, Suite 300
Dallas, TX 75201
Phone: 214-871-4000
Fax: 214-953-1218
e-mail: dkrauss@dalsym.com
Web Site: www.dallassymphony.com
Officers:
Administrator: Donna Krauss
Management:
Director: David Davidson
Mission: Supporting the Dallas Symphony Association; performing major choral works in conjunction with the symphony.
Founded: 1978
Specialized Field: Lyric Opera; Light Opera; Operetta; Choral; Ethnic; Folk
Status: Nonprofit
Paid Staff: 3
Volunteer Staff: 1
Non-paid Artists: 240
Performs At: Meyerson Symphony Center
Organization Type: Performing; Touring; Resident

2309 TURTLE CREEK CHORALE
PO Box 190137
Dallas, TX 75219
Phone: 214-526-3214
Fax: 214-528-0673
Toll-free: 800-746-4412
Web Site: www.turtlecreek.com
Officers:
Chairman: Ken Morris
President: Kirk Bradford
VP: Chuck Swattn
Secretary: John Henrickson
Treasurer: Franklin Reed
Management:
Artistic Director: Dr. Timothy Seelig
Managing Director: David Mitchell
Artistic Operations: Graig Gregory

Mission: To enhance the musical and cultural lives of our audiences through the presentation of male choral music and other musical activities.
Founded: 1980
Specialized Field: Choral
Status: Non-Professional; Nonprofit
Paid Staff: 8
Non-paid Artists: 200
Performs At: Meyerson Symphony Center
Annual Attendance: 30,000
Facility Category: Concert hall
Seating Capacity: 1875
Year Built: 1990
Organization Type: Performing

2310 FORT WORTH OPERA ASSOCIATION

3505 W Lancaster Avenue
Fort Worth, TX 76107
Phone: 817-731-0833
Fax: 817-731-0835
e-mail: mail@fwopera.org
Web Site: www.fwopera.org
Officers:
　　President: Whit Smith
　　President, Opera Guild of Ft. Worth: Petra Grimes
Management:
　　General Director: Darren Woods
Mission: Cultivating and promoting the love and understanding of opera.
Founded: 1946
Specialized Field: Grand Opera; Lyric Opera
Status: Professional; Nonprofit
Paid Staff: 10
Budget: $2,700,000
Income Sources: Opera America; Arts Council of Fort Worth & Tarrant County; Private Foundations and Businesses.
Performs At: Bass Performance Hall
Affiliations: Opera America; Arts Council of Forth Worth and Tarrant County
Facility Category: Opera performance hall
Stage Dimensions: 57x65
Seating Capacity: 2,000
Year Built: 1999
Rental Contact: Paul Beard
Organization Type: Performing; Resident; Educational

2311 SCHOLA CANTORUM OF TEXAS

3505 W Lancaster
Fort Worth, TX 76107
Phone: 817-737-5788
Fax: 817-737-0835
e-mail: voicebox@flash.net
Web Site: startext.net/homes/schola
Management:
　　Director: Gary Ebensberger
　　Executive Director: Pamela Wood
Mission: To provide outstanding choral music at the Metroplex; to provide a performance outlet for singers.
Founded: 1962
Specialized Field: Choral
Status: Semi-Professional; Nonprofit
Paid Staff: 60
Performs At: Kimbell Art Museum; Irons Recital Hall
Organization Type: Performing

2312 TEXAS GIRLS' CHOIR

4449 Camp Bowie Boulevard
Fort Worth, TX 76107-3834
Phone: 817-732-8161
Fax: 817-732-4774
e-mail: tgc@texasgirlschoir.org
Web Site: www.texasgirlschoir.org
Management:
　　Founder/Executive Director: Shirley Carter
　　Admin. Assistant/Handbell Director: Debi Weir
Mission: To develop girls' lives through excellence in music; girls, ages 8-14, come from 30 different North Texas cities and participate in music and leadership training throughout the year.
Founded: 1962
Specialized Field: Choral; Ethnic; Folk
Status: Non-Professional; Nonprofit
Paid Staff: 9
Volunteer Staff: 50
Budget: $622,370
Income Sources: Semester Fees; Donations; Concerts; Performances; Fundraisers
Performs At: Concert Hall; Auditorium
Facility Category: Former church
Type of Stage: Full width of auditorium
Seating Capacity: 600
Year Built: 1949
Rental Contact: Debi Weir
Organization Type: Performing; Touring; Educational

2313 HOUSTON CHAMBER CHOIR

PO Box 53388
Houston, TX 77052-3388
Phone: 713-224-5566
Fax: 713-222-2412
e-mail: hcc@net1.net
Web Site: www.houstonchamberchoir.org/
Officers:
　　President: David Scott
Management:
　　Director: Robert L Simpson
　　Board of Director: David Scott
Founded: 1996
Specialized Field: Music
Paid Staff: 2
Volunteer Staff: 20
Paid Artists: 24
Affiliations: Chorus America

2314 HOUSTON GRAND OPERA

510 Preston
Suite 500
Houston, TX 77002
Phone: 713-546-0260
Fax: 713-247-0906
Web Site: www.houstongrandopera.org
Officers:
　　President: Harry Pinson
　　Executive Vice President: David Gockley
Management:
　　General Director: David Gockley
　　Music Director: Patrick Summers

Mission: To produce opera of consistent excellence offering nontraditional and innovative works; to develop new forms, new artists and new audiences.
Founded: 1955
Specialized Field: Grand Opera; Lyric Opera; Light Opera; Operetta
Status: Professional; Nonprofit
Volunteer Staff: y
Budget: $20,000,000
Income Sources: Donations
Organization Type: Performing; Touring; Resident; Educational

2315 HOUSTON MASTERWORKS CHORUS
3131 W Alabama
Suite 302
Houston, TX 77098-2031
Phone: 713-529-8900
Fax: 713-529-7325
e-mail: houmast@winstarmail.com
Web Site: www.choral.org/hmc
Officers:
   President: Larry Collmann
   VP: Bev Raney
   Treasurer: Jennifer Harvey
Management:
   Executive Director: Grace Blair
   Chorus President: Velma Gleason
Mission: Dedicated to the presentation of great choral music, and to the continuation of the choral society tradition.
Founded: 1986
Specialized Field: Choral
Paid Staff: 3
Volunteer Staff: 150
Paid Artists: 25
Non-paid Artists: 129
Budget: 344,000
Income Sources: Endowment; Foundations; Individual Contributions

2316 HOUSTON SYMPHONY CHORUS
615 Louisiana Street
Suite 102
Houston, TX 77002-2798
Phone: 713-743-3160
Fax: 713-807-7824
e-mail: hausmann@bayou.uh.edu
Web Site: www.choral.org/grou/hsc/
Management:
   Director: Dr. Charles Hausmann
   Chorus Manager: Marilyn Dyess
   Accompanist: Scott Holshouser
   Assistant Director: Betsy Weber
Founded: 1946
Specialized Field: Choral
Status: Non-Professional; Nonprofit
Paid Staff: 170
Income Sources: Chorus America
Performs At: Jesse H. Jones Hall for the Performing Arts
Organization Type: Performing; Resident

2317 IRVING CHORALE
3613 Northgate
#121
Irving, TX 75062
Phone: 972-257-1417
Fax: 972-257-1417
Web Site:
www.ci.irving.tx.us/Arts/13ArtsGroups/Choral/
Management:
   Artistic Director: Dr. Harrell Lucky
   Managing Director: Lita Strubhar

2318 LONGVIEW OPERA COMPANY
PO Box 1175
Longview, TX 75606
Phone: 903-757-3199
Fax: 903-757-3199
Web Site: www.longviewtx.com/LOC/default.html
Management:
   Artistic Committee: Wes Gomer
   Music Director: Scott York
   General Manager: Miki Parris
Budget: $35,000-$60,000
Performs At: Longview Community Center
Seating Capacity: 265

2319 MIDLAND-ODESSA SYMPHONY AND CHORALE
3100 LaForce Boulevard
PO Box 60658
Midland, TX 79711
Phone: 915-563-0921
Fax: 915-498-9251
e-mail: symphony@mosc.org
Web Site: www.mosc.org
Management:
   Executive Director: Jeannine Donnelly
   Music Director/Conductor: Nyela Basney
Mission: To offer residents of the Permian Basin symphonic, chamber and choral music.
Founded: 1962
Specialized Field: Symphony; Orchestra; Chamber; Ensemble
Status: Nonprofit
Paid Staff: 6
Volunteer Staff: 100
Paid Artists: 65
Budget: $670,000
Income Sources: Tickets; Grants; Donations
Affiliations: ASOL
Annual Attendance: 10,000
Organization Type: Performing; Educational

2320 SAN ANGELO SYMPHONY ORCHESTRA AND CHORALE
PO Box 5922
San Angelo, TX 76902
Phone: 915-658-5877
Fax: 915-653-1045
e-mail: mercyla@sanangelosymphony.org
Web Site: www.sanangelosyphony.org
Officers:
   President: Fred Key

VP: Doris Rousselot
Secretary: Johnell Vincent
Treasurer: Bill McKinney
Past President: Teady George
Management:
   Music Director/Conductor: Hector Guzman
   Executive Director: Mercyla Sheiburne
Mission: To further cultural advancement and enjoyment of symphonic music in the San Angelo area.
Founded: 1948
Specialized Field: Symphony
Status: Professional; Non-Professional; Nonprofit
Paid Staff: 140
Income Sources: Broadcast Music Incorporated; American Society of Composers, Authors and Publishers; American Symphony Orchestra League
Performs At: City Auditorium
Annual Attendance: 50,000
Seating Capacity: 1,590
Organization Type: Performing

2321 TWIN MOUNTAIN TONESMEN

PO Box 2711
San Angelo, TX 76902
Phone: 915-949-0608
Web Site: www.geocites.com/Broadway/Stage/3010/
Management:
   Director: Mark E Clark
Mission: To present Barbershop Singing in our area and compete in contests.
Founded: 1979
Specialized Field: Barbershop Quartet
Status: Non-Professional; Nonprofit; Charitable
Volunteer Staff: 38
Performs At: City Auditorium
Affiliations: Cultural Affairs Council; SOEBSQSA
Organization Type: Performing; Resident

2322 TEXAS BACH CHOIR

11 St Lukes Lane
San Antonio, TX 78209
Phone: 210-821-5382
e-mail: tbc@prontomail.com
Web Site: www.texasbachchoir.org
Officers:
   President: Mary Beth Garay
   VP: Katya Thompson-Cantu
   President Elect: Steve Matteson
   Secretary: Don Peterson
   Treasurer: Jim Harnish
Management:
   Music Director: Daniel Long
   Accompanist: John Moore
   Administrator: Samantha A Beer
Mission: The performance of classical sacred choral works of all periods, with emphasis on Baroque.
Founded: 1976
Specialized Field: Choral
Status: Semi-Professional; Nonprofit
Paid Staff: 36
Income Sources: Chorus America
Organization Type: Performing; Touring; Resident

2323 UTAH FESTIVAL OPERA COMPANY

59 S 100 W
Logan, UT 84321
Phone: 435-750-0300
Fax: 435-753-5856
Toll-free: 800-262-0074
e-mail: opera@ufoc.org
Web Site: www.ufoc.org
Officers:
   Chairperson: Melanie Raymond
   Vice-Chair: Ralph Binns
   Treasurer: Brent Nyman
Management:
   General Director: Michael Ballam
   Artistic Administrator: Lynn Jemison-Keisker
   Development Director: Lila Geddes
   Marketing/Communications Director: Darla Seamons
Mission: Bringing people together to share ennobling artistic experiences.
Founded: 1992
Specialized Field: Opera; Operetta; Musical Theater
Paid Staff: 76
Volunteer Staff: 1
Paid Artists: 116
Budget: $2 million
Income Sources: Box Office; Foundations; Endowment; Government Grants; Private Contributors
Performs At: Ellen Eccles Theatre
Affiliations: Opera America
Annual Attendance: 23,000
Facility Category: Theater
Type of Stage: Proscenium
Stage Dimensions: 36'x 35'x 25'
Seating Capacity: 1,110
Year Built: 1923
Year Remodeled: 1993
Organization Type: Performing; Educational

2324 ORATORIO SOCIETY OF UTAH

PO Box 11714
Salt Lake City, UT 84147
Phone: 801-572-7464
Fax: 801-572-9398
Web Site: reality.sgi.com/csp/osutah/
Mission: Performing oratorio music and engaging in cultural exchanges with other countries.
Founded: 1915
Specialized Field: Choral
Status: Semi-Professional; Nonprofit
Paid Staff: 250
Organization Type: Performing; Touring

2325 SALT LAKE MORMON TABERNACLE CHOIR

50 E North Temple Street
20th Floor
Salt Lake City, UT 84150
Phone: 801-240-3221
Fax: 801-240-4886
e-mail: jessopcd@ldschurch.org
Web Site: www.ids.org

Officers:
President: Mac Christensen
Manager: Brent R Peterson
Administrative Assistant: Herold Gregory
Spokesperson: Lloyd Newell
Management:
Director: Craig Jessop
Associate Director: Mack Willberg
Organist: Richard Elliott
Organist: John Longhurst
Organist: Clay Christiansen
Associate Director: Barlow Bradford
Mission: To serve as a public relations organization of The Church of Jesus Christ of Latter-day Saints performing in Salt Lake City and on tours, both national and international; to represent the Latter-day Saints Church and, at times, the United States of America.
Founded: 1847
Specialized Field: Choral
Status: Non-Professional; Nonprofit
Paid Staff: 9
Volunteer Staff: 23
Non-paid Artists: 360
Income Sources: Church of Jesus Christ of Latter-day Saints
Performs At: Mormon Tabernacle
Annual Attendance: 55,000
Seating Capacity: 6100
Year Built: 1867
Organization Type: Performing; Touring; Resident

2326 SALT LAKE SYMPHONIC CHOIR
PO Box 45
Salt Lake City, UT 84110
Phone: 801-272-1663
Fax: 801-278-3828
e-mail: gbettinson@excite.com
Web Site: www.saltlakesymphonicchoir.com/
Officers:
President: Greg Bettinson
VP: Ron Houston
VP Public Relations: George Redd
Management:
Manager: Greg Bettinson
Choral Director: George Welch
Mission: Presenting choral concerts world-wide.
Founded: 1949
Specialized Field: Choral
Status: Professional; Nonprofit
Non-paid Artists: 100
Organization Type: Performing; Touring

2327 UTAH OPERA COMPANY
50 W 200 S
Salt Lake City, UT 84101
Phone: 801-736-6868
Fax: 801-736-6815
e-mail: info@utahopera.org
Web Site: www.utahopera.org
Officers:
Chairman: William C Bailey
Management:
Managing Director: Leslie Peterson
General Director: Anne Ewers
Artistic Administator: Christopher McBeth

Mission: To offer quality productions featuring standard opera repertoire; to educate the community.
Founded: 1978
Specialized Field: Grand Opera; Light Opera
Status: Professional; Nonprofit
Paid Staff: 30
Budget: $4,500,000
Income Sources: Opera America; American Arts Alliance; Utah Arts Council; Salt Lake City Arts Council
Performs At: Capitol Theatre
Annual Attendance: 9,000
Facility Category: Capitol Theatre
Type of Stage: Proscenium
Seating Capacity: 1,835
Year Built: 1913
Year Remodeled: 1976
Organization Type: Performing; Resident; Educational

2328 UTAH SYMPHONY CHORUS
Department Of Music
David Gardner Hall
Salt Lake City, UT 84112
Fax: 801-581-5683
Toll-free: 888-901-7464
e-mail: Ed.Thompson@music.utah.edu
Officers:
President: Bennett P Peterson
Chairman: Tom McFarland
Management:
Music Director: Ed Thompson
Associate Director: Kelly Dehaan
Paid Staff: 5
Volunteer Staff: 10
Budget: 55,000
Income Sources: Performances fees; Fundrasiers
Affiliations: Utah Symphony Orchestra

Vermont

2329 BRATTLEBORO MUSIC CENTER
36 Walnut Street
Brattleboro, VT 05301
Phone: 802-257-4523
Fax: 802-254-7355
e-mail: info@bmcvt.org
Web Site: www.bmcvt.org
Officers:
President: Beth-Ann Betz
Management:
Artistic Director: Blanche Honegge Moyse
Managing Director: Zon Eastes
Mission: To perform the music of J.S. Bach as the resident choral ensemble of the New England Bach Festival; to tour with programs of a cappella works from all periods.
Founded: 1976
Specialized Field: Choral
Status: Non-Professional; Nonprofit
Paid Staff: 36
Performs At: Persons Auditorium; Marlboro College
Organization Type: Performing; Touring; Resident

2330 NORTH COUNTRY CHORUS

PO Box 184
Wells River, VT 05081
Phone: 802-748-5027
Web Site: www.northcountrychorus.org
Officers:
   President: Marilyn Dempsey
Management:
   Music Director: Alan Rowe
Mission: To enrich the musical lives of North Country Area residents; to offer participation to anyone who loves singing.
Founded: 1948
Specialized Field: Choral
Status: Semi-Professional; Nonprofit
Season: June - August
Organization Type: Performing; Touring; Resident

Virginia

2331 OPERA THEATRE OF NORTHERN VIRGINIA

2700 S Lang Street
Arlington, VA 22206
Phone: 703-528-1433
Fax: 703-812-5039
Web Site: www.members.aol.com/lziluca/otnv.htm
Officers:
   VP/Production: Virginia D Martin
Management:
   Artistic Director/Conductor: John Edward Niles
Mission: To provide affordable opera in English to the Northern Virginia and Greater Metropolitan Washington Area; to sponsor educational programs and performances geared to young audiences; to provide stage experience.
Founded: 1961
Specialized Field: Grand Opera; Light Opera
Status: Professional; Nonprofit
Income Sources: Opera America; Cultural Alliance of Greater Washington
Performs At: Thomas Jefferson Community Theatre
Organization Type: Performing; Resident

2332 VIRGINIA CHORAL SOCIETY

Warwick Station
PO Box 1131
Newport News, VA 23601
Phone: 757-851-9114
e-mail: marketing@vachoralsociety.org
Web Site: www.vachoralsociety.org
Officers:
   Secretary: Ruth Sacks
   Treasurer: Al Schweizer II
Management:
   Director Of Programming: Charles Bump
   Managing Director: Charles Bump
   Acting Director Of Marketing: Jerry Cranfill
   Director Of Personnel: Victor Hollingsworth
   VCS Chorus President: William Tew
   Artistic Director: James Powers

Mission: The goal of the Virginia Choral Society is to foster a broader awareness of vocal music in the community; cooperate with other groups in support of the arts; and continue our long tradition of presenting only the finest compositions from our rich choral heritage.
Founded: 1931
Specialized Field: Choral
Status: Nonprofit
Paid Staff: 90
Organization Type: Performing

2333 VIRGINIA OPERA

160 E Virginia Beach Boulevard
Norfolk, VA 23501
Mailing Address: PO Box 2580, Norfolk, VA 23501
Phone: 757-623-1223
Fax: 757-622-0058
Toll-free: 866-003-7282
e-mail: press@vaopera.com
Web Site: www.vaopera.org
Officers:
   President: John Turbyfil
Management:
   Artistic Director: Peter Mark
   Executive Director: Keith Stava
   Production Manager: John Kenmelley
   Development Director: John Paul Schaefer
   Marketing Director: Lisa Jardanhazy
Mission: Mission is to create high quality productions of a broad range of opera.
Founded: 1974
Specialized Field: Opera
Status: Professional; Nonprofit
Budget: $6.5 million
Income Sources: Cultural Arts Alliance of Greater Hampton Roads; Opera America; American Arts Alliance; Patrons; Donors; Corporations; Grants
Performs At: Harrison Opera House; Carpenter Center; GMU
Organization Type: Performing; Touring; Educational

2334 VIRGINIA SYMPHONY CHORUS

880 N Military Highway
Suite 1064
Norfolk, VA 23502
Phone: 757-466-3060
Fax: 757-466-3046
e-mail: VSCSinger@aol.com
Web Site: www.virginiasymphony.org
Management:
   Chorus Master: Robert Shoup
   Chorus Manager: Dan Kooken
   Executive Director: David Gaylin
Mission: To perform symphonic choral repertoire.
Founded: 1990
Specialized Field: Choral Music

2335 OPERA ROANOKE

541 Luck Avenue
Suite 209
Roanoke, VA 24065

Phone: 540-982-2742
Fax: 540-982-3601
e-mail: mail@operaroanoke.org
Web Site: www.operaroanoke.org
Officers:
   President: Dana Maritn
   VP: Joseph Logan III
   Treasurer: Charles Troland
   Secretary: Mary Evelyn Tielking
Management:
   Artistic Director: Craig Fields
   Executive Director: Bill Krause
Mission: Providing Southwestern Virginia with professional opera.
Founded: 1977
Specialized Field: Grand Opera; Light Opera; Operetta
Status: Professional
Paid Staff: 4
Budget: $500,000
Income Sources: Box Office; Grants; Individual Donations
Performs At: Shaftman Performance Hall
Facility Category: Performance Hall
Type of Stage: Proscenium
Seating Capacity: 950
Year Remodeled: 2000
Cost: $9.5 Million
Organization Type: Performing; Resident

2336 WOLF TRAP OPERA COMPANY
1624 Trap Road
Vienna, VA 22182-2063
Phone: 703-255-1935
Fax: 703-255-1924
e-mail: wtoc@wolf-trap.org
Web Site: www.wolf-trap.org
Management:
   General Director: Kim Pensinger Witman
   Administrative Director: Lisa Ostrich
Founded: 1971
Specialized Field: Opera
Performs At: Barns of Wolf Trap; Filene Center
Seating Capacity: 350; 7,000

Washington

2337 CHASPEN OPERA THEATRE
27819 NE 49th Street
Redmond, WA 98053
Phone: 425-880-6035
Fax: 425-880-6035
e-mail: chaspen@aol.com
Web Site: www.hometown.aol.com/chaspen
Management:
   Music Director: Charles Long
Mission: To foster an appreciation of the musical arts in Seattle's Eastside communities, by producing top-quality, locally-accessible professional performances. To that end, the Foundation sponsors three first-rate ensembles.
Budget: $35,000-$60,000
Performs At: Bellevue Meydenbauer Theatre
Seating Capacity: 450 - 1,200

2338 ESOTERICS
1426 Harvard Avenue
#327
Seattle, WA 98122
Phone: 206-344-3327
Fax: 206-344-3327
e-mail: info@theesotemis.org
Web Site: www.theesoterics.org
Management:
   Executive Director: Eric Banks
   Production: Jacob Hunter
Mission: Contemporary a cappella art music.
Founded: 1993
Status: Nonprofit
Paid Staff: 1
Volunteer Staff: 1
Paid Artists: 4

2339 ORCHESTRA SEATTLE & SEATTLE CHAMBER SINGERS
1305 4th Avenue
Suite 402
Seattle, WA 98101
Phone: 206-682-5208
e-mail: osscs@osscs.org
Web Site: www.osscs.org
Management:
   Music Director: George Shangrow
   Executive Director: Leif-Ivar Pedersen
Founded: 1969
Specialized Field: Classical Music
Status: Nonprofit
Paid Staff: 10

2340 TACOMA OPERA ASSOCIATION
PO Box 7468
Tacoma, WA 98406
Phone: 235-627-7789
Fax: 253-627-1620
e-mail: info@tacomaopera.com
Web Site: www.tacomaopera.com
Officers:
   President: Sue Stibbe
   VP: Wendy Phillips
   VP: Heidi Madson
   Treasurer: Catherine Adams
   Secretary: Mickey Kramer
Management:
   Executive Director: Rod Gideons
   Artistic Director: David Bartholomew
Mission: To offer residents of the South Puget Sound area light opera performed in English.
Founded: 1968
Specialized Field: Opera
Status: Professional
Paid Staff: 4
Volunteer Staff: 4
Paid Artists: 100
Budget: $500,000
Performs At: Pantages Theater; Railto Theater
Affiliations: Opera America
Annual Attendance: 7,200
Facility Category: Renovated Vaudeville House
Type of Stage: Proscenium

Seating Capacity: 1,166
Year Built: 1920
Year Remodeled: 1983
Organization Type: Performing

West Virginia

2341 CHARLESTON CIVIC CHORUS

PO Box 2014
Charleston, WV 25327
Phone: 304-744-5078
Fax: 304-747-5448
e-mail: thedaltons@yahoo.com
Web Site: www.geocities.com/charleston_civic_chorus/
Officers:
President: C Conrad Haskell
VP: Michael W Lilly
Treasurer: Evan Buck
Management:
Music Director: J Truman Dalton
Mission: To perform high-quality choral classics as well as some lighter fare.
Founded: 1952
Specialized Field: Choral
Status: Non-Professional; Nonprofit
Performs At: The Baptist Temple
Organization Type: Performing; Resident

2342 WEST VIRGINIA SYMPHONY CHORUS

PO Box 2292
Charleston, WV 25304
Phone: 304-357-4903
Fax: 304-357-4715
e-mail: jjanisch@uchaswv.edu
Web Site: www.newwave.net/~wvso/chorus.htm
Management:
Director: Dr. Joseph Janisch

Wisconsin

2343 PAMIRO OPERA COMPANY

115 S Jefferson Street
#301-A
Green Bay, WI 54301-4534
Phone: 920-437-8331
Fax: 920-437-8352
e-mail: info@pamiro.org
Web Site: www.pamiro.org
Management:
Artistic/Musical Director: Miroslav Pansky
Managing Director: Eric T Strelow
Development Specialist: Edith Valentina
Founded: 1984
Paid Staff: 3
Budget: $200,000-$400,000
Performs At: Wiedner Center for the Performing Arts
Affiliations: Opera America
Seating Capacity: 2,019

2344 MADISON OPERA

333 Glenway Street
Madison, WI 53711
Phone: 608-238-8085
Fax: 608-233-3431
e-mail: stanke@madisonopera.org
Web Site: www.madisonopera.org/main.htm
Officers:
President: Karen Walsh
VP: Paul Shain
Secretary: Jo Greenhalgh
Treasurer: J Marshall Osborn
Management:
General Director: Ann Stanke
Director Development: Susan Buzby
Mission: To bring quality opera, locally produced, to the city of Madison.
Founded: 1962
Specialized Field: Grand Opera
Status: Professional; Nonprofit
Paid Staff: 10
Volunteer Staff: 25
Paid Artists: 175
Budget: $900,000
Income Sources: Opera America
Performs At: Oscar Meyer Theatre
Organization Type: Performing; Educational

2345 OPERA FOR THE YOUNG

6441 Enterprise Lane
Suite #207
Madison, WI 53719
Phone: 608-277-9560
Fax: 608-277-9570
e-mail: information@operafortheyoung.org
Web Site: www.operafortheyoung.org
Management:
General Director: David O'Dell
Artistic Director: Diane Garton Edie
Music Director: Jeffrey Sykes
Operations Director: Catherine McKenzie
Mission: To engage and educate children about opera with professional, affordable school-based performances; to involve students in performance and production; to provide professional opportunities for emerging artists; and to foster the creation of new operatic work expressly intended for young audiences.
Founded: 1970
Specialized Field: Opera
Status: Semi-Professional; Nonprofit
Paid Staff: 4
Paid Artists: 16
Budget: $235,000
Income Sources: School Fees; Grants
Performs At: Tour to elementary schools
Annual Attendance: 80,000
Organization Type: Performing; Touring; Educational

2346 BEL CANTO CHORUS

3195 S Superior Street
Milwaukee, WI 53207

Phone: 414-481-8801
Fax: 414-481-8807
e-mail: info@belcanto.org
Web Site: www.belcanto.org
Officers:
    President: Sally D Hoyt
    Treasurer: Susan R Connor
    Secretary: Adam J Wiensch
Management:
    Music Director: Richard Hynson
    Managing Director: Sarah Schwab
Mission: To enrich its members, its audiences and the community through the outstanding presentation of the finest choral music that appeals to the head and the heart.
Founded: 1931
Paid Staff: 3
Volunteer Staff: 10
Paid Artists: 12
Non-paid Artists: 140
Budget: $400,000
Performs At: Churches; Performing Arts Centers
Affiliations: Chorus America, UPAF
Facility Category: Various

2347 FLORENTINE OPERA COMPANY
700 N Water Street
Milwaukee, WI 53202
Phone: 414-291-5700
Fax: 414-291-5706
Toll-free: 800-320-7372
e-mail: info@florentineopera.org
Web Site: www.florentineopera.org
Management:
    General Director/Artistic Director: Dennis Hanthorn
    Director Marketing/Education: Ellen Hayward
    Director Production: Noele Stollmack
    Director Development: Ellen Lang
    Director Finance: Catherine Krekhofer
Mission: Producing Grand Opera for Wisconsin.
Founded: 1932
Specialized Field: Grand Opera
Status: Professional; Nonprofit
Paid Staff: 15
Paid Artists: 175
Budget: $3.7 million
Income Sources: Private foundations; Grants; Endowments; Business/Corporate Donations; Government grants; Individual donation
Performs At: Marcus Center for the Performing Arts
Affiliations: Opera America; Downtown Theatre District; UPAF
Annual Attendance: 23,000 - 24,000
Seating Capacity: 2,219
Organization Type: Performing; Touring; Educational

Alabama

2348 AUBURN UNIVERSITY THEATRE
Department of Theatre
School of Fine Arts, Auburn University
Auburn, AL 36849
Phone: 334-844-4748
Fax: 334-844-4939
Web Site: www.auburn.edu
Officers:
  Department Chair: Ralph E Miller
Budget: $3,000-5,000
Affiliations: NAST; ATHE
Seating Capacity: 370
Year Built: 1973

2349 BIRMINGHAM CHILDREN'S THEATRE
2130 Richard Arrington Jr Boulevard N
Birmingham, AL 35203
Mailing Address: PO Box 1362
Phone: 205-458-8181
Fax: 205-458-8895
e-mail: BERTB@BCT123.org
Web Site: www.BCT123.org
Officers:
  President: Clark Gillespy
  First VP: Robert M Lee
  Second VP: Betty McMahon
  Third VP: W. Wheeler Smith, Esquire
  Secretary: Larry Contri
  Treasurer: Jean P. Pierce
Management:
  Managing Director: Bert Brosowsky
  Associate Artisitic Director: Joe Zellner
  School Groups Coordinator: Teresa Shepperd
  Tour Coordinator: Darrell Revel
Mission: The Birmingham Children's Theatre is a
professional company providing quality theatre for young
people which incorporates literature, art, music and drama
into a medium that is both entertaining and educational.
Founded: 1947
Specialized Field: Theatrical Group
Status: Professional; Nonprofit
Paid Staff: 25
Paid Artists: 50
Budget: $1,425,0000
Income Sources: City, County, State, grants; Corporate;
Indiviuals, Ticket sales; Tour revenue
Performs At: Civic Center Theatre; Black Box; Studio
Theatre
Annual Attendance: 450,000
Facility Category: Civic Convention Center
Type of Stage: Flex Trust
Stage Dimensions: 140'w x 60'd
Seating Capacity: 250 - 1,100
Year Built: 1974
Year Remodeled: 1997
Organization Type: Performing; Touring; Resident;
Educational; Sponsoring

2350 GARDEN VARIETY SHAKESPEARE
Birmingham Botanical Gardens
2126 Lane Park Road
Birmingham, AL 35226
Mailing Address: PO Box 531034, Birnigham, AL.
35253
Phone: 205-879-1227
Web Site: www.thetre-resources.net/al.html

2351 UNIVERSITY OF ALABAMA, BIRMINGHAM: DEPARTMENT OF THEATRE
Department of Theatre
101 Bell Building, Univ. of AL-Birmingham
Birmingham, AL 35294
Phone: 205-934-3236
Fax: 205-934-8076
Toll-free: 800-421-8743
Web Site: www.uabtheatre.bhawn.net
Officers:
  Chair: Marc Powers
Budget: $7,000-25,000
Seating Capacity: 350
Year Built: 1999

2352 SOUTHEAST ALABAMA COMMUNITY THEATRE
PO Box 6065
Dothan, AL 36303
Phone: 334-794-0400
Web Site: www.downtown.ala.net/~seact
Management:
  Business Manager: Connie Miller
  General Manager: Marge Wein
Mission: To provide Southeast Alabama with performing
theatre.
Founded: 1974
Specialized Field: Summer Stock; Community
Status: Non-Professional; Nonprofit
Performs At: Dothan Opera House
Organization Type: Performing

2353 LOONEY'S TAVERN PRODUCTIONS
22400 Highway 278 E
Double Springs, AL 35553
Phone: 205-489-5000
Fax: 205-489-3500
Toll-free: 800-566-6397
e-mail: info@looneystavern.com
Web Site: www.looneystavern.com
Officers:
  President/CEO: Dwain Moody
Mission: To produce live performances of stage plays to
include drama, comedy, musical.
Founded: 1989
Specialized Field: Live Performance
Status: Non-Equity
Paid Staff: 8
Volunteer Staff: 10
Paid Artists: 50
Budget: $500,000
Income Sources: Sales
Season: Year-round
Performs At: Amphitheater; Indoor Theatre
Annual Attendance: 25,000
Type of Stage: Amphitheatre; Theatre
Stage Dimensions: 90'x 40'

Seating Capacity: 1500; 275
Rental Contact: President/CEO Dwain Moody

2354 UNIVERSITY OF NORTH ALABAMA: DEPARTMENT OF COMMUNICATIONS & THEATRE

Florence, AL
Mailing Address: PO Box 5007, University of North Alabama, Florence, AL 35632
Phone: 256-765-4247
Fax: 256-765-4839
Web Site: www.una.edu
Budget: $2,500-12,000
Seating Capacity: 1700
Year Built: 1969

2355 BROADWAY THEATRE

700 Monroe Street
Huntsville, AL 35801
Phone: 256-518-6155
Fax: 256-551-2990
e-mail: jwarren@btleague.org
Web Site: www.btleague.org
Management:
    Director: Jean S Warren

2356 SAENGER THEATRE

6 Joachim Street S
Mobile, AL 36602
Phone: 334-438-5686
Fax: 334-433-2087
e-mail: mike@mobilesaenger.com
Web Site: www.mobilesaenger.com
Management:
    General Manager: Mihael D Maxwell

2357 UNIVERSITY OF SOUTH ALABAMA

Department of Dramatic Arts
PAC 1052
Mobile, AL 36688
Phone: 334-460-6305
Fax: 334-461-1511
Web Site: www.southalabama.edu
Officers:
    Department Chair: Dr. Eugene R Jackson
Budget: $17,000-23,000
Affiliations: ATHE; Alabama Lyric Theatre
Seating Capacity: 180; 800
Year Built: 1999

2358 UNIVERSITY OF MONTEVALLO: DIVISION OF THEATRE

Montevallo, AL
Mailing Address: Box 6210, Univ. of Montevallo, Montevallo, AL 35115
Phone: 205-665-6210
Fax: 205-665-6211
Web Site: www.montevallo.edu/thea
Management:
    Director of Theatre: Luke Hart
Budget: $4,000-19,000
Seating Capacity: 1200

Year Built: 1931
Year Remodeled: 1978

2359 AUVURN UNIVERSITY MONTGOMERY THEATRE

Department of Communication and Dramatic Arts
Montgomery, AL 36124
Mailing Address: PO Box 244023
Phone: 334-244-3379
Fax: 334-244-3740
Management:
    Department Head: Dr. Robert A Gaines
Budget: $2,000
Affiliations: Alabama Shakespeare Festival
Seating Capacity: 180
Year Built: 1979

2360 UNIVERSITY OF ALABAMA, TUSCALOOSA: DEPARTMENT OF THEATRE AND DANCE

Tuscaloosa, AL
Mailing Address: Box 870239, Tuscaloosa, AL 35487
Phone: 205-348-5283
Fax: 205-348-9048
Toll-free: 800-933-2222
Web Site: www.as.ua.edu/theatre
Officers:
    Chair: Dr. Edmund Williams
Affiliations: NAST; U/RTA; Alabama Shakespeare Festival
Seating Capacity: 338
Year Built: 1958

Alaska

2361 ANCHORAGE COMMUNITY THEATRE

1133 E 70th Avenue
Anchorage, AK 99518-2353
Phone: 907-344-4713
Web Site: www.home.gci.net/~acthome
Management:
    Managing Director: Patty Star
Specialized Field: Theatrical Group
Status: Semi-Professional

2362 ECCENTRIC THEATRE COMPANY

413 D Street
Anchorage, AK 99501
Phone: 907-274-2599
Fax: 907-277-4698
e-mail: cyrano@ak.net
Web Site: www.cyrano.org
Management:
    Producer: Sandy Harper
Founded: 1992
Specialized Field: Theatre Company
Performs At: Cyrano's Off Center Playhouse
Type of Stage: Black Box
Seating Capacity: 86

2363 OUT NORTH CONTEMPORARY ART HOUSE
1325 Primrose
Anchorage, AK 99508-3000
Phone: 907-279-8099
Fax: 907-279-8100
e-mail: jay@outnorth.org
Web Site: www.outnorth.org
Officers:
   President: Rev. Dianne O'Connell
Management:
   Programs Director: Gene Dugan
   Project Director: Jay Brause
Mission: Out North exists to develop and present bold new work that challenges and changes the art, the artist, and the audience. We encourage artistic risk-taking and collaboration, examining today's world through diverse culturel perspectives, and creative community through the arts.
Founded: 1985
Specialized Field: Visual Arts; Education; Media Art
Status: Professional; Nonprofit
Paid Staff: 5
Volunteer Staff: 50
Budget: $300,000
Income Sources: Ticket Sales; Government Grants; Private Foundations; Individual Donations
Affiliations: National Alliance for Media Arts & Culture; National Performance Network; National Association of Artists Organizations
Annual Attendance: 8,000
Facility Category: Multidisciplinary
Type of Stage: Flexible black box
Seating Capacity: 99
Year Built: 1958
Year Remodeled: 1994
Organization Type: Performing; Educational

2364 UNIVERSITY OF ALASKA, ANCHORAGE: DEPARTMENT OF THEATRE AND DANCE
3211 Providence Drive
Anchorage, AK 99508
Phone: 907-786-1792
Fax: 907-786-1799
Web Site: www.uaa.alaska.edu/theatre
Officers:
   Department Chair: Fran Lautenberger
Budget: $11,000-26,000
Affiliations: ATHE
Seating Capacity: 171; 99
Year Built: 1986

2365 PERSEVERANCE THEATRE
914 Third Street
Douglas, AK 99824
Phone: 907-364-2421
Fax: 907-364-2603
e-mail: marketing@perseverancetheatre.org
Web Site: www.perseverancetheatre.org
Officers:
   President: Glenda Carino
Management:
   Artistic Director: Peter Dubois
Producing Director: Jeffrey Hermann
Founded: 1979

2366 UNIVERSITY OF ALASKA, FAIRBANKS: THEATRE DEPARTMENT
Fairbanks, AK
Mailing Address: PO Box 775700, Fairbanks, AK 99775
Phone: 907-474-6590
Fax: 907-474-7048
Web Site: www.uaf.edu/theatre
Officers:
   Theatre Department Chair: Tara Maginnis
Budget: $3,700-11,000
Affiliations: Fairbanks Drama Associates & Children's Theatre; Fairbanks Shakespeare Theatre; Fairbanks Light Opera Theatre Summer Fine Arts Camp
Seating Capacity: 480; 110;
Year Built: 1968

2367 LYNN CANAL COMMUNITY PLAYERS
PO Box 1030
Haines, AK 99827
Phone: 907-766-2708
Fax: 907-766-2425
Officers:
   Treasurer: Annette Smith
   Secretary: Jane Sebena
   President: Kathy Pashigan
   VP: Tod Sebens
Mission: Performing in and sponsoring all forms of theatre; hosting the biennial presentation of the Alaska Community Theatre Festival.
Founded: 1957
Specialized Field: Musical; Community
Status: Non-Professional
Volunteer Staff: 1
Income Sources: Arts Southeast
Performs At: Chilkat Center for the Arts
Organization Type: Performing

Arizona

2368 NORTHERN ARIZONA UNIVERSITY: THEATRE DIVISION, SCHOOL OF PERFORMING ARTS
Flafstaff, AZ
Mailing Address: Box 6040, Flagstaff, AZ 86011
Phone: 520-523-3731
Fax: 520-523-5111
Web Site: www.nau.edu/spa/theatre
Budget: $5,000-9,650
Affiliations: ATHE
Seating Capacity: 300; 120
Year Built: 1968
Year Remodeled: 1999

2369 THEATER WORKS
9850 W Peoria Avenue
Peoria, AZ 85345

Phone: 623-815-1791
Fax: 623-815-9043
Web Site: www.theaterworks.org
Officers:
  CEO: Michael Foulds
  President: Robert T Root
  VP: David Lunch
  Treasurer: Vicky Holly
  Secretary: Linda Kidwell
Management:
  Executive Director: Michael Foulds
  Artistic Director: Scott Campbell
Mission: To provide a diversified, strikingly creative performing arts program of the highest quality, accessible to all in the community.
Founded: 1986
Status: Non professional; Nonprofit
Paid Staff: 8
Volunteer Staff: 100
Non-paid Artists: 70
Income Sources: Local Corporations; Arts Commissions; Patrons; Donations
Annual Attendance: 30,000
Seating Capacity: 150

2370 ACTORS THEATRE OF PHOENIX
Stage West
Herberger Theater Center
222 E Monroe
Phoenix, AZ 85001
Mailing Address: PO Box 1924, Phoenix, AZ. 85001-1924
Phone: 602-253-6701
Fax: 602-254-9577
e-mail: info@atphx.org
Web Site: www.actorstheatrephx.org/main.htm
Management:
  Producing Artistic Director: Matthew Wiener
  General Manager: Linda Barry
  Marketing Director: Serena Torres Webbe
  Director Development: Pamela Reed Sanchez
  Production Manager: Adrienne Wohleen
Mission: Providing Phoenix with fine professional theatre; employing only local actors; building a resident company as well as a training program.
Founded: 1985
Specialized Field: Theatrical Group
Status: Professional; Nonprofit
Income Sources: Theatre Communications Group
Performs At: Herberger Theater Center; Stage West
Organization Type: Performing

2371 THEATRE DIVISION
33 S Third Street
Phoenix, AZ 85004
Phone: 602-534-9580
Fax: 602-495-3608
e-mail: baller@ci.phoenix.az.us
Management:
  Division Chair: Harold Herman
  Costume Design: Jennifer F Adams
  Box Office Manager: Mary Radciewicz

2372 ARIZONA STATE UNIVERSITY THEATRE
Tempe, AZ
Mailing Address: PO Box 872002, Tempe, AZ 85287
Phone: 480-965-5359
Fax: 480-965-5351
Web Site: www.asu.edu
Officers:
  Interim Chair: John Saldana
Budget: $5,500-10,000
Affiliations: U/RTA; ATHE; Arizona Theatre Company
Seating Capacity: 525; 166; 70
Year Built: 1989

2373 CHILDSPLAY
PO Box 517
Tempe, AZ 85280
Phone: 480-350-8101
Fax: 480-350-8584
e-mail: info@childsplayaz.org
Web Site: www.childsplayaz.org
Management:
  Artistic Director: David Saar
  Managing Director: Steve Martin
Mission: To create theatre so strikingly original in form, content, or both, that it instills in young people an enduring awe, love and respect for the medium, thus preserving imagination and wonder, the hallmarks of childhood, which are the keys to the future.
Founded: 1977
Specialized Field: Theater
Performs At: Herberger Theater, Scottsdale Center for the Arts, Stage West, Tempe Performing Arts Center
Type of Stage: Proscenium, Black Box
Seating Capacity: 800, 800, 350, 175

2374 ARIZONA THEATRE COMPANY
Tucson, AZ
Mailing Address: PO Box 1631, Tuscon, AZ 85702
Phone: 520-884-8210
Fax: 520-628-9129
Web Site: www.arizonatheatre.org
Officers:
  President: Aubra Spaulding-Gaston
  Board Chairman: Jack Davis
Management:
  Artistic Director: David Ira Goldstein
Mission: Creating outstanding professional theatre for Arizona; having an impact locally and nationally.
Founded: 1967
Specialized Field: Theatre
Status: Professional; Nonprofit
Paid Staff: 15
Paid Artists: 80
Budget: $6.9 million
Income Sources: Ticket Sales; Donations; Grants; Government
Performs At: Theatre
Affiliations: League of Resident Theatres
Annual Attendance: 80,000
Type of Stage: Proscenium
Seating Capacity: 600
Year Built: 1929
Year Remodeled: 1988

Cost: $4 million
Organization Type: Resident

2375 UAPRESENTS CENTENNIAL HALL
1020 E University Boulevard
PO Box 210029
Tucson, AZ 85721-0029
Phone: 520-621-3341
Fax: 520-621-8991
e-mail: uapresents@arizona.edu
Web Site: uapresents.arizona.edu/contact.html
Management:
   Executive Director: Ken Foster

2376 UNIVERSITY OF ARIZONA SCHOOL OF THEATRE ARTS
University of Arizona
Tucson, AZ 85721
Phone: 520-621-7008
Fax: 520-621-2412
Web Site: www.arts.arizona.edu/theatre
Officers:
   Chair: Albert D Tucci
Budget: $9,000-34,000
Affiliations: NAST; U/RTA; Arizona Theatre Company
Type of Stage: Proscenium
Seating Capacity: 332; 300
Year Built: 1957
Year Remodeled: 1992

Arkansas

2377 LYON COLLEGE THEATRE DEPARTMENT
Batesville, AR
Mailing Address: PO Box 2317, Batesville, AR 72503
Phone: 870-793-1750
Fax: 870-698-4622
Toll-free: 800-423-2542
Web Site: www.lyon.edu
Management:
   Director of Theatre: Dr. Michael L Counts
Budget: $2,000-3,600
Affiliations: ATHE; Arkansas Repertory Theatre
Type of Stage: Black Box
Seating Capacity: 200
Year Built: 1991
Year Remodeled: 1999

2378 UNIVERSITY OF CENTRAL ARKANSAS THEATRE PROGRAM
Conway, AR
Mailing Address: PO Box 4942, University of Central AR, Conway, AR 72035
Phone: 501-450-5608
Fax: 501-450-3296
Web Site: www.uca.edu/theatre
Management:
   Director: Bob Willenbrink
Budget: $3,100-17,500
Affiliations: NAST

Seating Capacity: 307; 1200; 80-120
Year Built: 1968
Year Remodeled: 1996

2379 UNIVERSITY OF ARKANSAS AT FAYETTEVILLE: DEPARTMENT OF DRAMA
619 Kimpel Hall
Fayetteville, AR 72701
Phone: 501-575-2953
Fax: 501-575-7602
Officers:
   Chair: Dr. Andrew Gibbs
Budget: $
Seating Capacity: 331; 1205; 75
Year Built: 1950

2380 FORT SMITH LITTLE THEATRE
401 N Sixth Street
PO Box 3752
Fort Smith, AR 72913
Phone: 479-783-1295
e-mail: billcovey@worldnet.att.net
Web Site: www.fslt.20fr.com
Officers:
   President: Michael Richardson
   VP: Clara Jane Rubarth
   Treasurer: Mike Tickler
   Secretary: Wendy Quick
Founded: 1947
Specialized Field: Theatrical Group
Status: Nonprofit
Income Sources: ticket sales
Performs At: Fort Smith Little Theatre
Organization Type: Performing

2381 FOUNDATION OF ARTS
115 W Monroe
PO Box 310
Jonesboro, AR 72403-0310
Phone: 870-935-2726
Fax: 870-933-9505
e-mail: foa@insolwwb.net
Web Site: www.insolwwb.net/-foa
Officers:
   Executive Director: Sherri Greuel
   Marketing Director/Box Office: Danita Martin
   Education Director: Lara Shelton
   Technical Director: Brett Kellett
Management:
   Music Director: Dr. Neale King Bartee
   Executive Director: Margaret Peacock
   Education Director: Lara Shelton
   Marketing/Box Office: Danita Martin-Wilkins
Mission: Education, Community Theatre Workshops, Guest Directors, etc. to conduct workshops. Emphasis on youth, but offered to all ages.
Founded: 1978
Paid Staff: 5
Budget: $35,000-$100,000
Income Sources: Box Office, Grants, Private Donation, Class Tuition
Annual Attendance: 25,000
Facility Category: Theatre

Type of Stage: Proscenium
Seating Capacity: 670
Year Built: 1940
Year Remodeled: 2000
Rental Contact: Executive Director Sherri Greuel
Resident Groups: Nea Symphony, Theatre on the Ridge, Act Experience, Jonesboro City Ballet

2382 ARKANSAS ARTS CENTER CHILDREN'S THEATER

Mac Arthur Park
9th + Commerce, PO Box 2137
Little Rock, AR 72203
Phone: 501-372-4000
Fax: 501-375-8053
Toll-free: 800-264-2787
e-mail: mpreble@arkarts.com
Web Site: www.arkarts.com
Officers:
   President: Terri Erwin
Management:
   Artistic Director: Bradley D Anderson
   Stage Manager: Cris Skinner
Mission: Family theater.
Founded: 1979
Specialized Field: Theatrical Group
Status: Professional; Nonprofit
Performs At: Arkansas Art Center Theater
Annual Attendance: 50,000
Facility Category: Auditorium
Type of Stage: Proscenium
Seating Capacity: 381
Year Built: 1930
Organization Type: Performing; Touring
Resident Groups: Resident Theatre Company

2383 ARKANSAS REPERATORY THEATRE

601 Main Street
PO Box 110
Little Rock, AR 72203
Phone: 501-378-0445
Fax: 501-378-0012
e-mail: tickets@therep.org
Web Site: www.therep.org
Officers:
   Chairman: Wyck Nisbet
   Treasurer: Steve Strickland
   Secretary: Ann Bradford
Management:
   Artistic Director: Robert Hupp
   Business Manager: Lynn Frazier
   Development Associate: Wanda Hoover
   General Manager: Michael McCurdy
   Marketing Director: Kelly Ford
Mission: To be a professional theatre of excellence that entertains and challenges local, regional, and national audiences. Through educational outreach, and as a creative forum for artists, The Rep strives to provide valuable services to the community and make significant contributions to the national theatre agenda.
Founded: 1976
Specialized Field: Theatrical Group
Status: Professional; Nonprofit
Paid Staff: 35

Volunteer Staff: 200
Non-paid Artists: 10
Income Sources: Corporations; Private; Government; Ticket Sales
Performs At: Arkansas Repertory Theatre
Affiliations: Actors Equity Association and Theatre Communication Group
Annual Attendance: 60,000
Type of Stage: Modified Proscenium
Stage Dimensions: 40' x 30'
Seating Capacity: 350
Year Remodeled: 1988
Rental Contact: Michael McCurdy
Organization Type: Performing; Touring; Resident; Educational; Sponsoring

2384 UNIVERSITY OF ARKANSAS AT LITTLE ROCK: DEPARTMENT OF THEATRE AND DANCE

2801 South University
Little Rock, AR 72204
Phone: 501-569-3291
Management:
   Director: Victor Ellsworth
Budget: $3,750-7,800
Affiliations: NAST; ATHE; Arkansas Repertory Theatre; Arkansas Arts Center Children's Theatre; Murray's Dinner Theatre
Seating Capacity: 680; 150

2385 SOUTHERN ARKANSAS UNIVERSITY THEATRE & MASS COMMUNICATIONS DEPARTMENT

Magnolia, AR
Mailing Address: Box 9203, Magnolia, AR 71754
Phone: 870-235-4257
Officers:
   Chair: David Murphy
Budget: $550-2,100
Affiliations: ATHE
Seating Capacity: 475
Year Built: 1975

2386 TWIN LAKES PLAYHOUSE

PO Box 482
Mountain Home, AR 72653
Phone: 870-481-5811
Web Site: www.dynamyx.com/playhouse
Mission: Providing live theater for the area.
Founded: 1971
Specialized Field: Community
Status: Semi-Professional; Non-Professional; Nonprofit
Paid Staff: 40
Organization Type: Performing

California

2387 HUMBOLT STATE UNIVERSITY: DEPARTMENT OF THEATRE, FILM AND DANCE

#1 Harpst Street
Arcata, CA 95521
Phone: 707-826-3566
Fax: 707-826-5494
Web Site: www.humbolt.edu/~records
Officers:
   Chair: Michael Goodman
Budget: $6,000-12,000
Affiliations: NAST; ATHE
Seating Capacity: 810; 140; 125
Year Built: 1959

2388 CALIFORNIA STATE UNIVERSITY, BAKERSFIELD: THEATRE PROGRAM

9001 Stockdale Highway
Bakersfield, CA 93311
Phone: 661-664-3093
Fax: 661-665-6901
Officers:
   Chair: Annie DuPratt
Budget: $6,500
Affiliations: ATHE
Seating Capacity: 500; 100
Year Built: 1980

2389 AURORA THEATRE COMPANY

2081 Addison Street
Berkeley, CA 94704
Mailing Address: PO Box 559, Berkeley, CA. 94701
Phone: 510-843-4822
Fax: 510-843-4826
e-mail: general@auroratheatre.org
Web Site: auroratheatre.org
Management:
   Artistic Director: Barbara Oliver
   Producing Director: Tom Ross
Mission: Produce five professional plays per season.
Founded: 1991
Specialized Field: Theatre
Paid Staff: 8
Paid Artists: 50
Performs At: Airpra Theatre
Affiliations: Actor's Equity Theatre Company; Theatre Communications Group; Theatre Bay Area
Type of Stage: Arena
Seating Capacity: 67

2390 BERKELEY COMMUNITY THEATRE

1930 Allstom Way
2134 Martin Luther King Jr. Way
Berkeley, CA 94703
Phone: 510-644-6863
Fax: 510-644-6363
Management:
   Theatre Manager: Judson H Owens
   Assistant Manager: Lance C James
   Facility Reservations: Yvonne Adams
Mission: To offer the community professional theatre.

Founded: 1950
Specialized Field: Musical; Community; Theatrical Group
Status: Professional; Non-Professional
Paid Staff: 4
Volunteer Staff: 60
Income Sources: Berkeley Unified School District
Performs At: Berkeley Community Theatre
Affiliations: Berkeley Unified School District
Seating Capacity: 3,500
Organization Type: Performing; Touring; Educational

2391 BERKELEY REPERTORY THEATRE

2025 Addison Street
Berkeley, CA 94704
Phone: 510-647-2900
Fax: 510-647-2976
Toll-free: 888-427-8849
e-mail: turg@berkeleyrep.org
Web Site: www.berkeleyrep.org
Officers:
   President: Nicholas M Graves
   VP: Phillip R Trapp
   Treasurerident: Kenneth P Avery
   Secretary: Jean Strunsky
Management:
   Artistic Director: Tony Taccone
   Managing Director: Susan Medak
   General Manager: Karen Racanelli
Mission: To set a national standard for ambitious programming, engagement with our audiences, and leadership within the community in which we reside. We endeavor to create a diverse body of work that expresses a rigorous, embracing aesthetic and relects the highest artistic standards, and seek to maintain an environment in which talented artists can do their best work.
Founded: 1968
Specialized Field: Theatrical Group
Status: Professional; Nonprofit
Paid Staff: 75
Budget: $8.9 Million
Income Sources: Tickets; Grants; Donations; Subscriptions
Performs At: Berkeley Repertory Theatre
Affiliations: San Francisco Convention and Visitor Bureau; Berkeley Convention and Visitor Bureau
Annual Attendance: 150,000
Type of Stage: Thrust Stage and Proscenium Stage
Seating Capacity: 400 and 600
Year Built: 1980
Cost: $20 Million
Rental Contact: Alisha Tonsic
Organization Type: Performing; Touring; Resident; Educational

2392 BLACK REPERTORY GROUP

3201 Adeline Street
Berkeley, CA 94703
Phone: 510-652-2120
Fax: 510-652-8030
Web Site: dwww.blackrepertorygroup.org
Officers:
   President: Ella Wiley
   VP: Pastor Earl Bill
   Secretary: Doreen Zayas

Management:
  Executive Director: Dr. Mona Vaughan Scott
  Development Director: Sean Scott
  Bookkeeper/Assistant to Director: Panda Martin
Mission: Building discipline and self-esteem in youth through drama. Showcasing the plays of black playwrights. Providing a folks arts venue for the community.
Founded: 1964
Specialized Field: Community; Theatrical Group; Community Cultural Center
Status: Non-Professional; Nonprofit
Paid Staff: 4
Organization Type: Resident

2393 DELL'ARTE INTERNATIONAL SCHOOL OF PHYSICAL THEATRE

131 H Street
PO Box 816
Blue Lake, CA 95525
Phone: 707-668-5663
Fax: 707-668-5665
e-mail: dellarte@aol.com
Web Site: www.dellarte.com
Officers:
  President: Mary Maloney
  Secretary/Treasurer: Bobbi Ricca
Management:
  Managing Director: Michael Fields
  Co-Artistic Director: Donald Forrest
  Co-Artistic Director: Joan Schirle
Mission: To give artists an opportunity to work and live in a rural setting.
Founded: 1971
Specialized Field: Theatrical Group
Status: Professional; Nonprofit
Budget: $900,000
Income Sources: Humboldt Arts Council; Theatre Communications Group, Theatre Bay Area
Performs At: Dell' Arte Theatre
Affiliations: NAST; ATHE
Facility Category: Black Box/Amphitheatre
Type of Stage: Sprung Floor
Seating Capacity: 113; 300
Year Remodeled: 1995
Organization Type: Performing; Touring
Resident Groups: Dell' Arte Company

2394 COLONY THEATRE COMPANY

555 N Third Street
Burbank, CA 91502-1103
Phone: 818-558-7000
Fax: 818-558-7110
e-mail: boxoffice@colonytheatre.org
Web Site: www.colonytheatre.org
Officers:
  President/Producing Director: Barbara Beckley
  VP: Michael Wadler
  Secretary: Priscilla Davis
  Treasurer: Nonie Lann
  Chairman: Keith Bardellini
Management:
  Managing Director: Amanda Diamond

Mission: To produce full productions of plays for the public recognized to be of significant artistic, social, and/or historical value.
Founded: 1975
Specialized Field: Live Theater
Status: Professional; Nonprofit
Paid Staff: 7
Volunteer Staff: 10
Budget: $800,000
Income Sources: Subscription & single ticket sales; Individual donations
Performs At: Burbank Center Stage
Affiliations: Actors Equity Association
Annual Attendance: 20,500
Facility Category: Theater
Type of Stage: Thrust
Stage Dimensions: 37.5 x 22.5
Seating Capacity: 276
Year Built: 2000
Cost: $1,500,000 (built)
Rental Contact: Managing Director Amanda Diamond
Organization Type: Performing; Resident
Resident Groups: Colony Theatre Company

2395 ROBEY THEATRE COMPANY

4444 Riverside Drive
Suite 110
Burbank, CA 91505
Phone: 818-567-3294
Fax: 818-567-3296
Management:
  Artistic Director: Bennet Guillory
  Grant Writer: Royce Herron
  Special Events Coordinator: Julie Serquinia
  Administrative Assistant: Lia Johnson

2396 CALIFORNIA STATE UNIVERSITY, DOMINGUEZ HILLS: DEPARTMENT OF THEATRE

California State University
Carson, CA 90747
Phone: 310-243-3588
Officers:
  Chairman: Peter Rodney
Budget: $8,550-12,100
Affiliations: NAST
Seating Capacity: 475; 80

2397 CHICO PRESENTS
California State University Chico

400 W First Street
Chico, CA 95929-0116
Phone: 530-898-5917
Fax: 530-898-6824
e-mail: pkopp@sc4chico.edu
Web Site: www.csuchico.edu/hfa
Management:
  Director: Patrick W Kopp

2398 POMONA COLLEGE DEPARTMENT OF THEATRE AND DANCE

Pomona College
Claremont, CA 91711

Phone: 909-621-8186
Fax: 909-621-8780
Web Site: www.pomona.edu
Officers:
    Chair: Sherry Linnell
Budget: $9,000-14,000
Affiliations: ATHE
Seating Capacity: 330; 150
Year Built: 1992
Year Remodeled: 1998

2399 LAMB'S PLAYERS THEATRE

1142 Orange Avenue
PO Box 18229
Coronado, CA 92178
Phone: 619-437-6050
Fax: 619-437-8904
Web Site: www.lambsplayers.org/Pages/overview.html
Officers:
    Chairman: Michael Roeder
Management:
    Producing Artistic Director: W Robert Smyth
    Associate Director: Kerry Meads
    Associate Director: Deborah Smyth
    Art/Marketing Director: Christian Turner
    Administrative Director: James Beaubeaux
    Director Education: Jeffrey S Miller
    Technical Director: Nathan Peirson
    Facilities Manager: David Cochran Heath
    Production Manager: Paul Eggington
Mission: To be a theatre that probes and questions the values and choices of contemporary culture. Celebrates the joys, strengths and diverse traditions of family and community. Explores the spiritual dimension of life.
Founded: 1973
Specialized Field: Theatrical Group
Status: Professional; Nonprofit
Income Sources: Theatre Communications Group; California Theatre Council
Performs At: Harder Stage; Hahn; Lyceum
Type of Stage: Thrust/Proscenium, Flexible
Seating Capacity: 350, 250, 200
Organization Type: Performing; Touring; Resident; Educational

2400 SOUTH COAST REPERTORY

655 Town Center Drive
Costa Mesa, CA 92626
Phone: 714-708-5500
Fax: 714-545-0391
e-mail: theatre@scr.org
Web Site: www.scr.org
Management:
    Producing Artistic Director: David Emmes
    Artistic Director: Martin Benson
    Managing Director: Paula Tomei
    Public Relations Director: Cristofer Gross
    Director Development: Patricia Graff-Falzon
    Director Marketing: John Mouledoux
Mission: To serve the art of theatre and Orange County audiences in a manner socially relevant and theatrically inventive.
Founded: 1964
Status: Professional; Nonprofit
Paid Staff: 70

Paid Artists: 150
Budget: $8,000,000
Income Sources: Ticket sales; annual fund campaign
Performs At: South Coast Repertory Theatre
Affiliations: League of Resident Theatres; Theatre Communications Group
Type of Stage: Flexible; Proscenium; End Stage
Seating Capacity: 507; 336; 95
Year Built: 1978
Year Remodeled: 2002
Cost: $29 million
Rental Contact: Nelson Denniston
Organization Type: Performing; Touring; Resident; Educational

2401 UNIVERSITY OF CALIFORNIA, DAVIS: DEPARTMENT OF DRAMATIC ART

University of California - Davis
Davis, CA 95616
Phone: 530-752-0888
Fax: 530-752-8818
Web Site: http://theatredance.ucdavis.edu
Officers:
    Chair: Barbara Sellers
Budget: $3,600-11,000
Affiliations: ATHE; Sacramento Theatre Company; Tahoe Shakespeare Festival; Magic Theatre; B Stret Theatre
Seating Capacity: 470; 250; 220; 150
Year Built: 1967

2402 CHRISTIAN COMMUNITY THEATER

1545 Pioneer Way
El Cajon, CA 92020
Phone: 619-588-0206
Fax: 619-588-4384
Toll-free: 800-696-1929
e-mail: info@cctcyt.org
Web Site: www.cctcyt.org
Management:
    Artistic Director: Paul Russell
    Executive Director: Sheryl Russell
    Production Director: Henry Laughman
    Marketing Director: Charles W Patmon, Jr
    Managing Director: Diane Mosce
    Operations Director: Mary Mwanger
    Development Director: Sharon Milligan
    Expansion Director: Justin Parks
    Graphic Designer: Lynette Fisk
Mission: To produce quality wholesome family entertainment and reflect Judeo-Christian values through training in the arts; to provide a children's theatre training program.
Founded: 1980
Specialized Field: Musical Theatre; Children's Theatre
Status: Nonprofit; Educational
Paid Staff: 25
Volunteer Staff: 50
Paid Artists: 5
Non-paid Artists: 200
Budget: $2,000,000
Income Sources: Box Office; Tuition; Grants; Private Donations

Performs At: Rented- Outdoor amphitheater and public performance center
Affiliations: American Alliance for Theatre and Education; Christians in Theater Arts
Annual Attendance: 50,000+

2403 WELK RESORT SAN DIEGO THEATRE
8860 Lawrence Walk Drive
Escondido, CA 92026
Phone: 760-749-3000
Fax: 760-749-9592
Toll-free: 800-802-7459
e-mail: theatre@welkresort.com
Web Site: www.welkresort.com
Management:
   Producer/Theatre Manager: Sean Coogan
Founded: 1981
Specialized Field: Equity Dinner Theatre
Status: Professional; Commercial
Income Sources: Actors' Equity Association
Performs At: The Welk Resort; San Diego Theatre
Facility Category: Broadway Style Dinner Theatre
Seating Capacity: 339
Organization Type: Performing

2404 FERNDALE REPERTORY THEATRE
447 Main Street
PO Box 892
Ferndale, CA 95536
Phone: 707-786-5483
Fax: 707-786-5480
e-mail: therep@northcoast.com
Web Site: www.ferndale-rep.org
Management:
   Director: Marilyn McCormick
Mission: To provide North Coast residents and visitors theatrical performances of the highest quality.
Founded: 1972
Specialized Field: Community
Status: Semi-Professional; Nonprofit
Paid Staff: 3
Budget: $160,000
Income Sources: Grants; Ticket sales; Membership
Performs At: Ferndale Repertory Theatre
Facility Category: Live Stage Productions
Type of Stage: Thrust Percenium
Seating Capacity: 265
Year Built: 1922
Year Remodeled: 1972
Organization Type: Performing

2405 CALIFORNIA STATE UNIVERSITY, FRESNO: THEATRE ARTS DEPARTMENT
5201 North Maple
Fresno, CA 93740
Phone: 559-278-3987
Fax: 559-278-7512
Web Site: http://csufresno.edu/Theatre
Officers:
   Chair: Kathleen McKinley
Budget: $2,900-4,900
Affiliations: NAST; ATHE
Seating Capacity: 360; 200; 100
Year Remodeled: 1991

2406 THEATRE THREE REPERTORY COMPANY
1544 Fulton Street
Fresno, CA 93721-1461
Phone: 559-486-3333
Fax: 559-486-4465
Web Site: www.theatre3.com
Management:
   Artistic Director: Gordon Goede
Status: Non-Equity

2407 CALIFORNIA STATE UNIVERSITY, FULLERTON: DEPARTMENT OF THEATRE AND DANCE
800 North College Boulevard - PA-157
Fullerton, CA 92835
Phone: 714-278-3628
Fax: 714-278-7549
Web Site: www.arts.fullerton.edu/events
Officers:
   Chair: Susan Hallman
Budget: $9000-23,650
Affiliations: NASD; NAST; ATHE; South Coast Repertory; A Noise Within
Seating Capacity: 500; 200; 100
Year Remodeled: 2000

2408 VANGUARD THEATRE ENSEMBLE
699-A S State College Boulevard
Fullerton, CA 92831
Phone: 714-526-8007
Fax: 714-526-8007
Management:
   Artistic Director: Wade Williamson
   Business Manager: Paulette Kendall

2409 GROVE THEATRE CENTER
12852 Main Street
Garden Grove, CA 92840-5207
Phone: 714-741-9555
Fax: 714-741-9560
e-mail: gabin@gtc.org
Web Site: www.grovetheatercenter.com
Management:
   Artistic Director: Kevin Cochran
   Executive Director: Charles Johanson
   Company Manager: Gigi Horowitz
   Casting Coordinator: Hunter Stevenson
   Production Manager: Gabin PanGriff
   Production Stage Manager: Zac Prostein
Status: Nonprofit
Budget: $350,000
Season: Year Round
Annual Attendance: 15,000
Stage Dimensions: 35'x45',60'x45',40'x35',30'x60'
Seating Capacity: 172, 548, 246, 98

2410 ACTORS' GANG THEATER
6201 Santa Monica Boulevard
Hollywood, CA 90038

Phone: 323-465-0566
Fax: 323-467-1246
e-mail: dactorsgng1@aol.com
Management:
    Literary Manager: Chris Wells
Performs At: Actors' Gang Theater, Actors' Gang El Centro
Type of Stage: Flexible Stage
Seating Capacity: 99, 40

2411 AMERICAN ACADEMY OF DRAMATIC ARTS/HOLLYWOOD

1336 North LaBrea Avenue
Hollywood, CA 90028
Phone: 323-464-2777
Fax: 323-464-1250
Web Site: www.aada.org
Management:
    Director of Instruction: Georgia Phillips
Affiliations: NAST; WASC

2412 BLANK THEATRE COMPANY

6500 Santa Monica Boulevard
Hollywood, CA 90026
Mailing Address: 1301 Lucile Avenue, Los Angeles, CA. 90026
Phone: 323-662-7734
Fax: 323-661-3903
e-mail: info@theblank.com
Web Site: www.theblank.com
Management:
    Artistic Director/Producer: Daniel Henning
    Artistic Producer: Noah Wyle
    Producer: Christopher Steele
Founded: 1990
Specialized Field: Theatre

2413 HUDSON THEATRE

6539 Santa Monica Boulevard
Hollywood, CA 90038
Phone: 323-856-4249
Fax: 323-856-4316
e-mail: info@hudsontheatre.com
Web Site: www.hudsontheatre.com
Management:
    Artistic Director: Elizabeth Reilly
    Artistic Director: Leigh McLeod Fortier
    Managing Director: Laila Karima
    Managing Director: Zeke Rettman
    Managing Director: Trevor Ysaguiree
Founded: 1991
Status: Professional; Nonprofit
Performs At: Hudson Theatre (Mainstage, Avenue Theatre, Guild Theatre)
Type of Stage: Modified Thrust; Proscenium
Seating Capacity: 99; 99; 43
Organization Type: Producing in House

2414 OPEN FIST THEATRE COMPANY

1625 La Brea Avenue
Hollywood, CA 90028
Phone: 323-882-6912
Web Site: www.openfist.org

Management:
    Artistic Director: Martha Demson
    Managing Director: David Castellani
    Managing Director: Chelsea Hackett
    Literary Manager: Dietrich Smith
    Publicity Manager: Amy Edlin
Mission: The Open Fist Theatre Company is a community of actors, playwrights, designers and directors.
Founded: 1989

2415 STAGES THEATRE CENTER

1540 N McCadden Place
210 S Westgate Avenue
Hollywood, CA 90028
Phone: 323-465-1010
Fax: 323-462-2176
e-mail: e-mail@stagestheatre.org
Web Site: www.staes.org//stages_frames.htm
Officers:
    Chairperson: Pompea Smith
    Treasurer: Sonia Lloveras
Management:
    Artistic Director: Paul Verdier
    Managing Director: Sonia Lloveras
Mission: To expose new or unfamiliar works or styles of theater to Los Angeles audiences; to host unique artists-in-residence who utilize distinctive theatrical styles, such as Theater of the Absurd and Commedia del' Arte.
Founded: 1981
Status: Professional; Nonprofit
Paid Staff: 3
Income Sources: Theatre Communications Group
Performs At: Stages Theatre
Stage Dimensions: 14'x14'
Organization Type: Performing

2416 HUNTINGTON BEACH PLAYHOUSE

7111 Talbert Avenue
Huntington Beach, CA 92648
Phone: 714-375-0696
Fax: 714-375-0698
e-mail: hbplay@earthlink.net
Web Site: www.hbph.com
Officers:
    President: Bettie Mullenberg
    Vice President: Catherine Stip
    Treasurer: Don Stanton
    Business Manager: Dawn Conant
    Secretary: BJ O'Rourke-Smith
Management:
    Business Manager: Dawn Conant
Mission: As a non-profit organization dedicated to community educational and cultural enrichment in dramatic arts, Huntington Beach Playhouse presents dramatic productions, sponsors student scholarships and offers stagecraft workshops.
Founded: 1963
Specialized Field: Musical; Community; Theatrical Group
Status: Non-Professional; Nonprofit
Paid Staff: 4
Volunteer Staff: 100
Non-paid Artists: 75

Income Sources: Ticket Sales
Performs At: Central Library Theatre
Annual Attendance: 27,000
Type of Stage: Proscenium
Seating Capacity: 319
Year Built: 1994
Organization Type: Performing

2417 UNIVERSITY OF CALIFORNIA-IRVINE: SCHOOL OF THE ARTS (DRAMA)

249 Drama
Irvine, CA 92697
Phone: 949-824-6614
Web Site: www.arts.uci.edu/drama
Officers:
  Chair: Cameron Harvey
Budget: $10,050-49,050
Affiliations: NAST; U/RTA;ATHE; South Coast Repertory
Seating Capacity: 420; 231; 165
Year Built: 1970

2418 JULIAN'S LIVE DINNER THEATRE

2960 La Posada Way
Julian, CA 92036
Phone: 760-765-1100
Web Site: www.pinehillslodge.com/theatre/
Founded: 1980

2419 KIDS 4 BROADWAY

PO Box 122
Kelseyville, CA 95451
Phone: 707-277-7550
Fax: 707-277-7557
e-mail: kidsplay@pacific.net
Web Site: www.pacificsites.com/~kidsplay
Mission: Offers a unique opportunity for a school or community to create love, laughter and magic in their childrens lives.

2420 LA JOLLA PLAYHOUSE

2910 La Jolla Villiage Drive
PO Box 12039
La Jolla, CA 92039
Phone: 858-550-1070
Fax: 858-550-1075
e-mail: ljplayhouse@ucsd.edu
Web Site: www.lajollaplayhouse.com
Management:
  Artistic Director: Des McAnuff
  Managing Director: Terrance Dwyer
  Literary Manager: Elizabeth Bennett
Mission: Producing bold, innovative, adventurous theater; offering a summer home to America's leading theater artists.
Founded: 1947
Status: Professional; Nonprofit
Income Sources: Actors' Equity Association; League of Resident Theatres; Theatre Communications Group
Season: April - December
Performs At: La Jolla Playhouse; Mandell Weiss Performing Arts
Type of Stage: Proscenium/Thrust

Seating Capacity: 500, 400
Organization Type: Touring; Resident; Educational

2421 UNIVERSITY OF CALIFORNIA-SAN DIEGO: DEPARTMENT OF THEATRE AND DANCE

La Jolla, CA 92093
Phone: 858-534-3791
Fax: 858-534-1080
Web Site: www.theatre.ucsd.edu
Officers:
  Chair: Walton Jones
Budget: $3,600-24,000
Performs At: Mandell Weiss Theater
Affiliations: ATHE; The La Jolla Playhouse
Seating Capacity: 500; 400; 100
Year Built: 1982

2422 UNIVERSITY OF LAVERNE

1950 Third Street
LaVerne, CA 91750
Phone: 909-593-3511
Fax: 909-392-2787
Web Site: www.ulaverne.edu/thart
Officers:
  Chair: Elizabeth Pietrzak
Budget: $550-14,000
Affiliations: U/RTA; ATHE; The Guilford School of Acting (England); The Split International Theatre Festival (Croatia)
Seating Capacity: 175-250; 60; 475
Year Built: 1972

2423 LAGUNA PLAYHOUSE

606 Laguna Canyon Road
PO Box 1747
Laguna Beach, CA 92651-1747
Phone: 949-497-5900
Fax: 949-497-8185
Web Site: www.lagunaplayhouse.com
Management:
  Executive Director: Richard Stein
  Artistic Director: Andrew Barnicle
  Youth Theatre Director: Joe Lauderdale
  Education Director: Donna Inglima
  Production Manager: Jim Ryan
  Business Manager: Kat Hiclklin
  Corporate Development Manager: Elaine Smith
  Systems Administrator: Deborah Purnell
  Telephone Sales Manager: June Rodgers
Mission: Committed to excellence in professional theatre.
Founded: 1920
Specialized Field: Professional; Children's Theatre
Status: Professional; Nonprofit
Paid Staff: 150
Income Sources: Inter-theatre Institute; American Association of Theatre Educators
Performs At: Moulton Theater
Organization Type: Performing; Educational

2424 CALIFORNIA REPERTORY COMPANY

1250 Bellflower Boulevard
Long Beach, CA 90840-2701

Phone: 562-432-1818
Fax: 562-985-2263
Web Site: www.calrep.org
Management:
   Artistic Producing Director: Howard Berman
   Managing Director: Paul Stuart Graham
Founded: 1989
Performs At: UT Theatre, Studio Theatre, Edison Theatre, Players Theatre
Type of Stage: Proscenium, Flexible
Seating Capacity: 400, 225, 99, 90

2425 CALIFORNIA STATE UNIVERSITY, LONG BEACH: DEPARTMENT OF THEATRE

Long Beach, CA 90840
Phone: 562-985-5357
Fax: 562-985-2263
Officers:
   Chairman: Howard Burman
Affiliations: NAST; California Repertory Company
Seating Capacity: 378; 250; 90; 99
Year Built: 1952
Year Remodeled: 1989

2426 FOUND THEATRE

251 E Seventh Street
Long Beach, CA 90813
Phone: 362-433-3363
Management:
   Artistic Managing Director: Cynthia Galles
   Literary Director: Virginia DeMoss
   Music Director: Alice Secrist
Mission: To provide professional-quality alternative theatre to the community as inexpensively as possible; to provide a place for actors, directors, and technicians to experiment, refine their craft, and grow as artists.
Founded: 1974
Specialized Field: Theatrical Group
Status: Professional; Nonprofit
Performs At: The Found Theatre
Organization Type: Performing

2427 BUS BARN STAGE COMPANY

97 Hillview Avenue
PO Box 151
Los Altos, CA 94023-0151
Phone: 650-941-0551
Fax: 650-941-0884
e-mail: busbarn@BUSBARN.ORG
Web Site: www.busbarn.org
Officers:
   President: Vicki Reeder
   Secretary: Roy Lave
   Treasure: Chet Frankenfield
Management:
   Business Manager: Kristin Reams
   Artistic Director: John Draginoff
   Technical Director: Fred Eiras
   Production Manager/Publicist: Geoff Fiorito

Mission: To engage the community and the artists in a shared experience of intimate, professional-quality theatre. BusBarn is a professionally managed, community based theatre company serving Los Altos, and the greater South Bay community.
Founded: 1995
Specialized Field: Performing Arts
Status: Nonprofit
Paid Staff: 5
Budget: $260,000
Income Sources: Box Office; Grants; Individual donations
Performs At: Bus Barn Theatre
Affiliations: Theatre Bay Area
Annual Attendance: 7,000
Type of Stage: Proscenium
Seating Capacity: 100
Year Built: 1965
Year Remodeled: 1980

2428 A NOISE WITHIN

3603 Seneca Avenue
Los Angeles, CA 90039
Phone: 818-240-0910
Fax: 323-953-7794
Web Site: www.anoisewithin.org
Management:
   Artistic Advisor: Sabin Epstein
   Artistic Director: Geoff Elliott
   Artistic Director: Julia Rodriquez
   General Manager: Todd Delliger
Mission: To present the classics of world literature in rotating repertory performed by a classically trained ensemble.
Founded: 1991
Type of Stage: Thrust
Seating Capacity: 200 - 300

2429 ACTORS ART THEATRE

6128 Wilshire Boulevard
Los Angeles, CA 90048
Phone: 323-969-4953
Fax: 323-857-5891
Management:
   Artistic Director: Jolene Adams
   Managing Director: Douglas Coler
   Facility Manager: Grady Lee Richmond

2430 ACTORS FOR THEMSELVES

Matrix Theatre
7657 Melrose Avenue
Los Angeles, CA 90048
Phone: 213-852-1445
Management:
   Artistic Director: Joe Stern
Mission: Giving actors a chance to hone their craft and affording them more opportunity to control the production process.
Founded: 1974
Specialized Field: Theatrical Group
Status: Professional; Nonprofit
Performs At: Matrix Theatre
Organization Type: Performing; Resident; Educational

2431 AHMANSON THEATRE
601 W Temple Street
Los Angeles, CA 90012
Phone: 213-628-2772
Fax: 213-628-2796
e-mail: tickets@ctgla.com
Web Site: www.taperahmanson.com
Management:
Artistic Director: Gordon Davidson
Managing Director: Charles Dillingham
Chairman: Phyllis Hennigan
Founded: 1967
Specialized Field: Theatre
Paid Staff: 350
Performs At: Music Center of Los Angeles
Affiliations: Mark Taper Forum
Facility Category: Theatre House
Type of Stage: Proscenium
Stage Dimensions: 190Wx47Dx67H; 40Wx28H
Seating Capacity: 2,100
Year Built: 1967
Year Remodeled: 1995
Rental Contact: Gordon Davidson

2432 ATTIC THEATRE CENTRE
2245 W 25th Street
Los Angeles, CA 90018
Phone: 323-734-8977
e-mail: info@attictheatre.org
Web Site: www.attictheatre.org
Management:
Artistic Director: James Carey
Business Manager: Denise Ragan
Mission: To provide a small theatre with its own resident
company which is also available for rental to outside
productions.
Founded: 1987
Specialized Field: Theatrical Group
Status: Professional; Semi-Professional; Commercial
Income Sources: Theatre Los Angeles
Organization Type: Performing; Resident; Sponsoring

**2433 BILINGUAL FOUNDATION OF THE
ARTS**
421 N Avenue 19
Los Angeles, CA 90031
Phone: 323-225-4044
Fax: 323-225-1250
Officers:
Chairman: Robert Gomez
President: Carmen Zapata
Management:
Producing Director: Carmen Zapata
Artistic Director: Margarita Galban
Los Angeles Theatre Alliance, Produ: Estela Scarlata
Business Manager: Aracelly Alvarcz
Dramaturg: Agustin Coppola
Mission: Celebrating the richness and diversity of
Hispanic Theater by offering theatre produced and
directed in English and Spanish.
Founded: 1973
Specialized Field: Theatrical Group
Status: Professional; Nonprofit

Performs At: The Bilingual Foundation of the Arts
Theatre
Affiliations: American Arts Alliance; Theatre
Communications Group; California Confederation of the
Arts
Annual Attendance: 125,000
Type of Stage: Thrust
Seating Capacity: 99 & 299
Organization Type: Performing; Touring; Educational

2434 BOB BAKER MARIONETTE THEATRE
1345 W First Street
Los Angeles, CA 90026
Phone: 215-250-9995
Fax: 213-250-1120
Mission: Marionette productions available for birthday
parties and shop tours.
Founded: 1963
Specialized Field: Puppet
Status: Professional
Income Sources: Admissions
Performs At: Marionette Theatre
Type of Stage: Proscenium; 3/4 Arena
Seating Capacity: 200
Year Built: 1950
Year Remodeled: 1963
Organization Type: Resident

2435 COLONY STUDIO THEATRE
1944 Riverside Drive
Los Angeles, CA 90039
Phone: 323-665-0280
Fax: 323-667-3235
Management:
Artistic Director: Ross Nelson
Managing Director: Anne Younan

2436 COMPLEX
6476 Santa Monica Boulevard
Los Angeles, CA 90038
Phone: 323-465-0383
Fax: 323-469-5408
Management:
Owner: Matt Chait
Assistant: Ryan Callahan
Founded: 1990
Specialized Field: Theatrical Group
Status: Professional; Non-Professional
Paid Staff: 3
Facility Category: 5 Theaters
Type of Stage: 4 Proscenium, 1 Black Box
Seating Capacity: 42-55
Cost: $150-225 per night
Rental Contact: Matt Ryan
Organization Type: Performing

2437 CORNERSTONE THEATER COMPANY
708 Traction Avenue
Los Angeles, CA 90013
Phone: 213-613-1700
Fax: 213-613-1714
e-mail: cornerstn@aol.com
Web Site: www.cornestonetheatre.org
Management:

Founding Director: Alison Carey
Program Associate: Teeko Parran
Founded: 1986
Status: Nonprofit
Season: Year Round

2438 EAST WEST PLAYERS
244 S Pedro Street
Suite 301
Los Angeles, CA 90012
Phone: 213-625-7000
Fax: 213-625-7111
e-mail: info@eastwestplayers.org
Web Site: www.eastwestplayers.org
Officers:
   Chairman: Lynn Fukuhara Arthurs
   Co-President: Dan M Mayon
   Co-President: Wendy Anderson
Management:
   Managing Directorc Director: Al Choy
   Producing Artistic Director: Tim Dang
Mission: To be a leader in creating engaging, and empowering theatre that gives voice to the Asian Pacific Islander community.
Founded: 1965
Specialized Field: Theatre
Status: Professional; Nonprofit
Paid Staff: 10
Volunteer Staff: 300
Paid Artists: 50
Non-paid Artists: 50
Budget: $1,000,000
Annual Attendance: 30,000
Facility Category: Theater
Type of Stage: Open/Modified Proscenium
Seating Capacity: 240
Year Built: 1922
Year Remodeled: 1997
Rental Contact: Meg Imamoto
Organization Type: Performing; Touring; Resident; Educational

2439 EBONY SHOWCASE THEATRE
1285 S La Brea Avenue
Los Angeles, CA 90019
Mailing Address: Suite 203
Phone: 323-965-8837
Fax: 323-965-0420
e-mail: talentscout@ebonyshowcase.org
Web Site: www.ebonyshowcase.org
Management:
   Founder/Managing Director: Nick Stewart
   Founder/Managing Director: Edna Stewart
Mission: To promote cultural enrichment and education through entertainment.
Founded: 1950
Specialized Field: Theatrical Group
Status: Semi-Professional; Nonprofit
Performs At: Ebony Showcase Theatre
Organization Type: Performing; Resident

2440 FOUNTAIN THEATRE
5060 Fountain Avenue
Los Angeles, CA 90029
Phone: 323-663-2235
Fax: 323-663-1629
e-mail: ftheatre@aol.com
Web Site: www.fountaintheatre.com
Management:
   Producing Director/Dramaturg: Simon Levy
   Producing Artistic Director: Deborah Lawlol
   Managing Artistic Director: Stephen Sachs
Mission: To present live theatre and dance.
Founded: 1990
Specialized Field: Theater
Budget: 450,000
Performs At: Fountain Theatre
Affiliations: TCG; Theatre
Type of Stage: Thrust
Seating Capacity: 78

2441 GEFFEN PLAYHOUSE
10886 Le Conte Avenue
Los Angeles, CA 90024
Phone: 310-208-6500
Fax: 310-208-0341
Web Site: www.geffenplayhouse.com
Officers:
   General Manager: Paul Morer
Management:
   Executive Director: Eric Krebs
   Literary Manager: Amy Levinson
Mission: To produce quality theatre in a broad range of presentations of many moods and characters; to present comedy, drama, musicals, new plays, revivals, classics, experimental children's theatre, special events, multimedia.
Founded: 1995
Specialized Field: Theater
Status: Professional; Commercial
Performs At: Geffen Playhouse
Type of Stage: Proscenium
Seating Capacity: 498
Organization Type: Performing; Resident

2442 GREEK THEATRE
2700 N Vermont Avenue
Los Angeles, CA 90027
Phone: 323-665-5857
Web Site: www.greektheatrela.com
Management:
   General Manager: Susan Rosenbluth
Mission: Presenting a variety of Broadway plays, concerts and comedy.
Founded: 1930
Specialized Field: Dance; Vocal Music; Instrumental Music; Theater
Status: Commercial
Performs At: Greek Theatre
Organization Type: Performing

2443 GROUNDLING THEATRE
7307 Melrose Avenue
Los Angeles, CA 90046
Phone: 323-934-4747
Fax: 323-934-8143
e-mail: staff@groundlings.com
Web Site: www.groundlings.com

Officers:
Business Director: Anesta Almonor
Management:
Executive Director: Eric Vennerbeck
Mission: To create new comedy talent and new comedy productions.
Founded: 1974
Specialized Field: Theatrical Group; Comedy; Improvisation
Status: Nonprofit
Paid Staff: 5
Volunteer Staff: 15
Non-paid Artists: 30
Income Sources: Shows; Donations; School of Improvitional Comedy
Performs At: The Groundling Theatre
Annual Attendance: 20,000
Seating Capacity: 99
Organization Type: Performing; Resident

2444 LOS ANGELES THEATRE ACADEMY

Los Angeles City College
855 North Vermont Avenue
Los Angeles, CA 90029
Phone: 323-953-4336
Management:
Chairman: Winston Butler
Theatre Manager: Dena M Paponis
Mission: Providing professional training to students in theatre arts and supporting this training through professional-level productions.
Founded: 1929
Specialized Field: Theatrical Group
Status: Nonprofit
Paid Staff: 100
Budget: 1,600-8,500
Income Sources: Equity-Waiver; Los Angeles Theatre Alliance; SCETA; American College Theatre Festival
Seating Capacity: 312; 99
Year Built: 1965
Organization Type: Performing; Educational

2445 LOS ANGELES THEATRE CENTER: MOVING ARTS

514 S Spring Street
Los Angeles, CA 90013-2304
Phone: 213-622-8906
Fax: 213-622-8946
e-mail: info@movingarts.org
Web Site: www.movingarts.org
Management:
Artistic Director: Lee Wochner
Artistic Director: Julie Briggs
Literary Director: Trey Nichols
Administrative Director: David Davidson
Mission: We produce new plays that challenge, illuminate, and reveal truths about the human condition in a fresh and startling way.
Founded: 1992
Specialized Field: Theatre
Paid Staff: 1
Volunteer Staff: 3
Non-paid Artists: 28

2446 LOYOLA MARYMOUNT UNIVERSITY THEATRE ARTS DEPARTMENT

Los Angeles, CA 90045
Phone: 310-338-2837
Officers:
Co-Chair: Katharine B Free
Affiliations: NAST; ATHE
Seating Capacity: 174; 100
Year Built: 1961

2447 MARK TAPER FORUM

601 W Temple Street
Los Angeles, CA 90012
Phone: 213-628-2772
Fax: 213-628-2796
e-mail: tickets@ctgla.com
Web Site: www.taperahmanson.com
Management:
Artistic Director: Gordon Davidson
Managing Director: Charles Dillingham
Chairman: Phyllis Hennigan
Founded: 1967
Paid Staff: 350
Performs At: Performing Arts Center of Los Angeles
Affiliations: Ahmanson Theatre
Annual Attendance: 250,000
Facility Category: Theatre House
Type of Stage: Thrust
Stage Dimensions: 190Wx47Dx67H; 40Wx28H
Seating Capacity: 750
Year Built: 1967
Rental Contact: Gordon Davidson

2448 MOVING ARTS AT THE LOS ANGELES THEATRE CENTER

514 S Spring Street
Los Angeles, CA 90013-2304
Phone: 925-938-3300
Fax: 925-938-3300
e-mail: info@movingarts.org
Web Site: www.movingarts.org
Officers:
VP: Connie Leonard
Secretary: Darrell Kunitomi
Management:
Artistic Director: Kimberley Glann
Literary Director: Terry Nichols
Mission: Moving Arts is committed to producing high quality presentations of orginal dramas and comedies that are bold, challenging, edgy and relevant to the community
Founded: 1992
Specialized Field: Theatre
Paid Staff: 1
Volunteer Staff: 6
Budget: $79,000
Income Sources: Ticket Sales; Individual Donars; Government Grants
Annual Attendance: 1200
Type of Stage: Black Box
Seating Capacity: 51

2449 NINE O'CLOCK PLAYERS
1367 N St. Andrews Place
Los Angeles, CA 90028
Phone: 323-469-1970
Fax: 323-469-3533
Officers:
   Chairman: Nanette Taylor
   First Vice Chairman: Heather Lee
   Second Vice Chairman: Shelia Swicker
   Third Vice Chairman/Production: Mary Ferrara
Mission: To provide free musical theater for culturally and physically disadvantaged children as well as paid performances for all children of Southern California; to donate proceeds to the services of the Assistance League of Southern California.
Founded: 1929
Specialized Field: Musical; Theatrical Group; Musical Theatre; Childrens classic fairy tales
Status: Semi-Professional; Nonprofit
Paid Staff: 4
Volunteer Staff: 145
Budget: $100,000
Income Sources: Donations; Tickets
Performs At: ALSC Playhouse
Affiliations: Assistance League of Southern California
Annual Attendance: 15,000
Facility Category: Theatre
Seating Capacity: 329
Year Built: 1939
Year Remodeled: 2000
Rental Contact: 323-469-1973 Janet Harrison
Organization Type: Performing; Touring

2450 OCCIDENTAL COLLEGE DEPARTMENT OF THEATRE
1600 Campus Road
Los Angeles, CA 90041
Phone: 213-259-2771
Fax: 213-341-4987
Web Site: www.oxy.edu
Officers:
   Chair: Susan Gratch
Budget: $4,400-6,800
Seating Capacity: 400; 400
Year Built: 1988

2451 ODYSSEY THEATRE ENSEMBLE
2055 S Sepulveda Boulevard
Los Angeles, CA 90025
Phone: 310-477-2055
Fax: 310-444-0455
e-mail: odyssey@odysseytheatre.com
Web Site: www.odysseytheatre.com
Officers:
   President: Sol Rabin
   Secretary: Ben Olan
   VP: David Simon
   Treasurer: Fred Mantner
Management:
   Artistic Director: Ron Sossi
   Production Manager: Christina Burck
   Managing Director: David A Mills
   Associate Artistic Director: Beth Hogan

Mission: The creation of a theatre centre which is experimental and alternative and houses an ensemble company; the development of an international theatre center.
Founded: 1969
Specialized Field: Musical; Theatrical Group
Status: Professional; Nonprofit
Paid Staff: 14
Volunteer Staff: 86
Paid Artists: 126
Budget: $700,000
Income Sources: Theatre Consortium (Los Angeles Theatre Pass); League of Producers; Theatres of Los Angeles; Los Angeles Theatre Alliance; Theatre Communications Group
Performs At: Odyssey Theatre
Annual Attendance: 2000
Seating Capacity: 99
Rental Contact: Stephanie Meyer
Organization Type: Performing; Resident; Sponsoring

2452 PLAYWRIGHTS' ARENA
514 S Spring Street
Los Angeles, CA 90013
Phone: 213-627-4473
Fax: 213-473-0620
e-mail: jrivera923@juno.com
Web Site: www.playwrightsarena.org
Management:
   Artistic Director: Jon Lawrence Rivera
Mission: Dedicated to discovering, nurturing and producing bold new works for the stage written exclusively by Los Angeles playwrights. Develops new materials through several series of readings, workshops and round table discussions. Local playwrights are encouraged to create original, adventurous, daring materials with the intent of challenging the mind touching the heart and provoking the spirit.
Founded: 1992
Status: Nonprofit
Season: January - December
Type of Stage: Proscenium
Seating Capacity: 35

2453 THEATRE WEST
3333 Cahuenga Boulevard W
Los Angeles, CA 90068
Phone: 323-851-4839
Fax: 323-851-5286
e-mail: theatrewest@theatrewest.org
Web Site: www.theatrewest.org
Management:
   Executive Director: John Gallogly
   Administrative Assistant: Molly Reynolds
   Artistic Moderator: Lou Antonio
Mission: Conducting weekly theater workshops; producing several plays annually; enhancing the cultural life of the community.
Founded: 1962
Specialized Field: Theatrical Group
Status: Professional; Nonprofit
Paid Staff: 2
Volunteer Staff: 100
Income Sources: Dues; fund-raisers; grants
Performs At: Theatre West

Annual Attendance: 9,000
Facility Category: Non-profit
Seating Capacity: 168
Organization Type: Performing; Resident; Educational

2454 UNIVERSITY OF CALIFORNIA-LOS ANGELES: DEPARTMENT OF THEATER

Los Angeles, CA 90095
Phone: 310-825-7008
Fax: 310-825-3383
Web Site: www.tft.ucla.edu
Officers:
   Chair: William D Ward
Budget: $7,100-22,500
Affiliations: Geffen Playhouse
Seating Capacity: 589; 200; 100
Year Built: 1963

2455 UNIVERSITY OF SOUTHERN CALIFORNIA: SCHOOL OF THEATRE

Los Angeles, CA 90089
Phone: 213-740-1285
Fax: 213-740-8888
Web Site: www.usc.edu/theatre
Management:
   Dean: Robert R Scales
Affiliations: 24th Street Theatre
Seating Capacity: 575; 99; 60
Year Built: 1965

2456 WEST COAST ENSEMBLE

Box 38728
Los Angeles, CA 90038
Phone: 323-876-9337
Fax: 323-876-8916
Management:
   Artistic Director: Les Hanson
Founded: 1982

2457 WILTERN THEATRE

3790 Wilshire Boulevard
Los Angeles, CA 90010
Phone: 213-388-4005
Fax: 213-388-1400
Management:
   General Manager: Rena Wasserman

2458 ZEPHYR THEATRE

7456 Melrose Avenue
Los Angeles, CA 90046
Phone: 323-653-4667
Fax: 323-852-9633
Management:
   General Manager: Linda Toliver
   Technical Director: Gary Guidinger
Mission: Producing new work; Providing a rental venue for independent producers to mount shows.
Founded: 1977
Status: Professional; Commercial
Income Sources: Los Angeles League of Theaters & Producers
Performs At: Zephyr Theatre
Organization Type: Performing

2459 MAMMOTH LAKES SUMMER REPERTORY THEATRE

Cerro Coso College
PO Box 1865, 100 College Parkway
Mammoth Lakes, CA 93546
Phone: 760-924-3650
Fax: 760-934-9568
e-mail: vmguder@gte.net
Management:
   Instructor: Vic Guder
Founded: 1998
Status: Nonprofit; Non-Equity
Season: July 9-August 19
Type of Stage: Flexible
Seating Capacity: 150

2460 MENDOCINO THEATRE COMPANY

45200 Little Lake Street
PO Box 800
Mendocino, CA 95460
Phone: 707-937-4477
e-mail: www.mcn.org/1/mtc
Web Site: mtc@mcn.orn
Officers:
   President: Raven Deerwater
   VP: Dorothy Wandruff
   Treasurer: Ferren Taylor
   Secretary: Lindsey Morin
Management:
   Producing Director: Doug Warner
   Business Manager: Dick Ahrens
   Program/Signage: Mervin Gibert
Mission: The mission of the Mendocino Theatre Company is to produce plays of substance and excitement ranging from classics to cutting edge; nurture local talent; and provide meaningful theatrical experiences for both local and visiting audiences.

2461 MENLO PLAYERS GUILD

601 Laurel Street
Menlo Park, CA 90028
Mailing Address: PO Box 301, Menlo Park, CA. 94026
Phone: 213-463-5336
Fax: 213-463-5356

2462 THEATREWORKS

1100 Hamilton Court
PO Box 50458
Menlo Park, CA 94303-0458
Phone: 650-463-7126
Fax: 650-463-1963
e-mail: jeannie@theatreworks.org
Web Site: www.theatreworks.org
Management:
   Literary Manager: Jeannie Barroga
   Artistic Director: Robert Kelley
   Managing Director: Randy Adams
Founded: 1969

2463 MARIN THEATRE COMPANY

397 Miller Avenue
Mill Valley, CA 94941

Phone: 415-388-5200
Fax: 415-381-3724
e-mail: info@marintheatre.org
Web Site: www.marintheatre.org
Officers:
 President: Thomas M Foster
 VP: Joseph Bodovitz
 Treasurer: Ivan Poutiatine
 Secretary: Susan Johann Gilardi
Management:
 Marketing Director: Ellie Madnick
 Artistic Director: Lee Sankowich
 Managing Director: James A Kleinmann
 Development Associate: Suzie Woodward-Morris
 Development Associate: Loretta Brice
Mission: Presenting a season of performances; nurturing new plays; providing theatrical training; presenting other art forms.
Founded: 1966
Specialized Field: Theatrical Group
Status: Professional; Nonprofit
Paid Staff: 12
Income Sources: Theatre Communications Group; Grants; Individual donations; Ticket sales; Corporate sponsorship; Special events
Performs At: Marin Theatre Company
Seating Capacity: 264
Organization Type: Performing; Resident; Educational; Sponsoring

2464 SADDLEBACK COLLEGE

28000 Marguerite Parkway
Mission Viejo, CA 92692-3635
Phone: 949-582-4763
Fax: 949-347-8653
e-mail: info@saddleback.cc.ca.us
Web Site: www.saddleback.cc.ca.us
Management:
 Director Performing Arts: Geof English
Performs At: McKinney Theatre; Cabaret Theatre

2465 ACTORS FORUM THEATRE

10655 Magnolia Boulevard
N. Hollywood, CA 91601
Phone: 818-506-0600
Fax: 818-506-0686
e-mail: Actorsamtheatre@aol.com
Management:
 Co-Artistic Director: Audrey Marlyn Singer
 Co-Artistic Director: Shawn Michael
Founded: 1975
Status: Nonprofit
Income Sources: Patrons; Classes; Rentals; Shows
Facility Category: Theatre
Type of Stage: Floor with curtain
Stage Dimensions: 24' x 20'
Seating Capacity: 49
Year Remodeled: 1994

2466 TEATRO SHALOM

1811 Monarch Drive
Napa, CA 94558
Phone: 707-226-9918
Fax: 707-224-8065

Management:
 Artistic Director: David Gassner
 Managing Director: David Acevedo
Specialized Field: Theater

2467 FOOTHILL THEATRE COMPANY

401 Broad Street
PO Box 1812
Nevada City, CA 95959
Phone: 530-265-9320
Fax: 530-265-9325
Toll-free: 888-730-8587
e-mail: info@foothilltheatre.org
Web Site: www.foothilltheatre.org
Management:
 Literary Manager: Gary Wright
 Artistic Director: Philip Charles Sneed
 Marketing Director: Karyn Casl
Founded: 1977
Specialized Field: Theater Company
Performs At: Nevada Theatre
Affiliations: AEA; CAC; TCG
Annual Attendance: 56,000
Facility Category: Historic Structure
Type of Stage: Proscenium
Seating Capacity: 246

2468 AMERICAN RENEGADE THEATRE COMPANY

11136 Magnolia Boulevard
North Hollywood, CA 91601
Phone: 818-763-4430
Management:
 Likterary Manager: Barry Thompson
Performs At: Front Theatre, Back Theatre(Black Box)
Type of Stage: Proscenium, Black Box
Seating Capacity: 99, 45

2469 EL PORTAL CENTER FOR THE ARTS

5269 Lankershim Boulevard
North Hollywood, CA 91601
Phone: 818-508-4234
Fax: 818-508-5113
Officers:
 President: Thomas H Cole
 Vice President: Carol Rowen
 Secretary: Sunny Caine
Management:
 Artistic Director: Jeremiah Morris
 Managing Director: Robert Caine
Mission: The challenge of a true regional theater is to create and enhance the development of all facets of theater arts within the community in which it lives. Actors Alley Repertory Theater is dedicated to meeting that challenge.
Founded: 1971
Status: Professional; Nonprofit
Paid Staff: 65
Income Sources: Los Angeles Theatre Alliance; California Theater Council
Performs At: Alley Theater (Pavilion, Circle Forum)
Type of Stage: Proscenium, Thrust, Flexible
Seating Capacity: 350, 99, 42
Organization Type: Performing; Resident

2470 GROUP REPERTORY THEATRE
10900 Burbank Boulevard
North Hollywood, CA 91601
Phone: 818-769-7529
Officers:
   President: Larry Eisenberg
   Treasurer: Geraldine Allen
Management:
   Artistic Director: Lonny Chapman
   Assistant Artistic Director: Burt Rosario
Mission: To stage five to six productions each year emphasizing new works by playwrights and young actors; to work with the Los Angeles Unified School District to produce theatrical presentations for those learning English as a second language.
Founded: 1973
Specialized Field: Theatrical Group
Status: Professional; Nonprofit
Income Sources: Valley Arts Council
Performs At: Group Repertory Theatre
Organization Type: Performing

2471 SYNTHAXIS THEATRE COMPANY
6310 Whitsett Avenue
North Hollywood, CA 91607
Phone: 213-877-4726
Management:
   Executive Director: Estelle Bush
Mission: Presenting new works as well as lesser-known works of renowned authors; emphasizing works by women; presenting benefit performances and shows for children.
Founded: 1972
Specialized Field: Theatrical Group
Status: Professional; Nonprofit
Income Sources: Los Angeles Theatre Alliance; San Fernando Valley Arts Council
Organization Type: Performing; Touring; Resident; Educational

2472 CALIFORNIA STATE UNIVERSITY, NORTHRIDGE: DEPARTMENT OF THEATRE
18111 Nordhoff Street
Northridge, CA 91330
Phone: 818-677-3086
Officers:
   Chair: Jerry Abbitt
Affiliations: NAST; ATHE; Mark Taper Forum
Seating Capacity: 400; 205; 100
Year Built: 1960

2473 MILLS COLLEGE DEPARTMENT OF DRAMATIC ARTS & COMMUNICATIONS
5000 MacArthur Boulevard
Oakland, CA 94613
Phone: 510-430-2327
Fax: 510-430-3314
Officers:
   Chair: Ken Burke
Budget: $1,050-3,200
Seating Capacity: 196; 63

Year Built: 1901
Year Remodeled: 1972

2474 GREAT AMERICAN MELODRAMA AND VAUDEVILLE
1863 Pacifiv Boulevard, Highway 1
PO Box 1026
Oceano, CA 93445
Phone: 805-489-2499
Fax: 805-489-5539
e-mail: jrslink@hotmail.com
Web Site: www.amiercanmelodrama.com
Management:
   Producer: John Schlenker
   Artistic Director: Eric Hoit
Mission: Produce 7 shows per year.
Founded: 1975
Status: 5on-Equity
Paid Staff: 8
Paid Artists: 12
Season: Year round
Type of Stage: Proscenium
Stage Dimensions: 20'x 25'
Seating Capacity: 260

2475 DELTA KING THEATRE
1000 Front Street
Old Sacramento, CA 95814
Phone: 916-995-5464
Fax: 916-444-5314
e-mail: sgularte@deltaking.com
Web Site: www.deltaking.com/theatre
Management:
   Artistic Director/Theatre Manager: Stephanie Gularte
   Theatre Assistant Manager: Amy Yan
Mission: To provide audiences with quality dinning/live theatre experience with contemporary plays performed by Sacramento top talent.
Founded: 2000
Specialized Field: Theatre/Dinner theatre
Paid Staff: 3

2476 SHAKESPEARE ORANGE COUNTY
301 E Palm Street
Orange, CA 92866
Mailing Address: PO Box 923, Orange, CA. 92856
Phone: 714-744-7016
Fax: 714-744-7015
Management:
   Artistic Director: Thomas F Bradac

2477 OROVILLE STATE THEATRE
1735 Montgomery Street
Oroville, CA 95965
Phone: 530-538-2471
Fax: 530-538-2468
Web Site: www.oroville-city.com
Management:
   Manager: Amelia Jennings
Performs At: State Theatre
Seating Capacity: 608

All listings are in alphabetical order by state, then city, then organization within the city.

2478 PALO ALTO CHILDREN'S THEATRE
1305 Middlefield Road
Palo Alto, CA 94301
Phone: 415-329-2216
Web Site: www.city.palo-alto.ca.us/theatre
Management:
    Director: Patricia Briggs
    Assistant Director: Michael Litfin
    Technical Director/Designer: Andy Hayes
    Costume Supervisor: Alison Williams
    Program Assistant: Sandy Rankin
Mission: To educate young people in all theatre arts including acting, dance, set design and construction, costuming and makeup, the design and use of sound and light systems, and performance direction and production.
Founded: 1932
Specialized Field: Musical; Theatrical Group
Status: Non-Professional; Nonprofit
Performs At: Palo Alto Children's Theatre
Organization Type: Performing; Educational

2479 THEATREWORKS
1305 Middlefield Road
Palo Alto, CA 94301
Phone: 415-323-8311
Fax: 415-323-3311
Web Site: www.theatreworks.org
Management:
    Artistic Director: Robert Kelley
    Managing Director: Randy Adams
Founded: 1970
Specialized Field: Musical; Theatrical Group
Status: Professional; Semi-Professional; Nonprofit
Income Sources: Theatre Communications Group
Performs At: The Lucy Stern Theatre; The Mountain View Center
Organization Type: Performing

2480 PASADENA PLAYHOUSE
39 S El Molino Avenue
80 S Lake Avenue, Suite 500
Pasadena, CA 91101
Phone: 626-692-8672
Fax: 626-792-7343
e-mail: patroninfo@pasadenaplayhouse.com
Web Site: www.pasadenaplayhouse.org
Management:
    Artistic Director: Sheldon Epps
    Executive Director: Lyla L White
    Producing Director: Thomas Ware
    General Manager: Brian Colburn
Founded: 1917

2481 CINNABAR THEATER
3333 Petaluma Boulevard N
Petaluma, CA 94952
Phone: 707-763-8920
Fax: 707-763-8929
Management:
    Director Artistic/Managing: Elly Lichenstein

2482 INDEPENDENT EYE
115 Arch Street
Philadelphia, CA 19106
Phone: 215-925-2838
Fax: 215-925-0839
Toll-free: 800-357-6016
e-mail: info@independenteye.org
Web Site: www.independenteye.org
Management:
    Associate Producing Director: Elizabeth Fuller
    Artistic Director: Donald Alsedek
Mission: The Independent Eye is a progressive theatre ensemble, now in its 27th year, devoted to creating new plays and new visions of classics. Based in Northern California, our work reaches a national audience.
Founded: 1974
Status: Nonprofit; Non-Equity
Season: Year Round

2483 THEATRE EL DORADO
El Dorado County Fairgrounds
100 Placerville Drive
Placerville, CA 95667
Phone: 530-626-5193
e-mail: email@theatreeldorado.com
Web Site: www.theatreeldorado.com

2484 CALIFORNIA STATE POLYTECHNIC UNIVERSITY: DEPARTMENT OF THEATRE
3801 West Temple Avenue
Pomona, CA 91768
Phone: 909-869-3900
Fax: 909-869-3184
Officers:
    Chair: Kathleen H Waln
Budget: $5,375-20,650
Affiliations: Mark Taper Forum; South Coast Repertory
Seating Capacity: 543; 300-500
Year Built: 1965
Year Remodeled: 1998

2485 GARBEAU'S DINNER THEATER
12401 Folsom Boulevard
Rancho Cordova, CA 95742-6413
Phone: 916-985-6361
Fax: 916-985-7375
e-mail: info@garbeaus.com
Web Site: www.garbeaus.com
Management:
    Managing Director: Mark Fahey
    House Manager: Raquel Pearson
    Artistic Director: Barbara Valente
Founded: 1981
Status: Non-Equity
Seating Capacity: 100
Year Remodeled: 1980

2486 PERFORMANCE RIVERSIDE
4800 Magnolia Avenue
Riverside, CA 92506
Phone: 909-222-8399
Fax: 909-222-8940

Management:
Executive Director: Steven A Glaudini
Founded: 1983

2487 UNIVERSITY OF CALIFORNIA-RIVERSIDE: DEPARTMENT OF THEATRE
Riverside, CA 92521
Phone: 909-787-3343
Fax: 909-787-4651
Web Site: www.performingarts.ucr.edu
Officers:
Chairperson: Eric Barr
Budget: $20,500-22,500
Affiliations: ATHE; U/RTA
Seating Capacity: 500; 150; 120; 50

2488 SONOMA STATE UNIVERSITY THEATER DEPARTMENT
1801 East Cotati Avenue
Rohnert Park, CA 94928
Phone: 707-664-2474
Web Site: www.sonoma.edu/Depts/PerformingArtsTheatre
Officers:
Chair: Jeff Langley
Budget: $14,250-62,000
Affiliations: ATHE
Seating Capacity: 500; 300; 99
Year Built: 1990

2489 MAGIC CIRCLE REPERTORY THEATER
241 Vernon Street
Roseville, CA 95678
Phone: 916-782-1777
Fax: 916-782-1766
e-mail: mcircle@mcircle.org
Web Site: www.mcircle.org
Officers:
President: Dave Woolridge
VP: Cindy Nichols-Kitchell
Secretary: Harry Crabb
Treasurer: Ted Parker
Management:
Executive Producer: Robert C Gerould
Artistic Director: Rosemarie Gerould
Administrative Assistant: Teri Heitman
Education Outreach Director: Michelle Pabst
Marketing Director: Kris Hunt
Mission: To offer a high quality, full performing arts center for production and performance in the fields of dance, acting, and music. Additionally, we offer superior education and training of new talent in the areas of acting, dancing, technical support, production, and theatre management skills for all age groups. We will continue to invest in the future of our craft, to grow with the communities surrounding us, and to listen to our patrons.
Founded: 1987
Specialized Field: Live Theater
Budget: $500,000

Income Sources: Ads in the Program; Grants; Donations; Ticket Sales; Concessions; Sponsorships; Workshop Fees; Acting Class Fees
Performs At: Community Theatre
Affiliations: Roseville Theatre
Facility Category: Community Theatre
Type of Stage: Proscenium
Seating Capacity: 500
Year Built: 1929
Year Remodeled: 2001
Rental Contact: Executive Director Robert Gerould

2490 B STREET THEATER
2711 B Street
Sacramento, CA 95816
Phone: 916-443-5300
Fax: 916-443-0874
e-mail: bstreetsac@aol.com
Founded: 1991
Specialized Field: New American Works
Paid Staff: 10
Income Sources: Ticket Sales; Donations; Grants
Performs At: 3/4 Thrust Stage
Facility Category: Small Theatre
Type of Stage: Thrust
Year Built: 1991

2491 BEST OF BROADWAY
4010 El Camino Avenue
Sacramento, CA 95821
Phone: 916-974-6280
Fax: 916-974-6281
e-mail: cathy@bestofbroadway.org
Web Site: www.bestofbroadway.org
Mission: Dedicated to bringing a live theatrical experience to the community of Sacramento. Through music, song and dance its goals are to educate, entertain and inspire local children, youth and adults.
Founded: 1973
Specialized Field: Musical theatre
Paid Staff: 2
Volunteer Staff: 100
Non-paid Artists: 250
Budget: $250,000
Income Sources: Grants; Ticket sales; Concessions
Annual Attendance: 12,000
Facility Category: High School Auditorium
Type of Stage: Proscenium
Seating Capacity: 1,400 per performance
Year Built: 1950
Year Remodeled: 1990

2492 BEYOND THE PROSCENIUM PRODUCTIONS
2030 Del Pado Boulevard
Sacramento, CA 95815
Phone: 916-922-9774
Fax: 916-922-9774
e-mail: beyondpro@aol.com
Web Site: www.shopgenerocity.com/beyond
Status: Nonprofit

2493 CALIFORNIA MUSICAL THEATRE
1510 J Street
Suite 200
Sacramento, CA 95801
Phone: 916-446-5880
Fax: 916-446-1370
e-mail: subscribers@calmt.com
Web Site: www.californiamusicaltheatre.com
Officers:
  President: Rick Frey
  Market President: David Galasso
  President: Cecilia Delury
Management:
  Producing Director: Leland Ball
  Managing Director: Richard Lewis
  Co-Manager: Marlene Shire
Founded: 1951
Status: Nonprofit
Paid Staff: 10
Season: June-August
Type of Stage: Arena
Seating Capacity: 2500

2494 CALIFORNIA STATE UNIVERSITY, SACRAMENTO: DEPARTMENT OF THEATRE OF DANCE
6000 J Street
Sacramento, CA 95819
Phone: 916-278-6368
Fax: 916-278-5681
Web Site: www.csus.edu/dram/index.html
Officers:
  Chair: Robert Pomo
Budget: $4,850-12,100
Affiliations: NAST
Seating Capacity: 438; 200
Year Built: 1957
Year Remodeled: 1970

2495 LAMBDA PLAYERS
1927 L Street
Sacramento, CA 95814
Phone: 916-442-0185
e-mail: lambdapl@pacbell.net
Web Site: www.lambdaplayers.org
Officers:
  President: West Ramsey
  Secretary: Maureen Gaynor
  VP: Tom Swanner
  Business Manager: Charles Peer
Management:
  Production Manager: Stephen Abate
  Secretary: Gregg Peterson
  Business Manager: Charles Peer
  Fund Development: West Ramesy
  President: Marsha Swayze
  VP: Greg Brooks
Affiliations: Sacramento Area Regional Theater Alliance and The League of Sacramento Theaters.

2496 RIVER STAGE
Cosumnes River College
Visual & Performing Arts Center
8401 Center Parkway
Sacramento, CA 95823-5799
Phone: 916-688-7364
Fax: 916-688-7181
Web Site: www.riverstage.org
Officers:
  President: Steve Macugenroth
  President: Willam Smith
  VP: Steve Macugenroth
Management:
  Artistic Director: Frank Condon
  Assistant Artistic Director: Kale Braden
  Managing Partner: Robert King Fong
  Design Director: Jim Love
  Features Editor: Nan Mahon
  Assistant Executvie Officer: Patricia Canterbury
  Principal: Blair Barton
  Theatre Arts Educator: Carolyn Elder
Status: Professional

2497 SACRAMENTO THEATRE COMPANY
1419 H Street
Sacramento, CA 95814
Phone: 916-443-6722
Fax: 916-446-4066
Web Site: www.sactheatre.org/
Management:
  Artistic Director: Peggy Shannon
  Company Manager: Shpritz Anthony
  Managine Directorr: Christine Begovich
  Group Sales Manager: Elaine Rodman
  Business Manager: Raj Badhan
  Box Office Manager: Keri Losche
  Marketing Manager: Nicole Schallig
  Managing Director: Christine Bedovich
  Director Development: Carol Davydova
Mission: To professionally produce contemporary and traditional theatrical works that are engaging to the hearts and minds of a diverse regional audience.
Founded: 1942
Status: Professional; Tax Exempt; Nonprofit
Performs At: McClatchy Mainstage Theatre
Seating Capacity: 300

2498 WESTERN STAGE
156 Homestead Avenue
Salinas, CA 93901
Phone: 831-755-6987
Fax: 831-755-6954
e-mail: mchin@hartnell.cc.ca.us
Web Site: www.westernstage.org
Officers:
  President: Raul Chavez
Management:
  Executive Director: Harvey Landa
  Associate Artistic Director: Melissa Chin
  Artistic Director: Tom Humphrey
  Development Director: John Light

Mission: To provide theatre programs that educate and enrich the lives of the people of the Central Coast of California by utilizing professional artists, teachers, students and the community.
Founded: 1973
Specialized Field: Theater
Status: Non-Equity; Nonprofit
Paid Staff: 16
Volunteer Staff: 18
Paid Artists: 41
Non-paid Artists: 11
Budget: $1,100,000
Income Sources: Ticket Sales; Donations; Contract Services
Season: June - August
Performs At: Main Theater; Black Box Studio
Affiliations: NAMT; TCG
Annual Attendance: 35,000
Type of Stage: Proscenium; Black Box
Seating Capacity: 501; 99
Year Built: 1973

2499   GLOBE THEATRES
1363 Old Globe Way
San Diego, CA 92112
Mailing Address: PO Box 122171, San Diego, CA. 92112-2171
Phone: 619-231-1941
Fax: 619-231-5879
Web Site: www.theglobetheatres.org
Officers:
   President: Paul Meyer
Management:
   Associated Artistic Director: Karen Carpenter
   Executive Director: Craig Noel
   Artistic Director: Jack O'Brien
Mission: To affirm its commitment to its survival in maintaining the integrity of theatre by producing the highest quality professional theatre; to undertake a wide spectrum of theatrical enterprises with continued emphasis on Shakespeare as well as other world classics and contemporary and new works; to provide theatrical professionals with a challenging and supportive environment.
Founded: 1935
Opened: 1982
Specialized Field: Theatrical Group
Status: Professional; Nonprofit
Paid Staff: 200+
Budget: $8.5 million
Income Sources: Theatre Communications Group; League of Resident Theatres; American Arts Alliance
Season: January - November
Performs At: Old Globe; Cassius Carter Centre; Lowell Davies Festival
Annual Attendance: 300,000+
Type of Stage: Proscenium, black box, 3/4 thrust
Seating Capacity: 543-649
Organization Type: Performing; Educational; Sponsoring

2500   HORTON GRAND THEATRE
444 Fourth Avenue
San Diego, CA 92101

Phone: 619-234-3588
Fax: 619-234-3587
e-mail: matt@tripleespresso.com
Web Site: www.tripleespresso.com
Management:
   General Manager: Matt Boden
Founded: 1985
Paid Staff: 20
Paid Artists: 20
Income Sources: Ticket Sales
Affiliations: San Diego Arts League; San Diego Regional Chamber of Commerce; San Diego Convention & Visitors Bureau
Annual Attendance: 50,000
Facility Category: Rental House
Type of Stage: Proscenium
Stage Dimensions: 29'9x18'x2s'6"
Organization Type: Performing; Educational; Sponsoring

2501   MARIE HITCHCOCK PUPPET THEATRE IN BALBOA
Balboa Park Management Office
2130 Pan American Plaza
San Diego, CA 92101
Phone: 619-685-5045
Fax: 619-235-1100
Affiliations: San Diego Guild of Puppetry
Facility Category: Puppet Theatre
Type of Stage: Proscenium

2502   PLAYWRIGHTS PROJECT
450 B Street
Suite 1020
San Diego, CA 92101-8093
Phone: 619-239-8222
Fax: 619-239-8225
e-mail: write@playwrightsproject.com
Web Site: www.playwrightsproject.com
Officers:
   Board President: David Carr
   Treasurer: Millie Basden
   Secretary: Kathleen Snyder
Management:
   Executive Director: Deborah Salzer
   Managing Director: Cecelia Kouma
Mission: The mission is to promote literacy, communication skills and creativity through drama-based activities, with an emphasis on inspiring youth and seniors
Founded: 1985
Paid Staff: 7

2503   SAN DIEGO JUNIOR THEATRE
Casa del Prado
#208, Balboa Park
San Diego, CA 92101
Phone: 619-239-1311
Fax: 619-239-4058
Web Site: www.juniortheatre.com
Management:
   Artistic Director: Wil Neblett
   Executive Director: Pat Rogers
   Education Director: Jennifer Nash
   Marketing/Public Relations: Deborah Sims

Mission: To offer instruction in theatre arts to youth, aged 8-18.
Founded: 1948
Specialized Field: Theatrical Group
Status: Non-Professional; Nonprofit
Paid Staff: 300
Income Sources: SCETA; San Diego Theatre League
Performs At: Casa del Prado Theatre
Organization Type: Performing; Educational

2504 SAN DIEGO REPERTORY THEATRE
79 Horton Plaza
San Diego, CA 92101
Phone: 619-231-3586
Fax: 619-235-0939
Web Site: www.sandiegorep.com/
Management:
   Managing Director: Karen Wood
   Artistic Director/Co-Founder: Sam Woodhouse
   Marketing Director: Laurie Malmstrom
   Public Relations Manager: Jill McIntyre
Mission: Adventurous theatre.
Founded: 1975
Paid Staff: 43

2505 SAN DIEGO STATE UNIVERSITY: DEPARTMENT OF THEATRE
San Diego, CA 92182
Phone: 619-594-6363
Officers:
   Chair: Alicia Annas
Budget: $11,347-12,747
Affiliations: NAST; ATHE
Seating Capacity: 500; 175
Year Built: 1969
Year Remodeled: 1989

2506 SOUTHEAST COMMUNITY THEATRE
5140 Solola Avenue
San Diego, CA 92114
Phone: 619-262-2817
Management:
   Artistic Director: Floyd Gaffney
   Production Manager: Bonnie J Ward
   Business Manager: Rufus DeWitt
Mission: Promoting African-American playwrights by showcasing non-professional, semi-professional and professional artists.
Founded: 1976
Specialized Field: Community; Theatrical Group
Status: Semi-Professional; Nonprofit
Income Sources: American Association of Community Theatres
Performs At: Educational Cultural Complex Performing Arts Thea
Organization Type: Performing; Resident; Sponsoring

2507 STARLIGHT MUSICAL THEATRE SAN DIEGO CIVIC LIGHT OPERA ASSOCIATION
1549 El Prado - Balboa Park
San Diego, CA 92101
Phone: 619-544-7800
Fax: 619-544-0496
Management:
   Executive Director: CE Bud Farnks
   Producing Artistic Director: Don Ward
   Producing Artistic Director: Bonnie Ward
Mission: The preservation and promotion of the art form of musical theatre.
Founded: 1946
Specialized Field: Light Opera; Musical Theatre
Status: Professional; Nonprofit
Performs At: Starlight Bowl; Civic Theatre; Spreckles Theatre
Organization Type: Performing; Educational

2508 AFRICAN AMERICAN DRAMA COMPANY
394 5th Avenue
San Francisco, CA 94118
Phone: 415-333-2232
Management:
   Executive Director: Phillip E Walker
   Executive Director: Ethel Pitts Walker
Mission: To offer American audiences Black history and African plays.
Founded: 1977
Specialized Field: Theatrical Group
Status: Professional
Organization Type: Touring

2509 AMERICAN CONSERVATORY THEATRE
30 Grant Avenue, 6th Floor
San Francisco, CA 94108-5800
Phone: 415-439-2350
Fax: 415-834-3300
Web Site: www.act-sfbay.org
Officers:
   General/Company Manager: Dianne F Prichard
   Associate Managing Director: Scott Ellis
   Executive Assistant/Managing: Kai Collins
   Company Management Assistant: Caresa Capaz
   Volunteer Coordinator: Barbara Gerber
   Finance Director: Jeffrey P. Malloy
   Marketing Director: Andrew Smith
Management:
   Director: Melissa Smith
   Dramaturg: Paul Walsh
   Associate Artistic Director: Margo Whitcomb
   Assistant/Artistic Director: Jennifer Caleshu
   Casting Assistant: Kathryn Clark
   Artistic Director: Carey Perloff
   Managing Director: Heather Kitchen
   Conservatory Director: Melissa Smith
   Producing Director: James Haire
Mission: Performing contemporary and classical plays in conjunction with theatre training.
Founded: 1965
Status: Professional; Nonprofit
Income Sources: League of Resident Theatres; Theatre Communications Group; American Arts Alliance; California Confederation of the Arts; National Corporation Theatre Fund
Performs At: Geary Theatre
Affiliations: American Conservatory Theatre

Type of Stage: Proscenium
Seating Capacity: 1014
Year Built: 1910
Year Remodeled: 1996
Rental Contact: Bob MacDonald (439-2392)
Organization Type: Performing; Resident; Educational

2510 ASIAN AMERICAN THEATER COMPANY

1840 Sutter Street
Suite 207
San Francisco, CA 94115
Phone: 415-440-5545
Fax: 415-440-5597
e-mail: aatc@wenet.net
Management:
    Producing Director: Pamela Wu

2511 BRAVA! FOR WOMEN IN THE ARTS

2781 24th Street
San Francisco, CA 94110
Phone: 415-641-7657
Fax: 415-641-7684
e-mail: ellen@brava.org
Web Site: www.brava.org
Management:
    Artistic/Executive Director: Ellen Gavin
Founded: 1986
Performs At: Brava Theatre Center, Barbie Stein Youth Theater
Type of Stage: Thrust, Black Box
Seating Capacity: 375, 100

2512 EL TEATRO DE LA ESPERANZA

PO Box 40578
San Francisco, CA 94140
Phone: 415-255-2320
Web Site: www.artsandlectures.ucsb.edu/
Management:
    Artistic Director: Rodrigo Durte Clark
    General Manager: Eve Donovan
Mission: To present bi-cultural, bilingual plays that further theatre in the Chicano community.
Specialized Field: Theatrical Group
Status: Professional; Nonprofit
Performs At: Mission Culture Center
Organization Type: Touring; Resident

2513 EUREKA THEATRE COMPANY

215 Jackson Street
San Francisco, CA 94111
Mailing Address: 555 Howard Street, Suite 201A, San Francisco, CA. 94105
Phone: 415-243-9899
Fax: 415-243-0789
Web Site: www.eurekatheatre.org
Management:
    Co-Artistic Director: Andrea Gordon
    Co-Artistic Director: Lane Nishikawa
    Co-Artistic Director: Benny Sato Ambush
Mission: Producing contemporary plays focusing on social and political issues.
Founded: 1972

Specialized Field: Theatrical Group
Status: Professional; Nonprofit
Income Sources: Actors' Equity Association; Coalition of Bay Area Theatres
Performs At: Eureka Theatre
Type of Stage: Proscenium
Stage Dimensions: 22' x 40'
Seating Capacity: 200
Organization Type: Performing; Resident; Educational

2514 GEORGE COATES PERFORMANCE WORKS

110 McAllister Street
San Francisco, CA 94102
Phone: 415-863-8520
Fax: 415-863-7939
e-mail: staff@georgecoates@org
Web Site: www.georgecoates.org
Officers:
    President: Craig Martin
    VP: Richard Cole
    Secretary: Cathy Elienberger-Ubell
    Treasurer: Michael McDonell
Management:
    Artistic Director: George Coates
    Managing Director: Friday Savathphoun
    Production Manager: Chris Read
Mission: To broaden the boundaries of contemporary performances and the creative experience itself; to explore new relationships between performer and audience; to develop new alliances between arts ensembles, individuals and emerging technology industries; emphasis on contemporary vocal expression and multimedia.
Founded: 1977
Specialized Field: New Music Theatre
Status: Nonprofit
Paid Staff: 4
Performs At: Performance Works
Organization Type: Performing; Touring; Resident

2515 ILLUSTRATED STAGE COMPANY

PO Box 640063
San Francisco, CA 94164
Phone: 415-861-6655
Management:
    General Manager: Barbara Malinowski
Founded: 1979
Specialized Field: Theatrical Group
Status: Professional; Nonprofit
Paid Staff: 1
Performs At: Alcazar Theatre
Organization Type: Performing; Resident

2516 JULIAN THEATRE

777 Valencia
San Francisco, CA 94110
Fax: 415-626-8986
Officers:
    Chairman: George Crowe
Management:
    Artistic/General Director: Richard Reineccius
    Library Manager: Veronica Masterson
    Development Director: Jackie Hayes
    Production Manager: Michael Dingle

Mission: To maintain interest in works that have a social or political sense of the times to serve as a multi-cultural theater working with new plays.
Founded: 1965
Specialized Field: Theatrical Group
Status: Professional; Nonprofit
Income Sources: Actors' Equity Association
Organization Type: Performing; Touring; Resident; Educational; Sponsoring

2517 LORRAINE HANSBERRY THEATRE

620 Sutter Street
555 Sutter Street, Suite 305
San Francisco, CA 94102
Phone: 415-288-0336
Fax: 415-288-0353
e-mail: lhtheatresf@cs.com
Web Site: www.lorrainehansberrytheatre.com
Management:
    Artistic Director: Stanley Williams
    Executive Director: Quentin Easter
    Adminstrative Associate: Amani Rashidi
    Administrative Director: Tod Green
    Production Associate: Marianella Macchiarini
Mission: To produce plays by America's and the world's leading Black writers; to foster the development of new Black writers through the ongoing activities of the playwrights workshop.
Founded: 1981
Status: Professional; Nonprofit
Paid Staff: 5
Volunteer Staff: 30
Paid Artists: 30
Performs At: Lorraine Hansberry Theater
Type of Stage: Modified, Proscenium Thrust
Seating Capacity: 300
Organization Type: Performing; Educational

2518 MAGIC THEATRE

Fort Mason Center
Building D
San Francisco, CA 94123
Phone: 415-441-8001
Fax: 415-771-5505
e-mail: info@magictheatre.org
Web Site: www.magictheatre.org
Management:
    General Manager: John Warren
Mission: Focused exclusively on developing new plays and playwrights and operating two professional theaters.
Founded: 1967
Specialized Field: Theatrical Group
Status: Professional; Nonprofit
Paid Staff: 20
Paid Artists: 150
Budget: 1.1 million
Income Sources: Actors' Equity Association
Season: June - August
Performs At: Northside Theatre; Southside Theatre
Annual Attendance: 20,000
Type of Stage: Proscenium
Stage Dimensions: 18'x 24'
Seating Capacity: 160
Rental Contact: General Manager John Warren
Organization Type: Performing; Resident; Sponsoring

2519 MAKE A CIRCUS

755 Frederick Street
San Francisco, CA 94117
Phone: 415-242-1414
Fax: 415-242-0579
e-mail: booking@makeacircus.org
Web Site: www.makeacircus.org
Management:
    Executive Director: Bill Ralhfuss
Mission: To provide opportunities for individuals, families and communities to experience self-empowerment through the magic of particapitory circus theatre.
Founded: 1974
Specialized Field: Musical; Community; Circus
Status: Nonprofit
Paid Staff: 5
Paid Artists: 25
Performs At: Any outdoor 100 x 100 flat, grassy area free of distractions
Annual Attendance: 40,000
Facility Category: Parks
Type of Stage: Outdoor
Stage Dimensions: 100' x 100'
Seating Capacity: 1,000
Organization Type: Performing; Touring; Educational; Participatory

2520 NEW CONSERVATORY CENTER THEATRE

25 Van Ness
Lower Lobby
San Francisco, CA 94102
Phone: 415-861-4914
Fax: 415-861-6988
e-mail: nctcsf@yahoo.com
Web Site: www.nctcsf.org
Officers:
    Chairman: Thomas Burke
    Chair Emeritus: George Vanberg Wolff
    Treasurer: Paul R Brody
    Secretary: Rich Kowalewski
Management:
    Artistic Director: Ed Decker
    Conservatory Director: Andrew Nance
    Business Manager: Brad Pence
    Managing Director: George Qureck
Mission: Through our work, we strive to make positive contributions to enrich the cultural and educational well-being of our world.
Founded: 1981
Specialized Field: Musical; Semi-Professional; Children's Theatre
Status: Professional; Nonprofit
Paid Staff: 9
Volunteer Staff: 5
Paid Artists: 20+
Budget: $950,000
Income Sources: 60% Earned; 40% Contributed
Performs At: The New Conservatory Theatre Center
Annual Attendance: 75,000
Facility Category: Multi-theatre; Art Gallery
Type of Stage: 2 Black Box; 1 Proscenium
Seating Capacity: 50 - 140
Year Built: 1904

All listings are in alphabetical order by state, then city, then organization within the city.

Year Remodeled: 1986
Organization Type: Performing; Touring; Educational

2521 PERSONA GRATA PRODUCTIONS

2 Alta Mar
San Francisco, CA 94121
Phone: 415-387-7898
Web Site: www.personagradaprod.org
Management:
   Executive Director: Paul Kwan
   Artistic Director: Arnold Iger
Mission: Educational and cross-cultural.
Founded: 1979
Specialized Field: Theatrical Group; Puppet
Status: Professional; Nonprofit
Paid Staff: 4
Organization Type: Performing; Educational

2522 PHOENIX ARTS ASSOCIATION THEATRE/WESTCOAST PLAYWRIGHTS ALLIANCE

Phoenix Theatre
414 Mason Street
San Francisco, CA 94117-3930
Mailing Address: 138 Carl Street
Phone: 415-759-7696
Fax: 415-664-5001
e-mail: lbaf23@aol.com
Management:
   Artistic Director/Managing Director: Linda B
   Ayres-Frederick
   Dramaturg: Eugene Price
   Technical Director: Michael Burg
Mission: To present new and often unperformed scripts and original adaptations of American, British, and European writers by Bay Area Artists as well as premiering the works of the West Coast Playwrights Alliance at their two intimate downtown San Francisco theatres.
Founded: 1985
Specialized Field: Theatre
Paid Staff: 4
Volunteer Staff: 10
Paid Artists: 15
Non-paid Artists: 3
Income Sources: Performances; Contributions; Rentals
Facility Category: Theatre
Type of Stage: Thrust
Stage Dimensions: 30x20
Seating Capacity: 47-75
Year Built: 2002
Rental Contact: Linda Ayros-Frederick

2523 SAN FRANCISCO STATE UNIVERSITY: DEPARTMENT OF THEATRE ARTS

1600 Holloway Avenue
San Francisco, CA 94132
Phone: 415-338-1341
Web Site: www.sfu.edu/~tha/
Officers:
   Chair: Ron Conboy
Budget: $1,000-5,500
Affiliations: NAST

Seating Capacity: 250; 95

2524 SAN FRANCISCO MIME TROUPE

855 Treat Avenue
San Francisco, CA 94110
Phone: 415-285-1717
Fax: 415-285-1290
e-mail: office@sfmt.org
Web Site: www.sfmt.org
Management:
   General Manager: Peggy Rose
   Office Marketing Manager: Miche Hall
   Production Manager: Natalie Saibel
Mission: Creating original, socially-relevant, musical theatre of high professional quality; performing for the broadest audience possible.
Founded: 1959
Status: Professional; Nonprofit
Paid Staff: 5
Volunteer Staff: 25
Paid Artists: 10
Budget: $700,000
Income Sources: Free shows in Bay Area Parks; International Touring Engagements; Youth Project for at-risk communities in San Francisco; Grants; Donations
Performs At: Varies (plays in parks for free in July)
Affiliations: Network of Ensemble Theaters, Theater Bay Area
Annual Attendance: 60,000
Type of Stage: Portable Raked Stage
Organization Type: Performing; Touring; Educational

2525 SHADOWLIGHT PRODUCTIONS

22 Chattanooga Street
San Francisco, CA 94114
Phone: 415-648-4461
Fax: 415-641-9734
Management:
   Artistic/Executive Director: Larry Reed
   Managing Director: Kate Sheehan

2526 SOON 3 THEATER

951 Church Street
PO Box 460298
San Francisco, CA 94114-3028
Phone: 415-558-8575
e-mail: soon3@sirius.com
Web Site: www.soon3.com
Management:
   Executive Director: Edward Doherty
   Founder Artistic Director: Alan Finneran
Mission: Developing innovative forms of presentation for socially significant theatrical works.
Founded: 1972
Specialized Field: Theatrical Group; Interdisciplinary Experimental
Status: Professional; Nonprofit
Income Sources: Theater Bay Area
Organization Type: Performing

2527 STEVE SILVER PRODUCTIONS

678 Green Street
San Francisco, CA 94133

Phone: 415-421-4284
Fax: 415-421-0518
e-mail: bbb@beachblanketbabylon.com
Web Site: www.beachblanketbabylon.com
Management:
  Producer: Jo Schuman Silver
Founded: 1974
Specialized Field: Musical
Status: Professional; Commercial
Paid Staff: 100
Paid Artists: 40
Income Sources: San Francisco & California Chambers of Commerce; Theater Bay Area
Performs At: Club Fugazi
Annual Attendance: 150,000
Organization Type: Performing; Resident

2528 THEATER RHINOCEROS

2926 16th Street
San Francisco, CA 94103
Phone: 415-552-4100
Fax: 415-558-9044
Web Site: www.therhino.org
Management:
  Artistic Director: Doug Holsalaw
  Managing Director: John Simpson
Mission: The presentation of Lesbian and Gay theatre.
Founded: 1977
Specialized Field: Theatrical Group
Status: Professional; Nonprofit
Paid Staff: 4
Budget: $600,000
Income Sources: Non-profit
Performs At: Main Stage; Studio Theater
Annual Attendance: 20,000
Facility Category: Mainstage + Studio
Type of Stage: Proscenium
Seating Capacity: 112/54
Organization Type: Performing; Resident

2529 THEATRE ARTAUD

450 Florida Street
499 Alabama Street #450
San Francisco, CA 94110
Phone: 415-437-2700
Fax: 415-437-2722
e-mail: info@theatretaud.org
Web Site: www.theatretaud.org
Management:
  General Director: Kim Cook
  Production Manager: David Szlasa
  Technical Director: Sean Riley
Founded: 1972
Specialized Field: Performing Arts / Theatre
Paid Staff: 7

2530 THICK DESCRIPTION

1695 18th Street
San Francisco, CA 94107
Phone: 415-401-8081
Web Site: www.thickdescription.org
Management:
  Artistic Collective: Karen Amano
  Artistic Collective: Tony Kelly

  Artistic Collective: Rick Martin
Mission: Thick Description is run by a collective of three theater artists who share the duties and responsibilities of traditional artistic director.

2531 TRAVELING JEWISH THEATRE

323 Geavy Street
Suite 415
San Francisco, CA 94102
Phone: 415-399-1809
Fax: 415-399-1844
Web Site: www.atjt.com
Officers:
  Associate Artistic Director: Corey Fisher
Management:
  Artistic Director: Aaron Davidman
Mission: To create and perform original works of theatre, as an ensemble and in collaboration with theatre artists from a variety of cultural and ethnic backgrounds, that contribute to a generous vision of the human condition.
Founded: 1978
Specialized Field: Theatrical Group
Status: Professional; Nonprofit
Income Sources: Theatre Communications Group
Organization Type: Performing; Touring; Educational

2532 CHILDREN'S MUSICAL THEATER-SAN JOSE

1401 Parkmoor Avenue
San Jose, CA 95128
Phone: 408-288-5437
Fax: 408-288-6241
e-mail: cmtsj@cmtsj.org
Web Site: www.cmtsj.org
Officers:
  President: David J Stock
  VP: Rose Froehlich
  Treasurer: G Ron Lester
  Secretary: Kathy Custanza
Management:
  Executive Director: Jennifer Sandretto Hull
  Artistic Director: Kevin R Hauge
  Marketing/PR Director: Micki Sever
  Educational/Outreach Director: Drew Chappell
Mission: Committed to providing excellent, accessible musical theater training for youth, with high-quality performances for families and the entire community.
Founded: 1968
Specialized Field: North Bay
Paid Staff: 9
Volunteer Staff: 35
Paid Artists: 86
Rental Contact: Facilities Manager/Rentals Timm Reinhart

2533 CITY LIGHTS THEATRE COMPANY

529 S 2nd Street
San Jose, CA 95112
Phone: 408-295-4200
Fax: 408-295-8318
e-mail: citylights@cltc.org
Web Site: www.cltc.org
Management:
  Artistic Director: Rose Nelson

Production Manager: Dorothy Cosby
Box Office Manager: Bobbi Kalmanash
Mission: City Lights is a resident non-profit company of theater artists dedicated to staging and hosting quality productions year round. This company prides itself on producing works you won't see at any other theater in the area.
Founded: 1982
Status: Nonprofit
Income Sources: Various
Annual Attendance: 10,000
Facility Category: Transformed Warehouse
Type of Stage: Flexible
Seating Capacity: 110
Rental Contact: Managing Director Lisa Mallette

2534 NORTHSIDE THEATRE COMPANY

848 E William Street
San Jose, CA 95116
Phone: 408-288-7820
e-mail: northside8@hotmail.com
Web Site: www.northsidetheatre.com
Officers:
  Chairperson: Dana Grover
  Vice Chairperson: Valerie Singer
  Treasurer: Matt Singer
  Secretary: Kathy Harwood
Management:
  Artistic Director: Richard T Orlando
  Communications Manager: Mertedith King
  Tech Director: Casey Snodgrass
  Production Manager: James Lucas
Mission: To provide high quality, theatrical opportunities for youth, regardless of economic, educational, cultural or physical limitations. Dedicated to the manifestation of the human spirit.
Founded: 1978
Specialized Field: Theatrical Group
Status: Nonprofit
Paid Staff: 6
Volunteer Staff: 12
Paid Artists: 25
Non-paid Artists: 50
Budget: $200,000
Income Sources: Community Foundation of Silicon Valley
Annual Attendance: 5,000
Type of Stage: Thurst
Stage Dimensions: 20x20
Year Built: 1965
Year Remodeled: 2000
Organization Type: Performing; Touring; Resident; Educational

2535 SAN JOSE REPERTORY THEATRE

101 Paseo de San Antonio
San Jose, CA 95113
Phone: 408-367-7255
Fax: 408-367-7237
e-mail: info@sjrep.com
Web Site: www.sjrep.com
Officers:
  President: John Michael Sobrato
Management:
  Artistic Director: Timothy Near

Managing Director: Alexandra Urbanowski
Mission: The theatre exists to produce seasons of visually exciting, challenging, entertaining and evocative plays selected from classical and contemporary periods; provide a creative environment for theatre artists and offer opportunities for innovative approaches to existing work and the development of new work; to reflect and enhance the community.
Founded: 1980
Specialized Field: South Bay Area
Status: Professional; Nonprofit
Paid Staff: 70
Volunteer Staff: 100
Budget: $5,900,000
Income Sources: League of Resident Theatres; Theatre Communications Group
Performs At: Performing Arts Complex
Annual Attendance: 110,000
Facility Category: Theater; Performing Arts
Seating Capacity: 533
Year Built: 1997
Cost: $24,000,000
Rental Contact: Drayton Foltz
Organization Type: Performing; Resident; Educational

2536 SAN JOSE STAGE COMPANY

490 S 1st Street
San Jose, CA 95112
Phone: 408-283-7142
Fax: 408-283-7146
e-mail: admin@sjstage.com
Web Site: www.sanjose-stage.com
Officers:
  President: Michael C Froncek
  VP: Faye Van Boxtel
  Secretary: Les Stevens
  Treasurer: Dr. Erik Cohen
Management:
  Executive Director: Cathleen King
  Artistic Director: Randall King
  Development Director: Mary Smith
  Production Manager: Scott Tukloff
  Technical Consultant: Scott Baker
Status: Nonprofit
Income Sources: Private Contributions; Ticket/Subscription Revenues

2537 SAN JOSE STATE UNIVERSITY: DEPARTMENT OF THEATRE ARTS

One Washington Square
San Jose, CA 95192
Phone: 408-924-4530
Web Site: http://www.theatre.sjsu.edu
Officers:
  Chair: Dr. Robert Jeenkins
Budget: $8,100-17,000
Affiliations: NAST; ATHE; San Jose Repertory Theatre; Theatreworks; KQED; Paramount Great America; American Musical Theatre; The Barn Theatre
Seating Capacity: 400; 160; 60
Year Built: 1954

2538 TEATRO VISION
Mexican Heritage Plaza
1700 Alum Rock Avenue, Suite 265
San Jose, CA 95116
Phone: 408-272-9926
Fax: 408-928-5589
e-mail: teatrovision@teatrovision.org
Web Site: www.teatrovision.org
Management:
　　Artistic Director: Elisa Marina Alvarado
　　Executive Director: Raul Lozano
　　Production Manager: Dianne Vega
Mission: A Chicago theater company that celebrates culture, nurtures community, and inspires vision. Our art serves to move people to feel, think and act to create a better world.
Founded: 1984
Specialized Field: Theatrical Group; Chicano Theatre
Status: Semi-Professional; Nonprofit
Income Sources: Movimiento de Arte y Cultura Latinoamericana; Theatre Bay Area
Organization Type: Performing; Touring

2539 EL TEATRO CAMPESINO
PO Box 1240
San Juan Bautista, CA 95045
Phone: 831-623-2444
Fax: 408-623-4127
Web Site: www.elteatrocampesino.com/campesin
Management:
　　Managing Director: Phillip Esparza
　　Education/Workdhop Director: Rosa Maria Escalante
　　Artistic Director: Luis Valdez
Mission: To be recognized as one of the country's leading Latino/Chicano theaters.
Specialized Field: Theatrical Group
Status: Professional; Nonprofit
Performs At: El Teatro
Organization Type: Touring; Resident; Educational; Sponsoring

2540 SOUTH ORANGE COUNTY COMMUNITY THEATRE
Camino Real Playhouse
31776 El Camino Real
San Juan Capistrano, CA 92675
Phone: 949-489-8082
Fax: 949-489-8082
Specialized Field: Live community theater

2541 MARIN SHAKESPEARE COMPANY
Forest Meadows Ampitheatre
Grand Avenuedominican University of CA
San Rafael, CA 94913
Phone: 415-499-1108
Fax: 415-499-1492
e-mail: management@marinshakesperare.org
Web Site: www.marinshakespeare.org
Management:
　　Managing Director: Lesley Schisgall Currier
　　Artistic Director: Robert Currier

Mission: Our mission is to acheive excellence in the staging of Shakespearean plays; to celebrate Shakespeare; and to serve as a cultural and educational resource for Marin County, the San Francisco Bay Area and beyond.
Founded: 1989
Specialized Field: Theatre
Status: Non-Equity; Nonprofit
Paid Staff: 4
Paid Artists: 35
Season: July-September
Affiliations: Shakespeare Theatre Association of America; Theatre Bay Area Chamber of Commerce; Marin Arts Council; San Rafael Chamber of Commerce
Annual Attendance: 10,000
Facility Category: Outdoor Amphitheatre
Seating Capacity: 600
Year Built: 1967

2542 RUDE GUERRILLA THEATER COMPANY
200 N Broadway
Santa Ana, CA 92701
Phone: 714-547-4688
Web Site: www.rudeguerilla.org
Management:
　　Artistic Director: Dave Barton
Mission: Art that provides its audience with an imaginative representation of the world both around and inside: Literate, exciting stories brimming with dynamic situations, sharp imagery, brutally honest acting and laugh-out-loud humor.

2543 STOP-GAP
1570 Brookhollow Drive #114
Santa Ana, CA 92705
Phone: 714-979-7061
Fax: 714-979-7065
e-mail: mstewart@stopgap.org
Web Site: www.stopgap.org
Management:
　　Executive Director: Don Laffoon
　　Managing Director: Victoria Bryan
Mission: To use theatre as an educational and therapeutic tool to make a positive difference in individual lives.
Founded: 1978
Specialized Field: Theatrical Group
Status: Professional; Nonprofit
Organization Type: Performing; Touring; Educational

2544 ENSEMBLE THEATRE COMPANY OF SANTA BARBARA
914 Santa Barbara Street
Santa Barbara, CA 93101
Mailing Address: PO Box 2307, Santa Barbara, CA. 93120-9946
Phone: 805-965-6252
Fax: 805-965-5322
Management:
　　Artistic Director: Robert Grande-Weiss
　　Managing Director: Patricia Baldwin

2545 SPEAKING OF STORIES

924 Anacapa Street
Suite 3-0
Santa Barbara, CA 93101
Mailing Address: PO Box 21143, Santa Barbara, CA. 93121
Phone: 805-966-3875
Fax: 805-966-1107
e-mail: info@speakingofstories.org
Web Site: www.speakingofstories.org
Officers:
   Board President: Carolyn Butcher
Management:
   Artistic/Outreach Director: Karin delaPena
   Managing Director: Teri Ball
Mission: Mission is to promote the appreciation of literature through live theatrical readings and community educational programs.
Founded: 1995
Specialized Field: Literature; Performance
Paid Staff: 5
Volunteer Staff: 1
Paid Artists: 25
Budget: 250,000
Income Sources: Volunteers; Contributors; Supporters; Tickets
Facility Category: Theater

2546 UNIVERSITY OF CALIFORNIA-SANTA BARBARA: DEPARTMENT OF DRAMATIC ART

Santa Barbara, CA 93106
Phone: 805-893-4895
Management:
   Professor: W. Davies King
Budget: $8,500-9,000
Affiliations: ATHE; Theatre Artists Group
Seating Capacity: 340; 110; 100
Year Built: 1964

2547 LYRIC THEATRE WAREHOUSE

860 Walsh Avenue
Santa Clara, CA 95050-2622
Phone: 408-986-8631
e-mail: lyricmail@yahoo.com
Web Site: www.lyrictheatre.org
Management:
   Managing Director: Angela Norlander
   Director: Jerald Enos
Mission: Lyric Theatre is a performing group of over 150 dedicated volunteers who have committed themselves to the art of stagecraft.
Income Sources: Donations
Season: june 6th - august

2548 SANTA CLARA UNIVERSITY THEATRE AND DANCE DEPARTMENT

Santa Clara, CA 95053
Phone: 408-554-4989
Fax: 408-554-5199
Budget: $4,650-10,200
Affiliations: NAST; ATHE; San Jose Repertory Theatre; TheatreWorks; SRI; AMT; PCPA

Seating Capacity: 388; 88-139
Year Built: 1975

2549 SHAKESPEARE SANTA CRUZ

University of California
1156 High Street
Santa Cruz, CA 95064
Phone: 831-459-2121
Fax: 831-459-3316
Web Site: www.shakespearesantacruz.org
Officers:
   President: Joe Denisola
   Co-Vice President: Liz Sandoud
   Secretary: Anita Elliot
Management:
   Artistic Director: Risa Brainin
   Managing Director: Marcus Cato
Mission: To produce Shakespeare and world drama in translation.
Founded: 1982
Specialized Field: Theatre
Paid Staff: 7
Paid Artists: 45
Budget: 1,800,000
Income Sources: Tickets; Grants; Donation
Season: July - August
Performs At: Outdoor, Stanley-Sinsheimer-Glen Theater; Indoor Mainstage
Affiliations: AEA; SSO & C; USA
Annual Attendance: 45,000
Type of Stage: Indoor-Thrust
Seating Capacity: Indoor, 540; Outdoor, 750+

2550 PCPA THEATERFEST

800 S College Drive
PO Box 1700
Santa Maria, CA 93456
Phone: 805-928-7731
Fax: 805-928-7506
Toll-free: 800-727-2123
e-mail: pcpa@pcpa.org
Web Site: www.pcpa.org
Management:
   Artistic Director: R Michael Grob
   Managing Director: Judy Frost
   Conservatory Dir/Actor Training: Mark Booher
   Conservatory Director Tech Theatre: Micheal J Dempsey
Mission: Professional theatre company of the California Central Coast. Through the work of its professional company and conservatory training programs
Founded: 1964
Specialized Field: Theatrical Group
Status: Professional; Semi-Professional; Non-Professional; Nonprofit
Paid Staff: 30
Volunteer Staff: 200
Paid Artists: 40
Non-paid Artists: 75
Budget: $2,500,000
Income Sources: Ticket Sales; State Education Monies; Grants; Sponsorships; Donations
Performs At: Marian Theatre, Santa Maria; Severson Theatre, Santa Maria; Festival Theatre, Solvang

Affiliations: TCG
Annual Attendance: 80,000
Type of Stage: Thrust; Black Box; Thrust
Seating Capacity: 450; 200; 700
Organization Type: Performing; Resident; Educational

2551 ACTORS REPERTORY THEATRE & SANTA MONICA GROUP

1211 4th Street
Santa Monica, CA 90401
Phone: 310-394-9779
Fax: 310-393-5573
e-mail: workshops@santamonicaplayhouse.com
Web Site: www.santamonicaplayhouse.com
Management:
    Artistic Director: Evelyn Rudie
    Artistic/Managing Director: Chris De Carlo
    Associate Producer: John Waroff
    Education Coordinator: Cammy Truong
Mission: To educate, enlighten and entertain. Providing comtemporary and classic new plays; touring, including internationally; offering educational workshops for all ages; maintaining a young professionals' company and resident acting company.
Founded: 1962
Specialized Field: Summer Stock; Musical; Theatrical Group; Family & Children's Theatre
Status: Professional; Nonprofit
Paid Staff: 10
Volunteer Staff: 20
Paid Artists: 50
Income Sources: Theatre Communications Group; Actors' Equity Association; Theatre Los Angeles
Performs At: Santa Monica Playhouse
Organization Type: Performing; Touring; Resident; Educational

2552 SANTA MONICA COLLEGE: MADISON THEATRE

1900 Pico Boulevard
Santa Monica, CA 90405
Phone: 310-434-3430
Fax: 310-434-3439
e-mail: franzen_dale@smc.edu
Management:
    Special Projects Director: Dale Franzen

2553 ACTORS' THEATRE

Luther Burbank Center for the Arts
50 Mark West Springs Road
Santa Rosa, CA 95403
Phone: 707-523-4185
Fax: 707-523-3544
e-mail: argo@actorstheatre.com
Web Site: www.actorstheatre.com
Officers:
    President: Eileen Carlisle
    VP: Spencer Flournoy
    Secretary: Nancy Humpries
    Director Of Finance: Kevin Lingener
Management:
    Artistic Director: Argo Thompson
    Production Stage Manager: April George
    Public Relations Director: Sheila Groves

Box Office Manager: Danielle Cain
Mission: The purpose of Actors Theatre is to provide to the public excellent live productions of contemporary and adventurous theatre at affordable prices, to create, train and maintain a professional theatre company within Sonoma County, and to provide a nurturing environment for its artists.
Founded: 1982
Paid Staff: 2
Paid Artists: 20
Budget: $150,000
Income Sources: Grants; Individual & Corporate contributions; program ads
Performs At: Outdoor amphitheatre
Annual Attendance: 30,000
Type of Stage: Proscenium
Stage Dimensions: 40 x 30
Seating Capacity: 850

2554 SUMMER REPERTORY THEATRE
Santa Rosa Junior College

Burbank Auditorium
Santa Rosa, CA 95401
Phone: 707-527-4221
Fax: 707-524-1689
e-mail: fzwolinski@santarosa.edu
Web Site: www.santarosa.edu/srt
Management:
    Artistic Director: Frank Zwolinski
Founded: 1972
Status: Non-Equity; Nonprofit
Season: May - August
Type of Stage: Proscenium
Stage Dimensions: 36'x 30'

2555 ANTENNA THEATER

Building 1057
Fort Cronkhite
Sausalito, CA 94965
Mailing Address: PO Box 939, Sausalito, CA. 94966
Phone: 415-332-8867
Fax: 415-332-8648
e-mail: sleon@antenna-theatre.org
Web Site: www.antenna-theatre.org/
Management:
    Artistic Director: Chris Hardman
    Administrative Director: Steven Leon
Mission: Antenna seeks to invent, discover, and explore ways of involving a variety of artistic disciplines and new technologies in the theatre experience.
Founded: 1980
Specialized Field: Theatrical Group
Status: Professional; Nonprofit
Budget: $500,000
Income Sources: Theatre Communications Group; California Confederaton of the Arts; Theatre Bay Area
Performs At: Site Specific
Organization Type: Performing; Touring

2556 LA CONNECTION COMEDY THEATRE

13442 Ventura Boulevard
Sherman Oaks, CA 91423

Phone: 818-710-1320
Fax: 818-710-8666
e-mail: madmovies@hotmail.com
Web Site: www.laconnectioncomedy.com
Management:
    Artistic Director: Kent Skov
Mission: To produce comedy productions for film, TV, industrial and theatrical shows. Live improvised comedy sketch, movie dubbing, year round. To become a member, performers may audition by appointment.
Founded: 1977
Status: Commercial
Paid Staff: 6
Volunteer Staff: 1
Season: Year Round
Type of Stage: Thrust
Seating Capacity: 99

2557 NORTH COAST REPERTORY THEATRE

987D Lomas Santa Fe Drive
Solana Beach, CA 92075
Phone: 858-481-1055
Fax: 858-481-1527
e-mail: ncrt@northcoastrep.org
Web Site: www.northcoastrep.org/CONTACT.html
Officers:
    President: Ira Epstein
    VP: Lorraine Stamoulis
    Treasurer: Michael Tedesco
    Secretary: Marvin Read
Management:
    Artistic Director: Olive Blakistone
    Director: Tom Blakistone
    Marketing Director: Lale Kumral
    Director of Public Relations/Media: Joru Guth
Mission: To produce artistically demanding plays of high quality, which include original works, neglected works of literary merit, both contemporary and classical and those which address social issues.
Founded: 1982
Specialized Field: Musical; Theatrical Group
Status: Non-Professional; Nonprofit
Volunteer Staff: 300
Paid Artists: 75
Budget: $750,000 +
Income Sources: San Diego Theatre League; California Arts Council
Performs At: Thomas Santa Fe Plaza
Annual Attendance: 35,000 +
Facility Category: Indoor
Type of Stage: 3/4 Thrust
Seating Capacity: 194
Year Built: 1982
Year Remodeled: 1988
Rental Contact: Sue Schaffner
Organization Type: Performing

2558 SIERRA REPERTORY THEATRE AT EAST SONORA

13891 Highway 108
PO Box 3030
Sonora, CA 95370
Phone: 209-532-3133
Fax: 209-532-7270
e-mail: srt@mlode.com
Web Site: www.sierrarep.com
Management:
    Producing Director: Dennis Jones
    Managing Director: Sara Jones
    Marketing Director: Jan Mangili
Founded: 1980
Specialized Field: Professional Live Theatre
Paid Staff: 30
Volunteer Staff: 2
Paid Artists: 140
Budget: $1,000,000
Income Sources: Ticket Sales; National Endowment for the Arts Grants; California Arts Council Grants; Fundraising & Sponsors
Season: Febuary - December
Performs At: Contemporary Live Theatre
Annual Attendance: 54,000
Facility Category: Live Theatre
Type of Stage: Proscenium
Stage Dimensions: 40x30
Seating Capacity: 202; 270
Year Built: 1980
Year Remodeled: 1992

2559 STAGE 3 THEATRE COMPANY

208 S Green Street
Sonora, CA 95370
Phone: 209-536-1778
e-mail: info@stage3.org
Web Site: www.stage3.org/tickets.htm
Management:
    Artistic Director: Barbara Segal-Mill
    Managing Director: Neil Mill
Mission: Stage 3 Theatre Company is dedicated to the development and production of new plays by new playwrights, and contemporary works by established playwrights.
Founded: 1993
Specialized Field: Theatre
Status: Nonprofit
Paid Staff: 3
Paid Artists: 6-30
Budget: $100,000
Income Sources: Ticket Sales; Grants; Contributions; Rentals; Touring; Classes; Advertising Revenue
Annual Attendance: 6,000
Type of Stage: Black Box
Stage Dimensions: 20'x20'
Seating Capacity: 80-100
Year Built: 1996
Rental Contact: Artistic Director Barbara Segal-Mill
Resident Groups: Stage 3 Theatre Company

2560 STOCKTON CIVIC THEATRE

2312 Rose Marie Lane
Stockton, CA 95207
Phone: 209-473-2400
Fax: 209-473-1502
Web Site: www.californiamall.com/SCT/Default.asp
Management:
    Producing Director: Paul Bengston
Mission: To provide the community with quality theatre.

Founded: 1951
Specialized Field: Musical; Community; Theatrical Group
Status: Non-Professional; Nonprofit
Paid Staff: 4
Volunteer Staff: 300
Non-paid Artists: 200
Income Sources: Patrons
Performs At: Civic Center
Annual Attendance: 25,000
Facility Category: Community Theatre
Type of Stage: Proscenium
Seating Capacity: 275
Year Built: 1980
Rental Contact: Producing Director Paul Bengston
Organization Type: Performing; Resident

2561 TILLIE LEWIS THEATER
Delta College
5151 Pacific Avenue
Stockton, CA 95207
Phone: 209-954-5209
Fax: 209-954-5600
Specialized Field: Theatre; Educational
Facility Category: Theatre
Type of Stage: Proscenium
Seating Capacity: 400
Year Built: 1973
Rental Contact: Dr. Charles Jennings

2562 UNIVERSITY OF THE PACIFIC: DEPARTMENT OF THEATRE ARTS
Drama Building
Stockton, CA 95211
Phone: 209-946-2116
Fax: 209-946-2118
Web Site: www.uop.edu/cop/theatrearts
Officers:
　Department Chair: W Wolak
Budget: $2,550-8,600
Affiliations: U/RTA
Seating Capacity: 400; 80-120
Year Built: 1956
Year Remodeled: 1999

2563 ARK THEATRE COMPANY
PO Box 1188
Studio City, CA 91614
Phone: 323-969-1707
e-mail: arltheatre@hotmail.com
Web Site: www.arktheatre.org
Management:
　Artistic Director: Paul Wagar
　Artistic Director: Derek Medina
　Associate Artistic Director: Richard Tatum
Mission: A new Los Angeles theatre company formed to produce and present a repertory season by an ongoing company of actors, writers, directors, and designers.

2564 LOS ANGELES DESIGNERS' THEATRE
PO Box 1883
Studio City, CA 91614-0883

Phone: 323-650-9600
Fax: 323-654-3260
e-mail: ladesigners@juno.com
Management:
　Artistic Director: Richard Niederberg
Founded: 1970
Status: Nonprofit

2565 THEATRE EAST
12655 Ventura Boulevard
Studio City, CA 91604
Phone: 818-760-4160
e-mail: theatreeast@yahoo.com
Web Site: www.angelfire.com/la/theatreeast
Officers:
　President: Michael Harrity
　VP: Linda DeMetrick
　Treasurer: Susan O'Sullivan
　Secretary: Jill Martin
Mission: Theatre East shall be an organization of dedicated professional artists in the theatrical and allied arts, banded together for the purpose of gaining artistic growth through performance and self-evaluation. We shall stimulate and encourage workshop activity that may be considered for public performance. We shall endeavor to make our influence felt as a creative force in the theatrical community.
Founded: 1960
Specialized Field: Theatrical Group
Status: Professional
Paid Staff: 125
Organization Type: Resident

2566 CALIFORNIA THEATRE CENTER
PO Box 2007
Sunnyvale, CA 94087
Phone: 408-245-2978
Fax: 408-245-0235
e-mail: ctc@ctcinc.org
Web Site: www.ctcinc.org
Management:
　General Director: Gayle Cornelison
　Resident Director: Will Huddleston
　Box Office: Diana Burnell
　Production Manager: Marley Morris
　Administrative Director: Susan Earle
　Tour Director: Lisa Mallette
Mission: Providing children and families with quality theatre.
Founded: 1976
Specialized Field: Theatrical Group
Status: Professional; Nonprofit
Paid Staff: 12
Paid Artists: 20
Budget: $1,750,000
Income Sources: Box Office; Touring; Education; Contributions
Performs At: The Performing Arts Center
Affiliations: Theatre Communications Group
Annual Attendance: 95,000; 150,000
Facility Category: Theatre
Type of Stage: Proscenium
Stage Dimensions: 34x25
Seating Capacity: 200
Year Built: 1974

Year Remodeled: 1991
Organization Type: Performing; Touring

2567 WILL GEER THEATRICUM BOTANICUM
1419 N Topanga Canyon Boulevard
Topanga Canyon, CA 90290
Phone: 310-455-2322
Fax: 310-455-3724
e-mail: theatricum@earthlink.net
Web Site: www.theatricum.com
Management:
General Manager: Jennifer Beale
Artistic Director: Ellen Geer
Mission: The Will Geer Theatricum Botanicum is dedicated to the belief that theatre, music and education are integral and necessary parts of life for all individuals to experience on a regular and inexpensive basis.
Founded: 1973
Specialized Field: Theatrical Group
Status: Professional; Nonprofit
Paid Staff: 50
Budget: $500,000
Income Sources: Tuitions; Ticket Sales; Donations
Season: April - September
Performs At: Repertory Theatre
Facility Category: Repertory Theatre
Type of Stage: Outdoor
Seating Capacity: 300
Organization Type: Performing; Resident; Educational

2568 CALIFORNIA STATE UNIVERSITY, STANISLAUS: DRAMA DEPARTMENT
CSUS
Turlock, CA 95832
Phone: 209-667-3451
Fax: 209-667-3782
Web Site: www.csustan.edu
Officers:
Chair: Dr. Jere D Wade
Budget: $5,000-9,000
Affiliations: NAST; ATHE
Seating Capacity: 300; 100
Year Built: 1970

2569 UKIAH PLAYERS THEATRE
1041 Low Gap Road
Ukiah, CA 95482
Phone: 707-462-1210
Fax: 707-462-1790
e-mail: players@pacific.net
Web Site: www.wkohplayerstheatre.org
Management:
Artistic Director: Michael Ducharme
Community/Cultural Dev Director: Kate Magruder
Production Manager: Jonathan Wipple
Publicity Manager: Dan Hibshman
Mission: Offering the general community a broad range of theatre experience; encouraging and educating theatre artists; providing a cultural venue.
Founded: 1977
Specialized Field: Community; Theatrical Group
Status: Semi-Professional; Nonprofit
Paid Staff: 4

Volunteer Staff: 200
Paid Artists: 20
Non-paid Artists: 100
Budget: $175,000
Performs At: Community Theatre
Affiliations: AACT, TCS, TBA
Annual Attendance: 10,000
Facility Category: Playhouse
Type of Stage: Proscenium
Stage Dimensions: 24'x38'
Seating Capacity: 120
Year Built: 1981
Year Remodeled: 1985
Rental Contact: Michael Ducharme
Organization Type: Performing; Touring; Resident; Educational; Sponsoring

2570 CALIFORNIA INSTITUTE OF THE ARTS: SCHOOL OF THEATER
24700 McBean Parkway
Valencia, CA 91355
Phone: 661-255-7834
Fax: 661-255-0462
Web Site: www.calarts.edu
Management:
Dean: Susan Solt
Budget: $6,600-12,800
Affiliations: NAST; U/RTA
Seating Capacity: 300; 30-100; 30-80
Year Built: 1971
Year Remodeled: 1994

2571 SIX FLAGS MAGIC MOUNTAIN
26101 Magic Mountain Parkway
Valencia, CA 91355
Mailing Address: PO Box 5500, Valencia, CA. 91385
Phone: 661-255-4100
Fax: 661-255-4171
Management:
Entertainment Manager: Scott Sterner
Founded: 1971
Status: Non-Equity; Commercial
Type of Stage: Proscenium; Thrust; Flex
Seating Capacity: 200-3000

2572 LOS ANGELES THEATRE WORKS
681 Venice Boulevard
Venice, CA 90291
Phone: 310-827-0808
Fax: 310-827-4949
Toll-free: 800-708-8863
e-mail: latw@latw.org
Web Site: www.latw.org
Officers:
President: Doug Jaffe
Vice President: Aviva Covitz
Secretary: Doris Blaizely
Treasurer: Alan Finkel
Management:
Producing Director: Susan Albert-Loewenberg
Mission: Los Angeles Theatre Works, a pioneering lab for playwrights, directors and other theatre artists, is committed to the exploration of contemporary work in theatre.

Founded: 1974
Status: Professional; Nonprofit
Income Sources: California Arts Council
Performs At: Skirball Cultural Center
Facility Category: Auditorium
Seating Capacity: 350
Rental Contact: 310-440-4595 Skirball Cultural Center
Organization Type: Touring; Producing

2573 CELEBRATION THEATRE
7985 Santa Monica Boulevard
Suite 109-1
West Hollywood, CA 90046
Phone: 323-957-1884
Fax: 323-957-1826
Web Site: www.celebrationtheatre.com
Management:
    Managing Artistic Director: Derek Charles
    Livingston
Mission: To illuminate all aspects of the gay and lesbian experience to the gay community and the community at large, while providing a safe and nurturing environment for gay and lesbian writers, directors, designers, and performers.
Founded: 1982
Specialized Field: Theatre
Status: Professional; Nonprofit
Paid Staff: 10
Income Sources: Grants; Ticket Sales; Indunderal Dancers
Performs At: Celebration Theatre
Annual Attendance: 4,000
Type of Stage: Three Quarter Stage
Seating Capacity: 64
Organization Type: Resident; Educational

2574 GROUP AT THE STRASBERG ACTING STUDIO
7936 Santa Monica Boulevard
West Hollywood, CA 90046
Phone: 323-650-7777
Fax: 323-650-7770
Web Site: www.strasberg.com
Management:
    Producer: David Strasberg
Founded: 2000
Specialized Field: Theater and Acting STudio
Performs At: Marilyn Monroe Theatre, Studio Stras, Stage Lee
Type of Stage: Endstage
Seating Capacity: 99, 49, 49

2575 WHITTIER JUNIOR THEATRE
7630 S Washington Avenue
Whittier, CA 90602
Phone: 562-464-3430
Fax: 562-464-3581
Management:
    Managing Supervisor: Dan Walker
    Theatre Manager/JT Director: Michael Eiden
Mission: Offering performance opportunities to children 9 through 18 years old; presenting three productions per year.
Founded: 1962

Specialized Field: Theatrical Group
Status: Non-Professional; Nonprofit
Paid Staff: 150
Budget: $18,000
Income Sources: Box Office; Class Registration
Performs At: The Center Theatre
Type of Stage: Proscenium
Seating Capacity: 400
Year Built: 1961
Year Remodeled: 1987
Rental Contact: Michael Eiden
Organization Type: Performing; Touring; Educational

2576 YREKA COMMUNITY THEATRE
810 N Oregon Street
Yreka, CA 96097
Phone: 530-841-2332
Fax: 530-841-2339
e-mail: yctheatre@hotmail.com
Management:
    Manager: Jeff Smith
Mission: To provide a venue for community performances and productions both in-house and private.
Founded: 1976
Paid Staff: 3
Volunteer Staff: 4
Performs At: Yreka Community Theatre
Seating Capacity: 300
Year Built: 1976
Cost: $2 million
Rental Contact: Jeff Shirn

Colorado

2577 AURORA FOX CHILDREN'S THEATRE COMPANY
9900 E Colfax Avenue
Aurora, CO 80010
Mailing Address: PO Box 9 Aurora, CO 80040
Phone: 303-361-2910
Fax: 303-361-2909
Management:
    Children's Theatre Coordinator: Thom Wise
Mission: To provide training and performance opportunities for young people.
Founded: 1979
Specialized Field: Community
Status: Non-Professional
Paid Staff: 8
Non-paid Artists: 60
Budget: $550,000
Income Sources: City of Aurora; SCFO
Performs At: Aurora Fox Arts Center
Annual Attendance: 30,000
Facility Category: Theatre
Type of Stage: Proscenium
Stage Dimensions: 50'w x 40' d x 14'
Seating Capacity: 245
Year Built: 1946
Year Remodeled: 1985
Cost: $1 million
Organization Type: Performing; Resident; Educational

2578 COLORADO SHAKESPEARE FESTIVAL
University of Colorado
277 UCB
Boulder, CO 80309-0277
Phone: 303-492-1527
Fax: 303-735-5140
e-mail: csfbo@colorado.edu
Web Site: www.coloradoshakes.org
Management:
  Artistic Director: Richard M Devin
  General Manager: Lynn Nichols
  Business Manager: Ray Kembles
Mission: To produce an aesthetically challenging mix of both traditional and innovative productions of Shakespeare's plays.
Founded: 1958
Specialized Field: Theater
Status: Professional; Nonprofit
Paid Staff: 150+
Volunteer Staff: 500
Paid Artists: 120
Budget: 1 million
Income Sources: Blue Mountain Arts
Season: June 27th - August 17th
Performs At: Mary Rippon Outdoor Theatre; University Mainstage Theatre
Annual Attendance: 41,000
Facility Category: Outdoor Theatre and Indoor Theatre
Type of Stage: Greco-Roman; Proscenium
Seating Capacity: 1,000; 400
Year Built: 1936
Organization Type: Performing

2579 LE CENTRE DU SILENCE MIME SCHOOL
PO Box 1015
Boulder, CO 80306-1015
Phone: 303-661-9271
Fax: 303-604-6046
e-mail: savital@concentric.net
Web Site: www.indranet.com/leds/html
Management:
  Founder/Director: Samuel Avital
Mission: To surpass the normal means of communication offered by the entertainment industry, and society's abuse of the spoken word; to perpetuate and educate in the Art of Silence - MIME.
Founded: 1971
Specialized Field: Mime; Movement Theatre; Masks; Acting

2580 UNIVERSITY OF COLORADO AT BOULDER: DEPARTMENT OF THEATRE AND DANCE
Campus Box 261
Boulder, CO 80309
Phone: 303-492-7355
Officers:
  Chair: Dr. Oliver Gerland
Budget: $3,500-5,500
Affiliations: ATHE; Colorado Shakespeare Festival
Seating Capacity: 416; 140; 1004
Year Built: 1902
Year Remodeled: 1989

2581 UPSTART CROW THEATRE COMPANY
2131 Arapahoe
Boulder, CO 80302
Phone: 303-442-1415
e-mail: info@theupstartcrow.org
Web Site: www.theupstartcrow.org
Mission: A dedicated core group of actors not only supplies stage talent, but backstage support as well.
Founded: 1980

2582 CREEDE REPERTORY THEATRE
124 N Main Street
PO Box 269
Creede, CO 81130
Phone: 719-658-2541
Fax: 719-658-2343
e-mail: art@creederep.com
Web Site: www.creederep.com
Officers:
  Chairman: Tom Templeton
  VP: Penny Coulson
  Secretary: Margaret Steffens
  Treasurer: Beverly Hettinger
Management:
  Artistic Director: Maurice La Mee
  Development Director: Kay Wyley
  Outreach Director: Julie Jackson
  Financial Director: Rhonda Jantzen
Mission: To produce a summer repertory season of eight plays; to promote knowledge of performing arts; to raise standards; to increase accessibility.
Founded: 1966
Specialized Field: Non-Musical; Musical; Children's Theater
Status: Professional; Nonprofit
Paid Staff: 6
Paid Artists: 40
Budget: $350,000
Income Sources: Donations; Grants; Box office
Season: Late May - early September
Performs At: Creede Repertory Theatre
Annual Attendance: 16,000
Facility Category: Performance center
Type of Stage: Proscenium
Seating Capacity: 234
Year Remodeled: 1991
Organization Type: Performing; Touring; Educational; Sponsoring

2583 AVENUE THEATER
2119 E 17th Avenue
Denver, CO 80206-1125
Phone: 303-321-5925

2584 CHANGING SCENE THEATER
1527 1/2 Champa Street
Denver, CO 80202
Phone: 303-893-5775
Management:
  President: Alfred Brooks
  VP: Maxine Munt
Mission: To offer experience and performing space to young artists. Specializes in new works.
Founded: 1968

All listings are in alphabetical order by state, then city, then organization within the city.

Specialized Field: Theatrical Group
Status: Nonprofit
Organization Type: Performing; Resident; Educational; Sponsoring

2585 DENVER CENTER THEATER COMPANY

1050 13th Street
Denver, CO 80204
Phone: 303-893-4000
Toll-free: 800-641-1222
Web Site: www.denvercenter.org
Management:
Artistic Director: Donovan Markey
Executive Director: Kevin Maifeld
Producing Director: Barbara Sellers
Dean Conservatory: Tony Church
Associate Artistic Director: Bruce K Sevy
Mission: Committed to providing the finest in performing arts for the Rocky Mountain Region.
Founded: 1979
Specialized Field: Musical; Theatrical Group
Status: Professional; Nonprofit
Income Sources: The Denver Center; Theatre Communications Group; League of Resident Theatres
Performs At: Denver Center Theatre
Type of Stage: Thrust, Arena, Proscenium
Seating Capacity: 642, 450, 250, 200
Organization Type: Performing; Touring; Resident; Educational

2586 DENVER CIVIC THEATRE

721 Sante Fe Drive
Denver, CO 80204
Phone: 303-595-3800
Fax: 303-265-9366
e-mail: info@denvercivic.com
Web Site: www.denvercivic.com
Founded: 1985
Opened: 1991
Status: Nonprofit; Professional

2587 DENVER PUPPET THEATRE

3156 W 38th Avenue
Denver, CO 80211-2004
Phone: 303-458-6446
e-mail: annie@hypermall.net
Web Site: www.denverpuppettheater.com
Officers:
President: Amiee Zock
Management:
Boss: Amiee Zock
Mission: Top quality puppet performance plus hands on puppet activities year round.
Founded: 1989
Specialized Field: Puppetry
Status: Professional; Profit
Paid Staff: 24
Paid Artists: 28
Budget: $90,000
Income Sources: Ticket Sales; Puppet Sales; Birthdays
Affiliations: Puppets of America; Theatre of Youth Coalition
Annual Attendance: 20,000
Stage Dimensions: 10'x20'

Seating Capacity: 100
Year Built: 1950
Year Remodeled: 1996
Resident Groups: Denver Puppet Theatre

2588 GERMINAL STAGE DENVER

2450 W 44th Avenue
Denver, CO 80211
Phone: 303-455-7108
e-mail: gsden@privatei.com
Web Site: www.germinalstage.com
Management:
Director/Manager: Ed Baierlein
Associate Producer: Sallie Diamond
Founded: 1973
Specialized Field: Theatrical
Status: Professional
Affiliations: Germinal Stage Denver
Stage Dimensions: 20'x15'
Orchestra Pit: 1
Architect: Ron Rinker

2589 IMPULSE THEATER

1634 18th Street
Lower Level
Denver, CO 80202
Phone: 303-297-2111
Fax: 303-297-1378
Toll-free: 877-467-8571
e-mail: info@impulsetheater.com
Web Site: www.impulsetheater.com
Management:
Producer/Director: John Bauers
Mission: Quick-witted cast of talented actors performing a funny mix of comedy, theater, and audience interaction.
Founded: 1987
Opened: 1987
Specialized Field: Comedy
Status: Professional
Seating Capacity: 178

2590 JAFRIKA

3230 Clay Street
Denver, CO 80211
Phone: 303-433-7163
Fax: 303-433-7163
e-mail: tingzen@juno.com
Web Site: www.interpacificnet.com
Management:
Dancer/Choreographer: Ricki Harada
Musician/Composer: Chris Macor
Mission: Japanese dancer, black poet, white musician.
Paid Artists: 3
Budget: $18,000
Income Sources: Paid by venue
Annual Attendance: 2,000
Facility Category: Schools, Libraries, Festivals

2591 METROPOLITAN STATE COLLEGE OF DENVER: DEPARTMENT OF THEATRE

Campus Box 34
Denver, CO 80217

Mailing Address: PO Box 173362
Phone: 303-556-3033
Management:
    Director of Theatre: Dr. Marilyn Hetzel
Budget: $4,000-7,000
Affiliations: Denver Civic Theatre; Denver Center for the Performing Arts
Seating Capacity: 99
Year Built: 1967

2592 NATIONAL THEATRE CONSERVATORY
1050 13th Street
Denver, CO 80204
Phone: 303-446-4855
Fax: 303-825-2117
Management:
    Director of Education: Daniel Renner
Budget: $30,000-46,000
Affiliations: Denver Centre Theatre Company
Seating Capacity: 550; 420; 150
Year Built: 1979

2593 SU TEATRO
4725 High Street
Denver, CO 80216
Phone: 303-296-0219
Fax: 303-296-4614
e-mail: elcentro@suteatro.org
Web Site: www.suteatro.org
Officers:
    Board Member: Debra Gallegos
Management:
    Artistic Director: Anthony J Garcia
    Managing Director: Valerie Bustos
    Development Director: Tonya Mote
Mission: Speaking to the struggles of the barrios of the Southwest; preserving and perpetuating Chicano culture and language.
Founded: 1971
Specialized Field: Community; Theatrical Group
Status: Semi-Professional; Nonprofit
Performs At: El Centro Su Teatro
Organization Type: Performing; Touring; Educational; Sponsoring

2594 UNIVERSITY OF COLORADO AT DENVER: DEPARTMENT OF PERFORMING ARTS
Denver, CO
Mailing Address: PO Box 173364, Denver, CO 80217
Phone: 303-556-4797
Fax: 303-556-2335
Budget: $5,000-7,000
Affiliations: ATHE; Curious Productions; The Denver Center for the Performing Arts
Seating Capacity: 350; 120
Year Built: 2000

2595 UNIVERSITY OF DENVER THEATRE DEPARTMENT
MRH 104
Denver, CO 80208

Phone: 303-871-2518
Fax: 303-871-2505
Web Site: www.du.edu/thea
Management:
    Assistant Professor: Paula Sperry
Budget: $2,700-4,900
Affiliations: ATHE; KC/ACTF
Seating Capacity: 200-450; 50
Year Built: 1938
Year Remodeled: 1991

2596 DIAMOND CIRCLE MELODRAMA
7th and Main
PO Box 3041
Durango, CO 81302
Phone: 970-247-3400
Fax: 970-259-2208
Toll-free: 877-325-3400
e-mail: info@diamondcirclemelodrama.com
Web Site: www.diamondcirclemelodrama.com
Management:
    Producer: Jeannie B Wheeldon
Mission: To present quality professional productions. We specialize in Authentic Melodrama and Vaudeville.
Founded: 1961
Specialized Field: Professional Theatre
Status: Non-Equity; Commercial
Paid Staff: 25
Paid Artists: 15
Season: June 2 - September 29
Type of Stage: Proscenium
Stage Dimensions: 30'x 20'
Seating Capacity: 250

2597 OPENSTAGE THEATRE AND COMPANY
PO Box 617
201 S College Avenue
Fort Collins, CO 80522
Phone: 303-484-5237
Fax: 303-454-5237
Web Site: www.openstage.com
Management:
    Executive Producer: Bruce K Freestone
    Artistic Director: Peter Anthony
    Office Manager: Lisa Rosenhagen
Mission: To develop and maintain a nationally recognized regional theatre company. Emphasis will be placed on providing the best in quality theatre for the public benefit, on providing educational outreach to the community, and on providing professional opportunities for company members.
Founded: 1973
Specialized Field: Theatrical Group
Status: Semi-Professional; Nonprofit
Paid Staff: 25
Income Sources: American Association of Community Theatres; Colorado Theatre Producers Guild; Fort Collins Convention & Visitors Bureau; Fort Collins Chamber of Commerce.
Performs At: Lincoln Center Mini-Theatre
Organization Type: Performing

2598 LITTLE THEATRE OF THE ROCKIES
University of Northern Colorado
Frasier 115
Greeley, CO 80639
Phone: 970-351-2194
Fax: 970-351-1923
e-mail: artsinfo@arts.unco.edu
Web Site: www.arts.unco.edu/theatredance/LTR.html
Management:
    Theatre Arts Chairman: Dan Guyette
Founded: 1934
Status: Nonprofit; Non-Equity
Season: Mid June - Early August
Type of Stage: Proscenium
Stage Dimensions: 34' x 32'
Seating Capacity: 600
Rental Contact: Diane Cays

2599 UNIVERSITY OF NORTHERN COLORADO: DEPARTMENT OF THEATRE ARTS & DANCE
Greeley, CO 8063
Phone: 970-351-2194
Officers:
    Chairman: Thomas P McNally
Budget: $2,050-3,650
Affiliations: ATHE; Little Theatre of the Rockies
Seating Capacity: 650; 100; 1,800

2600 COUNTRY DINNER PLAYHOUSE
6875 S Clinton
Greenwood Village, CO 80112
Phone: 303-799-1410
Fax: 303-790-2615
Web Site: www.countrydinnerplayhouse.com
Officers:
    President/Producer/CEO: David M Pritchard
    Executive VP: David Lovinggood
    VP/General Manager: Robert E Buffington
Management:
    Producer: David M Pritchard
    Associate Producer: Paul Dwyer
    Assistant CEO/Producer/Casting: Patrick Alan Kearns
Founded: 1970
Specialized Field: Dinner Theatre
Status: Professional; AEA
Paid Staff: 85
Paid Artists: 25
Income Sources: Ticket Sales
Affiliations: NDTA; NTA; CTG; Tour Colorado
Annual Attendance: 170,000
Type of Stage: Theater-in-the-round
Seating Capacity: 470
Year Built: 1970
Year Remodeled: 2000
Rental Contact: Technical Director Jacob Weler
Organization Type: Performing

2601 PICKETWIRE PLAYERS
Eighth and San Juan
La Junta, CO 81050
Phone: 719-384-8320
Web Site: www.ruralnet.net/~csn/business/picketwire
Management:
    Board of Directors:
Mission: To provide a showcase for Southeastern Colorado's regional talent.
Founded: 1968
Specialized Field: Community; Theatrical Group
Status: Non-Professional; Nonprofit
Income Sources: La Junta Chamber of Commerce; Colorado Community Theater Coalition
Performs At: Picketwire Center for the Performing and Visual Arts
Organization Type: Performing

2602 LONGMONT THEATRE COMPANY
513 Main Street
PO Box 573
Longmont, CO 80501
Phone: 303-772-5200
Fax: 303-651-0388
e-mail: manager@longmonttheatre.org
Web Site: www.longmonttheatre.org
Officers:
    President: Chris Curtis
    VP: Len Worland
    Treasurer: Mick Finnegan
    Secretary: Brain Curtiss
Management:
    Executive Director: Cheri E Friedman
Mission: To provide high quality entertainment with a strong educational component for and by the citizens of the Greater Boulder County area and to successfully manage a self-sufficient performing arts center.
Founded: 1957
Specialized Field: Theatre
Status: Nonprofit
Paid Staff: 1
Budget: $160,000
Income Sources: Ticket Sales; Advertising; Concessions; Grants; Donations; In Kind
Annual Attendance: 10,000
Type of Stage: Thurst
Seating Capacity: 294
Year Built: 1939
Year Remodeled: 1991

2603 BROADWAY THEATRE LEAGUE OF PUEBLO
PO Box 1394
Pueblo, CO 81002
Phone: 719-545-4721
Fax: 719-543-0134
Management:
    Manager: Maggie Divelbiss
    Administrative Assistant: Jen Owews
    Box Office Manager: Cheryl Califano
Mission: To bring professional theatre to the community.
Founded: 1960
Status: Professional; Nonprofit
Volunteer Staff: 20
Budget: $200,000
Income Sources: Ticket sales; Donations
Performs At: Pueblo Memorial Hall

Annual Attendance: 5,500
Type of Stage: Proscenium
Seating Capacity: 1,676
Year Built: 1920
Year Remodeled: 1960
Organization Type: Performing; Touring; Sponsoring

2604 IMPOSSIBLE PLAYERS

PO Box 1005
Pueblo, CO 81002
Phone: 719-542-6969
Officers:
 President: Marlene Schmidt
 Vice President: Bill Mattoon
 Secretary: Carol Martin
 Treasurer: Don Warren
Mission: To promote the enjoyment of the performing arts by the public; to further the education of both members and the public in the skills of those arts; to give people an opportunity to perform for the public.
Founded: 1966
Specialized Field: Community; Theatrical Group
Status: Non-Professional; Nonprofit
Performs At: Public Community College; The Hoag Theater
Organization Type: Performing; Resident; Educational

Connecticut

2605 RENAISSANCE THEATER COMPANY/ACTOR'S ENSEMBLE

45 Tabor Drive
Branford, CT
Mailing Address: 217 Greenwich Avenue New Haven, CT 06519
Phone: 203-772-2557
e-mail: actorsensemble@aol.com
Web Site: www.actorsensemble.com
Management:
 Artistic Director: Dana Sachs
 Company Manager: Joyce Tucker
Mission: For the purpose of providing quality theater for the general public and creative opportunities for local artists and technicians.
Founded: 1978
Specialized Field: Theatrical Group
Status: Professional; Nonprofit
Income Sources: New England Foundation for the Arts
Organization Type: Performing; Touring; Educational

2606 CHESHIRE COMMUNITY THEATRE

PO Box 149
Cheshire, CT 06410
Phone: 203-272-2787
e-mail: cct@cctonstage.org
Web Site: www.cctonstage.org
Officers:
 President: John Grabar
 VP: Kristen Hinckley
 Secretary: Gayle Barrett
 Treasurer: Kim Wantroba
 Membership: Dawn Reiss

Business Manager: Kurt Fusaris
Publicity: Aleta Looker
Play-Reading: Dorothy Brady
Technical Director: Richard Conrad
Mission: To develop amateur dramatic talent, to produce plays in which members shall take part as actors, producers, and managers, to encourage the writing of plays by its members, and to encourage dramatic art.
Founded: 1953
Specialized Field: Musical; Community; Theatrical Group
Status: Non-Professional; Nonprofit
Budget: $20,000
Income Sources: Ticket Sales; Program Ads; Membership Dues; Donations
Performs At: Cheshire High School
Annual Attendance: 1,800
Seating Capacity: 800
Rental Contact: Cheshire Board of Education
Organization Type: Performing; Resident

2607 EAST-WEST FUSION THEATRE

147 Kent Road
Cornwall Bridge, CT 06754
Phone: 860-672-3938
Fax: 860-672-3938
e-mail: eastwestarts@hotmail.com
Management:
 Artistic Director: Teviot Fairservis
Mission: International and fusion theatre collaborations with artists and scholars from around the world, multicultural arts education.
Founded: 1975
Specialized Field: Multicultural and International Fusion Theatre
Paid Staff: 6
Paid Artists: 6
Non-paid Artists: 25
Budget: $50,000
Income Sources: Tour Bookings; Grants; Corporate & Private Donors
Performs At: East-West Arts Retreat
Affiliations: AAP; UCTA
Annual Attendance: 500
Facility Category: Outdoor Spaces; Platforms; Grassy Areas
Stage Dimensions: 20x20 plus
Seating Capacity: 75-350
Year Built: 2001
Rental Contact: Teviot Fairservis

2608 WESTERN CONNECTICUT STATE UNIVERSITY: THEATRE ARTS DEPARTMENT

181 White Street
Danbury, CT 06810
Phone: 203-837-8250
Fax: 203-837-8611
Officers:
 Chairman: William Walton
Budget: $7,300-13,500
Affiliations: Circle Repertory; Barrow Group
Seating Capacity: 600; 200
Year Built: 1959

Year Remodeled: 1979

2609 AMERICAN MAGIC-LANTERN THEATER

Box 44
East Haddam, CT 06438
Phone: 860-345-2574
Fax: 860-345-7578
e-mail: jackiealvarez@earthlink.net
Web Site: www.magiclanternshows.com

2610 FAIRFIELD UNIVERSITY: DEPARTMENT OF VISUAL & PERFORMING ARTS

Fairfield, CT 06430
Phone: 203-254-4000
Management:
    Director Theatre Program: Dr. Martha LoMonaco
Budget: $10,250-20,500
Affiliations: ATHE
Type of Stage: Black Box
Seating Capacity: 150; 750
Year Built: 1989

2611 ARTISTS COLLECTIVE

1200 Albany Avenue
Hartford, CT 06112
Phone: 203-527-3205
Management:
    Executive Director: Dollie McLean
    Creative Consultant: Jackie McLean
Founded: 1970
Specialized Field: Theatrical Group
Status: Non-Professional; Nonprofit
Organization Type: Resident

2612 HARTFORD STAGE COMPANY

50 Church Street
Hartford, CT 06103-1298
Phone: 860-525-5601
Fax: 860-525-4420
e-mail: stagehartford@worldnet.att.net
Web Site: www.hartfordstage.org
Management:
    Director Marketing: Damon Caldwell
    Director Development: Dina Plapler
    Marketing Manager: Mark LaFleur
Mission: Founded in 1963, the theatre is internationally known for entertaining audiences with a wide range of the best of world drama, from classics to provocative new works and neglected works from the past.
Founded: 1963
Status: Not-for-profit
Affiliations: Hartford Stage Company
Type of Stage: Thrust
Stage Dimensions: 40'x90'x90'
Orchestra Pit: 1
Seating Capacity: 489
Architect: Venturi & Rauch
Rental Contact: Production Manager Candice Chirgotis

2613 NATIONAL THEATRE OF THE DEAF

55 Van Dyke Avenue
Suite 312
Hartford, CT 06412
Phone: 860-724-5179
Fax: 860-550-7974
Toll-free: 800-300-5179
e-mail: info@ntd.org
Web Site: www.ntd.org
Officers:
    Executive Director: Jerry Goehring
Management:
    Tour Director: Betty Beekman
    Artistic Manager: Mike Lamitola
Mission: To produce theatrically challenging work at a world class level, drawing from as wide a range of the world's literature as possible; to perform these original works in a style that links American Sign Language with the spoken work; to seek, train, and employ Deaf artists; to offer our work to as culturally diverse and inclusive an audience as possible; to provide community outreach activities.
Founded: 1967
Specialized Field: Theatrical Group
Status: Professional; Nonprofit
Organization Type: Performing; Touring; Educational

2614 THEATERWORKS

1 Gold Street
Hartford, CT 06103
Phone: 860-727-4027
Fax: 860-525-0758
Management:
    Executive Director: Steve Campo
Mission: To provide unique works, especially recent American plays. We strive to address a diversified range of socially relevant works by important active authors.
Founded: 1985
Status: Nonprofit
Season: Year Round
Annual Attendance: 30,000+
Type of Stage: Modified Thrust
Seating Capacity: 197
Year Built: 1927
Year Remodeled: 1996

2615 TRINITY COLLEGE THEATRE AND DANCE DEPARTMENT

Austin Arts Center
Hartford, CT 06106
Phone: 860-297-5122
Officers:
    Co-Chair: Judy Dworkin
    Co-Chair: Katharine Power
Budget: $12,550-17,600
Affiliations: La Mama (equity theatre company); National Theater Institute at the Eugene O'Neill Theater Center; Nikitsky-Gates Theater (Moscow)
Seating Capacity: 400; 100; 60
Year Built: 1967

2616 RIVER REP AT IVORYTON PLAYHOUSE

Box 637
Ivoryton, CT 06442

Phone: 212-674-8181
Fax: 212-780-0814
Web Site: www.riverrep.com
Management:
  Artistic Director: Jane Stanton
  Managing Director: Joan Shepard
Mission: To bring 11 weeks a year of fulfilling theatre to the shoreline of Eastern Connecticut.
Founded: 1987
Specialized Field: Professional Theatre
Status: Nonprofit
Paid Staff: 15
Volunteer Staff: 10
Paid Artists: 18
Non-paid Artists: 5
Season: June - September
Type of Stage: Proscenium
Stage Dimensions: 18' x 30'

2617 MANCHESTER MUSICAL PLAYERS

Cheney Hall
PO Box 626
Manchester, CT 06045
Phone: 860-649-9065
e-mail: mvkellyct@aol.com
Web Site: www.geocities.com/broadway
Officers:
  President: David Gorman
  Vice President of Finance: Ann Azevedo
  VP Production: Marge Kelly
  Treasurer: Chris Stone
  Secretary: Dianne Burnham
Mission: 50-year-old community theater organization presenting one major Broadway musical each spring and a cabaret fundraiser in September. Other activities include holiday performances and annual scholarship.
Founded: 1947
Specialized Field: Musical
Status: Semi-Professional; Nonprofit
Non-paid Artists: 60+
Budget: $40,000
Income Sources: Tickets; Grants; Donations; Dues; Annual Fundraiser; Stock rental; Fundraising sales
Performs At: Cheney Hall
Annual Attendance: 2,000
Facility Category: Theater
Type of Stage: Theatrical
Seating Capacity: 325
Year Built: 1867
Organization Type: Performing

2618 ODDFELLOWS PLAYHOUSE

128 Washington Street
Middletown, CT 06457
Phone: 860-347-6143
e-mail: oddfellows@wesleyan.edu
Web Site: www.oddfellows.org
Officers:
  Chair: Melissa Z Schilke
  Vice Chair: Alain Munkittrick
  Treasurer: Grady L Faulkner Jr
  Secretary: Robert Hoppenstedt
Management:
  Managing Director: Mimi Rich
  Artistic Director: Dic Wheeler

  Technical Director: Jesse Alford
  Development Director/PR Coordinator: Susan Brown
  Associate Artistic Director: Marcella Trowbridge
Mission: Oddfellows Playhouse is a non-profit youth theater and performing arts program that serves over 2,500 central CT young people, ages 6-20, each year through classes, workshops, mini-productions, mainstage shows, neighborhood-based troupes, and special events.
Status: Nonprofit

2619 WESLEYAN UNIVERSITY THEATER DEPARTMENT

Middletown, CT 06459
Phone: 860-685-2950
Fax: 860-685-2591
Web Site: www.wesleyan.edu
Officers:
  Chair: Ron Jenkins
Budget: $1,500-9,000
Affiliations: ATHE
Seating Capacity: 400; 150
Year Built: 1973
Year Remodeled: 1994

2620 CENTRAL CONNECTICUT STATE UNIVERSITY: DEPARTMENT OF THEATRE

1615 Stanley Drive
New Britain, CT 06050
Phone: 860-832-3151
Fax: 860-832-3164
Officers:
  Chair: Lani Beck Johnson
Budget: $9,000-23,000
Seating Capacity: 150; 300; 80
Year Built: 1989

2621 HOLE IN THE WALL THEATRE

10 Harvard Street
PO Box 942
New Britain, CT 06050-0942
Phone: 860-229-3049
e-mail: mail@hitw.org
Web Site: www.hitw.org
Mission: To allow anyone who walks through the door to enjoy theater at whatever level he or she desires.
Founded: 1972
Specialized Field: Musical; Community; Theatrical Group; Dance; Staged Readings
Status: Professional; Nonprofit
Non-paid Artists: all
Budget: $40,000
Income Sources: Box Office; Grants; Individual audience & member donations
Performs At: Black Box Studio Theatre
Affiliations: Greater New Britian Chamber of Commerce
Annual Attendance: 3,500
Facility Category: Thrust or 3/4 stage
Stage Dimensions: 42x30
Seating Capacity: 100
Year Remodeled: 1988
Rental Contact: Board of Directors

Organization Type: Performing; Resident

2622 ELM SHAKESPEARE COMPANY
PO Box 206029
New Haven, CT 06520-6029
Phone: 203-772-1474
Fax: 203-785-1569
e-mail: info@elmshakespeare.org
Web Site: www.elmshakespeare.org
Officers:
President: Cheever Tyler
VP: Frank Logue
Treasurer: John Conte
Secretary: Hyla Crane
Management:
Artistic Director: James Andreassi
Director Development: Barbara Schaffer
Founded: 1995
Specialized Field: Summer Theatre
Status: Nonprofit
Paid Staff: 3
Season: August 1 - September 1
Annual Attendance: 30,000
Facility Category: Outdoor
Seating Capacity: 3000

2623 LONG WHARF THEATRE
222 Sargent Drive
New Haven, CT 06511
Phone: 203-787-4284
Fax: 203-776-2287
Toll-free: 800-782-8497
Web Site: www.longwharf.org
Management:
General Manger: Deb Clapp
Managing Director: Michael Ross
Director Production: Jean Routt
Mission: Offering full production plays.
Founded: 1965
Status: Professional; Nonprofit
Budget: 120,000+
Income Sources: League of Resident Theatres; Theatre Communications Group; Connecticut Commission on the Arts; Actors' Equity Association
Performs At: Long Wharf Theatre
Facility Category: 2 stages
Seating Capacity: 487,199
Organization Type: Touring; Resident; Educational; Producing

2624 SOUTHERN CONNECTICUT STATE UNIVERSITY: DEPARTMENT OF THEATRE
501 Crescent Street
New Haven, CT 06515
Phone: 203-392-6100
Fax: 203-392-6105
Web Site: www.scsu.ctstateu.edu
Officers:
Chair: William R Ellwood
Budget: $29,000-40,000
Affiliations: ATHE; USITT; NETC; Long Wharf Theatre; Hartford Stage; Shubert Performing Arts Center; Goodspeed Opera; Circle in the Square

Seating Capacity: 1,550; 150; 125
Year Built: 1969
Year Remodeled: 1973

2625 YALE REPERTORY THEATRE
222 York Street
PO Box 208244
New Haven, CT 06520
Phone: 203-432-1591
Fax: 203-432-8332
Web Site: www.yale.edu/yalerep
Management:
Artistic Director: James Bundy
Managing Director: Victoria Nolan
Mission: Producing new American plays, as well as little-known works and classics revisited through contemporary metaphors.
Founded: 1966
Specialized Field: Theatrical Group
Status: Professional; Nonprofit
Income Sources: Actors' Equity Association; Theatre Communications Group; American Arts Alliance; League of Resident Theatres; Connecticut Advocates for the Arts
Performs At: Yale Repertory Theatre; University Theatre
Organization Type: Performing; Resident; Educational

2626 YALE SCHOOL OF DRAMA
New Haven, CT
Mailing Address: PO Box 208244, New Haven, CT 06520
Phone: 203-432-1507
Fax: 203-432-8337
Web Site: www.yale.edu/drama
Management:
Dean: Stan Wojewodski Jr.
Budget: 46,200-77,800
Affiliations: Yale Repertory Theatre
Seating Capacity: 487; 658; 200
Year Built: 1926
Year Remodeled: 2000

2627 CONNECTICUT COLLEGE DEPARTMENT OF THEATRE
New London, CT 06320
Phone: 860-439-2606
Officers:
Chair: Linda Herr
Seating Capacity: 1300; 130; 75
Year Built: 1941
Year Remodeled: 2000

2628 CONNECTICUT CONSERVATORY OF THE PERFORMING ARTS
79 W Street
New Milford, CT 06776
Phone: 860-354-2978
Fax: 860-350-0221
e-mail: ctconservatory@snet.net
Officers:
President: Jim Wilder
VP: Sarah Jane Chelminski
Treasurer: Shirley Waters
Secretary: Deborah Casey

Management:
Executive Director: Kristin Marks
Music Director: John Shackelford
Dance Department Chair: Robert Maiorano
Theatre Department Chair: Heather McNeil
Mission: Offers professional training in dance, music, theatre, and voice concurrently with an academic program for grades 7-12.
Founded: 1980
Paid Staff: 2
Paid Artists: 20
Performs At: Black Box
Facility Category: Small, informal
Seating Capacity: 75
Year Built: 1975
Resident Groups: Conservatory School

2629   GREENWOODS THEATRE AT NORFOLK
Route 44
Norfolk, CT 06058
Mailing Address: PO Box 490, Norfolk, CT. 06068-0569
Phone: 860-542-0026
Fax: 860-542-5205
Web Site: www.greenwoodstheatre.com
Founded: 1999
Specialized Field: Summer Theatre; Winter Vintage Films
Status: Nonprofit
Income Sources: Ticket Sales, Donations
Performs At: Classic 1880's Opera House with Shops
Annual Attendance: 8000
Facility Category: Opera House
Type of Stage: Proscenium with Balcony
Seating Capacity: 280
Year Built: 1983
Year Remodeled: 1999
Cost: $650,000
Rental Contact: Maura Cavanaugh

2630   CLOCKWORK REPERTORY THEATRE
133 Main Street
Oakville, CT 06779
Phone: 860-274-7247
Management:
Producer: Harold J Pantely
Artistic Director: Susan P Pantely
Mission: Producing plays, emphasizing new American plays dealing with controversial events.
Founded: 1977
Specialized Field: Theatrical Group
Status: Semi-Professional; Nonprofit
Income Sources: New England Theatre Conference
Organization Type: Performing; Resident

2631   TRI-ARTS AT THE SHARON PLAYHOUSE
49 Amenia Road
PO Box 1187
Sharon, CT 06069
Phone: 860-364-7469
Fax: 860-364-8043
e-mail: info@triarts.net
Web Site: www.triarts.net

Officers:
President: Patricia Best
VP: Ian Cadenhead
VP/Treasurer: William P Suter
Secretary: Helen Townsend
Secretary: Marilyn Buchenholz
Mission: To create and administer a dynamic and creative center for the arts, presenting live theatre and other cultural events to the residents of the Tri-State area (Connecticut, New York, and Massachusetts).
Founded: 1989
Specialized Field: Summer theater
Budget: 250,000
Income Sources: Donations; Tickets
Performs At: Theater; Gallery
Annual Attendance: 8,000-10,000
Facility Category: Barn style summer theater
Type of Stage: Proscenium
Seating Capacity: 370
Year Built: 1953
Year Remodeled: 1994
Resident Groups: Tri State Center for the Arts

2632   SHERMAN PLAYERS
Route 37 and Route 39
PO Box 471
Sherman, CT 06784
Phone: 860-354-3622
e-mail: ewscholze@aol.com
Web Site: www.geocities.com/~shermanplayers
Officers:
President: Elizabeth Scholze
VP: Glenn Anderson
Secretary: Jack Heidt
Treasurer: Bobbie Tiebout
Publicity: Jean Buoy
Membership: Larry Buoy
Board of Directors: Ellen Burnett
Wardrobe: Alpha Castro
Mission: To provide good theater and related artistic offerings to the CT area.
Founded: 1929
Specialized Field: Musical; Community; Theatrical Group
Status: Non-Professional; Nonprofit
Paid Staff: n
Paid Artists: y
Budget: $16,000 - 32,000
Income Sources: Membership; Playbill Advertising; Contributions; Occasional Fundraisers
Performs At: Sherman Playhouse
Annual Attendance: 3,200
Facility Category: Church, converted to a Theater
Type of Stage: Proscenium
Stage Dimensions: 15x36
Seating Capacity: 126
Year Built: 1837
Year Remodeled: 1961
Rental Contact: Town of Sherman
Organization Type: Performing; Sponsoring

2633   CENTENNIAL THEATER FESTIVAL
995 Hopmeadow Street
Simsbury, CT 06070

Phone: 860-408-5300
Fax: 860-408-5301
e-mail: deanadams@msn.com
Web Site: www.ctfestival.com
Management:
  Artistic Director: Dean Adams
Founded: 1990
Status: Nonprofit
Season: June 11 - August 1
Annual Attendance: 8,000
Facility Category: Theater; Air Conditioned, Handicap Access
Type of Stage: Proscenium
Stage Dimensions: 29' x 35'
Seating Capacity: 400
Year Built: 1989

2634   THEATRE PROJECT CONSULTANTS
25 Elizabeth Street
South Norwalk, CT 06854
Phone: 203-299-0835
Fax: 203-299-0835
e-mail: usa@tpcworld.com
Web Site: www.tpcworld.com
Officers:
  President: Victor Gotesman
Management:
  General Manager: Elissa Getto
Mission: We are stage managers, theatre technicians, designers, producers, arts administrators and architects.

2635   PALACE THEATRE OF THE ARTS
61 Atlantic Street
307 Atlantic Street
Stamford, CT 06901
Phone: 203-358-2305
Fax: 203-358-2313
Management:
  Facilities Manager: John Hiddlestone
  Marketing Director: Nancy Koffin
  House Manager: Vicki Kieffer
Founded: 1983
Specialized Field: Musical; Theatrical Group
Status: Professional; Commercial
Performs At: Palace Theatre
Affiliations: International Association of Theatrical Stage Employees
Seating Capacity: 1580
Year Built: 1927
Year Remodeled: 1983
Architect: Thomas Lamb
Organization Type: Sponsoring

2636   STAMFORD THEATRE WORKS
95 Atlantic Street
Strawberry Hill Avenue
Stamford, CT 06901
Phone: 203-359-4414
Fax: 203-356-1846
e-mail: stwct@aol.com
Web Site: www.stamfordartstheatreworks.org
Officers:
  President: Steve Karp
  VP: Marietta Morrelli

  Secretary: Charry Boris
Management:
  Producing Director: Steve Karp
  General Manager: Patrick Shea
  Press/Marketing Director: Patricia Blaufuss
  Box Office Manager: Valarie Howard
  Administrative Assistant: Peter Young
Mission: To produce plays of cultural and social significance for the benefit of the greater Stamford area; to build a theatre of regional and national prominence, acclaimed for its innovative productions of contemporary and classical plays.
Founded: 1988
Specialized Field: Theatre
Status: Professional; Nonprofit
Paid Staff: 10
Volunteer Staff: 75
Paid Artists: 125
Budget: 800,000
Income Sources: Actors' Equity Association; Society for Stage Directors and Choreographers
Annual Attendance: 16,000
Seating Capacity: 150
Organization Type: Performing

2637   PUPPET HOUSE THEATRE
128 Thimble Island Road
PO Box 3081
Stony Creek, CT 06405
Phone: 203-488-5752
Mission: Presenting theatrical programs of small professional and community groups.
Founded: 1972
Specialized Field: Summer Stock; Community; Folk; Puppet
Status: Professional; Non-Professional; Nonprofit
Paid Staff: 75
Year Built: 1903
Organization Type: Performing; Touring; Sponsoring

2638   CONNECTICUT REPERTORY THEATRE
802 Bolton Road, Unit 1127
University of Connecticut
Storrs, CT 06269-1127
Phone: 860-486-1628
Fax: 860-486-3110
Web Site: www.sfa.uconn.edu
Management:
  Artistic Director: Gary M English
Mission: Connecticut Repertory Theatre exists as the primary training mechanism for the Department of Dramatic Arts at the University of Connecticut, and as a nationally recognized professional theatre center for the University.
Founded: 1957
Specialized Field: Theatre
Status: Nonprofit
Season: June - July
Type of Stage: Proscenium
Stage Dimensions: 30'x 25'
Seating Capacity: 492

2639 UNIVERSITY OF CONNECTICUT: DEPARTMENT OF DRAMATIC ARTS

U-127, University of Connecticut
802 Bolton Road
Storrs, CT 06269
Phone: 860-486-4025
Fax: 860-486-3110
Web Site: www.uconn.edu
Management:
    Professor: Gary English
Budget: $8,500-18,800
Affiliations: NAST; U/RTA; Connecticut Repertory
Theatre
Seating Capacity: 500; 100; 90
Year Built: 1960

2640 STRATFORD FESTIVAL THEATER

1850 Elm Street
Stratford, CT 06615
Phone: 203-378-1200
Fax: 203-378-9777
Management:
    Dramaturg: J Wishnia
Founded: 1996

2641 SEVEN ANGELS THEATRE

Box 3358
Waterbury, CT 06705
Phone: 203-591-8223
Fax: 203-591-8223
Management:
    Artistic Director: Semina De Laurentis
Founded: 1991

2642 EUGENE O'NEILL THEATER CENTER

305 Great Neck Road
Waterford, CT 06385
Phone: 860-443-5378
Fax: 860-443-9653
e-mail: info@oneilltheatercenter.org
Web Site: www.oneilltheatercenter.org
Officers:
    Executive Director: Howard Sherman
    Chairman: Thomas Viertel
Management:
    Communications Director: Lex Leifheit
Mission: Dedicated to the development of new work for
the theater.
Founded: 1964
Status: Nonprofit
Season: July
Seating Capacity: 100-300

2643 NATIONAL THEATER INSTITUTE EUGENE O'NEILL THEATER CENTER

305 Great Neck Road
Waterford, CT 06385
Phone: 860-443-7139
Fax: 860-443-9653
Web Site: www.oneilltheatre.org
Officers:
    Chairman: Thomas Viertel
Management:

Executive Director: Howard Sherman
Artistic Director: Jim Houghton
Artistic Director: Paulette Hawpt
Director: David B Jaffe
Mission: To support the development and education of
theatrical artists, students and audiences.
Founded: 1964
Specialized Field: Theatrical Group
Status: Professional; Nonprofit
Performs At: The Rose Barn; The Edith Oliver Theatre;
The Amphitheatre
Affiliations: Theatre Communication Group; ATHE;
Moscow Art Theater
Seating Capacity: 300; 50
Year Built: 1964
Organization Type: Performing; Educational;
Sponsoring

2644 UNIVERSITY OF HARTFORD: DEPARTMENT OF ART HISTORY, CINEMA, DRAMA

200 Bloomfield Avenue
West Hartford, CT 06117
Phone: 860-768-4742
Fax: 860-768-4080
Web Site: www.hartford.edu
Budget: $6,000-9,000
Seating Capacity: 200
Year Built: 1960
Year Remodeled: 1996

2645 FAIRFIELD COUNTY STAGE COMPANY

25 Powers Court
Westport, CT 06880
Phone: 203-227-5137
Officers:
    Chairman: Rita Fredricks
    President: Marilyn Hersey
    Secretary: Christopher Cull
    Treasurer: Burry Fredrik
Management:
    Associate Artistic Director: Anne Ueefe
Mission: Professional regional theatre operating under the
Letter of Agreement/LORT 'D' Contract with Actors'
Equity Association.
Founded: 1981
Specialized Field: Theatrical Group
Status: Professional
Paid Staff: 40
Paid Artists: 70
Income Sources: Actors' Equity Association; Theatre
Communications Group
Organization Type: Performing; Resident

2646 WESTPORT COMMUNITY THEATRE

Town Hall
110 Myrtle Avenue
Westport, CT 06880
Phone: 203-226-1983
Management:
    Artistic Manager: H Edward Spires
Mission: Offering entertainment and instruction to the
community regarding theatre; developing appreciation of
theatre.

Founded: 1956
Specialized Field: Community; Theatrical Group
Status: Non-Professional; Nonprofit
Season: June - September
Organization Type: Performing

2647 WESTPORT COUNTRY PLAYHOUSE

25 Powers Court
PO Box 629
Westport, CT 06880
Phone: 203-227-5137
Fax: 203-221-7482
e-mail: westportplay@mindspring.com
Web Site: www.westportplayhouse.com
Management:
    Artistic Manager: Janice Muirhead
    General Manager: Julie Monahan
Mission: Offering professional theatre to Connecticut.
Founded: 1930
Specialized Field: Summer Stock
Status: Professional; Nonprofit
Income Sources: Council of Stock Theatres
Season: june-september
Performs At: Westport Summer Country Playhouse
Facility Category: Summer Theatre
Type of Stage: Proscenium
Seating Capacity: 707
Year Built: 1930
Rental Contact: Julie Monahan
Organization Type: Performing; Resident

2648 WHITE BARN THEATRE

Newton Turnpike
Westport, CT 06880
Phone: 203-227-3768
e-mail: whitebarntheatre@aol.com
Web Site: www.whitebarntheatre.org
Management:
    General Manager: Vincent Curcio
    Founder/Artistic Director: Lucille Lortel
Founded: 1947
Season: July - August
Type of Stage: Proscenium
Seating Capacity: 148

2649 WILTON PLAYSHOP

15 Lovers Lane
PO Box 363
Wilton, CT 06897
Phone: 203-762-7629
Fax: 203-544-8820
e-mail: skip.ploss@electricbruin.com
Web Site: www.wiltonplayshop.org
Officers:
    President: Skip Ploss
    VP: Jon Murray
    Chairman, Trustees: Karen Young
Management:
    President: Skip Ploss
    Secretary: Art Gallagher
    VP: Jon Murray
    Membership: Brenda Froehlich

Mission: The presentation of musicals and plays to the general public at an affordable price under high quality conditions.
Founded: 1937
Specialized Field: Theatrical Group
Status: Non-Professional
Volunteer Staff: 36
Non-paid Artists: 75
Budget: $50,000
Income Sources: Ticket Sales & Program Advertising
Performs At: Auditorium; Stage w/loft;
Annual Attendance: 3,000 - 4,000
Facility Category: Performing Arts Theatre
Type of Stage: Proscenium
Stage Dimensions: 18x32
Seating Capacity: 125
Year Built: 1870
Year Remodeled: 1977
Organization Type: Performing; Educational
Resident Groups: Community Theatre

Delaware

2650 KENT COUNTY THEATRE GUILD

140 E Roosevelt Avenue
PO Box 783
Dover, DE 19903-0783
Phone: 302-674-3568
e-mail: kctg@kctg.org
Web Site: www.kctg.org
Mission: Kent County has been providing quality theatre to the central Delaware community since 1953.

2651 POSSUM POINT PLAYERS

Old Laurel Highway
PO Box 96
Georgetown, DE 19947
Phone: 302-856-3460
Fax: 302-856-4560
Management:
    Executive Director: Andre Beaumont
    Adminstrative Assistant: Mary Cahill
Mission: Offering quality theatrical productions to Sussex County, Delaware.
Founded: 1973
Specialized Field: Musical; Dinner; Community; Theatrical Group
Status: Non-Professional; Nonprofit
Paid Staff: 50
Income Sources: Delaware Theater Association
Performs At: Possum Hall; Delaware Tech Theater
Organization Type: Performing; Educational

2652 UNIVERSITY OF DELAWARE: DEPARTMENT OF THEATRE

413 Academy Street
Newark, DE 19716
Phone: 302-831-2201
Fax: 302-831-3673
Web Site: www.udel.edu/theatre
Management:
    Director: Sanford Robbins

Performs At: Hartshorn Theatre
Affiliations: ATHE
Seating Capacity: 200-300
Year Built: 1930
Year Remodeled: 1989

2653 ARTISTS THEATRE ASSOCIATION

PO Box 7258
Wilmington, DE 19803
Phone: 302-798-8775
e-mail: artstheatr@aol.com
Web Site: www.dca.net/ata
Officers:
  President: L Jeffrey DiSabatino
  Vice-President: Claire Ennis
  Acting Treasurer: Claire Braun
  Secretary: Tina M. Sheing
  Past President: Tom Marshall
Mission: To further the dramatic arts; to encourage new plays; to present workshops in high schools.
Founded: 1968
Specialized Field: Musical; Community; Theatrical Group
Status: Non-Professional; Nonprofit
Paid Staff: 100
Income Sources: Delaware Theatre Association; Delaware Alliance for Arts Education
Organization Type: Performing

2654 DELAWARE THEATRE COMPANY

200 Water Street
Wilmington, DE 19801
Phone: 302-594-1104
Fax: 302-594-1107
e-mail: dtc@delawaretheatre.org
Web Site: www.delawaretheatre.com
Officers:
  Chairman: Gary Wilkinson
  President: William Shea
Management:
  Artistic Director: Fontaine Syer
  General Manager: Rebecca Frederick
  Marketing Director: Tom Kirkpatrick
  Development Director: Gail O'Donnell
Mission: To create high quality professional theatre in Delaware.
Founded: 1978
Specialized Field: Musical; Theatrical Group
Status: Professional; Nonprofit
Paid Staff: 35
Budget: $2.3 million
Performs At: The Delaware Theatre Company
Type of Stage: Semi-Thrust
Seating Capacity: 389
Year Built: 1985
Rental Contact: Tom Kirkpatrick
Organization Type: Performing; Educational

2655 SHOESTRING PRODUCTIONS LIMITED

214 W 18th Street
Wilmington, DE 19802
Phone: 302-655-0299
Management:
  Artistic Director: Deborah Dehart

Mission: Creating, producing and touring original musicals to entertain and educate young audiences.
Founded: 1978
Specialized Field: Musical; Theatrical Group
Status: Professional
Organization Type: Performing; Touring; Educational

2656 WILMINGTON DRAMA LEAGUE

10 W Lea Boulevard
Wilmington, DE 19808
Phone: 302-764-3396
e-mail: infowdl@wdl.org
Web Site: www.wdl.org
Officers:
  President: Kate Monaghan
  Secretary: Alicia Bader
  Treasurer: Dennis Williams
Management:
  Managing Director: Ted Wilson
Mission: To provide low-cost, quality theatre, theatrical activities, and education to the Greater Wilmington Region.
Founded: 1933
Specialized Field: Community; Theatrical Group
Status: Non-Professional; Nonprofit
Paid Staff: 1
Volunteer Staff: 300
Budget: $195,000
Income Sources: Ticket Sales; Contribution; State Arts Council
Annual Attendance: 8,000
Facility Category: Theatre
Seating Capacity: 256
Year Built: 1940
Year Remodeled: 1999
Organization Type: Performing; Educational

District of Columbia

2657 AFRICAN CONTINUUM THEATRE COMPANY (ACTCO)

3523 12th Street NE
2nd Floor
Washington, DC 20017-2545
Phone: 202-529-5763
Fax: 202-529-5782
Web Site: www.onwashingtons.com/groups-actco
Officers:
  President: William R Roberts
Management:
  Producing Artistic Director: Jennifer L Nelson
  Managing Director: Imani Droyton Hill
Founded: 1989
Specialized Field: Metro-Washington, D.C.
Paid Staff: 4
Volunteer Staff: 10

2658 ARENA STAGE

1101 6th Street SW
Washington, DC 20024

Phone: 202-554-9066
Fax: 202-488-4056
e-mail: info@arenastage.org
Web Site: www.arenastage.org
Officers:
  Chair: Wendy Farrow Raines
  VP: Stephen Richard
  President: James J Rouse
  VP: Riley K Temple
  Secretary: Helga Tarver
  Treasurer: Roger Williams
Management:
  Artistic Director: Molly Smith
  Executive Director: Stephen Richard
Mission: To offer huge plays that encompass all that is exuberant, passionate, deep, profound and dangerous in our American spirit. Arena Stage relentlessly pursues excellence and artistic process; flourishes by providing a dynamic and powerful artistic community; champions various diversities throughout our organization and in the community; is recognized as a leader throughout the world.
Founded: 1950
Status: Professional; Nonprofit
Income Sources: Actors' Equity Association; Society for Stage Directors and Choreographers
Performs At: Arena Theatre (Fichandler & Kreeger)
Organization Type: Performing; Educational
Notes: Box office 202-488-3300, TTY 202-484-0247

2659 DISCOVERY THEATER
Arts & Industries Building
900 Jefferson Drive, SW
Washington, DC 20560
Phone: 202-357-1500
Fax: 202-357-2588
e-mail: disc-th@tsa.si.edu
Web Site: www.discoverytheater.si.edu
Management:
  Director: Roberta Gasbarre
Mission: The Smithsonian's Discovery Theater, located in the Arts and Industries Building on the National Mall, is dedicated to offering the best in live performing arts for young people.
Founded: 1978
Status: Non-Equity
Season: September - August
Type of Stage: Thrust
Stage Dimensions: 25' x 10'
Seating Capacity: 175

2660 FOLGER SHAKESPEARE LIBRARY
201 E Capitol Street SE
Washington, DC 20003-1094
Phone: 202-544-7077
Fax: 202-608-1719
e-mail: webmaster@folger.edu
Web Site: www.folger.edu
Management:
  Head Public Relations: Garland Scott
  Director Education: Janet Alexander Griffin
  Production Manager: Janet Clark

Mission: Home of the world's largest Shakespeare collection, the Folger is a major international center for scholary research and a lively venue for exhibitions, literary programs, and the performing arts.
Founded: 1932
Specialized Field: Theatre; Music; Poetry; Literature; Exhibitions; Preformances and Programs
Status: Nonprofit
Paid Staff: 25
Volunteer Staff: 35
Paid Artists: 70
Budget: $9,000,000
Income Sources: Grants; Endowments
Performs At: Theater
Annual Attendance: 200,000
Type of Stage: Proscenium
Seating Capacity: 250
Year Built: 1932
Year Remodeled: 1992

2661 FORD'S THEATRE SOCIETY
511 10th Street NW
Washington, DC 20004
Phone: 202-638-2941
Fax: 202-737-3017
e-mail: bjlaczko@aol.com
Web Site: www.fordstheatre.org
Officers:
  Chairman: Hon. Joseph McDadeny
  Vice Chairman: Gerald M Lowrie
  Secretary: Mrs. Paul Laxalt
  Treasurer: Richard L. Thompson
Management:
  Producing Artistic Director: Frankie Hewitt
  Managing Director: Brian J Laczko
  General Manager: Patricia Humphery
Mission: Presenting live theatre productions to pay tribute to Abraham Lincoln's appreciation for the performing arts.
Founded: 1968
Specialized Field: Musical; Drama
Status: Professional; Nonprofit
Budget: $6,000,000
Performs At: Ford's Theatre
Annual Attendance: 150,000
Facility Category: Theatre House
Type of Stage: Proscenium/Thrust
Seating Capacity: 699
Year Built: 1860
Year Remodeled: 1968
Organization Type: Performing; Educational

2662 GALA HISPANIC THEATRE
PO Box 43209
Washington, DC 20010
Phone: 202-234-7174
Fax: 202-332-1247
e-mail: galadc@aol.com
Web Site: www.galadc.org
Management:
  Artistic Producing Director: Hugo Medrano
  Associate Producing Director: Abel Lopez
Mission: Expanding and promoting Hispanic culture.
Founded: 1976
Specialized Field: Theatrical Group

Status: Professional; Nonprofit
Performs At: GALA Hispanic Theatre
Type of Stage: Proscenium
Seating Capacity: 200
Organization Type: Resident; Educational

2663 KENNEDY CENTER AMERICAN COLLEGE THEATRE

John F Kennedy Center for the Performing Arts
Washington, DC 20566-0001
Phone: 202-416-8864
Fax: 202-416-8802
Web Site: www.kennedy-center.org/education/actf
Management:
   Artistic Director/Co-Manager: Gregg Henry
   Co-Manager/Administration: Susan Shaffer
Specialized Field: Plays, musicals
Paid Staff: 4
Volunteer Staff: 50
Non-paid Artists: 200
Season: April
Performs At: Kennedy Center [Festival Site]
Facility Category: Terrace Theatre; Theatre Lab
Seating Capacity: 513; 388

2664 LIVING STAGE

1101 6th Street SW
Washington, DC 20024
Phone: 202-234-5782
Fax: 202-797-1043
e-mail: info@livingstage.org
Web Site: www.arenastage.org
Management:
   Operations Manager: Catherine Lapinel
   Director: Ralph Rernington
Mission: Change through creative empowerment.
Founded: 1966
Specialized Field: Improvizational Theatre
Status: Professional; Nonprofit
Paid Staff: 8
Volunteer Staff: 3
Paid Artists: 6
Non-paid Artists: 1
Performs At: Performance Workshops
Affiliations: A division of Community Engagement at Arena Stage
Type of Stage: Black Box
Stage Dimensions: 45'x 37'
Seating Capacity: varies
Year Built: 1985
Year Remodeled: 1990
Rental Contact: Anne Theisen
Organization Type: Resident

2665 NATIONAL THEATRE

1321 Pennsylvania Avenue NW
Washington, DC 20004
Phone: 202-628-6161
Web Site: www.nationaltheatre.org
Officers:
   President: Donix Murphy
Management:
   General Manager: Harry Teter, Jr
   Theatre Manager: Carol M Hayes

   Box Office Treasurer: John Loomis
   Director Group Sales: Greg Flood
   Concession Manager: Bill Conn
Mission: The preservation of the historic playhouse; the presentation of top quality touring productions; the showcasing of professional and non-professional groups.
Founded: 1835
Specialized Field: Musical; Community; Folk; Puppet
Status: Professional; Nonprofit; Commercial
Paid Staff: 100
Paid Artists: 3
Income Sources: Actors' Equity Association; International Association of Theatrical Stage Employees; The Shubert Organization
Organization Type: Educational; Sponsoring

2666 SHAKESPEARE THEATRE

450 7th Street NW
Washington, DC 20004
Phone: 202-547-3230
Fax: 202-547-0226
e-mail: info@shakespearetheatre.com
Web Site: www.shakespearetheatre.com
Management:
   Artistic Director: Michael Kahn
   General Manager: Christine Dietze
   Production Manager: Michael Curry
Mission: To become the nation's leading force in producing and preserving the highest quality of classical theatre.
Founded: 1986
Specialized Field: Live Theatre
Status: Professional; Nonprofit
Paid Staff: 75
Volunteer Staff: 50
Paid Artists: 80
Income Sources: League of Washington Theatres; Cultural Alliance of Greater Washington
Performs At: The Shakespeare Theatre at the Lansburgh
Annual Attendance: 160,000
Facility Category: Theatre
Type of Stage: Proscenium
Seating Capacity: 451
Organization Type: Performing; Resident

2667 SOURCE THEATRE COMPANY

1835 14th Street NW
Washington, DC 20009
Phone: 202-462-1073
Fax: 202-462-2300
Web Site: www.sourcetheatre.org
Management:
   Artistic Director: Joe Banno
   Literary Manager: Keith Parker
   Managing Director: Delia Taylor
   Contact: Heather Pagella
Mission: To present innovative and exciting productions of new works and contemporary plays that have relevance to our community; to offer reinterpretations of the classics.
Founded: 1977
Specialized Field: Theatrical Group
Status: Professional; Nonprofit
Paid Staff: 4
Volunteer Staff: 40

Paid Artists: 20
Budget: $400,000
Income Sources: Ticket Sales, Grants
Performs At: Theatre
Affiliations: League of Washington Theatres; Theatre Communications Group; Actors' Equity Association
Annual Attendance: 15,000
Type of Stage: Black Box
Year Remodeled: 1998
Rental Contact: Heather Pagella
Organization Type: Performing; Touring; Resident

2668 STUDIO THEATRE

1333 P Street NW
Washington, DC 20005
Phone: 202-232-7267
Fax: 202-588-5262
e-mail: studio@studiotheatre.org
Web Site: www.studiotheatre.org
Officers:
 Chair of the Board of Trustees: Susan L Butler
 Vice Chair of the Board of Trustees: Janet L Dewar
 Chair Emeritus, Board of Trustees: Irene Harriet Blum
 Chair Emeritus, Board of Trustees: Jaylee M Mead
Management:
 Artistic Director/Managing Director: Joy Zinoman
 Assoc. Managing Dir/Artistic Dir: Keith Alan Baker
Mission: To produce the best in contemporary theatre and through its Secondstage and Acting Conservatory to provide opportunities for emerging artists and to offer rigorous theatre training. Our commitment to artistic excellence serves the diverse communities of the Nation's Capital.
Founded: 1978
Specialized Field: Theatrical Group
Status: Professional; Nonprofit
Paid Staff: 32
Budget: $3,000,000
Income Sources: Theatre Communications Group; Cultural Alliance of Greater Washington; League of Washington Theatres
Performs At: The Studio Theatre; The Secondstage
Facility Category: Theatre
Type of Stage: Proscenium
Seating Capacity: 182 Milton/218 Mead/50 Second Stage
Year Remodeled: 1997
Cost: to 5.5 million
Rental Contact: Roma Rogers
Organization Type: Performing; Educational; Sponsoring

2669 VSA ARTS

1300 Connecticut Avenue
Suite 700
Washington, DC 20036
Phone: 202-628-2800
Fax: 202-737-0725
e-mail: info@vsarts.org
Web Site: www.vsarts.org
Officers:
 Director Nation Programs/Events: Dani Fox
 Information Specialist: Johanna Bontwood

Specialized Field: Disability Arts Education Organization
Affiliations: John F Kennedy Center for the Performing Arts

2670 WASHINGTON STAGE GUILD

4048 7th Street NE
#4
Washington, DC 20017
Phone: 202-529-2084
Fax: 202-529-2740
Management:
 Producing Artistic Director: John MacDonald
 Executive Director: Ann Norton
 Dramaturge: William Largess
Mission: To perform plays that are often overlooked, including lesser-known works of famous playwrights, classics, and new plays of merit.
Founded: 1986
Specialized Field: Theatrical Group
Status: Professional; Nonprofit
Income Sources: Actors' Equity Association; League of Washington Theatres; Cultural Arts Alliance of DC
Performs At: Carroll Hall
Organization Type: Performing; Resident; Educational

2671 WOOLLY MAMMOTH THEATRE COMPANY

1401 Church Street NW
Washington, DC 20005
Phone: 202-393-3939
Fax: 202-667-0904
e-mail: info@woollymammoth.net
Web Site: www.woollymammoth.net
Management:
 Artistic Director: Howard Shalwitz
 Associate Director: Molly White
 Producing Associate: Nancy Turner Hensley
Mission: To present the most daring and experimental plays in the Washington, DC area.
Founded: 1980
Specialized Field: Musical; Theatrical Group
Status: Professional; Nonprofit
Paid Staff: 65
Income Sources: Theatre Communications Group
Performs At: Woolly Mammoth Theatre
Organization Type: Performing; Resident; Educational

2672 AMERICAN UNIVERSITY THEATRE PROGRAM

4400 Massachusetts Avenue
Washington, DC, DC 20016
Phone: 202-885-3429
Officers:
 Chair: Gail Humphries Breeskin
Affiliations: ATHE
Seating Capacity: 175-200; 175

2673 CATHOLIC UNIVERSITY OF AMERICA: THEATRE DEPARTMENT

105 Hartke
Washington, DC, DC 20064

Phone: 202-319-5351
Fax: 202-319-5359
Web Site: www.cua.edu/as/drama
Officers:
  Chair: Dr. Greta Honegger PhD
Budget: $10,100-15,500
Affiliations: Arena Stage
Seating Capacity: 590; 80; 40
Year Built: 1970
Year Remodeled: 1987

2674 CENTER FOR MOVEMENT THEATRE
Washington, DC, DC
Mailing Address: PO Box 11655, Washington, DC 20008
Phone: 301-495-8822
Fax: 301-495-4870
Management:
  School Director: Dody DiSanto

2675 GEORGE WASHINGTON UNIVERSITY: DEPARTMENT OF THEATRE AND DANCE
800 21st Street
Washington, DC, DC 20052
Phone: 202-994-8072
Officers:
  Chair: Leslie B Jacobson
Budget: $2,900
Affiliations: ATHE
Seating Capacity: 484; 50
Year Built: 1968

2676 HOWARD UNIVERSITY DEPARTMENT OF THEATRE ARTS
Division of Fine Arts
2455-6th Street Northwest
Washington, DC, DC 20059
Phone: 202-806-6100
Officers:
  Chair: Henriette Edmunds
Budget: $3,550-14,000
Affiliations: NAST; ATHE
Seating Capacity: 300; 75
Year Built: 1960
Year Remodeled: 1988

2677 NATIONAL CONSERVATORY OF DRAMATIC ARTS
1556 Wisconsin Avenue Northwest
Washington, DC, DC 20007
Phone: 202-333-2202
Management:
  Dean: Dennis Dulmage
Budget: $7,100-21,000
Type of Stage: Black Box
Seating Capacity: 60
Year Built: 1960

2678 ISLAND PLAYERS
PO Box 2059
Anna Maria, FL 34216
Phone: 941-778-5755
Mission: To present quality community theatre for the cultural enrichment of the area.
Founded: 1948
Specialized Field: Community
Status: Non-Professional; Nonprofit
Performs At: Island Players Theatre
Organization Type: Performing

2679 CALDWELL THEATRE COMPANY
7873 N Federal Highway
Levitz Plaza
Boca Raton, FL 33487
Mailing Address: PO Box 227 Boca Raton, FL 33429-0277
Phone: 561-241-7432
Fax: 561-997-6917
Web Site: www.caldwelltheatre.com
Management:
  Artistic And Managing Director: Michael Hall
  Company Manager: Patricia Burdett
  General Manager/Artistic Associate: Tom Salzman
Mission: To offer regional professional theater.
Founded: 1980
Specialized Field: Theatrical Group
Status: Professional; Nonprofit
Income Sources: Theatre Communications Group; Florida Professional Theatre Association
Organization Type: Performing; Touring; Resident

2680 FLORIDA ATLANTIC UNIVERSITY: DEPARTMENT OF THEATRE
777 Glade Road
Boca Raton, FL 33431
Phone: 561-297-3810
Fax: 561-297-2180
Officers:
  Chair: Jean Louis Baldet
Budget: $40,750-51,000
Affiliations: ATHE
Seating Capacity: 540; 150; 100
Year Built: 1996

2681 MANATEE PLAYERS/RIVERFRONT THEATRE
102 Old Main Street
Bradenton, FL 33505
Phone: 941-748-0111
Management:
  Managing Director: Nan Alderson
  Artistic Director: Peter Massey
  Technical Director: Dan Yerman
Mission: Improving the cultural and educational climate of our community through offering quality live theatre.
Founded: 1948
Specialized Field: Community
Status: Nonprofit
Paid Staff: 100

Income Sources: Festival of American Community Theatre; American Association of Community Theatres; Manatee County Cultural Alliance
Performs At: Riverfront Theatre
Organization Type: Performing; Educational

2682 CITY PLAYERS

Clearwater Parks and Recreation
PO Box 4748
Clearwater, FL 34618
Phone: 813-462-6035
Management:
    Cultural Arts Supervisor: Margo Walbolt
    Technical Director: Phillip Terry
    Music Director: B.J. Pucci
Mission: To offer the public quality theatre at nominal fees.
Founded: 1971
Specialized Field: Community; Theatrical Group
Status: Non-Professional; Nonprofit
Paid Staff: 4
Performs At: Ruth Eckerd Hall; Saint Petersburg Junior College
Organization Type: Performing; Educational

2683 SHOWBOAT DINNER THEATRE

3405 Ulmerton Road
Clearwater, FL 34622
Phone: 727-571-1200
Fax: 813-573-2735
Management:
    Owner/President/Producer: Virginia Sherwood
Founded: 1967
Specialized Field: Dinner
Status: Professional; Commercial
Organization Type: Performing

2684 SURFSIDE PLAYERS

PO Box 320053
Cocoa Beach, FL 32932-0053
Phone: 321-783-3127
e-mail: box.office@surfsideplayers.com
Web Site: www.surfsideplayers.com
Officers:
    President: Dave McFarland
    VP: Judy Bate
    Secretary: Kay Grinter
    Treasurer: Marilyn Rigerman
Management:
    General Manager: Lynea Adams
    Assistant General Manager: Jean Quigley
Mission: To produce high quality productions, and educate youth in the performing arts field.

2685 ACTORS' PLAYHOUSE AT THE MIRACLE THEATRE

280 Miracle Mile
Coral Gables, FL 33134
Phone: 305-444-9293
Fax: 305-444-4181
Web Site: www.actorsplayhouse.org
Officers:
    Chairman: Dr Lawrence Stein

Management:
    Executive Producing Director: Barbara S Stein
    Artistic Director: David Arisco
    Operations Director/Group Sales: Patricia Romeu
    Box Office Manager: Patricia Natter
    PR/Communications: Christi Soltz
    Company And Literary Manager: Javier Chacin
    Children And Education Sales: Sandra Perez
    Technical Director: Gene Seyffer
    Assistant Technical Director: Chris Jahn
Mission: Actors' Playhouse at the Miracle Theatre is one of Florida's major critically acclaimed non-profit cultural institutions and is dedicated to entertaining and culturally enriching South Florida audiences by producing quality live theatre for adults and children at affordable prices.
Founded: 1987
Status: Nonprofit
Season: October - June
Seating Capacity: 600

2686 GABLESTAGE

1200 Anastasia Avenue
Suite 230
Coral Gables, FL 33134
Phone: 305-446-1116
Fax: 305-445-8645
e-mail: gables22@bellsouth.net
Web Site: gablestage.org
Management:
    Producing Artistic Director: Joseph Adler
    Business Manager: Angelique del Mazo
Mission: To provide the South Florida community with classical contemporary theatrical productions of artistic excellence. FST hopes to challenge our multi-cultural audience with innovative productions that entertain as well as confront today's issues and ideas.
Founded: 1979
Specialized Field: Theater; Festivals
Status: Professional; Nonprofit
Paid Staff: 10
Budget: $1 million
Income Sources: Foundations; Government; Corporations; Individuals; Box Office
Performs At: Biltmore Hotel
Affiliations: Theatre Leader of South Florida
Annual Attendance: 30,000
Type of Stage: Proscenium
Seating Capacity: 150
Year Built: 1995
Organization Type: Performing; Touring; Resident; Educational

2687 UNIVERSITY OF MIAMI: DEPARTMENT OF THEATRE ARTS

Coral Gables, FL
Mailing Address: PO Box 248273, Coral Gables, FL 33124
Phone: 305-284-4474
Fax: 305-284-5702
Web Site: www.miami.edu/tha
Officers:
    Interim Chair: Bruce J Miller
Budget: $20,000-30,000
Affiliations: City Theatre

Seating Capacity: 300-400;45
Year Built: 1951
Year Remodeled: 1996

2688 DAYTONA PLAYHOUSE
100 Jessamine Boulevard
Daytona Beach, FL 32118
Phone: 386-255-2431
Fax: 386-255-2432
e-mail: info@daytonaplayhouse.com
Web Site: www.daytonaplayhouse.com
Management:
   Artistic Director: James F Sturgell
Mission: To provide enjoyment and entertainment.
Founded: 1947
Specialized Field: Community
Status: Nonprofit
Performs At: Daytona Playhouse
Organization Type: Performing; Resident

2689 SEASIDE MUSIC THEATER
901 6th Street
PO Box 2835
Daytona Beach, FL 32120
Phone: 904-252-3394
Fax: 904-252-8991
e-mail: lestermalizia@seasidemusictheater.org
Web Site: www.seasidemusictheater.org
Officers:
   Associate Producer: Julia Truild
Management:
   General Manager: Lester Malizia
   Director Marketing: Kelly Beasley
   Production Manager: Bob Fetterman
   Artistic Director/Producer: Tippen Davidson
   Company Manager: Jerry Lapidas
   Director Development: Monya Winzer
   Technical Director: Brian Kelley
Mission: To offer the finest examples of opera, operetta and musical theatre in repertory.
Founded: 1977
Specialized Field: Musical; Dinner; Theatrical Group
Status: Professional; Nonprofit
Paid Staff: 10
Paid Artists: 175
Budget: $2,800,000
Income Sources: Florida Professional Theatre Association; United States Institute for Theatre Technology; Southeastern Theatre Conference
Season: June - August
Annual Attendance: 40,000
Facility Category: Two theaters
Type of Stage: Proncenium
Stage Dimensions: 6'x30'; 47'x17'
Seating Capacity: 498; 576
Year Remodeled: 1999
Rental Contact: Director of Marketing Kelli Beasley
Organization Type: Performing; Touring; Educational

2690 DELRAY BEACH PLAYHOUSE
950 NW Ninth Street
Delray Beach, FL 33444

Phone: 561-272-1281
Fax: 561-272-5884
Web Site: www.delraybeachplayhouse.com
Management:
   Artistic Director: Randolph del Lago
   Box Office Manager: Cameron Penovi
   Technical Director: Chip Latimer
   Executive Director: Susan Easton
Mission: To increase community involvement in the performing arts.
Founded: 1948
Specialized Field: Community Theatre
Status: Non-Professional; Nonprofit
Paid Staff: 4
Volunteer Staff: 150
Non-paid Artists: 100
Income Sources: Florida Theatre Conference
Performs At: Delray Beach Playhouse
Facility Category: Non-profit community theatre
Organization Type: Performing; Educational

2691 BAY STREET PLAYERS
PO Box 1405
Eustis, FL 32726
Phone: 352-357-7777
Management:
   Executive Director: Dale R Carpenter
   Director: Deborah Carpenter
   Director: Lou Tally
   Managing Director: Michael Lake
Mission: To provide practical theater training through hands-on experience.
Founded: 1975
Specialized Field: Musical; Community; Theatrical Group
Status: Non-Professional; Nonprofit
Performs At: State Theatre
Organization Type: Performing; Touring; Educational

2692 FORT LAUDERDALE CHILDREN'S THEATRE
640 N Andrews Avenue
Fort Lauderdale, FL 33311
Phone: 954-763-6882
Fax: 954-523-0507
e-mail: FLCT@shadow.net
Web Site: www.flct.org
Management:
   Executive Artistic Director: Janet Erlick
   Education Director: Anthony Hubert
   Programming Director: Oliver Black
   Business Manager: Amy Rand
Mission: To develop the full potential of students as members of our community; to celebrate the diversity of Broward County's population through the arts; to nurture communication among various performing groups; to advance the highest possible standards of the theatre; to encourage public appreciation of the art form; to develop future audiences and supporters of the cultural arts.
Founded: 1952
Specialized Field: Community; Theatrical Group
Status: Nonprofit
Paid Staff: 10
Volunteer Staff: 25

Budget: $498,425
Income Sources: Classes; Plays; Outreach
Performs At: The Studio; Main Library Theatre
Affiliations: Florida Theatre Conference, Southeastern Theatre Conference, Florida Association for Theatre Educators, American Alliance for Theatre Education
Facility Category: Theatre
Type of Stage: Thrust, Proscenium
Seating Capacity: 132, 296
Rental Contact: Business Manager Amy Rand
Organization Type: Performing; Touring; Educational

2693 ONE WAY PUPPETS

PO Box 5346
Fort Lauderdale, FL 33310
Phone: 954-491-4221
Management:
    Director: Bob Dolan
Mission: Entertainment and education through puppetry.
Founded: 1971
Specialized Field: Theatrical Group; Puppet
Status: Professional
Organization Type: Performing; Educational

2694 BROADWAY PALM DINNER THEATRE

1380 Colonial Boulevard
Fort Myers, FL 33907
Phone: 239-278-4422
Fax: 239-278-5664
Toll-free: 800-475-7256
e-mail: tickets@broadwaypalm.com
Web Site: www.BroadwayPalm.com
Management:
    Owner/Executive Producer: William Prather
    General Manager: Susan Johnson
    Group Sales Coordinator: Joanna Lindsey
    Sales Manager: Becki Johnson
    Business Manager: Rob Ervin
    Marketing/Production Assistant: Beth Ellege
Mission: Year-round professional dinner theatre presenting Broadway's brightest musicals and comedies.
Founded: 1993
Specialized Field: Musical theatre, comedies
Status: Professional for profit
Paid Staff: 90
Paid Artists: 10
Income Sources: Ticket sales; Bar & gift shop revenue
Performs At: Broadway Palm Dinner Theatre
Affiliations: National Dinner Theatre Association
Annual Attendance: 150,000+
Facility Category: Dinner theatre
Type of Stage: Proscenium
Seating Capacity: 450
Year Remodeled: 1993
Rental Contact: Sales Manager Becki Johnson

2695 FLORIDA REPERTORY THEATRE

PO Box 2483
2267 1st Street
Fort Myers, FL 33902
Phone: 941-332-4665
Fax: 941-332-1808
e-mail: flrepertory@aol.com
Web Site: www.floridarep.org

Officers:
    Chairman: Gerald Laboda DMD
    Vice Chair: Sandra Stilwell
    Secretary: Janice Danzig
    Treasurer: Ken Nirenberg
Management:
    Producing Artistic Director: Robert Cacioppo
    Managing Director/Development: John W Martin
    Associate Producer/Education: Bari Newport
    Business Manager: Cheryl Ferrara
Mission: Providing a first class regional equity theatre for Southwest Florida; creating, nurturing, and developing an ensemble of theatre professionals who will develop long term relationships working on a wide variety of plays; helping improve the quality of life in our community through all arts, especially theatre, accessible to all while reflecting our growing commitment to the youth.
Founded: 1998
Specialized Field: Theatre
Paid Staff: 26
Volunteer Staff: 125
Paid Artists: 116
Non-paid Artists: 10

2696 PENINSULA PLAYERS

1436 Rosada Way
Fort Myers, FL 33901
Phone: 941-476-7305
Officers:
    President: James Zgoda
    VP: Ted Schirm
    Treasurer: Linda Jacobey
    Secretary: Suzanne Beeny
Management:
    Director: Al Richter
    Director: Dan Perry
    Director/Producer: Martha Richter
    General Manager: Tom Birmingham
    Executive Producer: James B McKenzie
Mission: To study, perform and promote choral works.
Founded: 1935
Specialized Field: Dinner; Community; Theatrical Group
Status: Nonprofit
Income Sources: Lee County Alliance of Arts
Performs At: Peninsula Playhouse
Organization Type: Performing

2697 UNIVERSITY OF FLORIDA: DEPARTMENT OF THEATRE

Hume Library, 4th Floor
University of Florida
Gainesville, FL 32611
Phone: 352-392-2038
Fax: 352-392-5114
Officers:
    Chair: Kevin Marshall
Budget: $5,100-7,200
Affiliations: NAST; U/RTA; ATHE; Hippodrome State Theatre
Seating Capacity: 460; 100; 50
Year Built: 1967
Year Remodeled: 1996

2698 GOLDEN THESPIANS
900 Tyler Street
Hollywood, FL 33019
Phone: 305-920-5492
Officers:
President: Ellen Bush
VP: Gloria Williams
Treasurer: Virginia Godfrey
Secretary: Madeline Barauskas
Management:
President/Director Shows: Ellen Bush
Mission: To bring together a senior group of men and women who were professional musicians, singers and dancers in their younger days to perform one-hour vaudeville shows in nursing homes, hospitals and at community affairs.
Founded: 1965
Specialized Field: Musical; Community; Folk; Theatrical Group
Status: Nonprofit
Paid Staff: 25
Income Sources: President's Council
Performs At: Recreation Center
Organization Type: Performing

2699 HOLLYWOOD PLAYHOUSE
2640 Washington Street
Hollywood, FL 33020
Phone: 954-922-0404
Fax: 954-922-0666
Web Site: www.hollywoodplayhouse.com
Officers:
President: Bea Yianilos
VP: Ivonne Morten
Secretary/Treasurer: Kothi Glist
Management:
Executive Artistic Director: Andy Rogow
Technical Director: David Sherman
Mission: Bringing culture to our community through theatre.
Founded: 1948
Specialized Field: Theatre; Plays; Musicals
Status: Professional regional theater
Paid Artists: 100
Budget: $750,000
Income Sources: Florida Theatre Conference
Affiliations: Theatre League of South Florida; Hollywood Chamber of Commerce
Facility Category: Prosenium theatre with ample fly and wing space
Type of Stage: Prosenium
Seating Capacity: 262
Year Built: 1960
Organization Type: Performing

2700 ALHAMBRA DINNER THEATRE
12000 Beach Boulevard
Jacksonville, FL 32216
Phone: 904-641-1212
Fax: 904-642-3505
Toll-free: 800-688-7469
e-mail: info@alhambradinnertheatre.com
Web Site: alhambradinnertheatre.com
Officers:
President: Tod Booth
Management:
Executive Producer: Tod Booth
Marketing Director: Jack Booth
Mission: Producing the finest professional theatrical productions.
Founded: 1967
Specialized Field: Dinner
Status: Professional; Commercial
Paid Staff: 100
Income Sources: Actors' Equity Association; American Dinner Theatre Institute; Society for Stage Directors and Choreographers; American Federation of Musicians
Performs At: Alhambra Dinner Theatre
Annual Attendance: 120,000
Facility Category: Dinner Theatre
Type of Stage: Thrust
Seating Capacity: 400
Year Built: 1967
Rental Contact: Director of Marketing Jack Booth
Organization Type: Performing

2701 RITZ THEATRE AND LA VILLA MUSEUM
829 N Davis Street
Jacksonville, FL 32202
Phone: 904-632-5555
Fax: 904-635-5553
Management:
Executive Director: Carol Alexander

2702 KEY WEST PLAYERS
Wall Street & Higgs Lane
PO Box 724
Key West, FL 33041
Phone: 305-294-5015
Fax: 305-294-1372
e-mail: pshilson@aol.com
Web Site: www.waterfrontplayhouse.com
Officers:
President: Paul Hilson
VP: Kelly Hedges-Peerman
Treasurer: Florence Recher
Mission: Presenting live professional and amateur entertainment; providing a teaching experience; teaching all of the aspects of theater.
Founded: 1940
Specialized Field: Live Performing Arts
Status: Nonprofit
Paid Staff: 5
Volunteer Staff: 12
Paid Artists: 150
Budget: $270,000
Income Sources: Box Office; Grants; Donations
Performs At: Waterfront Playhouse
Affiliations: FL. Professional Theater Association; League of South FL. Theaters; Theater Communications Group
Annual Attendance: 10,000
Facility Category: Live performing arts theatre
Type of Stage: Proscenium
Stage Dimensions: 25'x35'
Seating Capacity: 180
Year Built: 1853

Year Remodeled: 1960
Rental Contact: George Gugleotti
Organization Type: Performing; Educational

2703 RED BARN THEATRE

319 Duval Street
PO Box 707
Key West, FL 33041
Phone: 305-293-3035
Fax: 305-293-3035
Web Site: ww.redbarntheatre.org
Management:
 Co-Artistic Director: Joy Hawkins
 Managing Director: Mimi McDonald
Founded: 1981
Specialized Field: Theatrical Group
Status: Professional; Nonprofit
Paid Staff: 7
Paid Artists: 90
Income Sources: Theatre Communications Group
Performs At: Red Barn Theatre
Organization Type: Performing; Resident; Educational

2704 FLORIDA SOUTHERN COLLEGE: DEPARTMENT OF THEATRE ARTS

Buckner Theatre
111 Lake Hollingsworth Drive
Lakeland, FL 33801
Phone: 941-680-4226
Fax: 941-680-4457
Officers:
 Chairman: James F Beck
Budget: $600-5,000
Seating Capacity: 336; 75
Year Built: 1970

2705 KALEIDOSCOPE THEATRE

207 E 24th Street
Lynn Haven, FL 32444
Phone: 850-265-3226
Fax: 850-914-0846
Management:
 Board of Director: Lois Carter
 Board of Director: David Garcia
Mission: To increase knowledge of theatre and provide cultural enrichment.
Founded: 1972
Specialized Field: Musical; Dinner; Community
Status: Non-Professional; Nonprofit
Paid Staff: 300
Performs At: Kaleidoscope Theatre
Organization Type: Performing; Educational

2706 FLORIDA STAGE

262 S Ocean Boulevard
Manalapan, FL 33462
Phone: 561-585-3404
Fax: 561-588-4708
Toll-free: 800-514-3837
e-mail: info@floridastage.org
Web Site: www.floridastage.org
Officers:
 Chairman of the Board: Dennis Vlassis

Immediate Past Chairman: Laurie Gildan
Management:
 Producing Director: Louis Tyrrell
 Managing Director: Nancy Barnett
 Director Communications: Caroline Breder Watts
Mission: Dedicated to the production of new American plays by our finest contemporary playwrights.
Founded: 1987
Specialized Field: Theater
Status: Nonprofit
Paid Staff: 35
Budget: $2.5 Million
Season: October - August
Performs At: Florida Stage
Affiliations: AEA, SSDC, USA
Facility Category: Florida Stage
Type of Stage: Thrust
Seating Capacity: 258

2707 THEATRE CLUB OF THE PALM BEACHES

262 S Ocean Boulevard
Manalapan, FL 33462
Phone: 407-585-3404
Fax: 407-585-4708
Management:
 Producing Director: Louis Tyrrell
 Company Manager: Nancy Barnett
 Office Manager: Caroline Breder
 Marketing Director: Cheryl Dun
 Development Director: Alison Pruitt
Mission: To present the finest new works of young American playwrights.
Specialized Field: Theatrical Group
Status: Professional
Paid Artists: Yes
Income Sources: Actors' Equity Association; Society for Stage Directors and Choreographers
Organization Type: Performing

2708 MARATHON COMMUNITY THEATRE

PO Box 124
Marathon, FL 33050
Phone: 305-743-0994
Fax: 305-743-0408
Web Site: www.marathontheatre.org
Mission: To offer quality theatre events to adults in our community; to give cultural programs in schools.
Founded: 1957
Specialized Field: Musical; Dinner; Community; Theatrical Group; Puppet
Status: Nonprofit
Paid Staff: 60
Organization Type: Performing; Sponsoring

2709 MELBOURNE CIVIC THEATRE

3030 W New Haven Avenue
Melbourne, FL 32904
Phone: 321-723-1668
Fax: 321-723-6935
e-mail: yourmct@hotmail.com
Web Site: www.geocities.com/yourmct/index
Officers:
 President: June Borowski

Management:
  Business Manager: Anita Szczeciana
Mission: Entertaining, educating and enriching the community through the theatre arts.
Founded: 1952
Specialized Field: Community; Theatrical Group
Status: Non-Professional; Nonprofit
Volunteer Staff: 60
Non-paid Artists: 30
Budget: 120,000
Income Sources: Ticket Sales, Advertisments, Donations
Annual Attendance: 5,100
Facility Category: Theatre
Type of Stage: variable
Stage Dimensions: variable
Seating Capacity: 97
Rental Contact: Anita Saczeciana
Organization Type: Performing; Educational

2710 COCONUT GROVE PLAYHOUSE

3500 Main Highway
PO Box 616
Miami, FL 33133
Phone: 305-442-4000
Fax: 305-444-6437
Web Site: www.cgplayhouse.com
Officers:
  Chairperson: Vincent Post
  Vice Chairman: Judge Michael Chavies
  Secretary: Peggy Hollander
  Treasurer: Mitchell R. Less
Management:
  Producing Artistic Director: Arnold Mittelman
  Associate Producer: Earl Hughes
  Director Marketing: Debbie Eyerdan
  Director Finance/Operations: Bill Kerlin
Mission: Offering theater of quality to the community; expanding knowledge of theater.
Founded: 1956
Specialized Field: Theatrical Group
Status: Professional; Nonprofit
Budget: $5,000,000-$6,000,000
Income Sources: Theatre Communications Group
Performs At: Coconut Grove Playhouse
Affiliations: League of Resident Theatres, LORT B & D
Type of Stage: Proscenium/Black Box
Seating Capacity: 1000
Year Built: 1926
Organization Type: Performing; Touring; Educational

2711 FLORIDA INTERNATIONAL UNIVERSITY: DEPARTMENT OF THEATRE AND DANCE

Wertheim Performing Arts Center
Miami, FL 33199
Phone: 305-348-1684
Fax: 305-348-1803
Web Site: www.fiu.edu
Officers:
  Chairman: Dr. Leroy Clark
Budget: $7,100-11,900
Affiliations: NAST
Seating Capacity: 240; 150; 150
Year Built: 1996

2712 LAS MASCARAS THEATRE

2833 NW Seventh Street
Miami, FL 33125
Phone: 305-649-5301
Management:
  Artistic Director/Lead Actor: Alfonso Cremata
  Artistic Director/Lead Actor: Salvador Ugarte
Mission: To perform local and international plays in Spanish.
Founded: 1968
Specialized Field: Summer Stock; Musical; Theatrical Group
Status: Professional; Nonprofit
Performs At: Las Mascaras Theatre #1 & #2
Organization Type: Performing

2713 TEATRO AVANTE

742 SW 8th Street
Miami, FL 33130
Phone: 305-858-4155
Fax: 305-858-4155
Web Site: www.teatroavante.com
Management:
  Producing Artistic Director: Mario Ernesto Sanchez
  Resident Director/Designer: Rolando Moreno
  Technical Coordinator: Manelo Mina
Mission: To further Hispanic theatre.
Founded: 1979
Specialized Field: Summer Stock; Theatrical Group
Status: Professional; Nonprofit
Performs At: El Carruse Theatre
Organization Type: Performing; Touring; Educational

2714 GOLD COAST THEATRE

PO Box 402964
Miami Beach, FL 33140-0964
Phone: 305-538-5500
Fax: 305-538-6315
e-mail: judeparry@aol.com
Management:
  Director: Jude Parry
Mission: To bring professional theatre to people from all walks of life with multi-media, original shows featuring the art of mime
Founded: 1982
Specialized Field: Theatrical Group; Mime
Status: Professional
Paid Staff: 3
Volunteer Staff: 3
Paid Artists: 12
Budget: $100,000
Performs At: Touring Theatre Specializing in Mime
Annual Attendance: 100,000
Organization Type: Performing; Touring; Educational

2715 BERRY COLLEGE THEATRE PROGRAM

Berry College
Mount Berry, FL 30149
Phone: 706-232-5374
Management:
  Director: Dr. John Countryman
Affiliations: ATHE; SETC
Seating Capacity: 240; 115

Year Built: 1984

2716 ICEHOUSE THEATRE
PO Box 759
Mount Dora, FL 32756-0759
Phone: 352-383-3133
Fax: 352-383-7897
Management:
　Managing Director: Richard Traum
　Artistic Director: Terrence Shank
Mission: Enhance the cultural life of Central Florida with first-quality theatrical productions and programs designed to inspire and educate patrons and their children. The theatre is also dedicated to providing talented area artists with numerous opportunities to refine their craft.
Status: Nonprofit
Paid Staff: 5
Paid Artists: 2
Income Sources: Memberships; Corporate Sponsorships
Affiliations: CFTA; AACT
Facility Category: Performing Arts Theatre
Type of Stage: Thrust/Proscenium Combination
Seating Capacity: 274
Year Built: 1947
Year Remodeled: 1953

2717 ORANGE PARK COMMUNITY THEATRE
2900 Moody Avenue
PO Box 391
Orange Park, FL 32067-0391
Phone: 941-472-4109
Fax: 941-472-0055
e-mail: OPCTweb@yahoo.com
Web Site: www.OPCT.org
Officers:
　President: Betty Detamore
Mission: Provides five stage productions annually, including at least one Broadway style musical, to the residents and visitors to the Jacksonville area and Northeast Florida.
Founded: 1968
Specialized Field: Musical; Community
Status: Non-Professional; Nonprofit
Income Sources: Ticket Sales; Program Ads; Grants
Annual Attendance: 7,000
Facility Category: Community
Type of Stage: Proscenium
Stage Dimensions: 26x18
Seating Capacity: 101
Year Built: 1920
Year Remodeled: 1987
Organization Type: Performing; Educational

2718 MARK TWO DINNER THEATER
3376 Edgewater Drive
Orlando, FL 32804
Phone: 407-843-6275
Fax: 407-843-1510
Toll-free: 800-726-6275
e-mail: M2Orlando@AOL.com
Web Site: www.themarktwo.com
Management:
　Executive Producer/Director/Owner: Mark Howard

　General Manager: Scott A Reeder
　Marketing Director: Karen Good
Mission: Providing Orlando with full scale Broadway musicals and fine dining experience.
Founded: 1986
Specialized Field: Dinner Theater/Equity
Status: Professional
Paid Staff: 40
Paid Artists: 25
Income Sources: Actors' Equity Association; American Dinner Theatre Association
Performs At: Mark Two Dinner Theater
Organization Type: Performing

2719 THEATRE-IN-THE-WORKS
PO Box 532016
Orlando, FL 32853
Phone: 407-365-7235
Management:
　Producing Director: Edward Dilks
Mission: Developing original musicals, operas and plays primarily written by Floridians.
Founded: 1984
Specialized Field: Theatrical Group
Status: Professional; Nonprofit

2720 UCF CIVIC THEATRE
1001 E Princeton Street
Orlando, FL 32803
Phone: 407-896-7365
Fax: 407-897-3284
Management:
　Acting Executive Director: Kathryn Seidel
　Youth Program Coordinator: Jeff Revels
Mission: Providing entertainment, information, stimulation, education and an arena for artistic expression.
Founded: 1926
Specialized Field: Theatrical Group; Youth Theatre
Status: Professional; Non-Professional; Nonprofit
Paid Staff: 2
Income Sources: American Association of Community Theatres; Florida Theatre Conference; United Arts
Performs At: Civic Theatre Complex
Organization Type: Performing; Touring; Educational

2721 UNIVERSITY OF CENTRAL FLORIDA: DEPARTMENT OF THEATRE
Orlando, FL
Mailing Address: PO Box 162372, Orlando, FL 32816
Phone: 407-823-2861
Fax: 407-823-6446
Web Site: http://pegasus.cc.ucf.edu/~theatre
Officers:
　Chair: Dr. Donald W Seay
Budget: $7,000-15,000
Affiliations: ATHE
Seating Capacity: 300; 100
Year Built: 1982

2722 PENSACOLA LITTLE THEATRE
PO Box 415
Pensacola, FL 32592

Phone: 850-432-2042
Fax: 850-432-2787
Web Site: www.pensacolalittletheatre.com
Management:
   General Manager: Herman Fischer
Mission: To stimulate interest in performing arts; to provide community members a chance to participate in live theatre.
Founded: 1936
Specialized Field: Community; Children's Theatre
Status: Non-Professional; Nonprofit
Paid Staff: 100
Income Sources: Florida Theatre Conference; American Association of Community Theatres; Southeastern Theatre Conference
Performs At: Pensacola Little Theatre
Organization Type: Performing; Educational; Sponsoring

2723 UNIVERSITY OF WEST FLORIDA

Center for Fine and Performing Arts
11000 University Parkway
Pensacola, FL 32514
Phone: 850-474-2547
Fax: 850-474-3247
Web Site: www.uwf.edu
Management:
   Director: Jim Jipson
Budget: $13,000-33,000
Seating Capacity: 426; 120
Year Built: 1991

2724 PLANTATION THEATRE COMPANY

1829 N Pineland Road
Plantation, FL 33317
Phone: 954-424-9701
Fax: 954-424-0137
Mission: To afford community members an opportunity to participate in the arts.
Founded: 1975
Specialized Field: Musical; Community
Status: Semi-Professional; Non-Professional; Nonprofit
Performs At: Diecke Auditorium
Organization Type: Performing; Educational

2725 POMPANO PLAYERS

PO Box 2045
Pompano Beach, FL 33061
Phone: 305-946-4646
Management:
   Box Office: Penny Manwell
   Technical: David Stockton
   Technical: Jerry Sullivan
Mission: To offer live theatre.
Founded: 1956
Specialized Field: Musical; Community; Theatrical Group
Status: Semi-Professional; Nonprofit
Income Sources: Florida Theatre Conference
Performs At: Pompano Players Theatre
Organization Type: Performing; Resident; Educational

2726 CHARLOTTE PLAYERS

PO Box 2187
Port Charlotte, FL 33949
Phone: 941-255-1022
Mission: To offer a burgeoning retirement community live, community theater; to nurture a love of theatre in young people.
Founded: 1960
Specialized Field: Community; Theatrical Group
Status: Non-Professional; Nonprofit
Performs At: Cultural Center Theater
Organization Type: Performing

2727 AMERICAN STAGE COMPANY

211 3rd Street S
PO Box 1560
Saint Petersburg, FL 33731
Phone: 727-823-1600
Fax: 727-821-2444
Web Site: www.americanstage.org
Management:
   Managing Director: Lee Manwaring Lowry
Mission: To prosper physically, mentally and spiritually as a cultural establishment which represents and influences the life of its communitiy through the art of live professional theatre.
Founded: 1977
Specialized Field: Theatrical Group
Status: Professional; Nonprofit
Paid Staff: 13
Volunteer Staff: 300
Paid Artists: 60
Budget: $1.2 million
Income Sources: Actors' Equity Association; Theatre Communications Group; Florida Professional Theatre Association; Pinellas County Arts Council
Season: June - August
Performs At: American Stage Company Theatre;
Affiliations: Actor's Equity USA
Annual Attendance: 60,000
Type of Stage: Modified Trust
Seating Capacity: 140
Year Built: 1927
Organization Type: Performing; Touring; Resident; Educational

2728 VAUDEVILLE PALACE

7951 9th Street N
Saint Petersburg, FL 33702
Phone: 813-557-5515
Fax: 813-578-1024
Management:
   Producer/Director: Buddy Graf
   General Manager: Carol Graf
   Box Office Manager: Skip Lewis
Mission: To offer amusing entertainment.
Founded: 1991
Specialized Field: Dinner; Vaudeville
Status: Professional; Commercial
Performs At: Vaudeville Palace
Organization Type: Performing; Resident

2729 PIRATE PLAYHOUSE
2200k Periwinkle Way
PO Box 1459
Sanibel, FL 33957
Phone: 641-472-4109
Fax: 941-472-0055
Management:
    Producing Artistic Director: Ralph Elias
    General Manager: Kevin Mooney

2730 J HOWARD WOOD THEATRE
2200 Periwinkle Way
Sanibel Island, FL 33957
Phone: 941-472-0006
Fax: 941-472-0055
Web Site: www.thewoodtheatre.com
Officers:
    President: Winnie Donoghue
    Treasurer: Jim Lavelle
    Secretary: Carla Benninga
Management:
    Managing Director: Cindy Lee Overton
    Artistic Producer: Robert Schelhammer
    Marketing/Public Relations: Honey Larsen
Mission: To present live, professional theatre in
Southwest Florida.
Founded: 1991
Specialized Field: Professional Classis and Modern
Theatre, Musicals, New Plays Play Reading/ Playwrights
Festival, Children's Program
Status: Not-for-Profit
Paid Staff: 10
Budget: 750k
Income Sources: Grants, Donations, Ticket Sales
Performs At: Theatre
Facility Category: Theater
Type of Stage: Thrust Stage
Seating Capacity: 180
Year Built: 1990
Organization Type: Performing; Touring; Resident;
Educational; Sponsoring

**2731 ASOLO THEATRE COMPANY: FLORIDA
STATE UNIVERSITY**
FSU Center for the Performing Arts
5555 North Tamiami Trail
Sarasota, FL 34243
Phone: 941-351-9010
Fax: 941-351-5796
e-mail: bruce_rodgers@asolo.org
Web Site: www.asolo.org
Management:
    Director: Brant Pope
Founded: 1960
Performs At: Mertz Theatre, Cook Theatre
Affiliations: U/RTA; ATHE
Type of Stage: Proscenium
Seating Capacity: 499, 161

2732 ASOLO THEATRE FESTIVAL
5555 N Tamiami Trail
Sarasota, FL 34243

Phone: 941-351-9010
Fax: 941-351-5796
Toll-free: 800-361-8388
e-mail: asolo@asolo.org
Web Site: www.asolo.org
Officers:
    President: Ron Greenbaum
Management:
    Producing Artistic Director: Howard J Millman
    Managing Director: Linda M DiGabriele
Mission: To produce and present the highest quality
professional theatre in a fiscally responsible manner for its
community. The Asolo performs primarily in rotating
repertory with a resident company.
Founded: 1960
Specialized Field: Theatrical Group
Status: Professional; Nonprofit
Volunteer Staff: 300
Non-paid Artists: 60
Budget: $5 million
Income Sources: Theatre Communications Group;
American Arts Alliance; Actors' Equity Association;
League of Resident Theatres
Performs At: Harold E and Esther M Mertz Theatre; Jane
B Cook Theatre
Affiliations: Florida State University
Annual Attendance: 92,000
Organization Type: Performing; Educational

2733 FLORIDA STUDIO THEATRE
1241 N Palm Avenue
Sarasota, FL 34236
Phone: 941-366-9017
Fax: 941-955-4137
Web Site: www.fst2000.org
Management:
    Artistic Director: Richard Hopkins
    General Manager: Rebecca Langford
    Casting/Literary Coordinator: James Ashford
Mission: To produce contemporary theatre with an
emphasis on new plays and regional premieres.
Founded: 1973
Specialized Field: Theatrical Group
Status: Professional; Nonprofit
Performs At: Florida Studio Theatre
Affiliations: Small Professional Theatre Assoication;
Actors' Equity Association
Type of Stage: ThrustBox, Cabaret Space
Stage Dimensions: 30'x35'x25'
Seating Capacity: 173, 100
Rental Contact: John Jacobsen
Organization Type: Performing; Resident; Educational;
Touring

2734 GOLDEN APPLE DINNER THEATRE
25 N Pineapple Avenue
Sarasota, FL 34236
Phone: 941-366-5454
Fax: 941-364-9100
Management:
    Producer/Director/General Manager: Robert Turoff
Mission: To entertain, educate and enlighten.
Founded: 1971
Specialized Field: Musical; Dinner
Status: Professional; Commercial

Income Sources: Actors' Equity Association
Performs At: Golden Apple Dinner Theatre
Organization Type: Sponsoring

2735 PLAYERS OF SARASOTA
838 N Tamiami Trail
Sarasota, FL 34236
Phone: 941-365-2494
Fax: 941-954-0282
e-mail: info@theplayers.org
Web Site: www.theplayers.org
Officers:
  President: Maryann Shorin
  Vice President: Barry Miller
  Teasurer: Ray Suplee
  Secretary: Charlene Knopp
Management:
  Executive Director: Elizabeth J DeVivo
  Artistic Director: Peter Strader
Mission: To be the first and only community theatre in Sarasota offering live entertainment, full orchestra, professional direction and children's theatre.
Founded: 1930
Specialized Field: Musical; Community; Theatrical Group; Puppet
Status: Non-Professional; Nonprofit
Paid Staff: 215
Organization Type: Performing; Touring; Educational

2736 LIMELIGHT THEATRE
11 Old Mission Avenue
PO Box 1196
St. Augustine, FL 32085-1196
Phone: 904-825-1164
Fax: 904-825-4662
e-mail: limeligt@bellsouth.net
Web Site: www.limelight-theatre.com
Officers:
  President: Paul McGuire
  VP: Wayne George
  Treasurer: Wayne Farrell
Management:
  Co-Producer/Artistic Director: Jean Rahner
  Co-Producer/Administration: Anne Kraft
  Stage Manager: Linda Shamlian
  General Manager: Emma Lee Carpenter
Mission: To provide professional entertainment to visitors to the Saint Augustine area.
Founded: 1992
Specialized Field: Theatrical Group
Status: Professional; Nonprofit
Paid Staff: 4
Volunteer Staff: 80
Paid Artists: 55
Non-paid Artists: 10
Budget: 250,000
Income Sources: Admissions; Subsciptions; Individual and Corporate Donations and Grants
Performs At: Monson Resort
Affiliations: Flager College
Facility Category: main stage + black box
Type of Stage: Proscenium
Stage Dimensions: 36' x 20'
Seating Capacity: 99
Year Built: 1927

Year Remodeled: 2001
Rental Contact: General Manager Emma Lee Carpenter
Organization Type: Performing

2737 ECKERD COLLEGE THEATRE DEPARTMENT
4200 54th Avenue South
St. Petersburg, FL 33711
Phone: 813-864-8279
Fax: 813-864-7800
Web Site: www.eckerd.edu/academics/cra/theatre
Officers:
  Chair: Cynthia Totten
Budget: $2,000-4,000
Affiliations: ATHE; SETC
Seating Capacity: 350; 60-80
Year Built: 1970

2738 MAHAFFEY THEATER
400 First Street S
St. Petersburg, FL 33701
Phone: 727-892-5708
Fax: 727-892-5858
Toll-free: 800-874-9015
e-mail: laura.kleinfeld@stpete.org
Web Site: www.stpete.org/venues.htm
Management:
  Marketing/Booking Manager: Lauren Kleinfeld
Performs At: Mahaffey Theatre for the Performing Arts

2739 KINGS POINT THEATRE AT THE CLUBHOUSE
1900 Clubhouse Drive
Sun City Center, FL 33573
Phone: 813-634-9229
Fax: 813-633-3759
Management:
  Entertainment Director: Marvin Donner

2740 FLORIDA STATE UNIVERSITY: SCHOOL OF THEATRE
239 FAB
Florida State University
Tallahassee, FL 32306
Phone: 850-644-6795
Fax: 850-644-7408
Web Site: www.fsu.edu/~Theatre
Budget: $13,750-37,500
Affiliations: NAST; Asolo State Theatre
Seating Capacity: 500; 191; 200
Year Built: 1969

2741 YOUNG ACTORS THEATRE
609 Glenview Drive
Tallahassee, FL 32303
Phone: 850-386-6602
Fax: 850-422-2084
e-mail: yat@nettally.com
Web Site: www.nettally.com/YAT
Officers:
  President: Kevin W Smith
  Treasurer: Susie Andrews

All listings are in alphabetical order by state, then city, then organization within the city.

Management:
   Director: Cristina Williams
   Music Director: Alison Grimes
   Managing Director: Valerie Smith
Mission: The education of youth in performance and theatre arts.
Founded: 1975
Specialized Field: Musical; Community; Theatrical Group
Status: Semi-Professional; Nonprofit
Paid Staff: 25
Volunteer Staff: 300
Paid Artists: 15
Non-paid Artists: 250
Budget: $550,000
Income Sources: Southeastern Theatre Conference; American Association of Theatre Educators, State of Florida, City of Tallahassee
Performs At: Young Actors Theatre
Affiliations: American Association of Theatre Educators, Southeastern Theatre Conference
Annual Attendance: 10,000
Facility Category: Theatre, classrooms
Type of Stage: Proscenium
Seating Capacity: 215
Year Built: 1986
Year Remodeled: 1995
Cost: $150,000
Organization Type: Performing; Touring; Educational

2742 BITS 'N PIECES GIANT PUPPET THEATRE

PO Box 368
Tampa, FL 33601
Phone: 813-659-0659
Management:
   Executive Director: Jerry Bickel
   Artistic Director: Holli Rubin
   Business Director: Jackie Hiendlmayr
Mission: To offer original, educational musicals featuring unique nine-foot puppets.
Founded: 1976
Specialized Field: Puppet
Status: Professional; Nonprofit
Paid Staff: 6
Organization Type: Performing; Touring; Resident; Educational

2743 CARROLLWOOD PLAYERS COMMUNITY THEATER

4333 Gunn Highway
Tampa, FL 33624
Phone: 813-265-4000
e-mail: heleneb@aol.com
Web Site: www.members.aol.com/HeleneB
Officers:
   President: Nancy Stearns
Founded: 1981
Status: Not-for-profit

2744 CENTER THEATER COMPANY OF TAMPA BAY

1010 N W.C. MacInnes Place
Tampa, FL 33602
Phone: 813-222-1000
Fax: 813-222-1057
e-mail: rick.criswell@tbpac.org
Web Site: www.tbpac.org
Management:
   Production Stage Manager: Rick Criswell
Founded: 1995
Status: Nonprofit
Type of Stage: Thrust
Stage Dimensions: 40' x 24'
Seating Capacity: 300
Rental Contact: Bobbi Warnick

2745 FLORIDA SUNCOAST PUPPET GUILD

7107 N Howard Avenue
Tampa, FL 33604
Phone: 813-932-9252
Fax: 813-932-9252
e-mail: jodymcat@aol.com
Web Site: www.puppeteers.org/guilds/fla-sunc.htm
Officers:
   Gdild President: Jody Wren
Management:
   Festival Director: Jody Wren
Mission: Promoting puppetry through shows, lectures, workshops, demonstrations, festivals and meetings.
Founded: 1973
Specialized Field: Puppet
Status: Nonprofit
Income Sources: Puppeteers of America
Organization Type: Educational; Sponsoring

2746 SPANISH LYRIC THEATRE

2819 Safe Harbor Drive
Tampa, FL 33618
Phone: 813-936-0217
Fax: 813-936-0217
Management:
   Founder and Artistic Director: Rene J Gonzalez
Mission: To promote Spanish musicals, or Zarzuelas; to offer lyric theatre in Spanish and English.
Founded: 1959
Specialized Field: Musical; Theatrical Group
Status: Semi-Professional; Nonprofit
Paid Staff: 20
Performs At: Tampa Bay Performing Arts Center
Organization Type: Performing

2747 UNIVERSITY OF SOUTH FLORIDA: DEPARTMENT OF THEATRE

4202 East Fowler
Tampa, FL 33620
Phone: 813-974-2701
Fax: 813-974-4122
Web Site: www.arts.usf.edu/theater
Officers:
   Chair: Dr. Denis Calandra
Budget: $2,000-25,100
Affiliations: NAST; ATHE

Seating Capacity: 552; 100-200; 80-125
Year Built: 1986
Year Remodeled: 95

2748 VENICE LITTLE THEATRE
140 W Tampa Avenue
Venice, FL 34285
Phone: 941-488-1115
Fax: 941-444-9437
Web Site: www.venicestage.com
Management:
    Managing Director: Lee Linkous
Mission: To present intellectual and instructive entertainment in the performing arts.
Founded: 1950
Specialized Field: Community
Status: Non-Professional; Nonprofit
Organization Type: Performing

2749 ACTING COMPANY OF RIVERSIDE THEATRE
3250 Riverside Park Drive
Vero Beach, FL 32963
Phone: 561-231-5860
Fax: 561-234-5298
Officers:
    President: Marilyn Chenault
    VP: Pat Trimble
    Treasurer: Rebecca Allen
    Board Secretary: Judy Balph
Management:
    Artistic Director: Allen D Cornell
    Production Manager: John Moses
    Business Manager: Ida Spada
    Development Director: Lynn Potter
    Director Education: Linda Downey
Mission: To provide audiences of this region with productions that are relevant either by nature of their importance within a particular genre or as socially vital within the changing environment of our culture.
Founded: 1995
Specialized Field: Theatrical Group
Status: Professional; Nonprofit
Paid Staff: 10
Income Sources: Actors' Equity Association; Theatre Communications Group; Florida Performing Theatre Association
Performs At: Riverside Theatre
Organization Type: Performing

2750 VERO BEACH THEATRE GUILD
2020 San Juan Avenue
Vero Beach, FL 32960
Phone: 561-562-8300
Fax: 561-562-8304
e-mail: info@berobeachtheatreguild.com
Web Site: www.vero-beach.fl.us/vbtg
Officers:
    President: Norma Damp
    VP: Dan Sullivan
    CPA/Treasurer: Dominic J Lettiere
    Secretary: Barbara Barthelman

Mission: To enhance appreciation of dramatic and musical pieces through community theater; to offer residents of Florida's Treasure Coast theatrical arts.
Founded: 1958
Specialized Field: Community
Status: Non-Professional; Nonprofit
Paid Staff: 200
Performs At: Riverside Theatre
Organization Type: Performing; Educational

2751 PALM BEACH ATLANTIC COLLEGE: DEPARTMENT OF THEATRE
West Palm Beach, FL
Mailing Address: PO Box 24708, West Palm Beach, FL 33416
Phone: 561-803-2417
Fax: 561-803-2424
Web Site: http://www.pbac.edu
Officers:
    Chair: Dr. Deborah McEniry
Budget: $8,000-10,500
Affiliations: Florida Stage
Facility Category: Historical building
Seating Capacity: 220; 80

2752 THEATRE WINTER HAVEN
210 Cypress Gardens Boulevard
PO Drawer 1230
Winter Haven, FL 33882
Phone: 863-299-2672
Fax: 863-291-3299
e-mail: twh1970@aol.com
Web Site: www.theatrewinterhaven.com
Management:
    Producing Director: Norman M Small
    General Manager: Thom Altman
    Technical Director: Jeff Dillon
    Education Director: Molly Judy
    Office Manager: Lola Watson
Mission: Fostering the community's cultural growth by offering quality live theatre.
Founded: 1970
Specialized Field: Community; Theatrical Group
Status: Non-Professional; Nonprofit
Paid Staff: 8
Volunteer Staff: 160
Paid Artists: 11
Budget: $500,000
Income Sources: Various
Affiliations: AACT, FTC
Type of Stage: Proscenium
Stage Dimensions: 30wx16hx28d
Seating Capacity: 332
Year Built: 1977
Rental Contact: Jane Waters
Organization Type: Performing; Educational

2753 ANNIE RUSSELL THEATRE
Rollins College
1000 Holt Avenue-2735
Winter Park, FL 32789
Phone: 407-646-2145
Fax: 407-646-2600
Officers:

VP/Treasurer: George Herbst
Management:
   Producing Director: S Joseph Nassif, PhD
Mission: Providing educational theatre; booking touring events for dance and theatre.
Founded: 1931
Specialized Field: Musical; Theatrical Group; Academic Theatre Program
Status: Semi-Professional; Non-Professional; Nonprofit; Commercial
Paid Staff: 9
Volunteer Staff: 12
Paid Artists: 3
Income Sources: Association of Performing Arts Presenters; Southeastern Theatre Conference; Florida Theatre Conference
Performs At: Annie Russell Theatre
Organization Type: Performing; Resident; Educational; Sponsoring

2754 ROLLINS COLLEGE: DEPARTMENT OF THEATRE AND DANCE

1000 Holt Avenue 2735
Winter Park, FL 32789
Phone: 407-646-2501
Fax: 407-646-2257
Web Site: www.rollins.edu/theater/index.htm
Officers:
   Chair: S Joseph Nassif
Budget: $13,500-24,000
Seating Capacity: 400; 100
Year Built: 1931
Year Remodeled: 1978

Georgia

2755 THEATRE ALBANY

514 Pine Avenue
Albany, GA 31701
Phone: 229-439-7193
Management:
   Artistic Director: Mark Costello
   Technical Director: Walter Thompson
Mission: Fostering live theatre in our community.
Founded: 1932
Specialized Field: Musical; Community; Theatrical Group
Status: Non-Professional; Nonprofit
Paid Staff: 60
Income Sources: American Association of Community Theatres; Southeastern Theatre Conference; Georgia Theatre Conference
Performs At: Theatre Albany
Organization Type: Performing; Educational

2756 GABBIES PUPPETS

367 Lexington Heights
Athens, GA 30605
Phone: 706-353-2785
Management:
   Director: Carolyn S Gabb

Mission: Presenting and teaching language communication skills using puppets; storytelling; creative dramatics.
Founded: 1975
Specialized Field: Puppet
Status: Professional
Organization Type: Performing; Educational

2757 GEORGIA REPERTORY THEATRE

Dept. of Drama, Fine Arts Building
University of Georgia
Athens, GA 30602-3154
Phone: 706-542-2836
Fax: 706-542-2080
e-mail: longman@arches.uga.edu
Management:
   Producer: Stanley V Longman
   Dramaturg: Allen Partridge
Mission: The production of previously unproduced plays.
Founded: 1990
Specialized Field: Theater
Paid Staff: 6
Paid Artists: 5
Performs At: Fine Arts Theatre, Cellar Theatre, Seneyu Stovall Theatre
Type of Stage: Arena
Seating Capacity: 250
Year Built: 1941

2758 7 STAGES

1105 Euclid Avenue NE
Atlanta, GA 30307
Phone: 404-522-0911
Fax: 404-522-0913
Web Site: www.7stages.org
Management:
   Artistic Director: Del Hamilton
   Producing Director: Faye Allen
   Managing Director: Tori Howell
Founded: 1979
Paid Staff: 7

2759 ACADEMY THEATRE

501 Means Street NW
Atlanta, GA 30318
Phone: 404-525-4111
Fax: 404-525-5659
e-mail: academytheatre@mindspring.com
Web Site: http://academytheatre.home.mindspring.com
Officers:
   Chairman: Jerry Dibble
   President: Frank Wittow
Management:
   Founder/Producing Artistic Director: Frank Wittow
   Managing Director: Lorenne Fey
   Development Director: Nick Rhoton
Mission: Creating and perforing orginal plays about critical issues for children and young adults, training teachers in the use of innovative techniques to accelerate learning and retention of knowledge, introducing children to theatre as a measn of self-discovery and self-expression.
Founded: 1956
Status: Professional; Nonprofit

Paid Staff: 2
Volunteer Staff: 19
Paid Artists: 10
Budget: $370,000
Income Sources: NEA; Georgia Council for the Arts; Fulton County Arts Council; City of Atlanta and Foundations; Individuals
Affiliations: Theatre Communications Group; Atlanta Coalition of Performing Arts; Georgia Shares
Annual Attendance: 70,000
Organization Type: Performing; Touring; Resident; Educational; Sponsoring

2760 ACTOR'S EXPRESS
887 W Marietta Street
Suite J-107
Atlanta, GA 30318
Phone: 404-875-1606
Fax: 404-875-2791
e-mail: actorsexpress@mindspring.com
Web Site: www.actorsexpress.com
Management:
Artistic Director: Wier Harman
Managing Director: Kim Julian
Marketing Director: Yvette Zarod
Artistc Associate: Davis Crowe
Mission: We produce a wildly eclectic mix of classic, contemporary, and cutting edge plays.
Founded: 1988
Facility Category: Flexible Black Box
Seating Capacity: 120-160

2761 ALLIANCE THEATRE COMPANY
1280 Peachtree Street NE
Atlanta, GA 30309
Phone: 404-733-4650
Fax: 404-733-4625
Web Site: www.alliancetheatre.org
Officers:
Chairperson: Debbie Shelton
First Vice Chair: Rick Western
Treasurer: Candace Bell
Management:
Managing Director: Gus Stuhlreyer
Artistic Director: Susan V Booth
General Manager: Max Leventhal
Mission: Dedicated to celebrating diversity by building bridges that can connect us as human beings through the development and production of exciting, entertaining, and stimulating plays to nurture and enrich the art, the artists, and the audience
Founded: 1969
Specialized Field: Theatrical Group
Status: Professional; Nonprofit
Paid Staff: 225
Paid Artists: 245
Budget: $10 Million
Performs At: Alliance Theatre
Affiliations: Actors' Equity Association; Society for Stage Directors and Choreographers; League of Resident Theatres; USA
Annual Attendance: 225,000
Type of Stage: Proscenium; Flexible
Stage Dimensions: 40x96; 44x75
Seating Capacity: 800; 200

Year Built: 1968
Year Remodeled: 1996
Organization Type: Performing; Touring; Resident; Educational

2762 ATLANTA STREET THEATRE
1660 Moores Mill Road
Atlanta, GA 30327
Phone: 404-355-0020
Management:
Executive Artistic Director: Michele McNichols
Mission: Providing underprivileged youth relevant theatre; maintaining an interracial group; using theatre educationally.
Founded: 1976
Status: Professional; Nonprofit
Organization Type: Performing; Touring; Educational

2763 CENTER FOR PUPPETRY ARTS
1404 Spring Street @ 18th Street
Atlanta, GA 30309
Phone: 404-873-3089
Fax: 404-873-9907
e-mail: puppet@mindspring.com
Web Site: www.puppet.org
Management:
Executive Director: Vincent Anthony
Mission: To expand public awareness of puppetry.
Founded: 1978
Specialized Field: Puppet
Status: Professional; Nonprofit
Paid Staff: 59
Volunteer Staff: 30
Performs At: Mainstage Theater; Downstairs Theater
Annual Attendance: 900,000
Type of Stage: Mainstage
Seating Capacity: 345/Downstairs 170
Year Built: 1918
Year Remodeled: 96
Organization Type: Performing; Touring; Resident; Educational; Sponsoring

2764 DAD'S GARAGE THEATRE COMPANY
280 Elizabeth Street
Suite C-101
Atlanta, GA 30307
Phone: 404-523-3141
Fax: 404-688-6644
Management:
Artistic Director: Sean Daniels
Managing Director: Kathryn Colegrove
Improvisation Director: Chris Blair

2765 ESSENTIAL THEATRE
995 Greenwood Avenue
#6
Atlanta, GA 30306
Phone: 404-876-8471
Management:
Producing Artistic Director: Peter Hardy
Founded: 1987
Specialized Field: Theatre

2766 GATEWAY PERFORMANCE PRODUCTIONS
PO Box 8062
Atlanta, GA 31106
Phone: 404-982-9922
e-mail: info@masktheatre.org
Web Site: www.masktheatre.org
Officers:
 President: Sandra Hughes
 Chairperson: Chris Moser
 Treasurer: Michael Hickey
Management:
 Artistic Director: Sandra Hughes
 Company Coordinator: Michael E Hickey
Mission: To create and produce high-quality outreach arts programming for touring theatres, festivals, museums, libraries, colleges, universities, schools, and other community sites. Gateway carries out this mission through touring the following programs and productions- Mask Theatre, Mime, Cultural Arts Programs, Workshops, Classes, Residencies, Demonstrations, and Exhibits.
Founded: 1974
Specialized Field: Theatrical Group; MIME
Status: Professional; Nonprofit
Organization Type: Performing; Touring; Resident; Educational

2767 GEORGIA SHAKESPEARE FESTIVAL
Conant Performing Arts Center
4484 Peachtree Road Northeast
Atlanta, GA 30319
Phone: 404-264-0020
Fax: 404-504-3414
e-mail: boxoffice@gashakespeare.org
Web Site: www.gashakespeare.org/
Management:
 Artistic/Producing Director: Richard Garner
 Managing Director: Philip J Santora
 Education Director: Kathleen McManus
 Marketing Director: Stacey Colosa Lucas
 Production Manager: Rob Dillard
 Development Officer: Sarah Robinson
 Events/Volunteer Coordinator: Carla Hyman
 Company Manager: Christy Costello
 Box Office Manager: Thomas Pinckney
Mission: To produce professional plays written by Shakespeare and other enduring authors.
Founded: 1985
Specialized Field: Theater; Festivals
Status: Professional; Nonprofit
Paid Staff: 7
Income Sources: Southeastern Theatre Conference; Atlanta Theatre Coalition
Organization Type: Performing; Resident

2768 HORIZON THEATRE COMPANY
1083 Austin Avenue
Corner of Euclid & Austin Avenues
Atlanta, GA 31107

Mailing Address: PO Box 5376 Atlanta, GA 31107
Phone: 404-523-1477
Fax: 404-584-8815
e-mail: horizonco@mindspring.com
Web Site: www.horizontheatre.com
Management:
 Co-Artistic/Producing Director: Lisa Adler
 Co-Artistic/Technical Director: Jeff Adler
 Public Relations/Marketing Director: Michael VanOsch
 Box Office Manager: Suehyla El-Attar
 Managing Director: Alison Hayes
 House Manager: Denny Zartman
Mission: To be a leader in the production and development of contemporary theatre in the Southeast. We present professional area premieres of new and recent plays and develop new artists and audiences for contemporary theatre through education and outreach programs.
Founded: 1983
Specialized Field: Contemporary
Status: Professional; Nonprofit
Income Sources: Grants
Performs At: Horizon Theatre
Type of Stage: Flexible
Seating Capacity: 170

2769 JOMANDI PRODUCTIONS
675 Ponce De Leon Avenue
City Hall East, 8th Floor
Atlanta, GA 30308
Phone: 404-876-6346
Fax: 404-872-5764
e-mail: jomandi@bellsouth.net
Web Site: www.jomandi.com
Officers:
 Chairman/State Representative: Bob Holmes
Management:
 General Manager: Greg Stevens
 Artistic Director: Andrea Fry
 Public Relations/Marketing Director: Arnie Epps
 Production Manager: Lisa L Watson
Mission: Nurturing new works that reflect the African-American experience; providing theatre artists an opportunity for training and performance.
Founded: 1978
Specialized Field: Theatrical Group
Status: Professional; Nonprofit
Paid Staff: 10
Performs At: 14th Street Playhouse
Type of Stage: Proscenium/Thrust
Seating Capacity: 370
Organization Type: Performing; Touring; Resident

2770 JUST US THEATER COMPANY
PO Box 42271
Atlanta, GA 30311
Phone: 404-753-2399
Fax: 404-758-9200
Officers:
 President: Walter R Huntley
 Treasurer: Pearle Cleage
 Secretary: Zaron W Burnett, Jr
Management:
 Artistic Director: Pearl Cleage

Producing Director: Zaron Burnett, Jr.
Mission: Just Us Theater Company is a Black professional company dedicated to the development of minority artists and the presentation of quality arts programs that reflect the diversity of our community; focus on sexism and racism.
Founded: 1976
Specialized Field: Theatrical Group
Status: Professional
Organization Type: Performing; Touring; Resident; Educational

2771 NEW AMERICAN SHAKESPEARE TAVERN

499 Peachtree Street NE
Atlanta, GA 30308
Phone: 404-874-5299
e-mail: becky@shakespearetavern.com
Web Site: www.shakespearetavern.com
Mission: The New American Shakespeare Tavern is unlike other theaters. It is a place out of time; a place of live music, hand-crafted period costumes, outrageous sword fights with the entire experience centered on the passion and poetry of the spo

2772 OMILAMI PRODUCTIONS/PEOPLE'S SURVIVAL THEATRE

8 E Lake Drive NE
Atlanta, GA 30317
Phone: 404-377-6434
Fax: 404-584-9166
Management:
   Co-Artistic Director: Elizabeth Omilami
   Co-Artistic Director: Afemo Omilami
Mission: To produce, provide and encourage arts programming for impoverished areas that are not serviced by traditional groups; to stimulate and encourage new playwrights and directors to write and direct for the inner city and rural areas.
Founded: 1977
Specialized Field: Community; Theatrical Group
Status: Semi-Professional; Nonprofit
Paid Staff: 8
Organization Type: Performing; Touring; Educational

2773 SEVEN STAGES

1105 Euclid Avenue
Atlanta, GA 30307
Phone: 404-522-0911
Fax: 404-522-0913
e-mail: boxoffice@7stages.org
Web Site: www.7stages.org
Officers:
   Board Chair: Ranjan Dattagupta
   Board Secretary: Tobie Kranitz
   Board Treasurer: Chris Ames
Management:
   Artistic Director: Del Hamilton
   Producing Director: Faye Allen
   Managing Director: Raye Varney
   Marketing Director: Joe Gfaller
Mission: Producing new works and international collaborations as well as contemporary theatre and reinterpretations of classics.

Founded: 1978
Specialized Field: Musical; Community; Theatrical Group
Status: Professional; Nonprofit
Paid Staff: 7
Volunteer Staff: 2
Paid Artists: 65
Budget: $850,000
Income Sources: Theatre Communications Group; National Endowment for the Arts; Georgia Council of the Arts; City of Atlanta Bureau of Cultural Affairs; Trust for Mutual Understanding; AT&T
Affiliations: Theatre Communications Group; Atlanta Coalition for the Performing Arts
Annual Attendance: 15,000
Facility Category: 2 Performing Arts Theatres
Type of Stage: Black Boxes
Seating Capacity: 90; 200
Year Built: 1928
Year Remodeled: 1994
Cost: $1.6 million
Organization Type: Performing; Resident
Resident Groups: Seven Stages

2774 SIX FLAGS OVER GEORGIA

PO Box 43187
Atlanta, GA 30336
Phone: 770-739-3400
Fax: 770-739-3457
Management:
   Production Coordinator: Daniel Barr
Founded: 1967
Status: Non-Equity; Commercial
Season: March - November
Type of Stage: Semi-Thrust
Stage Dimensions: 45' x 30'
Seating Capacity: 750

2775 SOUTHEASTERN SAVOYARDS

3270 Ivanhoe Drive
Atlanta, GA 30327
Phone: 404-233-7002
Officers:
   President: Jonn H Stevens
   VP: Robert B Langdon
   Treasurer: Fern M Stevens
   Secretary: Marcia Lane
Management:
   Executive Producer: John H Stevens
   Music Director/Artistic: J Lynn Thompson
Mission: Gilbert & Sullivan repertory company.
Founded: 1980
Specialized Field: Musical Theatre
Status: Professional; Nonprofit
Performs At: Center Stage Theater Atlanta
Organization Type: Theatrical Group

2776 THEATER EMORY

Rich Building, Room 230
Emory University
Atlanta, GA 30322

Phone: 404-727-0524
Fax: 404-727-6253
e-mail: vmurphy@emory.edu
Web Site: www.emory.edu/arts/
Management:
   Artistic Producing Director: Vincent Murphy
   Managing Director: Pat Miller
Founded: 1985
Performs At: Mary Gray Munroe Theater at Emory University

2777 THEATER OF THE STARS

PO Box 11748
Atlanta, GA 30355
Phone: 404-252-8960
Fax: 404-252-1460
e-mail: theaterstars@mindspring.com
Web Site: www.theaterofthestars.com
Management:
   Producer: Christopher B Manos
   Managing Director: Nicholas F Manos
Founded: 1953
Specialized Field: Musicals
Status: Professional; Nonprofit
Paid Staff: 7
Organization Type: Performing; Touring; Sponsoring

2778 THEATRE GAEL

PO Box 77156
Atlanta, GA 30357
Phone: 404-876-1138
Fax: 404-876-1141
e-mail: theatregael@mindspring.com
Web Site: www.theatregael.com
Management:
   Managing Director: Beth Jansa
   Artistic Director: John Stephens
Mission: The performance of plays from Scotland, Ireland and Wales.
Founded: 1982
Specialized Field: Theatrical Group; Children's Theatre
Status: Professional; Nonprofit
Paid Staff: 3
Volunteer Staff: 10
Paid Artists: 25
Income Sources: American Alliance for Theatre Arts; Alternate Rural Organization of Theaters South
Seating Capacity: 90
Organization Type: Performing

2779 THEATRICAL OUTFIT

70 Fairlie Street
Suite 36098
Atlanta, GA 30303
Phone: 404-577-5257
Fax: 404-577-5259
e-mail: info@theatricaloutfit.org
Web Site: www.theatricaloutfit.org/
Officers:
   President: Bill Bolzer
Management:
   Producing Artistic Director: Tom Key
   Managing Director/Artistic Assoc: Kate Warner
   Marketing/Development Director: Beth Haynes

Mission: Produces contemporary and classical scripts with an emphasis on Southern themes.
Founded: 1976
Specialized Field: Contemporary & Classical Theatre
Status: Professional; Nonprofit
Paid Staff: 5
Paid Artists: 50
Budget: $700,000
Income Sources: Ticket Revenue; Private; Corporate; Foundations; Public
Performs At: Rialto Center for the Performing Arts
Organization Type: Performing; Educational

2780 AUGUSTA PLAYERS

PO Box 2352
Augusta, GA 30903-2352
Phone: 706-826-4707
Fax: 706-826-4709
e-mail: info@augustaplayers.com
Web Site: www.augustaplayers.com
Officers:
   President: Donna Hall
Management:
   Executive Director: Debi Ballas
   Artistic Director: Richard Justice
Founded: 1945
Specialized Field: Theatrical Group
Status: Non-Professional; Nonprofit
Paid Staff: 400
Income Sources: Georgia Theatre Conference; Southeastern Theatre Conference
Organization Type: Performing; Educational

2781 WEST GEORGIA THEATRE COMPANY SUMMER CLASSIC

Department of Mass Comm./Theatre
1600 Maple Street
Carrollton, GA 30118
Phone: 770-836-4792
Fax: 770-830-2322
e-mail: relman@westga.edu
Web Site: www.westga.edu/~theatre
Management:
   Theatre Director: Shelly Elman
   Design Faculty/ Technical Director: Tommy Cox
   Design Faculty/ Costumes: Alan Yoeng
Founded: 1991
Status: Non-Equity; Nonprofit
Budget: $35,000
Season: June - August
Performs At: Multi-Stage
Affiliations: Georgia Theatre Conference; Southeastern Theatre Conference; Association for the Theatre in Higher Education; USITT
Facility Category: Performing Arts Center
Type of Stage: Proscenium; Balck Box
Seating Capacity: 450; 100

2782 SPRINGER OPERA HOUSE THE STATE THEATER OF GEORGIA

103 Tenth Street
Columbus, GA 31901

Phone: 706-324-5714
Fax: 706-324-4681
Web Site: www.springeroperahouse.org
Management:
   Artistic Director: Paul R Pierce
   Executive Director: Porrin Trotter
   Associate Artistic Director: Ron Anderson
Mission: Offering the Southeastern United States high quality productions; representing Georgia as its official State Theatre.
Founded: 1871
Specialized Field: Theatre Company
Status: Professional; Nonprofit
Paid Staff: 19
Volunteer Staff: 240
Paid Artists: 145
Non-paid Artists: 40
Budget: 1.6 Million
Income Sources: Private, Foundation, State, Municipal, Ticket Sales
Performs At: 130 year old National Historic Landmark Theatre
Annual Attendance: 125,000
Facility Category: Theatre
Type of Stage: Proscenium & Studio Theatre
Stage Dimensions: 32 W x 42 Deep
Year Built: 1871
Year Remodeled: 1998
Cost: 12 Million
Rental Contact: Allison Kent
Organization Type: Performing; Touring; Producing

2783 AGNES SCOTT COLLEGE: DEPARTMENT OF THEATRE AND DANCE

East College Avenue
Decatur, GA 32514
Phone: 404-471-6251
Fax: 404-638-5369
Web Site: www.agnesscott.edu
Management:
   Associate Professor: Dudley W Sanders
Budget: $2,800-4,000
Performs At: Winter Theatre
Affiliations: ATHE
Type of Stage: Semi-Thrust
Seating Capacity: 310
Year Built: 1965

2784 NEIGHBORHOOD PLAYHOUSE

430 W Trinity Place
Decatur, GA 30030
Phone: 404-373-3904
Fax: 404-373-4130
e-mail: nplayhs@bellsouth.net
Web Site: www.nplayhouse.org
Management:
   Artistic/Executive Director: Ann Pavlik
   Managing Director: George Canady
   Operations Manager: Micki Hibbs
Mission: Providing professional quality theatre that entertains, educates and challenges our community.
Founded: 1980
Specialized Field: Theatrical Group

Status: Professional; Semi-Professional; Nonprofit
Income Sources: Box office, Grants, Donations
Annual Attendance: 15,000
Stage Dimensions: 50x25 and 23x20
Seating Capacity: 170 and 70
Year Built: 1980
Year Remodeled: 1999
Rental Contact: Micki Hibbs
Organization Type: Performing

2785 PICCADILLY PUPPETS COMPANY

621 Densley Drive
Decatur, GA 30033
Phone: 404-636-0022
Fax: 404-636-0616
e-mail: ppuppets@bellsouth.net
Web Site: www.piccadillypuppets.org
Officers:
   President: Dr. Pat Penn
   Secretary/Treasurer: Carol Daniel
Management:
   Director: Carol Daniel
Mission: Perform puppet shows for children and families.
Founded: 1969
Specialized Field: Puppet (touring company)
Status: Professional
Paid Staff: 1
Paid Artists: 4
Budget: $75,000
Income Sources: Arts councils; Presenters; Foundation support
Organization Type: Performing; Touring; Educational

2786 PARENTHESIS THEATRE CLUB

4336 Highborne Drive
Marietta, GA 30066
Phone: 404-977-8340
Management:
   Artistic Director: Gregory Blum
   Producing Director: Darrell Wofford
Mission: Producing ten minute plays that are socially relevant and original one acts.
Founded: 1991
Specialized Field: Dinner; Theatrical Group
Status: Semi-Professional
Performs At: Cabaret Space
Organization Type: Performing; Resident

2787 THEATRE IN THE SQUARE

11 Whitlock Avenue
Marietta, GA 30064
Phone: 770-422-8369
Fax: 770-424-2637
e-mail: boxoffice@theatreinthesquare.com
Web Site: www.theatreinthesquare.com
Management:
   Producing Director: Palmer D Wells
   Artistic Associate: Jessica West
Mission: Presenting a wide range of live theatre; providing theatre professionals with exciting material as well as optimal working conditions.
Founded: 1982
Specialized Field: Theatrical Group; Classical and New Work; Children's Productions; Play Readings; Classes

Status: Professional
Paid Staff: 17
Performs At: Theatre in the Square
Organization Type: Performing; Touring

2788 PERRY PLAYERS

909 Main Street
Perry, GA 31069
Phone: 912-987-5354
e-mail: perryplayers@hotmail.com
Web Site: www.perryplayers.com
Officers:
    President: Tom Saul
    Treasurer: Marshall Hutten
    Secretary: Bill Andrews
Management:
    VP Of Production: Anita Williams
    VP Of Business And Facilities: Bob Bailey
Mission: We offer high-quality entertainment and cultural activities to the citizens of middle Georgia. Individuals who enjoy acting, singing, dancing and producing cultural entertainment share and improve these skills in a welcoming environment of cooperation and enthusiasm.
Founded: 1982
Specialized Field: Musical; Community; Theatrical Group
Status: Non-Professional; Nonprofit
Paid Staff: 30
Income Sources: Houston County Arts Alliance; Macon Arts Alliance; Perry Chamber of Commerce

2789 GEORGIA ENSEMBLE THEATRE

950 Forest Street
PO Box 607
Rosewell, GA 30077-0607
Phone: 770-641-1260
Fax: 770-641-1360
Management:
    Artistic Director: Robert J Farley
    Managing Director: Anita Allen-Farley
    Marketing Director: Tess Kincaias
Paid Staff: 7
Volunteer Staff: 200

2790 ART STATION THEATRE

ART Station Contemporary Art Center
5384 Manor Drive
Stone Mountain, GA 30083
Phone: 770-469-1105
Fax: 770-469-0355
e-mail: info@artstation.org
Web Site: www.artsation.org
Officers:
    President: David Thomas
    Chairman: Gary Sekulow
    Vice Chairperson: Martha McCance
    Secretary: Michael Hidalgo
    Treasurer: Pam Culbersom
Management:
    President/Artistic Director: David Thomas
    Administrative Manager: Michael Hidalgo
Founded: 1986
Status: Nonprofit
Paid Staff: 6

Budget: $750,000
Income Sources: Government; Corporate; Foundations; Private
Season: September - June
Affiliations: AEA
Annual Attendance: 10,000+
Facility Category: Arts Center
Type of Stage: Proscenium
Stage Dimensions: 28' x 30'
Seating Capacity: 105
Year Built: 1900
Year Remodeled: 1990
Rental Contact: John Goldstein

2791 JEKYLL ISLAND MUSICAL THEATRE FESTIVAL

Department of Communication Arts
Valdosta, GA 31698
Phone: 912-333-5820
Fax: 912-245-3799
e-mail: dguthrie@valdosta.edu
Management:
    Managing Director: Duke Guthrie
    Dean School of the Arts: Dr. Lanny Milbrandt
Mission: Providing Georgia's Golden Isles residents and visitors with quality musical theatre; offering college interns professional training.
Founded: 1990
Specialized Field: Summer Stock; Musical
Status: Professional; Nonprofit
Paid Artists: 65
Income Sources: Valdosta State University
Season: June - August
Performs At: Jekyll Island Amphitheater
Annual Attendance: 10,000
Facility Category: Professional Summer Stock Theatre
Type of Stage: Wooden, uncovered amphitheatre
Seating Capacity: 500
Year Built: 1970
Organization Type: Performing; Touring

2792 SOUTHERN APPALACHIAN STAGES

PO Box 499
Young Harris, GA 30582
Phone: 706-379-1711
Fax: 706-379-1542
Toll-free: 800-262-7664
Web Site: www.reachofsong.org
Management:
    Executive Director: Philip Albert
    Artistic Director: Sharon Albert
Mission: Preservation and presentation of the culture and history of the Southern Appalachian Mountains through the performing arts.
Founded: 1989
Specialized Field: Theater
Status: Non-Equity; Nonprofit
Paid Staff: 12
Volunteer Staff: 30
Paid Artists: 25
Season: June 20 - August 19
Type of Stage: Proscenium
Seating Capacity: 750

Hawaii

2793 ARMY ENTERTAINMENT PROGRAM
USASCH, DPCA, CRD, CSDAB
Entertainment Section
Fort Shafter, HI 96858
Phone: 808-438-1980
Fax: 808-438-1980
Management:
  Chief Army Entertainment: Vanita Rae Smith
  Technical Director: Tom Giza
Mission: The goals of the Army Entertainment Program are to provide interested individuals with a constructive outlet for talents, to maintain a high level of morals and to promote good cultural relations with the local civilian community.
Founded: 1949
Specialized Field: Musical; Community; Theatrical Group
Status: Non-Professional; Nonprofit
Paid Staff: 30
Income Sources: American Association of Community Theatres; Hawaii State Theatre Council
Performs At: Richardson Performing Arts Center
Organization Type: Performing; Resident; Educational

2794 HILO COMMUNITY PLAYERS
141 Kalakaua Street
PO Box 46
Hilo, HI 96720
Phone: 808-935-9155
e-mail: players@aloha.net
Web Site: www.planet-hawaii.com/hilocommplayers
Officers:
  President: Gene Gold
  Secretary: Angie Baker
  Treasurer: Glen Swartwout
Management:
  Business Manager: Paul M Clark
  Equipment Manager: Peter Schickler
  Costume Manager: Sarah Hilliard
Mission: Organizing, promoting and conducting an educational amateur drama program on the Island of Hawaii.
Founded: 1938
Specialized Field: Community; Theatrical Group
Status: Non-Professional; Nonprofit
Paid Staff: 100
Organization Type: Performing; Educational

2795 DIAMOND HEAD THEATRE
520 Makapuu Avenue
Honolulu, HI 96816
Phone: 808-734-0274
Fax: 808-735-1250
Web Site: www.diamondheadtheatre.com
Officers:
  Chairman: Chris Kanazawa
Management:
  Artistic Director: John Rampage
  Managing Director: Deena Dray

Mission: To present plays and musicals to the community; to hold classes and workshops in acting for all ages; to offer opportunities for all persons interested to participate both on stage and backstage in theatre.
Founded: 1915
Specialized Field: Musical; Community; Theatrical Group
Status: Professional; Non-Professional; Nonprofit
Paid Staff: 12
Volunteer Staff: 400
Budget: $1,500,000
Income Sources: Tickets; Donations; State of Hawaii; Foundations
Performs At: Diamond Head Theatre
Annual Attendance: 50,000
Facility Category: Community Theatre
Type of Stage: Proscenium
Seating Capacity: 500
Year Built: 1940
Year Remodeled: 1980
Rental Contact: Managing Director Deena Dray
Organization Type: Performing; Educational

2796 HAWAII THEATRE
1130 Bethel Street
Honolulu, HI 96813-2201
Phone: 808-528-5535
Fax: 808-529-8505
e-mail: burtonwhite@hawaii.rr.com
Web Site: www.hawiitheatre.com
Officers:
  Chairman of the Board: Robert Midkiff
  Treasurer: Paul Schraff
  Vice Chairman: Mary Foster Weya
Management:
  Theatre Manager: Burton White
  Assistant Theatre Manager: Ryan Sueoka
  Assistant Box Office Manager: Dawn Keeley
  Stage Manager: Jude Lampitelli
Mission: Provide a professional venue for the celebration of cultures and the arts for the people of Hawaii and its visitors.
Founded: 1922
Specialized Field: Venue
Status: Nonprofit
Paid Staff: 13
Volunteer Staff: 300
Budget: $1.5 Million
Annual Attendance: 5,000
Type of Stage: Proscenium
Stage Dimensions: 30x18
Seating Capacity: 325

2797 HONOLULU THEATRE FOR YOUTH
2846 Ualena Street
Honolulu, HI 96819-1910
Phone: 808-839-9885
Fax: 808-839-7018
e-mail: hty@htyweb.org
Web Site: www.htyweb.org
Management:
  Artistic Director: Mark Lutwak
  Technical Director: Wade Kersey
  Managing Director: Louise Lanzilotti
  Director of Drama Education: Daniel A Kelin, II

Mission: To provide quality drama education and theatre to all children and their families in the state of Hawaii.
Founded: 1955
Status: Professional; Nonprofit
Paid Staff: 21
Volunteer Staff: 50
Paid Artists: 35
Budget: 1.4 million
Annual Attendance: 120,000

2798 KIMU KAHUA THEATRE

46 Merchant Street
Honolulu, HI 96813
Phone: 808-536-4222
Fax: 808-536-4226
Management:
    Artistic Director: Harry Wong III
Mission: To produce plays by Hawaiian writers writing about Hawaii and plays of interest to Hawaii's under served communites.
Founded: 1971
Paid Staff: 3
Performs At: Kahua Theatre
Type of Stage: Black Box
Seating Capacity: 100

2799 WINDWARD THEATRE GUILD

PO Box 624
Kailua, HI 96734
Phone: 808-234-1751
Management:
    Manager: Charles Brockman
Mission: Enhancing and promoting excellence in all aspects of theatrical production.
Founded: 1956
Specialized Field: Musical; Dinner; Community; Theatrical Group
Status: Nonprofit
Paid Staff: 60
Income Sources: Hawaii State Theatre Council; State Foundation for Culture & the Arts; Alliance for Drama Education
Performs At: Boondocker Theatre; Kaneohe Marine Corps Air State
Organization Type: Performing; Educational

2800 WAIMEA COMMUNITY THEATRE

PO Box 1660
Kamuela, HI 96743
Phone: 808-885-5818
Web Site: www.waimeacommunitytheatre.org
Officers:
    President: Andy Kunellis
    VP: JR Storment
    Secretary: Robyn Duquesne
    Treasurer: Michael Bray
Mission: Providing residents of North Hawaii with quality theatrical entertainment; offering community support and educational services in theatrical performance.
Founded: 1964
Specialized Field: Musical; Dinner; Community; Theatrical Group
Status: Non-Professional; Nonprofit

Paid Staff: 50
Income Sources: Hawaii State Theatre Council
Performs At: Parker School Auditorium
Organization Type: Performing; Educational

2801 KAUAI INTERNATIONAL THEATRE

Kauai Village
4-831 Kuhio Highway
Kapaa, Kauai, HI 96746
Phone: 808-821-1588
e-mail: thekit@GoKauai.org
Web Site: www.kauaitheatre.org
Management:
    Executive/Artistic Director: Gabriel Oberman
Status: Volunteer

2802 LEEWARD COMMUNITY COLLEGE THEATRE

96-045 Ala Ike
Pearl City, HI 96782
Phone: 808-455-0381
Fax: 808-455-0384
e-mail: sknox@hawaii.edu
Web Site: LCCTheatre.hawaii.edu
Management:
    Theatre Manager: Steve Knox

2803 MAUI ACADEMY OF PERFORMING ARTS

81 North Church Street
Wailuku, HI 96732
Phone: 808-244-8760
Fax: 808-244-6530
e-mail: mapa@ccmaui.com
Web Site: www.mauiacademy.org
Management:
    Managing Director: Frances A von Tempsky
    Artistic Director: David C Johnston
Mission: Offering educational performing arts to youths and adults.
Founded: 1974
Specialized Field: Community; Youth
Status: Nonprofit
Paid Staff: 500
Volunteer Staff: 200
Income Sources: Grants; Fundraising; Earned revenue
Performs At: Maui Academy of Performing Arts
Annual Attendance: 10,000 +
Facility Category: Performing Arts Classrooms/ Theatre
Type of Stage: Multi-forum
Seating Capacity: 150 - 200
Year Built: 2000
Cost: 3.1 million
Rental Contact: David Johnson
Organization Type: Performing; Touring; Educational

Idaho

2804 IDAHO SHAKESPEARE FESTIVAL

615 E 43rd Street
Boise, ID 83714

Phone: 208-323-9700
Fax: 208-323-0700
Web Site: www.idahoshakespeare.org
Management:
　Artistic Director: Charles Fee
　Managing Director: Mark Hofflund
Founded: 1976
Specialized Field: Theater
Status: Professional; Nonprofit
Paid Staff: 10
Season: May - September
Organization Type: Performing; Touring; Educational

2805　IDAHO THEATER FOR YOUTH

520 S 9th
Boise, ID 83702
Phone: 208-345-0060
Fax: 208-429-8798
e-mail: info@idahoshakespeare.org
Web Site: www.idahoshakespeare.org
Management:
　Educational Director: John O'Hagan
Mission: To provide live, professional theater for the
cultural enrichment and theater-arts education of children,
young adults and their families at a cost which makes the
programs easily accessible to all.
Founded: 1981
Specialized Field: Theatrical Group
Status: Professional; Nonprofit
Paid Staff: 5
Non-paid Artists: 15
Performs At: Morrison Center for the Performing Arts,
Fulton St. Theatre
Annual Attendance: 25,000 - 30,000
Seating Capacity: 200; 200
Organization Type: Performing; Touring; Educational

2806　COEUR D'ALENE SUMMER
THEATRE/CARROUSEL PLAYERS

Hall Box Office Boswell Hall
W 1000 Garden Avenue, PO Box 1119
Coeur d'Alene, ID 83816-1119
Phone: 208-769-7780
Fax: 208-769-7856
Toll-free: 800-423-2849
e-mail: nic_boxoffice@nic.edu
Web Site: www.nic.edu/summertheatre
Management:
　Artistic Director: Roger Welch
　Managing Director: David Hollingshead
　Development Director: Jim Speirs
　Box Office Manager: Maria Pileggi
Founded: 1968
Specialized Field: Musical Theatre
Status: Non-Equity; Nonprofit
Budget: $560,000
Income Sources: Patrons; Donors; Business Advertisers;
Grants
Season: July 1 - August 29
Performs At: U
Affiliations: F
Annual Attendance: 30,000
Facility Category: College Auditorium
Type of Stage: Proscenium

Stage Dimensions: 56'x 42'
Seating Capacity: 1100

2807　COMPANY OF FOOLS

PO Box 329
Hailey, ID 83333
Phone: 208-788-6520
Fax: 208-788-1053
e-mail: fools@svidaho.net
Web Site: www.companyoffools.org
Management:
　Artistic Director: Rusty Wilson
　Associate Artistic Director: Denise Simone
　Managing Director: RL Rowsey
Founded: 1992
Specialized Field: Theater
Performs At: Liberty Theatre, Mint
Type of Stage: Proscenium, Flexible
Seating Capacity: 240, 30-90

2808　IDAHO FALLS ARTS COUNCIL
COLONIAL THEATER

498 A Street
Idaho Falls, ID 83402
Phone: 208-522-0471
Fax: 208-522-0413
e-mail: ifac@idahofallsarts.org
Web Site: www.idahofallssarts.org
Management:
　Executive Director: Carrie Getty
　Technical Director: Chris Martin
　Ticket/Front House Manager: Linda Evans
Mission: To promote and present visual and performing
arts in Eastern Idaho.
Founded: 1990
Specialized Field: Performing & Visual Arts
Type of Stage: Wood
Seating Capacity: 969
Year Built: 1919
Year Remodeled: 1999
Rental Contact: Linda Evans

2809　IDAHO REPERTORY THEATRE
COMPANY

University of Idaho
PO Box 443074
Moscow, ID 83844-3074
Phone: 208-885-6465
Fax: 208-885-2558
e-mail: theatre@vidaho.edu
Web Site: www.uitheatre.com
Management:
　Producing Director: David Lee Painter
Mission: Providing North Idaho with quality summer
theatre.
Founded: 1953
Specialized Field: Theatrical Group
Status: Professional; Semi-Professional; Nonprofit
Paid Staff: 8
Volunteer Staff: 10
Paid Artists: 35
Non-paid Artists: 5
Income Sources: Individual contribution;
Business/corporate donations; Foundations

Season: May - August
Performs At: Hartung Theatre
Type of Stage: Semi-Thrust/Proscenium
Seating Capacity: 417
Year Built: 1973
Architect: $4.3 Million
Organization Type: Performing; Educational

2810 PANIDA THEATRE
300 N 1st Avenue
Sandpoint, ID 83864
Phone: 208-263-9191
e-mail: panida@netw.com
Web Site: www.panida.org
Management:
    Manager/Executive Director: Karen Bowers
    Technical Director: Bill Lewis
Mission: Providing beautiful, versatile space for the presentation of quality performances; continuing to aid in the revitalization of downtown Sandpoint.
Founded: 1927
Specialized Field: Musical; Community; Folk; Theatrical Group; Puppet; Dance; Film
Status: Professional; Nonprofit
Income Sources: Fundraising; grants
Performs At: Panida Theatre
Annual Attendance: 25,000
Seating Capacity: 550
Year Built: 1927
Organization Type: Performing; Resident; Educational; Sponsoring

Illinois

2811 ABOUT FACE THEATRE
3212 N Broadway
Chicago, IL 60657
Phone: 773-549-7943
Fax: 773-935-4483
e-mail: faceline1@aol.com
Web Site: www.aboutface.base.org
Management:
    Literary Manager: Carl Hippensteel
Founded: 1995
Specialized Field: Theatre
Type of Stage: Flexible Thrust Stage
Seating Capacity: 99

2812 AMERICAN BLUES THEATRE
1225 W Belmont
Chicago, IL 60657
Phone: 773-327-5252
Management:
    Co-Artistic Director: Jim Leaming
    Co-Artistic Director: Kate Buddeke
Mission: Developing and producing new plays written by and for Midwesterners.
Founded: 1985
Status: Professional; Nonprofit
Paid Staff: 125
Income Sources: League of Chicago Theatres
Organization Type: Performing

2813 AMERICAN THEATER COMPANY
1909 W Byron Street
Chicago, IL 60613
Phone: 773-929-1031
Fax: 773-929-5171
e-mail: atcfolk@aol.com
Web Site: www.atcweb.org
Officers:
    President: Dino Biris
    Vice President: Doug Diefanbach
    Treasurer: Larry Levin
Management:
    Producing Artistic Director: Damon Kiely
    Executive Director: Gregory Werstler
    Audience Services Manager: Michael Happ
Mission: ATC is an ensemble of artists committed to producing new and classic works that have contemporary resonances and engage the imagination of our audience.
Founded: 1985
Specialized Field: Theater
Paid Staff: 3
Paid Artists: 85
Non-paid Artists: 20
Budget: $385,000
Income Sources: Private Foundations; Grants; Government Grants; Individual Donations
Performs At: American Theater Company
Affiliations: Actors' Equity Association
Annual Attendance: 10,000
Type of Stage: Modifide Thrust
Seating Capacity: 137
Year Remodeled: 1993
Rental Contact: General Manager Gregory Werstler

2814 APOLLO THEATER CENTER
2540 N Lincoln Avenue
Chicago, IL 60614
Phone: 773-935-6100
Fax: 773-935-6214
e-mail: info@apollochicago.com
Web Site: www.apollochicago.com
Management:
    Managing Director/Producer: Rob Kolson
Mission: Presenting local productions of off-Broadway and Broadway shows; providing a transfer house to smaller off-loop theaters.
Founded: 1978
Status: Professional; Commercial
Income Sources: League of Chicago Theatres
Facility Category: Theater
Type of Stage: thrust
Seating Capacity: 450
Rental Contact: Rob Kolson
Organization Type: Sponsoring; Presenting

2815 AUDITORIUM THEATRE COUNCIL
50 E Congress Parkway
Chicago, IL 60605
Phone: 312-922-2110
Fax: 312-341-9668
e-mail: info@auditoriumtheatre.org
Web Site: www.auditoriumtheatre.org
Management:
    Executive Director: Jan Kallish

Theatre Manager: Morton Zolotow
Marketing/Group Sales Director: Barbara V Corrigan
Mission: Restoring the original architectural splendor of the Auditorium Theatre; presenting theatre, dance and music programs.
Founded: 1960
Specialized Field: Dance; Vocal Music; Theater
Status: Professional; Nonprofit
Performs At: Auditorium Theatre
Organization Type: Resident; Educational; Sponsoring

2816 BAILIWICK REPERTORY

Bailiwick Arts Center
1229 W Belmont
Chicago, IL 60657
Phone: 773-883-1090
Fax: 773-883-2017
e-mail: bailiwickr@aol.com
Web Site: www.bailiwick.org
Officers:
   President: Don Cortelyou
   Treasurer: Elliot Ferdland
   Secretary: Garth Person
   Board of Directors: Gary Skala
Management:
   Artistic director: David Zak
   Producer: Rusty Hernandez
   Box Office Manager: Brannen Daugherty
   General Manager: Jamie Axtell
Mission: To provide contemporary theater with a classical core; to produce vivid productions of the greatest dramatists of all times, alongside great works from our time; to serve as host or co-producer for other productions or attractions with similar artistic aims; to present festivals of one act plays; to showcase new directors and gay and lesbian plays.
Founded: 1982
Specialized Field: Theatrical Group
Status: Professional; Nonprofit
Paid Staff: 5
Volunteer Staff: 200
Paid Artists: 195
Budget: $975,000
Income Sources: League of Chicago Theatres; Theatre Communications Group; Illinois Theater Association
Performs At: Bailwell Arts Center
Affiliations: League of Chicago Theatre; Theatre Communications Group
Annual Attendance: 95,000
Facility Category: Performing Arts Center
Year Built: 1995
Organization Type: Performing; Sponsoring

2817 BLACK ENSEMBLE THEATER

4520 N Beacon
Chicago, IL 60640
Phone: 773-769-5516
Fax: 773-769-4533
Management:
   Artistic Director/Producer: Jackie Taylor
   Stage Manager: Ben Morgan
Mission: Supplying continual employment for the Black artist; adhering to a philosophy of excellence.
Founded: 1975
Specialized Field: Theatrical Group

Status: Professional; Nonprofit
Income Sources: Black Theater Alliance
Performs At: Leo Lerner Theater
Organization Type: Performing; Touring; Resident; Educational

2818 BLIND PARROT PRODUCTIONS

1446 W Berteau
Chicago, IL 60613
Phone: 312-549-3991
Officers:
   President: Fred Hachmeister
   Secretary: Sheri Jones
   Treasurer: Frank Tourangeau
Management:
   Co-Artistic Director: Clare Nolan-Long
   Co-Artistic Director: David Perkins
   Executive Director: Jane Molnar
Mission: To produce innovative, intelligent, thought-provoking writing for the stage with a focus on scripts which test the limits of theatrical form; to introduce new concepts; to pursue new relationships between artists and the audience.
Founded: 1983
Specialized Field: Theatrical Group
Status: Non-Professional
Paid Staff: 20
Income Sources: League of Chicago Theatres
Organization Type: Performing

2819 BODY POLITIC THEATRE

2261 N Lincoln Avenue
Chicago, IL 60614
Phone: 773-549-5788
Fax: 773-549-2777
Officers:
   President: Richard Wier
Management:
   Artistic Director: Albert Pertalion
   Administrative Director: Kim Patrick Bitz
   Business Director: Rick Sheingold
Mission: Provides an intimate forum for the best of classic and contemporary dramatic literature through thought-provoking and entertaining productions.
Founded: 1966
Status: Professional; Nonprofit
Paid Staff: 10
Income Sources: Actors' Equity Association; United Scenic Arts; League of Chicago Theatres; Theatre Communications Group; Producers Association of Chicago Area Theatres
Organization Type: Performing; Touring; Resident; Educational

2820 CENTER THEATER AND THE TRAINING CENTER

1346 W Devon
Chicago, IL 60660
Phone: 773-508-0200
Fax: 773-508-9584
Management:
   Artistic Director: Dan LaMorte
   General Manager: RJ Coleman

Mission: Educating, inspiring and cultivating theatre audiences; offering actors an ongoing training program.
Founded: 1985
Specialized Field: Theatrical Group
Status: Professional; Nonprofit
Paid Staff: 10
Income Sources: Theatre Communications Group; International Association of Theatre for Children and Youth
Performs At: Center Theater
Facility Category: Mainstage Theatre; Studio Theatre
Type of Stage: Thrust, Black Box
Seating Capacity: 60; 30
Organization Type: Performing; Touring; Resident; Educational

2821 CHICAGO ACTORS ENSEMBLE

941 W Lawrence Avenue
5th Floor
Chicago, IL 60642
Phone: 773-275-4463
Management:
   Artistic Director: Richard Helweg
Founded: 1984
Status: Professional; Nonprofit
Income Sources: League of Chicago Theatres
Organization Type: Performing; Touring; Resident

2822 CHICAGO DRAMATISTS

1105 W Chicago Avenue
Chicago, IL 60622
Phone: 312-633-0630
Fax: 312-633-0610
e-mail: newplays@aol.com
Web Site: www.chicagodramatists.org/home/index.html
Management:
   Artistic Director: Russ Tutterow
   Managing Director: Ann Fimer
Mission: Chicago Dramatists is a professional, non-profit theatre, dedicated to the development and advancement of playwrights and new plays.
Founded: 1979
Specialized Field: Theatrical Group
Status: Professional; Nonprofit
Paid Staff: 3
Volunteer Staff: 150
Paid Artists: 350
Budget: $250,000
Income Sources: Ticket Sales; Grant; Donations; Membership Fees; Class Fees
Performs At: Theatre
Affiliations: League of Chicago Theatre Actors' Equity Association; The Dramatists Guild; TCG
Annual Attendance: 8,000
Facility Category: Theatre
Type of Stage: Proscenium
Stage Dimensions: 24'x24'
Seating Capacity: 77
Year Built: 1884
Year Remodeled: 1998
Organization Type: Performing

2823 CHICAGO SHAKESPEARE THEATER ON NAVY PIER

800 E Grand Avenue
Navy Pier
Chicago, IL 60611
Phone: 312-595-5656
Fax: 312-595-5644
Web Site: www.chicagoshakes.com
Management:
   Artistic Director: Barbara Gaines
   Executive Director: Criss Henderson
Mission: Shakespeare offers countless paths of learning to students. Through one of the largest arts-in-education programs in the entire country, Team Shakespeare brings Shakespeare to life for middle school and secondary school students.
Founded: 1986
Specialized Field: Theatrical Group
Status: Professional; Nonprofit
Paid Staff: 93
Volunteer Staff: 50
Paid Artists: 42
Performs At: Chicago Shakespeare Theater; Seven Story on Navy Pier
Annual Attendance: 200,000
Facility Category: Courtyard-style Theater
Type of Stage: Modified Thrust; Studio
Seating Capacity: 510; 175
Year Remodeled: 1999
Organization Type: Performing; Touring; Resident; Educational; Sponsoring

2824 CHICAGO THEATRE COMPANY

500 E 67th Street
Chicago, IL 60637
Phone: 773-493-0901
Fax: 773-493-0360
Officers:
   Co-Chair: Arnie Harris
   Co-Chair: Delia Gray
   Secretary: Gwen Guy
   Secretary: Dr. Calvin Morris
Management:
   Managing Director: Luther Goins
Mission: To provide a professional and creative environment in which local artists may develop their talents, broaden the public's theatrical options, improve economic opportunities for minority artists, and enhance the cultural environment of the inner-city neighborhoods.
Founded: 1984
Status: Professional; Nonprofit
Paid Staff: 5
Paid Artists: 25
Budget: $275,000
Affiliations: Actors' Equity Association; League of Chicago Theatres
Type of Stage: Thrust stage
Seating Capacity: 90
Organization Type: Performing; Resident

2825 CHILD'S PLAY TOURING THEATRE

2518 W Armitage Avenue
Chicago, IL 60647-4325

Phone: 773-235-8911
Fax: 773-235-5478
Toll-free: 800-353-3402
e-mail: booking@cptt.org
Web Site: www.cptt.org
Officers:
   President: Bernard Garbo
   VP: June Podagrosi
   Secretary: Eve Moran
   Treasurer: Mark Ackerman
Management:
   Executive Director/Producer: Nicole Rohr
   Founder/Executive Director: June Podagrosi
Mission: Performing exclusively original literature authored by children; sharing, encouraging and validating children's creative writing; advancing children's literacy through theatre.
Founded: 1980
Specialized Field: Theatrical Group
Status: Professional; Nonprofit
Paid Staff: 6
Volunteer Staff: 2
Paid Artists: 12
Budget: $800,000
Income Sources: Government; Foundations; Corporations; Individuals; Box Office
Performs At: Seasonal run at the Goodman Theatre
Affiliations: Illinois Theater Association; Arts and Business Council; League of Chicago Theatres; NAPAMA; Donor's Forum of Chicago
Annual Attendance: 200,000
Facility Category: Off-site
Organization Type: Performing; Touring; Educational

2826 CITY LIT THEATER COMPANY

1020 W Bryn Mawr
Chicago, IL 60660
Phone: 773-293-3682
Fax: 773-293-3684
e-mail: metapage@aol.com
Web Site: www.citylit.org
Officers:
   President: Gary Redeker
Management:
   Managing Director: Page Hearn
Mission: City Lit Theater Company's presents both new adaptions of quality literature and extant with a literary bent.
Founded: 1979
Specialized Field: Theater
Status: Professional; Nonprofit
Paid Staff: 2
Volunteer Staff: 5
Paid Artists: 35
Budget: $176,000
Income Sources: Admissions; Grants
Annual Attendance: 5,526
Type of Stage: Thrust
Stage Dimensions: 16x25
Seating Capacity: 100
Year Remodeled: 2000
Organization Type: Performing; Touring; Resident; Educational

2827 CLASSICS ON STAGE!

PO Box 25365
Chicago, IL 60625
Phone: 773-989-0532
e-mail: classstage@aol.com
Web Site: www.classicsonstage.com
Management:
   Managing Director: Robert D Boburka
   Axtistic Director: Michele L Vacca
Mission: Developing future audiences for legitimate theatre through presentations of live professional theatre.
Founded: 1982
Specialized Field: Musical; Theatrical Group
Status: Professional; Commercial
Income Sources: Actors' Equity Association; Association of American Theatre for Youth; League of Chicago Theatres
Organization Type: Performing; Resident; Educational

2828 COURT THEATRE

5535 S Ellis Avenue
Chicago, IL 60637
Phone: 773-702-7005
Fax: 773-834-1897
Web Site: www.courttheater.org
Officers:
   Chairman: Jim Clark
Management:
   Artistic Director: Charles Newell
   Executive Director: Diane Claussen
Mission: To celebrate the immutable power and relevance of classic theatre.
Founded: 1954
Status: Professional; Nonprofit
Income Sources: Actors' Equity Association; League of Chicago Theatres; Theatre Communications Group; Producers Association of Chicago Area Theatres
Performs At: Court Theatre
Organization Type: Performing; Educational

2829 DEFIANT THEATRE

3540 N Southport Avenue
#162
Chicago, IL 60657
Phone: 312-409-0585
e-mail: defianttheatre@defianttheatre.org
Web Site: www.defianttheatre.org
Management:
   Artistic Director: Jim Slonina
   Literary Manager: Lisa Rothsciller
   Managing Director: Jennifer Gehr
   Media Relations Manager: Linda Gillum
   Production Manager: Joy Ronstadt
   Developement Coordinator: Will Schutz
Mission: We strive to subvert the social, moral, and aesthetic expectations of mainstream artistic expression.

2830 DEPAUL UNIVERSITY MERLE RESKIN THEATRE

60 E Balbo Drive
Chicago, IL 60605
Phone: 312-922-1999
Fax: 773-325-7967
Web Site: www.depaul.edu

Management:
Dean: John Culbert
Specialized Field: Theatre
Facility Category: Proscenium theatre
Seating Capacity: 1325
Year Built: 1910
Rental Contact: Leslie Shook (773-325-7965)

2831 DREISKE PERFORMANCE COMPANY

1517 W Fullerton Avenue
Chicago, IL 60614
Phone: 312-281-9075
Officers:
Chairman: David Edelberg
Secretary: Emilye Hunterfields
Management:
Artistic Director: Nicole Dreiske
Managing Director: Milos Stehlik
Literary Manager: Catherine Berkenstein
General Manager: John Dreiske
Mission: Professional touring ensemble, many of whose productions were developed in historic and on-location projects; The Book of Lear in the Sahara Desert, Macondo in Columbia, South America; currently developing new theater works for performance for international TV and tours.
Founded: 1975
Specialized Field: Theatrical Group
Status: Professional; Nonprofit
Income Sources: Association for Theatre in Higher Education; International Theatre Institute; League of Chicago Theatres
Performs At: International Performance Studio
Organization Type: Performing; Touring; Resident; Educational

2832 ENSEMBLE ESPANOL SPANISH DANCE THEATER

5500 N Saint Louis Avenue
Chicago, IL 60625
Phone: 773-583-4050
Fax: 773-794-5314
e-mail: ensemble-espanol@neiu.edu
Web Site: www.neiu.edu/~eespanol
Officers:
President: Dr. Angelina Pedroso
VP: Lou Altman
Treasurer: Elba Maisonet
Secretary: Lillian Heminover
Management:
Director: Libby Komaiko
Administrative Assistant: Jorge D Perez
Accountant: Flor Dumblao
Mission: The Ensemble Espanol Spanish Dance Theater is chartered to share the rich traditions of Spanish dance, music, art and literature with all of our communities as the Spanish Dance Center in the United States.
Founded: 1976
Specialized Field: Spanish Dance; Music; Art; Education; Folkoric
Status: Professional; Nonprofit
Paid Staff: 4
Volunteer Staff: 2
Paid Artists: 30

Non-paid Artists: 31
Budget: $400,000
Income Sources: Foundations; Corporations; Government; Private Donations
Annual Attendance: 90,000
Facility Category: Auditorium; Dance Studios
Type of Stage: Proscenium
Stage Dimensions: 25x25
Seating Capacity: 650
Year Built: 1975
Year Remodeled: 2000
Organization Type: Performing; Touring; Resident; Educational; Sponsoring

2833 ETA CREATIVE ARTS FOUNDATION

7558 S Chicago Avenue
Chicago, IL 60619
Phone: 773-752-3955
Fax: 773-752-8727
e-mail: email@etacreativearts.org
Web Site: www.etacreativearts.org
Officers:
Chairman: Milton Davis
President: Abena Joan Brown
Secretary/Treasurer: Velma Wilson
Finance: Wiley Moore
Management:
President/Producer: Abena Joan P Brown
Artistic Director: Runako Jahi
Business Manager: Teresa A White
Building Manager: Kenneth Simmons
Technical Director: Darryl Goodman
Mission: ETA provides training in the performing and technical aspects of the arts, encouraging the development and employment primarily of Black artists. ETA also works to encourage the development and propagation of the works of Black writers through its productions of original works.
Founded: 1971
Status: Professional; Nonprofit
Paid Staff: 6
Volunteer Staff: 50
Paid Artists: 8
Budget: $1.6 million
Income Sources: Earned funds; Corporate; Individuals
Performs At: ETA Square
Seating Capacity: 200
Organization Type: Performing; Touring; Resident; Educational

2834 FAMOUS DOOR THEATRE

Box 57029
Chicago, IL 60657
Phone: 773-404-8283
Fax: 773-404-8292
e-mail: info@famousdoortheatre.org
Web Site: www.famousdoortheatre.org
Officers:
Chair: Dan Rivkin
Vice-Chair: Don Copper
Secretary: Leo Aubel
Treasurer: Jeff Anderle
Management:
Managing Director: Amanda LaFollette
Artistic Director: Marc Grapey

General Manager: Hanna Dworkin
Founded: 1987
Specialized Field: Theatre
Paid Staff: 5
Volunteer Staff: 25
Paid Artists: 100
Non-paid Artists: 20
Budget: $500,000
Performs At: Victory Gardens Theatre
Affiliations: AEA; SSDC; TCG
Annual Attendance: 15,000
Type of Stage: Thrust
Seating Capacity: 200

2835 FREE STREET PROGRAMS

1419 W Blackhawk
Chicago, IL 60622
Phone: 773-772-7248
Web Site: www.freestreet.org
Management:
Artistic Director: Ron Bieganski
Director Of Marketing & PR: Anita Evans
Executive Director: David Schein
Mission: Free Street Programs is an arts outreach organization that uses the performing arts to enhance the literacy, self-esteem, creativity and employability of populations consistently excluded from mainstream cultural programming.
Founded: 1969
Specialized Field: Theatrical Group
Status: Professional; Nonprofit
Income Sources: Theatre Communications Group; Illinois Arts Alliance
Performs At: Free Street Teen Street Theater
Organization Type: Performing; Touring

2836 GOODMAN THEATRE

200 S Columbus Drive
Chicago, IL 60603
Phone: 312-443-3811
Fax: 312-263-6004
e-mail: staff@goodman-theatre.org
Web Site: www.goodman-theatre.org
Management:
Executive Director: Roche Schulfer
Artistic Director: Robert Falls
Associate Artistic Director: Michael Maggio
Mission: To present the classics of our theatre heritage with freshness and new vision; to create an audience that reflects the diversity of the Chicago community; to showcase the finest local, national, and international artists; to provide its staff and artists with the best working conditions possible; to operate with fiscal responsibility.
Founded: 1925
Specialized Field: Musical
Status: Professional; Nonprofit
Paid Staff: 100+
Budget: $12 Million
Income Sources: Foundation; Corporate & individual contributions; Ticket revenue
Performs At: Albert Iva Goodman, Owen Bruner Goodman Theater

Affiliations: TCG, Illinois Arts Alliance, League of Resident Theaters, American Arts Alliance, League of Chicago Theaters, Illinois Theater Association
Annual Attendance: 214,016
Type of Stage: Proscenium, flexible courtyard
Seating Capacity: 850 Albert, 345-467 Owen
Year Built: 2000
Organization Type: Performing; Educational; Sponsoring

2837 IMAGINATION THEATER

1801 W Bryon
Studio 2S
Chicago, IL 60613
Phone: 773-929-4100
Fax: 773-929-5603
Management:
Artistic Director: Warren W Baumgart, Jr
Mission: Committed to the value of creative drama as a tool for learning through two basic programs: participatory theater for children, the elderly, and the disabled; and Child Sexual Abuse Prevention Program, a comprehensive program for teachers, parents and students.
Founded: 1966
Status: Professional; Nonprofit
Organization Type: Performing; Touring; Educational

2838 INTERNATIONAL PERFORMANCE STUDIO

1517 W Fullerton Avenue
Chicago, IL 60614
Phone: 800-331-6197
Fax: 773-929-5437
e-mail: nicole@facets.org
Management:
Artistic Director: Nicole Dreiske
Founded: 1975
Status: Nonprofit
Season: Year Round

2839 LIFELINE THEATRE

6912 N Glenwood
Chicago, IL 60626
Phone: 773-761-4477
Fax: 773-761-4582
e-mail: lifeline@lifelinetheatre.com
Web Site: www.lifelinetheatre.com
Management:
Managing Director: Suzanne Plunkett
Artistic Director: Dorothy Milne
Mission: Lifeline Theatre entertains, educates and empowers our community using an ensemble drived process to bring literature and new works to life.
Founded: 1982
Specialized Field: Theatre Group
Status: Professional; Nonprofit
Paid Staff: 7
Volunteer Staff: 1
Budget: $500,000
Income Sources: League of Chicago Theatres, contributes, earned
Performs At: Lifeline Theatre

Affiliations: TGG, League of Chicago Theatres, AATE, PACT
Annual Attendance: 20,000
Facility Category: Theatre
Type of Stage: Flexible
Seating Capacity: 100
Year Built: 1930
Year Remodeled: 1992
Rental Contact: John Hildreth
Organization Type: Performing

2840 LIVE BAIT THEATRICAL COMPANY
3914 N Clark Street
Chicago, IL 60613
Phone: 773-871-1212
Fax: 773-871-3191
e-mail: info@livebaittheater.org
Web Site: www.livebaittheater.org
Management:
    Managing Director: Chad Eric Bergmans
Mission: We produce all new, orginal works by Chicago area playwrights and solo performers.
Founded: 1987
Specialized Field: Theatre
Paid Staff: 4
Performs At: Live Bait Theater
Type of Stage: Black Box
Seating Capacity: 70

2841 LOOKINGGLASS THEATRE COMPANY
2926 N Southport
3rd Floor
Chicago, IL 60657
Phone: 773-477-9257
Fax: 773-447-6932
Management:
    Artistic Director: David Kersnar
    Artistic Director: Heidi Stillman
    Managing Director: Michael Rysczek
    Literary Manager: Tom Park

2842 LOYOLA UNIVERSITY DEPARTMENT OF THEATRE
6525 N Sheridan Road
Chicago, IL 60626
Phone: 773-508-3830
Fax: 773-508-8748
e-mail: abrowni@luc.edu
Web Site: www.luc.edu/depts/theatre
Officers:
    Chairman: Sarah Gabel, PhD
Mission: To provide students with a well-rounded education in all aspects of theatre.
Performs At: Kathleen Mullady Theatre

2843 MAYFAIR THEATRE/SHEAR MADNESS
636 S Michigan Avenue
Chicago, IL 60605
Phone: 312-786-9120
Management:
    Company Manager: Deborah Gordon
    Producer: Marilyn Abrams
    Producer: Bruce Jordan

Mission: Mayfair Theatre presents 'Shear Madness,' the comedy whodunit that lets the audience play armchair detective. 'Shear Madness' is the longest running play in the history of Chicago theatre.
Founded: 1982
Specialized Field: Theatrical Group
Status: Professional; Commercial
Income Sources: League of Chicago Theatres
Performs At: Mayfair Theatre
Organization Type: Performing

2844 NEW TUNERS THEATRE
Performance Community
1225 W Belmont
Chicago, IL 60657
Phone: 773-929-7367
Fax: 312-327-1404
Web Site: www.adamczyk.com/newtuners
Management:
    Co-Producer: Ruth Higgins
    Co-Producer: Joan Mazzonelli
    Casting/Drama Director: Alan Chambers
Mission: To give exposure to new musicals; to support emerging artists in our Chicago area.
Specialized Field: Musical
Status: Professional; Nonprofit
Income Sources: League of Chicago Theatres; Theatre Communications Group; National Alliance of Theatre Producers
Performs At: New Tuners Theatre Building
Organization Type: Performing; Resident

2845 PEGASUS PLAYERS
Truman College
1145 W Wilson
Chicago, IL 60640
Phone: 773-878-9761
Fax: 773-271-8057
Web Site: www.pegasusplayers.com
Management:
    Artistic Director: Arlene Crewdson
    Managing Director: Alan Salzenstein
Mission: To produce the highest quality artistic work and to provide exemplary theatre, entertainment, and arts education at no charge to people who have little or no access to the arts.
Founded: 1979
Specialized Field: Theatrical Group
Status: Professional; Nonprofit
Income Sources: League of Chicago Theatres
Performs At: O'Rourke Center
Organization Type: Performing

2846 PERFORMING ARTS CHICAGO
410 S Michigan Avenue
#911
Chicago, IL 60605
Phone: 312-663-1628
Fax: 312-663-1043
e-mail: mail@pachicago.org
Web Site: www.pachicago.org
Officers:
    President: Judys Neisser
    Executive Director: Susan Lipman

Director: Christy Uchida
Operations Manager: Laurell Zahrobsky
Development Assistant: Brigid Flynn
Treasurer: David Ellis
Management:
  Executive Director: Susan Lipman
  Director Marketing/Public Relations: Heidi Feldman
Mission: To present artists who explore the creative tension between tradition and innovation, to nurture an environment for and bring to performance new works and new performers, and to remain accountable to its community, furthering support for local artists, engagement and education, not only for its direct audience, but for society at large.
Founded: 1960
Specialized Field: Chamber; Theater; Dance; Puppetry
Status: Professional; Nonprofit
Budget: $1,000,000
Performs At: The Civic Theater
Organization Type: Performing; Resident; Educational; Sponsoring

---

2847 RAVEN THEATRE COMPANY
6157 N Clark
Chicago, IL 60626
Mailing Address: 2549 W Fargo Chicago, IL 60645
Phone: 773-338-2177
Fax: 773-508-9794
e-mail: raventheatre@aol.com
Web Site: www.raventheatre.com
Officers:
  President: John Munson
  Vice President: Barbara King
  Secretary: Joni Gatz
  Treasurer: Ed Bray
Management:
  Executive/Artistic Director: Michael Menendian
  Technical Director: John Munson
  Production Manager: Joni Gatz
Mission: To provide professional theatre affordable and accessible to the broadest cross-section of the people of Chicagoland and to provide the opportunity for local theatre artists to develop a showcase for their talents.
Founded: 1983
Specialized Field: Theatrical Group
Status: Professional; Nonprofit
Paid Staff: 30
Income Sources: League of Chicago Theatres
Organization Type: Performing; Resident

2848 REMAINS THEATRE
1800 N Clybourn Avenue
Chicago, IL 60614
Phone: 312-335-9800
Fax: 312-335-0626
Officers:
  President: Valerie Hoffman
  Vice President: David Harvey
  Secretary: Elizabeth Hubbard
Management:
  Artistic Director: Larry Sloan
  Producing Director: RP Sekon
  General Manager: Janis Post

Mission: To establish and maintain a theatre company dedicated to presenting work focused in three areas: 1) ensemble-developed original works; 2) provocative contemporary plays; and 3) lesser-known works by eminent writers and playwrights.
Founded: 1979
Status: Professional; Nonprofit
Income Sources: Theatre Communications Group; League of Chicago Theatres
Performs At: Remains Theatre
Organization Type: Performing; Touring; Educational

2849 ROADWORKS PRODUCTIONS
1144 W Fulton Market
Suite 105
Chicago, IL 60607
Phone: 312-492-7150
Fax: 312-492-7155
e-mail: shade@roadworks.org
Web Site: www.roadworks.org
Officers:
  Chair: David Shaw
  Vice Chair: Jean de St. Aubin
  Treasurer: Adam Dewitt
  Secretary: Marc Fisher
Management:
  Artistic Director: Geoffrey Curley
  Managing Director: Jason Rissman
  Development Director: Jennifer Avery
  Outreach Coordinator: Kimberly Senior
Founded: 1992

2850 SAINT SEBASTIAN PLAYERS
St Bonaventure 1641 W Diversey
Chicago, IL 60614
Phone: 312-404-7922
Fax: 312-728-0496
e-mail: stsebplyrs@aol.com
Web Site: members.aol.com/stsebplyrs
Officers:
  President: Jonathan Hagloch
  Secretary: Jill Chuckerman
  Treasurer: Jim Masini
Management:
  Public Relations Director: Jill Cluckerman
  Industry Liaison: Connie Anderko
Mission: To present comedies, dramas, musicals, mysteries and other theatrical events to the Chicago community.
Founded: 1981
Specialized Field: Theatre
Status: Nonprofit
Paid Staff: 7
Income Sources: Ticket Revenue; Concessions Revenue; Playbill Ad Revenue; Donations
Performs At: Saint Bonaventure Parish
Annual Attendance: 1,200-1,500
Type of Stage: Flexible Proscenium
Seating Capacity: 70-100
Organization Type: Performing

2851 SEANACHAI THEATRE COMPANY
5108 N Ashland
#2
Chicago, IL 60640
Phone: 773-878-3727
Fax: 847-729-8274
Management:
   Artistic Director: Michael Grant
   Managing Director: John Dunleavy
   Literary Manager: Karen Tarjan

2852 SECOND CITY
1616 N Wells Street
Chicago, IL 60614
Phone: 312-664-4032
Fax: 312-664-9837
Web Site: www.secondcity.com
Officers:
   Executive Producer/CEO: Andrew Alexander
Management:
   Producer: Kelly Leonard
   Associate Producer: Beth Kligerman
Mission: Satirical revue.
Founded: 1959
Status: Professional; Commercial
Performs At: Second City Mainstatge; Second City, Ect.
Type of Stage: Proscenium
Seating Capacity: 350; 180
Organization Type: Performing; Touring; Resident; Educational

2853 SHATTERED GLOBE THEATER
2856 N Halsted
Chicago, IL 60657
Phone: 773-404-1237
Fax: 773-404-1237
Officers:
   President: Brian Pudil
   VP: Joe Forbrich
   Secretary: Leigh Horsley
   Treasurer: Linda Reiter
Management:
   General Manager: Brian Pudil
   Artistic Director: Roger Smart
   Associate Director: Joe Forbrich
Mission: The foundation of the Shattered Globe is a core of actors, directors, playwrights, designers and teachers working together as the result of having received similar training in the Sanford Meisner technique.
Founded: 1990
Specialized Field: Theatrical Group
Status: Semi-Professional; Commercial
Paid Staff: 15
Income Sources: League of Chicago Theatres
Performs At: Chicago Actors Project
Organization Type: Performing; Resident; Educational

2854 STAGE LEFT THEATRE
3408 N Sheffield
Chicago, IL 60657
Phone: 773-883-8830
e-mail: SLTChicago@aol.com
Web Site: www.stagelefttheatre.com
Officers:

President: Jay Tarshis
Treasurer: Wendy Istvanick
   Secretary: Dr Alice Martin
Management:
   Co-Artistic Director: Jessi D Hill
   Co-Artistic Directors: Kevin Heckman
   Development Director: Jacki Singleton
   Company Manager: Leigh Barrett
Mission: Producing plays that raise awareness of social and political issues.
Founded: 1982
Specialized Field: Theatrical Group
Status: Professional; Nonprofit
Volunteer Staff: 19
Income Sources: League of Chicago Theatres
Facility Category: Storefront
Type of Stage: Black Box
Seating Capacity: 50
Organization Type: Performing; Touring; Educational

2855 STEPPENWOLF THEATRE COMPANY
1650 N Halsted Street
Chicago, IL 60614
Phone: 312-335-1888
Fax: 312-335-0808
e-mail: theatre@steppenwolf.org
Web Site: www.steppenwolf.org
Management:
   Artistic Director: Martha Lavey
   Executive Director: Michael Gennaro
   Casting Director: Erica Daniels
   Internship Coordinator: Jessica Vmphress
Mission: Committed to an ensemble approach.
Founded: 1976
Status: Professional; Nonprofit
Paid Staff: 60
Income Sources: Theatre Communications Group; Actors' Equity Association; Producers Association of Chicago Theatres
Performs At: Steppenwolf Theater
Type of Stage: Removable Thrust
Seating Capacity: 510
Organization Type: Performing; Resident; Educational

2856 STRAWDOG THEATRE COMPANY
3829 N Broadway
Chicago, IL 60613
Phone: 773-528-9889
Fax: 773-528-7238
e-mail: tickets@strawdog.org
Web Site: www.strawdog.org
Management:
   Artistic Director: Jennifer Avery
   Artistic Director: Michael Dailey
   Artistic Director: Jess Hill
Mission: To inspire and provoke through ensemble based theatrical works.
Founded: 1988
Specialized Field: Live Theatre Performance
Status: Not-for-profit 501(c) tax emempt
Volunteer Staff: 15
Paid Artists: 15
Non-paid Artists: 15

2857 THEATRE FIRST

6656 Sioux Avenue
Chicago, IL 60646
Phone: 773-792-2226
Management:
    Executive Producer: Joanne Notz
    Business Manager: William Mages
Founded: 1952
Specialized Field: Theatrical Group
Status: Non-Professional
Income Sources: League of Chicago Theatres
Performs At: Athenaeum Theatre
Organization Type: Performing

2858 THEATRE II COMPANY

3700 W 103rd Street
Chicago, IL 60655
Phone: 773-298-3000
Management:
    Artistic Director: Steve Micotto
    Managing Director: JoAnne Fleming
Mission: Providing the Southwest Chicago community with quality live theater.
Founded: 1978
Specialized Field: Theatrical Group
Status: Professional; Nonprofit
Income Sources: League of Chicago Theatres; Saint Xavier University
Performs At: McGuire Hall
Organization Type: Performing

2859 TIMELINE THEATRE COMPANY

615 W Wellington Avenue
Chicago, IL 60657
Phone: 773-281-8463
e-mail: info@timelinetheatre.com
Web Site: www.timelinetheatre.com
Management:
    Artistic Director: PJ Powers
    Managing Director: Pat Tiedemann
    Literary Manager: Brian Voelker
    Marketing Director: Juliet Hart
    Producing Director: Lara Goetsch

2860 VICTORY GARDENS THEATER

2257 N Lincoln Avenue
Chicago, IL 60614
Phone: 773-549-5788
Fax: 773-549-2779
e-mail: vgtheater@aol.com
Web Site: www.victorygardens.org
Management:
    Managing Director: Marcelle McVay
    Artistic Director: Dennis Zacek
    General Manager: Elizabeth Auman
    Associate Artistic Director: Sandy Shinner
Mission: Developing Chicago theatre artists, particularly playwrights.
Founded: 1974
Specialized Field: Theatrical Group
Status: Professional
Paid Staff: 14
Budget: $1.6M
Performs At: Block Box

Annual Attendance: 60,000+
Type of Stage: Black Box
Seating Capacity: 195
Rental Contact: Elizabeth Auman
Organization Type: Performing; Touring; Resident; Educational

2861 WAX LIPS THEATRE COMPANY

1524 W Berteau Avenue
#3
Chicago, IL 60613
Phone: 773-525-6797
e-mail: waxlips@email.msn.com
Web Site: www.waxlipstheatre.org
Management:
    Artistic Director: John Corwin
    Artistic Director: Brendan Hunt
    Director Special Events: Anita Deely
    Publicity Director: Carla DeLio
    Literary Manager: Chris Hainsworth
    Director Fundraising: Kat McDonnell
    Facilities Director: Kurt Reynolds
Mission: The Wax Lips Theatre Company was built on the foundation of truthful acting and innovative storytelling. The company was established in 1994 by a group of Illinois State University graduates drawn together by a common artistic sensibility. Its members have gained professional experience working with such respected Chicago theatres as Steppenwolf and Victory Gardens.

2862 WISDOM BRIDGE THEATRE

1559 W Howard Street
Chicago, IL 60626
Phone: 312-743-0486
Fax: 312-743-1614
Management:
    Producing Director: Jefferey Ortmann
    Producing Manager: Karl Sullivan
    Director Program Administration: Sharon Phillips
    Resident Director: Terry McCabe
Mission: Exploring classic literature; addressing new works with emphasis on risk-taking and enlightenment.
Founded: 1974
Status: Professional; Nonprofit
Income Sources: Actors' Equity Association; League of Chicago Theatres; Theatre Communications Group
Performs At: Wisdom Bridge Theatre
Organization Type: Performing; Touring; Educational

2863 WOMEN'S THEATRE ALLIANCE

407 S Dearborn Avenue
Suite 1775
Chicago, IL 60602
Phone: 312-408-9910
Management:
    President: Janel Winter
    VP Programming: Jennifer Alber
    Treasurer: Ester Lebo

2864 DES PLAINES THEATRE GUILD

620 Lee Street
Des Plaines, IL 60016
Phone: 708-296-1211

All listings are in alphabetical order by state, then city, then organization within the city.

Mission: Offering Northwest Suburban Chicago professional level community theatre for the education and entertainment of audiences.
Founded: 1946
Specialized Field: Community; Theatrical Group
Status: Non-Professional; Nonprofit
Performs At: Prairie Lake Community Center
Organization Type: Performing

2865 UNIVERSITY THEATRE: SUMMER SHOW BIZ

Campus Box 1777, Southern Illinois University
Katherine Dunham Hall 1031
Edwardsville, IL 62026-1777
Phone: 618-650-2773
Fax: 618-650-3716
Toll-free: 888-328-5168
e-mail: djhasty@siue.edu
Web Site: www.siue.edu/theater
Management:
    Chairman: C Otis Sweezey
    Dance Director: J Calvin Jarrell
    Director Design/Technical: James Dorethy
    Director Performance: Peter Cocuzza
Founded: 1975
Status: Non-Equity; Nonprofit
Season: June - July
Type of Stage: Proscenium
Stage Dimensions: 50' x 30'
Seating Capacity: 360

2866 LIVE THEATRE

1234 Sherman Avenue
Evanston, IL 60201
Phone: 847-492-1774
Management:
    Artistic Director: AC Thomas
    Executive Director: Marcia Riegel
    Managing Director: Marjorie Cohn
    Director: Richard O'Connell
    Director: Michael E Myers
Mission: To create a nourishing and challenging environment for our actors and artists in our continued exploration of the human condition.
Founded: 1983
Status: Professional; Nonprofit
Income Sources: League of Chicago Theatres; Evanston Arts Council
Performs At: Live Theatre
Organization Type: Performing

2867 NEXT THEATRE COMPANY

927 Noyes Street
Evanston, IL 60201
Phone: 847-475-1875
Fax: 847-475-6767
e-mail: NextTheatre@aol.com
Web Site: www.NextTheatre.org
Officers:
    President: Judy Kemp
    VP: Angel Ysuguirre
    Secretary: Jeff Emrich
Management:
    Artistic Director: Jason Loewith

Interim General Manager: Michael Osinski
Communications Manager: Jamie Foltz
Production Manager: Brandon Wardell
Mission: We believe theatre promotes awarness and provokes change with more power than any other form of expression, and we are devoted to producing socially proactive artistically challenging entertainment.
Founded: 1981
Status: Professional; Nonprofit
Income Sources: Actors' Equity Association; Theatre Communications Group; League of Chicago Theatres; Producers Association of Chicago Area Theatres
Performs At: Noyes Cultural Arts Center
Type of Stage: Proscenium
Stage Dimensions: 24' x 33'
Seating Capacity: 167
Organization Type: Performing; Resident

2868 NORTHWESTERN UNIVERSITY THEATRE AND INTERPRETATION CENTER

1979 S Campus Drive
Evanston, IL 60208
Phone: 847-491-3232
Fax: 847-467-7135
e-mail: p-brohan@northwestern.edu

2869 NORTHWESTERN UNIVERSITY SUMMER DRAMA FESTIVAL

Theatre Department
1979 S Campus Drive
Evanston, IL 60208
Phone: 847-491-3232
Fax: 847-467-7135
Management:
    Producer: Paul Brohan
Founded: 1954
Status: Non-Equity; Nonprofit
Season: June - August
Type of Stage: Thrust
Stage Dimensions: 21' x 30'
Seating Capacity: 450

2870 ORGANIC THEATER COMPANY

1420 Maple Avenue
Evanston, IL 60201
Phone: 847-475-0600
Fax: 847-475-9200
e-mail: organictheater@aol.com
Web Site: www.organictheater.com
Officers:
    President: Holly I Myers
    VP/Secretary: Judith Thomson
    Treasurer: Mark Thomas
Management:
    Producing Artistic Director: Ina Marlowe
    Managing Director: Katie Klemme
Mission: To develop and produce new works of theatre and to nurture the artists involved in that process; interested in adventurous, challenging scripts that truly explore the theatrical medium and its possibilities.
Founded: 1969
Status: Professional; Nonprofit

Paid Staff: 5
Volunteer Staff: 15
Paid Artists: 40
Budget: $300,0000
Income Sources: League of Chicago Theatres; Theatre Communications Group
Affiliations: AEA CAT, TYA
Annual Attendance: 15,000
Facility Category: House
Type of Stage: Proscenium
Seating Capacity: 260
Organization Type: Performing; Educational

2871 PIVEN THEATRE WORKSHOP
927 Noyes Street
Evanston, IL 60201
Phone: 847-866-6597
Fax: 847-866-6614
e-mail: piventw@aol.com
Web Site: www.piventheatreworkship.com
Officers:
President: Marcia Cahn
Vice President: David Doyle
Treasurer: Eric Rubenstein
Secretary: Emily Neuberger
Management:
Administrative Director: Diane Leavitt
Mission: To provide professional theatre and an actors training center for children and adults.
Founded: 1972
Specialized Field: Theatrical Group
Status: Professional; Nonprofit
Budget: $600,000
Income Sources: Illinois Arts Council; Evanston Arts Council
Performs At: Noyes Cultural Arts Center
Annual Attendance: 7,500
Type of Stage: Black Box
Seating Capacity: 75
Organization Type: Performing; Educational

2872 ORPHEUM THEATRE
60 S Kellogg Street
Galesburg, IL 61401
Phone: 309-342-2299
Fax: 309-342-2515
e-mail: orpheum@knoxnet.net
Web Site: www.theorpheum.org
Management:
Managing Director: Amy Kelso
Mission: To promote and preserve the Orpheum Theatre as a premier presentation venue for the community.
Founded: 1915
Status: Nonprofit
Paid Staff: 2
Volunteer Staff: 30
Budget: $252,000
Income Sources: City of Galesburg; Illinois
Affiliations: American Society of Composers, Authors and Publishers
Facility Category: Performance Theatre
Type of Stage: Proscenium
Stage Dimensions: 59'x 40'
Seating Capacity: 952
Year Built: 1916

Year Remodeled: 1989
Rental Contact: Business Manager Danny Davis
Organization Type: Performing; Touring; Educational
Resident Groups: Prairie Players

2873 PRAIRIE PLAYERS CIVIC THEATRE
233 N Main
PO Box 831
Galesburg, IL 61401
Phone: 309-343-7728
Web Site: www.prairieplayers.com
Officers:
President: Dennis Clark
VP: Kenny Knox
Secretary: Anita Reese
Treasurer: Bob Gutermuth
Mission: To sustain live theatre arts in a rural setting.
Founded: 1914
Specialized Field: Dinner; Community; Theatrical Group; Puppet
Status: Non-Professional; Nonprofit
Income Sources: Association of Kansas Theatres
Organization Type: Performing; Resident

2874 WRITERS' THEATRE CHICAGO
Books on Vernon
664 Vernon Avenue
Glencoe, IL 60022
Phone: 847-835-7366
Fax: 847-835-5332
e-mail: writerstheatre@aol.com
Web Site: www.writerstheatre.org
Management:
Artistic Director: Michael Halberstam
Executive Director: John W Adams
Mission: The Writers Theatre is a professional company dedicated to a theatre of language and passion.
Founded: 1992
Paid Staff: 9
Performs At: Nichols Pennell Theatre

2875 CONKLIN PLAYERS DINNER THEATRE
PO Box 301
Conklin Court
Goodfield, IL 61742
Phone: 309-965-2545
Management:
Owner/Producer/Director: Chaunce Conklin
Manager: Mary Simon
Mission: To entertain, to educate and to promote live performance.
Specialized Field: Dinner; Children's Theatre
Status: Professional; Commercial
Organization Type: Performing; Resident

2876 APPLE TREE THEATRE
595 Elm Place
Suite 210
Highland Park, IL 60035
Phone: 847-432-8223
Fax: 847-432-5214
e-mail: appletreetheatre@yahoo.com
Web Site: www.appletreetheatre.com

Management:
    Executive/Artistic Director: Eileen Boevers
    Artistic Director: Ross Lehman
    Producing Director: Cecilie Keenan
    Director Development: Mary Ellen Mason
    Production Manager: Tim Stadler
    Workshop/TYA Artistic Directors: Barbara Harris
Mission: Is committed to producing a diverse and challenging selection of both dramas and musicals, from new works to classics, all of which illuminate the human condition.
Founded: 1983
Volunteer Staff: 15
Budget: $1,200,000
Income Sources: Grants; Donations; Ticket Sales
Annual Attendance: 30,000
Type of Stage: Thrust
Seating Capacity: 177+

2877 MARRIOTT'S THEATRE IN LINCOLNSHIRE
10 Marriott Drive
Lincolnshire, IL 60069
Phone: 847-634-0204
Fax: 847-634-7358
e-mail: producer@marriotttheatr.com
Web Site: marriotttheatre.com
Management:
    Artistic Director: Rick Boynton
    Executive Producer: Terry James
    Director Marketing: Lauren Johnson
Mission: Presenting five productions annually, including classic musicals, rarely-seen musicals, and premieres of new works.
Founded: 1975
Specialized Field: Musical
Status: Professional; Commercial
Income Sources: League of Chicago Theatres; American Dinner Theatre Institute
Performs At: Marriott's Lincolnshire Theatre
Affiliations: NAMT
Annual Attendance: 400,000
Type of Stage: In the Round
Seating Capacity: 882
Year Built: 1978
Organization Type: Performing; Resident

2878 ENCORE PLAYERS
222 E Sargent
Litchfield, IL 62056
Phone: 217-326-4414
Officers:
    President: Keith Purcell
    VP: Joel Schnur
    Treasurer: Dick Butler
    Secretary: Pauline Coughlan
Management:
    Director: Mae Morton
    Director: Dennis Plozizka
    Director: David Lewey
    Director: Tim Price
    Artistic Director: George Dawson

Mission: To promote art and the development of artistic ability as well as related theatrical skills; to encourage public appreciation of theatrical arts.
Founded: 1968
Specialized Field: Musical; Dinner; Community; Theatrical Group
Status: Non-Professional; Nonprofit
Performs At: Community Center
Organization Type: Performing

2879 SUMMER MUSIC THEATRE
Western Illinois University Theatre Dept.
Browne Hall 101
Macomb, IL 61455
Phone: 309-298-1543
Fax: 309-298-2695
e-mail: davidpatrick@ccmail.wiu.edu
Management:
    Managing Director: David Patrick
Mission: To offer musical theatre to the community; to provide training for students.
Founded: 1972
Specialized Field: Summer Stock; Musical
Status: Nonprofit
Paid Staff: 10
Income Sources: University/Resident Theatre Association
Season: June - August
Performs At: Hainline Theatre
Type of Stage: Proscenium
Seating Capacity: 387
Year Built: 1972
Organization Type: Performing; Resident; Educational

2880 COLEMAN PUPPET THEATRE
1516 S Second Avenue
Maywood, IL 60153
Phone: 708-344-2920
Management:
    Director: FR Coleman
    Director: Barbara Coleman
Mission: To preserve and perpetuate stories, both classic and modern through dramatization with puppets.
Founded: 1947
Specialized Field: Puppet
Status: Professional
Income Sources: Puppeteers of America; Chicagoland Puppetry Guild; Puppeteers of America
Organization Type: Performing; Touring

2881 TIMBER LAKE PLAYHOUSE
PO Box 29
Mt. Carroll, IL 61053
Phone: 815-244-2035
Fax: 815-244-2035
Web Site: www.artsaxis.com/tlp
Management:
    Artistic Director: Brad Lyons
Mission: Dedicated to providing a center for cultural opportunity for developing artists and a showcase of quality theatre for the residents of the Midwest, particularly in Northwestern Illinois and Eastern Iowa.
Founded: 1961
Status: Non-Equity; Nonprofit

Season: June - September
Type of Stage: Semi-Thrust
Seating Capacity: 375

2882 ILLINOIS SHAKESPEARE FESTIVAL

Illinois State University
Box 5700
Normal, IL 61790-5700
Phone: 309-438-8974
Fax: 309-438-5806
e-mail: shake@ilstu.edu
Web Site: www.thefestival.org
Management:
    Managing Director: Fergus G Currie
    Artistic Director: Calvin MacLean
    Assistant Managing Director: Paul Berg
Founded: 1978
Specialized Field: Festivals
Status: Nonprofit
Paid Staff: 100
Paid Artists: 85
Non-paid Artists: 15
Budget: $600,000
Income Sources: Box Office, Fund Raising
Season: June - August
Performs At: Ewing Manor
Affiliations: UARTA; Actors' Equity Association; SSOC
Annual Attendance: 15,000
Facility Category: Outdoor
Type of Stage: Thrust
Seating Capacity: 420
Year Built: 1999
Cost: $1.65 million
Organization Type: Performing; Educational

2883 OAK PARK FESTIVAL THEATRE

PO Box 4114
Oak Park, IL 60303
Phone: 708-524-2050
Fax: 708-524-4950
Web Site: www.oprf.com/festival
Management:
    Artistic Director: Dale Calandra
    Managing Director: Sandy Wredegreen
Founded: 1975
Specialized Field: Summer Stock
Status: Professional; Nonprofit
Paid Staff: 20
Volunteer Staff: 14
Budget: $160,000
Income Sources: Illinois Arts Council; Oak Park Area Arts Council; Foundations; Membership
Season: July - August
Performs At: Outside
Affiliations: Actors Equity Association; League of Chicago Theatres; Producers Association of Chicago
Facility Category: Outdoor
Type of Stage: Platform
Seating Capacity: 350
Organization Type: Performing

2884 VILLAGE PLAYERS THEATER

1006 W Madison Street
Oak Park, IL 60302

Phone: 708-524-1892
Fax: 708-524-9892
Web Site: www.angelfire.com/il/opup
Officers:
    President: Jack Crowe
    VP: Kevin Bry
    Secretary: Mardie Meegan
    Treasurer: Robby Robinson
Management:
    Artistic Dir/Theater School Manager: Maura Elizabeth Manning
Mission: Promoting community involvement in cultural arts; developing theatrical ability through public performances and education.
Founded: 1961
Specialized Field: Community; Theatrical Group for Young Audiences
Status: Professional; Non-Equity
Paid Staff: 90
Paid Artists: 10
Budget: 280K
Income Sources: Tickets; Tuition; Grants
Performs At: Persidium
Affiliations: Village Players Theater School
Annual Attendance: 20,000
Facility Category: Mainstage/Blackbox
Type of Stage: Proscenium
Seating Capacity: 222
Organization Type: Performing Resident; Educational

2885 DRURY LANE OAKBROOK TERRACE

100 Drury Lane
Oakbrook Terrace, IL 60181
Phone: 708-530-8300
Fax: 630-530-0436
Web Site: www.drurylaneoakbrook.com
Officers:
    President: Steve Bortolotti
    VP: Johanne Grewell
    Treasurer: Rex Yancey
    Secretary: Ginny Andrews
Management:
    Managing Director: Diane Van Lente
    General Manager: John Tapia
    Artistic Director: Ray Frewen
Mission: To present large-scale musicals and comedies that feature leading theatre artists.
Founded: 1984
Specialized Field: Musical; Dinner
Status: Professional; Non-Professional; Commercial
Income Sources: American Dinner Theatre Association
Performs At: Drury Lane Theater
Facility Category: Theatre House
Type of Stage: Proscenium
Seating Capacity: 972
Year Built: 1984
Organization Type: Performing; Touring

2886 ILLINOIS THEATRE CENTER

371 Artists' Walk
PO Box 397
Park Forest, IL 60466

Phone: 708-481-3510
Fax: 708-481-3693
e-mail: ilthetr@big planet.com
Web Site: www.ilthetr.org
Officers:
   President: Denyse Carreras
   Secretary: Candace Kleindorfer
Management:
   Producing Artistic Director: Etel Billig
   Music Director: Jonathan Roark Billing
   Administrative Assistant: Alexandra Murdoch
Mission: To bring professional, equity productions of new and award winning plays and musicals to residents of the Southland and surrounding communities; to provide a full season of seven productions, each running one month, and two summer specialized productions.
Founded: 1976
Specialized Field: Theatrical Group
Status: Professional; Nonprofit
Paid Staff: 8
Volunteer Staff: 6
Paid Artists: 42
Performs At: Illinois Theatre Center
Affiliations: Actors' Equity Association; Theatre Communications Group; League of Chicago Theatres
Annual Attendance: 32,000
Facility Category: Theatre
Type of Stage: Proscenium
Seating Capacity: 179
Year Remodeled: 1999
Cost: $265,000
Organization Type: Performing; Touring; Resident; Educational

2887 PEORIA CIVIC CENTER BROADWAY THEATER SERIES

201 SW Jefferson Street
Peoria, IL 61602-1448
Phone: 309-673-8900
Fax: 309-673-9223
Web Site: www.peoriaciviccenter.com
Management:
   Director Marketing: Marc Burnett
   General Manager: Deb Ritschel
   Director Operations: Bruce Ashley
   Director Event Services: Jim Weatherington
   Director Marketing: Marc Burnett
Mission: Public Assembly / Entertainment Facility
Founded: 1982
Paid Staff: 450
Annual Attendance: 20,000
Facility Category: Theater
Seating Capacity: 2127

2888 PEORIA PLAYERS THEATRE

4300 N University
Peoria, IL 61614
Phone: 309-688-4473
Fax: 309-688-4474
e-mail: players@ocslink.com
Web Site: www.peoriaplayers.com
Management:
   Business Administrator: Nicki Haschke

Mission: Enhances and promotes a tradition of excellence in community theatre by providing theatrical entertainment and by giving everyone an opportunity to participate in the theatre experience.
Founded: 1919
Specialized Field: Community
Status: Non-Professional; Nonprofit
Paid Staff: 2
Volunteer Staff: 50
Non-paid Artists: 100
Budget: $150,000
Income Sources: American Association of Community Theatres; Illinois Theatre Association
Performs At: Peoria Players Theatre
Annual Attendance: 13,000
Facility Category: Handicap-Accessible
Type of Stage: Proscenium
Stage Dimensions: 20x36
Seating Capacity: 350
Year Built: 1957
Year Remodeled: 2000
Rental Contact: Nicki Haschke
Organization Type: Performing; Resident; Educational

2889 CIRCA '21 DINNER PLAYHOUSE

1828 3rd Avenue
Rock Island, IL 61201
Phone: 309-786-2667
Fax: 309-786-4119
e-mail: dpjh@circa21.com
Web Site: www.circa21.com
Management:
   Producer: Dennis Hitchcock
Mission: To offer professional musicals and plays year-round along with the finest in dining.
Founded: 1976
Specialized Field: Dinner
Status: Professional; Commercial
Paid Staff: 65
Affiliations: Vaudeville House Converted
Annual Attendance: 70,000
Type of Stage: Proscenium with Thrust
Seating Capacity: 336
Year Built: 1920
Year Remodeled: 1977
Cost: $500,000
Organization Type: Performing; Touring; Resident

2890 NEW AMERICAN THEATER

118 N Main Street
Rockford, IL 61101
Phone: 815-963-9454
Fax: 815-963-7215
e-mail: webmaster@newamericantheater.com
Web Site: www.newamericantheater.com
Management:
   Artistic Director: Richard Raether
   Administrative Director: Mary L Beaver
Mission: Presenting classic and modern as well as new work.
Founded: 1972
Specialized Field: Theatrical Group
Status: Professional; Nonprofit
Paid Staff: 20
Volunteer Staff: 400

Income Sources: Theatre Communications Group
Performs At: New American Theater
Type of Stage: Main; Second
Seating Capacity: 280; 90
Organization Type: Performing; Touring; Resident; Educational

2891 PHEASANT RUN THEATRE

4051 E Mian
PO Box 64
Saint Charles, IL 60174
Phone: 708-584-6342
Management:
    Producer/Director: Diana Martinez
Founded: 1964
Specialized Field: Dinner
Status: Professional; Commercial
Organization Type: Performing

2892 NORTHLIGHT THEATRE AT THE CORONET

9501 Skokie Boulevard
Skokie, IL 60076
Phone: 847-679-9501
Fax: 847-679-1879
Management:
    Artistic Director: BJ Jones
    Managing Director: Richard Friedman
Mission: The theatre's objective is to challenge, as well as entertain its audiences with a focus to produce compelling new interpretations of contemporary plays drawn from an international repertoire and to create stage adaptions inspired by the full spectrum of artistic disciplines.
Founded: 1974
Status: Professional; Nonprofit
Income Sources: Theatre Communications Group; League of Resident Theatres; American Arts Alliance
Performs At: North Shore Center for the Performing Arts
Organization Type: Resident; Producing

2893 LITTLE THEATRE ON THE SQUARE

16 E Harrison Street
PO Box 288
Sullivan, IL 61951-0288
Phone: 217-728-2065
Fax: 217-728-7525
Toll-free: 888-261-9675
e-mail: theshow@one-eleven.net
Web Site: www.thelittletheatre.org
Management:
    Executive Director: Leonard A Anderson
    Artistic Director: M Seth Reines
Founded: 1957
Status: Nonprofit
Season: June - August
Type of Stage: Proscenium
Stage Dimensions: 28' x 27'
Seating Capacity: 450
Year Built: 1928
Year Remodeled: 1958

2894 UNIVERSITY OF ILLINOIS: SUMMERFEST

4-122 Krannert Center for Performing Arts
500 S Goodwin Avenue
Urbana, IL 61801
Phone: 217-333-0245
Fax: 217-244-1861
e-mail: j-harris@uiuc.edu
Web Site: www.theatre.uiuc.edu
Officers:
    Head: Robert Graves
Management:
    Production Director: JB Harris
Founded: 1991
Specialized Field: Theatre
Status: Non-Equity; Nonprofit
Paid Staff: 21
Volunteer Staff: 9
Paid Artists: 8
Season: June - August
Performs At: Performing Arts Center
Facility Category: Studio Theatre
Type of Stage: Flexible
Seating Capacity: 200

2895 BOWEN PARK THEATRE & OPERA

39 Jack Benny Drive
Waukegan, IL 60087
Phone: 847-360-4740
Fax: 847-662-0592
e-mail: wkarts@waukeganparks.org
Web Site: www.waukeganparks.org

2896 THEATRE OF WESTERN SPRINGS

4384 Hampton Avenue
Western Springs, IL 60558
Phone: 708-246-4043
Fax: 708-246-4015
Web Site: theatrewesternsprings.com
Management:
    Business Manager: Allison Burkharht
    Artistic Director: Tony Vezner
    Children's Theatre Director: Scott Illingwarth
Mission: Promoting, developing and maintaining a community theatre that produces interesting, significant plays; providing a forum for artists.
Founded: 1928
Specialized Field: Theatre
Status: Non-Professional; Nonprofit
Paid Staff: 17
Volunteer Staff: 400
Budget: $750,000
Facility Category: Two theatres
Type of Stage: One open proscenium, one black box
Seating Capacity: 410; 120
Year Built: 1962
Rental Contact: Jeff Arena
Organization Type: Performing; Educational; Sponsoring

2897 INVENTIONS

1047 Gage Street
Winnetka, IL 60093

Phone: 847-446-0183
Fax: 847-446-0183
e-mail: inventions4@earthlink.net
Web Site: http://home.earthlink.net/~inventions4
Management:
   Co-Founder: T Daniel
   Co-Founder: Laurie Willets
   Co-Founder: John Bruce Yeh
   Co-Founder: Teresa Reilly
Mission: An innovative foursome that strikes out in a new direction! A visual slant to cleverly interpret Classical Music and Mime for the new Century.
Founded: 2000
Specialized Field: Music Ensemble
Status: Professional
Paid Staff: 2
Volunteer Staff: 2
Organization Type: Performing; Touring

2898 T. DANIEL PRODUCTIONS
1047 Gage Street
Winnetka, IL 60093
Phone: 847-446-0183
Fax: 847-446-0183
e-mail: tdaniel@tdanielcreations.com
Web Site: tdanielcreations.com
Management:
   Artistic Co-Director/Co-Founder: T Daniel
   Artistic Co-Director/Co-Founder: Laurie Willets
Mission: To create, educate and tour theatrical productions, shows and concert programs dynamically based upon the Art of Mime for audiences of all ages.
Founded: 1971
Specialized Field: Visual Theatre Company
Status: Professional
Paid Staff: 2
Paid Artists: 2

2899 WOODSTOCK OPERA HOUSE
121 Van Buren Street
PO Box 190
Woodstock, IL 60098
Phone: 815-338-4212
Fax: 815-334-2287
e-mail: ophsedir@woodstock-il.com
Web Site: www.woodstock-il.com
Management:
   Managing Director: John H Scharres

2900 ZION PASSION PLAY
2500 Dowie Memorial Drive
Zion, IL 60099
Phone: 847-746-2221
Fax: 847-746-1452
Web Site: www.ourzion.com/passionplay
Management:
   Artistic Director: Ron Arden
Mission: Biblical production about the life of Jesus Christ.
Founded: 1935
Specialized Field: Musical; Community
Status: Non-Professional; Nonprofit
Paid Staff: 200
Income Sources: Christ Community Church

Performs At: Christian Arts Auditorium
Seating Capacity: 522
Organization Type: Performing; Resident; Educational

Indiana

2901 LITTLE THEATRE OF BEDFORD
1704 Brian Lane Way
PO Box 142
Bedford, IN 47421
Phone: 812-279-3009
e-mail: boxoffice@ltb.org
Web Site: www.ltb.org
Officers:
   Treasurer: Denny Underwood
   VP: Tom Taylor
   Secretary: Rachel Fishback
   President: Roger Manning
Management:
   Board of Directors/Executive Commi:
Mission: To offer an opportunity for amateur directors and performers to entertain our community.
Founded: 1960
Specialized Field: Musical; Community; Theatrical Group
Status: Nonprofit
Paid Staff: 150
Performs At: Little Theatre
Organization Type: Performing

2902 SHAWNEE THEATRE OF GREENE COUNTY
PO Box 22
Bloomfield, IN 47424
Phone: 812-384-4562
Fax: 812-659-3144
Officers:
   President: Mary Aiken
Management:
   Producing Director: Rockland Mars
Founded: 1960
Status: Non-Equity; Nonprofit
Paid Staff: 6
Volunteer Staff: 26
Paid Artists: 20
Season: June - July
Annual Attendance: 4,900
Type of Stage: Proscenium
Stage Dimensions: 36' x 20'
Seating Capacity: 360
Year Built: 1979

2903 BLOOMINGTON COUNTY PLAYHOUSE
Indiana University
Bloomington, IN 47405
Phone: 812-855-0074
e-mail: hkibbey@indiana.edu

2904 COMMUNITY THEATRE OF CLAY COUNTY
8 E National
Brazil, IN 47834

All listings are in alphabetical order by state, then city, then organization within the city.

Phone: 812-442-1059
Fax: 973-455-1607
Officers:
   President: Susan M Bradbury
   VP: John Berry
   Secretary/Treasurer: Lois Myers
Mission: To provide opportunities for involvement in the arts in Clay County for all ages, by presenting dinner theatre, musicals, children's workshops, senior citizens programs, and sponsoring drama scholarships.
Founded: 1983
Specialized Field: Musical; Dinner; Community; Theatrical Group
Status: Non-Professional; Nonprofit
Paid Staff: 200
Income Sources: Arts Indiana; Indiana Theatre Association
Organization Type: Performing; Educational

2905 ELKHART CIVIC THEATRE

Bristol Opera House
210 E Vistula, PO Box 252
Bristol, IN 46507-0252
Phone: 219-848-5853
Fax: 219-848-9726
e-mail: ECTinfo@aol.com
Officers:
   President: Cynthia Antonelli
   VP: Stephanie Yoder
   Treasurer: Timothy Yoder
   Secretary: Connie Deuschle
Management:
   Artistic Director: Leslie Torok
   Technical Director: John Shoup
Mission: To produce and present a high-quality and award-winning community theater.
Founded: 1946
Specialized Field: Theatre
Status: Non-Professional; Nonprofit
Paid Staff: 2
Paid Artists: 2
Non-paid Artists: 200
Budget: $125,000
Income Sources: Indiana Arts Commission; Local & Regional Government & Foundation Sources; Business Community; Private & Individual Sources
Performs At: Bristol Opera House
Affiliations: American Association of Community Theatres; ICTL; Performing Arts & Cultural Entertainment of Elkhart County
Annual Attendance: 13,000
Facility Category: Intimate Vaudeville style wood frame/historic
Type of Stage: Proscenium/thrust
Stage Dimensions: 17Wx25D
Seating Capacity: 192
Year Built: 1897
Year Remodeled: 1992
Organization Type: Performing; Resident; Educational

2906 JACKSON COUNTY COMMUNITY THEATRE

121 W Walnut Street
PO Box 65
Brownstown, IN 47220
e-mail: jcctonline@hotmail.com
Web Site: www.jcct.org
Management:
   Artistic Director: Marianne Green
Mission: Producing live plays; Bringing cultural programs to our community.
Founded: 1971
Specialized Field: Dinner; Community; Theatrical Group
Status: Non-Professional; Nonprofit
Income Sources: Indiana Theatre Association
Performs At: Royal Office Square Theatre
Organization Type: Performing; Educational

2907 BROADWAY SERIES: INDIANAPOLIS

200 Medical Drive
Suite D
Carmel, IN 46032
Phone: 317-818-3970
Fax: 317-818-3961
Toll-free: 800-793-7469
Web Site: www.broadwayseries.com

2908 DERBY DINNER PLAYHOUSE

525 Marriott Drive
Clarksville, IN 47129
Phone: 812-288-8281
Fax: 812-288-2636
Toll-free: 877-898-8577
e-mail: tickets@derbydinner.com
Web Site: www.derbydinner.com
Management:
   Producer: Bekki Jo Schneider
   General Manager: Carolyn Thomas
   Group Sales: Cindy Nevitt
Mission: Professional dinner theatre.
Founded: 1974
Specialized Field: Dinner
Status: Professional; Commercial
Paid Staff: 80
Volunteer Staff: 10
Paid Artists: 25
Budget: $4 million
Income Sources: Ticket Sales; Gift Shop, Food, Drink
Performs At: Derby Dinner Playhouse
Affiliations: NAMT, NDTA, ABA, NTA
Annual Attendance: 200,000
Facility Category: Dinner Theatre
Type of Stage: Theatre-in-the-round
Stage Dimensions: 20'x20'
Seating Capacity: 520
Year Remodeled: 1998
Rental Contact: Group Sales Cindy Nevitt
Organization Type: Performing

2909 RIVER CENTER/ADLER THEATRE

136 E 3rd Street
Davenport, IN 52801
Phone: 319-326-8500
Fax: 319-326-8505

Management:
 Executive Director: Mike Hartman

2910 LINCOLN AMPHITHEATRE: MUSICAL OUTDOOR DRAMA

University of Southern Indiana
8600 University Boulevard
Evansville, IN 47712-3596
Phone: 812-465-1668
Fax: 812-464-0029
Toll-free: 800-264-4223
e-mail: lincoln@usi.edu
Web Site: www.lincoln-amphitheatre.com
Officers:
 Marketing Coordinator: Stacy A Brown
Management:
 Choreographer: Barbara Brandt
 Artistic Director: Elliot H Wasserman
 Producer: Iain Crawford
 Producer: Tom Wilhelmus
Founded: 1987
Status: Non-Equity; Nonprofit
Paid Staff: 20
Volunteer Staff: 20
Paid Artists: 40
Non-paid Artists: 10
Season: June - August
Stage Dimensions: 150' x 80'
Seating Capacity: 150

2911 REPERTORY PEOPLE OF EVANSVILLE

Old Courthouse Building
Room 200
Evansville, IN 47708
Mailing Address: PO Box 3555, Evansville, IN 47734
Phone: 812-423-2060
e-mail: plays@repertorypeople.net
Web Site: www.repertorypeople.net
Officers:
 Founder: Tom Angermeier
Management:
 Director: Jim Jackson
 Executive Producer: Tom Angermeier
Mission: To present serious American dramas and occasionally comedies.
Founded: 1973
Specialized Field: Theatrical Group
Status: Non-Professional; Nonprofit
Organization Type: Performing; Resident

2912 ARENA DINNER THEATRE

719 Rockhill Street
Fort Wayne, IN 46835
Phone: 219-493-1384
Mission: To provide an additional option for actors and theatre-goers in the community.
Founded: 1974
Specialized Field: Dinner; Community
Status: Non-Professional
Paid Staff: 50
Income Sources: Fine Arts Foundation; Indiana Theatre Association
Organization Type: Performing

2913 FIRST PRESBYTERIAN THEATER

300 W Wayne Street
Fort Wayne, IN 46802
Phone: 260-422-6329
Fax: 260-422-5111
e-mail: thomhof@juno.com
Management:
 Artistic Director: Thom Hofrichter
Mission: To produce provocative contemporary and classical drama in a supportive atmosphere.
Founded: 1968
Specialized Field: Community
Status: Nonprofit
Paid Staff: 2
Volunteer Staff: 14
Non-paid Artists: 75
Income Sources: Fort Wayne Community Arts Council
Annual Attendance: 8000
Facility Category: 300 Seat Proscenium
Type of Stage: Proscenium
Stage Dimensions: 50 x 22
Seating Capacity: 300
Year Built: 1968
Year Remodeled: 2001
Organization Type: Performing; Educational

2914 FORT WAYNE CIVIC THEATRE

303 E Main Street
Fort Wayne, IN 46802
Phone: 219-422-8641
Fax: 219-422-6699
e-mail: civic@fwa.cioe.com
Web Site: www.fwcivic.org
Officers:
 President: Randall Steiner
 VP: John Burns
 Treasurer: Mark Rupp
 Secretary: Edward Kos
 VP: Ken Menefee
Management:
 Executive Director: Phillip Colglazier
 Business Manager: Carol Coles
 Marketing Director: Carolyn Myers
Mission: Dedicated to strengthening itself as a significant cultural force in the Fort Wayne area through excellence in programming, theatre education and development of talent in the disciplines of theatre and the related performing arts.
Founded: 1928
Specialized Field: Community
Status: Non-Professional; Nonprofit
Paid Staff: 11
Performs At: The Performing Arts Center
Annual Attendance: 50,000
Facility Category: Community Theatre
Type of Stage: Proscenium
Stage Dimensions: 60x30
Seating Capacity: 669
Year Built: 1973
Rental Contact: Shellie Englehart
Organization Type: Resident

2915 BRIDGEWORK THEATER
113 1/2 E Lincoln Avenue
Goshen, IN 46526
Phone: 219-534-1085
Fax: 219-534-9493
Toll-free: 800-200-1602
e-mail: info@bridgework.org
Web Site: www.bridgework.org
Officers:
   President: Ruth Hollinger
   VP: Shirley Lint
   Treasurer: Cheryl Cooper
   Secretary: Lynn Miller
Management:
   Director: Donald C Yost
Mission: To create and perform issue-oriented plays for children in the Great Lakes Region.
Founded: 1979
Specialized Field: Theatrical Group
Status: Professional; Nonprofit
Organization Type: Performing; Touring

2916 AMERICAN CABARET THEATRE
401 E Michigan Street
Indianapolis, IN 46204
Phone: 317-631-0334
Fax: 317-686-5443
Toll-free: 800-375-8887
e-mail: cabaret@americancabarettheatre.com
Web Site: www.americancabarettheatre.com
Management:
   Producing Artist Director/Founder: Claude McNeal
   Associate Director: Mary Lou Szczesiul
   Chairman: Barbara Weaver Smith
   Vice Chairman: Jow Newman
   Treasurer: David Mills
Founded: 1989
Annual Attendance: 60,000
Facility Category: Theatre
Type of Stage: Proscenium
Seating Capacity: 400
Year Remodeled: 2001
Rental Contact: Jeff Owen

2917 BEEF AND BOARDS DINNER THEATRE
9301 N Michigan Road
Indianapolis, IN 46268
Phone: 317-872-9664
Fax: 317-876-0510
Web Site: www.beefandboards.com
Management:
   Managing Director: Robert Zehr
   Artistic Director: Douglas Stark
   Associate Producer: Eddie Curry
   Media Relations: JoEllen Miller
Founded: 1971
Specialized Field: Dinner Theatre
Status: Professional
Paid Staff: 100
Income Sources: National Dinner Theatre Association; American Dinner Theatre Institute
Performs At: Beef and Boards Dinner Theatre
Facility Category: Dinner Theatre
Type of Stage: 3/4 Thrust

Seating Capacity: 480
Rental Contact: Pat Minneman
Organization Type: Performing

2918 EDYVEAN REPERTORY THEATRE
University of Indianapolis
PO Box 47509
Indianapolis, IN 46227-7509
Phone: 317-788-2072
Fax: 317-788-2079
Toll-free: 800-807-7732
e-mail: ert@indy.net
Web Site: www.edyvean.org
Management:
   Artistic Director: Rose Kleiman
   Managing Director: Bill Simmons
   Administrative Director: Frederick Marshall
   Market/Public Relations Director: Anne Penny
   Sales/Box Office Manager: Brandon Truax
   Tech Director/Production Manager: Michael Moffatt
   Scenic Artist: Christian McKinney
   Master Carpenter: Donald-Mac MacIntyre
   Costumer: Chistopher Arthur
Mission: Illuminates the human journey by exploring its many dimensions and celebrating its possibilities.
Founded: 1967
Specialized Field: Theatre
Status: Professional
Performs At: Ransburg Auditorium, University of Indianapolis
Annual Attendance: 12,000
Type of Stage: Proscenium
Seating Capacity: 750

2919 INDIANA REPERTORY THEATRE
140 W Washington Street
Indianapolis, IN 46204-3465
Phone: 317-635-5277
Fax: 317-236-0767
e-mail: indianarep@indianarep.com
Web Site: www.indianarep.com
Officers:
   President: William E Smith
   Vice President: David Klapper
   VP: Jane Schlegel
   Secretary: Marjorie Herald
   Treasurer: David L. Morgan
Management:
   Managing Director: Daniel Baker
   Artistic Director: Janet Allen
   Marketing Director: Richard Ferguson
   Development Director: Meg Gamage Tucker
Mission: Through innovative productions of classic and contemporary plays, the Indiana Repertory Theatre creates high quality, professional theatre of consistent artistic and cultural significance; the theatre also offers student programs.
Founded: 1972
Status: Professional; Nonprofit
Budget: $4,900,000
Income Sources: League of Resident Theatres; Grants from the National Endowment for the Arts; Lila Wallace-Reader's Digest Fund; Schubert Foundation; Ticket Sales
Performs At: Indiana Theatre

Annual Attendance: 124,000
Facility Category: Historic Theatre; Ballroom
Type of Stage: Mainstage; Upperstage; Cabaret
Year Built: 1927
Year Remodeled: 2001
Rental Contact: Erika Keller
Organization Type: Performing; Resident; Educational

2920 PHOENIX THEATRE

749 N Park Avenue
Indianapolis, IN 46202
Phone: 317-635-2381
Fax: 317-635-0010
Web Site: www.phoenixtheatre.org
Management:
Producing Director: Bryan Fonseca
Managing Director: Shannon Callahan
Founded: 1982
Status: Nonprofit
Budget: $400,000

2921 THEATRE ON THE SQUARE

627 Massachusetts Avenue
Indianapolis, IN 46204
Phone: 317-637-8085
Fax: 317-637-0302
e-mail: info@tots.org
Web Site: www.tots.org
Mission: To explore contemporary, classic plays and musicals in an intimate environment.

2922 STAR PLAZA THEATRE

I-65 & US 30
8001 Deleware Place
Merrillville, IN 46410
Phone: 219-757-3549
Fax: 219-756-0604
Officers:
President: Charles Blum
Seating Capacity: 3400

2923 CANTERBURY SUMMER THEATRE/THE FESTIVAL PLAYERS GUILD

PO Box 57
807 Franklin Street
Michigan City, IN 46360
Phone: 219-874-4269
Fax: 219-879-6377
Management:
Productions Administrator: Gerald E Peters
Founded: 1969
Status: Non-Equity; Nonprofit
Season: June - August
Type of Stage: Proscenium
Stage Dimensions: 26'x 26'

2924 RIDGEWOOD ARTS FOUNDATION: THEATRE AT THE CENTER

1040 Ridge Road
Munster, IN 46321-1850

Phone: 219-836-0422
Fax: 219-836-0159
Web Site: www.theatreatthecenter.com
Management:
Artistic Director: Michael Weber
Founded: 1991
Status: Nonprofit
Season: January - December
Type of Stage: Thrust; Flexible
Stage Dimensions: 12' x 8'
Seating Capacity: 454

2925 ROUND BARN THEATRE AT AMISH ACRES

1600 W Market Street
Nappanee, IN 46550
Phone: 219-773-4188
Fax: 219-773-4180
Toll-free: 800-800-4942
e-mail: amishacres@amishacres.com
Web Site: www.amishacres.com
Management:
Producer: Richard Pletcher
Founded: 1986
Status: Non-Equity; Commercial
Season: April - December
Type of Stage: Proscenium
Stage Dimensions: 25' x 35'
Seating Capacity: 360

2926 BROWN COUNTY PLAYHOUSE

70 Buren Street S
Nashville, IN 47448
Mailing Address: PO Box 1187 Nashville, IN 47448
Phone: 812-988-2123
Fax: 812-855-4244
e-mail: jkinzer@indiana.edu
Web Site: www.indiana.edu/~thtr/bcplay.html
Mission: The Brown County Playhouse, a professional theatre operated in conjunction with the Indiana University Department of Theatre and Drama, is located in the center of scenic Nashville.
Status: Not-for-Profit

2927 UNIVERSITY OF NOTRE DAME DEPARTMENT OF FILM, TELEVISION & THEATRE

125 Washington Hall
Norte Dame, IN 46556
Phone: 219-631-5956
Fax: 219-631-3566
e-mail: thtrmail@nd.edu
Web Site: nd.edu/-cothweb/wwwhomepage.html
Management:
Manager-Washington Hall: Tom Barkes

2928 OLE OLSEN MEMORIAL THEATRE

154 S Broadway
PO Box 580
Peru, IN 46970
Phone: 765-472-3680
Web Site: www.oleolsen.org
Officers:

President: Jim Walker
Executive VP: Cheryl Jaquay
Secretary: Michelle Boswell
Treasurer: Sue Malloy
Management:
  Director Of Ticket Sales: Kathy Yeoman
  Producer: Dick Schaffhausen
  Publicity: Kelly Voss
Mission: Purpose of this organization shall be to promote and encourage interest in the theatrical arts on a non-profit basis.
Founded: 1964
Specialized Field: Community; Theatrical Group
Status: Non-Professional; Nonprofit
Income Sources: Indiana Community Theatre League; Division of Indiana Theaters
Performs At: High School Auditorium
Organization Type: Performing

2929 BROADWAY THEATRE LEAGUE OF SOUTH BEND

PO Box 866
South Bend, IN 46624-0866
Phone: 219-234-4044
Fax: 219-288-0290
e-mail: leahwhitebtl@aol.com
Web Site: www.btlsbn.com
Management:
  Executive Director: Leah White
Founded: 1959
Specialized Field: Northern Indiana/Southwest Michigan
Performs At: Morris Performing Arts Center

2930 INDIANA STATE UNIVERSITY SUMMER STAGE

Indiana State University
540 N 7th Street
Terre Haute, IN 47809
Phone: 812-237-3336
Fax: 812-237-3954
e-mail: tharthur@isugw.indstate.edu
Web Site: www.theatre.indstate.edu/
Management:
  Chairman/Artistic Director: Arthur Feinsod
  Production/Business Manager: David Del Colletti
Founded: 1965
Status: Non-Equity; Nonprofit
Paid Staff: 20
Paid Artists: 20
Season: June 15 - July 28
Type of Stage: Thrust; Arena
Seating Capacity: 250

2931 VINCENNES UNIVERSITY SUMMER THEATRE

1002 N First
Vincennes, IN 47591
Phone: 812-885-4256
Fax: 812-885-5868
Management:
  Managing/Artistic Director: James J Spurrier, PhD
Mission: Offering quality theatrical entertainment to Vincennes and surrounding areas in the summer months.

Founded: 1968
Specialized Field: Summer Stock; Musical
Status: Semi-Professional; Nonprofit
Performs At: Shircliff Theatre
Organization Type: Performing; Resident; Educational

2932 WAGON WHEEL THEATRE

PO Box 804
2517 E Center Street
Warsaw, IN 46580
Phone: 219-267-8041
Fax: 219-269-7996
Toll-free: 866-823-2618
Web Site: www.wagonwheeltheatre.com
Officers:
  Business Manger: Carol Craig
  Director Marketing: Carla Robinson
Management:
  Artistic Director: Roy Hine
Founded: 1956
Status: Non-Equity; Commercial
Season: June - September
Type of Stage: Arena
Stage Dimensions: 32' x 35'
Seating Capacity: 835

2933 PURDUE PROFESSIONAL SUMMER THEATRE

1376 Stewart Center
Room 85
West Lafayette, IN 47907
Phone: 317-494-3082
Fax: 317-494-3660
Management:
  Division Theater: Jim O'Connor
  Associate Professor Of Theatre: Russ Jones
  Scenic Construction Supervisor: Ron Clark
  Secretary/Account Clerk: Darlene Flook
  Costume Shop Manager: Shauna Meador
  Operations Manager: Rosie Starks
  Marketing/Public Relations Director: Lori Sparger
Mission: To present more recent American plays both dramatic and comedic.
Founded: 1958
Status: Professional; Nonprofit
Income Sources: Purdue University
Performs At: Experimental Theater
Organization Type: Performing

Iowa

2934 OLD CREAMERY THEATRE COMPANY

39 39th Avenue
Suite 200
Amana, IA 52203
Phone: 319-622-6034
Fax: 319-622-6187
e-mail: octc@netins.net
Web Site: www.oldcreamery.com
Officers:
  President: Bruce Eichacker
  VP: Richard Welch

Treasurer: Vic Rathje
Secretary: Ron Baldwin
Management:
    Producing Director: Thomas Peter Johnson
    Associate Artistic Director: Meg Merckens
    Associate Artistic Director: Sean McCall
Mission: To bring live theater to as many people as possible in rural Iowa.
Founded: 1971
Specialized Field: Theatrical Group
Status: Professional; Nonprofit
Season: March - December
Performs At: Main Stage; Courtyard Stage; The Old Creamery Theatre-Amana
Affiliations: Actors' Equity Association
Annual Attendance: 30,000
Type of Stage: Proscenium; Courtyard Stage
Seating Capacity: 300
Year Built: 1988
Organization Type: Performing; Touring; Resident; Educational

2935 CLINTON AREA SHOWBOAT THEATRE

PO Box 764
Clinton, IA 52733-0764
Phone: 563-242-6760
Fax: 563-242-9247
e-mail: boxoffice@clintonshowboat.org
Season: May - August

2936 BROADWAY THEATRE LEAGUE OF THE QUAD-CITIES

PO Box 130
Davenport, IA 52805
Phone: 319-326-1916
Mission: Supporting New York tours featuring Broadway theatre productions.
Founded: 1960
Status: Nonprofit
Performs At: Adler Theatre
Organization Type: Sponsoring

2937 JUNIOR THEATRE

2822 Eastern Avenue
Davenport, IA 52803
Phone: 563-326-7862
Fax: 563-888-2216
Management:
    Parks/Recreation Department: Bonnie F Guenther
Mission: To offer classes in dance play production and creative drama to students in kindergarten through high school; To present five major productions and twenty eight touring productions.
Founded: 1951
Specialized Field: Community; Dance, Children's Theatre
Status: Nonprofit
Paid Staff: 15
Volunteer Staff: 12
Paid Artists: 4
Income Sources: Local grants/class fees
Performs At: Mary Fluhrer Nighswander Junior Theatre
Affiliations: AATE
Annual Attendance: Classrooms

Facility Category: Theatre, Dance Studio
Type of Stage: Proscenium
Stage Dimensions: 46 W x 30 D with thrust
Seating Capacity: 440
Year Remodeled: 1981
Organization Type: Performing; Touring; Educational
Resident Groups: Professional Modern Dance Company

2938 GRAND OPERA HOUSE

135 8th Street
PO Box 632
Dubuque, IA 52001
Phone: 563-588-4356
Fax: 563-588-3497
e-mail: richgoh@aol.com
Web Site: www.thegrandoperahouse.com
Management:
    Theatre Manager: Richard Hill
    Office Manager: Sheri Eichhorn
    Box Office Manager: William Hoerstman
Mission: To offer quality entertainment and contribute to the community's cultural growth.
Founded: 1971
Specialized Field: Musical; Community
Status: Non-Professional; Nonprofit
Paid Staff: 200
Income Sources: Iowa Community Theatre Association; Dubuque Arts Alliance; Dubuque, Galena & Dyersville Area Chambers of Commerce
Performs At: Grand Opera House
Seating Capacity: 640
Year Built: 1989
Rental Contact: Sheri Eichhorn
Organization Type: Performing; Educational

2939 IOWA SUMMER REPERTORY

University Theatre
N Riverside Drive
Iowa City, IA 52242
Phone: 319-335-2700
Fax: 319-335-3568
e-mail: eric-forsythe@uiowa.edu
Web Site: www.uiowa.edu/theatre
Management:
    Artistic Director: Eric Forsythe
Mission: Retrospective of plays by a single contemporary playwright each season and the development of new scripts.
Founded: 1920
Status: Equity; Nonprofit
Paid Artists: 50
Budget: $170,000
Income Sources: Box office, grants
Season: May - July
Affiliations: AEA; URTA
Type of Stage: Proscenium; Flexible; Black Box
Seating Capacity: 477, 165, 135
Year Remodeled: 1986

2940 RIVERSIDE THEATRE

213 N Gilbert Street
Iowa City, IA 52245

Phone: 772-231-5860
Fax: 772-234-5298
e-mail: companymanager@riversidetheatre.com
Web Site: www.riversidetheatre.org
Officers:
President: Bob Bauchman
VP: Gay Bain
Treasurer: Bob Kingston
Secretary: Craig Marshall
Management:
Artistic Director: Allen D Cornell
Production Manager: Jon Moses
Executive Director: Chuck Still
General Manager: Paul Cazzolla
Mission: Riverside Theatre is committed to providing a broad spectrum of high quality professional theatre on Flordia's Treasure Coast, theatre which explores the sensibilities of the artists without losing sight of the audience. Education plays an integral role in this mission, strengthening the Theatre's ties to the community while at the same time introducing young people to live theatre.
Founded: 1985
Specialized Field: Theatrical Group
Status: Nonprofit
Paid Staff: 35
Volunteer Staff: 20
Paid Artists: 60
Budget: $3 million
Income Sources: Ticket Sales; Annual Giving; Rentals; Special Events
Affiliations: Actors' Equity Association; Florida Professional Theatre Association; LORT
Annual Attendance: 110,000
Facility Category: Theatre
Type of Stage: Proscenium; Black Box
Stage Dimensions: 40x30
Seating Capacity: 610; 300
Year Built: 1973
Year Remodeled: 1990
Rental Contact: Jon Moses
Organization Type: Performing; Touring; Resident; Educational; Sponsoring

2941　SIOUX CITY COMMUNITY THEATRE

1401 Riverside Boulevard
Sioux City, IA 51102
Mailing Address: PO Box 512
Phone: 712-233-2719
Fax: 712-233-1611
e-mail: scctia@aol.com
Web Site: www.scct.org
Officers:
President: Ken Biggerstaff
Vice President: Dave Happe
Secretary: Kristi Quinn
Treasurer: Don Klynsma
Management:
Executive Director: Kelly Hasner
Office Manager: Christina Luther
Building Managers: Deb & Jerry Morgan
Box Office Manager: Julie Ferris
Youth Theatre Director: Kristy Tremayne
Concession Manager: Michelle Foster
Concession Manager: Rick Myers

Mission: To provide an opportunity for people interested in participating in theatrical productions, as well as an educational tool for teaching theatre crafts.
Founded: 1948
Specialized Field: Community; Theatrical Group
Status: Non-Professional
Paid Staff: 12
Volunteer Staff: 500
Paid Artists: 20
Non-paid Artists: 100
Income Sources: Iowa Community Theatre Association
Performs At: Shore Acres
Organization Type: Performing

2942　WATERLOO COMMUNITY PLAYHOUSE & BLACK HAWK CHILDRENS THEATRE

4 Commercial Street
PO Box 433
Waterloo, IA 50704
Phone: 319-235-0367
Fax: 319-235-7489
e-mail: wcpbhct@cedarnet.org
Web Site: www.cedarnet.org/wcpbhet
Officers:
President: Beverly McCuster
President Elect/VP Fund Development: H James Potter
Secretary: Marina Olson
Treasurer: Brad Carter
Management:
Artistic Director: Charles Stilwill
Development Director: Mary Beth O'Brian
Business Manager: Erica Andorf
Children's Theatre Director: Greg Holt
BHCT Director: Gregory Holt
Designer/Production Manager: Steve Stabenow
Costume Director: Patricia Stilwill
Marketing/Development Director: Mary Beth O'Brien
Buisness Manager: Lori Kammerdiner
Mission: Providing quality theatre productions; enhancing the cultural growth of Northeast Iowa.
Founded: 1916
Specialized Field: Theatre
Status: Non-Professional; Nonprofit
Paid Staff: 9
Non-paid Artists: 400
Budget: $552,450
Income Sources: American Association of Community Theatres; Association of American Theatre for Youth; Waterloo, Cedar Falls & Waverly Chambers of Commerce; Iowa Community Theatre Association
Performs At: American Association of Community Theatres; Association of American Theatre for Youth; Waterloo/Cedar Falls/Waverly Chambers
Annual Attendance: 31,640
Facility Category: Arts Center
Type of Stage: Proscenium
Seating Capacity: 367
Year Built: 1965
Year Remodeled: 1977
Organization Type: Performing; Educational; Sponsoring

Kansas

2943 AUGUSTA ARTS COUNCIL/AUGUSTA HISTORICAL THEATRE
PO Box 561
523 State Street
Augusta, KS 67010
Phone: 316-775-2900
Fax: 316-775-7475
e-mail: aacht@worldnet.att.net
Management:
   Executive Manager: Mindy Heusinkveld
Performs At: Auditorium

2944 CHANUTE COMMUNITY THEATRE
PO Box 371
Chanute, KS 66720
Phone: 620-431-1628
e-mail: bushnelln@usct413.k12.ka.us
Mission: To offer the community wide-ranging theatrical entertainment.
Founded: 1978
Specialized Field: Musical; Dinner; Community; Theatrical Group
Status: Non-Professional; Nonprofit
Income Sources: Association of Kansas Theatres
Performs At: Memorial Auditorium; Chanute Country Club
Organization Type: Performing; Resident; Educational

2945 COFFEYVILLE COMMUNITY THEATRE
PO Box 317
Coffeyville, KS 67337
Phone: 316-251-1194
Mission: Providing live theatre for the community.
Founded: 1945
Specialized Field: Musical; Dinner; Community; Theatrical Group
Status: Non-Professional; Nonprofit
Paid Staff: 35
Income Sources: Association of Kansas Theatres; Kansas Arts Council
Performs At: Floral Hall
Organization Type: Performing

2946 BROWN GRAND THEATRE
PO Box 341
310 W 6th Street
Concordia, KS 66901
Phone: 785-243-2553
e-mail: browngrand@dustdevil.com
Web Site: browngrand.org
Officers:
   President: Susan Sutton
   VP: Luann Miller
   Secretary/Treasurer: Wonda Brunkow
Management:
   Theatre Manager: Susan Haver
Mission: Maintaining the historic Brown Grand Theatre; enhancing the cultural life of the area by providing quality theatre.
Founded: 1907
Specialized Field: Musical; Community; Folk; Theatrical Group; Puppet

Status: Professional; Nonprofit
Income Sources: Mid-America Arts Alliance
Organization Type: Performing; Educational; Sponsoring

2947 SALINA COMMUNITY THEATRE
303 E Iron
PO Box 2305
Salina, KS 67401
Phone: 785-827-6126
e-mail: staff@salinatheatre.com
Web Site: www.salinatheatre.com
Management:
   Managing Director: Charles Kephart
Mission: To offer entertainment to the community; to provide recreation for those who would like to participate in theatrical productions.
Founded: 1960
Specialized Field: Musical; Community; Theatrical Group
Status: Non-Professional; Nonprofit
Paid Staff: 50
Organization Type: Performing; Sponsoring

2948 BARN PLAYERS THEATRE
PO Box 12767
Shawnee Mission, KS 66282
Phone: 913-381-4004
Officers:
   President: Margaret Godfrey
   VP: Shirley Wagner
   Secretary: Martha Coulter
Management:
   Managing Director: Margaret Godfrey
   Artistic Director: Max Beatty
   Webmaster/Director: Richard Buswellk
   Marketing Director/House Manager: Tricia Kyler
   Webmaster/Developer/Technical Dir: Scott Bowling
   Graphic Artist/Stage Manager: Bryan Colley
   Co-Founder/Actor/Mistress Elec.: Diane Bulan
Mission: To promote artistic excellence through theatre; to produce community theatre productions; to encourage participation by interested persons; to promote theatre interest in the community.
Founded: 1956
Specialized Field: Community; Theatrical Group
Status: Nonprofit
Income Sources: Association of Kansas Theatres; American Association of Community Theatres
Performs At: Overland Theatre
Organization Type: Performing

2949 TOPEKA CIVIC THEATRE & ACADEMY
3028 SW 8th Street
Topeka, KS 66606
Phone: 785-357-5211
Fax: 913-357-0719
e-mail: carol@topekacivictheatre.com
Web Site: www.topekacivichteatre.com
Management:
   Producing Artistic Director: Michael Wainstein
   Business Manager: Brett Landow
   Box Office Manager: Donna Jenks

All listings are in alphabetical order by state, then city, then organization within the city.

Mission: Stimulating, entertaining, educating and serving our community; providing opportunities for performing and developing theatrical skills.
Founded: 1936
Specialized Field: Musical; Dinner; Community
Status: Non-Professional; Nonprofit
Paid Staff: 100
Income Sources: American Association of Community Theatres; Association of Kansas Theatres; Kansas Community Theatre Conference
Performs At: Topeka Civic Theatre
Type of Stage: Proscenium
Seating Capacity: 286
Organization Type: Performing

2950 COLUMBIAN THEATRE: MUSEUM & ART CENTER

521 Lincoln Avenue
PO Box 72
Wamego, KS 66547-0072
Phone: 785-456-2029
Fax: 785-456-9498
e-mail: ctheatre@wamego.net
Web Site: www.wamego.com
Management:
  Artistic Director: Scott Kickhaefer
Performs At: Peddicord Playhouse

2951 MUSIC THEATRE OF WICHITA

225 West Douglas
Suite 202
Wichita, KS 67202
Phone: 316-265-3107
Fax: 316-265-8708
e-mail: wayne@musictheatreofwichita.org
Web Site: www.musictheatreofwichita.org
Management:
  Producing Director: Wayne Bryan
  Administative Director: David Frain
Mission: Dedicated to stimulating and nurturing interest in musical theatre by producing and or presenting Broadway quality productions, while entertaining and educating patrons, the community, and the theatrical artists.
Founded: 1972
Specialized Field: Theater
Status: Professional; Nonprofit
Paid Staff: 6
Volunteer Staff: 200
Paid Artists: 250
Budget: $2,000,000
Income Sources: Ticket Sales; Fundraisers; Set Rentals; State Funding
Season: June - August
Performs At: Century II Concert Hall
Affiliations: National Alliance for Musical Theatre
Annual Attendance: 70,000
Facility Category: Civic Arts Center
Type of Stage: Proscenium
Stage Dimensions: 44'Wx45'Dx22'H
Seating Capacity: 2,100
Year Built: 1969
Organization Type: Performing; Educational

2952 TAPESTRY PERFORMING ARTS

831 Buffum
Wichita, KS 67203
Phone: 316-265-4405
Fax: 316-265-4405
Management:
  Artistic Director: Nicole Brocksieck
  Music/Marketing Director: Kevin Brocksieck

2953 WICHITA COMMUNITY THEATRE

258 N Fountain
Wichita, KS 67208
Phone: 620-686-1282
e-mail: shortysboy69@cs.com
Web Site: www.wichitacommunitytheatre.com
Officers:
  President: Dona Lancaster
  VP: Terri Ingram
  Secretary: Deanne Zogleman
  Treasurer: Bob Lancaster
Management:
  Business Manager: Scott Marshall
Mission: Providing the community with a wide range of theatrical entertainment; offering opportunities to amateur performers and technicians.
Founded: 1946
Specialized Field: Theatrical Group
Status: Non-Professional; Nonprofit
Income Sources: Association of Kansas Theatres
Performs At: Century II Civic Center; Workshop
Organization Type: Performing

2954 HORSEFEATHERS & APPLESAUCE SUMMER DINNER THEATRE

Southwestern College
100 College Street
Winfield, KS 67156-2499
Phone: 620-229-6328
Fax: 620-229-6335
e-mail: amoon@sckans.edu
Web Site: www.sckans.edu
Management:
  Director Theatre: Roger Moon
Founded: 1973
Status: Non-Equity; Nonprofit
Paid Staff: 35
Volunteer Staff: 10
Season: June 1 - July 31
Type of Stage: Proscenium
Seating Capacity: 240

Kentucky

2955 STEPHEN FOSTER DRAMA ASSOCIATION

US 150 E
PO Box 546
Bardstown, KY 40004

All listings are in alphabetical order by state, then city, then organization within the city.

Phone: 502-348-5971
Fax: 502-349-0574
Toll-free: 800-626-1563
e-mail: info@stephenfoster.com
Web Site: www.stephenfoster.com
Officers:
   Chairman: Richard Heaton
   Vice Chairman: Marylin Dick
   Secretary/Treasurer: Jack Barnes
   Trustee: Steve Hamilton
   Trustee: Howard Keene
   Trustee: Nicky Rapier
   Trustee: Diane Thompson
Management:
   Executive Producer: Bill Coleman
   Director/Choreographer: Scott Holsclaw
   Music Director: David Brown
Mission: Fostering area cultural activities.
Founded: 1959
Specialized Field: Dance; Vocal Music; Theater
Status: Professional; Semi-Professional; Nonprofit
Paid Staff: 45
Paid Artists: 60
Budget: $900,000
Performs At: J. Dan Talbott Amphitheatre
Annual Attendance: 60,000+
Facility Category: Outdoor Amphitheatre
Seating Capacity: 1,500
Year Built: 1958
Year Remodeled: 1997
Organization Type: Amphitheatre

2956 FOUNTAIN SQUARE PLAYERS

414 Main Street
Bowling Green, KY 42101
Phone: 207-782-2787
Web Site: www.geocities.com/fountainsquareplayers
Officers:
   President: Mike Grubbs
   VP: Robyn Murphy
   Secretary: Jennifer Hicklin
   Treasurer: Dr. William B. Russell
Mission: To promote appreciation and enjoyment of theatre.
Founded: 1978
Specialized Field: Community; Theatrical Group
Status: Non-Professional; Nonprofit
Paid Staff: 150
Income Sources: American Arts Alliance
Performs At: Capitol Arts Center
Organization Type: Performing

2957 PIONEER PLAYHOUSE OF KENTUCKY

840 Stanford Road
Danville, KY 40422
Phone: 859-236-2747
Fax: 859-236-4321
e-mail: pioneer@mis.net
Web Site: www.pioneerplayhouse.com
Management:
   Founder/Producer: Colonel Eben Henson
   Artistic Director: Holly Henson
   Director: Robby Henson
Mission: Maintaining an arts vocational training center with professionals as performers and teachers.

Founded: 1950
Specialized Field: Summer Stock; Musical; Dinner
Status: Professional; Nonprofit
Paid Staff: 30
Income Sources: Southeastern Theatre Conference; Kentucky Theatre Association
Season: June - August
Performs At: Colonel Eben Henson Amphitheatre
Organization Type: Performing; Resident; Educational

2958 HARDIN COUNTY PLAYHOUSE

102 W Dixie Avenue
Elizabethtown, KY 42701
Phone: 270-351-0577
Management:
   Board of Directors:
Mission: To provide performing arts for the community.
Founded: 1969
Specialized Field: Musical; Community; Theatrical Group
Status: Semi-Professional; Non-Professional; Nonprofit
Income Sources: Grants
Performs At: Hardin County Playhouse
Annual Attendance: varies
Organization Type: Performing

2959 KINCAID REGIONAL THEATRE

Chapel Street
Falmouth, KY 41040
Phone: 859-654-2636
Toll-free: 800-647-7469
Management:
   Artistic Director: Charles Kondek
   Production Manager: Terry Lee Stump
   Music Director: Bob Myers
   Public Relations: Linda Dietrich
Mission: Employing talented actors and offering quality entertainment to the region.
Founded: 1983
Specialized Field: Musical; Theatrical Group
Status: Professional; Nonprofit
Income Sources: Southeastern Theatre Conference
Performs At: Falmouth Auditorium
Organization Type: Performing; Resident; Educational; Sponsoring

2960 FAR-OFF BROADWAY PLAYERS

2110 Hall Street
Glasgow, KY 42141
Phone: 270-651-8612
Officers:
   President: Eve Harris
   VP: Louise Bachelor
   Secretary: Pat Hazelip
   Treasurer: Phillip Patton
Mission: To study and perform amateur drama.
Founded: 1980
Specialized Field: Community; Theatrical Group
Status: Non-Professional; Nonprofit
Paid Staff: 40
Organization Type: Performing; Resident

2961 MUHLENBERG COMMUNITY THEATRE
119 N Main Street
Greenville, KY 42345-7165
Phone: 270-338-7165
e-mail: weartslady@muhlon.com
Web Site: www.mctiky.com
Officers:
   President: Jeff Dickinson
   VP: Onalee Kidd
   Recording Secretary: Karen Willis
   Corresponding Secretary: David Eplett
   Treasurer: Sherry Lorenzen
   Assistant Treasurer: Daven Edmonds
Management:
   Managing Director: Karen Willis
Mission: Promoting the theatrical arts.
Founded: 1980
Specialized Field: Musical; Dinner; Community; Theatrical Group
Status: Professional; Semi-Professional; Nonprofit
Paid Staff: 20
Income Sources: American Association of Community Theatres
Performs At: Palace Theatre
Year Remodeled: 1999
Organization Type: Performing; Touring; Resident; Educational

2962 LEGEND OF DANIEL BOONE/JAMES HARROD AMPHITHEATRE
Box 365
Harrodsburg, KY 40330
Phone: 606-734-3346
Fax: 602-734-3348
Management:
   General Manager: Maureen Daly
Founded: 1963
Status: Non-Equity; Nonprofit
Season: Mid June - Late August
Type of Stage: Amphitheatre
Stage Dimensions: 60'x 40'
Seating Capacity: 600

2963 HORSE CAVE THEATRE
107 E Main Street
PO Box 215
Horse Cave, KY 42749
Phone: 270-786-1200
Fax: 270-786-5298
Toll-free: 800-342-2177
e-mail: hctstaff@scrtc.com
Web Site: www.horsecavetheatre.org
Officers:
   President: Carla Wertzer
Management:
   Director: Robert Brock
   Development Director: Ann T Baker
   Education Associate: Lynn Gilcrease
   Marketing Director: Melissa McGoire
   Development Director: Kim Harrison

Mission: To be the only resident professional theater outside of metropolitan Louisville that provides a forum for Kentucky writers to produce their works; to present an annual Shakespeare production that assists in meeting the needs of students.
Founded: 1977
Specialized Field: Professional Theatrical Group
Status: Professional; Nonprofit
Paid Staff: 30
Budget: $625,000
Income Sources: Kentucky Arts Council; KY Tourism Cabinet; Corporations; Foundations; Businesses & Individuals
Season: June - December
Performs At: Horse Cave Theatre
Annual Attendance: 30,000
Facility Category: Theatre
Type of Stage: Thrust
Seating Capacity: 346
Year Built: 1977
Year Remodeled: 1993
Architect: Tate Jacobs
Cost: $1,500,000
Organization Type: Performing; Touring; Resident; Educational

2964 ACTORS' GUILD OF LEXINGTON
141 E Main Street
Lexington, KY 40507
Phone: 859-233-7330
Fax: 859-233-3773
e-mail: aguild@qx.net
Web Site: www.actorsguildoflexington.org
Management:
   Artistic Director: Kevin Hardesty
   Managing Director: Tom Hayward
Mission: To produce compelling contemporary theatre for the region.
Founded: 1984

2965 ACTORS' THEATRE OF LEXINGTON
139 W Short Street
Lexington, KY 40507
Phone: 858-233-7330
Fax: 858-233-3773
Management:
   Producing Director: Deb Shoss
   Associate Producing Director: Kevin Hardesty

2966 BROADWAY LIVE AT THE OPERA HOUSE
430 W Vine
Lexington, KY 40507
Phone: 859-233-4567
Fax: 859-253-2718
e-mail: mail@lexingtonoperahouse.com
Web Site: www.lexingtonoperahouse.com
Officers:
   CEO: William B Owen
Management:
   Program Director: Luanne A Franklin
   Marketing Coordinator: Shelia Kenny
   Events Manager: Tom Hagermann
   Technical Director: Bob Stoors

Founded: 1976
Performs At: Broadway Live Series; Variety Series;
Local Artist Groups
Affiliations: APAP; WTAT
Facility Category: Theatre
Type of Stage: Proscenium
Stage Dimensions: 37'3"x21'
Seating Capacity: 1,000
Year Built: 1886
Year Remodeled: 1976
Rental Contact: Program Director Luanne Franklin

2967 LEXINGTON CHILDREN'S THEATRE
418 W Short Street
Lexington, KY 40507
Phone: 859-254-4546
Fax: 859-254-9512
Toll-free: 800-928-4545
Management:
Producing Director: Larry Snipes
General Manager: Ronald K Schull
Production Manager: Vivian R Snipes
Audience Development: Ronlad Smith
Education Director: Jeremy Kisling
Production Stage Manager: Dawn Crabtree
Resident Designer: Eric Morris
Technical Director: Thomas Taylor

2968 STUDIO PLAYERS
West Bell Court
Lexington, KY 40508
Mailing Address: PO Box 23252, Lexington, KY. 40523
Phone: 859-253-2512
Web Site: www.studioplayers.org
Officers:
President: Ashley S Barbour
Past President: Ellen Hellard
President Elect: Gary McCormick
Secretary: Ed Hager
Treasurer: Bob Kinstle
Mission: Studio Players has presented plays since 1953.
Founded: 1953
Status: Nonprofit

2969 ACTORS THEATRE OF LOUISVILLE
316-320 West Main Street
Louisville, KY 40202-4218
Phone: 502-584-1265
Fax: 502-561-3300
e-mail: mail@actorstheatre.org
Web Site: www.actorstheatre.org
Officers:
President: Bruce C Merrick
VP Finance: Frederic H Davis
Treasurer: Bruce K Dudley
Secretary: Sarah D. Fuller
Management:
Artistic Director: Marc Masterson
Executive Director: Alexander Speer
Production Manager: Frazier Marsh
Mission: To offer the finest in professional entertainment
to a wide audience at reasonable prices; to maintain fiscal
responsibility.
Founded: 1964

Status: Professional; Nonprofit
Budget: $8 Million
Income Sources: Ticket sales; grants; contributions
Affiliations: League of Resident Theatres
Annual Attendance: 240,000
Facility Category: 3 theatre complex
Type of Stage: 2 thrust stages and an arena
Seating Capacity: 637; 318; 159
Year Built: 1972
Year Remodeled: 1994
Rental Contact: Mike Brooks
Organization Type: Performing; Resident

2970 KENTUCKY SHAKESPEARE FESTIVAL
1114 S 3rd Street
Louisville, KY 40203
Phone: 502-583-8738
Fax: 502-583-8751
e-mail: tofter@aol.com
Web Site: www.kyshakes.org
Management:
Producing Director: Curt L Tofteland
Director Education: Doug Sumey
Mission: To provide accessible, professional, classical
theatre and quality education touring programs.
Founded: 1960
Status: Professional
Budget: $600,000
Income Sources: Corporate, Foundation, Individuals,
Government, Fund, Earned
Season: May - August
Performs At: C. Douglas Ramey Amphitheater
Annual Attendance: 10,000
Facility Category: Outdoor Ampitheatre
Type of Stage: Thrust
Seating Capacity: 1000
Year Built: 1963
Year Remodeled: 1993
Organization Type: Performing; Resident; Touring;
Educational

2971 MUSIC THEATRE LOUISVILLE
624 W Main Street
Suite 402
Louisville, KY 40202
Phone: 502-589-4060
Fax: 502-589-0741
e-mail: info@musictheatrelouisville.com
Web Site: www.musictheaterlouisville.com
Management:
Artistic Director: Jim Hesselman
Executive Director: Diane Tobin Bennett
Artistic Director: Jim Hesselman
General Manager: Eric Frantz
Director Marketing: Kara Brown
Director Education: Sharon Kinnison
Operations Supervisor: Bill Beauchamp
Box Office Manager: Michelle Kaelin
Administrative Coordinator: Greg Wood
Founded: 1981
Status: Non-Equity; Nonprofit
Season: May - August
Type of Stage: Proscenium
Stage Dimensions: 60' x 50'
Seating Capacity: 1600

2972 STAGE ONE: THE LOUISVILLE CHILDREN'S THEATRE
501 W Main Street
Louisville, KY 40202
Phone: 502-589-5946
Fax: 502-588-5910
Toll-free: 800-989-5946
e-mail: stageone@stageone.org
Web Site: www.stageone.org
Management:
    Producing Director: Moses Goldberg
Mission: To provide high-quality, professional live theatre for young audiences that develops the whole child, supports the learning environment and builds strong family bonds.
Founded: 1946
Specialized Field: Professional theatre
Status: Professional
Paid Staff: 25
Paid Artists: 15
Budget: 1.8 Million
Income Sources: Ticket sales; Grants; Donations
Performs At: Kentucky Center for the Arts; Brown Theatre
Affiliations: The Kentucky Center for the Arts
Annual Attendance: 150,000
Organization Type: Performing; Touring; Educational

2973 THEATRE WORKSHOP OF OWENSBORO
407 W 5th Street
PO Box 644
Owensboro, KY 42302
Phone: 270-683-5003
Fax: 270-683-5003
e-mail: twodrama@bellsouth.net
Web Site: www.theatreworkshop.org
Management:
    Executive Director: John Bryenton
    Assistant: Sandy Self
    Education Director: Sean Dysinger
    House Manager: Tom Mudd
Mission: To offer quality amateur theatre to the Owensboro area; to provide area performers and technicians with opportunities to practice their crafts.
Founded: 1955
Specialized Field: Community
Status: Non-Professional; Nonprofit
Paid Staff: 4
Non-paid Artists: 350
Budget: 140,000
Income Sources: Corporate; Indivdual; Grants
Performs At: Old Trinity Centre; River Park Center
Annual Attendance: 4000
Facility Category: church
Stage Dimensions: 20' x 22'
Seating Capacity: 100
Year Remodeled: 1999
Organization Type: Performing; Resident

2974 MARKET HOUSE THEATRE
141 Kentucky Avenue
Paducah, KY 42003
Phone: 270-444-6829
Fax: 270-575-9321
e-mail: info@mhtplay.com
Management:
    Artistic/Executive Director: April S Cochran
    Technical Director: Michael L Cochran
    Business Manager: Marsha Cash
    Technical Director: Joe Searcy
Mission: To enrich the cultural and artistic life of the community through the presentation of a diverse season; touring; providing educational programs.
Founded: 1964
Specialized Field: Community
Status: Non-Professional; Nonprofit
Paid Staff: 120
Performs At: Market House Theatre
Organization Type: Performing; Touring; Educational

2975 JENNY WILEY THEATRE
PO Box 22
Prestonburg, KY 41653-0022
Phone: 606-886-9274
Fax: 606-886-8875
e-mail: justcasting@aol.com
Web Site: www.jwtheatre.com
Management:
    Managing Director: Martin Childers
    Artistic Coordinator: Scott Bradley
Mission: To enrich our regional community through the performing arts, namely large scale stagings of music theatre classics.
Founded: 1964
Status: Nonprofit; Non-Equity
Paid Staff: 20
Volunteer Staff: 15
Paid Artists: 30
Non-paid Artists: 10
Season: May 30 - August 24
Type of Stage: Proscenium
Stage Dimensions: 44' x 28'
Seating Capacity: 580

2976 RICHMOND CHILDREN'S THEATRE
321 N 2nd Street
Richmond, KY 40475
Phone: 859-254-4546
Fax: 859-254-9512
Mission: To provide young people, ages 8-18, an opportunity to become involved in theatre arts through participation in performances, workhops, stagecraft and crew.
Founded: 1978
Specialized Field: Musical; Community; Theatrical Group
Status: Non-Professional; Nonprofit
Income Sources: Richmond Parks & Recreation Department
Performs At: Eastern Kentucky University Campus Theatre
Organization Type: Performing; Touring; Educational

2977 ROADSIDE THEATER
91 Madison Avenue
Whitesburg, KY 41858

Phone: 606-633-0108
Fax: 606-633-1009
e-mail: roadside@appalshop.org
Web Site: www.appalshop.org/rst
Management:
    Administrative/Producing Director: Tamara Coffey
Mission: Creating original plays concerned with Central Appalachian Mountains home, and collaborating with artists and communities in other marginalized areas.
Founded: 1975
Specialized Field: Theatre/Musical; Theatre/Storytelling Theatre; Community-Building and Arts-In-Education Residencies
Status: Professional; Nonprofit
Paid Staff: 3
Paid Artists: 7
Performs At: Appalshop Theatre
Affiliations: Theatre Communications Group; Alternate ROOTS; American Festical Project; Global Network for Cultural Rights
Seating Capacity: 150
Rental Contact: Barbara Church
Organization Type: Performing; Touring; Educational

Louisiana

2978 BATON ROUGE LITTLE THEATER

7155 Florida Boulevard
PO Box 64967
Baton Rouge, LA 70806
Phone: 225-924-6496
Fax: 225-924-9972
e-mail: brlt@premier.net
Web Site: www.brlt.org
Officers:
    President: Sara Downing
    Vice President Administration: David Kiesel
    VP Publicity: Diane Mayer
    VP Production: Lynn Noland
    Treasurer: Louis LoBue
    Secretary: Gary Schaefer
Management:
    Theater Manager: Jody Banta
Mission: Entertaining, educating and providing an artistic outlet.
Founded: 1946
Specialized Field: Musical; Community
Status: Non-Professional; Nonprofit
Paid Staff: 8
Volunteer Staff: 100
Non-paid Artists: 200
Organization Type: Performing; Educational

2979 SWINE PALACE PRODUCTIONS

PO Box 18699
Baton Rouge, LA 70803
Phone: 504-388-3533
Fax: 504-388-4135
Web Site: www.swinepalace.com
Management:
    Founding Artistic Director: Barry Kyle
    Executive Director: Marilyn Hersey
    Executive Producing Director: Michael Tick

Founded: 1992
Status: Nonprofit
Performs At: Claude L. Shaver Theatre
Type of Stage: Traverse
Stage Dimensions: 111' x 47'
Seating Capacity: 488

2980 COLUMBIA THEATRE/FANFARE

220 E Thomas Street
SLU 10797
Hammond, LA 70402
Phone: 985-543-4366
Fax: 985-543-4369
e-mail: kcouret@selu.edu
Web Site: www.selu.edu
Management:
    Director: Donna Gay Anderson
    Associate Director/Programming: Kerion Couret
    Associate Director/Marketing: Pamela Mills
    Associate Director/Operations: Pete Pfeil
Mission: The mission and purpose of the Columbia Theatre for the Performing arts is to enhance and support Southeastern Louisiana University serves the educational, economic and cultural needs of Southeastern Louisiana.
Founded: 1986
Specialized Field: Performing Arts
Paid Staff: 8
Volunteer Staff: 55
Paid Artists: 25
Non-paid Artists: 10
Budget: $305,811
Income Sources: Ticket Renue; Rental Income; Sorporate Sponsorships; Business and Individual Donations; Poster Sales; Merchandise Commissions
Affiliations: Association of Performing Arts Presenters
Annual Attendance: 51,000
Stage Dimensions: 31'x6'x22'
Seating Capacity: 889
Year Built: 1928
Year Remodeled: 2001
Rental Contact: Pete Pfeil

2981 ARTISTS' CIVIC THEATRE AND STUDIO

One Reid Street
PO Box 278
Lake Charles, LA 70602
Phone: 337-433-2287
Fax: 337-436-5908
e-mail: marcpettaway@aol.com
Management:
    Executive Director: Marc Pettaway
Mission: To give local talent a place to work under the direction of a trained professional director where production values are maintained at a high level; to offer formal classes in various aspects of theatre.
Founded: 1966
Specialized Field: Musical; Dinner; Community; Theatrical Group; Children's
Status: Non-Professional; Nonprofit
Paid Staff: 1
Volunteer Staff: 70+
Non-paid Artists: 50-
Income Sources: Ticket sales; Grants

Performs At: ACTS' One Reid Street Theatre
Facility Category: Community Theatre
Seating Capacity: 125
Organization Type: Performing; Touring; Resident; Educational

2982 LAKE CHARLES LITTLE THEATRE
Canal Place
PO Box 13586
Lake Charles, LA 70185
Phone: 504-522-6545
Web Site: www.southernrep.com
Officers:
   President: Miriam Schulingkamp
   Executive VP: James George
   VP-Development: Gregory Curtis
   Treasurer: Christie Johnsen
   Secretary: Barry Cooper
Management:
   Executive Director: Dick O'Neill
   Artistic Director: Ryan Rilette
Mission: Recognizing a need for professional theater in New Orleans, Dr. Rosary Hartel O'Neill, Dick O'Neill, Nancy Mendard and Clydia Davenport founded Southern Rep Theatre in 1986 with the goal of creating a leading center for Southern playwrights and plays.
Founded: 1926
Specialized Field: Theater
Status: Non-Professional; Nonprofit
Organization Type: Performing

2983 NORTH STAR THEATRE
347 Gerard Street
Mandeville, LA 70448
Phone: 504-624-5266
Fax: 504-626-1692
Management:
   Producing Director: Lori Bennett
Founded: 1991

2984 JUNEBUG PRODUCTIONS
PO Box 2331
New Orleans, LA 70176
Phone: 504-524-8257
Fax: 504-529-5403
e-mail: jpi@artswire.org
Web Site: www.gnofn.org/~junebug
Officers:
   Chairman: Wallace Young
   President: John O'Neal
   VP:
   Treasurer: Theresa Holden
   Secretary: John T. Scott
Management:
   Artistic Director: John O'Neal
   Managing Director: Theresa Holden
Mission: To produce, present and support the development of high-quality theater, dance, music, storytelling and other artistic work that represents, supports and encourages African Americans in the Black Belt South.
Founded: 1980
Status: Professional; Nonprofit
Budget: $300,000

Affiliations: Alternate ROOTs, National Performance Network
Facility Category: Touring theater
Organization Type: Performing; Touring; Educational; Sponsoring

2985 NEW ORLEANS RECREATION DEPARTMENT THEATRE
545 St. Charles Avenue, PO Box 791344
Lafayette Street Entrance
New Orleans, LA 70179
Phone: 504-565-7860
Fax: 504-565-6084
Mission: To present musical comedy productions three times yearly and to involve children, teenagers, and adults.
Founded: 1960
Paid Staff: 4
Non-paid Artists: Var
Budget: Varies
Performs At: NORD Theatre
Annual Attendance: 5,000
Facility Category: Recreation Center
Type of Stage: Proscenium
Seating Capacity: 99

2986 SAENGER THEATRE
143 N Rampart Street
New Orleans, LA 70112
Phone: 504-524-2490
Fax: 504-569-1533
e-mail: mail@saengertheatre.com
Management:
   Booking/Special Sevents Manager: Patricia Baham

2987 SHAKESPEARE FESTIVAL AT TULANE
Tulane University
Department of Theatre & Dance
New Orleans, LA 70118
Phone: 504-865-5105
Fax: 504-865-6737
e-mail: brobbert@tulane.edu
Web Site: www.NewOrleansShakespeare.com
Management:
   Artistic Director: Aimee K Michel
   Managing Director: Clare Moncrief
   Production Manager: Brad Robbert
Mission: To provide professional Shakespeare productions to the Greater New Orleans and surrounding Gulf South area along with educational programs to the schools.
Founded: 1993
Specialized Field: Classical Theatre; Shakespeare; New Works; Modern Classics
Status: Professional; Nonprofit
Paid Staff: 6
Paid Artists: 60
Budget: $250,000
Income Sources: Public; Private; Corporate; Foundation; Box Office; Tuition
Facility Category: Equity Small Professional Theatre
Type of Stage: Black Box; Laboratory
Seating Capacity: 150; 60

2988 SOUTHERN REPERTORY THEATRE

7214 St. Charles
Box 912, Broadway Campus
New Orleans, LA 70118
Phone: 504-861-8163
Web Site: www.southernrep.com/contact.htm
Management:
   Founding Artistic Director: Rosary H O'Neill, PhD
Mission: Professional theatre created for the audience by paying the actors, stage manager, and designers for their art, as contrasted to community and educational theatres which create for educational and social experiences with volunteers. Selections for each season strive to include one masterpiece adapted to a Southern setting; a classic Southern play; and a play which addresses a Southern issue.
Founded: 1986
Specialized Field: Drama
Status: Professional regional theatre
Organization Type: Performing; Educational

2989 TULANE UNIVERSITY THEATRE
Newcomb Dance Program

Department of Theatre and Dance
215 McWilliams Hall
New Orleans, LA 70118
Phone: 504-862-8000
Fax: 504-865-6737
Web Site: www.tulane.edu/~theatre
Management:
   Chairman: Barbara Hayley
Founded: 1937
Performs At: Albert J. Lupin Experimental Theatre, Dixon Hall

2990 ST. JOHN THEATRE

103-205 W 4th Street
Reserve, LA 70084
Phone: 504-536-6630
Web Site: www.stjohntheatre.org
Officers:
   President: Ralph Romaguera, Jr.
   VP: Sterling Snowdy
   Treasurer: Karen Duffy
   Secretary: Robert Beadle
Management:
   Managing Director: Beverly Beard
Mission: Providing live theatre for the community, with particular emphasis on schools and students.
Founded: 1980
Specialized Field: Musical; Community
Status: Non-Professional; Nonprofit; Corporation
Paid Staff: 50
Performs At: St. John Theatre Stage
Organization Type: Performing; Educational

2991 SHREVEPORT LITTLE THEATRE

812 Margaret Place/71101
Shreveport, LA 71134
Mailing Address: PO Box 4853
Phone: 318-424-4439
Fax: 318-424-4440
Web Site: www.shreveportlittletheatre.org
Officers:

President: Dr. David Pov
VP: Jan Pov
Treasurer: Janice Nelson
Secretary: Marcia Cassanova
Management:
   Managing Director: John-Michael Strange
   Artistic Director: Robert K. Darrow
Mission: Committed to producing a variety of quality live theatre with predominantly volunteer participation from the community, with the guidance of trained artistic and managerial leadership, for entertainment, enlightenment and growth of audience awareness and pride.
Founded: 1921
Specialized Field: Community Theatre
Status: Non-Professional; Nonprofit
Budget: $165,000
Income Sources: Memberships; Ticket Sales; Contributions; Annual Fund; Grants
Affiliations: American Association of Community Theatres
Annual Attendance: 10,000+
Facility Category: Theater
Seating Capacity: 140
Year Built: 1925
Year Remodeled: 2002
Cost: $125,000
Organization Type: Performing; Touring

Maine

2992 ARUNDEL BARN PLAYHOUSE

53 Old Post Road
Arundel, ME 04046
Phone: 207-985-5552
e-mail: majordomo@arundelbarnplayhouse.com
Web Site: www.arundelbarnplayhouse.com
Management:
   Production Artistic Director: Adrienne Wilson Grant
Founded: 1998
Season: June - September
Type of Stage: Proscenium
Stage Dimensions: 25' x 22'
Seating Capacity: 225

2993 PUBLIC THEATRE

Two Great Falls Plaza
Box 7
Auburn, ME 04210
Phone: 207-782-2211
Fax: 207-784-3856
Toll-free: 800-639-9575
e-mail: thepublictheatre@aol.com
Web Site: www.thepublictheatre.org
Officers:
   President: Linda S Gretta
   VP: Marilyn Clausson
   Treasurer: Thomas H Platz
   Secretary: Barbara Livingston
Management:
   Artistic Director: Christopher Schario
   Associate Artistic Director: Janet Mitchko
   Development Director: Alice P Chamberlin
   Technical Director: Duper Berry

Mission: Was founded to bring high quality professional theatre to the people of Maine, at affordable prices. We strive to make our presentations accessible to all, especially those less likely by tradition or inclination to attend live theatre.
Founded: 1991
Status: Nonprofit
Paid Staff: 7
Volunteer Staff: 65
Budget: $450,000
Income Sources: Ticket Sales
Annual Attendance: 20,000
Facility Category: Theatre
Type of Stage: Proscenium
Stage Dimensions: 36' x 33'
Seating Capacity: 307

2994 PENOBSCOT THEATRE COMPANY

183 Main Street
Bangor, ME 04401
Phone: 207-947-6618
Fax: 207-947-6678
e-mail: ptcmsf@mint.net
Web Site: www.penobscotTheatre.com
Management:
   Producing/Artistic Director: Mark Torres
   Marketing Director: Judy L Hanscom
Mission: To offer high quality, professional theatre experiences staged throughout the year; to provide educational outreach programs, and to develop and enrich new and existing audiences and artists.
Founded: 1974
Status: Professional; Nonprofit
Paid Staff: 8
Type of Stage: Proscenium
Seating Capacity: 132
Organization Type: Performing; Touring; Resident; Sponsoring

2995 HACKMATACK PLAYHOUSE

538 Route 9
Beaver Dam
Berwick, ME 03901
Phone: 207-698-1807
Fax: 207-698-1162
Web Site: www.members.tripos.com/hackmatack
Management:
   Artistic/Production Director: Sam Scalamoni
Founded: 1971
Status: Non-Equity; Nonprofit
Season: June 27 - September 2
Seating Capacity: 200

2996 CAROUSEL MUSIC THEATRE

Townsend Avenue
PO Box 358
Boothbay Harbor, ME 04538
Phone: 207-633-6440
e-mail: carousel@mint.net
Web Site: www.boothbaydinnertheatre.com/
Management:
   Artistic Director: Dominic Garvey
Founded: 1978
Status: Non-Equity; Commercial

Season: May - October
Type of Stage: Proscenium; Thrust

2997 MAINE STATE MUSIC THEATER

14 Main Street
Suite 109
Brunswick, ME 04011
Phone: 207-725-8769
Fax: 207-725-1199
e-mail: info@msmt.org
Web Site: www.msmt.org
Officers:
   President: Kathy Greason
   Vice President: Doug Niven
   Secretary: Susan Sharpan
   Treasurer: Thomas Pierle
Management:
   Artistic Director: Chuck Abbott
   Managing Director: Raymond M Dumontre
   Company Manager: Kathi Kacinski
Mission: Educating young theatre professionals; presenting quality musical theatre; preserving the American musical.
Founded: 1959
Specialized Field: Summer Stock; Musical
Status: Professional; Nonprofit
Paid Staff: 15
Volunteer Staff: 100
Income Sources: Actors' Equity Association
Season: May - August
Performs At: AEA summer musical theatre
Annual Attendance: 60,000+
Type of Stage: Proscenium
Stage Dimensions: 36 x 32, 5'5 R 5'5 L
Seating Capacity: 600
Organization Type: Performing; Resident; Educational

2998 FIGURES OF SPEECH THEATRE

77 Durham Road
Freeport, ME 04032
Phone: 207-865-6355
Fax: 207-865-6355
e-mail: figures@concentric.net
Web Site: figures.org
Management:
   Co-Director: Carol Farrell
Mission: Tours nationally and internationally. Award winning adult productions as well as family shows. Presenters include Kennedy Center, New Victory Theatre, Jim Henson festival.
Founded: 1982
Specialized Field: Theater
Paid Staff: 2
Volunteer Staff: 3
Paid Artists: 8
Non-paid Artists: 1
Income Sources: Earned & contributed
Annual Attendance: 25,000

2999 DOWNRIVER THEATRE COMPANY

9 O'Brien Avenue
Machias, ME 04654-1397

Phone: 207-255-1200
Fax: 207-255-4864
Toll-free: 888-468-6866
e-mail: ummadmissions@maine.edu
Web Site: www.umm.maine.edu/whatsnew/downriver
Officers:
   President: Skip Cole
Management:
   President: Wendy Schors
Mission: The Downriver Theatre Company will present its 2003 bill of fare in the spacious and well-appointed Performing Arts Center at the University of Maine and Machias.
Founded: 1990
Status: Non-Equity; Nonprofit
Season: June 15 - August 15

3000 THEATRE AT MONMOUTH

PO Box 385
Monmouth, ME 04259-0385
Phone: 207-933-9999
Fax: 207-933-2952
e-mail: tamoffice@theatreatmomouth.org
Web Site: www.theatreatmonmouth.org

3001 ACADIA REPERTORY THEATRE

PO Box 106
Mount Desert, ME 04660
Phone: 207-244-7260
Toll-free: 888-362-7480
e-mail: arep@acadia.net
Web Site: www.acadiarep.com
Management:
   Artistic Director: Kenneth Stack
Mission: In our quaint performance space which seats 148, we have presented an impressive mix of comedies, dramas, mysteries, and children's theatre for over a quarter of a century.
Founded: 1973
Status: Non-Equity; Commercial
Season: July - September
Type of Stage: Flexible; Thrust
Stage Dimensions: 20'x 25'
Seating Capacity: 148

3002 MARITIME PRODUCTIONS

PO Box 2400
Ogunquit, ME 03907
Phone: 207-641-2313
Fax: 207-641-2314
e-mail: maritimeprod@cybertorus.com
Management:
   Artistic Director: Rene Risher
Founded: 1993
Status: Non-Equity; Commercial
Season: June - October

3003 OGUNQUIT PLAYHOUSE

PO Box 915
Ogunquit, ME 03907
Phone: 207-646-2402
Fax: 207-646-4732
e-mail: mail@ogunquitplauhouse.org
Web Site: www.ogunquitplayhouse.org

Officers:
   President: Larry Smith
Management:
   Producer: Roy Rogosin
   General Manager: Henry Weller
   Assistant Producer: Jean Benda
   Director Operations: Kimberly Starling
Founded: 1933
Specialized Field: Summer Theatre
Status: Professional; Commercial
Paid Staff: 29
Volunteer Staff: 10
Paid Artists: 50
Season: June - September
Performs At: Ogunquit Playhouse
Annual Attendance: 40,000
Facility Category: Summer Theatre
Type of Stage: Proscenium
Seating Capacity: 750
Rental Contact: Kemberly Starling
Organization Type: Sponsoring

3004 PORTLAND STAGE COMPANY

25A Forest Avenue
Box 1458
Portland, ME 04104
Phone: 207-774-1043
Fax: 207-774-0576
e-mail: portstage@aol.com
Web Site: www.portlandstage.com
Management:
   Artistic Director: Anita Stewzut
   Managing Director: Joel Thuyer
   Director Marketing/Development: Kippy Rudy
   Director Literacy/Education: Lisa DiFranza
Mission: To produce high-quality work that explores human issues; to entertain, engage and educate the audience.
Founded: 1974
Specialized Field: Theatrical Group
Status: Professional; Nonprofit
Paid Staff: 20
Volunteer Staff: 100
Paid Artists: 60
Budget: $1,200,000
Income Sources: Ticket Sales; Donations
Performs At: Portland Performing Arts Center
Annual Attendance: 45,000
Facility Category: Theater
Type of Stage: Proscenium
Seating Capacity: 290
Year Built: 1920
Year Remodeled: 1979
Rental Contact: Peter Brown
Organization Type: Performing; Resident; Educational

3005 LAKEWOOD THEATER

PO Box 331
Skowhegan, ME 04976
Phone: 207-474-7176
Web Site: www.lakewoodtheater.org
Management:
   Treasurer: Jeffrey Quinn

Mission: Standing in a high grove of stately white birch, Lakewood Theater, the State Theater of Maine, presents high quality entertainment and stage education at a unique and beautiful site that is particularly Maine.
Founded: 1901
Status: Non-Equity; Nonprofit
Season: May - September
Type of Stage: Proscenium
Seating Capacity: 300

3006 SANFORD MAINE STAGE COMPANY

PO Box 486
Springvale, ME 04086
Phone: 207-324-9691
e-mail: peacefreak@webtv.net
Web Site: www.sanfordmainestage.com
Officers:
   President: Leo Lunser
   Secretary: Melanie Emmons
Management:
   Buisness Manager: Mary Stair
Mission: We are a community theater located on Beaver Hill in Springvale, Maine. We offer quality, affordable entertainment for Southern Maine.
Founded: 1984
Status: Non-Equity; Nonprofit
Season: April - December
Type of Stage: Proscenium
Stage Dimensions: 30' x 30'
Seating Capacity: 160

Maryland

3007 ANNAPOLIS SUMMER GARDEN THEATRE

143 Compromise Street
Annapolis, MD 21401
Phone: 410-268-9212
e-mail: info@summergarden.com
Web Site: www.summergarden.com
Management:
   Technical Director: Peter O'Malley

3008 ARENA PLAYERS

801 McCulloh Street
Baltimore, MD 21201
Phone: 410-728-6500
Fax: 410-728-6503
Management:
   Artistic Director: Ed Terry
   Managing Director: Rodney Orange, Jr
   Youth Program Director: Catherine B Orange
Mission: Discovering, fostering and showcasing community talent.
Founded: 1953
Specialized Field: Community; Theatrical Group
Status: Non-Professional; Nonprofit
Paid Staff: 1
Volunteer Staff: 20
Non-paid Artists: all
Income Sources: National Endowment for the Arts; Maryland State Arts Council; Mayor's Committee

Annual Attendance: 12,000
Facility Category: Community Theatre
Type of Stage: Thrust
Stage Dimensions: 22x14
Seating Capacity: 300
Year Remodeled: 1975
Organization Type: Performing; Touring; Educational

3009 AXIS THEATRE

3600 Clipper Mill Road
#114
Baltimore, MD 21211
Phone: 410-243-5237
Fax: 410-243-1294
Web Site: www.axistheatre.org
Management:
   Artistic Director: Brian Klaas
Founded: 1992
Performs At: Axis Theatre
Type of Stage: Proscenium
Seating Capacity: 68

3010 BALTIMORE ACTORS' THEATRE

The Dumbarton House
300 Dumbarton Road
Baltimore, MD 21212
Phone: 410-337-8519
Fax: 410-337-8582
Management:
   Artistic Director: Helen M Grigal
   Executive Director: Walter E Anderson
Mission: Teaching and performing at a professional level.
Founded: 1959
Specialized Field: Musical; Dinner; Theatrical Group; Children's
Status: Semi-Professional; Nonprofit
Performs At: Oregon Ridge Dinner Theatre
Organization Type: Performing; Touring; Educational

3011 CENTER STAGE

700 N Calvert Street
Baltimore, MD 21202-3686
Phone: 410-685-3200
Fax: 410-539-3912
e-mail: info@centerstage.org
Web Site: www.centerstage.org
Management:
   Artistic Director: Irene Lewis
   Managing Director: Michael Ross
   Dramaturg: Jim Magruder
   Director of Audience Development: Barbara Watson
   Media Relations Director: Steve Lickteig
Mission: To serve as Maryland's official theatrical company.
Founded: 1963
Specialized Field: Theatrical Group
Status: Professional; Nonprofit
Paid Staff: 60
Volunteer Staff: 800
Paid Artists: 100
Performs At: Pearlstone Theater, Head Theater
Affiliations: BACVA; Baltimore Tourism Association; Baltimore Theatre Alliance; TCG; AEA
Annual Attendance: 106,462

Type of Stage: Thrust, Flexible
Stage Dimensions: 40' x 36'; 67' x 118'
Seating Capacity: 541, 100-400
Organization Type: Performing; Resident; Educational

3012 CHILDREN'S THEATER ASSOCIATION

100 W 22nd Street
Baltimore, MD 21218-3597
Phone: 612-874-0500
Fax: 410-366-6404
Toll-free: 877-789-0409
e-mail: info@childrenstheatre.org
Web Site: www.childrenstheatre.org
Officers:
   Chairperson: Rebecca Roloff
   Vice Chair: Kenneth Piper
   Vice Chair: Rusty Cohen
   Secretary: Michael Marqulies
   Treasurer: Mary K. Stern
Management:
   Managing Director: Kevin R Daly
   Administrative Assistant: Roz Byus
   Artistic Director: Peter C Brosivs
   Managing Director: Teresa Eyring
Mission: Offering young people creative drama classes and theatre performances that will stimulate creativity.
Founded: 1943
Specialized Field: Children's Theatre
Status: Professional; Nonprofit
Paid Staff: 200
Season: June - August
Organization Type: Performing; Touring; Educational

3013 COCKPIT IN COURT SUMMER THEATRE

CCBC, Essex Campus
7201 Rossville Boulevard
Baltimore, MD 21237-3899
Phone: 410-780-6644
Fax: 410-682-6871
e-mail: fblack@ccbc.cc.md.us
Management:
   Managing Director: Carl Freundel
   Artistic Director: F Scott Black
Mission: Community-based performing arts organization dedicated to providing a variety of quality live theatre opportunities to our performers and audiences including musicals, Shakespeare, drama and children's theatre.
Founded: 1972
Specialized Field: Theatre
Status: Non-Equity; Nonprofit
Paid Staff: 5
Volunteer Staff: 50
Paid Artists: 20
Non-paid Artists: 75
Season: June - August
Type of Stage: Proscenium

3014 DUNDALK COMMUNITY THEATRE

7200 Soillers Point Road
Baltimore, MD 21222
Phone: 410-285-9667
Fax: 410-285-2626
e-mail: sgruhn@ccbc.cc.md.us

Officers:
   President: Charlotte Hayes
   VP: Kevin Ecker
   Secretary: Sue Gruhn
Management:
   Managing Director: Tom Colanna
   Technical Director: Marc Smith
Mission: Community-based performing arts organization of a professional quality at a reasonable ticket price and to be a resource for expanding the cultural experiences of the community
Founded: 1974
Specialized Field: Theatre
Status: Nonprofit
Paid Staff: 3
Paid Artists: 25
Non-paid Artists: 104
Budget: $90,000
Income Sources: Ticket sales; Subscription sales; Private donations; Grants
Performs At: Dundalk Community Theatre
Annual Attendance: 6,800
Seating Capacity: 388
Year Built: 1981
Rental Contact: 410-285-9822 Mary Huffman

3015 THEATRE HOPKINS

The Merrick Barn
The Johns Hopkins University
Baltimore, MD 21218
Phone: 410-516-7159
Fax: 410-516-8198
e-mail: thehop@jhu.edu
Web Site: www.jhu.edu/~theatre/info.html
Management:
   Artistic Director: Suzanne Straughn Pratt
   Box Office Manager: Graham Yearley
Mission: Theatre Hopkins presents a four-play season.
Founded: 1921

3016 THEATRE PROJECT

45 W Preston Street
Baltimore, MD 21201
Phone: 410-752-8558
Fax: 410-539-3091
Management:
   Director: Philip Arnoult
Mission: To support national and international new works and innovative forms of expression; to continue as the entry point for international performing companies; to further promote new performance opportunities for them throughout North America.
Founded: 1971
Specialized Field: Musical; Theatrical Group; Puppet
Status: Professional; Nonprofit
Income Sources: Theatre Communications Group; International Theatre Institute; Towson State University
Performs At: Theatre Project
Organization Type: Sponsoring

3017 ROUND HOUSE THEATRE

EW Highway & Waverly Street
Bethesda, MD 20902

Mailing Address: PO Box 30688 Bethesda, MD 20824-0688
Phone: 240-644-1099
Fax: 240-644-1090
e-mail: roundhouse@roundhousetheatre.org
Web Site: www.roundhousetheatre.org
Officers:
   President: Peter A Jablow
   VP: Judith H Zickler
Management:
   Producing Artistic Director: Jerry Whiddon
   Director Marketing: Mark Robert Blackmon
   Director Production: Danshia Crosby
   Managing Director: Ira Hillman
Mission: To vitalize an ever increasing circle of individuals and communities with a multitude of compelling theatre expirences through performance and education.
Founded: 1978
Specialized Field: Theatrical Group
Status: Professional; Nonprofit
Income Sources: Actors' Equity Association
Performs At: Professional LORT-D Theatre
Organization Type: Performing; Touring; Resident Educational

3018   NEW THEATRE

PO Box 173
Boston, MD 02117
Phone: 617-247-7388
Management:
   Artistic Director: Rick DesRochers
Founded: 1980
Status: Non-Equity; Nonprofit
Season: September - June

3019   REP STAGE

10901 Little Patuxent Parkway
Columbia, MD 21044
Phone: 410-772-4940
Fax: 410-772-4040
e-mail: marietta@howardcc.edu
Web Site: www.howardcc.edu/repstage
Management:
   Artistic Director: Valerie Costantini
   Associate Artistic Director: Kasi Campbell
   Production Manager: Robert Marietta
Founded: 1993
Status: Nonprofit
Paid Staff: 5
Volunteer Staff: 100
Paid Artists: 75
Season: September - March
Affiliations: LOW7, BTA
Annual Attendance: 10,000
Facility Category: Two theatres
Type of Stage: Proscenium; Flexible
Stage Dimensions: 36' x 30'
Seating Capacity: 250; 150
Rental Contact: Sue Kramer

3020   CUMBERLAND THEATRE

101 Johnson Street
Cumberland
Cumberland, MD 21502
Phone: 301-759-4990
Fax: 301-777-7189
e-mail: ctdon@mindspring.com
Management:
   Artistic Director: Don Whitsted
Founded: 1987
Status: Nonprofit
Season: June - December
Type of Stage: Proscenium; Thrust
Stage Dimensions: 40' x 28'
Seating Capacity: 197

3021   ADVENTURE THEATRE: GLEN ECHO PARK

7300 MacArthur Boulevard
Glen Echo, MD 20812
Phone: 301-320-5331
Fax: 301-320-3108

3022   PETRUCCI'S DINNER THEATRE

312 Main Street
Laurel, MD 20707
Phone: 301-490-1993
Management:
   Producer: C David Petrucci
   Producer: Angela Jo Leonard
Founded: 1977
Specialized Field: Dinner
Status: Commercial
Income Sources: National Dinner Theatre Association
Organization Type: Performing

3023   YOUNG ARTISTS THEATER

Route 29 & 216
Cherry Tree Center
Laurel, MD 20723
Phone: 301-604-2844
e-mail: info@youngartiststheater.com
Web Site: www.youngartiststheater.com
Officers:
   Chairman: William P Furr
   Vice Chairman: Henry Mitchell
   Secretary: Carolyn Turner
   Treasurer: Wade Reece
Management:
   Director: Kathy Kurichh
Mission: Presenting live orchestral music for residents of North Carolina; providing music education programs in the schools.
Founded: 1994

3024   SMALLBEER THEATRE COMPANY

4107 33rd Street
Mt. Rainier, MD 20712-1947
Phone: 301-277-8117
Fax: 703-993-2191
e-mail: lraybuck@posf1.gmu.edu
Management:
   Artistic Director: Lynnie Raybuck

Status: Non-Equity; Nonprofit
Season: September - June

3025 OLNEY THEATRE CENTER NATIONAL PLAYERS

2001 Olney-Sandy Spring Road
Olney, MD 20832
Phone: 301-924-3400
Fax: 301-924-2654
e-mail: cbenjamin@olneytheatre.org
Web Site: www.olneytheatre.org
Management:
  Artistic Director: James A Petosa
  Managing Director: Debra L Kraft
  Director Communications: Chuck Benjamin
  General Manager: Bill Snyder
Mission: Mission is to create professional theater productions and other programs to nurture the artist, student, technician, administrator and audience member; to develop each of these individual's potenial and skills using comprehensive possibilities of theater and the performing arts.
Founded: 1938
Specialized Field: Year-round Family Theater
Status: Professional; Nonprofit
Paid Staff: 25
Volunteer Staff: 300
Paid Artists: 200
Budget: 2.5 Million
Income Sources: Actors' Equity Association; Society for Stage Directors and Choreographer
Season: March - Decembers
Performs At: Mainstage; Theatre Lab; Amphitheater
Annual Attendance: 70,000+
Seating Capacity: 450
Year Built: 1938
Year Remodeled: 1992
Rental Contact: Bill Synder
Organization Type: Performing; Touring; Educational

3026 WASHINGTON JEWISH THEATRE

6125 Montrose Road
Rockville, MD 20852
Phone: 301-230-3775
Fax: 301-881-5512
Officers:
  President: Eric Slipp
  Vice President: Dr. Jean Owener
  Secretary: Jameser Pannabecker
  Treasurer: Cynthis A. Thomas
Management:
  Executive Director: Missy Shives
Founded: 1969
Status: Nonprofit

3027 SILVER SPRING STAGE

10145 Colesville Road
Silver Spring, MD 20901
Mailing Address: PO Box 3086 Silver Spring, MD 20918-3086
Phone: 301-593-6036
e-mail: sss@dancinman.com
Web Site: www.ssstage.org
Officers:

Chairperson: Barry Hoffman
Vice-Chairperson: Carol Leahy
Treasurer: Christopher Carey
Secretary: Judie Chaimson
Vice-Chairperson: Norm Seltzer
Management:
  Executive Producer: John Sciarretto
  Technical Director: Don Slater
  Marketing/Publicity Director: Michael Kharfen
  Box Office/House Manager: Chris Kashuba
  Facilities Coordinator: Bill Strein
  External/Community Affairs: Norm Seltzer
  Grants/Fund Raising: Judie Chaimson
  Membership Director: Neil Edgell
  Volunteer Development: Leon Levenson
Mission: Silver Spring Stage Board of Directors

3028 F SCOTT BLACK'S DINNER THEATRE

100 East Chesapeake Avenue
Towson, MD 21286
Phone: 410-321-6595
Fax: 410-823-4390
Web Site: www.fscottblacks.com
Officers:
  President: John R Stike
  Treasurer: Ralph Godwin
Founded: 1982

3029 THEATRE ON THE HILL

McDaniel College
2 College Hill
Westminster, MD 21157
Phone: 410-386-4637
Fax: 410-857-2447
e-mail: jselzer@mcdaniel.edu
Web Site: www.theatreonthehill.com
Management:
  Producer: Ira Domser
  Arts Manager: Josh Selzer
Founded: 1982
Status: Non-Equity; Nonprofit
Paid Staff: 10
Volunteer Staff: 2
Paid Artists: 50
Budget: $125,000
Season: June 10 - August 12
Annual Attendance: 10000
Facility Category: Theatre; Black Box
Type of Stage: Proscenium
Stage Dimensions: 46' x 40'
Seating Capacity: 550; 150
Year Built: 1895
Year Remodeled: 1977

Massachusetts

3030 UNDERGROUND RAILWAY THEATER

41 Foster Street
Arlington, MA 02474
Phone: 781-643-6916
Fax: 781-643-7539
e-mail: info@undergroundrailwaytheatre.org
Web Site: www.undergroundrailwaytheatre.org

Management:
Business Manager: Tracey Clarke
Artistic Director: Debra Wise
Mission: Underground Railway Theater explores a changing landscape of artistic forms and social concerns, combining puppetry, music and acting to engage diverse audiences with images that challenge and delight, inform and celebrate.
Founded: 1976
Specialized Field: Musical; Puppet
Status: Professional; Nonprofit
Paid Staff: 5
Type of Stage: Proscenium
Stage Dimensions: 30' x 18'
Seating Capacity: 140
Organization Type: Performing; Touring; Educational

3031 PILGRAM THEATER RESEARCH & PERFORMANCE COLLABORATION

1948 Conway Road
Ashfield, MA 01330
Phone: 413-628-0112
Fax: 413-628-0112
e-mail: pilgram@mit.edu

3032 BELMONT DRAMATIC CLUB

123 D Sycamore Street
Apartment 4
Belmont, MA 02478
Phone: 617-484-9174
Web Site: www.belmontdramaticclub.org
Officers:
President: Vern Gerig
Vice President: Clifford Grubb
Secretary: Roy Johnson
Treasurer: Carter Lehmann
Mission: Providing quality drama for the community.
Founded: 1903
Specialized Field: Musical; Community; Theatrical Group
Status: Non-Professional; Nonprofit
Paid Staff: var
Volunteer Staff: 10
Paid Artists: var
Non-paid Artists: var
Income Sources: Ticket Sales
Performs At: Payson Park Church
Organization Type: Performing

3033 NORTH SHORE MUSIC THEATRE

PO Box 62
62 Dunham Road
Beverly, MA 01915
Phone: 978-232-7203
Fax: 978-921-0793
Toll-free: 800-926-9220
e-mail: pr@nsmt.org
Web Site: www.nsmt.org
Officers:
President: John P Drislane
Vice President: Donald J Short
Treasurer: Wendell P Wood
Management:
Executive Producer: Jon Kimbell

General Manager: Robert Sweibel
Executive Director: James K Polese
Marketing Director: Joesph Amaral
Chairman: Kevin Bottomley
Vice Chairman: Thomas S Barenboim
Vice Chairman: David Fellows
Secretary/Clerk: Marcia Ruderman
Director Marketing: Joseph Amaral
Mission: To emphasize the development of new musical works and the expansion of educational programming to capture the interest of all age groups in the creative process.
Founded: 1955
Specialized Field: Musical; Theatrical Group
Status: Professional; Nonprofit
Paid Staff: 220
Volunteer Staff: 500
Paid Artists: 400
Non-paid Artists: 0
Budget: 11,000,000.00
Income Sources: Ticket Sales; Contributions
Season: April - December
Performs At: North Shore Music Theatre
Annual Attendance: 350,000
Type of Stage: In-the-Round
Seating Capacity: 1800
Year Built: 1955
Year Remodeled: 1990
Organization Type: Performing; Touring; Educational

3034 BOSTON CHILDREN'S THEATRE

321 Columbus Avenue
Boston, MA 02116
Phone: 617-424-6634
Fax: 617-424-7108
Management:
Executive Director: Patricia M Gleeson
Mission: To promote live theatre for children, by children; Enchanted Forest. Hosted at the Franklin Park Zoo in October.
Founded: 1951
Specialized Field: Theatrical Group
Status: Professional; Nonprofit
Paid Staff: 20
Income Sources: New England Theatre Conference; Association of American Theatre for Youth; Massachusetts Cultural Alliance
Performs At: New England Life Hall
Organization Type: Performing

3035 HUNTINGTON THEATRE COMPANY

264 Huntington Avenue
Boston, MA 02115
Phone: 617-226-7900
e-mail: info@bu.edu
Web Site: www.huntingtonthetre.org
Management:
Managing Director: Michael Maso
Artistic Director: Nicholas Martin
Mission: Remaining faithful to the spirit of classic works; speaking to today's issues through the presentation of trenchant, literate contemporary works new to Boston.
Founded: 1982
Specialized Field: Theatre; Performing Arts
Status: Professional; Nonprofit

Budget: $8 milliom
Income Sources: Ticket Sales; Donations
Season: September - June
Performs At: Boston University Theatre
Annual Attendance: 175,000
Facility Category: Theatre
Type of Stage: Proscenium
Seating Capacity: 890
Rental Contact: Roger Meeker
Organization Type: Performing; Resident

3036 LYRIC STAGE COMPANY OF BOSTON

140 Clarendon Street
Boston, MA 02116
Phone: 617-437-7172
Fax: 617-536-2830
e-mail: lyricmz@aol.com
Web Site: www.lyricstage.com
Management:
   Producing Artistic Director: Spiro Veloudos
   Box Office Manager: Tasmin Elias
   Marketing/Public Relations: MaryAnn Zschau
Mission: Offering high-quality, professional theatre to audiences at low prices, so that they can appreciate their theatrical heritage.
Founded: 1973
Specialized Field: Theatrical Group
Status: Professional; Nonprofit
Paid Staff: 5
Volunteer Staff: 50
Paid Artists: 55
Budget: $750,000
Income Sources: Actors' Equity Association; New England Area Theatres
Season: September - May
Affiliations: AEA, SSOC
Type of Stage: 3/4 Thrust
Seating Capacity: 236
Organization Type: Performing

3037 PUBLICK THEATRE

165 Friend Street
Boston, MA 02134
Phone: 617-782-5425
e-mail: heydiego@aol.com
Web Site: www.publick.org
Officers:
   President: Michael McDermott
   Treasurer: Randall Filer
Management:
   Artistic Director: Spiro Veloudos
   Marketing/Development Director: Deborah Schoenberg
   Artistic Director: Diego Arciniegas
   Artistic Associate: Susanne Nitter
   Production Manager: Maureen Heakey
Mission: To discover, develop and showcase Boston-area theatrical talent in programs of professional quality that are accessible to a diverse audience.
Founded: 1970
Specialized Field: Musical; Theatrical Group
Status: Professional; Nonprofit
Season: June - September
Performs At: The Publick Theatre

Organization Type: Performing; Touring; Resident; Sponsoring

3038 WHEELOCK FAMILY THEATRE

200 The Riverway
Boston, MA 02215
Phone: 617-873-2147
Web Site: www.wheelock.edu/wft/wft.htm
Management:
   Artistic Director: Jane Staab
Mission: The Wheelock Family Theatre is conveniently on The Riverway in Boston, near the museums, Longwood Medical Area, College Corner and Fenway Park.
Founded: 1981
Status: Nonprofit
Season: October - November
Type of Stage: Proscenium
Seating Capacity: 650

3039 PUPPET SHOWPLACE THEATRE

32 Station Street
Brookline, MA 02445
Phone: 617-731-6400
Fax: 617-731-0526
e-mail: info@puppetshowplace.org
Web Site: www.puppetshowplace.org
Officers:
   Board Chairperson: Kym Williams
Management:
   Executive Director: Jovonna Van Pelt
   Artistic Director: Karen Larsen
   Artist-In-Residence: Paul Vincent Davis
   Office Manager: Heather Balchunas
Mission: A non-profit performing arts organization committed to excellence in puppetry for all audiences.
Founded: 1974
Specialized Field: Puppet
Status: Professional; Nonprofit
Income Sources: Puppeteers of America; United International Marionette Association
Organization Type: Performing; Touring; Resident; Sponsoring

3040 AMERICAN REPERTORY THEATRE

64 Brattle Street
Cambridge, MA 02138
Phone: 617-495-2668
e-mail: info@amrep.org
Web Site: www.amrep.org
Management:
   Executive Director: Robert J Orchard
   Artistic Director: Robert Woodruff
   Associate Artistic Director: Gideon Lester
   Founding Director/Creative Cons.: Robert Brustein
Founded: 1966
Status: Nonprofit
Income Sources: Major Grants, Andrew W. Mellon Foundation; The Harold and Mimi Steir Charitable Trust; National Endowment for the Arts; Shubert Foundation; Massachusetts Cultural Council
Season: October - July
Type of Stage: Flexible Prosc.; Proscenium
Seating Capacity: 556; 353

3041 AMERICAN REPERTORY THEATRE
Loeb Drama Center, Harvard University
64 Brattle Street
Cambridge, MA 02138
Phone: 617-495-2668
Fax: 617-495-1705
e-mail: info@amrep.org
Web Site: www.amrep.org
Management:
  Artistic Director: Robert Woodruff
  Executive Director: Robert J Orchard
  General Manager: Jonathan Seth Miller
  Associate Director: Francois Rochaix
  Associate Director: Marcus Stern
  Director Development: Jan Geidt
  Production Manager: Patricia Quinlan
  Marketing Director: Henry Lussier
  Associate Artistic Director: Gideon Lester
Mission: The American Repertory Theatre is a separately incorporated not-for-profit organization chartered to provide a service to the widest possible public in the Boston/Cambridge community and to the theatre world in general.
Founded: 1966
Status: Professional; Nonprofit
Paid Staff: 7
Income Sources: Actors' Equity Association; League of Resident Theatres; Subscriptions; Massachusetts Cultural Councils
Performs At: Loeb Drama Center; A.R.T New Stages
Affiliations: Andrew W. Mellon Foundation; Harold and Mimi Steinberg Charitable Trust; National Endowment for the Arts; Shubert Foundation; PaineWebber Group
Organization Type: Performing; Touring; Resident; Educational

3042 SNAPPY DANCE THEATER
PO Box 400075
Cambridge, MA 02140
Phone: 617-718-2497
e-mail: snappy@snappydance.com
Web Site: www.snappydance.com
Officers:
  Co-Founder: Martha Mason
  Co-Founder: Marjorie Morgan
  Co-Founder: George Whiteside
  President: Barry Chaiken
  Clerk: Gary Sclar
  Treasurer: Philippe Wells
Management:
  Artistic Director: Martha Mason
  Executive Director: Jurgen Weiss
Mission: The group is dedicated to creating compelling performances which work the edge of oxymoron-emotions and images which contradict themselves in art, as in real life.
Founded: 1996

3043 KING RICHARD'S FAIRE
PO Box 419
Carver, MA 02330
Phone: 508-866-5391
Fax: 508-866-8600
Web Site: www.kingrichardsfaire.net

Management:
  Producer: Bonnie Shapiro
  General Manager: Aimee Sedley
Founded: 1982
Status: Non-Equity; Commercial
Season: september - october
Performs At: Outdoor with 10 stages and a tourney field
Annual Attendance: 200,000

3044 CHARLESTOWN WORKING THEATER
442 Bunker Hill Street
Charlestown, MA 02129
Phone: 617-242-3285
Management:
  Managing Director: Kristen Johnson
Mission: To enhance the quality of life through the artistic process.
Founded: 1972
Specialized Field: Summer Stock; Community; Theatrical Group; Puppet
Status: Professional; Semi-Professional; Non-Professional; Nonprofit
Income Sources: Massachusetts Council on the Arts & Humanities
Organization Type: Performing; Touring; Resident; Educational; Sponsoring

3045 MINIATURE THEATRE OF CHESTER
PO Box 722
Chester, MA 01011
Phone: 413-354-7770
Fax: 413-354-7825
Web Site: www.miniaturetheatre.org
Management:
  Artistic Director: Byam Stevens
Founded: 1990
Status: Nonprofit
Budget: $175,000
Season: July - September
Performs At: Theatre
Annual Attendance: 5,500
Facility Category: Town Hall
Type of Stage: Proscenium
Stage Dimensions: 25' x 15'
Seating Capacity: 150

3046 STRAWBERRY PRODUCTIONS
PO Box 12
Chicopee, MA 01021
Phone: 413-592-4184
Fax: 413-594-7758
e-mail: info@strawberryproductions.com
Web Site: www.strawberryproductions.com/
Officers:
  President: Jack Desroches
Management:
  Producer: Jack Desroches
  Division Manager: Nancy J Floyd
  Technical Director: Gary Bessett
Founded: 1976
Specialized Field: Theatre
Status: Commercial; Non-Equity
Season: Year Round

3047 YARD

Box 405
Chilmark, MA 02535
Phone: 508-645-9662
Fax: 508-645-3176
e-mail: theyard@tiac.net
Web Site: home.tiac.net/~theyard
Management:
    Executive Director: DiAnn Ray
    Founder/Artistic Director: Patricia N Nanon
    Administrative Associate/Production: Ernest W Iannaccone
Mission: Stives to promote growth and experimentation in theatre arts with its mission to give professional artists the time and space to create and perform dance, music, theatre pieces in a concentrated and supported environment.
Founded: 1973
Specialized Field: Dance
Status: Non-Equity; Nonprofit
Paid Staff: 2
Season: Summer
Type of Stage: Black Box
Stage Dimensions: 34'x 28'
Seating Capacity: 100

3048 CAPE PLAYHOUSE

820 Main Street
Route 6A
Dennis, MA 02638
Mailing Address: PO Box 2001 Dennis, MA 02638
Phone: 508-385-3838
Fax: 508-385-8162
Toll-free: 877-385-3911
Web Site: www.capeplayhouse.com
Officers:
    President: James Wilson
    VP: Avard Craig
    Treasurer: Katherine Dorshimer
    Secretary: Robert Oek
Management:
    Managing Director: Kathleen A Fahle
    Artistic Director: Evans Haile
Mission: Established by the Raymond Moore Foundation and chartered by the Commonwealth of Massachusetts in 1948, Cape Playhouse operates for educational and charitable purposes as well as presenting top summer entertainment with stars of stage, screen and television.
Founded: 1927
Specialized Field: Summer Stock
Status: Professional; Nonprofit
Season: June - September
Performs At: Cape Playhouse
Organization Type: Performing

3049 GLOUCESTER STAGE COMPANY

267 E Main Street
Gloucester, MA 01930
Phone: 508-281-4099
Fax: 508-283-5150
e-mail: info@intermktg.com
Management:
    Business Director: Mary John Boylan
    Publicity Director: Heidi J Dallin
    Production Stage Manager: Janet Howes
    Artistic Director: Israel Horovitz
    Production Coordinator: Keri Ellis Cahill
    Assistant Artistic Director: Robbie Chasitz
    Technical Director: Rob Duggan
Mission: To support contemporary playwrights through staged readings and productions of important new plays.
Founded: 1979
Specialized Field: Theatrical Group
Status: Professional; Nonprofit
Organization Type: Performing; Resident; Educational; Sponsoring; Producing

3050 ARENA CIVIC THEATRE

PO Box 744
Greenfield, MA 01302
Phone: 413-774-5898
Web Site: www.arenacivictheatre.org
Officers:
    President: Jerry Marcanio
    VP (External): Phyllis Roy
    VP (Internal): Steve Woodard
    Secretary: Elisa Martin
    Treasurer: Sondra Radosh
Mission: To recognize the unique ability of theatre to provide spiritual fulfillment and personal growth for its participants.
Founded: 1971
Specialized Field: Community; Theatrical Group
Status: Non-Professional; Nonprofit
Paid Staff: 70
Income Sources: National Association of Local Arts Agencies; Mohawk Trail Association
Performs At: Shea Theater; Turner Falls, MA
Organization Type: Performing

3051 HINGHAM CIVIC MUSIC THEATRE

Box 50
Hingham, MA 02043
Phone: 781-749-0083
Mission: To foster theatre arts and music in the community.
Founded: 1935
Specialized Field: Musical; Dinner; Community; Theatrical Group
Status: Non-Professional; Nonprofit
Performs At: Hingham High School Auditorium
Organization Type: Performing; Resident; Educational

3052 CAPE COD MELODY TENT

21 W Main Street
Hyannis, MA 02601
Phone: 508-775-9100
Fax: 508-778-0899
e-mail: info@musiccircus.com
Web Site: www.melodytent.com
Management:
    General Manager: Vince Longo
Founded: 1950
Status: Not-for-Profit
Season: June 1 - September
Seating Capacity: 2300

3053 VILLAGE PLAYERS
PO Box 81
Hyannis, MA 69350
Phone: 308-458-2701
Management:
    Artistic Director: Al Davis
Mission: To present and sponsor theatre.
Founded: 1980
Specialized Field: Summer Stock; Musical; Dinner;
Community; Theatrical Group
Status: Professional; Semi-Professional; Nonprofit;
Commercial
Organization Type: Performing; Touring; Sponsoring

3054 FOOTLIGHT CLUB
Eliot Hall
7A Eliot Street
Jamaica Plain, MA 02130
Phone: 617-524-6506
e-mail: boxoffice@footlight.org
Web Site: www.footlight.org
Officers:
    President: Paul Campbell
    VP: Jane Yoffe
    Secretary: Derek Clark
    Treasurer: Jason Sheehan
Management:
    Box Office Manager: Bill Shamlian
    House Management Director: Tom Brady
    Producations Director: Gail Debiak
    Technical Director: Paul O'Shaughnessy
    Volunteers Director: Sarah Kary
Mission: To provide quality theatre as an integral
component of a vital arts community and to offer
involvement to anyone interested in theatre.
Founded: 1877
Specialized Field: Community; Theatrical Group
Status: Non-Professional; Nonprofit
Paid Staff: 200
Performs At: Eliot Hall
Organization Type: Performing; Resident

3055 SHAKESPEARE & COMPANY
70 Kemble Street
Lenox, MA 01240-2813
Phone: 413-637-3353
Fax: 413-637-4274
e-mail: general@shakespeare.org
Web Site: www.shakespeare.org
Officers:
    President/Artistic Director: Tina Packer
    Chairman: Michael A Miller
Management:
    Artistic Director: Tina Packer
    Managing Director: Christopher Sink
    General Manager: Steve Ball
    Artistic Associate/Communications: Dan McCleery
Mission: To create a theatre of unprecedented excellence
in the Elizabethan ideals of inquiry, balance and harmony.
To establish a theatre company which, by its commitment
to the creative impulse, is a revolutionary force in society,
which connects the truths of the past to the challenges and
possibilities of today, which finds its source in the
performance of Shakespeare's plays and reaches the wides
possible audience through trainig and education.
Founded: 1978
Specialized Field: Theatre, Theatre Training/Education
Paid Staff: 33
Volunteer Staff: 250
Paid Artists: 100
Budget: $3.8 million
Income Sources: Earned Income; Contributions
Season: May - January
Performs At: Founders' Theatre, SpringLawn Theatre
and outdoor space at 70 Kemble Street.
Annual Attendance: 45,000
Notes: Wheelchair accessible.

3056 MERRIMACK REPERTORY THEATRE
Liberty Hall
50 E Merrimack Street
Lowell, MA 01852
Phone: 978-454-6324
Fax: 978-934-0166
e-mail: info@merrimackrep.org
Web Site: www.merrimackrep.org
Management:
    Artistic Director: Charles Towers
    General Manager: Edgar Cyrus
    Managing Director: Lisa B Merrill-Buttzak
Mission: To present engaging, vital theatre that
communicates to the audience.
Founded: 1979
Specialized Field: Theatrical Group
Status: Professional; Nonprofit
Paid Staff: 20
Paid Artists: 50
Budget: $1.8 million
Season: September - June
Performs At: Liberty Hall
Affiliations: Society for Stage Directors and
Choreographers; Actors' Equity Association; USA;
Dramatists Guild
Annual Attendance: 60,000
Type of Stage: 3/4 Thrust
Stage Dimensions: 34x30
Seating Capacity: 384
Year Built: 1900
Year Remodeled: 1984
Organization Type: Performing; Resident

3057 ACTORS THEATRE OF NANTUCKET
The Historic Methodist Church
2 Centre Street
Nantucket, MA 02554-4100
Phone: 508-228-6325
e-mail: actors@nantucket.net
Web Site: www.nantuckettheatre.com
Management:
    Artistic Director/Founder: Richard Cary
    Associate Director: Jane Karakula
Mission: To offer professional theatre to Nantucket
Island.
Founded: 1985
Specialized Field: Musical; Theatrical Group; Children's
Theatre
Status: Professional; Nonprofit; Non-Equity

Organization Type: Performing; Resident; Educational; Sponsoring

3058 THEATRE WORKSHOP OF NANTUCKET

PO Box 1297
Nantucket, MA 02554
Phone: 508-228-4305
e-mail: johnmillar@attbi.net
Web Site: www.theatreworkshop.com
Officers:
    President: Elizabeth Gilbert
    Treasurer: Marie Giffin
Management:
    Business Manager: Edgar A Anderson
    Artistic Director: S. Warren Krebs
Mission: To bring theatrical stage entertainment to the community using local talent; to offer year-round productions.
Founded: 1956
Specialized Field: Community
Status: Non-Professional; Nonprofit
Paid Staff: 25
Performs At: Bennett Hall
Organization Type: Performing; Educational

3059 ZEITERION THEATRE

PO Box 4084
684 Purchase Street
New Bedford, MA 02741-4084
Phone: 508-997-5664
Fax: 508-999-5956
e-mail: zeiterion@usa.net
Web Site: www.zeiterion.com
Officers:
    President: Philip M Carney
    Vice President: Ben Baker
    Treasurer: Doug Rodrigues
Management:
    Executive Director: Christopher J Le Blanc
Mission: To provide the community with a wide range of quality programs in the performing arts.
Founded: 1982
Status: Professional; Nonprofit
Income Sources: New England Presenters
Performs At: Zeiterion Theatre
Seating Capacity: 1,057
Organization Type: Performing; Touring; Sponsoring

3060 NEW REPERTORY THEATRE

54 Lincoln Street
PO Box 610418
Newton, MA 02161-0418
Phone: 617-332-7058
Fax: 617-527-5217
e-mail: info@newrep.org
Web Site: www.newrep.org
Management:
    Producing Artistic Director: Rick Lombardo
    Producing Associate: Adam Zahler
    Marketing Director: Harriet Sheels
Mission: Producing 5 professional theatre productions each year with an emphasis on area premieres and the classics.

Founded: 1984
Specialized Field: Theatre
Status: Nonprofit
Paid Staff: 5
Volunteer Staff: 100
Paid Artists: 75
Season: September - June
Affiliations: TCG; NEAT; NETC; MASSK
Type of Stage: Thrust
Stage Dimensions: 20' x 30'
Seating Capacity: 160

3061 JEWISH THEATRE OF NEW ENGLAND

Leventhal-Sidman Jewish Community Center
333 Nahanton Street
Newton Center, MA 02459-3213
Phone: 617-558-6480
Fax: 617-244-8290
e-mail: Pgoldman@jccgb.org
Web Site: www.lsjcc.org/cultural_arts/
Management:
    Performance Artistic Director: Barrie Keller
Founded: 1984
Status: Nonprofit
Season: Fall & Spring
Type of Stage: Thrust
Stage Dimensions: 48' x 30'
Seating Capacity: 250-450

3062 AVAILABLE POTENTIAL ENTERPRISES

150 Main Street
Northampton, MA 01060
Phone: 413-586-5553
Fax: 413-586-7313
Officers:
    President: Gordon G Thorne
Management:
    Executive Director: Gordon G Thorne
    Association Director: Lisa Thompson
Mission: To support the work of local and guest artists.
Founded: 1975
Specialized Field: Visual and Performing Arts
Status: Professional; Nonprofit
Paid Staff: 3
Volunteer Staff: 15
Performs At: Third Floor Thornes
Annual Attendance: 4,000
Facility Category: Open loft space for Theatre and two Art Galleries
Type of Stage: Open Loft
Seating Capacity: 100
Year Built: 1975
Organization Type: Touring; Resident; Sponsoring

3063 CALVIN THEATER

136 W Street
Northampton, MA 01060
Phone: 413-586-2632
Fax: 413-586-1162
e-mail: jordi@shortstreet.com
Web Site: iheg.com
Management:
    Creative Director: Jordi Herold

3064 NEW CENTURY THEATRE
PO Box 186
Northampton, MA 01061-0186
Phone: 413-537-3933
Fax: 413-585-3354
e-mail: NCTheatre@aol.com
Web Site: www.smith.edu/theatre/nct
Management:
   Producing Director: Sam Rush
Mission: Produces four productions from June-August and are beginning to produce productions in the fall and spring.
Founded: 1991
Status: Nonprofit
Season: June - August
Type of Stage: Black Box
Seating Capacity: 134

3065 FIDDLEHEAD THEATRE COMPANY
109 Central Street
Norwood, MA 02062
Phone: 781-762-4060
e-mail: fiddleheaddrama@aol.com
Web Site: www.fiddleheadtheatre.com
Officers:
   President: Meg Fofonoff
Management:
   Artistic Director: Meg Fofonoff
   Associate Producer: Stacie Moye
   Business Manager: Darrell Moye
Mission: The Fiddlehead Theatre Company in Norwood, MA is a non-profit orginazation which draws its strength from the rich talents of local amateurs and volunteers as well as gifted professionals, and has already brought pleasures to thousands of Boston area residents.

3066 ACADEMY OF PERFORMING ARTS
PO Box 1843
120 Main Street
Orleans, MA 02653
Phone: 508-255-3075
Fax: 508-255-8704
Officers:
   President: Edward Lewis
   Vice President, Production: Dick Hatch
   Treasurer: C Page McMahan
Management:
   Director: Carol Demas
   Director: Raymond Froso
   Director: Marcia Galazzi
Mission: To provide an educational opportunity for students and people of all ages and backgrounds to further their abilities, understanding and appreciation for jazz. To increase public awareness and appreciation for jazz as an American art form. To preserve the history and foster the development of this unique music. To bring world class performers and educators to greater Cleveland audiences.
Founded: 1975
Specialized Field: Musical; Community; Theatrical Group; Education
Status: Professional; Semi-Professional; Non-Professional; Nonprofit
Paid Staff: 800
Paid Artists: y

Non-paid Artists: y
Income Sources: Productions; Memberships; Fundraising & Events; Private Donation
Performs At: Academy Playhouse
Affiliations: Orleans Chamber of Commerce
Annual Attendance: 21,000
Facility Category: Playhouse
Type of Stage: Arena
Seating Capacity: 162
Rental Contact: Artistic Director Peter Bartle
Organization Type: Performing; Touring; Educational; Sponsoring

3067 PROVINCETOWN REPERTORY THEATRE
PO Box 812
Provincetown, MA 02657
Phone: 508-487-0600
Management:
   Artistic Director: Ken Hoyt
   General Director: Ted Vitale
   Administrative Director: Margie Mahrdt
Performs At: Pilgrim Monument

3068 ROBBINS-ZUST FAMILY MARIONETTES
20 Reservoir Road
Richmond, MA 01254
Phone: 413-698-2591
Fax: 413-698-2080
e-mail: genieszust@aol.com
Web Site: www.berkshireweb.com/zust
Management:
   Actor/Designer: Genie Zust
   Actor/Designer: Maia Robbins-Zust
   Actor/Designer: Dion Robbins-Zust
   Actor/Designer: Anne Undeland
   Actor/Director: Genie Zust
Mission: To pass on to the next generations the ancient stories and the art and craft of puppetry and to delight all ages.
Founded: 1971
Specialized Field: Puppetry
Status: Professional
Budget: $30,000
Income Sources: Performances
Performs At: Theatres; Homes; Stores; Schools throughout New England/New York
Annual Attendance: 10,000+
Type of Stage: Marionette
Stage Dimensions: 14'x8'x10'
Organization Type: Performing; Touring

3069 SHARON COMMUNITY THEATRE
53 High Street
Sharon, MA 02067
Phone: 617-784-3721
Management:
   Business Manager: Tina Koppel
   Publicity: Dick Leemon
Mission: To present family-oriented, high quality, local entertainment consisting mainly of play productions to the South Shore area at reasonable prices.
Founded: 1975

Specialized Field: Community; Theatrical Group
Status: Nonprofit
Paid Staff: 60
Income Sources: New England Theatre Conference
Performs At: Sharon Recreation Department
Mini-Theatre
Organization Type: Performing; Educational

3070 BARRINGTON STAGE COMPANY

Box 1205
Sheffield, MA 01257
Phone: 413-528-8888
Fax: 413-528-8807
e-mail: marketing@barringtonstageco.org
Web Site: www.barringtonstageco.org
Management:
Artistic Director: Julianna Boyd
Director Education: Mira Hilbert
General Manager: Bonnie English
Director Marketing: Eric Shamie
Founded: 1994
Specialized Field: Summer theatre
Performs At: Consolati Performing Arts Center
Seating Capacity: 500
Notes: Wheelchair accessible, assisted-hearing devices
available

3071 STUDEBAKER MOVEMENT THEATER COMPANY

1 Fitchburg Street
B450
Somerville, MA 02143
Phone: 617-782-6226
Management:
Tour Manager: John Bay
Mission: Creating new performance works.
Founded: 1978
Specialized Field: Theatrical Group; Performance
Status: Professional
Paid Staff: 10
Income Sources: National Movement Theatre
Association
Performs At: Performance Place
Organization Type: Performing; Touring; Resident;
Sponsoring

3072 SUMMER THEATRE AT MT. HOLYOKE COLLEGE

50 College Street
South Hadley, MA 01075
Phone: 413-538-2632
Fax: 413-538-3036
e-mail: sdaniels@summertheatre.net
Web Site: www.summertheatre.net
Officers:
President: Debra Guston
VP: Jennifer Symington
Treasurer: Roger Allard
Management:
Artistic Director: Susan Daniels
Production Manager: Christopher Paul
Director/Education: Van Farrier

Mission: To provide Western Massachusetts with the
highest quality summerstock entertainment while
educating and nurturing a new genetration of theatre
artists.
Founded: 1970
Specialized Field: Theatre
Status: Professional; Nonprofit
Budget: $425,000
Income Sources: Ticket Sales; Sponsors; Donors;
Businesses; Grants
Season: June - August
Annual Attendance: 15,000
Facility Category: Mainstage
Type of Stage: Thrust
Stage Dimensions: 36'x36'
Seating Capacity: 400
Year Remodeled: 2000

3073 STAGEWEST

One Columbus Center
Springfield, MA 01103
Phone: 413-781-4470
Fax: 413-781-3741
Web Site: www.springfieldweb.com/stagewest/
Management:
Artistic Director: Eric Hill
Managing Director: Martha Richards
Artistic Administrator: Catherine Mandel
Marketing/Public Relations: Rebecca Strang
Mission: The presentation of resident professional
theatre, education and outreach programs, research, and
the development of revitalized classics and new work.
Founded: 1967
Status: Professional; Nonprofit
Paid Staff: 10
Income Sources: Theatre Communications Group;
American Arts Alliance; League of Resident Theatres
Performs At: S. Prestley Blake Theatre; Winifred Arms
Studio Theatre
Organization Type: Performing; Resident; Educational

3074 VINEYARD PLAYHOUSE

24 Church Street
Box 2452
Vineyard Haven, MA 02568
Phone: 508-693-6450
Fax: 508-696-9299
e-mail: info@vineyardplayhouse.org
Web Site: www.vineyardplayhouse.org
Officers:
Chairperson: George L Cohn
Clerk: Gerald Yukevich
Treasurer: Ted E Desrosiers
Management:
Artistic Director: MJ Bruder Munafo
Managing Director: Josh Sommers
Mission: Community based professional theater dedicated
to developing, producing and presenting exceptional live
theater for adults and children; to providing educational
programs; and to encourage and supporting the work of
theater artists of all ages, abilities and ethnic and social
background.
Founded: 1982
Specialized Field: Professional Theater (AEA)
Status: Nonprofit

Paid Staff: 6
Paid Artists: 100
Budget: $450,000
Season: June - October
Type of Stage: Black Box
Seating Capacity: 120

3075 SPINGOLD THEATER CENTER

PO Box 9110
Brandeis University
Waltham, MA 02254
Phone: 781-736-3400
Fax: 617-736-3389
e-mail: theater@brandeis.edu
Web Site: www.brandeis.edu/theater/
Management:
    General Manager: John-Edward Hill
    Theatre Arts Program Director: Michael Murray
    Production Manager: Mark Stevens
Mission: To offer an educational program blending booked programming with resident professionals; to provide a broad training program.
Founded: 1964
Specialized Field: Theater
Status: Professional; Nonprofit
Income Sources: New England Theatre Conference; Massachusetts Cultural Alliance
Performs At: Spingold Theater Center
Organization Type: Performing; Educational

3076 HISTORY MAKING PRODUCTIONS

100 Summer
Suite 3-6
Watertown, MA 02172
Phone: 617-924-4430
Officers:
    Chairperson: Lisa Gregory
    Secretary Clerk: Judith Einach
    Treasurer: Richard Freedberg
Management:
    Director: Linda Myer
Mission: To tour live, professional plays which dramatize historical events and people; to bring literature to life; to spark critical thinking and thoughtful discussion on gender, race, social diversity and social change.
Founded: 1976
Specialized Field: Theatrical Group
Status: Professional; Nonprofit
Income Sources: Massachusetts Advocates for Arts; Sciences & Humanities; Stage Source
Organization Type: Performing; Touring; Educational

3077 WELLFLEET HARBOR ACTORS THEATER

PO Box 797
Wellfleet, MA 02667
Phone: 508-349-3011
Toll-free: 866-282-9428
e-mail: info@what.org
Web Site: www.what.org
Officers:
    President: Carol Green
Management:
    Co-Artistic Director: Gip Hoppe

Producing Artistic Director: Jeff Zinn
Mission: To present most adventurous professional theater company.
Founded: 1985
Status: Nonprofit; Equity
Season: May - October
Type of Stage: Proscenium
Seating Capacity: 90

3078 HARWICH JUNIOR THEATRE

105 Division Street
PO Box 168
West Harwich, MA 02671
Phone: 508-432-0934
Fax: 508-432-0726
e-mail: hjt@capecod.net
Web Site: www.hjtcapecod.org
Management:
    Business Manager: Mary Jane Byrne
    Artistic Director: Nina Schuessler
Mission: To provide young people with the opportunity to explore and expand their creative talents and aspirations; to entertain, develop, and foster a love and full appreciation of theatre and the enrich lives through the theatrical experience.
Founded: 1951
Specialized Field: Theater; Education and Production
Status: Non-Equity; Nonprofit
Paid Staff: 3
Season: June - August
Type of Stage: Thrust
Stage Dimensions: 20' x 30'
Seating Capacity: 210

3079 NEW PHOENIX

42 Cold Spring Road
Williamstown, MA 01267
Phone: 413-458-2411
Officers:
    President: Ralph Hamman
    Vice President: Dana Swanson
Management:
    Artistic Director/Producer: Ralph Hammann
    Associate Director: Douglas Bradburd
Mission: To produce a diversity of small-cast, transportable theatre pieces; special interest in Samuel Beckett, mono dramas, psychological thrillers and black comedies.
Founded: 1975
Specialized Field: Theatrical Group
Status: Professional; Semi-Professional; Nonprofit
Organization Type: Performing; Touring; Educational; Sponsoring

3080 FOOTHILLS THEATRE COMPANY

100 Front Street
Suite 137
Worcester, MA 01608
Phone: 508-754-3314
Fax: 508-767-0676
e-mail: info@foothillstheatre.com
Web Site: www.foothillstheatre.com
Officers:
    President: Guy Jones

Treasurer: James F Goulet
Clerk: Hon Mel Greenberg
Management:
Artistic Director: Brad Kenney
General Manager: Virginia Chojnicki
Mission: To provide professional regional theatre for Worcester and the Central New England Region and serve the region by providing many ancillary services including a theatre conservatory, intern/apprentice programs, youth services, services for the communicatively and physically disabled and more.
Founded: 1974
Specialized Field: Theatrical Group
Status: Professional; Nonprofit
Income Sources: Actors' Equity Association
Season: October - May
Performs At: Foothills Theatre Company
Type of Stage: Proscenium
Seating Capacity: 349
Organization Type: Performing

3081 WORCESTER CHILDREN'S THEATRE

6 Chatman Street
Worcester, MA 01609
Phone: 404-315-0235
Management:
Director Programs/Development: Mary Pantano
Managing Director: Liz Humphreys
Artistic Director: Steven Braddock
Mission: Providing performances and educational programming that educates children about theatre.
Founded: 1968
Specialized Field: Children's Theatre
Status: Professional; Semi-Professional; Nonprofit
Performs At: Worcester State College; Administration Building
Organization Type: Performing; Touring; Educational

3082 WORCESTER FORUM THEATER

6 Chatham Street
Worcester, MA 01609
Phone: 508-799-9166
Fax: 508-799-9166
Management:
Artistic Director: Brian T Tivnan
Founded: 1985
Status: Nonprofit
Season: Year Round
Type of Stage: Black Box; Amphitheatre
Seating Capacity: 110; 400+

Michigan

3083 COMMUNITY THEATRE ASSOCIATION OF MICHIGAN

4619 W Van Buren Road
Alma, MI 49441
Phone: 616-927-1492
e-mail: peska@cmsinter.net
Officers:
President: Terry Jolink
VP: Harry Johnson

Treasurer: Kevin Arnett
Secretary: Bill Haycook
Executive Secretary: Nancy Peska
Mission: To foster cooperation and communication among all community theatre groups in Michigan; to Provide educational programs.
Founded: 1951
Status: Nonprofit
Affiliations: Arts Council For Chautauqa County
Annual Attendance: 5000
Organization Type: Service Organization

3084 THUNDER BAY THEATRE

400 N Second Avenue
Alpena, MI 49707
Phone: 989-354-2264
e-mail: TBT@deepnet.com
Web Site: www.oweb.com/upnorth/tbt
Officers:
President: Kathryn Kunze
Management:
Artistic Director: Chip Lavely
Mission: To enhance the cultural life of Northeast Michigan.
Founded: 1967
Specialized Field: Summer Stock; Musical; Theatrical Group
Status: Professional; Nonprofit; Non-Equity
Season: May - September
Performs At: Thunder Bay Theatre
Type of Stage: Proscenium
Stage Dimensions: 33' x 15'
Seating Capacity: 180
Year Built: 1930
Organization Type: Performing; Resident; Educational

3085 PERFORMANCE NETWORK OF ANN ARBOR

120 E Huron
An Arbor, MI 48104
Phone: 734-663-0696
Fax: 734-663-7367
e-mail: pnetwork@bizserve.com
Management:
Artistic Director: Dan Walker
Marketing/Sales Director: David Wolber
Development Director: Carla Milarch
Executive Director: Johanna Broughton
Founded: 1981
Specialized Field: Theatre
Paid Staff: 10
Paid Artists: 70

3086 UNIVERSITY PRODUCTIONS: UNIVERSITY OF MICHIGAN

Department of Theatre & Drama
2550 Frieze Building
Ann Arbor, MI 48109-1265
Phone: 734-764-5350
Fax: 734-747-2282
Web Site: www.theatre.music.umich.edu
Management:
Managing Director: Jeffrey Kuras
Dean School of Music: Paul Boylan

Mission: To create 10 productions annually through the departments of Musical Theatre, Opera and Theatre and Dance.
Founded: 1973
Specialized Field: Musical; University
Status: Professional; Nonprofit
Paid Staff: 200
Performs At: Power Center for the Performing Arts; Trueblood Theatre
Type of Stage: Flexible; Proscenium; Arena
Seating Capacity: 1414; 650; 200
Organization Type: Performing; Educational

3087 BARN THEATRE
13351 W Michigan 96
Augusta, MI 49012
Phone: 616-731-4545
Fax: 616-731-2306
e-mail: barntheatre@aol.com
Web Site: www.barntheatre.com
Management:
  Founder/Producer: Jack P Ragotzy
  Co-Producer: Brendan Ragotzy
  Apprentice Coordinator: Penelope Aalex Ragotzy
  General Manager: Howard McBride
  Resident Manager: James B Knox
  Assistant Producer: Brendan Ragotzy
Mission: To offer high-quality professional summer theatre to Southwestern Michigan.
Founded: 1946
Specialized Field: Summer Stock; Musical; Plays
Status: Professional; Commercial
Paid Staff: 14
Paid Artists: 40
Income Sources: Actors' Equity Association
Organization Type: Performing; Resident

3088 BAY CITY PLAYERS
1214 Colombus Avenue
Bay City, MI 48708
Phone: 989-893-5555
e-mail: bcplayers@chartermi.net
Web Site: www.baycityplayers.com
Mission: To provide quality theatrical productions for our area.
Founded: 1917
Specialized Field: Musical; Community; Theatrical Group
Status: Nonprofit
Income Sources: Community Theatre Association of Michigan
Facility Category: Theatre
Organization Type: Performing

3089 CALUMET THEATRE COMPANY
340 Sixth Street
PO Box 167
Calumet, MI 49913
Phone: 906-337-2166
Fax: 906-337-4073
e-mail: calumettheartre@chartermi.net
Web Site: www.calumettheatre.com
Officers:
  Board Director: Johnnie De Bernard

Board Director: Andrew Gryuruch
Management:
  Executive Director: James F O'Brien, III
  Technical Director: James Jacobson
Mission: Hosting and sponsoring performing events.
Founded: 1900
Specialized Field: Musical; Dinner; Community; Folk; Theatrical Group
Status: Professional; Nonprofit
Income Sources: Michigan Association of Community Arts Agencies
Organization Type: Educational; Sponsoring

3090 PURPLE ROSE THEATRE COMPANY
137 Park Street
Chelsea, MI 48118
Phone: 734-475-5817
Fax: 734-475-0802
e-mail: purplerose@earthlink.net
Web Site: www.purplerosetheatre.org
Officers:
  VP: Gail Bauer
  Treasurer: John Mann
  Secretary: William Holmes
Management:
  Artistic Director: Guy Sanville
  Managing Director: Alan Ribant
  Company Manager: Christine Purchis
  Associate Artistic Director: Anthony Caselli
  Executive Director/President: Jeff Daniels
Founded: 1991
Specialized Field: Professional Theater
Status: Nonprofit
Paid Staff: 24
Paid Artists: 75
Season: September - August
Type of Stage: Thrust
Seating Capacity: 160

3091 ATTIC / NEW CENTER THEATRE
2990 W Grand Boulevard
Suite 308
Detroit, MI 48202
Phone: 313-875-8285
Officers:
  Chairman: Andy Soffel
  President: Lavinia Moyer
  Treasurer: Peter C Gray
  Secretary: Paul R. Retenbach
Management:
  Artistic Director: Lavinia Moyer
  Managing Director: Jim Moran
Mission: Attic/New Center Theatre is a resident, professional theatre company committed to the development of actors, directors, playwrights, and technicians as craftsmen in the art of theatre. It exists to create new works and to present new and challenging plays by contemporary playwrights.
Founded: 1975
Specialized Field: Musical; Theatrical Group
Status: Professional; Nonprofit
Income Sources: Theatre Communications Group; Foundation for the Extension and Development of American Professional Theatre
Performs At: The New Center Theatre

Organization Type: Performing; Touring; Resident; Educational

3092 DETROIT REPERTORY THEATRE

13103 Woodrow Wilson
Detroit, MI 48238
Phone: 313-868-1347
Fax: 313-868-1705
e-mail: detrepth@aol.com
Officers:
    Chairperson: Frances Beeman
Management:
    Artistic Director/Managing Director: Bruce E Millan
Mission: The Detroit Repertory Theatre has demonstrated that racial harmony and non-traditional casting (casting without racial distinction) can produce an artistic vitality and quality second to none and win over an audience in sufficient numbers to prove viability.
Founded: 1956
Specialized Field: SE Michigan
Status: Professional; Nonprofit
Paid Staff: 7
Volunteer Staff: 6
Budget: $800,000
Income Sources: Box Office; Grants; Contributors
Season: November - June
Performs At: Theatre
Affiliations: TCG, AFA, DMCVB
Annual Attendance: 30,000+
Type of Stage: Proscenium
Stage Dimensions: 28' x 26'
Seating Capacity: 194
Year Remodeled: 1990
Organization Type: Performing
Resident Groups: Hire only indigenous professional artists.

3093 HILBERRY THEATRE, WAYNE STATE UNIVERSITY

Cass and Hancock
Detroit, MI 48202
Phone: 313-577-3340
Fax: 313-577-5495
Toll-free: 888-457-8357
e-mail: ac8806@wayne.edu
Management:
    Chairman/Director: Blair Anderson
    Director Public Relations: Shawn Seuell
    Assistant Director Public Relations: Beth Thibault
Founded: 1963
Status: Non-Professional; Nonprofit
Paid Staff: 60
Volunteer Staff: 100
Budget: $2.5 Million
Income Sources: Box Office; Fundraising; Grants; University
Performs At: Hilberry Theatre
Affiliations: Association for Theatre in Higher Education; U/RTA; National Association of Schools of Theatre
Annual Attendance: 50,000
Facility Category: Theatre
Type of Stage: Thrust
Seating Capacity: 530
Year Remodeled: 1963

Organization Type: Performing; Touring; Resident; Educational; Sponsoring
Resident Groups: Repertory Company

3094 MASONIC TEMPLE THEATRE

500 Temple Avenue
Detroit, MI 48201
Phone: 313-832-2232
Fax: 313-832-1047
Web Site: www.masonicdetroit.com
Management:
    Managing Director: Alan N Lichtenstein
Mission: Presents broadway productions.
Opened: 1926
Specialized Field: Grand Opera; Ballet; Musical and Comedy Concerts
Status: Professional
Affiliations: Fisher Theatre
Facility Category: Live Stage Theatre
Type of Stage: Proscenium
Seating Capacity: 4,404
Year Remodeled: 1990

3095 PLOWSHARES THEATRE COMPANY

2870 Grand Boulevard
Suite 600
Detroit, MI 48202-3146
Phone: 313-872-0279
Fax: 313-872-0067
e-mail: plowshares@earthlink.net
Web Site: www.plowshares.org
Officers:
    President: Justin Klimko
    VP: Mildred Morton Cross
    Secretary: Johnnie Hunter
    Treasurer: Bessie Burden
Management:
    Producing Artistic Director: Gary Anderson
    Office Manager: Pearl Kali
    Production Manager: Janet Cleveland
    Managing Director: Addell Anderson
Mission: To produce relevant, high quality African American theatre for a culturally and socially diverse audience through the establishment of supportive relationships within the civic, religious and business communities.
Founded: 1989
Specialized Field: Theatrical Group
Status: Professional; Nonprofit
Paid Staff: 4
Volunteer Staff: 140
Paid Artists: 30
Budget: $500,000
Affiliations: BTN; TCG; NCAAT; MAPT; DMVCB
Organization Type: Performing; Touring

3096 THEATER GROTTESCO

PO Box 32658
Detroit, MI 48232
Phone: 313-961-5880
Management:
    Co-Artistic Director: John Flax
    Co-Artistic Director: Elizabeth Wiseman

Mission: To create modern original plays; to conduct master classes and training workshops.
Founded: 1983
Specialized Field: Theatrical Group
Status: Professional; Nonprofit
Income Sources: Association of Performing Arts Presenters; Theatre Communications Group; Arts Midwest; National Association for Campus Activities
Organization Type: Performing; Touring; Educational

3097 CIVIC THEATRE & SCHOOL OF THEATRE

30 North Division
Grand Rapids, MI 49503
Phone: 616-222-6650
Fax: 616-222-6660
Web Site: www.grct.org
Management:
Executive Director: Bruce Tinker
Founded: 1925

3098 COMMUNITY CIRCLE THEATRE

161 Ottawa NW
Suite 408
Grand Rapids, MI 49503
Phone: 616-456-5535
Fax: 616-456-8540
Management:
Managing Director: Joe Dulin

3099 URBAN INSTITUTE FOR CONTEMPORARY ARTS

41 Sheldon Boulevard SE
Grand Rapids, MI 49503
Phone: 616-454-7000
Fax: 616-454-7013
e-mail: uica@iserv.net
Web Site: www.uica.org
Officers:
President: Tom Clinton
Vice President: Daryl Fischer
Second VP/Secretary: Heidi Holst Leeestma
Treasurer: David J. Everett
Management:
Executive Director: Jill Donabauer
Program Manager: Gail Philbin
Administrative Coordinator: Brenda Cain
Facilities Manager: Aaron Smith
Special Events Coordinator: Carole Walters
Mission: To foster cultural dialogue and creative activity through innovative and diverse events and services.
Founded: 1977
Seating Capacity: 170

3100 HOPE SUMMER REPERTORY THEATRE

PO Box 9000
Hope College
Holland, MI 49422-9000
Phone: 616-395-7600
Fax: 616-395-7180
e-mail: arts@hope.edu
Web Site: www.hope.edu
Management:

Producing Director: Mary Schakel
Founded: 1972
Status: Non-Equity; Nonprofit
Season: June - August
Type of Stage: Thrust
Seating Capacity: 500

3101 IRONWOOD THEATRE

109 E Aurora Street
Ironwood, MI 49938
Phone: 906-932-0618
Fax: 906-932-0457
e-mail: office@ironwoodtheatre.org
Web Site: www.ironwoodtheatre.org
Officers:
President: Dale Ballone
VP: Tom Brown
Secretary: Lee Brown
Treasurer: David Sauter
Management:
Administrative Assistant: Andrea Soltis
Mission: To provide cultural entertainment of the highest possible quality to the greatest number of people in the Western Upper Peninsula of Michigan and Northern Wisconsin.
Founded: 1928
Budget: $125,000
Income Sources: Grants; State of Michigan; Fund Raisers
Performs At: Auditorium
Affiliations: Michigan Council for Arts-Cultural Affairs
Annual Attendance: 20,000
Facility Category: Performing Arts Center
Type of Stage: Proscenium
Stage Dimensions: 28'6"w x 23'l
Seating Capacity: 732
Year Built: 1928
Year Remodeled: 1983
Cost: $160,000
Rental Contact: Managing Director Kaye Johnson

3102 ACTORS & PLAYWRIGHTS' INITIATIVE

359 S Burdick Street
Suite 205, Epic Center
Kalamazoo, MI 49007
Phone: 616-343-8090
Fax: 616-343-8450
e-mail: theaterapi@aol.com
Management:
Artistic Director: Robert C Walker
Marketing Director: Jeremy M Morris
Founded: 1989
Specialized Field: Southwest Michigan
Paid Staff: 6
Volunteer Staff: 12
Paid Artists: 20
Non-paid Artists: 12
Performs At: Epic Center
Facility Category: Theatre
Type of Stage: Black Box
Seating Capacity: 120

All listings are in alphabetical order by state, then city, then organization within the city.

3103 KALAMAZOO CIVIC PLAYERS

329 S Park Street
Kalamazoo, MI 49007
Phone: 616-343-2280
Fax: 616-343-0532
Web Site: www.kazoocivic.com
Management:
    Managing Director: James C Carver
Mission: Offering the finest possible dramatic experience
to the area.
Founded: 1929
Specialized Field: Theatrical Group
Status: Nonprofit
Paid Staff: 250
Income Sources: American Association of Community
Theatres; Community Theatre Association of Michigan
Performs At: Civic Auditorium; Carver Center
Organization Type: Performing

3104 WHOLE ART THEATER

326 W Kalamazoo
Kalamazoo, MI 49007
Phone: 616-344-0182
e-mail: wholeart@net-link.net
Management:
    Artistic Director: Sniedze Rungis
    Educational Director: Daniel Runyan
    Managing Director: Francis Bilancio
    Office Manager: Matthew Clysdale
Mission: To offer experimental theater to all; to maintain
a touring schedule throughout the Midwest.
Founded: 1976
Specialized Field: Theatrical Group
Status: Professional; Nonprofit
Income Sources: Great Lakes Performing Arts
Association
Organization Type: Performing; Touring; Educational

3105 BOARSHEAD THEATER

425 S Grand Avenue
Lansing, MI 48933
Phone: 517-484-7800
Fax: 517-484-2564
e-mail: boarshead@boarshead.org
Web Site: www.boarshead.org
Management:
    Founding Artistic Director: John Peakes
    Managing Director: Judith Peakes
    Director Public Relation/Market: Carey McConkey
    Director Education: Nancy Rominger
Mission: Boarshead theater exists to entertain, educate
and inspire audiences of all ages throughout Michigan.
Founded: 1966
Specialized Field: Professional theater company
Status: Professional
Paid Staff: 14
Paid Artists: 75
Budget: $1,000,000
Income Sources: Michigan Council of Arts & Cultural
Affairs; National Endowment for the Arts
Performs At: Lansing Center for the Arts
Affiliations: TCG; Actors' Equity Association;
International Alliance of Theatrical Stage Employees;
Lansing Chamber of Commerce

Annual Attendance: 25,000
Type of Stage: Semicircular Thrust
Seating Capacity: 250
Year Remodeled: 1975
Organization Type: Performing; Touring; Resident;
Educational; Sponsoring

3106 CHERRY COUNTY PLAYHOUSE

425 W Western
Suite 406
Muskegon, MI 49440
Phone: 231-727-8888
Fax: 231-722-0549
Toll-free: 800-686-9666
e-mail: wmccp@aol.com
Web Site: www.cherrycountyplayhouse.org
Management:
    Producing Director: Bill Castellino
    General Manager: Gwen W Nelson
Mission: To preserve the art of musical theater by
presenting the most exciting classical and contemporary
musicals while also creating new works that expand the
range of the audience's experience.
Founded: 1955
Specialized Field: Summer Stock
Status: Professional; Commercial
Paid Staff: 3
Paid Artists: 120
Budget: $1,000,000
Income Sources: Box Office; Grants; Private Donations
Performs At: Performance Center
Annual Attendance: 35,000
Facility Category: Performing Arts Center
Type of Stage: Proscenium
Stage Dimensions: 41'6" x 29'
Seating Capacity: 1750
Year Built: 1930
Year Remodeled: 1998
Cost: 8.2 million
Rental Contact: Susan McGarry
Organization Type: Performing

3107 PORT HURON CIVIC THEATRE

701 Me Morran Boulevard
PO Box 821
Port Huron, MI 48060
Phone: 810-985-6166
Fax: 810-985-3358
e-mail: webmaster@mcmorran.com
Web Site: www.memorran.com
Officers:
    President: Ernest Werth
    1st Vice President: Bryan Shelby
    Second VP: Denise Selby
    Secretary: Chris Hendrickson
    Treasurer: Jennifer Dent
Management:
    General Manager: Larry Krabach
    Administrative Director: Lynn Hines
    Box Office Manager: Pat David
    Marketing Director: Karen Pennewell
Mission: To offer a theatre season each year; to train and
educate; to promote theatre arts.
Founded: 1957
Specialized Field: Community; Theatrical Group

Status: Semi-Professional; Nonprofit
Paid Staff: 200
Income Sources: Saint Clair County Community College
Performs At: McMorran Place Theatre
Organization Type: Performing; Educational

3108 SHELDON THEATRE

443 W 3rd Street
PO Box 34
Red Wing, MI 55066
Phone: 651-385-3664
Fax: 651-385-3663
e-mail: sdowse@ci..red-wing.mn.us
Web Site: www.sheldontheatre.org
Management:
    Executive Director: Sean Dowse

3109 MEADOW BROOK THEATRE

Oakland University
Rochester, MI 48309-4401
Phone: 248-370-3310
Fax: 248-370-3108
e-mail: mbrkthea@oakland.edu
Web Site: www.mbtheatre.com
Management:
    Interim Artistic Director: Debra Wicks
    Managing Director: Gregg Bloomfield
    Director Marketing: Rob Gold
Mission: To present a broad variety of top-quality live theatre, ranging from classic to contemporary works; to offer seven plays each season.
Founded: 1967
Specialized Field: Theatrical Group
Status: Professional; Nonprofit
Income Sources: Oakland University; Concerned Citizens for the Arts in Michigan
Season: September - May
Affiliations: LORT
Annual Attendance: 100,000+
Facility Category: Theatre
Type of Stage: Proscenium
Seating Capacity: 584
Year Built: 1963
Organization Type: Performing; Touring

3110 RED BARN PLAYHOUSE

PO Box 670
Saugatuck, MI 49453
Phone: 616-857-7707
Fax: 616-857-7803
Web Site: www.redbarnplayhouse.com
Season: June - September

3111 YOUTHEATRE

Michigan Performing Arts

15600 JL Hudson Drive
Box B
Southfield, MI 48075
Phone: 248-557-7529
Fax: 248-557-4415
e-mail: dkempskie@youtheatre.org
Web Site: www.youtheatre.org

Mission: Youtheatre is a program of Michigan Performing arts, organization dedicated to providing the best in professional, family entertainment to its audience.
Income Sources: Michigan Council of Arts & Cultural Affairs; City of Detroit Cultural Affairs Department; National Endowment for the Arts; McGregor Fund
Seating Capacity: 1,100
Cost: $900,000 (message)

3112 OLD TOWN PLAYHOUSE

148 E 8th
PO Box 262
Traverse City, MI 49685
Phone: 231-947-2210
Fax: 231-947-4955
e-mail: otp@traverse.net
Web Site: oldtownplayhouse.com
Officers:
    President: John Dew
    VP: Tracey Towner
    Secretary: Edson Shephard
    Treasurer: Peg Brace
    Board of Artistic Directors Chair: Steve Morse
    Chairman: George Beebx
Management:
    Executive Director: Mary Bevans Gillett
Mission: Assisting, encouraging, promoting and improving the cultural development of our community through education and entertainment.
Founded: 1960
Specialized Field: Community
Status: Non-Professional; Nonprofit
Paid Staff: 3.5
Volunteer Staff: 150
Budget: $300,000
Income Sources: Ticket Sales; Season Subscribers; Donors, Fund Devlopment and Grants
Affiliations: CTAM; AACT; MACAA
Annual Attendance: 18,000
Facility Category: Community Theatre
Type of Stage: Mainstage; Black Box
Stage Dimensions: 350; 80
Seating Capacity: 350
Year Built: 1903
Year Remodeled: 1999
Organization Type: Performing; Educational
Resident Groups: Traverse City Civic Players

3113 BLUE LAKE REPERTORY THEATRE

Route #2
300 E
Twin Lake, MI 49457
Phone: 616-894-2540
Fax: 231-893-5123
Management:
    President: Fritz Stansell
    Treasurer: Reverend Walter Marek
Mission: To present summer-stock theatre of quality for our community.
Founded: 1966
Specialized Field: Summer Stock; Musical; Theatrical Group
Status: Semi-Professional
Income Sources: Blue Lake Fine Arts Camp
Performs At: Howmet Playhouse

Organization Type: Performing; Resident; Educational

3114 JET THEATRE
6600 W Maple Road
West Bloomfield, MI 48322-3002
Phone: 248-788-2900
Fax: 248-788-5160
Management:
   Artistic Director: Evelyn Orbach
   Literary Manager: Pearl Orbach

3115 JEWISH ENSEMBLE THEATRE
6600 W Maple Road
West Bloomfield, MI 48322-3002
Phone: 248-788-2900
Fax: 248-788-5160
e-mail: jetplay@aol.com
Web Site: www.comnet.org/jet
Management:
   Artistic Director: Evelyn Orbach
Founded: 1989
Performs At: Aaron DeRoy Theatre
Type of Stage: Thrust
Seating Capacity: 193

Minnesota

3116 THEATRE L'HOMME DIEU
PO Box 1086
Alexandria, MN 56308
Phone: 320-255-3229
Fax: 320-255-2902
e-mail: lhd@rea-alp.com
Web Site: www.alexweb.net/theatrelhommedieu
Officers:
   President: Linda Roles
   Secretary: Barbara Kleeper
Management:
   Artistic Director: Dave Borron
   Marketing Director: Janelle Sladek
Founded: 1960
Specialized Field: Theatre
Status: Non-Equity; Nonprofit
Paid Staff: 15
Volunteer Staff: 15
Paid Artists: 30
Budget: $125,000
Income Sources: Grants; Box Office; University Subsidy
Season: June-August
Affiliations: St. Claude State University
Annual Attendance: 8,000
Facility Category: Theatre
Type of Stage: Proscenium
Stage Dimensions: 40' x 18'
Seating Capacity: 265
Year Built: 1961
Year Remodeled: 2000
Cost: $50,000

3117 MATCHBOX CHILDREN'S THEATRE
407 1/2 N Main Street
PO Box 576
Austin, MN 55912
Phone: 507-437-9078
e-mail: matchboxtheatre@hotmail.com
Web Site: matchboxtheatre.tripod.com
Officers:
   President: Carrie Parker
   VP: Sarah Lenn
   Treasurer: Linda Sistek
   Secretary: Cindy Bellrichard
Mission: To consistently offer quality theatre experiences to families and young audiences.
Founded: 1975
Specialized Field: Musical; Community; Theatrical Group
Status: Nonprofit
Performs At: Austin Community College Theatre
Organization Type: Performing; Resident

3118 PAUL BUNYAN PLAYHOUSE
314 Beltrami Avenue
Bemidji, MN 56601
Phone: 218-444-8591
e-mail: pbphouse@paulbunyan.net
Web Site: www.paulbunyan.net
Officers:
   President: Becky Lueben
   VP: Kristine Cannon
   Treasurer: Karen Moe
   Secretary: Sandy Johnson
Management:
   Artistic Director: Curtiss Grittner
Mission: To produce the best possible theatre utilizing local and regional talent as well as interns from Bemidji State University.
Founded: 1951
Specialized Field: Summer Stock; Musical; Theatrical Group
Status: Professional; Nonprofit
Paid Staff: 15
Performs At: Paul Bunyan Playhouse; Old Chief Theatre
Organization Type: Performing; Educational

3119 CHANHASSEN DINNER THEATRE
501 W 78th
PO Box 100
Chanhassen, MN 55317
Phone: 612-934-1500
Fax: 612-952-1511
Toll-free: 800-362-3515
e-mail: information@chanassentheatres.com
Web Site: www.chanassentheatres.com
Officers:
   VP: Michael Brindisi
Management:
   Managing Director: Solveig Huseth
   Artistic Director: Michael Brindisi
   Director Marketing: Margo Gisselman
   Director Public Relations: Kris Howland
Mission: To present fine theatre and dining.
Founded: 1968
Specialized Field: Dinner; Theatrical Group

Status: Professional
Paid Staff: 250
Paid Artists: 75
Income Sources: American Dinner Theatre Institute
Performs At: Chanhassen Dinner Theatres
Annual Attendance: 250,000
Facility Category: Professional Dinner Theater
Seating Capacity: 600
Organization Type: Performing

3120 COLDER BY THE LAKE

PO Box 3473
Duluth, MN 55803-3473
Phone: 218-722-8867
e-mail: colder@colderbythelake.com
Web Site: www.colderbythelake.com
Officers:
   President: Mary Anderson
   VP: Dr Scott Wolf
   Secretary/Treasurer: Mary Treuer
Management:
   Artistic Director: Jean M Sramek
Mission: Colder by the Lake presents all original theater, specifically: satire, comedy and the offbeat.
Founded: 1983
Specialized Field: Theatrical Group
Status: Nonprofit
Organization Type: Performing; Touring

3121 UNIVERSITY OF MINNESOTA DULUTH: DEPARTMENT OF THEATRE

University of Minnesota at Duluth
141 MPAC
Duluth, MN 55812
Phone: 218-726-8562
Fax: 218-726-6798
e-mail: pdennis@d.umn.edu
Management:
   Department Head: Patricia Dennis
   Associate Professor: Mark Harvey
   Directing The Dance: Ann A Bergeron
Performs At: Marshall Performing Arts Center

3122 OLD LOG THEATER

5175 Meadville Street
PO Box 250
Excelsior, MN 55331
Phone: 952-474-5951
Fax: 952-474-1290
e-mail: oldlog@uswest.net
Web Site: www.oldlog.com
Management:
   Manager: Don Stolz
Mission: To offer entertainment to the public.
Founded: 1940
Specialized Field: Dinner; Theatrical Group
Status: Professional
Paid Staff: 30
Income Sources: Ticket sales
Performs At: Old Log Theatre
Affiliations: Actors' Equity
Type of Stage: Proscenium
Stage Dimensions: 70x80x24
Seating Capacity: 655

Year Built: 1960
Rental Contact: Don Stocz
Organization Type: Performing; Touring; Resident

3123 STAGES THEATRE COMPANY

1111 Main Street
Hopkins, MN 55343
Phone: 952-979-1111
Fax: 952-979-1124
Web Site: www.stagestheatre.org
Management:
   Producing Director: Steve Barberio
Mission: To provide entertainment and theatre education for families and young people.
Founded: 1984
Specialized Field: Musical; Theatrical Group
Status: Semi-Professional; Nonprofit
Paid Staff: 30
Performs At: Eisenhower Community Center; Hopkins
Organization Type: Performing; Resident; Educational

3124 CLIMB THEATRE

6415 Carmen Avenue E
Inner Grove Heights, MN 55076
Phone: 651-453-9275
Fax: 651-453-9274
e-mail: mail@climb.org
Web Site: www.climb.org
Management:
   Executive/Artistic Director: Peg Wetli
Founded: 1975
Status: Non-Equity; Nonprofit
Season: July - May

3125 COMMONWEAL THEATRE COMPANY

206 Parkway Avenue N
PO Box 15
Lanesboro, MN 55949
Phone: 507-467-2905
Fax: 507-467-2468
Toll-free: 800-657-7025
e-mail: info@commonwealtheatre.org
Web Site: www.commonwealtheatre.org
Officers:
   Chairman of the Board: M Judith Schmidt
   VP: David Ruen
   Secretary/Treasurer: Eric L bunge
Management:
   Executive Director: Harold N Cropp
   Founding Core Artist: Eric L Bunge ood
   Resident Company Member: Chirstine Winkler
   Resident Company Member: Jill Underwood
Mission: The Commonwealth is a non profit professional thatre company dedicated to delighting and challenging the audiences of our region.
Founded: 1989
Specialized Field: Live Theatre
Status: Non-Equity; Nonprofit
Paid Staff: 7
Paid Artists: 30
Budget: $500,000
Income Sources: 64% Contributed Income
Season: February - December
Annual Attendance: 18,000

Facility Category: Silent Movie House
Type of Stage: Proscenium
Stage Dimensions: 23' x 30'
Seating Capacity: 126
Year Built: 1896

3126 GREEN EARTH PLAYERS
216 W Main Street
Luverne, MN 56156
Phone: 507-283-9891
Mission: To bring live theatre to the area.
Founded: 1978
Specialized Field: Musical; Community; Theatrical Group
Status: Nonprofit
Income Sources: Minnesota Arts Council; Southern Minnesota Arts & Humanities Council
Performs At: Palace Theatre
Organization Type: Performing

3127 HIGHLAND SUMMER THEATRE
Minnesota State University
201 Performing Arts Center
Mankato, MN 56001
Phone: 507-389-2118
Fax: 507-389-2922
e-mail: paul.hustoles@mnsu.edu
Web Site: www.msutheatre.com
Management:
    Artistic Director: Paul J Hustoles
Mission: Summer stock theatre in its 37th season
Founded: 1967
Specialized Field: Theatre
Status: Non-Equity; Nonprofit
Paid Staff: 15
Volunteer Staff: 4
Paid Artists: 15
Non-paid Artists: 20
Season: May - July
Affiliations: Minnesota State University Mankato
Annual Attendance: 40,000
Type of Stage: Proscenium; Black Box
Stage Dimensions: 38' x 38'; 60' x 70'
Seating Capacity: 529; 250

3128 ZORONGO FLAMENCO DANCE THEATRE
3012 Minnehaha Avenue
Minneapolis, MN 55406
Phone: 612-724-2000
e-mail: flamenco@zorongo.org
Web Site: www.zorongo.org

3129 ARTS MIDWEST
2908 Hennepin Avenue
Suite 200
Minneapolis, MN 55408
Phone: 612-341-0755
Fax: 612-341-0902
e-mail: dfraher@artsmidwest.org
Web Site: www.artsmidwest.org
Management:
    Executive Director: David Fraher

3130 CHILDREN'S THEATER COMPANY
2400 3rd Avenue S
Minneapolis, MN 55404-3597
Phone: 612-874-0500
Fax: 612-874-8119
Officers:
    Chairman: Ken Piper
    Co-Vice Chair: Rusty Cohen
    Co-Vice Chair: Michael Margulies
    Secretary: Kathleen Flynn Peterson
Management:
    Artistic Director: Peter C Brosius
    Managing Director: Teresa Eyring
    Literary Manager: Elissa Adams
Mission: To produce significant theatre experiences for young people and their families through nuturing a creative ensemble of the highest professional quality.
Founded: 1965
Specialized Field: Musical; Theatrical Group
Status: Professional
Budget: $9 million
Income Sources: Theatre Communications Group; International Association of Theatre for Children and Youth; Actors' Equity Association
Performs At: Children's Theatre Company
Annual Attendance: 350,000
Facility Category: Theater
Type of Stage: Proscenium
Seating Capacity: 745
Organization Type: Performing; Touring; Educational

3131 COMMEDIA THEATER COMPANY
3040 10th Avenue S
Minneapolis, MN 55407
Phone: 612-788-2157
Management:
    General Manager: Linda Bruning
    Office/Booking Manager: Rudd Rayfield
Mission: To bring improvisational comedy with direct audience contact, into communities unfamiliar with live theater.
Founded: 1975
Specialized Field: Theatrical Group
Status: Professional
Organization Type: Performing; Touring; Educational

3132 GUTHRIE THEATER
725 Vineland Place
Minneapolis, MN 55403
Phone: 612-377-2224
Fax: 612-347-1188
Toll-free: 877-447-8243
e-mail: webmaster@guthrietheater.org
Web Site: www.guthrietheater.org
Officers:
    President: Charles Zelle
    VP: Susan Engel
    Treasurer: Jay Kiedrowski
    Secretary: M. Joahn Jundt
Management:
    Artistic Director: Joe Dowling
    Managing Director: Susan Trapnell
    General Manager: Thomas C Proehl

Mission: To serve as a vital artistic resource for the people of Minnesota and the region; to celebrate, through theatrical performances, the common humanity binding us all together; devoted to the traditional classical repertoire.
Founded: 1963
Status: Professional; Nonprofit
Season: June - February/March
Performs At: The Guthrie Theater
Affiliations: League of Resident Theatres
Type of Stage: Modified Thrust
Seating Capacity: 1300
Year Built: 1963
Year Remodeled: 1993
Cost: 3.5 Million
Organization Type: Performing; Touring; Resident

3133 HIDDEN THEATRE

2301 Franklin Avenue E
Minneapolis, MN 55406
Phone: 612-339-4949
Fax: 612-332-6037
Web Site: www.hiddentheatre.org
Management:
    Audience Services Manager: David Pisa
Founded: 1994

3134 HISTORIC ORPHEUM THEATRE

910 Hennepin Avenue
Minneapolis, MN 55403
Phone: 612-339-0075
Fax: 612-339-5917
Web Site: www.state-orpheum.com
Founded: 1921
Paid Staff: 27
Budget: $2,000,000
Income Sources: Ticket Sales; Rent; Concessions Revenues
Annual Attendance: 500,000
Type of Stage: Proscenium
Stage Dimensions: 54'5'Wx28'8'Hx58'D
Seating Capacity: 2,600
Year Built: 1921
Year Remodeled: 1994
Cost: $10,000,000
Rental Contact: Joe Duca

3135 HISTORIC STATE THEATRE

805 Hennepin Avenue
Minneapolis, MN 55403
Phone: 612-373-5600
Fax: 612-339-0601
e-mail: education@orpheum.com
Web Site: www.state-orpheum.com
Founded: 1921
Paid Staff: 27
Budget: $2,000,000
Income Sources: Ticket Sales; Rent; Concessions Revenues
Annual Attendance: 600,000
Type of Stage: Proscenium
Stage Dimensions: 45'7'Wx25'7'Hx35'7'D
Seating Capacity: 2,150
Year Built: 1921
Year Remodeled: 1991

Cost: $8,800,000
Rental Contact: Joe Duca

3136 ILLUSION THEATER

528 Hennepin Avenue
Suite 704
Minneapolis, MN 55403
Phone: 612-339-4944
Fax: 612-337-8042
e-mail: info@illusiontheater.org
Web Site: www.illusiontheater.org
Management:
    Executive Director: Michael Robins
    Education Director: Karen Gundlach
    Producing Director: Bonnie Morris
    Communications Director: Delta Giordano
Founded: 1974
Specialized Field: Theatrical Group
Status: Professional; Nonprofit
Paid Staff: 15
Paid Artists: 100
Budget: $1,500,000
Income Sources: Actors' Equity Association; Small Professional Theatre Association; Grants; Box Office
Season: September - August
Performs At: Hennepin Center for the Arts
Annual Attendance: 15,000
Facility Category: Theater
Type of Stage: Proscenium
Seating Capacity: 225
Year Remodeled: 1999
Organization Type: Performing; Touring; Resident; Educational; Sponsoring

3137 IN THE HEART OF THE BEAST PUPPET AND MASK THEATRE

1500 E Lake Street
Minneapolis, MN 55407
Phone: 612-721-2535
Fax: 612-721-7174
e-mail: info@hobt.org
Web Site: www.hobt.org
Officers:
    Chairman: Paul Halverson
    Vice Chairman: Jack Fistler
    Secretary: Lynet Norris
    Treasurer: Jon Weesk
Management:
    Artistic Director: Sandy Spieler
    Associate Artistic Director: Beth Peterson
    Executive Director: Kathleen Foran
Mission: To entertain and enrich audiences of all ages and cultures through puppetry and mask; to build a relationship between artist and audience; to be an active participant in the dialogue of our times.
Founded: 1973
Specialized Field: Theatrical Group; Puppet
Status: Professional; Nonprofit
Paid Staff: 13
Volunteer Staff: 350
Paid Artists: 80
Non-paid Artists: 20
Income Sources: Grants from Private and Public Sectors; Ticket Revenue and Earned Fees

Performs At: Restored Movie Theater
Annual Attendance: 100,000
Facility Category: Theatre
Type of Stage: Proscenium
Seating Capacity: 300
Year Built: 1937
Year Remodeled: 1997
Rental Contact: Executive Director K Foran
Organization Type: Performing; Touring; Resident;
Educational; Sponsoring

3138 INTERNATIONAL THEATRES CORPORATION

4701 IDS Center
Minneapolis, MN 55402
Phone: 612-340-1900
Fax: 612-340-9919
Management:
   President: Tom Scallen

3139 JACKSON MARIONETTE PRODUCTIONS

1500 E Lake Street
Minneapolis, MN 55407
Phone: 612-721-2535
Management:
   Manager: Sara Jackson
Specialized Field: Puppet
Status: Professional
Income Sources: Puppeteers of America; United
International Marionette Association; Twin City
Puppeteers
Organization Type: Performing; Touring

3140 JUNGLE THEATER

2951 S Lyndale Avenue
Minneapolis, MN 55408
Phone: 612-822-7063
Fax: 612-822-9408
e-mail: info@jungletheater.com
Web Site: www.jungletheater.com
Officers:
   Marketing Director: Sonja Wahlberg
Management:
   Artistic Director: Bain Boehlke
   Managing Director: Julia Sand
   Development Director: Don Sommer
   Community Programs Manager: Charles Bethel
   Board Chair: Eric Galatz
   Vice Chair: Julie Umbarger
Mission: To produce high quality theatre in an intimate
setting.
Founded: 1991
Specialized Field: Theatre
Paid Staff: 15
Volunteer Staff: 80
Paid Artists: 200
Budget: $1.1 million
Income Sources: Earned; Contributions
Performs At: Theater
Affiliations: Theatre Communications Group
Annual Attendance: 26,000
Facility Category: Theater
Type of Stage: Proscenium

Seating Capacity: 135
Year Built: 1911
Year Remodeled: 1999
Rental Contact: Charlie Bethel

3141 MARGOLIS BROWN THEATRE COMPANY

3112 17th Avenue S
Minneapolis, MN 55407
Phone: 612-722-2333
e-mail: margolisbrown@aol.com
Web Site: www.margolisbrown.org
Management:
   Director Of Education & Outreach: Kym Longhi
   Artistic/Executive Director: Tony Brown
   Artistic/Executive Director: Karl Margolis
Mission: To create original multimedia productions of
movement theatre; to share our facilities with other artists.
Founded: 1983
Specialized Field: Theatrical Group; Multimedia
Movement Theatre
Status: Professional; Nonprofit
Income Sources: National Movement Theatre
Association
Organization Type: Performing; Touring; Resident;
Educational; Sponsoring; Dramatic Movement School

3142 MIXED BLOOD THEATRE COMPANY

1501 S 4th Street
Minneapolis, MN 55454
Phone: 612-338-0937
Fax: 612-338-1851
Web Site: www.mixedblood.com
Management:
   Managing Artistic Director: Jack Reuler
   Marketing Director: Charlie Moore
   Technical Director: Christine Nelson
Mission: A multiracial, professional theatre ensemble
employing colorblind casting, and dedicated to fostering
the spirit of Dr. Martin Luther King's dream.
Founded: 1976
Specialized Field: Theatrical Group
Status: Professional; Nonprofit
Paid Staff: 6
Budget: $1 million
Income Sources: Society for Stage Directors and
Choreographers
Season: September - May
Annual Attendance: varies
Type of Stage: Flexible
Seating Capacity: 200
Organization Type: Performing; Touring; Educational

3143 PANGEA WORLD THEATER

2509 Dupont Avenue S
#209
Minneapolis, MN 55405
Phone: 612-377-1728
Fax: 612-377-1728
e-mail: quest@pangeaworldtheater.org
Web Site: www.pangeaworldtheater.org
Management:
   Executive/Literary Director: Meena Natarajan

3144 PILLSBURY HOUSE THEATRE

3501 Chicago Avenue S
Minneapolis, MN 55407
Phone: 612-824-0708
Fax: 612-827-5818
Management:
   Co-Artistic Director: Faye Price
   Managing Director: Noel Raymond
Founded: 1992

3145 PLAYWRIGHTS' CENTER

2301 Franklin Avenue E
Minneapolis, MN 55406-1099
Phone: 612-332-7481
Fax: 612-332-6037
e-mail: info@pweenter.org
Web Site: www.pwcenter.org
Officers:
   President: Roy Close
   VP: Jeff Keyes
   Treasurer: Joyce Bevning
   Secretary: Paula Anderson
Management:
   Director External Affairs: Dawn Mikkelson
   Director Playwright Services: Megan Monaghan
   Membership Coordinator: Ronnell Wheeland
   Executive Director: Carlo Cuesta
Mission: To fuel contemporary theatre by providing services that support the development and public appreciation of playwrights and playwriting.
Founded: 1971
Specialized Field: Playwright Service Organization
Status: Nonprofit
Paid Staff: 10+
Paid Artists: 20+
Income Sources: Actors' Equity Association; Theatre Communications Group
Season: July - August
Year Built: 1900
Year Remodeled: 2000
Cost: $1,100,000
Organization Type: Touring; Educational; Sponsoring; Developmental Workshops; Reading

3146 RED EYE

15 W 14th Street
Minneapolis, MN 55403
Phone: 612-870-7531
e-mail: staff@theredeye.org
Web Site: www.theredeye.org
Management:
   Managing Director: Miriam Must
   Artistic Director: Steve Busa
   Marketing Director: Karen Sauro
   Production and Facility Manager: Tim Heins
Mission: To provide experimental theatre; to develop multimedia theater productions.
Founded: 1983
Specialized Field: Theatrical Group
Status: Professional; Nonprofit
Income Sources: National Endowment for the Arts; Dayton Hudson Foundation; Jerome Foundation; McKnight Foundation; United Artists; Metropolitan Regional Arts Council

Performs At: Red Eye's 14th Street Theatre
Organization Type: Performing; Touring; Resident; Educational

3147 THEATER MU

711 W Lake Street
Suite 212
Minneapolis, MN 55408
Phone: 612-824-4804
Fax: 612-824-3396
e-mail: info@theatermu.org
Web Site: www.theatermu.org
Management:
   Artistic Director: Rick Shiomi
Founded: 1992

3148 THEATRE DE LA JEUNE LUNE

105 1st Street N
Minneapolis, MN 55401
Phone: 612-332-3968
Fax: 612-332-0048
e-mail: info@junelune.org
Web Site: www.jeunelune.org
Management:
   Artistic Director: Robert Rosen
   Artistic Director: Barbra Berlovitz-Desbois
   Artistic Director: Dominique Serrand
   Artistic Director: Vincent Gracieux
   Business Director: Kit Waickman
   Development Director: Jennifer Halcrow
   Marketing Director: Steve Richardson
Mission: The production of immediate, energetic, dynamic, theatre through company creations and scripted material.
Founded: 1978
Specialized Field: Theatrical Group
Status: Professional; Nonprofit
Paid Staff: 10
Income Sources: Foundation for the Extension and Development of American Professional Theatre
Season: September - June
Type of Stage: Mobile
Stage Dimensions: 60' x 100'; 47' x 30'
Seating Capacity: 500;100-150
Organization Type: Performing; Touring

3149 THEATRE IN THE ROUND

245 Cedar Avenue
Minneapolis, MN 55454-1054
Phone: 612-333-3010
e-mail: editorial@theatremania.com
Web Site: www.theatreintheround.org
Management:
   Managing Director: Steve Antenucci
Mission: To bridge the gap between professional and amateur theatre with quality drama; to entertain the community; to educate.
Founded: 1952
Specialized Field: Community
Status: Non-Professional; Nonprofit
Paid Staff: 250
Income Sources: American Association of Community Theatres; Minnesota Association of Community Theatres
Performs At: Theatre-in-the-Round

All listings are in alphabetical order by state, then city, then organization within the city.

Organization Type: Performing; Resident; Educational

3150 TROUPE AMERICA

528 Hennepin Avenue
Suite 206
Minneapolis, MN 55403
Phone: 612-333-3302
Fax: 612-333-4337
e-mail: johnt@naninter.net
Web Site: www.TroupeAmerica.com
Officers:
    President: Curtis N Wollan
    Secretary/Treasurer: Jane Wollan
Management:
    Producing Director: Curtis N Wollan
    Associate Producer: John Tsafoyannis
    Production Manager: Scott Herbst
    Publicist: Linda Twiss
Mission: To provide top quality theatrical experiences for our audiences, on the road and in the Twin Cities.
Founded: 1972
Specialized Field: Musical; Theatrical Group
Status: Professional; Commercial
Paid Staff: 23
Paid Artists: 100
Budget: $1,750,000
Income Sources: Ticket Sales; Concessions; Touring Fees
Season: September - August
Performs At: Plymouth Playhouse; and Touring Venues
Affiliations: Southeastern Theatre Conference; United Professional Theatre Association; National Alliance of American Theatre
Annual Attendance: 50,000
Facility Category: Theatre of Touring
Type of Stage: Semi Thrust
Stage Dimensions: 30x24
Seating Capacity: 211
Year Built: 1973
Year Remodeled: 1998
Cost: $150,000
Rental Contact: Production Manager Scott Herbst
Organization Type: Performing; Touring; Resident; Sponsoring

3151 WALKER ART CENTER

Vineland Place
Minneapolis, MN 55403
Phone: 612-375-7624
Fax: 612-375-7618
Web Site: www.walkerart.org
Management:
    Director: Kathy Halbreich
    Curator Performing Arts: Philip Bither
Mission: To serve as a catalyst regionally and internationally for emerging forms of expression; to engage the audience in contemporary arts issues.
Specialized Field: Visual; Performing and Media Arts
Status: Professional; Nonprofit
Paid Staff: 150
Income Sources: Endowment; Grants; Ticket Revenue; Donations
Performs At: Walker Art Center Auditorium
Facility Category: Multidiscliplinary Arts Center
Seating Capacity: 350

Organization Type: Performing; Touring; Resident; Educational; Sponsoring; Exhibition

3152 WORLD TREE PUPPET THEATER

3305 E Calhoun Parkway
Minneapolis, MN 55408
Phone: 612-824-3112
Management:
    Director: Joan Mickelson
Mission: To use the traditions of puppetry and adaptations of folklore to entertain families and children; to employ experimental uses of puppets, dolls and masks for adult theater.
Founded: 1982
Specialized Field: Puppet
Status: Professional
Organization Type: Performing; Touring; Resident

3153 GOOSEBERRY PARK PLAYERS

901 8th Street S
Moorhead, MN 56562
Phone: 218-299-4000
Web Site: www.gooseberryparkplayers.org
Officers:
    President: Ann Vandermaten
Management:
    Director: Ann Vandermaten
    Director: John Vandermaten
    Managing Artistic Director: Jim Cermack
Mission: Provide a summer outdoor theatre for and by children for family entertainment providing a fun, educational experience for young people.
Founded: 1984
Specialized Field: Theatrical Group
Status: Nonprofit
Income Sources: Moorhead Parks & Recreational Department
Organization Type: Performing

3154 STRAW HAT PLAYERS

Center for the Arts
Moorhead, MN 56560
Phone: 218-236-2271
e-mail: bartruff@mnstate.edu
Web Site: www.mnstate.edu/speech/strawhat
Management:
    Director: Jim Bartruff
Founded: 1963
Status: Non-Equity; Nonprofit
Season: May - July
Type of Stage: Thrust
Seating Capacity: 900

3155 OFF-BROADWAY MUSICAL THEATRE

3243 Flag Avenue N
New Hope, MN 55427
Phone: 612-544-3810
Fax: 612-545-3622
Mission: To offer major musicals employing local talent of all ages and degrees of proficiency.
Founded: 1979
Specialized Field: Community
Status: Nonprofit
Income Sources: Minnesota State Arts Council

Performs At: New Hope Outdoor Theatre; Brooklyn Center Civic
Organization Type: Performing

3156 LITTLE THEATRE OF OWATONNA
Dunell Drive
PO Box 64
Owatonna, MN 55060
Phone: 507-451-0764
Management:
   Executive Secretary: Sharon Stark
Mission: To bring performing arts, particularly theatre, to the community.
Founded: 1966
Specialized Field: Theatrical Group
Status: Non-Professional; Nonprofit
Organization Type: Performing

3157 ROCHESTER CIVIC THEATRE
220 E Center Street
Rochester, MN 55904
Phone: 507-282-8481
Fax: 507-282-0608
Management:
   Artistic Director: Greg Millern
   Technical Director: Doug Sween
   Costume Designer: Tracy Van Voorst
   Managing Director: Mark Colbenson
Mission: Promoting interest in and appreciation of dramatic arts through programs and productions.
Founded: 1951
Specialized Field: Community
Status: Non-Professional; Nonprofit
Income Sources: Minnesota Association of Community Theatres
Organization Type: Performing; Touring; Educational

3158 CLIMB THEATRE - CREATIVE LEARNING IDEAS
500 N Robert Street
Suite 220
Saint Paul, MN 55101
Phone: 800-767-9660
Fax: 612-227-9730
Officers:
   President: Peg Wetli
   Secretary: D Joe Haller
   Treasurer: Greg Rybak
Management:
   Executive Director: Peg Wetli
   Residency Company Manager: Peg Endres
   Performance Company Sales Rep.: Susan Lund
   Performance Company Director: Leigh Anne Adams
Mission: To harness and direct the creative power and artistic talents of its writers, directors, actors and educators to create and perform plays, classes and other creative works which communicate matters of social or educational significance to all citizens.
Founded: 1975
Specialized Field: Theatrical Group
Status: Professional; Nonprofit
Organization Type: Performing; Touring; Educational

3159 GREAT AMERICAN HISTORY THEATRE
30 E 10th Street
Saint Paul, MN 55101
Phone: 651-292-4323
Fax: 651-292-4322
Officers:
   President: Susan Hawken
   VP: John Apitz
   Treasurer: Elizabeth Alberts
Management:
   Artistic Director: Ron Peluso
   Managing Director: Virgina Nugent
Mission: To create new plays about Minnesota the Midwest and the diverse American experience.
Founded: 1978
Specialized Field: Musical; Theatrical Group
Status: Professional; Nonprofit
Paid Artists: 40
Income Sources: 70% Earned; 30% Contributed
Performs At: Crawford Livingston Theatre
Annual Attendance: 54,000
Type of Stage: Thrust
Seating Capacity: 597
Rental Contact: Erik Paulson
Organization Type: Performing; Touring; Resident; Educational; Sponsoring

---

3160 NAUTILUS MUSIC GROUP
620 N 1st Street
Saint Paul, MN 55401
Phone: 651-298-9913
Fax: 612-333-0869
Management:
   Co-Artistic Director: Ben Krywosz
   Co-Artistic Director: Karen Miller
   Managing Director: Marge Betley
Mission: To develop and produce new musical theater works; to nurture the creative artist.
Status: Professional; Nonprofit
Organization Type: Performing; Educational

3161 PARK SQUARE THEATRE COMPANY
408 St. Peter Street
Suite 110
Saint Paul, MN 55102-1130
Phone: 651-291-7005
Fax: 651-291-9180
e-mail: production@parksquaretheatre.org
Web Site: www.parksquaretheatre.org
Management:
   Artistic Director: Richard G Cook
   Executive Director: Steven Kent Lockwood
   Audience Services Director: Eric M Herr
   Education Director: Mary Finnerty
Mission: Entertaining and enriching area audiences with quality productions of the classics.
Founded: 1975
Specialized Field: Theatrical Group
Status: Professional; Nonprofit
Paid Staff: 10
Paid Artists: 100
Budget: $1.2 million
Income Sources: Sales; Contributions

Season: January - August
Annual Attendance: 54,000
Facility Category: Rental
Type of Stage: Proscenium
Stage Dimensions: 34' x 30'
Seating Capacity: 340
Organization Type: Performing

3162 PENUMBRA THEATRE COMPANY

270 N Kent Street
Saint Paul, MN 55102
Phone: 612-224-4601
Fax: 612-224-7074
Management:
 Artistic Director: Lou Bellamy
 General Manager: Jayne Khalifa
Mission: To present high quality theatre from the Pan African/American viewpoint.
Founded: 1976
Specialized Field: Musical; Folk
Status: Professional; Nonprofit
Income Sources: Actors' Equity Association
Season: August - June
Type of Stage: Proscenium/Thrust
Stage Dimensions: 27' x 41'
Seating Capacity: 260
Organization Type: Performing; Touring; Educational

3163 RAINBO CHILDREN'S THEATRE COMPANY

688 Selby Avenue
Saint Paul, MN 55104
Phone: 651-293-9043
Management:
 Founder/Managing Artistic Director: Merline Batiste Doty
Mission: To bring children together for cultural exchange through participation in the performing arts.
Founded: 1979
Specialized Field: Community; Folk; Theatrical Group
Status: Professional; Nonprofit
Paid Staff: 10
Organization Type: Performing; Touring; Resident; Educational; Sponsoring

3164 DUDLEY RIGGS INSTANT THEATRE COMPANY

1586 Burton Street
St. Paul, MN 55108
Phone: 612-647-6748
Fax: 612-647-5637
Management:
 Producing Director: Dudley Riggs
Founded: 1954
Specialized Field: Theatre Company
Performs At: Dudley Riggs Theatre
Type of Stage: Modified Thrust
Seating Capacity: 260

3165 LAKESHORE PLAYERS

PO Box 10564
White Bear Lake, MN 55110

Phone: 651-426-3275
e-mail: info@lakeshoreplayers.com
Web Site: www.lakeshoreplayers.com
Management:
 Business Manager: Sherrie Tarble
Mission: To provide entertainment for the community.
Founded: 1953
Specialized Field: Musical; Theatrical Group
Status: Nonprofit
Paid Staff: 25
Income Sources: Minnesota Association of Community Theatres
Performs At: Lakeshore Playhouse
Organization Type: Performing; Educational

3166 SHAKESPEARE & COMPANY

Century College, W Campus
3300 Century Avenue N
White Bear Lake, MN 55110
Phone: 651-779-5818
e-mail: info@shakespeare-company.org
Web Site: www.shakespeare-company.org
Management:
 Artistic Director: George M Roesler
Mission: To provide an environment where families can come and enjoy an informal picnic atmosphere and see performances of Shakespeare and other classical plays.
Founded: 1976
Performs At: Outdoor Theatre Complex, West Campus of Century College

Mississippi

3167 CORINTH THEATRE-ARTS

303 Fulton Drive
PO Box 127
Corinth, MS 38834
Phone: 662-287-2995
Fax: 662-287-6272
e-mail: cta@dixie-net.com
Web Site: www.corinththeatrearts.com
Officers:
 Chairman: John Treadway
 Vice Chairman: Paul Schumacher
 Secretary: Laurie Prichett
 Treasurer: Jimmy Deaton
Management:
 Office Manager: Haven Young
 Artistic Director: Katie Simons
 VP Production: Timothy Hodges
Mission: To offer theatrical performances, arts education, economic stimulation and quality arts entertainment.
Founded: 1967
Specialized Field: Community theater
Status: Nonprofit
Paid Staff: 2
Volunteer Staff: 2
Paid Artists: 10
Non-paid Artists: 500
Budget: $105,000
Income Sources: Theatre Patrons; Box Office; Grants
Performs At: Crossroads Playhouse; Coliseum Civic Center

Annual Attendance: 8500
Type of Stage: Proscenium
Stage Dimensions: 19 x 30
Seating Capacity: 204
Organization Type: Resident

3168 NEW STAGE THEATRE
PO Box 4792
1100 Carlisle Street
Jackson, MS 39202
Phone: 601-948-3533
Fax: 601-948-3538
e-mail: mail@newstagetheatre.com
Web Site: www.newstagetheatre.com
Management:
  Business Manager: Dawn Buck
  Artistic Director: Patrick Benton
  General Manager: Bill McCarty
Founded: 1965
Status: Professional; Nonprofit
Paid Staff: 10
Volunteer Staff: 10
Paid Artists: 25
Non-paid Artists: 10
Budget: $500,000
Season: September - June
Performs At: New Stage Theatre
Affiliations: Actors' Equity Association
Type of Stage: Proscenium
Seating Capacity: 364
Organization Type: Resident; Educational; Producing

3169 PUPPET ARTS THEATRE
1927 Springridge Drive
Jackson, MS 39211
Phone: 601-956-3414
Fax: 601-432-6746
e-mail: pupperarts@hotmail.com
Management:
  Artistic Director: Peter Zapletal
  Business Manager: Jarmila Zapletal
Mission: To offer entertainment and education in the Southeast through programs featuring puppets and classical music.
Founded: 1968
Specialized Field: Puppet
Status: Professional; Commercial
Organization Type: Performing; Touring

Missouri

3170 ARROW ROCK LYCEUM THEATRE
High Street
Arrow Rock, MO 65320
Phone: 660-837-3311
Fax: 660-837-3112
Web Site: www.lyceumtheatre.org
Officers:
  President: Vicki Russell
Management:
  Artistic Producing Director: Michael Bollinger
  Associate Artistic Director: Philip Coffield

Mission: To touch, enrich and entertain human beings with live professional theatre.
Founded: 1961
Specialized Field: Professional Theatre
Status: Professional; Nonprofit
Paid Staff: 25
Volunteer Staff: 80
Paid Artists: 35
Non-paid Artists: 80
Budget: $750,000
Income Sources: Actors' Equity Association
Season: June - August
Performs At: Lyceum Theatre
Annual Attendance: 35,000
Facility Category: Indoor A/C Theatre
Type of Stage: Proscenium w/thrust
Seating Capacity: 408
Year Remodeled: 1993
Rental Contact: Business Manager Elizabeth Ostrin
Organization Type: Performing; Touring; Resident

3171 SHEPHERD OF THE HILLS
W Highway 76
Branson, MO 65616-0000
Phone: 417-334-4191
Toll-free: 800-653-6288
e-mail: groups@tablerock.net
Web Site: www.theshepherdofthehills.com
Management:
  Director: Keith Thurman
Mission: In 1907, a novel was published that forever changed the way of life for Branson area residents. That novel, The Shepherd of the Hills, sold millions of copies and attracts many people to the Ozark hills around which its story is centered.
Founded: 1960
Status: Non-Equity; Commercial
Season: April - October
Type of Stage: Outdoor
Seating Capacity: 1100

3172 TRILAKES COMMUNITY THEATRE
PO Box 1301
Branson, MO 65616
Phone: 417-335-4241
Mission: To foster the Performing Arts; To entertain the community.
Founded: 1983
Specialized Field: Musical; Community; Theatrical Group
Status: Nonprofit
Paid Staff: 30
Income Sources: Missouri Arts Council
Organization Type: Performing

3173 SIX FLAGS ST. LOUIS
PO Box 60
Eureka, MO 63025
Phone: 636-938-5300
Fax: 314-938-9006
Management:
  Entertainment Manager: Theresa Bargman
Status: Non-Equity; Commercial
Season: April - October

All listings are in alphabetical order by state, then city, then organization within the city.

Type of Stage: Amphitheatre
Seating Capacity: 10000

3174 FLORISSANT CIVIC CENTER THEATER
1 James J Eagan Drive
Florissant, MO 63033
Phone: 314-921-5678
Fax: 314-921-5666
Management:
   Manager: Gary Gaydos

3175 CITY THEATRE OF INDEPENDENCE
Roger T Sermon Center
201 N Dodgion Street
Independence, MO 64050
Phone: 816-325-7367
e-mail: marciabrownlee@sbcglobal.net
Web Site: www.citytheatreofindependence.org
Officers:
   President: Steve Kennedy
   Treasurer: Carolyn Putsch
   Secretary: Sarah Schmidt
Management:
   VP Production: Nancy Madsen
   VP Marketing: Sharon Propst
   VP Fundraising: Nancy Eppert
   Season Production Manager: RJ Parish

3176 COTERIE THEATRE
2450 Grand Avenue
Suite 144
Kansas City, MO 64108-2520
Phone: 816-474-6785
Fax: 816-474-7112
e-mail: jeffchurch@aol.com
Web Site: www.thecoterie.com
Officers:
   President: Karen Weltner
   Vice President: Bob Inerman
   Secretary: Mark Gilgus
   Treasurer: LJ Buckner
Management:
   Executive Director: Jolette M Pelster
   Producing Artistic Director: Jeff Church
   Marketing Manager: Beth Norman
   Business/Box Office Manager: Gayle Sumbroff
Mission: To provide professional classic and contemporary theater which challenges the audience as well as the artist; to provide educational dramatic outreach programs in the community.
Founded: 1979
Specialized Field: Musical; Theatrical Group
Status: Professional; Nonprofit
Paid Staff: 8
Paid Artists: 100
Income Sources: Theatre Communications Group; International Association of Theatre for Children and Youth
Performs At: Coterie Theatre
Type of Stage: Flexible
Seating Capacity: 240
Organization Type: Performing; Touring; Resident; Educational

3177 FOLLY THEATER
300 W 12th Street
PO Box 26505
Kansas City, MO 64196
Phone: 816-842-5500
Fax: 816-842-8709
e-mail: follytheater@swbell.net
Management:
   Executive Director: Douglas Tatum
   Events Manager: Kate Egan
Founded: 1900
Specialized Field: Music; Dance; Theater
Paid Staff: 4
Volunteer Staff: 380
Budget: $60,000-150,000
Annual Attendance: 55,000
Type of Stage: Proscenium
Stage Dimensions: 34'x31'
Seating Capacity: 1,078
Year Built: 1900
Year Remodeled: 2000
Cost: $2,500,000
Rental Contact: Events Manager Kate Egan

3178 MID-AMERICA ARTS ALLIANCE
912 Baltimore Avenue
#700
Kansas City, MO 64105
Phone: 816-421-1388
Fax: 816-421-3918
Web Site: www.maaa.org
Management:
   Program Manager/Performing Arts: Diane Green

3179 MISSOURI REPERTORY THEATRE
4949 Cherry Street
Kansas City, MO 64110-2499
Phone: 816-235-2727
Fax: 816-235-5367
Toll-free: 888-502-2700
e-mail: theatre@vmkc.edu
Web Site: www.missourirep.org
Management:
   Producing Artistic Director: Peter Altman
   Managing Director: William Preacvost
Founded: 1964
Specialized Field: theatre
Status: Professional; Nonprofit
Paid Staff: 25
Volunteer Staff: 10
Paid Artists: 30
Budget: $5,000,000
Season: August - May
Performs At: Helen F. Spencer Theatre
Type of Stage: Proscenium
Seating Capacity: 700
Organization Type: Performing; Resident; Educational

3180 QUALITY HILL PLAYHOUSE
303 W Tenth Street
Kansas City, MO 64105-1615

Phone: 816-421-1700
Fax: 816-221-6556
e-mail: info@qualityhillplayhouse.com
Web Site: www.qualityhillplayhouse.com
Officers:
   President: Dale Wassergord
   VP: Jack Rosenfield
   Secretary: Jeaneane KO Bla
   Treasurer: Kent Maughan
Management:
   Executive Director: J Kent Barnhart
   Assistant Executive Director: Nancy Nail
Specialized Field: Cabaret Revue, Musical Theatre
Status: Professional
Paid Staff: 8
Volunteer Staff: 98
Paid Artists: 30
Budget: $650,000
Income Sources: Ticket Sales; Contributions
Performs At: Quality Hill Playhouse
Annual Attendance: 30,000
Facility Category: Theatre
Type of Stage: Thrust
Stage Dimensions: 12' x 28'
Seating Capacity: 153
Year Built: 1989
Rental Contact: Nancy Nail
Comments: Handicapped Accessible

3181   STARLIGHT THEATRE

6601 Swope Parkway
Kansas City, MO 64132
Phone: 816-363-7827
Fax: 816-361-6398
Toll-free: 800-776-1730
e-mail: starlight@kcstarlight.com
Web Site: www.kcstarlight.com
Management:
   Executive VP/Producer: Robert M Rohlf
   Director Marketing: Manon Eihs
   Company Manager: Courtney Adler
   VP Events/Entertainment: Bill Hartnett
Founded: 1950
Specialized Field: Kansas City
Season: June - August

3182   UNICORN THEATRE

3828 Main Street
Kansas City, MO 64111
Phone: 816-531-7529
Fax: 816-531-0421
Web Site: www.unicorntheatre.org
Management:
   Producing Artistic Director: Cynthia Levin
   Business Manager: Jeffrey Blaha
   Marketing: David Golston
   Development Director: Yvonne Jameson
Mission: To enhance the cultural life of Kansas City by producing professional contemporary, thought-provoking theater which inspires emotional response and stimulates discussion.
Founded: 1974
Specialized Field: Musical; Theatrical Group
Status: Professional
Paid Staff: 7

Income Sources: Actors' Equity Association; Theatre Communications Group
Season: September - June
Performs At: Unicorn Theatre
Affiliations: Actors' Equity Association; National New Play Network; Arts Council of Metropolitan Kansas City; Realtors For the Arts
Type of Stage: Thrust
Seating Capacity: 180
Organization Type: Performing
Comments: Discounts for students, seniors and working artists

3183   CHARACTERS & COMPANY

338 S Kirkwood Road
Kirkwood, MO
Phone: 314-822-6228
e-mail: mdvaugh@aol.com
Web Site: www.charactersandcompany.org
Management:
   Artistic Director: Mark D Vaughan
   Media Support: Randy Hastings
Mission: Began as a children's group, but today provides an intergenerational experience for cast members from age 3 to 80-plus, who learn from each other as they work on a common goal. We have no participation fees so that members of all socioeconomic levels can participate. The cast and crew are strictly bound by contract to maintain an atmosphere free of drugs, alcohol and smoking and violence.
Founded: 1985

3184   MEMPHIS COMMUNITY PLAYERS

125 S Main
Memphis, MO 63555
Phone: 660-465-7770
Mission: To offer summer musical theatre to our area.
Founded: 1974
Specialized Field: Musical; Community; Theatrical Group
Status: Non-Professional; Nonprofit
Performs At: Memphis Cinema
Organization Type: Performing; Resident; Educational

3185   MOBERLY COMMUNITY THEATRE

212 Crest Drive
Moberly, MO 65270
Phone: 660-263-3345
Management:
   Producer/Director: Carolee Hazlet
Mission: Working together as a community to promote the performing arts.
Founded: 1979
Specialized Field: Musical; Dinner; Community
Status: Nonprofit
Paid Staff: 50
Performs At: Moberly Municipal Auditorium; Peppermint Loft
Organization Type: Performing; Sponsoring

3186   MARK TWAIN OUTDOOR THEATRE

12665 Fox Run Place
New London, MO 63459
Phone: 573-221-2945

Management:
   Managing Director: Sharon Donegan
Founded: 1979
Status: Non-Equity; Commercial
Season: May - September
Type of Stage: Outdoor
Stage Dimensions: 150' x 20'
Seating Capacity: 500+

3187 OZARK ACTORS THEATRE

PO Box K
Rolla, MO 65402
Phone: 573-364-9523
Fax: 573-364-9523
e-mail: oat@rollanet.org
Web Site: www.ozarkactorstheatre.org
Management:
   Artistic Director: F Reed Brown
Mission: Ozark Actors Theatre is a professional, summer stock theatre. Professional actors, directors, technicians, and designers are employed by OAT on a seasonal basis.
Founded: 1988
Status: Professional; Nonprofit
Season: July - August
Type of Stage: Proscenium
Stage Dimensions: 36' x 24'
Seating Capacity: 188

3188 EDISON THEATRE

Campus Box 1119
One Brookings Drive
Saint Louis, MO 63130-4899
Phone: 314-935-6518
Fax: 314-935-7362
e-mail: crobin@artsci.wustl.edu
Web Site: www.artsci.wustl.edu/edison
Management:
   Managing Director: Charles E Robin
   Operations Manager: Melinda Compton
   Marketing Manager: Aly Abrams
   Technical Director: Clinton McLanghlin
Founded: 1973
Specialized Field: Dance; Vocal Music; Instrumental Music; Theater
Status: Professional; Nonprofit
Paid Staff: 12
Budget: $150,000-400,000
Performs At: Edison Theatre; Mallinckrodt Drama Studio
Facility Category: Concert Hall; Performance Theatre
Type of Stage: proscenium
Seating Capacity: 656
Rental Contact: Melinda Compton
Organization Type: Performing; Touring; Educational; Sponsoring; Presenting

3189 METRO THEATER COMPANY

8308 Olive Boulevard
Saint Louis, MO 63132-2814
Phone: 314-997-6777
Fax: 314-997-1811
e-mail: mail@metrotheatrecompany.org
Web Site: www.metrotheatercompany.org
Officers:

President: Janet Schoedinger
VP: Kathe Rasch
CFO/Treasurer: John Weil
Secretary: Peggy O'Brien
Management:
   Artistic Director: Carol North
   Managing Director: Joan T Briccetti
   Booking Director: Rita Mocek
Mission: Metro Theater Company is a professional touring ensemble that develops and produces original theater pieces that respect the intelligence and emotional wisdom of young people, blend drama, movement, music, and design, and challenge both the artists who develop the work and the audience who receive it.
Founded: 1973
Specialized Field: Theatrical for young people
Status: Professional; Nonprofit
Paid Staff: 7
Paid Artists: 7
Budget: $535,000
Income Sources: Contributions; NEA; Missouri Arts Council; Regional Arts Commission of St. Louis; Arts & Education Council of Greater St. Louis
Season: August - May
Affiliations: American Alliance for Theatre & Education; International Association of Theatre for Children and Youth/USA; Theatre Communications Group, Inc.
Annual Attendance: 60,000+
Type of Stage: Proscenium
Stage Dimensions: 30x25x15
Rental Contact: Managing Director Joan T. Briccetti
Organization Type: Performing; Touring; Resident; Educational

3190 MUNICIPAL THEATER ASSOCIATION OF SAINT LOUIS

Forest Park
Saint Louis, MO 63112
Phone: 314-361-1900
Fax: 314-361-0009
Web Site: www.muny.com
Management:
   General Manager/CEO: Dennis M Reagan
Mission: To perform and produce musical theater shows 7 nights a week, during the summer only.
Founded: 1919
Specialized Field: Theater
Status: Professional; Nonprofit
Income Sources: NAMTP; Arts & Education Council of Greater Saint Louis
Performs At: The MUNY; Forest Park
Organization Type: Performing; Educational

3191 NEW THEATRE

634 N Grand Boulevard
Suite 10-C
Saint Louis, MO 63103
Phone: 314-531-8330
Fax: 314-533-3345
Officers:
   President: DeLancey Smith
   VP: Suzanne Couch
   Treasurer: James F O'Donnell
   Secretary: Agnes Wilcox

Management:
Artistic Director: Agnes Wilcox
Production Manager: Amy Allen
Director Public Relations: Dean Minderman
Office Manager: Joan Duggan
Mission: To provide innovative professional theatre in accessible locations for Saint Louis audiences.
Founded: 1985
Specialized Field: Theatrical Group
Status: Professional; Nonprofit
Income Sources: Theatre Communications Group: League of Saint Louis Theatres
Organization Type: Performing

3192 REPERTORY THEATRE OF SAINT LOUIS

130 Edgar Road
Box 191730
Saint Louis, MO 63119
Phone: 314-968-7340
Fax: 314-968-9638
e-mail: ecoffield@repstl.org
Web Site: www.repstl.org
Officers:
President: Gretta Forrester
Management:
Artistic Director: Steven Woolf
Mission: Dedicated to producing live theatre of superior quality. In celebrating the joy of live performance, this theatre is committed to building and sustaining a vital connection among all its stakeholders.
Founded: 1966
Specialized Field: Theatrical Group
Status: Professional
Income Sources: Actors' Equity Association; Society for Stage Directors and Choreographers; American Federation of Musicians; International Association of Theatrical Stage Employees
Season: September - April
Performs At: Loretto-Hilton Center for the Performing Arts
Type of Stage: Thrust; Flexible
Seating Capacity: 734; 125
Organization Type: Performing
Notes: Services for the hearing impaired, sight impaired and handicapped accessibility.

3193 SAINT LOUIS BLACK REPERTORY COMPANY

634 N Grand- 10F
Saint Louis, MO 63103
Phone: 314-534-3807
Fax: 314-534-8456
e-mail: stlouisblackrep@hotmail.com
Web Site: www.stlouisblackrep.org
Management:
Producing Director: Ron Himes
General Manager: Donna Adams
Managing Director: Maria Bradford
Mission: To provide platforms for theatre, dance and other creative expressions from the African-American perspective that heighten the social and cultural awareness of its audiences.
Founded: 1976

Specialized Field: Musical; Community; Theatrical Group
Status: Professional; Nonprofit
Paid Staff: 12
Volunteer Staff: 50
Performs At: Grandel Square Theatre
Affiliations: Theatre Communications Group; Actors' Equity Association
Annual Attendance: 75,000
Seating Capacity: 467
Organization Type: Performing; Touring; Educational; Sponsoring

3194 STAGES ST. LOUIS

104 N Clay
Saint Louis, MO 63122
Phone: 314-821-2412
Fax: 314-821-2191
e-mail: mailbox@stagesslouis.com
Web Site: www.stagesstlouis.com
Officers:
Chairman: Betty Von Hoffmann
President: Dory Poholsky
VP: Susan Svejkosky
Secretary: Philip S. Roush
Treasurer: Carl O. Trautman
Management:
Artistic Director: Michael Hamilton
Executive Producer: Jack Lane
General Manager: Steve Bertani
Production Stage Manager: Judith Grothe Cullen
Production Manager: John Cattanach
Mission: To produce the indigenous American art form of musical theatre which artfully combines the three disciplines of music, dance and drama. Through vital and unique interpretations of classic musicals, Stages strives to keep this threatened art form alive.
Founded: 1987
Paid Staff: 10
Paid Artists: 100
Budget: $1,200,000
Income Sources: Ticket Revenue; Private Donors; Corporations and Foundations
Performs At: Reim Theatre
Annual Attendance: 46,000
Facility Category: Theatre
Type of Stage: Proscenium
Stage Dimensions: 24'Dx34'W
Seating Capacity: 380
Year Built: 1960
Rental Contact: Kirkwood Civic Center
Resident Groups: Kirkwood Civic Center

3195 THEATER FACTORY SAINT LOUIS

4265 Shaw Avenue
Saint Louis, MO 63110
Phone: 314-771-0780
Management:
Managing Director: Earl D Weaver
Artistic Director: Hope Wurdack
Business Manager: Cindy Vahle
Founded: 1982
Specialized Field: Summer Stock; Theatrical Group
Status: Professional
Income Sources: League of St. Louis Theatres

Organization Type: Performing; Educational

3196 WEST END PLAYERS GUILD
Union Avenue Christian Church
Union Boulevard
Saint Louis, MO 63108
Phone: 314-367-0025
Web Site: www.westendplayers.org
Mission: Compromises two groups, the Players Guild and the West End Players, both of which originated and prospered in the city's Central West End.
Founded: 1911
Status: Non-professional

3197 LIBERTY CENTER
111 W 5th
Sedalia, MO 65301
Phone: 816-827-3228
Fax: 816-827-3103
Management:
   Administrator: Patti McFatrich
Mission: Promoting the Arts and cultural activities in the community.
Founded: 1981
Specialized Field: Musical; Dinner; Community; Folk; Theatrical Group; Puppet
Status: Professional; Non-Professional; Nonprofit
Paid Staff: 100
Performs At: Liberty Center
Organization Type: Performing; Touring; Educational; Sponsoring

3198 SIKESTON LITTLE THEATRE
PO Box 126
Sikeston, MO 63801
Phone: 573-681-9400
Management:
   Administrator: Lynn A Colley
Mission: To nurture theatrical arts in the Sikeston area; to provide theatre experience for students.
Founded: 1959
Specialized Field: Musical; Community; Theatrical Group
Status: Non-Professional; Nonprofit
Paid Staff: 150
Income Sources: Missouri Community Theatre Association
Performs At: Chaney-Harris Cultural Center
Organization Type: Performing; Resident

3199 GOLDENROD SHOWBOAT DINNER THEATRE
1000 Riverside Drive
St. Charles, MO 63301
Phone: 636-946-2020
Fax: 636-946-0946

3200 HOTHOUSE THEATRE COMPANY
1527-29 Washington Avenue
PO Box 43021
St. Louis, MO 63143
Phone: 314-241-1517
e-mail: info@hothousetheatre.org
Web Site: www.hothousetheatre.org
Management:
   Managing Director: Donna M Parrone
   Artistic Director: Marty Stanberry
Mission: HotHouse's mission is to produce thought-provoking theatre dedicated to cultural enhancement.
Founded: 1997
Status: Nonprofit
Season: October - May
Type of Stage: Flexible Black Box
Seating Capacity: 90

3201 MULE BARN THEATRE OF TARKIO COLLEGE
PO Box 114
224 Main Street
Tarkio, MO 64491
Phone: 816-736-4185
Mission: To provide cultural and educational enrichment for the area featuring the American musical and children's theatre, theatre for area residents and training for young professionals in theatre.
Founded: 1967
Specialized Field: Theater
Status: Professional; Nonprofit
Paid Staff: 15
Performs At: Mule Barn Theatre
Organization Type: Performing

3202 ROYAL ARTS COUNCIL
PO Box 273
107 S Monroe
Versailles, MO 65084
Phone: 573-378-6226
e-mail: royalart@advertisnet.com
Officers:
   President: Richard Williott
   VP: Kevin Schehr
   Secretary: Michelle Gerlt
   Treasurer: Cindy Davenport
Management:
   Executive Director: Pam Voth
   Director: Steve Bannon
   Director: Mary Jo Jackson
   Director: Lana James
   Director: Lois Viebrock
Mission: Promote the appreciation of various art disciplines through education, presentation, organization and the provision of an appropriate facility.
Founded: 1984
Specialized Field: Musical; Community; Theatrical Group
Status: Non-Professional; Nonprofit
Paid Staff: 1
Budget: $60,000
Income Sources: Ticket Sales; MAC Funding; Corporate Funding; Concessions; Program Advertising; Donations
Performs At: Royal Theatre
Annual Attendance: 4,000
Facility Category: Converted movie theatre with enlarged stage

Stage Dimensions: 34'x5 1/2'x22'
Seating Capacity: 294
Year Built: 1931
Year Remodeled: 2000
Rental Contact: Executive Director Pam Voth
Organization Type: Performing; Educational;
Sponsoring

Montana

3203 BIGFORK SUMMER PLAYHOUSE
PO Box 456
Bigfork, MT 59911
Phone: 406-837-4886
Fax: 406-837-2432
Web Site: www.digisys.net/playhouse/
Season: May - August

3204 ALBERTA BAIR THEATER
2801 3rd Avenue
Billings, MT 59101
Mailing Address: PO Box 1556, Billings, MO. 59103
Phone: 406-256-8915
Fax: 406-256-5060
e-mail: bfisher@albertabairtheater.org
Web Site: www.albertabairtheater.org
Management:
  Executive Director: Bill Fisher
  Program/Marketing Director: Corby Skinner
  Technical Director: Tom Lund
Paid Staff: 15
Volunteer Staff: 200
Budget: $1.2 million
Income Sources: Ticket income
Annual Attendance: 123,000

3205 MONTANA SHAKESPEARE IN THE PARKS
Montana State University
PO Box 174120
Bozeman, MT 59717-4120
Phone: 406-994-3901
Fax: 406-994-4591
e-mail: ggibk@aol.cpm
Web Site: www.montana.edu/shakespeare
Management:
  Artistic Director: Joel Jahnke
  Developemnt/Marketing Director: Moira Keshishian
  Business Director: Jolee Barry
  Marketing Assistant: JoDee Palin
Founded: 1973
Specialized Field: Outdoor Theatre
Status: Non-Equity; Nonprofit
Paid Staff: 4
Volunteer Staff: 82
Paid Artists: 35
Budget: $400,000
Income Sources: Grants; Corporate Sponsorship;
Montana State University; Indidvidual Donations; Earned
Income
Season: June - September
Affiliations: Montana State University

Annual Attendance: 26,000
Facility Category: Portable Elizabethan-style wood stage

3206 VIGILANTE THEATRE COMPANY
PO Box 507
Bozeman, MT 59771
Phone: 406-994-5884
e-mail: vigilante@in-touch.com
Web Site: www.vigilantetheatre.com
Management:
  Artistic Director: John Hosking
  Marketing Director: Celia Styren
  Office Manager: Chavon Kautzman
Mission: To stimulate, cultivate and promote interest in
theatre; to tour original, professional-level theatre in the
Northwest.
Founded: 1981
Specialized Field: Dinner; Theatrical Group; Comedy
Dinner Theatre; Main Stage Production; Montana's
Touring Repretory Theatre
Status: Professional; Nonprofit
Paid Staff: 2
Paid Artists: 4
Income Sources: Bookings; Ticket Sales; Grants;
Membership; Contributors
Season: January - December
Annual Attendance: 14,000
Organization Type: Performing; Touring; Educational

3207 ALEPH MOVEMENT THEATRE
822 E 6th Avenue
Helena, MT 59601
Phone: 406-443-1274
Mission: To perform movement theatre; to provide an
opportunity for education; to foster cultural exchange.
Founded: 1985
Specialized Field: Theatrical Group
Status: Professional; Nonprofit
Income Sources: National Mime Association
Organization Type: Performing; Touring; Educational

3208 MISSOULA CHILDREN'S THEATRE
200 N Adams Street
Missoula, MT 59802
Phone: 406-728-1911
Fax: 406-721-0637
e-mail: tour@mctinc.org
Web Site: www.mctinc.org
Management:
  Tour Marketing Director: Jonna Miller-Michelson
Mission: The development of lifeskills through
participation in the performing arts
Founded: 1971
Specialized Field: Musical Theatre/ Family
Entertainment

3209 MONTANA REPERTORY THEATRE
Performing Arts Center
University of Montana
Missoula, MT 59812
Phone: 406-243-6809
Fax: 406-243-5726
e-mail: mrt@selway.umt.edu
Web Site: www.umt.edu/mrt/mrt.html

Management:
    Artistic Director: Greg Johnson
    Production Manager: Steve Wing
    Administrative Assistant: Mary Ann Riddle
    Booking Agent: Rena Shagan Associates
Mission: To tell the great stories of our world to an ever expanding community.
Founded: 1976
Specialized Field: Theatrical Group
Status: Professional; Nonprofit
Paid Staff: 4
Budget: $900,000
Income Sources: Box Office; Grants; State Aid
Season: November - April
Performs At: Montana Theatre; University of Montana
Affiliations: Society for Stage Directors and Choreographers; Actors' Equity Association; International Alliance of Theatrical Stage Employees
Annual Attendance: varies
Facility Category: Educational
Type of Stage: Proscenium
Seating Capacity: 499
Year Built: 1985
Organization Type: Performing; Touring; Resident; Educational

3210 WHITEFISH THEATRE COMPANY

One Central Avenue
Whitefish, MT 59937
Phone: 406-862-5371
Fax: 406-863-9200
Web Site: www.whitefishtheatreco.org

Nebraska

3211 BELLEVUE LITTLE THEATRE

PO Box 162
Bellevue, NE 68005
Phone: 402-291-1554
e-mail: cyberma609@ao.com
Web Site: www.hometown.aol.com/bellelittle
Management:
    Board of Directors: Bobb Topp
Mission: To create a superior environment for the promotion of the performing arts through the presentation of comedy, drama, and musical theatre productions; and to stimulate educational and recreational programs in the technical and artistic venues of the performing arts for the citizens of the city of Bellevue, Sarpy County, and the Greater Omaha Metropolitan Area.
Founded: 1968
Specialized Field: Musical; Community; Theatrical Group; Puppet
Status: Non-Professional; Nonprofit
Volunteer Staff: all
Seating Capacity: 244
Year Built: 1942
Organization Type: Performing; Educational

3212 POST PLAYHOUSE INCORPORATED

PO Box 271
Crawford, NE 69339

Phone: 308-665-1976
Fax: 308-432-6396
e-mail: lmacneill@csc.edu
Management:
    Executive Director: Loree MacNeill
Mission: A Summer Repertory Theatre for tourists and residents.
Founded: 1966
Specialized Field: Theater
Status: Non-Equity; Nonprofit
Paid Staff: 15
Budget: $80,000
Income Sources: Ticket Sales; Nebraska Arts Council; Chadron stage College
Season: May - August
Performs At: Proscenium Theater
Annual Attendance: 9-12,000
Type of Stage: Proscenium
Stage Dimensions: 24' x 30'
Seating Capacity: 182
Year Remodeled: 1991

3213 GOTHENBURG COMMUNITY PLAYHOUSE

10th and D Street
PO Box 15
Gothenburg, NE 69138
Phone: 308-537-3235
Management:
    Manager: LaVon Pape
Mission: To offer cultural, literary and educational opportunities to residents of the community and region.
Founded: 1967
Specialized Field: Dinner; Community
Status: Non-Professional; Nonprofit
Performs At: Sun Theatre
Organization Type: Performing; Resident; Sponsoring

3214 KEARNEY COMMUNITY THEATRE

83 Plaza Boulevard
Kearney, NE 68845
Phone: 308-234-1529
e-mail: kct@kearney.net
Web Site: www.kctonline.com
Officers:
    President: Richard Jussel
    VP: Mary Haeberle
    Treasurer: Pat Munro
    Secretary: Maria Beucke
Management:
    Executive Director: Bradley J Driml
    President: Michael Johnson
    VP: Larry Nickles
Mission: To present five shows annually, as well as a summer children's workshop.
Founded: 1977
Specialized Field: Musical; Dinner; Community; Theatrical Group
Status: Non-Professional; Nonprofit
Income Sources: Nebraska Arts Council; Nebraska Association of Community Theatres; American Association of Community Theatres
Performs At: Kearney Community Theatre

Organization Type: Performing; Educational;
Sponsoring

3215 LINCOLN COMMUNITY PLAYHOUSE
2500 S 56th Street
Lincoln, NE 68506
Phone: 402-489-7529
Fax: 402-489-1035
Web Site: lincolnplayhouse.com
Officers:
President: Gary Hall
Secretary: Olinda Boslau
Treasurer: Shannon Meyerer
President Elect: Randal Hawthorne
Management:
Business Manager: Lettie Van Hemert
Artistic Director: Rob McKercher
Mission: To offer quality theatrical experiences to the
community.
Founded: 1946
Specialized Field: Community
Status: Nonprofit
Paid Staff: 10
Volunteer Staff: 400
Income Sources: NE Arts Council
Performs At: Oliver T. Joy Mainstage; L.L. Coryell &
Sons
Affiliations: American Association of Community
Theatres; Nebraska Association of Community Theatres
Organization Type: Performing

3216 NEBRASKA REPERTORY THEATRE
215 Temple Building
12th and R Streets
Lincoln, NE 68588-0201
Phone: 402-472-2072
Fax: 402-472-9055
Toll-free: 800-432-3231
e-mail: jhagemeier1@unl.edu
Web Site: www.unl.edu/rep
Officers:
President: Larry Frederick
Past President: Joyce Cartmill
Management:
Executive Director: Jeffery Scott Elwell
General Manager: Julie Hagemeier
Production Stage Manager: Brad Buffum
Founded: 1968
Specialized Field: Theatrical Group
Status: Professional; Semi-Professional; Nonprofit
Paid Staff: 30
Volunteer Staff: 30
Budget: $176,000
Income Sources: Ticket Sales; University; Contributions
Season: June - August
Performs At: Howell Theatre; Studio Theatre; Carson
Theatre
Affiliations: TCG, ATHE, KC/ACTF, NAST, UIRTA
Annual Attendance: 6,000
Type of Stage: Proscenium; Black Box
Seating Capacity: 320; 240
Year Built: 1908
Year Remodeled: 1980
Rental Contact: Brad Buffum
Organization Type: Performing; Resident

3217 CENTER STAGE
3010 R Street
Omaha, NE 68107
Phone: 402-444-6230
Management:
Executive Director: Linda Runice
Mission: The presentation of ethnic performances.
Founded: 1980
Specialized Field: Community; Theatrical Group
Status: Non-Professional; Nonprofit
Performs At: LaFerne Williams Center
Organization Type: Performing

3218 CIRCLE THEATRE
2015 S 60th Street
Omaha, NE 68106
Phone: 402-553-4715
Fax: 402-553-4715
Officers:
President: Ward Peters
VP: Robert Bradley
Treasurer: Karen Dowell
Secretary: Nancy Ross
Management:
Executive Director: Laura Marr
Artistic Director: Doug Marr
Mission: Developing and producing new plays by
Nebraska playwrights, employing Nebraska artists.
Founded: 1983
Specialized Field: Dinner; Theatrical Group
Status: Semi-Professional; Nonprofit
Paid Staff: 10
Budget: $120,000
Income Sources: Nebraska Arts Council; Local
Foundation; Private Support
Annual Attendance: 10,000
Type of Stage: Black Box
Seating Capacity: 100
Year Built: 1945
Organization Type: Performing; Touring; Resident

3219 GRANDE OLDE PLAYERS THEATRE COMPANY
2339 N 90th
Omaha, NE 68134
Phone: 402-397-5262
Fax: 402-573-7532
e-mail: LensArtCPP@aol.com
Officers:
President: David Kistler
VP: Kieth Homan
Treasurer: Jack Kincaid
Secretary: Riza Breen
Management:
Executive Director: Warren H Johnson
Mission: Provide live community theatre experience with
and for senior citizens.
Founded: 1984
Specialized Field: Live Theatre
Status: Non-Professional; Nonprofit
Non-paid Artists: 125
Budget: $59,000
Income Sources: Ticket Sales
Annual Attendance: 5,000

Facility Category: Live Theatre
Type of Stage: Proscenium
Stage Dimensions: 43'x17'
Seating Capacity: 141
Year Remodeled: 1993
Rental Contact: Executive Director Warren H. Johnson
Organization Type: Performing; Touring; Educational

3220 OMAHA COMMUNITY PLAYHOUSE

6915 Cass Street
Omaha, NE 68132-2696
Phone: 402-553-4890
Fax: 402-553-6288
Toll-free: 800-964-0990
Web Site: www.omahaplayhouse.com
Officers:
  President: Dennis O'Neal
  Executive VP: Lucia Milone Williams
  Secretary: Dee Owen
  Treasurer: Dan Hassel
Management:
  Artistic Director: Carl Beck
  Marketing Director: Betsye Poragas
  Man. Dir., Nebraska Theatre Caravan: Rick Scott
Mission: To offer the finest possible theatre to our audiences; to provide a performance outlet for amateur actors.
Founded: 1924
Specialized Field: Theatrical Group
Status: Professional; Non-Professional; Nonprofit
Paid Staff: 45
Paid Artists: 120
Budget: $4,000,000
Income Sources: Donations; Subscribers; Single Ticket Revenue
Season: September - June
Performs At: Omaha Community Playhouse
Annual Attendance: 110,000
Facility Category: Theatre
Type of Stage: Traditional Proscenium & Black Box
Seating Capacity: 600; 235
Year Built: 1959
Year Remodeled: 1986
Organization Type: Performing; Touring

3221 OMAHA THEATER COMPANY FOR YOUNG PEOPLE

2001 Farnam Street
Omaha, NE 68102
Phone: 402-345-4852
Fax: 402-344-7255
Management:
  Artistic Director: James Larson
Founded: 1949

3222 OMAHA THEATRE COMPANY FOR YOUNG PEOPLE

2001 Farnam Street
Omaha, NE 68102
Phone: 402-345-4852
Fax: 402-344-7255
e-mail: boxoffice@otcmail.org
Web Site: www.otcyp.org
Officers:

President: Richard Heyman
VP Marketing: Stephen Zubrod
Past President: Tracy Stanko
Foundation Representative: Susie Buffett
Management:
  Executive Director: Roberta Wilhelm
  Artisitic Director: James Larson
Mission: Providing quality theater for Omaha children and their families.
Specialized Field: Theatrical Group
Status: Professional; Nonprofit
Paid Staff: 32
Volunteer Staff: 15
Paid Artists: 10
Budget: $2.4 million
Income Sources: Theatre Communications Group; Nebraska Arts Council; Douglas County; National Endowment for the Arts; Corporations; Private Donations
Facility Category: Live theatre for children and their families
Type of Stage: Proscenium; Black Box
Stage Dimensions: 48'& 31' deep. Pit 11'x6'/11'X 6'
Year Built: 1927
Year Remodeled: 1994
Cost: $5.9 million
Rental Contact: Stan Kiepke
Organization Type: Performing; Touring; Resident; Educational

3223 SHAKESPEARE ON THE GREEN

Department of Fine Arts
Creighton University
Omaha, NE 68178
Phone: 402-280-2391
Fax: 402-280-2320
e-mail: neshakes@creighton.edu
Web Site: www.neshakespeare.creighton.edu
Management:
  Artistic Director: Michael Markey
Founded: 1986
Status: Non-Equity
Season: May - July
Type of Stage: Outdoor
Stage Dimensions: 100' x 300'
Seating Capacity: 5000

Nevada

3224 BREWERY ARTS CENTER

449 W King Street
Carson City, NV 89703
Phone: 702-883-1976
Fax: 702-883-1922
e-mail: ann@breweryarts.org
Web Site: www.breweryarts.org
Management:
  Executive Director: Joe McCarthy
  Development Director: Bill Cowee
Mission: To provide and promote the arts and culture in Carson City.
Founded: 1976
Specialized Field: Musical; Community; Folk; Theatrical Group

Status: Non-Professional; Nonprofit
Paid Staff: 8
Volunteer Staff: 100
Performs At: Carson City Community Center; Brewery Arts Center
Organization Type: Performing; Sponsoring

3225 ACTORS REPERTORY THEATRE
1824 Palo Alto Circle
Las Vegas, NV 89108
Phone: 702-647-7469
Fax: 702-647-3130
Web Site: www.actorsrep.com
Officers:
   President: Michael Levy
Management:
   Artistic Director: Georgia Neu
   Managing Director: Rob Gubbins
Mission: Dedicated to training for, and the performance of, the classics, and the best in modern and musical theatre, with special emphasis given to new works of exceptional merit.
Performs At: Summerlin Performing Arts Center
Comments: Summerlin Theatre is accesible to the mobility impaired and listening assistance devices are available.

3226 LAS VEGAS LITTLE THEATRE
3844 Schiff Drive
Las Vegas, NV 89103
Phone: 702-362-7996
Web Site: www.lvlt.org
Management:
   Executive Producer: Jack Bell
   Managing Director: Paul A Thornton
Mission: To educate and entertain the community; to provide hands-on training for interested artists.
Founded: 1978
Specialized Field: Musical; Community; Theatrical Group
Status: Semi-Professional; Nonprofit
Income Sources: Nevada Community Theatre Association; Allied Arts Council of Southern Nevada; American Association of Community Theatres
Organization Type: Performing; Educational

3227 NEVADA THEATRE COMPANY
6130 W Flamingo
Suite 228
Las Vegas, NV 89103
Phone: 702-873-0191
Management:
   Artistic Director: Deanna Duplechain
Founded: 1997
Status: Non-Equity; Nonprofit
Season: September - June

3228 THEATER COALITION/THE LEAR THEATER
528 W 1st Street
Reno, NV 89503

Phone: 775-786-2278
Fax: 775-786-4350
e-mail: theatercoalition@theatercoalition.org
Web Site: www.theatercoalition.org
Management:
   Executive Director: Susan Mayes-Smith
   Office Administrator: Rhonda Hernandez
   Capital Campaign Coordinator: Angela Rodriquez-Cao
Founded: 1994
Specialized Field: All
Paid Staff: 5
Volunteer Staff: 50

New Hampshire

3229 MAINSTAGE CENTER FOR THE ARTS
100 S Black Horse Pike
Blackwood, NH 08012
Phone: 856-232-1012
Fax: 856-401-1776
e-mail: stage3091@snip.net
Web Site: www.mainstage.org
Management:
   President: Edward P Fiscella

3230 COMMUNITY PLAYERS OF CONCORD
PO Box 681
Concord, NH 03302-0681
Phone: 603-224-4905
Web Site: www.newww.com/org/players
Officers:
   President: Abby Lange
   VP: Paul Bacon
   Secretary: Kevin Barrett
   Treasurer: Doris Ballard
Mission: To nurture interest in all aspects of community theater.
Founded: 1927
Specialized Field: Community; Theatrical Group
Status: Nonprofit
Income Sources: New Hampshire Community Theater Association
Performs At: Concord City Auditorium
Organization Type: Performing

3231 HAMPTON PLAYHOUSE
Winnacunnet Road
Hampton, NH 03842
Phone: 603-926-3076
Management:
   Producing/Artistic Director: Alfred Christie
   Producer: John Vari
Founded: 1948
Specialized Field: Summer Stock; Musical
Status: Professional; Commercial
Income Sources: Actors' Equity Association; Society for Stage Directors and Choreographers; Council of Resident Summer Theatres
Season: June - September
Performs At: Hampton Playhouse Theatre Arts Workshop
Organization Type: Performing; Resident; Educational

3232 PAPERMILL THEATRE/NORTH COUNTY CENTER FOR THE ARTS
Box 1060
Lincoln, NH 03251
Phone: 706-880-8324
Fax: 706-880-8041
e-mail: kbarber@papermilltheatre.org
Web Site: www.papermilltheatre.org
Management:
Artistic Director: Kim Barber
Founded: 1986
Specialized Field: New England
Status: Non-Equity; Nonprofit
Paid Staff: 12
Paid Artists: 20
Season: June - August
Type of Stage: Proscenium
Stage Dimensions: 36' x 40'
Seating Capacity: 250

3233 LAKES REGION SUMMER THEATRE
Route 25
Meredith, NH 03253
Phone: 603-279-9933
Fax: 603-279-4525
e-mail: meredith@lr.net
Season: June - September

3234 MOUNT WASHINGTON VALLEY THEATRE COMPANY
Box 265
North Conway, NH 03860
Phone: 603-356-5425
Fax: 603-356-8357
e-mail: pinkham@pinkhamrealestate.com
Management:
President: Linda Pinkham
Founded: 1971
Status: Nonprofit
Season: June - August
Type of Stage: Proscenium
Seating Capacity: 183

3235 PETERBOROUGH PLAYERS
PO Box 118
Peterborough, NH 03458
Phone: 603-924-9344
Fax: 603-924-6359
Management:
Artistic Director: Gus Kaikkonen
Managing Director: Keith Stevens
Founded: 1933
Specialized Field: Theatrical Group
Status: Professional; Nonprofit
Income Sources: Actors' Equity Association; Council of Resident Summer Theatres
Season: June - September
Organization Type: Performing; Resident; Educational

3236 PONTINE MOVEMENT THEATRE
The McDonough St. Studio
135 McDonough Street
Portsmouth, NH 03801
Phone: 603-436-6660
Fax: 603-436-1577
e-mail: info@pontine.org
Web Site: www.pontine.org
Officers:
President: Anne Salzer
VP: Tina Marcoux
Secretary/Treasurer: Heather Ashton
Management:
Co-Artistic Director: Marguerite Mathews
Co-Artistic Director: Greg Gathers
Mission: Dedicated to the cultural enhancements of its various publics, its performances and educational programs are offered to inform the public in the art of corporeal mime and to the preservation and development of this exciting theatrical form
Founded: 1977
Status: Professional; Nonprofit
Paid Staff: 4
Paid Artists: 4
Budget: $101,000
Performs At: McDonough Street Theater
Affiliations: New Hampshire State Council on the Arts
Annual Attendance: 1,200
Facility Category: Studio/theatre
Type of Stage: Black Box
Stage Dimensions: 20'x20'
Seating Capacity: 48
Year Built: 1900
Year Remodeled: 1987
Rental Contact: Greg Gathers
Organization Type: Performing; Touring; Resident; Educational; Sponsoring
Resident Groups: Pontine Movement Theatre

3237 SEACOAST REPERTORY THEATRE
125 Bow Street
Portsmouth, NH 03801
Phone: 603-433-4793
Fax: 603-431-7818
Toll-free: 800-639-7650
e-mail: info@seacoastrep.org
Web Site: www.seacoastrep.org
Officers:
President: Martin Lessard
VP: John Bosen
Secretary: John Colliander, Esquire
Treasurer: Steven Scott
Management:
Producing Artistic Director: Roy Rogosin
Associate Director/Producer: Eileen Rogosin
Assistant Artistic Director: Jean Benda
Director Marketing/Publicity: Stacy Baker
Mission: To provide a safe haven for performers and audiences.
Founded: 1986
Specialized Field: Northern New England
Status: Professional; Nonprofit
Paid Staff: 15
Volunteer Staff: 6
Budget: $1,100,000
Income Sources: Ticket Sales; Sponsorships; Fundraising Events
Season: Summer and All - Year
Annual Attendance: 50,000

Facility Category: Live Theatre
Type of Stage: 3/4 Thrust
Seating Capacity: 235
Year Built: 1890
Year Remodeled: 1970
Rental Contact: Sandi Clark
Organization Type: Performing; Resident; Educational

3238 BARNSTORMERS

PO Box 434
Tamworth, NH 03886
Phone: 603-323-8661
Fax: 603-323-3351
e-mail: info@barnstormerstheatre.com
Web Site: www.barnstormerstheatre.com
Officers:
　Secretary: Helen Steele
　Treasurer: Bob Lloyd
　Co-Chair: Kate Thompson
　Co-Chair: Dana Steele
　Board Chair: Shirley Ganem
Management:
　Artistic Director: Cope Murray
　Executive Director: Dan Rowe
Mission: To provide a summer theatre program featuring old—and some new—plays.
Founded: 1931
Specialized Field: Summer Stock
Status: Professional; Nonprofit
Income Sources: Actors' Equity Association
Season: June - August
Performs At: The Barnstormers Theatre
Organization Type: Performing; Resident

3239 WEATHERVANE THEATRE

53 Jefferson Road
Whitefield, NH 03598
Phone: 603-837-9010
Fax: 603-837-3333
e-mail: wvtheatreaol.com
Web Site: www.weathervanetheatre.org
Officers:
　COO: Richard Portner
Management:
　Producing Director: Gibbs Murray
　Artistic Director: Jacques Stewart
Mission: To present 7-8 shows each season, including musicals.
Founded: 1965
Specialized Field: Summer Stock; Musical; Professional; Alternating Repertory
Status: Professional; Commercial
Paid Staff: 5
Paid Artists: 20
Non-paid Artists: 15
Budget: $300,000
Income Sources: Box Office; Grants; Donor Appeal
Season: July - August
Performs At: Barn Theatre
Affiliations: Actors' Equity Association
Annual Attendance: 10,000
Type of Stage: Open Thrust
Seating Capacity: 250
Year Built: 2002
Organization Type: Performing

3240 ANDY'S SUMMER PLAYHOUSE

Issac Frye Highway
PO Box 601
Wilton, NH 03086
Phone: 603-654-2613
e-mail: andyssummerplayhouse@yahoo.com
Web Site: www.andyssummerplayhouse.org
Management:
　Artistic Director: Robert Lawson
　Managing Director: Lizzie Harris
Mission: Andy's Summer Playhouse is innovative theater by children for people of all ages. We serve all of Southern New Hampshire from Nashua to Keene, and from Concord to Massachusetts.
Founded: 1970
Season: June - August
Type of Stage: Flexible
Stage Dimensions: 40' x 50'
Seating Capacity: 152

New Jersey

3241 SURFLIGHT THEATRE

Beach & Engleside
PO Box 1155
Beach Haven, NJ 08008
Phone: 609-492-9477
Fax: 609-492-4469
e-mail: surflight@dandy.net
Web Site: www.lbinet.com\surflight
Officers:
　President: Patricia Offerman
　VP: Suzethe Whiting
Management:
　Executive Producer: T Scott Henderson
　Artistic Director: Steve Steiner
　Production Manager: Gail Steiner
Founded: 1950
Specialized Field: Stock; Musical; Dramatic
Status: Professional
Paid Staff: 25
Volunteer Staff: 25
Paid Artists: 60
Non-paid Artists: 20
Budget: $1,500,000
Income Sources: Box Office; NJSCA; Donations
Affiliations: New Jersey Theatre Alliance
Annual Attendance: 60,000
Facility Category: Theatre House
Type of Stage: Proscenium
Stage Dimensions: 24x35
Seating Capacity: 450
Year Built: 1987
Rental Contact: Gail Anderson Steiner
Organization Type: Performing; Resident

3242 CAPE MAY STAGE

Theatre in the Welcome Center
Bank and Lafayette Streets
Cape May, NJ
Phone: 609-884-1341
e-mail: michael@capemaystage.com
Web Site: www.capemaystage.com

Management:
   Director: Michael Laird
Mission: To be a professional theatre company with a spirit of community. Places emphasis on acting, directing and playwriting excellence.
Season: May - December

3243 CRANFORD DRAMATIC CLUB
78 Winans Avenue
PO Box 511
Cranford, NJ 07016
Phone: 908-276-7611
Mission: To stimulate interest in theatre.
Founded: 1919
Specialized Field: Community
Status: Non-Professional; Nonprofit
Performs At: Cranford Dramatic Club
Organization Type: Performing

3244 PLAYS-IN-THE-PARK
Middlesex County Department of Parks and Recreation
Pine Drive/Roosevelt Park
PO Box 661
Edison, NJ 08903
Phone: 732-548-2884
Fax: 732-548-1484
e-mail: pipoffice@playsinthepark.com
Web Site: www.playsinthepark.com
Management:
   Office Manager: Jackie Neill
   Producer: Gary Cohen
Founded: 1963
Status: Nonprofit
Paid Staff: 30
Volunteer Staff: 75
Non-paid Artists: 100
Budget: $405,000
Income Sources: Middlesex County Department of Parks and Recreation; Middlesex County Taxpayers; Patrons
Season: June - August
Performs At: Indoor/Outdoor Amphitheater
Annual Attendance: 60,000
Type of Stage: Proscenium
Stage Dimensions: 40'x20'
Year Built: 1963
Year Remodeled: 1975

3245 NEW GLOBE THEATER
166 Fairview Avenue
High Bridge, NJ 08829
Phone: 908-638-4942
Fax: 908-638-4715
e-mail: stuartvaughan@sprintmail.com
Management:
   Associate Producer: Anne Vaughan

3246 HOLMDEL THEATRE COMPANY
PO Box 182
Holmdel, NJ 07733
Phone: 732-946-0427
Web Site: www.holmdeltheatrecompany.org
Management:

Artistic Director: Gregg W Brevoort
Managing Director: Carl J Nolan
Mission: To provide artistic/theatrical opportunities for community residents to perform and create in a professional environment.
Founded: 1985
Status: Semi-Professional
Performs At: Duncan Smith Theatre

3247 NEW JERSEY REPERTORY COMPANY
179 Broadway
Long Branch, NJ 07740
Phone: 732-229-3166
Fax: 732-229-3167
e-mail: info@njrep.org
Web Site: www.njrep.org
Officers:
   Director Marketing: Debbie Mura
Management:
   Artistic Director: SuzAnne Barabas
   Executive Director: Gabor Barabas
Mission: The primary mission of the theater is to develop and produce new plays with diverse themes. It is also devoted to creating an atmosphere where classics can take on a fresh look and forgotten plays can find a home.
Founded: 1997
Status: Professional
Income Sources: Donations, Grants
Facility Category: Theater
Type of Stage: Black Box
Year Remodeled: 1998

3248 PLAYWRIGHTS THEATRE OF NEW JERSEY
33 Green Village Road
PO Box 1295
Madison, NJ 07940
Phone: 973-514-1787
Fax: 973-514-2060
e-mail: info@ptnj.org
Web Site: www.ptnj.org
Management:
   Artistic Director: John Pietrowski
   Producing Director: Elizabeth Murphy
Mission: Provides opportunities for writers to develop their work in a nurturing environment and connect with new audiences. Four step process through which playwrights, theatre artists and audiences collaborate to bring selected texts from rough draft to finished production. Education programs for students of all ages and backgrounds.
Founded: 1986
Status: Nonprofit
Paid Staff: 10
Volunteer Staff: 30
Paid Artists: 100
Budget: 900,000
Income Sources: Earned; Government; Corporate Foundation; Individuals
Season: September - June
Affiliations: AEA; SSDC; USA
Annual Attendance: 6,000
Type of Stage: Black Blox
Stage Dimensions: 30' x 18'

Seating Capacity: 125
Year Built: 1985

3249 SIMULATIONS

PO Box 399
Martinsville, NJ 08836
Phone: 732-356-7800
Web Site: www.simulationsincl.com
Founded: 1979
Status: Commercial

3250 FORUM THEATRE

314 Main Street
Metuchen, NJ 08840
Phone: 732-548-4670
Management:
   Artistic Director: Peter Loewy
Founded: 1983
Status: Nonprofit
Season: October - June
Type of Stage: Proscenium/Thrust

3251 PAPER MILL PLAYHOUSE

Brookside Drive
Millburn, NJ 07041
Phone: 973-379-3636
Fax: 973-376-0825
e-mail: NMarino@papermill.org
Web Site: www.papermill.org
Management:
   Executive Producer: Angelo Del Rossi
   Artistic Director: Robert Johanson
   General Manager: Peter Croken
   Marketing Manager: Nancy Marino
Mission: To enrich the cultural lives of a wide and diverse audience. A nationally recognized professional arts center committed to excellence and to preserving the rich heritage of plays and musicals through productions of the highest quality; to develop new works; collaborating with established and emerging artists, providing arts education for all ages; and to maintaining a leadership role in the community.
Founded: 1934
Specialized Field: Musical Equity Theater
Status: Professional; Not-for-Profit
Paid Staff: 60
Income Sources: AEA; Council of Stock Theatres; Society for Stage Directors and Choreographers; American Federation of Musicians; International Association of Theaters
Season: September - June
Performs At: Paper Mill Playhouse
Annual Attendance: 450,000
Type of Stage: Proscenium
Seating Capacity: 1192
Organization Type: Performing; Touring; Resident; Educational; Sponsoring

3252 ARTSPOWER NATIONAL TOURING THEATRE

39 S Fullerton Avenue
Montclair, NJ 07042-3354
Phone: 973-744-0909
Fax: 973-744-3609
e-mail: info@artspower.org
Web Site: www.artspower.org
Officers:
   Production Manager: Ginny Bowers Coleman
Management:
   Managing Director: Gary Blackman
   Director Development: Mark Blackman
   Artistic Director: Greg Gunning
   Senior Booking Associate: Stacey Sander Higgins
Founded: 1985
Specialized Field: Theatre for young audiences
Status: Nonprofit
Paid Staff: 9
Paid Artists: 32
Budget: $1.7 million
Income Sources: Ticket Sales; Presenting Fees; Grants
Season: October - June
Performs At: Performs in 40 states across US
Affiliations: AEA
Facility Category: Touring Theatre
Organization Type: varies

3253 YASS HAKOSHIMA MIME THEATRE

239 Midland Avenue
Montclair, NJ 07042
Phone: 973-783-9845
Fax: 973-783-0001
e-mail: yass@bellatlantic.net
Web Site: www.yasshakoshima.com
Officers:
   Artistic Director: Yass Hakoshima
   Assistant Director: Renate A Boue
Management:
   Business Manager Danmari Ltd.: Lynn K Palmer
   Chairperson: Anne Benbow
   Artistic Director: Yass Hakoshima
   Assistant Director: Renate A Boue
Mission: To present the highest form of the art of mime through performances, master classes, lecture demonstrations and workshops worldwide.
Founded: 1976
Specialized Field: Mime
Status: Professional; Nonprofit
Paid Staff: 4
Organization Type: Performing; Touring; Resident; Educational

3254 CROSSROADS THEATRE COMPANY

7 Livingston Avenue
New Brunswick, NJ 08901
Phone: 732-249-5581
Fax: 908-249-1861
Web Site: www.crossroadstheatre.org
Officers:
   President: Dale Caldwell
   VP: James Norfleet
   Secretary: Dee Henock
   Treasurer: Melanie A. Nicholson
Management:
   Artistic Director: Ricardo Khan
   Executive Director: Andre Robinson, Jr
   Literary Manager: Lenora Inez Brown

Mission: To provide a professional environment to encourage public interest of all backgrounds; to present honest portrayals and uphold the highest standard of artistic excellence of professional Black Theatre.
Founded: 1978
Specialized Field: Theatrical Group; Afro-American Theatre Company
Status: Professional; Nonprofit
Income Sources: Private Foundations/Grants; Business/Corporate Donations; Box Office; Government Grants; Individual Donations
Season: September - May
Performs At: Crossroads Theatre
Type of Stage: Modified Thrust
Seating Capacity: 300
Organization Type: Touring; Resident; Educational

3255 GEORGE STREET PLAYHOUSE

9 Livingston Avenue
New Brunswick, NJ 08901-1903
Phone: 732-846-2895
Fax: 732-247-9151
Web Site: www.georgestplayhouse.org
Management:
 Artistic Director: David Saint
 Managing Director: Michael Stotts
 Producer: George Ryan
 Business Manager: Karen Price
Mission: To produce new musicals and world premieres; to revitalize contemporary classics.
Founded: 1974
Specialized Field: Musical; Theatrical Group
Status: Professional; Nonprofit
Income Sources: Theatre Communications Group
Season: September - May
Performs At: George Street Playhouse
Type of Stage: Proscenium/Thrust
Seating Capacity: 367
Organization Type: Performing; Touring; Resident; Producing

3256 NEWARK PERFORMING ARTS CORPORATION/NEWARK SYMPHONY HALL

1030 Broad Street
Newark, NJ 07102
Phone: 973-643-4550
Fax: 973-643-6722
Officers:
 Chairman: Miquel E Rodriguez
 Treasurer: Julian Marsh
 Secretary: J Barry Washington
Management:
 Acting Executive Director: Roslyn L Lightfoot
 General Manager: Oscar James
 Marketing/Development Director: Catherine J Lenix-Hooker
Mission: To enhance the cultural and community life of the citizens of the greater Newark area by presenting a program of the highest quality and artistic integrity and to complement that activity by providing first class facilities for classical, ethnic, popular and community arts groups, for arts education, and civic/social organizations.
Founded: 1986

Specialized Field: Musical; Community; Theatrical Group
Status: Professional; Nonprofit
Paid Staff: 16
Budget: $1,400,000
Income Sources: Box Office Receipts; State & City Government Grants; Space Rental Fees; Concessions; Foundation & Corporation Grants
Performs At: Newark Symphony Hall
Affiliations: American Society of Composers, Authors, & Publishers; Garden State Theatrical Organ Society; Broadcast Music, Inc.
Annual Attendance: 250,000+
Facility Category: Performing Arts Center
Type of Stage: Proscenium
Stage Dimensions: 63'x40'
Seating Capacity: 2,800
Year Built: 1925
Rental Contact: General Manager Oscar N. James
Organization Type: Performing; Presenting
Resident Groups: African Globe Theatre Works Company; Kabu Okai-Davies

3257 THEATRE OF UNIVERSAL IMAGES

360 Central Avenue
Newark, NJ 07103
Phone: 201-645-6930
Fax: 201-642-6013
Management:
 Executive Producer: Clarence C Lilley
Mission: Providing education in the performing arts and telecommunications to the Greater Newark Community, the priority of TUI is to increase opportunities and cultural enrichment of African-Americans in Greater Essex County.
Founded: 1970
Status: Professional; Nonprofit
Income Sources: National Endowment for the Arts; Dodge Foundation; Victoria Foundation; Black United Foundation
Performs At: Theatre of Universal Images
Organization Type: Performing; Touring; Resident

3258 THEATRE OF RARITAN VALLEY COMMUNITY COLLEGE

Route 28 & Lamington Road
North Branch, NJ 08876
Mailing Address: PO Box 3300, Somerville, NJ. 08876-1265
Phone: 908-526-1200
Fax: 908-526-7890
e-mail: theatre@raritanval.edu
Web Site: www.raritanval.edu/theatre
Officers:
 President: G Jeremiah Ryan
 VP: Marie Gnage
Management:
 Theatre Director: Alan Liddell
 Communications Assistant: Cristina Lankay
 Theatre Manager: Jacinthia Alexander
 Production Assistant: John Widemann
Founded: 1985

3259 FOUNDATION THEATRE
Burlington County College
Route 530
Pemberton, NJ 08068
Phone: 609-894-9311
Fax: 609-894-9440
Management:
    Interim Production Director: Daniel Aubrey
Founded: 1975
Status: Nonprofit
Season: June - August
Type of Stage: Proscenium
Seating Capacity: 244

3260 CREATIVE THEATRE
102 Witherspoon Street
Princeton, NJ 08540
Phone: 609-924-8777
Management:
    Executive Director: Carly Tilton
    Artistic Director: Eloise Bruce
    Education Director: Jean Prall
Mission: To provide theatre and creative drama for children.
Founded: 1969
Specialized Field: Children's Theatre
Status: Professional; Nonprofit
Organization Type: Performing; Touring; Resident; Educational

3261 MCCARTER THEATRE
91 University Place
Princeton, NJ 08540
Phone: 609-258-6500
Fax: 609-497-0369
Toll-free: 888-278-7932
e-mail: admin@mccarter.org
Web Site: www.mccarter.org
Management:
    Artistic Director: Emily Mann
    Managing Director: Jeffrey Woodward
    Special Programming Director: William W Lockwood
Founded: 1930
Specialized Field: Classical Music and Dance; Jazz; World Music; Modern Dance; Theatre
Status: Nonprofit
Season: September - May
Affiliations: McCarter Theatre Company
Annual Attendance: 200,000+
Facility Category: Performing Arts Center
Type of Stage: Proscenium
Stage Dimensions: 42' x 36'
Orchestra Pit: 1
Seating Capacity: 1078
Year Built: 1930
Architect: DK Este Fisher
Rental Contact: General Manager Kathleen Nolan

3262 PRINCETON REPERTORY COMPANY
1 Palmer Square
Suite 541
Princeton, NJ 08542

Phone: 609-921-3682
e-mail: PRCRepRap@aol.com
Web Site: www.princetonrep.org
Management:
    Artistic Director: Victoria Liberatori
    Executive Producer: Anne Reiss
    Press Contact: Carol Fineman
Mission: Princeton Repertory Company was founded in 1984 and is a professional theatre company operating under a Small Professional Theatre Contract with Actors' Equity Association.
Founded: 1984
Status: Professional; Not-for-Profit
Season: June - August

3263 PRINCETON SHAKESPEARE FESTIVAL
1 Palmer Square
Suite 541
Princeton, NJ 08542
Phone: 609-921-3682
e-mail: PRCRepRap@aol.com
Web Site: www.princetonrep.org
Management:
    Artistic Director: Victoria Liberatori
    Executive Producer: Anne Reiss
    Press Contact: Carol Fineman
Mission: The impressive growth of the Princeton Rep Shakespeare Festival is due in part to the sustained lead sponsorship.
Founded: 1995
Status: Professional; Not-for-Profit

3264 TWO RIVER THEATRE COMPANY
223 Maple Avenue
PO Box 8035
Red Bank, NJ 07701
Phone: 732-345-1400
Fax: 732-345-1414
e-mail: info@tworivertheatre.org
Web Site: www.tworivertheatre.org
Management:
    Artistic Director: Jonathan Fox
Mission: Dedicated to presenting works, which most richly direct our gaze to the life of the human spirit. Our mission is to produce works, from the classical and contemporary canons, which are literary and intelligent. Two River's programs include not only mainstage productions, but special performances including a student matinee series (for high school classes), singles nights and sign-interpretation and audio-described performances.
Founded: 1993
Status: Nonprofit
Season: September - May
Affiliations: AEA
Annual Attendance: 10,000
Type of Stage: Proscenium
Stage Dimensions: 35' x 35'
Seating Capacity: 300

3265 THEATRE AT RARITAN VALLEY COMMUNITY COLLEGE
Route 28 & Lamingdon Road
PO Box 3300
Somerville, NJ 08876-1265

Phone: 908-725-3420
Fax: 908-526-7890
e-mail: theatre@raritanval.edu
Web Site: www.raritanval.edu/theatre
Officers:
  President: G Jeremiah Ryan
  Senior VP: Marie Gnage
  VP Finance/Administration: Thomas Carroll
Management:
  Director of Theatre: Alan Liddell
  Communications Assistant: Cristina Lankay
  Theatre Manager: Jacinthia Alexander
  Production Assistant: John Wiedermann
Founded: 1985
Status: Nonprofit
Paid Staff: 7
Volunteer Staff: 60
Paid Artists: 100
Budget: $600,000
Income Sources: Ticket Sales, Facility Rental;
Contributions; Concessions
Performs At: Edward Nash Theatre; Welpe Theatre
Affiliations: APAP; IPAY; IAAM
Annual Attendance: 30,000
Stage Dimensions: 46'x40'
Seating Capacity: 984
Year Built: 1985

3266 AMERICAN STAGE COMPANY

Box 336
Teaneck, NJ 07666

Management:
  Producing Artistic Director: Matthew Parent
Performs At: American Stage in Residence, Fairleigh
Dickinson University
Type of Stage: Proscenium
Seating Capacity: 290

3267 TEANECK NEW THEATRE

PO Box 213
Teaneck, NJ 07666
Phone: 201-836-6384
e-mail: tnthattie@aol.com
Web Site: www.njtheater.com
Management:
  Secretary: Harriet Gottlieb
  Artistic Director: C Edwin Shade
Mission: We try to introduce our audience to new
playwrights while continuing to present classics along
with current well known plays.
Founded: 1990
Volunteer Staff: 20
Non-paid Artists: var
Budget: $10,000
Income Sources: Tickets; Local Support
Performs At: Bogart Memorial Church
Annual Attendance: 900
Facility Category: Auditorium
Type of Stage: Raised Proscenium
Seating Capacity: 100

3268 PASSAGE THEATRE COMPANY

PO Box 967
Trenton, NJ 08605-0967
Phone: 609-392-0318
e-mail: jamie@trentondowntowner.com
Web Site: www.passagetheatre.org
Management:
  Production Artistic Director: June Ballinger
Mission: Committed to staging dynamic works that
celebrate the human experience across cultural lines.
Founded: 1985
Status: Nonprofit
Season: September - June
Stage Dimensions: 30' x 22'
Seating Capacity: 125

3269 THE WAR MEMORIAL THEATRE

PO Box 232
W Lafayette Street
Trenton, NJ 08625
Phone: 609-984-8484
Fax: 609-777-0581
Web Site: www.thewarmemorial.com
Management:
  Executive Manager: Molly S McDonough
Founded: 1932
Specialized Field: Performing arts

3270 THEATREFEST

Montclair State University
Upper Montclair, NJ 07043-9987
Phone: 973-655-7071
Fax: 973-655-5335
e-mail: wootenj@mail.montclair.edu
Web Site: www.montclair.edu
Management:
  Artistic Director: John Wooten
  Artistic Director: Laura Kelly
Mission: Evolving theatre featuring new works and
American standards.
Founded: 1986
Specialized Field: Metropolitan, 14 Miles West of
Manhattan
Status: Nonprofit
Paid Staff: 50
Volunteer Staff: 15
Paid Artists: 40
Budget: $550,000
Income Sources: Grants; Ticket Revenue; Individuals
Season: June - August
Affiliations: LOA; SPT
Annual Attendance: 15,000
Facility Category: Equity Theater
Type of Stage: 2 Prosceniums and Flexible
Stage Dimensions: 40' x 36'
Seating Capacity: 950 + 99
Year Remodeled: 2002
Rental Contact: John Wooten

3271 PUSHCART PLAYERS

197 Bloomfield Avenue
Verona, NJ 07044
Phone: 973-857-1115
Fax: 973-857-4366

Management:
Artistic Director: Paul Whelihan
Founded: 1974
Status: Nonprofit
Season: September - June

3272 CUMBERLAND PLAYERS
The Little Theatre
Sherman Avenue & SE Boulevard
PO Box 494
Vineland, NJ 08362
Phone: 856-692-5626
e-mail: theatre@cumberlandplayers.com
Web Site: www.cumberlandplayers.com
Officers:
President: Richard Curcio
VP Finance: Mary Wijsmuller
Management:
VP Production: Brian Garrison
Mission: Promoting opportunities for grassroots participation amoung young and old theatre lovers. Dedicated to enriching the culture life, spirit of volunteerism, community service and love for the theatre.
Founded: 1946
Status: Volunteer; Non-Professional
Income Sources: New Jersey Council on the Arts; The Cumberland County Cuultural & Heritage Commisssion; Bridgeton Exchange Club

3273 SHADOW LAWN SUMMER STAGE
Woods Theatre
Monmouth University
West Long Branch, NJ 07764
Phone: 732-571-3442
Fax: 732-263-5330
e-mail: jburke@manmouth.edu
Management:
Chairman: John J Burke
Founded: 1979
Status: Nonprofit
Season: June - August
Type of Stage: Thrust
Stage Dimensions: 35' x 20'
Seating Capacity: 148

3274 MAURICE LEVIN THEATER SEASON
760 Northfield Avenue
West Orange, NJ 07052
Phone: 973-736-3200
Fax: 973-736-6871
e-mail: dnitzberg@vjfmetravest.org
Management:
Arts/Education Director: Isabel Margolin
Budget: $500,000 - $600,000
Performs At: Maurice Levin Theater

New Mexico

3275 ADOBE THEATER
9813 4th Street NW
Albuquerque, NM 87102

Mailing Address: PO Box 276, Corrales, NM. 87048
Phone: 505-892-0697
Fax: 505-892-9761
e-mail: Adobeact@aol.com
Web Site: www.adobetheater.com
Officers:
President: Erin K Moots
VP/Technical Director: Jeff Kuykendall
Secretary: Ninetter S Mordaunt
Treasurer: Beverly Herring
Management:
Chairman-Artistic Committee: Phil Bock
Chairman-Business/Publicity: Drew Carlin
Mission: To provide an educational vehicle to produce plays, musicals and other entertainments, primarily for the Westside and Greater Albuquerque Communities, including Bernalillo, Sandoval, Valencia and Cibola Counties. To furnish an opportunity for learning experiences for theater enthusiasts of all ages with any degree of experience.
Founded: 1960
Budget: $40 Million
Income Sources: Box Office; Individual Donations
Season: Year-round
Performs At: Adobe Theatre
Annual Attendance: 9,000
Type of Stage: Thrust
Stage Dimensions: 24 x 24
Seating Capacity: 90
Year Built: 1960

3276 ALBUQUERQUE LITTLE THEATRE
224 San Pasquale SW
Albuquerque, NM 87102
Phone: 505-242-4750
e-mail: alt@swcp.com
Officers:
President: Jean Block
VP: Jan Alvidrez
Secretary: Karen Patterson
Treasurer: Wesley Daniels, CPA
Management:
Executive Director: Larry D Parker
Technical Director: Andew McHarney
Sales/Box Office: David A Rivera
Director Development: Marie G Hamitlon
House Manager: Deborah Dickey
Business Manager: Kristi Gore
Founded: 1930
Status: Not-for-profit
Affiliations: Albuquerque Children's Theatre

3277 CITY OF ALBUQUERQUE KIMO THEATRE
423 Central NW
Albuquerque, NM 87102
Phone: 505-768-3522
Fax: 505-768-3542
e-mail: crivera@cabq.gov
Web Site: www.cabq.gov/kimo
Management:
Operations/Events Manager: Craig Rivera
Technical Manager: Dennis Potter
Business Manager: Lauren Griego

Founded: 1927
Status: Rental House
Paid Staff: 5
Budget: $55,000
Type of Stage: Proscenium
Seating Capacity: 650
Year Built: 1927
Year Remodeled: 2000

3278 LA COMPANIA DE TEATRO DE ALBUQUERQUE

La Compania North Albuquerque
PO Box 884
Albuquerque, NM 87103-0884
Phone: 505-242-7929
Management:
Artistic Director: Ramon A Flores
Mission: To reflect, preserve and empower the New Mexican society and culture through professional production; Southwest bilingual theatre.
Founded: 1977
Specialized Field: Theatrical Group
Status: Semi-Professional; Nonprofit
Budget: $95,000
Performs At: KiMo Theatre; South Broadway Cutural Center
Annual Attendance: 10,000
Seating Capacity: 700; 309
Organization Type: Performing; Touring; Resident; Educational

3279 SANDSTONE PRODUCTIONS

901 Fairgrounds Road
Framington, NM 87401
Phone: 505-327-9336
Management:
Producer: Shawn F Lyle
Founded: 1993
Status: Non-Equity; Nonprofit
Season: June - August
Type of Stage: Outdoor
Stage Dimensions: 150' x 100'
Seating Capacity: 600

3280 LAS CRUCES COMMUNITY THEATRE

313 N Downtown Mall
Las Cruces, NM 88001
Phone: 505-523-1200
Web Site: www.zianet.com/lcct
Officers:
President: Michael Mandel
Secretary: Cindy Pitts
Treasurer: Ray Carter
Management:
VP Membership: Larry Fisher
VP Development: Paula Leighton
VP Public Relations: Heather Moore
Mission: Las Cruces Community Theatre is an all volunteer non-profit organiation with many opportunities for involvement.
Founded: 1963
Specialized Field: Theatrical Group
Status: Non-Professional; Nonprofit
Organization Type: Performing

3281 SHAKESPEARE IN SANTA FE

The Pink Church Art Space
1516 Pacheco Street, Rear Suite
Santa Fe, NM 87505
Phone: 505-982-2910
Fax: 505-982-5001
e-mail: shakespeareinsf@mindspring.com
Web Site: www.shakespearesantafe.org
Officers:
President: Patricia Pipkin
VP: Reverdy Johnson
Treasurer: David Burling
Secretary: Sarah Lawless
Management:
Managing Director: Janey Potts
Production Manager: Terri Ross
Mission: To present classical theatre to the entire Santa Fe community and its visitors; to present classical theatre specifically to young people through our Education & Outreach programs, Shakespeare in the Schools touring program and the Internship Training Program.
Founded: 1987
Paid Staff: 3
Paid Artists: 50
Budget: $500,000
Income Sources: Ticket Income; Grants; Corporate (individual gifts)
Annual Attendance: 15,000
Facility Category: Outdoors
Type of Stage: Elevated
Stage Dimensions: varies
Seating Capacity: 350+

New York

3282 BLACK EXPERIENCE ENSEMBLE

5 Homestead Avenue
Albany, NY 12203
Phone: 518-482-6683
Officers:
President/Founder: Mars Hill
Mission: To provide cultural exposure and enrichment to the minority community through the performing arts.
Founded: 1968
Specialized Field: Community; Theatrical Group
Status: Professional; Nonprofit
Paid Staff: 5
Income Sources: Albany League of Arts
Organization Type: Performing; Touring; Sponsoring

3283 PARK PLAYHOUSE INCORPORATED

60 Orange Street
Albany, NY 12210
Phone: 518-434-2035
Fax: 518-434-1048
e-mail: hrhven@aol.com
Web Site: www.parkplayhouse.com
Management:
Producer: Venustiano Borromeo
Founded: 1989
Status: Nonprofit
Season: July - August
Type of Stage: Proscenium

Stage Dimensions: 56' x 36'
Seating Capacity: 900

3284 2 TEXANS
21-22 43rd Street
Astoria, NY 11105
Phone: 212-561-1815
Management:
    Artistic Director: Sonnet Blanton

3285 AUBURN PLAYERS COMMUNITY THEATRE
PO Box 543
Auburn, NY 13021
Phone: 315-258-8275
e-mail: mgmword@twcny.rr.com
Web Site: www.community.syracuse.com/cc/auburnplays
Officers:
    President: Deborah Scott
    Secretary: Cynthia Nagle
    Administrative Treasurer: Ellie Beck
    Production Treasurer: Dia Carabajal
Management:
    Administrative VP: Elisa Hunt
    Production VP: Andrew Rankin
Mission: To be a non-profit, educational and cultural organization; to present dramatic productions; to increase appreciation for the theatre.
Founded: 1961
Specialized Field: Community
Status: Nonprofit
Paid Staff: 100
Organization Type: Performing

3286 MERRY-GO-ROUND PLAYHOUSE
PO Box 506
Auburn, NY 13021
Phone: 315-255-1305
e-mail: mgrplays@dreamscape.com
Web Site: www.merry-go-round.com
Officers:
    President: Robert Nethercott
    1st VP: Sally Reutlinger
    2nd VP: Barbara Clary
    Treasurer: Brenda Holland
    Secretary: Laurel Ullyette
Management:
    Producing Director: Edward Sayles
    Business Manager: Kathlene Carr
    Youth Theatre Company Manager: Michael Deforrest
    Secretary: Cheri Downes
    Youth Theatre Production Manager: Mark Goodloe
Mission: The Merry-Go-Round Playhouse is a professional theatre providing a Summer Season of Broadway quality musicals.
Founded: 1975
Status: Not-for-profit
Season: June - August
Annual Attendance: 17,000
Seating Capacity: 325

3287 MOHAWK PLAYERS
PO Box 382
Babylon, NY 11702
Phone: 516-669-7605
Mission: To present live theatre to diverse groups at libraries.
Founded: 1954
Specialized Field: Community
Status: Nonprofit
Paid Staff: 10
Income Sources: New York State Coucil on Arts
Organization Type: Performing; Touring

3288 RIVER ARTS REPERTORY
Route 212
Bearsville, NY 12409
Phone: 914-679-7693
Fax: 845-679-9239
Management:
    Co-Artistic Director: Lawrence Sacharow
    Co-Artistic Director: Michael Cristofer
    Managing Director: Albert Idhe
Mission: To offer new interpretations of the classics; to create innovative new works.
Founded: 1979
Specialized Field: Summer Stock; Theatrical Group; Puppet
Status: Professional; Nonprofit
Income Sources: Actors' Equity Association; Theatre Communications Group
Performs At: Bearsville Theatre
Organization Type: Performing; Sponsoring

3289 GATEWAY PLAYHOUSE
215 S Country Road
Box 5
Bellport, NY 11713
Phone: 631-286-1133
Fax: 631-286-5806
Toll-free: 888-484-9669
Web Site: www.gatewayplayhouse.com
Management:
    Producer: Paul Allan
Founded: 1950
Status: Commercial
Season: May - December
Type of Stage: Proscenium
Stage Dimensions: 30' x 8'
Seating Capacity: 500

3290 AIRPORT PLAYHOUSE
218 Knickerbocker Avenue
PO Box 162
Bohemia, NY 11716-0162
Phone: 631-589-7588
e-mail: airportplayhouse@aol.com
Web Site: www.airportplayhouse.com
Management:
    Managing Director: Kim Dufrenoy
Mission: The Airport Playhouse is a year-round professional, not-for-profit theater offering an annual roster of 10 full scale productions and an array of children's programs, fund-raising activities, special events, dinner theater packages and theater classes.

Founded: 1977
Status: Non-Equity; Commercial
Season: Year-Round
Type of Stage: Proscenium
Stage Dimensions: 38' x 38'
Seating Capacity: 270

3291 BELMONT PLAYHOUSE

2385 Arthur Avenue
Bronx, NY 10458
Phone: 718-364-4700
Fax: 718-563-5053
e-mail: thebelmont@hotmail.com
Management:
    Artistic Director: Dante Albertie
Founded: 1991
Performs At: Belmont Playhouse
Type of Stage: Black Box, Platform
Seating Capacity: 75, 25-100

3292 PREGONES THEATER

571-575 Walton Avenue
Bronx, NY 10451
Phone: 718-585-1202
Fax: 718-585-1608
e-mail: pregones@aol.com
Web Site: www.pregones.org
Management:
    Artistic Director: Rosalba Rolon
    Associate Artistic Director: Alvan Colon Lespier
    Associate Artistic Director: Jorge Merced
    Associate Director: Jorge Merced
Mission: To offer bilingual theatre mainly for Latino audiences; to present a broad range of professional performers.
Founded: 1979
Specialized Field: Theatrical Group
Status: Professional; Nonprofit
Organization Type: Performing; Touring

3293 ADELPHIAN PLAYERS

8515 Ridge Boulevard
Brooklyn, NY 11209
Phone: 718-238-3308
Fax: 718-238-2894
Web Site: www.adelphianacademy.org
Management:
    Artistic Director: Russell E Bonanno
    Business Manager: Philip Stone
    Director Advancement: Albert C Corham
Mission: To provide quality theatre for the residents of Brooklyn.
Founded: 1964
Specialized Field: Summer Stock; Theatrical Group
Status: Non-Professional
Paid Staff: 25
Volunteer Staff: 10
Performs At: Adelphi Academy
Organization Type: Performing; Educational

3294 BILLIE HOLIDAY THEATRE

1368 Fulton Street
PO Box 470131
Brooklyn, NY 11247-0131

Phone: 718-636-0919
Fax: 622-202-2956
Management:
    Executive Director: Marjorie Moon
Mission: To offer trained Black artists a professional environment; to provide theatre that enlightens and educates the community.
Founded: 1972
Specialized Field: Theatrical Group
Status: Professional; Nonprofit
Stage Dimensions: Proscenium
Seating Capacity: 200
Organization Type: Performing; Resident

3295 CHEKHOV THEATRE ENSEMBLE

138 S Oxford Street
Suite 1B
Brooklyn, NY 11217
Phone: 718-398-2494
Fax: 718-398-2494
e-mail: floyd@chekhov-theatre.com
Web Site: www.chekhovtheatre.org
Management:
    Artistic Director: Floyd Rumohr
    Stages of Learning Program Manager: Terry Hofler
    Administrative Assistant: Mike Halverson
Mission: To improve the educational success, social well-being and potential for happiness of children, ages 8-13, through kinesthetic, theatre-based activities guided by the artistic principles of Michael Chekhov and to inspire and unite artists, teachers, children and families through theatre experiences.
Founded: 1994
Specialized Field: Theatre
Paid Staff: 6
Volunteer Staff: 15
Paid Artists: 20
Non-paid Artists: 3

3296 CONEY ISLAND USA

1208 Surf Avenue
Brooklyn, NY 11224
Phone: 718-372-5159
Fax: 718-372-5101
e-mail: info@coneyisland.com
Web Site: www.coneyisland.com
Management:
    Artistic Director: Dick D Zigun
    Managing Director: Jennifer Upchurch
Mission: To present America's popular art forms in innovative sideshow parades, performances and exhibitions.
Founded: 1980
Specialized Field: Sideshow Theatrical Group
Status: Professional; Nonprofit
Paid Staff: 12
Volunteer Staff: 4
Budget: 250,000
Income Sources: Alliance of Resident Theatres/New York
Performs At: Sideshows by the Seashore, Coney Island Museum
Annual Attendance: 75,000+
Facility Category: Sideshows by the seashore, Coney Island Museum

---

All listings are in alphabetical order by state, then city, then organization within the city.

Type of Stage: Arena, Cabaret
Seating Capacity: 99; 74
Organization Type: Performing; Educational;
Sponsoring

3297 RYAN REPERTORY COMPANY AT HARRY WARREN THEATRE

2445 Bath Avenue
Brooklyn, NY 11214
Phone: 718-996-4800
Fax: 718-996-4800
e-mail: ryanrep@juno.com
Management:
   Executive Director: Barbara Parisi
   Technical Director: Michael Pasterneck
   Artistic Director: John Sannuto
Mission: Developing new musicals and working on new plays.
Founded: 1972
Specialized Field: Musical; Theatrical Group
Status: Professional; Nonprofit
Volunteer Staff: 18
Non-paid Artists: 200
Budget: $60,000
Performs At: Harry Warren Theatre
Annual Attendance: 2000
Stage Dimensions: 12 x 12
Seating Capacity: 40
Year Built: 1990
Organization Type: Performing; Resident

3298 ALLEYWAY THEATRE

One Curtain Up Alley
Buffalo, NY 14202-1911
Phone: 716-852-2600
Fax: 716-852-2266
e-mail: email@alleyway.com
Web Site: www.alleway.com
Management:
   Executive Director: Neal Radice
   Director Public Relations: Joyce Stilson
   Director Marketing: Todd Warfield
Mission: To develop and produce new theatre.
Founded: 1980
Specialized Field: New plays
Annual Attendance: 17,000
Type of Stage: Black Box
Seating Capacity: 100

3299 IRISH CLASSICAL THEATRE COMPANY

625 Main Street
Buffalo, NY 14203
Phone: 716-853-4282
Fax: 716-853-0592
e-mail: iclassical@aol.com
Web Site: www.irishclassicaltheatre.com
Management:
   Artistic Director: Vincent O'Neill
   Associate Artistic Director: Fortunato Pezzimenti
Mission: To present the greatest works of dramatic literture, international classics, modern plays of exceptional merit, and Irish plays, both traditional and contemporary; to produce them at the highest level of artistic excellence; to offer them to the public of Buffalo, Western New York and Southern Ontario, and subsequently, for national and international audiences.
Founded: 1990
Specialized Field: Theatre
Annual Attendance: 25,000+
Type of Stage: In The Round
Seating Capacity: 200
Year Built: 1998

3300 KAVINOKY THEATRE

320 Porter Avenue
Buffalo, NY 14201
Phone: 716-881-7652
Fax: 716-881-7790
Web Site: kavinokytheatre.com
Management:
   Artistic Director: David Lamb
   Managing Director: Steve Cooper
Founded: 1981
Specialized Field: Performing Arts
Paid Staff: 4
Volunteer Staff: 300
Paid Artists: 50
Performs At: D'Youville College campus
Type of Stage: Proscenium/Thrust
Seating Capacity: 260

3301 PANDORA'S BOX THEATRE COMPANY

One Curtain Up Alley
Buffalo, NY 14202
Phone: 716-852-2600
Fax: 716-852-2266
Web Site: www.alleyway.com/pandorasbox/
Management:
   Artistic Director: Ellen Opiela
Mission: To produce plays about women and their experiences.
Founded: 1995

3302 PAUL ROBESON THEATRE

350 Masten Avenue
Buffalo, NY 14209
Phone: 716-884-2013
Fax: 716-885-2590
Management:
   Executive Director: Agnes M Bain
Mission: To develop and nurture an appreciation for Black Theatre in the Black community, especially among Black youth.
Founded: 1958
Specialized Field: Theatrical Group
Status: Semi-Professional; Nonprofit
Performs At: Paul Robeson Theatre
Organization Type: Performing; Educational

3303 SHAKESPEARE IN DELAWARE PARK

PO Box 716
Buffalo, NY
Phone: 716-515-3960
Web Site: www.shakespeareindelawarepark.com
Officers:
   Chair: Scott L Sroka
   Vice Chair: Melissa R Grainger

Treasurer: Anne K Kyzmir
Secretary: Marita Ronald
Management:
Artistic Director: Saul Elkin
Program Director: Roger Keicher
Mission: Shakespeare in Delaware Park is a not-for-profit, professional theatre company dedicated to providing free, high-quality public theatre to the widest possible audience by performing Shakespearean plays outdoors.
Founded: 1976
Specialized Field: Classical Material
Status: Professional; Nonprofit
Season: June - August

3304 STUDIO ARENA THEATRE

710 Main Street
Buffalo, NY 14202
Phone: 716-856-8025
Fax: 716-856-3415
Toll-free: 800-777-8243
Web Site: www.studioarena.org
Officers:
President: James Anderson
Management:
Artistic Director: Gavin Cameron-Webb
Executive Director: Ken Neufeld
Director Development: Wendy Sanders
Director Marketing: Roberta Mackey
Mission: To provide Western New York with a varied theatre season of the finest quality.
Founded: 1927
Status: Professional; Nonprofit
Budget: 4.5 Million
Income Sources: League of Resident Theatres; Theatre Communications Group; Actors' Equity Association
Season: September - May
Affiliations: Theatre Communications Group; League of Resident Theatres
Annual Attendance: 100,000
Type of Stage: Semi-Thrust
Seating Capacity: 637
Year Remodeled: 2001
Organization Type: Performing; Educational

3305 THEATRE OF YOUTH COMPANY

203 Allen Street
Buffalo, NY 14201
Phone: 716-884-4400
Fax: 716-819-9653
e-mail: theatreofyouth@hotmail.com
Web Site: www.buffalo.com/toy
Officers:
President: Lynn Edelmam
VP: Kevin Brady
Secretary: Janice Dearing
Treasurer: Richard D'Arcy
Management:
Artistic Director: Meg Quinn
Director Marketing/Sales: Robert Brunschmid
Business Manager: Linda D'Agostino
Founded: 1972
Specialized Field: Children's Theatre
Status: Professional; Nonprofit
Annual Attendance: 53,000

Facility Category: Theatre
Type of Stage: Proscenium
Year Built: 1913
Year Remodeled: 1999
Organization Type: Performing; Touring; Educational

3306 MAC-HAYDN THEATRE

PO Box 204
Route 203
Chatham, NY 12037
Phone: 518-392-9292
Fax: 518-392-4547
Management:
Artistic Producing Director: Lynne Hayden
Artistic Producing Director: Linda MacNish
Founded: 1969
Specialized Field: Summer Theatre
Season: May - September
Annual Attendance: 40,000+
Facility Category: Theatre
Type of Stage: In the Round
Seating Capacity: 350

3307 HUDSON VALLEY SHAKESPEARE FESTIVAL

155 Main Street
Cold Spring, NY 10516
Phone: 845-265-7858
Fax: 845-265-7865
e-mail: info@shakespeare.org
Web Site: www.hvshakespeare.org
Officers:
President: Carol Manguard
Vice President: Betsy Simons
Treasurer: Nathaniel Peutice
Management:
Executive Director: Susan Landstreet
Artistic Director: Terrence O'Brien
Director Marketing: Abigail Adams
Founded: 1987
Specialized Field: Summer Theater
Status: Nonprofit
Paid Staff: 25
Volunteer Staff: 50
Paid Artists: 34
Budget: $955,000
Income Sources: Ticket Sales and Fundraising
Season: June, July, August
Performs At: Tent Theater
Annual Attendance: 24,000
Type of Stage: Thrust
Seating Capacity: 450

3308 LEATHERSTOCKING THEATRE COMPANY

Box 711
Cooperstown, NY 13326
Phone: 607-547-1363
Fax: 607-547-6144
Management:
Artistic Director: Mercedes Gotwald
Founded: 1991
Status: Nonprofit
Season: July - September

Type of Stage: Proscenium
Seating Capacity: 150

3309 CORTLAND REPERTORY THEATRE

PO Box 783
37 Franklin Street
Cortland, NY 13045
Phone: 607-753-6161
Fax: 607-753-0047
Toll-free: 800-427-6160
e-mail: cortlandrep@hotmail.com
Web Site: www.cortlandrep.org
Officers:
   President: Christine Snyder
   VP: Peter O'Connell
   Secretary: Clayton Alcorn
   Treasurer: Matt Banazek
Management:
   Producing Director: Kerby Thompson
   General Manager: Barclay Kuske
   Managing Director Educational: Chad Sweet
Mission: To offer residents of Central New York an opportunity to experience, at an accessible price, the range and scope of excellent professional theatre.
Founded: 1971
Specialized Field: Summer Stock; Musical
Status: Professional; Nonprofit
Paid Staff: 2
Volunteer Staff: 60
Paid Artists: 30
Budget: $237,000
Income Sources: NYSCA; Grants; Corporate Sponsors; Individual Donations
Season: June - August
Performs At: Pavilion Theatre
Annual Attendance: 15,000
Facility Category: Summer Stock
Type of Stage: 3/4 Thrust
Seating Capacity: 249
Year Built: 1904
Year Remodeled: 1971
Organization Type: Performing

3310 ARENA PLAYERS REPERTORY COMPANY OF LONG ISLAND

296 Route 109
East Farmingdale, NY 11735
Phone: 516-293-0674
Fax: 516-777-8688
Web Site: arena109.com
Officers:
   President: Frederic De Feis
   VP: Joanne Gobrick
   Secretary: Carolyn Poppadin
   Treasurer: Christie Zummo
Management:
   Artistic Director: Frederic De Feis
   Production Coordinator: Joanne Gobrick
   Administrative Assistant: Joseph Yoga
Mission: To develop and encourage a love of arena theatre; to assist new playwrights as they develop original scripts.
Founded: 1955
Specialized Field: Theatrical Group

Status: Professional; Nonprofit
Paid Staff: 3
Volunteer Staff: 5
Paid Artists: 7
Non-paid Artists: 5
Budget: $450,000
Income Sources: Theatre Communications Group
Season: Year-Round
Performs At: Arena Players Repertory Theater
Annual Attendance: 30,000
Facility Category: 2 stages
Type of Stage: Arena
Seating Capacity: 240; 100
Year Remodeled: 1970
Organization Type: Performing; Touring

3311 JOHN DREW THEATER OF GUILD HALL

158 Main Street
East Hampton, NY 11937
Phone: 631-324-4051
Fax: 631-324-2722
e-mail: joshgladstone@guildhall.org
Web Site: www.guildhall.org
Management:
   Executive Director: Dr. Ruth Appelhof
   Program Director: Pamela Calvert
   Artistic Director: Josh Gladstone
Mission: The John Drew Theater of Guild Hall operates under an educational/arts charter; dedicated to the presentation of the finest in the performing arts.
Founded: 1931
Specialized Field: Dance; Instrumental Music; Theater
Status: Professional; Nonprofit
Paid Staff: 50
Paid Artists: 100
Non-paid Artists: 200
Budget: $350,000
Income Sources: Actors' Equity Association
Season: May-September
Performs At: John Drew Theater
Affiliations: Film Society Lincoln Center; Hamptons International Film Festival; Playwrights Theatre of the Hampton
Annual Attendance: 20,000
Seating Capacity: 382
Rental Contact: Josh Gladstone
Organization Type: Performing; Educational

3312 SHADOWLAND ARTISTS

157 Canal Street
Ellenville, NY 12428
Phone: 845-647-3510
Fax: 845-647-5511
Management:
   Executive Artistic Director: Bill Lelbach
Founded: 1985
Status: Nonprofit
Season: May - September
Type of Stage: Thrust
Stage Dimensions: 36' x 24'
Seating Capacity: 148

All listings are in alphabetical order by state, then city, then organization within the city.

3313 QUEENS COLLEGE SUMMER THEATRE

Rathaus Hall 213
65-30 Kissena Boulevard
Flushing, NY 11367
Phone: 718-997-3185
Fax: 718-997-3095
Web Site: www.sunv.edu
Management:
    Production Manager: Barbara Codd
    Technical Director: Ike Rathbone
Mission: Educational setting presenting diverse
productions and programs in the arts. Three theatre
complex with seating for 100 to 500.
Founded: 1970
Specialized Field: Drama, Theatre and Dance
Status: Non-Equity; Nonprofit
Season: July - August
Type of Stage: Proscenium; Thrust
Stage Dimensions: 45' x 45'; 30' x 25'
Seating Capacity: 476

3314 FORESTBURGH PLAYHOUSE

39 Forestburgh Road
Forestburgh, NY 12777
Phone: 845-794-2005
Fax: 845-794-3747
e-mail: info@fbplayhouse.com
Web Site: www.fbplayhouse.com
Management:
    Producer: Norman Duttweiler
Founded: 1947
Status: Equity; Commercial
Season: June - September
Type of Stage: Proscenium
Seating Capacity: 150

3315 ADIRONDACK THEATRE FESTIVAL

PO Box 3203
Glens Falls, NY 12801
Phone: 518-798-7479
Fax: 518-793-1334
e-mail: atf@atfestival.org
Web Site: www.atfestival.org
Management:
    Artistic Director: Martha Banta
    Producing Director: David Turner
Mission: To present a season of new and contemporary
theater.
Founded: 1994
Specialized Field: Summer Theater
Status: Nonprofit
Paid Staff: 10
Volunteer Staff: 10
Paid Artists: 24
Budget: $150,000
Season: June - July
Performs At: Temporary theater in an old Woolworths
Store
Annual Attendance: 5,000
Type of Stage: Black Box
Seating Capacity: 150

3316 STAGEWORKS

133 Warren Street
Hudson, NY 12534
Phone: 518-828-7843
Fax: 518-828-4026
e-mail: contact@stageworkstheater.org
Web Site: www.stageworktheater.org
Management:
    Production Artistic Director: Laura Margolis
    Administrative Director: Phil Gliman
Founded: 1993
Status: Nonprofit
Budget: $190,000
Income Sources: Earned and Unearned
Season: April - November
Affiliations: Theater Communications; Hudson Valley
East Consortium of Professional Theaters
Facility Category: North Point in Kinderhook, NY
Type of Stage: Thrust
Stage Dimensions: 40' x 20'
Seating Capacity: 100-125

3317 CORNELL UNIVERSITY THEATRE, FILM & DANCE DEPARTMENT

Cornell University
Ithaca, NY 14853-6902
Phone: 607-254-2733
Fax: 607-254-2700
Affiliations: Cornell Concert Series
Facility Category: Dance Hall
Resident Groups: Cornell Savoyards

3318 HANGAR THEATRE

116 N Cayuga Street
Ithaca, NY 14850
Mailing Address: PO Box 205 Ithaca NY, 14851
Phone: 607-273-8588
Fax: 607-273-4516
e-mail: rhoan@hangartheatre.org
Web Site: www.hangartheatre.org
Officers:
    President: Laurel Southard
    VP: Roy Decheimer
    Secretary: Jeol Zumoff
    Treasurer: Raymond M Schlath
Management:
    Executive Director: Lisa Bushlow
    Artistic Director: Kevin Mariarty
    Business Director: Maryann Summer
    Marketing Director: Rhoan Morgan
Mission: As a professional theatre the Hangar hires
Equity and non equity actors, designers and directors for
each play the theatre produces during the summer.
Founded: 1964
Specialized Field: Theater
Status: Professional; Nonprofit
Paid Staff: 20
Paid Artists: 20
Budget: $900,000
Income Sources: Foundation; Individual; Grant; Earned
Season: May - August
Performs At: Hangar Theatre; Cass Park

Affiliations: Actors Equity Association; United Scenic Artists; Society of Stage Directors and Choregography; Drama League
Annual Attendance: 20,000
Type of Stage: Thrust
Seating Capacity: 349
Organization Type: Performing; Educational

3319 KITCHEN THEATRE COMPANY
116 N Cayuga Street
Ithaca, NY 14850
Phone: 607-272-0403
Fax: 607-273-4816
e-mail: kitchenithaca@aol.com
Web Site: www.kitchentheatre.com
Management:
   Artistic Director: Rachel Lampert
Founded: 1992
Status: Nonprofit
Volunteer Staff: 50
Season: August - May
Annual Attendance: 10,000
Type of Stage: 3/4 Thrust
Seating Capacity: 73

3320 CHINESE THEATRE WORKSHOP
37-45 84th Street
Suite 31
Jackson Heights, NY 11372
Phone: 718-457-1627
Management:
   President: Kuang Yu Fong
Founded: 1975
Status: Non-Equity; Nonprofit
Season: Year-Round

3321 YUEH LUNG SHADOW THEATRE
34-41 74th Street
Jackson Heights, NY 11372
Phone: 718-457-1627
Fax: 718-457-1627
Management:
   Executive/Artistic Director: Joe Humphrey
   Assistant Director: Sarah Jonker-Burke
Mission: To preserve and perpetuate the art of shadow theatre, which began in China 2000 years ago.
Founded: 1976
Specialized Field: Folk; Puppet
Status: Professional; Nonprofit
Income Sources: Alliance of Resident Theatres/New York; United International Marionette Association; Queens Council on Arts; Puppeteers of America; UNIMA
Organization Type: Performing; Touring; Educational

3322 AFRIKAN POETRY THEATRE
176-03 Jamaica Avenue
Jamaica, NY 11432
Phone: 718-523-3312
Fax: 718-523-1054
e-mail: jwatusi@aol.com
Web Site: www.afrikanpoetrytheatre.com
Management:
   Executive Director: John Watusi Branch
   Administrative Assistant: Byron W Perry

Administrative Assistant: Ronald Burwell
   Program Director: Shadiyah Waliyaya
Mission: To offer performances, classes, workshops, cultural reference sources and exhibits to the community.
Founded: 1976
Specialized Field: Musical; Community; Folk
Status: Professional; Nonprofit
Paid Staff: 20
Budget: $450,000
Income Sources: Grants; Contributions; Tickets
Performs At: Afrikan Poetry Theatre
Annual Attendance: 10,000
Type of Stage: Platform
Stage Dimensions: 18 x 20
Seating Capacity: 125
Year Built: 1930
Year Remodeled: 1979
Rental Contact: John Watusi Branch
Organization Type: Performing; Touring; Educational; Sponsoring

3323 NEW YORK STREET THEATRE CARAVAN
8705 Chelsea Street
Jamaica Estates, NY 11432
Phone: 718-657-8070
Management:
   Artistic Director of the Collective: Marketa Kimbrell
Founded: 1968
Specialized Field: Theatrical Group
Status: Professional
Organization Type: Performing

3324 COACH HOUSE PLAYERS
12 Augusta Street
PO Box 3481
Kingston, NY 12401
Phone: 845-338-7097
Management:
   Business Manager: Kay Finn
Mission: To offer the finest possible productions in every aspect of theatre.
Founded: 1950
Specialized Field: Musical; Community; Theatrical Group
Status: Nonprofit
Performs At: J. Watson Bailey School
Organization Type: Performing; Educational

3325 CONTEMPORARY THEATRE OF SYRACUSE
2888 Eager Road
Lafayette, NY 13084
Phone: 315-425-0405
Fax: 315-425-0405
Management:
   Producer: Kristi McKay
   Summer Producer: Jo Lynn Stressing
   New Plays Artistic Director: David Feldman
   New Plays Production Director: Shirley Myrls
Mission: To offer contemporary drama; to encourage works-in-progress through stage readings; to provide programs in schools.
Founded: 1980

Specialized Field: Theatrical Group
Status: Semi-Professional
Paid Staff: 35
Organization Type: Performing

3326 LAKE GEORGE DINNER THEATRE
Canada Street
Lake George, NY 12845
Mailing Address: PO Box 4623, Queensbury, NY. 12804
Phone: 518-761-1092
Fax: 518-798-0735
e-mail: lgot@nycap.com
Management:
   Producer: Vicky Eastwood
Founded: 1968
Specialized Field: Seasonal Theatre
Status: Professional Equity
Paid Staff: 8
Season: June - October
Organization Type: Performing

3327 OPEN EYE THEATER
Box 959
Margaretville, NY 12455
Phone: 845-586-1660
Fax: 845-586-1660
e-mail: openeye@catskill.net
Web Site: www.theopeneye.com
Management:
   Producing Artistic Director: Amie Brockway
   Literacy Associate: Sharone Stacy
Founded: 1972
Specialized Field: Theater
Paid Staff: 6
Volunteer Staff: 30
Paid Artists: 30
Affiliations: TCG; ART/NY; ASS/TEJ/USA; AATE
Annual Attendance: 1,000
Facility Category: Church and Community Hall
Type of Stage: Flexible
Stage Dimensions: 12x16
Seating Capacity: 75
Year Built: 1943

3328 PERIWINKLE NATIONAL THEATRE
19 Clinton Avenue
Monticello, NY 12701
Phone: 845-794-1666
Fax: 845-794-0304
Toll-free: 800-888-8271
e-mail: perwinkle@fcc.net
Web Site: www.periwinkle.org
Officers:
   President: Robert S Kapito
   VP: Patricia Sternberg
   Secretary/Treasurer: Julie Hoffman
   Secretary: Joel Lerber
Management:
   Executive Director: Sunna Rasch
   Managing Director: Sarah Lynn Hazatrd
   Director Education: Scott Laughead

Mission: To provide quality programing with a unique blend of preliminary materials, original productions and workshops designed to challenge students intellectually, imaginatively and artistically.
Founded: 1963
Specialized Field: Theatrical Group
Status: Professional; Nonprofit
Paid Staff: 7
Volunteer Staff: 3
Paid Artists: 28
Budget: $650,000
Income Sources: Program Fees ; Grants
Season: Feburary - May; September - December
Affiliations: AATE
Annual Attendance: 100,000
Organization Type: Performing; Touring; Educational

3329 BRISTOL VALLEY THEATER
151 S Main Street
PO Box 218
Naples, NY 14512
Phone: 716-374-9032
Fax: 716-374-8520
e-mail: bvt.bvtnaples.org
Web Site: www.bvtnaples.org
Management:
   Artistic Director: Michael Perreca
Mission: Professional summer stock theater.
Founded: 1986
Status: Non-Equity; Nonprofit
Season: June - September
Annual Attendance: 10,000
Type of Stage: Proscenium
Seating Capacity: 200

3330 THEATER BARN
PO Box 390
New Lebanon, NY 12125
Phone: 518-794-8989
Management:
   Co-Producer: Abe Phelps
Founded: 1984
Status: Non-Equity; Nonprofit
Season: June - October
Type of Stage: Proscenium
Stage Dimensions: 30' x 16'
Seating Capacity: 134

3331 NEW PALTZ SUMMER REPERTORY THEATRE
Department of Theatre, CT 102
SUNY at New Paltz, 75 S Manheim Boulevard
New Paltz, NY 12561-2499
Phone: 914-257-3870
Fax: 914-257-3882
Management:
   Producer: Yoan Kaddar
Founded: 1973
Status: Non-Equity; Nonprofit
Season: June - August
Type of Stage: Thrust
Stage Dimensions: 20' x 24'
Seating Capacity: 212

3332 FLEETWOOD STAGE
44 Wildcliff Drive
New Rochelle, NY 10805
Phone: 914-654-8533
Fax: 914-235-4459
Management:
  Producing Director: Lewis Arlt
Founded: 1993
Specialized Field: Theater
Performs At: Playhouse at Wildcliff
Type of Stage: Proscenium
Seating Capacity: 100

3333 SARATOGA INTERNATIONAL THEATER INSTITUTE
1922 Old Chelsea Station
New Tork, NY 10011
Phone: 212-477-1469
Fax: 212-477-0564
e-mail: TheSITICo@aol.com
Web Site: www.siti.org
Management:
  Artistic Director: Anne Bogart
  Associate Artistic Director: Ellen Lauren
  Managing Director: Megan Wanlass Szalla
  Development Associate: Erika Green
Mission: SITI exemplifies the disciplines it practices and the artistic values it develops in its work; to create new works for the theater; to perform and tour these productions nationally and internationally; to provide ongoing training for young theater professionals in an approach to acting that forges unique and highly disciplined artists for the theater; to foster opportunities for cultural exchange.
Founded: 1992
Specialized Field: Theater
Status: Nonprofit
Paid Staff: 5
Volunteer Staff: 3
Paid Artists: 16

3334 52ND STREET PROJECT
500 W 52nd Street
2nd Floor
New York, NY 10019
Phone: 212-333-5252
Fax: 212-333-5598
Management:
  Artistic Director: Gus Rogerson
  Executive Director: Carol Ochs

3335 A.V. PRODUCTIONS AND THEATRE GUILD
116 Central Park S
Apartment 11N
New York, NY 10019
Phone: 212-977-5937
Fax: 212-765-5145
e-mail: tcacci@aol.com
Management:
  President: Tony Cacciotti

3336 ABINGDON THEATRE COMPANY
432 W 42nd Street
4th Floor
New York, NY 10036
Phone: 212-736-6604
Fax: 212-736-6608
e-mail: atcnyc@aol.com
Management:
  Artistic Director: Jan Buttram
  Artistic Director: Pamela Paul
  Managing Director: Samuel J Bellinger

3337 ABOUTFACE THEATRE COMPANY
835 Broadway, Suite 1516
Box 210
New York, NY 10003
Phone: 212-268-9638
Management:
  Artistic Director: Sean Burke
  Managing Director: Allison Jones
  Resident Director: Martin Fluger
  General Manager: Michael Herz
  Development: Ron O'Conner
  Development: Barry Rowell
  Development: Ralph Lewis
Mission: To create and present original plays that explore American idealogy and mythology.
Founded: 1984
Specialized Field: Musical; Theatrical Group
Status: Professional; Nonprofit
Income Sources: Alliance of Resident Theatres/New York; New York Foundation for the Arts
Performs At: Nat Horne Theatre and Studios
Organization Type: Resident; Sponsoring

3338 ACTING COMPANY
630 Ninth Avenue
Suite 214
New York, NY
Mailing Address: PO Box 898 New York, NY 10108-0898
Phone: 212-258-3111
Fax: 212-258-3299
e-mail: mail@theactingcompany.org
Web Site: www.theactingcompany.org
Officers:
  Chairman: Edgar Lansbury
  President: Joan M Warburg
  Vice Chairman: Earl D Weiner
  VP: Robert T Goldman
  VP: John C McDonald
  VP: Elinor A Seevak
  Treasurer: Mark Levenfus
  Secretary: Wade Nichols
Management:
  Producing Artistic Director: Margot Harley
Mission: Dedicated to the development of classical repertory actors and a national audience for the theatre.
Founded: 1972
Specialized Field: Classical
Status: Professional; Nonprofit
Paid Staff: 17
Volunteer Staff: 2
Paid Artists: 25

Budget: $2,500,000
Income Sources: Foundations; Corporations; Individuals
Season: September - May
Affiliations: Actor's Equity; USA; SSDC
Annual Attendance: 65,000
Organization Type: Performing; Touring; Resident; Educational

**3339 ACTING STUDIO
CHELSEA REPERTORY COMPANY**
PO Box 230389
New York, NY 10023
Phone: 212-580-6600
e-mail: info@actingstudio.com
Web Site: www.actingstudio.com
Management:
    Studio Director: James Price
    Associate Director: John Grabowski
Mission: To serve as a training institution; to develop new scripts; to provide a resident theatre company.
Founded: 1983
Specialized Field: Theatrical Group; School
Status: Professional; Semi-Professional
Organization Type: Performing; Resident; Educational

3340 ACTORS STUDIO
165 W 46th Street
Suite 509
New York, NY 10036
Phone: 212-302-1900
Fax: 212-302-1926
Toll-free: 800-884-2772
Officers:
    Founder/CEO: Alan S Nusbaum
Management:
    Artistic Director: Estelle Parsons
    Administrator: Rebecca L Scott
Mission: Provide actors with a center where they can focus on the business of their careers in addition to learning the necessary skills to compete as an actor.
Founded: 1986
Specialized Field: Theatre
Status: Professional; Nonprofit
Performs At: Actors Studio
Organization Type: Resident

3341 ACTORS' ALLIANCE
JAF PO Box 7370
New York, NY 10116
Phone: 718-768-6110
Management:
    Artistic Director: Melanie Sutherland
Mission: To offer classical and contemporary plays developed by theatre artists of a resident company.
Founded: 1976
Status: Professional; Nonprofit
Paid Staff: 8
Organization Type: Performing; Touring; Resident

3342 ADOBE THEATRE COMPANY
453 W 16th Street
New York, NY 10011

Phone: 212-352-0441
Fax: 212-352-0441
Web Site: www.adobe.org
Management:
    Literary Manager: Jordan Schildcrout
    Artistic Director: Jeremy Dobrish
    Producing Director: Christopher Roberts
Founded: 1991
Performs At: Ohio Theatre
Type of Stage: Flexible Stage
Seating Capacity: 75

**3343 ALLAN ALBERT PRODUCTIONS
INCORPORATED**
665 Broadway
4th Floor
New York, NY 10012
Phone: 212-398-9500
Fax: 212-388-9848
Toll-free: 800-966-8881
e-mail: kcaap@aol.com
Web Site: www.allan-albert.com
Management:
    Senior Producer: Kathy Carney
Founded: 1980
Status: Non-Equity; Commercial
Season: May - September
Type of Stage: Amphitheatre
Seating Capacity: 3000

3344 AMAS MUSICAL THEATRE
450 W 42nd Street
Suite 2J
New York, NY 10036
Phone: 212-563-2565
e-mail: amas@amasmusical.org
Web Site: www.amasmusical.org
Officers:
    Chairman: Erik Krebs
Management:
    Founder: Rosetta LeNoire
    Business Manager/Administrator: Donna Trinkoff
Mission: To provide a starting place for new American theatrical pieces in a multi-racial environment which instills creative professionalism.
Founded: 1968
Specialized Field: Summer Stock; Musical; Folk
Status: Professional; Nonprofit
Paid Staff: 5
Volunteer Staff: 4
Budget: $200,000 - 300,000
Organization Type: Performing; Touring; Resident; Educational; Sponsoring

**3345 AMERICAN CENTER FOR
STANISLAVSKI THEATRE ART**
485 Park Avenue
New York, NY 10022
Phone: 212-308-5458
Management:
    Artistic Director: Sonia Moore
    Executive Director: Thalia White
    Development Consultant: Marie Lou Catalano

All listings are in alphabetical order by state, then city, then organization within the city.

Mission: Bringing Stanislavski's ultimate acting technique and solution to spontaneity, the method of Physical Actions, to American theatre.
Founded: 1964
Status: Professional; Nonprofit
Paid Staff: 15
Income Sources: Alliance of Resident Theatres/New York
Performs At: Trinity Presbyterian Church
Organization Type: Performing; Touring; Educational

3346 AMERICAN ENSEMBLE COMPANY
PO Box 972
Peck Slip Station
New York, NY 10272
Phone: 212-684-7766
Fax: 212-684-7857
Management:
   Artistic Director: Robert Petito
   General Manager: Robert Dominguez
Mission: Production of plays and musicals of literary merit and development of a working ensemble of actors, directors, designers, and writers.
Founded: 1967
Specialized Field: Musical; Theatrical Group
Status: Professional; Nonprofit
Organization Type: Performing; Touring; Resident; Educational

---

3347 AMERICAN PLACE THEATRE
111 W 46th Street
New York, NY 10036
Phone: 212-840-2960
Fax: 212-391-4019
e-mail: apt@americanplacetheatre.org
Web Site: www.americanplacetheatre.org
Officers:
   Chairman: Wynn Handman
Management:
   Artistic Director: Wynn Handman
   General Manager: Zafra Whitcomb
Mission: To produce new plays by living American writers.
Founded: 1963
Specialized Field: Theatrical Group
Status: Professional; Nonprofit
Paid Staff: 20
Paid Artists: 25
Budget: $1,200,000
Season: Year-Round
Performs At: Main Stage; Subplot Theatre; First Floor Theatre
Affiliations: AEA; IATSE
Annual Attendance: 10,000
Type of Stage: Proscenium; Black Box
Stage Dimensions: 55' x 35'; 40'x 30'
Seating Capacity: 199-349; 74
Year Built: 1970
Rental Contact: Genral Manager Zafra Whitcomb
Organization Type: Performing

3348 AMERICAN THEATRE OF ACTORS
314 W 54th Street
New York, NY 10019

Phone: 212-581-3044
Management:
   Artistic Director: James Jennings
   Technical Director: James Lynn
   Press Agent: David Lipsky
Mission: To help to develop new actors, playwrights and directors; to produce new plays.
Founded: 1977
Specialized Field: Theatrical Group
Status: Professional; Nonprofit
Organization Type: Performing

3349 ATLANTIC THEATER COMPANY
453 W 16th Street
New York, NY 10011
Phone: 212-691-5919
Fax: 212-691-6280
Management:
   Literary Manager: Toni Amicarella
Performs At: Atlantic Theater Mainstage, Black Box
Type of Stage: Proscenium
Seating Capacity: 160, 70

3350 BARROW GROUP
Box 5112
New York, NY 10185
Phone: 212-253-2001
Fax: 212-253-1909
Founded: 1986

3351 BAT THEATRE COMPANY
Flea Theater
41 White Street
New York, NY 10013
Phone: 212-226-0051
Fax: 212-965-1808
e-mail: theflea@thebat.com
Web Site: www.theflea.org
Management:
   Artistic Director: Jim Simpson
   Literary Manager: Gary Winter
   Technical Director: Ben Struck
   Producing Director: Carol Ostrow
   Associate Producer: Nella Vera
   General Manager: Todd Rosen
   Office Manager: Jen McKenna
   Stage Manager: Rebecca Gura
Founded: 1996
Specialized Field: Theatre, Dance, Music

3352 BIG LEAGUE THEATRICALS, INC.
1501 Broadway
Suite 2015
New York, NY 10036
Phone: 212-575-1601
Fax: 212-575-9817
e-mail: generalinfo@bigleague.org
Web Site: www.bigleague.org
   Booking Associate: Christiane Cayea
   Director Booking: John Starr

3353 BLACK SPECTRUM

119-07 Merrick Boulevard
New York, NY 11434
Phone: 718-723-1800
Fax: 718-723-1806
Web Site: www.blackspectrum.com
Management:
   Founder/Producer: Carl Clay
Mission: To present socially significant Black classical as well as contemporary works.
Founded: 1970
Specialized Field: Musical; Dinner; Theatrical Group
Status: Professional; Nonprofit
Organization Type: Performing; Touring; Educational

3354 BOND STREET THEATRE COALITION

2 Bond Street
New York, NY 10012
Phone: 212-254-4614
Fax: 212-254-4614
e-mail: info@bondst.org
Web Site: www.bondst.org
Officers:
   President: Patrick Sciarratta
   VP: Joanna Sherman
Management:
   Artistic Director: Joanna Sherman
   Managing Director: Michael McGuigan
   Music Director: Sean Nowell
Mission: To develop new works of theatre employing an imagistic and physical vocabulary; to explore politically relevant themes for diverse audiences.
Founded: 1978
Specialized Field: Theatrical Group
Status: Professional; Nonprofit
Paid Staff: 3
Volunteer Staff: 4
Paid Artists: 12
Budget: $150,000
Income Sources: Trust for Mutual Understanding; Art Link; Arts International
Affiliations: ART/NY; NPCC
Organization Type: Performing; Touring; Sponsoring; Artists' Colony

3355 BRIDGE STATE OF THE ARTS

101 W 78th Street
Suite 21
New York, NY 10024
Phone: 212-887-3362
Fax: 212-887-3362
Management:
   Founder/Artistic Director: Avra Petrides

3356 BROADWAY TOMORROW

191 Claremont Avenue
Suite 53
New York, NY 10027
Phone: 212-531-2447
Fax: 212-531-2447
e-mail: solight@aorldnet.att.net
Web Site: http://home.att/~solight
Officers:
   President: Elyse Curtis PhD
   VP: Mitchell Robinson
   Secretary/Treasurer: Norman Curtis
Management:
   Artistic Director: Elyse Curtis
   Music Director: Norman Curtis
Mission: To foster new musicals.
Founded: 1983
Specialized Field: Musical
Status: Professional; Nonprofit
Budget: $25,000
Income Sources: Donations
Organization Type: Performing

3357 CASTILLO THEATRE

500 Greenwich Street
Suite 201
New York, NY 10013
Phone: 212-941-5800
Fax: 212-941-8340
e-mail: castilloth@aol.com
Web Site: www.castillo.org
Management:
   Managing Director: Diane Stiles
   Artistic Director: Fred Newman
   Dramaturg: Dan Friedman
Founded: 1983
Paid Staff: 2
Volunteer Staff: 70
Non-paid Artists: 18
Performs At: Castillo Theatre
Affiliations: TCG; ART; NY
Type of Stage: Thrust
Seating Capacity: 71
Year Built: 1989

3358 CHICAGO CITY LIMITS

1105 First Avenue at 61st Street
New York, NY 10021
Phone: 212-888-5233
Fax: 212-888-0810
e-mail: info@chicagocitylimits.com
Web Site: www.chicagocitylimits.com
Management:
   Director/Executive Producer: Paul Zuckerman
   Music Director: Frank Spitznagel
   Producer: Linda Gelman
   Producer: Jay Stern
   Production Coordinator: Susie Pierce
   House Manager: Elliott Lipsey
   Associate: Austin Cadore
Mission: To offer satirical comedy revues that incorporate audience suggestions for an evening of improvisation, comedy and song.
Founded: 1977
Specialized Field: Improvisational theater
Status: Professional; Commercial
Paid Staff: 3
Paid Artists: 10
Season: Year-Round
Performs At: Chicago City Limits Theater
Type of Stage: Proscenium
Seating Capacity: 190
Year Built: 1971
Rental Contact: Producer Jay Stern

Organization Type: Performing; Touring; Resident; Educational
Resident Groups: Chicago City Limits

3359 CIRCLE-IN-THE-SQUARE
Broadway and 50th Street
New York, NY 10019
Phone: 212-239-6200
Fax: 212-581-6371
Toll-free: 800-432-7250
Officers:
   President: Paul Libin
Management:
   Artistic Director: Theodore Mann
   Executive Director: E Colin O'Leary
Mission: To produce new plays, classics and little-seen works deserving of a second look.
Founded: 1961
Status: Professional; Nonprofit
Performs At: Circle In The Square
Affiliations: League of Resident Theatres; Theatre Communications Group; League of American Theatres & Producers
Organization Type: Performing

3360 CLASSIC STAGE COMPANY
136 E 13th Street
New York, NY 10003
Phone: 212-677-4210
Fax: 212-477-7504
e-mail: info@classicstage.org
Web Site: www.classicstage.org
Officers:
   President: Donald Donovan
Management:
   Artistic Director: Barry Edelstein
   Producing Director: Beth Emelson
   General Manager: Rachel Tischler
Mission: To produce classics with a relevance to today's audience.
Founded: 1967
Specialized Field: Theatrical Group
Status: Professional; Nonprofit
Paid Staff: 8
Paid Artists: 100
Budget: $1,300,000
Income Sources: Various
Season: September - May
Performs At: Theater
Affiliations: Actors Equity; USA; American Guild of Musical Artists
Annual Attendance: 17,000
Facility Category: Theater
Type of Stage: 3/4 Thrust
Stage Dimensions: 30'x30'
Seating Capacity: 180
Year Built: 1800
Year Remodeled: 2000
Rental Contact: Rachel Tischler
Organization Type: Performing; Resident

3361 CREATION PRODUCTION COMPANY
127 Greene Street
New York, NY 10012

Phone: 212-674-5593
Management:
   Director: Anne Hemenway
   Managing Director: Jennifer McDowall
   Co-Artistic Director: Susan Mosakowski
   Co-Artistic Director: Matthew Maguire
Mission: To create experimental theatre.
Founded: 1977
Specialized Field: Theatrical Group
Status: Professional; Nonprofit
Season: Year-Round
Organization Type: Performing; Touring; Educational

3362 CREATIVE ARTS TEAM
715 Broadway, 5th Floor
New York University
New York, NY 10003
Phone: 212-998-7380
Fax: 212-995-4151
Management:
   Executive Director: Lynda Zimmerman
   Playwright-in-Residence: Jim Mirrione
   Managing Director: Dr. Leslie White
   Program Director: Mark Riherd
Founded: 1974
Specialized Field: Theatrical Group
Status: Professional; Nonprofit
Income Sources: New York State Council on Arts; Theatre Communications Group; New York University
Organization Type: Performing; Touring; Resident; Educational

---

3363 DISNEY THEATRICAL PRODUCTIONS
1450 Broadway
#300
New York, NY 10018
Phone: 212-827-5400
Fax: 212-703-1048
e-mail: michele.gold@disney.com
Web Site: www.disneyonbroadway.com
   Booking Assistant/Domestic Touring: Jim Lanahan

3364 DIXON PLACE
258 Bowery
New York, NY 10012
Phone: 212-219-3088
Fax: 212-274-9114
Management:
   Curators of New Play Reading Series: Andrew J. Mellen
   Curators of New Play Reading Series: Micah Schraft
Founded: 1986
Specialized Field: Theater
Performs At: Dixon Place
Type of Stage: Thrust
Seating Capacity: 70

3365 DO GOODER PRODUCTIONS
359 W 54th Street
Suite 4FS
New York, NY 10019

Phone: 212-581-8852
Fax: 212-541-7928
e-mail: dogooder@panix.com
Web Site: www.panix.com/~dogooder
Management:
   Founding Artistic Director: Mark Robert Gordon
   Managing Producer: Joel Feltman
Mission: An off broadway theater company dedicated to new play development and charitable endeavors.
Founded: 1994
Specialized Field: Theater Productions
Paid Staff: 2

3366 DON QUIJOTE CHILDREN'S THEATRE

250 W 65th Street
New York, NY 10023
Phone: 212-579-2358
Management:
   Artistic Director: Oswaldo Pradere
   Resident Director: Stefanie Scott
   Administrator: Jim Finn
   Administrative Assistant: Wendy Samuel
Mission: To inspire, entertain and educate children through theatre.
Founded: 1972
Specialized Field: Musical; Theatrical Group; Puppet
Status: Professional; Nonprofit
Organization Type: Performing; Touring; Resident; Educational

3367 DOWLING ENTERTAINMENT CORPORATION

226 W 47th Street
Suite 700
New York, NY 10036
Phone: 212-719-3090
Fax: 212-719-2987
Management:
   Office Manager: Doreen Chila
Mission: Business management
Founded: 1984
Status: Professional; Commercial
Performs At: The Cherry Lane Theatre
Organization Type: Performing

3368 DOWNTOWN ART COMPANY

64 E 4th Street
New York, NY 10003
Phone: 212-732-1227
Management:
   Artistic Director: Ryan Gilliam
   Producing Director: Cliff Scott
   Artistic Associate: Dan Hurlin
   Artistic Associate: Dan Froot
Mission: To support the development of contemporary performance works.
Founded: 1987
Specialized Field: Theatrical Group
Status: Professional; Nonprofit
Income Sources: National Association of Artists; Alliance of Resident Theatres/New York
Organization Type: Performing; Touring; Sponsoring

3369 DRAMA DEPARTMENT

27 Barron Street
New York, NY 10014
Phone: 212-633-9108
Fax: 212-633-9578
e-mail: info@dramadept.org
Web Site: www.dramadept.org
Officers:
   Development Director: Clinton Cargill
   Ticketing Director: Cheryl French
Management:
   Artistic Director: Douglas Carter Beane
   Managing Director: Michael S Rosenberg
   Head Production: Ilene Rosen
   Director Operations: Alexis Rehrmann
   Director Development: Clinton Cargill
   Director Ticketing: Cheryl French
Mission: A collective of actors, directors, designers, writers and stage managers who collaborate to create new works and revive neglected classics.
Founded: 1995
Specialized Field: New works & Neglected classics
Status: Nonprofit
Paid Staff: 2
Volunteer Staff: 2
Budget: $1,000,000
Income Sources: Ticket sales; Grants; Private contributions
Season: July - June
Annual Attendance: 10,000+
Facility Category: Great theatre in old settlement house
Type of Stage: Proscenium
Stage Dimensions: 35'x20'
Seating Capacity: 99
Year Built: 1916
Year Remodeled: 2001
Cost: $3,000,000+
Rental Contact: Alexis Rehrmann

3370 EMERGING ARTISTS THEATRE COMPANY

518 9th Avenue
Suite 2
New York, NY 10018
Phone: 212-627-5792
e-mail: info@eatheatre.org
Web Site: www.eatheatre.org
Officers:
   President: Roland Dib
   Senior VP: Brad Punty
   VP: Leigh Giroux
   Treasurer: Dara Falco
Management:
   Artistic Director: Paul Adams
   Manager For Directors: Blake Lawrence
   Manager For Playwrights: Johnathan Reuing
   Managing Director: Brad Punty
   Sales And Marketing: Ilona Lima
   Development Director: Donna Moreau
Mission: Emerging Artists Theatre Company exists to provide a safe and secure home for new playwrights to develop their work from an idea to fully realized production and where the playwright remains the key component in the creation and birth of t
Founded: 1993

3371 EN GARDE ARTS
225 Rector Place
Suite 3A
New York, NY 10280
Phone: 212-941-9793
Fax: 212-274-8123
Management:
Producer: Anne Hamburger
Managing Director: Ron Aja
Director Development: Mary McBride
Mission: To commission artists for the purpose of creating theatrical productions that are inspired by socially, historically or architecturally significant sites.
Status: Professional; Nonprofit
Organization Type: Performing

3372 ENSEMBLE STUDIO THEATRE
549 W 52nd Street
New York, NY 10019
Phone: 212-247-4982
Fax: 212-664-0041
e-mail: postmaster@ensemblestudiotheatre
Web Site: www.ensembloestudiotheatre.org
Management:
Artistic Director: Curt Dempster
Executive Director: Jamie Richards
Mission: To nurture and develop the American theatre artist.
Founded: 1972
Specialized Field: Theatrical Group
Status: Professional; Nonprofit
Paid Staff: 14
Volunteer Staff: 25
Budget: $ 1.3 Million
Season: October - June
Performs At: The Ensemble Studio Theatre
Type of Stage: Black Box; Proscenium
Seating Capacity: 99; 60
Organization Type: Performing

3373 ERGO THEATRE COMPANY
PO Box 290
Times Square Station
New York, NY 10108
Phone: 212-501-2710
e-mail: info@ergotheatre.org
Web Site: www.ergotheatre.org
Management:
Artistic Director: Robert Jay Cronin
Managing Director: Johanna Pinzler
Business Manager: Katherine Clark Helzer
Mission: Ergo Theatre Company is making a new home for bright rising talent in the New York theatre community.

3374 FIJI COMPANY
47 Great Jones Street
New York, NY 10012
Phone: 212-254-7228
Management:
Artistic Director: Ping Chong
Managing Director: Joe Jeffcoat

Mission: Created out of a desire to incorporate the visual arts (dance, film, video and theater) into a multimedia show questioning the syntax of global theater.
Founded: 1972
Specialized Field: Theatrical Group
Status: Professional; Nonprofit
Income Sources: Theatre Communications Group; Alliance of Resident Theatres/New York
Organization Type: Performing; Touring; Resident; Educational

3375 FREDERICK DOUGLASS CREATIVE ARTS CENTER
168 W 46th Street
New York, NY 10036
Phone: 212-864-3375
Fax: 212-864-3474
Management:
Artistic Director: Fred Hudson
Executive Administrator: Yvonne Hudson
Mission: A writers development organization which includes a performance component.
Founded: 1971
Specialized Field: Theatrical Group; Literary
Status: Professional; Nonprofit
Organization Type: Resident

3376 GLINES
240 W 44th Street
New York, NY 10036
Phone: 212-354-8899
e-mail: theglines@aol.com
Officers:
President/Treasurer: John Glines
VP: Steve Carpenter
Secretary: Malcolm Wexchler
Board of Director: Mark Hostetter
Management:
Artistic Director: John Glines
Mission: To promote positive gay images and dispel negative stereotyping.
Founded: 1976
Specialized Field: Theatrical Group
Status: Nonprofit
Organization Type: Performing

3377 HARBOR THEATRE
160 W 71st Street
PHA
New York, NY 10023
Phone: 212-787-1945
Web Site: www.harbortheatre.org
Management:
Artistic Director: Stuart Warmflash
Webmaster: Mark E Lang
Artistic Associate: Amanda Sewlyn
Artistic Associate: Marc Gellar
Mission: In 1994 a group of writers, under that artistic leadership of Stuart Warmflash, began a theatre workshop that would focus on the written word. Its purpose was to provide a safe haven for a few dedicated playwrights to express and refine their personal vision.
Founded: 1994

3378 HARLEM ARTISTS' DEVELOPMENT LEAGUE
207 W 133rd Street
New York, NY 10030
Phone: 212-368-9314
Officers:
Chairman: Dr. Nathan A Wright
Management:
Artistic Director: Gertrude Jeannette
Business/Company Manager: Ajene Washington
Secretary/Treasurer: Murphree Johnson
Training Supervisor: Louise Mike
Mission: To offer professional theatre to residents of the Harlem community at modest prices; to train artists in speech, acting and dance.
Specialized Field: Community; Theatrical Group
Status: Professional; Semi-Professional; Nonprofit
Paid Staff: 25
Income Sources: Community Service Council of Greater Harlem
Performs At: Saint Philips Church
Organization Type: Performing; Resident; Educational

3379 HENSON INTERNATIONAL FESTIVAL OF PUPPET THEATRE
117 E 69th Street
New York, NY 10021
Phone: 212-794-2400
Fax: 212-439-6036
e-mail: info@hensonfestival.org
Web Site: www.hensonfestival.org
Management:
Executive Producer: Cherly Henson
Generla Manager: Heidi Wilenius
Development Officer: Meg Daniel
Mission: To provide some of the finest international puppetry performers for American audiences. To present the finest international puppet artists to American audiences.
Specialized Field: Puppet theatre
Status: Nonprofit
Performs At: Joseph Papp Public Theater
Organization Type: Sponsoring

3380 HERE ARTS CENTER
145 6th Avenue
New York, NY 10013
Phone: 212-647-0202
Fax: 212-647-0257
e-mail: info@here.org
Web Site: www.here.org
Management:
Founder/Producer: Barbara Busackijno
Founder/Executive Producer: Kristen Marting
Founder: Randy Rollison
Execuktive Director: Kristin Marting
Mission: To support emerging and mid-career artist in all disciplines.
Founded: 1993
Specialized Field: Multidisciplinary
Status: Nonprofit
Paid Staff: 21
Volunteer Staff: 6
Budget: $1.2 million

Income Sources: Earned; Contributions
Affiliations: Art NY Member
Annual Attendance: 75,000
Facility Category: Multi-Arts Center
Type of Stage: Flexible
Seating Capacity: 99
Year Built: 1993

3381 HISPANIC ORGANIZATION OF LATIN ACTORS
250 W 65th Street
New York, NY 10023
Phone: 212-253-1015
Fax: 212-799-6718
Management:
Executive Director: Francisco G Rivela
Managing Director: Manny Alfaro
Board Member: Arnold E Rivera
Mission: To offer workshops, advocacy-training and referrals.
Founded: 1977
Specialized Field: Community; Theatrical Group
Status: Professional; Nonprofit
Organization Type: Arts Service Organization

3382 HUDSON GUILD THEATRE
441 W 26th Street
New York, NY 10001
Phone: 212-760-9800
Fax: 212-268-9983
Management:
Theatre Director: Jim Furlong
Founded: 1895
Specialized Field: Theatrical Group; Community
Status: Profesional; Nonprofit
Paid Staff: 1
Budget: $35,000
Facility Category: Theatre
Stage Dimensions: 28'x29'
Seating Capacity: 104
Rental Contact: Jim Furlong
Organization Type: Performing

3383 HYPOTHETICAL THEATRE COMPANY
344 E 14th Street
New York, NY 10003
Phone: 212-780-0800
Fax: 212-780-0859
e-mail: htcd@nyc.rr.com
Web Site: hypotheatrical@bigfoot.com
Founded: 1992
Performs At: Hypothetical Theatre
Type of Stage: Proscenium
Seating Capacity: 99

3384 IGLOO, THE THEATRICAL GROUP
225 E 4th Street
Apartment 6
New York, NY 10009
Phone: 212-460-9055
Management:
Artistic Director: Maria Taribassi
Artistic Director: Chris Peditto

Artistic Director: Paul Peditto
Mission: Dedicated to ensemble production of new and rarely seen works.
Founded: 1985
Specialized Field: Musical; Theatrical Group
Status: Professional; Nonprofit
Paid Staff: 10
Organization Type: Performing; Resident

3385 INTAR HISPANIC AMERICAN ARTS CENTER

International Arts Relations
508 W 53rd Street
New York, NY 10019
Mailing Address: PO Box 756, New York, NY, 10108
Phone: 212-695-6134
Fax: 212-268-0102
e-mail: intarnewyork@aol.com
Management:
   Artistic Director: Max Ferra
   Artistic Associate: Lorenzo Mans
Mission: To identify, develop and present the work of Hispanic-American theatre artists and visual artists, as well as to introduce outstanding works by internationally respected Latin artists to American audiences.
Founded: 1966
Status: Professional; Nonprofit
Income Sources: Non-profit funding
Season: October - June
Performs At: Black Box
Affiliations: Theatre Communications Group, Alliance of Resident Theatres (NY)
Facility Category: Off-Broadway Theater / Visual Arts Gallery
Type of Stage: Proscenium
Seating Capacity: 74
Year Remodeled: 1999
Rental Contact: Ext. 12 Jose Sanchez
Organization Type: Performing

3386 INTERBOROUGH REPERTORY THEATER

154 Christopher Street
Suite 3B
New York, NY 10014
Phone: 212-206-6875
Fax: 212-206-7037
Web Site: www.bd-studios.com/IRTonline
Officers:
   President: Mimi Craig
   Secretary: Pamala L La Bonne
Management:
   Artistic Director: Luane Davis
   Executive Director: Jonathan Fluck
Mission: To offer adaptations of literature and history as well as issues of interest to disenfranchised audiences; to provide standard repertory for general audiences.
Founded: 1986
Specialized Field: Musical; Theatrical Group
Status: Semi-Professional; Nonprofit
Income Sources: Brooklyn Arts & Cultural Association; Actors' Equity Association; Encore; Saturday Theater for Children; Division of American Theater Wing
Organization Type: Performing; Touring; Educational

3387 IRISH ARTS CENTRE THEATRE

553 W 51st Street
New York, NY 10019
Phone: 212-757-3318
Fax: 212-247-0930
Management:
   Artistic Director: Neal Jones
   Executive Director: Pauline Turley
Mission: Preserving, celebrating and developing Irish culture in America through producing New Irish, Classic Irish, and Irish-American plays.
Founded: 1972
Status: Professional; Nonprofit
Paid Staff: 50
Volunteer Staff: 30
Season: Year-Round
Performs At: Irish Arts Center Theatre
Stage Dimensions: 23x15x1000
Seating Capacity: 99
Year Built: 1972
Year Remodeled: 1995
Organization Type: Performing; Resident

3388 IRONDALE ENSEMBLE PROJECT

Box 1314
Old Chelsea Station
New York, NY 10011-1314
Phone: 212-633-1292
Fax: 212-633-2078
e-mail: irondalert@aol.com
Web Site: www.irondale.org
Management:
   Artistic Director: Jim Niesen
   Executive Director: Terry Greiss
Founded: 1983

3389 JAM AND COMPANY

331 W 38th Street
#5
New York, NY 10018
Phone: 212-714-2263
Fax: 212-594-1245
Management:
   Artistic Director: John Amudd
Founded: 1985
Specialized Field: Theatrical Group
Status: Semi-Professional
Organization Type: Performing

3390 JEAN COCTEAU REPERTORY

330 Bowery
New York, NY 10012
Phone: 212-677-0060
Fax: 212-777-6151
e-mail: cocteau@jeancocteaurep.org
Web Site: www.jeancocteaurep.org
Officers:
   President: David Jiranek
   VP: John Horn
   Secretary: Carmen Anthony
Management:
   Producing Artistic Director: David Fuller
   Director Development: Ryan Teller
   General Manager: Amy Wagner

Marketing/Promotions Manager: Denise R Zeiler
Mission: Committed to presenting innovative productions of the world's classics; dedicated to sustaining a resident company presenting rotating repertory.
Founded: 1971
Specialized Field: Theatrical Ensemble
Status: Professional; Nonprofit
Paid Staff: 10
Volunteer Staff: 5
Paid Artists: 20
Budget: $850,000
Income Sources: Box Office; Individuals; Corporations; Foundation
Performs At: Bouwerie Lane Theatre
Affiliations: Theatre Communications Group; Alliance of Resident Theatres/New York
Annual Attendance: 22,000
Facility Category: Theatre
Type of Stage: Proscenium
Stage Dimensions: 17'x22'x13'
Seating Capacity: 140
Year Built: 1960
Year Remodeled: 1996
Rental Contact: Ernest Johns
Organization Type: Performing; Resident; Educational
Resident Groups: Jean Cocteau Repertory

3391 JEWISH REPERTORY THEATRE

92nd Street Y
1395 Lexington Avenue
New York, NY 10128
Phone: 212-831-2001
Fax: 212-831-0082
e-mail: jrep@echo.nyc.com
Web Site: www.jrt.org
Management:
   Artistic Director: Rau Avni
   Managing Director: Kathleen Germann
   Assoc. Artistic Director/Literary: Richard Sabellico
Mission: To present works in English which relate to Jewish experience.
Status: Professional; Nonprofit
Income Sources: Actors' Equity Association
Performs At: Jewish Repertory Theatre
Organization Type: Performing

3392 KATHRYN BACHE MILLER THEATRE

Columbia University
Mail Code 1801, 2960 Broadway
New York, NY 10027
Phone: 212-854-1633
Fax: 212-854-7740
e-mail: miller-arts@columbia.edu
Web Site: www.millertheatre.com
Management:
   Executive Director: George Steel
   General Manager: Melisa Smey
Mission: To provide high quality presentations of contemporary, classical and early music to the greater New York City audience.
Founded: 1998
Facility Category: Concert Hall
Seating Capacity: 688
Rental Contact: Gary Caruana

3393 KOHAV THEATRE FOUNDATION

118 Riverside Drive
New York, NY 10024
Phone: 212-877-1667
Management:
   Director: Hava Kohav Beller
   Production Assistant: Kathleen Greene
   Counsel: Herbert C Kantor
Founded: 1959
Specialized Field: Theater
Status: Professional; Nonprofit
Organization Type: Performing

3394 LA MAMA EXPERIMENTAL THEATRE

74A E 4th Street
New York, NY 10003
Phone: 212-254-6468
Fax: 212-254-7597
e-mail: lamama@lamama.org
Web Site: www.lamama.org
Management:
   Founder/Director: Ellen Stewart
   Associate Director: Beverly Petty
   Business Manager: Gretchen Green
Founded: 1961
Specialized Field: Theatrical Group; Multi-Art
Status: Professional; Nonprofit
Budget: $1,500,000
Income Sources: Foundations; Government; Ticket Revenue; Playwright Royalties
Performs At: Experimantal Theatre; Dance; Opera
Annual Attendance: 30,000
Facility Category: Theatre (3 venues) 1 Gallery
Seating Capacity: 100; 400
Organization Type: Performing; Producing

3395 LAMB'S THEATRE COMPANY

130 W 44th Street
New York, NY 10036
Phone: 212-997-1780
Officers:
   Chairman: Kendyl K Monroe
   Secretary: Patricia McCorkle
Management:
   Producing Director: Carolyn Rossi-Copeland
   Production Manager: Clark Cameron
   Administrative Coordinator: Carl H Jaynes
   Box Office Treasurer: Larry Staroff
Mission: To develop and present the work of new American theatre artists hoping to offer positive solutions to modern ethical problems.
Founded: 1980
Status: Professional; Nonprofit
Income Sources: Theatre Communications Group; Alliance of Resident Theatres/New York
Performs At: Lamb's Theatre; Lamb's Little Theatre
Organization Type: Performing; Touring; Educational

3396 LATIN AMERICAN THEATRE EXPERIMENT & ASSOCIATES

107 Suffolk Street
New York, NY 10002
Phone: 212-529-1948
Management:

Executive Director: Margarita Toirac
Founder: Mario Pena
Mission: Our purpose is to expand the theatre movement to the Spanish and English communities.
Founded: 1970
Specialized Field: Theatrical Group
Status: Professional; Nonprofit
Type of Stage: Proscenium
Stage Dimensions: 25'x20'x14'
Seating Capacity: 150
Organization Type: Performing; Touring; Resident; Educational

3397 LES BALLETS GRANDIVA

101 W 67th Street
Suite 49 E
New York, NY 10023
Phone: 212-595-3675
Fax: 212-336-5646
e-mail: grandiva01@aol.com
Web Site: www.balletsgrandiva.com
Officers:
  President: Suguru Aito
Management:
  Artistic Director: Victor Trevino
Mission: To develop sance audiences by performing comedic parodies of a wide range of choreographic styles both classical and contemporary.
Founded: 1996
Specialized Field: Ballet; Dance Comedy
Paid Staff: 2
Paid Artists: 19
Budget: $600,000
Income Sources: Performance Fees; Donations
Annual Attendance: 80,000

3398 LIGHTNING STRIKES THEATRE COMPANY

PO Box 1545
New York, NY 10028
Phone: 212-713-5335
Management:
  Artistic Director: John McDermott
  Managing Director: Lori Funk
  Literary Manager: DL Shroder

3399 LINCOLN CENTER THEATER

150 W 65th Street
New York, NY 10023
Phone: 212-362-7600
Fax: 212-873-0761
Web Site: www.lct.org
Officers:
  Chairman: John B Beinecke
  President: John S Chalsty
  Vice Chairman: Joan Straus Cullman
  Vice Chairman: J Tomilson Hill
  Vice Chairman: Daryl Roth
  Treasurer: Constance L Clapp
  Secretary: William D Zabel
Management:
  Associate General Manager: Melanie Weinraub
  Box Office Treasurer: Fred Bonis
  Production Manager: Jeff Hamlin

Director Development: Hattie K Jutagir
Manager Special Events/Corp. Rel.: Karin Schall
Associate Director: Graciela Daniele
Associate Director: Gerald Gutierrez
Associate Director: Susan Stroman
Associate Director: Daniel Sullivan
Founded: 1966
Performs At: Vivian Beaumont, Mitzi E. Newhouse
Type of Stage: Thrust
Seating Capacity: 1000, 300

3400 LIVING THEATRE

272 E 3rd Street
New York, NY 10009
Phone: 212-982-2335
Fax: 212-865-3234
Officers:
  President: Hanon Reznikov
Management:
  Executive Director: Hanon Reznikov
  Artistic Director: Judith Malina
  Managing Director: Joanie Fritz
  Managing Associate: Isha Manna Beck
Mission: To create socially relevant theatre to be performed by an artistic ensemble of the highest calibre.
Founded: 1947
Specialized Field: Theatrical Group
Status: Nonprofit
Income Sources: Alliance of Resident Theatres/New York; Theatre Communications Group
Organization Type: Performing; Touring; Resident; Educational

3401 MABOU MINES

150 1st Avenue
2nd Floor
New York, NY 10009
Phone: 212-473-0559
Fax: 212-473-2410
e-mail: office@maboumines.org
Web Site: www.maboumines.org
Management:
  Company Manager: Joe Stackell
  Co-Artistic Director: Sharon Fogarty
  Co-Artistic Director: Ruth Malecaech
  Artistic Director: Sharon Fogarty
  Artistic Director: Ruth Maleczech
  Artistic Director: Frederick Neumann
  Artistic Director: Terry O'Reilly
Mission: To look at theater in fresh ways by re-exploring existing theatrical works and creating new ones.
Founded: 1970
Specialized Field: Theatrical Group
Status: Professional; Nonprofit
Affiliations: Theatre Communications Group; Alliance of Resident Theatres/New York
Type of Stage: Block Box
Organization Type: Performing; Touring; Educational

3402 MANHATTAN THEATRE CLUB

311 W 43rd Street
8th Floor
New York, NY 10036

Phone: 212-399-3000
Fax: 212-399-4329
e-mail: questions@mtc-nyc.org
Web Site: www.manhattantheatreclub.com
Management:
  Artistic Director: Lynne Meadow
  Executive Producer: Barry Grove
  General Manager: Harold Woltert
Mission: Encouraging, developing, and presenting important new American and international work that provides insight into culture, life and conflict.
Founded: 1970
Specialized Field: Theatre
Status: Professional; Nonprofit
Paid Staff: 335
Volunteer Staff: 25
Paid Artists: 348
Income Sources: Theatre Communications Group; Alliance of Resident Theatres/New York; Foundation for the Extension and Development of American Professional Theatre
Organization Type: Performing

3403 MARCEL MARCEAU

253 W 73rd Street
Suite 8G
New York, NY 10023
Phone: 212-874-2030
Fax: 212-874-1175
e-mail: staff@micocci.com
Web Site: www.micocci.com

3404 MCC THEATER

120 W 28th Street
New York, NY 10001
Phone: 212-727-7722
Fax: 212-727-7780
e-mail: mcc@mcctheater.org
Web Site: www.mcctheater.org
Management:
  Literary Manager: Stephen Willems
  Artistic Director: Robert Lupone
  Artistic Director: Bernard Tesley
  Associate Artistic Director: William Cantler
  Office Manager: Greta Rothman
  General Manager: Jodi Schoenbrun
Founded: 1986
Paid Staff: 9

3405 METRO PLAYHOUSE

220 E 4th Street
New York, NY 10009
Phone: 212-995-5302
e-mail: groups@mertoplayhouse.com
Web Site: www.metropolitianplayhouse.org
Management:
  Artistic Director: David Zarko
  Comapany Manager: Ed Chemaly
  Literary Manager: Kim Wadsworth

3406 MIRROR REPERTORY COMPANY

PO Box 286186
New York, NY 10128

Phone: 212-427-7393
Toll-free: 866-647-7371
e-mail: info@mirrorrepertoryco.com
Web Site: www.mirrorrepertoryco.com
Management:
  Artistic Director: Sabra Jones
Mission: The Mirror Repertory Company, aka Mirror Theatre Ltd., was founded in 1983. It was a daring return to the European theatre style of alternating repertory theatre—a different play each night as in the ballet and the opera.
Founded: 1982
Specialized Field: Theatrical Group
Status: Professional; Nonprofit
Income Sources: Actors' Equity Association
Performs At: Mirror Repertory Theater
Organization Type: Performing; Resident; Educational

3407 MUSIC THEATRE ASSOCIATES

1841 Broadway
Suite 914
New York, NY 10019
Phone: 212-841-9690
Fax: 212-841-9542
e-mail: jsimpson@cami.com
Web Site: www.camitheatricals.com
Founded: 1981
Specialized Field: Musical Theatre; Theatrical Dance; Plays; Dance

3408 MUSIC THEATRE GROUP AT LENOX ARTS CENTER

30 W 26th Street #1001
New York, NY 10010
Phone: 212-366-5260
Fax: 212-366-5265
Officers:
  Co- Chairman: Katheryn Walker
  Co- Chairman: Charles Hollerith
  President: Lyn Austin
  VP: Lynda Sthrner Traum
Management:
  Producing Director: Lyn Austin
  General Director: Diane Wondisford
  Associate Producer: Charlotte Kreutz
  Development: Peter Krasny
Mission: Exclusively engaged in and dedicated to the creation of new musical theatre works with distinctive focus on developing new forms and artists through unique combinations of music, theatre, dance and visual arts.
Founded: 1970
Specialized Field: Theatrical Group; Musical Theatre
Status: Professional; Nonprofit
Budget: $80,000
Income Sources: Box Office, Grants, Private Donations
Organization Type: Performing; Touring

3409 MUSICAL THEATRE WORKS

440 Lafayette Street
New York, NY 10003
Phone: 212-677-0040
Fax: 212-598-0105
e-mail: jsiegel@akula.com
Management:

Artistic Director: Anthony Stimack
General Manager: Marilyn Stimack
Managing Director: Mike Teel
Mission: Developing and producing new works for American musical theatre.
Founded: 1983
Specialized Field: Musical; Theatrical Group
Status: Professional; Nonprofit
Income Sources: Actors' Equity Association; Theatre Communications Group; Alliance of Resident Theatres/New York
Organization Type: Performing; Resident

3410 NATIONAL BLACK THEATRE

2033 5th Avenue
New York, NY 10035
Phone: 212-722-3800
Fax: 212-926-1571
Management:
Founder/CEO: Barbara Ann Teer
Executive Director: Shirley Faison
Performing Program Director: Tunde Samuel
Action Arts Director: Ade Faison
Rental Program Director: Nabi Faison
Mission: To enhance human dignity by increasing the unity, appreciation and availability of Black Theatre.
Founded: 1968
Specialized Field: Theatrical Group
Status: Professional; Nonprofit
Performs At: National Black Institute of Communication
Organization Type: Performing; Touring; Resident

3411 NATIONAL BLACK TOURING CIRCUIT

790 Riverside Drive
Suite 3E
New York, NY 10032
Phone: 212-283-0974
Fax: 212-283-0983
Officers:
Co-Chairman: Shaunielle Perry
Management:
Producer/Director: Woodie King Jr
Associate Producer: Ashia Dervisa
Mission: To tour plays to colleges, festivals, and black cultural institutions across the USA, Europe, and Africa.
Founded: 1976
Specialized Field: Theatre
Status: Professional; Nonprofit
Paid Staff: 3
Paid Artists: 25
Non-paid Artists: 2
Budget: $240,000
Income Sources: Contracted Services
Organization Type: Performing; Touring; Resident; Educational

3412 NATIONAL IMPROVISATIONAL THEATRE

223 8th Avenue
New York, NY 10011
Phone: 212-243-7224
Fax: 212-366-4312
Management:
Executive Director: Christopher Smith

Artistic Director: Tamara Wilcox-Smith
VP Public Relations: Robert Martin
VP Operations: Eva Mahoney
Mission: To bring art improvisation to the highest possible level.
Founded: 1984
Specialized Field: Theatrical Group
Status: Professional; Nonprofit
Paid Staff: 30
Organization Type: Performing; Educational

3413 NATIONAL SHAKESPEARE COMPANY

353 W 48th Street
3rd Floor
New York, NY 10036
Phone: 212-265-1340
Fax: 212-265-1258
e-mail: nsc62@aol.com
Management:
Producing Director: Deborah Teller
Tour Director: Val Sherman
Education Director: Heather Drastal
Mission: Nurturing and developing performing arts through touring professional, live theatre to American communities.
Founded: 1963
Status: Professional
Season: September - May
Organization Type: Performing; Touring

3414 NEGRO ENSEMBLE COMPANY

154 Christopher Street
#2A-A
New York, NY 10014
Phone: 212-691-6730
Fax: 212-691-6798
e-mail: newgroup1@earthlink.net
Web Site: www.newgrouptheatre.com
Management:
Artistic Director: Scott Elliot
Executive Director: Geoffrey Rich
Literary Manager: Ian Morgan
Associate Executive Director: Josh Boggioni
Mission: To offer plays about the Black experience.
Founded: 1967
Specialized Field: Theatrical Group
Status: Professional; Nonprofit
Performs At: Theatre Four
Organization Type: Performing; Touring

3415 NEW DRAMATISTS

424 W 44th Street
New York, NY 10036
Phone: 212-757-6960
Fax: 212-265-4738
e-mail: newdramatists@newdramatists.org
Web Site: www.newdramatists.org
Officers:
Chairman: Seth Gelblum
President: Isobel Robins Koneccy
Management:
Artistic Director: Todd London
Executive Director: Joel K Rukark
Mission: To develop plays and playwrights.

Founded: 1949
Specialized Field: Theatrical Group
Status: Semi-Professional; Nonprofit
Paid Staff: 7
Volunteer Staff: 50
Paid Artists: 200
Non-paid Artists: 55
Income Sources: National Endowment for the Arts
Performs At: New Dramatists Theater
Organization Type: Resident; Educational

3416 NEW FEDERAL THEATRE
292 Henry Street
New York, NY 10002
Phone: 212-353-1176
Fax: 212-353-1088
e-mail: newfederal@aol.com
Web Site: www.newfederaltheatre.org
Management:
   Producing Director: Woodie King Jr
   Company Director: Pat White
   Marketing Director: Shea Douglas
   Office Administrator: Andrena Hale
Mission: To present both new and unknown works; to allow unknown and known directors and actors the opportunity to work together.
Founded: 1970
Specialized Field: Theatrical Group
Status: Professional; Nonprofit
Income Sources: Actors' Equity Association; Alliance of Resident Theatres/New York; Theatre Communications Group; Foundations; Corporate and Private Individuals
Season: September 30 - June 30
Performs At: Henry Street Settlement; New Federal Theater
Organization Type: Performing; Resident

3417 NEW GEORGES
90 Hudson Street
#2E
New York, NY 10013
Phone: 212-620-0113
Fax: 212-334-9239
e-mail: newgeorges@aol.com
Web Site: www.newgeorges.org
Management:
   Artistic Director: Susan Bernfield
Founded: 1992

3418 NEW RAFT THEATER COMPANY
450 W 42nd Street
Suite 2J
New York, NY 10036
Phone: 212-268-5501
Fax: 212-967-1458
Officers:
   Artistic Director: Avi Ber Haffman
Management:
   Artistic Director: Avi Ber Hoffman
   Associate Producer: Mary Ellen Ashley
   Executive Director: Eric Krebs
Mission: To find and develop original plays and musicals.
Founded: 1976
Specialized Field: Musical; Theatrical Group

Status: Professional; Nonprofit
Performs At: Houseman Theatre Complex
Organization Type: Performing

3419 NEW VICTORY THEATER
229 W 42nd Street
10th Floor
New York, NY 10036
Phone: 212-564-4222
Fax: 212-239-4298
e-mail: mrose@new42ndstreet.org
Web Site: www.newvictory.org

3420 NEW YORK SHAKESPEARE FESTIVAL/PUBLIC THEATER
425 Lafayette Street
New York, NY 10003
Phone: 212-539-8500
Fax: 212-539-8505
Management:
   Producer: George C Wolfe
   Excutive Director: Fran Reiter
   Marketing Director: Ed Leibman

3421 NEW YORK STAGE & FILM
151 W 30th Street
Suite 905
New York, NY 10001
Phone: 212-239-2334
Fax: 212-239-2996
Management:
   Managing Producer: Johanna Pfaelzer
Founded: 1984

3422 NEW YORK THEATRE WORKSHOP
79 E 4th Street
New York, NY 10003
Phone: 212-780-9037
Fax: 212-460-8996
e-mail: info@nytw.org
Web Site: www.nytw.org
Management:
   Managing Director: Lynn Moffat
   Artistic Director: James C Nicola
Mission: To offer inventive new plays; to showcase new directors.
Founded: 1980
Status: Professional; Nonprofit
Paid Staff: 25
Volunteer Staff: 25
Paid Artists: 150
Non-paid Artists: 300
Income Sources: Actors' Equity Association; Theatre Communications Group; Alliance of Resident Theatres/New York
Performs At: New York Theatre Workshop
Type of Stage: Proscenium
Seating Capacity: 189
Organization Type: Performing

3423 OHIO THEATRE
66 Wooster
New York, NY 10012

Phone: 212-966-4844
Management:
    Artistic Director: Robert Lyons
Mission: To offer experimental theatre.
Founded: 1977
Specialized Field: Theatrical Group
Status: Professional
Income Sources: Downtown Theatre Coalition
Performs At: Ohio Theatre
Organization Type: Performing; Sponsoring

3424 ONTOLOGICAL-HYSTERIC THEATRE

260 W Broadway
New York, NY 10013
Phone: 212-941-8911
Fax: 212-334-5149
e-mail: ontological@mindspring.com
Web Site: www.ontological.com
Management:
    Artistic Director: Richard Foreman
    Administrator: Mimi Johnson
    Production Manager: Patricia Ybarra
Mission: Producing and presenting the works of playwright, director and designer Richard Foreman.
Founded: 1970
Specialized Field: Theatre
Status: Professional; Nonprofit
Paid Staff: 1
Paid Artists: 8
Performs At: Ontological at St. Mark's Theater
Type of Stage: Black box
Seating Capacity: 85
Organization Type: Performing

3425 OPEN BOOK

525 W End Avenue
12E
New York, NY 10024-3207
Phone: 212-362-9014
e-mail: theopenbook@juno.com
Officers:
    CEO: Bill Bonham
    CFO: Saralee Kaye
    Board: Jay Broad
    Board: Mary Higgins Clark
    Board: Mario Fratti
    Board: Rev. Kathleen L Camera
    Board: Marc Lewis
    Board: Beverly Penberthy
    Board: Eugenia Rawls
Management:
    Artistic Director: Marvin Kaye
    Public Relations Director: Nancy Temple
    Director Development: Pat Costello
Mission: Producing new and little-known literature of quality in readers theatre format.
Founded: 1975
Specialized Field: Theatrical Group; Authors Reading Series; Readers Theatre
Status: Professional; Nonprofit
Income Sources: Various
Performs At: Various
Annual Attendance: 300 - 500
Facility Category: NY Performing Arts Spaces
Type of Stage: Modified Platform

Stage Dimensions: Varies
Seating Capacity: 70 - 100
Organization Type: Performing; Touring; Resident

3426 OPEN EYE: NEW STAGINGS

270 W 89th Street
New York, NY 10024
Fax: 212-769-4141
Officers:
    Chairman: Stephen Graham
    VP: Joan Stein
    Secretary: Elliot Brown
Management:
    Founding Director: Jean Erdman
    Artistic Director: Amie Brockway
    Production Manager/Business Manager: Adrienne Brockway
Mission: Presents productions of new and rare plays, plays geared for family audiences and provides playwrights the opportunity to develop new works through the New Stagings Lab.
Founded: 1972
Specialized Field: Theatrical Group
Status: Professional; Nonprofit
Income Sources: Theatre Communications Group; Alliance of Resident Theatres/New York; International Association of Theatre for Children and Youth
Performs At: The Open Eye; New Stagings
Organization Type: Performing; Touting; Educational

3427 PAN ASIAN REPERTORY THEATRE

263 W 86th Street
W End Theatre
New York, NY 10024
Mailing Address: 47 Great Jones Street, New York, NY, 10012
Phone: 212-868-4030
Fax: 212-868-4033
e-mail: panasian@aol.com
Web Site: www.panasianrep.org
Officers:
    Chairman: Sybil Nadel
    Vice Chairman: Muzaffar Chishti
Management:
    Artistic/Producing Manager: Tisa Chang
    Communications Director: Sylvia Fan
    Education Coordinator: Erika Hirokawa
    Artistic Associate: Ron Nakahara
Mission: To offer new Asian-American plays of the highest artistic standards, as well as adaptations of classics from around the world; to premiere Asian masterworks in America.
Founded: 1977
Specialized Field: Theatrical Group
Status: Professional; Nonprofit
Paid Staff: 4
Volunteer Staff: 10
Paid Artists: 50
Income Sources: Theatre Communications Group: Alliance of Resident Theatres/New York
Performs At: West End Theatre
Type of Stage: Proscenium
Organization Type: Performing; Touring; Resident; Educational

3428 PAPER BAG PLAYERS
50 Riverside Drive
New York, NY 10024
Phone: 212-362-0431
Fax: 212-362-0431
Officers:
   President: Huroco Nurasz
   VP: Kathy Mele
Management:
   Managing Director: Judith Liss
   Managing Director: Judith Martin
Mission: To create a contemporary theatre for children with shows based on a child's everyday experiences and perceptions of the world.
Founded: 1958
Specialized Field: Theatrical Group
Status: Professional; Nonprofit
Organization Type: Performing; Touring; Resident; Educational

3429 PARK AVENUE THEATRICAL GROUP
404 Park Avenue S
10th Floor
New York, NY 10016
Phone: 212-213-5270
Fax: 212-689-9140
e-mail: obresner@parny.com
Web Site: www.parny.com
Management:
   Director Sales: Carol Bresner

3430 PEARL THEATRE COMPANY
80 St. Mark's Place
New York, NY 10003
Phone: 212-505-3401
Fax: 212-505-3404
e-mail: mbeals@pearltheatre.org
Web Site: www.pearltheatre.org
Officers:
   Chairperson: Brian Heidtke
   President: Ellen Hirsch
   Treasurer: Jean Cheever
   Secretary: Ellen Jakobson
Management:
   Associate Director: Joanne Camp
   Director Development: Margaret Benson
   Director Marketing: Michelle Brandon
   Programs Manager/Casting: Meghan Beals
   Business Manager: Amy Kaiser
   Production Manager: Dale Smallwood
Mission: To present a full-range repertory strongly rooted in the classics with a resident acting company, guest artists and theatre staff.
Founded: 1982
Specialized Field: Theatrical Group
Status: Professional; Nonprofit
Paid Staff: 9
Volunteer Staff: 50
Paid Artists: 35
Budget: $1.5 million
Income Sources: Foundations; Individual Giving; Earned Income
Performs At: Theatre
Annual Attendance: 27,000

Facility Category: Theatre with Lobby, Box Office and Dressing Rooms
Type of Stage: Proscenium
Stage Dimensions: 22' x 44'
Seating Capacity: 160
Rental Contact: Production Manager Dale Smallwood
Organization Type: Performing; Resident; Educational

3431 PECULIAR WORKS PROJECT
595 Broadway
2nd Floor
New York, NY 10012-3222
Phone: 212-529-3626
e-mail: info@peculiarworks.org
Web Site: www.peculiarworks.org
Management:
   Director: Ralph Lewis
Mission: Peculiar Works Project generates original, multi-disciplinary performance that is accessible and fun for diverse audiences.

3432 PING CHONG & COMPANY
47 Great Jones Street
New York, NY 10012
Phone: 212-529-1557
Fax: 212-529-1703
Management:
   Artistic Director: Ping Chong
   Managing Director: Bruce Allardice

3433 PLAYWRIGHTS HORIZONS
630 9th Avenue
Suite 708
New York, NY 10036
Phone: 212-564-1235
Fax: 212-594-0296
Web Site: www.playwrightshorizons.org
Management:
   Artistic Director: Tim Sanford
   Managing Director: Leslie Marcus
   General Manager: William Russo
   Literary Manager: Sonya Sobieski
   Casting Director: James Callen
Mission: Developing American composers, lyricists and playwrights; offering internships and training programs.
Founded: 1971
Status: Professional; Nonprofit
Income Sources: Actors' Equity Association; Alliance of Resident Theatres/New York; New York University
Performs At: Mainstage Theatre; Studio Theatre
Facility Category: Theater
Type of Stage: Proscenium
Seating Capacity: 141
Organization Type: Performing; Educational

3434 PRIMARY STAGES COMPANY
131 W 45th Street
New York, NY 10036
Phone: 212-840-9705
Fax: 212-840-9725
e-mail: primary@ix.netcom.com
Web Site: www.primarystages.commary.htm
Management:
   Artistic Director: Casey Childs

General Manager: Peg Schuler
Associate Artistic Director: Tyler Marchant
Literary Manager: Seth Gordon
Casting Director: Gina Gionfriddo
Mission: Discovering and producing the finest new American plays.
Founded: 1983
Specialized Field: Theatrical Group
Status: Professional; Nonprofit
Paid Staff: 5
Paid Artists: 4
Organization Type: Performing

3435 PROCESS STUDIO THEATRE

257 Church Street
New York, NY 10007
Phone: 212-271-0410
Management:
    Artistic Director: Bonnie Loren
    Technical Director: Anthony Sandkamp
Mission: Promoting new artists and works; offering a home to professional artists.
Founded: 1977
Specialized Field: Musical; Theatrical Group
Status: Professional; Nonprofit
Organization Type: Performing; Touring; Resident; Educational; Sponsoring; Outreach

3436 PROTEAN THEATRE COMPANY

484 W 43rd Street
Suite 31-O
New York, NY 10036
Phone: 212-290-1595
Web Site: www.proteantheatre.com
Management:
    Artistic Director: Owen Thompson
Mission: The Protean Theatre Company was founded in 1996 and prides itself on producing lost, undervalued, or even unpublished plays that deserve an exciting, professional New York production.
Founded: 1996
Status: Not-For-Profit

3437 PUERTO RICAN TRAVELING THEATRE COMPANY

141 W 94th Street
New York, NY 10025
Phone: 212-354-1293
Fax: 212-307-2769
Management:
    Artistic Director: Miriam Colon
    Managing Director: Michael Palma
Mission: Presenting bilingual plays; conducting workshops for underprivileged youth; providing training for playwrights.
Founded: 1967
Status: Professional; Nonprofit
Performs At: Puerto Rican Travelling Theatre
Organization Type: Performing; Touring; Educational

3438 RAJECKAS AND INTRAUB MOVEMENT THEATRE

AKA Theatremoves Inc.
New York, NY 10009
Mailing Address: PO Box 1333
Phone: 212-529-8068
Fax: 212-529-8068
e-mail: NINTRAUB@aol.com
Web Site: www.theatremoves.com
Management:
    Co-Artistic Director: Neil Intraub

3439 REPERTORIO ESPANOL

138 E 27th Street
New York, NY 10016
Phone: 212-889-2850
Fax: 212-686-3732
Management:
    Artistic Director: Rene Buch
    Associate Artistic Producer: Robert Federico
    Producer: Gilberto Zaldivar

3440 RIDGE THEATER

141 Ridge Street
Suite 8
New York, NY 10002
Phone: 212-674-5485
Fax: 212-674-5485
e-mail: laobob@aol.com
Web Site: www.ridgetheater.org
Management:
    Artistic Director: Bob McGrath
Mission: Exploring the boundaries of theatre and opera.
Status: Professional; Nonprofit
Facility Category: Theatre
Organization Type: Performing

3441 RIVERSIDE SHAKESPEARE COMPANY

Shakespeare Center
165 W 86th Street
New York, NY 10024
Phone: 212-505-2021
Fax: 212-505-2054
Management:
    Artistic Director: Gus Kaikkonen
    Executive Director: Ann Harvey
    Academy Director: Robert Mooney
Mission: Bringing classic works to life and making them more accessible.
Founded: 1976
Specialized Field: Theatrical Group
Status: Professional
Organization Type: Performing; Touring; Resident; Educational

3442 ROGER FURMAN THEATRE

60 E 42nd Street
Suite 1336
New York, NY 10017
Phone: 212-599-1922
Fax: 212-599-2414
Management:
    Executive Director: Voza Rivers

Mission: Encouraging cultural pluralism in New York City through the presentation of high-quality, professional Black theatre.
Founded: 1964
Specialized Field: Theatrical Group
Status: Professional; Nonprofit
Paid Staff: 5
Income Sources: National Endowment for the Arts; Department of Cultural Affairs
Performs At: Roger Furman Theater; B Smiths Rooftop Cafe
Organization Type: Performing; Touring; Resident; Educational

3443 ROUNDABOUT THEATRE COMPANY

231 W 39th Street
Suite 1200
New York, NY 10018
Phone: 212-719-9393
Fax: 212-869-8817
Web Site: www.roundabouttheatre.org
Management:
    Artistic Director: Todd Haimes
    Managing Director: Ellen Richard
Mission: To produce the classics, both ancient and modern.
Founded: 1965
Specialized Field: Theatrical Group
Status: Professional; Nonprofit
Affiliations: Actors' Equity Association; League of Resident Theatres; Society for Stage Directors and Choreographers
Facility Category: Theatre
Type of Stage: Proscenium
Seating Capacity: 700
Rental Contact: Christine Vall
Organization Type: Performing; Resident

3444 SAINT BART'S PLAYHOUSE

109 E 50th Street
New York, NY 10022
Phone: 212-751-1616
Fax: 212-378-0251
Founded: 1927
Specialized Field: Musical; Theatrical Group; Revival
Status: Semi-Professional; Nonprofit
Paid Staff: 75
Income Sources: Theatre Communications Group
Performs At: Saint Bartholomew's Community House
Organization Type: Performing; Resident; Educational

3445 SALT AND PEPPER MIME COMPANY

320 E 90th
#1B
New York, NY 10128
Phone: 212-262-4989
Fax: 212-262-4989
Management:
    Artistic Manager/Producer: Scottie Davis
    Director: Chuck Wise
    Resident Playwright: Mark Pearce
Mission: Preserving the art forms of vaudeville and mime through performances, exhibitions and workshops.
Founded: 1978

Specialized Field: Musical; Community; Theatrical Group; Drama; Variety; Children's
Status: Professional; Nonprofit
Income Sources: Alliance of Resident Theatres/New York; Westside Arts Coalition
Performs At: Lincoln Square Theatre; Studio Theatre
Organization Type: Performing; Touring; Educational

3446 SECOND STAGE THEATRE

301 W 43rd Street
New York, NY 10036
Phone: 212-787-8302
Fax: 212-877-9886
e-mail: info@secondstagetheatre.com
Web Site: www.secondstagetheatree.com
Management:
    Artistic Director: Carole Rothman
    Managing Director: Carol Fishman
    General Manager: Barrack Evans
    Producing Manager: Peter Davis
    Director Marketing: David Henderson
    Marketing Assistant/Promotions: Nicole Ruskin
Mission: To produce plays of the recent past which we feel deserve a second production; to produce world and New York premieres by emerging authors, with emphasis on women authors and authors of color.
Founded: 1979
Specialized Field: Theatrical Group
Status: Professional; Nonprofit
Paid Staff: 20
Annual Attendance: 67,000
Facility Category: Theatre
Seating Capacity: 296
Year Built: 1999
Rental Contact: Producing Manager Peter Davis
Organization Type: Performing

3447 SHADOW BOX THEATRE

325 W End Avenue
New York, NY 10023
Phone: 212-724-0677
Fax: 212-724-0767
e-mail: sbt@shadowboxtheatre.org
Web Site: www.shadowboxtheatre.org
Management:
    Executive Director: Sandra Robbins
    Managing Director: Marlyn Baum
    Administrator: Elaine Brand
Mission: To serve inner city disadvantaged children with a high quality art-in-education program.
Specialized Field: Musical; Folk; Puppet
Status: Professional; Nonprofit
Paid Staff: 5
Paid Artists: 10
Affiliations: NYC Board of Education Vendor
Organization Type: Performing; Touring; Resident; Educational; Sponsoring

3448 SIGNATURE THEATRE COMPANY

534 W 42nd Street
New York, NY 10036
Phone: 212-967-1913
Fax: 212-967-2957
Web Site: www.signaturetheatre.org

Officers:
  Chairman: Peter Norton
  President: Molly O'Neil Frank
  VP: Christine M Millen
  VP: Marika Blades
Management:
  Founding Artistic Director: James Houghton
  Director Development: Kathryn M Lipuma
  Director Marketing: Rick Berube
  Production Manager: Bill Kneissl
  General Manager: Karalee Dawn
Founded: 1991
Specialized Field: Theatre
Paid Staff: 13
Volunteer Staff: 1
Paid Artists: 150
Affiliations: Alliance of Resident Theatres, NY; Theatre Communications Group
Type of Stage: Proscenium
Seating Capacity: 160

3449 SOHO REPERTORY THEATRE

86 Franklin Street
5th Floor
New York, NY 10013
Phone: 212-941-8632
Fax: 212-941-7148
Web Site: www.sohorep.org
Management:
  Executive Director: Alexandra Conley
  Artistic Director: Daniel Aukin
  Associate Director: Linsay Firman
  Administrative Manager: Young Jean Lee
  Facility Manager: Noah Hall
Founded: 1975
Specialized Field: Theater
Seating Capacity: 70

3450 SOUPSTONE PROJECT

309 E 5th Street
Suite 19
New York, NY 10003
Phone: 212-473-7584
Management:
  Director/Literary Manager: Neile Weissman
Mission: To expand the theatergoing audience through free, trilingually-accessible presentations of new American plays.
Founded: 1985
Specialized Field: Theatrical Group
Status: Professional
Performs At: Henry Street Settlement; Louis Abrons Art Center
Organization Type: Performing

3451 SPANISH THEATRE REPERTORY COMPANY

138 E 27th Street
New York, NY 10016
Phone: 212-889-2850
Fax: 212-686-3732
Management:
  Producer: Gilbert Zaldivar
  Associate Producer: Robert Federico

Press Agent: Ellen Jacobs
Mission: To offer Spanish-language professional theatre; to promote Hispanic culture.
Founded: 1969
Specialized Field: Musical; Community; Theatrical Group
Status: Professional
Income Sources: Theatre Communications Group; American Arts Alliance; Alliance of Resident Theatres/New York
Performs At: Gramercy Arts Theatre; Equitable Tower Auditorium
Organization Type: Performing

3452 STAGEWRIGHTS

PO Box 4745
Rockefeller Center Station
New York, NY 10185
Phone: 212-768-8964
Mission: To develop scripts.
Founded: 1983
Specialized Field: Theatrical Group
Status: Semi-Professional; Nonprofit
Paid Staff: 100
Organization Type: Writer's Theatre

3453 TADA!

120 W 28th Street
2nd Floor
New York, NY 10001
Phone: 212-627-1732
Fax: 212-243-6736
e-mail: tada@tadatheater.com
Web Site: www.tadatheater.com
Management:
  Artistic Director: Janine Nina Trevens
Founded: 1984

3454 TAIPEI THEATER OF CHINESE INFORMATION & CULTURE

1230 Avenue of the Americas
New York, NY 10020
Phone: 212-373-1852
Fax: 212-373-1878
e-mail: utheatre@tpts8.seednet.net
Web Site: www.taipei.org

3455 TALKING BAND

PO Box 293
Prince Street Station
New York, NY 10012
Phone: 212-295-0371
Management:
  Artistic Director: Paul Zinet
Mission: The creation and performance of new theatre works.
Specialized Field: Theatrical Group
Status: Professional; Nonprofit
Organization Type: Performing; Touring

3456 TARGET MARGIN THEATER

1879 Murray Hill Station
New York, NY 10156

Phone: 212-725-4617
Fax: 212-725-4627
Management:
   Artistic Director: David Herskovits
   Managing Director: Meredith Palin
   Development Director: Tonya Canada

3457 THEATER BY THE BLIND

306 W 18th Street
New York, NY 10011
Phone: 212-243-4337
Fax: 212-243-4337
e-mail: ashiotis@panix.com
Web Site: www.tbtb.org
Management:
   Artistic Director: Ike Schambelan
Mission: To change the image of the blind from one of dependence to independence.
Founded: 1979
Paid Staff: 4
Paid Artists: 70

3458 THEATER FOR THE NEW CITY

155 1st Avenue
Between 9th & 10th
New York, NY 10003
Phone: 212-245-1109
Fax: 212-979-6570
e-mail: info@theaterforthenewcity.org
Web Site: www.theaterforthenewcity.org
Management:
   Executive Director: Crystal Field
   Production Manager: Mark Marcante
   Administrator: Jerry Jaffe
   Development Director: Victoria Linchon
Mission: To embody the vision of a center for new and innovative theater arts that would be truly accessible to the community and its experimental theater artists; to discover relevant new writing and to nurture new playwrights; to be a bridge between playwright, experimental theater artist, and the ever growing audiences in the community; to create spaces where a new vision can breathe and be nourished by a working process.
Founded: 1970
Specialized Field: Theatrical Group
Status: Professional; Nonprofit
Paid Staff: 5
Volunteer Staff: 20
Performs At: Four Theatre Complex
Affiliations: Alliance of Resident Theatres/New York; Theatre Communications Group; American Arts Alliance
Annual Attendance: 30,000
Facility Category: Multi-theater complex
Type of Stage: Black Box; Cabaret; Flexible Stage
Seating Capacity: 270; 99; 74; 104
Organization Type: Performing; Touring

3459 THEATERMANIA.COM

1501 Broadway
Suite 1510
New York, NY 10036

Phone: 212-398-8625
Fax: 212-398-8622
e-mail: interactiveartists@worldnet.att.net
Web Site: www.theatermania.com

3460 THEATRE DU GRAND-GUIGNOL DE PARIS

310 E 70th Street
New York, NY 10021
Phone: 212-861-1813
Fax: 212-861-1813
Management:
   Embassy of Montmartre: Barry Alan Richmond
Mission: Specializing in grotesquerie, shock, terror, the macabre and earthy laughter.
Founded: 1896
Specialized Field: Worlds largest repertoire in one of the world's oldest theatres.
Status: Professional; National Theatre of Montmartre
Income Sources: State Theatre of the Republic of Montmartre
Organization Type: Performing; Touring; Resident

3461 THEATRE FANTASTIQUE

Arthur Shafman
163 Amsterdam Avenue #121
New York, NY 10023-5001
Phone: 212-799-4814
Fax: 212-874-3613
e-mail: ashafman@aol.com
Web Site: www.arthurshafman.com
Officers:
   President: Arthur Shafman
Management:
   Director: Richard Zachary
Founded: 1984
Specialized Field: Mime
Status: Professional; Commercial
Organization Type: Performing; Touring; Resident; Educational; Sponsoring

3462 THEATRE FOR A NEW AUDIENCE

154 Christopher Street
Suite 3D
New York, NY 10014
Phone: 212-229-2819
Fax: 212-229-2911
e-mail: info@tfana.org
Web Site: www.tfana.org
Management:
   Artistic/Production Director: Jeffrey Horowitz
   General Manager: Erika Feldman
   Education Director: Joseph Giardina
   Development Director: Louisa Benton
   Executive Director: M Edgar Rosenblum
Mission: Producing works of poetic imagination; building a diverse audience.
Founded: 1979
Specialized Field: Theatrical Group
Status: Professional; Nonprofit
Income Sources: Theatre Communications Group
Performs At: Lucille Lortel Theatre
Organization Type: Performing; Educational

3463 **THEATRE OFF PARK**
224 Waverly Place
New York, NY 10014
Phone: 212-627-2556
Management:
Artistic Director: Albert Harris
Mission: The production of new works; the presentation of neglected works by established writers.
Founded: 1975
Specialized Field: Musical; Theatrical Group
Status: Professional; Nonprofit
Income Sources: Actors' Equity Association; Alliance of Resident Theatres/New York
Performs At: Theatre Off Park
Organization Type: Educational

3464 **RAJECKAS AND INTRAUB - MOVEMENT THEATRE**
PO Box 1333
New York, NY 10009
Phone: 212-529-8068
Fax: 212-529-8068
e-mail: nintraub@aol.com
Management:
Co-Artistic Director: Neil Intraub
Co-Artistic Director: Paul Rajeckas
Mission: Increasing public exposure to the art form of movement theatre.
Specialized Field: Community; Theatrical Group; Movement Theatre
Status: Professional; Nonprofit
Organization Type: Performing; Touring; Educational

3465 **THEATREWORKS USA**
151 W 26th Street
New York, NY 10001
Phone: 212-647-1100
Fax: 212-924-5377
e-mail: info@theatreworksusa.org
Web Site: www.theatreworksusa.org
Officers:
Chairman: Ellen Weiss
President: Ken Arthur
VP: Barbara Pasternack
Secretary: Richard Darmise
Treasurer: Charles Hull
Management:
Managing Director: Ken Arthur
Marketing Director: Barbara Sandek
Mission: Theatreworks/USA, a nonprofit organization and America's largest theatre creating, producing, and touring plays for young audiences, has presented more than 27,000 performances to well over 22 million young people in schools, art centers, museums and theatres, in 49 states.
Founded: 1961
Specialized Field: Musical; Folk; Theatrical Group; Puppet
Status: Professional; Nonprofit
Paid Staff: 21
Paid Artists: 211
Budget: $10 million
Performs At: Town Hall; Promenade Theatre; Variety Arts Theatre

Affiliations: AEA, SSDC, USA, AGG, IAPAYP, APAP
Annual Attendance: 4.6 million
Organization Type: Performing; Touring; Resident; Educational; Sponsoring

3466 **THERESA LANG THEATRE**
Marymount Manhattan College
221 E 71 Street
New York, NY 10021
Phone: 212-774-0760
Fax: 212-774-0770
Management:
Managing Director: Mary Fleischer
Operations Coordinator: Ross Chappell

3467 **THUNDER BAY ENSEMBLE**
350 Central Park W
Apartment 14H
New York, NY 10025
Phone: 413-269-4201

3468 **TURNIP THEATRE COMPANY**
145 W 46th Street
New York, NY 10036
Phone: 212-768-4016
Founded: 1991

3469 **UNION SQUARE THEATRE**
100 E 17th Street
New York, NY 10003
Phone: 212-505-0700
Fax: 212-505-0709
Type of Stage: Proscenium
Seating Capacity: 499
Rental Contact: Margaret Cotter

3470 **UBU REPERTORY THEATER**
95 Wall Street
21st Floor
New York, NY 10005
Phone: 212-509-1455
Fax: 212-509-1635
e-mail: uburep@spacelab.net
Management:
Founder/Artistic Director: Francoise Kourilsky
General Manager: Robin Gilette

3471 **VINEYARD THEATRE**
108 E 15th Street
New York, NY 10003
Phone: 212-353-3366
Fax: 212-353-3803
Web Site: www.vineyardtheatre.org
Management:
Artistic Director: Douglas Aibel
Executive Director: Barbara Zinn Krieger
General Manageror: Jody Schornbrun
Managing Director: Barda Ramirez
Mission: Developing musical theatre and new plays.
Founded: 1981
Specialized Field: Musical; Theatrical Group
Status: Professional; Nonprofit
Budget: 1.2 Million

Income Sources: Theatre Communications Group; Opera America
Season: Late-Fall - Spring
Affiliations: AEA, AFM, SSDC
Type of Stage: Flexible; Thrust
Seating Capacity: 129; 71
Organization Type: Performing

3472 VIVIAN BEAUMONT THEATER

150 W 65th Street
New York, NY 10023
Phone: 212-362-7600
Fax: 212-873-0761
Web Site: www.lct.org
Officers:
  Assistant Treasurer: Robert A Belkin
  Box Office Treasurer: Fred Bonis
Management:
  Director Development: Hattie K Jutagir
  Associate Director Development: Rachel Norton
  Production Manager: Jeff Hamlin
  Assistant Production Manager: Paul Smithyman
  Associate General Manager: Mala Yee Mosher
  Management Assistant: Melanie Weiner
  Company Manager: Adam Siegal
  Assistant Company Manager: Anthony LaTorella
Founded: 1985
Specialized Field: Theatrical Group
Status: Professional; Nonprofit
Performs At: Vivian Beaumont Theater; Mitzi E Newhouse Theater
Facility Category: Theater
Organization Type: Performing

3473 WEISSBERGER THEATER GROUP

909 3rd Avenue
27th Floor
New York, NY 10022-9998
Phone: 212-339-5529
Fax: 212-486-8996
Management:
  Producer: Jay Harris
Founded: 1992

3474 WINGS THEATRE COMPANY

154 Christopher Street
New York, NY 10014
Phone: 212-617-2960
Fax: 212-462-0024
e-mail: jcorrick@wingstheatre.com
Web Site: www.wingstheatre.com
Management:
  Literary Manager: Tricia Gilbert
  Artistic Director: Jeffery Corrick
  Managing Director: Robert Mooney
Founded: 1986
Specialized Field: Theatre
Paid Staff: 3
Volunteer Staff: 3
Paid Artists: 0
Non-paid Artists: 20
Type of Stage: Proscenium
Stage Dimensions: 20 x 20
Seating Capacity: 74

Year Built: 1990

3475 WOMEN'S INTERART CENTER

549 W 52nd Street
New York, NY 10019
Phone: 212-246-1050
Management:
  Artistic Director: Margot Lewitin
  Dramaturge: Jean Rowan
  Development Director: Susan Waring Morris
Mission: To explore all avenues of theatrical expression; to emphasize the work of new playwrights.
Founded: 1971
Specialized Field: Theatrical Group
Status: Professional; Nonprofit
Income Sources: Actors' Equity Association
Performs At: Interart Theater
Organization Type: Performing

3476 WOMEN'S PROJECT & PRODUCTIONS

55 W End Avenue
New York, NY 10023
Phone: 212-765-1706
Fax: 212-765-2024
e-mail: info@womensproject.org
Management:
  Artistic Director: Julia Miles
  Artistic Associate: Suzanne Bennett
  Managing Director: Patricia Taylor
  Literary Manager: Karen Keagle
Mission: Promoting and developing women directors and playwrights in the theatre.
Founded: 1978
Specialized Field: Theatrical Group
Status: Professional; Nonprofit
Income Sources: Theatre Communications Group; Alliance of Resident Theatres/New York
Organization Type: Performing; Resident; Educational; Sponsoring

3477 WOOSTER GROUP

PO Box 654
Canal Street Station
New York, NY 10013
Phone: 212-966-9796
Fax: 212-226-6576
e-mail: mail@thewoostergroup.org
Web Site: www.thewoostergroup.org
Officers:
  President: Kate Valk
Management:
  Artistic Director: Elizabeth LeCompte
  Managing Director: Joel Bassin
Mission: An artists collective working together on live performances.
Founded: 1967
Specialized Field: Theatrical Group
Status: Nonprofit
Paid Staff: 17
Budget: $1 Million
Income Sources: Ticket Sales; Touring; Grants & Contributions
Performs At: The Performing Garage
Annual Attendance: 15,000

Facility Category: Flexible black box
Type of Stage: Flexible floor
Seating Capacity: 100
Year Built: 1950
Organization Type: Performing; Touring; Resident; Sponsoring

3478 WORKING THEATRE COMPANY

400 W 40th Street
New York, NY 10018
Phone: 212-967-5464
Officers:
  Chairman: Larry Beers
Management:
  Artistic Director: Bill Mitchelson
  Development Director: Honour Molloy
Mission: America's only professional theatre company dedicated to producing new plays of cultural diversities that reflect the issues and concerns that working people face in the modern world.
Status: Professional; Nonprofit
Organization Type: Performing; Educational

3479 WPA THEATRE

159 W 23rd Street
Suite 301
New York, NY 10001
Phone: 212-206-0523
Fax: 212-637-7154
Management:
  Artistic Director: Kyle Renick
  Managing Director: Donna Lieberman
Mission: Committed to fostering realistic writing, acting and design in American repertory.
Founded: 1977
Status: Professional; Nonprofit
Income Sources: Alliance of Resident Theatres/New York; Theatre Communications Group
Season: September - June
Performs At: Chelsea Playhouse
Type of Stage: Proscenium
Seating Capacity: 160
Organization Type: Performing

3480 YORK THEATRE COMPANY

619 Lexington Avenue @ 54th Street
New York, NY 10022-4610
Phone: 212-935-5820
Fax: 212-832-0037
Web Site: www.yorktheatre.org
Management:
  Artistic Director: Jim Morgan
  Consulting Managing Director: Louis Chiodo
Mission: A professional equity off-Broadway company dedicated to presenting great classical works as well as revivals and/or premieres of unusual, avant-garde musicals.
Founded: 1969
Specialized Field: Musical; Theatrical Group
Status: Professional; Nonprofit
Affiliations: Actors' Equity Association
Organization Type: Performing

3481 YOUNG PLAYWRIGHTS

321 W 44th Street
Suite 906
New York, NY 10036
Phone: 212-307-1140
Fax: 212-307-1454
Management:
  Artistic Director: Sheri Goldhirsch
  Managing Director: Brett Reynolds
  Project Administrator: Rebecca Sheir
  Literary Associate: Ruth McKee

3482 PUPPET THEATRE: DANCE AND MUSIC FROM INDONESIA

1 Sir Kenneth Court
Northport, NY 11768
Phone: 631-754-5035
Fax: 631-754-2341
e-mail: javapuppets@aol.com
Web Site: www.indonesianshadowplay.com
Management:
  Artistic Director: Tamara Fielding
Founded: 1975
Specialized Field: Indonesian Traditional Arts

3483 TAMARA AND THE SHADOW THEATRE OF JAVA

1 Sir Kenneth Court
Northport, NY 11768
Phone: 631-754-5035
Fax: 631-754-2341
e-mail: javapuppets@aol.com
Web Site: www.indonesianshadowplay.com
Management:
  Artistic Director: Tamara Fielding
Founded: 1975
Specialized Field: Indonesian Puppet theatre
Paid Staff: 2
Volunteer Staff: 1

3484 ELMWOOD PLAYHOUSE

16 Park Street
Nyack, NY 10960
Phone: 845-353-1313
Founded: 1946
Specialized Field: Community
Status: Non-Professional; Nonprofit
Income Sources: Art Council of Rockland County
Performs At: Elmwood Playhouse
Organization Type: Performing; Educational

3485 MAIN STREET ARTS

94 Main Street
Nyack, NY 10960
Phone: 914-358-7701
Fax: 914-358-7701
e-mail: msapaul@cs.com
Founded: 1993

All listings are in alphabetical order by state, then city, then organization within the city.

3486 OGDENSBURG COMMAND PERFORMANCES
1100 State Street
Ogdensburg, NY 13669
Phone: 315-393-2625
Fax: 315-393-2625
e-mail: mcpalao@internetusa.net
Mission: To offer theatrical productions, drama and music for the enjoyment and inspiration of the residents of Ogdensburg and the North Country.
Founded: 1963
Specialized Field: Theater
Status: Professional; Nonprofit
Paid Staff: 2
Performs At: George Hall Auditorium; Ogdensburg Free Academy
Organization Type: Sponsoring

3487 ORPHEUS THEATRE
31 Maple Street
PO Box 1014
Oneonta, NY 13820
Phone: 607-432-1800
Fax: 607-436-9682
e-mail: orpheus@stny.rr.com
Web Site: www.orpheustheatre.org
Officers:
President: Carolyn Anderson
1st VP: Arnold Drogen
2nd VP: Duncan Smith
Secretary: Carol Detweiler
Treasurer: Rosalie Benson
CEO: Sammy Dallas Bayes
Management:
Co-Producers: Peter Macris
Founded: 1983
Status: Nonprofit; Non-Equity
Season: September - August
Type of Stage: Proscenium
Stage Dimensions: 49' x 35'
Seating Capacity: 497

3488 IMAGO, THE THEATRE MASK ENSEMBLE
163 Amsterdam Avenue #121
Pawling, NY 10023
Phone: 212-799-4814
Fax: 212-874-3613
Management:
Artistic Director: Carol Trifle
Artistic Director: Jerry Mouwad
Mission: To present our unique art form.
Founded: 1981
Specialized Field: Summer Stock; Community; Theatrical Group
Status: Professional
Income Sources: Westaff Touring Program; North Carolina Touring Program; Arts Midwest; Performing Arts Touring Program of Oregon
Organization Type: Performing; Touring; Resident; Educational

3489 THEATRE THREE PRODUCTIONS
412 Main Street
PO Box 512
Port Jefferson, NY 11777
Phone: 631-928-9202
Fax: 631-928-9120
e-mail: md@theatrethree.org
Web Site: www.theatrethree.org
Management:
Associate Artistic Director: Clayton Phyllips
Managing Director: Ronald Peierls
Mission: To offer Central Long Island the highest quality professional theatre.
Founded: 1969
Specialized Field: Musical; Theatrical Group
Status: Professional; Nonprofit
Paid Staff: 10
Volunteer Staff: 5
Paid Artists: 7
Non-paid Artists: 25
Income Sources: Port Jefferson Arts Council
Season: July - June
Type of Stage: Thrust
Seating Capacity: 247
Organization Type: Performing; Touring; Resident; Educational

3490 NEW DAY REPERTORY COMPANY
29 N Hamilton Street
PO Box 269
Poughkeepsie, NY 12602
Phone: 845-485-7399
Fax: 845-485-6544
e-mail: newdayrep@netzero.com
Officers:
Chairman: Al Coley
Treasurer: Dr. Tansukh Dorawala
Secretary: Dorothy Paulin
Management:
Producer/Artistic Director: Rodney K Douglas
Mission: Make quality life theatre accessible to culturally/socially diverse, economically disadvantaged, and underserved audiences of all ages
Founded: 1963
Specialized Field: Community
Status: Professional; Nonprofit
Paid Staff: 2
Budget: $160,000
Performs At: Vassar Institute Theatre
Facility Category: Schools; Colleges; Community Centers; Churches
Type of Stage: Proscenium
Seating Capacity: 1,100
Year Remodeled: 1997
Organization Type: Performing; Touring; Resident; Educational

3491 POWERHOUSE THEATER AT VASSAR
Vassar College
124 Raymond Avenue
Poughkeepsie, NY 12604
Phone: 845-437-5902
e-mail: powerhouse@vassar.edu
Web Site: www.vassar.edu/powerhouse

All listings are in alphabetical order by state, then city, then organization within the city.

Mission: Since its founding in 1985, the Powerhouse summer theater program at Vassar has fostered emerging artists, produced new works by some of the nation's most innovative young playwrights, and trained aspiring actors, directors, and designers for theater careers.
Founded: 1985
Status: Nonprofit
Season: June - August
Type of Stage: Black Box
Seating Capacity: 130

3492 BLACKFRIARS THEATRE

248 E Avenue
Rochester, NY 14604
Phone: 585-454-1260
e-mail: mail@blackfriars.org
Web Site: www.blackfriars.org
Management:
 Artistic Director: John Halboupis
Mission: A professional oriented community theater.
Founded: 1950
Facility Category: Theatre
Type of Stage: Thrust Stage; Flexible
Stage Dimensions: 20'x40'
Seating Capacity: 99-165
Year Remodeled: 1997

3493 GEVA THEATRE

75 Woodbury Boulevard
Rochester, NY 14607-1717
Phone: 716-232-1366
Fax: 716-232-4031
e-mail: gevatalk@gevatheatre.org
Web Site: www.gevatheatre.org
Officers:
 Chairman: John F Kraushaar
 Vice Chairman at Large: Susan Mascette Brandt
 Secretary: James C Moore
 Treasurer: Nannette Nocon
Management:
 Artistic Director: Mark Cuddy
 Managing Director: John Quinlivan
 Literary Manager: Marge Betley
 Director Marketing: Bob Russell
Mission: To produce work that celebrates the human spirit.
Founded: 1972
Specialized Field: Regional Theatre
Status: Professional; Nonprofit
Paid Staff: 85
Volunteer Staff: 120
Paid Artists: 125
Income Sources: Theatre Communications Group; American Arts Alliance; League of Resident Theatres
Season: September - June
Performs At: Elaine Wilson Theatre, Ronald and Donna Fielding Nextstage
Annual Attendance: 15,000
Type of Stage: Thrust, Proscenium
Stage Dimensions: 50' x 40'
Seating Capacity: 552, 180
Organization Type: Performing; Resident; Educational

3494 ROCHESTER BROADWAY THEATRE LEAGUE

100 E Avenue
Rochester, NY 14604
Phone: 716-325-7760
e-mail: info@rbtl.org
Web Site: www.rbtl.org
Officers:
 Chief Administrative Officer: Nancy B Calocerinos
 COO: John C Parkhurst
 Director of Outreach/Commun.: Debra Jansen
Mission: The Rochester Broadway Theatre League was founded in 1957 by a small group of volunteers to stimulate, promote and develop interest in the dramatic and musical arts for the cultural benefit of the community.
Founded: 1957

3495 THEATRE ON THE RIDGE

200 Ridge Road W
Building 28
Rochester, NY 14652
Phone: 716-722-9449
Fax: 716-477-8041
Management:
 Manager: David R Dunn
Mission: To provide entertainment for Eastman Kodak Company as well as the local community.
Specialized Field: Musical; Dinner; Community
Status: Professional; Commercial
Organization Type: Performing; Resident; Sponsoring

3496 UNIVERSITY OF ROCHESTER THEATRE PROGRAM

107 Todd Union
Rochester, NY 14627
Phone: 716-275-4088
Fax: 716-461-4547
Management:
 Artistic Director: Mervyn Willis
 Administrator: Katherine Mcgill
 Associate Director: Nigel Maister
 Technical Director: John Gilfus
Mission: To offer modern, contemporary and classical plays; to provide professional training.
Founded: 1968
Specialized Field: Theater
Status: Semi-Professional; Nonprofit
Paid Staff: 4
Paid Artists: 10
Performs At: Black Box Theatre
Organization Type: Performing; Resident; Educational

3497 CAPITOL THEATRE SUMMERSTAGE

220 W Dominick Street
Rome, NY 13440
Phone: 315-337-6277
Officers:
 President: Peter Ehrnstrum
Management:
 Executive Director: Meg McNeeley
Mission: Offering the community an opportuniity for participation in quality music performances.
Founded: 1990

Status: Non-Equity; Nonprofit
Season: July - August
Type of Stage: Proscenium
Stage Dimensions: 40' x 25'
Seating Capacity: 1700

3498 BROADHOLLOW PLAYERS LIMITED
80 13th Avenue
Building 5, Unit 6
Ronkonkoma, NY 11779
Phone: 631-471-0064
Fax: 631-471-8276
Web Site: www.broadhollow.org
Management:
   Executive Producer: Jerry Zaback
Founded: 1973
Status: Nonprofit
Season: Year-Round
Seating Capacity: 175; 288; 250;

3499 BAY STREET THEATRE
PO Box 810
Sag Harbor, NY 11963
Phone: 631-725-0818
Fax: 631-725-0906
Web Site: www.baystreet.org
Management:
   Literary Manager: Mia Emlen Grosjean
   Artistic Director: Sybil Christopher
   Artistic Director: Emma Walton
   Executive Director: Stephen Hamilton
   General Manager: Norman Kline
Founded: 1991
Facility Category: Theater
Type of Stage: Thrust Stage
Seating Capacity: 299

3500 FORT SALEM THEATRE
Box 10
Salem, NY 12865
Phone: 518-854-9200
Fax: 518-854-9200
Management:
   Producer: Kathy Beaver
Mission: Bring professional theatre to the Washington county and Saratoga springs area.
Founded: 1972
Status: Non-Equity; Nonprofit Professional
Paid Staff: 10
Volunteer Staff: 10
Paid Artists: 35
Non-paid Artists: 10
Season: June - September
Type of Stage: Proscenium
Stage Dimensions: 41' x 25'
Seating Capacity: 200

3501 METTAWEE THEATRE COMPANY
209 Dunnigan Road
Salem, NY 12865
Phone: 518-854-9357
Fax: 518-854-9321
Web Site: www.mettawee.org
Officers:

President: Stephanie Gallas
Management:
   Artistic Director: Ralph Lee
   Managing Director: Casey Compton
Mission: To offer original theatre works incorporating masks, live music and figures that are larger than life to illustrate the myths and legends of different cultures.
Founded: 1975
Status: Professional; Nonprofit
Organization Type: Performing; Touring

3502 PENDRAGON THEATRE
148 River Street
Saranac Lake, NY 12983
Phone: 518-891-1854
Fax: 518-891-7012
e-mail: pdragon@northnet.org
Web Site: www.pendragontheatre.com
Management:
   Artistic Director: Susan Neal
   Managing Director: Bob Pettee
Mission: To produce a full range of theatrical material and educational services and presentations like festival of the lakes
Founded: 1980
Specialized Field: Theatre
Status: Non-Equity; Nonprofit
Paid Staff: 5
Volunteer Staff: 15
Paid Artists: 30
Season: June - September
Type of Stage: Proscenium
Stage Dimensions: 30' x 24'
Seating Capacity: 132

3503 SARATOGA PERFORMING ARTS CENTER
Saratoga Spa State Park
Saratoga Springs, NY 12866
Phone: 518-587-9330
Fax: 518-587-3330
e-mail: info@spar.org
Web Site: www.spac.org
Officers:
   Honorary Chairman: Cornelius Whitney
   Chairman: Charles V Wait
   President: Herbert A Chesbrough
   Secretary: Walter M. Jeffords, Jr
   Treasurer: Harold N. Langlitz
Mission: To host performing arts events.
Founded: 1966
Specialized Field: Dance; Vocal Music; Instrumental Music; Theater; Grand Opera
Status: Professional; Nonprofit
Budget: $11 Million
Income Sources: International Association of Auditorium Managers; New York Performing Arts Association; membership ticket sales
Affiliations: Summer home of New York City Ballet, Philadelphia Orchestra and Saratoga Chamber Music Festival
Annual Attendance: 350,000
Facility Category: Ampitheatre
Type of Stage: Proscenium

Stage Dimensions: 80 W x 60 D
Seating Capacity: 5100
Year Built: 1966
Organization Type: Performing; Educational;
Sponsoring

3504 PROCTOR'S THEATRE

432 State Street
Schenectady, NY 12305
Phone: 518-382-3884
Fax: 518-346-2468
e-mail: boxoffice@proctors.org
Web Site: www.proctors.org
Management:
 General Manager: Fred Daniels
 Executive Director: Gloria Lamere
Mission: Presenting Broadway, opera, popular music,
dance and classical
Founded: 1926
Specialized Field: Performance, Live
Paid Staff: 30
Volunteer Staff: 900
Paid Artists: 35

3505 SCHENECTADY CIVIC PLAYERS

12 S Church Street
Schenectady, NY 12305
Phone: 518-382-2081
e-mail: postmaster@civicplayers.org
Web Site: www.civicplayers.org
Officers:
 President: Charles Hepburn
 VP: Laura Houlihan
 Secretary: Gail Kitchen
 Treasurer: Melissa Brown
Management:
 Business Manager: Robin Hackett
Mission: Continuation of long tradition of providing
non-profit community theatre.
Founded: 1928
Specialized Field: Community
Status: Non-Professional; Nonprofit
Income Sources: New York State Community Theatre
Association; New York State Theater Festival Association
Organization Type: Performing; Resident

3506 STERLING RENAISSANCE FESTIVAL

15385 Farden Road
Sterling, NY 13156
Phone: 315-947-5783
Fax: 315-947-6905
Toll-free: 800-879-4446
e-mail: office@sterlingfestival.com
Web Site: www.sterlingfestival.com
Officers:
 President: Alisa Cook
 VP: John Kissler
 Secretary: Phil Holding
 Treasurer: Marylee Pangman
Management:
 Office Manager/Sales Director: Kelli Raymond
Mission: To present interactive and staged performances.
Paid Staff: 10
Paid Artists: 80

Season: June - August
Annual Attendance: 100,000
Facility Category: Outdoor
Type of Stage: 8 Stages
Year Built: 1977

3507 PENGUIN REPERTORY COMPANY

Crickettown Road
Box 91
Stony Point, NY 10980
Phone: 845-786-2873
Fax: 914-786-3638
Officers:
 President: Glen Kerslake
 VP: Bob Patrick
 Treasurer: Lorette Peto
 Secretary: Thomas Wilson
Management:
 Artistic Director: Joe Brancato
 Executive Director: Andrew Horn
Mission: To give new playwrights opportunities through
mounting new plays; to stage works that are tried and
true.
Founded: 1977
Status: Professional; Nonprofit
Paid Staff: 25
Paid Artists: 20
Income Sources: Actors' Equity Association; Society for
Stage Directors and Choreographers
Season: May - October
Annual Attendance: 7,000-10,000
Type of Stage: Proscenium
Stage Dimensions: 23'x 25'
Seating Capacity: 108
Year Built: 1830
Year Remodeled: 1986
Organization Type: Performing

3508 THALIA SPANISH THEATRE

41-17 Greenpoint Avenue
PO Box 4368
Sunnyside, NY 11104
Phone: 718-729-3880
Fax: 718-729-3388
e-mail: info@thaliatheatre.org
Web Site: www.thaliatheatre.org
Officers:
 Chairperson/Treasurer: Soledad Lopez
 President: Angel Gil Orrios
 VP: Odon Betanzos
 Secretary: Jose Vazquez
Management:
 Artistic/Executive Director: Angel Gil Orrios
 Administrative Director: Kathryn A Giaimo
 Managing Director: Soledad Lopez
 Technical Director: Hector Palacios
Mission: To offer New York City's Hispanic communities
the highest quality productions.
Founded: 1969
Specialized Field: Musical; Community; Theatrical
Group
Status: Professional; Nonprofit
Paid Staff: 4
Volunteer Staff: 6
Paid Artists: 90

Budget: $561,000
Income Sources: National Endowment for the Arts; New York State Coucil on Arts; New York City - Department of Cultural Affairs; NY Community Trust; JP Morgan; Chase Manhattan
Annual Attendance: 10,000
Facility Category: Theatre
Type of Stage: Proscenium
Seating Capacity: 75
Year Remodeled: 1992
Organization Type: Performing; Touring; Resident

3509 OPEN HAND THEATER

518 Prospect Avenue
Syracuse, NY 13208
Phone: 315-476-0466
Fax: 315-472-2578
e-mail: openhandtheater@aol.com
Web Site: www.openhandtheater.org
Officers:
    President: Susan Wadley
Management:
    Artistic Director: Geoffrey Navias
    Producer: Leslie Archer
    Administrativ Assistant: Kathy Ferro
    Development Director: Ellen Schwartz
Founded: 1980
Paid Staff: 2
Volunteer Staff: 85
Paid Artists: 4
Non-paid Artists: 4

3510 SYRACUSE STAGE

820 E Genesee Street
Syracuse, NY 13210-1508
Phone: 315-443-4008
Fax: 315-443-9846
e-mail: syrstage@syr.edu
Web Site: www.syracusestage.org
Officers:
    President: Mark Russell
Management:
    Producing Director: James A Clark
    Assistant Production Manager: Dianna Angell
    Director Marketing/Development: Barbara Beckos
    Technical Director: Randy Steffen
    Artistic Director: Robert Moss
    Dir Communications/Special Event: Heidi Holtz
Mission: To enrich, empower and entertain our community through the creation of professional theatre and to be an essential element in affecting the lives of thoughts in our community.ceptions of the world.
Founded: 1974
Specialized Field: Theatrical Group
Status: Professional; Nonprofit
Budget: $3.3 million
Income Sources: Theatre Communications Group; League of Resident Theatres; Actors' Equity Association
Season: September - May
Performs At: The John D Archbold Theatre
Annual Attendance: 90,000
Type of Stage: Proscenium
Seating Capacity: 499
Organization Type: Performing; Touring; Educational

3511 NEW YORK STATE THEATRE INSTITUTE

37 1st Street
Troy, NY 12180
Phone: 518-274-3200
Fax: 518-274-3815
e-mail: nysti@capital.net
Web Site: www.nysti.org
Officers:
    Chairman: David Morris
Management:
    Producing Artistic Director: Patricia D Benedette Snyder
Mission: To provide production of a high quality professional theatre; extensive arts in education programs; new play development; international cultural exchange.
Founded: 1976
Specialized Field: Family Theatre
Status: Professional
Paid Staff: 33
Volunteer Staff: 250
Annual Attendance: 50,000
Facility Category: Theatre
Type of Stage: Proscenium
Stage Dimensions: 48'x30'
Seating Capacity: 850

3512 NEW YORK RENAISSANCE FAIRE

600 Route 17A
Tuxedo, NY 10987
Phone: 845-351-5171
Fax: 845-351-5646
Web Site: www.renfair.com
Management:
    General Manager/Entertainment Dir: David Casey
    Crafts Director/Merchandise: Bob Corsette
    Asst. Entertainment Director/PR: Kevin Dunn
    Finance Manager: Douglas DeTroy
    Art Director/Web Mistress: Joni Massengale
    Office Manager: Melissa McKeever
Specialized Field: Renaissance theater
Season: July - September

3513 BROADWAY THEATRE LEAGUE OF UTICA

259 Genesee Street
Utica, NY 13501-3402
Phone: 315-724-7196
Fax: 315-724-1227
e-mail: btlutica@dreamscape.com
Management:
    Executive Director: Robert A Lewis

3514 WATERTOWN LYRIC THEATER PRODUCTIONS

1333 Holcomb Street
Watertown, NY 13601
Phone: 315-788-6492
Fax: 315-779-8002
e-mail: lyric_theatre@yahoo.com
Officers:
    President: James S Williams Jr
    Treasurer: Steve Hunt

Management:
Artistic Director: Barry Pratt
Business Manager: Joan Jones
Mission: To offer the community live theatre employing local talent; to provide young people with training in musical theatre.
Founded: 1959
Specialized Field: Musical; Community; Theatrical Group
Status: Non-Professional; Nonprofit
Volunteer Staff: 360
Non-paid Artists: 150
Performs At: State Office Building Auditorium
Organization Type: Performing; Educational

3515 DAS PUPPENSPIEL PUPPET THEATER
1 1/2 E Main Street
Westfield, NY 14787
Phone: 716-326-2611
Fax: 716-326-6625
Toll-free: 877-326-2611
e-mail: sadpupp@puppets.org
Management:
Managing Director: Kevin Kuhlman
Founded: 1974
Specialized Field: Theatrical Group; Puppet
Status: Professional; Nonprofit
Paid Staff: 1
Income Sources: United International Marionette Association; Puppeteers of America; Children's Theatre Association of America
Organization Type: Performing; Touring; Educational

3516 STREET THEATER
228 Fisher Avenue
White Plains, NY 10606
Phone: 914-761-3307
Fax: 914-422-2340
e-mail: thestreettheater@aollll.com
Management:
Artistic Director: Gray Smith
Mission: Committed to educational programs. Mission: to insure success in school for disadvantaged students through early literacy programs. Program components: weekly performance-based instruction by professional actors, teacher training, curriculum materials, parent participation, professional touring company.
Founded: 1970
Specialized Field: Theatrical Group
Status: Professional; Semi-Professional; Nonprofit
Income Sources: Actors' Equity Association
Organization Type: Performing; Touring; Educational

3517 COMMON STAGE THEATRE COMPANY
PO Box 1028
Woodstock, NY 12498
Phone: 845-679-9256
Mission: Developing and producing plays by women.
Founded: 1989
Specialized Field: Theatrical Group; Women Playwrights Only
Status: Semi-Professional; Nonprofit
Paid Staff: 10

3518 BLACK SWAN THEATER
166 W Haywood #1
Asheville, NC 28801
Phone: 828-254-6057
Fax: 828-251-6603
e-mail: swantheatre@aol.com
Management:
Director: David B Hopes
Mission: To produce original contemporary scripts and reinterpret the classics.
Founded: 1988
Specialized Field: Theatrical Group
Status: Non-Professional; Nonprofit
Paid Staff: 70
Income Sources: University of North Carolina at Asheville Creative Writing Department; Ticket Sales
Organization Type: Performing; Touring; Sponsoring

3519 DIANA WORTHAM THEATRE AT PACK PLACE
2 S Pack Square
Asheville, NC 28801
Phone: 828-257-4544
Fax: 828-251-5652
e-mail: jellis@dwtheatre.com
Web Site: www.main.nc.us/packplace
Management:
Manager: John Ellis
Paid Staff: 3
Volunteer Staff: 30
Budget: $400,000
Annual Attendance: 40,000
Facility Category: Performing Arts Center
Type of Stage: Proscenium
Stage Dimensions: 40x40
Seating Capacity: 500
Year Built: 1992

3520 SMOKY MOUNTAIN REPERTORY THEATRE
26 S Lexington Street
Asheville, NC 28801
Phone: 704-252-9661
Management:
Managing Director: H Byron Ballard
Business Manager: Joe Fioccola
Technical Director: M Michael Hyatt
Youth Director: Vivienne Conjura
Mission: Producing new works and adaptations with particular emphasis on plays of regional significance.
Founded: 1981
Specialized Field: Folk; Theatrical Group
Status: Professional; Semi-Professional; Nonprofit
Paid Staff: 10
Performs At: First Artists Studio Theater
Organization Type: Performing; Touring; Resident; Educational

3521 LEES-MCRAE COLLEGE SUMMER THEATRE

PO Box 128
Banner Elk, NC 28604
Phone: 828-898-5241
Toll-free: 800-280-4562
Web Site:
www.lmc.edu/lmcPerformingArts/LMSTinfo.htm
Mission: LMST is a professional company that shows three musicals each summer.
Season: June - August

3522 BLOWING ROCK STAGE COMPANY

PO Box 2170
Blowing Rock, NC 28605
Phone: 828-295-9168
Fax: 828-295-9104
e-mail: theatre@blowingrock.com
Web Site: www.blowingrockstage.com
Officers:
   President: Connie Baird
   VP: Rebecca Wright
   Treasurer: Jerry Burns
   Secretary: Yvonne Myers
Management:
   Artistic Director: Kenneth Kay
   General Manager: Chip Taylor
Founded: 1986
Specialized Field: Professional Summer Theatre
Status: Nonprofit
Paid Staff: 2
Paid Artists: 20
Season: June - September
Type of Stage: Proscenium
Stage Dimensions: 28'x 36'
Seating Capacity: 240

3523 ARTSCENTER

300-G E Main Street
Carrboro, NC 27510
Phone: 919-929-2787
Fax: 919-969-8574
e-mail: Artscenter@aol.com
Web Site: www.artscenterlive.com
Officers:
   Chairman: Steve Benezra
Management:
   Executive Director: Colin Bissett
   Booking Manager: Bo Osborne
Mission: To inspire a love of the arts through presentation of a broad range of artists and educational programs, and by supporting the development of young artists; to create an environment for exploring and appreciating artistic expression.
Founded: 1973
Specialized Field: Musical; Community; Theatrical Group
Status: Professional; Non-Professional; Nonprofit
Paid Staff: 12
Volunteer Staff: 30
Paid Artists: 250
Income Sources: Grants; Ticket Sales; Class Tuitions; Donars; Foundations
Performs At: Earl Wynn Theatre

Annual Attendance: 83,750
Seating Capacity: 350
Year Built: 1972
Year Remodeled: 1986
Organization Type: Performing; Touting; Resident; Educational; Sponsoring

3524 INSTITUTE OF OUTDOOR DRAMA

CB 3240, 1700 Airport Road
UNC
Chapel Hill, NC 27599-3240
Phone: 919-962-1328
Fax: 919-962-4212
e-mail: outdoor@unc.edu
Web Site: www.unc.edu/depts/outdoor/
Management:
   Director: Scott J Parker
Mission: Sponsors regional auditions for performers and technicians in outdoor dramas; hosts management conference annually; conducts feasibility studies.
Founded: 1963
Specialized Field: Theater; Outdoor
Status: Nonprofit
Paid Staff: 3
Organization Type: Educational; Sponsoring

3525 PLAYMAKERS REPERTORY COMPANY

Center for Dramatic Art UNC Campus
CB #3235
Chapel Hill, NC 27599-3235
Phone: 919-962-1122
Fax: 919-962-4069
e-mail: prcboxoffice@unc.edu
Web Site: www.playmakersrep.org
Management:
   Artistic Director: David Hammond
   Managing Director: Donna Heins
   Production Manager: Jerry Genochio
Mission: To engage our community in an ongoing exploration of and significance of theatre in contemporary life; to investigate the theatrical events and the methods used for its realization in performance.
Founded: 1976
Specialized Field: Theatrical Group
Status: Professional
Paid Staff: 7
Budget: 1.3 million
Income Sources: Private Foundations; Grants; Endowments; Business; Ccorporte Donations; Box Office; Government Grant; Individual Donors
Performs At: Paul Green Theatre
Affiliations: League of Resident Theatres; Actors' Equity Association; Society for Stage Directors and Choreographers
Type of Stage: Thrust
Seating Capacity: 499
Organization Type: Performing; Educational

3526 ACTOR'S THEATRE OF CHARLOTTE

PO Box 12325
Charlotte, NC 28220-2325

All listings are in alphabetical order by state, then city, then organization within the city.

Phone: 704-342-2251
Fax: 704-342-1229
e-mail: actorstheatre@mindspring.com
Web Site: www.actorstheatrecharlotte.org
Management:
　　Executive/Artistic Director: Dan Shoemaker
　　Producing Artistic Director: Chip Decker
Mission: The mission of Actor's Theatre of Charlotte is to produce bold and innovative new works by contemporary playwrights.
Founded: 1989
Specialized Field: Performing - Theatre
Paid Staff: 2
Volunteer Staff: 6
Paid Artists: 37
Budget: $197,000
Type of Stage: Proscenium

3527　CENTRAL PIEDMONT COMMUNITY THEATRE
1201 Elizabeth Avenue
Charlotte, NC 28204
Phone: 704-330-6534
Fax: 704-342-5934
Management:
　　Producer/Director: Tom Vance
　　Director: Tom Hollis
Mission: To offer quality entertainment to the community; to provide training for students aspiring to careers in professional theatre.
Founded: 1974
Specialized Field: Musical; Theatrical Group
Status: Semi-Professional
Paid Staff: 40
Income Sources: North Carolina Theatre Conference; Southeastern Theatre Conference
Performs At: Pease Auditorium
Organization Type: Performing; Educational

3528　CHARLOTTE REPERTORY THEATRE
129 W Trade Street
Suite 401
Charlotte, NC 28202
Phone: 704-333-8587
Fax: 704-333-0224
e-mail: info@charlotterep.org
Web Site: www.charlotterep.org
Officers:
　　President: Mike McGuire
　　Treasurer: Neil Glenn
　　Secretary: Anita Doran
Management:
　　Producer/Managing Director: Matt Olin
　　Founder/Artistic Director: Steve Umberger
　　Literary Manager: Claudia Carter Covington
　　General Manager: Debbie Fitts
Mission: Presenting contemporary plays, developing and presenting new works and reviving modern drama classics.
Founded: 1976
Specialized Field: Theatrical Group
Status: Professional; Nonprofit
Income Sources: Actors' Equity Association

Performs At: Booth Theatre at North Carolina Blumenthal Performing Arts Center
Type of Stage: Flexible
Seating Capacity: 450
Organization Type: Performing; Resident

3529　CHILDREN'S THEATRE OF CHARLOTTE
1017 E Morehead Street
Charlotte, NC 28204
Phone: 704-376-5745
Fax: 704-376-3774
Web Site: www.ctcharlotte.org
Management:
　　Director: April Jones
　　Director: Alan Poindexter
Mission: To enrich the lives of young people, ages 3-18, of all cultures, through theatre and education experiences of the highest quality.
Specialized Field: Theatre; Drama
Income Sources: Arts and Science Council; Cultural Education Collaborative; North Carolina Arts Council; National Endowment for the Arts

3530　THEATRE CHARLOTTE
501 Queens Road
Charlotte, NC 28207
Phone: 704-376-3777
Fax: 704-347-5216
Web Site: www.theatrecharlotte.org
Mission: To offer community members an opportunity to participate in or attend amateur theatre productions.
Founded: 1927
Specialized Field: Community; Theatrical Group
Status: Nonprofit
Paid Staff: 6
Income Sources: First Nighters
Facility Category: Community Theatre
Type of Stage: Proscenium
Seating Capacity: 221
Year Built: 1941
Year Remodeled: 1998
Cost: $100,000
Organization Type: Performing; Educational

3531　CAROLINA THEATRE OF DURHAM
309 W Morgan Street
Durham, NC 27701-2119
Phone: 919-560-3040
Fax: 919-560-3065
e-mail: connie@carolinatheatre.org
Web Site: www.carolinatheatre.org
Management:
　　Executive Director: Connie Campanero
　　Programming Rentals Director: Jim Carl
Mission: To manage, operate and program the creative theater for the city of Durham.
Founded: 1992
Paid Staff: 60
Volunteer Staff: 200
Paid Artists: 30
Budget: $1,000,000
Performs At: Fletcher Hall
Annual Attendance: 150,000

Facility Category: Performance Center/Cinemas
Type of Stage: Proscenium
Stage Dimensions: 30'x 60'
Seating Capacity: 1,015
Year Built: 1926
Year Remodeled: 1994
Rental Contact: Jim Carl

3532 THEATRE PREVIEWS AT DUKE
209 Bivins Building
Box 90680
Durham, NC 27708-0680
Phone: 919-660-3343
Fax: 919-684-8906
e-mail: zannie@duke.edu
Management:
    Producing Director: Zannie Giraud Voss
Founded: 1986
Specialized Field: Professional Theatre

3533 BROADWAY AT DUKE COMMITTEE
101-2 Bryan Center
Box 90834
Durham, NC 27708
Phone: 919-684-2911
e-mail: calis.smith@duke.edu
Web Site: www.duke.edu/web/duu/broadway.htm
Management:
    Associate Dean: Peter Coyle
    Chairperson: Calisa Smith
Mission: To bring Broadway caliber shows to the campus of Duke University and the Durham community.
Founded: 1968
Specialized Field: Performing Arts
Paid Staff: 1
Budget: $150,000-400,000
Performs At: Page Auditorium
Seating Capacity: 1,232

3534 CHILDREN'S THEATRE OF EDEN
PO Box 547
Eden, NC 27288
Phone: 336-725-4531
Fax: 336-725-4531
Mission: To provide professional plays for all children in Eden City schools at no cost.
Founded: 1971
Specialized Field: Musical; Folk; Theatrical Group; Puppet
Status: Professional; Nonprofit
Performs At: High School Auditorium
Organization Type: Sponsoring

3535 CAPE FEAR REGIONAL THEATRE
1209 Hay Street
Fayetteville, NC 28305
Phone: 919-323-4234
Fax: 919-323-0898
Web Site: www.cfrt.org
Management:
    Artistic Director: Bo Thorp
    Associate Director: Deborah Martin-Mintz
Mission: To offer a diverse program of plays to the Cape Fear Region.

Founded: 1962
Specialized Field: Musical; Community; Puppet; Drama
Status: Professional; Semi-Professional; Nonprofit
Income Sources: North Carolina Theatre Conference; Southeastern Theatre Conference; Arts Council
Seating Capacity: 327
Organization Type: Performing

3536 GILBERT THEATER
647 Brandts Lane
Fayetteville, NC 28301
Phone: 910-678-7186
Web Site: www.theartscouncil.com/gilbert
Management:
    Artistic Director: Lynn Pryer
Mission: Our purpose is to use our creativity and enthusiasm to support and inspire others as we all freely express our talents in joyfulness, harmony and love.

3537 FLAT ROCK PLAYHOUSE
PO Box 310
2661 Greenville Highway
Flat Rock, NC 28731
Phone: 828-693-0403
Fax: 828-693-795
e-mail: frp@flatrockplayhouse.org
Web Site: www.flatrockplayhouse.org
Management:
    Executive/Artistic Director: Robin R Farquhar
Mission: To offer a summer stock season lasting 16 weeks combined with The Vagabond School of Drama Workshops; to tour productions in schools throughout North Carolina.
Founded: 1937
Specialized Field: Summer Stock; Musical; Theatrical Group
Status: Professional; Nonprofit; Commercial
Paid Staff: 20
Income Sources: Actors' Equity Association; Southeastern Theatre Conference
Season: May - October
Performs At: Flat Rock Playhouse
Organization Type: Performing; Touring; Resident; Educational; Sponsoring

3538 LITTLE THEATER OF GASTONIA
238 Clay Street
PO Box 302
Gastonia, NC 28053
Phone: 704-865-0160
e-mail: ewixson@prodigy.net
Web Site: www.ncsmartfinder.com/littletheater
Mission: To offer entertainment as well as education in the theatre arts.
Founded: 1950
Specialized Field: Musical; Community
Status: Non-Professional; Nonprofit
Paid Staff: 50
Volunteer Staff: 6
Income Sources: Ticket Sales; Season Memberships
Performs At: The Little Theatre of Gastonia
Organization Type: Performing; Educational

3539 COMMUNITY THEATRE OF GREENSBORO
200 N Davie Street
#9
Greensboro, NC 27401
Phone: 336-333-7470
Fax: 336-333-2607
e-mail: CTGEmail@aol.com
Web Site: www.ctgso.com
Officers:
President: Scott Brewington
VP: Randy Hanson
Secretary: Brett Brackett
Treasurer: Dennis Duquette
Management:
Executive Director: Mitchel Sommers
Administrative Assistant: Rozalynn Taylor
Director Marketing/Development: Robert Ankrom
Director Education: Pauline Cobrda
Mission: To provide an outlet in the community whereby persons may participate avocationally in a live theatrical experience of high calibre, both as talent and audience under professional guidance.
Specialized Field: Musical; Dinner; Community; Theatrical Group
Status: Non-Professional; Nonprofit
Paid Staff: 5
Budget: $552,000
Income Sources: United Arts Council of Greensboro; Fundraising
Performs At: Carolina Theatre; GSO Cultural Center
Annual Attendance: 35,000
Organization Type: Performing; Resident; Educational

3540 GREENSBORO CHILDREN'S THEATRE
200 N Davie Street
Greensboro, NC 27401
Phone: 336-373-2728
Fax: 336-373-2659
e-mail: barbara.britton@ci.greensboro.nc.us
Web Site:
www.ci.greensboro.nc.us/leisure/drama/gct.htm
Management:
Director: Barbara Britton
Mission: To offer a series of drama classes and three quality plays annually by and for children and families as part of a recreation program.
Founded: 1971
Specialized Field: Musical; Community; Theatrical Group
Status: Non-Professional; Nonprofit
Paid Staff: 2
Volunteer Staff: 10
Paid Artists: 50
Income Sources: City of Greensboro NC Parks and Recreation Depertment; Ticket Sales
Performs At: Weaver Education Center Theatre
Affiliations: Southeastern Theatre Conference; City Arts Drama; NC Theatre Conference
Annual Attendance: 2,500-3,000
Facility Category: Rented
Type of Stage: Proscenium Stage
Organization Type: Performing

3541 LIVESTOCK PLAYERS MUSICAL THEATRE
200 N Davie Street
Greensboro, NC 27401
Phone: 336-373-2728
Fax: 336-333-2607
e-mail: barbara.britton@ci.greensboro.nc.us
Web Site: www.ci.greensboro.nc.us/leisure/drama/lpmt.ht
Management:
Director: Barbara Britton
Mission: To present six musicals annually.
Founded: 1971
Specialized Field: Musical; Dinner; Community; Theatrical Group
Status: Non-Professional; Nonprofit
Paid Staff: 200
Income Sources: Southeastern Theatre Conference
Performs At: Carolina Theatre
Organization Type: Performing

3542 HICKORY COMMUNITY THEATRE
30 3rd Street NW
Hickory, NC 28601
Phone: 828-327-3855
Fax: 828-328-2284
Web Site: www.hct.org
Management:
Managing Artistic Director: Pamela Livingstone
Mission: To offer quality theatre to the community; to provide a performance outlet for talented local performers.
Founded: 1949
Specialized Field: Musical; Community; Dramatic
Status: Non-Professional; Nonprofit
Paid Staff: 26
Budget: $412,000
Income Sources: Catawba County Council for the Arts; Box Office; Grants; Donatios
Performs At: Old City Hall
Affiliations: AACT; NCTC; SETA
Facility Category: Community Theatre
Type of Stage: Proscenium/Cabaret
Seating Capacity: 382; 72
Organization Type: Performing; Touring; Resident; Educational

3543 YOUTHEATRE
810 8th Street NE
Hickory, NC 28601
Phone: 828-324-5354
Management:
Owner/Executive Director: Sylvia B Hoffmire
Mission: To provide an arena for the creative expression of young people through performance and study.
Founded: 1976
Specialized Field: Community; Theatrical Group
Status: Professional; Semi-Professional; Commercial
Income Sources: Catawba County Council for the Arts
Organization Type: Performing; Touring; Educational; Sponsoring

3544 HIGH POINT COMMUNITY THEATRE

1014 Mill Avenue
Suite 190
High Point, NC 27260
Mailing Address: PO Box 1152, High Point, NC 27261
Phone: 336-882-2542
Fax: 336-882-4178
Web Site: hpct.netmcr.com/
Management:
    Executive Director: Jennifer Blevins
Mission: To promote community involvement in performing arts; to provide high quality entertainment for citizens in our area.
Founded: 1976
Specialized Field: Community; Theatrical Group
Status: Non-Professional; Nonprofit
Paid Staff: 100
Income Sources: High Point Arts Council
Performs At: High Point Theatre
Affiliations: High Point Area Arts Council
Organization Type: Performing

3545 NORTH CAROLINA SHAKESPEARE FESTIVAL

220 E Commerce Avenue
PO Box 6066
High Point, NC 27262
Phone: 336-841-2273
Fax: 336-841-8627
e-mail: bjatncsf@nr.infi.net
Web Site: www.ncshakes.org
Officers:
    Chairman: Christine Green
Management:
    Artistic Director: Louis Rackoff
    Marketing/Public Relations Director: Laura Ward
    Managing Director: Thomas G Gaffney
Mission: Seeks to serve the cultural and educational needs of North Carolina audiences through traditional and nontraditional staging of the plays of Shakespeare and other classic playwrights.
Founded: 1977
Specialized Field: Theater
Status: Professional; Nonprofit
Paid Staff: 10
Paid Artists: 55
Budget: $1,400,000
Income Sources: Ticket Sales; Touring Fees; Contributors
Season: Late August - December
Performs At: High Point Theatre
Organization Type: Performing; Touring; Resident; Educational

3546 LOST COLONY

1409 National Park Drive
Manteo, NC 27954
Phone: 252-473-2127
Fax: 252-473-6000
Toll-free: 866-468-7630
Web Site: www.thelostcolony.org
Founded: 1937
Status: Non-Equity; Nonprofit
Season: June - August

Type of Stage: Amphitheatre
Stage Dimensions: 80' x 40'
Seating Capacity: 1650
Year Built: 1937
Year Remodeled: 1998

3547 FOOTHILLS COMMUNITY THEATRE

24 S Main Street
PO Box 1387
Marion, NC 28752
Phone: 828-659-7529
Management:
    Artistic Director: Sandra Epperson
Mission: To offer opportunities for participation in the performing arts; to enhance cultural life and provide entertainment.
Founded: 1972
Specialized Field: Community
Status: Non-Professional; Nonprofit
Income Sources: McDowell Arts & Craft Association
Performs At: McDowell East Junior High; McDowell Technical Company
Organization Type: Performing

3548 SOUTHERN APPALACHIAN REPERTORY THEATRE

Mars Hill College
PO Box 1720
Mars Hill, NC 28754
Phone: 828-689-1384
Fax: 828-689-1272
e-mail: sart@mhc.edu
Web Site: www.sartheatre.com
Management:
    Artistic Director: Willaim Gregg
    Production Manager: Neil St Clair
Mission: From the beginning, SART's purpose has been to produce quality theatre by a professional non-profit company in an area considered economically and culturally deprived, to present plays concerning Applachia that portray the rich culture and heritage of its people.
Founded: 1975
Specialized Field: Summer Stock; Musical; Professional
Status: Professional; Nonprofit
Paid Staff: 15
Volunteer Staff: 3
Paid Artists: 30
Non-paid Artists: 4
Income Sources: Mars Hill College; Ticket Sales
Performs At: Owen Theatre
Year Built: 1887
Organization Type: Performing; Touring; Resident

3549 MOORESVILLE COMMUNITY THEATRE

PO Box 194
Mooresville, NC 28115
Phone: 704-664-5254
Fax: 704-662-3344
Officers:
    President: Larry Gambill
    VP: Julian D'Amico
    Secretary/Treasurer: Clayton Miller

Mission: To provide live theatre for the Mooresville area.
Founded: 1973
Specialized Field: Community; Theatrical Group
Status: Non-Professional; Nonprofit
Volunteer Staff: 10
Paid Artists: 4
Income Sources: Box; Office Receipts
Performs At: Joe V Knox Auditorium
Organization Type: Performing

3550 UNTO THESE HILLS

PO Box 398
Pittsboro, NC 27312
Phone: 828-497-2111
Toll-free: 866-554-4557
e-mail: info@westernncattractions.com
Web Site: www.untothesehills.com/
Mission: America's most popular outdoor drama, Unto These Hills, is the tragic and triumphant story of the Cherokee.
Founded: 1950
Season: May - August

3551 ACTORS COMEDY LAB

1610 Midtown Place
Raleigh, NC 27609
Phone: 919-873-1333
Fax: 919-875-0703
e-mail: nancy@seriousrobots.com
Officers:
   Board Member: Nancy Rich
Status: Nonprofit

3552 BURNING COAL THEATRE COMPANY

1620 Glenwood Avenue
PO Box 90904
Raleigh, NC 27675-0904
Phone: 919-388-0066
Fax: 919-388-0065
e-mail: burning_coal@ipass.net
Web Site: www.burningcoal.org
Officers:
   Board of Directors: Kate Day
   Board of Directors: William Lightfoot
   Board of Directors: Marvin Swirsky
   Board of Advisors: Wiliam Peeples
Management:
   Artistic Director: Jerome Davis
   Managing Director: Simmie Kastner
Mission: To produce, literate, visceral, affecting theatre that is experienced, not simply seen.
Status: Incorporated; Nonprofit
Income Sources: City of Raleigh Arts Commission; United Arts

3553 NORTH CAROLINA THEATRE

One E S Street
Raleigh, NC 27601
Phone: 919-831-6941
Fax: 919-831-6951
e-mail: cymnct@aol.com
Web Site: www.nctheatre.com
Officers:
   President: Duke Fentress

Management:
   Executive Director/Founder: De Ann S Jones
   Producer: William Jones
Mission: To provide Broadway-quality professional theatre at an affordable price as well as provide available employment to theatre artists and craftsmen.
Founded: 1983
Specialized Field: Musical; Theatrical Group
Status: Professional
Paid Staff: 10
Budget: $678,000
Income Sources: Grants; Sponsors; Donations; Ticket Sales; Kids' Programs
Facility Category: Auditorium
Seating Capacity: 2000-2500
Year Remodeled: 2002
Organization Type: Performing

3554 RALEIGH ENSEMBLE PLAYERS

201 E Davie Street
Raleigh, NC 27601
Phone: 919-832-9607
Fax: 919-821-0383
e-mail: gorep@juno.com
Web Site: www.realtheatre.org
Founded: 1983

3555 SIDE BY SIDE

150 Fayetteville Street
PO Box 19416
Raleigh, NC 27601
Phone: 919-833-1141
Management:
   Director: Paul B Conway
Mission: To provide entertainment.
Founded: 1981
Specialized Field: Musical; Dinner; Community; Folk
Status: Semi-Professional; Nonprofit
Organization Type: Performing

3556 THEATRE IN THE PARK

107 Pullen Road
Raleigh, NC 27607-7367
Phone: 919-831-6936
Fax: 919-831-9475
Web Site: www.theatreinthepark.com
Officers:
   President: Bill Parmelee
   VP: G Troy Page
   Secretary: Camille Patterson
   Treasurer: Johy Taylor
Management:
   Executive Director: Ira David Wood III
Mission: North Carolina's largest community theatre. Each year, theatre in the park produces humorous productions, Shakepeare and original plays.
Founded: 1973
Specialized Field: Musical; Community; Theatrical Group
Status: Non-Professional; Nonprofit
Paid Staff: 6
Volunteer Staff: 10
Non-paid Artists: 120

Income Sources: American Alliance for Theatre Arts; North Carolina Community Theatre
Performs At: Theatre In The Park
Organization Type: Performing; Touring; Resident; Educational; Sponsoring

3557 PIEDMONT PLAYERS THEATRE

213 S Main Street
PO Box 762
Salisbury, NC 28145
Phone: 704-633-5471
Fax: 704-633-4653
e-mail: BM@piedmontplayers.com
Web Site: www.piedmontplayers.com
Officers:
  President: David Crook
  VP: John Sofley
  Treasurer: John Brincefield
Management:
  Business Manager: Diana Moghrabi
  Resident Director: Reid Leonard
  Box Office Manager: Laura Sandridge
  Volunteer Coordinator: Suzanne Burgess
Mission: To entertain and educate the community.
Founded: 1961
Specialized Field: Community; Theatrical Group
Status: Non-Professional; Nonprofit
Paid Staff: 2
Volunteer Staff: 100
Budget: $255,700
Income Sources: Season Memberships; Ticket Sales; Donations
Performs At: The Meroney Theatre
Affiliations: NC Center for Non-Profits
Annual Attendance: 16,000
Facility Category: Performing Arts Center
Type of Stage: Proscenium
Stage Dimensions: 24'x32'x30' deep, 12' wings
Seating Capacity: 361
Year Built: 1906
Year Remodeled: 1995
Architect: Newman & Jones
Cost: $1,800,000
Rental Contact: Faculty Manager Diana Moghrabi
Organization Type: Performing

3558 TEMPLE THEATRE COMPANY

120 Carthage Street
PO Box 1391
Sanford, NC 27330
Phone: 919-774-4512
Fax: 919-774-7531
e-mail: templetheatre@mindspring.com
Web Site: www.transoftinc.com/temple/
Officers:
  President: Cindy Boggs
  VP: Mary Dossenbath
  Secretary: Martha Ragsdale
  Treasurer: Kathi Smith
Management:
  Artistic Director: Jerry Sipp
  Technical Director: Brad Sizemore
  Office Manager: Sheila Brewer
  Box Office Manager: Bonnie Sexton

Mission: To entertain, enlighten, educate, and enrich lives through the performing arts.
Founded: 1925
Specialized Field: Performing Arts
Status: Professional; Semi-Professional; Nonprofit
Paid Staff: 5
Volunteer Staff: 30
Paid Artists: 55
Budget: $330,000
Income Sources: State; Local Government; Corporate; Individuala Theatre Conference
Performs At: Temple Theatre
Affiliations: SETC, NCTC
Annual Attendance: 21,000
Facility Category: Theatre
Type of Stage: Proscenium
Seating Capacity: 339
Year Built: 1925
Year Remodeled: 1984
Cost: $500,000
Rental Contact: Jerry Sipp
Organization Type: Performing; Educational; Sponsoring

3559 SNOW CAMP HISTORICAL DRAMA SOCIETY

1 Drama Road
PO Box 535
Snow Camp, NC 27349
Phone: 336-376-6948
Fax: 910-376-6849
Toll-free: 800-726-5115
e-mail: snowcampot@aol.com
Web Site: www.snowcampdrama.com
Management:
  General Manager: James Wilson
Founded: 1974
Status: Non-Equity; Nonprofit
Season: Year Round
Type of Stage: Amphitheater
Stage Dimensions: 100' x 400'
Seating Capacity: 500

3560 SANDHILLS LITTLE THEATRE

250 NW Broad Street
Southern Pines, NC 28387
Phone: 910-692-3340
Fax: 910-692-9821
e-mail: slt@pinehurst.net
Web Site: web2.sandhillsonline.com
Management:
  Administrator: Paula Reeder
Mission: To please audiences.
Founded: 1981
Specialized Field: Community
Status: Non-Professional; Nonprofit
Paid Staff: 200
Income Sources: New England Theatre Conference; Southeastern Theatre Conference
Performs At: Performing Arts Center
Organization Type: Performing; Resident; Sponsoring

3561 OLD COLONY PLAYERS

PO Box 112
Valdese, NC 28690
Phone: 828-874-0176
Fax: 828-874-2311
Web Site: www.hci.net/~ocp.
Officers:
  President: Marvin Folger
  VP: Chuck Moseley
  Treasurer: Mark Rostan
  Secretary: Nancy McFadden
Management:
  General Manager: Martin R Rice
  Business Manager: Knolan Benfield
Mission: To produce the historical outdoor drama from this day forward annually; to produce Dickens' A Christmas Carol annually; to produce other dramas, engage in outreach activities, and sponser workshops and cultural events.
Founded: 1968
Specialized Field: Musical; Dinner; Community; Theatrical Group; Choral Society
Status: Professional; Nonprofit
Income Sources: Southeastern Theatre Conference; North Carolina Theatre Conference; North Carolina Association of Professional Theatres; Burke County Chamber of Commerce; Burke Arts Council
Season: July - August
Performs At: Old Colony Players Amphitheater; Old Rock School
Organization Type: Performing; Touring; Resident; Educational

3562 MARTIN COMMUNITY PLAYERS

300 North Watts Street
Williamston, NC 278922099
Phone: 252-792-1521
Fax: 252-792-0826
Management:
  Artistic Director: Allan Osborne
Mission: To offer theatre to all citizens in our county, primarily through the schools, providing one selected offering annually.
Founded: 1974
Specialized Field: Musical; Community; Theatrical Group
Status: Non-Professional; Nonprofit
Performs At: Martin County Auditorium
Organization Type: Performing; Resident

3563 OPERA HOUSE THEATRE COMPANY

2011 Carolina Beach Road
Wilmington, NC 28401
Phone: 910-762-4234
Fax: 910-251-9800
e-mail: ohte@wilmington.net
Management:
  Executive Director/Founder: Lou Criscuolo
Mission: To produce and promote high quality, accessible, professional theatre; to train and develop the talents of musicians, actors and technicians.
Founded: 1985
Specialized Field: Summer Stock; Musical; Theatrical Group

Status: Professional
Paid Staff: 20
Performs At: Thalian Hall Center for the Performing Arts
Organization Type: Performing; Educational

3564 CHILDREN'S THEATRE BOARD

610 Coliseum Drive
Winston-Salem, NC 27106
Phone: 336-725-4531
Fax: 336-725-4531
Officers:
  President: Mary Harper
  President Elect: Libby Noah
  Treasurer: Leslie Madigan
  Treasurer-Elect: Ernestine Worley
  Immediate Past President: Janet Bondurant
Management:
  Executive Director: Pat Land
  Director Marketing/ Development: Jennifer Lewis
Mission: To provide opportunities for students, educators and families to experience and participate in the performing arts; to offer multidisciplinary, culturally diverse programs to foster sensitivity and acceptance of others. Our programs are accessible and entertaining, our vision is to reach young people through experimental learning.
Founded: 1940
Specialized Field: Theatrical Group
Status: Professional; Nonprofit
Performs At: The Arts Council Theatre; W-S/FC Schools
Organization Type: Performing; Educational; Sponsoring

3565 LITTLE THEATRE OF WINSTON-SALEM

610 Coliseum Drive
Winston-Salem, NC 27106
Phone: 336-748-0857
Fax: 336-748-0857
e-mail: theatre@littletheatreonline.com
Web Site: www.littletheatreonline.com
Officers:
  President: Eva Wu
Management:
  Executive Director: Whit Andrews
  Box Office Manager: Elizabeth Brooks
  Marketing Director: Patricia Oldis
  Director Finance/Development: Mike Orsillo
  Education Director: Angela Chance
Mission: To provide for all within the community an avenue for education and development in all aspects of theatrical arts and to provide entertainment for the community by offering a series of well-staged performances of live theatre.
Founded: 1935
Specialized Field: Community
Status: Non-Professional; Nonprofit
Income Sources: Winston-Salem Arts Council
Performs At: Hanes Community Center; Arts Council Theatre
Organization Type: Performing; Educational

**3566 NORTH CAROLINA BLACK
REPERTORY COMPANY**
610 Coliseum Drive
PO Box 2793
Winston-Salem, NC 27106
Phone: 336-723-7907
Fax: 336-723-2223
Web Site: www.nbtf.org/history.htm
Management:
  Founder Executive/Artistic Director: Larry Leon
  Hamlin
  Resident Playwright: Nathan Ross Freeman
  Administrative Assistant: Chena Sulley
Mission: To offer professional productions of musicals
and plays including original and renowned works with
universal as well as ethnic (African-American) themes.
Founded: 1979
Specialized Field: Musical; Theatrical Group
Status: Professional; Nonprofit
Season: September - June
Performs At: Winston-Salem Arts Council Theatre
Type of Stage: Proscenium
Seating Capacity: 541
Organization Type: Performing; Touring; Resident;
Educational; Sponsoring

3567 YADKIN PLAYERS
108 E Elm Street
PO Box 667
Yadkinville, NC 27055
Phone: 336-679-2941
Fax: 336-679-2941
e-mail: yadkinarts@yadtel.net
Web Site: www.yadkinarts.com
Management:
  Executive Director: Deborah C Davis
Founded: 1975
Specialized Field: Community
Status: Nonprofit
Paid Staff: 1
Organization Type: Performing; Touring; Educational

North Dakota

**3568 FARGO-MOORHEAD COMMUNITY
THEATRE**
333 S 4th Street
Fargo, ND 58103
Phone: 701-235-1901
Fax: 701-235-2685
Web Site: www.fmct.org
Officers:
  President: Dawn Duncan
  VP: Robin Hoffer
  Treasurer: Dave Stende
  Secretary: Kim Horab
Management:
  Artistic Director: Charlene Hudgins
  Business Director: Marsha Schalek
  Development Director: Sherry Shadley
  Technical Director: Don Santer

Mission: To provide quality avocational theatre
opportunities to the cities of Fargo and Moorhead, as well
as the region.
Founded: 1946
Specialized Field: Community
Status: Nonprofit
Paid Staff: 12
Volunteer Staff: 500
Paid Artists: 20
Income Sources: American Association of Community
Theater; Lake Agassiz Arts Council; North Dakota
Community Theatre Association; Minnesota Association
of Community Theaters
Performs At: Emma K. Herbst Playhouse
Annual Attendance: 28,000
Facility Category: Theatre
Type of Stage: Thrust
Seating Capacity: 302-380
Year Built: 1965
Year Remodeled: 1994
Organization Type: Resident

3569 LITTLE COUNTRY THEATRE
PO Box 5691
Fargo, ND 58102-5691
Phone: 701-231-9442
Web Site: www.ndsu.edu/finearts/theatre_arts/lct.shtml
Management:
  Director Division Fine Arts: Don Stowell Jr
  Artistic Director: Don Larew
  Managing Director: M Joy Erickson
Mission: To produce theatrical productions reflecting a
high degree of professionalism; to develop artists in the
theatre as well as responsive audiences.
Founded: 1914
Specialized Field: Theatrical Group
Status: Nonprofit
Paid Staff: 50
Income Sources: American College Theatre Festival;
United States Institute for Theatre Technology
Performs At: Askanase Auditorium; Walsh Studio
Theatre
Organization Type: Educational

3570 FORT TOTTEN LITTLE THEATRE
PO Box 97
Fort Totten, ND 58335
Phone: 701-766-4473
Web Site: www2.stellarnet.com
Officers:
  President: Carol Leevers
  VP: Jane Traynor
  Treasurer/Secretary: Dean Petska
  Artistic Director: Judy Ryan
Management:
  Community Relation: Carol Leevers
  Community Relation: Jane Traynor
  Attorney: John Traynor
  Advanced Ticket Drive: Chuck Jerome
  Publicity: Armin Hanson
Mission: Provide an opportunity for talented people to
have theatre experience; attract tourists to a state historic
site; entertainment for the citizens of rural areas.
Founded: 1962

Specialized Field: Musical; Community; Theatrical Group
Status: Semi-Professional; Non-Professional; Nonprofit
Paid Staff: 20
Income Sources: North Dakota Council of Arts; Council of Lake Region
Season: June - August
Performs At: Cavalry Square; Historic Site
Organization Type: Performing; Resident

3571 MEDORA MUSICAL

528 Hennepin Avenue, Suite 206
Minneapolis, ND 55403
Phone: 612-333-3302
Fax: 612-333-4337
Toll-free: 800-633-0721
e-mail: cwollan@mninter.net
Web Site: www.troupeamerica.com
Management:
   Producer/Director: Curt Wollan
   Co-Manager: John Tsafoyanni
Founded: 1965
Status: Non-Equity; Commercial
Paid Staff: 18
Paid Artists: 30
Budget: $500,000
Income Sources: Ticket Sales; Grants; Donations
Season: June - September
Annual Attendance: 115,000
Facility Category: Ampitheatre
Type of Stage: Outdoor
Stage Dimensions: 90' x 60'
Seating Capacity: 3000
Year Built: 1992
Cost: $4 Million

Ohio

3572 CAROUSEL DINNER THEATRE

1275 E Waterloo Road
PO Box 7530
Akron, OH 44306
Phone: 330-724-9855
Fax: 330-724-2232
Toll-free: 800-362-4100
e-mail: carousel@carouseldinnertheatre.com
Web Site: www.carouseldinnertheatre.com
Officers:
   President/Owner/Executive Producer: Prescott F Griffith
Management:
   Director Sales/Marketing: Jeffrey Lynch
Mission: Elegant Dinner Theatre featuring live Broadway musical productions with prosfessional New York talent.
Founded: 1973
Paid Staff: 175
Income Sources: Box Office; Ticket Sales
Affiliations: National Dinner Theatre Association; Actors' Equity Association
Annual Attendance: 200,000
Facility Category: Dinner Theatre
Type of Stage: Proscenium
Stage Dimensions: 60'x40'x18'

Seating Capacity: 1,130
Year Built: 1988
Year Remodeled: 1988
Rental Contact: Producer Marc A Resnik
Resident Groups: Sheila A Fetterman

3573 MAGICAL THEATRE COMPANY

565 W Tuscarawas Avenue
PO Box 386
Barberton, OH 44203
Phone: 330-848-3708
Fax: 330-848-5768
e-mail: magicaltheatre@core.com
Web Site: www.oac.state.oh.us/
Management:
   Co-Producing Director: Holly Barkdoll
   Co-Producing Director: Dennis O'Connell
   Development Director: Phyllis Griffith
Mission: Resident and touring, educational and entertainment resource for young audiences. In partnership with schools and other organizations, we are leaders in providing a positive cultural service as a strong and energetic professional theatre serving Northeast Ohio. We enhance learning, growth and civic improvement through live theatre.
Founded: 1973
Specialized Field: Theatrical Group
Status: Professional; Nonprofit
Paid Staff: 4
Paid Artists: 40
Budget: $350,000
Income Sources: Foundations; Corporate Donors; Ticket Sales
Affiliations: Ohio Theatre Asssociation; Acron Area Arts Alliance; Professional Association of Cleveland Theatres
Annual Attendance: 50,000
Facility Category: Renovated Movie House
Type of Stage: Proscenium; Thrust
Seating Capacity: 285
Year Built: 1919
Year Remodeled: 2000
Cost: $500,000
Rental Contact: Dennis O'Connell
Organization Type: Performing; Touring; Resident; Educational

3574 HUNTINGTON THEATRE

28601 Lake Road
Bay Village, OH 44140
Phone: 216-871-8333
Mission: To maintain a community theatre.
Founded: 1958
Specialized Field: Musical; Community; Theatrical Group
Status: Non-Professional; Nonprofit
Paid Staff: 100
Performs At: Huntington Playhouse
Organization Type: Performing; Educational

3575 HURON PLAYHOUSE

Bowling Green State University
Theatre Department
338 S Hall
Bowling Green, OH 43403

Phone: 419-372-0370
Fax: 419-372-7186
e-mail: jglann@bgnet.bgsu.edu
Web Site: www.bgsu.edu/departments/huron_playhouse
Officers:
    President: Dr. Sydney Ribeau
Management:
    Chairman Theatre Department: Dr. Ron Shields
    Managing/Artistic Director: Dr. Jann Graham Glann
    Business/Operations Manager: Shaun W Moorman
Mission: To provide a unique educational theatre experience for company members; to extend services of Bowling Green State University; to provide live theatre to a large area.
Founded: 1949
Specialized Field: Summer Stock; Musical
Status: Non-Professional; Nonprofit
Paid Staff: 50
Paid Artists: 25
Income Sources: University; Grants; Corporate Sponsors
Season: June - August
Performs At: McCormick High School Auditorium
Annual Attendance: 11,000
Facility Category: Proscenium
Type of Stage: 34x26
Stage Dimensions: 507
Seating Capacity: 2535
Organization Type: Performing; Educational
Resident Groups: Huron Playhouse

3576   BRECKSVILLE LITTLE THEATRE

Box 41131
Brecksville, OH 44141
Phone: 440-526-4477
e-mail: jpfuthey@earthlink.net
Web Site: www.brecksville.oh.us
Mission: To offer good theatre; to provide performance opportunities.
Founded: 1941
Specialized Field: Musical; Community; Theatrical Group
Status: Non-Professional; Nonprofit
Paid Staff: 100
Performs At: Old Towne Hall; Brecksville Square
Organization Type: Performing; Resident; Educational

3577   THEATRE ON THE SQUARE

49 Public Square
Brecksville, OH 94102
Phone: 404-526-6436
Fax: 404-526-6591
Toll-free: 800-895-4708
e-mail: theatre@btots.org
Web Site: www.btots.org
Management:
    Owner: Jonathan Reinis
    Theatre Manager: Hillary Reinis
    Manager: Dana Dizon
    House Manager: Judy Karwan
Mission: Presenting touring and original plays.
Founded: 1981
Specialized Field: Musical/straight plays
Status: Professional; Commercial
Performs At: Theatre on the Square
Stage Dimensions: 40x32

Seating Capacity: 750
Year Built: 1924
Organization Type: Performing; Touring

3578   PLAYERS GUILD OF CANTON

1001 Market Avenue N
Canton, OH 44702
Phone: 330-453-7619
Fax: 330-453-8368
e-mail: playersguild@netzero.net
Web Site: www.playersguildtheatre.com
Officers:
    President: Susan Steiner
    President Elect: Tony Snyder
    VP: Norm Warren
    Secretary: Byran Fetty
    Treasurer: Jeff Sutton
Management:
    Producing Artistic Director: Bil Pfuderer
    Technical Director/Designer: Joe Carmola
    Business Manager: Jan Clark
    Costumer: Joshua Erichsen
Mission: A charitable and educational institution which produces and exhibits plays and provides instruction of the theatre arts for the purpose of fostering and advancing education in and appreciation of the theatre by and among the people of the Greater Canton Area.
Founded: 1932
Specialized Field: Community
Status: Non-Professional; Nonprofit
Paid Staff: 5
Volunteer Staff: 500
Non-paid Artists: 150
Budget: $700,000
Facility Category: Community Theatre
Type of Stage: Proscenium; Thrust
Stage Dimensions: 60'x40'; 30'x20'
Seating Capacity: 478; 139
Year Built: 1970
Rental Contact: Bil Pfuderer
Organization Type: Performing

3579   CHAGRIN VALLEY LITTLE THEATRE

40 River Street
Chagrin Falls, OH 44022
Phone: 216-247-8955
Web Site: www.cvlt.org
Management:
    Business Manager: Rollin DeVere
Mission: To provide community theater.
Founded: 1929
Specialized Field: Theatrical Group
Status: Non-Professional; Nonprofit
Paid Staff: 150
Seating Capacity: 262
Organization Type: Performing

3580   TECUMSEH!

PO Box 73
Chilicothe, OH 45601

Phone: 740-775-4100
Fax: 740-775-4349
Toll-free: 866-775-0700
e-mail: tecumseh@bright.net
Web Site: www.tecumsehdrama.com
Management:
    Producer: Marion Waggoner
Founded: 1973
Status: Nonprofit
Paid Staff: 115
Paid Artists: 65
Season: June - September
Annual Attendance: 70,000
Facility Category: Outdoors
Type of Stage: Amphitheater
Stage Dimensions: 150'x50'
Seating Capacity: 1,700
Year Built: 1971
Year Remodeled: 1998
Cost: $ 1.4 million

3581 CINCINNATI PLAYHOUSE IN THE PARK

962 Mt. Adams Circle
PO Box 6537
Cincinnati, OH 45202
Phone: 513-345-2242
Fax: 513-345-2254
Toll-free: 800-582-3208
e-mail: admin@cincyplay.com
Web Site: www.cincyplay.com
Officers:
    Board of Trustees President: Jack D Osborn
    Boarf of Trustees VP: Richard Curry
Management:
    Producing Artistic Director: Ed Stern
    Executive Director: Buzz Ward
    Public Relations Director: Christa Skiles
Mission: Produced on stage in a fiscally responsible manner, and through stimulating educational and outreach programs.
Founded: 1960
Status: Professional; Nonprofit
Paid Staff: 74
Budget: $9 million
Performs At: Robert S Marx Theatre; Thompson Shelterhouse Theatre
Affiliations: League of Cincinnati Theatres
Annual Attendance: 250,000
Facility Category: Robert S Marx Theatre; Thomson Shelterhouse Theat
Type of Stage: Thrust
Seating Capacity: 626; 225
Rental Contact: 513-345-2242 Norma Niinemets
Organization Type: Performing; Resident

3582 ENSEMBLE THEATRE OF CINCINNATI

1127 Vine Street
Cincinnati, OH 45210
Phone: 513-421-3555
Fax: 513-562-4104
Web Site: www.cincyetc.com
Management:
    Producing Artistic Director: D Lynn Meyers

Managing Director: David Adams
Director Development: Sarah Basch
Director Public Relations: Sue Cohen
Mission: Professional equity theatre dedicated to the production and development of new works and works new to the region.
Founded: 1986
Specialized Field: Theatre
Paid Staff: 15
Volunteer Staff: 50
Performs At: Ensemble Theatre
Type of Stage: Thrust
Seating Capacity: 202

3583 HOT SUMMER NIGHTS

University of Cincinnati, PO Box 210003
College-Conservatory of Music
Cincinnati, OH 45221-0003
Phone: 513-556-4183
Fax: 513-556-3399
e-mail: finnely@ucmail.uc.edu
Web Site: www.ccm.uc.edu/musicaltheatre
Management:
    Producer: R Terrell Finney Jr
    Artistic Director: Richard Hess
Founded: 1980
Status: Non-Equity; Nonprofit
Paid Staff: 15
Volunteer Staff: 10
Paid Artists: 20
Budget: 300,000
Income Sources: Box Office
Season: June-August
Affiliations: Univeristy
Annual Attendance: 15,314
Type of Stage: Thrust
Stage Dimensions: 42' x 27'
Seating Capacity: 380

3584 MADCAP PRODUCTIONS PUPPET THEATRE

3316 Glenmore Avenue
Cincinnati, OH 45211
Phone: 513-921-5965
Fax: 513-921-3845
e-mail: info@madcappuppets.com
Web Site: www.madcappuppets.com
Officers:
    President: Rosemary Schlachter
    VP: Maroene Johnson
    Secretary/Treasurer: Paul Rattermann
Management:
    Artistic Director: Jerry Handorf
    Puppet Center Manager: Karey Kattelman
    Managing Director: Vickie Francis
    Booking Manager: Jim Lepscomb, JR
Mission: To present educational theatre experiences and further the art of puppet theatre.
Founded: 1981
Specialized Field: Touring Children's Theatre Company
Status: Professional; Nonprofit
Paid Staff: 9
Paid Artists: 12

Performs At: Touring Company; Resident Theatre at Cincinnati Art Museum
Affiliations: Puppeteers of America; Ohio Theatre Alliance; League of Cincinnati Theatres
Annual Attendance: 450,000
Organization Type: Performing; Touring; Educational

3585 MARIEMONT PLAYERS
4101 Walton Creek Road
Cincinnati, OH 45227
Phone: 513-271-1661
Web Site: wwwk.geocities.com/mariemontplayers
Mission: To produce plays for the enrichment and enjoyment of area audiences.
Founded: 1936
Specialized Field: Community; Theatrical Group
Status: Non-Professional; Nonprofit
Income Sources: American Association of Community Theatres-Cincinnati; Ohio Community Theatre Alliance
Performs At: Walton Creek Theater
Organization Type: Performing

3586 SHOWBOAT MAJESTIC
PO Box 5255
Cincinnati, OH 45205-0255
Phone: 513-241-6550
e-mail: info.crc@rcc.org
Season: April - October

3587 STAGECRAFTERS
1580 Summit Road
Cincinnati, OH 45237
Phone: 513-761-7500
Fax: 513-761-0084
Mission: To provide a performance outlet and entertainment for the community.
Founded: 1952
Specialized Field: Community
Status: Non-Professional
Paid Staff: 25
Income Sources: American Association of Community Theatres; Ohio Community Theatre Alliance
Performs At: Jewish Community Center
Organization Type: Performing; Resident

3588 TALENT CENTER
PO Box 23220
Cincinnati, OH 45223
Fax: 513-542-7858
Toll-free: 800-878-2287
e-mail: center@iac.net
Web Site: www.talentcenter.com
Management:
    Director: Brain Eastman
Mission: To perform original theatre for children and adults using mime, movement, clown, improvisation and music; to specialize in music, storytellers, variety acts, troubadours, acting troupes, dance troupes, school shows, comedians, holiday shows, and nostalgia groups.
Founded: 1981
Specialized Field: Booking Agency-Performing Arts
Status: Professional; Nonprofit
Income Sources: National Mime Association
Organization Type: Performing; Touring; Resident

3589 THEATRE IV
3567 Edwards Road
Suite 5
Cincinnati, OH 45208
Phone: 513-871-2300
Fax: 513-533-1295
Toll-free: 800-235-8687
e-mail: theatreIV@zoomtown.com
Web Site: www.theatreiv.org
Officers:
    President: Joel Belsky
Management:
    Artistic Director: Kelly Germain
    Managing Director: Daniel Bayer
    Development Director: Jon Ashton
    Arts Education Manager: Elizabeth Harris
    Technical Manager: Josh Neumever
Mission: To provide quality, theatrical presentations to family audiences in schools and theatres across the nation.
Founded: 1976
Status: Non-Equity; Nonprofit
Paid Staff: 5
Paid Artists: 30
Income Sources: Theatre Communications Group; Association of Performing Arts Presenters; American Association of Theatre Educators; Arts Midwest
Season: September - May
Performs At: Touring

3590 BAD EPITAPH THEATER COMPANY
PO Box 6794
Cleveland, OH 44101-1794
Phone: 216-556-4490
Fax: 216-382-2993
Management:
    Artistic Director: David Hansen
    Managing Director: Brain Pedaci

3591 CLEVELAND PLAY HOUSE
8500 Euclid Avenue
Cleveland, OH 44106
Phone: 216-795-7000
Fax: 216-795-7005
Web Site: www.clevelandplayhouse.com
Officers:
    President: Robert Paul
    Chairman: Robert Trombly
Management:
    Managing Director: Dean R Gladden
    Artistic Director: Peter Hackett
    Director Communications: Peter Cambariere
    Director Development: Joyce Braun
Mission: To provide the experience of a complete performing arts environment through its varied repertoire of classical and contemporary theatre, facilities and the continuance of young people's theatre training.
Founded: 1915
Status: Professional; Nonprofit
Paid Staff: 150
Volunteer Staff: 300
Budget: $6.5 million
Income Sources: Ticket Sales; Grants; Donations
Performs At: Bolton Theatre; Drury Theatre; Brooks Theatre

Affiliations: League of Resident Theatres; Theatre Communications Group; Ohio Arts Council
Annual Attendance: 300,000
Type of Stage: Proscenium;
Seating Capacity: 504; 500; 120
Year Built: 1916
Year Remodeled: 1991
Rental Contact: Managing Director Dean R Gladden
Organization Type: Performing; Educational

3592 CLEVELAND PUBLIC THEATRE

6415 Detroit Avenue
Cleveland, OH 44102-3011
Phone: 216-631-2727
Fax: 216-631-2575
e-mail: info@cptonline.org
Web Site: www.cptonline.org
Officers:
   President: George H Carr
   VP: Jillian Davis
Management:
   Director Marketing/Public Relations: Jeffery Syroney
   Artistic Director: Randy Rollison
   Executive Director: James Levin
   General Manager: Deidre Lauer
Mission: To inspire, nurture, challenge, amaze, educate and empower artists and audiences in order to make the Cleveland public a more conscious and compassionate community.
Founded: 1981
Specialized Field: Expirimental; Theatrical Group; Musical; Dance; Film; Performing Art
Status: Semi-Professional; Nonprofit
Paid Staff: 23
Volunteer Staff: 40
Paid Artists: 170
Budget: $1.2 Million
Income Sources: Foundations; Government; Individual; Corporate
Affiliations: Ohio Theatre Association; Theatre Communications Group; Ohio Arts Council; National Endowment for the Arts
Annual Attendance: 20,000
Facility Category: Multi Theatre
Type of Stage: Proscenium; Black Box
Year Built: 1920
Year Remodeled: 2000
Rental Contact: James Levin
Organization Type: Performing; Touring; Resident; Educational; Sponsoring

3593 CLEVELAND SIGNSTAGE THEATRE

8500 Euclid Avenue
Cleveland, OH 44106
Phone: 216-229-2838
Fax: 216-229-2769
e-mail: deaftheatre@signstage.org
Web Site: www.signstage.org
Officers:
   President: Richard Slosar
Management:
   Artistic Director: James Burton
   Education: Rebecca Spencer

Mission: FTD accepts the unique responsibility for providing theatrical and educational performances and workshops for deaf, hearing impaired and hearing people.
Founded: 1975
Specialized Field: Theatrical Group; Sign Language Translators
Status: Professional; Nonprofit
Paid Staff: 7
Volunteer Staff: 2
Paid Artists: 7
Budget: $800,000
Performs At: Cleveland Play House
Facility Category: Resident Theatre
Stage Dimensions: 25'x25'
Seating Capacity: 139
Organization Type: Performing; Touring; Resident; Educational

3594 KARAMU HOUSE

2355 E 89th Street
Cleveland, OH 44106
Phone: 216-795-7070
Fax: 216-795-7073
e-mail: info@karamu.com
Web Site: www.karamu.com
Officers:
   President: Constance Hagg
   VP: Andrew Jackson
Management:
   Marketing Manager: Vivian C Wilson
   Executive Director: Gerry McClamy
Mission: To support and encourage the preservation, celebration and evaluation of African American culture and provide a vehicle for social, eccnomic and educational development.
Founded: 1915
Specialized Field: Cultural Arts (Dance, Drama, Music, Visual)
Status: Semi-Professional; Nonprofit
Paid Staff: 38
Volunteer Staff: 20
Paid Artists: 20
Affiliations: American Alliance for Theatre Arts
Annual Attendance: 60,000
Facility Category: Outdoor; Theater House; Amphitheatre
Type of Stage: Arena; Proscenium
Seating Capacity: 100/225
Organization Type: Performing; Educational

3595 PLAYHOUSE SQUARE FOUNDATION

1501 Euclid Avenue
Suite 200
Cleveland, OH 44115
Phone: 216-771-4444
Fax: 216-771-0217
Toll-free: 800-492-6048
Web Site: www.playhousesquare.com
Officers:
   President: Art J Falco
Management:
   Technical Director: Bob Rody
   Director of Marketing: Jim Szakacs
   Director Programming: Gina Vernael

Mission: The renovation and operation of five theatres in the Playhouse Square Center.
Founded: 1970
Specialized Field: Great Lakes Theater Festival, Ohio Ballet
Status: Professional; Nonprofit
Paid Staff: 250
Budget: $34 Million
Income Sources: Ticket Sales; Contributions
Performs At: Five historic theatres ranging in size from 750 to 3100.
Annual Attendance: 1,200,000
Facility Category: Performing Arts Center
Type of Stage: Proscenium
Rental Contact: Hallie Yavitch 216-348-5257
Organization Type: Performing; Touring; Resident; Educational

3596 CAIN PARK THEATRE
Lee and Superior Road
Cleveland Heights, OH 44118
Phone: 216-371-3000
Fax: 216-371-6995
Season: June - August
Facility Category: Amphitheater

3597 DOBAMA THEATRE
1846 Coventry Road
Cleveland Heights, OH 44118
Phone: 216-932-6838
Fax: 216-932-3259
e-mail: sledel@dobama.org
Web Site: www.dobama.org
Management:
   Literary Manager: Jean Cummins
   Public Relations Director: Owen Kelly
   Artistic/Managing Director: Joyce Casey
   Development Director: Deborah Bradlin
   Technical Director: Ron Newell
   House Manager: Dave Morris
Mission: Produce five plays not yet available to Cleveland Heights audiences; encourage new American playwrights by offering staged readings and full world premiere productions of their work; encourage creative expression in children through annual Marilyn Biarchi Kids Playwriting Festival.
Founded: 1959
Specialized Field: Theatrical Group
Status: Non-Professional; Nonprofit
Paid Staff: 70
Income Sources: Ohio Theatre Association
Performs At: Dobama Theatre
Type of Stage: Thrust
Seating Capacity: 200
Organization Type: Performing; Resident; Educational

3598 ACTORS' THEATRE COMPANY
1000 City Park
Columbus, OH 43206
Phone: 614-444-6888
e-mail: ghoffmanoh@columbus.rr.com
Web Site: www.theactorstheatre.org
Officers:
   President: Joel M Winston

1st VP: Debbie Matan
2nd VP: Noel C Shepard
Treasurer: Eric A Carlson
Secretary: Kara L Miller
Management:
   Artistic Director: Patricia B Ellson
   Designer/Technical Director: Scott Skiles
Mission: To make quality theatre accessible by providing free outdoor plays, particularly entertaining Shakespeare productions.
Founded: 1982
Specialized Field: Shakespeare Plays
Status: Semi-Professional; Nonprofit
Paid Staff: 100
Performs At: Schiller Park Amphitheatre
Organization Type: Performing; Touring; Resident; Educational

3599 CATCO (CONTEMPORARY AMERICAN THEATRE COMPANY)
77 S High Street
2nd Floor
Columbus, OH 43215
Phone: 614-461-1382
Fax: 614-461-4917
e-mail: administator@catco.org
Web Site: www.catco.org
Management:
   Artistic Director: Geoffrey Nelson
   Development Director: Patrick Roehrenbeck
   Executive Director: David Edelman
   Executive Assistant: Jerry Matheny
Mission: Entertaining theatre company, dramatically different.
Founded: 1985
Specialized Field: Theatre
Status: Nonprofit
Paid Staff: 25
Volunteer Staff: 4
Paid Artists: 7
Income Sources: Organizations; Individuals; Foundations

3600 COLUMBUS CHILDREN'S THEATRE
512 N Park Street
Columbus, OH 43215-2224
Phone: 614-224-6672
e-mail: cctcolsoh@aol.com
Web Site: www.colschildrenstheatre.org
Officers:
   President: Olga Lucia
   VP: Linda Cochran
   Treasurer: Sue Zazon
   Secretary: Dawn Farrell
Management:
   Executive/Artistic Director: William Goldsmith
   Managing Director: Patricia R Shannon
   Education Director: Mark Mann
   Office/Touring Manager: Kathy Hyland
Mission: CCT is committed to the proposition that the best way for young people to understand and appreciate the theatre arts is through direct participation. Our focus is on professionally directed, interactive, hands-on programs

that celebrate young people's spirit, creativity and fresh perspective... to provide creative outlets, structure and discipline for young people to progress in the theatre arts.
Founded: 1963
Annual Attendance: 100,000

3601 OHIO STATE UNIVERSITY-DEPARTMENT OF THEATRE

1089 Drake Union
1849 Cannon Drive
Columbus, OH 43210-5821
Phone: 614-292-5821
Fax: 614-292-3222
Web Site: www.the.ohio-state.edu
Management:
　Chairperson: Lesley Ferris
Status: Non-Professional
Performs At: Thuber Theatre; Bowen Theatre
Type of Stage: Proscenium; Thrust
Seating Capacity: 600; 250

3602 PHOENIX THEATRE FOR CHILDREN

PO Box 06238
Columbus, OH 43206-0238
Phone: 614-481-4360
Fax: 614-481-4363
e-mail: mail@thepheonixonline.org
Web Site: www.thepheonixonline.org
Management:
　Artistic Director: Steven C Anderson
　Marketing Associate: Lonelle Yoder
Mission: We are a non-profit theatre for young audiences dedicated to providing quality arts opportunities and arts education programs for Central Ohio.
Founded: 1993
Specialized Field: Children's Theatre
Status: Professional; Nonprofit
Paid Staff: 8
Paid Artists: 10
Performs At: Vern Riffg Center for Government and the Arts
Facility Category: Government Run Facility
Type of Stage: 3/4 Thrust and Proscenium
Seating Capacity: 180 and 240
Organization Type: Performing; Educational

3603 PLAYERS THEATRE COLUMBUS

77 S High Street
Columbus, OH 43215
Mailing Address: PO Box 18185, Columbus, OH 43218-0185
Phone: 614-228-9456
Fax: 614-621-2338
Management:
　Artistic Director: Ed Graczyk
　Managing Director: Jean Ann Klaus
　Associate Artistic Director: Steven C Anderson
　Marketing Director: Lenore P Kaler
　Public Relations Manager: P Susan Sharrock
　Production Manager: John York
　Production Manager: Carol Dultigg

Mission: Dedicated to providing a broad range of quality theatrical productions to audiences of all ages in Central Ohio.
Founded: 1923
Status: Professional; Nonprofit
Income Sources: League of Resident Theatres; Ohio Theatre Association; Actors' Equity Association; United Scenic Arts; Theatre Communications Group; Cols Area Chamber of Commerce
Performs At: Vein Rifle Center for Government and the Arts
Organization Type: Performing; Touring; Resident; Educational

3604 REALITY THEATRE

736 N Pearl Street
Columbus, OH 43215
Phone: 614-294-7541
e-mail: info@realitytheatre.com
Web Site: www.realitytheatre.com
Management:
　Producer/Artistic Director: Frank A Barnhart
　Producer/Artistic Director: Daneta Shepherd
Mission: Primarily dedicated to the development of experimental plays and also the presentation of original scripts written by Ohio playwrights.
Founded: 1985
Specialized Field: Theatrical Group
Status: Semi-Professional; Nonprofit
Organization Type: Performing; Resident

3605 RED HERRING THEATRE COMPANY

736 N Pearl Street
Columbus, OH 43215
Phone: 614-291-8252
Fax: 614-291-8654
e-mail: info@redherring.org
Web Site: www.redherring.org
Mission: To provide unique theatre experience for audiences of central Ohio.

3606 ROSEBRIAR SHAKESPEARE COMPANY

3211 Indianola Avenue #3
Columbus, OH 43202
Phone: 614-470-1616
e-mail: sdvavies@ohiohistory.org
Web Site: www.wiliqueen.com/rosebriar/
Management:
　Managing Director: Sandra Davies
Founded: 1990
Income Sources: Grants from the Ohio Arts Council; Jefferson Center for Learning and the Arts
Performs At: Davis Discovery Center's Van Fleet Theatre

3607 SHADOWBOX CABARET

164 Easton Town Center
Columbus, OH 43219
Phone: 614-416-7625
Fax: 614-416-7630
Toll-free: 888-887-4230
e-mail: info@shadowboxcabaret.com
Web Site: www.shadowboxcabaret.com
Management:

Artistic Director: Rebecca Gentile
Managing Director: Julie Klein
Literary Manager: Jimmy Makofsky
Director Public Relations: Katy Psenicka
Mission: To change the face of live entertainment so that it meets our standards and to create a self-perpetuating organization that acts as a virus by breeding change and dynamism.
Founded: 1992
Specialized Field: Theatre; Comedy; Rock-n-Roll
Paid Staff: 97
Volunteer Staff: 3
Budget: $2.5 million
Income Sources: Tickets Sales
Annual Attendance: 100,000
Facility Category: Multi-stage Theaters

3608 SRO THEATRE COMPANY
Grandparents' Living Theatre Company
51 Jefferson Avenue
Columbus, OH 43215
Phone: 614-228-7458
Fax: 614-228-2052
e-mail: gplt@glt-theatre.org
Web Site: www.glt-theatre.org
Officers:
   President: Toni Tinsley
   Board Member: Ruth Fullen
   Treasurer: Tom Giusti
Management:
   Executive/Artistic Director: Nancy S Nocks
   Operations Director: Pat Craff
   Touring Director: Ronald E Nocks
Mission: Five original shows and a home season emphatically shatters myths about aging and celebrates life experience. Create theatre that joyously takes risks, is sometimes provacative, but always truthful and unafraid.
Founded: 1985
Specialized Field: Theatre (senior and intergenerational)
Status: Semi-professional; Nonprofit
Paid Staff: 4
Volunteer Staff: 43
Paid Artists: 30
Non-paid Artists: 47
Budget: $150,000
Income Sources: Private Foundations; Grants; Business & Corporate Donations; Box Office; Government Grants; Individual Donations
Affiliations: Ohio Arts Presenters Network; Greater Columbus Convention and Visitors Bureau; Greater Theatre Round Table

3609 STROLLERS THEATRICS
1739 N High Street
Box 36, Ohio Union
Columbus, OH 43201
Phone: 419-841-0007
e-mail: stollers@osu.edu
Web Site: www.osu.edu/students/sst
Mission: Offering Ohio State University students and community members an opportunity for participation in all areas of performing arts.
Founded: 1892

Specialized Field: Musical; Community; Theatrical Group
Status: Non-Professional; Nonprofit
Organization Type: Performing

3610 DAYTON PLAYHOUSE
1301 E Siebenthaler Avenue
Dayton, OH 45414
Phone: 937-333-7469
Fax: 937-333-2827
e-mail: dave@daytonplayhouse.com
Web Site: www.daytonplayhouse.com
Officers:
   Chair: Betty Gould
   Treasurer: Gwen Eberly
Management:
   Executive Director: David Seyer
   Box Office Manager: Marilyn Knox
Founded: 1959
Specialized Field: Musical; Community; Theatrical Group
Status: Non-Professional; Nonprofit
Paid Staff: 2
Volunteer Staff: 600
Income Sources: Membership; MCACD, Culture Works
Performs At: Dayton Playhouse
Affiliations: OCTA; Culture Works
Annual Attendance: 3,000
Seating Capacity: 200
Year Built: 1987
Organization Type: Performing

3611 HUMAN RACE THEATRE COMPANY
126 N Main Street
Suite 300
Dayton, OH 45402-1710
Phone: 937-461-3823
Fax: 937-461-7223
e-mail: contact@humanracetheatre.org
Web Site: www.humanracetheatre.org
Management:
   Artistic Director: Marsha Hanna
   Executive Director: Kevin Moore
Mission: Works to affect the conscience of our community, to see our audience as our partner in the creative experience, to provide a platform for our artists to evolve and explore and to be educational resource for our community. As our name suggests, we present universal themes that explore the human condition and startle us all into a renewed awareness of ourselves.
Founded: 1986
Specialized Field: Theatre
Status: Nonprofit
Paid Staff: 9
Paid Artists: 200
Budget: $1.2 million
Season: September - June
Performs At: The Loft Theatre; Victoria Theatre
Affiliations: AEA
Annual Attendance: 85,000
Type of Stage: Proscenium
Seating Capacity: 1139

3612 SUMMER STOCK AT THE UNIVERSITY OF FINDLAY
1000 N Main Street
Findlay, OH 45840
Phone: 419-424-6924
Fax: 419-424-4822
e-mail: hayes@findlay.edu
Web Site: www.findlay.edu
Management:
   Producing Artistic Director: Scott Hayes
   Curtain Raiser Advisory Chair: Anne Hermiller
Mission: Provide professional theatre opportunities for pre professional thatre students, and produce quality. affordable thatre for northwest Ohio.
Founded: 1977
Specialized Field: Classical Music
Status: Non-Equity; Nonprofit
Paid Staff: 5
Volunteer Staff: 10
Paid Artists: 6
Non-paid Artists: 15
Season: June - August
Type of Stage: Proscenium
Stage Dimensions: 28' x 30'
Seating Capacity: 222
Year Built: 1964
Year Remodeled: 2001

3613 FOSTORIA FOOTLIGHTERS
225 S Poplar Street
PO Box 542
Fostoria, OH 44830
Phone: 419-435-7501
Web Site: www.noguska.net/footlighters
Founded: 1959
Specialized Field: Musical; Community; Theatrical Group
Status: Non-Professional; Nonprofit
Paid Staff: 100
Income Sources: Ohio Community Theatre Alliance
Performs At: Fostoria Footlighters
Organization Type: Performing; Resident; Educational

3614 CURTAIN PLAYERS
5691 Harlem Road
Galena, OH 43086
Mailing Address: PO Box 1143 Westerville, OH 43086
Phone: 614-885-7000
Fax: 614-470-4809
e-mail: curtainplayers@mail.com
Web Site: www.curtainplayers.com
Officers:
   President: Sherry Erickson
   VP: Douglas Browell
   Secretary: Joyce Prochaska
   Treasurer: David Erickson
Management:
   Business Manager: Linda Sopp
   Production Manager: Deborah Singer
   Artistic Director: Michael Schacherbauer
Founded: 1963
Seating Capacity: 76

3615 PORTHOUSE THEATRE COMPANY
PO Box 5190
Kent, OH 44242
Phone: 330-672-3884
Fax: 330-672-2889
Web Site: www.theatre.kent.edu/porthouse/index.htm
Management:
   Producing Director: John R Crawford
   Producing Manager: Karl Erdmann
   Production Stage Manager: Rebbeca M Balogh
   Artistic Director: Terri Kent
   Managing Director: Jeff Cruszewski
Founded: 1968
Specialized Field: Summer Stock; Musical; Theatrical Group
Status: Professional; Semi-Professional; Nonprofit
Income Sources: Kent State University
Season: June - August
Performs At: Porthouse Theatre of Blossom Music Center
Type of Stage: Outdoor, Covered Pavilion Theatre
Seating Capacity: 450
Organization Type: Performing; Educational

3616 BECK CENTER FOR THE CULTURAL ARTS
17801 Detroit Avenue
Lakewood, OH 44107
Phone: 216-521-2540
Fax: 216-228-6050
Web Site: www.lkwdpl.org/beck
Officers:
   President: Rosemary Corcoran
   VP: Brian King
   Treasurer: Marjorie Wiess
Management:
   Acting Artistic Director: Scott Spencer
   Managing Director: Andrea Krist
   Executive Director: Bill Beckenbach
   Director Education: Linda Sackett
   Production/Design: Don McBride
Mission: To be a comprehensive community arts center focusing on theater, arts education, and gallery exhibitions.
Founded: 1930
Specialized Field: Dance; Theater; Visual Arts and Music
Status: Non-Professional
Paid Staff: 200
Annual Attendance: 12,000
Organization Type: Performing; Touring; Resident; Educational

3617 CLEVELAND SHAKESPEARE FESTIVAL
PO Box 771430
Lakewood, OH 44107
Phone: 216-732-3311
e-mail: info@cleveshakes.org
Web Site: www.cleveshakes.org
Management:
   Managing Director: Joshua Brown
   Co-Artistic Director: Kelly Elliot
   Co-Artistic Director: Larry Nehring
   Education Director: Tonya Beckman Ross

Mission: Committed to producing the plays of Shakespeare in the way that the author intened—fun, at the speed of thought, and in the midst of a vibrant community. To that end, they are committed to free admission, a festive atmosphere, and an earned attention to the work of the play.

3618 MANSFIELD PLAYHOUSE
95 E Third Street
Mansfield, OH 44902
Phone: 419-522-8140
Fax: 419-522-8446
Web Site: www.mansfieldplayhouse.com
Officers:
   President: Char Hutchison
   First VP: Mark Jordan
   Second VP: Dan Fetertag
   Secretary: Dauphne Maloney
   Treasurer: Hugh Maxwell
Management:
   Business Manager: Cliff Mears
   Theatre Manager: Susie Schaus
Mission: Providing entertainment and encouraging all branches of theatre arts.
Founded: 1929
Specialized Field: Musical; Community; Theatrical Group
Status: Non-Professional
Income Sources: Ohio Theatre Association; Ohio Arts Council; Ohio Community Theatre Alliance
Organization Type: Performing; Touring; Resident; Educational

3619 RENAISSANCE THEATRE
138 Park Avenue W
PO Box 789
Mansfield, OH 44901-0789
Phone: 419-522-2726
Fax: 419-524-7098
e-mail: rpaa@rparts.org
Web Site: www.rparts.org
Officers:
   President/CEO: Dr. Thomas J Carto
Management:
   Development Director: Shelley A Mauk
   Operations Manager: Darlene Taylor
   Technical Director: Scott Gross
   Marketing Director: Martha Fort
Mission: To operate a community and regional entertainment, cultural, educational and civic center; to preserve and restore the Renaissance Theatre.
Founded: 1979
Specialized Field: Community
Status: Professional; Semi-Professional; Nonprofit; Commercial
Paid Staff: 25
Volunteer Staff: 300
Budget: $1.4 Million
Income Sources: Association of Performing Arts Presenters; ORACLE; Ohio Theatre Association
Performs At: Renaissance Theatre
Affiliations: American Symphony Orchestra league, Association of Performing Arts Presenters
Annual Attendance: 65,000
Facility Category: Performing arts theatre

Type of Stage: proscenium
Stage Dimensions: 47 x 26
Seating Capacity: 1,406
Year Built: 1928
Year Remodeled: 1982
Cost: $2.5 Million
Rental Contact: Operations Manager Darlene Taylor
Organization Type: Performing; Educational; Sponsoring

3620 SHOWBOAT BECKY THATCHER
237 Front Street
PO Box 572
Marietta, OH 45750
Phone: 740-373-6033
Fax: 740-373-6084
Toll-free: 877-746-2628
e-mail: showboat@axces.com
Web Site: www.marietta-ohio.com/becky thatcher
Management:
   Executive Director: Jena L Blair
Founded: 1975
Status: Non-Equity; Nonprofit
Paid Staff: 6
Volunteer Staff: 25
Paid Artists: 30
Non-paid Artists: 10
Season: June - August
Type of Stage: Proscenium
Stage Dimensions: 26' x 14'
Seating Capacity: 200
Year Built: 1926

3621 PALACE THEATRE
276 W Center Street
Marion, OH 43302
Phone: 740-383-2101
Fax: 740-387-3425
e-mail: marionpalace@marion.net
Web Site: www.marionpalace.org
Officers:
   Board President: Sue Jacob
   Board VP: Mike Greeley
Management:
   Operations Director: Bev Ford
   Executive Director: Elaine Merchant
   Stage Manager: Steve Beltz
   Business Manager: Veronica Bodine
Mission: To stimulate, promote and develop interest in the dramatic arts by operation of a permanent theatre.
Founded: 1976
Specialized Field: Musical; Theatrical Group
Status: Nonprofit
Paid Staff: 8
Income Sources: Ohio Arts Council; Private Foundations; Donations
Performs At: Palace Theatre
Affiliations: League of Historic American Theatres
Annual Attendance: 77,650
Seating Capacity: 1420
Year Built: 1928
Year Remodeled: 1976
Organization Type: Performing; Educational

3622 TRUMPET IN THE LAND
Schoenbrunn Amphitheatre
PO Box 450
New Philadelphia, OH 44663
Phone: 330-364-5111
Fax: 330-339-1132
e-mail: trumpet@tusco.net
Web Site: www.tusco.net/trumpet
Management:
    General Manager: Margaret M Bonamico
Founded: 1965
Status: Nonprofit
Season: June - August
Type of Stage: Proscenium
Stage Dimensions: 40' x 30'
Seating Capacity: 1400

3623 LICKING COUNTY PLAYERS
131 W Main Street
PO Box 945
Newark, OH 43058-0945
Phone: 740-349-2287
e-mail: hobbit275@adelphia.net
Web Site: lcp.tripod.com
Officers:
    President: John Roberts
    VP: Aara Chapman
    Treasurer: Joe Higginbotham
    Secretary: Sue Salina
Mission: To preserve, promote, and perform all types of living theater in the community.

3624 WEATHERVANE PLAYHOUSE
100 Price Road
PO Box 607
Newark, OH 43058-0607
Phone: 330-366-4616
Fax: 330-344-3185
e-mail: email@weathervaneplayhouse.org
Web Site: www.weathervaneplayhouse.com
Management:
    Managing/Artistic Director: Tony Mata
Founded: 1968
Status: Non-Equity; Nonprofit
Season: June - August
Type of Stage: Thrust
Stage Dimensions: 30' x 30'
Seating Capacity: 333

3625 TOWNE AND COUNTRY PLAYERS
PO Box 117
Norwalk, OH 45380
Phone: 937-526-5566
e-mail: info@tcplayers.com
Web Site: www.tcplayers.com
Management:
    Executive Director: Ronn Koerper
Mission: Providing family entertainment.
Founded: 1973
Specialized Field: Musical; Dinner; Community; Theatrical Group
Status: Semi-Professional; Nonprofit
Paid Staff: 2
Performs At: Historic Shrine Theatre

Annual Attendance: 40,000
Year Remodeled: 1941
Organization Type: Performing

3626 CEDAR POINT LIVE ENTERTAINMENT
One Cedar Point Drive
Sandusky, OH 44870-5259
Phone: 419-627-2390
Fax: 419-627-2389
e-mail: liveshows@cedarpoint.com
Web Site: www.cedarpoint.com
Management:
    Manager: Herbe Donald English
Founded: 1870
Status: Non-Equity; Commercial
Paid Staff: 100
Season: May - October
Annual Attendance: 3 million
Facility Category: Theme Park

3627 SANDUSKY STATE THEATRE
107 Columbus Avenue
Sandusky, OH 44870
Phone: 419-626-1950
Fax: 419-626-2994
e-mail: rdipple@state-theatre.com
Management:
    Executive Director: Rob Dippel
Mission: Performing Arts Center.
Founded: 1988
Paid Staff: 9
Volunteer Staff: 150
Budget: $150,000-400,000
Income Sources: Ticket Sales; Sponsorship; Grants
Type of Stage: Proscenium
Seating Capacity: 1,600

3628 TOLEDO CULTURAL ARTS CENTER VALENTINE THEATRE
425 N Saint Clair Street
Springfield, OH 43604-1407
Phone: 419-242-3490
Fax: 419-242-2791
e-mail: valentine@glasscity.net
Web Site: www.valentinetheatre.comil.org
Management:
    Executive Director: Dale Vivirito
    Director Devolpment: Roseann Buck
    Technical Director: Tim Durham
    Special Events Coordinator: Dan Heberling
Paid Staff: 20
Volunteer Staff: 185
Paid Artists: 20

3629 RITZ THEATRE
PO Box 289
30 S Washington Street
Tiffin, OH 44883
Phone: 419-448-8544
Fax: 419-448-7410
e-mail: dennis@ritztheatre.org
Web Site: www.ritztheatre.org
Management:

Executive Director: Dennis Sankovich
Budget: $400,000-1,000,000
Performs At: Studio Theatre
Seating Capacity: 1,260

3630 OHIO THEATRE
3114 Lagrange Street
Toledo, OH 43608-1802
Phone: 419-241-6785
Fax: 419-241-2151
e-mail: info@theohiotheatre.org
Web Site: www.theohiotheatre.org
Management:
  President/Manager: Geraldine Simpson
Mission: To preserve the historic neighborhood theatre.
Founded: 1921
Paid Staff: 1
Volunteer Staff: 50
Budget: $35,000-60,000
Type of Stage: Thrust
Seating Capacity: 964
Year Built: 1921

3631 TOLEDO REPERTOIRE THEATRE
1717 Adams Street
Toledo, OH 43624
Phone: 419-243-9277
Fax: 419-243-0454
Web Site: www.toledorep.org
Officers:
  Chairman: Douglas Braun
  President: Michael Calabrese
  Second VP: Carlane Miller
Management:
  Artistic Director/CEO: Brian D Bethune
  Marketing/Development Director: Matthew Kizaur
  Resident Tech Director/Lighting Des: Michael Oesch
Mission: To entertain, educate, and provide services to Toledo and the surrounding region through the disciplines of theatre.
Founded: 1933
Specialized Field: Theatrical Group
Status: Semi-Professional; Nonprofit
Income Sources: Ohio Concerned Citizens for the Arts
Organization Type: Performing; Educational

3632 MAD RIVER THEATER WORKS
PO Box 248
West Liberty, OH 43357
Phone: 937-465-6751
e-mail: madriver@bright.net
Web Site: www.madrivertheater.org
Management:
  Marketing Director: Jeff Hooper
  Administrative Director: Laurie Collins
  Composer/Musical Director: Bob Lucas
Mission: Our purpose is to create and produce plays that explore the concerns of rural people and to perform these works for multi-generational, primarily rural audiences.
Founded: 1978
Specialized Field: Musical; Theatrical Group
Status: Professional; Nonprofit
Income Sources: Theatre Communications Group

Organization Type: Performing; Touring; Resident; Educational

3633 BLUE JACKET, FIRST FRONTIER
PO Box C
Xenia, OH 45385-0692
Phone: 937-376-4358
Fax: 937-376-5364
Toll-free: 877-465-2583
e-mail: bjacket@aol.com
Web Site: www.bluejacketdrama.com
Management:
  Executive Producer: Jan Abel
  Associate Producer: Ron Gray
  Marketing Director/Public Relations: Scott Galbraith
  Business Manager: Tina Neff
Founded: 1982
Status: Nonprofit
Season: June - August
Annual Attendance: 50,000
Facility Category: Outdoor Amphitheatre
Type of Stage: Amphitheater
Seating Capacity: 1,500

3634 YOUNGSTOWN PLAYHOUSE
600 Playhouse Lane
Youngstown, OH 44511
Phone: 330-788-8739
Fax: 330-788-1208
e-mail: playhouselane@hotmail.com
Web Site: www.youngstownplayhouse.com
Management:
  Artistic Director: David Vosburgh
  Managing Director: Robert Vargo
Budget: $10,000
Seating Capacity: 400

Oklahoma

3635 BULLSHED THEATRE PROJECT
5501 E Mountain View Road
Edmond, OK 73034
Phone: 405-341-0928
e-mail: bullshedtheatre@aol.com
Web Site: www.geocities.com/bullshedtheatre
Mission: Using a minimalist approach without sacrificing the artistic intent. From Shakespeare to Shepard, we produce gypsy/guerilla theatre fare. Minimal design, minimal cast equals maximum overdrive.

3636 OKLAHOMA SHAKESPEARE IN THE PARK
PO Box 1171
Edmond, OK 73083
Phone: 405-340-1222
Fax: 405-340-1222
e-mail: okshakespr@aol.com
Management:
  Managing Director: Sue Ellen Reiman
  Artistic Director: Kathryn McGill
Mission: To produce works of Shakespeare; to teach Shakespeare in school.

Founded: 1985
Status: Non-Equity; Nonprofit
Paid Staff: 10
Volunteer Staff: 20
Paid Artists: 40
Non-paid Artists: 12
Budget: $120,000
Income Sources: Ticket Sales; Donations
Season: June - September
Affiliations: University of Oklahoma
Annual Attendance: 10,000
Facility Category: Ampitheatre
Type of Stage: Amphitheatre
Stage Dimensions: 50' x 25'
Seating Capacity: 1000
Year Built: 1990
Year Remodeled: 2002
Cost: $50,000

3637 POLLARD THEATRE

120 W Harrison
PO Box 38
Guthrie, OK 73044
Phone: 405-282-2802
Fax: 405-282-0061
Management:
    Artistic Director: W Jerome Stevenson
    General Manager: Donna Dickson
    Managing Director: Robert D Thompson
Founded: 1987
Status: Nonprofit; Non-Equity
Season: July - June
Type of Stage: Proscenium
Stage Dimensions: 50' x 50'
Seating Capacity: 277

3638 CAMERON UNIVERSITY: THEATRE ARTS DEPARTMENT

2800 W Gore Boulevard
Lawton, OK 73505
Phone: 580-581-2211
e-mail: thescoop@cameron.edu
Web Site: www.cameron.edu
Officers:
    Chair: Scott Richard Klein
Facility Category: Auditorium; Studio Performance; Theatre House
Type of Stage: Flexible; Proscenium
Rental Contact: Scott Hofmann

3639 SOONER THEATRE OF NORMAN

101 E Main
PO Box 6565
Norman, OK 73070
Phone: 405-321-9600
Fax: 405-321-8091
e-mail: stnormanok@aol.com
Web Site: members.aol.com/stnormanok
Management:
    Managing Director: Kelly E Kelsay

3640 LYRIC THEATRE OF OKLAHOMA

1727 NW 16th Street
Civic Center Music Hall-Performance Venue
Oklahoma City, OK 73106
Phone: 405-524-9310
Fax: 405-524-9316
e-mail: lyrictheatreokc.com
Web Site: www.lyrictheatreokc.com
Officers:
    Business Manager: Deborah Minard
Management:
    Artistic Director: Nick Demos
    Executive Director: Paula Stover
    Ticket Operations: Ben Williams
    Public Relations/Marketing Director: Paula Love
    Director Education: Chris Harrod
Mission: Oklahoma's only professional Musical Theatre for 4 years.
Founded: 1962
Specialized Field: Musical Theatre
Status: Professional; Nonprofit
Paid Staff: 9
Budget: $1.7 million
Income Sources: Ticket Sales; Donations from Foundations; Corporations; Individuals
Performs At: The Civic Center Music Hall
Affiliations: AEA; SSDC; IATSE
Annual Attendance: 50,000
Facility Category: Theatre
Type of Stage: Proscenium
Seating Capacity: 1,396
Year Built: 1932
Year Remodeled: 1999
Rental Contact: Bob Lawrence
Organization Type: Performing; Resident

3641 OKLAHOMA CHILDREN'S THEATRE

Fair Park
3000 General Pershing Boulevard
Oklahoma City, OK 73107-6202
Phone: 405-951-0000
Fax: 405-951-0003
e-mail: cacoct@swbell.net
Web Site: www.okchildrenstheatre.com
Officers:
    President: Tim Berney
    Past President: Pat Burns
    Secretary: Carmelita Shinn
    Tresurer: Paul Lienhard
Management:
    Executive Director: Lyn Adams
    Artistic Director: Ellen Webster
    Public Relations Director: Shoshanna Wasserman
    Development Director: Lisa Kibblewhite
Mission: To provide entertaining, educational and accessible experiences through theatrical productions, creative programming and events.
Founded: 1986
Specialized Field: Theatre productions; Touring productions; Children's classes/camps; City Arts Center
Paid Staff: 6
Volunteer Staff: 3
Paid Artists: 40
Performs At: City Arts Center

3642 OKLAHOMA OPERA & MUSICAL THEATER COMPANY
2501 N Blackwelder
Oklahoma City, OK 73106
Phone: 405-521-5315
Fax: 405-521-5971
e-mail: mparker@okcu.edu
Web Site: www.okcu.edu
Management:
   Dean: Mark Edward Parker
Budget: $10,000-20,000
Performs At: Kirkpatrick Fine Arts Auditorium; Burg Theater; Wymberly

3643 STAGE CENTER
400 W California Street
Oklahoma City, OK 73102-5021
Phone: 405-270-4800
Fax: 405-270-4806
e-mail: rmartn@artscouncilokc.com
Web Site: www.artscouncilokc.com
Management:
   Director: Ron Martin
   Operations Manager: Don Lusk
Mission: Provides a facility that bring the arts and community together.
Founded: 1970
Budget: $60,000-150,000
Income Sources: Grants
Performs At: Mary Noble Tolbert Theatre; Arena Theatre
Annual Attendance: 79,000
Facility Category: Multi-use Facility
Type of Stage: Round; Thrust stage
Seating Capacity: 210-580
Year Built: 1970
Year Remodeled: 1987

3644 PONCA PLAYHOUSE
Ponca Playhouse Box Office
107 E Central Avenue
Ponca City, OK 74601
Mailing Address: PO Box 1414 Ponca City, OK 74602
Phone: 580-765-5360
Mission: To offer interested area amateurs opportunities to participate in producing live theatre for the benefit of a discriminating audience.
Founded: 1959
Specialized Field: Musical; Community; Theatrical Group
Status: Non-Professional; Nonprofit; Commercial
Income Sources: American Association of Community Theatres; Oklahoma Community Theatre Association; Southwest Theatre Association
Organization Type: Performing; Touring; Resident

3645 CHEROKEE NATIONAL HISTORICAL SOCIETY
PO Box 515
Tahlequah, OK 74465

Phone: 918-456-6007
Fax: 918-456-6165
Toll-free: 888-999-6007
e-mail: tourism@cherokeeheritage.org
Web Site: www.cherokeeheritage.org
Officers:
   President: Charles/Chief Boyd
   VP: Mary Ellen Meredith
Management:
   Interim Executive Director: Mary Ellen Meredith
   Drama Producer: Patrick Whelan
   Marketing Director: Marilyn Craig
Mission: Seeks to preserve the history and traditions of the Cherokee Indian tribe and to educate the public concerning the Cherokee story through the presentation of the Trail of Tears drama and other cultural presentations.
Founded: 1964
Specialized Field: Theatrical Group
Status: Professional; Nonprofit
Paid Staff: 30
Volunteer Staff: 25
Income Sources: Tourism and Recreation Department, State of Oklahoma
Performs At: Cherokee Heritage Center Tsa La Gi Amphitheater
Annual Attendance: 16,000
Facility Category: Amphitheater
Stage Dimensions: 80'x40'
Seating Capacity: 1,800
Year Built: 1969
Cost: 500,000
Rental Contact: Seth Hecht
Organization Type: Resident; Educational

3646 NORTHEASTERN STATE UNIVERSITY SIZZLIN' SUMMER SHOWCASE
Northeastern State University
College of Arts & Letters
609 N Grand Avenue
Tahlequah, OK 74464
Phone: 918-456-5511
Fax: 918-458-2348
e-mail: robinska@nsuok.edu
Web Site: www.nsuok.edu
Management:
   Producer: Charles Seat
   Technical Director: Ecott Pursley
Founded: 1983
Specialized Field: Musical Theatre
Status: Non-Equity; Commercial
Paid Staff: 50
Volunteer Staff: 1
Paid Artists: 35
Season: June - August
Type of Stage: Proscenium
Stage Dimensions: 35' x 40'
Seating Capacity: 200

3647 AMERICAN THEATRE COMPANY
PO Box 1265
Tulsa, OK 74101
Phone: 914-747-9494
Management:
   Producing Artistis Director: Kitty Roberts

Managing Director: Linda Kidd

3648 DISCOVERYLAND!
W 41st Street
Tulsa, OK 74136
Phone: 918-742-6552
Fax: 918-743-7059
Management:
    Casting Director: Rosemary Beckham
Founded: 1976
Status: Non-Equity; Commercial
Season: June - August
Type of Stage: Arena
Seating Capacity: 2200

3649 THEATRE TULSA
207 N Main
Tulsa, OK 74103
Phone: 918-587-8402
Fax: 918-592-0848
e-mail: theatretul@aol.com
Web Site: www.theatretulsa.org
Management:
    Office Manager: Kelly Jackson
Mission: To provide enrichment, entertainment and
education to all sectors of the community by facilitating
participation in the theatre arts.
Founded: 1922
Specialized Field: Community; Theatrical Group
Status: Non-Professional; Nonprofit
Paid Staff: 100
Income Sources: Oklahoma Community Theatre
Association; State Arts Council of Oklahoma
Performs At: Performing Arts Center
Organization Type: Performing; Touring; Resident;
Educational; Sponsoring

**3650 WOODWARD ARTS AND THEATRE
COUNCIL**
818 Main
PO Box 1523
Woodward, OK 73802-1523
Phone: 580-256-7120
Fax: 580-256-7120
Management:
    Executive Director: Jeanie K Raymer
Mission: To foster and promote cultural arts activities in
Woodward and surrounding areas; to own and operate
Woodward Arts Theatre.
Founded: 1981
Specialized Field: Musical; Community; Theatrical
Group
Status: Nonprofit
Income Sources: State Arts Council of Oklahoma
Organization Type: Performing; Sponsoring

**3651 OREGON SHAKESPEAREAN FESTIVAL
ASSOCIATION**
15 S Pioneer
PO Box 158
Ashland, OR 97520
Phone: 541-482-4331
Fax: 541-482-0446
Web Site: www.osfashland.org
Management:
    Artistic Director: Libby Appel
    Executive Director: Paul Nicholson
    Director Marketing/Communications: Janeen Olsen
Mission: To create bold new interpretations of
contemporary and classic plays in repertory, influenced by
American diversity and inspired by the high standard of
Shakespeare.
Founded: 1935
Specialized Field: Performance Arts/Shakespeare
Status: Professional; Nonprofit
Paid Staff: 450
Volunteer Staff: 750
Budget: 23,000,000
Income Sources: Earned; Contributed
Season: June - August
Performs At: Angus Bowmer Theatre; New Theatre;
Elizabethan Theatre
Affiliations: Actors' Equity Association; ATA;
University/Resident Theatre Association; Theatre
Communications Group
Annual Attendance: 375,000
Type of Stage: Thrust Stage; Black Box; Outdoors
Seating Capacity: 601; 250; 1188
Organization Type: Performing; Touring; Resident;
Educational

3652 QUARTZ THEATRE
392 Taylor
Ashland, OR 97520
Phone: 513-482-8119
Management:
    Artistic Director: Robert Spira
Mission: The development of playwrights.
Founded: 1976
Specialized Field: Theatrical Group
Status: Nonprofit
Organization Type: Performing

**3653 COMMUNITY THEATRE OF THE
CASCADES**
148 NW Greenwood
Bend, OR 97701
Phone: 541-389-0803
Management:
    Business Manager: Barbara Matlick
Mission: To offer quality live theatre to the community.
Founded: 1978
Specialized Field: Musical; Community; Theatrical
Group
Status: Non-Professional; Nonprofit
Paid Staff: 50
Income Sources: Oregon Theatre Association
Organization Type: Performing

3654 MAINSTAGE THEATRE COMPANY

996 Willamette Street
Eugene, OR 97401
Phone: 541-683-4368
Management:
   Producer/Executive Director: Jim Roberts
   Artistic Director: Joe Zingo
Mission: To offer a broad range of experiences to participants and audiences in both a professional theater and community theatre atmosphere.
Founded: 1979
Specialized Field: Musical; Dinner; Community; Theatrical Group
Status: Professional; Semi-Professional; Non-Professional; Nonprofit
Paid Staff: 100
Performs At: Downtown Cabaret; Eugene Downtown Mall
Organization Type: Performing

3655 OREGON FANTASY THEATRE

Celeste Rose
820 E 36th Avenue
Eugene, OR 97405
Phone: 541-686-1574
Management:
   Director: Celeste Rose
Mission: Producing and performing puppet shows which combine live actors with hand puppets, marionettes, shadows and masks.
Founded: 1978
Specialized Field: Musical; Community; Theatrical Group; Puppet
Status: Professional; Non-Professional; Commercial
Paid Staff: 3
Income Sources: Puppeteers of America
Performs At: Hult Center for the Performing Arts
Organization Type: Performing; Touring; Educational

3656 ROGUE MUSIC THEATRE

PO Box 862
980 SW 6th Street
Grants Pass, OR 97526
Phone: 541-479-2559
Fax: 541-471-0919
Web Site: www.rogueweb.com
Management:
   Artistic Director: Richard Jessup
Mission: To provide the highest quality musical theatre to the home region and beyond.
Specialized Field: Musical Theatre, Education
Status: Non-profit
Paid Staff: 4
Volunteer Staff: 100
Paid Artists: 110
Non-paid Artists: 10
Budget: $150,000-400,000
Annual Attendance: 11,000
Facility Category: Outdoor ampitheatre
Type of Stage: Proscenium
Stage Dimensions: 35'x70'
Seating Capacity: 1,385
Year Built: 1915
Year Remodeled: 1978

3657 ROSS RAGLAND THEATRE

218 N 7th Street
Klamath Falls, OR 97601-6017
Phone: 541-884-0651
Fax: 541-884-8574
e-mail: rrt@rrtheatre.org
Web Site: www.rrtheatre.org
Management:
   Executive Director: Susan Malins
Founded: 1990
Specialized Field: Multidisciplinary
Status: Non-Profit
Paid Staff: 7
Volunteer Staff: 80
Paid Artists: 35
Non-paid Artists: 20
Budget: $600,000

3658 ROSS RAGLAND THEATER

218 N 7th Street
Klamath Falls, OR 97601-6017
Phone: 541-884-5483
Fax: 541-884-8574
e-mail: rrt@kfalls.net
Web Site: www.rrtheater.org
Management:
   Executive Director: Steve Lents
Paid Staff: 11
Volunteer Staff: 80
Paid Artists: 40
Non-paid Artists: 40
Facility Category: Performing Arts Center
Type of Stage: Proscenium
Stage Dimensions: 51x45
Seating Capacity: 700
Year Remodeled: 1989
Rental Contact: Kelly Buckles

3659 LAKEWOOD THEATRE COMPANY

368 S State Street
PO Box 274
Lake Oswego, OR 97034
Phone: 503-635-3901
Fax: 503-635-2002
e-mail: center.info@lakewood-center.org
Web Site: www.lakewood-center.org
Officers:
   President: Malcolm Mathes
Management:
   Executive Director: Andrew Edwards
   Executive Producer: Kay Vega
Mission: Establishment and maintenance of a permanent multi-arts and theatre facility; the sponsorship and coordination of education and cultural programming in visual arts, theatre and community events.
Founded: 1952
Specialized Field: Musical; Community; Theatrical Group
Status: Non-Professional; Nonprofit
Paid Staff: 10
Volunteer Staff: 150
Paid Artists: 150
Non-paid Artists: 100
Budget: $700,000

Income Sources: Oregon Theatre Association; Oregon Advocates for the Arts; Portland Area Theatre Alliance
Season: June - September
Annual Attendance: 30,000
Facility Category: Arts Facility
Type of Stage: Thrust
Stage Dimensions: 30'x30'
Seating Capacity: 196
Year Built: 1980
Cost: $80,000
Organization Type: Performing; Resident; Educational; Sponsoring

3660 GALLERY THEATRE OF OREGON
210 N Ford
PO Box 245
McMinnville, OR 97128
Phone: 503-472-2227
Fax: 503-434-1394
Web Site: gallerytheatre.com
Officers:
President: Ken Moore
VP: Lea New
Secretary: Barbara Knutson
Treasurer: Ken Myers
Management:
Managing Director: Jane Maddox
Mission: To provide a performing arts center in Yamhill County.
Founded: 1968
Specialized Field: Musical; Community
Status: Nonprofit
Paid Staff: 2
Type of Stage: Black Box; Mainstage
Stage Dimensions: 20'x40'
Seating Capacity: 240-100
Year Built: 1968
Year Remodeled: 1992
Organization Type: Performing; Educational

3661 BRITT FESTIVALS
PO Box 1124
Medford, OR 97501
Phone: 541-779-0847
Fax: 541-776-3712
e-mail: info@brittfest.org
Web Site: www.brittfest.org
Management:
Executive Director: Ron McUne
Music Director: Peter Bay
Marketing/Public Relations Director: Kelly Gonzales
Development Director: Ed Foss
Booking/Production Director: Mike Sturgill
Education Director: David MacKenzie
Mission: To present and sponsor, in Southern Oregon, performing arts of the highest quality for the education, enrichment and enjoyment of all.
Founded: 1963
Specialized Field: Classical; Jazz; Blues; Pop/Rock; Country; Folk; Bluegrass; World Music; Dance; Musical Theater; Comedy
Status: Professional; Nonprofit
Paid Staff: 12
Volunteer Staff: 600
Performs At: The Britt Gardens

Annual Attendance: 70,000
Facility Category: Outdoor Amphitheatre
Seating Capacity: 2200
Year Built: 1963
Year Remodeled: 1992
Organization Type: Performing; Touring; Resident; Educational; Sponsoring

3662 DOLPHIN PLAYERS
2540 Union
North Bend, OR 97459
Phone: 503-756-7088
Mission: Presenting quality theater in a comfortable intimate setting.
Founded: 1980
Specialized Field: Musical; Dinner; Community; Theatrical Group
Status: Non-Professional; Nonprofit
Paid Staff: 50
Organization Type: Performing; Resident; Educational; Sponsoring

3663 ARLENE SCHNITZER CONCERT HALL
1111 SW Broadway
Portland, OR 97205
Phone: 503-248-4335
Fax: 503-274-7490
e-mail: lori@pcpa.com
Web Site: www.pcpa.com
Management:
Booking: Lori Kramer
Director: Robyn Williams
Operations Manager: Don Scorby
Box Office Manager: Ron Sanders
Event Services Manager: Patricia Iron
Booking Coordinator: Judy Siemssen
Paid Staff: 130
Volunteer Staff: 600
Budget: $8 Million
Income Sources: Hotel/Motel Tax; City; County & Regional Government
Affiliations: Oregon Symphony
Annual Attendance: 300,000
Facility Category: Concert Hall
Type of Stage: Proscenium
Stage Dimensions: 54'x40'
Seating Capacity: 2,992
Year Built: 1928
Year Remodeled: 1984
Cost: $10,000,000
Rental Contact: Lori Kramer
Resident Groups: Oregon Symphony Orchestra

3664 ARTISTS REPERTORY THEATRE
1516 SW Alder Street
Portland, OR 97205
Phone: 503-241-1278
Fax: 503-241-8268
e-mail: allen@artistsrep.org
Web Site: www.artistsrep.org
Management:
Artistic Director: Allen Nause
Founded: 1981
Performs At: Reiersgaard Theatre

Type of Stage: Flexible Black Box
Seating Capacity: 170

3665 BRODY THEATER
1904 NW 27th Avenue
Portland, OR 97210
Phone: 503-224-0688
e-mail: info@brodytheater.com
Web Site: www.brodytheater.com
Mission: The Brody's double focus on entertainment and experiment, marks it as a showcase for both audience-pleasing performances and cutting edge theatrical presentation.
Founded: 1996
Specialized Field: Focuses on entertainment and experiment

3666 DOLORES WINNING STAD THEATRE
1111 SW Broadway
Portland, OR 97205
Phone: 503-248-1335
Fax: 503-274-7490
e-mail: lori@pcpa.com
Web Site: www.pcpa.com
Management:
    Booking Manager: Lori Kramer
    Booking Coordinator: Judy Siemssen
    Operations Manager: Don Scorby
    Box Office Manage: Ron Sanders
    Director: Robyn Williams
    Event Services Manager: Patricia Iron
Paid Staff: 130
Volunteer Staff: 600
Budget: $8 Million
Income Sources: City; County; Regional Government; Hotel-Motel Tax
Annual Attendance: 200,000
Facility Category: Black box
Type of Stage: Black Box
Seating Capacity: 292
Year Built: 1987

3667 MIRACLE THEATRE GROUP
425 SE 6th Avenue
Portland, OR 97214
Phone: 503-236-7253
Fax: 503-236-4174
e-mail: miracle@milagro.org
Web Site: www.milagro.org
Officers:
    Chair Board of Directors: Ann Marcus
Management:
    Artistic Director/Founder: Danielle Malan
    Dance Director: Rebecca Martinez
    Director Dance Education: Catherine Evleshin
Mission: Provides programming that includes public performances as well as specialized touring and education projects that currently encompass all of the Western states and the countries of Mexico and Canada. Incorporated as a nonprofit organization in 1985. The Miracle Theatre Group oversees three professional performance companies: Miracle Mainstate, Teatro Milagro, and the Milagro Bailadores.
Founded: 1985

Specialized Field: Hispanic Theater; Arts
Status: Nonprofit
Performs At: Miracle Theatre; 525 SE Stark
Rental Contact: Alice Snyder

3668 NEWMARK THEATRE
1111 SW Broadway
Portland, OR 97205
Phone: 503-248-4335
Fax: 503-274-7490
e-mail: lori@pcpa.com
Web Site: www.pcpa.com
Management:
    Booking Manager: Lori Kramer
    Booking Coordinator: Judy Siemssen
    Operations Manager: Don Scorby
    Box Office Manager: Ron Sandersr
    Director: Robyn Williams
    Event Services Manager: Patricia Iron
Paid Staff: 130
Volunteer Staff: 600
Budget: $8 Million
Income Sources: City; County; Regional Government; Hotel-Motel Tax
Performs At: Theatre, dance, choral, chamber music
Affiliations: Oregon Symphony Orchestra
Annual Attendance: 200,000
Facility Category: Concert Hall
Type of Stage: Proscenium
Stage Dimensions: 48'6" x 56'
Orchestra Pit: 1
Seating Capacity: 880
Year Built: 1987
Architect: Rapp & Rapp
Cost: $18,000,000

3669 OREGON CHILDREN'S THEATRE
600 SW 10th
Suite 501
Portland, OR 97205-2723
Phone: 503-228-9571
Fax: 503-228-3545
e-mail: info@octc.org
Web Site: www.octc.org
Officers:
    Board President: Mark Wilcox
Management:
    Executive Producer: Sondra Pearlman
    Director Marketing: Sharon Martell
Mission: To present professional live theatre for youth at a price affordable to schools and families; to educate young people to the wonders of live theatre.
Specialized Field: Contemporary Children's Literature
Performs At: Keller Auditorium
Annual Attendance: 100,000

3670 PORTLAND ACTORS ENSEMBLE
PO Box 8671
Portland, OR 97207
Phone: 503-321-0710
Web Site: www.portlandactors.org
Mission: To bring financially accessible classical theatre to Portland communities in a non-traditional environment.
Founded: 1970

Specialized Field: Shakespeare-in-the-parks program

3671 PORTLAND CENTER STAGE

1111 SW Broadway
PO Box 9008
Portland, OR 97207
Phone: 503-274-6588
Fax: 503-228-7058
e-mail: webmaster@pcs.org
Web Site: www.pcs.org
Management:
    Artistic Director: Chris Coleman
Founded: 1988
Status: Nonprofit
Season: October - April
Type of Stage: Partial Thrust
Seating Capacity: 860

3672 STARK RAVING THEATRE

3430 SE Belmont Street
Portland, OR 97214
Phone: 503-232-7072
Web Site: www.starkravingtheatre.org/resident.htm
Officers:
    President: Lani Miller
    Treasurer: Catherine Scheidler
    Secretary: Jane Davies
Management:
    Artistic Director: Dave Demke
    Associate Artistic Director: Jim Davis
    Outreach Coordinator: Adrienne Flagg
    Marketing Manager: David Seitz
    Business Manager: Steve Alexander
    Box Office Manager: Jim Wilhite
    Production Manager/Technical: Ian Smith
Founded: 1988

3673 TYGRES HEART SHAKESPEARE COMPANY

PO Box 12650
Portland, OR 97212-0650
Phone: 503-288-8400
Fax: 503-288-8401
e-mail: tygre@teleport.com
Web Site: www.tygresheart.org
Founded: 1989
Status: Non-Equity; Nonprofit
Paid Staff: 5
Season: September - May
Type of Stage: Black Box; Elizabethan
Seating Capacity: 292

3674 PENTACLE THEATRE

324 52nd Avenue
PO Box 186
Salem, OR 97308
Phone: 503-364-7121
Fax: 503-362-6393
e-mail: Pentacle@open.org
Web Site: www.pentacletheatre.org
Officers:
    Founder: Robert Putnam
Management:

General Manager: Lee Ann Reed
Mission: Pentacle's History begin in the early 1950's when a small group of theatre enthusiasts rented a barn (that subsequently became known as The Old Barn) and mounted a four production summer season.
Founded: 1954
Specialized Field: Quality Live Theatre
Paid Staff: 4
Volunteer Staff: 350
Non-paid Artists: 200
Budget: $275,000
Affiliations: AACT

3675 ACTORS THEATRE

Box 780
Talent, OR 97540
Phone: 541-535-5250
e-mail: alzado47@aol.com
Management:
    Artistic Director: Peter Alzado
Founded: 1983
Season: June - August
Performs At: Actors' Theatre
Facility Category: Theatre
Type of Stage: Thrust Stage
Seating Capacity: 108

3676 BROADWAY ROSE THEATRE COMPANY

PO Box 231004
Tigard, OR 97281
Phone: 503-620-5262
Fax: 503-670-8512
e-mail: info@bwayrose.com
Web Site: www.bwayrose.com
Management:
    General Manager: Dan Murphy
Mission: Broadway Rose has been producing live, fun, professional summer stock theater since 1992. As the only professional theater company in Washington County, we provide accessible, quality entertainment.
Founded: 1992
Specialized Field: Theater
Status: Professional; Nonprofit
Season: June - August
Performs At: Deb Fennell Auditorium

3677 ENCHANTED FOREST SUMMER THEATRE

8462 Enchanted Way SE
Turner, OR 97392
Phone: 503-371-4242
Fax: 503-371-6462
e-mail: museact@aol.com
Web Site: www.enchantedforest.com
Management:
    Artistic Director: Susan Vaslev
Mission: To make people of all ages laugh and leave our theatre with wonderful memories.
Founded: 1972
Status: Non-Equity; Commercial
Paid Staff: 2
Paid Artists: 9
Income Sources: Paid Admission

Season: May - September
Annual Attendance: 100,000
Type of Stage: Proscenium
Stage Dimensions: 22' x 25'
Seating Capacity: 300

Pennsylvania

3678 ARDEN THEATRE COMPANY
40 N 2nd Street
PA 19106
Phone: 215-922-8900
Fax: 215-922-7011
Web Site: www.ardentheatre.org
Management:
    Producing Artistic Director: Terrence J Nolen
    Managing Director: Amy L Murphy
    Associate Artistic Director: Amy Lincoln
Founded: 1988
Budget: $3,000,000.00
Performs At: Hass Stage/Mainstage; Arcadia
Stage/Studio Theatre
Affiliations: LORT; AEA
Type of Stage: Flexible Stage
Seating Capacity: 400-175

3679 THEATRE OUTLET
29 N 9th Street
Allentown, PA 18101
Phone: 610-820-9270
Fax: 610-820-9130
Management:
    Artistic Director: George Miller
    Executive Director: Kate Scuffle

3680 ACT II PLAYHOUSE
56 E Butler Pike
Ambler, PA 19002
Phone: 215-654-0200
Fax: 215-654-5001
e-mail: act@libertine.org
Management:
    Artistic Director: Steve Blumethal
    Managing Director: Alan Blumenthal
Founded: 1999

3681 SOUTH PARK THEATRE
PO Box 254
Bethel Park, PA 15102
Phone: 412-831-8552
Fax: 412-831-1647
e-mail: sopktheat@aol.com
Web Site: www.southparktheatre.com
Officers:
    President: Robert H Craft Jr
Management:
    Executive Director: Audrey Castracane
Mission: To provide highest quality opera; to broaden public awareness and understanding of opera through education and comunity programming; to support

development of young American singers; to encourage work of new composers to maintain oper as a living arts form.
Founded: 1995
Status: Non-Equity; Nonprofit
Season: May - September
Type of Stage: Proscenium
Stage Dimensions: 24' x 36'
Seating Capacity: 136

3682 TOUCHSTONE THEATRE
321 E 4th Street
Bethlehem, PA 18015
Phone: 610-867-1689
Fax: 610-867-0561
e-mail: touchstone@nni.com
Web Site: www.touchstone.org
Officers:
    President: Paul Pierponit
Management:
    Administrative Director: Jeannette MacDonald
    Artistic Director: Mark McKenna
    Marketing Director: Mary Wright
    Office Manager: Wendy Caskie
Mission: Dedicated to being an active force in the renewal of theatre as a vital art form. At our center is a resident professional acting ensemble rooted both in the local community of Bethlehem, Pennsylvania and the international community.
Founded: 1981
Specialized Field: Professional Theatre Ensemple
Status: Professional; Nonprofit
Paid Staff: 3
Volunteer Staff: 50
Paid Artists: 5
Income Sources: Theatre Communications Group; Theatre Association of Pennsylvania; National Mime Association
Performs At: Touchstone Theatre
Seating Capacity: 72
Year Built: 1980
Organization Type: Performing; Touring; Resident; Educational; Sponsoring

3683 PENN AVENUE THEATRE
4809 Penn Avenue
Bloomfield, PA 15224
Phone: 412-661-7366
Web Site: www.pennavetheatre.com
Management:
    Artistic Director: Michael E Moats
    Box Office Manager: Maria L Moats
    Managing Director: Carla Delaney
    Technical Director: Adolf Hundertmark
    Webmaster: David Stefanac
    Photographer: Meg Stefanac
Mission: They employ local talent, producing high quality, contemporary drama, which is thought-provoking and entertaining for the theatergoer on a budget.
Founded: 1998
Seating Capacity: 100

3684 BLOOMSBURG THEATRE ENSEMBLE
226 Center Street
PO Box 66
Bloomsburg, PA 17815
Phone: 570-784-5530
Fax: 570-784-4912
Toll-free: 800-282-0283
e-mail: bte@bte.org
Web Site: www.bte.org
Officers:
President: Nancy Coulmas
VP: Mike Sigler
Secretary: Dianne Peeling
Treasurer: Harry Ward
Management:
Ensemble Director: James Good
Managing Director: Jon White-Spunner
Director Development: J Scott Atherton
Stage Manager: Jerry Matheny
Founded: 1978
Specialized Field: Professional Regional Theatre Company
Status: Nonprofit
Paid Staff: 25
Volunteer Staff: 4
Paid Artists: 7
Budget: $650,000
Performs At: Alvina Krause Theatre
Type of Stage: Proscenium
Seating Capacity: 350
Rental Contact: Jon White Spunner
Organization Type: Performing; Touring; Resident; Educational; Sponsoring

3685 STATE COLLEGE COMMUNITY THEATRE
Boal Barn Playhouse
Route 322
PO Box 23
Boalsburg, PA 16804
Phone: 814-466-7141
e-mail: info@scctonline.org
Web Site: www.scctonline.org
Officers:
President: Mark Comly
VP: Susanna Ritti
Treasurer: Charlie Wilson
Secretary: Bonnie Spetzer
Management:
Producer: Deborah M Meder
Founded: 1955
Status: Non-Equity; Nonprofit
Season: June - August
Annual Attendance: 2,000
Type of Stage: Arena
Seating Capacity: 201

3686 ALLENBERRY PLAYHOUSE
Route 174
PO Box 7
Boiling Springs, PA 17007
Phone: 717-258-3211
Fax: 717-960-5236
Web Site: www.allenberry.com

Management:
Managing Director: Cate Van Wickler
Artistic Director: Richard I Frost
Producer: Joan I Heinze
Mission: A repertory equity theatre with a season running from April-November.
Founded: 1949
Specialized Field: Theatrical Group
Status: Professional; Commercial
Paid Staff: 15
Paid Artists: 30
Income Sources: Actors' Equity Association; Society for Stage Directors and Choreographers
Season: April - November
Performs At: Allenberry Playhouse
Affiliations: AEA, SSDC, USSA
Annual Attendance: 60,000
Type of Stage: Proscenium
Stage Dimensions: 28'x60'x28'
Seating Capacity: 400
Year Built: 1949
Year Remodeled: 1988
Organization Type: Performing; Resident

3687 BRISTOL RIVERSIDE THEATRE
PO Box 1250
120 Radcliffe Street
Bristol, PA 19007
Phone: 215-785-6664
Fax: 215-785-2762
e-mail: brtboss@aol.com
Web Site: www.brtstage.org
Management:
Producing Artistic Director: Susan D Atkinson
Founded: 1983
Status: Nonprofit
Budget: $35,000-60,000
Performs At: Bristol Riverside Theatre
Type of Stage: Flexible
Seating Capacity: 302

3688 PENNSYLVANIA SHAKESPEARE FESTIVAL
2755 Station Avenue
Center Valley, PA 18034
Phone: 610-282-9455
Fax: 610-282-2084
e-mail: Kathryn.Cousar@desales.edu
Web Site: www.pashakespeare.org
Management:
Artistic Director: Jack Young
Managing Director: Kathryn Cousar
Managing Associate: Robyn Brady
Director Educational Outreach: Sandy Marino
Endowment Director: Gerard J Schubert OSFS
Business Manager: Janice Hein
Founded: 1991
Specialized Field: Professional (Actor's Equity Association) summer repertory festival dedicated to staging quality productions of William Shakespeare and classics.
Status: Nonprofit; Equity
Paid Staff: 6
Volunteer Staff: 200

Paid Artists: 100
Season: May - August
Type of Stage: Thrust
Stage Dimensions: 38' x 40'
Seating Capacity: 473

3689 ROBERT MORRIS COLONIAL THEATRE
Narrows Run Road
Coraopolis, PA 15108
Phone: 412-262-8336
e-mail: cscopp@stargate.net
Management:
    Contact: Craig Coppaway
Mission: To provide our Western Pennsylvania Community with a high standard of community theater in light summer fare and winter classics.
Founded: 1967
Specialized Field: Community
Status: Non-Professional; Nonprofit
Paid Staff: 1
Income Sources: Fundraising
Performs At: Massey Theatre
Annual Attendance: 1,200
Organization Type: Performing; Educational

3690 PENNSYLVANIA RENAISSANCE FAIRE
Box 685
Cornwall, PA 17016
Phone: 717-665-7021
Fax: 717-664-3466
e-mail: royalspk@parenfaire.com
Web Site: www.parenfaire.com
Management:
    Associate Producer: Thomas Roy
Founded: 1980
Status: Non-Equity; Commercial
Season: August - October
Annual Attendance: 200,000
Facility Category: Outdoor Festival
Type of Stage: Outdoor
Year Built: 1980

3691 UPPER DARBY SUMMER STAGE
601 N Lansdowne Avenue
Drexel Hill, PA 19026
Phone: 610-394-1570
Fax: 610-622-6960
e-mail: hdietzler@rcn.com
Web Site: www.udpac.org
Management:
    Executive/Artistic Director: Harry Dietzler
Mission: One of the nations most sucessfully youth theater programs, producing sic children's musicals and a mainstage Broadway show. We involve more than 600 youth ages 11 through 25 and employ more than 70 professionals and staff.
Founded: 1976
Specialized Field: Theater; Music; Dance
Status: Non-Equity; Nonprofit
Paid Staff: 80
Paid Artists: 25
Budget: $300,000
Income Sources: Government; Fundraising; Ticket Sales

Season: July - August
Facility Category: Performing Arts Center
Type of Stage: Thrust
Stage Dimensions: 50' x 40'
Year Built: 1960
Year Remodeled: 1974

3692 STATE THEATER CENTER FOR THE ARTS
453 Northhampton Street
Easton, PA 18042
Phone: 610-258-7766
Fax: 610-258-2570
Web Site: www.state3thatre.org
Management:
    Executive Director: Shelley Brown

3693 ALLEGHENY HIGHLANDS REGIONAL THEATRE AT CRESSON LAKE
526 W Ogle Street
Ebensburg, PA 15931-1824
Phone: 814-472-4333
Fax: 814-472-4419
e-mail: ahrtclp@aol.com
Web Site: www.geocites.com/cressonlakeplayhouse
Officers:
    President: James Dugan
    Treasurer: Gary Bradley
Management:
    Business Director: Elaine Mastalski
    Artistic Director: Jim Ledford
Mission: AHRT is governed by a Board of Directors. It is a non- profit organization sponsored in a part by Pennsylvania Council on the Arts. The theatre's mission since 1974 is to bring quality entertainment at an affordable price to the rural communities of Central Pennsylvania.
Founded: 1974
Status: Nonprofit
Paid Staff: 50
Volunteer Staff: 30
Non-paid Artists: 100
Season: May-October
Performs At: Pre-Civil War Barn
Annual Attendance: 12,000-14,000
Facility Category: Barn Theatre
Type of Stage: Thrust
Seating Capacity: 199
Year Built: 1850
Year Remodeled: 1974
Rental Contact: Office Manager Elaine Mastalski

3694 TOTEM POLE PLAYHOUSE
9555 Golf Course Road
PO Box 603
Fayetteville, PA 17222-0603
Phone: 717-352-2164
Fax: 717-352-8870
Toll-free: 888-805-7056
e-mail: boxoffice@totempoleplayhouse.org
Web Site: www.totempoleplayhouse.org
Officers:
    President/Treasurer: Carl Schurr
    Secretary: Sue McMurtray

Management:
Managing Director: Sue McMurtray
Producing Artistic Director: Carl Schutt
Associate Artistic Director: Wil Love
Mission: To offer the finest professional theater to our local area.
Founded: 1954
Specialized Field: Summer Stock
Status: Professional; Commercial
Paid Staff: 80
Budget: $600,000
Income Sources: Actors' Equity Association
Season: June - August
Performs At: Totem Pole Playhouse
Annual Attendance: 33,300
Facility Category: Summer Theatre
Type of Stage: Proscenium
Seating Capacity: 453
Year Built: 1970
Organization Type: Performing; Resident

3695 BARROW-CIVIC THEATRE

1223 Liberty Street
PO Box 1089
Franklin, PA 16323
Phone: 814-432-5196
Fax: 814-432-6608
Toll-free: 800-537-7769
e-mail: john@barrowtheatre.com
Web Site: www.barrowtheatre.com
Management:
General Manager: John McConnell
Mission: Committed to providing leadership and education in cultural development and performing arts to the region, striving to create a legacy of quality entertainment by tapping the resources of all age group and encouraging the pursuit of artist
Specialized Field: Performing Arts
Seating Capacity: 497

3696 OPEN STAGE OF HARRISBURG

223 Walnut Street
Harrisburg, PA 17101-1711
Phone: 717-232-6736
Fax: 717-232-1505
e-mail: management@openstagehbg.org
Web Site: www.openstagehbg.com
Officers:
President: Marianne M Fisher
Management:
Artistic Director/CEO: Donald L Alsedek
Associate Director: Clair Myers
Educational Director: Anne L Alsedek
Mission: To develop and support an ensemble of theatre artists for the purpose of presenting modern, contemporary and original dramatic literature in close relationship with its audiences; to provide educational opportunites through a school and outreach program.
Founded: 1983
Specialized Field: Theatre
Status: Professional; Nonprofit
Budget: $406,315

Income Sources: Theatre Communications Group; Citizens for the Arts in Pennsylvania; Theatre Association of Pennsylvania; Box Office; Student Tuition; Individual, Public and Private Fundings.
Performs At: Citizens for the Arts in PA
Affiliations: Theatre Communications Group
Annual Attendance: 9000
Facility Category: Theatre
Type of Stage: Black Box
Stage Dimensions: 18x24
Seating Capacity: 99
Year Remodeled: 1991
Rental Contact: Donald L Alscolk
Organization Type: Performing; Touring; Resident; Educational; Sponsoring

3697 THEATRE HARRISBURG

513 Hurlock Street
Harrisburg, PA 17110
Phone: 717-232-5501
Fax: 717-232-5912
e-mail: email@theatreharrisburg.com
Web Site: www.theatreharrisburg.com
Officers:
President: Brian Tyler
VP: Lyle Shughart
Secretary: Linda Matter
Management:
Artistic Director: Thomas G Hostetter
Executive Director: Samuel Kuba
Mission: To provide quality theatrical experiences, opportunities and education to the Capital Region.
Founded: 1926
Specialized Field: Musical; Community; Theatrical Group
Status: Non-Professional; Nonprofit
Paid Staff: 7
Income Sources: Grants
Performs At: Whitaker Center
Annual Attendance: 21,000
Organization Type: Performing; Educational

3698 HERSHEY THEATRE

15 E Caracas Avenue
PO Box 395
Hershey, PA 17033
Phone: 717-534-3411
Fax: 717-533-2882
e-mail: htheatre@hersheytheatre.com
Web Site: www.hersheytheatre.com
Management:
Executive Director: Susan R Fowler
Box Office Manager: Millie Morris
Assistant Box Office Manager: Dennis Norton
Mission: Premiere performing arts center presenting the finest in touring Broadway shows, classical music and dance attractions, and world-renowned entertainers.
Founded: 1933
Specialized Field: Dance; Vocal Music; Instrumental Music; Theater; Grand Opera
Status: Professional; Nonprofit
Paid Staff: 5
Volunteer Staff: 400
Performs At: Hershey Theatre
Annual Attendance: 75,000

Facility Category: Theatre
Type of Stage: Proscenium
Seating Capacity: 1,904
Year Built: 1933
Year Remodeled: 2002
Cost: $3,000,000
Rental Contact: Executive Director Susan Fowler
Organization Type: Touring; Sponsoring

3699 HERSHEYPARK ENTERTAINMENT
100 W Hersheypark Drive
Hershey, PA 17033
Phone: 717-534-3349
Fax: 717-534-3336
e-mail: audition@hersheypa.com
Management:
Manager Resident Shows: Cherie Lingle
Founded: 1976
Status: Non-Equity; Commercial
Season: May - September

3700 KEYSTONE REPERTORY THEATER
104 Waller Hall
Indiana, PA 15705
Mailing Address: 401 S 11th Street Indiana, PA 15705
Phone: 412-357-2965
Fax: 412-357-7899
e-mail: bblackle@grove.iup.edu
Web Site: www.arts.iup.edu/krt
Officers:
Preisdent: George Fender
Management:
Artistic Director: Barbara Blackledge
Associate Artistic Director: Brain Jones
Mission: Professional summer theater bringing theater to rural western PA.
Founded: 1981
Specialized Field: Theater
Status: Nonprofit
Paid Staff: 22
Volunteer Staff: 5
Paid Artists: 15
Budget: $45,000-60,000
Income Sources: Grants; Tickets; Subscriptions; Advertising; Donations
Season: June - July
Affiliations: AEA Special Appearence Contracts
Annual Attendance: 2000-2500
Type of Stage: Black Box
Seating Capacity: 199
Year Built: 1915
Year Remodeled: 1989
Cost: $2 Million

3701 MOUNTAIN PLAYHOUSE
PO Box 205
Jennerstown, PA 15547
Phone: 814-629-9201
Fax: 814-629-6221
e-mail: boxoffice@mountainplayhouse.com
Web Site: www.mountainplayhouse.com
Management:
Artistic Director: Teresa Stoughton Marafino
Resident Director: Henry Scott Baron

Music Director: David Garwood
Founded: 1939
Specialized Field: Dinner Theater; Comedy; Musical; Drama; Classical
Status: Professional; Commercial
Season: May - October
Performs At: Mountain Playhouse
Facility Category: Resident; Educational
Organization Type: Resident; Educational

3702 FULTON OPERA HOUSE/ACTOR'S COMPANY OF PENNSYLVANIA
Box 1865
Lancaster, PA 17608-1865
Phone: 717-394-7133
Fax: 717-397-3780
e-mail: artdir@fultontheatre.org
Web Site: www.fultontheatre.org
Management:
Artistic Director: Michael Mitchell
Founded: 1963
Specialized Field: Theater
Performs At: Fulton Opera House; Studio Theatre
Type of Stage: Proscenium, Black Box
Seating Capacity: 630, 100

3703 SESAME PLACE
100 Sesame Road
Langhome, PA 19047
Phone: 215-752-7070
Fax: 215-741-5300
e-mail: michael.joyce@anhuerserbusch.com
Web Site: www.sesameplace.com
Officers:
Chairman: Jan Cavanaugh
Vice-Chairman: Ann Marie Boweyer
Treasurer: Michael Eiser
Secretary: Joanne Bujnoski
Management:
Director Entertainment: Michael Joyce
Founded: 1980
Status: Non-Equity; Commercial
Season: May - October
Stage Dimensions: 30' x 32'
Seating Capacity: 1000

3704 SAINT VINCENT THEATRE
Saint Vincent College
300 Fraser Purchase Road
Latrobe, PA 15650-2690
Phone: 724-537-8900
Toll-free: 800-782-5549
Web Site: www.stvincent.edu
Management:
Producer: Fr. Thomas Devereux
Co-Chairman: Leo M Rogers
Co-Chairman: David Pomier
Mission: To continue to bring quality opera to out community and to showcase it in out own opera house; to educate the general community in an appreciation of opera and send our outreach programs into the schools of both Manatee and Sarasota counties; to offer statewide touring programs.
Founded: 1969

Status: Nonprofit
Season: May - August
Type of Stage: Half-Round
Stage Dimensions: 32' x 20'
Seating Capacity: 280

3705 PEOPLE'S LIGHT AND THEATRE COMPANY

39 Conestoga Road
Malvern, PA 19355
Phone: 610-647-1900
Fax: 610-640-9521
Officers:
    President: L Frederick Sutherland
    Vice President: Carole F Haas Gravagno
    Treasurer: Sally S Bullard
    Secretary: Hal Real
Management:
    Producing Director: Danny S Fruchter
    Managing Director: Grace E Grillet
    Literary Manager: Alda Cortese
    Communications Director: Mary Bashaw
    Artistic Director: Abigail Adams
    Marketing Director: Wendy E Worthington
    Communications Assistant: Sara Montgomery
Mission: To help unify a culturally diverse society by giving the community barrier-free access to drama that celebrates our joys, terrors and dreams as we struggle to live together in difficult times.
Founded: 1974
Specialized Field: Theatrical Group
Status: Professional; Nonprofit
Income Sources: Actors' Equity Association; League of Resident Theatres
Season: Year-round
Performs At: The People's Light Theater
Organization Type: Performing; Resident; Educational

3706 HEDGEROW THEATRE

64 Rose Valley Road
Media, PA 19063
Phone: 610-565-4211
Web Site: www.hedgerowtheatre.org
Officers:
    Founder: Jasper Deeter
Management:
    Artistic Director: Penelope Reed
    General Manager: John Gallagher
    Fiscal Director: Gay Kuhn
    Literary Manager: Walt Vail
Mission: Hedgerow Theatre is passionately dedicated to producing and performing quality artistic work and is committed to the development of actors, students, and patrons.
Founded: 1923
Specialized Field: Theatre Group
Status: Professional; Non-Equity
Paid Staff: 70
Performs At: Hedgerow Theatre
Type of Stage: Proscenium
Seating Capacity: 144
Organization Type: Performing; Touring; Resident; Educational

3707 MEDIA THEATRE FOR THE PERFORMING ARTS

104 E State Street
323 W State Street
Media, PA 19063
Phone: 610-891-0100
Fax: 610-891-0247
Web Site: www.mediatheatre.com
Management:
    Executive Director: Patrick Ward
    Artistic Director: Jesse Cline
Founded: 1994
Specialized Field: Theatre
Budget: $2,000,000
Income Sources: Grants; Membership; Ticket Sales
Performs At: Proscenium
Affiliations: AEA
Annual Attendance: 80,000
Facility Category: Theatre
Type of Stage: Proscenium
Seating Capacity: 632
Year Built: 1927
Year Remodeled: 1993
Cost: $1,500,000
Rental Contact: Artistic Director Jesse Cline

3708 VAGABOND ACTING TROUPE

PO Box 355
Morgantown, PA 19543
Phone: 610-286-5567
Fax: 610-286-5567
e-mail: Inthelime@aol.com
Web Site: http://hometown.aol.com
Officers:
    President: Ty Furman
    Secretary: April Sandor
    Treasurer: Gavin McCulloch
Management:
    Managing Artistic Director: Aileen McCulloch
    Executive Director: Ty Furman
    Resident Director: Leonard Kelly
    Resident Director: Charlie DelMarcelle
Mission: Family and adult theatre utilizing an intense physical style.
Founded: 1993
Specialized Field: Theatre
Paid Staff: 3
Paid Artists: 15
Budget: $50,000
Income Sources: Ticket Sales; Advertising; Individual Donors; Government and Corporate Sponsorships
Performs At: Contro Thoatra; Montgomery County Cultural Center
Affiliations: Theatre Alliance of Greater Philadelphia
Annual Attendance: 3,000
Type of Stage: Proscenium
Seating Capacity: 70
Year Built: 1995
Rental Contact: Executive Director (610-279-1013 Fran Doyle

3709 GRETNA PRODUCTIONS
Mount Gretna Playhouse
PO Box 578
Mount Gretna, PA 17064
Phone: 717-964-3322
Fax: 717-964-2189
Management:
   Managing Director: Robin Wray
   Producing Director: Al Franklin
   Composer: Allen Krantz
Mission: Is to provide excellent classical music and emphasis on communication and audience.
Founded: 1978
Specialized Field: Theatrical Group
Status: Professional; Nonprofit
Paid Staff: 3
Income Sources: League of Resident Theatres; Actors' Equity Association; Theatre Association of Pennsylvania; Metro Arts of Harrisburg
Performs At: Mt. Gretna Playhouse
Organization Type: Performing; Touring

3710 TIMBERS DINNER THEATRE
Timber Road
PO Box 10
Mount Gretna, PA 17064
Phone: 717-964-3601
Web Site: www.mtgretna.com
Management:
   Production Manager: Katheleen Briody
Mission: Family entertainment, affordable price.
Founded: 1975
Specialized Field: Musical; Dinner
Status: Professional; Commercial
Paid Staff: 25
Paid Artists: 10
Season: June - September
Performs At: Timbers Summer Dinner Theatre
Facility Category: Outdoor/Under Roof (semi-enclosed)
Type of Stage: Proscenium
Seating Capacity: 450
Year Built: 1950
Year Remodeled: 1976
Organization Type: Performing

3711 POCONO PLAYHOUSE
Playhouse Lane
Mountainhome, PA 18342
Phone: 570-595-7456
Fax: 570-595-7465
Management:
   Owner/Producer: Hubert Fryman
   General Manager: Donna McMicken
Founded: 1947
Specialized Field: Musical; Theatrical Group
Status: Professional; Commercial
Season: June - October
Performs At: Pocono Playhouse
Organization Type: Performing; Educational

3712 BUCKS COUNTY PLAYHOUSE
70 S Main
PO Box 313
New Hope, PA 18938
Phone: 215-862-2041
Fax: 215-862-0220
e-mail: mail@buckscountyplayhouse.com
Web Site: www.buckscountyplayhouse.com
Management:
   Artistic Director: Stephen Casey
Founded: 1939
Specialized Field: Musical; Theatrical Group
Status: Professional; Commercial
Performs At: Bucks County Playhouse
Organization Type: Performing; Educational; Partial-Equity Season

3713 AMERICAN FAMILY THEATER
1429 Walnut Street
4th Floor
Philadelphia, PA 19102
Phone: 215-563-3501
Fax: 215-563-1588
Toll-free: 800-822-8487
e-mail: jkneppervp@aol.com
Management:
   Managing Director: Joan L Knepper
   Account Executive: Amy Wozniak
Founded: 1971
Specialized Field: Musical Theatre

3714 AMERICAN MUSIC THEATER FESTIVAL/PRINCE MUSIC THEATER
100 S Broad Street
Suite 650
Philadelphia, PA 19110
Phone: 215-972-1000
Fax: 215-972-1020
Web Site: www.amtf.org
Management:
   Artistic Director: Ben Levit
Founded: 1984
Performs At: Prince Music Theater
Facility Category: Theater
Type of Stage: Proscenium
Seating Capacity: 450

3715 AMERICAN THEATER ARTS FOR YOUTH
1429 Walnut Street
Philadelphia, PA 19102
Phone: 800-822-8487
Fax: 215-563-3501
e-mail: atafy@aol.com
Web Site: www.atafy.org
Management:
   Artistic Director: Don Kersey
Founded: 1971
Status: Nonprofit; Non-Equity
Season: October - May

3716 BIG MESS THEATRE
1112 Manning Street
Philadelphia, PA 19107
Phone: 215-829-8333
e-mail: bigmessthr@aol.com
Web Site: www.members.aol.com/bigmessthr

Management:
Artistic Director: Greg Giovanni
Mission: Big Mess Theatre dedicates itself to visionary forms of theatre and theatrical experience.

3717 BUSHFIRE THEATRE OF PERFORMING ARTS

224 S 52nd Street
Philadelphia, PA 19139
Phone: 215-747-9230
Fax: 215-747-9236
e-mail: thebushfire@earthlink.net
Management:
Artistic Director: Al Simpkins
Executive Director: Verlina Dawson
Mission: Is to offer greater opportunity for black professional and non-professional actors, playwrights and other theatre personnel to develop their skills and careers.
Founded: 1977
Specialized Field: Musical; Theatrical Group
Status: Professional; Nonprofit
Income Sources: Actors' Equity Association
Performs At: Bushfire Theatre of Performing Arts; Writers Works
Organization Type: Performing; Educational

3718 FREEDOM REPERTORY THEATRE

1346 N Broad Street
Philadelphia, PA 19121
Phone: 215-765-2793
Fax: 215-765-4191
Web Site: www.freedomtheatre.org
Management:
Managing Director: Jamie Brunson
Artistic Director: Walter Dallas
Founded: 1966
Specialized Field: Theater; Performing Arts Training Program
Performs At: John E Allen Theatre, Freedom Cabaret Theatre
Type of Stage: Proscenium; Flexible
Seating Capacity: 299-120

3719 GERMANTOWN THEATRE GUILD

4821 Germantown Avenue
Philadelphia, PA 19144
Phone: 215-991-0419
Fax: 215-991-0419
e-mail: gtc@germantowntheatre.org
Web Site: www.germantowntheatre.org
Management:
Artistic Director: Mark Hallen
Managing Director: Darla Max
Technical Director: GA Carafelli
Mission: Germantown Theatre Center is a place for arts education in the northwest neighborhood of Philedelphia, providing classes, residencies and performances which excite and inspire a diverse economic, ethnic and racial population and enhance cultural and community revitalization.
Founded: 1933
Specialized Field: Theatrical Group
Status: Professional; Nonprofit

Income Sources: Theatre Alliance of Pennsylvania; Greater Philadelphia Cultural Alliance; Citizens for the Performing Arts in Pennsylvania; Performing Arts League of Philadelphia
Organization Type: Performing; Touring; Educational; Sponsoring

---

3720 INDIAN RIVER THEATRE OF THE PERFORMING ARTS

32925 US Route 11
Philadelphia, PA 13673
Phone: 315-642-5521
Fax: 315-642-5658
e-mail: pdixon@mail.ircsd.org
Web Site: www.ircsd.org
Management:
Theatre Secretary: Pamela Dixon
Technical Director: Rob Drader
Assistant Principal: Tray Decker
Mission: Community Theatre arts education theatre.
Founded: 1995
Facility Category: Community School Theatre
Type of Stage: Proscenium
Stage Dimensions: 60'x24'
Seating Capacity: 1400
Year Built: 1995
Rental Contact: Theatre Secretary Pamela Dixon

3721 INTERACT THEATRE COMPANY

2030 Sansom Street
Philadelphia, PA 19103
Phone: 215-568-8077
Fax: 215-568-8095
e-mail: interact@interacttheatre.org
Web Site: www.interacttheatre.org
Management:
Producing Artistic Director: Seth Rozin
Managing Director: James Haskins
Education Director: Tom Reing
Mission: Believes in developing and producing important new plays that represent our time and place, and introducing new writers to local audiences.
Founded: 1988
Specialized Field: Theatre
Paid Staff: 8
Paid Artists: 75
Performs At: Adrienne
Type of Stage: Proscenium
Seating Capacity: 106

3722 PHILADELPHIA THEATRE COMPANY

230 S 15th Street
4th Floor
Philadelphia, PA 19102
Phone: 215-985-1400
Fax: 215-985-5800
e-mail: info@phillytheatreco.com
Web Site: www.phillytheatreco.com
Officers:
President: Sheldon Thompson
VP: E Gerald Riesenbach Esq
VP: Carol Saline
VP: Anita I Steen
VP: Harriet Weiss

Treasurer: Robert A Brown
Secretary: Julia Ericksen PhD
Management:
 Producing Artistic Director: Sara Garonzik
 General Manager: Ada Coppock
Mission: Dedicated to producing the Philadelphia and world premieres of major works by contemporary American playwrights.
Founded: 1975
Specialized Field: Theatrical Group
Status: Professional; Nonprofit
Paid Staff: 14
Volunteer Staff: 200
Budget: $1.7 million
Income Sources: Foundations; Corporations; Individuals
Performs At: Plays and Players Theater
Affiliations: AEA; LORT; TCG; PCVB; TAGP; GPCA; Philadelphia Chamber of Commerce
Annual Attendance: 40,000
Facility Category: Historic
Type of Stage: Proscenium
Stage Dimensions: 25'x25'
Seating Capacity: 324
Year Built: 1919
Organization Type: Performing; Resident

3723   PRINCE MUSIC THEATER

1412 Chestnut Street
100 S Broad Street
Philadelphia, PA 19110
Phone: 215-972-1000
Fax: 215-972-1020
Web Site: www.princemusictheater.org
Management:
 Managing Director: Joe Farina
 Producing Director: Marjorie Samoff
 Dramaturg: Julie Felise Dubiner
Mission: Dedicated to developing music theatre in its various forms.
Founded: 1983
Specialized Field: Festivals; Musical Theater
Status: Nonprofit
Annual Attendance: 100,000
Seating Capacity: 450
Year Built: 1999
Rental Contact: Managing Director Joe Farina
Organization Type: Sponsoring

3724   SOCIETY HILL PLAYHOUSE

507 S Eighth Street
Philadelphia, PA 19147
Phone: 215-923-0210
Fax: 215-923-1789
e-mail: shp@erols.com
Web Site: www.societyhillplayhouse.com
 Managing Artistic Director: Deen Kogan
 Director Play Development: Walter Vail
Mission: To present works of the finest contemporary American and European writers.
Founded: 1959
Specialized Field: Theatrical Group
Status: Professional; Nonprofit
Performs At: Society Hill Playhouse
Affiliations: Theatre Communications Group; American Arts Alliance; Theatre Alliance

Annual Attendance: 100,000
Facility Category: Historic Building
Seating Capacity: 250; 99
Year Built: 1900
Year Remodeled: 1979
Rental Contact: Ray Buffington
Organization Type: Performing; Touring; Educational

3725   WILMA THEATER

265 S Broad Street
Philadelphia, PA 19107
Phone: 215-893-9456
Fax: 215-546-7824
e-mail: info@wilmatheatre.org
Web Site: www.wilmatheatre.org
Management:
 Artistic Director: Blanka Zizka
 Artistic Director: Jiri Zizka
 Managing Director: Naomi Grabel
 Production Manager: Patrick Heydenburg
 Technical Director: Douglas Marshall
 Director Development: Brian Moore
 Director Marketing: Liz Walsh
Mission: To produce innovative theatre of the highest artistic quality from international and contemporary American repertoires.
Founded: 1973
Status: Professional; Nonprofit
Paid Staff: 21
Budget: $1.5 Million
Income Sources: Theatre Communications Group
Facility Category: 1 Stage Studio
Type of Stage: Proscenium
Stage Dimensions: 44'x46'
Seating Capacity: 296
Year Built: 1996
Architect: Hugh Hardy
Rental Contact: Neal Racioppo
Organization Type: Performing

3726   WALNUT STREET THEATRE

825 Walnut Street
Philadelphia, PA 19107
Phone: 215-574-3550
Fax: 215-574-3598
e-mail: wstpc@erols.com
Web Site: www.wstonline.org
Officers:
 President: Louis Fryman
Management:
 Producing Artistic Director: Bernard Harvard
 Managing Director: Mark Sylvester
 Director Development: Rebekah A Sassi
 Director Marketing/Public Relations: Cristian E David
Mission: The mission of the Walnut Street Theatre Company is to sustain the tradition of professional theatre and contribute to its future viability and vitality. It does so through: the production and presentation of professional theatre; the encouragement, training and development of artists; the development of diverse audiences; the preservation and chronicling of its theatre building, a National Historic Landmark.
Founded: 1809
Specialized Field: Live Theatre

Status: Nonprofit
Paid Staff: 100
Budget: $10 million
Income Sources: Tickets; Grants; Funders
Affiliations: Greater Philadelphia Cultural Alliance;
National Alliance of Musical Theaters; Theatre
Community Group; League of Historic American
Theatres
Annual Attendance: 300,000
Facility Category: Mainstage; Studio
Type of Stage: Proscenium; Black Box
Seating Capacity: 1,075; 80
Year Built: 1809
Year Remodeled: 1969
Rental Contact: D Jadico

3727　MUM PUPPETTHEATRE
115 Arch Street
Phildelphia, PA 19106-2000
Phone: 215-952-8686
Fax: 215-922-5184
e-mail: heather@mumpuppet.org
Web Site: www.mumpuppet.org
Management:
　General Manager: Heather Rogers
　Artistic Director: Robert Smythe
Founded: 1985
Status: Nonprofit
Rental Contact: Heather Rogers

3728　CITY THEATRE COMPANY
1300 Bingham Street
Pittsburgh, PA 15203
Phone: 412-431-4400
Fax: 412-431-5535
e-mail: caquiline@citytheatrecompany.org
Web Site: www.citytheatrecompany.org
Management:
　Literary Manager/Dramature: Carlyn Ann Aquiline
　Managing Director: David Jobin
Mission: To provide an artistic home for the development
and production of contemporary plays of substance and
ideas that engage and challenge diverse audiences.
Founded: 1974
Specialized Field: Theatrical Group
Status: Professional; Nonprofit
Paid Staff: 50
Volunteer Staff: 5
Income Sources: Theatre Communications Group
Performs At: City Theatre
Type of Stage: Flexible; Black Box
Seating Capacity: 272; 99
Organization Type: Performing; Resident; Educational

**3729　PITTSBURGH INTERNATIONAL
CHILDREN'S THEATER**
182 Allegheny Center Mall
Pittsburgh, PA 15212
Phone: 412-321-5520
Fax: 412-321-5212
e-mail: pictheater@aol.com
Web Site: www.pghkids.org
Officers:
　Board Chair: M E Zmuda

Vice Chair: Karen Flam
Management:
　Founding Artistic Director: Maranne Purcell Welch
　Executive Director: Sara Jane Lowry
Founded: 1969
Specialized Field: Performing Series; Theater; Music;
Dance; Circus
Paid Artists: 40
Budget: $615,000
Income Sources: Ticket Sales; Contributions;
Concession; Special Events; Program Ads
Performs At: Byham Theatre; Area Schools
Affiliations: IPAY (International Performing Arts for
Youth)
Annual Attendance: 56,000

**3730　PITTSBURGH IRISH & CLASSICAL
THEATRE**
PO Box 23607
Pittsburgh, PA 15222
Phone: 412-396-6426
Fax: 412-396-4792
Web Site: www.picttheatre.org
Officers:
　President: Ray Werner
　VP: Andrew S Paul
　VP: Stephanie Riso
　CPA/Treasurer: Michael Regan
　Secretary: Sr. Michele O'Leary
Management:
　General Manager: Stephanie Riso
　Development/Marketing Director: Maureen
McGranaghan
Mission: To challenge, educate and entertain Pittsburgh
audiences by providing quality, professional, text-driven
theatre at a reasonable price, while respectfully utilizing
and compensating local talent, and by encouraging
collaborative efforts with other successful theatres and
individuals, particularly focusing on theatre of an Irish,
English and Classical nature.
Founded: 1996
Specialized Field: Classical Theatre
Status: Professional

**3731　PITTSBURGH PLAYHOUSE OF POINT
PARK COLLEGE**
222 Craft Avenue
Pittsburgh, PA 15213
Phone: 412-621-4445
Fax: 412-621-4762
Web Site: www.ppc.edu
Management:
　Artistic Producing Director: Ronald A Lindblom

3732　PITTSBURGH PUBLIC THEATER
621 Penn Avenue
Pittsburgh, PA 15222
Phone: 412-316-8200
Fax: 412-316-8216
e-mail: info@ppt.org
Web Site: www.ppt.org
Officers:
　President: Tony Bucci
　Secretary: Edward L Linder

Treasurer: Richard L Crouch
Counsel: Thomas M. Thompson
Management:
Artistic Director: Ted Pappas
Managing Director: Stephen Klein
Mission: To provide artistically diverse experiences of the highest quality, thereby holding a preeminent position among American theaters. We strive to serve, challenge, stimulate, and entertain an expanding audience while operating in a fiscally responsible manner.
Founded: 1974
Specialized Field: Theatrical Group
Status: Professional; Nonprofit
Paid Staff: 44
Volunteer Staff: 400
Paid Artists: 100
Budget: $6.3 Million
Income Sources: Actors' Equity Association; League of Resident Theatres
Performs At: O'Reilly Theater
Affiliations: AEA, SSDC, USA, IATSE
Annual Attendance: 110,000
Type of Stage: Thrust
Seating Capacity: 650
Year Built: 1999
Cost: 25 Million
Rental Contact: Jason Hassell
Organization Type: Performing; Educational

3733 PRIME STAGE

PO Box 1849
Pittsburgh, PA 15230
Phone: 412-771-7373
Fax: 412-771-8585
e-mail: producerinfo@primestage.com
Web Site: www.primestage.com/
Officers:
Chairman: Thomas Wettach Esquire
VP: Jerry Weinand Esquire
Management:
Producing Director: Wayne Brindag
Assistant Producer: Lynn DeBree
Mission: We are commited to exposing and engaging young people and families in the discovery of live theatre. We accomplish this by producing new plays and other works, which celebrate the achievements of young people and adults.
Founded: 1996
Specialized Field: Theatre for young audiences
Status: Professional; Nonprofit; Non-Equity
Affiliations: American Alliance for Theatre and Education.
Annual Attendance: 9,000

3734 VERONICA'S VEIL PLAYERS

44 Puis Street
Pittsburgh, PA 15203-1897
Phone: 412-431-5550
Fax: 412-431-3463
e-mail: vvplayers@aol.com
Web Site: www.trfn.clpgh.org/vvp
Management:
Managing Director: Dennis M Thompston

Mission: We are dedicated to continuing the tradition of presenting the Lenten drama Veronica's Veil as well as presenting other quality theatrical productions at affordable prices.
Founded: 1910
Specialized Field: Theater
Status: Nonprofit
Volunteer Staff: 5
Non-paid Artists: 200
Performs At: Theater
Seating Capacity: 833
Year Built: 1900
Year Remodeled: 1925

3735 READING COMMUNITY PLAYERS

403 N 11th Street
Reading, PA 19604
Mailing Address: PO Box 1032 Reading, PA 19603-1032
Phone: 610-375-9106
e-mail: noisesoff@prodigy.net
Web Site: www.rcptheatre.org
Management:
Business Manager: Terry Fullmer
Mission: To develop the community's interest in theatrical arts.
Founded: 1920
Specialized Field: Community; Theatrical Group
Status: Non-Professional; Nonprofit
Paid Staff: 114
Affiliations: American Association of Community Theatre; Berks Arts Council
Organization Type: Performing; Educational

3736 NORTHEASTERN THEATRE

Box 765
Scranton, PA 18501-0765
Phone: 570-969-1770
e-mail: tnttheatre@excite.com
Management:
Producer: Alicia Grega-Pikul
Founded: 1992

3737 SHAWNEE PLAYHOUSE

PO Box 159
Shawnee-on-Delaware, PA 18356
Fax: 570-421-4914
Toll-free: 800-742-9633
e-mail: playhouse@shawneeinn.com
Web Site: www.shawneeplayhouse.com
Management:
General Manager: Rob Howell
Founded: 1978
Status: Non-Equity; Commercial
Season: June - December
Type of Stage: Proscenium
Seating Capacity: 200

3738 STRUTHERS LIBRARY THEATRE

302 3rd Avenue W
PO Box 844
Warren, PA 16365

Phone: 814-723-7231
Fax: 814-723-3856
e-mail: info@srutherslibrarytheatre.com
Web Site: www.sruthersibrarytheatre.com
Management:
   Executive Director: Charles R Tranter
Founded: 1883
Status: Equity; Nonprofit
Season: June - August
Type of Stage: Proscenium
Stage Dimensions: 35' x 26'
Seating Capacity: 989

3739 SALTWORKS THEATRE COMPANY
2553 Brandt School Road
Wexford, PA 15090-7931
Phone: 724-934-2820
Fax: 724-934-2815
e-mail: stc@lm.com
Web Site: www.saltworks.org
Management:
   Director of Marketing: Barbara Baun
Mission: To perform plays for youth and families that
address social issues.
Founded: 1981
Specialized Field: Theatrical Group
Status: Professional; Semi-Professional; Nonprofit
Paid Staff: 12
Budget: $450,000
Affiliations: ARAD; Tix for Teachers
Annual Attendance: 7,000
Seating Capacity: 150-250
Year Built: 1986
Organization Type: Performing; Touring; Educational

3740 ARENA SUMMER THEATRE
700 Academy Street
Lycoming College, Theatre Department
Williamsport, PA 17701
Phone: 570-321-4000
Fax: 570-321-4090
e-mail: stanley@lycoming.edu
Management:
   Production Director: NJ Stanley
   Associate Director: Jerry D Allen
Founded: 1964
Specialized Field: Theatre
Status: Non-Equity; Nonprofit
Paid Staff: 7
Paid Artists: 2
Non-paid Artists: 5
Budget: $45,000
Income Sources: Ticket Sales
Season: June - July
Affiliations: Actor Equity Association; TCG
Type of Stage: Thrust
Seating Capacity: 204
Year Built: 1964

3741 MOVEMENT THEATRE INTERNATIONAL
50 Bernard Drive
Yardley, PA 19067

Phone: 215-337-9100
Fax: 215-337-9100
e-mail: MAPedretti@aol.com
Mission: Provide space for area troupes and general
services to mime field.
Founded: 1979
Specialized Field: Movement Theater
Paid Staff: 1
Volunteer Staff: 3
Budget: $20,000-35,000
Income Sources: Retails, Box Office, Gifts
Type of Stage: Proscenuim
Seating Capacity: 299
Year Built: 1890
Year Remodeled: 1986
Cost: 1,000,000

Rhode Island

3742 THEATRE-BY-THE-SEA
364 Cards Pond Road
Matunuck, RI 02879
Phone: 401-782-8587
Fax: 401-783-9452
e-mail: fourquest@ids.com
Web Site: www.theatrebythesea.com
Management:
   Artistic Producer: Laura Harris
   Managing Producer: Renny Serrz
   Associate Producer: Marcy Simpson
   Marketing/Sales/Public Relations: Karen Gail
   Kessler
Mission: To provide summer theatre entertainment.
Founded: 1933
Specialized Field: Summer Stock; Musical
Status: Professional; Commercial
Performs At: Theatre-by-the-Sea
Facility Category: Summer Theatre
Seating Capacity: 505
Year Built: 1935
Year Remodeled: 1988
Organization Type: Performing; Resident

3743 ASTORS BEECHWOOD MANSION
580 Bellevue Avenue
Newport, RI 02840
Phone: 401-846-3772
Fax: 401-849-6998
e-mail: casting@astors-beechwood.com
Web Site: www.astors-beechwood.com
Management:
   Executive Director: Charlotte C Lee
Mission: Victorian Living History
Founded: 1981
Paid Staff: 10
Paid Artists: 18
Season: year round
Year Built: 1851

3744 BROWN SUMMER THEATRE
77 Waterman Street
Box 1897
Providence, RI 02912

Phone: 401-863-3284
Fax: 401-862-7529
e-mail: laura-e-smith@brown.edu
Web Site: www.brown.edu
Management:
    Producer: Laura E Smith
Founded: 1969
Season: June - August
Type of Stage: Arena
Stage Dimensions: 22' x 16'
Seating Capacity: 200

3745 BROWN UNIVERSITY THEATRE
77 Waterman Street
Box 1897
Providence, RI 02912
Phone: 401-863-2838
Fax: 401-863-7529
Web Site: www.brown.edu
Officers:
    Chairman: Spencer Golub
Management:
    Box Office Manager/Summer Theatre: Karen
    Longest
    Production Manager: Laura Smith
Mission: To offer a balanced theatrical season during the
academic year and in the summer for the university
community and Providence area; to train students.
Founded: 1901
Specialized Field: Summer Stock; Theatrical Group
Status: Non-Professional; Nonprofit
Paid Staff: 20
Performs At: Stuart Theatre; Leeds Theatre
Organization Type: Performing; Resident; Educational;
Sponsoring

3746 LOOKING GLASS THEATRE
312 Wickenden Street
Providence, RI 02093
Phone: 401-331-9080
Fax: 401-351-2051
e-mail: LGTinc@msn.com
Web Site: www.lookingglasstouringtheatre.org
Management:
    Managing Director: Pat McDougal
    Executive/Artistic Director: Diane Postoian
Mission: To enlighten and educate children and their
families through audience participation, theater and
follow-up workshops; to present new productions
annually focusing on the classics and topical issues.
Founded: 1965
Status: Professional; Nonprofit
Income Sources: Theatre Communications Group
Performs At: Looking Glass Theatre
Facility Category: Touring Theatre
Organization Type: Touring; Educational; Sponsoring

3747 NEWGATE THEATER
134 Mathewson Street
Providence, RI 02903
Phone: 401-421-9680
e-mail: brien@newgatetheatre.org
Web Site: www.newgatetheatre.org
Management:

Artistic Director: Brien Lang
Managing Director: Pam Fearn
Webmaster: Peter Gogol
Mission: Committed to producing new and established
works which challenge both artists and audiences.
Founded: 1982
Status: Semi-Professional; Nonprofit
Income Sources: New England Theatre Conference
Organization Type: Performing; Resident; Producing

3748 RITES AND REASON
Brown University
PO Box 1148
Providence, RI 02912
Phone: 401-863-3558
Fax: 401-863-3559
Management:
    Artistic Director: Elmo Terry-Morgan
    Managing Director: Karen Allen Baxter
    Research Director: Rhett S Jones
    Administrative Manager: Donna Mitchell
Mission: Developmental research theatre committed to
offering new plays celebrating and exploring Africana
culture and history.
Founded: 1970
Specialized Field: Theatrical Group
Status: Professional; Nonprofit
Income Sources: University/Resident Theatre
Affiliations: Black Theatre Network; National Alliance
for Music Theatre
Annual Attendance: 2,000
Type of Stage: Black Box
Seating Capacity: 125
Organization Type: Performing; Touring; Resident;
Educational

3749 SANDRA FEINSTEIN-GAMM THEATER
31 Elbow Street
Providence, RI 02903
Phone: 401-831-2919
Fax: 401-831-8635
e-mail: sfgt@earthlink.net
Web Site: www.sfgt.org
Officers:
    President: Samuel Babbitt
Management:
    Artistic Associate: Eric Tucker
Mission: To create intimate, professional, actor-centered
theater which delights and inspires through the communal
experience of the telling of great stories.
Founded: 1984
Specialized Field: Theatre
Status: Professional; Semi-Professional; Nonprofit
Paid Staff: 5
Volunteer Staff: 10
Paid Artists: 15
Organization Type: Performing

3750 TRINITY REPERTORY COMPANY
201 Washington Street
Providence, RI 02903-3226

All listings are in alphabetical order by state, then city, then organization within the city.

Phone: 401-521-1100
Fax: 401-751-5577
e-mail: info@trinityrep.com
Web Site: www.trinityrep.com/
Officers:
  Chairman: Arnold B Chace Jr
Management:
  Artistic Director: Oskar Eustis
  Managing Director: Edgar Dobie
  Marketing Director: Yvonne Seggerman
  General Manager: Chris Jennings
  Communications Director: Emily Atkinson
  Production Manager: Ruth Sternberg
Mission: Providing theatrical performances as well as educational services for Rhode Island and surrounding New England audiences.
Founded: 1964
Specialized Field: Theatrical Group
Status: Professional; Nonprofit
Paid Staff: 130
Budget: 7.2 million
Income Sources: League of Resident Theatres
Performs At: Trinity Repertory Company
Affiliations: AEA, LORT, TEG, SSD&C
Annual Attendance: 145,000
Facility Category: Theater
Type of Stage: Two
Stage Dimensions: Flexible
Seating Capacity: 300;600
Year Built: 1917
Year Remodeled: 1973
Rental Contact: Bob Whitney
Organization Type: Performing; Touring; Educational

South Carolina

3751 AIKEN COMMUNITY PLAYHOUSE

124 Newberry Street
Aiken, SC 29801
Phone: 803-648-1438
Web Site: members.atlantic.net/~acp/
Management:
  Publicity: Elizabeth Mouser
Mission: To offer community members an opportunity to participate in legitimate theatre; to encourage the public's appreciation of theatre arts.
Founded: 1953
Specialized Field: Community
Status: Nonprofit
Income Sources: South Carolina Theatre Association
Performs At: Aiken Community Playhouse
Organization Type: Performing

3752 FOOTLIGHT PLAYERS

1705 Franklin Street
PO Box 46
Charleston, SC 46360
Phone: 219-874-4035
Web Site: www.footlightplayers.org
Management:
  General Manager: Kit Lyons
  Designer/Technical Director: Richard Heffner
  Artistic Director: Dorothy D'Anna

Director: Jacqueline Verdeyen
Mission: To offer community members an opportunity for self-expression through amateur theatre; to provide education in drama and related subjects.
Founded: 1931
Specialized Field: Musical; Community; Theatrical Group
Status: Non-Professional; Nonprofit
Paid Staff: 100
Income Sources: South Carolina Theatre Association; Charleston Area Arts Council; Southeastern Theatre Conference; American Association of Community Theatres
Performs At: Footlight Players Theatre
Organization Type: Performing; Resident

3753 SPOLETO FESTIVAL USA

478 E Bay Street
Suite 200
Charleston, SC 29403
Mailing Address: PO Box 157 Charleston, SC 29402
Phone: 843-579-3100
Fax: 843-723-6383
e-mail: receptionist@spoletousa.org
Web Site: www.spoletousa.org
Officers:
  Director Finance: Tasha Gandy
  Chairman of the Board: William B Hewitt
  President: Eric G Friberg
Management:
  Artistic Director: Joesph Flummerfrlt
  Music Director: Emmanuel Villaume
  General Director: Nigel Redden
  Producer: Nunally Kersh
Mission: To present opera, dance, theater, symphonic, choral and chamber music, jazz and visual arts exhibits of the highest quality; to serve as an educational environment for young artists and audiences alike.
Founded: 1977
Specialized Field: Opera; Chamber; Choral & Symphonic Music; Jazz; Theater; Dance
Status: Professional; Semi-Professional; Nonprofit
Paid Staff: 21
Income Sources: Opera America; Dance USA; Theatre Communications Group; National Institute for Music Theater; American Arts Alliance
Performs At: Gaillard Municipal Auditorium; Dock Street Theater
Organization Type: Performing; Educational; Sponsoring

3754 COLUMBIA STAGE SOCIETY AT TOWN THEATRE

1012 Sumter Street
Columbia, SC 29201
Phone: 803-799-2510
Fax: 803-799-6463
e-mail: info@towntheatre.com
Web Site: www.towntheatre.com
Officers:
  President: Robert R Russell Jr
  Vice President: E Warner Wells
  Treasurer: Thomas P Monahan
  Secretary: David M Dunlap

Management:
    Manager: WJ Arvay
    Executive Director: Sandra Willis
    Technical Director: John WK Young
    Assistant Manager: Ann B Fogle
Mission: The advancement in the community, both city and state, of the experimental arts of the little theatre, including spoken drama, pantomime, music, musical drama, and promotion of such literary and artistic objects as will foster and develop the cultural aspects of our community life.
Founded: 1919
Specialized Field: Community; Theatrical Group
Status: Non-Professional; Nonprofit
Income Sources: South Carolina Theatre Association
Performs At: The Town Theatre
Annual Attendance: 20,000
Year Built: 1924
Year Remodeled: 1993
Cost: $1,200,000
Organization Type: Performing; Educational

3755   TRUSTUS

PO Box 11721
Columbia, SC 29211
Phone: 803-254-9732
Fax: 803-771-9153
e-mail: trustus@trustus.org
Web Site: www.trustus.org
Management:
    Artistic Director: Jim Thigpen
    Producing Director: Kay Thigpen
    Box Office Manager: Steve Levine
    Technical Director: Brian Riley
Mission: To bring to the area a professional theatre dedicated to new works, plays of literary and artistic merit, and quality mainstream theatre in an environment that allows us to reach a broad spectrum of patrons.
Founded: 1985
Status: Professional; Nonprofit
Income Sources: Theatre Communications Group; South Carolina Theatre Association
Organization Type: Performing; Resident; Educational

3756   SWAMP FOX PLAYERS

710 Front Street
PO Box 911
Georgetown, SC 29442
Phone: 843-527-2924
Mission: To offer a cultural center to the area; to provide dramatic presentations for area citizens.
Founded: 1971
Specialized Field: Community
Status: Non-Professional; Nonprofit
Paid Staff: 60
Performs At: Strand Theatre
Year Built: 1937
Organization Type: Performing; Resident

3757   BOB JONES UNIVERSITY CONCERT, OPERA & DRAMA SERIES

Bob Jones University
Greenville, SC 29614

Phone: 864-242-5100
Fax: 864-233-9829
e-mail: finearts@bju.edu
Web Site: www.bju.edu
Officers:
    President: Dr. Bob Jones III
Budget: $35,000-60,000
Performs At: Founder's Memorial Auditorium

3758   CENTRE STAGE-SOUTH CAROLINA

501 River Street
Greenville, SC 29604-8951
Phone: 864-233-6733
Fax: 864-233-3901
Web Site: www.centrestage.org
Officers:
    President: Steven D Bichel
    VP: Caroline B Stewart
    Treasurer: Scott Frierson
    Secretary: Robyn Zimmerman
Management:
    Administrative Director: Claude W Blakely
    Executive/Artistic Director: Douglas McCoy
    Literary Manager: Barbara Hackett
Mission: To bring the most current critically acclaimed works to upstate SC with emphasis on Pulizer and Tony winners.
Founded: 1983
Specialized Field: Theater
Paid Staff: 2
Volunteer Staff: 200
Type of Stage: Thrust
Seating Capacity: 292

3759   WAREHOUSE THEATRE

37 Augusta Street
Greenville, SC 29601
Phone: 864-235-6948
Web Site: www.warehousetheatre.com
Management:
    Business Manager: Connie Jenkins
Mission: To excite the imagination; to examine the signposts/symbols of our time; to test the old, explore the new; to allow our audience to test-drive parts of the human experience.
Founded: 1974
Specialized Field: Professional Theatre Company
Status: Nonprofit
Paid Staff: 4
Volunteer Staff: 50
Paid Artists: 20
Non-paid Artists: 50
Budget: $260,000
Season: September - June
Type of Stage: Flexible; Proscenium
Seating Capacity: 170; 349

3760   NEWBERRY COLLEGE THEATRE

Newberry College
2000 College Street
Newberry, SC 29108

Phone: 803-276-5010
Fax: 803-321-5627
Toll-free: 800-845-4955
Web Site: www.newberry.edu
Officers:
   Director Theatre/Dept. Chair: Patrick Gagliano
   Technical Director: Rupert Gaddy
Mission: To provide a performing arts program of quality in the environment of a liberal arts college.
Founded: 1856
Specialized Field: Musical; Theatrical Group
Status: College
Paid Staff: 3
Type of Stage: Proscenium; Thrust; Flexible
Seating Capacity: 100-200
Organization Type: Performing; Educational

South Dakota

3761   ABERDEEN COMMUNITY THEATRE
417 S Main
PO Box 813
Aberdeen, SD 57402-0813
Phone: 605-225-2228
Fax: 605-226-5494
e-mail: actheatre@home.com
Web Site: www.pclan-sd.com/act
Management:
   Artistic/Managing Director: James L Walker
   Administrative Assistant: Rhonda Jo Anderson
Mission: To educate, entertain and further performing arts through community involvement.
Founded: 1979
Specialized Field: Musical; Dinner; Community; Theatrical Group
Status: Non-Professional; Nonprofit
Paid Staff: 2
Volunteer Staff: 300
Income Sources: American Association of Community Theatres; South Dakota Theatre Association
Performs At: Capitol Theatre
Seating Capacity: 450
Organization Type: Performing; Educational; Sponsoring

3762   BLACK HILLS PLAYHOUSE
HC 83 Box 68
Custer, SD 57730
Phone: 605-255-4141
e-mail: bhphq@aol.com
Web Site: www.blackhillsplayhouse.com
Officers:
   President: Dr. John Barlow
   VP: Steven McCarthy
   Secretary: Pat Stofft
   Treasurer: Jo Anna Warder
   Founder: Doc Lee
Management:
   Managing Artistic Director: Jan D Swank
   Business Manager: Jill Swank
Mission: To offer high quality performances to audiences; to provide theatre students with intensive professional training.

Founded: 1955
Specialized Field: Summer Stock; Theatrical Group
Status: Professional; Semi-Professional; Nonprofit
Paid Staff: 2
Paid Artists: 70
Budget: $400,000
Income Sources: Box Office; Grants; Donations
Season: May - August
Performs At: Black Hills Playhouse (Custer State Park)
Affiliations: University of South Dakota
Annual Attendance: 16,000
Facility Category: Theatre
Type of Stage: Modified Thrust
Seating Capacity: 360
Year Built: 1955
Organization Type: Performing; Resident; Educational

3763   BLACK HILLS COMMUNITY THEATRE
713 7th Street
Rapid City, SD 57701
Phone: 605-394-1786
Management:
   Manager: Merritt Olsen
Mission: To offer quality theatre employing community talent.
Founded: 1968
Specialized Field: Community
Status: Nonprofit
Paid Staff: 150
Income Sources: South Dakota Arts Council; Allied Arts Fund
Organization Type: Performing

3764   SIOUX FALLS COMMUNITY PLAYHOUSE
315 N Phillips Avenue
PO Box 600
Sioux Falls, SD 57101
Phone: 605-336-7418
Fax: 605-336-0926
e-mail: sfcp@sfcp.org
Web Site: www.sfcp.org
Management:
   Executive Director: Larae Blanker
   Technical Director: Dion Denevan
   Artistic Assoc/Education Director: Lee Shackelford
Mission: To offer the community and the area opportunities for experiencing live theatre through participation on a variety of levels.
Founded: 1930
Specialized Field: Community
Status: Nonprofit
Paid Staff: 8
Non-paid Artists: 200
Budget: $250,000
Income Sources: American Association of Community Theatres; South Dakota Arts Council
Performs At: Sioux Falls Community Playhouse
Annual Attendance: 10,000
Seating Capacity: 262
Year Remodeled: 1999
Cost: $1,200,000
Organization Type: Performing; Touring; Resident; Educational; Sponsoring

3765 BLACK HILLS PASSION PLAY

PO Box 489
Spearfish, SD 57783
Phone: 605-642-2646
Fax: 605-642-7993
Toll-free: 800-457-0160
e-mail: bhpp@blackhills.com
Web Site: www.blackhills.com/bhpp
Management:
    Producer/Director: Johanna Meier
Founded: 1932
Status: Non-Equity; Commercial
Paid Staff: 76
Volunteer Staff: 150
Paid Artists: 24
Season: June - August
Type of Stage: Amphitheatre
Seating Capacity: 5600

3766 MATTHEWS OPERA HOUSE SOCIETY

614 Main Street
Spearfish, SD 57783
Phone: 605-642-7973
Fax: 605-642-3477
e-mail: scah@rushmore.com
Web Site: www.moh-scah.com
Management:
    Administrative Director: Ardis Golay
    Artsitc Director: David Whitlock
Mission: To provide quality programming while preserving the Matthews Opera House.
Founded: 1989
Specialized Field: Musical; Community; Theatrical Group; Visual Arts; Humanities
Status: Non-Professional; Nonprofit
Paid Staff: 2
Volunteer Staff: 20
Budget: $300,000
Income Sources: Show Fees; Festival Fees; Grants; Memberships Fees
Performs At: Senior High Theatre; Matthews Opera House
Annual Attendance: 12,000 - 15,000
Seating Capacity: 230
Year Built: 1906
Year Remodeled: 1997
Rental Contact: Ardis Golay
Organization Type: Performing; Educational

3767 MATTHEWS OPERA HOUSE SOCIETY

614 Main Street
Spearfish, SD 57783
Phone: 605-642-7973
Fax: 605-642-3477
e-mail: scah@rushmore.com
Web Site: www.matthewsoperahousetheater.com
Management:
    Administrative Director: Ardis Golay
    Managing Artistic Director: R David Whitlock
Mission: To offer opportunities for talented people interested in theatre; to continue restoration of the Opera House.
Founded: 1906
Specialized Field: Theater, Visual, Humanities

Status: Non-Professional; Nonprofit
Paid Staff: 2
Volunteer Staff: 12
Budget: $300,000
Income Sources: Show Fees; Festival Fees; Grants
Performs At: Senior High Theatre; Matthews Opera House
Annual Attendance: 12,000 - 15,000
Seating Capacity: 230
Year Built: 1906
Year Remodeled: 1997
Rental Contact: Ardis Golay
Organization Type: Performing; Educational

3768 TOWN PLAYERS

5 S Broadway
Watertown, SD 57201
Phone: 605-882-2076
Fax: 605-882-2076
Management:
    Manager: Nancy Johnson
Mission: To promote appreciation of dramatic arts.
Founded: 1940
Specialized Field: Musical; Community; Theatrical Group
Status: Non-Professional; Nonprofit
Paid Staff: 45
Organization Type: Performing; Touting; Resident

3769 LEWIS & CLARK THEATRE COMPANY

328 Walnut Street
PO Box 836
Yankton, SD 57078
Phone: 605-665-4711
e-mail: lctheatr@byelectric.com
Web Site: www.lewisandclarktheatre.com
Management:
    Executive Director: Michael Kohn
Founded: 1961
Status: Non-Equity; Nonprofit
Season: June - August
Type of Stage: Proscenium
Stage Dimensions: 60' x 36'
Seating Capacity: 640

Tennessee

3770 THEATRE BRISTOL

512 State Street
Bristol, TN 37620
Phone: 423-968-4977
Fax: 423-968-4978
e-mail: theatreb@3wave.com
Web Site: www.theatrebristol.org
Officers:
    President: Dorothy Havlik
    VP: Anne Koehner
    Treasurer: Holly Whitley
    Secretary: Ann Christ
Management:
    Executive Director: Russ Bralley
    General Manager: Emily Anne Thompson
    Technical Director: Jim Quensenberry

Director Education: Amy Bussey
Mission: Theatre Bristol is a regional theatre that uses the arts to inspire educate and entertain.
Founded: 1965
Specialized Field: Musical; Community; Theatrical Group
Status: Non-Professional; Nonprofit
Paid Staff: 6
Volunteer Staff: 20
Performs At: Paramount Center for the Arts; Theatre Bristol Artspace
Seating Capacity: 756; 95
Organization Type: Performing; Resident; Educational; Sponsoring

3771 ROXY THEATER

100 Franklin Street
Clarksville, TN 37040
Phone: 931-645-7699
Management:
   General Manager: Tom Thayer
   Artistic Director: John McDonald
Mission: To promote and produce the performing and visual arts.
Founded: 1983
Specialized Field: Musical; Community; Theatrical Group
Status: Professional; Nonprofit
Paid Staff: 2
Organization Type: Performing; Educational

3772 CUMBERLAND COUNTY PLAYHOUSE

221 Tennessee Avenue
PO Box 484
Crossville, TN 38557
Phone: 931-484-5000
Fax: 931-484-6299
e-mail: info@ccplayhouse.com
Web Site: www.ccplayhouse.com
Management:
   Producing Director: Jim Crabtree
   Associate Producer: John Briggs
Mission: To provide cultural enrichment for the area and beyond.
Founded: 1965
Specialized Field: Theatrical Group
Status: Professional; Nonprofit
Paid Staff: 20
Paid Artists: 35
Budget: $2.1 million
Income Sources: 80% Earned Income; Grants; Donations
Season: Year-round
Performs At: Cumberland County Playhouse
Annual Attendance: 145,000
Type of Stage: 2 indoor; 1 outdoor
Year Built: 1965
Year Remodeled: 1992
Rental Contact: Producing Director Jim Crabtree
Organization Type: Performing; Touring; Resident; Educational; Sponsoring

3773 PULL-TIGHT PLAYERS

PO Box 105
Franklin, TN 37065-0105

Phone: 615-790-3204
e-mail: thespian@pull-tight.com
Web Site: www.pull-tight.com
Officers:
   President: Marianne Clark
   VP: Jeanne Drone
   Secretary: Heather Bottoms
   Tresurer: Iain MacPhearson
   Founder: Vance Ormes
Management:
   Executive Producer: John Kitson
   Executive Technical Director: Kenny Van Hook
   House Manager: Laurie Sackett
Mission: To provide quality community theatre for Williamson County and the surrounding area.
Founded: 1968
Specialized Field: Community; Theatrical Group
Status: Non-Professional; Nonprofit
Paid Staff: 60
Organization Type: Performing; Resident

3774 SWEET FANNY ADAMS THEATRE & MUSIC HALL

461 Parkway
Gatlinburg, TN 37738
Phone: 865-436-4039
Fax: 865-436-4038
Toll-free: 877-388-5784
e-mail: sfatheatre@aol.com
Web Site: www.sweetfannyadams.com
Management:
   Producer/Co-Owner: Pat MacPherson
   Director/Co-Owner: Don MacPherson
Founded: 1977
Status: Non-Equity; Commercial
Paid Staff: 6
Paid Artists: 8
Season: May - October
Annual Attendance: 20,000
Facility Category: Theatre
Type of Stage: Thrust
Stage Dimensions: 12'x13'
Seating Capacity: 184
Year Built: 1877
Year Remodeled: 1996
Rental Contact: Don MacPherson

3775 GERMANTOWN COMMUNITY THEATRE

3037 Forest Hill Road
Germantown, TN 38138
Phone: 901-754-2680
Fax: 901-755-1185
Web Site: www.germantownchamber.com
Management:
   Executive Producer: Leigh Walden
Founded: 1972
Income Sources: Memphis Arts Council; Germantown Arts Alliance

3776 POPLAR PIKE PLAYHOUSE

7653 Old Poplar Pike
Germantown, TN 38138

Phone: 901-755-7775
Fax: 901-755-6951
e-mail: poppikeplayhouse@aol.com
Web Site: www.ppp.org
Management:
    Managing Director: Frank Bluestein
    Business Manager: Gail Ridenhour
Mission: To present educational theatre at Germantown High School.
Founded: 1976
Specialized Field: Musical; Community; Theatrical Group
Status: Nonprofit
Paid Staff: 10
Volunteer Staff: 5
Paid Artists: 3
Budget: $50,000
Income Sources: Shelby County Schools; Germaston Arts Alliance
Annual Attendance: 5,000
Facility Category: Theatre
Type of Stage: Proscenium
Stage Dimensions: 55'x40'
Seating Capacity: 300
Year Built: 1975
Year Remodeled: 1998
Rental Contact: E Frank Bluestein
Organization Type: Performing; Educational

3777   JACKSON THEATRE GUILD

314 E Main Street
PO Box 7041
Jackson, TN 38301
Phone: 901-427-3200
Fax: 901-425-8674
e-mail: info@jtonline.com
Web Site: www.jtgonline.com
Officers:
    President: Bill Worboys
    VP: Brenda Poteet
    Secretary: Ann Bailey
    Treasurer: Sue Barnes
Management:
    Office Manager: Charlotte Bork
Mission: To promote public education appreciation and enjoyment of dramatic literature, current stage craft, and theatre by the presentation of quality productions. Also, by conducting other related activities, we reflect our diverse community.
Founded: 1966
Specialized Field: Musical; Community; Theatrical Group
Status: Nonprofit
Income Sources: Tickets; Grants
Annual Attendance: 6,900
Seating Capacity: 400
Organization Type: Performing; Resident; Educational

3778   ACTORS CO-OP

406 11th Street
2nd Floor
Knoxville, TN 37916
Phone: 423-523-0900
Fax: 423-523-0900
e-mail: actoop@aol.com

Management:
    Artistic Director: Amy Hubbard
    Managing Director: Kara Kemp

3779   ARTS & CULTURE ALLIANCE OF GREATER KNOXVILLE

PO Box 2506
Knoxville, TN 37901
Phone: 615-523-7543
Fax: 615-523-7312
e-mail: alliance@esper.com
Web Site: www.koxarts.com
Officers:
    President: Patrick Roddy
    Treasurer: Kathy Hamilton
    VP: Jefferson Hcapma
    VP: Lila Plfleger
Management:
    Executive Director: Liza Zenni
Mission: To unite, strenghen, and promote arts and culture activities in East Tennessee.
Founded: 1976
Specialized Field: Dance; Music; Theatre; Visual Arts
Status: Nonprofit
Organization Type: Educational

3780   BIJOU THEATRE

PO Box 1746
803 S Gan Street
Knoxville, TN 37901
Phone: 865-523-4211
Fax: 865-522-0238
Toll-free: 800-738-0832
e-mail: bijoutc@aol.com
Web Site: bijoutheater.com
Management:
    Director: Beverly Snukals
Founded: 1984
Paid Staff: 7
Volunteer Staff: 60
Paid Artists: 40
Budget: $35,000-60,000
Facility Category: Performing Arts
Type of Stage: Proscenium
Stage Dimensions: 35'x 51'
Seating Capacity: 750
Year Built: 1909
Year Remodeled: 1998

3781   CARPETBAG THEATRE

3018 E 5th Avenue
Knoxville, TN 37914
Phone: 423-524-6629
Fax: 423-524-6631
Management:
    Executive/Artistic Director: Linda Parris-Bailey
    Managing/Technical Director: Jeff Cody
Mission: To give artistic voice to the underserved. We address the issues and dreams of people who have historically been silenced by racism, classism, sexism and ageism; tell stories of empowerment; celebrate our culture; and reveal hidden stories
Founded: 1970
Status: Professional; Nonprofit

Income Sources: National Endowment for the Arts; Tennessee Arts Commision; East Tennessee Community Foundation
Organization Type: Touring

3782 CLARENCE BROWN THEATRE COMPANY
University of Tennessee
206 McClung Tower
Knoxville, TN 37996-0420
Phone: 423-974-6011
Fax: 423-974-4867
e-mail: cbt@utk.edu
Web Site: www.clarencebrowntheatre.org
Officers:
   Chairperson: Andrew White
Management:
   Company Manager: Thomas Adkins
   Producing Director: Blake Robison
   Marketing Director: Sarah Patterson
   Managing Director: Thomas A Cervone
   Outreach Coordinator: Carol Cruzan
   Public Relations Coordinator: Sandra Van Winkle Campbell
   Production Manager: Laura Sims
Founded: 1974
Specialized Field: Theatrical Group
Status: Professional; Nonprofit
Budget: $1.5 million
Income Sources: League of Resident Theatres; Theatre Communications Group; Knoxville Arts Council; University of Tennessee
Performs At: Clarence Brown Theatre, Carousel Theatre
Affiliations: Actors' Equity Association; League of Resident Theatres; SSOC
Annual Attendance: 34,000
Facility Category: Theatre
Type of Stage: Proscenium; Arena
Stage Dimensions: 60'x32'
Seating Capacity: 600; 250
Year Built: 1970
Rental Contact: Product Manager Laura Sims
Organization Type: Performing; Touring; Resident

3783 TENNESSEE STAGE COMPANY
1060 World's Fair Park Drive
PO Box 1186
Knoxville, TN 37996
Phone: 865-546-4280
Fax: 865-546-9677
e-mail: gparkhill@juno.com
Web Site: www.korrnet.org/tnstage/
Management:
   Artistic Director/Producer: Tom Parkhill
Mission: To serve the Knoxville and East Tennessee area by producing exciting, high quality, productions of primarily American plays, both classical and current, with a strong Southern regional emphasis (both in material and emphasis), and with special attention given to finding and producing new works.
Founded: 1989
Specialized Field: Plays; Reading; Acting Classes; Community Outreach Programs
Status: Non-Equity; Nonprofit

Income Sources: Arts Council of Greater Knoxville; Community Televison of Knoxville; Comcast
Season: August
Stage Dimensions: 24' x 24'
Seating Capacity: 1,300

3784 THEATER KNOXVILLE
Bijou Theater
803 S Gay Street
PO Box 1746
Knoxville, TN 37901
Phone: 865-523-4211
Fax: 865-524-0821
Mission: To provide quality productions employing community members as actors and technicians.
Founded: 1976
Specialized Field: Community
Status: Non-Professional; Nonprofit
Performs At: The Bijou Theater
Organization Type: Performing; Touring; Educational

3785 TENNESSEE PLAYERS
304 W Due West Avenue
Madison, TN 37115
Phone: 615-868-3738
Fax: 615-868-3738
e-mail: symposium2000@webtv.net
Management:
   Executive Director: Thurston Moore
Mission: To create something beautiful for somebody else.
Founded: 1986
Status: Non-Professional; Nonprofit
Annual Attendance: 15,000
Organization Type: Performing; Touring; Educational

3786 CIRCUIT PLAYHOUSE
51 S Cooper Street
Memphis, TN 38104
Phone: 901-725-0776
Fax: 901-272-7530
e-mail: info@playhouseonthesquare.org
Web Site: www.playhouseonthesquare.org
Officers:
   President: PJ Smoot
   VP: Leigh McLean
Management:
   Executive Producer: Jackie Nichols
   Administrative Director: Kittianne Velloff
   Technical Director: Carin Orr
   Managing Director: Whitney Jo
Founded: 1969
Income Sources: Southeastern Theatre Conference; Theatre Communications Group; Tennessee Theatre Association; Playhouse on the Square
Performs At: Circuit Playhouse; Playhouse on the Square

3787 EWING CHILDREN'S THEATRE
2635 Avery Avenue
Memphis, TN 38112
Phone: 901-452-3968
Fax: 901-452-3805
e-mail: ewingct1949@aol.com

Officers:
President: June Scudder
Secretary/Treasurer: Pat Barnes
Management:
Theatre Director: Kay Lighffoot
Mission: Memphis Children's Theatre uses children, ages 5-17, and involves them in all aspects of theatre.
Founded: 1949
Specialized Field: Community
Status: Nonprofit
Paid Staff: 6
Income Sources: Memphis Park Services; American Children's Theatre Association; Tennessee Theatre Association; Southeastern Theatre Conference
Annual Attendance: 10,000
Facility Category: Theatre
Seating Capacity: 200
Year Remodeled: 1979
Organization Type: Performing; Educational

3788 PLAYHOUSE ON THE SQUARE

51 S Cooper Street
Memphis, TN 38104
Phone: 901-725-0776
Fax: 901-272-7530
e-mail: info@playhouseonthesquare.org
Web Site: www.playhouseonthesquare.org
Management:
Executive Director: Jackie Nichols
Administrative Director: Elizabeth Howard
Public Relations Director: Patty McNaulty
Mission: Producing live theatrical productions including new plays, Broadway and off-Broadway shows.
Founded: 1968
Specialized Field: Theatrical Group
Status: Professional; Nonprofit
Income Sources: Theatre Communications Group; Circuit Playhouse
Season: Year round
Performs At: Playhouse on the Square
Organization Type: Performing; Touring; Resident; Educational

3789 MORRISTOWN THEATRE GUILD

314 S Hill Street
PO Box 1502
Morristown, TN 37816
Phone: 423-586-9260
Officers:
Chairman: Ralph Ozmun
Vice-Chairman: Candice Durman
Secretary: Angela Marshall
Treasurer: Susan Christophel
Management:
Artistic Director: David Horton
Mission: To provide exposure to live theatre; to offer school-age children educational training.
Founded: 1934
Specialized Field: Musical; Dinner; Community
Status: Non-Professional; Nonprofit
Paid Staff: 50
Income Sources: Tennessee Theatre Association
Performs At: Theatre Guild
Organization Type: Performing; Educational

3790 CHAFFIN'S BARN - A DINNER THEATRE

8204 Highway 100
Nashville, TN 37221
Phone: 615-646-9977
Fax: 615-662-5439
Toll-free: 800-282-2276
e-mail: info@dinnertheatre.com
Web Site: www.dinnertheatre.com
Management:
Producer: John P Chaffin
Manager: Angela Burnett
Mission: Package price for professional non-equity theatre and buffet dining.
Founded: 1967
Specialized Field: Musical; Dinner
Status: Professional
Performs At: Chaffin's Barn
Organization Type: Performing

3791 CORPORATE MAGIC

2802 Opryland Drive
Nashville, TN 37214
Phone: 615-871-5662
Fax: 615-871-6297
Toll-free: 800-275-7026
e-mail: info@corpmagic.com
Web Site: www.oprylandproductions.com
Founded: 1972
Status: Non-Equity; Commercial
Season: January - December

3792 DARKHORSE THEATER

4610 Charlotte Avenue
Nashville, TN 37209
Phone: 615-297-7113
Fax: 615-665-3336
e-mail: info@darkhorsetheater.com
Web Site: www.darkhorsetheater.com
Management:
Managing Director: Shannon Wood
Mission: To provide home to the Nashville creative performance community. Darkhouse theater presents aneclectic mix of original, classic, alternative, collorative, controversial and relevant theater and dance.
Founded: 1990
Specialized Field: Theater,Dance,Music

3793 DAVID LIPSCOMB UNIVERSITY THEATER

3901 Granny White Pike
Nashville, TN 37204-3951
Phone: 615-279-5715
Fax: 615-279-6516
e-mail: larry.brown@lipscomb.edu
Web Site: www.theatre.Lipscomb.edu
Management:
Professor/Theater Director: Dr. Larry Brown
Type of Stage: Black Box
Seating Capacity: 140

3794 MOCKINGBIRD PUBLIC THEATRE

PO Box 24002
Nashville, TN 37202
Phone: 615-242-6704
Fax: 615-242-7201
e-mail: mockingbirdtheatre@prodigy.net
Web Site: dr
Officers:
   Chairman: Chris Chamberlin
   Treasurer: Rueben Buck
   Secratery: Pamela Crosby
Management:
   Artistic Director: David Alford
   Associate Artistic Director: Rene Copeland
   General Manager: Kara V Kindall
Mission: To produce theatre that is relevant to the life of our community, maintain artistic integrity and pursue a standard of excellence; to promote, develop and support the culture and artists of our region.
Founded: 1994
Status: Professional; Nonprofit
Paid Artists: 40
Budget: $250,000-$300,000
Income Sources: Foundation; Private; Government
Performs At: Tennesee Performing Arts Center
Annual Attendance: 9,000-10,000

3795 NASHVILLE CHILDREN'S THEATRE

724 2nd Avenue S
Nashville, TN 37210
Phone: 615-254-9103
Fax: 615-254-3255
e-mail: adillon@nct-dragonsite.org
Web Site: www.nashvillechildrenstheatre.org
Officers:
   Chair: Paul Meyers
   Vice Chair: Chris Chamberlain
   Secretary: Sue Mendes
   Treasurer: Joel Goldberg
Management:
   Producing Director: Scot Copeland
   Financial Administration: Jean Johnson
   Managing Director: Allison Dillon
   Marketing/PR Director: Sharon Armstrong
   Education Director: Martha Goodman
   Office/House Manager: Lorna Turner
Mission: An ensemble of professional artists who bring unique vision and compelling voice to the creation of meaningful theatre for young audiences at NCT. We strive to make live theatre a vital part of the childhood experience for all young people in Nashville and Middle Tennessee.
Founded: 1931
Specialized Field: Theatrical Group
Status: Professional; Nonprofit
Paid Staff: 12
Paid Artists: 60
Income Sources: Box Office; Government Grants & Individual; Corporate & Foundation Support
Performs At: Hill Theatre, Cooney Playhouse
Affiliations: ASSITEJ/USA; AEA:TYA
Type of Stage: Main Stage; Black Box
Seating Capacity: 690; 300
Year Built: 1960
Organization Type: Performing; Resident; Educational

3796 NASHVILLE SHAKESPEARE FESTIVAL

800 4th Avenue S
Nashville, TN 37210
Phone: 615-255-2273
Fax: 615-248-2273
Web Site: www.brotherswest.com/nsf
Officers:
   Chairman: Donald Capparella
   Secretary/Treasurer: Denah Shabal
Management:
   Artistic Director: Denice Hickes
   Managing Director: Denah Shabal
Mission: Dedicated to community enrichment and arts in education through innovative and relevant presentations of the works of William Shakespeare and other curriculum-based programming. We focus our work to stimulate imagination and inspire conversation, which are essential elements to a healthy society.
Founded: 1988
Specialized Field: Central Park
Status: Professional
Season: August
Performs At: Centennial Park Bandshell
Affiliations: Shakespeare Theatre Association of America
Annual Attendance: 14,000
Organization Type: Performing; Resident; Touring; Educational

3797 TENNESSEE REPERTORY THEATRE

427 Chestnut Street
Nashville, TN 37203
Phone: 615-244-4878
Fax: 615-244-1232
e-mail: david@tnrep.oeg
Web Site: www.tnrep.org
Officers:
   President: Kerry Graham
Management:
   Director Operations: Donna Center
   Artistic Director: David Grapes
   Production Coordinator: Elizabeth Evert
   Director Public Relations/Market: Jayne Rogavin
   Associate Artistic Director: Todd Olson
Mission: The presentation of quality, professional theatre and a complete season of plays.
Founded: 1985
Specialized Field: Theatrical Group
Status: Professional
Paid Staff: 18
Volunteer Staff: 20
Paid Artists: 40
Income Sources: Ticket Sales; Fund-raising
Performs At: James K. Polk Theater; Tennessee Performing Arts Center
Affiliations: League of Resident Theatres; Actors' Equity Association; SSD&C
Annual Attendance: 70,000
Facility Category: Performing Arts Center
Type of Stage: Proscenium
Seating Capacity: 1,000
Year Built: 1980
Organization Type: Performing; Resident

3798 OAK RIDGE PLAYHOUSE
27 E Tennessee Avenue at Jackson Square
PO Box 5705
Oak Ridge, TN 37831
Phone: 865-482-9999
Fax: 865-482-0945
e-mail: playhouse@orplayhouse.com
Web Site: www.orplayhouse.com
Officers:
   President: Robert Wham
   VP: Em Way
   Secretary: John E Gunning
   Treasurer: Eugene Spejewski
Management:
   Managing Artistic Director: Reggie Law
   Technical Director: Jim Prodger
   Public Relations Director: Karen Brunner
   Costume Shop Manager: Jennifer Taylor-Smith
Mission: To provide quality theatre for the community while maintaining volunteer status.
Founded: 1943
Specialized Field: Theatre
Status: Nonprofit
Paid Staff: 3
Volunteer Staff: 100
Paid Artists: 15
Non-paid Artists: 10
Budget: $250,000
Income Sources: Box Office; Grants; Private Donations; Corporate Donations & Sponsors; Subscription
Performs At: Oak Ridge Playhouse in Jackson Square
Affiliations: SE Theatre Conference; Knoxville Area Theatre Coalition; Arts Council of Oak Ridge; American Assoc of Community Theatres; Knoxville Arts Council
Annual Attendance: 25,000
Facility Category: Community Theatre; Children's Theatre
Type of Stage: Proscenium
Stage Dimensions: 40'x25'
Seating Capacity: 344
Year Built: 1943
Year Remodeled: 1988
Rental Contact: Reggie Law
Organization Type: Performing

3799 DIXIE STAMPEDE
3849 Parkway
PO Box 58
Pigeon Forge, TN 37868
Phone: 865-453-9473
Fax: 865-908-7061
Toll-free: 800-356-1676
Management:
   General Manager: John Shaver
Founded: 1988
Status: Non-Equity; Commercial
Season: March - December
Type of Stage: Arena
Stage Dimensions: 75' x 150'
Seating Capacity: 1000

3800 LIFE OF CHRIST PASSION PLAY
329 Bethel Church Road
Townsend, TN 37882
Phone: 423-448-9080

Texas

3801 WATERTOWER THEATRE
15650 Addison Road
Addison, TX 75001
Phone: 972-450-6220
Fax: 972-450-6244
e-mail: info@watertowertheatre.com
Web Site: www.watertowertheatre.com
Management:
   Producing Artistic Director: Terry Martin
Founded: 1976
Annual Attendance: 20,800

3802 FORT GRIFFIN FANDANGLE ASSOCIATION
1 Railroad Street
PO Box 155
Albany, TX 76430
Phone: 915-762-3838
Fax: 915-762-3125
Officers:
   President: John Matthews
   VP: Harold Law
   VP/Treasurer: Winifred Waller
   Executive Secretary: Debbie Hudman
Mission: To present historical narration with song and dance.
Founded: 1937
Specialized Field: Theatrical Group
Status: Non-Professional; Nonprofit
Paid Staff: 250
Season: June
Performs At: Fort Griffin Fandangle Outdoor Theatre
Facility Category: Outdoor Ampitheater
Type of Stage: Grass
Seating Capacity: 1,800
Year Built: 1951
Organization Type: Performing

3803 THEATRE ARLINGTON
305 W Main Street
Arlington, TX 76010
Phone: 817-275-7661
Fax: 817-275-3370
e-mail: mail@theatrearlington.org
Web Site: www.theatrearlington.org
Management:
   Managing/Producing Director: Penny Patrick
   Artistic Director: BJ Cleveland
Founded: 1973
Specialized Field: Community; Theatrical Group
Status: Semi-Professional; Nonprofit
Paid Staff: 6
Income Sources: Texas Nonprofit Theatre
Performs At: Theatre Arlington
Organization Type: Performing; Resident; Educational

3804 AUSTIN MUSICAL THEATRE

2011 E Riverside Drive
Suite C
Austin, TX 78741
Phone: 512-428-9696
Fax: 512-428-9699
e-mail: jhammond@amtpresents.org
Web Site: www.amtpresents.com
Management:
  Producing Artistic Director: Scott Thompson
  Managing Artistic Director: Richard Byron
  Company Manager: Stuart Moultan
  Production Manager: Jeanine Lisa
  Executive Director: Jared Hammond
  Academy Coordinator: Ginger Morris
  Academy Assistant: Kevin Archambealt
  Marketing Director: Suzie Harriamn
Founded: 1996
Specialized Field: Music; Production; Training
Paid Staff: 10
Paid Artists: 100
Budget: $3,500,000
Income Sources: Donations; Grants; Academy Revenue;
Ticket Sales
Performs At: The Paramount Theatre
Affiliations: Actors' Equity Association; International
Alliance of Theatrical Stage Employees
Annual Attendance: 50,000
Type of Stage: Proscenium
Seating Capacity: 1,200
Year Built: 1915
Year Remodeled: 1975

3805 AUSTIN SHAKESPEARE FESTIVAL

PO Box 683
Austin, TX 78767-0683
Phone: 512-454-2273
e-mail: asf@austinshakespeare.org
Web Site: www.austinshakespeare.org
Officers:
  President: Daniel B Wilson
  VP: Susan Threadgill
  Treasurer: Jill K Sawnson
  Secretary: Sylvester L. Ruffin
Mission: To produce professional quality productions of
Classical theatre with an emphasis on the plays of William
Shakespeare and to entertain and enrich the theatre-going
public by presenting productions that are accessible,
imaginative, and stimulating, while remaining true to the
integrity of the plays and the author.
Founded: 1984
Status: Non-Equity; Nonprofit
Season: September - October
Type of Stage: Outdoor
Stage Dimensions: 50' x 40'
Seating Capacity: 3000

3806 AUSTIN THEATRE ALLIANCE

713 Congress
PO Box 1566
Austin, TX 78767

Phone: 512-472-2901
Fax: 512-472-5824
e-mail: jclearman@austintheatrealliance.org
Web Site: www.theparamount.org
Management:
  Program Director: Paul Beutel
Mission: To present and produce the best in theatre, film
and the performing arts. To own and operate the histroic
Paramount and State Theatres.
Founded: 1975
Paid Staff: 25
Paid Artists: 100

3807 FRONTERA

511 W 43rd Street
Austin, TX 78751
Phone: 512-302-4933
Fax: 512-302-5041
Management:
  Artistic Director: Vicky Boone
Founded: 1992
Specialized Field: Theater
Performs At: Hyde Park Theatre
Type of Stage: Flexible
Seating Capacity: 90

3808 PROJECT INTERACT - ZACHARY SCOTT THEATRE CENTER

1510 Toomey Road
Austin, TX 78704
Phone: 512-476-0594
Fax: 512-476-0314
Management:
  Artistic Director: Jeff Frank
  Business Manager: Alex B Alford
Mission: To offer the finest contemporary and classical
scripts and original works for young people; to maintain a
multicultural company.
Founded: 1977
Specialized Field: Theatrical Group
Status: Professional
Income Sources: Theatre Communications Group;
American Association of Theatre Educators; Theatre in
Disability; Austin Circle of Theatres
Performs At: ZSTC Arena; ZSTC Kleberg
Organization Type: Performing; Touring; Educational

3809 RUDE MECHANICALS

2211-A Hidalgo Street
Suite 220
Austin, TX 78702
Phone: 512-476-7833
Fax: 512-477-3157
e-mail: info@rudemech.com
Web Site: www.rudemech.com
Officers:
  President: Paul Drown
  VP: Ron Marks
  Treasurer: Alex Alford
  Secretary: Jonathan Tamez
Management:
  Venue Manager: Madge Darlington
  Development Director: Mike Henry
  Business Manager: Lana Lesley

Marketing Director: Sarah Richardson
Resident Producer: Shawn Sides

3810 STATE THEATER COMPANY

719 Congress Avenue
Austin, TX 78701
Phone: 512-472-5143
Fax: 512-472-7199
Web Site: www.statetheatercompany.com
Officers:
   CEO: Dan Fallon
Management:
   Producing Artistic Director: Scott Kanoff
Founded: 1982
Status: Professional
Paid Staff: 5
Paid Artists: 75
Income Sources: Corporations; Foundations; Individual Gifts
Season: March - August

3811 VORTEX REPERTORY COMPANY

2307 Manor Road
PO Box 33125
Austin, TX 78722
Phone: 512-478-5282
e-mail: ponty@jollylox.com
Web Site: www.jollylox.com/vortex/
Management:
   Managing Director: Steve Bacher
   Producing Artistic Director: Bonnie Cullum
Mission: To create new, innovative performances, including original works, new plays, revitalized classics, and to present nationally-recognized, cutting edge touring artists.
Founded: 1988
Specialized Field: Theatrical Group
Status: Professional; Nonprofit
Paid Staff: 200
Performs At: Vortex Performance Care
Organization Type: Performing; Touring; Resident; Educational; Sponsoring

3812 BASTROP OPERA HOUSE

711 Spring Street
PO Box 691
Bastrop, TX 78602
Phone: 512-321-6283
e-mail: info@bastropoperahouse.com
Web Site: www.bastropoperahouse.com
Management:
   Executive Director: Chester Eitze
Mission: To present dance, music and theatre in a performing arts center at the restored Old Bastrop Opera House.
Founded: 1889
Specialized Field: Summer Stock; Musical; Dinner; Community; Theatrical Group
Status: Semi-Professional; Non-Professional; Nonprofit
Performs At: Old Bastrop Opera House
Organization Type: Performing; Sponsoring

3813 CAMILLE PLAYERS

1 Dean Porter Park
Brownsville, TX 78520
Phone: 956-542-8900
Fax: 956-986-0639
e-mail: camillight@aol.com
Web Site: www.camilleplayhouse.utl.com
Officers:
   President: John P Kinch
   VP: Ben Salinas
   Second VP: Fidencio Zavala
   Treasurer: Dan Anderson
Management:
   Executive Artistic Director: Ben Agresti
   Business Manager: Carla Reynolds
Mission: To stimulate interest in drama through presenting plays.
Founded: 1964
Specialized Field: Musical; Community; Children's Theatre
Status: Non-Professional; Nonprofit
Paid Staff: 2
Volunteer Staff: 3
Budget: $9,000
Performs At: Camille Lightner Playhouse
Annual Attendance: 5,000
Facility Category: Theatre
Type of Stage: Proscenium
Stage Dimensions: 30'x25'
Seating Capacity: 301
Year Built: 1964
Year Remodeled: 1995
Organization Type: Performing

3814 TEXAS MUSICAL DRAMA

Palo Duro Canyon State Park
1514 5th Street
Canyon, TX 79015
Phone: 806-655-2181
Fax: 806-655-4730
Web Site: www.texasmusicaldrama.com
Officers:
   President: Blaine Bertrand
   President of the Executive Board: Lorene Lacer
Management:
   General Manager: Blaine Burtrand
   Marketing Director: Sheila Blackburn
   Office Manager: Nancy McClendon
Mission: To perpetuate the heritage of the area by presenting a historical drama about the 1880's settling of the Texas Panhandle.
Founded: 1965
Specialized Field: Dance; Vocal Music; Instrumental Music; Theater
Status: Professional; Nonprofit
Paid Staff: 11
Paid Artists: 140
Income Sources: Texas Panhandle Heritage Foundation
Performs At: Pioneer Amphitheatre
Annual Attendance: 85,000
Facility Category: Outdoor Amphitheater
Seating Capacity: 1723
Year Built: 1965
Rental Contact: Blaine Bertrand
Organization Type: Performing; Educational

3815 STAGECENTER
701 N Main Street
PO Box 9475
College Station, TX 77842
Phone: 979-823-4297
Management:
Business Manager: Winnie Nelson
Mission: To offer community members an opportunity for participation in theatre.
Founded: 1966
Specialized Field: Community
Status: Nonprofit
Paid Staff: 50
Income Sources: Arts Council of Brazos Valley
Organization Type: Performing; Educational

3816 BRAVVO! PRODUCTIONS
701 S Main Street
PO Box 314
Corsicana, TX 75110
Phone: 903-872-0559
Fax: 903-872-0636
Management:
Director: Cranston Dodds
Founded: 1990
Status: Non-Equity; Commercial
Season: August - April

3817 CORSICANA COMMUNITY PLAYHOUSE
119 W 6th Avenue
Corsicana, TX 75110
Phone: 903-872-5421
Management:
Executive Director: Sandra McCluremahood
Mission: To provide quality theatrical performances for Corsicana and the north and east Texas regions.
Founded: 1971
Specialized Field: Community; Theatrical Group
Status: Semi-Professional; Nonprofit
Income Sources: Texas Nonprofit Theatre
Performs At: Warehouse Living Arts Center
Organization Type: Performing; Touring

3818 CABBAGES AND KINGS
7436 Kenshine Lane
Dallas, TX 75230
Phone: 214-363-7292
Fax: 214-867-7615
Management:
Founder/Artistic Director: Linda Comess
Business Manager: Tricia Avery
Mission: To entertain and enlighten families and children; to present original plays which are based on mythology and stories and are relevant to modern life.
Founded: 1984
Specialized Field: Theatrical Group
Status: Professional; Nonprofit
Income Sources: Actors' Equity Association
Performs At: Addison Centre Theatre
Organization Type: Performing; Touring

3819 DALLAS CHILDREN'S THEATER
2215 Cedar Springs
Dallas, TX 75201
Phone: 214-978-0110
Fax: 214-978-0118
e-mail: family@dct.org
Web Site: www.dct.org
Management:
Executive/Artistic Director: Robyn Flatt
Associate Artistic Director: Artie Claisen
Education Director: Nancy Schaeffer
Tour Director: Sally Fiorello
Mission: To enrich children's lives through theater arts.
Founded: 1984
Specialized Field: Theatrical Group; Educational Programming
Status: Professional; Nonprofit
Paid Staff: 22
Volunteer Staff: 100
Paid Artists: 175
Budget: $2,500,000
Income Sources: International Association of Theatre for Children and Youth; Corporate; Foundation; Individuals; Grants; Ticket Purchases
Performs At: El Centre College Theatre; Crescent Theatre
Affiliations: TGG; AEA; AATE; TNT; ASSITEJ
Annual Attendance: 245,00
Organization Type: Performing; Touring; Educational

3820 DALLAS PUPPET THEATER
3905 Main Street
Dallas, TX 75226
Phone: 214-515-0004
Web Site: www.puppetry.org
Management:
Founding Artistic Director: James Smith
Technical Director: Michael Robinson
Mission: Dedicated to promoting and advancing the performing, visual, and creative art of puppetry.
Founded: 1982
Specialized Field: Puppet
Status: Professional; Not-for-Profit
Organization Type: Performing; Touring; Resident; Educational; Sponsoring

3821 DALLAS THEATER CENTER
3636 Turtle Creek Boulevard
Dallas, TX 75219-5598
Phone: 214-526-8210
Fax: 214-521-7666
Web Site: www.dallastheatercenter.org
Management:
Artistic Director: Richard Hamburger
Managing Director: Edith Love
Literary Office: Allison Horsley
Artistic Associate: Claudia Zelavansky
Mission: To offer excellent professional theatre that produces classic, contemporary and new plays of the highest artistic quality.
Founded: 1959
Specialized Field: Theatrical Group
Status: Professional; Nonprofit

Income Sources: Theatre Communications Group; League of Resident Theatres; American Arts Alliance
Performs At: Kalita Humphreys Theater; Arts District Theater
Type of Stage: Flexible; Thrust
Seating Capacity: 530; 466
Organization Type: Performing; Resident; Educational

3822   DRAMA CIRCLE THEATRE
2929 Mayhew
Dallas, TX 75228
Phone: 972-270-9255
Management:
   Managing Director: Linda Boatman
   Founder: Bill Green
   Co-Founder: Nan Truax
Mission: To promote the theatre arts.
Founded: 1971
Specialized Field: Theatrical Group
Status: Semi-Professional; Nonprofit
Paid Staff: 30
Organization Type: Performing; Touring; Educational

3823   ECHO THEATRE
PO Box 820698
Dallas, TX 75328
Phone: 214-904-0500
e-mail: mail@echotheatre.org
Web Site: www.echotheatre.org
Officers:
   Co-Founder: Linda Marie Ford
   Co-Founder: Pam Myers-Morgan
   Co-Founder: Suzy Blaylock
Mission: For years, theatre seasons at all levels of production have been programmed mainly wiht works by male playwrights, often resulting in an absence of the female voice.
Founded: 1997

3824   KATHY BURKS MARIONETTES
2979 Ladybird Lane
Dallas, TX 75229
Phone: 214-353-9277
e-mail: saltee@flash.net
Web Site: www.flash.net/~saltee
Management:
   Artistic Director: Kathy Burks
   Managing Director: Sarah Jayne Fiorello
   Master Puppeteer/Co-Artistic Direct: Douglas Burks
   Composer/Lyricist: Beatrice Wolf
Mission: To perpetuate the art of puppetry; to cover the spectrum of the art itself.
Founded: 1973
Specialized Field: Theatrical Group; Puppet
Status: Professional; Nonprofit
Income Sources: Puppeteers of America; Lone Star Puppet Guild
Performs At: The Loft Puppet Theatre at Fairview Farms
Organization Type: Performing; Resident; Educational

3825   KITCHEN DOG THEATER
3120 McKinney Avenue
Dallas, TX 75204
Phone: 214-953-1055
Fax: 214-953-1873
e-mail: admin@kitchendogtheater.org
Web Site: www.kitchendogtheater.org
Officers:
   Co-President/Board Director: Jason Ankele
   Co-President/Board Director: Susan Albritton
Management:
   Artistic Director: Dan Day
   Administrative Director: Tina Parker
   Development/Marketing Manager: Heidi Shen
Mission: It is the mission of Kitchen Dog Theater to provide a place where questions of justice, morality, and human freedom can be explored. We choose plays that challenge our moral and social consciences, and invite our audiences to be provoked, challenged, and amazed. We believe that the theater is a site of individual discovery as well as a force against conventional views of the self and experience.
Founded: 1990
Performs At: McKinney Avenue Contemporary
Affiliations: National New Play Network; Dallas Theatre League; Theater Communications Group
Type of Stage: Thrust; Black Box
Seating Capacity: 150; 75-100
Year Built: 1994

3826   PEGASUS THEATRE
3916 Main Street
Dallas, TX 75226
Phone: 214-821-6005
Web Site: www.pegasustheatre.com
Management:
   Artistic Director: Kurt Kleinmann
   General Manager: Barbara Weinberger
Mission: A professional live stage theatre specializing in new and original comedies. They offer four main stage productions each season.
Founded: 1985
Specialized Field: Musical; Theatrical Group
Status: Professional; Nonprofit
Income Sources: Stage
Performs At: Pegasus Theatre
Organization Type: Performing; Touring

3827   POCKET SANDWICH THEATRE
5400 E Mockingbird Lane
Suite 119
Dallas, TX 75206
Phone: 214-821-1860
e-mail: pst@dallas.net
Web Site: www.pocketsandwich.com
Management:
   Owner/Technical Director: Rodney Dobbs
   Owner/Artistic Director: Joe Dickinson
Mission: To offer variety in live theatre performances.
Founded: 1980
Specialized Field: Musical; Dinner
Status: Professional; Commercial
Performs At: Pocket Sandwich Theatre
Organization Type: Performing

3828 SHAKESPEARE FESTIVAL OF DALLAS
3630 Harry Hine Boulevard
4th Floor
Dallas, TX 75219
Phone: 214-559-2778
Fax: 214-559-2782
e-mail: sgreenway@shakespearedallas.org
Web Site: www.shakespearedallas.org
Management:
   Managing Director: Sandra L Greenway
Founded: 1972
Status: Professional; Nonprofit
Paid Staff: 3
Performs At: Fair Park Band Shell
Organization Type: Performing; Educational

3829 TEATRO HISPANO DE DALLAS
2204 Commerce Street
Dallas, TX 75201
Phone: 214-741-6833
Fax: 214-946-5820
e-mail: teatro@airmail.net
Web Site: web2.airmail.net/teatro
Officers:
   President: Phillip Fiqueroa
   VP: Priscilla Diaz
Management:
   Artistic Director/Producer: Cora Cardona
   Executive Director: Christie Hernandez
Founded: 1985
Specialized Field: Community; Theatrical Group
Status: Professional; Semi-Professional; Nonprofit
Paid Staff: 3
Paid Artists: 20
Budget: $250,000
Performs At: Teatro Dallas
Annual Attendance: 15,000
Facility Category: Leases various venues
Organization Type: Performing

3830 TEXAS INTERNATIONAL THEATRICAL ARTS SOCIETY
3101 N Fitzhugh Avenue
Suite 301
Dallas, TX 75204
Phone: 214-528-6112
Fax: 214-528-2617
e-mail: dthompson@titas.org
Web Site: www.titas.org
Officers:
   President: William P Benac
Management:
   Executive Director: Charles Santos
   Director Finance: Doug Thompsom
   Director Development: Lynne Richardson
Mission: To create opportunities otherwise unavailable in Dallas and North Texas for our community to experience an abundant mixture of the best American and international dance, performance art, and music through performances and cultural and educational outreach activities.
Founded: 1982
Specialized Field: Dance; Performance Art; Music
Status: Nonprofit

Paid Staff: 15
Volunteer Staff: 70
Budget: $2,100,000
Income Sources: Private; Corporate; Foundation; Individual; Box Office
Performs At: McFarlin Auditorium; Southern Methodist University
Affiliations: Association of Performing Arts Presenters; International Society of Performing Arts
Annual Attendance: 52,000
Facility Category: Auditorium
Seating Capacity: 2,383
Rental Contact: Director Melissa Berry
Organization Type: Presenting; Educational

3831 THEATRE GEMINI
PO Box 191225
Dallas, TX 75219
Phone: 214-521-6331
Management:
   General Manager: Craig Hess
Founded: 1984
Specialized Field: Community; Theatrical Group
Status: Non-Professional; Nonprofit
Paid Staff: 60
Organization Type: Performing; Educational

3832 THEATRE THREE
2800 Routh Street
Dallas, TX 75201
Phone: 214-871-2933
Fax: 214-871-3139
e-mail: theatre3@airmail.net
Web Site: www.theatre3dallas.com
Management:
   Executive Producer: Jac Alder
   Co-Manager: Terry Dawson
Mission: To offer professional theatre as well as related activities to the Dallas-Ft. Worth area and to further the artistic careers of theatre artists who reside in North Texas.
Founded: 1961
Specialized Field: Musical; Comedy; Drama
Status: Nonprofit
Paid Staff: 30
Budget: $1.4 million
Income Sources: Admission Earnings; Miscellaneous Earnings; Government; Corporate; Foundation; Individual Grants/Donations
Performs At: Theatre in the round
Affiliations: AEA; Southwest Theatre Association; Texas Non Profit Theatres
Facility Category: Theatre
Seating Capacity: 242; 70
Year Built: 1969
Year Remodeled: 1986
Organization Type: Performing; Touring; Resident; Educational; Sponsoring

3833 UNDERMAIN THEATRE
3200 Main Street
PO Box 144466
Dallas, TX 75214

Phone: 214-747-5515
Fax: 214-747-1863
e-mail: undermain@aol.com
Web Site: www.undermain.com
Management:
   Artistic Director: Katherine Owens
   Operations Manager: Victor Ruiz
Mission: To focus on regionally and nationally premiering work that is challenging intellectually, emotionally and philosphically.
Founded: 1984
Status: Professional; Nonprofit
Performs At: Undermain Theatre Basement
Affiliations: Actors' Equity Association; TCG; National Endowment for the Arts
Facility Category: Basement Theatre
Type of Stage: Flexible
Seating Capacity: 90
Year Built: 1900
Organization Type: Performing

3834 BREAD AND CIRCUS THEATRE

1009 Bull Run
Denton, TX 76201
Phone: 817-387-2408
Management:
   Managing Director: Connie Whitt-Lambert
Mission: To offer fun theatrical experiences to children and adults through audience participation.
Founded: 1982
Specialized Field: Theatrical Group; Summer Stock; Community; Musical
Status: Professional; Semi-Professional
Organization Type: Performing; Touring

3835 DENTON COMMUNITY THEATRE

214 W Hickory
PO Box 1931
Denton, TX 76202
Phone: 940-382-7014
Fax: 940-891-1691
e-mail: dct@campustheatre.com
Web Site: www.campustheatre.com
Officers:
   President: Steve Plunkett
Management:
   Executive Director: Scott Wilkinson
Mission: To offer artistic, educational experiences to participants; to provide quality theatre for audiences.
Founded: 1969
Specialized Field: Community; Theatrical Group
Status: Non-Professional; Nonprofit
Paid Staff: 5
Volunteer Staff: 50
Paid Artists: 300
Non-paid Artists: 300
Budget: $450,000
Income Sources: City of Denton
Performs At: Campus Theatre
Affiliations: ACT; SWTC; TNT
Annual Attendance: 30,000
Type of Stage: Proscenium
Stage Dimensions: 40'x40'
Seating Capacity: 299
Year Built: 1949

Year Remodeled: 1985
Cost: $2 million
Organization Type: Performing; Educational

3836 EL PASO ASSOCIATION FOR THE PERFORMING ARTS/VIVA EL PASO!

PO Box 31340
El Paso, TX 79931-0340
Phone: 915-565-6900
Fax: 915-565-6999
Web Site: www.viva-ep.org
Management:
   Managing Director: David Mills
   Director of Marketing: Mario A Duron
Founded: 1978
Status: Non-Equity; Nonprofit
Season: June - August
Type of Stage: Amphitheatre
Stage Dimensions: 80' x 40'
Seating Capacity: 1500

3837 SOUTHWEST REPERTORY ORGANIZATION

1301 Texas Avenue
El Paso, TX 79901
Phone: 915-534-7653
Management:
   Interim Executive/Artistic Director: Ed Hamilton
   Technical Director: Glen O Brooks
   Office Manager: Glenda Nevarez
Mission: To provide a main season including musicals, comedies and contemporary dramas; to offer a summer repertory featuring contemporary plays as well as classes in directing, acting and the technical aspects of theatre.
Founded: 1978
Specialized Field: Musical; Community; Theatrical Group
Status: Non-Professional; Nonprofit
Organization Type: Performing; Touring

3838 ALLIED THEATRE GROUP/STAGE WEST

3053-55 S University Drive
Fort Worth, TX 76109
Phone: 817-924-9454
Fax: 817-926-8650
e-mail: stagewest@gbronline.com
Web Site: www.stagewest.org
Officers:
   President: Charles Reid
   VP: Sharon Harrelson
   Treasurer: Janie Frank
   Past President: Maggie Knapp
Management:
   Producing Artistic Director: Jim Covault
   Administrative Associate: Jenae Yerger
   Literary Associate: Natalie Gaupp
Mission: To produce a minimum of six major productions annually, including some musicals; to offer a broad range of works from classical to new and contemporary.
Founded: 1979
Specialized Field: Theatrical Group
Status: Professional; Nonprofit

Paid Staff: 10
Volunteer Staff: 100
Non-paid Artists: 20
Income Sources: Actors' Equity Association; Theatre Communications Group; Texas Nonprofit Theatre; Live Theatre League of Tarrant County; Arts Council of Fort Worth & Tarrant County
Performs At: Stage West
Facility Category: Theatre-in-the-Round
Seating Capacity: 200
Year Remodeled: 1993
Organization Type: Performing

3839 CASA MANANA MUSICALS

300 W 3rd Street
Suite 1715
Fort Worth, TX 76102
Phone: 817-332-2272
Fax: 817-332-5711
Web Site: www.casamanana.org
Management:
Executive Producer: Denton Vockey
Founded: 1958
Specialized Field: Musical Theatre
Status: Professional; Nonprofit
Performs At: Casa Manana Theatre; Bass Performance Hall
Affiliations: National Alliance for Musical Theatre; Live Theatre League of Tarrant County; Texas Nonprofit Theatre Association
Organization Type: Performing; Touring; Resident; Educational

3840 CASA MANANA PLAYHOUSE

3101 W Lancaster
Fort Worth, TX 76107
Phone: 817-332-9319
Fax: 817-332-5711
Officers:
Chairman: Bob Bolen
President: Ted B Bevan
VP Finance/Budget: David Walker
Secretary: D'Ann Reed Dagen
Management:
Executive Producer: Van Kaplan
Director Playhouse: Deborah Brown
Mission: To present plays for children Fridays and Saturday with special weekday performances for local schools; to present Casa Kids, 15 children who provide free performances for area civic and nonprofit organizations.
Founded: 1962
Specialized Field: Musical
Status: Professional; Nonprofit
Income Sources: International Association of Theatre for Children and Youth; Actors' Equity Association; American Federation of Musicians
Performs At: Casa Manana Theatre
Organization Type: Performing; Resident; Educational

3841 CIRCLE THEATRE

230 W 4th Street
PO Box 470456
Fort Worth, TX 76147-0456

Phone: 817-921-3040
Fax: 817-877-3848
Officers:
President: Joan Kline
VP: Robert I Fenandez
VP: Tom Gaffney
Corresponding Secretary: Kim Kirk
Recording Secretary: Sherry Jackson
Treasurer: Marilyn Austin
Management:
Executive Director: Rose Pearson
Managing Director: Bill Newberry
Director Public Relations/Marketing: Carlo Cuesta
Mission: Our mission is the advocacy of contemporary plays rarely seen in this community. We are commited to presenting professional, innovative theatre in an intimate setting.
Founded: 1981
Specialized Field: Theatrical Group
Status: Semi-Professional; Nonprofit
Organization Type: Performing; Resident

3842 FORT WORTH THEATRE

4401 Trail, Ake Drive
Fort Worth, TX 76109
Phone: 817-921-5300
Web Site: fwtheatre.homestead.com
Management:
Artistic Director: William Garber
Administrative Director: Brynn Bristol
Mission: To offer quality theatre to Fort Worth; to provide an outlet for talented amateurs.
Founded: 1955
Specialized Field: Theatrical Group
Status: Non-Professional; Nonprofit
Performs At: William Edrington Scott Theatre
Organization Type: Performing; Resident

3843 HIP POCKET THEATRE

PO Box 136758
Fort Worth, TX 76136
Phone: 817-246-9775
Fax: 817-246-5651
e-mail: dsimons@hippocket.org
Web Site: www.hippocket.org
Officers:
President: Judy Clark
President Elect: Ralph Watterson
Secretary: Judy Golden
Treasurer: Jessica Weaver
Management:
Producer: Diane Simons
Artistic Director: Johnny Simons
Mission: Showcasing the original work of regional composers and playwrights, as well as works rarely seen in this area.
Founded: 1977
Specialized Field: Musical; Folk; Theatrical Group; Puppet
Status: Professional; Nonprofit
Paid Staff: 4
Volunteer Staff: 2
Paid Artists: 45
Non-paid Artists: 30
Budget: $165,000

Income Sources: Texas Commission on the Arts; National Endowment
Performs At: Oak Acres Amphitheatre
Affiliations: Live Theatre League Arts Council at Fort Worth
Facility Category: Outdoor Amphitheatre
Type of Stage: Multi-leveled tree house
Seating Capacity: 175
Year Built: 1978
Rental Contact: Diene Simons
Organization Type: Performing; Touring; Resident; Educational

3844 STAGE WEST

3055 S University
Fort Worth, TX 76109
Phone: 817-923-6698
Fax: 817-926-8650
e-mail: stgwest@ix.netcom.com
Web Site: www.alliedtheatre.org
Management:
   Box Office Manager: Natalie Gaupp
   Artistic Director: Jim Covault
Mission: To provide Shakespeare-in-the-Park for Fort Worth residents at no cost.
Founded: 1977
Specialized Field: Theater; Festivals
Status: Professional; Nonprofit
Paid Staff: 12
Income Sources: Texas Christian University; City of Fort Worth
Performs At: Indoor venue; Outdoor venue
Annual Attendance: 125,000
Facility Category: Park Site Fort Worth's Trinity Park, Stagewest
Rental Contact: Managing Director Mark Waltz
Organization Type: Performing; Touring

3845 GALVESTON OUTDOOR MUSICALS

PO Box 5253
Galveston, TX 77554
Phone: 409-737-1744
Fax: 409-737-2033
Web Site: www.galveston.com
Founded: 1977
Status: Nonprofit
Season: June - August
Type of Stage: Amphitheatre
Stage Dimensions: 150' x 150'
Seating Capacity: 1766

3846 GARLAND CIVIC THEATRE

108 N 6th Street
Garland, TX 75040
Phone: 972-485-8884
Fax: 214-553-0081
Management:
   Producing Director: James Weir
   Administrative Assistant: Linda White
   Technical Director: Dwight Swanson
Mission: To offer quality entertainment to our audiences; to provide space for community performers; to advance theatre.
Founded: 1967

Specialized Field: Musical; Theatrical Group
Status: Semi-Professional; Nonprofit
Income Sources: Texas Nonprofit Theatre; Theatre Communications Group
Performs At: Garland Center for the Performing Arts
Organization Type: Performing; Resident

3847 TEXAS AMPHITHEATRE

PO Box 8
202 Bo Gibbs Boulevard
Glen Rose, TX 76043
Phone: 254-897-4509
Fax: 254-897-7713
Web Site: www.glenrose.org
Management:
   Facilities Manager: Mike Dooley
Founded: 1989
Status: Non-Equity; Nonprofit
Season: June - October
Type of Stage: Amphitheatre
Stage Dimensions: 130' x 64'
Seating Capacity: 3200

3848 GRANBURY OPERA HOUSE

116 E Pearl Street
PO Box 297
Granbury, TX 76048
Phone: 817-573-9191
Fax: 817-579-5529
Web Site: www.granburyoperahouse.org
Management:
   Managing Director: Marty Van Kleeck
   Technical Director: Adam Puglielli
   Costume Designer: Drenda Lewis
   Facilities Manager: Jake Jacobs
Founded: 1974
Specialized Field: Year-round Stock
Status: Nonprofit
Income Sources: Box Office; Texas Commission for the Arts Grant; Individual Donors
Season: Year round
Performs At: Granbury Opera House
Annual Attendance: 63,000
Organization Type: Performing; Educational

3849 ACTORS THEATRE OF HOUSTON

2506 S Boulevard
Houston, TX 77098
Phone: 713-529-6606
e-mail: kgeorgeb@flash.net
Web Site: actorstheatre.hypermart.net
Management:
   Producing Director: Chris Wilson
Founded: 1986

3850 AD PLAYERS

2710 W Alabama Street
Houston, TX 77098
Phone: 713-526-2721
Fax: 713-439-0905
e-mail: adplayer@hern.org
Web Site: www.adplayers.org
Management:
   Director: Dan Bunch

Assistant Director: Brenda Fager
TAA Assistant: Mindy Hines
Mission: To offer a complete season featuring Christian theatrical productions for Houston audiences; to tour repertory and concert presentations nationally and internationally.
Founded: 1967
Specialized Field: Theatrical Group
Status: Professional; Semi-Professional; Nonprofit
Income Sources: Texas Nonprofit Theatre; Theatre Communications Group; Houston Theatre Association; Cultural Arts Council of Houston
Season: September - August
Performs At: Grace Theatre
Type of Stage: Proscenium; Arena; Round
Seating Capacity: 220; 200; 75
Organization Type: Performing; Touring; Resident; Educational

3851 ALLEY THEATRE

615 Texas Avenue
Houston, TX 77002
Phone: 713-228-8421
Fax: 713-222-6542
Web Site: www.alleytheatre.org or www.teatroalley.org
Management:
  Artistic Director: Gregory Boyd
  Managing Director: Paul Tetreanlt
  General Manager: Sean Skeehan
Mission: Promoting the presentation of theatrical literature.
Founded: 1947
Specialized Field: Theatrical Group
Status: Professional; Nonprofit
Income Sources: Sponsors; Corporations
Performs At: Alley Theatre
Affiliations: League of Resident Theatres; Actors' Equity Association; USA; Society for Stage Directors and Choreographers
Organization Type: Performing; Touring; Resident; Educational; Sponsoring

3852 CHANNING PLAYERS

PO Box 631363
Houston, TX 77263
Phone: 713-785-9492
Management:
  Artistic Director: Janis Halliday
  Technical Director: Donald Williams
Mission: Producing quality plays.
Founded: 1955
Specialized Field: Community
Status: Nonprofit
Paid Staff: 50
Income Sources: Cultural Arts Council of Houston; Texas Nonprofit Theatre
Organization Type: Performing; Educational

3853 CHILDREN'S THEATRE FESTIVAL

School of Theatre
University of Houston
Houston, TX 77204-4016
Phone: 713-743-3003
e-mail: sjudice@uh.edu
Web Site: www.hfac.uh.edu/theatre/ctf.htm
Management:
  Production Director: Sidney Berger
Founded: 1978
Status: Non-Equity; Nonprofit
Season: June - August
Type of Stage: Proscenium
Stage Dimensions: 40' x 33'
Seating Capacity: 566

3854 ENSEMBLE THEATRE

3535 Main
Houston, TX 77002
Phone: 713-520-0055
Fax: 713-520-1269
Management:
  Producing Artistic Director: Marsha Jacobson Randolph
  Production Manager: Sara Sturtevant
Mission: The Ensemble Theatre is the Southwest's largest African American theatre presenting a season of classic and contemporary works featuring local and national artists.
Founded: 1976
Specialized Field: Theatrical Group
Status: Professional; Nonprofit
Paid Staff: 9
Paid Artists: 115
Performs At: The Ensemble Theatre
Organization Type: Performing; Touring; Resident; Educational

3855 HOUSTON SHAKESPEARE FESTIVAL

School of Theatre
University of Houston
Houston, TX 77204-5071
Phone: 713-743-3003
Fax: 713-749-1420
Web Site: www.hfac.uh.edu/theatre/hsf.htm
Management:
  Producing Director: Sidney L Berger
  Secretary: Sandy Judice
  Business Administrator: Jerry Aven
Mission: To provide classical theater at no cost to citizens of Houston and surrounding areas.
Founded: 1975
Specialized Field: Theater; Festivals
Status: Professional; Nonprofit
Income Sources: University of Houston
Performs At: Miller Outdoor Theatre
Organization Type: Performing

3856 INFERNAL BRIDEGROOM PRODUCTIONS

2524 McKinney
Houston, TX 77003
Mailing Address: PO Box 131004 Houston, TX 77219-1004
Phone: 713-522-8443
Fax: 713-630-5208
e-mail: infernalbridegroom@hotmail.com
Management:

Associate Director: Anthony Barilla
Artistic Director: Jason Nodler
Managing Director: Lisa Haymes
Founded: 1993

3857 MAIN STREET THEATER

2540 Times Boulevard
Houston, TX 77005
Phone: 713-524-3622
Fax: 713-524-3977
e-mail: info@mainstreettheater.com
Web Site: www.mainstreettheater.com
Management:
  Artistic Director: Rebecca Greene Udden
  Production Manager: Andrew Ruthven
  Managing Director: Robbye Floyd-Archibald
  Marketing Associate: Misty Johnson
  Director Education: Angela Harris
Mission: To offer a lively year-round repertory of classic and contemporary plays for audiences of all ages; to provide a much-needed showcase for Houston theatre professionals. Main Street Theatre is a member of Theatre Communications Group, the national organization of professional not-for-profit theatres and produces under an agreement with Actors' Equity Association, the union of professional actors.
Founded: 1975
Specialized Field: Theatrical Group
Status: Professional; Semi-Professional; Non-Professional
Organization Type: Performing; Touring; Resident

3858 STAGES REPERTORY THEATRE

3201 Allen Parkway
Suite 101
Houston, TX 77019
Phone: 713-527-0220
Fax: 713-527-8669
e-mail: kmlaughlin@stagestheatre.com
Web Site: www.stagestheatre.com
Management:
  Artistic Director: Rob Bundy
  Managing Director: Kenn McLaughlin
  Early Stages Artistic Director: Chesley Krohn
Mission: To present plays that are challenging to a developing company and are of social value and that set a standard of excellence.
Founded: 1978
Specialized Field: Theatrical Group
Status: Professional; Nonprofit
Paid Staff: 27
Volunteer Staff: 2
Paid Artists: 128
Budget: $1.5 Million
Income Sources: Ticket Sales; Private Foundations; Corparations; Local and State Funding
Season: Year round
Performs At: Arena Theatre; Thrust Theatre
Affiliations: Actors' Equity Association; TCG; ASSITJ
Annual Attendance: 60,000
Facility Category: Dual Stages
Stage Dimensions: 19'x 20'; 23'x 30'
Seating Capacity: 229;171
Year Built: 1933
Year Remodeled: 1983

Rental Contact: Managing Director Thomas M. Smith
Organization Type: Performing; Touring; Resident; Educational; Sponsoring

3859 TALENTO BILINGUE DE HOUSTON

333 S Jenson
Houston, TX 77003
Phone: 713-222-1213
Web Site: www.tbhcenter.com
Management:
  Artistic/Project Director: Richard E Reyes
  Manager: Fernando Gonzales
  Technical Director: Rodney Becerra
  Publicity: Jim Bratton
  Special Events: Rick Camargo
  Program Manager: Fernando Perez
Mission: A non-profit cultural and educational organization.
Founded: 1977
Specialized Field: Musical; Community; Theatrical Group
Status: Nonprofit
Paid Staff: 40
Organization Type: Performing; Touring; Educational; Sponsoring

3860 THEATRE SUBURBIA

1410 W 43rd
Houston, TX 77018
Phone: 713-682-3525
Management:
  Box Office: CR Glover
  Technical Director: Keith Ross
  Back Stage Coordinator: Melissa Merten
Mission: To provide the public with quality entertainment consisting of light comedy through heavy drama; to achieve recognition as a producer of the finest quality original scripts.
Founded: 1960
Specialized Field: Theatrical Group
Status: Non-Professional; Nonprofit
Performs At: Theatre Suburbia
Organization Type: Performing

3861 THEATRE UNDER THE STARS

4235 San Felipe
Houston, TX 77002
Phone: 713-622-1626
Fax: 713-622-0025
Web Site: www.tuts.com
Management:
  Executive Director/Founder: Frank M Young
  Producing Director: John Holly
  Managing Director: Cissy Segall
  General Manager: Vivian Flynn
Mission: To present light opera regionally as well as on tour; to operate a school for aspiring artists; to foster the development of new musical theatre works.
Specialized Field: Musical; Theatrical Group
Status: Professional; Nonprofit
Performs At: The Music Hall
Organization Type: Performing; Touring; Educational

3862 SMITH-RITCH POINT THEATRE

Highway 39
PO Box 176
Ingram, TX 78025
Phone: 830-367-5121
Fax: 830-367-5724
Toll-free: 800-459-4223
Web Site: www.hcaf.com
Management:
   Theatre Director: Susan Balentine
   Executive Director: Lane Tait
   Technical Director: Douglas Balentine
Mission: Dedicated to the performing and visual arts.
Founded: 1959
Specialized Field: Community
Status: Non-Professional; Nonprofit
Income Sources: Texas Nonprofit Theatre; Texas Educators Theatre Association
Performs At: Smith-Ritch Point Theater
Affiliations: Hill Country Arts Foundation
Type of Stage: Outside Amphitheater; Pavilion
Seating Capacity: 722; 140
Organization Type: Performing; Touring; Educational

3863 IRVING COMMUNITY THEATER

2333 Rochelle
Irving, TX 75062
Phone: 972-594-6104
e-mail: info@irvingtheatre.org
Web Site: www.irvingtheatre.org/ict.htm
Mission: To promote the cultural, educational, and literary advancement of the residents of Irving and surrounding areas.
Founded: 1971
Specialized Field: Musical; Community; Theatrical Group
Status: Non-Professional; Nonprofit
Income Sources: Cultural Affairs Council
Performs At: Irving Center for Cultural Arts
Organization Type: Performing; Resident

3864 TEXAS SHAKESPEARE FESTIVAL

Kilgore College
1100 Broadway
Kilgore, TX 75662
Mailing Address: PO Box 2788 Kilgore, TX 75663
Phone: 903-983-8117
Fax: 903-983-8124
e-mail: info@texasshakespeare.co
Web Site: www.texasshakespeare.com
Management:
   Artistic Director: Raymond Caldwell
   Managing Director: John Dodd
Founded: 1986
Status: Non-Equity; Nonprofit
Season: June - July
Type of Stage: Flexible
Stage Dimensions: 30' x 30'
Seating Capacity: 240

3865 VIVE LES ARTS THEATRE

3401 S WS Young Drive
PO Box 10657
Killeen, TX 76547
Phone: 254-526-9090
Fax: 254-526-6906
e-mail: vh@desklink.com
Web Site: www.vlattheatre.com
Officers:
   Chairman: Mary Kliewer
Management:
   Director: Eric Shephard
   Administration: Tami Young
   WebMaster: Linda McMurray
   Children's Theatre Director: Amy Ball
Mission: To provide artistic and cultural activities in the areas of Killeen, Fort Hood, Copperas Cove and Harker Heights.
Founded: 1976
Specialized Field: Musical; Community; Theatrical Group; Children's Theatre
Status: Professional; Non-Professional; Nonprofit
Paid Staff: 4
Income Sources: City of Killeen Hotel Motel Occupancy Tax; Meadows Foundation
Performs At: Vive Les Arts Center for the Arts
Type of Stage: Thrust
Seating Capacity: 400
Year Built: 1991
Rental Contact: Tam Young
Organization Type: Performing; Touring; Sponsoring

3866 MESQUITE COMMUNITY THEATRE

1527 N Galleway
Mesquite, TX 75149
Mailing Address: PO Box 870431 Mesquite, TX 75187-0431
Phone: 972-216-6444
Web Site: www.mindspring.com/~jsfrank/mainframe
Mission: To offer quality live theatre to the Mesquite Community.
Founded: 1983
Specialized Field: Community; Theatrical Group
Status: Professional; Semi-Professional; Nonprofit
Performs At: East Ridge Park Christian Church
Type of Stage: Black Box
Seating Capacity: 492
Year Built: 1995
Organization Type: Performing

3867 LAMP-LITE THEATER

224 Old Tyler Road
PO Box 630446
Nacogdoches, TX 75963
Phone: 936-564-8300
Management:
   Director: Sarah McMullan
Mission: To provide quality live theatre for the East Texas region; to offer a dynamic creative experience for actors and related artists.
Founded: 1971
Specialized Field: Musical; Community
Status: Non-Professional; Nonprofit
Volunteer Staff: 120
Income Sources: Ticket sales
Performs At: Lamp-Lite Theater
Annual Attendance: 1,500
Seating Capacity: 237
Year Built: 1979

Organization Type: Performing; Touring; Educational

3868 GLOBE OF THE GREAT SOUTHWEST THEATRE
2308 Shakespeare Road
Odessa, TX 79761
Phone: 915-332-1586
Fax: 915-332-1587
e-mail: hamlet@globesw.org
Web Site: www.globesw.org
Officers:
   President: G William Fowler
   Treasurer: La Doyce Lambert
   Secretary: Jerri Nickel
Management:
   Artistic Director: Anthony Ridley
   Office Manager: Ann Wilson
Mission: To provide Shakespearean and classical plays that are educational; to present contemporary and religious plays and musicals; to present an annual Shakespeare Festival; to advance the enjoyment, appreciation and study of great literature; to make available the Globe Building and grounds to the community for all the arts.
Founded: 1958
Specialized Field: Community; Theatrical Group; Professional Shakespeare Festival
Status: Professional; Nonprofit
Paid Staff: 4
Volunteer Staff: 100
Paid Artists: 6
Non-paid Artists: 150
Income Sources: Grants; Patron Membership Ffees; Ssponsorships
Performs At: An authentic replica of an Elizabethan Theatre
Affiliations: Shakespeare Theatre Association of America; Texas Nonprofit Theatres
Annual Attendance: 15,000
Facility Category: Elizabethan Theatre
Type of Stage: Thrust
Seating Capacity: 400
Year Built: 1968
Rental Contact: Anthony Ridley
Organization Type: Performing; Educational

3869 PERMIAN PLAYHOUSE OF ODESSA
310 W 42nd
PO Box 13374
Odessa, TX 79768-3374
Phone: 915-362-2329
Fax: 915-362-2678
e-mail: pph@permianplayhouse.org
Web Site: www.permianplayhouse.org
Officers:
   Board President: Vicki Gomez
   First VP: Melissa Hirsch
   Second VP: Vonnie Downey
Management:
   Artistic Director: Hank Belilove
   Educational Director: Laura Bond
Mission: To provide high quality, culturally diverse theatrical experiences and educational programs to enrich the lives of the people in the Permian Basin.

Founded: 1939
Specialized Field: Community; Theatrical Group
Status: Non-Professional; Nonprofit
Paid Staff: 5
Volunteer Staff: 25
Income Sources: American Association of Community Theatres; Southwest Theatre Association; Texas Nonprofit Theater; Season Membership; Ticket Sales
Performs At: Permian Playhouse of Odessa
Facility Category: Community Theatre
Seating Capacity: 400
Year Built: 1966
Organization Type: Performing; Touring; Educational

3870 LUTCHER THEATER
707 West Main
Box 2310
Orange, TX 77630
Phone: 409-886-5535
Fax: 409-886-5537
e-mail: lutcher@exp.net
Web Site: www.lutcher.org
Management:
   Director: James Clark
Budget: $150,000-400,000

3871 PLANO REPERTORY THEATRE
1028 E 15th Place
Plano, TX 75074
Mailing Address: PO Box 86185 Plano, TX 75086
Phone: 214-422-7460
Fax: 972-578-7072
e-mail: info@planorep.org
Web Site: www.planorep.org
Officers:
   Board President: Craig McKinney
   VP: Tiffany Kellerman
   Treasurer: Howard Danziger
   Secretary: Christine Henry
Management:
   Director Marketing/Development: David James
   Patron Services Manager: Ryan Pointer
Mission: To bring audiences and artists together through innovative productions and theatrical outreach, creating opportunities to experience our shared humanity.
Founded: 1975
Status: Nonprofit
Paid Staff: 6
Volunteer Staff: 325
Paid Artists: 100
Budget: $720,000
Income Sources: Earned 75%; Contributed 25%
Performs At: Courtyard Theatre
Affiliations: Actor's Equity Association
Annual Attendance: 32,000
Facility Category: Theater
Type of Stage: Proscenium
Stage Dimensions: 51'x28'
Seating Capacity: 319
Year Built: 1935
Year Remodeled: 2002
Organization Type: Performing; Educational

3872 GUADALUPE CULTURAL ARTS CENTER

1300 Guadalupe Street
San Antonio, TX 78207
Phone: 210-271-3151
Fax: 210-271-3480
e-mail: mariat@guadalupeculturalarts.org
Web Site: www.guadalupeculturalarts.org
Officers:
    Chairman: Hector Fransto
Management:
    Executive Director: Marie Elena Torrelva Alonso
Mission: To present and promote Mexican-American arts; to facilitate a deeper knowledge and appreciation of Native American and Latino cultures as well as their artistic expressions.
Founded: 1980
Specialized Field: Musical; Community; Folk; Comedy; Multi-Cultural Events
Status: Professional; Nonprofit
Paid Staff: 23
Budget: $1,500,000
Income Sources: Corporations; Foundations; City & Federal funding
Performs At: Guadalupe Theater
Annual Attendance: 190,000
Facility Category: Theater; Gallery
Seating Capacity: 372
Year Built: 1940
Year Remodeled: 1984
Organization Type: Performing; Touring; Resident; Educational; Sponsoring; Presenting
Resident Groups: Grupo Animo Youth Theatre; Folk Flamenco Dance Company

3873 JUMP-START PERFORMANCE COMPANY

108 Blue Star
San Antonio, TX 78204
Phone: 210-227-5867
Fax: 210-322-2231
Web Site: www.arts.texas.us/rosters/aiersource.asp
Management:
    Artistic Director: Steve Bailey
    Administrator: Sterling Houston
    Technical Director: Max Parrilla
Mission: Committed to the creation of art that is a lasting voice of many diverse cultures.
Founded: 1985
Specialized Field: Community; Theatrical Group
Status: Professional; Semi-Professional; Nonprofit
Income Sources: American Association of Community Theatres; Rural Organization of Theaters South
Performs At: Jump-Start Theater
Organization Type: Performing; Touring; Resident; Educational; Sponsoring; Commissioning

3874 MAGIK THEATRE

420 S Alamo
San Antonio, TX 78205
Phone: 210-227-2751
Fax: 210-227-2753
e-mail: info@magiktheatre.org
Web Site: www.magiktheatre.org
Officers:
    Marketing Director: Erin Fernandes
Management:
    Executive Director: Richard Rosen
    Music Director: Mark G Johnson
    Operations Manager: David Ankrom
Mission: To promote literacy and learning, strengthen family life; to create tomorrow's live theater audience.
Founded: 1984
Specialized Field: Theatre
Paid Staff: 13
Paid Artists: 11
Budget: $900,000
Income Sources: Box Office; Classes; Tours; Contributed Income
Performs At: Theatre
Affiliations: ASSITES/USA; SATCO; TNT, ATHE
Annual Attendance: 155,000
Facility Category: Theatre
Type of Stage: Thrust
Stage Dimensions: 30'x42'
Seating Capacity: 600
Year Built: 1899
Year Remodeled: 1939
Rental Contact: Operations Manager David Ankrom
Resident Groups: Magik Theatre Company

3875 SAN PEDRO PLAYHOUSE

800 W Ashby
PO Box 12356
San Antonio, TX 78212
Phone: 210-733-7258
Fax: 210-734-2651
e-mail: sanpedplay@aol.com
Web Site: www.members.tripod.com/san_pedro_playhouse
Officers:
    President: Janet Nevenschwander
    1st VP: Joe Medina
    Second VP: Rickard Archer
    Secretary: Susan Lelauren
Management:
    Executive Director: Diann Sweed
    Office Manager: Yvette Oakes
    Artistic Director: Vivienne Elborne
Mission: Literary and educational community theatre.
Founded: 1912
Specialized Field: Community
Status: Nonprofit
Paid Staff: 8
Budget: $450,000
Income Sources: Private Donations; Business Donations
Annual Attendance: 35,000
Type of Stage: Proscenium; Thrust
Seating Capacity: 400; 60
Year Built: 1929
Year Remodeled: 2000
Rental Contact: Yvette Oakes
Organization Type: Performing; Educational

3876 SHOESTRING SHAKESPEARE COMPANY

PO Box 15012
San Antonio, TX 78212

Phone: 210-212-3948
Management:
   Artistic Director: Laurie Dietrich
   Managing Director: John Poole
   Literary Manager: Alicia Sternberg

3877 TEMPLE CIVIC THEATRE
2413 S 13th Street
Temple, TX 76504
Phone: 254-778-4751
Fax: 254-778-4980
e-mail: tct@artstemple.com
Web Site: www.vvm.com
Management:
   Artistic/Managing Director: C Suzanne
   Hudson-Smith
   Technical Director: Roger Daniels
Mission: To promote community involvement in theatre arts; to offer an outlet for talent in the community.
Founded: 1965
Specialized Field: Community; Theatrical Group
Status: Non-Professional; Nonprofit
Affiliations: Texas Non-Profit Theatre's; Southwest Teatre Association
Organization Type: Performing; Educational

3878 WICHITA FALLS BACKDOOR PLAYERS
501 Indiana
PO Box 896
Wichita Falls, TX 76307
Phone: 940-322-5000
Fax: 940-322-8167
e-mail: backdoor@wf.net
Management:
   Managing Director: Linda Bates
Mission: To offer participation in all areas of theatre to anyone interested regardless of experience.
Founded: 1971
Specialized Field: Community Theatrical Group
Status: Nonprofit
Paid Staff: 2
Volunteer Staff: 200
Non-paid Artists: 20
Organization Type: Performing

Utah

3879 UTAH SHAKESPEAREAN FESTIVAL
351 W Center Street
Cedar City, UT 84720
Phone: 435-586-7880
Fax: 435-865-8003
Toll-free: 800-752-9849
e-mail: bahr@suu.edu
Web Site: www.bard.org
Officers:
   Development Director: Jyl Shuler
   Marketing Director: Donna Law
   Education Director: Michael Bahr
   Publications Director: Bruce Lee
Management:
   Executive Producer: Fred C Adams
   Managing Director: R. Scott Phillips

   Producing Artistic Director: Cameron Harvey
   Associate Artistic Director: JR Sullivan
   Marketing Director: Donna Law
   Production Manager: Ran Inkel
   Director Plays-in-Progress: George Judy
   Education Director: Michael Don Bahr
   Publications Director: Bruce Lee
Mission: To present six classic and Shakespearean works in repertory each summer and fall.
Founded: 1961
Specialized Field: Theater
Status: Professional; Nonprofit
Paid Staff: 25
Volunteer Staff: 250
Paid Artists: 200
Budget: $5 Million
Income Sources: Box Office Sales; Contributed Income; Endowment Income; Merchandise Sales
Season: June - August
Performs At: Adams Memorial Stage; Randall L. Jones Theatre; University Stage
Affiliations: USA; SSD&C; Actors' Equity Association; LORT; TCG
Annual Attendance: 155,000
Facility Category: Outdoor/Indoor
Type of Stage: Thrust; Proscenium
Stage Dimensions: 50Wx30D; 22Hx42Wx25D; 18Hx44Wx39D
Seating Capacity: 887; 769; 981
Year Remodeled: 1989
Rental Contact: Production Manager Ray Inkel
Organization Type: Performing; Resident; Educational

3880 OLD LYRIC REPERTORY COMPANY
Theatre Arts Department
Utah State University
Logan, UT 84322-4035
Phone: 435-797-0085
Fax: 435-797-0086
e-mail: vicki@hass.usu.edu
Management:
   Artistic Director: Colin Johnson
   Business Asst: Vicki Fowler
Mission: Advanced student training; community outreach.
Founded: 1967
Status: Non-Equity; Nonprofit
Season: May - August
Performs At: Legitimate Theatre
Type of Stage: Proscenium
Stage Dimensions: 22' x 18'
Seating Capacity: 380

3881 PEERY'S EGYPTIAN THEATER
2415 Washington Boulevard
Ogden, UT 84401
Phone: 801-395-3222
Fax: 801-395-3201
e-mail: klmaguet@weber.edu
Web Site: www.oecenter.com
Management:
   Director: David Rowell
Paid Staff: 8
Budget: $60,000-150,000
Facility Category: Historic Theater

Type of Stage: Proscenium
Seating Capacity: 800
Year Built: 1924
Year Remodeled: 1997
Rental Contact: Director Kathryn Maguet

3882 PERRY'S EGYPTIAN THEATRE
Utah Musical Theatre
2415 Washington Boulevard
1902 University Circle
Ogden, UT 84408-1902
Phone: 801-626-7775
Web Site: www.weber.edu/umt
Officers:
   UMT Association President: Pam Higginson
Management:
   Artistic Director: Jerry P O'Connor
   Managing Director: Timothy Gibson
   Marketing Director: Debra Francis
   Manager/ Administrative Assistant: Brad Crews
Mission: A professional based, educational, founded and community support stock theater serving the artistic and cultural needs in Northern Utah. Seeks to preserve and advance the musical theatre genre as well as expand its audience in both theatrical scope and artistic integrity. Strives to serve the community by entertaining, enlightening and celebrating the best of the human spirit.
Founded: 1980
Status: Non-Equity; Nonprofit
Season: June - August
Type of Stage: Proscenium
Stage Dimensions: 36' x 40'
Seating Capacity: 800

3883 EMILY COMPANY
737 N Hilltop Road
Salt Lake City, UT 84103
Phone: 801-799-0559
Fax: 801-799-0660
e-mail: emilyco@msn.com
Web Site: www.emilycompany.org
Management:
   Producing Artistic Director: Katharine Reilly
Mission: To produce three to four plays a year, with emphasis on continuing education, also plays a key role. Pay-what-you-can performances are offered to the public.

3884 OFF BROADWAY THEATRE
272 S Main Street
Salt Lake City, UT 84101
Phone: 801-355-4628
Fax: 801-355-4641
e-mail: melissa@theobt.com
Web Site: www.theobt.com
Management:
   Owner: Melissa Porter
   Owner: Eric Jensen
   Owner: Ben Poter
   Owner: Sandy Jensen
Founded: 1994
Specialized Field: Theater; Comedy
Paid Staff: 6
Volunteer Staff: 8
Paid Artists: 20

3885 PIONEER THEATRE COMPANY
University of Utah
300 S 1400
Salt Lake City, UT 84112-0660
Phone: 801-581-6961
Fax: 801-581-5472
e-mail: kpeterson@ptc.utah.edu
Web Site: www.ptc.utah.edu/
Management:
   Artistic Director: Charles Morey
   Managing Director: Christopher Lino
   Business Manager: Pat Wells
   Development Director: Diane Parisi
   Marketing Director: Kwin Peterson
Mission: Dedicated to offering high quality professional theater to Utah as well as the Northwestern United States.
Founded: 1962
Specialized Field: Theatrical Group
Status: Professional; Nonprofit
Budget: 3.5 million
Income Sources: Ticket Sales; Donations; Grants
Performs At: Pioneer Memorial Theater
Affiliations: Theatre Communications Group
Annual Attendance: 94,000
Type of Stage: Proscenium
Seating Capacity: 932
Year Built: 1962
Year Remodeled: 2000
Organization Type: Performing; Educational

3886 PLAN - B THEATRE COMPANY
617 E Wilson Avenue
Salt Lake City, UT 84105
Phone: 801-487-8291
Management:
   Producing Director: Morgan Ludlow
   Managing Director: Cheryl Ann Cluff
   Company Manager: Jennifer Freed

3887 SALT LAKE ACTING COMPANY
168 West 500 N
Salt Lake City, UT 84103
Phone: 801-363-0526
Fax: 801-532-8513
Management:
   Producing Artistic Director: Edward J Gryska
   Managing Director: Victoria Panella
Mission: To present a unique and innovative repertoire of plays and regional premieres to the city; to support new works and develop a community of artists; to make a contribution to the American professional theater.
Founded: 1970
Specialized Field: Theatrical Group
Status: Professional; Nonprofit
Income Sources: Theatre Communications Group
Performs At: The Salt Lake Acting Company Theater
Organization Type: Performing

3888 SUNDANCE INSTITUTE
PO Box 3630
Salt Lake City, UT 84110

Phone: 801-328-3456
Fax: 801-575-5175
e-mail: institute@sundance.org
Web Site: www.sundance.org
Officers:
    President: Robert Redford
    Chairman: Walter Weisman
Management:
    Artistic Director: Phillip Himberg
    Director Programming: Geoff Gilmore
    Managing Director: Aaron Young
    Dir Feature Film Programming: Michelle Satter
    Press Contact: Patrick Hubley
Mission: Dedicated to the development of artists of independent vision and the exhibition of their new work.
Founded: 1981
Specialized Field: Film; Theatre
Status: Professional; Nonprofit
Budget: $10,600,000
Income Sources: 35% Earned; 65% Contributed Income
Organization Type: Educational

3889 SUNDANCE THEATRE PROGRAM

PO Box 3630
Salt Lake City, UT 84110-3630
Phone: 801-328-3456
Fax: 801-575-5175
Web Site: www.sundance.org
Officers:
    Chairman: Walter Weisman
Management:
    Managing Director: Aaron Young
    Press Contact: Patrick Hubley
Founded: 1990
Status: Nonprofit
Budget: $10,600,000
Type of Stage: Outdoor; Indoor
Seating Capacity: 880; 250

3890 TUACAHN CENTER FOR THE ARTS

PO Box 1996
St. George, UT 84771
Phone: 435-652-3300
Fax: 435-652-3227
Toll-free: 800-746-9882
e-mail: tuacahn@infowest.com
Web Site: www.tuacahn.org
Officers:
    CEO: Kevin Smith
    COO: Kevin Warnick
Mission: Was established to awaken the mobility of the hman soul and transmit light and hope to people everywhere through the arts and education. The theatre wishes to preserve and project the legacy of the American Musical into the 21st century.
Founded: 1992
Status: Nonprofit
Season: June - September
Facility Category: Ampitheatre; Highschool
Type of Stage: Proscenium
Stage Dimensions: 75' x 60'
Seating Capacity: 1920

3891 SUNDANCE CHILDREN'S THEATRE

Rural Route 3
PO Box 624-D
Sundance, UT 84604
Phone: 801-328-3456
Fax: 801-225-3096
Officers:
    Chairman: Walter Weisman
Management:
    Managing Director: David Kirk Chambers
    Artistic Director: Jerry Parch
    Press Contact: Patrick Hubley
Mission: To develop and produce new plays for young audiences.
Founded: 1990
Specialized Field: Theatrical Group
Status: Professional; Semi-Professional; Nonprofit
Organization Type: Performing; Touring

3892 HALE CENTRE THEATRE AT HARMAN HALL

3333 S Decker Lake Drive
2200 W
West Valley City, UT 84119
Phone: 801-984-9000
Fax: 801-984-9009
e-mail: info@halecentretheatre.com
Web Site: www.halecentretheatre.com
Management:
    Executive Producer: Mark Dietlein
    Executive Producer: Sally Dietlein
    Executive Producer: Sally Hale
    Technical Director: Andrew Barrus
    Costumer Rentals: Amy Glaser
    Office Manager: Tammy Morgan
    Marketing Director/Building Rentals: JaceSon Barrus
Performs At: Comedies; Musicals
Rental Contact: Marketing Director JaceSon Barrus

Vermont

3893 OLDCASTLE THEATRE COMPANY
Bennington Center for the Arts

Route 9 & Gypsy Lane
PO Box 1555
Bennington, VT 05201
Phone: 802-447-0564
Fax: 802-442-3704
e-mail: espach@oldcastle.org
Web Site: www.oldcastle.org
Management:
    Producing Artistic Director: Eric Peterson
    Associate Artistic Director: Richard Howe
    Managing Director: Steven R Espach
    Director Production: Kenneth Mooney
    Marketing Director: Daryl Kenny
    House/Box Office Manager: Jana Lillie
Mission: Resident professional theatre company.
Founded: 1972
Specialized Field: Drama; Comedy; Musicals; New Plays
Status: Professional; Nonprofit

Paid Staff: 5
Budget: $400,000
Income Sources: Ticket Revenue; Donations; Special Events; Corporate Underwriting; Grants
Season: March - October
Performs At: Bennington Center for the Arts
Affiliations: Actors' Equity Association; Society for Stage Directors and Choreographers
Annual Attendance: 10,000
Facility Category: Auditorium & Art Gallery
Type of Stage: Proscenium
Seating Capacity: 313
Year Built: 1994
Rental Contact: Oldcastle Theatre Company Eric Peterson
Organization Type: Performing; Touring; Resident; Educational; Sponsoring

3894 NATIONAL MARIONETTE THEATRE
350 Putney Road
Brattleboro, VT 05301
Phone: 802-257-3090
Fax: 802-257-4079
Web Site: www.nationalmarionette.com
Management:
   Artistic Director: David Syrotiak
Founded: 1968
Specialized Field: Theatrical Group; Puppet
Status: Professional; Nonprofit
Income Sources: Association of Performing Arts Presenters; NECA; New England Arts Foundation
Organization Type: Performing; Touring

3895 VERMONT STAGE COMPANY
PO Box 874
Burlington, VT 05402
Phone: 802-862-1497
Fax: 802-862-1257
e-mail: vsc@vtstage.org
Web Site: www.vtstage.org
Management:
   Producing Artistic Director: Mark Nash
   Managing Director: Jamie Kornstein
Mission: Theatre gives us the oppurtunity to fulfill one of our deepest longings' the need to connect. The intimacy of our theatre, the closeness of the actors, the honesty and simplicity and passion of the acting, compels us to engage ina way that few theatrical expirences can.
Founded: 1994
Status: Nonprofit
Paid Staff: 2
Volunteer Staff: 50
Budget: $275,000
Income Sources: Ticket Sales; Corporate Sponsorships; Program Advertising; Private Contributions
Season: September - May
Affiliations: Flynn Center for the Performing Arts
Annual Attendance: 6,000-7,000
Type of Stage: Flexible; Black Box
Seating Capacity: 150

3896 AMERICAN THEATRE WORKS
PO Box 510
Dorset, VT 05251
Phone: 802-867-2223
Fax: 802-867-0144
e-mail: theatre@sover.net
Web Site: www.theatredirectories.com
Officers:
   President: Robert G Bushell Jr
   VP: Jean Miller
   Treasurer: Ben Weil
Management:
   Producing/Artistic Director: John Nassivera
   General Manager: Barbara Ax
Mission: To offer a season of five plays each summer, as well as a writers' colony.
Founded: 1976
Specialized Field: Summer Stock
Status: Professional; Nonprofit
Income Sources: Theatre Communications Group
Performs At: Dorset Playhouse
Seating Capacity: 290
Year Remodeled: 2001
Organization Type: Performing; Resident; Educational; Publishing

3897 POTOMAC THEATRE PROJECT
4 Nedde Lane
Middlebury, VT 05753
Phone: 802-388-3318
e-mail: info@olneytheatre.org
Management:
   Director: Cheryl Faraone
   Director: James Petosa
   Director: Richard Romagnoli
Mission: Producing highly theatrical new works; Providing professional theatre training.
Founded: 1977
Specialized Field: Theatrical Group
Status: Professional; Nonprofit
Paid Staff: 15
Income Sources: Alliance of Resident Theatres/New York; Vermont Council on the Arts
Performs At: Hall of Nations
Organization Type: Performing; Resident; Educational

3898 LOST NATION THEATER
39 Main Street
Montpelier, VT 05602
Phone: 802-229-0492
Fax: 802-223-9608
e-mail: info@lostnationtheater.org
Web Site: lostnationtheater.org
Management:
   Co-Artistic Producing Director: Kim Bent
Founded: 1977
Specialized Field: Performing
Status: Nonprofit
Season: June - October
Type of Stage: Flexible Thrust
Stage Dimensions: 32' x 28'
Seating Capacity: 124

3899 GREEN MOUNTAIN GUILD
PO Box 659
Pittsfield, VT 05762
Phone: 802-746-8320

Management:
 Program Coordinator/Managing Dir: Marjorie
O'Neill-Butler
 Artistic Director: Robert O'Neill-Butler
 Associate Artistic Director: Jay Berkow
Mission: Developing and promoting excellence in
Northern New England's performing arts.
Founded: 1971
Specialized Field: Summer Stock; Musical; Theatre for
Children
Status: Professional
Paid Staff: 3
Income Sources: New England Theatre Conference;
Vermont Council on the Arts; New England Touring
Foundation
Season: July - August
Performs At: Killington Playhouse
Organization Type: Performing; Touring; Resident

3900 CATAMOUNT FILM AND ARTS COMPANY
139 Eastern Avenue
PO Box 324
Saint Johnsbury, VT 05819
Phone: 802-748-2600
Fax: 802-748-0852
Toll-free: 888-757-5559
e-mail: catamount@kingcon.com
Management:
 Executive Director: Reg Ainsworth
 Executive Director: Brenda Sherman
Mission: To perform community-based multidisciplinary
presentations.
Founded: 1975
Specialized Field: Modern; Mime; Ballet; Jazz; Ethnic;
Folk
Status: Professional; Nonprofit
Paid Staff: 3
Volunteer Staff: 15
Organization Type: Performing; Educational

3901 SAXTONS RIVER PLAYHOUSE
Westminster W Road
Box 727
Saxtons River, VT 05154
Phone: 802-869-2030
Web Site: www.sover.net/~falklorn/srp.html
Management:
 Producer: Falko Schilling
Founded: 1988
Status: Non-Equity; Nonprofit
Season: June - September
Type of Stage: Proscenium
Seating Capacity: 149

3902 WESTON PLAYHOUSE
703 Main Street
Weston, VT 05161
Phone: 802-824-8167
Fax: 802-824-5099
e-mail: mail@westplay.com
Web Site: www.westplay.com
Management:
 Producing Director: Malcolm Ewen

General Manager: Stuart Duke
Founded: 1937
Status: Nonprofit
Season: June - September
Type of Stage: Proscenium
Seating Capacity: 285

3903 NORTHERN STAGE
PO Box 4287
White River Junction, VT 05001
Phone: 802-296-7000
Fax: 802-291-9156
e-mail: northern.stage@valley.net
Web Site: www.northernstage.org
Officers:
 Board President: Hunt Whitcare
 Treasurer: Byron Hathorn Jr
Management:
 Artistic Director: Brooke Wetzel
 Director Media/Marketing: Charlie Glazer
 Fiscal Manager: Catherine Lyndes
 Production Manager: Angelina Giudice
Mission: Dedicated to presenting new interpretations of
classics, regional premires of recent and new works, and
professioanl theater education.
Founded: 1992
Specialized Field: Theater
Status: Nonprofit
Paid Staff: 25
Volunteer Staff: 60
Paid Artists: 8
Income Sources: Donations
Season: September - December
Affiliations: TCG
Annual Attendance: 12,000
Facility Category: Theater
Type of Stage: 3/4 Thrust
Stage Dimensions: 50' x 24'
Seating Capacity: 245
Year Built: 1885
Year Remodeled: 1972
Rental Contact: Charlie Glazer

Virginia

3904 BARTER THEATRE - STATE THEATRE OF VIRGINIA
Main Street
PO Box 867
Abingdon, VA 24210
Phone: 276-628-2281
Fax: 276-628-4551
e-mail: info@bartertheatre.com
Web Site: www.bartertheatre.com
Management:
 Artistic Director/Producer: Rex Partington
 Producing Artistic Director: Richard Rose
 Business Manager: Joan Ballou
 Development Director: Lisa Alderman
 Marketing Director: Debbie Addison
 Associate Artistic Director: John Hardy
 Group Sales Reservationist: Linda Pruner
 Media Specialist/Web/Graphics: Stacy Fine

Mission: Performing the finest in contemporary and classical theatre for residents as well as visitors to our region.
Founded: 1933
Status: Professional; Nonprofit
Income Sources: Actors' Equity Association; League of Resident Theatres; Theatre Communications Group
Performs At: Barter Playhouse; Barter Theatre House
Type of Stage: Proscenium, Flexible Stage
Seating Capacity: 508, 140
Organization Type: Performing; Touring; Resident; Educational

3905 KATHY HARTY GRAY DANCE THEATRE
PO Box 3291
Alexandria, VA 22302
Phone: 703-413-3811
Fax: 703-413-4198
e-mail: slandess@stratsight.com
Web Site: www.khgdt.org
Management:
    Executive Director: Susan E Landess
Mission: Mondern dance company providing concerts, school shows, residencies and master classes.
Founded: 1978
Specialized Field: Modern Dance
Paid Staff: 1
Volunteer Staff: 1
Paid Artists: 10

3906 METROSTAGE
1201 N Royal Street
Alexandria, VA 22314
Phone: 703-548-9044
Fax: 703-548-9089
e-mail: info@metrostage.org
Web Site: www.metrostage.org
Management:
    Producing Artistic Director: Carolyn Griffin
Mission: To offer a season of mainstage productions, staged readings, cabarets, and new-plays
Founded: 1984
Specialized Field: Theatrical Group
Status: Professional; Nonprofit
Paid Staff: 2
Volunteer Staff: 2
Non-paid Artists: 0
Budget: $500,000
Income Sources: Box Office
Performs At: Theatre
Affiliations: League of Washington Theatres; Alexandria Chamber of Commerce; Cultural Alliance of Greater Washington; King Street Metro Enterprise Team
Annual Attendance: 4,000
Facility Category: Theatre
Type of Stage: Modified Thrust
Seating Capacity: 130
Year Remodeled: 2001
Organization Type: Performing; Touring; Educational

3907 HORIZONS THEATRE
4350 N Fairfax Drive
Suite 127
Arlington, VA 22203
Phone: 703-243-8550
Fax: 703-243-4561
e-mail: info@horizonstheatre.org
Management:
    Artistic Director: Leslie B Jacobson
    Managing Director: Joan Kelley
Founded: 1976
Status: Non-Equity; Nonprofit

3908 SIGNATURE THEATRE
3806 S Four Mile Run Drive
Arlington, VA 22206
Phone: 703-820-9771
Fax: 703-820-7790
Web Site: www.sig-online.org
Management:
    Literary Manager: Marcia Gardner
    Artistic Director: Eric D Schaeffer
    Program Marketing Coordinator: Lisa Hanson
Mission: To reinvent musical classics and premiere groundbreaking new work by today's best writers
Founded: 1990
Specialized Field: Theatre
Status: Nonprofit

3909 ASHLAWN-HIGHLAND SUMMER FESTIVAL
1941 James Monroe Parkway
Charlottesville, VA 22902
Phone: 804-293-4500
Fax: 804-293-0736
e-mail: summerfestival@avenue.gen.va.us
Web Site: www.avenue.org/summerfestival
Management:
    General Director: Judith H Walker
Founded: 1978
Status: Non-Equity; Nonprofit
Paid Staff: 4
Volunteer Staff: 100
Paid Artists: 80
Non-paid Artists: 25
Season: June - August
Stage Dimensions: 24' x 16'
Seating Capacity: 450

3910 OFFSTAGE THEATRE
PO Box 131
Charlottesville, VA 22902
Phone: 804-295-7249
Management:
    Co-Artistic Director: Tom Coash
    Co-Artistic Director: Doug Grissom
    Resident Director: John Quinn
    Public Relations Director: Amy Lowenstein
Mission: Producing new plays of high quality in nontraditional, low-cost theatre environments.
Founded: 1989
Specialized Field: Theatrical Group; Independent Theatre
Status: Professional; Semi-Professional; Nonprofit

Organization Type: Performing; Touring; Resident; Educational

3911 SWIFT CREEK MILL PLAYHOUSE

PO Box 41
Colonial Heights, VA 23834
Phone: 804-748-5203
e-mail: RONeill@SwiftCreekMill.com
Web Site: www.swiftcreekmill.com
Management:
   Artistic Director: Tom Width
Founded: 1965
Status: Dinner Theatre
Paid Staff: 3
Paid Artists: 25

3912 THEATER OF THE FIRST AMENDMENT

George Mason University
Mail Stop 3E6
Fairfax, VA 22030-4444
Phone: 703-993-2195
Fax: 703-993-2191
e-mail: rdavi4@gmu.edu
Web Site: www.gmu/edu/cfa
Management:
   Managing Director: Kevin Murray
Mission: Is dedicated to the discovery, development, and production of exciting new york work and both adult and multigenerational audiences, along with explorations of the less well known areas of classical repertory.
Founded: 1990
Status: Nonprofit
Paid Staff: 7
Budget: $350,000
Income Sources: George Mason University; Box Office
Season: September - April
Affiliations: AEA, SSDC, USA
Annual Attendance: 6,000
Type of Stage: Flexible
Stage Dimensions: 40' x 30'
Seating Capacity: 150
Year Built: 1975

3913 RIVERSIDE CENTER DINNER THEATER

95 Riverside Parkway
Fredericksburg, VA 22406
Phone: 540-370-4300
Fax: 540-370-4304
e-mail: riversided@aol.com
Web Site: www.riversidedt.com
Management:
   Music Director: Rollin Wehman
   Producer Assistant: Stephen R Hayes
   Artistic Director/General Manager: Rollin E Wehman
Mission: Presentation of Broadway musicals, children's theatre musicals, and education of youth and adults in all aspects of the performing arts, while providing an outlet for the diverse talents of area actors, musicians, and dancers.
Founded: 1998
Specialized Field: Musicals - Main Stage and Children's Theatre

Paid Staff: 12
Volunteer Staff: 8
Paid Artists: 35
Non-paid Artists: 6
Budget: $2.4 million
Income Sources: Group Sales; General Public; Bus-Tour Companies; Season Subscribers
Annual Attendance: 50,000
Type of Stage: Proscenium
Stage Dimensions: 35' x 30'
Year Built: 1998
Cost: $30 million

3914 LIME KILN ARTS

14 S Randolph Street
Lexington, VA 24450
Phone: 540-463-7088
Fax: 540-463-1082
e-mail: limekiln@cfw.com
Web Site: www.thetheatreatlimekiln.com
Officers:
   President: Paul Belo
Management:
   Executive Director: Jennifer Anderson
   Marketing Director: Alysia Graber
   Artistic Associate: Zach Hanks
   Artistic Director: John Heeley
   Touring Coordinator: Scott Fix
Mission: Promoting and preserving the traditions of the Southern Appalachian Mountains and exploring their myths as well as their potential.
Founded: 1982
Specialized Field: Summer Stock; Musical; Folk; Theatrical Group
Status: Professional; Nonprofit
Paid Staff: 6
Volunteer Staff: 100
Paid Artists: 50
Budget: $500,000
Income Sources: Private; earned; government
Season: May - September
Performs At: Lime Kiln Theater-Outdoor
Annual Attendance: 17,000
Facility Category: Theatre and Concert Venue
Type of Stage: Outdoor
Seating Capacity: 388; 700
Rental Contact: Jennifer D. Anderson
Organization Type: Performing; Touring; Resident; Educational; Sponsoring
Resident Groups: Artists-in-Residence

3915 THEATER AT LIME KILN

14 S Randolph Street
Lexington, VA 24450
Phone: 540-463-7088
Fax: 540-463-1082
e-mail: limekiln@cfw.com
Web Site: www.theateratlimekiln.com
Management:
   Artistic Director: John Healey
   Executive Director: Jennifer D Anderson
   Marketing Director: Gail Abbott
   Development Director: Cydney Davis
   Touring Coordinator: Ron Smith

Mission: To promote entertainment and education in the arts while exploring Appalachian traditions and culture.
Founded: 1983
Specialized Field: Summer Stock; Touring; Musical; Folk; Theatrical Group
Status: AEA-LOA/Outdoor Drama; Professional; Nonprofit
Paid Staff: 5
Volunteer Staff: 100
Paid Artists: 50
Non-paid Artists: 4
Budget: $629,000
Income Sources: Private; Earned; Foundation; Government
Performs At: Lime Kiln Theater
Affiliations: AEA; Institute of Outdoor Drama
Annual Attendance: 17,000
Facility Category: Outdoor Theater and Concert Venue
Seating Capacity: 388; 700
Year Built: 1983
Rental Contact: Jennifer D Anderson

3916   SPENCERS: THEATER OF ILLUSION

PO Box 10396
Lynchburg, VA 24506
Phone: 434-384-4740
Fax: 434-384-8032
e-mail: office@inmind.com
Web Site: www.TheatreOfIllusion.com
Management:
   Artist: Kevin Spencer
Founded: 1982

3917   ALDEN THEATRE SERIES

1234 Ingleside Avenue
McLean, VA 22101-2817
Phone: 703-790-0123
Fax: 703-556-0547
Web Site: www.mcleancenter.org
Management:
   Performing Arts Director: Clare M Kiley
Founded: 1975
Paid Staff: 20
Volunteer Staff: 30
Budget: $400,000
Type of Stage: Proscenium
Stage Dimensions: 28 x 35
Seating Capacity: 424
Year Built: 1975
Year Remodeled: 1988
Rental Contact: Performing Arts Director Clare Kiley

3918   WAYSIDE THEATRE

7853 Main Street
PO Box 260
Middletown, VA 22645
Phone: 540-869-1776
Fax: 540-869-1746
e-mail: info@waysidetheatre.org
Web Site: www.waysidetheatre.org
Officers:
   President: John Norton
   VP: Martha Ingram
   Secretary: Sara Cohen

Treasurer: John Costello
Management:
   Artistic Director: Warner Crocker
   General Manager: Betsy Blauvelt
   Sales/Outreach Coordinator: Cephe Place
   Company Manager: Becca Cintron
Mission: Community based professional theatre which strives to enrich the lives of the people of our community through a broad spectrum of live professional theatre and performance opportunities that are entertaining, challenging, educational and accessible, and which effectively transmits that wonder to future generations.
Founded: 1962
Status: Professional; Nonprofit
Paid Staff: 5
Paid Artists: 26
Budget: $500,000
Income Sources: Ticket Sales; Corporate/Foundation Grants; Government Grants; Program Advertising, Concession Sales
Season: May - December
Affiliations: Actors Equity Association
Annual Attendance: 15,000
Type of Stage: Proscenium
Stage Dimensions: 24'x22'
Seating Capacity: 180
Year Built: 1942
Year Remodeled: 1962
Rental Contact: Artistic Director Warner Crocker
Organization Type: Performing; Touring; Resident

3919   2ND STORY THEATRE COMPANY

809 Brandon Avenue
Suite 210
Norfolk, VA 23517
Phone: 757-623-1776
Fax: 757-623-1777
e-mail: 2ndstory@brucehartmandesign.com
Web Site: www.brucehartmandesign.com
Management:
   Co-Owner/Producer: Ethan Marten
   Co-Owner/Producer: Richard Marten
   Webmaster/Advertising Design: Bruce Hartman
   Lighting Design: Yoni Charry
   Stage Manager: Sheri Beyrau
   Graphic/Web/Print Designer: Bruce Hartman
Mission: 2nd Story Theatre has functioned as a community resource encouraging the development and employment of local and regional talent, and activly fostering the performance of sister arts in Tidewater, Virginia. Committed to the concept of training and developing the talents of aspiring theatre professionals.
Specialized Field: Comedy Talent

3920   GENERIC THEATER

912 W 21st Street
PO Box 11071
Norfolk, VA 23517
Phone: 757-441-2160
Fax: 757-441-2729
e-mail: generic@whro.net
Web Site: www.generictheater.org
Officers:
   President: GF Rowe
   VP: Sarah Jane Ward

Treasurer: Elisabeth Burgess
Secretary: Carin Cowell
Mission: To produce innovative productions of contemporary works, new plays, and reinterpretations of the classics.
Founded: 1981
Paid Staff: 2
Paid Artists: 50
Non-paid Artists: 50
Budget: $100,000
Income Sources: Ticket Sales; State and Local Grant Organizations; Contributions
Performs At: Theater
Affiliations: Generic Theatre
Annual Attendance: 4,000 - 5,000
Facility Category: Black Box
Type of Stage: Proscenium
Stage Dimensions: 28'x56'
Seating Capacity: 80
Rental Contact: Artistic Director (757-441-2729) Steven Harders

3921   LITTLE THEATRE OF NORFOLK

801 Claremont Avenue
Norfolk, VA 23507
Phone: 804-627-8551
e-mail: itn@norfolk-little-theatre
Mission: To offer excellent amateur theatre and give non-professionals an opportunity to utilize their talents.
Founded: 1926
Specialized Field: Community
Status: Nonprofit
Performs At: Little Theatre of Norfolk
Organization Type: Performing

3922   VIRGINIA STAGE COMPANY

254 Granby Street
PO Box 3770
Norfolk, VA 23514
Phone: 757-627-6988
Fax: 757-628-5958
Web Site: www.vastage.com
Officers:
   President: Philip Campbell
   Secretary: Katherine Willis
Management:
   Artistic Director: Charlie Hensley
   Interim Managinng Director: Faye Bailey Timm
   Production Manager: Randy Foster
   Assistant to Directors: Patricia Darden
   Strategic Planning: Kerry Jahnou
   Production Manager: Randy Foster
   Production Management Aapprentice: Gretchen Schaefer
   Company Manager: Kerry Jahn
   Box Office Manager: Mary T Hassan
Mission: To develop and sustain a fully professional theatre serving Southeastern Virginia which enriches the region and the field through the production of theatrical art of the highest quality.
Founded: 1980
Specialized Field: Theatrical Group
Status: Professional; Nonprofit
Paid Staff: 44
Budget: $1,900,000

Income Sources: League of Resident Theatres; Theatre Communications Group
Performs At: Wells Theatre
Annual Attendance: 55,000
Facility Category: Theatre
Type of Stage: Prosecnium
Stage Dimensions: 36'x36'
Seating Capacity: 677
Year Built: 1913
Year Remodeled: 1986
Rental Contact: Beth Spangler
Organization Type: Performing; Resident; Educational; Sponsoring

3923   LONG WAY HOME

PO Box 711
Radford, VA 24141
Phone: 540-639-0679
Fax: 540-731-8306
Management:
   Technical Director: Al Shumate
Founded: 1971
Status: Nonprofit
Season: June - August
Type of Stage: Amphitheatre, Open Stage
Seating Capacity: 500

3924   BARKSDALE THEATRE

1601 Willow Lawn Drive
Suite 301-E
Richmond, VA 23230
Phone: 804-282-2620
Fax: 804-288-6470
e-mail: development@barksdalerichmond.org
Web Site: www.barksdalerichmond.org
Management:
   Managing Director: Phil Whiteway
   Artistic Director: Bruce Miller
   Director Development: Victoria McClure Mautinko
   Box Office Manager: Pam Northrup
Mission: To produce diverse and outstanding contemporary plays to a growing regional audience.
Founded: 1953
Specialized Field: Musical; Theatrical Group
Status: Professional; Nonprofit
Paid Staff: 7
Volunteer Staff: 50
Budget: $750,000
Income Sources: Ticket Sales; Program Advertising; Charitable Contributions
Performs At: 214 Theatre-in-the-Round
Affiliations: TCG; Richmond Alliance of Professional Theatres
Annual Attendance: 30-40,000
Type of Stage: 3/4 Thrust
Seating Capacity: 190
Organization Type: Performing; Touring

3925   MYSTERY DINNER PLAYHOUSE

2025 E Main Street
Suite 206
Richmond, VA 23223

Phone: 804-649-2583
Fax: 804-649-7419
Toll-free: 888-471-4802
e-mail: info@mysterydinner.com
Web Site: www.mysterydinner.com
Management:
   Producer/Director: James Daab
Founded: 1993
Paid Staff: 6
Paid Artists: 21
Budget: $800,000
Income Sources: Ticket Sales
Performs At: Best Western Governor's; Ramada Central; Double Tree
Affiliations: National Dinner Theatre Association
Annual Attendance: 50,000
Facility Category: Hotel
Type of Stage: Promenade
Seating Capacity: 100; 150; 150
Organization Type: Commercial

3926   THEATRE IV

114 W Broad Street
Richmond, VA 23220
Phone: 804-783-1688
Fax: 804-775-2325
Toll-free: 800-235-8687
e-mail: ewilliams@theatreIV.org
Web Site: www.theatreIV.org
Management:
   Director Tour Operations: Eric Williams
Mission: To create exciting and innovative professional theatrical productions of high quality.
Founded: 1975
Specialized Field: Theatrical Group
Status: Professional; Nonprofit
Income Sources: Theatre Communications Group
Performs At: The Empire Theatre; The Little Theatre
Type of Stage: Proscenium; Flexible
Seating Capacity: 604; 84
Organization Type: Performing; Touring; Resident; Educational

3927   THEATREVIRGINIA

Virginia Museum of Fine Arts
2800 Grove Avenue
Richmond, VA 23221-2466
Phone: 804-353-6161
Fax: 804-353-8799
Toll-free: 877-353-6161
e-mail: info@theatreva.com
Web Site: www.theatreva.com
Management:
   Producing Artistic Director: Benny Sato Ambush
Founded: 1955
Status: Professional; Nonprofit
Income Sources: League of Resident Theatres; Actors' Equity Association; Society for Stage Directors and Choreographers
Organization Type: Performing; Resident

3928   JEFFERSON THEATRE CENTER

541 Luck Avenue
Roanoke, VA 24016

Phone: 540-343-2624
Fax: 540-343-3744
e-mail: info@jeffcenter.org
Web Site: www.jeffcenter.org
Management:
   Managing Director: Geoffrey Woodward
Mission: Strives to be the destination of choice in the Blue Ridge for cultural and artistic opportunities within a dynamic environment that nurtures creativity, facilitates community events and presents diverse programming.

3929   MILL MOUNTAIN THEATRE

One Market Square
Roanoke, VA 24011
Phone: 540-342-5730
Fax: 540-342-5745
Toll-free: 800-317-6455
e-mail: mmtmail@millmountain.org
Web Site: www.millmountain.org
Officers:
   President: Howard Beck Jr
   VP: John Jessee
   Treasurer: John Light
   Secretary: Ted Feinour
Management:
   Producing Artistic Director: Jere Lee Hodgin
   General Manager: Mary C Knapp
   Director Development: John Levin
   Youth Ensemble Director: David Dvorscak
   General Manager: Mary Knapp
   Director Finance: Jim Ayers
   Director Audience Services: Dick Vipperman
   Group Sales Coordinator: John Whitney
   Production Manager: Doug Flinchum
Mission: Professional production of musicals, dramas and comedies with particular emphasis on the production and development of original works.
Founded: 1964
Specialized Field: Musical; Theatrical Group
Status: Professional; Nonprofit
Paid Staff: 35
Volunteer Staff: 300
Budget: $2,000,000
Income Sources: Box Office Sales; Private & Public Support
Season: October - August
Performs At: Mill Mountain Theatre; Trinkle Main Stage; Waldron Stage
Affiliations: Theatre Communications Group; Southeastern Theatre Conference; Society for Stage Directors and Choreographers; Actors Equity
Annual Attendance: 60,000
Facility Category: Performing; Touring
Type of Stage: Proscenium; Black Box
Stage Dimensions: 44'x34'; 15'x20'
Seating Capacity: 400; 110
Year Built: 1983
Rental Contact: Doug Flinchum
Organization Type: Performing; Resident; Educational

3930   SHENANDOAH SHAKESPEARE

11 E Beverley Street
Suite 31
Staunton, VA 24401

All listings are in alphabetical order by state, then city, then organization within the city.

Phone: 540-885-5588
Fax: 540-885-4886
Toll-free: 877-682-4236
e-mail: shsh@shenandoahshakespeare
Web Site: www.shenandoahshakespeare
Management:
   Executive Director: Ralph Alan Cohen
   Artistic Director: Jim Warren
   Director Development: Martha P Farmer
   Director Marketing: Deona Houff
   Director Tour Operations: Bill Gordon
   Director Community Relations: Susan Hawthorne
   Managing Director: Sandie Nelson
Mission: Shenandoah shakespeare through its performances, its theatres, its exhibitions, and its educational programs, seeks to make Shakespeare, the joys of theatre and language, and the communal experience of the Renaissance stage accessible to a
Income Sources: Sponsors; Donor

3931 BABCOCK SEASON

Box AU
Sweet Briar College
Sweet Briar, VA 24595
Phone: 804-381-6100
Fax: 804-381-6263
e-mail: Wittman@sbc.edu
Web Site: www.scene.sbc.edu
Management:
   Babcock Theatre Manager: Loretta Wittman
Budget: $39,000
Income Sources: College Budget, Grants
Performs At: Babcock Auditorium
Affiliations: Association of Performing Arts Presenters; Virginia Arts Presenters
Annual Attendance: 5,000
Facility Category: General Purpose Theatre
Type of Stage: Proscenium
Seating Capacity: 652
Year Built: 1962

3932 VIRGINIA MUSICAL THEATRE

228 N Lynnhaven Road
Suite 114
Virginia Beach, VA 23452-7514
Phone: 757-340-5446
Fax: 757-340-5398
e-mail: vmtheatr@pinn.net
Web Site: www.ymtheatre.org
Management:
   Executive Producing Director: Jeff Meredith
Founded: 1991
Status: Nonprofit
Paid Staff: 4
Volunteer Staff: 40
Paid Artists: 300
Season: October - July
Type of Stage: Proscenium
Stage Dimensions: 50' x 35'
Seating Capacity: 964

3933 VIRGINIA SHAKESPEARE FESTIVAL

College of William and Mary
PO Box 8795
Williamsburg, VA 23187
Phone: 757-221-4563
Management:
   Executive Director: Jerry H Bledsoe
Mission: To offer quality Shakespeare performed in the classical manner.
Founded: 1978
Specialized Field: Theater; Festivals
Status: Professional; Nonprofit
Paid Staff: 20
Income Sources: The College of William & Mary
Season: July - August
Performs At: Phi Beta Kappa Memorial Hall; The College of Williamsburg
Organization Type: Performing; Educational

Washington

3934 BAINBRIDGE PERFORMING ARTS

200 Madison Aveneu N
Bainbridge Island, WA 98110
Phone: 206-482-8578
Fax: 206-842-0195

3935 THEATRE AT MEYDENBAUER

11100 NE 6th Street
Bellevue, WA 98004
Phone: 425-450-3810
Fax: 425-637-0166
e-mail: selliott@meydenbauer.com
Web Site: www.meydenbauer.com

3936 MOUNT BAKER THEATRE

104 N Commercial Street
PO Box 2329
Bellingham, WA 98225
Phone: 360-733-5793
Fax: 306-671-0114
e-mail: baker@cnw.net
Web Site: www.mtbakertheatre.com
Management:
   Executive Director: Brad Burdick
   Marketing Director: Kim Lastkey
Status: Nonprofit
Budget: $150,000-400,000
Seating Capacity: 1,509
Year Built: 1927
Year Remodeled: 1995
Cost: $1.6 million
Rental Contact: Sharon Cassidy

3937 WWU SUMMER STOCK

MS-9108
Bellingham, WA 98225
Phone: 360-650-3876
Fax: 360-650-3028
e-mail: theatre@cc.wwu.edu
Web Site: www.as.wwu.edu/~theatre/
Season: Jule - August

3938 ADMIRAL THEATRE FOUNDATION

515 Pacific Avenue
Bremerton, WA 98337
Phone: 360-373-6810
Fax: 360-405-0673
e-mail: admiraltheatre@msn.com
Web Site: www.admiraltheatre.org
Management:
    Executive Director: Ruth Enderle
    Business Manager: Brian Johnson
    Technical Director: Jeff Vaughan
    Music/Box Office Manager: Tim Walbel
Specialized Field: Presenting Performing Arts
Paid Staff: 5

3939 BERMERTON COMMUNITY THEATRE

599 Lebo Boulevard
Bremerton, WA 98310
Phone: 360-373-5152
Fax: 360-373-6754
e-mail: bet@silverlink.net
Web Site: www.silver.net/bet
Management:
    Treasurer: R Bruce Hankins
Mission: Production of amateur dramas, comedies,
mysteries and musicals for the local community.
Founded: 1945
Specialized Field: Musical; Community; Theatrical
Group
Status: Non-Professional; Nonprofit
Volunteer Staff: 12
Non-paid Artists: 100
Organization Type: Performing

3940 EVERETT THEATRE

2911 Colby
Everett, WA 98201
Mailing Address: PO Box 12 Everett, WA 98206
Phone: 425-258-6766
e-mail: boxoffice@everetttheatre.org
Officers:
    President: Randy Mather
    Finance: Terry Klett
Management:
    Executive Director: Kenn Wessel
Founded: 1901

3941 VILLAGE THEATRE

2710 Wetmore Avenue
Everett, WA 98201
Phone: 425-257-6363
Fax: 425-257-6393
Web Site: www.villagetheatre.org
Mission: The mission of Village Theatre is to be a
regionally recognized and nationally influenced center of
excelent in family theatre.
Founded: 1979
Specialized Field: Musical Theatre
Budget: $6.1 million
Performs At: Francis J Gaudette Theatre; Everett
Performing Arts Center

3942 KNUTZEN FAMILY THEATRE - CITY OF FEDERAL WAY

3200 SW Dash Point Road
Federal Way, WA 98023
Phone: 253-835-2025
Fax: 253-835-2010
e-mail: johng@fedway.org

3943 SAN JUAN COMMUNITY THEATRE AND ARTS CENTER

100 Second Street
PO Box 1063
Friday Harbor, WA 98250
Phone: 360-378-3211
Fax: 360-378-2398
e-mail: sjarts@rockusland.com
Web Site: www.sanjuanarts.org
Officers:
    President: David Bayley
Management:
    Executive Director: Merritt Olsen
Mission: To maintain a center for visual and performing
arts for the residents of the island.
Founded: 1989
Specialized Field: Community
Status: Non-Professional; Nonprofit
Paid Staff: 6
Volunteer Staff: 350
Organization Type: Performing; Educational;
Sponsoring

3944 PARADISE THEATRE

9916 Peacock Hilll NW
Gig Harbor, WA 98332
Phone: 253-851-7529
Fax: 253-851-7503
e-mail: vrichards@paradisetheatre.org
Web Site: www.paradisetheatre.org
Officers:
    President: Bob Flynn
    Treasurer: Lynn Bromley
    Secretary: Gus Berry
Management:
    Artistic Director: Jeff Richards
Mission: To promote theatre arts and cultural enrichment
through performances as well as educational workshops
and classes.
Founded: 2000
Specialized Field: Musical; Theatrical Group
Status: Semi-Professional; Nonprofit
Paid Staff: 4
Volunteer Staff: 15
Paid Artists: 16
Non-paid Artists: 15
Income Sources: Grants; Individual Donations; Ticket
Sales
Performs At: Paradise Theatre
Type of Stage: Proscenium
Seating Capacity: 50 indoor; 800 outdoor
Year Built: 1900
Year Remodeled: 2000
Organization Type: Performing; Touring; Educational

3945 VILLAGE THEATRE
303 Front Street N
Issaquah, WA 98027
Phone: 425-392-1942
Fax: 425-391-3242
Web Site: www.villagetheatre.org
Mission: The mission of Village Theatre is to be a regionally recognized and nationally influenced center of excelent in family theatre.
Founded: 1979
Specialized Field: Musical Theatre
Budget: $6.1 million
Performs At: Francis J Gaudette Theatre; Everett Performing Arts Center

3946 COLUMBIA THEATRE FOR THE PERFORMING ARTS
1231 Vandercook Way
Longview, WA 98632-4001
Phone: 360-423-1011
Fax: 360-423-8626
e-mail: info@columbiatheatre.com
Web Site: www.columbiatheatre.com
Mission: To provide engaging theatre experience of the highest quality that we always strive to uplift and entertain; to instill in audience and theatre members the value of our integrity as a source of inspiration and hope.
Specialized Field: Musical; Community; Theatrical Group
Status: Nonprofit
Annual Attendance: 60,000
Facility Category: Performing Arts Center
Type of Stage: Proscenium
Seating Capacity: 1,000
Year Built: 1925
Organization Type: Performing; Sponsoring

3947 CUTTER THEATRE
PO Box 133
Metaline Falls, WA 99153-0133
Phone: 509-446-4108
Fax: 509-446-3037
e-mail: cutter@iomet.com
Web Site: www.povn.com/cutter

3948 HARLEQUIN PRODUCTIONS
State Theater
204 4th Avenue
Olympia, WA 98501
Phone: 360-705-3215
Fax: 360-534-9859
e-mail: whitney@orcalink.com
Web Site: www.orcalink.com/whitney
Management:
    Artistic Director: Linda Whitney
    Executive Director: Jon Engelman
    Costume Designer: Monique Anderson
    Technical Director: Mark Bujeaud
    Lighting Designer: Jill Carter
    Costume Designer: Lucy Gentry
    Scenic Designer: Ariel Goldberger
    Production Manager: Nick Shellman
    Composer/Sound Designer/Operator: Karl Welty
Founded: 1990

Status: Nonprofit
Season: May - December
Type of Stage: Thrust
Stage Dimensions: 48'6" x 32'
Seating Capacity: 218

3949 BEASLEY PERFORMING ARTS COLISEUM
PO Box 641710
Pullman, WA 99146-1710
Phone: 509-335-2241
Fax: 509-335-3853
e-mail: kerrjf@wsu.edu

3950 PULLMAN SUMMER PALACE
Theatre Program
Washington State University
Pullman, WA 99164-2432
Phone: 509-335-5682
Fax: 509-335-7447
e-mail: caldwell@wsu.edu
Management:
    Managing Director: George Caldwell
Founded: 1977
Status: Non-Equity; Nonprofit
Season: July - August
Type of Stage: Proscenium
Stage Dimensions: 45' x 45'
Seating Capacity: 460

3951 RAYMOND THEATER
230 2nd Street
Raymond, WA 98577
Phone: 360-942-5536
Fax: 360-942-5616
e-mail: raymond@willapabay.org
Web Site: www.visit.willapabay.com

3952 ACT THEATRE
Kreielsheimer Place
700 Union Street
Seattle, WA 98101-4037
Phone: 206-292-7660
Fax: 206-292-7670
e-mail: act@acttheatre.org
Web Site: www.acttheatre.org
Officers:
    Chairman: Philip M Condit
    President: Andrew Fallat
    VP: Lawton Henry Humphrey
    Secretary: Bruce T Goto
Management:
    Managing Director: Jim Loder
    Producing Director: Vito Zingarelli
    Founding Director: Gregory A Falls
    Public Relations Director: Barry Allar
Mission: To offer the best in contemporary theater.
Founded: 1965
Specialized Field: Theatrical Group
Status: Professional; Nonprofit
Paid Staff: 75
Paid Artists: 170
Budget: 5,000,000

Income Sources: Actors' Equity Association; League of Resident Theatres; American Arts Alliance; Washington State Arts Alliance
Season: March - December
Performs At: A Contemporary Theatre
Annual Attendance: 125,000
Facility Category: 4 Venue Performance Facility
Type of Stage: 3/4 Thrust; Arena; Caberat
Year Built: 1925
Year Remodeled: 1996
Rental Contact: Adam Moomey
Organization Type: Resident

3953 BATHHOUSE THEATRE
7312 W Greenlake Drive N
Seattle, WA 98103
Phone: 206-524-9108
Fax: 206-527-1942
Management:
   Artistic Director: Arne Zaslove
   Managing Director: Steven Lerian
Mission: To develop our full potential as a resident theatre company; to put excellent theatre within reach of the widest possible audience.
Founded: 1970
Specialized Field: Theatrical Group
Status: Professional; Nonprofit
Income Sources: Theatre Communications Group; Actors' Equity Association; Small Professional Theatre Association
Performs At: Bathhouse Theatre
Organization Type: Performing; Touring; Resident

3954 EMPTY SPACE THEATRE
3509 Fremont Avenue N
Seattle, WA 98103
Phone: 206-547-7500
Fax: 206-547-7635
e-mail: emptyspace@emptyspace.org
Web Site: www.emptyspace.org
Officers:
   Chairman: David R Perry
   VP: Margaret Lane
   VP: Susan Takemoto
   Treasurer: Jacqueline Lorenz
Management:
   Artistic Director: Allison Narver
   Managing Director: John Bradshaw
   Communications Director: Terri Hiroshima
   Development Director: Cindy Reynolds
Mission: Strives to make theater an event - bold, provocative, celebratory - bringing audiences and artists to a common ground through an uncommon experience.
Founded: 1970
Specialized Field: Musical; Theatrical Group
Status: Professional; Nonprofit
Paid Staff: 20
Volunteer Staff: 4
Paid Artists: 80
Non-paid Artists: 4
Budget: $1,000,000
Income Sources: Ticket Sales; Donations; Grants
Performs At: Empty Space Theatre
Affiliations: TCG; TPS
Annual Attendance: 25,000

Facility Category: Theater
Type of Stage: Thrust
Seating Capacity: 150
Year Built: 1928
Rental Contact: 206-57-47-7633 Ext 169 Rod Pillous
Organization Type: Performing; Resident; Educational

3955 HYPERION THEATRE
7512 34th Avenue NW
Seattle, WA 98117
Phone: 206-781-0022
Management:
   Artistic Director: Joe Seabeck

3956 INTIMAN THEATRE COMPANY
201 Mercer Street, Seattle Center
PO Box 19760
Seattle, WA 98109
Phone: 206-269-1901
Fax: 206-269-1928
e-mail: scripts@intiman.org
Web Site: www.intiman.org
Management:
   Artistic Director: Bartlett Sher
   Dramaturg: Mame Hunt
   Artistic Administrator: Kate Godman
   Community Programs Manager: Liza Comtois
   Managing Director: Laura Penn
   General Manager: Art Bridenstine
   Associate Managing Director: Rebecca Sherr
   Assistant/Managing Director: Precious Butiu
   Production Manager: David A Mulligan
Mission: To produce engaging dramatic work that celebrates the intimate relationship among audience and language and, through the exploration of enduring themes, illuminates the shared human experience of our diverse community.
Founded: 1972
Specialized Field: Theatrical Group
Season: May - December
Performs At: Intiman Playhouse
Type of Stage: Modified Thrust
Seating Capacity: 480
Year Remodeled: 1987
Cost: $1,200,000

3957 NEW CITY THEATER
1703 13th Avenue
Seattle, WA 98122
Phone: 206-328-4683
Fax: 206-328-4683
Management:
   Artistic Director: John Kazanjian
   Theater Manager: Alan Horton
Mission: Dedicated to research and development in the contemporary arts.
Founded: 1982
Specialized Field: Theatrical Group
Status: Professional; Nonprofit
Income Sources: Theatre Communications Group
Performs At: The New City Theatre
Organization Type: Performing; Resident

3958 NORTHWEST PUPPET

9123 15th Avenue NE
Seattle, WA 98103
Phone: 206-523-2579
Fax: 206-783-0851
e-mail: info@nwpup
Web Site: www.nwpuppet.org
Management:
    Executive Co-Director: Stephen Carter
    Executive Co-Director: Chris Carter
Mission: To create professional puppet theater; to present top quality puppet theater; to teach puppet skills and cultural knowledge; to serve children and adults by providing entertainment and education.
Founded: 1985
Specialized Field: Puppet
Status: Professional; Nonprofit
Paid Staff: 2
Income Sources: Puppeteers of America; United International Marionette Association
Organization Type: Performing; Touring; Resident; Educational; Sponsoring

3959 SEATTLE CHILDREN'S THEATRE

201 Thomas Street
Seattle, WA 98109
Phone: 206-443-0807
Fax: 206-443-0442
e-mail: sctpr@sct.org
Web Site: www.sct.org
Officers:
    President: Lauie Oki
    First VP: Richard Bendix
    Second VP: Judy Bunnell
    Secretary: Marty Chilberg
Management:
    Artistic Director: Linda Hartzell
    General Manager: Shelley Saunders
    Managing Director: Kevin Maifeld
    Public Relations: Taryn Essinger
Mission: To produce professional theater for the young with appeal to people of all ages; to provide theater education and theater arts training; to develop scripts and musical scores for new theater works.
Founded: 1975
Specialized Field: Theatrical Group
Status: Professional; Nonprofit
Budget: $5,300,000
Performs At: Charlotte Martin Theatre; Eve Alvovd Theatre
Affiliations: ASSITES/USA; Actors' Equity Association/TYA; American Association of Theatre Educators; International Alliance of Theatrical Stage Employees; TCG
Annual Attendance: 250,000
Seating Capacity: 480; 285
Year Built: 1993
Rental Contact: General Manager Shelley Sanders
Organization Type: Performing; Touring; Resident; Educational

3960 SEATTLE MIME THEATRE

915 E Pine Street
#419
Seattle, WA 98122
Phone: 206-324-8788
Fax: 206-322-5569
e-mail: smt@halcyon.com
Web Site: www.seattlemime.org
Mission: Dedicated to enlivening the imaginations of minds and bodies of people of all ages with its unique form of physical theater through the interlaced processes of creation, teaching and performances.
Founded: 1977
Specialized Field: Theatrical Group
Status: Nonprofit
Paid Staff: 1
Paid Artists: 4
Facility Category: Offices and Theater
Type of Stage: Black Box
Stage Dimensions: 55'x40'
Seating Capacity: 49
Rental Contact: Richard Davidson
Organization Type: Performing; Touring; Educational

3961 SEATTLE REPERTORY THEATRE

155 Mercer Street
Seattle, WA 98109
Phone: 206-443-2210
Fax: 206-443-2379
Toll-free: 877-960-9235
e-mail: info@seattlerep.org
Web Site: www.seattlerep.org
Management:
    Artistic Director: Sharon Ott
    Managing Director: Benjamin Moore
Mission: To offer professional live theatre and education for residents of the Pacific Northwest.
Founded: 1963
Specialized Field: Theatrical Group
Status: Professional; Nonprofit
Income Sources: Actors' Equity Association; League of Resident Theatres
Performs At: Bagley Wright Theatre
Facility Category: Theatre
Type of Stage: Proscenium
Seating Capacity: 856 and 286
Year Built: 1983
Year Remodeled: 1996
Rental Contact: Ten Eyck Swackharner
Organization Type: Performing; Resident

3962 TAPROOT THEATRE COMPANY

204 N 85th Street
PO Box 30946
Seattle, WA 98103
Phone: 206-781-9705
Fax: 206-706-1502
e-mail: taproot@taproottheatre.org
Web Site: www.taproottheatre.org
Officers:
    President: Scott Hardman
    Secretary: Stephen Schertzinger
    Treasurer: Sharon Morrison
Management:

Producing Artistic Director: Scott Nolte
Managing Director: M Christopher Boyer
Associate Artistic Director: Karen Lund
Public Relations/Marketing Director: Pamela Nolte
Mission: Preserving Christian values and maintaining excellence in diverse production activities.
Founded: 1976
Specialized Field: Theatrical Group
Status: Professional; Semi-Professional; Nonprofit
Paid Staff: 24
Volunteer Staff: 285
Paid Artists: 98
Budget: $880,000
Affiliations: TCG; CITA; Greenwood Chamber of Commerce
Annual Attendance: 85,000
Facility Category: Renovated historic cinema
Type of Stage: Thrust
Stage Dimensions: 15'x22'
Seating Capacity: 226
Year Built: 1915
Year Remodeled: 1996
Rental Contact: Jennifer Matthews
Organization Type: Performing; Touring; Resident

3963 THEATER SCHMEATER

1500 Summit Avenue
Seattle, WA 98122-3622
Phone: 206-324-5621
Management:
Artistic Director: Shelia Daniels
Managing Director: Andrew Hanies

3964 SPOKANE CIVIC THEATRE

1020 Howard
PO Box 5222
Spokane, WA 99205
Phone: 509-325-1413
Fax: 509-325-9287
Toll-free: 800-446-9576
e-mail: civictheatre@mindspring.com
Web Site: www.spokanecivictheatre.com
Management:
Executive Producer: John G Phillips
Marketing Director: Marilyn Langbehn
Develoment Director: Susan Hammond
Office Administrator: Shirley Deranleau
Technical Director: Peter Hardie
Mission: To offer opportunities for participation in the art of theatre; to promote new plays.
Founded: 1947
Specialized Field: Community; Theatrical Group
Status: Non-Professional; Nonprofit
Budget: $625,000
Income Sources: Washington State Arts Commission; Allen Foundation; Box Office
Performs At: Spokane Civic Theatres
Affiliations: American Association of Community Theatres; WA Arts Alliance; TCG
Annual Attendance: 35,000
Facility Category: Theatre
Type of Stage: Proscenium; Black Box
Seating Capacity: 339; 100
Year Built: 1966
Year Remodeled: 1999

Rental Contact: Jack Phillips
Organization Type: Performing; Educational

3965 SPOKANE INTERPLAYERS ENSEMBLE

174 S Howard Street
Spokane, WA 99204
Phone: 509-455-7529
Fax: 509-624-9348
e-mail: interplayers@interplayers.com
Web Site: www.interplayers.com
Management:
Producing Artistic Director: Robin Stanton
Associate Artistic Director: Michael Weaver
Marketing/Development: Grant Smith
Production Manager: Jason Lewis
Box Office Manager: Jennifer Laws
Mission: To maintain a resident non-profit, professional theatre company offering an annual season ranging from contemporary and classic to original works.
Founded: 1980
Specialized Field: Theatrical Group
Status: Professional; Nonprofit
Paid Staff: 14
Volunteer Staff: 150
Paid Artists: 100
Budget: $485,000
Income Sources: Ticket Sales; Grants
Performs At: Spokane Interplayers Ensemble Theatre
Affiliations: Theatre Communications Group
Annual Attendance: 25,000
Type of Stage: Thrust
Seating Capacity: 253
Year Built: 1926
Year Remodeled: 1980
Organization Type: Performing; Resident; Educational

3966 TACOMA ACTORS GUILD

901 Broadway
Suite 600
Tacoma, WA 98402
Phone: 253-272-3107
Fax: 253-272-3358
Web Site: www.tacomaactorsguild.org
Management:
General Manager: Chris Shelton
Artistic Director: Pat Petttan
Mission: To offer quality theatre and to entertain and enrich the South Puget Sound area.
Founded: 1978
Specialized Field: Theatrical Group
Status: Professional; Nonprofit
Income Sources: Theatre Communications Group
Performs At: Tacoma Actors Guild
Annual Attendance: 35,000
Seating Capacity: 302
Year Built: 1998
Cost: $8,000,000
Organization Type: Performing; Resident

3967 OLD SLOCUM HOUSE THEATRE COMPANY

605 Esther Street
Vancouver, WA 98660
Web Site: www.slocumhouse.com

Management:
    Board of Directors:
Mission: The restoration of the Slocum House Theatre and the production of 19th-century plays.
Founded: 1969
Specialized Field: Musical; Community
Status: Nonprofit
Organization Type: Resident

3968 COLUMBIA GORGE REPERTORY THEATRE
72 Staats Road
White Salmon, WA 98672
Phone: 509-493-1213
Fax: 509-493-1501
Toll-free: 800-405-3450
e-mail: cgrep@aol.com
Web Site: www.cgrep.com
Management:
    Artistic Director: Jesse Merz
    Executive Director: Jan Merz
    Youth Director: G Arwen Nichols
Founded: 1996
Status: Non-Equity; Commercial
Season: June - September
Type of Stage: Proscenium
Stage Dimensions: 30' x 40'
Seating Capacity: 150

3969 CAPITOL THEATRE
19 S 3rd Street
PO Box 102
Yakima, WA 98907
Phone: 509-575-6267
Fax: 509-575-6251
e-mail: arts@capitoltheatre.org
Web Site: www.capitoltheatre.org
Management:
    Executive Director: Steven J Caffery
Budget: $400,000-1,000,000

West Virginia

3970 THEATRE WEST VIRGINIA
PO Box 1205
Beckley, WV 25802
Phone: 304-256-6800
Fax: 304-256-6807
Toll-free: 800-666-9142
e-mail: contact@theatrewestvirginia.com
Web Site: www.theatrewestvirginia.com
Officers:
    President: John Rist
    VP: Alice Cox
    Secretary: Colleen McCalhoah
    Treasurer: Brad Wartella
    Marketing Director: Lola Rizer
Management:
    General Manager: Gayle Bowling
    Artistic Director: Marina Dolinger
Mission: To provide theatre of the highest quality to community and state residents as well as tourists.

Founded: 1955
Specialized Field: Theatrical Group; Touring Marionettes and Touring Educational Programs
Status: Professional
Paid Staff: 20
Paid Artists: 70
Season: June - August
Annual Attendance: 120,000
Facility Category: Amphitheatre; Touring
Stage Dimensions: 60'x60'
Seating Capacity: 1,259
Year Built: 1960
Year Remodeled: 1991
Organization Type: Performing; Touring; Educational; Sponsoring

---

3971 KANAWHA PLAYERS
5315 MacCorkle Avenue
PO Box 4575
Charleston, WV 25304
Phone: 304-925-5051
Officers:
    President: Stephen E Kawash
Management:
    Company Administrator: Kathie M Frank
    Historian: Betsy Stuart
Founded: 1922
Specialized Field: Dinner; Community; Theatrical Group
Status: Non-Professional; Nonprofit
Paid Staff: 175
Income Sources: Arts Advocacy of West Virginia
Performs At: Charleston Civic Center-Little Theatre
Organization Type: Performing; Touring; Educational

3972 APPLE ALLEY PLAYERS
PO Box 144
Keyser, WV 26726
Phone: 304-788-1105
Fax: 304-788-5883
e-mail: lymyersaap@yahoo.com
Officers:
    President: Annette Favara
    VP: Bob Shadier
    Secretary: Alexa Fazenbaker
    Treasurer: Sandy Shadler
Mission: To provide quality theatre for the surrounding area.
Founded: 1980
Specialized Field: Community
Status: Nonprofit
Performs At: McKee Art Center; Potomac State College
Organization Type: Resident; Sponsoring

3973 GREENBRIER VALLEY THEATRE
113 E Washington Street
PO Box 494
Lewisburg, WV 24901
Phone: 304-645-3838
Fax: 304-645-3818
e-mail: cathey@gvtheatre.org
Web Site: www.gvtheatre.org
Officers:
    President: Claire LaRocco
    Secretary: Carolyn Rudley

Treasurer: Stephen P King
Management:
  Artistic Director: Cathey Crowell Sawyer
  Equity Stage Manager: Alan Porch
  Public Relations Director: Claudia O'Keefe
  Business Manager: Mary Buskirk
  Technical Director: Devin Preston
  Volunteer Director: Jane Matheny
Mission: To provide a vehicle for bringing live, professional-quality theatre experiences to our community; to explore all practical means of encouraging the performing arts and artists in our area.
Founded: 1966
Specialized Field: Year Round Theatre; Mix of Contemporary; Classical/Musical Plays; Childrens Theatre; Educational Programs
Status: Non-Professional
Paid Staff: 18
Budget: $400,000
Income Sources: Private Donations; Foundation
Performs At: Hollowell Theatre; Black Box Flexible Seating
Annual Attendance: 10,000
Facility Category: Black Box
Type of Stage: Flexable-Sprung Floor
Stage Dimensions: Fexible
Seating Capacity: 150; 200
Year Built: 1953
Year Remodeled: 2000
Cost: $1,700,000
Rental Contact: Cathy Sawyer
Organization Type: Performing; Touring; Educational

3974 ARACOMA STORY

311 Main Street
PO Box 2016
Logan, WV 25601
Phone: 304-752-0253
Fax: 304-752-0253
e-mail: scfossco@mail.wvnet.edu
Web Site: www.thearacomastory.com
Management:
  Office Manager: Jeannie Gore
Founded: 1976
Status: Non-Equity; Nonprofit
Paid Staff: 4
Volunteer Staff: 5
Paid Artists: 5
Non-paid Artists: 50
Season: June - August
Annual Attendance: 3,000
Facility Category: Amphitheatre
Type of Stage: Proscenium-Wood Walls
Stage Dimensions: 60' x 40'
Seating Capacity: 650
Year Built: 1982
Year Remodeled: 2002

3975 VIVIAN DAVIS MICHAEL LABORATORY THEATRE- COLLEGE OF CREATIVE ARTS

PO Box 6111
1 Evandale Drive
Morgantown, WV 26506-6111
Phone: 304-296-4841
Fax: 304-293-6896
e-mail: msoreskovich@mail.wvu.edu
Web Site: www.wvu.edu/nccarts/
Management:
  Dean/Director: J Bernard Schultz
  Chair Division Theatre/Dance: Margaret McKowen
  Chairman Division of Art: Sergio Soave
  Chair, Division Music: David Bess
  Associate Director/Finance: Linda Queen
  Director Operations: Mark S Oresicovich
Mission: Educational facility
Specialized Field: Visual Art; Music Theatre; Dance
Income Sources: Stage; Private
Performs At: Vivian Davis Michael Laboratory Theatre
Affiliations: NASM - National Association of Schools of Theatre; NASAD - National Association of Schools of Art and Design
Annual Attendance: 1,000
Facility Category: Educational
Type of Stage: Proscenium
Stage Dimensions: 16'x32'
Seating Capacity: 75
Year Built: 1968
Year Remodeled: 1998
Cost: $50,000

3976 WEST VIRGINIA PUBLIC THEATRE

PO Box 4270
Morgantown, WV 26504-4270
Phone: 304-598-0144
Fax: 304-594-0145
e-mail: info@wvpublictheatre.org
Web Site: www.wvpt.org
Management:
  Founder/Production Artistic Dir: Ron Iannone
Founded: 1985
Status: Nonprofit
Season: June - August
Seating Capacity: 650

3977 CONTEMPORARY AMERICAN THEATER FESTIVAL

Box 429
Shepherdstown, WV 25443
Phone: 304-876-3473
Fax: 304-876-0955
Web Site: www.catf.org
Management:
  Producing Director: Ed Herendeen
  Managing Director: Catherine Irwin
Founded: 1991
Specialized Field: Theater Festival
Performs At: Main Stage; Studio Theater
Type of Stage: Proscenium, Black Box
Seating Capacity: 350; 99

3978 BROOKE HILLS PLAYHOUSE

PO Box 186
140 Gist Drive
Wellsburg, WV 26070
Phone: 304-737-3344
Fax: 304-737-4247
Management:

President: Paula Welch
Founded: 1972
Specialized Field: Theatre
Status: Nonprofit; Non-Equity
Paid Staff: 1
Volunteer Staff: 6
Income Sources: Ticket Sales
Season: June - August
Annual Attendance: 4,000
Facility Category: Barn
Type of Stage: Proscenium
Stage Dimensions: 26' x 22'
Seating Capacity: 195

Wisconsin

3979 AL RINGLING THEATRE LIVELY ARTS SERIES

136 4th Avenue
PO Box 381
Baraboo, WI 53913
Phone: 608-356-8864
Fax: 608-356-0976
e-mail: ringling@baraboo.com
Web Site: www.alringling.com
Management:
   Managing Director: Larry McCoy
Paid Staff: 2-4
Volunteer Staff: 80
Budget: $20,000-35,000
Type of Stage: Proscenium
Stage Dimensions: 37' x 27'
Seating Capacity: 800
Year Built: 1915

3980 CHIPPEWA VALLEY THEATRE GUILD

316 Eau Claire Street
Eau Claire, WI 54701
Phone: 715-832-7529
Fax: 715-832-0828
Web Site: www.cvtg.org
Officers:
   President: Sara Antonson
   Vice President: Cathy Statz
   Treasurer: Jim Mueller
   Secretary: Sue Frederick
Management:
   Executive Director: Kurt Majkowski
   Executive Director: Ann Sessions
   Volunteer Coordinator: Emily McPeck
Mission: To bring quality theatre productions to our area, as well as allowing community members to perform in a theatrical production.
Founded: 1982
Specialized Field: Community
Status: Nonprofit
Paid Staff: 2
Volunteer Staff: 300
Income Sources: Eau Claire Parks & Recreation
Performs At: The State Regional Arts Center
Annual Attendance: 10,500
Seating Capacity: 1,117
Organization Type: Performing; Educational

3981 SUNSET PLAYHOUSE

800 N Elm Grove Road
Elm Grove, WI 53122
Phone: 262-782-4430
Management:
   Artistic Director: Tom Somerville
   Technical Director: John Kleis
Mission: To introduce as many new people as possible to live entertainment.
Founded: 1954
Specialized Field: Community; Theatrical Group
Status: Non-Professional; Nonprofit
Performs At: Sunset Playhouse
Organization Type: Performing; Open Auditions

3982 AMERICAN FOLKLORE THEATRE

PO Box 273
Fish Creek, WI 54212
Phone: 920-854-6117
Fax: 920-854-9106
e-mail: gen@folkloretheatre.com
Web Site: www.folkloretheatre.com
Officers:
   Chairman of Board: Mary Seeberg
Management:
   Managing Director: M Kaye Christman
   Artistic Director: Jeffrey Herbst
   Technical Director: David Colby
Mission: To develop and present professional dramatic productions of a cultural and/or educational nature which will futher the knowledge and appreciation of the heritage of the United States.
Founded: 1990
Specialized Field: Original Musical Theatre
Status: Nonprofit
Budget: 850,000
Income Sources: Box Office; Donations; Sponsorships; Grants
Season: May - September
Affiliations: TCG; NAMT; Theatre Wisconsin
Annual Attendance: 50,000
Facility Category: Indoor and Outdoor
Type of Stage: Proscenium
Stage Dimensions: 35' x 15'
Seating Capacity: 750
Year Built: 1962
Year Remodeled: 2003

3983 PENINSULA PLAYERS

W 4351 Peninsula Players Road
Fish Creek, WI 54212
Phone: 920-868-3287
Fax: 920-868-3288
Management:
   General Manager: Tom Birmingham
   Executive Producer: James B McKenzie
Mission: As America's oldest professional resident summer theatre, our purpose is to present the latest of Broadway fare.
Founded: 1935
Specialized Field: Summer Stock; Theatrical Group
Status: Professional; Nonprofit
Income Sources: Council of Resident Summer Theatres; Actors' Equity Association

Season: June - October
Performs At: Theatre in a Garden; Open Air Pavilion
Organization Type: Performing; Resident; Educational

3984 NORTHERN LIGHTS PLAYHOUSE
PO Box 256
Hazelhurst, WI 54531-0256
Phone: 715-356-7173
Fax: 715-356-1851
e-mail: nlplays@newnorth.net
Management:
General Manager: Randall Clure
Founded: 1976
Status: Non-Equity; Commercial
Season: May - October
Type of Stage: Proscenium
Seating Capacity: 299

3985 BROOM STREET THEATER
1119 Williamson Street
Madison, WI 53703
Phone: 608-241-2345
Officers:
Chairperson: Rod Clark
Acting Chairperson/Vice Chairperson: Kurt Meyer
Treasurer: Tracy Will
Management:
Artistic Director: Joel Gersmann
Technical Director: Gary Cleven
Mission: Produces eight original plays by Madison playwrights per year. The shows are directed or supervised by the play-wrights. Our work is highly visual and physical. We are one of the oldest experimental theaters in the United States, and occasionally tour.
Founded: 1968
Specialized Field: Theatrical Group
Status: Professional; Nonprofit
Paid Staff: 150
Organization Type: Performing

3986 MADISON REPERTORY THEATRE
122 State Street
#201
Madison, WI 53703-2500
Phone: 608-256-0029
Fax: 608-256-7433
e-mail: postmaster@madisonrep.org
Web Site: madisonrep.org
Officers:
President: Tim Christen
President Elect: Robert Birkhauser
Management:
Artistic Director: Richard Corley
Managing Director: Tony Forman
Mission: Mission is to produce, in an intimate setting, both new and classical work for a diverse audience.
Founded: 1969
Status: Professional
Paid Staff: 20
Volunteer Staff: 350
Paid Artists: 18
Budget: $1,300,000
Income Sources: 60% Earned; 40% Conutributed
Affiliations: Actors' Equity Association; TCG

Annual Attendance: 35,000
Type of Stage: Thrust Stage
Stage Dimensions: 24'x30'
Seating Capacity: 335
Year Built: 1978
Year Remodeled: 2004
Rental Contact: Madison Civic Center
Organization Type: Performing; Resident

3987 MADISON THEATRE GUILD
2410 Monroe Street
Madison, WI 53711
Phone: 608-238-9322
Officers:
President: Jay Rath
Treasurer: Carol Pierick
Management:
Costume Shop Manager: Robby Sonzogi
Mission: To provide education and recreation through theatrical production.
Founded: 1946
Specialized Field: Community; Theatrical Group
Status: Nonprofit
Paid Staff: 150
Income Sources: Wisconsin Theatre Association
Performs At: McDaniels Auditorium
Organization Type: Performing; Educational

3988 WISCONSIN UNION THEATER
800 Langdon Street
Madison, WI 53706
Phone: 608-262-2202
Fax: 608-265-5084
Web Site: www.wisc.edu/union/theater
Management:
Director: Michael Goldberg
Operations Manager: Bruce Ehlinger
Mission: Cultural, entertainment and educational programming for university and community audiences.
Founded: 1939
Specialized Field: Musical; Community; Folk; Theatrical Group
Status: Professional; Nonprofit
Paid Staff: 30
Volunteer Staff: 80
Budget: $900,000
Income Sources: Ticket Reserves
Performs At: Wisconsin Union Theater
Annual Attendance: 120,000
Type of Stage: Proscenium
Stage Dimensions: 36x24
Seating Capacity: 1,300
Year Built: 1934
Organization Type: Sponsoring

3989 MABEL TAINTER MEMORIAL THEATER
205 Main Street
PO Box 250
Menomonie, WI 54751
Phone: 715-235-9726
Fax: 715-235-9736
e-mail: mtainter@mabeltainter.com
Web Site: www.mabeltainter.com

Management:
Executive Director: Laura Reisinger
Facility Manager/Technical Director: Jeff Torgerson
General Manager: Maxine Terry
Box Office Manager: Kate Donicht
Mission: Historic 1890's theater with a performing arts season.. Our mission is dedicated to promoting and enhancing the region's cultural life.
Founded: 1890
Specialized Field: Musical; Community; Folk; Blues; Jazz; Classical
Status: Professional; Nonprofit
Paid Staff: 12
Volunteer Staff: 51
Paid Artists: 30
Budget: $330,000
Income Sources: Tickets; Tours; Rentals; Donations; City and County
Performs At: Mabel Tainter Memorial Theater
Facility Category: Theater and Gift Shop
Type of Stage: Opera House w/orchestra pit
Stage Dimensions: 26'6'x20'
Seating Capacity: 313
Year Built: 1889
Cost: $106,000
Rental Contact: Jeff Torgorson
Organization Type: Sponsoring

3990 ACACIA THEATRE

3300 N Sherman Boulevard
Suite 227
Milwaukee, WI 53202
Phone: 414-769-3200
Management:
Artistic Director: Jon Layton
Marketing Director: Jeffrey Bohmann
Mission: To produce plays with a Christian viewpoint.
Founded: 1980
Specialized Field: Theatrical Group
Status: Semi-Professional; Nonprofit
Paid Staff: 10
Organization Type: Touring; Resident; Educational

3991 FIRST STAGE CHILDREN'S THEATER

929 N Water Street
Milwaukee, WI 53202
Phone: 414-273-2314
Fax: 414-273-5595
e-mail: rgoodman@firststage.org
Web Site: www.firststage.org
Management:
Producer/Artistic Director: Rob Goodman
Founded: 1987
Specialized Field: Theater
Performs At: Marcus Center for the Performing Arts's Todd Wehr Theater
Type of Stage: Thrust
Seating Capacity: 500

3992 GREAT AMERICAN CHILDREN'S THEATRE COMPANY

PO Box 92123
Milwaukee, WI 53202

Phone: 414-276-4230
Fax: 414-276-2214
Officers:
President: Paul Medved
VP Development: Danita Medved
Secretary/Treasurer: Thomas Balgeman
Management:
Producer: Teri Solomon Mitze
Managing Director: Annie Jurczyk
Mission: To provide quality theatre for young audiences.
Founded: 1975
Status: Professional; Nonprofit
Performs At: Pabst Theatre
Organization Type: Performing; Touring; Educational; Sponsoring

3993 MILWAUKEE CHAMBER THEATRE

158 N Broadway
Milwaukee, WI 53202
Phone: 414-276-8842
Fax: 414-277-4474
e-mail: mail@chamber-theatre.com
Web Site: www.chamber-theatre.com
Management:
Managing Director: Lisa B Merrill
Artistic Director: Montgomery Davis
Subscription Manager: Sharon Middleton
Mission: To produce the only annual Shaw festival in the nation and is committed to employing primarily Wisconsin actors and artists. Each season Chamber Theatre offers a wide variety of plays with strong literary and philosophical merit and produces World and regional premieres.
Founded: 1975
Specialized Field: Theatrical Group
Status: Professional; Nonprofit
Paid Staff: 6
Volunteer Staff: var
Paid Artists: var
Non-paid Artists: var
Income Sources: Individual Ticket Revenue; Foundation; Corporation; Goverment Grants
Performs At: Broadway Theatre Center
Annual Attendance: 12,500
Facility Category: 2 Theatres (Cabot; Studio)
Stage Dimensions: 358; 96
Organization Type: Performing; Touring; Resident

3994 MILWAUKEE PUBLIC THEATRE

626 E Kilbourn
Suite 802
Milwaukee, WI 53202
Phone: 414-347-1685
Officers:
Secretary: Mary Scholle
Treasurer: Kathy Ramirez
VP: Jack Keyes
President: John Korsmo
Management:
Co-Founder: Mike Moynihan
Co-Founder: Barbara Leigh
Production Manager: Melinda Boyd
Mission: To create and present theatre, performance and video, as well as celebrations and festivals.
Founded: 1973

Specialized Field: Musical; Theatrical Group; Puppet
Status: Professional
Paid Staff: 5
Income Sources: Theatre Communications Group; WTA
Season: June - August
Organization Type: Performing; Touring; Resident; Educational; Sponsoring

3995 MILWAUKEE REPERTORY THEATER

108 E Wells Street
Milwaukee, WI 53202
Phone: 414-224-1761
Fax: 414-224-9097
e-mail: mailrep@milwaukeerep.com
Web Site: www.milwaukeerep.com
Officers:
    President: Susan Lueger
Management:
    Artistic Director: Joe Hanreddy
    Managing Director: Timothy Shields
    Public Relations Manager: Annie Jurczyk
Mission: To play a vital role in the cultural life of our region through: creating theatrical productions of the highest standard which explore and illuminate the human condition; providing an artistic home for a diverse company of theater professionals; and providing a variety of educational programs for all ages.
Founded: 1954
Specialized Field: Theatrical Group
Status: Professional; Nonprofit
Paid Staff: 120
Volunteer Staff: 8
Paid Artists: 170
Non-paid Artists: 30
Budget: $8,800,000
Income Sources: Ticket Sales; Foundations; Corporations; Individuals; Merchandise
Performs At: Milwaukee Repertory Theater
Affiliations: Actors' Equity Association; Lort; TCG
Annual Attendance: 225,000
Type of Stage: Thrust; Black Box; Cabaret
Stage Dimensions: 3 theater complex and full support
Year Built: 1900
Year Remodeled: 1987
Rental Contact: Associate Manager Rebecca Stibbe
Organization Type: Performing; Resident; Educational

3996 NEXT ACT THEATRE

PO Box 394
342 N Water Street
Milwaukee, WI 53201
Phone: 414-278-7780
Fax: 414-278-5930
e-mail: nextact@exeupc.com
Web Site: www.nextact.org
Management:
    Producing Director: David Cecsarini
    General Manager: Charles Kakuk
    Associate Artistic Director: Michael Wright
    Marketing/Development Manager: Amy Geyser
Mission: To produce engaging and thought-provoking up close and personal theatre, highlighting the Milwaukee area's finest talent.
Founded: 1990
Specialized Field: Theatrical Group

Status: Professional; Nonprofit
Income Sources: Wisconsin Professional Community Theatre Association
Performs At: Off Broadway Theatre; Stiemke Theater
Affiliations: Corporate member of the United Performing Arts Fund; Wisconsin Arts Board
Organization Type: Performing

3997 RENAISSANCE THEATERWORKS

342 N Water Street
4th Floor
Milwaukee, WI 53202
Phone: 414-273-0800
Fax: 414-273-0801
Web Site: www.renaissancetheaterworks.com
Management:
    Marketing Director: Liesl Thorton
    Co-Artistic Director: Marie Kohler
    Producing Director: Julie Swenson Petras
Mission: To produce classical and contemporary theater of the highest artistic quality, rooted in the humanist tradition and with particular interest in the feminine voice.
Founded: 1993
Status: Professional; Nonprofit
Paid Staff: 2
Volunteer Staff: 35
Paid Artists: 15

3998 SKYLIGHT OPERA THEATRE

158 N Broadway
Milwaukee, WI 53202
Phone: 414-291-7811
Fax: 414-271-8896
Web Site: www.skylightopera.com
Management:
    Managing Director: Christopher Libby
    Artistic Director: Richard Carsey
Mission: To bring the full spectrum of music theatre works to a wide and diverse audience in a celebration of the musical and theatrical arts and their reflection of the human condition.
Founded: 1959
Specialized Field: Theatrical Group; Musical; Opera; Operetta; Gilbert and Sullivan; Contemporary Chamber Opera; Original Musical Revues
Status: Professional
Budget: $2.2 million
Income Sources: Box Office; Rentals; Private Foundations/Grants/Endowments; Business/Corporate Donations; Government Grants; Individual Donations
Performs At: Cabot Theatre
Affiliations: Skylight Opera Theatre
Facility Category: Theatre House; Opera House; Room
Type of Stage: Flexible; Platform
Stage Dimensions: 12'x24' Expandable
Orchestra Pit: 1
Architect: Wenzler & Associates
Rental Contact: Artistic Administrator John VandeWalle

3999 THEATRE X

158 N Broadway
Milwaukee, WI 53202
Phone: 414-278-0555
Fax: 414-278-8233

Management:
Producing Director: David Ravel
Founded: 1969
Status: Non-Equity; Nonprofit
Season: September - May
Type of Stage: Black Box
Stage Dimensions: 27' x 70'
Seating Capacity: 99

4000 PORTAGE AREA COMMUNITY THEATRE

PO Box 263
Portage, WI 53901
Phone: 608-742-6942
Officers:
President: Pat Madoni
VP: Lisa Piekarski
Secretary/Registered Agent: Fran Malone
Treasurer: Hans Jensen
Mission: To promote, encourage and increase the public's knowledge and appreciation of the arts, especially theatre, and to provide an outlet for the above.
Founded: 1971
Specialized Field: Community; Theatrical Group
Status: Non-Professional; Nonprofit
Paid Staff: 300
Income Sources: Wisconsin Theatre Association; Wisconsin Council on the Arts
Organization Type: Performing

4001 SHAWANO COUNTY ARTS COUNCIL

PO Box 213
Shawano, WI 54166
Phone: 715-526-2525
Officers:
President: Rusty Mitchell
VP: Deb Lonick
Treasurer: Jaquee Salzman
Founded: 1967
Specialized Field: Musical; Community; Folk; Theatrical Group
Status: Nonprofit
Performs At: Mielke Theatre
Organization Type: Resident; Sponsoring

4002 SHEBOYGAN THEATRE COMPANY

607 S Water Street
Sheboygan, WI 53081
Phone: 920-459-3779
Fax: 920-459-4021
e-mail: rmaffongeli@sheboygan.k12.wi.us
Web Site: www.sheboygan.k12.wi.us
Officers:
President: Karin Gunderson
First VP: Mike Roehl
Second VP: Kevin Heling
Secretary: Steve Flook
Treasurer: Stan Seagren
Management:
Director Theatre: Ralph Maffongelli
Business Manager: Steven Stauber
Technical Director: Dustin L Vhl

Mission: The advancement of and involvement in quality community theatre from the classical to contemporary, that afford entertainment and education for both audience and participants.
Founded: 1934
Specialized Field: Community; Theatrical Group
Status: Non-Professional; Nonprofit
Paid Staff: 2
Volunteer Staff: 250
Budget: $250,000
Income Sources: Tickets; Donations; Concessions; Program Advertisements; Rentals
Performs At: Leslie W Johnson Theatre; Horace Mann Middle School
Affiliations: Sheboygan Area School District
Annual Attendance: 18,000-20,000
Facility Category: Standard Theatre
Type of Stage: Thrust; Proscenium
Seating Capacity: 750
Year Built: 1970
Organization Type: Performing; Resident; Educational

4003 AMERICAN PLAYERS THEATRE

PO Box 819
Spring Green, WI 53588
Phone: 608-588-7401
Fax: 608-588-7085
e-mail: broth@americanplayers.org
Web Site: www.playinthewoods.org
Management:
Managing Director: Sheldon Wilner
Artistic Director: David Frank
Associate Artistic Director: Roseann Sheridan
Production Manager: Michael Broh
Founded: 1980
Specialized Field: Theatrical Group
Status: Professional; Nonprofit
Paid Staff: 96
Paid Artists: 45
Budget: $ 3.2 Million
Income Sources: Ticket Sales; Consessions; Giftshop; Individual Giving; Corporate Giving; Grants
Season: June - October
Performs At: Classical Outdoor Repertory
Affiliations: Actors' Equity Association; TCG
Annual Attendance: 100,000
Facility Category: Outdoor Arena
Type of Stage: Thrust
Seating Capacity: 1,133
Year Built: 1980
Rental Contact: Production Manager Michael Broh
Organization Type: Performing; Touring; Resident; Educational
Resident Groups: Lort C Special

4004 ST. CROIX FESTIVAL THEATRE

PO Box 801
St. Croix Falls, WI 54024
Phone: 715-294-2991
Founded: 1990
Status: Non-Equity; Nonprofit
Season: July - December
Type of Stage: Thrust
Seating Capacity: 260

4005 REED MARIONETTES
700 Llambaris Pass
Wales, WI 53183
Phone: 414-968-3277
Toll-free: 877-803-6575
e-mail: treed@execpc.com
Web Site: www.execpc.com/~treed/
Officers:
   President: Robin Reed
Management:
   Managing Director: Robin Reed
Mission: A professional touring company presenting colorful, entertaining and faithful versions of children's classics, combining the best of the arts of puppetry and theatre.
Founded: 1950
Specialized Field: Puppet
Status: Professional
Income Sources: Puppeteers of America; Wisconsin Puppetry Guild
Organization Type: Performing; Touring

4006 WAUKESHA CIVIC THEATRE
Margaret Brate Bryant Civic Theatre
264 W Main Street
PO Box 221
Waukesha, WI 53187
Phone: 262-547-4911
Fax: 262-547-8454
e-mail: kthoule@waukeshacivictheatre.com
Web Site: www.waukeshacivictheatre.com
Management:
   Managing Artistic Director: Kevin Houle
   Office Manager: Katie Stevens
Mission: Mission is to enrich, challenge and entertain participants through the performance of live theatre.
Founded: 1957
Organization Type: Performing; Educational

Wyoming

4007 CHEYENNE LITTLE THEATRE PLAYERS
2706 E Pershing Boulevard
PO Box 1086
Cheyenne, WY 82001
Phone: 307-638-6543
Fax: 307-638-6430
Management:
   Managing Director: Patrick Brien
Mission: To entertain and educate through theatre; to promote creativity among volunteers.
Founded: 1930
Specialized Field: Musical; Dinner; Community
Status: Non-Professional; Nonprofit
Paid Staff: 100
Income Sources: American Association of Community Theatres
Performs At: Mary Godfrey Playhouse; Atlas Theatre
Organization Type: Performing; Educational

4008 SHERIDAN CIVIC THEATRE GUILD
PO Box 1
Sheridan, WY 82801
Phone: 307-672-9886
Officers:
   President: Chip King
   VP: Ken Thorpe
   Secretary: Diana McGahan
   Treasurer: Tracy Thorpe
Management:
   Manager: Judi O'Neal
Mission: To foster community theatre in our area; to involve community members in all areas of theatre; to entertain.
Founded: 1953
Specialized Field: Musical; Community; Theatrical Group
Status: Nonprofit
Performs At: Carriage House Theatre
Organization Type: Performing; Resident

Alabama

4009 BIRMINGHAM INTERNATIONAL FESTIVAL

Frank Nelson Building, Suite 423
205 N 20th Street
Birmingham, AL 35203
Phone: 205-252-7652
Fax: 205-252-7656
e-mail: bifstaff@bellsouth.net
Web Site: www.bifsalutes.org
Officers:
    President: Catherine Sloss Crenshaw
    VP: Lawrence J Lemak, MD
    Treasurer: C Matthew Lusco
    Legal Advisor: Robert Bauch, Esquire
Management:
    Executive Director: Iris Gross
Mission: Seeks to present an international festival of arts, education, and economic development programs that build bridges of understanding with nations of the world.
Founded: 1951
Specialized Field: Chamber Music; Contemporary Classical; Light Orchestral; Multi-Media; Band; Jazz; Pops; Dance; Theatre; Childrens'; Ethnic
Paid Staff: 4
Volunteer Staff: 1k+
Income Sources: Grants; Donations
Season: April 4 - 20
Performs At: Various venues throughout Alabama
Annual Attendance: 50,000
Facility Category: Public park
Seating Capacity: 1,200

4010 INDEPENDENT PRESBYTERIAN CHURCH-NOVEMBER ORGAN RECITAL SERIES

3100 Highland Aveune S
Birmingham, AL 35205
Phone: 205-933-1830
Fax: 205-933-1836
e-mail: bfillmer@bellsouth.net

4011 PRINCESS THEATRE PROFESSIONAL SERIES

112 2nd Avenue NE
Decatur, AL 35601
Phone: 256-350-1745
Fax: 256-350-1712
e-mail: lindy@princess.org
Web Site: www.princesstheatre.org
Officers:
    Executive Director: Lindy Ashwander
Mission: To present and promote a variety of performing-arts events.
Founded: 1983
Specialized Field: Dance; Vocal Music; Instrumental Music; Theater
Status: Nonprofit
Paid Staff: 5
Volunteer Staff: 250
Budget: $570,000
Income Sources: Tickets; Rental; Contribution

Performs At: Princess Theatre
Annual Attendance: 50,000
Facility Category: Performing Arts Center
Type of Stage: Proscenium
Stage Dimensions: 40'x35'x18'.6"
Seating Capacity: 700
Year Built: 1919
Year Remodeled: 2000
Cost: $6 million
Rental Contact: Penny Linville
Organization Type: Performing; Educational

4012 COFFEE COUNTY ARTS ALLIANCE

PO Box 310447
Enterprise, AL 36330
Phone: 334-347-1249
Officers:
    President: Suzanne Sawyer

4013 WC HANDY MUSIC FESTIVAL

PO Box 1827
Florence, AL 35631
Phone: 256-766-7642
Fax: 256-776-7549
Web Site: www.wchandyfest.org
Management:
    Executive Director: Nancy C Gonce

4014 CITY OF GULF SHORES ENTERTAINMENT SERIES

Erie H Meyer Civic Center
1930 W 2nd Street, PO Box 299
Gulf Shores, AL 36542
Phone: 334-968-1173
e-mail: events@ci.gulf-shores.al.us
Web Site: www.ci.gulf-shores.al.us
Management:
    Special Events Director: Patsy Hollingsworth
Rental Contact: Kathy Van Cor

4015 OAKWOOD COLLEGE ARTS & LECTURES

Oakwood College Music Department
7000 Adventist Boulevard
Huntsville, AL 35896
Phone: 256-726-7279
Fax: 256-726-7481
e-mail: llacy@oakwood.edu
Web Site: oakwood.edu
Management:
    Chair/Music Department: Lucile Lacy
Mission: Music education & performances.
Founded: 1896
Specialized Field: Music; Music Education; Music Performance
Status: Full Time Music Facility
Budget: 8,000
Income Sources: Tuition
Performs At: Seventh-Day Adventist Church
Annual Attendance: 12,000
Facility Category: Auditorium
Seating Capacity: 400
Year Built: 1899

Year Remodeled: 1998

4016 PANOPLY ARTS FESTIVAL

Von Braun Civic Center
700 Monroe Street, Suite 2
Huntsville, AL 35801-5599
Phone: 256-519-2787
Fax: 256-533-3811
e-mail: tac@panoply.org
Web Site: www.panoply.org
Management:
    Executive Director: Lea McIntosh Ellison
    Festival Director: Jo Ann Henderson
    Production Assistant: Gaby Clark
    Production Coordinator: Shannon Magers
Founded: 1982
Specialized Field: Instrumental; Multi-Media; Opera;
Choral; Jazz; Folk; Dance; Theatre; Educational;
Children's; Ethnic
Performs At: Big Spring Park
Annual Attendance: 90,000
Facility Category: Three outdoor tents with stages;
Concert Hall

4017 ALABAMA SHAKESPEARE FESTIVAL

One Festival Drive
Montgomery, AL 36117
Phone: 334-271-5300
Fax: 334-271-5348
Web Site: www.asf.net
Management:
    Managing Director: Alan Harrison
    Artistic Director: Kent Thompson
    Marketing Director: Catherine Gwin
Mission: Dedicated to artistic excellence in the
production and performance of the classics and the best of
contemporary plays, with the plays of Shakespeare
forming the core of our repertoire. Through the Southern
Writer's Project, ASF commissions, develops, and
produces new plays that reflect the rich, diverse cultures
of the South.
Specialized Field: Dance; Vocal Music; Instrumental
Music; Theater; Festivals
Status: Professional; Nonprofit
Performs At: Alabama Shakespeare Festival
Organization Type: Performing; Touring; Resident;
Educational; Sponsoring

4018 JASMINE HILL ARTS COUNCIL

PO Box 6001
Montgomery, AL 36106
Phone: 334-567-6463
Fax: 334-263-5715
e-mail: jasminehill@mindspring.com
Web Site: www.jasminehill.org
Management:
    Manager: Jim Inscoe
Founded: 1976
Budget: $35,000-60,000
Performs At: Amphitheatre
Type of Stage: Concrete
Seating Capacity: 1500
Year Built: 1977

4019 OPELIKA ARTS ASSOCIATION

1032 South Railroad Avenue
Opelika, AL 36801
Phone: 334-705-5545
Fax: 334-749-8105
e-mail: opelika.arts@mindspring.com
Web Site: www.opelika.org

4020 SELMA COMMUNITY CONCERT ASSOCIATION

1034 Dawson Avenue
PO Box 310
Selma, AL 36701
Phone: 334-872-3527
Fax: 334-872-3504
Officers:
    President: Doris Holland
Mission: Dedicated to providing classical and popular
performances.

4021 TROY STATE UNIVERSITY-LYCEUM SERIES

Adams Center 125
Troy, AL 36082
Phone: 334-670-3714
Web Site: www.troyst.edu
Officers:
    Chairman: Dr. Jim Vickrey
Budget: Under $10,000
Performs At: Adams Center Theatre for the Performing
Arts; Claudia Crosby
Annual Attendance: 700
Facility Category: Fully equipped theatres
Seating Capacity: 350; 900
Year Remodeled: 1999

4022 ARTS COUNCIL OF TUSCALOOSA FANFARE

PO Box 1117
Tuscaloosa, AL 35403-1117
Phone: 205-758-5195
Fax: 205-345-2787
e-mail: education@tuscarts.org
Web Site: www.tuscarts.org
Management:
    Education Programs Director: Sandra Wolfe
Budget: $20,000-35,000
Performs At: Bama Theatre
Annual Attendance: 7,500-10,000
Facility Category: Presentation House
Seating Capacity: 1000
Year Built: 1938
Year Remodeled: 1976

4023 HORIZONS PERFORMING ARTS SERIES

PO Box 6689
Tuscaloosa, AL 35486-6689
Phone: 205-348-7525
Fax: 205-348-8251
Web Site: www.up.ua.edu
Management:

Assistant Director: Steven McCuller
Mission: To provide a variety of performing art to the University of Alabama.
Paid Staff: 4
Volunteer Staff: 100

4024 UNIVERSITY OF ALABAMA SCHOOL OF MUSIC CELEBRITIES
PO Box 870366
Tuscaloosa, AL 35487-0366
Phone: 205-348-7110
Fax: 205-348-1473
e-mail: jgrant@music.ua.edu
Web Site: www.music.ua.edu
Management:
Director School of Music: Bruce Murray
Assistant Director: Daniel Drill
Budget: $60,000-150,000
Performs At: Concert Hall, Moody Music Building
Seating Capacity: 934

Alaska

4025 ANCHORAGE CONCERT ASSOCIATION
430 W 7th Avenue
Suite 200
Anchorage, AK 99501
Phone: 907-272-1471
Fax: 917-272-2519
e-mail: executive@anchorageconcerts.org
Web Site: www.anchorageconcerts.org
Management:
Acting Executive Director: Ruth Glenn
Founded: 1950
Specialized Field: Performing Arts Presenter
Status: Nonprofit
Paid Staff: 7
Volunteer Staff: 82

4026 ANCHORAGE FESTIVAL OF MUSIC
PO Box 103251
Anchorage, AK 99510
Phone: 907-276-2465
Fax: 907-276-2540
e-mail: anchfest@alaska.net
Web Site: www.alaska.net/~anchfest
Management:
Executive Director: Steven Alvarez
Artistic Director: Grant Cooper
Mission: Promoting diverse musical events in Anchorage and the surrounding area.
Founded: 1976
Specialized Field: Instrumental; Choral; Educational
Status: Professional; Nonprofit
Paid Staff: 30
Season: June
Performs At: Anchorage (Festival Site)
Affiliations: Alaska Center for the Performing Arts
Seating Capacity: 300; 800; 2,200
Organization Type: Performing

4027 FAIRBANKS ARTS ASSOCIATION
PO Box 72786
Fairbanks, AK 99707
Phone: 907-456-6485
Fax: 907-456-4112
e-mail: fairbanksarts@mosquitonet.com
Officers:
President: Bob Dempsey
Vice-President: Carol Hilgeman
Secretary: Jan Stitt
Treasurer: Douglas Leggett
Management:
Executive Director: June Rogers
Budget: $35,000-60,000
Performs At: Auditorium
Seating Capacity: 1300

4028 FAIRBANKS CONCERT ASSOCIATION MASTER SERIES
794 University Avenue, Suite 104
PO Box 80547
Fairbanks, AK 99709
Phone: 907-474-8081
Fax: 907-474-0266
e-mail: concert@ptialaska.net
Web Site: www.fairbanksconcert.org
Management:
Executive Director: Herta Prechtel
Budget: $60,000-150,000
Performs At: Hering Auditorium; Charles W Davis Concert Hall
Annual Attendance: 13,000
Facility Category: Rented
Type of Stage: Proscenium
Stage Dimensions: 47'10x22'x36'6"
Seating Capacity: 1305; 967

4029 FAIRBANKS SUMMER ARTS FESTIVAL
PO Box 80845
Fairbanks, AK 99708
Phone: 907-474-8869
Fax: 907-479-4329
e-mail: festival@ptialaska.net
Web Site: www.fsaf.org
Officers:
Chairman: Patty Kastelic
Vice Chairman: Theresa Reed
Recording Secretary: Joy McDougal
Treasurer: David B. Stephenson
Management:
Producing Director/Founder: Jo Ryman Scott
Artistic Director: Gianna Drogheo
Mission: To offer a two-week residency with approximately 70 professional guest performers/master teachers.
Founded: 1980
Specialized Field: Instrumental; Opera; Choral; Jazz; Dance; Theatre;Educational
Status: Professional; Semi-Professional; Non-Professional; Nonprofit
Paid Staff: 2
Volunteer Staff: 100
Paid Artists: 70
Budget: $150,000-$400,000

Season: July - August
Performs At: University of Alaska at Fairbanks
Affiliations: UAF Concert Hall
Seating Capacity: 1,000
Year Built: 1917
Organization Type: Performing; Educational

4030 HAINES ARTS COUNCIL

PO Box 505
Haines, AK 99827
Phone: 907-766-2592
Officers:
  VP: Len Feldman
Management:
  Music Director: Dr. Suzanne Summerville
  Contact: Tom Morphet
  Staff Director: Theodora Mann
  Staff Conductor: Robert Luther
Mission: To provide performing arts resources for local artists; to offer concerts and festivals.
Founded: 1983
Specialized Field: Dance; Vocal Music; Instrumental Music; Theater; Festivals; Lyric Opera
Status: Non-Professional; Nonprofit
Income Sources: Lynn Community Players
Performs At: Chilkat Center for the Arts
Organization Type: Performing; Touring; Resident; Educational; Sponsoring

4031 KENAI PENINSULA ORCHESTRA STRING FESTIVAL

315 W Pioneer Avenue
Homer, AK 99603
Phone: 907-235-6318
Fax: 907-235-7333
e-mail: norton@xyz.net
Web Site: www.xyz.net/~smokybay/festival.html
Management:
  Music Director: Mark Robinson
  Festival Manager: Laura Norton
Mission: To provide an opportunity for sting players from greater Alaska and points beyond to join the Kenai Peninsula Orchestra in workshops and concerts with world-class clinicians.
Budget: $35,000
Seating Capacity: 200-450

4032 CROSSSOUND

1109 C Street
Juneau, AK 99801
Phone: 907-586-9601
e-mail: directors@crosssound.com
Web Site: www.crosssound.com
Management:
  Co-Director: Jocelyn Clark
  Co-Director: Stefan Hakenberg
Mission: To commission new works for musicians from Southeast Alaska and beyond that stretch the boundaries of the planets of chamber music
Founded: 1999
Specialized Field: New Music; Chamber; Multi Media
Status: Nonprofit
Volunteer Staff: 10
Paid Artists: 30

Income Sources: Donations

4033 JUNEAU ARTS & HUMANITIES COUNCIL

PO Box 20562
Juneau, AK 99802-0562
Phone: 907-586-2787
Fax: 907-586-2148
e-mail: jahc@gci.net
Web Site: www.juneauartscouncil.org
Management:
  Executive Director: Sybil Davis
Founded: 1973
Specialized Field: Performing Arts; Visual Arts; Literary Arts
Paid Staff: 2
Volunteer Staff: 40
Budget: For concert series $56,000
Performs At: Juneau-Douglas H.S. Auditorium; ANB Community Hall
Facility Category: High School Auditorium
Type of Stage: Proscenium
Stage Dimensions: 40 x 50
Seating Capacity: 1,000

4034 KODIAK ARTS COUNCIL

PO Box 1792
Kodiak, AK 99615
Phone: 907-486-5391
Fax: 907-486-2148
e-mail: kac@kodiak.alaska.edu
Management:
  Director: Nancy Kemp
Budget: $35,000-60,000
Performs At: Gerald C Wilson Auditorium

4035 SITKA SUMMER MUSIC FESTIVAL

PO Box 3333
Sitka, AK 99835
Phone: 907-747-6774
Fax: 907-747-6853
e-mail: director@sitkamusicfestival.org
Web Site: www.sitkamusicfestival.org
Management:
  Festival Director: Heather MacLean
Mission: To present chamber music festivals throughout Alaska
Founded: 1972
Specialized Field: Classical
Status: Professional; Nonprofit
Volunteer Staff: 80
Paid Artists: 15
Non-paid Artists: 30
Budget: $250,000
Season: June
Performs At: Harrigan Centennial Hall
Annual Attendance: 8,000
Facility Category: Performance Hall
Seating Capacity: 500
Year Built: 1970
Year Remodeled: 1998
Organization Type: Performing; Touring

Arizona

4036 DESERT FOOTHILLS MUSICFEST
PO Box 5254
Carefree, AZ 85377
Phone: 480-488-0806
Fax: 480-488-1401
e-mail: roberta@azmusicfest.org
Web Site: www.azmusicfest.org
Management:
   Music Director/Conductor: Paul Perry
   Chairman Musicfest: John Gosule
   Managing Director: Roberta Pappas
Mission: To assist in making the Arizona High Desert area a major winter cultural center.
Founded: 1992
Specialized Field: Instrumental; Jazz; Classical
Status: Professional; Nonprofit
Paid Staff: 5
Paid Artists: 30
Budget: $400,000
Income Sources: Individual Contributions; Corporate Sponsors; Grants; Ticket Revenue
Season: February
Performs At: Carefree; Cave Creek; North Scottsdale
Annual Attendance: 4,500
Seating Capacity: 250 - 700
Organization Type: Performing; Educational

4037 PINAL COUNTY FINE ARTS COUNCIL: ARTS IN THE DESERT
8470 N Overfield Road
Central Arizona College
Coolidge, AZ 85228
Phone: 520-426-4223
Fax: 520-426-4224
e-mail: community_services@central.az.edu
Web Site: www.centralaz.edu
Management:
   Cultural Events Coordinator: Cheryl Ragsdale Sanborn
   Technical Director: Norm Wigton
Founded: 1975
Paid Staff: 1
Volunteer Staff: 15
Paid Artists: 135
Budget: $44,000
Income Sources: Series Subscribers
Performs At: Pence Auditorium, Central Arizona College
Annual Attendance: 6,000-7,000
Facility Category: Auditorium
Type of Stage: Proscenium
Stage Dimensions: 45'x20'
Seating Capacity: 735
Year Built: 1969
Rental Contact: Cheryl Ragsdale

4038 VERDE VALLEY CONCERT ASSOCIATION
14 S Main Street
PO Box 26
Cottonwood, AZ 86326-0026

Phone: 928-639-0636
Fax: 928-639-2185
e-mail: vvca@wildapache.net
Officers:
   President: Anna May Cory
Founded: 1952
Paid Staff: 1
Performs At: Mingus Union High School Auditorium
Seating Capacity: 852

4039 FLAGSTAFF FESTIVAL OF THE ARTS
PO Box 1607
Flagstaff, AZ 86002
Phone: 520-774-7750
Fax: 520-774-2600
Web Site: www.flagstaffguide.com/festival
Management:
   Managing Director: Larry Reid
   Orchestra Conductor: Irwin Hoffman
   Theatre Artistic Director: Tal Russell
Mission: Offering professional arts programs to the Flagstaff community.
Founded: 1966
Specialized Field: Dance; Vocal Music; Instrumental Music; Theater; Festivals
Status: Professional; Semi-Professional; Nonprofit
Income Sources: Northern Arizona University
Performs At: Ardrey Auditorium; Creative Arts Theatre
Organization Type: Performing; Educational

4040 NORTHERN ARIZONA UNIVERSITY SPECTRUM SERIES
PO Box 6040
Flagstaff, AZ 86011
Phone: 520-523-8780
Fax: 520-523-5111
e-mail: Kathryn.Maloney@nau.edu
Management:
   Co-ordinator: Kathy Battali
Budget: $60,000-150,000
Performs At: Ardrey Auditorium
Seating Capacity: 1500

4041 GRAND CANYON MUSIC FESTIVAL
PO Box 1332
Grand Canyon, AZ 86023
Phone: 520-638-9215
Fax: 520-638-3373
Toll-free: 800-997-8285
e-mail: gcmf@thecanyon.com
Web Site: www.grandcanyonmusicfest.org
Officers:
   President: Kenneth Bacher
   VP/Secretary: Clare Hoffman
Management:
   Executive Director: Frances Joseph
   Artistic Director: Clare Hoffman
Mission: To present a series of concerts in Grand Canyon National Park each September, maintaining high musical standards and diversity of programming; to commission new chamber music from American composers; to give a public service tour to schools in Northern Arizona.
Founded: 1984
Specialized Field: Instrumental; Jazz

Status: Nonprofit
Budget: $20,000-$35,000
Season: September
Performs At: Grand Canyon National Park (Festival Site)
Affiliations: Shrine of the Ages
Seating Capacity: 310
Organization Type: Presenting

4042 WEST VALLEY FINE ARTS COUNCIL

PO Box 754
387 Wigwam Boulevard
Litchfield Park, AZ 85340
Phone: 623-935-6384
Fax: 623-935-4327
e-mail: info@wvfac.org
Web Site: www.wvfac.org
Management:
   Executive Director: Marcia Ellis
Mission: To develop, enhance and promote quality arts opportunities and arts education for everyone in the West Valley
Performs At: Various Community Spaces

4043 PARADISE VALLEY JAZZ PARTY

6014 N Nauni Valley Drive
Paradise Valley, AZ 85253
Phone: 480-948-7993
Fax: 480-991-5732
e-mail: dzmiller@cox.net
Web Site: www.paradisevalleyjazz.com
Founded: 1978
Volunteer Staff: 5

4044 ARIZONA EXPOSITION & STATE FAIR

1826 W McDowell Road
Phoenix, AZ 85007
Phone: 602-252-6771
Fax: 602-495-1302
Web Site: www.azstatefair.com
Management:
   Executive Director: Gary D Montgomery

4045 SOUTHWEST ARTS & ENTERTAINMENT

PO Box 55566
Phoenix, AZ 85078-5566
Phone: 602-482-6410
Fax: 602-482-0939
e-mail: swac@southwestac.com
Web Site: www.southwestac.com
Management:
   President: Charles Fischil
Founded: 1992
Status: Nonprofit
Paid Staff: 2
Budget: $555,000
Income Sources: Arts Commissions; Foundations; Corporations
Affiliations: WAA; AZ Presenters; CA Presenters
Annual Attendance: 60,000
Facility Category: Orphium Theatre
Type of Stage: Proscenium
Stage Dimensions: 30'x50'
Seating Capacity: 1,300
Year Built: 1929
Year Remodeled: 1994

4046 PRESCOTT FINE ARTS

The Corner of Marina and Willis
208 N Marina
Prescott, AZ 86301
Phone: 928-445-3286
Fax: 928-778-7888
e-mail: pfaadirector@qwest.net
Web Site: www.pfaa.net
Officers:
   President: Ralph Hess
   Secretary: Sandy Moss
   Treasurer: John Cargill
Management:
   Executive Director: Dee R Toci
   Operations Manager: Suzy Campbell
   Box Office: Sue Lord
   Associate Director: Casey Knight
Mission: To offer cultural and artistic activities.
Founded: 1969
Specialized Field: Theatre and Music
Status: Nonprofit
Paid Staff: 4
Non-paid Artists: 600
Budget: $225,000
Income Sources: Ticket sales, Grants, Donations
Annual Attendance: 20,000
Facility Category: Historic Church
Type of Stage: Proscenium
Seating Capacity: 194
Year Built: 1894
Resident Groups: Yavapai County, North central Arizona

4047 GILA VALLEY ARTS COUNCIL

PO Box 1022
Safford, AZ 85548-1022
Phone: 520-428-1009
Fax: 520-428-2772
e-mail: pizarro@zakes.com
Web Site: www.zakes.com
Officers:
   President: Joann Mortensen
   Treasurer: Dorine Chancellor
   Residency Chair: Cecilia Roudenbush
   Recording Secretary: Mary Ann Ripplinger
Management:
   Artistic Director: Jack Kukuk
   Executive Director: Shelly Williams
Mission: To promote, support, and sponsor performing arts in Southeaster Arizona through the School Residency Program and Public Performance.
Budget: $35,000-60,000
Performs At: Eastern Arizona College of Fine Arts Studio
Seating Capacity: 941+; 300

4048 RAGTYME-JAZZTYME SOCIETY

6835 E Kings Avenue
Scottsdale, AZ 85254-1512

Phone: 480-951-8339
Fax: 480-348-3702
Toll-free: 800-473-5396
e-mail: AZragtime2001@aol.com
Officers:
   President: Robert Lynn
Management:
   Managing Director: Robert Lynn
   Newsletter Editor: Patricia Gray
   Chairman: Ross Dunshee
Mission: To preserve, promote and promulgate Ragtime and Early American Jazz Music. To provide educational activities and benefits to our younger generation of musicians and music lovers.
Founded: 2001
Specialized Field: Ragime and Early American Jazz Music
Volunteer Staff: 12

4049   SCOTTSDALE ARTS FESTIVAL

Scottsdale Center for the Arts
7380 E 2nd Street
Scottsdale, AZ 85251
Phone: 480-994-2787
Fax: 480-874-4699
e-mail: JaniceB@sccarts.org
Web Site: www.scottsdalearts.org
Management:
   Festival Manager: Janice Bartczak

4050   SEDONA CHAMBER MUSIC SOCIETY & FESTIVAL

PO Box 153
Sedona, AZ 86339-0153
Phone: 928-204-2415
Fax: 928-282-0893
e-mail: sedonacms@aol.com
Web Site: www.chambermusicsedona.org
Officers:
   President: Jim Pease
Management:
   Executive Director: Bert Harclerode
Founded: 1983
Budget: $200,000
Performs At: St. John Vianney Church; Museum of Northern Arizona
Affiliations: CMA, ACA
Annual Attendance: 4000
Seating Capacity: 250; 200

4051   SEDONA JAZZ ON THE ROCKS

PO Box 889
Sedona, AZ 86339
Phone: 520-282-1985
Fax: 520-282-0590
Web Site: www.sedonajazz.com
Officers:
   President: Gina Lohrey
Management:
   Executive Director: Chris Irish
Mission: To preserve and promote jazz for the next generation.
Founded: 1982
Specialized Field: Jazz

Status: Nonprofit
Paid Staff: 3
Volunteer Staff: 200
Paid Artists: 50
Non-paid Artists: 4
Budget: $400,000
Income Sources: Box Office; Corporate Sponsors; Grants
Season: September
Performs At: Sedona Cultural Park (Festival Site)
Annual Attendance: 6,000
Facility Category: Various Venues
Seating Capacity: 200-4,500
Organization Type: Performing; Sponsoring

4052   ARIZONA STATE UNIVERSITY PUBLIC EVENTS

Arizona State University
PO Box 870205
Tempe, AZ 85287-0205
Phone: 480-965-5062
Fax: 480-965-7663
e-mail: Shpotter@asu.edu
Web Site: www.asu.edu/ia/publicevents
Management:
   Program Manager: Stephen Potter
   Executive Director: Colleen Jennings-Roggensack
Mission: To connect communities through performing arts.
Founded: 1967
Specialized Field: Performing Arts
Paid Staff: 54
Volunteer Staff: 400
Budget: $1,000,000+
Performs At: Grady Gammage Memorial Auditorium; Sundome Center
Affiliations: Arts Presenters, ISPAA, WAA
Annual Attendance: 500,000
Facility Category: Auditorium
Type of Stage: Prosenium Sprungwood
Seating Capacity: 3017; 7034
Year Built: 1967
Rental Contact: Paul Abe

4053   MICHELOB COOL SUMMER JAZZ SERIES

730 N Mill Avenue
Tempe, AZ 85281
Fax: 480-829-1552
Toll-free: 800-466-6779
Web Site: www.redrivermusichall.com

4054   GREATER ORO VALLEY ARTS COUNCIL

7400 N Oracle Road
Suite 100R
Tucson, AZ 85704
Phone: 520-797-3959
Fax: 520-531-9225
Management:
   Executive Director: Carmen Feriend

4055 PIMA COMMUNITY COLLEGE FOR THE ARTS
2202 W Anklam Road
Tucson, AZ 85709-0225
Phone: 520-206-6986
Fax: 520-206-6670
e-mail: cfa@pimacc.pima.edu
Management:
   Dean of Performing/Visual Arts: Frank Pickard
Budget: $20,000-35,000
Performs At: Proscenium Theatre; Black Box Theatre; Recital Hall
Seating Capacity: 425;170;120

4056 ST. PHILIP'S IN THE HILLS FRIENDS OF MUSIC
4440 N Campbell Avenue
PO Box 65840
Tucson, AZ 85728
Phone: 520-299-6421
Fax: 520-299-0712
e-mail: stphilips@juno.com
Web Site: stphipipstucon.org
Management:
   Association Music Director: Dr. Jeffery I Campbell
Mission: To present concert series.
Budget: $10,000-20,000
Performs At: St. Philip's in the Hills Episcopal Church
Seating Capacity: 500

4057 TUCSON WINTER CHAMBER MUSIC FESTIVAL
6429 E Calle de San Alberto
Tucson, AZ 85710-2115
Phone: 520-577-3769
Fax: 520-881-2009
e-mail: friends@arizonachambermusic.org
Web Site: www.arizonachambermusic.org/
Management:
   Artistic Director: Peter Rejto
   Executive Director: Dr. Jean Paul Bierny
Specialized Field: Instrumental
Budget: $60,000-$150,000
Season: February - March
Affiliations: Leo Rich Theatre; Tucson Convention Center
Seating Capacity: 550

4058 UNIVERSITY OF ARIZONA PRESENTS
1020 E University Boulevard
PO Box 210029
Tucson, AZ 85721-0029
Phone: 520-621-3341
Fax: 520-621-8991
e-mail: uapresents@arizona.edu
Web Site: uapresents.arizona.edu/contact.html
Management:
   Executive Director: Ken Foster
Performs At: Centennial Hall

Arkansas

4059 OUACHITA BAPTIST UNIVERSITY: ARTISTS SERIES
Box 3771
Ouachita Baptist University
Arkadelphia, AR 71998-0001
Phone: 870-246-4531
Fax: 870-245-5500
e-mail: wrightc@alpha.obu.edu
Officers:
   School of Fine Arts Dean: Charles W Wright
Performs At: Jones Performing Arts Center; Recital Hall
Seating Capacity: 1500; 300

4060 WALTON ARTS AND IDEAS
University of the Ozarks
Clarksville, AR 72830
Phone: 501-979-1346
Fax: 501-979-1349
e-mail: gemyers@ozarks.edu
Web Site: www.ozarks.edu
Management:
   Director: Ginny Myers
Performs At: Seay Thaetre
Seating Capacity: 699

4061 UNIVERSITY OF CENTRAL ARKANSAS PUBLIC APPEARANCES
201 Donaghey
Conway, AR 72035-0001
Phone: 501-450-3293
Fax: 501-450-3296
e-mail: gucch@aol.com
Web Site: www.uca.edu/reynolds
Management:
   Public Appearances Director: Guy Couch
Performs At: Ida Waldran Auditorium; Conway Public Schools Auditorium
Seating Capacity: 1100-1500

4062 EUREKA SPRINGS JAZZ FESTIVAL
PO Box 1
Eureka Springs, AR 72632
Phone: 501-253-6258
e-mail: jazz@eurekaweb.com
Web Site: www.eurekaweb.com/jazz

4063 INSPIRATION POINT FINE ARTS COLONY
16311 Highway 62 W
PO Box 127
Eureka Springs, AR 72632-3160
Phone: 501-253-8595
Mission: To provide local students with exposure to professional opera.
Founded: 1950
Specialized Field: Instrumental Music; Lyric Opera; Grand Opera
Status: Non-Professional; Nonprofit
Paid Staff: 50
Income Sources: National Federation of Music Clubs
Performs At: Inspiration Point Fine Arts Colony

Organization Type: Performing; Educational; Sponsoring

4064   NORTH ARKANSAS SYMPHONY

PO Box 1243
Fayetteville, AR 72702
Phone: 501-521-4166
Fax: 501-582-4252
Management:
    Executive Director: Stephen Olans
    Music Director: Jeannine Wagar
Founded: 1982
Specialized Field: Vocal Music; Instrumental Music; Lyric Opera
Status: Professional; Nonprofit
Performs At: Walton Arts Center
Organization Type: Educational; Sponsoring

4065   WESTARK COLLEGE SEASON OF ENTERTAINMENT

PO Box 3649
Fort Smith, AR 72913
Phone: 501-788-7301
Fax: 501-788-7016
e-mail: sjones@systema.westark.edu
Management:
    Associate Dean/Operations: Stacey Jones
Performs At: Breedlove Fine Arts Auditorium; Fort Smith Civic Center
Seating Capacity: 440; 1,300

4066   NORTH CENTRAL ARKANSAS CONCERT ASSOCIATION

PO Box 2117
Harrison, AR 72602-2117
Phone: 870-741-5058
Management:
    Contractor/President: Charles Butler
Mission: To promote arts in Northwest Arkansas.
Founded: 1965
Specialized Field: Performance
Volunteer Staff: 15
Budget: $25,000
Income Sources: Patrons; Grants
Performs At: Harrison High Scholl Auditorium
Affiliations: Ozark Arts Council
Annual Attendance: 2,500
Seating Capacity: 600

4067   WARFIELD CONCERTS

129 Stonebrook Road
Helena, AR 72342
Phone: 870-572-2665
Fax: 870-572-5870
e-mail: stonebrook@aol.com
Officers:
    Chairperson: Betty M Faust
    Treasurer: Bettye W Hendrix
Management:
    Director: Cassie Brothers
Founded: 1968
Specialized Field: Instrumental; Multi-Media; Opera; Choral; Jazz; Dance; Theatre; Childrens'; Educational

Paid Staff: 1
Volunteer Staff: 3
Paid Artists: 160
Budget: $20,000-$35,000
Season: Late April - Early May
Performs At: Philips Colliseum Fine Arts Center (Festival Site)
Affiliations: Lily Peter Auditorium
Seating Capacity: 1,250

4068   HOT SPRINGS MUSIC FESTIVAL CHAMBER ORCHESTRA

634 Prospect Avenue
Hot Springs, AR 71901-3918
Phone: 501-623-4763
Fax: 501-624-6440
e-mail: hsmusfest@prodig.com
Web Site: www.hotmusic.org
Management:
    Artistic Director: Richard Rosenberg
    Executive Director: Laura S Rosenberg

4069   HOT SPRINGS MUSIC FESTIVAL

634 Prospect Avenue
Hot Springs National Park
Hot Springs, AR 71901-3918
Phone: 501-623-4763
Fax: 501-624-6440
e-mail: festival@hotmusic.org
Web Site: www.hotmusic.org
Officers:
    Chairman: W C Hitt
    Secretary/Treasurer: Kenneth Wheatley III
    Vice Chairman: Helen Selig
Management:
    Artistic Director: Richard Rosenberg
    Executive Director: Laura S Rosenberg
Founded: 1996
Specialized Field: Orchestral and Chamber Music Mentorship and Performance
Budget: $60,000-$150,000
Season: Early June
Performs At: Hot Springs National Park (Festival Site)
Affiliations: Variuos Historic Venues
Seating Capacity: 1,100 - 2,200

4070   FOWLER CENTER AT ARKANSAS STATE UNIVERSITY

201 Olympic Drive
Jonesboro, AR 72401
Mailing Address: PO Box 2339 State University, AR 72467
Phone: 870-910-8115
Fax: 870-910-8118
e-mail: fowlercenter@astate.edu
Web Site: www.fowlercenter.astate.edu
Management:
    Director: Jerome Biebesheimer
    Director: Lee Christensen
    Technical Director: Albert Juhrend

Mission: The mission is to present to the students, faculty and staff of Arkansas State University and the citizens of Northeast Arkansas an opportunity to exprience visual and performing arts events of national and international stature.
Founded: 2001
Specialized Field: Music; Theatre; Visual Art
Status: Nonprofit
Paid Staff: 5
Budget: $400,000
Income Sources: Arkansas State University; Endowments; Ticket Sales
Performs At: Fine Arts Recital Hall; Wilson Auditorium
Facility Category: Concert Hall, Drama Theatre
Type of Stage: Proscenium
Seating Capacity: 975; 342
Year Built: 2000
Rental Contact: Manager Jerry Biebesheimer

4071 ARTSPREE
University of Arkansas At Little Rock

164 Fine Arts Building
2801 S University
Little Rock, AR 72204-1099
Phone: 501-569-3288
Fax: 501-569-8775
e-mail: fwmartin@ualr.edu
Management:
   Director: Floyd Martin
Performs At: University Theatre; Stella Boyle Smith Concert Hall
Seating Capacity: 679; 312

4072 HARDING UNIVERSITY CONCERT & LYCEUM SERIES

PO Box 15767
Harding University
Searcy, AR 72149
Phone: 501-279-4311
Fax: 501-279-4086
e-mail: ganus@harding.edu
Management:
   Chairman: Dr. Clifton L Ganus
Budget: $10,000
Performs At: Benson Auditorium; Administration Auditorium
Seating Capacity: 3000; 990
Rental Contact: David Briggs

4073 JOHN BROWN UNIVERSITY LYCEUM ARTISTS SERIES

PO Box 3142, JBU
Siloam Springs, AR 72761
Phone: 501-524-7265
Fax: 501-524-9548
e-mail: nnethert@acc.jbu.edu
Management:
   Manager: Nancy Netherton
Paid Staff: 1
Volunteer Staff: 3
Budget: $9,000
Income Sources: Fees (student); grants
Performs At: Jones Recital Hall; Cathedral of the Ozarks

Annual Attendance: 500-600
Facility Category: Small recital hall; large sanctuary with platform
Seating Capacity: 159; 1000
Year Built: 1991

4074 GRAND PRAIRIE FESTIVAL OF THE ARTS

PO Box 65
Stuttgart, AR 72160
Phone: 870-673-1781
Fax: 870-673-1781
Management:
   Director: Wanda Loudermilk
Mission: To provide a diverse program of performing arts for the Grand Prairie community.
Founded: 1956
Specialized Field: Vocal Music; Instrumental Music; Theater
Status: Professional; Non-Professional
Income Sources: Grand Prairie Arts Council
Performs At: Grand Prairie War Memorial Auditorium
Organization Type: Educational; Sponsoring

California

4075 KELSONARTS PERFORMANCES

315 Crest Avenue
Alamo, CA 94507
Phone: 925-934-4566
Fax: 925-934-4536
e-mail: info@kelsonarts.com
Web Site: www.kelsonarts.com
Management:
   Managing Director: Linus Eukel
Performs At: Various Sites
Seating Capacity: 200-750

4076 ALHAMBRA PERFORMING ARTS

111 S First Street
Alhambra, CA 91801
Phone: 626-570-3242
Fax: 626-284-0310
Management:
   Cultural Arts Co-ordinator: Rick C Crawford
   Community Programs Supervisor: Mike Macias
Performs At: Outdoor Bandshell
Seating Capacity: 750-1000

4077 OLD PASADENA JAZZ FESTIVAL

27101 Aliso Creek Road
Suite 154
Aliso Viejo, CA 92656
Phone: 949-362-3366
Fax: 949-362-5366
e-mail: info@omegaevents.com
Web Site: www.omegaevents.com

All listings are in alphabetical order by state, then city, then organization within the city.

4078 NORTH ORANGE COUNTY COMMUNITY CONCERTS ASSOCIATION
623 S Clara Street
Anaheim, CA 92804
Phone: 714-535-8925
Officers:
 VP Memberships: John Jackson
Performs At: Fullerton First United Methodist Church
Seating Capacity: 700

4079 SHASTA COMMUNITY CONCERT ASSOCIATION
6396 Vista del Sierra Drive
Anderson, CA 96007
Phone: 530-365-2664
Officers:
 President: Jane G Wittmann

4080 PACIFIC UNION COLLEGE FINE ARTS SERIES
Music Department
Pacific Union College
Angwin, CA 94508
Phone: 707-965-6202
Fax: 707-965-6390
Management:
 Manager: Del Case
Performs At: Paulin Hall
Seating Capacity: 465

4081 BEAR VALLEY MUSIC FESTIVAL
PO Box 5068
Bear Valley, CA 95223
Phone: 209-753-2574
Fax: 209-753-2576
e-mail: music@bearvalleymusic.org
Web Site: www.bearvalleymusic.org
Management:
 Music Director: Carter Nice
 Executive Director: Ardelle Fellows
Specialized Field: Instrumental; Opera; Jazz; Childrens'
Budget: $20,000-$35,000
Season: July - August
Performs At: Bear Valley (Festival Site)
Facility Category: Festival Tent
Seating Capacity: 1,200

4082 COLLEGE OF NOTRE DAME RALSTON CONCERT SERIES
1500 Ralston Avenue
Belmont, CA 94002
Phone: 650-508-3597
Fax: 650-637-0493
e-mail: bmoyer@cnd.edu
Web Site: www.cndarts.com
Officers:
 President: Christopher Clausen
Management:
 Chairman Music Department: Dr. Brigitte Moyer
Performs At: Ralston Ballroom
Seating Capacity: 200

4083 BERKELEY FESTIVAL & EXHIBITION
UC Berkeley, Cal Performances
101 Zellerbach Hall, #4800
Berkeley, CA 94720-4800
Phone: 510-642-0212
Fax: 510-643-6707
e-mail: rcole@calperfs.berkeley.edu
Web Site: www.calperfs.berkeley.edu
Management:
 General Director: Robert W Cole
Specialized Field: Instrumental
Budget: $150,000-$400,000
Season: June
Performs At: Berkeley; University of California (Festival Site)
Affiliations: Various Bay Locations
Seating Capacity: 400 - 2,000

4084 CALIFORNIA SHAKESPEARE FESTIVAL
701 Heinz Avenue
Berkeley, CA 94710
Phone: 510-548-3422
Fax: 510-843-9921
e-mail: letters@calshake.org
Web Site: www.calshakes.org
Officers:
 President: Jim Roethe
Management:
 Managing Director: Debbie Chin
 Artistic Director: Jonathan Moscone
 Development Director: Michael Stephens
 Production Manager: John Anderson
 Publicity/Publications Manager: Sunny Grettinger
 Associate Producer: Marcy Straw
Mission: Committed to innovative productions of Shakespearean plays.
Founded: 1973
Specialized Field: Theater
Status: Professional; Nonprofit
Paid Staff: 13
Budget: $2,300,000
Income Sources: Ticket Sales; Government; Individuals; Corporations; Foundations
Season: June - October
Performs At: Bruns Memorial Amphitheater
Annual Attendance: 43,000
Facility Category: Outdoor Amphitheater
Seating Capacity: 545
Year Built: 1990
Organization Type: Performing; Touring; Educational

4085 EARLY MUSIC IN MARIN
PO Box 9313
Berkeley, CA 94709
Phone: 510-549-9799
e-mail: AGSugden@aol.com
Web Site: www.sfems.org
Management:
 Coordinator: Alisa Gould Sugden
Specialized Field: Instrumental
Budget: $10,000
Season: June - July

All listings are in alphabetical order by state, then city, then organization within the city.

Performs At: Dominican Colliseum; San Rafael (Festival Site)
Affiliations: Angelico Hall; Meadowlands Assembly Hall
Seating Capacity: 500; 100

4086 FOUR SEASONS CONCERTS
PO Box 507
Berkeley, CA 94701
Phone: 510-601-6184
Fax: 510-549-3504
e-mail: info@fourseasonsconcerts.com
Web Site: www.fourseasonsconcerts.com
Officers:
President: Jesse Anthony
Performs At: Scottish Rite Auditorium; Herbst Theatre; Opera House
Seating Capacity: 1497; 915; 3176

4087 SAN FRANCISCO EARLY MUSIC SOCIETY
PO Box 10151
Berkeley, CA 94709
Phone: 510-845-1440
e-mail: sfems@sfems.org
Web Site: www.sfems.org
Management:
General Manager: Robin Lockert
Performs At: St. Johns Presbytarian Church
Seating Capacity: 400

4088 UNIVERSITY OF CALIFORNIA-BERKELEY CALIFORNIA
101 Zellerbach Hall
#4800
Berkeley, CA 94720-4800
Phone: 510-642-0212
Fax: 510-643-6707
e-mail: rcole@calperfs.berkeley.edu
Web Site: www.calperfs.berkeley.edu
Officers:
CEO: Lori Cripps
Management:
Director: Robert W Cole
Assistant/Director: Susan Hamblen
Associate Director: Hollis Ashby
General Manager: Mark Heiser
Director/Marketing/Sales: Mary Dixon
Mission: To offer professional performances in the performing arts to students.
Founded: 1904
Specialized Field: Dance; Vocal Music; Instrumental Music; Theater; Classical Music
Status: Nonprofit
Income Sources: Association of Performing Arts Presenters; International Society of Performing Arts Administrators; Western Alliance of Arts Administrators
Performs At: Zellerbach Auditorium; University of California
Organization Type: Educational; Sponsoring

4089 INTERNATIONAL CONCERTS EXCHANGE
1124 Summit Drive
Beverly Hills, CA 90210
Phone: 213-272-5539
Fax: 213-272-5539
Management:
Producer/Managing Director: Dr. Irwin Paones
Founded: 1942
Specialized Field: Festivals
Status: Professional; Semi-Professional; Non-Professional; Nonprofit
Organization Type: Performing; Educational

4090 BIG SUR JAZZ FEST
PO Box 459
Big Sur, CA 93920
Phone: 831-667-1530
Fax: 831-667-1530
Web Site: www.bigsurjazz.org
Management:
Director: Ron Birmingham

4091 MUSIC AT KOHL MANSION
2750 Adeline Drive
Burlingame, CA 94010
Phone: 650-343-8463
Fax: 650-343-2316
Management:
Executive Director: Carol Eggers
Mission: To offer chamber music performance and music education.
Performs At: Great Hall; Kohl Mansion
Seating Capacity: 200

4092 CATALINA ISLAND JAZZTRAX FESTIVAL
23679 Calabasas Road
#401
Calabasas, CA 91302
Phone: 818-347-5299
Fax: 818-340-2676
Toll-free: 888-330-5252
e-mail: info@jazztrax.com
Web Site: www.jazztrax.com
Management:
Director: Art Good

4093 CARMEL BACH FESTIVAL
PO Box 575
Carmel, CA 93921
Phone: 831-624-1521
Fax: 831-624-2788
e-mail: info@bachfestival.org
Web Site: www.bachfestival.org
Officers:
President: Natalie Stewart
Management:
Music Director: Bruno Weil
Artistic Director: Nana Faridany
Executive Managing Director/VP: William Witnbergen

Mission: Performing the works of Johann Sebastian Bach, as well as other classical compositions.
Founded: 1935
Specialized Field: Instrumental; Opera; Choral; Childrens'; Educational
Status: Professional; Nonprofit
Paid Staff: 35
Paid Artists: 100
Non-paid Artists: 30
Budget: $2,300,000
Income Sources: Private Donations
Season: July - August
Performs At: Carmel (Festival Site)
Affiliations: Various Sites in the vicinity of Carmel-by-the-Sea
Annual Attendance: 17,000
Facility Category: Community Auditorium
Type of Stage: Proscenium
Seating Capacity: 733; 400; 250; 200
Year Built: 1928
Organization Type: Performing; Educational

4094 CARMEL MUSIC SOCIETY

PO Box 1144
Carmel, CA 93921
Phone: 831-625-9938
Fax: 831-625-6823
e-mail: info@carmelmusic.org
Web Site: www.carmelmusic.org
Management:
  Booking Chairman: Sam Trust
Founded: 1927
Specialized Field: Music
Budget: $60,000-150,000
Performs At: Various
Seating Capacity: 300-1,200

4095 PACIFIC REPERTORY THEATRE/CARMEL SHAKESPEARE FESTIVAL

PO Box 222035
Carmel, CA 93922
Phone: 408-622-0700
Fax: 831-622-0703
Management:
  Artistic Director: Stephen Moorer
Status: Non-Equity; Nonprofit
Season: February-October
Type of Stage: Proscenium; Thrust; Arena

4096 PACIFIC REPERTORY THEATRE

Monte Verde between 8th and 9th Streets
Carmel by the Sea, CA 93922
Phone: 831-622-0700
Fax: 831-622-0703
e-mail: prdebby@aol.com
Officers:
  President: Lee Cox
  VP: Harriet Middledorf
  VP: Shirley Loomis
  Treasurer: Alan Brenner
  Secretary: Barbara Brooks
Management:
  Producing Artistic Director: Stephen Moorer

Managing Director: Geoffrey C Shaley
Mission: To present theatre at its best for residents of and visitors to the Central California Coast. It offers dynamic experiences of professional live theatre which challenge and enrich the lives of audiences and actors. Operates in a variety of venues, presenting great plays from the world stage, contemporary theatre, classic, children's theatre and outreach to diverse communities.
Founded: 1982
Specialized Field: Theatre
Paid Staff: 20
Volunteer Staff: 100
Paid Artists: 100
Season: Year Round

4097 LA GUITARRA CALIFORNIA

2275 Cass Avenue
Cayucos, CA 93430
Phone: 805-995-0987
Fax: 805-995-0987
e-mail: reedandchic@earthlink.net
Web Site: www.reedgilchrist.com
Management:
  Director: Reed Gilchrist
Mission: To offer classical guitar festival.
Founded: 1999
Specialized Field: Classical Guitar
Paid Staff: 1
Volunteer Staff: 30
Paid Artists: 14

4098 BESSIE BARTLETT FRANKEL FESTIVAL OF CHAMBER MUSIC

Scripps College, Music Department
1030 Columbia
Claremont, CA 91711
Phone: 909-607-3266
Fax: 909-621-8323
e-mail: kkosakow@scrippscol.edu
Web Site: www.scrippscol.edu/~dept/Music/music.html
Management:
  Music Department: Jane O'Donnell
Specialized Field: Instrumental
Season: September - March
Performs At: Balch Auditorium; Scripps College; Claremont (Festival Site)
Affiliations: Balch Auditorium; Humanities Auditorium
Facility Category: Auditorium
Seating Capacity: 300

4099 FUTITSU CONCORD JAZZ FESTIVAL

PO Box 845
Concord, CA 94522
Phone: 925-682-6770
Fax: 925-682-3508
e-mail: info@concordrecords.com
Web Site: www.concordpavilion.org

4100 ORANGE COAST COLLEGE COMMUNITY EDUCATION

2701 Fairview Road
PO Box 5005
Costa Mesa, CA 92628-0120

All listings are in alphabetical order by state, then city, then organization within the city.

Phone: 714-432-5916
Fax: 714-432-5902
e-mail: gblanc@cccd.edu
Web Site: occtickets.com
Management:
   Administative Dean: George Blanc
   Lead Technician: Brock Cilley
   Administrative Secretary: Helen McGinley
Mission: To offer an enriching and affordable quality performing arts season for adults and school children.
Founded: 1947
Specialized Field: Band
Status: Semi-Professional
Paid Staff: 3
Budget: $350,000 Artist Fees
Income Sources: Orange Coast College
Performs At: Robert B Moore Theatre; Fine Arts Recital Hall; Drama Lab
Affiliations: WAA
Annual Attendance: 55,000
Facility Category: Concert Hall
Stage Dimensions: 40'x 50'
Seating Capacity: 916
Year Built: 1950
Year Remodeled: 1996
Rental Contact: Brock Cilley
Organization Type: Performing; Touring; Educational

4101 DEL NORTE ASSOCIATION FOR CULTURAL AWARENESS

595 G Street
PO Box 1480
Crescent City, CA 95531
Phone: 707-464-1336
Fax: 707-464-1336
e-mail: dnaca@northcoast.com
Management:
   Executive Director: Holly O Autin
Performs At: Crescent Elk Auditorium
Seating Capacity: 530

4102 UC DAVIS PRESENTS

200 B Street
Suite A
Davis, CA 95616-8561
Phone: 530-757-3488
Fax: 530-757-6815
Web Site: www.ucdavispresents.ucdavis.edu
Performs At: Freeborn Hall
Seating Capacity: 1280

4103 REDWOOD COAST DIXIELAND JAZZ FESTIVAL

PO Box 314
Eureka, CA 95502
Phone: 707-445-3378
Web Site: www.redwoodjazz.org/pages/dixieland

4104 FAIRFIELD CITY ARTS

CityArts Fairfield
1000 Webster Street
Fairfield, CA 94533

Phone: 707-428-7662
Fax: 707-428-7780
e-mail: kswett@ci.fairfield.ca.us
Performs At: Fairfield Center for Creative Arts
Seating Capacity: 368

4105 LIVELY ARTS FOUNDATION

3637 Wishon Avenue
Fresno, CA 93704
Phone: 559-222-3129
Fax: 559-222-1977
e-mail: LivelyArts@aol.com
Web Site: www.livelyartsfoundation.com
Management:
   Artistic Director: Diane K Mosler
Performs At: William Saroyan Theatre
Seating Capacity: 2300

4106 FULLERTON FRIENDS OF MUSIC

1417 Kensington Drive
Fullerton, CA 92631
Phone: 714-525-8617
Fax: 714-529-1512
e-mail: lynnsr@pacbell.net
Web Site: www.webpan.com/fullerton-friends-of-music
Management:
   Artistic Director: Beulah Strickler
Performs At: Sunny Hills High School Performing Arts Center
Seating Capacity: 350

4107 FULLERTON PROFESSSIONAL ARTISTS IN RESIDENCE

PO Box 6850
Fullerton, CA 92834-6850
Phone: 714-278-3347
Fax: 714-278-1488
e-mail: wfarrelly@fullerton.edu
Web Site: www.arts.fullerton.edu
Management:
   Cultural Events Director: Wallace Farrelly
   Marketing/Public Relations: Elizabeth Chmpion
   Box Office Administrator: Laura Trotter
Founded: 1976
Specialized Field: Music; Theatre; Dance
Status: Nonprofit
Budget: $35,000-60,000
Performs At: Plummer Auditorium
Seating Capacity: 1,308
Year Built: 1930

4108 CITRUS COLLEGE HAUGH PERFORMING ARTS CENTER

1000 W Foothill Boulevard
Glendora, CA 91741-1899
Phone: 626-852-8047
Fax: 626-335-4715
e-mail: ghinrichsen@citrus.cc.ca.us
Web Site: www.haughpac.com
Management:
   Executive Director: Greg Hinrichsen
Founded: 1971
Status: Nonprofit

Paid Staff: 30
Paid Artists: 100
Non-paid Artists: 300
Income Sources: Ticket Sales; College Budget; Foundations
Performs At: Proscenium Theatre
Annual Attendance: 150,000
Type of Stage: Proscenium
Seating Capacity: 1440
Year Built: 1971
Rental Contact: Greg Hinrichsen

4109 RUSSIAN RIVER JAZZ FESTIVAL
3rd Street
PO Box 1913
Guerneville, CA 95446
Phone: 707-869-3940
Fax: 707-869-0147
Management:
Office Manager: Kathryn Marceau
Mission: Bringing top name jazz and related performers to perform in an outdoor venue while benefitting local programs for the community and its youth.
Founded: 1976
Specialized Field: Vocal Music; Instrumental Music; Festivals
Status: Nonprofit
Paid Staff: 5
Organization Type: Performing

4110 CALIFORNIA STATE UNIVERSITY: HAYWARD
CSUH Theatre and Dance Department
25800 Carlos Bee Boulevard
Hayward, CA 94542
Phone: 510-885-3118
Fax: 510-885-4748
e-mail: third@csuhayward.edu
Web Site: www.isis.csuhayward.edu
Management:
Chairman: Tom Hird
Music Chairman: Bill Wohlmacher
Production Manager: Ed Wright
Mission: To offer instructional programs in theatre and dance, with professional guest artists.
Founded: 1964
Specialized Field: Theatre; Dance
Paid Staff: 3
Paid Artists: 7
Budget: $12,000
Performs At: University Theatre; Studio Theatre
Annual Attendance: 70,000
Facility Category: University Theatre; Studio Theatre
Type of Stage: Proscenium and Modular
Stage Dimensions: 36'x40'; 20'x25'
Seating Capacity: 481; 130
Year Built: 1971
Rental Contact: University Facilities Reservations Barbara Aro-Valle

4111 HEALDSBURG JAZZ FESTIVAL
PO Box 266
Healdsburg, CA 95448

Phone: 707-433-4633
e-mail: info@healdsburgjazzfestival.com
Web Site: www.healdsburgjazzfestival.com
Management:
Artistic Director: Jessica Felix

4112 RAMONA HILLSIDE PLAYERS
27402 Ramona Bowl Road
PO Box 462
Hemet, CA 92546
Phone: 909-658-5300
e-mail: info@hillsideplayers.org
Web Site: www.hillsideplayers.org
Officers:
President: Amanda Burr
VP: Arlene McNair
Treasurer: Carey McLain
Secretary: Kim Negrete
Management:
Contact Person: Peggy L McQuown
Technical Supervisor: Kim Negrete
Mission: To offer professional education in theatre performance and a series of performances.
Founded: 1941
Specialized Field: Vocal Music; Instrumental Music; Theater
Status: Non-Professional; Nonprofit
Performs At: Ramona Hillside Playhouse
Organization Type: Performing; Resident; Educational

4113 RAMONA PAGEANT ASSOCIATION
27400 Ramona Bowl Road
Hemet, CA 92544
Phone: 909-658-3111
Fax: 909-658-2695
Toll-free: 800-645-4465
e-mail: ramona@ramonapageant.com
Web Site: www.ramonapageant.com
Officers:
President: Don Meek
Management:
General Manager: Roger Vitaich
Secretary: Kathy Long
Marketing/ Communications Manager: Janine Mundwiler
Historian: Phil Bligandi
Box Office Supervisor: Lori West
Events Coordinator: Stephany Borders
Mission: To bring California history to life through performances highlighting the region's Indian and Spanish cultures.
Founded: 1923
Specialized Field: Dance; Vocal Music; Theater; Community
Status: Professional; Non-Professional; Nonprofit
Paid Staff: 8
Non-paid Artists: 600
Income Sources: Box Office; Private Donations; Grants
Performs At: Ramona Bowl Outdoor Amphitheatre
Affiliations: NTA; INTIX; Institute of Outdoor Drama; California Arts Council
Rental Contact: Events Coordinator Stephany Borders
Organization Type: Performing; Resident; Educational

4114 HOLLYWOOD BOWL SUMMER FESTIVAL

Los Angeles Philharmonic Association
135 N Grand Avenue
Hollywood, CA 90078
Phone: 323-850-2000
Fax: 323-850-5376
e-mail: leasly@laphil.org
Web Site: www.hollywoodbowl.org
Officers:
  VP: Deborah Borda
Management:
  Conductor: John Mauceri
  General Manager: Lindsey Nelson
  Program Director, World Music: Tom Schnabel
  Music Director: Esa-Pekka Salonen
  Conductor: John Mauceri
Mission: To provide summer home to both the Hollywood Bowl Orchestra and the Los Angeles Philharmonic, which offers pop, classical and jazz performances.
Specialized Field: Instrumental; Multi-Media; Opera; Choral; Jazz; Folk; Dance; Theatre; Ethnic; Educational
Status: Professional; Nonprofit
Budget: $1,000,000
Income Sources: Los Angeles Philharmonic
Season: June - September
Performs At: Hollywood (Festival Site)
Facility Category: Hollywood Bowl
Seating Capacity: 17,400
Organization Type: Performing; Touring; Resident; Educational; Sponsoring

4115 IDYLLWILD ARTS-ACADEMY & SUMMER PROGRAM

52500 Temecula Drive
PO Box 38
Idyllwild, CA 92549
Phone: 909-659-2171
Fax: 909-659-4383
e-mail: admission@idyllwildarts.org
Web Site: www.idyllwildarts.org
Management:
  Director Summer Program: Steven Fraider
  Headmaster: William Lowman
  Dean of Admission: Anne Behnke
  Director Public Relations: Darren Schilling
Mission: To provide pre-professional training in the arts and a comprehensive college preparatory curriculum in an environment conducive to positive personal development for gifted young artists from all over the world.
Founded: 1950
Specialized Field: Dance; Vocal Music; Instrumental Music; Theater; Festivals; Chamber Music Festival
Status: Professional; Non-Professional; Nonprofit
Performs At: Idyllwild Arts Foundation Theatre; Holmes Amphith
Organization Type: Performing; Educational

4116 ECLECTIC ORANGE FESTIVAL

2082 Business Center Drive
Suite 100
Irvine, CA 92612
Phone: 949-553-2422
Fax: 949-553-2421
e-mail: contactus@philharmonicsociety.org
Web Site: www.eclecticorange.org
Management:
  Executive Director: Dean Corey
Mission: As a project of the Philharmonic Society of Orange County, to foster, promote and increase the knowledge and appreciation of music and the arts through the presentation of performances of national and international stature; to development and implementation of a wide variety of education outreach programs.
Founded: 1947
Specialized Field: Classical Music
Paid Staff: 25
Volunteer Staff: 999

4117 UCI CULTURAL EVENTS

320 University Tower
University of California
Irvine, CA 92717
Phone: 714-856-5589
Fax: 714-725-2201
Management:
  Manager Cultural Events: Desiree Mallory
Mission: To provide professional performances for students and residents of the surrounding area.
Founded: 1965
Specialized Field: Dance; Instrumental Music; Theater
Status: Professional; Nonprofit
Performs At: Irvine Barclay Theatre; Bren Events Center
Organization Type: Educational; Sponsoring; Presenting

4118 TAHOE JAZZ FESTIVAL

PO Box 2390
Kings Beach, CA 96143
e-mail: info@tahoejazz.org
Web Site: www.tahoejazz.org

4119 CELEBRITY PRESENTATIONS

PO Box 457
La Canada, CA 91012
Phone: 818-790-3944
Fax: 818-790-2544
Management:
  Director: Sunny Charla Asch
Budget: $60,000-150,000
Type of Stage: Proscenium

4120 LA JOLLA CHAMBER MUSIC SOCIETY'S - SUMMERFEST LA JOLLA

PO Box 2168
La Jolla, CA 92038
Phone: 858-459-3724
Fax: 858-459-3727
e-mail: ljcms@aol.com
Web Site: www.ljcms.org
Management:
  General Manager: Kathryn Martin

4121 UNIVERSITY EVENTS OFFICE
9500 Gilman Drive
UCSD Campus
La Jolla, CA 92093-0078
Phone: 858-534-4090
Fax: 858-534-7665
e-mail: knlee@ucsd.edu
Web Site: http://ueo.ucsd.edu
Management:
   Production Manager: Steve Evans
   Assistant Director: Kathy Lee
Mission: University Events Office, a department of
Student Affairs at UC San Diego, is dedicated to
presenting entertaining performing artists and film to
expose the campus and community of the various art
forms and diverse cultures of the world.
Founded: 1965
Paid Staff: 8
Volunteer Staff: 25
Paid Artists: 30
Budget: $120,000 presenting only
Income Sources: Student Registration Fees; Ticket Sales;
Patrons
Performs At: Mandeville Center
Affiliations: California Presenters
Annual Attendance: 20,000-30,000
Facility Category: Concert
Type of Stage: Proscenium
Stage Dimensions: 100'x40'
Seating Capacity: 788
Year Built: 1968
Rental Contact: Russell King

4122 DEL VALLE FINE ARTS CONCERT SERIES
PO Box 2335
Livermore, CA 94550
Phone: 925-447-3564
Officers:
   Jr President: Ervin C Woodward
   President: Jeffrey B Garberson
Performs At: First Presbyterian Church
Seating Capacity: 450

4123 CITY OF LOS ANGELES CULTURAL AFFAIRS DEPARTMENT
433 S Spring Street
10th Floor
Los Angeles, CA 90013
Phone: 213-473-7700
Fax: 213-485-6835
Web Site: www.culturela.org
Management:
   General Manager: Adolfo Nodal
   Assistant General Manager: Rodney Punt
   Assistant General Manager: Ann Giagmi
Mission: To promote varied performing arts performances
in the Los Angeles community.
Founded: 1980
Specialized Field: Dance; Vocal Music; Instrumental
Music; Theater; Festivals
Status: Nonprofit
Organization Type: Performing

4124 GRAND PERFORMANCES
350 S Grand Avenue
Suite A-4
Los Angeles, CA 90071
Phone: 213-687-2190
Fax: 213-687-2191
e-mail: booking@grandperformances.org
Web Site: www.grandperformances.org
Management:
   Executive Director: Michael Alexander
   Associate Director: Leigh Ann Hahn
   Development Director: Alice Platt
   Business Manager: Paula Jones
   Development Associate: Karlee Decima
   Office Adminstrator: Michelle Diaz
   Production Manager: Fred Stites
   Technical Director: Mark Baker
   Office Administrator: Johnny Tu
Founded: 1987
Specialized Field: Multi Disciplinary Performing Arts
Presenter
Status: Nonprofit
Paid Staff: 10
Volunteer Staff: 2
Paid Artists: 504
Budget: $1.3 million
Income Sources: Contracts; Grants
Affiliations: APAP; WAA; California Presenters;
California Arts Advocates
Annual Attendance: 65,000
Facility Category: Outdoor Plaza
Type of Stage: Thrust
Seating Capacity: 2,000; 6,500
Year Built: 1992

4125 JAZZ AT DREW LEGACY MUSIC & CULTURAL MARKETPLACE
1730 E 120th Street
Charles Drew University of Medicine & Science
Los Angeles, CA 90059
Phone: 323-563-5850
Fax: 323-563-4919
e-mail: toabdul@cdrewu.edu
Management:
   Executive Producer/Founder: Roland H Betts
   Producer Assistant: Toni Abdul-Hanson
Mission: To offer jazz performances as public relation
events and fundraisers.
Founded: 1991
Specialized Field: Instrumental Music (Jazz)
Paid Staff: 2
Volunteer Staff: 125
Paid Artists: 11

4126 LMU GUITAR CONCERT & MASTERCLASS SERIES
LMU Music Department
One LUM Drive
Los Angeles, CA 90045-8347
Phone: 310-338-5158
Fax: 310-338-5046
e-mail: mmiranda@lmumail.lmu.edu
Web Site: www.lmu.edu/colleges/cfa/music/guitarseries
Management:

Assistant Professional of Music: Michael Miranda
Founded: 1999

4127 LOS ANGELES COUNTY MUSEUM OF ART
5905 Wilshire Boulevard
Los Angeles, CA 90036
Phone: 323-857-6000
Fax: 213-931-7347
e-mail: membership@lacma.org
Web Site: www.lacma.org
Management:
   Director Music Programs: Dorrance Stalvey
   Administration/Promotion: Cheryl Tiano
   President/Director: Andrea Rich
Mission: To produce concerts of chamber music and jazz.
Founded: 1939
Specialized Field: Vocal Music; Instrumental Music
Status: Professional; Nonprofit
Income Sources: Los Angeles County Museum of Art
Performs At: Leo S. Bing Theatre
Organization Type: Performing

4128 MONDAY EVENING CONCERTS
5905 Wilshire Boulevard
Los Angeles, CA 90036
Phone: 323-857-6115
Fax: 323-857-6214
e-mail: dstalvey@lacma.org
Web Site: www.lacma.org
Management:
   Music Director: Dorrance Stalvey
Founded: 1957
Specialized Field: Chamber Music
Paid Staff: 2
Volunteer Staff: 5
Paid Artists: 60
Performs At: Leo S. Bing Theatre
Seating Capacity: 600

4129 MOUNT SAINT MARY'S COLLEGE - THE DA CAMERA SOCIETY
10 Chester Place
Los Angeles, CA 90007
Phone: 213-477-2953
Fax: 213-477-2959
e-mail: mbonino@msmc.la.edu
Web Site: www.dacamera.org
Management:
   Founder/Artistic Director: Dr. MaryAnn Bonino
   Managing Director: Kelly Garrison
   Production Manager: Bruce Williaims
   Outreach And Education Manager: Susan Helfter
Performs At: Doheny Mansion; Los Angeles' Union Station; The Queen Mary; The former Bullocks Wilshire
Seating Capacity: 50-2000

4130 MUSIC CENTER OF LOS ANGELES COUNTY/EDUCATION DIVISION
717 W Temple Street
Suite 400
Los Angeles, CA 90012

Phone: 213-977-9555
Fax: 213-481-7597
e-mail: msolomon@pacla.org
Web Site: www.performingartscenterla.org
Management:
   Managing Director: Michael Solomon

4131 MUSIC GUILD
6022 Wilshire Boulevard
Suite 203
Los Angeles, CA 90067
Phone: 323-954-0404
Fax: 323-954-0303
e-mail: themusicguild@aol.com
Management:
   Executive Director: Eugene Golden
Mission: To present chamber music groups to our audiences at Cal State Long Beach and the Beverly Hills High School.
Founded: 1948
Paid Staff: 2
Income Sources: Ticket Sales; Donations
Performs At: Cal State Northridge Performing Arts Center
Affiliations: Chamber Music of America
Annual Attendance: 1,500
Seating Capacity: 1294

4132 OCCIDENTAL COLLEGE ARTIST SERIES
1600 Campus Road
Los Angeles, CA 90041
Phone: 323-259-2737
Fax: 323-341-4987
Management:
   Marketing Consultant: Sandy Robertson
   Technical Director for Theatres: Terri Gens
Founded: 1887
Specialized Field: Dance; Vocal Music; Instrumental Music; Theater; World Music
Status: Nonprofit
Performs At: Thorne Hall; Keck Theater
Organization Type: Sponsoring

4133 ROSALINDE GILBERT CONCERTS
5905 Wilshire Boulevard
Los Angeles, CA 90036
Phone: 323-857-6115
Fax: 323-857-6214
e-mail: dstalvey@lacma.org
Web Site: www.lacma.org
Management:
   Music Director: Dorrance Stalvey
Founded: 1996
Specialized Field: Chamber Music
Performs At: Leo S Bing Thaetre; LA County Museum of Art
Seating Capacity: 600

4134 SWEET & HOT SUMMER MUSIC FESTIVAL
PO Box 642269
Los Angeles, CA 90064-2269

e-mail: sweethot@sweethot.org
Web Site: www.sweethot.org

4135 MASS ENSEMBLE
3525 Coast View Drive
Malibu, CA 90265
Phone: 312-243-2366
Fax: 312-243-2366
e-mail: closesound@aol.com
Web Site: www.MASSEnsemble.com
Management:
    Artist: Bill Close

4136 MAMMOTH LAKES JAZZ JUBILEE
PO Box 909
Mammoth Lakes, CA 93456
Phone: 760-934-2478
Fax: 760-934-2478
e-mail: mljj@qnet.com
Web Site: www.mammothjazz.org
Management:
    Director: Ken Coulter
    Director: Flossie Coulter
Mission: To bring to a small town-big time entertainment. To keep America's true art form alive.
Founded: 1989
Specialized Field: Music; Jazz
Paid Staff: 3
Volunteer Staff: 500
Paid Artists: 140
Facility Category: 10 Venues in Tents

4137 YUBA COUNTY-SUTTER COUNTY REGIONAL ARTS COUNCIL TOURING/PRESENTING PROGRAM
PO Box 468
Marysville, CA 95901
Phone: 530-742-2787
Fax: 530-742-1171
Management:
    Executive Director: Lee Burrows
Performs At: Marysville Auditorium
Seating Capacity: 1,083

4138 MENDOCINO MUSIC FESTIVAL
PO Box 1808
Mendocino, CA 95460
Phone: 707-937-2044
Fax: 707-937-1045
e-mail: music@mendocinomusic.com
Web Site: www.mendocinomusic.com
Officers:
    President: Lisa Orselli
Management:
    Managing Director: Nancy Harrisr
    Artistic Director: Allan Pollack
Mission: To bring classical, chamber, world music and dance, jazz and blues to the spectacular, rural Mendocino coast.
Founded: 1986
Specialized Field: Instrumental; Opera; Choral; Jazz; Childrens'; Educational
Status: Professional; Nonprofit

Paid Staff: 10
Volunteer Staff: 200
Paid Artists: 100
Budget: $500,000
Season: July
Performs At: Mendocino Headlands State Park (Festival Site)
Annual Attendance: 9,800
Facility Category: Festival Tent
Seating Capacity: 808
Organization Type: Performing

4139 SADDLEBACK COLLEGE GUEST ARTISTS SERIES
Division of Fine Arts
28000 Marguerite Parkway
Mission Viejo, CA 92692-3635
Phone: 949-582-4763
Fax: 949-347-8653
e-mail: info@saddleback.cc.ca.us
Web Site: www.saddleback.cc.ca.us/
Management:
    Director Performing Arts: Geofrey English
Performs At: McKinney Theatre
Seating Capacity: 401; 1500

4140 STARLITE PATIO THEATER SUMMER SERIES
Montclair Civic Center
Benito and Fremont
Montclair, CA 91763
Phone: 909-625-9460
Fax: 909-399-9751
Management:
    Manager/Program Director: Harve Edwards
    Facility Supervisor: Shirley Wofford
Mission: Offering summer cultural entertainment (eight programs) at no charge on Tuesdays.
Founded: 1963
Specialized Field: Dance; Theater
Status: Nonprofit
Paid Staff: 3
Paid Artists: 16
Budget: $2,400
Performs At: The Starlite Patio Theater
Facility Category: Outdoor Patio
Type of Stage: Small Outdoor; Covered
Seating Capacity: 200
Organization Type: Performing

4141 DIXIELAND MONTEREY
177 Webster Street
A-206
Monterey, CA 93940
Fax: 831-656-9560
Toll-free: 888-349-6879
Web Site: www.dixiejazz.com/montery.html

4142 MONTEREY JAZZ FESTIVAL
2000 Fairgrounds Road
Monterey, CA 93940

Mailing Address: PO Box Jazz Monterey, CA 93942
Phone: 831-373-3366
Fax: 831-373-0244
e-mail: jazzinfo@montereyjazzfestival.org
Web Site: www.montereyjazzfestival.org
Management:
   Director: Tim Jackson
   Director: Paul S Fingerote
Mission: To perpetuate jazz and further jazz education.
Founded: 1958
Specialized Field: Jazz
Paid Artists: 500

4143 **MUSIC IN THE VINEYARDS**
NAPA VALLEY CHAMBER MUSIC
FESTIVAL
PO Box 432
Mt. Helena, CA 94574
Phone: 707-578-5656
Fax: 707-578-5699
e-mail: gadams@sonic.net
Web Site: www.napavalleymusic.org
Officers:
   President: David Marsten
   VP: Robilee F Deane
Management:
   Executive Director: Gail V Adams
   Artistic Director: Michael Adams
   Music Director: Daria Adams
   Development Director: Melinda Mendelson
Mission: Dedicated to bringing together outstanding artists to perform in the vineyard settings of the Napa Valley so that performers and audience alike can experience the intimacy of chamber music as it was intended to be performed.
Founded: 1995
Specialized Field: Instrumental
Budget: $140,000
Season: August
Performs At: Napa Valley (Festival Site)
Affiliations: Various vineyards and related venues
Seating Capacity: 150 - 250

4144 **MUSIC IN THE MOUNTAINS**
530 Searls Avenue, Suite A
PO Box 1451
Nevada City, CA 95959
Phone: 530-265-6173
Fax: 530-265-6810
Toll-free: 800-218-2188
e-mail: mim@musicinthemountains.org
Web Site: www.musicinthemountains.org
Officers:
   President: Hazel Shewell
Management:
   Artistic Director: Paul Perry
   Executive Director: Barry Bonifas
Mission: To present high-quality classical, jazz and Broadway music at affordable prices.
Founded: 1981
Specialized Field: Instrumental; Choral; Jazz; Educational; Childrens'
Status: Professional; Nonprofit
Paid Staff: 6

Volunteer Staff: 300
Paid Artists: 175
Budget: $700,000-$1,000,000
Income Sources: Donation; Grants; Ticket Sales; Benefit Events; Advertising; Sponsoring
Season: November; December; April; June; July
Performs At: Festival sites around Nevada City & Grass Valley
Affiliations: Chamber Music America; American Symphony Orchestra League; Association of California Symphony Orchestras; BMI; ASCAP
Annual Attendance: 17,000
Facility Category: Renovated Concert Hall; Outdoor Tent
Stage Dimensions: 48'x56'
Seating Capacity: 550 inside; 4,000 outside
Year Remodeled: 2001
Organization Type: Performing; Resident; Educational; Sponsoring

---

4145 **CENTER FOR THE VISUAL AND**
PERFORMING ARTS
California State University, Northbridge
18111 Nordhoff, ARTS
Northridge, CA 91330-8398
Phone: 818-677-5768
Fax: 818-677-5472
e-mail: cvpa@csun.com
Web Site: www.cvpa.csun.com
Officers:
   Dean: William Toultant
   Associate Dean: Cynthia Raywrtch
Management:
   Interim Artistic Director: William C Martin
   Interim Managing Director: Kathy Anthony
Mission: Provide quality arts programming for the San Fernando Valley and surrounding areas of Los Angeles, California.
Founded: 1996
Specialized Field: Jazz Series; Dance Series; Celebrity Shows Series
Paid Staff: 10
Volunteer Staff: 75
Budget: $300,000
Income Sources: University Subsidy; Tickets Sales; Contributions
Performs At: USU Performing Arts Center; Campus Theatre; Little Theatre
Annual Attendance: 50,000
Type of Stage: Proscenium
Seating Capacity: 500/150
Year Built: 1994
Rental Contact: Kathy Anthony

4146 **MULTI-CULTURAL MUSIC AND ART**
FOUNDATION OF NORTHRIDGE
(MCMAFN)
PO Box 280101
Northridge, CA 91328
Phone: 818-349-3400
Fax: 818-349-0716
e-mail: romil@mcmaf.j.org
Web Site: www.mcmafn.org
Officers:

VP/Historian: Paul A Dentzel
Accountant: William V King
President: WM Paulin
Social/Arts Coordinator: Julia Jones
Management:
    Program Coordinator/Creative Dir: Elizabeth Waldo
    Music: Barry Turchen
    Composer-Violinist/Conductor: Elisabeth Waldo
Mission: Supporting a wide range of performing and visual arts, particularly music and dance.
Founded: 1990
Specialized Field: Dance; Vocal Music; Instrumental Music; Festivals
Status: Nonprofit
Paid Staff: 2
Budget: $100,000
Income Sources: Memberships, Grants, Admissions to Theatre
Performs At: New Mission Theatre
Affiliations: All Los Angeles Museums, ASCAP, Local 47 AIF
Type of Stage: Expandable
Seating Capacity: 150, outdoors; 300 seats
Year Remodeled: 1995
Rental Contact: Booking Calendar Hengamett
Organization Type: Performing; Educational

4147 FOUR SEASONS CONCERTS, NEW YORK SERIES

5701 Broadway
Oakland, CA 94618
Mailing Address: PO Box 507 Berkeley, CA 94701
Phone: 510-451-0775
Fax: 510-549-3504
e-mail: fourseasonsconcerts@juno.com
Web Site: www.fourseasonsconcerts.com
Officers:
    President: Jesse W Anthony
Performs At: Carnegie Hall; Alice Tully Hall

4148 MILLS COLLEGE MUSIC DEPARTMENT

5000 MacArthur Boulevard
Oakland, CA 94613
Phone: 510-430-2334
Fax: 510-430-3228
e-mail: steed@mills.edu
Web Site: www.mills.edu
Management:
    Concert Coordinator: Steed Cowart

4149 REDWOOD ART COUNCIL

PO Box 449
Occidental, CA 95465
Phone: 707-874-1124
Fax: 707-874-1516
e-mail: racmusic@monitor.net
Web Site: www.redwoodarts.org
Officers:
    President/Director: Kathryn Neustadter
Mission: To present exceptional chamber music.
Founded: 1980
Specialized Field: Chamber Music
Paid Staff: 1

Volunteer Staff: 15
Paid Artists: 35
Budget: $50,000
Income Sources: Tickets, Donations, Grants
Performs At: Occidental Community Church
Annual Attendance: 1,500-2,000
Facility Category: Mostly Churches
Type of Stage: Platform
Stage Dimensions: 8' x 20'
Seating Capacity: 150
Year Built: 1876

4150 OJAI FESTIVALS

201 S Signal Street
PO Box 185
Ojai, CA 93024
Phone: 805-646-2094
Fax: 805-646-6037
e-mail: info@ojaifestival.org
Web Site: www.ojaifestival.org
Management:
    Artistic Director: Ernest Fleischmann
    Executive Director: Jacqueline Saunders
Mission: Promoting contemporary music and dance performances, from artists such as Emerson Quartet.
Founded: 1947
Specialized Field: Instrumental; Choral; Childrens'; Ethnic
Status: Professional; Nonprofit
Paid Staff: 5
Budget: $600,000
Income Sources: American Symphony Orchestra League; California Confederation of the Arts
Season: May - June
Performs At: Ojai Festival; Libbey Bowl
Affiliations: Libbey Bowl
Seating Capacity: 1,500
Organization Type: Educational; Sponsoring

4151 OJAI MUSIC FESTIVAL

PO Box 185
201 S Signal Street
Ojai, CA 93024
Phone: 805-646-2094
Fax: 805-646-6037
e-mail: info@ojaifestival.org
Web Site: www.ojaifestival.org
Management:
    Executive Director: Jacqueline Saunders

4152 OJAI SHAKESPEARE FESTIVAL

PO Box 575
Ojai, CA 93024
Phone: 805-646-9455
Fax: 805-646-9455
e-mail: jaye@ojaishakespeare.org
Web Site: www.ojaishakespeare.org
Officers:
    VP: Bruce Wallace
    Treasurer: Wayne Francis
    Secretary: Marilyn Wallace
    Madrigali Representative: Dave Farber
Management:
    Artistic Director: Jaye Hersh

Executive Director: Phil Casanta
Artistic Advisor: Paul Backer
Marketing/Public Relations: Amy Jones
Marketing/Public Relations: Dina Pielaet
Founded: 1982
Status: Non-Equity; Nonprofit
Season: June - August
Type of Stage: Amphitheatre
Stage Dimensions: 38'x32'
Seating Capacity: 650

4153 OROVILLE CONCERT ASSOCIATION

29 Orchard Hill Drive
Oroville, CA 95966
Phone: 530-589-0836
e-mail: swedin@cncnet.com
Officers:
President: Sharon Wedin
Performs At: State Theatre
Seating Capacity: 612

4154 CANYON INDUSTRIES

PO Box 256
Palm Springs, CA 92263.
Phone: 760-778-7966
Fax: 760-778-4890
e-mail: sheffield@juno.com
Web Site: www.canyonentertainment.com
Management:
President: Simone Sheffield
Paid Staff: 30
Volunteer Staff: 100
Paid Artists: 10
Non-paid Artists: 10
Budget: $400,000-1,000,000

4155 CALTECH PUBLIC EVENTS SERIES

Caltech Public Events
Mail Code 332-92
Pasadena, CA 91125
Phone: 626-395-4638
Fax: 626-577-0130
e-mail: events@caltech.edu
Web Site: www.events.caltech.edu
Management:
Director: Denise Nelson Nash
Associate Director: Chris Harcourt
Technical Operations Manager: Louis Lind
Marketing/Outreach Manager: Cara Steven
Stage Technician: Erick Ferguson
Budget: $60,000-150,000
Performs At: Beckman Auditorium; Ramo Auditorium; Dabney Lounge
Seating Capacity: 1165; 423; 200

4156 MONTICELLO MEDICI PERFORMING ARTS ACADEMY

200 Fern Drive
Pasadena, CA 91105-1216
Phone: 626-792-3096
Fax: 626-792-5049
e-mail: vburner@juno.com
Officers:

President: Dr. Victor Burner
Performs At: Monticello Medici Recital Hall
Seating Capacity: 25-75

4157 SONGFEST

703 Lakewood Place
Pasadena, CA 91106
Phone: 626-449-7146
Fax: 626-405-0151
e-mail: songfest@earthlink.net
Management:
Executive Director: Rosemary Hyler Ritter
Development: Elaine Chow
Mission: To advance the art of song by cultivating its musical literary traditions and promoting its contemporary development, with both artists and audiences. To provide both professional and pre-professional artists with unique opportunity of close working association with some of the world's most distinguished artists.
Founded: 1996
Specialized Field: Classical Voice and Piano
Status: Non-Profit
Paid Staff: 1
Volunteer Staff: 7
Paid Artists: 10
Budget: $110,000
Income Sources: Private Donors; Tuitions
Affiliations: Chapman University
Facility Category: Music School

4158 GOLDEN GATE INTERNATIONAL CHILDREN'S CHORAL FESTIVAL

401-A Highland Avenue
Piedmont, CA 94611
Phone: 510-547-7721
Fax: 510-547-7449
e-mail: akelly@piedmontchoirs.org
Web Site: www.piedmontchoirs.org
Management:
Director/Founder: Robert Geary

4159 RUSTAVI COMPANY

IAI Presentations, Inc
PO Box 4
Pismo Beach, CA 93448-0004
Phone: 805-476-8422
Fax: 805-476-8426
Toll-free: 800-424-3454
e-mail: don@iaipresentations.com
Web Site: www.iaipresentations.com

4160 SHANGRI - LA CHINESE ACROBATS

IAI Presentations, Inc.
PO Box 4
Pismo Beach, CA 93448-0004
Phone: 805-476-8422
Fax: 805-476-8426
Toll-free: 800-424-3454
e-mail: don@iaipresentations.com
Web Site: www.iaipresentations.com

4161 ART OF RECITAL
PO Box 9401
Rancho Santa Fe, CA 92067
Phone: 858-259-2503
Fax: 858-259-5508
e-mail: iim_imf@hotmail.com
Web Site: www.fairbanksartscenter.com
Officers:
   President: Michael Tseitlin
Performs At: California Center for the Arts; Horizon
Auditorium
Seating Capacity: 1600; 650

**4162 CARMEL VALLEY LIBRARY CONCERT
SERIES**
PO Box 9401
Rancho Santa Fe, CA 92067
Phone: 858-259-2503
Fax: 858-259-5508
e-mail: iim_imf@hotmail.com
Web Site: www.fairbankartscenter.com
Management:
   Artistic Director: Michael Tseitlin
Budget: $35,000-60,000
Performs At: Concert Hall
Seating Capacity: 300

**4163 INTERNATIONAL INSTITUTE OF
MUSIC FESTIVAL**
PO Box 9401
Rancho Santa Fe, CA 92067
Phone: 858-259-2503
Fax: 858-259-5508
e-mail: iim_imf@hotmail.com
Web Site: www.fairbankscenter.com
Management:
   Executive Director: Michael Tseitlin
   Administrative Director: Paul Lindenauer
   Artistic Advisor: Giuseppe Nova
Specialized Field: Instrumental; Educational
Budget: $35,000-$60,000
Season: July
Performs At: Bayerische Musikakademie; Marktoberdorf
(Festival Site)
Seating Capacity: 400 - 800

4164 SHASTA JAZZ FESTIVAL
3336 Wilshire Drive
Redding, CA 96002
Fax: 530-223-0301
Toll-free: 800-874-7562
e-mail: chet@shasta.com
Web Site: www.shastajazzfestival.com
Management:
   Festival Director: Dr. Chet Moore

**4165 REDLANDS BOWL SUMMER MUSIC
FESTIVAL**
PO Box 466
Redlands, CA 92373
Phone: 909-793-7316
Fax: 909-793-5086
e-mail: redlandsbowl@aol.com
Web Site: www.redlandsbowl.org
Officers:
   Executive Director: Beverly Noerr
Management:
   Program Director/VP: Marsha Gebara
   Artistic Advisor: Frank Fetta
Mission: Providing a range of performing arts to residents
of Redlands at no admission charge.
Founded: 1923
Specialized Field: Instrumental; Opera; Choral;
Traditional Jazz; Dance; Childrens'
Status: Professional; Nonprofit
Paid Staff: 2
Volunteer Staff: 100
Budget: $150,000-$400,000
Income Sources: Freewill Donations; Underwriting;
Grants
Season: Late June - Late August
Performs At: Redlands Open-air Amphitheatre (Festival
Site)
Affiliations: Redlands Bowl
Annual Attendance: 80,000 to 100,000
Seating Capacity: 3,750
Organization Type: Performing; Sponsoring

4166 JAZZ ON THE LAKE
176 Rusk Lane
PO Box 962
Redway, CA 95560
Phone: 707-923-4599
Fax: 707-923-4509
e-mail: people@humboldt.net
Management:
   Director: Carol Bruno
Founded: 1985

4167 SUMMER ARTS & MUSIC FESTIVAL
Mateel Community Center
PO Box 1910
Redway, CA 95560
Phone: 707-923-3368
Fax: 707-923-3370
e-mail: mateel@humboldt.net
Web Site: www.mateel.org/samf.html
Management:
   Talent Coordiantor: Justin Crellin
   Craft Booth Coordinator: Eva Evans
Specialized Field: Instrumental; Jazz; Folk; Dance;
Theatre; Childrens'
Paid Artists: 20
Non-paid Artists: 40
Season: Late June
Performs At: Benbow Lake State Recreation Area
(Festival Site)
Facility Category: Outdoor venue
Seating Capacity: 6,000

4168 WINTER ARTS FESTIVAL
PO Box 1910
Redway, CA 95560

Phone: 707-923-3368
Fax: 707-923-3370
e-mail: justcrel@hotmail.com
Management:
    Winter Arts Coordinator: Justin Crellin
    Craft Booth Coordinator: Eva Evans
    Executive Director: Kathryn Manspeaker
    Hall Manager: Leo Valladeres
Specialized Field: Instrumental; Jazz
Season: December, second weekend
Affiliations: Mateel Community Center; Redway
Annual Attendance: 1,500 per day
Facility Category: Community Center/Performance Hall

4169 INDIAN WELLS VALLEY CONCERT ASSOCIATION

PO Box 1802
Ridgcrest, CA 93556-1802
Phone: 760-375-5600
Management:
    Business Manager: Carl N Helmick Jr
Performs At: China Lake Auditorium
Seating Capacity: 1018

4170 PERFORMING ARTS PRESENTATIONS

University of California Music Department
1339 Olmsted Hall
Riverside, CA 92521
Phone: 909-787-3343
Fax: 909-787-4651
Web Site: www.performingarts.ucr.edu
Management:
    Management Services Officer: Andrea Jones
    Student Affairs Assistant: Cindy L Roulette
    Administrative Assistant: Darline Starling
    Production Assistant: Kathleen DeAtley
Mission: Providing educational and cultural resources for students and area residents.
Founded: 1973
Specialized Field: Dance; Vocal Music; Instrumental Music; Theater
Status: Professional; Nonprofit
Income Sources: Western Alliance of Arts Administrators; Association of Performing Arts Presenters; California Presenters
Performs At: University Theatre
Organization Type: Sponsoring

4171 UNIVERSITY OF CALIFORNIA AT RIVERSIDE: CULTURAL EVENTS

133 Costo Hall
Riverside, CA 92521-0406
Phone: 909-787-4629
Fax: 909-787-2221
e-mail: todd.wingate@ucr.edu
Web Site: www.cultural.eventsucr.edu
Performs At: University Theatre
Seating Capacity: 500

4172 CALIFORNIA STATE SUMMER SCHOOL FOR THE ARTS

4825 J Street
Suite 120
Sacramento, CA 95819-3747
Mailing Address: PO Box 1077 Sacramento, CA 98512-1077
Phone: 916-227-9320
Fax: 916-227-9455
e-mail: rjaffe@csssa.org
Web Site: www.csssa.org/
Officers:
    Chair: Susan Dolgen
    VP: Megan Chernin
    VP Finance: Bret Magpiong
    Secretary: Donna Miller Casey
Management:
    Director: Robert M Jaffe
    Deputy Director: Joseph Alameida
    Program Analyst: Katrina Dolenga
    Office Assistant: Cynthia Glenn
    Development Director: Joan Newberg
Mission: The California State Summer School for the Arts is a rigorous, preprofeesional, month long training program in the visual and performing arts, creative writing, animation and film for talented artists of high school age.
Founded: 1987
Budget: $1.9 million
Performs At: Various Auditoriums
Facility Category: Rented College Campus

4173 FESTIVAL OF NEW AMERICAN MUSIC

Music Department
CSU Sacramento
Sacramento, CA 95819-6015
Phone: 916-278-7988
Fax: 916-278-7217
Web Site: www.csus.edu/music
Management:
    Co-Director: Daniel Kennedy
    Co-Director: Ernie Hills
Mission: To showcase the works of contemporary American composers.
Specialized Field: Instrumental; Multi-Media; Jazz; Dance; Childrens'
Status: Nonprofit
Budget: $60,000-$150,000
Season: Early-mid November, 12 days
Performs At: Sacremento (Festival Site)
Facility Category: Music Recital Hall
Seating Capacity: 350
Organization Type: Performing; Educational; Sponsoring

4174 FINEST ASIAN PERFORMING ARTS

PO Box 162163
Sacramento, CA 95816
Phone: 916-924-1212
Fax: 916-924-7212
Management:
    Executive Director: Anna Y Mayo
    Secretary: Lucy Nemac
    Music Director/Advisor: Yan Zhang

Mission: To expose the Western community to Eastern culture works.
Founded: 1988
Specialized Field: Dance; Vocal Music; Instrumental Music; Festivals
Status: Professional; Semi-Professional
Paid Staff: 12
Income Sources: Finest Asian Music Festival
Organization Type: Performing; Sponsoring

4175 HUGHES STADIUM
3835 Freeport Boulevard
Sacramento, CA 95822
Phone: 916-558-2197
Fax: 916-558-2030
Management:
    Facility Manager: Vicki Byers

4176 SALINAS CONCERT ASSOCIATION
14260 Mountian Quail Road
Salinas, CA 93908
Phone: 831-484-5099
Fax: 831-484-5843
e-mail: mmimibob@aol.com
Officers:
    President: Carl Christensen
Performs At: Performing Arts Centre
Seating Capacity: 550

4177 LAPINSKY FAMILY SAN DIEGO JEWISH ARTS FESTIVAL
San Diego Repertory Theatre
79 Horton Plaza
San Diego, CA 92101
Phone: 619-231-3586
Fax: 619-235-0939
Web Site: www.sandiegorep.com
Management:
    Artistic Director: Todd Salovey

4178 MAINLY MOZART FESTIVAL
121 Broadway
Suite 374
San Diego, CA 92101
Mailing Address: PO Box 124705 San Diego, CA 92112-4705
Phone: 619-239-0100
Fax: 619-233-4292
e-mail: admin@mainlymozart.org
Web Site: www.mainlymozart.org
Officers:
    Chairman: Edward Richards
    President: Christopher Weil
    Treasurer: Jim Rosenfield
    Secretary: Linda Satz
Management:
    Artistic Director: David Atherton
    Executive Director: Nancy S Laturno
    Development Director: Alexandra Pearson
    Director Administration: Dalouge Smith
Founded: 1989
Specialized Field: Classical Music; Jazz; Education
Status: Nonprofit

Paid Staff: 7
Paid Artists: 80
Budget: $700,000 - 800,000
Income Sources: Box Office Receipts; Grants; Donations; Memberships; Special Events; Retail
Affiliations: Spreckels Theatre; Neurosciences Institution; St Pauls Cathedral; US Grant Hotel; East County Performing Arts Center; Lambs Theatre
Annual Attendance: 26,000
Seating Capacity: 1,500

4179 POINT LOMA NAZARENE UNIVERSITY CULTURAL EVENTS SERIES
3900 Lomaland Drive
San Diego, CA 92106
Phone: 619-849-2559
Fax: 619-849-2668
e-mail: paulkenyon@ptloma.edu
Web Site: www.ptloma.edu
Management:
    Chairman: Dr. Paul Kenyon
Performs At: Chapel
Seating Capacity: 1800

4180 SAN DIEGO STATE UNIVERSITY-SCHOOL OF MUSIC AND DANCE
San Diego State University
San Diego, CA 92182-7902
Phone: 619-594-6031
Fax: 619-594-1692
e-mail: sbazirji@mail.sdsu.edu
Web Site: www.musicdance.sdsu.edu
Management:
    Administrative Support Coordinator: Stephanie Bazirjian, BA
    Receptionist/Student Coordinator: Sandra Konar
    Publicity/Events Coordinator: Rhoda Nevins, BA
Mission: To provide the highest quality education for performers, choreographers, educators, researchers and those who may be in fields related to music and dance.
Founded: 1897
Specialized Field: Music; Dance

4181 SAN DIEGO THANKSGIVING, DIXIELAND JAZZ FESTIVAL
PO Box 880387
San Diego, CA 92168-0387
Phone: 619-297-5277
Fax: 619-297-5281
e-mail: info@dixielandjazzfestival.org
Web Site: www.dixielandjazzfestival.org
Management:
    Director: Alan D Adams

4182 CHAMBER MUSIC WEST FESTIVAL
San Francisco Conservatory of Music
1201 Ortega Street
San Francisco, CA 94122
Phone: 415-564-8086
Fax: 415-759-3499
Management:
    Artistic Director: Colin Murdoch

Festival Coordinator: Timothy Bach
Mission: Offering advanced students and faculty the opportunity to perform with outstanding guest artists and providing Bay Area audiences with concerts featuring highly imaginative programming.
Specialized Field: Chamber
Status: Professional; Nonprofit
Performs At: Hellman Hall
Organization Type: Performing; Educational

4183 GRACE CATHEDRAL CONCERTS

Grace Cathedral
1100 California Street
San Francisco, CA 94108
Phone: 415-749-6355
Fax: 415-749-6349
e-mail: concerts@gracecathedral.org
Web Site: www.gracecathedral.org
Management:
   Concerts Manager: Louis Weiner
Paid Staff: 1
Performs At: Grace Cathedral
Facility Category: Church
Seating Capacity: 1309
Year Built: 1934

4184 MASSENKOFF RUSSIAN FOLK FESTIVAL

357 Howth Street
San Francisco, CA 94117
Phone: 415-586-9654
Fax: 415-586-7987
e-mail: RussianFok@aol.com
Web Site: www.members.aol.com/russianfok/music1/index.
Management:
   Singer/Director: Nikolai Massenkoff
   Artist Representative: Sandra Calvin
Mission: To provide entertainment and expand knowledge of Russian culture and people.
Founded: 1975
Specialized Field: Russian Music; Song; Dance
Facility Category: Flexible
Type of Stage: Flexible
Seating Capacity: 500-50,000

4185 MIDSUMMER MOZART FESTIVAL

World Trade Center
#250G
San Francisco, CA 94111
Phone: 415-292-9620
Fax: 415-954-0852
e-mail: wolfgang@midsummermozart.org
Web Site: www.midsummermozart.org
Officers:
   Chairman: James M Rockett
   President: Wendell Rider
   Treasurer: Richard Heath
Management:
   Music Director/Conductor: George Cleve
   Executive Director: Helena Zaludova
   Librarian: Marta Tobey
   Public Relations Manager: Alexandra Ivanoff
   Associate Advisory Administrator: Clark Griffith

Mission: To present the music of Wolfgang Amadeus Mozart to expanding Bay Area audiences through performances of unparalleled excellence.
Founded: 1975
Specialized Field: Instrumental
Status: Professional; Nonprofit
Budget: $10,000
Income Sources: American Symphony Orchestra League; California Confederation of the Arts; Association of California Symphony Orchestras
Season: July
Affiliations: Various venues throughout California
Seating Capacity: 928; 700; 315; 600; 300
Organization Type: Performing

4186 MORRISON ARTIST SERIES

San Francisco State University Music Dep.
1600 Holloway Avenue
San Francisco, CA 94123
Phone: 415-338-1442
Fax: 415-338-3294
e-mail: alarts@sfsu.edu
Web Site: www.sfsu.edu/~allarts/morrisonartist.html
Management:
   Artistic Director: Saul Gropman
Performs At: McKenna Theatre
Seating Capacity: 700

4187 NEW LANGTON ARTS

1246 Folsom Street
San Francisco, CA 94103-3817
Phone: 415-626-5416
Fax: 415-255-1453
e-mail: nla@newlangtonarts.org
Web Site: www.newlangtonarts.org
Officers:
   President: Evie Davis
   VP: Ell Crews
   Secretary: Simon J Frankel
   Treasurer: Lisette Sell
   VP: Margaret Tedesco
Management:
   Executive Director: Susan Miller
   Communications Director: Robyn Wise
   Program Director: James Bewley
   Grant Writer/Financial Manager: Sharon Maidenberg
   Operations Manager: Michael Smoler
   Gallery Coordinator/Executive Asst: Sara Ayazi
Founded: 1975
Specialized Field: Visual & Media Arts; Music Performance; Literature; Interdesciplnary Projects
Paid Staff: 6
Performs At: Auditorium
Seating Capacity: 80

4188 NOONTIME CONCERTS-SAN FRANCISCO'S MUSICAL LUNCH BREAK

756 Mission Street
San Francisco, CA 94103

Phone: 415-288-3840
Fax: 415-288-3838
e-mail: dsalslav@us.oracle.com
Web Site: www.sfcv.org
Management:
   Director: Alexandra Ivanoff
Performs At: St. Patrick's Church; Giannini Auditorium
Seating Capacity: 900

4189 OLD FIRST CONCERTS

1751 Sacramento Street
San Francisco, CA 94109
Phone: 415-474-1608
e-mail: staff@oldfirstconcerts.org
Web Site: www.oldfirstconcerts.org
Management:
   Administrative Manager: Domenic Pullano
Mission: To present emerging and under-recognized artists, as well as mid-career performers; to offer the orchestral musician a venue to express their musical individuality; to provide audiences with high quality chamber/new/worls/jazz music at an affordable price.
Founded: 1970
Performs At: Old First Church
Facility Category: Presbyterian Church
Type of Stage: Raised; Wooden
Seating Capacity: 450

4190 OMNI FOUNDATION FOR THE PERFORMING ARTS

236 W Portal Avenue
PMB 1
San Francisco, CA 94127
Phone: 650-726-1203
Fax: 650-726-9440
Toll-free: 888-400-6664
e-mail: director@omniconcerts.com
Web Site: www.omniconcerts.com
Management:
   Director: Richard Patterson
Founded: 1981
Specialized Field: Classical; Acoustic; Guitar Recitals
Paid Staff: 2
Paid Artists: 2
Budget: $125,000
Performs At: Herbst Theatre, San Francisco
Annual Attendance: 6,000
Seating Capacity: 915

4191 OTHER MINDS FESTIVAL

303 Valencia Street
#303
San Francisco, CA 94103
Phone: 510-934-8134
Fax: 510-934-8136
e-mail: otherminds@otherminds.org
Web Site: www.otherminds.org
Management:
   Executive Director: Charles Amirkhanian
Specialized Field: Instrumental; Multi-Media; Jazz; Dance; Ethnic
Budget: $35,000-$60,000
Season: Late March
Seating Capacity: 400 - 1,000

4192 SAN FRANCISCO BLUES FESTIVAL

PO Box 460608
San Francisco, CA 94146
Phone: 415-979-5588
Fax: 415-826-6958
e-mail: SFblues@earthlink.net
Web Site: www.sfblues.com
Management:
   Director: Tom Mazzolini
Founded: 1973
Annual Attendance: 18,000-20,000
Facility Category: Outdoors Lawns

4193 SAN FRANCISCO ETHNIC DANCE FESTIVAL

Fort Mason
Building D
San Francisco, CA 94123-1382
Phone: 415-474-3914
Fax: 415-474-3922
e-mail: wawstaff@worldartswest.org
Web Site: www.worldartswest.org
Management:
   Executive Director: Sarah Shelley
Specialized Field: Dance; Ethnic
Budget: $60,000-$150,000
Season: June
Affiliations: Palace of Fine Arts
Seating Capacity: 1,000

4194 SAN FRANCISCO FRINGE FESTIVAL

156 Eddy Street
San Francisco, CA 94102
Phone: 415-931-1094
Fax: 416-931-2699
e-mail: mail@sffringe.org
Web Site: www.sffringe.org
Founded: 1992
Volunteer Staff: 100

4195 SAN FRANCISCO PERFORMANCES

500 Sutter Street
Suite 710
San Francisco, CA 94102
Phone: 415-398-6449
Fax: 415-398-6439
e-mail: info@performances.org
Web Site: www.sfperformances.org
Officers:
   Chairman: Victor L Hymes
   Vice Chair: Gussie Stewart
   Secretary: Joan Burtzel
   Treasurer: C. William Criss, Jr
Management:
   President/Executive Director: Ruth A Felt
   Director Public Relations: Marian Kohlstedt
   Finance/Administration: Christian A Jessen
   Director Development: Maggie Pico
   Director Education Programs: Melanie Smith
   Director Marketing: Millicent Jones
Mission: To present outstanding national, international and emerging artists; to introduce innovative programs; to build new and diversified audiences for the arts.
Founded: 1979

Specialized Field: Chamber Music; Jazz; Contemporary Dance
Status: Professional
Paid Staff: 13
Budget: $2 million
Income Sources: Ticket Sales; Grants & Contributions
Performs At: Herbst Theatre; Cowell Theater at Fort Mason; Davies Symph.
Affiliations: Association of Performing Arts Presenters; International Society of Performing Arts Administrators; Western Arts Alliance
Annual Attendance: 48,000
Organization Type: Sponsoring
Resident Groups: Alexander String Quartet; Guitarist, Manuel Barrueco; Jazz Violin, Regina Clark

4196 SAN FRANCISCO SHAKESPEARE FESTIVAL

PO Box 590479
San Francisco, CA 941590479
Phone: 415-422-2222
Fax: 415-221-0643
e-mail: mccue@usfca.edu
Web Site: www.sfshakes.org
Management:
　Producing Director: Charlie McCue
Founded: 1982
Status: Nonprofit
Season: July - October
Seating Capacity: 1100

4197 SFJAZZ

3 Embarcadero Center
Lower Lobby
San Francisco, CA 94111
Phone: 415-398-5655
Fax: 415-398-5569
e-mail: mailbox@sfjazz.org
Web Site: www.sfjazz.org
Management:
　Executive Director: Randall Kline
　Development Director: Holly Kaslewicz

4198 STERN GROVE FESTIVAL ASSOCIATION

44 Page Street
Suite 600
San Francisco, CA 94102
Phone: 415-252-6252
Fax: 415-252-6250
e-mail: info@sterngrove.org
Web Site: www.sterngrove.org
Officers:
　Chairman: Douglas Goldman
　Treasurer: Robin Michel
　Program Chairman: Queenie Taylor
　Vice-Chairman: Dennis Wu
　Governance Chair: Wendy Bingham
　Development Chair: Glenn C Perry
　Secretary: Sandra Hernandez
Management:
　Executive Director: Corrina Marshall
　Director Programming: Hannah Bader
　Director Operations: Peter Palermo

Director Development: Rachel Fine
Mission: To present the highest quality performances, free of admission charge, to all Bay Area residents and visitors.
Founded: 1938
Specialized Field: Intsrumental Music; Vocal Music; Dance
Status: Professional; Nonprofit
Paid Staff: 8
Volunteer Staff: 300
Paid Artists: 15
Budget: $1.1 million
Income Sources: Foundations; Individuals; Government; Corporate
Season: June - August
Performs At: Sigmund Stern Grove (Festival Site)
Annual Attendance: 95,000
Facility Category: Ampitheatre
Seating Capacity: 8,000 - 10,000
Year Built: 1932
Organization Type: Sponsoring

4199 WORLD ARTS WEST

Fort Mason, Building D
San Francisco, CA 94123-1382
Phone: 415-474-3914
Fax: 415-474-3922
e-mail: wawstaff@worldartswest.org
Web Site: www.worldartswest.org
Management:
　Executive Director: Sarah Shelley
　Program Director: Antigone Trimis
　Adminiastractor Coordinator: Rob Taylor
Performs At: Palace of Fine Arts
Seating Capacity: 1000

4200 CAL POLY ARTS PRESENTS & GREAT PERFORMANCES

One Grand Avenue
San Luis Obispo, CA 93407
Phone: 805-756-7111
Fax: 805-756-5656
Toll-free: 888-233-2787
e-mail: cparts@polymail.calpoly.edu
Web Site: www.calpolyarts.org
Officers:
　President: Harry Heilenbrond
Management:
　Program Manager: Peter Wilt
　Director: Ralph Hoskins
　Marketing Director: Lira Woske
　Interim Director Development: Evie Globerman
Mission: To provide a broad program of high quality, professional touring performances, exhibitions, and readings while also assisting with the educational needs of students through various artist-residency activities.
Paid Staff: 6
Volunteer Staff: 175
Budget: $1 million
Income Sources: Box Office; Grants; Private Donations; Corporate Donations
Performs At: Harman Hall; Cal Poly Theatre
Affiliations: California Presenters; Association of Performing Arts Presenters; Western Arts Alliance

Annual Attendance: 75,000
Facility Category: Performing Arts Center; Theatre
Type of Stage: Proscenium
Stage Dimensions: 49'x23'
Seating Capacity: 1,300; 497
Year Built: 1996
Cost: 34 million
Rental Contact: 805-756-7222 Ron Regier

4201 CUESTA COLLEGE PUBLIC EVENTS

PO Box 8106
San Luis Obispo, CA 93403-8106
Phone: 805-546-3132
Fax: 805-546-3968
e-mail: sblattn@bass.cuesta.cc.ca.us
Web Site: www.communityprograms.com
Management:
    Manager: Sharon Blattner
Performs At: College Auditorium; Cuesta Interact
Theatre
Seating Capacity: 810; 150

4202 SAN LUIS OBISPO MOZART FESTIVAL

PO Box 311
San Luis Obispo, CA 93406
Phone: 805-781-3008
Fax: 805-781-3011
e-mail: info@mozartfestival.com
Web Site: www.mozartfestival.com
Officers:
    Associate Conductor: Jeffrey Kahane
Management:
    Music Director: Clifton Swanson
    Executive Director: Curtis Pendleton
Mission: To present a classical music festival highlighting
Mozart and other classical and contemporary composers.
Founded: 1970
Specialized Field: Instrumental; Opera; Choral; Jazz;
Childrens'; Ethnic; Educational
Status: Professional; Nonprofit
Budget: $150,000-$400,000
Season: July - August
Performs At: Throughout San Luis Obispo County
(Festival Sites)
Affiliations: San Luis Performing Arts Center; Wineries;
Chapels
Seating Capacity: 1,300
Organization Type: Performing; Educational

4203 CENTERSTAGE, OSHER MARIN JCC

200 N San Pedro Road
San Rafael, CA 94903
Phone: 415-444-8000
Fax: 415-491-1235
e-mail: centerstage1@marinjcc.org
Web Site: www.marinjcc.org
Management:
    Artistic Director: Greg Phillips
    Managing Director: Larry Fishkin
    Marketing Director: Mike Tekulsky
Performs At: Auditorium
Seating Capacity: 500

4204 COMMUNITY ARTS AND MUSIC ASSOCIATION OF SANTA BARBARA

111 E Yanonali Street
Santa Barbara, CA 93101-1822
Phone: 805-966-4324
Fax: 805-932-2014
e-mail: info@camasb.org
Web Site: www.camasb.org
Officers:
    Executive Director: Mark Truebllod
    President: Judith Lynn Hopkinson
    Director Development: Nancy Lynn
Management:
    Concert/Publicity Manager: Justin Weaver
Mission: To bring the world's greatest orchestras and
soloists to Santa Barbara and enrich the cultural aspect of
our community.
Founded: 1919
Specialized Field: Instrumental Music
Status: Nonprofit
Paid Staff: 4
Budget: $1,200,000
Income Sources: Grants; Foundations; Individual
Donations; Investment Income
Performs At: Arlington Theatre; Lobero Theatre
Annual Attendance: 18,000
Facility Category: Historic Movie House and Concert
Hall; Historic Opera House
Type of Stage: Theatre Stage; Opera Stage
Seating Capacity: 2,018
Year Built: 1923
Year Remodeled: 1976
Rental Contact: Karen Killingworth
Organization Type: Sponsoring

4205 MUSIC ACADEMY OF THE WEST FESTIVAL

1070 Fairway Road
Santa Barbara, CA 93108-2899
Phone: 805-969-4726
Fax: 805-969-0686
e-mail: festival@musicacademy.org
Web Site: www.musicacademy.org
Officers:
    Chairman: Carole E Halsted
    First Vice Chairman: Judith W Bartholomew
    Treasurer: Richard A Archer
    Second Vice Chairman: Benjamin J Cohen Jr
Management:
    President: David L Kuehn, DMA
    VP/Artistic Operations: Samuel Dixon
    Director Communications: Diane Eagle Kataoka
Mission: To maintain a pre-professional instrumental
company with vocal instruction.
Founded: 1947
Specialized Field: Instrumental; Opera; Educational
Status: Professional; Non-Professional; Nonprofit
Paid Staff: 30
Volunteer Staff: 90
Paid Artists: 40
Budget: $1,050,000 - 3,600,000
Income Sources: Individual Contributions; Foundations;
Corporations
Season: June - August

All listings are in alphabetical order by state, then city, then organization within the city.

Performs At: Santa Barbara (Festival Site)
Affiliations: Lobero Theatre
Annual Attendance: 17,000
Seating Capacity: 680
Year Built: 1909
Organization Type: Performing; Educational; Sponsoring
Resident Groups: The Canadian Brass

4206 SANTA BARBARA FESTIVAL BALLET
29 W Calle Laureles
PO Box 2327
Santa Barbara, CA 93105
Phone: 805-560-8883
Fax: 805-966-9521
Management:
Artistic Director: Michele Rinaldi
Co-Artistic Director: Denise Rinaldi
Co-Artistic Director: Michele Anderson

4207 UCSB ARTS & LECTURES
University of California
Santa Barbara, CA 93106-5030
Phone: 805-893-2080
Fax: 805-893-8637
e-mail: a&l-info@sa.ucsb.edu
Web Site: www.artsandlectures.ucsb.edu
Management:
Performing Arts Manager: Cathy Oliverson
Marketing Director: Susan Gwyane
Director Operations: Robert King
Director: Celesta Billeci
Mission: To present a wide variety of professional touring artists and ensembles in dance, theater, classical music, ethnic and traditional arts, film and literature for campus and community audiences.
Founded: 1959
Specialized Field: Dance; Vocal Music; Instrumental Music; Theater
Status: Professional; Nonprofit
Paid Staff: 12
Income Sources: Western Alliance of Arts Administrators; Arts Presenters; California Presenters
Performs At: Campbell Hall
Seating Capacity: 860
Organization Type: Performing; Educational; Presenting

4208 ARTS & LECTURES
University of California at Santa Cruz
D106 Porter
1156 High Street
Santa Cruz, CA 95064
Phone: 831-459-3861
Fax: 831-459-4521
e-mail: artslecs@cats.ucsc.edu
Web Site: events.ucsc.edu/artslecs
Management:
Arts/Lectures Manager: Michelle Witt
Publicity/Production Coordinator: Moon Rinaldo
Specialized Field: Dance; Theater; Spoken Word/Lectures; World Music; Classical; Jazz
Performs At: Performing Arts Theater
Seating Capacity: 528

4209 CABRILLO FESTIVAL OF CONTEMPORARY MUSIC
104 Walnut Avenue
Suite 206
Santa Cruz, CA 95060
Phone: 831-426-6966
Fax: 831-426-6968
e-mail: info@cabrillomusic.org
Web Site: www.cabrillomusic.org
Management:
Music Director: Marin Alsop
Development Director: Tom Fredricks
Executive Director: Ellen Primack
Founded: 1963
Specialized Field: Instrumental
Budget: $480,000
Season: July
Performs At: S. Cruz Civic Auditorium; Mission San Juan Bautista
Seating Capacity: 1,000

4210 SANTA CRUZ BAROQUE FESTIVAL
PO Box 482
Santa Cruz, CA 95061
Phone: 831-457-9693
e-mail: s.c.baroque@juno.com
Web Site: www.scbaroque.org
Management:
General Manager: Linda K Fawcett
Artistic Director: Linda Burman-Hall
Mission: Offering a series of early music concerts each spring.
Founded: 1974
Specialized Field: Instrumental
Status: Professional; Nonprofit
Budget: $10,000-$20,000
Season: February - May
Facility Category: Various auditoriums
Seating Capacity: 400
Organization Type: Performing; Sponsoring

4211 CONCERTS WEST
630 San Vicente Boulevard
Unit T
Santa Monica, CA 90402
Phone: 310-393-1155
Fax: 310-393-1155
e-mail: mpreston@ix.netcom.com
Management:
Artistic Director: Howard Colf
Performs At: Unitarian Universalist Community Church of Santa Monica
Seating Capacity: 225

4212 MUSIC AT OAKMONT CONCERT SERIES
444 Crestridge Place
Santa Rosa, CA 95409
Phone: 707-539-7066
Fax: 707-539-0894
e-mail: bartok2@sonic.net
Officers:
VP: Victor Spear

Secretary/Treasurer: Maureen Christ
Management:
   Artistic Director: Robert Hayden
   Assistant Artistic Director: Rosemarie Waller
   Associate Artistic Director: Victor Spear
   Programs: Judy Burness
Founded: 1990
Specialized Field: Classical Vocal and Instrumental
Solos; Chamber Music
Budget: $14,000
Income Sources: Entrance Fees
Performs At: Oakmont Auditorium
Seating Capacity: 650
Year Built: 1990
Year Remodeled: 2002

4213 REDWOODS FESTIVAL

PO Box 1766
Santa Rosa, CA 95402
Phone: 707-542-2995
Fax: 707-542-2995
e-mail: operalafayette@operalafayette.org
Web Site: www.operalafayette.org
Management:
   Artistic Director: Ryan Brown
   Administrative Assistant: Michelle Sikora
Mission: To present historically-informed performances
from the 17th and 18th centruy repertoire on period
instruments with the finest musicians/interpreters of this
genre. To educate children and adults in this period.
Specialized Field: Opera, Chamber Music, Summer
Season Redwoods Festival
Paid Staff: 4
Budget: $35,000-$60,000
Season: August, weekends
Performs At: Sonoma County (Festival Site)
Affiliations: Various Sonoma County wineries and
mansions
Seating Capacity: 1,300

4214 SANTA ROSA COMMUNITY CONCERT ASSOCIATION

PO Box 4821
Santa Rosa, CA 95402
Phone: 707-546-1152
Officers:
   President: John Lawrence
Performs At: Burbank Center for the Performing Arts
Seating Capacity: 1500

4215 MOUNTAIN WINERY

14837 Pierce Road
PO Box 2279
Saratoga, CA 95070
Phone: 408-741-0763
Fax: 408-741-0733
e-mail: events@mountainwinery
Web Site: www.mountainwinery.com
Mission: To enhance the cultural atmosphere of the San
Francisco Bay Area
Founded: 1957
Specialized Field: Vocal Music; Instrumental Music;
Theater
Status: Professional

Paid Staff: 70
Paid Artists: 70
Performs At: Mountain Winery
Annual Attendance: 100,000
Facility Category: Winerey
Type of Stage: Open Air
Stage Dimensions: 27'x24'
Seating Capacity: 1,700
Year Built: 1902
Rental Contact: Mark Karakas
Organization Type: Performing; Sponsoring

4216 TAHOE ARTS PROJECT

1156 Ski Run Boulevard
PO Box 14281
South Lake Tahoe, CA 96151
Phone: 530-542-3632
Fax: 530-542-4792
e-mail: tahoearts@aol.com
Management:
   Executive Director: Peggy Aguilar-Thompson
Mission: To provide cultural enrichment and diversity for
the community through the arts and education, with
particular focus on our youth.
Founded: 1987
Status: Nonprofit
Paid Staff: 2
Paid Artists: 5
Budget: $100,000
Income Sources: Grants; Donations; Fundraising Events
Facility Category: Schools
Seating Capacity: 200-1,200

4217 STANFORD JAZZ FESTIVAL & WORKSHOP

PO Box 20454
Stanford, CA 94309
Phone: 650-736-0324
e-mail: info@stanfordjazz.org
Web Site: www.stanfordjazz.org
Management:
   Director: Jim Nadel

4218 STANFORD LIVELY ARTS

537 Lomita Mall, MC 2250
Stanford University
Stanford, CA 94305-2250
Phone: 650-723-2551
Fax: 650-723-8231
e-mail: livelyarts@stanford.edu
Web Site: www.livelyarts.stanford.edu
Management:
   Executive Director: Lois Wagner
   Director Education/Programming: Martin Wolesen
Mission: To create unique expirecnces for diverse
communities and artists to share paaion, knowledge,
creative inspiration, and cultural traditions through live
performance and arts education.
Founded: 1969
Performs At: Memorial Auditorium
Annual Attendance: 55,000
Facility Category: Theater
Type of Stage: Proscenium
Stage Dimensions: 40'x50'

Seating Capacity: 1710

4219 UNIVERSITY OF THE PACIFIC CONSERVATORY OF MUSIC - RESIDENT ARTIST SERIES

3601 Pacific Avenue
Stockton, CA 95211
Phone: 209-946-2417
Fax: 209-946-2770
e-mail: sanderson@uop.edu
Web Site: www.uop.edu/conservatory/index.html
Management:
    DMA Dean: Stephen C Anderson
Performs At: Faye Spanos Concert Hall
Seating Capacity: 1000

4220 ARTS FOR THE SCHOOLS

PO Box 230
Tahoe Vista, CA 96148
Phone: 530-546-4602
e-mail: kyagura@sierra.net
Web Site: www.brainclick.com/afts
Management:
    Director: Terry Yagura
Mission: To provide artistic, educational and cultural opportunies for students, residents, and guests in Lake Tahoe.
Founded: 1984
Status: Nonprofit; Volunteer
Performs At: School Auditorium; Cal-Neva
Seating Capacity: 300; 350

4221 CALIFORNIA LUTHERAN UNIVERSITY MUSIC SERIES

60 W Olsen Road
Thousand Oaks, CA 91360-2787
Phone: 805-492-2411
Fax: 805-493-3479
e-mail: morton@clunet.edu
Web Site: www.clunet.edu
Management:
    Orchestra Conductor: Daniel Geeting
    Chair Music Department: Wyant Morton
Budget: $10,000
Performs At: Samuelson Chapel; Forum
Seating Capacity: 650; 250

4222 CONEJO RECREATION & PARK DISTRICT SUMMER CONCERT SERIES

155 E Wilbur Road
Thousand Oaks, CA 91360-5565
Phone: 805-495-6471
Fax: 805-497-3199
e-mail: recadmin@crpd.org
Web Site: www.crpd.org
Management:
    Administrator: Jesse Washington
    Recreation Services Manager: Steve Wiley
Performs At: Outdoors
Annual Attendance: 12,000-15,000
Type of Stage: Stage
Seating Capacity: 4600

4223 SPRING MUSIC FESTIVAL

California Institute of the Arts, School
24700 McBean Pkwy
Valencia, CA 91355
Phone: 661-225-1050
Fax: 805-254-8352
Web Site: www.music.calarts.edu
Management:
    Dean School of Music: David Rosenboom
    Production Manager: Bob Clendenen
Mission: To present contemporary music celebrating global traditions.
Status: Professional; Nonprofit
Performs At: California Institute of the Arts; Japan American
Organization Type: Performing; Educational

4224 VENTURA CHAPTER MUSIC FESTIVAL

89 South California Street
Suite D
Ventura, CA 93001
Phone: 805-648-3146
Fax: 805-648-4103
Toll-free: 888-882-8263
e-mail: nemfadir@aol.com
Web Site: www.vcmfa.org
Officers:
    President: Donna De Paola
Management:
    Artistic Director: Dr. E Burns Taft
    Executive Director: Patricia Young
Mission: Annual music festival
Founded: 1994
Specialized Field: Instrumental; Opera; Choral; Dance; Childrens'; Educational
Paid Staff: 1
Volunteer Staff: 300
Paid Artists: 40
Budget: $60,000-$400,000
Season: May
Affiliations: American Symphony League; Chamber Music America
Annual Attendance: 4,000
Facility Category: Historic buildings in downtown Ventura
Seating Capacity: 100 - 1,100

4225 VISALIA CULTURAL PROGRAMS-ON STAGE VISALIA

303 E Acequia
Visalia, CA 93291
Phone: 559-730-7000
Fax: 559-738-3579
e-mail: vcc@ci.visalia.ca.us
Web Site: www.visalia.org
Management:
    General Manager: Jim Thompson

4226 MOUNT SAN ANTONIO COLLEGE SERIES

1100 N Grand Avenue
Walnut, CA 91789

Phone: 909-594-5611
Fax: 909-468-3937
e-mail: kmeyers@mtsac.edu
Web Site: www.mtsac.edu
Officers:
   VP Community Education/Economic Dev: Karen Meyers
Management:
   Public Information/Event Specialist: Brian Yokoyama
Founded: 1946
Specialized Field: Music, Dance, Theater
Paid Staff: 2

4227 COLLEGE OF THE SISKIYOUS PERFORMING ARTS SERIES

800 College Avenue
Weed, CA 96094
Phone: 530-938-5373
Fax: 530-938-5570
e-mail: cozzalio@siskiyous.edu
Web Site: www.siskiyous.edu
Management:
   Public Relations Director: Dawna Cozzalio
Performs At: College Theatre
Seating Capacity: 584

4228 WHITTIER COLLEGE BACH FESTIVAL

PO Box 634
13406 E Philadelphia Street
Whittier, CA 90608
Phone: 562-907-4237
Fax: 562-907-4237
e-mail: dlozano@whittier.edu
Management:
   Director: Danilo Lozano
Specialized Field: Instrumental
Budget: $10,000
Season: March
Performs At: Whittier College Campus (Festival Site)
Facility Category: Whittier College Memorial Chapel & other venues
Seating Capacity: 300

4229 VALLEY CULTURAL CENTER CONCERTS IN THE PARK

21550 Oxnard Street
#470
Woodland Hills, CA 91367-7110
Phone: 818-704-1358
Fax: 818-704-1604
Web Site: www.valleycultural.org
Management:
   Executive Director: James W Kinsey III
Performs At: Lou Bredlow Pavillion; Warner Park

Colorado

4230 ASPEN MUSIC FESTIVAL AND SCHOOL

2 Music School Road
Aspen, CO 81611

Phone: 970-925-3254
Fax: 970-920-1643
e-mail: festival@aspenmusic.org
Web Site: www.aspenmusicfestival.com
Officers:
   President/CEO: Don Roth
Management:
   Music Director: David Zinman
   General Manager: James Berdahl
Founded: 1949
Budget: $11,000,000
Performs At: Joan & Irving Harris Concert Hall; Benedict Music Tent
Seating Capacity: 500; 2,050
Year Built: 2000

4231 JAZZ ASPEN SNOWMASS

110 E Hallam Street
Suite 104
Aspen, CO 81611
Phone: 970-920-4996
Fax: 970-920-9135
e-mail: jazzaspen@jazzaspen.com
Web Site: www.jazzaspen.com
Officers:
   Executive Producer: James Honowitz
   Executive VP/Sales/Marketing: Marc Breslin
Mission: To create world-class programing of jazz, American and world music, to educate and entertain audiences of diverse tastes and backgrounds, to preserve America's musical heritage.
Founded: 1991
Specialized Field: Music; Jazz
Income Sources: Ticket Sales; Grants; Donations

4232 BOULDER BACH FESTIVAL

PO Box 1896
Boulder, CO 80306
Phone: 303-494-3159
Fax: 303-494-4940
e-mail: BolderBach@aol.com
Web Site: www.boulderbachfest.org
Management:
   Music Director: Robert Spillman
   Executive Director: Cheryl Staats
Specialized Field: Instrumental; Choral
Paid Staff: 1
Volunteer Staff: 200
Paid Artists: 40
Budget: $100,000
Income Sources: Admissions; Donations; Grants
Season: January
Performs At: Boulder (Festival Site)
Affiliations: First Prebytery Church
Annual Attendance: 2,500
Seating Capacity: 800

4233 BOULDER INTERNATIONAL MUSIC FESTIVAL FOR YOUNG PERFORMERS

2955 Dover Drive
Boulder, CO 80303
Phone: 303-494-6975
Fax: 303-494-8225
e-mail: bimfya@uswestmail.net

Management:
Festival Director: Elena Mathys
Specialized Field: Instrumental; Recital/Workshops; Educational
Season: June
Facility Category: Saint Paul United Methodist Church

4234 COLORADO MAHLERFEST

PO Box 1314
Boulder, CO 80306-1314
Phone: 303-447-0513
Fax: 303-447-0514
e-mail: stanrutt@aol.com
Web Site: www.mahlerfest.org
Officers:
President: Stan Ruttenberg
VP: Barry G Knapp
Management:
Artistic Director: Robert Olson
Mission: To perform all the music of Gustav Mahler.
Founded: 1988
Specialized Field: Instrumental; Multi-Media; Choral
Budget: $45,000
Income Sources: Box Office; Grants; Donations
Season: July
Performs At: University of Colorado; Boulder (Festival Site)
Facility Category: University Auditorium
Seating Capacity: 2,000
Year Built: 1896
Year Remodeled: 1982

4235 COLORADO MUSIC FESTIVAL

1525 Spruce Street
Suite 101
Boulder, CO 80302
Phone: 303-449-1397
Fax: 303-449-0071
e-mail: cmf@coloradomusicfest.org
Web Site: www.coloradomusicfest.org
Officers:
President: Patricia Magette
Management:
Music Director: Michael Christie
Executive Director: Michael A Smith
Mission: To develop and promote an appreciation and love for the musical arts through the operation of an international professional orchestra; to present traditional symphonic literature; to challenge audiences with new or contemporary compositions; to stimulate an intellectual experience.
Founded: 1977
Specialized Field: Instrumental; Childrens'
Status: Professional; Nonprofit
Budget: $400,000-$1,000,000
Income Sources: American Symphony Orchestra League
Season: June - August
Performs At: Boulder (Festival Site)
Facility Category: Chautauqua Auditorium, Boulder
Seating Capacity: 1,250
Year Built: 1898
Organization Type: Performing

4236 COLORADO SHAKESPEARE FESTIVAL

University of Colorado
277 UCB
Boulder, CO 80309-0277
Phone: 303-492-1527
Fax: 303-735-5140
e-mail: csfbo@colorado.edu
Web Site: www.coloradoshakes.org
Management:
Artistic Director: Richard M Devin
General Manager: Lynn Nichols
Business Manager: Ray Kembles
Mission: To produce an aesthetically challenging mix of both traditional and innovative productions of Shakespeare's plays.
Founded: 1958
Specialized Field: Theater
Status: Professional; Nonprofit
Paid Staff: 150
Volunteer Staff: 500
Paid Artists: 120
Budget: $1 million
Income Sources: Blue Mountain Arts
Season: June - August
Performs At: Mary Rippon Outdoor Theatre; University Mainstage Theatre
Annual Attendance: 41,000
Facility Category: Outdoor Theatre; Indoor Theatre
Type of Stage: Greco-Roman; Proscenium
Seating Capacity: 1,000; 400
Year Built: 1936
Organization Type: Performing

4237 CU COORS EVENTS
Conference Center

University of Colorado
Regent Drive
Boulder, CO 80309
Phone: 303-492-5316
Fax: 303-492-4801
e-mail: eggertk@spot.colorado.edu
Web Site: www.colorado.edu
Management:
Director: Steven Wells

4238 EARLY MUSIC COLORADO FALL FESTIVAL OF EARLY MUSIC

PO Box 19078
Boulder, CO 80308-2078
Phone: 303-509-6039
e-mail: nurseholiday@uswest.net
Web Site: www.EarlyMusicColorado.org
Officers:
President: Leland G Hoover
Ex-Officio: Rebecca Beshore
Founded: 1992
Specialized Field: Instrumental; Choral
Status: Nonprofit; Tax-Exempt
Paid Artists: 50
Non-paid Artists: 50
Budget: $10,000
Season: February, May, July, October
Affiliations: Denver Aqmerican Recorder Society
Facility Category: Boulder Public Library

Seating Capacity: 500-700

4239 PEAK ASSOCIATION OF THE ARTS
Dairy Center for the Arts
2590 Walnut Street, Suite 6
Boulder, CO 80302-5700
Phone: 303-449-1343
Fax: 303-443-9203
e-mail: info@peakarts.org
Web Site: www.peakarts.org
Officers:
    President: Robert McAllister
Management:
    Music Director/Conductor: Theodore Kuchar
    Operations Director: Ed Williams
    Personel Manager: Nancy Headlee
    Chorale Director: Timothy Kreuger
Mission: To offer music, classical dance and arts education experiences.
Status: Nonprofit

4240 UNIVERSITY OF COLORADO CONCERTS
31 UCB
University of Colorado
Boulder, CO 80309-0301
Phone: 303-492-8008
Fax: 303-492-5619
e-mail: braunj@colorado.edu
Web Site: www.colorado.edu/music
Management:
    Executive Director: Joan McLean Braun
    Marketing Manager: Laima Gaigalas
    Operations Manager: Sandra Miller
Mission: The Artsist Series offers the highest quality emerging and internationally acclaimed soloists and ensembles with related educational programs and residency activities.
Founded: 1937
Paid Staff: 5
Performs At: Macky Auditorium

4241 BRECKENRIDGE MUSIC FESTIVAL
PO Box 1254
217 S Ridge Street
Breckenridge, CO 80424
Phone: 970-453-9142
Fax: 970-453-9143
e-mail: bmynro@breckenridgemusicfestival.net
Web Site: www.breckenridgemusicfestival.net
Management:
    BMI Conductor: Gerhardt Zimmermann
    NRO Director: Carl Topilow
    Executive Director: Jeff Baum
    Administrator/Marketing/Programs: Sara Anton
Specialized Field: Instrumental; Multi-Media; Opera; Choral; Jazz; Folk; Theatre; Educational
Paid Staff: 16
Volunteer Staff: 36
Budget: $150,000-$400,000
Season: Late June - Mid August
Performs At: Breckenridge (Festival Site)
Facility Category: Riverwalk Center Amphitheater
Seating Capacity: 750

4242 BRECKENRIDGE MUSIC INSTITUTE
130 Ski Hill Road
PO Box 1254
Breckenridge, CO 80424
Phone: 303-453-9142
Fax: 303-453-1423
Officers:
    President: RH VanDenburg
    VP: Charles Simpson
    Secretary: James Robertson
    Treasurer: Richard L Thomas
Management:
    Executive Director: Pamela G Miller
    Music Advisor: Peter Bay
    Festival Administrator: Daniel Schmidt
    Administrative Assistant: Allison Rouse
Mission: To provide cultural and educational growth and enrichment in music for Summit County residents and visitors.
Founded: 1980
Specialized Field: Vocal Music; Instrumental Music; Festivals
Status: Professional; Nonprofit
Performs At: Breckenridge Event Tent
Organization Type: Performing; Educational

4243 COLORADO COLLEGE SUMMER MUSIC FESTIVAL
The Colorado College
14 East Cache La Poudre Street
Colorado Springs, CO 80903
Phone: 719-389-6655
Fax: 719-389-6955
e-mail: festival@coloradocollege.edu
Web Site: www.coloradocollege.edu/summersession
Management:
    Summer Programs Coordinator: Paula Thomas
Mission: The Colorado College Summer Music Festival was founded in 1984, originally as the Summer Conservatory, to bring the highest level of chamber music performance to Colorado Springs and to offer a unique kind of intense training to promising young musicians.
Founded: 1984
Specialized Field: Chamber Music; Chamber Orchestra
Paid Staff: 4
Paid Artists: 16
Budget: $60,000-$150,000
Income Sources: Colorado College; Private Donors; Corporations; Foundations
Season: June - July
Performs At: Colorado College; Colorado Springs (Festival Site)
Affiliations: The Colorado Music Alliance
Annual Attendance: 2,500
Facility Category: Packard Hall
Seating Capacity: 350

4244 COLORADO SPRINGS FINE ARTS CENTER PERFORMING ARTS SERIES
30 West Dale
Colorado Springs, CO 80903
Phone: 719-643-5581
Fax: 719-634-0570
e-mail: rgeers@aol.com

Management:
   Performing Arts Program Director: Robert Geers
   Executive Director: Fran Holden
   Deputy Director: Nancy Sullivan
Performs At: Theatre
Seating Capacity: 450

4245 CRESTED BUTTE CHAMBER MUSIC FESTIVAL
PO Box 992
Crested Butte, CO 81224
Phone: 970-349-5864
Fax: 970-349-5864
Management:
   Artistic Director: Claire Jolivet
   Administrative Director: Karrie Tenley
Specialized Field: Instrumental; Choral; Folk; Ethnic
Budget: $20,000-$35,000
Season: July - August
Performs At: Crested Butte, CO (Festival Site)
Facility Category: Crested Butte Chamber Music Festival
Seating Capacity: 250

4246 CHERRY CREEK ARTS FESTIVAL
2 Steele Street
#B-100
Denver, CO 80206-5728
Phone: 303-355-2787
Fax: 303-355-2788
e-mail: management@cherryarts.org
Web Site: www.cherryarts.org
Officers:
   President/CEO: Bruce Storey
Founded: 1990
Specialized Field: Instrumental; Folk; Dance; Theatre
Paid Staff: 8
Volunteer Staff: 800
Non-paid Artists: 200
Budget: $60,000-$150,000
Season: July
Performs At: Cherry Creek North Business District (Festival Site)
Annual Attendance: 350,000
Facility Category: Outdoor
Stage Dimensions: 24'x 32'; 20'x16'; 20'x16'
Seating Capacity: 3,000; 1,000; 450

4247 COLORADO COUNCIL ON THE ARTS
750 Pennsylvania Street
Denver, CO 80203-3699
Phone: 303-894-2617
Fax: 303-894-2615
e-mail: fran.holden@state.co.us
Web Site: www.coloarts.state.co.us
Officers:
   Chairman: Donald K Bain
Management:
   Executive Director: Fran Holden
   Associate Director: Kelleen Zubick
   Associate Director: Maryo Ewell
Mission: To stimulate arts development in the state, to assist and encourage artists and arts organizations, and to help make the arts more accessible statewide.

Founded: 1967
Specialized Field: Visual; Performing; Literary Arts.
Status: Professional; Nonprofit; State Agency
Paid Staff: 7
Budget: $1,900,000
Income Sources: Annual State Appropriation; Federal Grants; Foundation Grants
Affiliations: National Endowment for the Arts; Western States Arts Federation; National Association of Local Arts Agencies
Organization Type: Sponsoring; Grant Making

4248 MUSIC IN THE MOUNTAINS INTERNATIONAL FESTIVAL
PO Box 3751
Durango, CO 81302
Phone: 970-385-6820
Fax: 970-259-9867
e-mail: showcase@rmi.net
Web Site: www.musicinthemountains.com
Management:
   Music Director: Mischa Semanitzky
   Festival Manager: Kay Ulwelling
Specialized Field: Instrumental; Childrens'
Budget: $10,000 - 20,000
Season: July - August
Performs At: Purgatory Ski Resort, Durango (Festival Site)
Facility Category: Tent
Seating Capacity: 600

4249 MUSIC IN THE MOUNTAINS
465 Longs Peak Road
Estes Park, CO 80517-6422
Phone: 970-586-4031
Fax: 970-586-4031
e-mail: rrmcoffice@aol.com
Officers:
   President: Mary Jane Clark
Management:
   Music Director: Elizabeth Mueller Grace
Mission: To provide live classical music of the highest quality to the Four Corners of Colorado, New Mexico, Utah and Arizona.
Founded: 1986
Specialized Field: Instrumental
Status: Professional; Nonprofit
Budget: $20,000 - 35,000
Season: Late June - Late August, Sundays
Performs At: Estes Park, CO (Festival Site)
Facility Category: Rocky Ridge Music Center
Seating Capacity: 250
Organization Type: Performing; Educational

4250 ROCKY RIDGE MUSIC CENTER
465 Longs Peak Road
Estes Park, CO 80517
Phone: 970-586-4031
Fax: 970-586-3962
e-mail: RRmcoffice@aol.com
Web Site: www.rockyridge.org
Officers:
   Founder: Beth Miller Harrod
   President: Madison Casey

VP: Miriam Reitz Baer
Management:
   Music Director: Elizabeth Grace
   Director Student Activities: Sandie Anderson
Mission: To offer summer programs of conservatory-level music training for young people, with emphasis on Youth Orchestra, young pianists, chamber music and composition; to offer this program simultaneously with the summer concert series, Music in the Mountains.
Founded: 1942
Specialized Field: Instrumental Music; Festivals
Status: Nonprofit
Paid Staff: 4
Annual Attendance: 300
Facility Category: Log cabins - historical
Seating Capacity: 150
Year Built: 1900
Year Remodeled: 1990
Organization Type: Performing; Educational

4251 SUMMIT JAZZ SWINGING JAZZ CONCERTS

PO Box 1150
Evergreen, CO 80437
Phone: 303-674-4190
Fax: 303-674-2122
e-mail: summitjazz@cs.com
Web Site: www.summitjazz.org
Officers:
   President: Alan P Frederickson
   Secretary/Treasurer: Juanita P Greenwood
Mission: to foster awareness and appreciation of traditional jazz through public concert performances by internationally recognized artists who have earned their reputation as dedicated exponents of this musical genre.

4252 MESA COUNTY COMMUNITY CONCERT ASSOCIATION

1220 Main Street
Grand Junction, CO 81501
Phone: 970-245-2083
Officers:
   Secretary: Jackie Porter
Performs At: Grand Junction High School Auditorium

4253 MESA SUMMER THEATRE FESTIVAL
Mesa State College

PO Box 2647
Grand Junction, CO 81502
Phone: 970-248-1540
Fax: 970-248-1159
Web Site: www.mesa7.mesa.colorado.edu/fpa/thea/
Management:
   Production Manager: David M Cox
   Production Director: Peter Ivanov
Founded: 1970
Specialized Field: Musicals, Non-Musicals
Status: Non-Equity; Nonprofit
Season: June - August
Type of Stage: Proscenium
Stage Dimensions: 50' x 34'
Seating Capacity: 625

4254 LOVELAND FRIENDS OF CHAMBER MUSIC

1000 King Drive
Loveland, CO 80537
Phone: 970-663-7928
Management:
   Music Director: Ruth J Hale
Performs At: Private Homes

4255 MUSIC IN OURAY

PO Box 14
Ouray, CO 81427
Phone: 970-626-5506
Fax: 970-626-4341
e-mail: chimney@rmi.net
Web Site: www.musicinouray.com
Management:
   Director: Soozie Arnold
Specialized Field: Instrumental
Budget: $35,000 - 60,000
Season: Early June
Facility Category: Wright Opera House, Ouray
Seating Capacity: 200

4256 SANGRE DE CRISTO ARTS AND CONFERENCE CENTER

210 North Santa Fe Avenue
Pueblo, CO 81003
Phone: 719-543-0130
Fax: 719-543-0134
e-mail: mail@solc-arts.org
Web Site: www.solc-arts.org
Management:
   Director: Maggie Divelbiss
   Associate Director: Jennifer Cook
   Technical Director: Timothy F Gately
Mission: Supporting diverse visual and performing arts in the Southeastern Colorado area.
Founded: 1972
Specialized Field: Dance; Vocal Music; Instrumental Music; Theater; Festivals; Lyric Opera
Status: Professional; Nonprofit
Paid Staff: 40
Volunteer Staff: 50
Income Sources: Association of Performing Arts Presenters; Western Alliance of Arts Administrators; Rocky Mountain Theatre Guild
Performs At: Sangre de Cristo Arts and Conference Center
Annual Attendance: 10,000
Facility Category: Arts Center
Type of Stage: Proscenium
Stage Dimensions: 35'x20'x22'
Seating Capacity: 496
Year Built: 1972
Rental Contact: Lorrie Marquez
Organization Type: Performing; Touring; Resident; Educational; Sponsoring

4257 TELLURIDE JAZZ CELEBRATION
Telluride Society for Jazz

PO Box 2132
Telluride, CO 81435

Phone: 970-728-7009
Fax: 970-728-5834
e-mail: paul@telluridejazz.com
Web Site: www.telluridejazz.com
Management:
   Director: Paul Machado
   President: John Burchmore
Mission: Jazz music
Founded: 1977
Specialized Field: Music Education
Paid Staff: 12
Volunteer Staff: 125
Paid Artists: 100
Non-paid Artists: 60
Budget: $ 300,000
Seating Capacity: 3,000

4258 TYER CHAMBER MUSIC FESTIVAL
PO Box 115
Telluride, CO 81435
Phone: 970-728-8686
Fax: 970-728-8686
Toll-free: 800-525-3455
e-mail: klangs@rmi.net
Web Site: www.telluride.com/chamber.html
Management:
   Director: Roy Malan
   Director: Robin Sutherford
   President: Kay Langstaff
Specialized Field: Instrumental
Budget: $10,000
Season: August
Performs At: Telluride (Festival Site)
Facility Category: Sheridan Opera House
Seating Capacity: 240

4259 ACADEMY CONCERTS
USAFA/34TRW/SDAE
2302 Cadet Drive, Suite 12
USAF Acadamy, CO 80840-6000
Phone: 719-333-4497
Fax: 719-333-4597
Management:
   Cultural Arts/Entertainment Dir: Candyce Thomas
Mission: To offer the Cadet Wing cultural enhancements, entertaining rock concerts, and comedians; to offer our military personnel and community cultural events.
Founded: 1959
Paid Staff: 4
Performs At: Arnold Hall Theater
Annual Attendance: 28,000
Facility Category: Theater; Concert Hall
Type of Stage: Proscenium
Seating Capacity: 2,809
Year Built: 1957
Year Remodeled: 1999

4260 BRAVO! VAIL VALLEY MUSIC FESTIVAL
PO Box 2270
Vail, CO 81658

Phone: 970-827-5700
Fax: 970-827-5707
Toll-free: 877-827-5700
e-mail: bravo@vail.net
Web Site: www.vailmusicfestival.org
Management:
   Executive Director: John W Giovando
   Artistic Director: Eugenia Zukerman
Specialized Field: Instrumental; Opera; Choral; Childrens'; Ethnic; Educational
Budget: $2,000,000
Season: June - August
Performs At: Venues throughout Vail, Beaver Creek (Festival Site)
Annual Attendance: 48,000
Seating Capacity: 2,500; 250

4261 VAIL JAZZ FESTIVAL
PO Box 3035
Vail, CO 81658
Fax: 970-477-0866
Toll-free: 800-824-5526
e-mail: vjf@vailjazz.org
Web Site: www.vailjazz.org
Mission: Dedicated to the perpetuation of jazz through th presentation of jazz performances and jazz education, with special emphasis on young musicians and young audiences.
Founded: 1995
Status: Nonprofit

4262 JAZZ IN THE SANGRES
PO Box 327
Westcliffe, CO 81252
Phone: 719-783-3785
e-mail: design@creativeminds.com
Web Site: www.custerguide.com/jazz

4263 WESTMINSTER COMMUNITY ARTIST SERIES
7380 Lowell Boulevard
Westminster, CO 80030
Phone: 303-429-1999
Fax: 303-469-4599
Mission: To bring world class visual and performing artists to audiences in the Westminster Area.
Founded: 1983
Specialized Field: Dance; Vocal Music; Instrumental Music; Grand Opera
Status: Nonprofit
Organization Type: Performing

Connecticut

4264 GREAT CONNECTICUT JAZZ FEST
PO Box 2426
Branford, CT 06510
Phone: 203-469-8592
Fax: 203-481-2603
Toll-free: 800-468-3836
e-mail: ct.traditional.jazz@snet.net
Web Site: www.ctjazz.org

Founded: 1986
Specialized Field: Dixieland Jazz; Swing Jazz
Volunteer Staff: 375
Paid Artists: 138
Non-paid Artists: 46
Annual Attendance: 10,000
Facility Category: Tent

4265 GOODSPEED MUSICALS

Route 82
PO Box A
East Haddam, CT 06423
Phone: 860-873-8664
Fax: 860-873-2329
e-mail: webmaster@goodspeed.org
Web Site: www.goodspeed.org
Management:
    Production Manager: R Glen Grusmark
    Technical Director: Jason W Harshaw
    Assistant Technical Director: Meredith Lidstone
    Production Stage Manager: Donna Lynn Cooper Hilton
Mission: Preserving and advancing the American musical as an art form; developing new works to be added to the repertoire.
Founded: 1963
Specialized Field: Musical
Status: Professional; Nonprofit
Performs At: Goodspeed Opera House
Type of Stage: Proscenium
Stage Dimensions: 27'x18'
Orchestra Pit: 1
Architect: William H Goodspeed
Organization Type: Performing; Equity Theater

4266 GOODSPEED OPERA HOUSE

Route 82
PO Box A
East Haddam, CT 06423
Phone: 860-873-8664
Fax: 860-873-2329
e-mail: info@goodspeed.org
Web Site: www.goodspeed.org
Management:
    Executive Director: Michael P Price
    Associate Producer: Sue Frost
Founded: 1963
Specialized Field: Opera
Performs At: Goodspeed Opera House; Goodspeed-at-Chester
Type of Stage: Proscenium; Adaptable Proscenium
Seating Capacity: 400; 200

4267 ENFIELD CULTURAL ARTS COMMISSION

9 Hemlock Drive
Enfield, CT 06082-2705
Phone: 860-253-6421
Fax: 860-253-6310
Officers:
    Chairman: Priscilla D McManus

4268 HOT STEAMED JAZZ FESTIVAL

Valley Railroad
PO Box 293
Essex, CT 06426
Phone: 860-767-3968
Fax: 860-767-3968
Toll-free: 800-348-0003
e-mail: info@hotsteamedjazz.com
Web Site: www.hotsteamedjazz.com
Officers:
    President: Joseph Bombaci
    Tresurer: Peter Tizzie
Management:
    Band Contact: Dick Moore
    Band Contact: Bob Bruwmostt
    President: JB Bombac
Mission: Providing good jazz for the Whole in the Wall Camp.
Founded: 1992
Specialized Field: Traditional Jazz
Volunteer Staff: 30
Budget: $35,000
Income Sources: Ticket Sales; Donations
Annual Attendance: 22,000

4269 CHESTNUT HILL CONCERTS

PO Box 183
Guilford, CT 06437
Phone: 203-245-5736
Web Site: www.madisonct.com
Officers:
    President: John Posner
Management:
    Artistic Director: Ronald Thomas
    Administrative Director: Denise Meyer
Specialized Field: Instrumental
Budget: $10,000
Season: August
Performs At: Madison, CT (Festival Site)
Facility Category: First Congregational Church of Madison
Seating Capacity: 500

4270 SHORELINE ARTS ALLIANCE

725 Boston Post Road
Guilford, CT 06437
Phone: 203-453-3890
Fax: 203-453-0611
Web Site: www.shorelinearts.org
Officers:
    President: Julie McClenan
    VP: Deborah Abildsoe
    Treasurer: Armand Rossi
Management:
    Program Coordinator: Donita Aruny
    Administrative Coordinator: Jennifer Zeliff Kearney
Mission: A performance and service organization offering juried competitions for artists, photographers and writers; student scholarships within the local region; and a performance series.
Status: Nonprofit
Budget: $100,000
Income Sources: Grants; Foundations; Memberships
Resident Groups: Connecticut Commission on the Arts

4271 FIRST NIGHT HARTFORD
750 Main Street
Suite 514
Hartford, CT 06103
Phone: 860-722-9546
Fax: 860-722-9627
e-mail: firstnighthartford@msn.com
Web Site: www.firstnighthartford.com
Management:
    Executive Director: Pamela Amodio
Mission: Offering downtown Hartford an alcohol-free
New Year's Eve celebration.
Founded: 1988
Specialized Field: Instrumental; Multi-Media; Opera;
Choral; Jazz; Folk; Dance; Theatre; Childrens'; Ethnic;
Educational
Status: Nonprofit
Paid Staff: 1
Volunteer Staff: 200
Paid Artists: 45
Budget: $250,000
Income Sources: Corporate Sponsorships; Foundation
Grants; Admissions
Season: December - January
Performs At: Downtown Hartford (Festival Site)
Annual Attendance: 30,000
Organization Type: Performing

**4272 TALCOTT MOUNTAIN MUSIC
FESTIVAL, SUMMER SERIES**
Hartford Symphony
228 Farmington Avenue
Hartford, CT 06105
Phone: 860-246-8742
Fax: 860-247-1720
e-mail: info@hartfordsymphony.org
Web Site: www.hartfordsymphony.org
Officers:
    President: Millard H Pryor Jr
    VP Finance: Thomas R Wildman, Esquire
    VP Marketing: Robinson A Grover
    VP Administration: John H Beers
Management:
    Executive Director: Charles Owens
    Orchestra Manager: Keith Powell
Specialized Field: Instrumental
Season: July
Performs At: Simsbury (Festival Site); Iron Horse
Boulevard; Simsbury
Annual Attendance: 21,300

4273 WOODLAND CONCERT SERIES
10 Woodland Street
Hartford, CT 06105
Phone: 860-527-8121
Fax: 860-293-1404
e-mail: immanvel@iccucc.org
Web Site: www.iccucc.org
Management:
    Manager: Kathleen Keith
Performs At: Immanuel Congregational Church
Seating Capacity: 700

4274 LITCHFIELD JAZZ FESTIVAL
174 W Street
PO Box 69
Litchfield, CT 06759
Phone: 860-567-4162
Fax: 860-567-3592
e-mail: phurley@litchfieldjazzfest.com
Management:
    Executive Director: Vita West Muir

**4275 LITCHFIELD PERFORMING ARTS
SERIES**
40 W Street
PO Box 69
Litchfield, CT 06759
Phone: 860-567-4162
Fax: 860-567-3592
e-mail: lpai@ct1.nai.net
Management:
    Executive Director: Vita West Muir
Performs At: Church

**4276 SILVERMINE GUILD ART CENTER
SERIES**
1037 Silvermine Road
New Canaan, CT 06840-4398
Phone: 203-966-9700
Fax: 203-966-2763
e-mail: sgac@silvermineart.org
Web Site: www.silvermineart.org/staff.htm
Management:
    Executive Director: Cynthia Clair
    Program Director: Carol Nordgren
Mission: Arts, education and appreciation.
Founded: 1927
Specialized Field: Visual Art; Concerts
Paid Staff: 13
Volunteer Staff: 15
Budget: $1.6 Million
Income Sources: Tuition; Private Donations; Art Sales
Performs At: Multi-Purpose
Facility Category: Galleries; Auditorium
Seating Capacity: 125
Year Remodeled: 2000

**4277 INTERNATIONAL FESTIVAL OF ARTS
& IDEAS**
195 Church Street
12th Floor
New Haven, CT 06510
Phone: 203-498-1212
Fax: 203-498-2220
Toll-free: 888-278-4332
e-mail: chedstrom@artidea.org
Web Site: www.artidea.org
Management:
    Program Director: Cynthia Hedstrom
Specialized Field: Instrumental; Dance; Theatre;
Childrens'; Ethnic
Season: June - July

4278 NEW HAVEN JAZZ FESTIVAL
New Haven Office of Cultural Affairs
165 Church Street
New Haven, CT 06510
Phone: 203-946-7821
Fax: 203-946-7174
Web Site: www.newhavenjazz.com
Management:
    Director: Barbara Lamb
Founded: 1982
Specialized Field: Music

4279 CONNECTICUT COLLEGE: ON STAGE
270 Mohegan Avenue
PO Box 5216
New London, CT 06320-4196
Phone: 860-439-2787
Fax: 860-439-2595
e-mail: onstage@conncoll.edu
Web Site: http://onstage.connoll.edu
Management:
    Director: Robert A Richter
Mission: To present a varied annual series of the world's great performing artists thereby enriching and enhancing the cultural life of our community.
Founded: 1939
Specialized Field: Dance; Vocal Music; Instrumental Music; Theater
Status: Professional; Nonprofit
Paid Staff: 2
Budget: $139,000
Performs At: Palmer Auditorium; Evans Hall
Organization Type: Performing; Presenting

4280 CONNECTICUT EARLY MUSIC FESTIVAL
PO Box 329
New London, CT 06320
Phone: 860-444-2419
Web Site: www.ctearlymusic.org
Management:
    Artistic Director: John Metz
Mission: To provide performances of music from the 16th-19th centuries on period instruments.
Founded: 1983
Specialized Field: Instrumental
Status: Professional; Nonprofit
Season: Mid June
Performs At: New London; Noank; Niantic; Waterford
Seating Capacity: 125; 500
Organization Type: Performing

4281 SUMMER MUSIC
300 State Street
Suite 400
New London, CT 06320
Phone: 860-442-9199
Fax: 860-442-9290
Management:
    Executive Director: Paul R Bunker

4282 NEWTOWN FRIENDS OF MUSIC
PO Box 295
Newtown, CT 06470-0295
Phone: 203-426-6470
Fax: 203-426-4587
e-mail: friendsofmusic@snet.net
Officers:
    President: Ellen Parrella
Founded: 1978
Specialized Field: Chamber Music; Recitals; Chamber Orchestra
Volunteer Staff: 16
Paid Artists: 22
Performs At: Edmond Town Hall
Annual Attendance: 2,500
Seating Capacity: 450

4283 NORFOLK CHAMBER MUSIC FESTIVAL/YALE SUMMER SCHOOL OF MUSIC
Ellen Battell Stoeckel Estate
Route 44 & 272
Norfolk, CT 06058-0545
Phone: 860-542-3000
Fax: 860-542-3004
e-mail: norfolk@yale.edu
Web Site: www.yale.edu/norfolk
Management:
    Director: Joan Panetti
    Operations Manager: Deanne Chin
Mission: To provide chamber-music performances and professional training.
Founded: 1941
Specialized Field: Instrumental; Folk; Educational
Status: Professional; Nonprofit
Paid Staff: 12
Paid Artists: 70
Budget: $60,000 - 150,000
Season: Late June - late August
Performs At: The Music Shed
Annual Attendance: 17,500
Facility Category: Indoor
Seating Capacity: 1,000
Rental Contact: Elaine C Carroll
Organization Type: Performing; Educational

4284 PROJECT TROUBADOR
374 Taconic Road
Salisbury, CT 06068
Phone: 860-435-0561
Fax: 860-435-0561
e-mail: louise@projecttroubador.org
Web Site: www.projecttroubador.org
Management:
    Executive Director: Louise Lindenmeyr
    Artistic Director: Eliot Osborn
Mission: Music, theatre and humor are powerful universal vehicles of communication yet there is little opportunity for cross-cultural sharing to take place on a person-to-person level around the world. Project Troubador is unique in its fulfillment of this need-offering a way for both performing artists and audiences to meet on common ground in celebration.

4285 FALCON RIDGE FOLK FESTIVAL

74 Modley Road
Sharon, CT 06069
Phone: 860-364-0366
Fax: 860-364-8081
e-mail: info@falconridgefolk.com
Web Site: www.falconridgefolk.com
Management:
   Artistic Director: Anne Saunders
Founded: 1988
Specialized Field: Folk Music; Dance
Paid Staff: 5-6
Paid Artists: 50
Income Sources: Ticket Sales
Performs At: Long Hill Farm
Affiliations: National Folk Alliance; International
Bluegrass; Americana Music Association
Annual Attendance: 10-15,000
Facility Category: Corporation

4286 MUSIC MOUNTAIN

PO Box 1739
Sharon, CT 06069
Phone: 860-824-7126
Fax: 860-364-2090
e-mail: ngordon@snet.net
Web Site: www.musicmountain.org
Officers:
   President: Nicholas Gordon
Mission: To provide professional chamber music to
western Connecticut through a Summer Chamber Music
Festival, as well as broadcasts to over 200 radio stations
and 220 foriegn countries.
Founded: 1930
Specialized Field: String Quartets; Jazz
Status: Professional; Nonprofit
Paid Staff: 1
Volunteer Staff: 10
Income Sources: Ticket Sales; Donations; Bequests;
Foundations; Government Grants
Season: June - September
Performs At: Gordon Hall; Falls Village
Facility Category: Colonial Concert Hall
Stage Dimensions: 18'x36'
Seating Capacity: 335
Year Built: 1930
Rental Contact: President Nicholas Gordon
Organization Type: Performing; Educational;
Sponsoring

4287 NORTHWEST CORNER YOUNG ARTISTS SERIES

18 Old Sharon Road
#3
Sharon, CT 06069
Phone: 860-364-0253
Management:
   Artistic Director: DeeAnne Hunstien
Performs At: Private Homes

4288 WINTERHAWK - BLUEGRASS & BEYOND

74 Modley Road
Sharon, CT 06069
Phone: 860-364-0366
Fax: 860-364-8081
e-mail: info@winterhawk2000.com
Web Site: www.winterhawk2000.com
Management:
   Artistic Director: Anne Saunders
Founded: 1983
Paid Staff: 4-6
Paid Artists: 50
Income Sources: Ticket Sales
Performs At: Long Hill Farm
Affiliations: National Folk Alliance; Interntional
Bluegrass; Americana Music Association
Annual Attendance: 2,500-7,000
Facility Category: Corporation

4289 CENTENNIAL THEATER FESTIVAL

995 Hopmeadow Street
Simsbury, CT 06070
Phone: 860-408-5300
Fax: 860-408-5301
e-mail: deanadams@msn.com
Web Site: www.ctfestival.com
Management:
   Artistic Director: Dean Adams
Founded: 1990
Status: Nonprofit
Season: June 11 - August 1
Annual Attendance: 8,000
Facility Category: Theater; Air Conditioned, Handicap
Access
Type of Stage: Proscenium
Stage Dimensions: 29' x 35'
Seating Capacity: 400
Year Built: 1989

4290 STRATFORD FESTIVAL THEATER

1850 Elm Street
Stratford, CT 06615
Phone: 203-378-1200
Fax: 203-378-9777
Management:
   Dramaturg: J Wishnia
Founded: 1996

4291 ARMSTRONG CHAMBER CONCERTS

86 Church Hill Road
PO Box 367
Washington Depot, CT 06794
Phone: 860-868-0522
Fax: 860-868-0522
e-mail: accnct@aol.com
Web Site: www.accnct.org
Officers:
   President/Treasurer: Helen Armstrong
   VP: Ajit Hutheesing
   Secretary: Greta Pofcher
   Secretary: Ann Wade
   Secretary: Suzanne Geiss-Robbins
Management:

Artistic Director: Helen Armstrong
Operations Manager: Lynelle Kyasky
Grant Writer: Carol Mallquist
Mission: To provide concerts of professional chamber music to diverse audiences.
Founded: 1983
Specialized Field: Instrumental Music; Chamber Music
Status: Professional; Nonprofit
Paid Staff: 2
Paid Artists: 15
Income Sources: Grants; Donations; Box Office
Performs At: Litchfield
Affiliations: Chamber Music America; Ulenfield Hills Visitors Bureau; American Symphony League
Annual Attendance: 5-6,000
Organization Type: Performing; Touring; Resident; Educational

4292 HARTT SCHOOL CONCERT SERIES

200 Bloomfield Avenue
West Hartford, CT 06117
Phone: 860-768-4454
Fax: 860-768-4441
Web Site: www.hartford.edu/hartt
Management:
Manager: Jessica Levine Pizano
Founded: 1920
Specialized Field: Music; Dance; Theatre
Performs At: Millard Auditorium; Lincoln Theater
Rental Contact: DaVid Bell

4293 SOUTH SHORE MUSIC

PO Box 403
Westport, CT 06881
Phone: 203-227-0695
Fax: 203-454-3682
e-mail: southshoremusic@bigplanet.com
Web Site: www.southshoremusic.com
Officers:
President/Program Chairman: Marianne Liberatore
Mission: To present chamber music concerts
Founded: 1933
Specialized Field: Classical Chamber Music
Volunteer Staff: 6
Budget: $100,000
Income Sources: Tickets; Ads; Contributions
Season: June-September
Performs At: Saugatuck Congregational Church

4294 TEMPLE ISRAEL OF WESTPORT SERIES

14 Coleytown Road
Westport, CT 06880
Phone: 203-227-1293
Fax: 203-454-2292
e-mail: rsilv3636@aol.com
Performs At: Temple Israel

Delaware

4295 UNIVERSITY OF DELAWARE PERFORMING ARTS SERIES

Alumni Hall
24 E Main Street
Newark, DE 19716-7101
Phone: 302-831-8741
Fax: 302-831-2045
e-mail: pas@mvs.udel.edu
Web Site: www.vdel.edu
Management:
Assistant Director: Robert Snyder
Mission: A public service for local community.
Founded: 1979
Paid Staff: 3
Volunteer Staff: 20
Paid Artists: 20
Performs At: Mitchell Hall

4296 DELAWARE CHAMBER MUSIC FESTIVAL

PO Box 3537
Wilmington, DE 19807-3537
Phone: 302-636-9400
Fax: 302-636-9400
Web Site: www.dcmf.org
Officers:
President: Mary P Richards
VP: Tamara Lyn Smith
Treasurer: Roger Cuson
Secretary: Marcia Peoples Halio
Management:
Music Director: Barbara Govatos
Co-Administrator: Cher Astolfi
Co-Administrator: Tracy Ann Smith
Paid Staff: 3
Volunteer Staff: 20
Paid Artists: 25

District of Columbia

4297 AMERICAN COLLEGE THEATER FESTIVAL

John F Kennedy Center
for the Performing Arts
Washington, DC 20566-0001
Phone: 202-416-8864
Fax: 202-416-8802
e-mail: ghenry@kennedy-center.org
Management:
Director: Gregg Henry

4298 AMERICAN MUSIC FESTIVAL

National Gallery of Art
6th Street & Constitution Avenue NW
Washington, DC 20565
Phone: 202-842-6941
Fax: 202-842-2407
e-mail: g-manos@nga.gov
Web Site: www.nga.gov
Management:

Music Director: George Manos
Music Program Specialist: Stephen Ackert
Specialized Field: Instrumental; Choral; Jazz; Educational
Season: May, Sundays only
Performs At: Washington, DC (Festival Site)
Seating Capacity: 500

4299 ARTS IN THE ACADEMY, NATIONAL ACADEMY OF SCIENCES

2101 Constitution Avenue NW
Washington, DC 20418
Phone: 202-334-2439
Fax: 202-334-1687
e-mail: jtomlins@nas.edu
Web Site: www.national-acadamies.org/arts
Officers:
    Administrative Assistant: Marsha Barrett
Management:
    Director: Janis Tomlinson
Performs At: Auditorium
Seating Capacity: 670

4300 CHILDREN'S NATIONAL MEDICAL CENTER, NEW HORIZONS PROGRAM

111 Michigan Avenue NW
Washington, DC 20010-2970
Phone: 202-884-3465
Fax: 202-884-3489
e-mail: tlassite@cnmc.org
Management:
    Manager: Tina S Lassiter
    Performance Coordinator: Arabella Johnson
Mission: To provide multi-disciplined high quality arts programming to patients at bedside, in playrooms and, in the Atrium space in order to expedite the healing process.
Founded: 1978

4301 DC SPORTS & ENTERTAINMENT COMMISSION

2400 E Capitol Street
SE RFK, 4th Floor
Washington, DC 20003
Phone: 202-547-0977
Fax: 202-547-7460
e-mail: nevwa@aol.com
Web Site: www.dcsec.dcgov.org
Management:
    Executive Director: James Dalrymple
    Marketing Director: Neville Waters
    Stadium Manager: Anthony Burnett
Mission: To promote Washington, DC as a location for holding sporting events to enhanve the city's economic development and welfare, and expand the city's national and international exposure. The Commission also creates opportunities for community outreach and local recreation for all residents of the district, particularly youths.
Seating Capacity: 56; 692

4302 DISTRICT CURATORS

PO Box 14197
Washington, DC 20044

Phone: 202-783-0360
Fax: 202-783-4185
Management:
    Executive Director: Bill Warrell
    Producer: Katea Stitt
Mission: Presenting the finest new performing arts to Washington DC and mid-Atlantic audiences; advancing cultural opportunities world-wide for artists and audiences.
Specialized Field: Ethnic
Status: Nonprofit
Organization Type: Presenting

4303 DUMBARTON CONCERT SERIES

3133 Dumbarton Street NW
Washington, DC 20007
Phone: 202-965-2000
Fax: 202-965-2004
e-mail: dumbartonc@aol.com
Web Site: www.dumbartonconcerts.org
Management:
    Executive Director: Connie Zimmer
    Managing Director: Mimi Newcastle
Mission: To provide a venue for the world's finest young musicians in the US capital.
Founded: 1978
Specialized Field: Instrumental Music
Status: Nonprofit
Income Sources: Box Office; Grants; Private Donations
Performs At: Dumbarton Church
Facility Category: Historic Church
Seating Capacity: 350
Organization Type: Presenting

4304 EMBASSY SERIES

PO Box 9871
Washington, DC 20016
Phone: 202-625-2361
Fax: 301-588-6445
e-mail: EmbSeries@aol.com
Web Site: www.embassyseries.com
Management:
    Director: Jerome Barry
Mission: Presents programs at embassies with local international artists and musicians.
Founded: 1981
Specialized Field: Chamber; Vocal Music

4305 FOLGER THEATRE

201 E Capitol Street SE
Washington, DC 20003-1094
Phone: 202-544-7077
Fax: 202-544-7520
e-mail: jpisano@folger.edu
Web Site: www.folger.edu
Management:
    Manager: Jane Pisano
    Production Manager: Janet Clark
    Events Publicist: Annalisa Rosmarin
Performs At: The Elizabethan Theatre at the Folger
Facility Category: Theatre
Type of Stage: Elizabethan indoor
Seating Capacity: 240
Year Built: 1930

4306 FREER GALLERY OF ART, BILL & MARY MEYER CONCERT SERIES
Smithsonian Institute
Washington, DC 20560-0707
Phone: 202-357-4880
Fax: 202-633-9026
Web Site: www.si.edu/asia
Management:
  Director: Milo C Beach
Performs At: Eugene & Agnus E Meyer Auditorium

4307 GEORGE WASHINGTON'S SERIES AT MOUNT VERNON COLLEGE
2100 Foxhall Road NW
Washington, DC 20007
Phone: 202-242-6600
Fax: 202-338-1089
e-mail: mvcfw@gwu.edu
Web Site: www.gwu.edu
Management:
  Artistic Director: Carla Hubner
Performs At: Hand Chapel

4308 IMAGINATION CELEBRATION - KENNEDY CENTER PERFORMANCES FOR YOUNG PEOPLE
John F Kennedy Center
for the Performing Arts
Washington, DC 20566-0001
Phone: 202-416-8807
Fax: 202-416-8802
Web Site: www.kennedy-center.org
Officers:
  VP Education: Derek Gordon

4309 KENNEDY CENTER ANNUAL OPEN HOUSE ARTS FESTIVAL
Kennedy Center for the Performing Arts
Washington, DC 20566-0003
Phone: 202-467-4600
Fax: 202-416-8205
Toll-free: 800-444-1324
Web Site: www.kennedy-center.org
Officers:
  Chairman: James A Johnson
  President: Laurence J Wilker
  Founding Chairman: Roger L Stevens
Management:
  Music Director/Orchestra: Leonard Slatkin
  Programming Coordinator: Tammie Ward
Specialized Field: Instrumental; Multi-Media; Opera; Choral; Jazz; Folk; Dance; Theatre; Childrens'; Ethnic; Educational
Season: September
Performs At: Kennedy Center (Festival Site)

4310 KENNEDY CENTER/MARY LOU WILLIAMS WOMEN IN JAZZ FESTIVAL
2700 F Street NW
Washington, DC 20566
Phone: 202-416-8824
Fax: 202-416-8802
e-mail: struthers@kennedy-center.org
Web Site: www.kennedy-center.org/womeninjazz
Management:
  Kennedy Center Program Manager: Kevin A Struthers

4311 LIBRARY OF CONGRESS CHAMBER MUSIC CONCERT SERIES
Library of Congress
Music Division
Washington, DC 20540-4710
Phone: 202-707-5503
Fax: 202-707-0621
Web Site: www.lcweb.loc.gov/rr/perform/concert
Management:
  Chief Music Division: Jon Newsom
  Producer: Anne McLean
Mission: To present free concerts of the highest artistic caliber, with a special emphasis on american music and musicians.
Founded: 1925
Specialized Field: Chamber Music; Jazz; America Music Theatre; Dance
Paid Staff: 6
Volunteer Staff: 6
Paid Artists: 120

4312 NATIONAL ACADEMY OF SCIENCES CONCERTS
500 Fifht Avenue NW
Washington, DC 20001
Phone: 202-334-2436
e-mail: arts@nas.edu
Management:
  Exhibitions/Events Coordinator: JD Talasek
Seating Capacity: 670

4313 NATIONAL GALLERY OF ART/CONCERT SERIES
National Art Gallery
Washington, DC 20565
Phone: 202-842-6941
Fax: 202-842-2407
e-mail: G-Manos@nga.gov
Web Site: www.nga.gov
Management:
  Music Director: George Manos
  Music Program Specialist: Stephen Ackert
Mission: To provide the public with free concerts at the National Gallery of Art.
Founded: 1941
Specialized Field: Symphony; Orchestra; Chamber; Ensemble
Status: Nonprofit
Paid Staff: 8
Performs At: Museum Garden Courts; National Gallery
Annual Attendance: 14,000
Seating Capacity: 500
Organization Type: Performing

4314 OPERA LAFAYETTE
10 4th Street NE
Washington, DC 20002
Phone: 202-546-9332
e-mail: washington@operalafayette.org
Web Site: www.operalafayette.org
Management:
   Artistic Director: Ryan Brown
   Administrative Assistant: Michelle Sikora
Mission: To present historically-informed performances
from the 17th and 18th century repertoire on period
instruments with the finest musicians/interpreters of this
period. To educate children and adults in this period.
Specialized Field: Opera, Chamber Music, Summer
Season Redwoods Festival, Winter Season Opera
Lafayette
Status: Nonprofit
Paid Staff: 4
Budget: $35,000-$60,000
Season: August
Performs At: Sonoma County (Festival Site)
Affiliations: Various Sonoma County Wineries and
Mansions
Seating Capacity: 1,300

**4315 PHILLIPS COLLECTION SUNDAY
AFTERNOON CONCERT SERIES**
1600 21st Street NW
Washington, DC 20009-1090
Phone: 202-387-2151
Fax: 202-387-3350
Management:
   Music Director: Mark Carrington

**4316 SMITHSONIAN INSTITUTION: THE
SMITHSONIAN ASSOCIATES**
1100 Jefferson Drive SW
Ripley Center, Suite 3077
Washington, DC 20560-0701
Phone: 202-357-3030
Fax: 202-786-2536
e-mail: rap@tsa.si.edu
Web Site: www.SmithsonianAssociates.org
Management:
   Director: Mara Mayor
   Program Manager: Brigitte Blachere
   Public Affairs: Mami Tamayo
   Deputy Director: Barbara Tuceling
   Associate Director: Carol Bogash
   Associate Director/Marketing: Robert Anastasio
   Webmaster: Dennis R Smoot
Mission: Encouraging and supporting the participation of
the Washington DC community in Smithsonian Institution
performing arts events.
Founded: 1974
Specialized Field: Dance; Vocal Music; Instrumental
Music; Theater
Status: Professional; Nonprofit
Paid Staff: 100
Volunteer Staff: 200
Performs At: Hirshhorn Museum Auditorium; Baird
Auditorium
Organization Type: Educational; Sponsoring
Resident Groups: Smithsonian Chamber Music Society

**4317 SOCIETY OF THE CINCINNATI
CONCERTS AT ANDERSON HOUSE**
2118 Massachusetts Avenue NW
Washington, DC 20008-2810
Phone: 202-785-2040
Fax: 202-293-3350
Management:
   Museum Director: Kathleen Betts
Performs At: Ballroom

**4318 WASHINGTON PERFORMING ARTS
SOCIETY**
2000 L Street NW
Suite 510
Washington, DC 20036-4907
Phone: 202-833-9800
Fax: 202-331-7678
e-mail: wpas@wpas.org
Web Site: www.wpas.org
Officers:
   Chairman: Lena Ingegerd Scott
   Vice Chairman: James F Lafond
   Vice Chairman: AW Smith Jr
   Vice Chairman: Paul Martin Wolff
   Secretary: Benjamin L Palumbo
   President: Douglas H Wheeler
Management:
   Managing Director: Douglas H Wheeler
   VP/General Manager: William F Reeder
   Director/Marketing/Communications: Trish Shuman
   Public Relations/Marketing Director: Liza Holtmeier
   Program Director: Kim Chan
   President: Douglas H Wheeler
Mission: To present the world's finest artists in the
nation's capital; to present over 100 concerts annually on
the major stages, as well as over 800 concerts each year in
the schools of the metropolitan Washington area using
resident artists.
Founded: 1966
Specialized Field: Dance; Vocal Music; Instrumental
Music; Festivals
Status: Professional; Nonprofit
Income Sources: International Society of Performing
Arts Administrators
Performs At: John F Kennedy Center for the Performing
Arts
Organization Type: Educational; Sponsoring
Notes: Access for persons with disabilities

Florida

**4319 MIAMI INTERNATIONAL PIANO
FESTIVAL**
20191 E Country Club Drive
Suite 709
Aventura, FL 33180
Phone: 305-935-5115
Fax: 305-935-9087
e-mail: giselle@miamipianofest.com
Web Site: www.miamipianofest.com
Management:
   Artistic Director: Gisela Brodsky

Executive Director: Anges Youngblood
Founded: 1997
Specialized Field: Music; Piano
Status: Nonprofit
Paid Staff: 2
Volunteer Staff: 10
Paid Artists: 15

4320 SOUTH FLORIDA COMMUNITY COLLEGE CULTURAL SERIES

600 W College Drive
Avon Park, FL 33825
Phone: 813-453-6661
Fax: 813-452-6042
e-mail: andrdo23@sfcc.cc.fl.us
Web Site: www.sfcc.cc.fl.us
Officers:
   Chairman Cultural Affairs: Douglas Andrews
Performs At: College Auditorium

4321 CLEARWATER JAZZ HOLIDAY

201 Drew Street
Clearwater, FL 33755
Mailing Address: PO Box 7278 Clearwater, FL 33758-7287
Phone: 727-461-5200
Fax: 727-461-1292
e-mail: clearjazz@aol.com
Web Site: www.clearwaterjazz.com
Management:
   Executive Director: Karen S Vann

4322 FESTIVAL MIAMI

University of Miami, School of Music
PO Box 248165
Coral Gables, FL 33124-7610
Phone: 305-284-3941
Fax: 305-284-3901
e-mail: whipp@miami.edu
Web Site: www.music.miami.edu
Management:
   Director: Barbara Muze
Founded: 1984
Budget: $60,000 - 250,000
Season: Mid September - Mid October
Performs At: University of Miami, Gusman Concert Hall
Seating Capacity: 600

4323 MIAMI BACH SOCIETY/TROPICAL BAROQUE MUSIC FESTIVAL

PO Box 4034
Coral Gables, FL 33114
Phone: 305-669-1376
Fax: 305-669-1376
e-mail: JGaubatz@msn.com
Web Site: miamibachsociety.org
Officers:
   President: Mark Hart
   VP: George Berberian
   Secretary: Claire Veater
   Treasurer: Myriam Ribenborm
Management:
   Artistic Director: Donald Oglesby

Executive Director: Kathy Gaubatz
Artistic Director: Robert Heath
Mission: To perform and present the music of Johann Sebastian Bach and his baroque composer contemporaries to the people and visitors of the sociable Florida community.
Founded: 1984
Paid Staff: 4
Budget: $300,000
Income Sources: Corporations; Government; Indivdual Donations; Ticket Sales
Annual Attendance: 5,000
Organization Type: Performing and Presenting Musical Organization
Resident Groups: MBS Chorus and Orchestra

4324 CENTRAL FLORIDA CULTURAL ENDEAVORS

901 6th Street
Daytona Beach, FL 32117-8099
Mailing Address: PO Box 1310 Daytona Beach, FL 32115-1310
Phone: 904-252-1511
Fax: 904-238-1663
e-mail: fifcfce@n-jcenter.com
Web Site: www.fif-lso.org
Officers:
   President: Tippen Davidson
   Treasurer: Georgia Kaney
Management:
   General Manager: Dewey Anderson
   Operations Manager: Erin Bailey
Mission: To provide world class chamber music and orchestra concerts for Daytona Beach audiences.
Founded: 1982
Specialized Field: Dance; Vocal Music; Instrumental Music; Festivals
Status: Professional; Nonprofit
Paid Staff: 5
Budget: $240,000
Income Sources: Individuals; Corporations; City; County; State; Grants
Performs At: Peabody Auditorium
Affiliations: Association of Performing Arts Presenters; FL Arts Presenters; INTIX
Facility Category: Churches
Seating Capacity: 600-1,200
Organization Type: Sponsoring

4325 FLORIDA INTERNATIONAL FESTIVAL
Central Florida Cultural Endeavors

PO Box 1310
Daytona Beach, FL 32115-1310
Phone: 904-257-7790
Fax: 904-238-1663
e-mail: fifcfce@fif-lfo.org
Web Site: www.fif-lso.org
Officers:
   President: Tippen Davidson
Management:
   Founder/Director: Tippen Davidson
   General Manager: Dewey Anderson
   Operations Manager: Erin Baileyts
   Business Manager: Terri Evans

All listings are in alphabetical order by state, then city, then organization within the city.

Mission: To provide the citizens of Volusia County and its visitors with a high quality, broadly based performing arts series built around the biennial residency of the London Symphony Orchestra, thereby promoting Daytona Beach as a culturally diverse and informed area.
Founded: 1966
Specialized Field: Dance; Vocal Music; Instrumental Music; Festivals
Status: Professional; Nonprofit
Budget: $2,400,700
Income Sources: Local Individuals, Corporations; City, County, State & other Grants
Performs At: Peabody Auditorium; Ocean Center; Ormond Beach, PA
Affiliations: Association of Performing Arts Presenters; FL Arts Presenters; INTIX
Seating Capacity: 200-9,000
Organization Type: Performing; Educational; Sponsoring

4326 FLORIDA INTERNATIONAL FESTIVAL FEATURING THE LONDON SYMPHONY ORCHESTRA

901 6th Street
Daytona Beach, FL 32115-1310
Mailing Address: PO Box 1310 Daytona Beach, FL 32115-1310
Phone: 386-252-1511
Fax: 386-238-1663
e-mail: fifcfce@fif-lso.org
Web Site: www.fif-lso.org
Management:
    General Manager: Dewey Anderson
Founded: 1974
Specialized Field: Music
Paid Staff: 6
Volunteer Staff: 100
Paid Artists: 200
Budget: $400,000 - 1,000,000
Income Sources: Ticket Sales; Contributions; Grants
Season: July
Performs At: Daytona Beach area [Festival Site]; Various
Annual Attendance: 2,000-40,000
Facility Category: Peabody Aud; Ocean Cntr; Ormond Beach Cntr; etc.
Seating Capacity: 250 - 8,000

4327 BEETHOVEN BY THE BEACH

Florida Philharmonic Orchestra
3401 NW 9th Avenue
Fort Lauderdale, FL 33309-5903
Phone: 954-561-2997
Fax: 954-561-1390
Toll-free: 800-930-1812
Web Site: www.floridaphilharmonic.org
Management:
    Music Director: James Judd
Specialized Field: Instrumental; Childrens'
Budget: $60,000 - 150,000
Season: July
Performs At: Fort Lauderdale [Festival Site]

4328 CORAL RIDGE PRESBYTARIAN CHURCH CONCERT SERIES

5555 N Federal Highway
Fort Lauderdale, FL 33308
Phone: 954-491-1103
Fax: 954-491-7374
e-mail: mcaulk@crpc.org
Web Site: www.crpc.org
Management:
    Concert Series Director: Martha Caulk
Paid Staff: 3
Volunteer Staff: 2
Performs At: Coral Ridge Presbytarian Church
Annual Attendance: 50,000
Facility Category: Church
Type of Stage: Chancel
Seating Capacity: 2000
Year Built: 1971

4329 FORT LAUDERDALE BROADWAY SERIES / PARKER PLAYHOUSE

PO Box 4603
Fort Lauderdale, FL 33338-4603
Phone: 954-764-0700
Fax: 954-764-0708

4330 FLORIDA ARTS CONCERT SERIES

146 Riverview Road
Fort Myers, FL 33905
Phone: 941-823-3758
Fax: 941-694-2787
e-mail: jimflarts@earthlink.net
Management:
    Executive Director/Chairman: James Griffith

4331 FORT MYERS COMMUNITY CONCERT ASSOCIATION SERIES

3934 W Riverside Drive
PO Box 606
Fort Myers, FL 33902
Phone: 813-936-5848
Officers:
    President: George T Mann
Performs At: Barbara B Mann Performing Arts Hall

4332 FIRST ARTS SERIES

103 1st Street SE
Fort Walton, FL 32548
Phone: 850-243-9292
Fax: 850-243-0905
e-mail: ktindall@iname.com
Web Site: www.fa2.org
Management:
    Director: Karen Tindall
    Concert Hospitality: Nancy Smith
    Treasurer: Joan Moody
    Artist Hospitality: Kay Walker
    Computer Support: Marylaide Newell
    Tickets/Membership: Judy Arrowsmith
    Special Projects: Nancy Ross
    Marketing and Publicity: Robbynne Raupers
    Grant Development: Beth Arrington
Performs At: First United Methodist Church

4333 NYK PRODUCTIONS
1747 Van Buren Street
Suite 700
Hollywood, FL 33028
Phone: 954-929-6010
Fax: 954-929-6399
Management:
 Chief Officer: Arie Kaduri
Performs At: Various Auditoriums

4334 DELIUS FESTIVAL
PO Box 5621
Jacksonville, FL 32247-5621
Phone: 904-384-3956
Management:
 Director: Jeff Driggers
 Director: Michael Blachly
 Education Coordinator: Elizabeth Auer
 Receptionist: Mary Monroe
 Assistant Director: Kay Holcomb
 Operations Manager: Matt Koropeckyj-Cox
 Assistant Director: Deborah C Rossi
 Accountant: Gay Hale
 Technical Director: Steve Schell
Specialized Field: Instrumental; Choral
Budget: $10,000
Season: April
Performs At: Jacksonville (Festival Site)
Facility Category: Terry Concert Hall; Friday Musicale
Auditorium
Seating Capacity: 450; 250

**4335 FLORIDA THEATRE PERFORMING
ARTS SERIES**
128 E 40th Street
Jacksonville, FL 32202
Phone: 904-355-5661
Fax: 904-358-1874
e-mail: stillcool@flordiatheatre.com
Web Site: www.flordiatheatre.com
Management:
 Executive Director: J Erik Hart
Performs At: Flordia Theatre

**4336 JACKSONVILLE UNIVERSITY
MASTER-CLASS & ARTISTS SERIES**
College of Fine Arts, Jacksonville University
2800 University Boulevard, North
Jacksonville, FL 32211
Phone: 904-256-7371
Fax: 904-256-7375
Toll-free: 800-225-2027
e-mail: tnetter@ju.edu
Web Site: www.ju.edu
Management:
 Dean College Fine Arts: D Terence Netter
 Fine Arts Coordinator: January Walker
Mission: Cultural enrichment of the university
community and the community at large.
Founded: 1958
Specialized Field: Art; Dance; Music; Theatre
Paid Staff: 12
Paid Artists: 20

Performs At: Terry Concert Hall

4337 KUUMBA FEST
PO Box 12001
Jacksonville, FL 92101
Phone: 904-353-2270
Fax: 904-355-0567
e-mail: kuumbafest@hotmail.com
Web Site: kuumbafestival.tripod.com

4338 WJCT JACKSONVILLE JAZZ FESTIVAL
100 Festival Park Avenue
Jacksonville, FL 32202-1397
Phone: 904-353-7770
Fax: 904-358-6344
e-mail: vic_digenti@wjct.pbs.org
Web Site: www.jaxjazzfest.com
Management:
 Executive Producer: Vic DiGenti

4339 BEACHES FINE ARTS SERIES
PO Box 51171
Jacksonville Beach, FL 32240-1171
Phone: 904-270-2074
Fax: 904-220-2327
e-mail: beachesfinearts@aol.com
Management:
 Executive Director: Kathy Wallis
Performs At: St. Pauls By-the-Sea Episcopal Church

**4340 KEY WEST COUNCIL ON THE ARTS
SERIES**
2932 Seidenberg Avenue
Key West, FL 33040

Management:
 Artistic Director: RJ Weiss

**4341 BACH FESTIVAL OF CENTRAL
FLORIDA**
PO Box 2764
Lakeland, FL 33806-2764
Phone: 863-605-2200
Fax: 863-439-0759
e-mail: mhas80@aol.com
Web Site: www.bachfestivalpolkcounty.com
Officers:
 President/Treasurer: Mark Stolz
 VP: Marie Hasse
 Secretary: Dave Otten
Management:
 Music Director: Andrew Walker

4342 FLORIDA SOUTHERN COLLEGE
111 Lake Hollingsworth Drive
Lakeland, FL 33801
Phone: 863-680-4218
Fax: 863-680-3758
Toll-free: 800-274-4131
e-mail: fla@flsouthern.edu
Web Site: www.flsouthern.edu
Management:

All listings are in alphabetical order by state, then city, then organization within the city.

Coordinator: Robert MacDonald

4343 LAKELAND CENTER ENTERTAINMENT SERIES & BROADWAY SERIES
700 W Lemon Street
Lakeland, FL 33815
Phone: 863-834-8100
Fax: 863-834-8101
e-mail: allen.johnson@lakelandgov.net
Web Site: www.thelakelandcenter.com
Management:
   Executive Director: Allen Johnson
   Client Services Manager: Tim Holloway
   Assistant Director: Scott Sioman
Performs At: The Lakeland Center
Facility Category: Event, Sports & Convention complex
Stage Dimensions: 78'x47'
Seating Capacity: 2,246 w/pit seats 2,296
Year Built: 1974
Year Remodeled: 1996
Rental Contact: Lisa Palas

4344 SUNCOAST DIXIELAND JAZZ CLASSIC
PO Box 1945
Largo, FL 33779-1945
Phone: 727-536-0064
Web Site: www.jazzclassic.com
Management:
   Director: Dave Fanning
Mission: Our charter, established to promote the further interest to Dixieland Jazz in our schools, continues through Scholarships and volunteer teachers in the public school system in addition to the formation of a Youth oriented to Dixieland Jazz
Founded: 1990
Specialized Field: Dixieland Jazz Festival
Status: Nonprofit
Paid Staff: 1
Volunteer Staff: 100
Paid Artists: 60
Performs At: Sheraton Sand Key Hotel
Affiliations: Suncoast Dixieland Jazz Society
Annual Attendance: 4,000

4345 NORTH FLORIDA COMMUNITY COLLEGE
100 Turner Davis Drive
Madison, FL 32340
Phone: 850-973-1606
Fax: 850-973-1685
e-mail: artistseries@nfcc.cc
Web Site: www.nfcc.cc
Officers:
   Artists Series Chairman: Patricia M Hinton
Management:
   Director Institutional Advancement: Patricia Hinton
Mission: To provide cultural enrichment through live performances for audiences of all ages residing in th North Florida area.
Founded: 1980
Specialized Field: Performing Arts; Concerts; Plays; Dance
Paid Staff: 3
Volunteer Staff: 5

Paid Artists: 7
Non-paid Artists: 11
Budget: $40,000
Income Sources: Ticket Sales; Private & Corporate Donations; Grants
Performs At: Priest Auditorium
Annual Attendance: 6,000
Facility Category: Auditorium
Type of Stage: Resilient Wood
Stage Dimensions: 29'x40'
Seating Capacity: 580
Year Built: 1992

4346 CHIPOLA JUNIOR COLLEGE SERIES
3094 Indian Circle
Marianna, FL 32446-2206
Phone: 850-718-2301
Fax: 850-718-2344
e-mail: stadsklevj@chipola.cc.fl.us
Management:
   Fine/Performing Arts Director: Joan Stadsklev
Performs At: Chipola Junior College Auditorium
Facility Category: Theatre
Type of Stage: Proscenium
Seating Capacity: 355

4347 KEY WEST MUSIC FESTIVAL
1057 NE 210 Terrace
Miami, FL 33179
Phone: 305-651-5525
Fax: 305-651-0885
e-mail: kwmfestival@aol.com
Web Site: www.keywestmusicfestival.com/
Budget: $10,000 - 20,000
Season: May
Performs At: Key West (Festival Site)
Facility Category: San Carlos Institute
Seating Capacity: 400

4348 MIAMI CIVIC MUSIC ASSOCIATION SERIES
5360 SW 87th Avenue
Miami, FL 33165
Phone: 305-271-8449
Fax: 305-595-9597
e-mail: miamicivic@aol.com
Management:
   Artistic Director: Dr. Rosalina Sackstein
Performs At: Gusman Hall, University of Miami

4349 MIAMI DADE COMMUNITY COLLEGE
300 NE 2nd Avenue
Suite 1467
Miami, FL 33132
Phone: 305-237-3010
Fax: 305-237-7559
Management:
   Cultural Affairs Director: Dr. Michelle Heffner Hayes
Paid Staff: 5
Paid Artists: 75
Budget: $1,000,000

Income Sources: Miami-Dade Community College; Miami-Dade County; State of Florida
Performs At: Auditorium
Annual Attendance: 10,000
Facility Category: Various

4350 TEMPLE BETH AM SERIES
5950 North Kendall Drive
Miami, FL 33156
Phone: 305-667-6667
Fax: 305-662-8619
Officers:
  President: Michael Bittel
  Executive VP: Bea Citron
  Corresponding Secretary: Randy Fisher
  Recording Secretary: Debbie Rosenthal
  Treasurer/Financial Secretary: Irwin Katz
Management:
  Executive Director: Irene Warner
  Finance Director: Hellene Strul
  Operations: Lori Solomon
  Commmunications Director: Helene Layne
  Administration Secretary: Rita Diaz
  Administration Assistant: Marylin Harrison
  Donations: Barbara Hoffman
  Receptionist: Sandy Morrison
Performs At: Temple Sanctuary

4351 CONCERT ASSOCIATION OF FLORIDA SERIES
555 17th Street
Miami Beach, FL 33139
Phone: 305-532-3491
Fax: 305-532-2119
Toll-free: 877-433-3200
e-mail: info@concertfla.org
Web Site: www.concertfla.org
Officers:
  President: Judith Drucker
Management:
  Marketing Director: Craig Hall
Performs At: Dade County Auditorium

4352 PERFORMING ARTS SOCIETY OF SOUTH FLORIDA
PO Box 6304
Miami Beach, FL 33141
Phone: 305-682-4999
e-mail: passouth@earthlink.net
Web Site: www.cdg.org
Management:
  Managing Director: Darrell Calvin
Mission: To bring the best entertainment to a diverse community.
Founded: 1984
Specialized Field: Dance; Music; Theatre; Pop
Status: Nonprofit
Paid Staff: 2
Volunteer Staff: 6
Budget: $200,000
Income Sources: Box Office; Grants; Gifts; In Kind Services
Affiliations: APAP; IEG
Annual Attendance: 5,500

4353 ORLANDO-UCF SHAKESPEARE FESTIVAL
812 E Rollins Street
Suite 100
Orlando, FL 32803
Phone: 407-893-4600
Fax: 407-893-5643
e-mail: shakesinfo@mpinet.net
Web Site: www.shakespearefest.org
Management:
  Artistic Director: Jim Helsinger
Mission: Will serve as a cultural resource to the community by presenting the plays of Shakespeare and other theatrical works, as well as the artistic and educational activities inspired by them. Festival presentations will reflect the highest possible artistic, educational and ethical values. We will strive fore artistic and educational excellence and innovation.

4354 SOCIETY OF THE FOUR ARTS
2 Four Arts Plaza
Palm Beach, FL 33480
Phone: 561-655-7227
Fax: 561-655-7233
e-mail: sfourarts@aol.com
Web Site: www.fourarts.org
Officers:
  President: Ervin Duggan
  Executive VP: Nancy Mato
  Director Public Relations: Paula Law
Founded: 1936
Specialized Field: Library; Childrens Library; Gardens; Concerts; Films
Paid Staff: 20
Volunteer Staff: 5
Performs At: Four Arts Auditorium

4355 TREASURE COAST CONCERT ASSOCIATION
2394 SW Foxpoint Way
Palm City, FL 34990
Phone: 772-220-8400
Fax: 772-220-8401
Officers:
  President: Ernest Berlin
Performs At: Lyric Theatre

4356 BAY ARTS ALLIANCE
PO Box 1153
Panama City, FL 32402
Phone: 850-769-1217
Fax: 850-785-5165
e-mail: thebigBA@prodigy.net
Web Site: www.bayarts.org
Management:
  Executive Director: Jan Benjamin
Performs At: Marina Civic Theatre

4357 PANAMA CITY MUSIC ASSOCIATION SERIES
PO Box 133
Panama City, FL 32402

Phone: 850-769-2707
Fax: 850-913-0498
e-mail: CoxJB@worldnet.att.net
Officers:
    Talent Chairman: Joanne B Cox
Performs At: Municipal Auditorium

4358 CLASSICFEST, PENSACOLA SUMMER MUSIC FESTIVAL

PO Box 12683
Pensacola, FL 32574
Phone: 850-432-5118
Fax: 850-434-8700
e-mail: ccpns@aol.com
Web Site: www.christchurchpns.org
Management:
    Executive Director: Kenneth Karadin

4359 MUSIC HALL ARTIST SERIES
University of West Florida

11000 University Parkway
Pensacola, FL 32514
Phone: 850-474-2541
Fax: 850-474-3247
e-mail: lmay0@uwf.edu
Web Site: www.uwf.edu/cfpa
Management:
    Assistant Director: Linda May
Mission: To provide the Pensacola community with world-class performances of chamber music.
Founded: 1970
Status: Professional
Paid Staff: 1
Paid Artists: 6
Budget: $10,000
Income Sources: SGA; University President; Private Funding
Performs At: Music Hall
Annual Attendance: 1,000
Facility Category: Education
Type of Stage: Proscenium; Arena; Concert Hall
Seating Capacity: 426; 120; 307
Year Built: 1992
Rental Contact: Linda May
Organization Type: Sponsoring

4360 HOLLYWOOD JAZZ FESTIVAL

10885 NW Fifth Street
Plantation, FL 33324
Phone: 954-236-0175
Fax: 954-236-0176
e-mail: rw@southfloridajazz.org
Web Site: www.southfloridajazz.org
Management:
    Artistic Director: Dr. Ronald B Weber

4361 FRIENDS OF MUSIC OF CHARLOTTE COUNTY CONCERT SERIES

533 Skylark Lane
Port Charlotte, FL 33952
Phone: 941-625-3177
Management:
    Concert Series Director: Mauriel Van Patten

Performs At: Port Charlotte Cultural Center Theatre
Facility Category: Concert Hall
Seating Capacity: 418

4362 BIG ARTS GREAT PERFORMERS SERIES

900 Dunlop Road
Sanibel, FL 33957
Phone: 941-395-0900
Fax: 941-395-0330
e-mail: email@bigarts.org
Web Site: www.bigarts.org
Management:
    Executive Director: Liz Fowler
Founded: 1979
Specialized Field: Performing Arts; Visual Arts; Arts Education; Films
Status: Nonprofit
Paid Staff: 4
Volunteer Staff: 40
Budget: $700,000
Facility Category: Cultural Center
Seating Capacity: 414
Year Built: 1979
Year Remodeled: 1997

4363 SANIBEL MUSIC FESTIVAL

PO Box 1623
Sanibel, FL 33957-1623
Phone: 941-336-7999
Fax: 941-395-1375
Web Site: www.sanibelmusicfestival.org
Management:
    Artistic Director: Mary Jaqua
Season: March
Performs At: Sanibel Island (Festival Site)
Facility Category: Sanibel Congregational Church
Seating Capacity: 350

4364 ASOLO THEATRE FESTIVAL

5555 N Tamiami Trail
Sarasota, FL 34243
Phone: 813-351-9010
Fax: 813-351-5796
Toll-free: 800-361-8388
e-mail: asolo@asolo.org
Web Site: www.asolo.org
Officers:
    Co-President: J Robert Peterson
    Co-President: Lee M Peterson
Management:
    Producing Artistic Director: Howard J Millman
    Managing Director: Linda M DiGabriele
Mission: To foster an appreciation for the performing arts in the community, state and country by utilizing live performances as to educate students by placing them with professional actors with whom they may learn the theatrical trade.
Founded: 1960
Specialized Field: Theatrical Group
Status: Professional; Nonprofit
Volunteer Staff: 200

Income Sources: Theatre Communications Group; American Arts Alliance; Actors' Equity Association; League of Resident Theatres
Performs At: Harold E and Esther M Mertz Theatre; Jane B Cook Theatre
Organization Type: Performing; Educational

4365   BONK FESTIVAL OF NEW MUSIC
New College of USF, Humanities Division
5700 N Tamiami Trail
Sarasota, FL 34243-2197
Phone: 813-930-8440
Fax: 941-359-4479
e-mail: info@bonkfest.org
Web Site: www.bonkfest.org
Specialized Field: Instrumental; Multi-Media; Dance; Educational
Budget: $10,000
Season: February - March
Performs At: Tampa, Sarasota, St. Petersburg (Festival Site)
Facility Category: Theatres; Auditoriums; Museums

4366   FLORIDA WEST COAST SYMPHONY SERIES
709 N Tamiami Trail
Sarasota, FL 34236
Phone: 941-953-4252
Fax: 941-953-3059
Toll-free: 800-287-9634
e-mail: symphony@fwcs.org
Web Site: www.fwcs.org
Officers:
   President: Jack Jost
   Vice President: Beatrice Friedman
   VP: Susan Weinkle
   Secretary: Ronald Jurgens
   Treasurer: Ernest Rice
Management:
   Executive Director: Joseph McKenna
   General Manager: Trevor Cramer
   Business Manager: Susan May-Lagg
   Educational Director: Elizabeth Power
Mission: To present Florida symphonies, festivals, orchestras and youth orchestra.
Founded: 1949
Specialized Field: Instrumental Music; Festivals
Status: Professional; Nonprofit
Paid Staff: 25
Paid Artists: 100
Budget: $3,800,000
Income Sources: Ticket Sales; Donations
Performs At: Holley Hall; Van Wezel Performing Arts Hall
Annual Attendance: 100,000
Facility Category: Concert Hall
Type of Stage: Raised Open
Stage Dimensions: 16'x32'
Seating Capacity: 500
Year Remodeled: 1985
Architect: Garry Hoyt
Cost: $800,000
Organization Type: Performing; Resident; Educational; Sponsoring

---

4367   LA MUSICA FESTIVAL
1741 Main Street
Suite 101
Sarasota, FL 34236
Mailing Address: PO Box 5442 Sarasota, FL 34277
Phone: 941-364-8802
Fax: 941-346-2414
Management:
   Executive Director: Sally R Faron
Founded: 1987
Specialized Field: Chamber Music Festival
Paid Staff: 4
Volunteer Staff: 4
Paid Artists: 11
Budget: $200,000
Income Sources: Tickets; Sponsorships; Gifts
Season: April
Performs At: University of South Florida, Sainer Center (Festival Site)
Annual Attendance: 4,500
Facility Category: Sarasota Opera House
Seating Capacity: 1,100

4368   SARASOTA CONCERT ASSOCIATION
4346 Bryant's Pond Lane
Sarasota, FL 34233
Phone: 941-925-7811
Fax: 941-925-7811
e-mail: streetleit@aol.com
Officers:
   President: Martha Leiter
Management:
   Artistic Selection Chairman: Martha Leiter
Performs At: Van Wezel Performing Arts Hall

4369   SARASOTA JAZZ FESTIVAL
330 S Pineapple Avenue
#111
Sarasota, FL 34236
Phone: 941-366-1552
Fax: 941-366-1553
e-mail: mail@jazzclubsarasota.com
Web Site: www.jazzclubsarasota.com
Officers:
   President: Bobby Prince

4370   SARASOTA MUSIC FESTIVAL
709 N Tamiami Trail
Sarasota, FL 34236
Phone: 941-953-4252
Fax: 941-953-3059
e-mail: smf@fwcs.org
Web Site: www.fwcs.org
Officers:
   President: Jack L Frost
   VP: Beatrice Friedman
   VP: Bryan Langton
   VP: Hope Leuchter
   Secretary: Ronald Jurgens
   Treasurer: Douglas Shanley
Management:
   Artistic Director: Paul Wolfe
   Administrative Director: RoseAnne McCabe
   Executive Director: Joseph McKenna

All listings are in alphabetical order by state, then city, then organization within the city.

General Manager: Trevor Cramer
Business Manager: Susan Lagg-May
Marketing Director: Linda Joffe
Development Director: Kristina Kelly
Mission: The Sarasota Music Festival, strives to promote and nurture the study and performance of chamber music; present the finest chamber music performances for residents and visitors; provide the highest quality music education for the nation's most talented music students; and establishes Sarasota as a national and international tourist destination.
Founded: 1965
Specialized Field: Festivals
Status: Educational; Nonprofit
Income Sources: Chamber Music America
Performs At: Holley Hall; Sarasota Opera House
Facility Category: Chamber Music; Music Education
Organization Type: Performing; Educational

4371 SEASIDE INSTITUTE SERIES

30 Smolian Circle, 2nd Floor
PO Box 4730
Seaside, FL 32459
Phone: 850-231-2421
Fax: 850-231-1884
e-mail: institute@seasidefl.org
Web Site: www.theseasideinstitute.org
Management:
Executive Director: Phyllis Bleiweis
Performs At: Seaside Meeting Hall

4372 MUSEUM OF FINE ARTS SERIES

255 Beach Drive NE
St. Petersburg, FL 33701
Phone: 727-896-2667
Fax: 727-894-4638
e-mail: gale@fine-arts.org
Web Site: www.fine-arts.org
Management:
AV Tech-Stage: Tom Gessler
Mission: To present classical concerts.
Founded: 1961
Specialized Field: Tampa Bay
Paid Staff: 4
Volunteer Staff: 6
Paid Artists: 12

4373 ST. PETERSBURG COLLEGE

6605 5th Avenue N
St. Petersburg, FL 33710
Mailing Address: PO Box 13489 St. Petersburg, FL 33733
Phone: 727-341-4360
Fax: 727-341-4744
e-mail: steelej@spcollege.edu
Web Site: www.spcollege.du/spg/music
Management:
Program Director: Jonathan E Steele
Mission: Education
Founded: 1927
Specialized Field: Music; Choral; Instrumental; Piano; Vocal; Guitar
Paid Staff: 60

4374 TALLAHASSEE MUSEUM

3945 Museum Drive
Tallahassee, FL 32310-6325
Phone: 850-575-8684
Fax: 850-574-8243
e-mail: karen@tallahasseemuseum.org
Web Site: www.tallahasseemuseum.org/jazz.html
Management:
Director: Russell Daws

4375 ATLANTIC SHAKESPEARE FESTIVAL

1435 22nd Avenue
Vero Beach, FL 32085-1975
Phone: 772-559-0556
e-mail: AtlanticShakes@yahoo.com
Web Site: www.geocities.com
Management:
Artistic Director: John A Putzke
Mission: Was founded to provide classical theatrical works, with an emphasis on the works of William Shakespeare, to the residents and visitors to St. Augustine, Florida.
Founded: 1997
Income Sources: Program Ad Sales; Production Sponsors; Grants; Private Donations
Facility Category: Outdoor Amphitheatre
Type of Stage: Proscenium
Stage Dimensions: 60;x30'
Seating Capacity: 2200
Year Built: 1995

4376 REGIONAL ARTS MUSIC AT THE KRAVIS CENTER FOR THE PERFORMING ARTS

701 Okeechobee Boulevard
West Palm Beach, FL 33401
Phone: 561-835-4141
Fax: 561-833-3901
e-mail: tilley@kravis.org
Management:
Administator: Susan Tilley
Performs At: Kravis Center for the Arts

4377 SUNFEST OF PALM BEACH COUNTY

319 Clematis Street
West Palm Beach, FL 33401
Phone: 561-659-5980
Fax: 561-659-3567
e-mail: sunfest@sunfest.org
Web Site: www.sunfest.org
Management:
Executive Director: Paul Jamieson
Communications Coordinator: Susan Grubbs
Marketing Manager: Terri Neil
Mission: To support a variety of quality visual and performing arts festivals and entertainment events meeting the highest degree of excellence.
Founded: 1982
Specialized Field: Festivals
Status: Nonprofit
Paid Staff: 10
Paid Artists: 210
Income Sources: International Festival Association

All listings are in alphabetical order by state, then city, then organization within the city.

Performs At: Along the Intracoastal Waterway; Flagler Drive
Organization Type: Resident

4378 POLK COMMUNITY COLLEGE SPECIAL PERFORMANCE SERIES
999 Avenue H NE
Winter Haven, FL 33881-4299
Phone: 863-297-1050
Fax: 863-297-1053
e-mail: sbevis@polk.cc.fl.us
Web Site: www.polk.cc.fl.us
Management:
    Cultural Events Assistant: Sharon Bevis
Paid Staff: 2
Volunteer Staff: 4
Paid Artists: 6

4379 BACH FESTIVAL SOCIETY
1000 Holt Avenue-2763
Winter Park, FL 32789-4499
Phone: 407-646-2182
Fax: 407-646-2692
e-mail: info@bachfestivalflorida.org
Web Site: www.bachfestivalflorida.org
Officers:
    President: John M Tiedtice
Management:
    Executive Director: J Joshua Garrick
    Conductor/Music Director: Dr. John V Sinclair
Founded: 1935
Specialized Field: Performing Arts; Education
Paid Staff: 11
Volunteer Staff: 215
Paid Artists: 40
Income Sources: Box Office; Grants; Private Donations
Performs At: Annie Russell Theatre; Knowles Memorial Chapel
Affiliations: Rollins College
Annual Attendance: 26,000
Facility Category: Theatre; Chapel
Type of Stage: Proscenium
Seating Capacity: 1,500; 375

4380 FESTIVAL OF ORCHESTRAS
1353 Palmetto Avenue
Suite 100
Winter Park, FL 32789
Phone: 407-539-0295
Fax: 407-539-0525
Toll-free: 800-738-8188
e-mail: greatorchs@cfl.rr.com
Web Site: www.festivaloforchestras.com
Officers:
    CEO: Joseph J Rizzo
Mission: The mission of the Festival of Orchestras (FOI) is to present premier live performances to the world's great symphony orchestras to the Central Florida public, and at a reasonable price for all. Introducing young children and their teachers, from local schools to world-class orchestral concerts. We also encourage support from the local business community, by providing introductions to international business leaders.
Founded: 1984

Paid Staff: 4
Volunteer Staff: 3
Performs At: Bob Carr Performing Arts Center
Affiliations: OCCA

4381 WINTER PARK BACH FESTIVAL
1000 Holt Avenue - 2763
Winter Park, FL 32789-4499
Phone: 407-646-2182
Fax: 407-656-2533
Officers:
    President: John Tiedtke
Management:
    Director/Conductor: Dr. John V Sinclair
Season: February
Performs At: Rollins Colliseum, Winter Park (Festival Site)
Facility Category: Knowles Memorial Chapel
Seating Capacity: 500

Georgia

4382 PORTERFIELD MEMORIAL UNITED METHODIST CHURCH - DISTINGUISHED ARTIST SERIES
2200 Dawson Road
Albany, GA 31707
Phone: 229-436-6336
Fax: 229-439-9141
e-mail: mikekeeley@porterfieldchurch.org
Web Site: www.porterfieldchurch.org
Management:
    Music Ministries Director: Michael Keeley
Seating Capacity: 850

4383 ARTS FESTIVAL OF ATLANTA
34 Peachtree Street NW
Suite 250
Altanta, GA 30303
Phone: 404-589-8777
Fax: 404-589-8161
e-mail: burgessafa@aol.com
Management:
    Artistic Director: Leslie Gordon
Season: June
Performs At: Centennial Olympic Park (Festival Site)
Seating Capacity: 1,000

4384 GEORGIA SOUTHWESTERN STATE UNIVERSITY CHAMBER CONCERT SERIES
800 Wheatley Street
Americus, GA 31709-4693
Phone: 229-931-2204
Fax: 229-931-2927
e-mail: jem@canes.gsw.edu
Officers:
    Fine Arts Department Chairman: Julie Megginson
Specialized Field: Music
Performs At: Fine Arts Theatre
Seating Capacity: 250

4385 FORTE: THE UNIVERSITY UNION PERFORMING ARTS SERIES

Tate Center, Room 153
University of Georgia
Athens, GA 30602-3401
Phone: 706-542-6396
Fax: 706-542-5584
e-mail: joslyn@arches.uga.edu
Web Site: www.uga.edu/stuart
Management:
   Program Advisor: Joslyn Diramio
   Student Coordinator: Nathan Copeland
Mission: To deliver a culturally and artistically diverse programming schedule to the University community.
Paid Staff: 1
Volunteer Staff: 15
Paid Artists: 6
Budget: $143,850
Income Sources: Student Activity Fees; Ticket Sales

4386 ATLANTA JAZZ FESTIVAL
Atlantic Bureau of Cultural Affairs

675 Ponce De Leon
Atlanta, GA 30308
Phone: 404-817-6851
Fax: 404-658-6945
Management:
   Bureau Director: Barbara Bowser
   Festivals Manager: Jackie Davis
Mission: To offer a showcase for talented local and national performers; to provide Atlanta citizens with jazz music.
Specialized Field: Dance; Vocal Music; Instrumental Music
Status: Professional; Nonprofit
Performs At: Grant Park
Organization Type: Performing; Educational

4387 GEORGIA SHAKESPEARE FESTIVAL

Conant Performing Arts Center
4484 Peachtree Road Northeast
Atlanta, GA 30319
Phone: 404-264-0020
Fax: 404-504-3414
e-mail: boxoffice@gashakespeare.org
Web Site: www.gashakespeare.org/
Management:
   Artistic/Producing Director: Richard Garner
   Managing Director: Philip J Santora
   Education Director: Kathleen McManus
   Marketing Director: Stacey Colosa Lucas
   Production Manager: Rob Dillard
   Development Officer: Sarah Robinson
   Events/Volunteer Coordinator: Carla Hyman
   Company Manager: Christy Costello
   Box Office Manager: Thomas Pinckney
Mission: To produce professional plays written by Shakespeare and other enduring authors.
Founded: 1985
Specialized Field: Theater; Festivals
Status: Professional; Nonprofit
Paid Staff: 7
Income Sources: Southeastern Theatre Conference; Atlanta Theatre Coalition

Organization Type: Performing; Resident

4388 NATIONAL BLACK ARTS FESTIVAL

659 Auburn Avenue
Studioplex Suite 254
Atlanta, GA 30312
Phone: 404-730-7315
Fax: 404-730-7104
Web Site: www.nbaf.org
Officers:
   Chairperson: Nancy A Boxill PhD
   Vice Chairperson: Curley M Dossman
   Treasurer: M Erwin Carter
Management:
   Executive Producer: Stephanie Hughley
   Associate Producer: Laura Greer
   Director Marketing/Development: Judith Service Montier
Mission: To develop, expose and educate audiences to the arts and culture of the African Diaspora and provide diverse opportunities for artistic and creative expression.
Founded: 1987
Specialized Field: Dance; Vocal Music; Instrumental Music; Theater; Festivals
Status: Nonprofit
Paid Staff: 10
Volunteer Staff: 200
Paid Artists: 150
Budget: $2 Million
Income Sources: Fulton County Arts Council; Ticket Sales; Corporate Sponsors; Foundations
Organization Type: Presenting

4389 OGLETHORPE UNIVERSITY- ARTS AND IDEAS AT OGLETHORPE

4484 Peachtree Road NE
Atlanta, GA 30319-4487
Phone: 404-364-8429
Fax: 404-364-8442
Toll-free: 800-428-4484
e-mail: IRAY@Oglethorpe.edu
Web Site: www.oglethorpe.edu
Officers:
   President: Larry D Large
Management:
   Music Director: Dr. W Irwin Ray
Mission: To support the programming of the university.
Founded: 1835
Specialized Field: Classical Concerts
Paid Staff: 1
Volunteer Staff: 4
Performs At: Conant Center for the Performing Arts

4390 SCHWARTZ CENTER FOR PERFORMING ARTS AT EMORY

1700 N Decatur Road
Atlanta, GA 30322
Phone: 404-727-8769
Fax: 404-727-4763
e-mail: dlayend@emory.edu
Web Site: www.emory.edu/arts/
Management:
   Managing Director: Robert McKay
   Assistant Marketing/PR Director: Sally Corbett

All listings are in alphabetical order by state, then city, then organization within the city.

Assistant Director Programming: Debbie Joyal
Box Office Manager: Piper Phillips
Specialized Field: Music; Dance; Theatre
Paid Staff: 9
Performs At: Glenn Memorial Auditorium; Munroe Theater; Dance Studio; Music; Dance; Theater; Schwartz Center for Performing Arts
Annual Attendance: 30,000
Facility Category: Multiple Facilities

4391 SPELMAN COLLEGE FRESH IMAGES CHAMBER MUSIC SERIES
PO Box 246
350 Spelman Lane Southwest
Atlanta, GA 30314
Phone: 404-223-7680
Fax: 404-215-7771
e-mail: kjohns10@spelman.edu
Web Site: www.spelman.edu
Officers:
   Chairman Music Department: Kevin Johnson
Specialized Field: Music
Performs At: Sisters Chapel

4392 GREATER AUGUSTA ARTS COUNCIL
PO Box 1776
Augusta, GA 30903
Phone: 706-826-4723
Fax: 706-826-4702
Web Site: www.augustaarts.com
Management:
   Events Director: Leslie Fletcher

4393 GEORGIA PERIMETER COLLEGE GUEST ARTIST SERIES
555 N Indian Creek Drive
Clarkston, GA 30021
Phone: 404-299-4150
Fax: 404-299-4271
Management:
   Music Performance Coordinator: Susan Sigmon
Performs At: Marvin Cole Auditorium

4394 ARTS ASSOCIATION IN NEWTON COUNTY
PO Box 1586
Covington, GA 30015
Phone: 770-786-8188
Fax: 770-784-1692
e-mail: info@concertasso.com
Web Site: www.artsassoc.org
Management:
   Executive Director: Bunny Lanners
Performs At: Olive Swann Porter Hall

4395 NORTH GEORGIA COLLEGE & STATE UNIVERSITY MUSIC SERIES
Student Center
101 College Circle
Dahlonega, GA 30597
Phone: 706-864-1643
Fax: 706-864-1647
e-mail: wthomas@ngcsu.edu
Web Site: www.ngc.peachnet.edu
Management:
   Student Activities Director: Wesley Thomas
   Professor Music/Keyboarding: Joe Chapman
   Director Choral Activities: John Broman
   Director Bands/Music Education: Kirk Weller
Performs At: Student Center Auditorium

4396 GILMER ARTS & HERITAGE ASSOCIATION SERIES
200 Industrial Boulevard
Suite 103-B
Ellijay, GA 30540-3335
Phone: 706-635-5605
Fax: 706-636-5606
e-mail: gaha@ellijay.com
Web Site: www.gilmercounty.com/gaha
Management:
   Director: Diana Gregory
   Administrative Assistant: Heather Herold
Founded: 1979
Paid Staff: 2
Volunteer Staff: 30
Non-paid Artists: 35
Performs At: Ellijay Elementary School Theatre
Seating Capacity: 600

4397 ARTS COUNCIL
PO Box 1632
331 Spring Street Southwest
Gainesville, GA 30503
Phone: 770-534-2787
Fax: 770-534-2973
e-mail: gladys@theartscouncil.net
Web Site: www.theartscouncil.net
Management:
   Executive Director: Gladys Wyant
Mission: To further the appreciation and participation in various art forms; to encourage high standards and public interest in the arts.
Founded: 1970
Paid Staff: 4
Volunteer Staff: 300
Paid Artists: 200
Non-paid Artists: 20
Budget: $420,000
Performs At: Pearce Auditorium
Affiliations: Brenau University; Crawford W Lang Museum; Elachee Nature Science Center; Gainesville Ballet Company; Gainesville Chorale; Gainesville Theatre
Seating Capacity: 720
Rental Contact: Gladys Wyant

4398 MACON CONCERT ASSOCIATION
3140 Ingleside Avenue
Macon, GA 31204
Phone: 478-743-6039
Officers:
   VP: Edward Eikner
Performs At: Porter Auditorium

4399 MUSIC MERCER SERIES
Mercer University
1400 Coleman Avenue
Music Department
Macon, GA 31207
Phone: 478-301-2748
Fax: 478-301-5633
e-mail: Roberts_JN@mercer.edu
Officers:
　Music Department Chairman: Dr. John Roberts
Performs At: McCorkle Music Building; Recital Hall
Affiliations: NASM
Seating Capacity: 190
Year Built: 2001
Cost: 7,000,000

4400 BREWTON-PARKER COLLEGE FINE ARTS COUNCIL
US 280
Mount Vernon, GA 30445
Phone: 912-583-3133
Fax: 912-583-3136
e-mail: pdickens@bpc.edu
Officers:
　Chairman: Pierce Dickens
Performs At: Gilder Recital Hall

4401 ARMSTRONG ATLANTIC STATE UNIVERSITY
11935 Abercorn Street
Savannah, GA 31419
Phone: 912-927-5325
Fax: 912-921-5492
Web Site: www.finearts.armstrong.edu
Founded: 1935
Specialized Field: Art; Music; Theatre
Performs At: AASU Fine Arts Auditorium
Seating Capacity: 960
Year Built: 1975

4402 SAVANNAH CONCERT ASSOCIATION
701 3 44th Street
Savannah, GA 31405
Phone: 912-356-8193
Officers:
　President: Martin Greenburg

4403 SAVANNAH MUSIC FESTIVAL
Stevens Shipping
26 E Bay Street
Savannah, GA 31401
Mailing Address: PO Box 8105 Savannah, GA 31412-8105
Phone: 912-236-5745
Fax: 912-236-1989
Toll-free: 800-868-3378
e-mail: atc@savannahonstage.org
Web Site: www.savannahonstage.org
Management:
　Executive/Artistic Director: Rob Gibson
Mission: Music festival in historic Savannah, Georgia.
Specialized Field: Presenting; Music
Paid Staff: 6

Volunteer Staff: 260
Paid Artists: 231
Non-paid Artists: 78
Budget: $866,000
Income Sources: Box Office; Grants; Corporate; Foundation; Individuals; Government
Season: March
Performs At: Historic District of Savannah (Festival Site)
Annual Attendance: 20,000
Facility Category: Historic Churches; Synagogues; Recital Halls
Seating Capacity: 400 - 1,200 (indoors); 3,000 (outdoors)

4404 THOMASTON-UPSON ARTS COUNCIL PERFORMING SERIES
201 S Center Street
PO Box 211
Thomaston, GA 30286
Phone: 706-647-1605
Fax: 706-647-2187
Management:
　Executive Director: Tempy Hoylal
Founded: 1986
Specialized Field: Dance; Vocal Music; Instrumental Music; Theater
Status: Nonprofit
Organization Type: Performing; Educational; Sponsoring

4405 THOMASVILLE ENTERTAINMENT FOUNDATION
600 East Washington Street
Thomasville, GA 31792
Mailing Address: PO Box 1976 Thomasville, GA 31799
Phone: 229-226-6130
Fax: 229-226-0599
e-mail: jpfga@rose.net
Web Site: tccarts.com/tef.htm
Management:
　Executive Director: Janice Faircloth
Performs At: Thomasville Cultural Center
Seating Capacity: 500

4406 JEKYLL ISLAND MUSICAL THEATRE FESTIVAL
Department of Communication Arts
Valdosta, GA 31698
Phone: 912-333-5820
Fax: 912-245-3799
e-mail: dguthrie@valdosta.edu
Management:
　Managing Director: Duke Guthrie
　Dean School of the Arts: Dr. Lanny Milbrandt
Mission: Providing Georgia's Golden Isles residents and visitors with quality musical theatre; offering college interns professional training.
Founded: 1990
Specialized Field: Summer Stock; Musical
Status: Professional; Nonprofit
Paid Artists: 65
Income Sources: Valdosta State University

Season: June - August
Performs At: Jekyll Island Amphitheater
Annual Attendance: 10,000
Facility Category: Professional Summer Stock Theatre
Type of Stage: Wooden, uncovered amphitheatre
Seating Capacity: 500
Year Built: 1970
Organization Type: Performing; Touring

**4407 LOWNDES/VALDOSTA ARTS
COMMISSION**
1204 N Patterson
PO Box 1966
Valdosta, GA 31603
Phone: 229-247-2787
Fax: 229-242-6690
e-mail: l/vac@surfsouth.com
Management:
    Executive Director: Roberta George
Performs At: Mathis Municipal Auditorium

Hawaii

4408 HAWAII CONCERT SERIES
PO Box 233
Hilo, HI 96721
Phone: 808-935-5831
e-mail: jwakely@hialoha
Officers:
    VP: Judith Wakely
Performs At: University of Hawaii at Hilo Theatre
Seating Capacity: 600

4409 HONOLULU CHAMBER MUSIC SERIES
Box 2233
Honolulu, HI 96804
Phone: 808-528-8226
Fax: 808-956-9422
e-mail: tslaught@outreach.hawaii.edu
Officers:
    President: Andrew Bunn
Performs At: Orvis Auditorium

4410 UNIVERSITY OF HAWAII SERIES
2530 Dole Street
Room D-406
Honolulu, HI 96822
Phone: 808-956-2036
Fax: 808-956-9422
e-mail: tslaught@outreach.hawaii.edu
Web Site: www.outreach.hawaii.edu
Management:
    Community Services Director: Tim Slaughter
Mission: Presenting organization
Performs At: Various Auditoriums

4411 MAUI COMMUNITY COLLEGE SERIES
310 Kaahumanu Avenue
Kahului, HI 96732

Phone: 808-984-3273
Fax: 808-244-9632
e-mail: Barbara.Bitner@mauicc.hawaii.edu
Management:
    Special Programs Coordinator: Barbara Bitner
Performs At: Maui Arts & Cultural Center

**4412 HALAU HULA KA NO'EAU
Hawai'i Arts Ensemble**
Kamuela, HI 96743-1907
Mailing Address: PO Box 1907
Phone: 808-885-6525
Fax: 808-885-9018
e-mail: HULA@artofhula.com
Web Site: www.artofhula.com
Management:
    Booking/Tour Coordinator: Virginia Ptaff
    Director: Michael Pili Pang
    Technical: Barbara Thompson
Mission: To promote and sustain the inherent cultural and
artistic values of Hawaiian Dance.
Founded: 1986
Specialized Field: Hula; Hawaiian Chant and Music

**4413 BRIGHAM YOUNG UNIVERSITY:
HAWAII PERFORMANCE SERIES**
PO Box 1924
Laie, HI 96762
Phone: 808-293-3551
Fax: 808-293-3374
e-mail: sagisis@byuh.edu
Web Site: www.byuh.edu
Management:
    Director: Sandra Sagisi
Performs At: David O. McKay Auditorium
Seating Capacity: 649

Idaho

4414 BOISE CHAMBER MUSIC SERIES
1910 University Drive
Boise, ID 83725-1560
Phone: 208-426-1216
Fax: 208-426-1771
e-mail: jbelfy@boisestate.edu
Management:
    Manager: Jeanne Belfy
Performs At: Morrison Center Recital Hall

4415 IDAHO SHAKESPEARE FESTIVAL
615 East 43rd Street
Boise, ID 83714
Phone: 208-323-9700
Fax: 208-323-0700
Web Site: www.idahoshakespeare.org
Management:
    Artistic Director: Charles Fee
    Managing Director: Mark Hofflund
Founded: 1976
Specialized Field: Theater
Status: Professional; Nonprofit
Paid Staff: 10

Season: May - September
Organization Type: Performing; Touring; Educational

4416 CALDWELL FINE ARTS SERIES

2112 Cleveland Boulevard
Caldwell, ID 83605
Phone: 208-454-1376
Fax: 208-459-2077
e-mail: cfa@acofi.edu
Web Site: www.albertson.edu/cfa
Management:
    Manager: Sylvia Hunt
Mission: To offer professional performances in the performing arts; to provide local industry groups and schools with training and support.
Founded: 1961
Specialized Field: Dance; Vocal Music; Instrumental Music; Theater; Grand Opera
Status: Nonprofit
Income Sources: Pacific Northwest Presenters
Performs At: Jewett Auditorium
Organization Type: Educational; Sponsoring

4417 LIONEL HAMPTON JAZZ FESTIVAL

University of Idaho
PO Box 444257
Moscow, ID 83844-4257
Phone: 208-885-6765
Fax: 208-885-6513
e-mail: jazzinfo@uidaho.edu
Web Site: www.jazz.uidaho.edu
Management:
    Executive Director: Dr. Lynn J Skinner
    Program Advisor: Christopher Peters
Mission: Through four days of student competitions, artist workshops and world class concerts, the Lionel Hampton Jazz Festival keeps the magic, music and spirit of jazz alive for generations to come by inspiring students, teachers and artists of all ages and abilities to support music education in schools and colleges throughout the US and Canada and very directly at the University of Idaho.
Founded: 1967
Specialized Field: Music Jazz Festival
Paid Staff: 6
Volunteer Staff: 400
Paid Artists: 84
Budget: $ 1 Million
Income Sources: Ticket Sales; Sponsorships; Registration Fees
Affiliations: University of Idaho
Annual Attendance: 25,000-30,000
Facility Category: University
Stage Dimensions: 50x100
Seating Capacity: 10,000

4418 PERFORMING ARTS SERIES OF MOUNTAIN HOME

935 N 12 E
Mountain Home, ID 83647
Phone: 208-587-4821
Management:
    Executive Director: Laurie Unrein

Mission: To offer diverse professional, performing arts presentations to the Mountain Home community.
Specialized Field: Dance; Vocal Music; Instrumental Music; Theater
Status: Non-Professional
Organization Type: Performing; Educational

4419 IDAHO STATE UNIVERSITY THEATRE DEPARTMENT

5th and Carter
PO Box 8115
Pocatello, ID 83209
Phone: 208-282-3695
Fax: 208-282-4598
e-mail: diensher@isu.edu
Web Site: cwis.isu.edu/departments/theater
Management:
    Director of Theatre: Sherri R Dienstfrey
Founded: 1901
Paid Staff: 2
Performs At: Student Union Ballroom
Affiliations: Alpha Psa Omega
Type of Stage: Proscenium Thurst

4420 BRIGHAM YOUNG UNIVERSITY: IDAHO

Brigham Young University-Idaho
Rexburg, ID 83460-1660
Phone: 208-496-1152
e-mail: sparhawkd@byui.edu
Web Site: www.byui.edu
Management:
    Coordinator: Don Sparhawk
Mission: Our year round series of more than 20 performance offers a variety of music, dance and theater that is intended to entertain, uplift and enlighten both our students and the surrounding community.
Founded: 1888
Performs At: Hart Auditorium; Barrus Concert Hall; Kirkham Auditorium

4421 SALMON ARTS COUNCIL

200 Main Street
Salmon, ID 83467
Phone: 208-756-2987
Fax: 208-756-4840
e-mail: sac1@ida.net
Web Site: www.salmonidaho.com
Management:
    Executive Director: Janice Torrey
Performs At: Salmon High School Gymnasium

4422 FESTIVAL AT SANDPOINT

PO Box 695
Sandpoint, ID 83864
Phone: 208-265-4554
Fax: 208-263-6858
e-mail: efstival@sandpoint.net
Web Site: www.sandpoint.org/festival
Management:
    Executive Director: Dyno Wahl
Performs At: Memorial Field; Schweitzer Mountain Resort (Festival Site)

Facility Category: Memorial Field
Seating Capacity: 2,500

4423 PEND OREILLE ARTS COUNCIL
PO Box 1694
Sandpoint, ID 83864
Phone: 208-263-0712
Fax: 208-265-2490
e-mail: msabella@dmi.net
Management:
   Artistic Director: Marilyn Sabella
Mission: Exists to facilitate and present the finest quality experiences in the arts for the people of the Sandpoint area.
Performs At: Panida Theatre

4424 SUN VALLEY SUMMER SYMPHONY
PO Box 1914
Sun Valley, ID 83353
Phone: 208-622-5607
Fax: 208-622-9149
e-mail: svss@sunvalley.net
Web Site: svsummersymphony.org
Officers:
   President: Harriet Parker-Bass
   VP: Jon Thorson
   VP: Preston Strazza
   Treasurer: Dick Porter
   Secretary: Preston Strazza
Management:
   Music Director: Alasdair Neale
   Founder: Carl Eberl
   Executive Director: Jaci Wilkins
Mission: To provide quality free, classical music performances that have cultural, educational, and artistic relevance.
Founded: 1985
Paid Staff: 1.5
Paid Artists: 90
Budget: $860,000
Income Sources: Individual; Business; Private Donations
Season: Late July - Mid August
Performs At: Sun Valley (Festival Site)
Facility Category: Sun Valley Esplanade Tent
Stage Dimensions: 60'x 40'
Seating Capacity: 1,000

4425 ARTS ON TOUR SERIES
PO Box 1158
Twin Falls, ID 83303
Phone: 208-734-2787
Fax: 208-736-3015
e-mail: mvac@micron.net
Performs At: Auditorium

Illinois

4426 ARTS AT ARGONNE MUSIC SERIES
Argonne National Laboratory, Building 221
9700 S Cass Avenue
Argonne, IL 60439

Phone: 630-252-7160
Fax: 630-252-5986
e-mail: arts@anl.gov
Web Site: www.anl.gov/ARTS/intro.html
Officers:
   Chairman: Dr. Hans Kaper
Mission: Supporting world class cultural presentations for employees of Argonne National laboratory and their families and for residents of neighboring communities.
Founded: 1988
Specialized Field: Instrumental Music
Status: Non-Professional
Volunteer Staff: 15
Budget: $20,000-$35,000
Income Sources: Ticket Sales; Illinois Arts Council
Performs At: Auditorium
Affiliations: Chicago Music Alliance
Facility Category: Auditorium
Seating Capacity: 400
Organization Type: Sponsoring

4427 PARAMOUNT ARTS CENTRE PERFORMING ARTS SERIES
8 E Galena Boulevard
Suite 230
Aurora, IL 60506
Phone: 630-896-7676
Fax: 630-892-1084
Web Site: www.paramountarts.com
Officers:
   Chairman: MW Meyer
   Vice Chairman: Richard Hawks
   Treasurer: Donna Williams
   Secretary: Gyda Stoner
Management:
   General Manager: Diana Martinez
   Theatre Services Coordinator: Jeff Wells
   Marketing Director: Julie Gann
   Box Office Manager: Jonnell Crawford
   Executive Director: Janet R Bean
Mission: To present a variety of quality performances at moderate prices in a convenient location, plus educational opportunities and activities; supports other not-for-profit performing arts organizations.
Founded: 1976
Status: Not-for-profit
Budget: $3.0 million
Income Sources: Ticket Sales; Theatre Rentals; Grants; Donations; Sponsors; Program Ads; Fundraisers
Annual Attendance: 100,000
Facility Category: Performance Center
Type of Stage: Proscenium
Stage Dimensions: 48'x2" x 38'
Seating Capacity: 1888
Year Built: 1931
Year Remodeled: 1975
Rental Contact: Theatre Center Coordinator Jeff Wells (630-264-7202)

4428 FERMILAB ARTS SERIES
PO Box 500
Batavia, IL 60510-0500

Phone: 630-840-2059
Fax: 630-840-5501
Web Site: www.fnal.gov/culture
Management:
    Arts Coordinator: Janet MacKay-Galbraith
    Box Office Manager: Colleen Choy
    Cultural Arts Supervisor: Denise M Adducci
Mission: To provide professional performing arts for the Batavia community.
Specialized Field: Dance; Instrumental Music; Theater; Comedy; Jazz
Status: Nonprofit
Paid Staff: 3
Budget: $35,000-$60,000
Income Sources: Fermi National Accel Laboratories
Performs At: Ramsey Auditorium
Organization Type: Sponsoring

4429 UNIVERSITY OF ILLINOIS: ASSEMBLY HALL

18005 First Street
Champaign, IL 61820
Phone: 217-333-2923
Fax: 217-244-8888
Web Site: www.uofiassemblyhall.com
Management:
    Director: Kevin Ullestad

4430 CHICAGO COLLEGE OF PERFORMING ARTS MUSIC CONSERVATORY SERIES

430 S Michigan Avenue
Chicago, IL 60605
Phone: 312-341-3785
Fax: 312-341-6358
e-mail: lberna@roosevelt.edu
Management:
    Director/Music Conservatory/Dean: Linda Berna
    Performance Activities Manager: Thomas Ballentine
Performs At: Rudolph Ganz Memorial Hall

4431 CHICAGO INTERNATIONAL ORGAN FESTIVAL

Fourth Presbyterian Church
126 E Chestnut Street
Chicago, IL 60611-2094
Phone: 312-787-4570
Fax: 312-787-4584
e-mail: ccole@fourthchurch.org
Web Site: www.fourthchurch.org
Management:
    Artistic Administrator: C Carroll Cole

4432 CHICAGO JAZZ FESTIVAL

Mayor's Office of Special Events
121 N LaSalle, Room 703
Chicago, IL 60602
Phone: 312-427-1676
Fax: 312-744-8523
e-mail: specialevents@ci.chi.il.us
Web Site: www.ci.chi.il.ns/wm/specialevents
Specialized Field: Jazz
Season: Labor Day Weekend
Performs At: Grant Park, Chicago (Festival Site)

Facility Category: Perillo Band Shell & Jazz on Jackson Stage
Seating Capacity: 5,000 seats, 100,000 lawn seating

4433 CHICAGO STUDIO OF PROFESSIONAL SINGING PERFORMANCE SERIES

Berger Cultural Center
6205 N Sheridan Road
Chicago, IL 60660
Phone: 773-764-5022
Fax: 773-764-5742
e-mail: Jtpsing@aol.com
Web Site: www.professionalsinging.com
Management:
    Director/Master Voice Teacher: Janice Pantazelos
    Assistant Marketing Director: Joyce Chacko
    Voice Teacher: Monique Robertson
    Voice Teacher: Grace Sanchez
Mission: CSPS performance series showcase top professional singers from the Chicagoland area.
Specialized Field: Edgewater
Paid Staff: 3
Income Sources: Tickets; Advertising
Affiliations: NATS

4434 CRYSTAL BALLROOM CONCERT ASSOCIATION SERIES

410 S Michigan Avenue
#521
Chicago, IL 60605
Phone: 312-595-5434
Management:
    Executive Secretary/Program Dir: Beverly DeFries-D'Albert
Mission: To provide performances of local and international artists for the Chicago community.
Founded: 1984
Specialized Field: Dance; Vocal Music; Instrumental Music; Festivals
Status: Professional; Nonprofit
Paid Staff: 50
Income Sources: Zoltan Kodaly Academy & Institute
Performs At: Crystal Ballroom
Organization Type: Performing; Educational; Sponsoring

4435 DAME MYRA HESS MEMORIAL CONCERT SERIES

650 N Dearborn
Suite 350
Chicago, IL 60610
Phone: 312-670-6888
Fax: 312-670-9166
e-mail: info@imfchicago.org
Web Site: www.imfchicago.org
Management:
    Director: Ann Murray
Founded: 1978
Specialized Field: Music
Performs At: Preston Bradley Hall

4436 GRANT PARK MUSIC FESTIVAL
Chicago Park District Administration Bldg
425 E McFetridge Drive
Chicago, IL 60605
Phone: 312-742-7638
Fax: 312-742-7662
Web Site: www.grantparkmusicfestival.com
Management:
    General Manager/Artistic Director: James W
Palermo
Mission: To offer symphonic concerts at no cost to
Chicago residents.
Founded: 1934
Status: Professional; Nonprofit
Paid Staff: 100
Season: June - August
Performs At: Grant Park, Chicago
Organization Type: Performing; Resident; Educational

**4437 ILLINOIS INSTITUTE OF
TECHNOLOGY, UNION BOARD
CONCERTS**
3241 S Federal Street
Chicago, IL 60616
Phone: 312-567-3075
Fax: 312-567-8930
e-mail: dicesare@alpha1.iit.edu
Management:
    Student Activities Director: Daniel DiCesare
Performs At: Grover M. Hermann Hall

**4438 LOYOLA UNIVERSITY OF CHICAGO
SEASON SUBSCRIPTION SERIES**
6525 N Sheridan Road
Chicago, IL 60626
Phone: 773-508-3833
Fax: 773-508-7126
e-mail: abrowni@luc.edu
Web Site: www.luc.edu/depts/theatre
Management:
    Managing Director: April Browning
Performs At: Kathleen Mullady Theatre

4439 NEWBERRY CONSORT
60 W Walton
Chicago, IL 60610
Phone: 312-255-3610
Fax: 312-255-3680
e-mail: consort@newberryorg
Web Site: www.newberry.org
Management:
    General Manager: Alex Bonus
Founded: 1987
Seating Capacity: 310

4440 PERFORMING ARTS CHICAGO SERIES
410 S Michigan Avenue
#911
Chicago, IL 60605
Phone: 312-663-1628
Fax: 312-663-1043
e-mail: mail@pachicago.org
Web Site: www.pachicago.org

Officers:
    President: Judys Neisser
    Executive Director: Susan Lipman
    Director: Christy Uchida
    Operations Manager: Laurell Zahrobsky
    Development Assistant: Brigid Flynn
    Treasurer: David Ellis
Management:
    Executive Director: Susan Lipman
    Director Marketing/Public Relation: Heidi Feldman
Mission: To present artists who explore the creative
tension between tradition and innovation, to nurture an
environment for and bring to performance new works and
new performers, and to remain accountable to its
community, furthering support for local artists,
engagement and education, not only for its direct
audience, but for society at large.
Founded: 1960
Specialized Field: Chamber; Theater; Dance; Puppetry
Status: Professional; Nonprofit
Budget: $1,000,000
Performs At: The Civic Theater
Organization Type: Performing; Resident; Educational;
Sponsoring

4441 PERFORMING ARTS ASSOCIATION
180 E Pearson Street
#5702
Chicago, IL 60611
Phone: 312-932-9566
Fax: 312-932-9566
Officers:
    President: Frederic W Schwartz
Founded: 1954

**4442 ROOSEVELT UNIVERSITY GUEST
RECITALS**
430 S Michigan Avenue
Chicago, IL 60605
Phone: 312-341-3785
Fax: 312-341-6358
e-mail: lberna@roosevelt.edu
Management:
    Associate Dean: Linda Berna

**4443 ROOSEVELT UNIVERSITY
PERFORMING ARTS SERIES**
430 S Michigan Avenue
Chicago, IL 60605
Phone: 312-341-3785
Fax: 312-341-6358
e-mail: lberna@roosevelt.edu
Officers:
    Director/Music Conservatory/Dean: Linda Berna
Management:
    Performance Activities Manager: Thomas Ballentine
Performs At: Rudolph Ganz Memorial Hall

**4444 UNIVERSITY OF CHICAGO
PERFORMING ARTISTS SERIES**
PRISM Series
1212 E 59th Street
Chicago, IL 60637-1604

Phone: 773-955-9339
Fax: 773-702-1195
e-mail: epstein@cs.uchicago.edu
Management:
   Managing Director: Farobag Homi Cooper

4445 UNIVERSITY OF CHICAGO PROFESSIONAL INSTRUMENTAL MUSIC SERIES

The PRISM Series
1212 E 59th Street
Chicago, IL 60637-1604
Phone: 773-955-9339
Fax: 773-702-1195
e-mail: epstein@cs.uchicago.edu
Management:
   Artistic Advisor: Charles Pikler
Performs At: Mandel Hall

4446 UNIVERSITY OF ILLINOIS AT CHICAGO FINE ARTS SERIES

Campus Programs, Room 50
828 S Wolcott
Chicago, IL 60612
Phone: 312-413-5070
Management:
   Union Programs Coordinator: Jill Rothamer

4447 URBAN GATEWAYS SERIES: CENTER FOR ARTS EDUCATION

200 W Jackson Boulevard
#300
Chicago, IL 60606-6910
Phone: 312-922-0440
Fax: 312-922-2740
e-mail: tsauers@urbangateways.org
Web Site: www.urbangateways.org
Management:
   Producing Director: Tim Sauers
   Assistant Producing Director: Carolann Fleming
Mission: To provide comprehensive arts education programs, to serve locally as a resource, and nationally as a model for incorporating the arts in all levels of education for aesthetic, academic, cultural and personal development.
Founded: 1961
Specialized Field: Literary; Performing; Visual Arts
Status: Nonprofit
Paid Staff: 18
Paid Artists: 160
Budget: $2.3 million
Income Sources: Ticket Sales; Fees for Service; Grants; Corporation; Government; Contributions

4448 WILBUR COLLEGE CULTURAL EVENTS SERIES

4300 N Narragansett
Chicago, IL 60634
Phone: 773-481-8144
Fax: 773-481-8147
Seating Capacity: 200
Year Built: 1993
Rental Contact: Director Student Affairs Betty Gilbert

4449 NORTHERN ILLINOIS UNIVERSITY FINE ARTS SERIES

NIU, University Programming
Campus Life Building 150
De Kalb, IL 60115
Phone: 815-753-1421
Fax: 815-753-2905
Web Site: www.niu.edu/cab/
Management:
   Assistant Director: Mary Tosch
Performs At: Carl Sandburg Auditorium; Duke Ellington Ballroom

4450 PERFORMING ARTS SERIES FOR STUDENTS

145 N Main
PO Box 1607
Decatur, IL 62525
Phone: 217-423-3189
Fax: 217-423-3194
e-mail: arts4all1@aol.com
Management:
   Executive Director: Susan Smith
Performs At: Kirkland Fine Arts Center

4451 TRINITY COLLEGE ARTIST SERIES

2065 Half Day Road
Deerfield, IL 60015
Phone: 847-317-8021
Fax: 847-317-4786
Management:
   Event Coordinator: Jane Victor
Performs At: Arnold T. Olson Chapel

4452 MAINE TOWNSHIP COMMUNITY CONCERT ASSOCIATION

986 Jeannette Street
Des Plaines, IL 60016
Phone: 847-824-2591
Officers:
   President: Anne Evans
Performs At: High School Auditorium

4453 ARTISTS SHOWCASE WEST
Downers Grove Concert Association

731 59th Street
Downers Grove, IL 60516
Phone: 630-252-7160
Fax: 630-252-5986
e-mail: kaper@mcs.anl.gov
Officers:
   Chairman: Dr. Hans G Kaper

4454 DOWNERS GROVE CONCERT ASSOCIATION SERIES

731 59th Street
Downers Grove, IL 60516
Phone: 630-252-7160
Fax: 630-252-5986
e-mail: kaper@mcs.anl.gov
Web Site: www.dgconcerts.org
Officers:

President: Tom Hamernik
Concert Impresario: Hans G Kaper
Mission: To increase public support for performing arts in Downers Grove through the presentation of professional dancers and musicians.
Founded: 1947
Specialized Field: Dance; Instrumental Music
Status: Non-Professional
Volunteer Staff: 20
Budget: $20,000-$35,000
Income Sources: Ticket Sales; Village of Downers Grove; Illinois Art Council
Performs At: Downers Grove North High School Auditorium
Affiliations: Chicago Music Alliance
Facility Category: Auditorium
Seating Capacity: 1,000
Organization Type: Sponsoring

4455 ILLINOIS CENTRAL COLLEGE SUBSCRIPTION SERIES

Illinois Central College
Performing Arts Center
East Peoria, IL 61635
Phone: 309-694-5138
Fax: 309-694-8505
e-mail: drademaker@icc.cc.il.us
Web Site: www.icc.cc.il.us
Management:
  PAC Assistant Manager: Dana Rademaker
  Fine Arts Department: Jefferey Hoover
Founded: 1967
Paid Staff: 20
Volunteer Staff: 20
Budget: $35,000
Income Sources: Funded by the School
Performs At: Performing Arts Center
Affiliations: Illinois Presenters Network
Annual Attendance: 25,000
Type of Stage: Prosceium; Thurst
Stage Dimensions: 40'x36'
Seating Capacity: 500
Year Built: 1979
Cost: $4,000,000

4456 SOUTHERN ILLINOIS UNIVERSITY-EDWARDSVILLE SERIES

Campus Box 1083
Edwardsville, IL 62026
Phone: 618-650-2626
Fax: 618-650-2000
Management:
  Series Coordinator: Rich Walker
Mission: To offer diverse performances and speakers to students and to the Southern Illinois area.
Specialized Field: Dance; Instrumental Music; Theater
Status: Nonprofit
Income Sources: Association of Performing Arts Presenters
Performs At: University Center and Communications Theater
Organization Type: Educational; Sponsoring

4457 ELMHURST COLLEGE JAZZ FESTIVAL

190 Prospect Avenue
Elmhurst, IL 60126
Phone: 630-617-3515
Fax: 630-617-3738
e-mail: barbv@elmhurst.edu
Web Site: www.elmhurst.edu
Management:
  Director: Doug Beach
  Coordinator: Barbara Vandergrift
Mission: To offer both jazz performances and the opportunity for artists to give constructive critiques, advice, demonstration of skills and guest band appearences.
Founded: 1967
Specialized Field: Jazz
Volunteer Staff: 150
Paid Artists: 3
Affiliations: UCC, Community
Facility Category: Chapel-Multi Purpose
Type of Stage: Indoor Elevated
Seating Capacity: 850
Year Remodeled: 1994

4458 PRINCIPIA COLLEGE CONCERT SERIES

Principia College
Elsah, IL 62028
Phone: 618-374-5004
Fax: 618-374-5911
Management:
  Concert Coordinator: Dr. Maric Garritson
Performs At: Cox Auditorium

4459 BACH WEEK FESTIVAL IN EVANSTON

PO Box 6133
Evanston, IL 60204-6133
Phone: 847-945-7929
Fax: 847-945-1106
e-mail: bachwk@aol.com
Web Site: www.bachweek.org
Management:
  Music Director: Richard R Webster
  General Manager: Anne Harris
Season: May
Facility Category: Saint Luke's Episcopal Church, Evanston
Seating Capacity: 450

4460 NORTHWESTERN UNIVERSITY SUMMER DRAMA FESTIVAL

Theatre Department
1979 S Campus Drive
Evanston, IL 60208
Phone: 847-491-3232
Fax: 847-467-7135
Management:
  Producer: Paul Brohan
Founded: 1954
Status: Non-Equity; Nonprofit
Season: June - August
Type of Stage: Thrust
Stage Dimensions: 21' x 30'

Seating Capacity: 450

4461 KNOX-ROOTABAGA JAMM JAZZ FESTIVAL

Knox College
2 E South Street, Box 4
Galesburg, IL 61401
Phone: 309-341-7265
Fax: 309-289-2823
e-mail: sgarlock@knox.edu
Web Site: www.knox.edu/knoxjazzrootabaga
Management:
   Director: Dr. Scott Garlock
Mission: Entertainment and education.
Founded: 1989
Paid Staff: 1
Volunteer Staff: 50
Paid Artists: 20
Non-paid Artists: 40

4462 COLLEGE OF LAKE COUNTY - PERFORMING ARTS BUILDING

19351 W Washington Street
Graylake, IL 60030-1198
Phone: 847-543-2077
Fax: 847-543-2629
e-mail: gbronner@clc.cc.il.us
Web Site: www.clc.cc.il.us
Management:
   Director: Gwethalyn Bronner
   Box Office Supervisor: Randall Otrembiak
   Technical Coordinator: Jeremy Eiden
   Media Coordinator: Lyla Maclean
Founded: 1997
Specialized Field: Music,Theatre, Dance
Performs At: Mainstage

4463 GREENVILLE COLLEGE GUEST ARTIST SERIES

315 E College Avenue
Greenville, IL 62246
Phone: 618-664-6582
Fax: 618-664-6580
e-mail: achaussee@greenville.edu
Management:
   Manager: Andrea Chaussee
Mission: Acts enrichment in a small community
Performs At: LaDue Auditorium

4464 SOUTHEASTERN ILLINOIS COLLEGE CULTURAL ARTS SERIES

3575 College Road
Harrisburg, IL 62946-0000
Phone: 618-252-5400
Fax: 618-252-3156
Web Site: www.sic.cc.il.us
Management:
   Executive Director: Kelli Whitler

4465 RAVINIA FESTIVAL

400 Iris Lane
PO Box 896
Highland Park, IL 60035
Phone: 847-266-5100
Fax: 847-433-7983
e-mail: ravinia@mail.ravinia.org
Web Site: www.ravinia.org
Officers:
   President/CEO: Welz Kauffman
Management:
   Artistic Director: Ramsey Lewis
   Music Director: Christopher Eschenbach
Mission: To present, at low cost, quality classical, jazz, folk, and pop music to the public.
Founded: 1935
Status: Professional; Nonprofit
Paid Staff: 50
Volunteer Staff: 50
Non-paid Artists: 100
Season: June - September
Performs At: Ravinia Park, Highland Park (Festival Site)
Annual Attendance: 500,000
Facility Category: Ravinia Pavilion; Martin Theatre; Bennet-Gordon Hall
Seating Capacity: 3,200; 850; 450
Year Built: 1955
Year Remodeled: 1995
Organization Type: Performing; Educational

4466 STARRY NIGHTS SUMMER CONCERT SERIES

18120 Highland Avenue
Homewood, IL 60430
Phone: 708-957-7275
Fax: 708-957-0267
Web Site: www.lincolnnet.net/hfparkdistrict
Management:
   Recreation Supervisor: Jodi Gosse
Season: June - July
Performs At: Homewood (Festival Site)
Facility Category: Marie Irwin Community Center Bandshell, Homewood
Seating Capacity: 4,000

4467 MYSTERY CAFE SERIES

231 S College Avenue
Indianapolis, IL
Phone: 317-684-0668
e-mail: info@themysterycafeindy.com
Web Site: www.mysterycafeonline.com
Founded: 1990

4468 BARAT COLLEGE PERFORMING ARTS CENTER SEASON

700 E Westleigh Road
Lake Forest, IL 60045
Phone: 847-604-6344
Fax: 847-604-6342
e-mail: drakethe@barat.edu
Web Site: www.barat.edu
Management:
   Theatre Department Chair: Steve Carmichael

Assistant Producer: Jeannie Petkewicz
Budget: $10,000-$20,000
Performs At: Drake Theatre
Facility Category: College
Type of Stage: Proscenium
Seating Capacity: 625

4469 MCKENDREE COLLEGE FINE ARTS SERIES

McKendree College
701 College Road
Lebanon, IL 62254
Phone: 618-537-6922
Fax: 618-537-6259
Toll-free: 800-232-7268
e-mail: nypma@mckendree.edu
Web Site: www.mckendree.edu
Officers:
   Chairperson Music Department: Dr. Nancy Ypma
Mission: For education of students and community.
Paid Staff: 2
Paid Artists: 5
Performs At: Bothwell Chapel; Pearsons Hall

4470 WESTERN ILLINOIS UNIVERSITY BCA PERFORMING ARTIST SERIES

University Union
Macomb, IL 61455
Phone: 309-298-3232
Fax: 309-298-2879
e-mail: K-Kohberger@wiu.edu
Management:
   Performing Arts Assistant Director: Christi Oquendo
Performs At: Western Hall

4471 QUAD-CITIES JAZZ FESTIVAL

PO Box 399
Moline, IL 61266
Phone: 563-324-0049
Officers:
   Chairman: Josef Fackel
Founded: 1994

4472 NAPERVILLE-NORTH CENTRAL COLLEGE PERFORMING ARTS SERIES

30 N Brainard Street
Naperville, IL 60566
Phone: 630-637-5100
Fax: 630-637-5121
Management:
   Director Fine Arts: Brian Lynch
Founded: 1974
Specialized Field: Dance; Vocal Music; Instrumental Music; Theater
Status: Non-Professional; Nonprofit
Income Sources: North Central College
Performs At: Pfeiffer Hall
Organization Type: Sponsoring

4473 ILLINOIS SHAKESPEARE FESTIVAL

Illinois State University
Box 5700
Normal, IL 61790-5700
Phone: 309-438-8974
Fax: 309-438-5806
e-mail: shake@ilstu.edu
Web Site: www.thefestival.org
Management:
   Managing Director: Fergus G Currie
   Artistic Director: Calvin MacLean
   Assistant Managing Director: Paul Berg
Founded: 1978
Specialized Field: Festivals
Status: Nonprofit
Paid Staff: 100
Paid Artists: 85
Non-paid Artists: 15
Budget: $600,000
Income Sources: Box Office, Fund Raising
Season: June - August
Performs At: Ewing Manor
Affiliations: UARTA; Actors' Equity Association; SSOC
Annual Attendance: 15,000
Facility Category: Outdoor
Type of Stage: Thrust
Seating Capacity: 420
Year Built: 1999
Cost: $1.65 million
Organization Type: Performing; Educational

4474 ILLINOIS STATE UNIVERSITY MUSIC SERIES

100 N University Street
Campus Box 2640
Normal, IL 61790-2640
Phone: 309-438-2222
Fax: 309-438-5167
e-mail: ccarte@ilstu.edu
Web Site: www.bsc.ilstu.edu/bsc
Management:
   Manager: Cassandra Carter
Founded: 1973
Specialized Field: Classical; Contemporary Performances
Paid Staff: 100
Volunteer Staff: 20
Paid Artists: 100
Non-paid Artists: 200
Performs At: Braden Auditorium

4475 FIRST FOLIO SHAKESPEARE FESTIVAL

1717 W 31st Street
Oak Brook, IL 60514
Mailing Address: 146 Juliet Center Claredon Hill, IL 06514
Phone: 630-986-8067
Fax: 630-455-0071
e-mail: firstfolio@firstfolio.org
Web Site: www.firstfolio.org
Management:
   Artistic Director: Alison C Vesely
   Producer: David Rice

All listings are in alphabetical order by state, then city, then organization within the city.

Mission: Bring attention to the historic and environmental site here. Mission emphasizes a training intiative for young theatre artists, including a college intern program.
Founded: 1996
Specialized Field: Theatre
Status: Nonprofit; Non-Equity
Paid Staff: 2
Volunteer Staff: 60
Paid Artists: 30
Season: July - September
Type of Stage: Thrust
Stage Dimensions: 40' x 30'

4476 COMMUNITY CHILDREN'S THEATRE OF PEORIA PARK DISTRICT
2218 N Prospect Road
Peoria, IL 61603-2193
Phone: 309-688-3667
Fax: 309-686-3384
Web Site: www.peoriaparks.org
Officers:
    President: Lisa Voyles
    Vice President: Ellen Wertz
Management:
    Fine Arts Coordinator: Linda Elegant Huff
Mission: To foster participation among the young people in the community in children's theatre activity; to present educational programs, with the purpose of raising awareness and standards of such programs.
Founded: 1958
Specialized Field: Children's Theatre. Performance by children for children.
Paid Staff: 1
Volunteer Staff: 200
Paid Artists: 5
Non-paid Artists: 65
Budget: $20,000
Income Sources: Tickets Sales and Concessions; Donations; Grants
Performs At: Theatre; Schools
Affiliations: Illinois Theatre Association
Annual Attendance: 5,000
Facility Category: Theatre
Type of Stage: Proscenium
Seating Capacity: 360

4477 MIDWEST JAZZ HERITAGE FESTIVAL
2206 N Prospect Road
Peoria, IL 61603
Phone: 309-685-4276
e-mail: bduffy@bigplanet.com
Web Site: www.midil.com/jazzpeoria.html
Management:
    Prducer/Promoter: B Duffy

4478 PEORIA CIVIC CENTER BROADWAY THEATER SERIES
201 SW Jefferson Street
Peoria, IL 61602-1448
Phone: 309-673-8900
Fax: 309-673-9223
Web Site: www.peoriaciviccenter.com
Management:
    Director Marketing: Marc Burnett

Annual Attendance: 20,000
Facility Category: Theater
Seating Capacity: 2127

4479 QUINCY CIVIC MUSIC ASSOCIATION
PO Box 1165
Quincy, IL 62306-1165
Phone: 217-224-5499
e-mail: qcma@hotmail.com

4480 DOMINICAN UNIVERSITY CENTER STAGE GUEST ARTIST SERIES
7900 W Division Street
River Forest, IL 60305
Phone: 708-524-6515
Fax: 708-524-6517
e-mail: raymond@dom.edu
Web Site: www.dom.edu
Management:
    Exec Dir Fine/Performing Arts: Dr. Jill Poehlman
    Artistic Director: Michael Poehlman
    Associate Director: Laura K Wolf
    Administrative Manager: Meghan Maxwell
Founded: 1901
Specialized Field: All
Performs At: Lund Auditorium; Martin Hall
Annual Attendance: 45,000
Facility Category: Fine Arts Building
Type of Stage: Proscenium
Seating Capacity: 1,182; 212
Year Built: 1952
Year Remodeled: 1992
Rental Contact: Jill Poehlman

4481 QUAD CITY ARTS
1715 2nd Avenue
Rock Island, IL 61201
Phone: 309-793-1213
Fax: 309-793-1265
e-mail: info@quadcityarts.com
Web Site: www.quadcityarts.com
Management:
    Director Programming: John Vogt
    Executive Director: Judi Holderf
Mission: To offer professional concerts by area performing artists.
Founded: 1988
Specialized Field: Dance; Vocal Music; Instrumental Music; Theater
Status: Nonprofit
Paid Staff: 10
Budget: $200,000
Income Sources: Grants; Foundations; Fund Drive
Performs At: Deere and Company; St. Ambrose University; Augustana College
Affiliations: Association of Performing Arts Presenters
Facility Category: Arts Center
Year Remodeled: 1988
Organization Type: Performing; Educational

4482 ROCK VALLEY COLLEGE LECTURE/CONCERT SERIES
3301 N Mulford Road
Rockford, IL 61114
Phone: 815-654-4290
Fax: 815-654-4402
e-mail: m.sink@rvc.cc.il.us
Management:
   Program Director: Monique Aduddell
Performs At: Performing Arts Room

4483 UNIVERSITY OF ILLINOIS AT SPRINGFIELD SANGAMON PERFORMING ARTS SERIES
Sangamon Auditorium
PAC397, UIS, PO Box 19243
Springfield, IL 62794-9243
Phone: 217-206-6150
Fax: 217-206-6391
e-mail: kennedy.john@uis.edu
Web Site: www.sangamonauditorium.org
Management:
   University Auditorium Director: John Dale Kennedy
Mission: To present a varied professional performing arts program to audiences in central illinois.
Founded: 1981
Paid Staff: 16
Volunteer Staff: 400

4484 ST. CHARLES ART & MUSIC FESTIVAL
103 W Main Street
Suite 2A
St. Charles, IL 60174
Phone: 630-584-3378
Fax: 630-377-3105
e-mail: robbm@ameritech.net
Management:
   Executive Director: Robert Murphy
Performs At: St. Charles & Tri-City Area (Festival Site)
Facility Category: Norris Cultural Arts Center
Seating Capacity: 980

4485 KRANNERT CENTER MARQUEE SERIES, UNIVERSITY OF ILLINOIS
500 S Goodwin Avenue
Urbana, IL 61801
Phone: 217-333-6700
Fax: 217-244-0810
e-mail: Kran-tix@uiuc.edu
Web Site: www.krannertcenter.com
Performs At: Foellinger Great Hall

4486 ARTIST SERIES AT WHEATON COLLEGE
Wheaton Conservatory of Music
501 College Avenue
Wheaton, IL 60187-5593
Phone: 630-752-5099
Fax: 630-752-5341
e-mail: artistseries@wheaton.edu
Web Site: www.wheaton.edu/TicketOffice
Management:

   Manager: Tony Payne
   Promotion Manager: Rhonda Sisson
Founded: 1950
Specialized Field: Classical
Paid Staff: 4
Volunteer Staff: 10
Paid Artists: 7
Budget: $300,000
Income Sources: Box Office; Private Donationas; Corporate Donations
Performs At: Edman Memorial Chapel
Affiliations: Wheaton College
Annual Attendance: 12,500
Facility Category: Auditorium/Hall
Type of Stage: Proscenium
Stage Dimensions: 35'x 60'
Seating Capacity: 2,350
Year Built: 1960

4487 MUSIC INSTITUTE OF CHICAGO SERIES
300 Green Bay Road
Winnetka, IL 60093
Phone: 847-446-3822
Fax: 847-446-3876
e-mail: info@musicinst.com
Web Site: www.musicinst.com
Officers:
   Chairman: William J Eichar
   President: Frank Little
   VP: Gilda Barston
Mission: To provide the foundation for a lifelong enjoyment of music.
Founded: 1931
Specialized Field: Music Education and Creative Arts Therapy
Paid Staff: 150
Budget: 4 million
Income Sources: Tuition; Donations
Performs At: Recital Hall
Annual Attendance: 1,000+
Facility Category: Recital Hall
Seating Capacity: 150
Year Built: 1956
Rental Contact: Jim Brown

4488 WOODSTOCK FINE ARTS ASSOCIATION - MUSIC FOR A SUNDAY AFTERNOON SERIES
PO Box 225
Woodstock, IL 60098
Phone: 815-338-0175
Management:
   Contact: Mary Sircar
Performs At: Auditorium

4489 WOODSTOCK MOZART FESTIVAL
PO Box 734
Woodstock, IL 60098
Phone: 630-983-7072
Fax: 630-717-7782
e-mail: mozartfest@aol.com
Web Site: www.mozartfest.org

All listings are in alphabetical order by state, then city, then organization within the city.

Officers:
    President: Louis La Coque
Management:
    General Director: Anita Whelan
    Artistic Advisor: Mark Peskanov
Founded: 1987
Paid Staff: 3
Paid Artists: 40
Budget: $130,000
Income Sources: Individuals, Corporations, Foundations
Facility Category: Woodstock Opera House
Seating Capacity: 412
Year Built: 1889
Year Remodeled: 1977

Indiana

4490 **FOUNTAIN/WARREN MUSICAL ARTS SERIES**
PO Box 6
Attica, IN 47918
Phone: 765-762-2481
Fax: 765-762-2487
e-mail: wrghthsm@hscast.com
Officers:
    Secretary: Mike Wrighthouse
Budget: $11,000
Performs At: Harrison Hills Country Club

4491 **DEARBORN HIGHLANDS ARTS COUNCIL SERIES**
406 Second Street
PO Box 193
Aurora, IN 47001-0193
Phone: 812-926-1778
Fax: 812-926-4700
Toll-free: 866-818-2787
e-mail: dhac@seidata.com
Management:
    Executive Director: Marilyn Bower
Mission: To serve, expand and enrich the lives of residents of Dearborn County and adjacent areas through education, exposure, diversity, enjoyment and participation in the performing and visual arts.
Founded: 1982
Paid Staff: 1
Volunteer Staff: 215
Budget: $100,000
Income Sources: Grants; Memberships; Ticket Sales; Corporate; Private Support
Performs At: Lawrenceburg HS Auditorium; South Dearborn HS Auditorium; Public Libraries
Annual Attendance: 4800
Facility Category: Auditorium, city park

4492 **BLOOMINGTON EARLY MUSIC FESTIVAL**
PO Box 734
Bloomington, IN 47402
Phone: 812-331-1263
Fax: 812-331-1263
e-mail: info@blemf.org
Web Site: www.blemf.org
Officers:
    President: Mary Tilton
    Chair, Program Commitee: Gesa Kordes
Management:
    Executive Director: Alain Barker
Founded: 1992
Paid Staff: 1
Volunteer Staff: 25
Paid Artists: 30
Non-paid Artists: 50
Season: May
Performs At: Bloomington (Festival Site)
Facility Category: Concert Halls, Opera Theatre
Seating Capacity: 230; 450

4493 **INDIANA UNIVERSITY PERFORMING ARTS SERIES**
Indiana University Auditorium
1211 E 7th Street
Bloomington, IN 47405
Phone: 812-855-9528
Fax: 812-855-4522
Web Site: www.iuauditorium.com
Management:
    Director: James Holland
Mission: To provide a program of professional performing arts events for students and community members.
Founded: 1820
Specialized Field: Dance; Instrumental Music; Theater
Status: Professional; Nonprofit
Income Sources: International Association of Auditorium Managers; Association of Performing Arts Presenters
Performs At: Indiana University Auditorium
Organization Type: Educational; Sponsoring

4494 **INDIANA UNIVERSITY SCHOOL OF MUSIC SUMMER FESTIVAL**
Indiana University School of Music
Bloomington, IN 47405
Phone: 812-855-9846
Fax: 812-855-4936
e-mail: jkosovsk@indiana.edu
Web Site: www.music.indiana.edu
Management:
    Special Programs Coordinator: Helena Walsh
Season: Mid June - Mid August
Performs At: Bloomington (Festival Site)
Annual Attendance: 12,000
Facility Category: Musical Arts Center; Auer Concert Hall
Seating Capacity: 1,460; 480

4495 **CREATIVE ARTS COUNCIL OF WELLS COUNTY**
110 W Washington Street
Bluffton, IN 46714
Phone: 219-824-5222
e-mail: cac@parlorcity.com

Management:
   Executive Director: Maureen Butler
Performs At: Auditorium

4496 BROADWAY SERIES: INDIANAPOLIS
200 Medical Drive
Suite D
Carmel, IN 46032
Phone: 317-818-3970
Fax: 317-818-3961
Toll-free: 800-793-7469
Web Site: www.broadwayseries.com

4497 COLUMBUS AREA ARTS COUNCIL
302 Washington Street
Columbus, IN 47201
Phone: 812-376-2539
Fax: 812-376-2589
Web Site: www.artsincolumbus.org
Management:
   Executive Director: Robert B Burnett Jr
Performs At: The Commons

4498 CONNERSVILLE AREA ARTISTS SERIES
3006 W 400 N
Connersville, IN 47331
Phone: 317-825-2427
Management:
   Manager: David Caldwell
Performs At: Robert Wise Auditorium

4499 CULVER MILITARY ACADEMY CONCERT SERIES
Culver Academies
CEF Suite 79
Culver, IN 46511
Phone: 219-842-8255
Fax: 219-842-7994
Management:
   Theatre Director: Richard Coven
Performs At: Eppley Auditorium

4500 FORT WAYNE PARKS & RECREATION FESTIVAL
705 E State Street
Fort Wayne, IN 46805
Phone: 219-427-6715
Fax: 219-427-6020
Management:
   Manager: Michael Thompson
Paid Staff: 7
Income Sources: Budget, Grants, Donations
Affiliations: Fort Wayne Parts and Recreation
Annual Attendance: 52,000
Facility Category: Outdoor Theatre
Seating Capacity: 2,500
Year Built: 1949
Year Remodeled: 1976
Rental Contact: Mike Thompson

4501 DEPAUW UNIVERSITY PERFORMING ARTS SERIES
DePauw University
709 Locust Street
Greencastle, IN 46135
Phone: 765-658-4689
Fax: 765-658-4356
e-mail: rdye@depauw.edu
Management:
   Coordinator: Ron Dye
Performs At: Auditoriums

4502 HANOVER COLLEGE COMMUNITY ARTIST SERIES
Hanover College
PO Box 108
Hanover, IN 47243-0108
Phone: 812-866-7185
Fax: 812-866-6879
e-mail: morrill@hanover.edu
Web Site: www.hanover.edu
Performs At: Fitzgibbon Recital Hall

4503 CLOWES MEMORIAL HALL SERIES
4600 Sunset Avenue
Indianapolis, IN 46208
Phone: 317-940-9697
Fax: 317-940-9820
Toll-free: 800-732-0800
e-mail: ekushigi@butler.edu
Web Site: www.cloweshall.org
Management:
   Executive Director: Elise J Kushigian
Resident Groups: Indianapolis Opera; Jordan College of Fine Arts; Town Hall Lecture Series

4504 CONCESCO FIELDHOUSE
125 S Pennsylvania Street
Indianapolis, IN 46204
Phone: 317-917-2500
Fax: 317-917-2799
e-mail: jjjohnson@pacers.com
Web Site: www.consecofieldhouse.com
Management:
   VP/General Manager: Rick Fuson
   VP Booking/Schedule: Jeff Bowen
Specialized Field: Home of the Indiana Pacers and downtown home of the Indianpolis Ice (IHL)
Seating Capacity: 18,000
Year Built: 1999

4505 ENSEMBLE MUSIC SOCIETY OF INDIANAPOLIS SERIES
PO Box 40188
Indianapolis, IN 46240
Phone: 317-254-8915
Fax: 317-254-8915
e-mail: pamelasteele@earthlink.net
Officers:
   President: Pamela Steele
Founded: 1944
Specialized Field: Chamber Music Concerts
Paid Artists: 15

Non-paid Artists: 36
Performs At: Indiana Historical Society
Seating Capacity: 300
Year Built: 1999

4506 FESTIVAL MUSIC SOCIETY OF INDIANA
6471 Central Avenue
Indianapolis, IN 46220
Phone: 317-251-5190
Fax: 317-251-8027
e-mail: merfms@msn.com
Web Site: www.emimdy.org
Officers:
　President: Richard A Johnson
　VP: David A Garrett
　Treasurer: Dorit S Paul
Management:
　Director: Frank Cooper
　Executive Secretary: Mary Ellen Roberts
Mission: To present early music including educational programs to diverse audiences at affordable prices.
Founded: 1969
Specialized Field: Early Music; Baroque; Renaissance
Paid Staff: 2
Volunteer Staff: 27
Income Sources: Contributions; Grants; Ticket Sales
Season: June - July
Performs At: Inside Auditorium, Indianapolis (Fesitval Site)
Annual Attendance: 1,200
Facility Category: Indianapolis Art Center
Stage Dimensions: 16'x32'
Seating Capacity: 300
Year Built: 1940
Year Remodeled: 1996

4507 INDY JAZZ FESTIVAL
22 E Washington Street
Suite 103
Indianapolis, IN 46204
Phone: 317-635-6630
Fax: 317-635-2010
Toll-free: 800-983-4639
e-mail: info@indyjazzfest.org
Web Site: www.indyjazzfest.org

4508 NATIONAL WOMEN'S MUSIC FESTIVAL
1800 N Meridan
#412
Indianapolis, IN 46202
Mailing Address: PO Box 1427, Indianapolis, IN. 46206
Phone: 317-927-9355
Fax: 317-923-4995
e-mail: wia@indy.net
Web Site: www.a1.com/wia
Management:
　Producer: Joyce Plummer
Season: June
Performs At: Muncie (Festival Site)
Facility Category: Emens Auditorium
Seating Capacity: 2,500

4509 PERFORMERS SERIES, BACKSTAGE SERIES, IU SERIES
951 College Avenue
Jasper, IN 47546-9382
Phone: 812-482-3070
Fax: 812-634-6997
e-mail: jasperarts@psci.net
Management:
　Executive Director: Darla Blazey
Performs At: Jasper Civic Auditorium

4510 BETHEL COLLEGE FINE ARTS SERIES
1001 W Mckinley Avenue
Mishawaka, IN 46545
Phone: 219-257-7623
Fax: 219-257-2678
e-mail: saboj@bethel-in.edu
Web Site: www.bethel-in.edu
Management:
　Operations Manager: Jonathan Sabo
Performs At: Everest-Rohrer Auditorium

4511 EMENS AUDITORIUM
Emens Auditorium
Ball State University
Muncie, IN 47306-0750
Phone: 765-285-1539
Fax: 765-285-3719
Toll-free: 877-993-6367
Web Site: www.bsu.edu/emens
Management:
　Manager: Robert Myers
　Assistant Manager: Julie Strider
Founded: 1964
Status: Nonprofit

4512 MANCHESTER COLLEGE PUBLIC PROGRAM SERIES
604 E College Avenue
North Manchester, IN 46962
Phone: 219-982-5000
Fax: 219-982-5043
e-mail: KLBatdorf@manchester.edu
Web Site: www.manchester.edu
Management:
　Manager: Kay L Batdorf
Performs At: Cordier Auditorium

4513 SAINT MARY'S COLLEGE CULTURAL ARTS SEASON
Saint Mary's College
Moreau Center For The Arts
Notre Dame, IN 46556-5001
Phone: 219-284-4625
Fax: 219-284-4784
e-mail: eckstein@saintmarys.edu
Web Site: www.saintmarys.edu
Management:
　Interim Director: Stacy Eckstein
Performs At: O'Laughlin Auditorium

4514 JAY COUNTY ARTS COUNCIL
PO Box 804
131 East Walnut Street
Portland, IN 47371
Phone: 219-726-4809
Fax: 219-726-2081
e-mail: artsland@jayco.net
Management:
Executive Director: Eric Rogers
Performs At: Hall Memorial Theatre

4515 EARLHAM COLLEGE GUEST ARTIST SERIES
801 National Road W
Richmond, IN 47374
Phone: 765-983-1323
Performs At: Goddard Auditorium

4516 FIREFLY FESTIVAL FOR THE PERFORMING ARTS
112 W Jefferson Boulevard
Suite 511
South Bend, IN 46601-1920
Phone: 219-288-3472
Fax: 219-288-3478
e-mail: firefly@fireflyfestival.com
Web Site: www.fireflyfestival.com
Management:
Executive Director: Carol Weiss Rosenberg
Promotion Director: Lisa Bitting
Office Assistant: Judy West
Mission: To promote and present to the general public artistic performanaces which have as their general theme music, dance, drama, and other arts.
Founded: 1981
Specialized Field: Dance; Vocal Music; Instrumental Music; Theater; Festivals
Status: Professional; Semi-Professional; Non-Professional; Nonprofit
Paid Staff: 3
Volunteer Staff: 140
Paid Artists: 12
Budget: $330,000
Income Sources: Grants; Sponsors; Advertisers; Ticket Sales; In-kind Donations; Private Donations; Business Donations
Season: June - August
Performs At: St. Patrick's County Park, South Bend (Festival Site)
Annual Attendance: 18,000
Facility Category: Robert J Fischgrund Center for the Performing Arts
Type of Stage: Proscenium
Stage Dimensions: 30x60
Seating Capacity: 6,000
Year Built: 1986
Rental Contact: St. Patrick's County Park
Organization Type: Performing; Educational

4517 CONVOCATION SERIES OF INDIANA STATE UNIVERSITY
Erickson Hall
Room 125
Terre Haute, IN 47809
Phone: 812-237-2336
Fax: 812-237-2347
Toll-free: 800-234-1639
e-mail: extvarner@ruby.indstate.edu
Management:
Manager: Allen D Varner
Specialized Field: Music; Device; Theater
Paid Staff: 1
Performs At: Tilson Auditorium
Seating Capacity: 1,684

4518 VALPARAISO UNIVERSITY GUEST ARTISTS SERIES
VU Center for the Arts
Valparaiso, IN 46383
Phone: 219-464-6932
Fax: 219-464-5244
e-mail: sarah.rothaar@valpo.edu
Web Site: www.valpo.edu
Management:
Arts Development Director: Sarah Rothaar
Performs At: Chapel of the Resurrection

4519 VINCENNES UNIVERSITY COMMUNITY SERIES
1002 N 1st Street
DC-38
Vincennes, IN 47591
Phone: 812-888-4354
Fax: 812-888-5942
e-mail: dclinken@indian.vinu.edu
Management:
Manager: Donna Clinkenbeard
Performs At: Auditorium
Facility Category: High School Auditorium
Seating Capacity: 900

4520 PURDUE UNIVERSITY CONVOCATIONS & LECTURES
1821 ENAD
Room S-103
West Lafayette, IN 47907
Phone: 765-494-9712
Fax: 765-494-0540
Web Site: www.convos.purdue.edu
Management:
Director: Todd E Wetzel
Performs At: Edward C. Elliot Hall of Music

Iowa

4521 IOWA STATE UNIVERSITY PERFORMING ARTS COUNCIL SERIES
Iowa State Center, ISU
Ames, IA 50011

Phone: 515-294-3347
Fax: 515-294-3349
e-mail: center@center.iastate.edu
Web Site: www.center.iastate.edu
Management:
   Director: Mark North
   Performing Arts Program Manager: Patti Cotter
Founded: 1969
Specialized Field: Multi
Paid Staff: 30
Performs At: Stephens Auditorium
Annual Attendance: 30,000
Facility Category: Auditorium
Type of Stage: Proscenium
Seating Capacity: 2720
Year Built: 1969

4522 CASS COUNTY ARTS COUNCIL

Box 255
Atlantic, IA 50022
Phone: 712-243-2527
Fax: 712-243-4182

4523 BURLINGTON CIVIC MUSIC ASSOCIATION

Box 324
Burlington, IA 52601
Fax: 319-754-6824
Toll-free: 800-397-1708
e-mail: bwilson@thehawkeye.com
Officers:
   Program Chairman: Bobby Wilson
Performs At: Memorial Auditorium

4524 UNIVERSITY OF NORTHERN IOWA ARTISTS SERIES

University of Northern Iowa
Gallagher Performing Arts Center
Cedar Falls, IA 50614-0801
Phone: 319-273-3660
Fax: 319-273-7470
Toll-free: 877-549-5469
e-mail: steve.carignan@uni.edu
Web Site: www.uni.edu/gbpac
Management:
   Director: Steve Carignan
Paid Staff: 11
Volunteer Staff: 350
Budget: 1.8 Million
Income Sources: Tickets; Grants; Fundraising; State Support
Performs At: Theatre/Concert Hall
Affiliations: APAP
Annual Attendance: 120,000
Facility Category: Multi-Venue, Performing Arts Center
Type of Stage: Proscenium/Thrust
Stage Dimensions: 30'x 40'
Seating Capacity: 1,700
Year Built: 2000
Cost: $27,000
Rental Contact: Director Steve Carignan

4525 CEDAR RAPIDS COMMUNITY CONCERTS ASSOCIATION

1017 F Avenue NW
Cedar Rapids, IA 52405
Phone: 319-362-4093
Officers:
   President: George Baldwin
   VP: Len D Staab
Performs At: Paramount Theatre for the Performing Arts

4526 COE COLLEGE JAZZ SUMMIT

Coe College
Marquis 104
Cedar Rapids, IA 52402
Phone: 319-399-8520
Fax: 319-399-8209
e-mail: Jazz Summit@coe.edu
Web Site: www.coe.edu
Management:
   Chair Department of Music: Dr. William S Carson
   Director Jaz Band: Steve Shanley
Mission: To offer student musicians the opportunity to work with renowned professional players/teachers.
Founded: 1992
Specialized Field: Jazz
Status: Nonprofit
Paid Staff: 5
Volunteer Staff: 40
Paid Artists: 6
Non-paid Artists: 20
Annual Attendance: 1,500

4527 COE COLLEGE MARQUIS SERIES

1220 1st Avenue NW
Cedar Rapids, IA 52402
Phone: 319-399-8682
e-mail: GCross@coe.edu
Web Site: www.coe.edu
Officers:
   Chairman: Dr. Maria Dean
   Marquis Series Committee Chair: Dr. Gavin Cross
Performs At: Sinclair Auditorium

4528 LEGION ARTS

CSPS
1103 3rd Street SE
Cedar Rapids, IA 52401
Phone: 319-364-1580
Fax: 319-362-9156
e-mail: info@legionarts.org
Web Site: www.legionarts.org
Management:
   Artistic Director: Mel Andringa
   Executive Director: F John Herbert
Mission: Promotes new and innovative expression in the visual, performing, literary and electronic arts; fosters creative interaction between artists, their communities and society; and encourages the imaginative exploration of contemporary ideas and experience.
Founded: 1981
Specialized Field: Folk; World Music; Performance Art; Theatre
Status: Professional; Nonprofit
Paid Staff: 4

Budget: $250,000
Income Sources: Association of Performing Arts Presenters; National Association of Artists Organizations
Performs At: Proscenium; Black Box; Concert Halls; Cabaret
Affiliations: National Performance Network; National Association of Artists Organizations
Annual Attendance: 10,000
Facility Category: Contemporary Arts Center
Type of Stage: Black Box
Seating Capacity: 75
Year Built: 1893
Year Remodeled: 1991
Rental Contact: Mel Andrinca
Organization Type: Performing; Touring; Sponsoring

4529 GLENN MILLER FESTIVAL

PO Box 61
107 E Main Street
Clarinda, IA 51632
Phone: 712-542-2461
Fax: 712-542-2461
e-mail: gmbs@clarinda.heartland.net
Web Site: www.glennmiller.org
Officers:
   President: Marvin Negley
Management:
   Office Manager: Jodi Eberly
   Secretary Of Board: Arlene Leonard
Paid Staff: 1
Volunteer Staff: 15

4530 BIX BIEDERBECKE MEMORIAL JAZZ FESTIVAL

311 N Ripley Street
PO Box 3688
Davenport, IA 52808
Phone: 563-324-7170
Fax: 563-326-1732
Toll-free: 888-249-5487
e-mail: info@bixsociety.org
Web Site: www.bixsociety.org
Officers:
   President: Don Estes
   Secretary: Muriel Voss
   Treasurer: Annette J Peart
Management:
   Festival Director: Ray Voss
   Music Director: Rich Johnson
Mission: To honor the memory and perpetuate the music of Leon Bix Beiderbecke, a Davenport native son, who was a world-renowned jazz cornetist, pianist and composer.
Founded: 1972
Volunteer Staff: 450
Paid Artists: 100
Season: July
Annual Attendance: 10,000

4531 MISSISSIPPI VALLEY BLUES FESTIVAL

102 S Harrison
Davenport, IA 52801

Phone: 319-322-5837
Fax: 319-322-5832
e-mail: mvbs@revealed.net
Web Site: www.mvbs.org
Management:
   Director: Steve Brundies

4532 LUTHER COLLEGE CENTER STAGE SERIES

Luther College
700 College Drive
Decorah, IA 52101
Phone: 319-387-1291
Fax: 319-387-1766
e-mail: Kuhlmayv@luther.edu
Web Site: www.luther.edu
Management:
   Campus Programming Director: Yvonne Kuhlman
Founded: 1977
Specialized Field: Performing Arts
Paid Staff: 6
Volunteer Staff: 25
Performs At: Center for Faith & Life
Facility Category: Performing Arts Facility
Type of Stage: Thrust
Stage Dimensions: 48'x 32'
Seating Capacity: 1,463
Year Built: 1977

4533 CIVIC MUSIC ASSOCIATION OF DES MOINES

221 Walnut Street
Des Moines, IA 50309
Phone: 515-288-8918
Fax: 515-243-1588
e-mail: info@civicmusic.org
Web Site: www.civicmusic.org
Management:
   Executive Director: Debra Peckumn
Seating Capacity: 2735

4534 GRAND VIEW COLLEGE-NIELSEN CONCERT SERIES

1200 Grand View Avenue
Des Moines, IA 50316
Phone: 515-263-2958
Fax: 515-263-6192
e-mail: kduffy@gvc.edu
Management:
   Director: Dr. Katherine Pohlmann Duffy
Performs At: College Center Theatre

4535 CLARKE COLLEGE CULTURAL EVENTS SERIES

1550 Clark Drive
Dubuque, IA 52001-3198
Phone: 319-588-6405
Fax: 319-588-6789
Web Site: www.clarke.edu

4536 LORAS COLLEGE ARTS & LECTURE SERIES
1450 Alta Vista
Dubuque, IA 52004-0178
Phone: 319-588-7153
Fax: 319-557-4086
e-mail: bhughes@loras.edu
Web Site: www.loras.edu
Officers:
   Chairman: Brian Hughes
Management:
   Chairman: Brain Hughes
Mission: To bring high quality cultural activity to the college and community.
Founded: 1985
Specialized Field: Insturmental Music, Vocal Music, Dance, Multi-Cultural, Theatre, Lecture
Volunteer Staff: 10
Performs At: St. Joseph Auditorium

4537 WALDORF COMMUNITY ARTISTS SERIES
Waldorf College
106 S 6th Street
Forest City, IA 50436
Phone: 641-582-8179
Fax: 641-582-8194
e-mail: thompsons@waldorf.edu
Management:
   Manager: Steven B Thompson
Mission: To offer the finest in performing arts events to the Forest City and Waldorf communities.
Founded: 1988
Specialized Field: Dance; Vocal Music; Instrumental Music; Theater; Lyric Opera; Grand Opera
Status: Nonprofit
Income Sources: Waldorf College
Organization Type: Sponsoring

4538 GRINNELL COLLEGE MUSIC DEPARTMENT CONCERT SERIES
Music Department
Grinnell, IA 50112
Phone: 641-269-3064
Fax: 641-269-4420
Web Site: www.grinnell.edu/music/
Officers:
   Music Department Chairman: Jonathan Chenette
Performs At: Sebring-Lewis Hall

4539 IOWA ARTS FESTIVAL
PO Box 3128
Iowa City, IA 52244
Phone: 319-337-7944
Fax: 319-351-6409
e-mail: iowaarts@avalon.net
Management:
   Executive Director: Vicki Jennings

4540 IOWA CITY JAZZ FESTIVAL
PO Box 10054
Iowa City, IA 52240
Phone: 319-358-9346
e-mail: gizmojazz@aol.com
Web Site: www.iowacityjazzfestival.com

4541 JACKSON CONCERT SERIES
400 Iowa Avenue
Muscatine, IA 52761
Phone: 319-263-1596
Fax: 319-263-1631
e-mail: wesumc@muscanet.com
Performs At: Wesely United Methodist Church

4542 ORANGE CITY ARTS COUNCIL
Box 202
Orange City, IA 51041
Phone: 712-737-4885
Fax: 712-737-4351
e-mail: ocarts@juno.com
Management:
   Program Director: Joyce Bloemendaal
Performs At: Christ Chapel

4543 BUENA VISTA UNIVERSITY ACADEMIC & CULTURAL EVENTS SERIES
Buena Vista University
610 W 4th Street
Storm Lake, IA 50588
Phone: 712-749-2401
Fax: 712-749-2404
e-mail: wagner@bvu.edu
Web Site: www.bvu.edu/~aces
Management:
   Cultural Events Director: Lisa Wagner
Founded: 1988
Paid Staff: 1
Budget: $140,000
Performs At: Anderson Auditorium
Affiliations: APAP
Annual Attendance: 3,500-4,000
Facility Category: Multi Use
Type of Stage: Proscenium
Seating Capacity: 822
Year Built: 1999
Rental Contact: Katie Schwint

4544 AMERICAFEST: INTERNATIONAL SINGING FESTIVAL FOR WOMEN
34 Fox Creek Drive
Waukee, IA 50263
Phone: 515-987-1405
Fax: 515-987-5480
e-mail: amfst98@aol.com
Management:
   Artistic Director: Carol Stewart
Season: October
Performs At: St. John's University (Festival Site)
Facility Category: Abbey Cathedral
Seating Capacity: 2,000

4545 LADYSING FESTIVAL FOR WOMEN
34 Fox Creek Drive
Waukee, IA 50263

All listings are in alphabetical order by state, then city, then organization within the city.

Phone: 515-987-1405
Fax: 515-987-5480
e-mail: amfst98@aol.com
Management:
    Artistic Director: Carol Stewart
Season: October
Performs At: St. John's University [Festival Site]
Facility Category: Abbey Cathedral
Seating Capacity: 2,000

4546 WARTBURG COLLEGE ARTISTS SERIES
100 Wartburg Boulevard
PO Box 1003
Waverly, IA 50677-1003
Phone: 319-352-8409
Fax: 319-352-8501
e-mail: artistseries@wartburg.edu
Web Site: www.wartburg.edu
Management:
    Director: Myrna Culbertson
    Technical Director: Tony Lutz
Mission: To provide diverse performing artists with community service and educational venues.
Founded: 1920
Specialized Field: Dance; Vocal Music; Instrumental Music; Theater; Lyric Opera; Grand Opera
Status: Nonprofit; College
Performs At: Neumann Auditorium
Organization Type: Sponsoring

Kansas

4547 GREAT PLAINS THEATRE FESTIVAL
PO Box 476
Abilene, KS 62410
Phone: 785-263-2903
Fax: 785-263-9960
e-mail: gptheatre@aol.com
Web Site: www.gptickets.org
Management:
    Executive Artistic Director: Richard Esvang
    Associate Artistic Director: Michelle Meade
Founded: 1994
Status: Nonprofit
Performs At: Remodeled Stone Church; State of the Art Theatre.
Affiliations: Equity
Facility Category: Theatre
Type of Stage: Proscenium
Stage Dimensions: 45' x 26'
Seating Capacity: 199
Year Built: 1880
Year Remodeled: 1994

4548 COMMUNITY CONCERTS ASSOCIATION OF ATCHISON SERIES
St. Benedict's Abbey
1020 N 2nd Street
Atchison, KS 66002

Phone: 913-367-7853
Fax: 913-367-6230
e-mail: blaine@benedictine.edu
Officers:
    President: Reverand Blaine Schultz
Performs At: Mount Community Center Auditorium

4549 COFFEYVILLE CULTURAL ARTS COUNCIL
PO Box 487
Coffeyville, KS 67337
Phone: 316-251-0088
Management:
    Executive Director: Kenneth Burchinal
Performs At: JH Benefiel Auditorium

4550 EMPORIA ARTS COUNCIL PERFORMING ARTS/CONCERT/CHILDREN'S SERIES
Box 1227
Emporia, KS 66801
Phone: 316-343-6473
Management:
    Executive Director: Catherine Rickbone
Performs At: Albert Taylor Hall

4551 GOODLAND ARTS COUNCIL
120 W 12
PO Box 526
Goodland, KS 67735
Phone: 785-899-6442
Fax: 785-899-6335
e-mail: gac@goodland.ixks.com
Web Site: www.goodlandnet.com/artcenter/
Management:
    Director: Rebecca J Downs
Performs At: Auditorium

4552 FORT HAYS STATE UNIVERSITY ENCORE SERIES
Memeorial Union
Hays, KS 67601
Phone: 785-628-5801
Fax: 785-628-4007
e-mail: cbrock@fhsu.edu
Management:
    Special Events Coordinator: Carol Brock
Performs At: Felton-Start Theatre

4553 HESSTON/BETHEL PERFORMING ARTS SERIES
PO Box 3000
Hesston, KS 67062
Phone: 316-327-8158
Fax: 316-327-8300
Officers:
    Chairman: Jacob Rittenhouse
    Executive Secretary: David W Rhodes
    Administrative Assistant: Krista Murray
Mission: To provide high quality cultural programming for the Hesston College/Bethel College student bodies and the immediate Hesston and Newton communities

Founded: 1982
Specialized Field: Vocal Music; Instrumental Music
Status: Nonprofit
Budget: $45,000
Income Sources: Season Tickets; Single Ticket Sales; Patrons; City Support
Performs At: Yost Center, Hesston College; Memorial Hall, Bethel College
Annual Attendance: 500
Facility Category: Gymnasium/Field House
Seating Capacity: 1,000
Year Built: 1983
Organization Type: Sponsoring

4554 MESSIAH FESTIVAL OF MUSIC

Bethany College
421 N 1st Street
Lindsborg, KS 67456
Phone: 913-227-3311
Fax: 913-721-2110
Management:
    Conductor: Gregory Aune
    Public Relations/Ticket Information: Jud Barclay
    Music Director: Daniel Mahraun
Founded: 1882
Specialized Field: Vocal Music; Instrumental Music
Status: Nonprofit
Income Sources: Bethany College
Performs At: Presser Hall Auditorium
Organization Type: Performing; Sponsoring

4555 BOWLUS CULTURAL ATTRACTIONS SERIES

PO Box 705
205 E Madison
Lola, KS 66749
Phone: 316-365-4765
Fax: 316-365-4767
e-mail: mary.bowlus@iolaks.com
Web Site: www.bowluscenter.com
Management:
    Director: Mary Martin
Seating Capacity: 752

4556 KANSAS STATE UNIVERSITY MCCAIN PERFORMANCE SERIES

McCain Auditorium
Manhattan, KS 66506-4711
Phone: 785-532-6425
Fax: 785-532-5870
e-mail: rpm@ksu.edu
Web Site: www.ksu.edu/mccain
Management:
    Director: Richard Martin
Seating Capacity: 1800

4557 OTTAWA MUNICIPAL AUDITORIUM ENTERTAINMENT SERIES

PO Box 462
301 S Hickory
Ottawa, KS 66067

Phone: 785-242-8810
Fax: 785-229-3760
e-mail: omalive@grapevine.net
Web Site: www.grapevine.net/~omalive
Management:
    Director: Dick Smith

4558 OVERLAND PARK ARTS COMMISSION

6300 W 87th Street
Overland Park, KS 66212
Phone: 913-895-6357
Fax: 913-895-6365
e-mail: jkbilyea@opkansas.org
Management:
    Arts Coordinator: Julie K Bilyea

4559 PITTSBURG ARTS COUNCIL

PO Box 1838
Pittsburg, KS 66762
Phone: 316-231-1230
Fax: 316-231-2340
e-mail: pittart@sunnetworks.net
Management:
    Executive Director: Karen Brady

4560 PITTSBURG STATE UNIVERSITY SOLO & CHAMBER MUSIC SERIES

PSU Department of Music
1701 S Broadway
Pittsburg, KS 66762
Phone: 620-235-4476
Fax: 620-235-4468
e-mail: music@pittstate.edu
Web Site: www.pittstate.edu/music
Management:
    Series Director: Susan Marchant
Specialized Field: Solo & Chamber Music Performances

4561 SALINA ARTS & HUMANITIES COMMISSION

PO Box 2181
Salina, KS 67402-2181
Phone: 785-826-7410
Fax: 785-826-7444
e-mail: sahc@midusa.net
Web Site: www.riverfestival.com
Management:
    Executive Director: Martha Rhea

4562 STERLING COLLEGE ARTIST SERIES

Sterling College
Sterling, KS 67579
Phone: 316-278-2173
Management:
    Artists Series Dirctor: Prof. Gordon King
Performs At: Culbertson Auditorium

4563 TOPEKA JAZZ FESTIVAL

214 SE 8th Street
Topeka, KS 66603

Phone: 785-297-9000
Fax: 785-234-2307
Web Site: www.tpactix.org/jazzfestival-2002.htm
Management:
    Artistic Director: Jim Moore
Mission: To promote and preserve jazz.
Founded: 1998
Specialized Field: Jazz Performance
Paid Staff: 6
Volunteer Staff: 60
Paid Artists: 36

4564 FRIENDS UNIVERSITY MILLER FINE ARTS SERIES

2100 University
Wichita, KS 67213
Phone: 316-295-5849
Fax: 316-295-5593
e-mail: riney@friends.edu
Officers:
    Fine Arts Division Chairman: Cecil J Riney
Performs At: Alexander Auditorium

4565 WICHITA STATE UNIVERSITY CONNOISSEUR SERIES

College of Fine Arts, 415 Jardine Hall
1845 Fairmount
Wichita, KS 67260-0151
Phone: 316-978-3389
Fax: 316-978-3951

Kentucky

4566 ARTISTS IN CONCERT SERIES

Ashland Community College
1400 College Drive
Ashland, KY 41101-3683
Phone: 606-325-1132
Fax: 606-326-2173
Management:
    Fiscal Agent: Robert Ross
Performs At: Ashland Community College Auditorium

4567 BEREA COLLEGE CONVOCATION SERIES

CPO 2160
Berea, KY 40404-2160
Phone: 859-985-3171
Fax: 859-985-3912
e-mail: John_Crowden@berea.edu
Web Site: www.berea.edu/medunews.html
Management:
    Coordinator: John Crowden
Performs At: Phelps - Stokes Auditorium

4568 CAPITOL ARTS ALLIANCE

416 E Main Street
Bowling Green, KY 42101-2241
Phone: 270-782-2787
Fax: 270-782-2804
e-mail: Johna.@capitol.ky.net
Web Site: www.capitolartscenter.com
Management:
    Manager: Carrie Barnett
    Managing Director: Jane Mercer
Seating Capacity: 840

4569 CENTRAL KENTUCKY ARTS SERIES

PO Box 383
Campbellsville, KY 42719
Phone: 270-789-5287
Fax: 270-789-5524
e-mail: wroberts@campbellsvil.edu
Officers:
    President: Wesley Roberts
Mission: To provide professional programs in all the arts.
Founded: 1967
Income Sources: Individual and Corporate Donations
Facility Category: Recital Hall; Auditoriums

4570 GREAT AMERICAN BRASS BAND FESTIVAL

PO Box 429
Danville, KY 40423-0429
Phone: 859-236-4692
Fax: 859-236-9610
Management:
    Director: George Foreman

4571 FOUST ARTIST SERIES

Georgetown College
Georgetown, KY 40324-1696
Phone: 502-863-8112
e-mail: sburnett@georgetowncollege.edu
Management:
    Cultural Programs Director: Dr. Sonny Burnette
Performs At: John L. Hill Chapel

4572 GREATER HAZARD AREA PERFORMING ARTS SERIES

Hazard Community College
1 Community College Drive
Hazard, KY 41702
Mailing Address: PO Box 1052 Hazard, KY 41702
Phone: 606-436-5721
Fax: 606-439-3821
Toll-free: 800-246-7521
e-mail: Tammy.Duff@kctcs.edu
Web Site: www.hazcc.kctcs.net/arts
Management:
    Performing Arts Series Coordinator: Tammy Duff
    Staff Assistant: Sandy Campbell
Founded: 1974
Paid Staff: 2
Volunteer Staff: 20
Paid Artists: 12
Non-paid Artists: 20
Budget: $100,000+
Income Sources: Ticket Sales; Corporate/Private Support; Grants
Performs At: First Federal Center

Affiliations: Hazard Community College
Facility Category: Flexible Conference Center; Smaller Auditorium
Type of Stage: Proscenium/Flexible
Seating Capacity: 800; 200-700
Year Built: 2002

4573 PENNYROYAL ARTS COUNCIL SERIES

425 E 9th Street
PO Box 1038
Hopkinsville, KY 42241
Phone: 270-887-4295
Fax: 270-887-4027
e-mail: paci@bellsouth.net
Management:
   Director: Jennifer Maddux
Performs At: Alhambra Theatre

4574 UNIVERSITY OF KENTUCKY ARTISTS SERIES

University of Kentucky
Singletary Center for the Arts
Lexington, KY 40506-0241
Phone: 859-257-1706
Fax: 859-323-9991
e-mail: hbsali00@pop.uky.edu
Web Site: www.uky.edu/SCFA/
Management:
   Center for the Arts Director: Holly Salisbury
Performs At: Otis A. Singletary Center for the Arts Concert Hall

4575 SUE BENNETT COLLEGE, APPALACHIAN FOLK FESTIVAL

151 College Street
London, KY 40741
Phone: 606-864-2238
Fax: 606-539-4404
Management:
   Chairperson: Madge Chestnut
Mission: To offer arts, performances and events showcasing Appalachian heritage.
Founded: 1973
Specialized Field: Vocal Music; Festivals
Status: Nonprofit
Performs At: Sue Bennett College Auditorium
Organization Type: Performing; Educational

4576 KENTUCKY SHAKESPEARE FESTIVAL

1114 S 3rd Street
Louisville, KY 40203
Phone: 502-583-8738
Fax: 502-583-8751
e-mail: tofter@aol.com
Web Site: www.kyshakes.org
Management:
   Producing Director: Curt L Tofteland
   Director Education: Doug Sumey
Mission: To provide accessible, professional, classical theatre and quality education touring programs.
Founded: 1960
Status: Professional
Budget: $750,000

Income Sources: Corporate; Foundation; Individuals; Government; Fund; Earned
Season: May - August
Performs At: C Douglas Ramey Amphitheater
Annual Attendance: 67,500
Facility Category: Outdoor Ampitheatre
Type of Stage: Thrust
Seating Capacity: 1,000
Year Built: 1963
Year Remodeled: 1993
Cost: $1,000,000
Organization Type: Performing; Resident; Touring; Educational

4577 SOUTHERN BAPTIST THEOLOGICAL SEMINARY-INMAN JOHNSON GUEST ARTIST SERIES

2825 Lexington Road
Louisville, KY 40280
Phone: 502-897-4115
Fax: 502-897-4066
Toll-free: 800-626-5525
e-mail: chmusic@sbts.edu
Web Site: www.sbts.edu
Officers:
   Manager: Linda Lancaster
Specialized Field: Music
Budget: $23,000
Income Sources: Endowment
Performs At: Recital Hall
Seating Capacity: 230

4578 MURRAY CIVIC MUSIC ASSOCIATION SERIES

Murray State University, Music Department
527 Fine Arts Center
Murray, KY 42071-3342
Phone: 270-762-6337
Fax: 270-762-3965
e-mail: robert.murray@murraystate.edu
Officers:
   VP Programming: Robert Murray
Mission: To provide Murray with the finest in performing arts events.
Founded: 1959
Specialized Field: Dance; Vocal Music; Instrumental Music; Theater; Lyric Opera; Grand Opera
Status: Nonprofit
Performs At: Lovett Auditorium; Murray State University
Organization Type: Sponsoring

4579 PIKEVILLE CONCERT ASSOCIATION SERIES

190 3rd Street
Pikeville, KY 41501
Phone: 606-437-7878
e-mail: jperry@eastky.com
Performs At: Auditorium

4580 ALICE LLOYD COLLEGE CANEY CONVOCATION SERIES
Purpose Road
Pippa Passes, KY 41844
Phone: 606-360-6136
Fax: 606-368-6217
Performs At: Estelle Campbell Center for the Arts

4581 ASBURY COLLEGE ARTIST SERIES
Asbury College
1 Macklem Drive
Wilmore, KY 40390
Phone: 606-858-3511
Fax: 606-858-3921
e-mail: kevin.sparks@asbury.edu
Web Site: www.asbury.edu
Officers:
    Chairman: Kevin Sparks
Performs At: Hughes Memorial Auditorium

4582 WINCHESTER COUNCIL FOR THE ARTS SERIES
PO Box 836
Winchester, KY 40392-0836
Phone: 859-744-6437
Fax: 859-744-1606
e-mail: leedswac@meginc.com
Web Site: www.leedscenter.com
Management:
    Executive Director: Bill Oliver
Performs At: Leeds Theatre & Performing Arts Center

Louisiana

4583 L.S.U. UNION GREAT PERFORMANCES THEATER SERIES
Box 25123 LSU
Baton Rouge, LA 70894
Phone: 225-578-5118
Fax: 225-578-9311
e-mail: rdunaw1@lsu.edu
Management:
    Program Coordinator: Rhonda Dunaway
Founded: 1963
Annual Attendance: 5,028
Seating Capacity: 1250
Rental Contact: Cason Duke

4584 LSU UNION GREAT PERFORMANCES THEATER SERIES
Box 25123
Baton Rouge, LA 70894
Phone: 225-578-5118
Fax: 225-578-9311
e-mail: rdunaw1@lsu.edu
Management:
    Program Coordinator: Rhonda R Dunaway
Founded: 1963

4585 FANFARE FESTIVAL
SLU 10797
500 Western Avenue
Hammond, LA 70402
Phone: 985-549-2333
Fax: 985-549-2868
e-mail: kcouret@selu.edu
Web Site: www.selu.edu/fanfare
Management:
    Artistic Director: Donna Gay Anderson
    Associate Director/Programming: Keiron Covrest
    Associate Director/Marketing: Pamela Mills
    Secretary: Betsy Creed
Founded: 1986
Paid Staff: 8
Volunteer Staff: 22
Paid Artists: 25
Non-paid Artists: 10

4586 SOUTHEASTERN LOUISIANA UNIVERSITY ARTS & LECTURES SERIES
SLU 346
Hammond, LA 70402
Phone: 504-549-3792
Fax: 504-549-5647
e-mail: jmchodgkins@selu.edu
Officers:
    Chairman: Jim McHodgkins

4587 JEFF DAVIS ARTS COUNCIL
PO Box 1068
Jennings, LA 70546
Phone: 337-824-5060
Fax: 337-824-1070

4588 FESTIVAL INTERNATIONAL DE LOUISIANE
PO Box 4008
Lafayette, LA 70502
Phone: 337-232-8086
Fax: 337-233-7536
e-mail: info@festivalinternational.com
Web Site: www.festivalinternational.com
Management:
    Marketing Director: Dana Canedo
    Programming Director: Lisa Stafford
    Marketing Coordinator: Rhon Barras
Mission: Free family event celebrating the French cultural heritage of southern Louisiana - a combination of French, African, Caribbean and Hispanic influences.
Founded: 1986
Specialized Field: Visual, Performing and Culinary Arts
Paid Staff: 4
Volunteer Staff: 950
Season: April
Performs At: Kimmel Center for the Performing Arts

4589 LAFAYETTE COMMUNITY CONCERTS SERIES
PO Box 2465
Lafayette, LA 70502

Phone: 337-233-1035
Officers:
President: George E Arceneaux

4590 PERFORMING ARTS SOCIETY OF ACADIANA SERIES

PO Box 52979
Lafayette, LA 70505
Phone: 337-237-2787
Fax: 337-237-3974
e-mail: pasajll@aol.com
Web Site: www.pasa.online.org
Performs At: Heymann Performing Arts - Convention Center

4591 UNIVERSITY OF LOUISIANA AT LAFAYETTE CONCERT SERIES

ULL Drawer 41207
Lafayette, LA 70504-1207
Phone: 337-482-5216
Fax: 337-482-5017
e-mail: pdm0677@louisiana.edu
Officers:
University Concert Committee Chair: Dr. Paul Morton

4592 UNIVERSITY OF SOUTHWESTERN LOUISIANA CONCERT SERIES

USL Drawer 41207
Lafayette, LA 70504
Phone: 337-482-5216
Fax: 337-482-5017
Officers:
Chairman: Andrea Loewy
Management:
Assistant Professor: Paul Morton
Performs At: Angelle Hall Auditorium

4593 MAMOU CAJUN MUSIC FESTIVAL ASSOCIATION

420 E Street
Apartment 1
Mamou, LA 70554
Phone: 337-468-2258
Mission: To offer traditional Cajun music, as well as related events.
Founded: 1972
Specialized Field: Vocal Music; Festivals
Status: Nonprofit
Organization Type: Performing; Resident; Educational

4594 JEFFERSON PERFORMING ARTS SOCIETY

1118 Clearview Parkway
Metairie, LA 70001
Phone: 504-885-2000
Fax: 504-885-3437
e-mail: info@jpas.org
Web Site: www.jpas.org
Officers:
Chairman: Hannah Cunningham
President: Wayne Keating

Past President: Dr. Bud Willis
Secretary: Subhash Kulkarni
Management:
Founder/Executive Director/Artistic: Dennis G Assaf
Director: Claudia Garofolo
Mission: Supporting performance and education in the performing arts.
Founded: 1978
Specialized Field: All Performing Arts
Status: Professional; Semi-Professional; Non-Professional; Nonprofit
Paid Staff: 14
Volunteer Staff: 100
Paid Artists: 100+
Budget: 1.2 million
Income Sources: Box Office; Ads; Sponsorships; Grants
Affiliations: APAP; ACDA; ASOL; Conductor's Guild
Annual Attendance: 30,000
Facility Category: Theater
Type of Stage: Proscenium Arch
Stage Dimensions: 42'x 35'
Seating Capacity: 1,350
Year Built: 1952
Year Remodeled: 1999
Organization Type: Performing; Educational

4595 ULM PERFORMING ARTS SERIES

University of Louisiana in Monroe
700 University Avenue
Monroe, LA 71209
Phone: 318-342-3600
Fax: 318-342-5425
e-mail: enhaedicke@uca.edu
Management:
Chairman: Dr. Janet Haddicke
Mission: To bring to students and townspeople the best in professional cultural entertainment.
Specialized Field: Dance; Vocal Music; Instrumental Music; Theater
Status: Nonprofit
Paid Staff: 1
Budget: $120,000
Income Sources: Season Ticket Sales
Performs At: Civic Center Theater; Brown Auditorium
Organization Type: Performing; Sponsoring

4596 UNIVERSITY OF LOUISIANA AT MONROE PERFORMING ARTS SERIES

700 University Avenue
Monroe, LA 71209
Phone: 318-342-1494
Fax: 318-342-1491
e-mail: Enhaedicke@ulm.edu
Officers:
University Concert Committee Chair: Dr. Paul Morton
Management:
Director: Dr. Janet V Haedicke
Paid Staff: 1
Volunteer Staff: 2
Paid Artists: 50

4597 NORTHWESTERN STATE UNIVERSITY CONCERT SERIES
CAPA
Northwestern State University of Louisiana
Natchitoches, LA 71497
Phone: 318-357-4522
Fax: 318-357-5906
e-mail: bandcamps@nsula.edu
Web Site: www.nsula.edu
Officers:
   Chairman: Bill Brent
Performs At: Fine Arts Auditorium

4598 NEW ORLEANS FRIENDS OF MUSIC SERIES
940 Turquoise Street
New Orleans, LA 70124
Phone: 504-887-1133
Fax: 504-282-4008
Officers:
   President: Dr. Stuart Farber
Performs At: Dixon Hall

4599 NEW ORLEANS INTERNATIONAL PIANO COMPETITION & KEYBOARD FESTIVAL
PO Drawer 19599
New Orleans, LA 70179-0599
Phone: 504-895-0700
Fax: 504-895-0700
e-mail: director@noipc.org
Web Site: www.noipc.org
Management:
   Director: Danial Weilbaecher
Founded: 1989
Specialized Field: Classical Piano Music

4600 NEW ORLEANS JAZZ & HERITAGE FOUNDATION
1205 N Rampart Street
New Orleans, LA 70116
Phone: 504-522-4786
Fax: 504-522-5456
Web Site: www.nojazzfest.com
Management:
   Director: Quint Davis

4601 SHAKESPEARE FESTIVAL AT TULANE
Tulane University
Department of Theatre & Dance
New Orleans, LA 70118
Phone: 504-865-5105
Fax: 504-865-6737
e-mail: SFTProdMgr@aol.com
Web Site: www.NewOrleansShakespeare.com
Management:
   Artistic Director: Aimee K Michel
   Managing Director: Clare Moncrief
   Production Manager: Brad Robbert

Mission: To provide professional Shakespeare productions to the Greater New Orleans and surrounding Gulf South area along with educational programs to the schools.
Founded: 1993
Specialized Field: Classical Theatre; Shakespeare; New Works; Modern Classics
Status: Professional; Nonprofit
Paid Staff: 6
Paid Artists: 60
Budget: $250,000
Income Sources: Public; Private; Corporate; Foundation; Box Office; Tuition
Facility Category: Equity Small Professional Theatre
Type of Stage: Black Box; Laboratory
Seating Capacity: 150; 60

4602 LOUISIANA TECH CONCERT ASSOCIATION SERIES
Tech Station
PO Bx 8608
Ruston, LA 71272
Phone: 318-257-2930
Fax: 318-257-4571
Toll-free: 800-528-3241
e-mail: ltca_latech@yahoo.com
Web Site: www.performingarts.iatech.edu
Management:
   Co-Director: Alan Goldspiel
   Co-Director: Cherrie Sciro
Founded: 1945
Specialized Field: Music; Drama
Budget: $133,000
Income Sources: Ticket Sales
Performs At: Howard Center for the Performing Arts
Annual Attendance: 6,000
Type of Stage: Proscenium
Seating Capacity: 1,051

4603 FRIENDS OF MUSIC SERIES
Hurley School of Music, Centenary College
2911 Centenary Boulevard
Shreveport, LA 71104
Phone: 318-869-5235
Fax: 318-869-5248
e-mail: godom@centenary.edu
Web Site:
www.centenary.edu/departme/music/music.html
Management:
   Manager: Dr. Gale Odom
Performs At: Hurley Recital Hall

4604 RED RIVER REVEL ARTS FESTIVAL
101 Crockett Street
Shreveport, LA 71101
Phone: 318-424-4000
Fax: 318-226-9559
e-mail: RRR@RedRiverRevel.com
Web Site: www.RedRiverRevel.com
Management:
   Executive Director: CL Holloway
Mission: Eight day celebration of the Arts.
Founded: 1976
Paid Staff: 4

Volunteer Staff: 6
Paid Artists: 160
Income Sources: Corporate Sponsors; Underwriters; State; Local Grants
Annual Attendance: 180,000-200,000
Facility Category: Outdoor Festival

4605 SLIDELL DEPARTMENT OF CULTURAL AFFAIRS

444 Erlanger Street
PO Box 828
Slidell, LA 70459
Phone: 504-646-4375
Fax: 504-646-4231
Web Site: www.slidell.la.us
Management:
   Director: Kelli Gustafson
Performs At: Auditorium

4606 IMPRESARIO'S CHOICE-THE BROADWAY SERIES AT THE MONROE CIVIC THEATRE

267 Verhagen Road
PO Box 828
Tallulah, LA 71284-0828
Phone: 318-574-0440
Fax: 318-574-0440
Toll-free: 888-822-0440
e-mail: impresariosmail@aol.com
Web Site: www.impresarioschoice.com
Officers:
   President: Raymond E Poliquit
   VP: Mark Henderson
   Secretary: Douglas Leporati
   Trasurer: Sherry Free
   Public Realtions: Ruby James
Management:
   Artistic Director: Raymond E Poliquit
   Executive Director: Ezekial J Moore
Mission: It is our mission to bring high quality national touring Broadway musicals to Northeast Louisiana, and to expand the theatregoing audience, both in number and diversity.
Founded: 1988
Specialized Field: Musical Theatre
Status: Nonprofit
Paid Staff: 1
Volunteer Staff: 1
Budget: $275,000
Income Sources: Corporate Sponsorship
Affiliations: Impresario's Friends
Annual Attendance: 6,200
Facility Category: Civic Center
Type of Stage: Procenium
Seating Capacity: 2,100

4607 NICHOLLS STATE UNIVERSITY ARTISTS & LECTURE SERIES

PO Box 2038
Thibodaux, LA 70301
Phone: 985-448-4273
Fax: 985-448-4926
Management:

Director: Angela Hammerli
Performs At: Auditorium

Maine

4608 NEW MUSIK DIRECTIONS SERIES

67 Green Street
Augusta, ME 04330
Phone: 207-623-1941
Fax: 207-623-1941
Management:
   Director: Joseph Baltar
Mission: To provide a network for artists in film, video and new music.
Founded: 1981
Specialized Field: Festivals
Status: Professional; Commercial
Organization Type: Performing; Educational; Sponsoring

4609 BAR HARBOR FESTIVAL

Rodick Building
59 Cottage Street
Bar Harbor, ME 04609-1800
Phone: 207-288-5744
Web Site: www.arcadia.net/bhcoc

4610 CHOCOLATE CHURCH ARTS CENTER FESTIVAL

804 Washington Street
Bath, ME 04530-2617
Phone: 207-442-8455
Fax: 207-442-8455
e-mail: chocolatechurch@gwi.net
Management:
   Executive Director: Suzanne Lufkin Weiss
Seating Capacity: 294

4611 KNEISEL HALL CHAMBER MUSIC FESTIVAL

PO Box 648
Blue Hill, ME 04614
Phone: 207-374-2811
Fax: 207-374-2811
e-mail: festival@kneisel.org
Web Site: www.kneisel.org
Management:
   Executive Director: Ellen Werner
   Artistic Director: Seymour Lipkin
Mission: To foster the art of chamber music through teaching and performance.
Founded: 1902
Paid Staff: 5
Paid Artists: 14
Budget: $485,000
Income Sources: Donations; Grants; Ticket Sales
Annual Attendance: 2,500
Facility Category: Historic Hall
Seating Capacity: 175
Year Built: 1922
Rental Contact: Ellen Werner

4612 BOWDOIN COLLEGE CONCERT SERIES

Music Department, Gibson Hall
9200 College Station
Brunswick, ME 04011-8492
Phone: 207-725-3747
Fax: 207-725-3748
e-mail: dsmall@bowdoin.edu
Management:
   Administrator: Delmar D Small
Specialized Field: College Music Department
Performs At: Kresge Auditorium, Pickard Theater and Chapel

4613 BOWDOIN SUMMER MUSIC FESTIVAL

6300 College Station
Bowdoin College
Brunswick, ME 04011
Phone: 207-373-1400
Fax: 207-373-1441
e-mail: bsmf@blazenetme.net
Web Site: www.summermusic.org
Officers:
   Chairman of the Board: Hugh Phelps
   Vice Chair: William A Rogers
   Treasurer: Lester Hodgdon
   Secretary: Nancy R Connery
Management:
   Artistic Director: Lewis Kaplan
   Executive Director: Peter Simmons
   Admissions Director: Jen Means
   Business Manager: Chris Murray
Mission: To provide the most promising music students from around the world with opportunities to further their musical development, and to present chamber music performed to the highest standards by distinguished professional musicians.
Founded: 1964
Specialized Field: Chamber
Status: Nonprofit
Budget: $1,100,000
Income Sources: Contributions; Ticket Sales; Tution
Performs At: Crooker Theater, Brunswick High School
Affiliations: Chamber Music America; Major Conservatories; Maine Performing Arts Network
Annual Attendance: 10,000
Seating Capacity: 600
Year Built: 1995
Organization Type: Educational; Presenting

4614 GAMPER FESTIVAL OF CONTEMPORARY MUSIC

Bowdoin Summer Music Festival
Bowdoin College, 6300 College Station
Brunswick, ME 04011-8463
Phone: 207-725-3322
Fax: 207-725-3047
e-mail: bsmf@blazenetme.net
Web Site: www.summermusic.org
Management:
   Director: Lewis Kaplan

4615 UNIVERSITY OF MAINE AT FORT KENT, INTERNATIONAL PERFORMERS SERIES

University of Maine at Fort Kent
25 Pleasant Street
Fort Kent, ME 04743
Phone: 207-834-7513
Fax: 207-834-7503

4616 BATES DANCE FESTIVAL

163 Wood Street
Lewiston, ME 04240-6016
Phone: 207-786-6381
Fax: 207-786-8282
e-mail: dancefest@bates.edu
Web Site: www.bates.edu/dancefest
Management:
   Director: Laura Faure
   Associate Director/Registrar: Alison Hart
Mission: The Bates Dance Festival fosters a cooperative community in which choreographers, performers, educators, and students come together to study, perform, and create new work.
Founded: 1982
Specialized Field: Dance
Status: Professional
Paid Staff: 5
Volunteer Staff: 24
Paid Artists: 20
Budget: over $500,000
Income Sources: Public; Private; and Earned Income
Performs At: Schaeffer Theatre
Affiliations: Bates College
Annual Attendance: 4,000
Type of Stage: Sprung
Stage Dimensions: 28'x35'
Seating Capacity: 300
Year Built: 1952
Organization Type: Resident; Educational; Sponsoring

4617 L/A ARTS

221 Lisbon Street
Lewiston, ME 04240
Phone: 207-782-7228
Fax: 207-782-8192
e-mail: mail@laarts.org
Web Site: www.laarts.org
Management:
   Executive Director: Richard Willing
Mission: To offer diverse performing arts to Central Maine communities.
Founded: 1973
Specialized Field: Dance; Vocal Music; Instrumental Music; Theater; Festivals
Status: Professional; Nonprofit
Paid Staff: 3
Income Sources: Association of Performing Arts Presenters; Maine Arts Sponsor Association
Organization Type: Performing; Educational; Sponsoring

4618 MT DESERT FESTIVAL OF CHAMBER MUSIC
Box 862
Northeast Harbor, ME 04662
Phone: 207-288-4144
Management:
    Executive Director: Natalie Raimondi
    Music Director: Todd Crow

4619 SACO RIVER FESTIVAL
PO Box 610
Parsonsfield, ME 04047
Phone: 207-625-7116
e-mail: maple_rock@cs.com
Web Site: www.psouth.net/~mapleroc/srfa.htm
Management:
    Executive Director: James O'Neil

4620 LARK SOCIETY FOR CHAMBER MUSIC
PO Box 11
Portland, ME 04112
Phone: 207-761-1522
Fax: 207-780-6554
e-mail: larksq@ctel.net
Mission: Committed to supporting and presenting a Portland concert series and educational presentations by the Portland String Quartet. Presenters of the Portland Concert Series, and supporters of the PSQ's outreach activities, we promote chamber music and music education in the state of Maine.
Specialized Field: Chamber; Ensemble
Status: Professional
Income Sources: Chamber Music America
Organization Type: Performing; Touring; Resident; Educational

4621 MAINE ARTS SERIES
582 Congress Street
Portland, ME 04101
Phone: 207-772-9012
Fax: 207-772-3995
e-mail: info@mainearts.org
Web Site: www.mainearts.org
Management:
    Executive Director: Mike Miclon
Mission: To provide artistic opportunities and to encourage the advancement of the performing and the visual arts in Maine through the presentation of a public program of services to artists.
Founded: 1977
Specialized Field: Dance; Vocal Music; Instrumental Music; Theater; Festivals
Status: Professional; Nonprofit
Performs At: Downtown Portland; Thomas Point Beach
Organization Type: Sponsoring

4622 MAINE FESTIVAL
582 Congress Street
Portland, ME 04101
Phone: 207-772-9012
Fax: 207-772-3995
e-mail: nbloom@mainearts.org
Web Site: www.mainearts.org

Management:
    Director: Nicolaus Bloom

4623 PCA GREAT PERFORMANCES
477 Congress Street
Portland, ME 04101
Phone: 207-773-3150
Fax: 207-774-1018
e-mail: pcabox@pcagreatperformances.org
Web Site: www.pcagreatperformances.org
Management:
    Executive Director: Judith Adams
Founded: 1931
Paid Staff: 6
Volunteer Staff: 200
Annual Attendance: 35,000-50,000
Seating Capacity: 1,908
Year Remodeled: 1997

4624 PORTLAND CHAMBER MUSIC FESTIVAL
135 Marginal Way #277
Portland, ME 04104-5015
Mailing Address: PO Box 9715 Portland, ME 04104
Toll-free: 800-320-0257
e-mail: jenelo@aol.com
Web Site: www.pcmf.org
Management:
    Artistic Co-Director: Jennifer Elowitch
    Artistic Co-Director: Dena Levine
    Managing Director: Timothy Paradis
Mission: Annual summer chamber music festival presenting concerts by nationally renowned performers and composers.
Founded: 1994
Specialized Field: Performing Arts; Classical Music; Summer Festival
Paid Staff: 3
Paid Artists: 20
Budget: $71,000
Income Sources: Individual; Corporate; Grants
Performs At: Concert Hall; Ludcke Auditorium; University of New England
Annual Attendance: 1,000
Seating Capacity: 250

4625 PORTLAND STRING QUARTET CONCERT SERIES
PO Box 11
Portland, ME 04112
Phone: 207-761-1522
Fax: 207-780-6554
e-mail: larkpsq@ctel.net
Web Site: www.portlandstringquartet.org
Management:
    LARK Society Executive Director: Giselle A Auger

4626 FORUM SERIES
84 Mechanic Street
PO Box 784
Presque Isle, ME 04769

Phone: 207-764-0491
Fax: 207-764-2525
e-mail: theforum@mfx.net
Web Site: www.maino.com/fourm
Management:
  Director: James F Kaiser
  Administrative Assistant: Sandra Bonville
Founded: 1978
Paid Staff: 18

4627 COLBY MUSIC SERIES
Colby College
5670 Mayflower Hill
Waterville, ME 04901
Phone: 207-872-3236
Fax: 207-872-3141
e-mail: dlkadyk@colby.edu
Web Site: www.colby.edu/music
Management:
  Music Department Chairman: Steve Saunders
Founded: 1987
Specialized Field: Music
Performs At: Given Auditorium; Lorimer Chapel

Maryland

4628 ST. JOHN'S COLLEGE CONCERT SERIES
St. John's College
Music Library, Box 2800
Annapolis, MD 21404
Phone: 410-269-6904
Fax: 410-626-2886
Management:
  Music Librarian: Eric Stolzfus
Performs At: Francis Scott Key Auditorium

4629 ARTSCAPE-BALTIMORE'S FESTIVAL OF THE ARTS
21 S Eutaw Street
Baltimore, MD 21201
Phone: 410-396-4575
Fax: 410-727-4840
e-mail: ask@macac.org
Web Site: www.artscape.org
Management:
  Director: Clair Zamoiski Segal
Specialized Field: Three day regional festival of the literary, visual and performing arts.

4630 BALTIMORE SYMPHONY ORCHESTRA SUMMER MUSIC FEST: OREGON RIDGE CONCERT SERIES
1212 Cathedral Street
Baltimore, MD 21201-5545
Phone: 410-783-8100
Fax: 410-783-8004
e-mail: tickets@baltimoresymphony.com
Web Site: www.baltimoresymphony.com
Officers:
  President: John Gidwitz

Management:
  Artistic Director: Mario Venzago

4631 COLLEGE OF NOTRE DAME OF MARYLAND CONCERTS
4701 N Charles Street
Baltimore, MD 21210
Phone: 410-532-5386
Fax: 410-435-5937
e-mail: eragogini@ndm.edu
Management:
  Manager: Ernest Ragogini
Performs At: LeClerc Auditorium

4632 CONCERT ARTISTS OF BALTIMORE
1114 St. Paul Street
Baltimore, MD 21022615
Phone: 410-625-3525
Fax: 410-625-9343
e-mail: fhomann@earthlink.net
Web Site: www.cabalto.org
Management:
  Artistic Director: Edward Polochick
  Managing Director: Felice Homann
Mission: To present chamber orchestra and vocal ensemble works in the clasical music genre.
Founded: 1987
Specialized Field: Calssical Music
Status: Nonprofit
Paid Staff: 4
Volunteer Staff: 65
Budget: $275,000
Income Sources: Ticket Sales; Contracted Services; Sate abd City Grants; Foundation Grants; Corporate and Individual Donations
Type of Stage: Proscenium
Seating Capacity: 250-2,500

4633 JOHNS HOPKINS UNIVERSITY OFFICE OF SPECIAL EVENTS
Shriver Hall
3400 N Charles Street
Baltimore, MD 21218-2696
Phone: 410-516-7157
Fax: 410-516-4494
e-mail: specialevents@jhu.edu
Web Site: www.jhu.edu/~special
Management:
  Director: Deborah Panky-Mebane
Mission: To enrich the cultural life of the University and the general community by initiating and presenting a variety of lectures, performances, and workshops.
Founded: 1966
Specialized Field: Dance; Music; Drama; Literary Readings; Lectures
Paid Staff: 3
Volunteer Staff: 2
Paid Artists: 17
Non-paid Artists: 2
Income Sources: University funding; ticket sales; audience donors; private foundations; grants; sponsors
Season: October - April
Affiliations: Association of Performing Arts Presenters
Annual Attendance: 6000+

Facility Category: Auditorium
Type of Stage: Proscenium arch stage
Stage Dimensions: 40 x 28
Seating Capacity: 1118
Year Built: 1954

4634 MARYLAND INTERNATIONAL CHAMBER MUSIC FESTIVAL

PO Box 28060
Baltimore, MD 21239
Phone: 410-830-2838
Fax: 410-426-6062
e-mail: intermuse@email.com
Web Site: www.internmusearts.org
Management:
   Coordinator: Barry Goldstein
   Director: Cathy Jones
Mission: To promote classical music in Maryland.
Founded: 1985
Specialized Field: Classical Music

4635 RES MUSICAMERICA SERIES

211 Goodwood Gardens
Baltimore, MD 21210
Phone: 410-889-3939
Management:
   Artistic Director: Vivian Adelberg Rudow
Performs At: Various Auditoriums

4636 SHRIVER HALL CONCERT SERIES

The Johns Hopkins University
3400 N Charles Street
Baltimore, MD 21218-2680
Phone: 410-516-7164
Fax: 410-516-7165
e-mail: info@shriverconcerts.org
Web Site: www.shriverconcerts.org
Officers:
   President: Jephta Drachman
   VP: Harriet Panitz
   Secretary: Douglas Fambrough
   Treasurer: Helmut Jenkner
Management:
   Executive Director: Sel Kardan
Mission: Present sob and chamber music concerts.
Founded: 1965
Specialized Field: Chamber Music, Recitals
Status: Nonprofit
Paid Staff: 1
Budget: $350,000
Income Sources: Ticket sales, contributions, ads, grants
Annual Attendance: 8,000+
Facility Category: Auditorium
Type of Stage: Proscenium
Stage Dimensions: 40x80
Seating Capacity: 1,100
Year Built: 1953
Rental Contact: 410-516-2224 Pat Forrester

4637 WORLD MUSIC CONGRESSES

Towson University
8000 York Road, Administration Building 423
Baltimore, MD 21252-0001
Phone: 410-704-3451
Fax: 410-704-4012
e-mail: hbreazeale@towson.edu
Web Site: www.towson.edu/worldmusiccongresses
Management:
   Executive Director: Dr. Helene Breazeale
   Associate Director: Dr. Sergei Zverev
Mission: To provide a celebration of music with an international gathering of the world's greatest musicians, composers, conductors and instrument manufacturers, plus students and music lovers from around the globe
Founded: 1995
Specialized Field: Music, specifically cello and guitar
Paid Staff: 2
Volunteer Staff: 100
Income Sources: Corporations; Foundations; Individuals
Affiliations: Towson University
Annual Attendance: 20,000
Seating Capacity: 2,500 concert hall; 700 theatre; 5,000 arena

4638 YOUNG AUDIENCES OF MARYLAND

927 N Calvert Street
Baltimore, MD 21202
Phone: 410-837-7577
Fax: 410-837-7579
e-mail: info@yamd.org
Web Site: www.yamd.org
Officers:
   President: Norris Brodsky
   VP: Jennifer Carr
   Treasurer: Eric M Pripstein
   Secretary: Ellen Stokes
Management:
   Executive Director: Patricia M Thomas
   Education Director: Caitlin Bell
   Director Development: Ann McIntosh
   Director Administration: Nancy Gracie
   Marketing/Special Events: Christine Kramer
   Scheduling Manager: Donna Sherman
Mission: To present performing arts-in-education programs in schools and throughout the community to both children and adults—Young Audiences of Maryland presents 2,000 programs annually.
Founded: 1950
Specialized Field: Vocal Music, Instrumental Music, Theater
Status: Professional; Nonprofit
Paid Staff: 7
Volunteer Staff: 1
Paid Artists: 100
Budget: $700,000
Income Sources: Special Events; Corporate; Foundations; Individual Contributions
Performs At: Maryland Schools; Libraries; Festivals
Affiliations: National Young Audiences
Annual Attendance: 200,000
Facility Category: School
Organization Type: Performing; Educational; Sponsoring

4639 MUSIC IN THE GREAT HALL SERIES

6607 Altamont Avenue
Catonsville, MD 21228
Phone: 410-747-6012

All listings are in alphabetical order by state, then city, then organization within the city.

Management:
   Artistic Director: Virginia Reinecke

4640 WASHINGTON COLLEGE CONCERT SERIES

300 Washington Avenue
Chestertown, MD 21620
Phone: 410-778-7839
Management:
   Director: Kate Bennett
Performs At: Tawes Theater

4641 LEONARD ROSE INTERNATIONL CELLO COMPETITION

Clarice Smith Performing Arts Center
University of Maryland
College Park, MD 20742-1625
Phone: 301-405-7794
Fax: 301-405-5977
Web Site: www.claricesmithcenter.umd.edu
Season: May - June
Notes: $50,000 in cash awards and performance opportunities to the First Prize Winner.

4642 MARYLAND PRESENTS

Clarice Smith Performing Arts Center
University of Maryland
College Park, MD 20742-5611
Phone: 301-405-7846
Fax: 301-405-5977
e-mail: rclevela@deans.umd.edu
Web Site: www.claricesmithcenter.umd.edu
Management:
   Executive Director: Susan Farr
   Associate Director Communications: Amy Harrison
   Director of Cultural Participation: Ruth Waalkes
Founded: 2001
Paid Staff: 50
Performs At: The Inn and Conference Center
Annual Attendance: 250,000
Facility Category: Performing Arts Center with 6 stages
Year Built: 2001
Rental Contact: Claudia Telliho

4643 UNIVERSITY OF MARYLAND: INTERNATIONAL MARIAN ANDERSON VOCAL COMPETITION & FESTIVAL

Clarice Smith Performing Arts Center
University of Maryland
College Park, MD 20742
Phone: 301-405-8174
Fax: 301-405-5977
e-mail: gmoquin@deans.umd.edu
Web Site: www.claricesmithcenter.umd.edu
Management:
   Director: George Moquin

4644 UNIVERSITY OF MARYLAND INTERNATIONAL WILLIAM KAPELL PIANO COMPETITION & FESTIVAL

Clarice Smith Performing Arts Center
University of Maryland
College Park, MD 20742
Phone: 301-405-8174
Fax: 301-405-5977
e-mail: gmoquin@deans.umd.edu
Web Site: www.claricesmithcenter.umd.edu
Management:
   Director: George Moquin
Mission: Sponsoring a major international festival biennially which features recitals, lecture-recitals, master classes and symposia as well as the William Kapell Piano Competition.
Founded: 1971
Specialized Field: Instrumental Music; Festivals
Status: Nonprofit
Income Sources: University of Maryland
Performs At: Tawes Fine Arts Center
Organization Type: Educational; Sponsoring

4645 BALTIMORE-WASHINGTON JAZZFEST

PO Box 1105
Columbia, MD 21044-0105
Phone: 410-730-7106
Fax: 410-715-7105
e-mail: africanartmuseum@erols.com
Web Site: www.baltowashjazzfest.org
Officers:
   Chairman: Claude M Ligon
Specialized Field: Jazz

4646 COLUMBIA FESTIVAL OF THE ARTS

9861 Broken Land Parkway
Suite 300
Columbia, MD 21117
Phone: 410-715-3089
Fax: 401-381-4530
Web Site: www.columbiafestival.com
Officers:
   President: Padraic M Kennedy
   VP: Jean F Moon
   Secretary: Lynne Nemeth
   Treasurer: Richard G. McCauley, Esquire
   Counsel: Harvey B. Steinman, Esquire
Management:
   Managing Director: Lynne Nemeth
   Artistic Director: Septime Webre
   Assistant Managing Director: Alexandria Lippincott
   Executive Director: Katherine Knowles
Mission: To present a variety of art forms and to make these accessible to the public.
Founded: 1988
Specialized Field: Dance; Vocal Music; Instrumental Music; Theater; Festivals
Status: Nonprofit
Volunteer Staff: 350
Paid Artists: 250
Budget: $750,000
Income Sources: Major business sponsors; individual & corporate support
Performs At: Merriweather Post Pavilion

Affiliations: The Baltimore Sun; Columbia Association; Columbia Flier
Organization Type: Presenting

4647 EASTERN SHORE CHAMBER MUSIC FESTIVAL

PO Box 461
Easton, MD 21601
Phone: 410-819-0380
e-mail: dbuxton@skipjack.bluecrab.org
Web Site: www.musicontheshore.org
Management:
   Director: Lawrie Bloom
   Managing Director: Donald C Buxton

4648 FREDERICK COMMUNITY COLLEGE ARTS SERIES

Arts Center
Frederick Community College
Frederick, MD 21702
Phone: 301-846-2513
Fax: 301-846-2498
e-mail: wpoindexter@frederick.edu
Web Site: www.frederick.edu
Management:
   Director: Wendell Poindexter
Founded: 1989
Specialized Field: Visual And Performing Arts
Paid Staff: 12
Performs At: Jack B. Kussmaul Theatre
Seating Capacity: 409

4649 FROSTBURG STATE UNIVERSITY CULTURAL EVENTS SERIES

Lane Center
Frostburg State University
Frostburg, MD 21532
Phone: 301-687-4151
Fax: 301-687-7049
e-mail: wmandicott@frostburg.edu
Officers:
   Chairman: Bill Mandicott
Performs At: Physical Education Center

4650 CITY OF GAITHERSBURG CULTURAL ARTS DIVISION

506 S Frederick Road
Gaithersburg, MD 20877
Phone: 301-258-6350
Fax: 301-948-8364
e-mail: dkayser@ci.gaithersburg.md.us
Management:
   Cultural Arts Director: Denise Kayser
   Arts Barn Director: Marty Willey
Mission: To promote, present, and support rge arts and hummanties.
Founded: 1989
Specialized Field: All areas
Performs At: Various Auditoriums

4651 CAPITAL JAZZ FESTIVAL

1400 Mercantile Lane
Suite 184
Largo, MD 20774
Phone: 301-218-0404
e-mail: mail@capitaljazz.com
Web Site: www.capitaljazz.com

Massachusetts

4652 BRIGHT MOMENTS FESTIVAL

UMass
15 Campus Center
Amherst, MA 01003
Phone: 413-545-2876
Fax: 413-545-0682
e-mail: gsiegel@stuaf.umass.edu
Web Site: www.umass.edu/fac
Management:
   Managing Director: Glenn Siegel

4653 MUSIC AT AMHERST SERIES

Music Department At Amherst College
Amherst, MA 01002-5000
Phone: 413-542-2195
Fax: 413-542-2678
e-mail: concerts@unix.amherst.edu
Web Site: www.amherst.edu/~concerts
Management:
   Concert Manager: Ellen Keel
Performs At: Buckley Recital Hall

4654 ANN ARBOR SUMMER FESTIVAL

400 4th Street #150
Ann Arbor, MA 48103-4816
Phone: 734-763-6780
Fax: 734-936-3393
e-mail: evyw@umich.edu
Web Site: www.mlive.com/aasf/
Management:
   Executive Director: Evy Warshawski

4655 ELECTRIC SYMPHONY FESTIVAL

PO Box 1316
Arlington, MA 02474
Phone: 877-646-1304
Fax: 877-646-1304
e-mail: mail@wildflowerpublishers.com
Web Site: www.electricsymphony.com
Management:
   Director: James Forte
Mission: Exploring the spirit in music since 1988

4656 JACOB'S PILLOW DANCE FESTIVAL: SCHOOL/ARCHIVES/COMMUNITY PROGRAMS

358 George Carter Road
Becket, MA 01223

Mailing Address: PO Box 287, Lee, MA 01238
Phone: 413-637-1322
Fax: 413-243-4744
e-mail: info@jacobspillow.org
Web Site: www.jacobspillow.org
Management:
 Executive Director: Ella Baff
 General Manager: Charlotte Wooldridge
Mission: To support dance creation, presentation, education and preservation; and to engage and deepen public appreciation and support for dance.
Founded: 1933
Specialized Field: Ballet; Jazz; Modern; and Culturally Specific Dance
Status: Professional; Nonprofit
Budget: $3,800,000
Performs At: Doris Duke Studio Theatre; Ted Shawn Theatre
Annual Attendance: 70,000
Organization Type: Performing; Resident; Educational; Sponsoring

4657 BOSTON CONSERVATORY

8 The Fenway
Boston, MA 02215
Phone: 617-536-6340
Fax: 617-536-3176
e-mail: admissions@bostonconservatory.edu
Web Site: www.bostonconservatory.edu
Officers:
 President: Richard Ortner
Founded: 1867
Specialized Field: Music, Dance, And Theater

4658 BOSTON UNIVERSITY EARLY MUSIC SERIES

855 Commonwealth Avenue
Boston, MA 02215
Phone: 617-353-6885
e-mail: mkroll@acs.bu.edu
Management:
 Series Director: Mark Kroll
Seating Capacity: 400

4659 CHARLES RIVER CONCERT SERIES

262 Beacon Street
3rd Floor
Boston, MA 02116
Phone: 617-262-0650
Fax: 617-267-6539
Management:
 Manager: Kathleen Fay
Performs At: Jordan Hall, New England Conservatory of Music

4660 EMMANUEL MUSIC SERIES

15 Newbury Street
Boston, MA 02116
Phone: 617-536-3356
Fax: 617-536-3315
e-mail: emmanmsc@aol.com
Web Site: www.emmanuelmusic.org
Management:

Executive Director: Leonard Matczynski
Artistic Director: Craig Smith
Seating Capacity: 1000

4661 FIRST NIGHT BOSTON

20 Park Plaza
Suite 1000
Boston, MA 02116
Phone: 617-542-1399
Fax: 617-426-9531
e-mail: info@firstnight.org
Web Site: www.firstnight.org
Officers:
 Co-Chairman: Eric Schwarz
 Co-Chairman: Edwin P Tiffany
 Clerk: Royal Dunham Jr
 Treasurer: Charles A Ansbacher
Management:
 Executive Director: Geri Guardino
 Marketing Director: Amy Havwood
 Production Director: Gina Mullen
 Marketing Assistant: Barbara Wojslawowicz
Mission: To use a street fair venue to broaden and deepen the public's appreciation for the visual and performing arts.
Founded: 1976
Specialized Field: Dance; Vocal Music; Theater
Status: Nonprofit
Paid Staff: 12
Volunteer Staff: 400
Paid Artists: 1000
Budget: $1,600,000
Annual Attendance: 2,000,000
Organization Type: Art Presenter

4662 FLEETBOSTON CELEBRITY SERIES

20 Park Plaza
Suite 1032
Boston, MA 02116-4303
Phone: 617-482-2595
Fax: 617-482-3208
e-mail: info@celebrityseries.org
Web Site: www.celebrityseries.org
Officers:
 President: Martha Jones
 Chairman: Harris A Berman
 Treasurer: Norman C Nicholson, Jr
 Clerk: Joseph D Steinfield
Management:
 President/Executive Director: Martha Jones
 CFO: Michael Botte
 VP Development/Board Relations: Alice Bruce
 VP Programming/Operations: Amy W Lam
 Director Marketing: David A Dalena
 Director Education: Suzanne Wilson
Mission: To bring Boston the world's greatest performing artists.
Founded: 1933
Specialized Field: Dance; Vocal Music; Instrumental Music; Theater
Status: Nonprofit
Paid Staff: 22
Budget: 6.3 Million
Income Sources: Ticket Sales; Sponsorship; Fundraising
Season: October - January

Performs At: Symphony Hall; Wang Center; Jordan Hall; Shubert Theatre
Affiliations: Association of Performing Arts Presenters; International Society of Performing Arts Dance USA
Annual Attendance: 100,000+
Organization Type: Presenting

4663 HARVARD MUSICAL ASSOCIATION IN BOSTON

57A Chesnut Street
Boston, MA 02108
Phone: 617-523-2897
Seating Capacity: 100

4664 KING'S CHAPEL CONCERT SERIES

58 Tremont Street
Boston, MA 02108
Phone: 617-227-2155
Management:
   Music Director: Daniel Pinkham
Mission: To offer chamber music, particularly Baroque and contemporary works.
Founded: 1958
Specialized Field: Vocal Music; Instrumental Music
Status: Professional
Performs At: King's Chapel
Organization Type: Performing

4665 MUSEUM OF FINE ARTS CONCERTS & PERFORMANCES

465 Huntington Avenue
Boston, MA 02115
Phone: 617-369-3291
Fax: 617-267-9328
Web Site: www.mfa.org
Management:
   Concert Co-ordinator: Laurie Thomas
Performs At: Remis Auditorium

4666 BRIDGEWATER STATE COLLEGE PROGRAM COMMITTEE

Bridgewater State College
109 Campus Center
Bridgewater, MA 02325
Phone: 508-531-1273
Fax: 508-531-1786
e-mail: mthorp@bridgew.edu
Management:
   Assistant Director: Mike Throp

4667 MASSASOIT COMMUNITY COLLEGE BUCKLEY ARTS CENTER PERFORMANCE SERIES

1 Massasoit Boulevard
Brockton, MA 02302
Phone: 508-427-1234
Fax: 508-427-1267
Management:
   Director: Michael Pevzner
Founded: 1983
Paid Staff: 3

4668 BOSTON EARLY MUSIC FESTIVAL AND EXHIBITION

PO Box 2632
Cambridge, MA 02238-2632
Phone: 617-661-1812
Fax: 617-267-6539
e-mail: bemf@bemf.org
Web Site: www.bemf.org
Officers:
   President: ES Whitney Thompson
   VP: Richard Hester
   Treasurer: Howard V Wagner
   Clerk: Richard Portars
Management:
   Executive Director: Kathleen Fay
   Director: Andrew Manze
Mission: To discover and reproduce how early music originally sounded to a composer and his audience; to produce a biennial international festival in Boston; to educate youth.
Founded: 1980
Specialized Field: Dance; Vocal Music; Instrumental Music; Festivals; Lyric Opera; Grand Opera; Early Music Festival
Status: Nonprofit
Seating Capacity: 557
Organization Type: Performing; Touring; Educational; Sponsoring

4669 BOSTON GLOBE JAZZ & BLUES FESTIVAL

36 Bay State Road
Cambridge, MA 02138
Web Site: www.boston.com/jazzfest
Management:
   Booker/Talent Buyer: Jodi Goodman

4670 MIT GUEST ARTISTS SERIES

77 Massachusetts Avenue
14N-207
Cambridge, MA 02139
Phone: 617-253-2906
Fax: 617-253-4523
e-mail: csnyder@mit.edu
Web Site: www.mit.edu/mta/www/
Management:
   Director: Clarise Snyder
Performs At: Kresge Auditorium

4671 REGATTABAR JAZZ FESTIVAL AT THE CHARLES HOTEL

Charles Hotel
1 Bennett Street
Cambridge, MA 02138-5780
Phone: 617-876-7777
Fax: 617-864-5715
e-mail: JeffKeyes@CharlesHotel.com
Web Site: www.concertix.com
Management:
   Lounge Manager: Jeffrey Keyes

4672 WORLD MUSIC FESTIVAL
720 Massachusetts Avenue
Cambridge, MA 02139
Phone: 617-876-4275
Fax: 617-876-9170
e-mail: worldmus@star.net
Web Site: www.worldmusic.org.html
Management:
   Executive Director: Maure Aronson
   Associate Director: Susan Weiler
Performs At: Auditoriums

4673 FRIENDS OF THE PERFORMING ARTS
51 Walden Street
PO Box 251
Concord, MA 01742
Phone: 978-369-7911
e-mail: fopac@tiac.net
Web Site: www.tiac.net/users/fopac
Management:
   Manager: Kathleen Chick
Performs At: Auditorium

4674 ASTON MAGNA FESTIVAL
323 Main Street
PO Box 28
Great Barrington, MA 01230
Phone: 732-572-5119
Fax: 732-572-5119
Toll-free: 800-875-7156
e-mail: info@astonmagna.org
Web Site: www.astonmagna.org
Management:
   Executive Director: Ronnie Boriskin
   Festival Director: Joseph Orchard
Founded: 1972
Specialized Field: Classical Music, Primarily Baroque, on Period Instruments

4675 CLOSE ENCOUNTERS WITH MUSIC SERIES
PO Box 34
Great Barrington, MA 01230
Phone: 413-392-6677
Fax: 413-392-9782
Management:
   Artistic Director: Yehunda Hanani
Performs At: St. James Church, Great Barrington

4676 HUDSON COMMUNITY ARTS SERIES
155 Apsley Street
Hudson, MA 01749-1697
Phone: 978-562-1646
Management:
   Executive Director: Jan Patterson
Performs At: Hudson High School Auditorium

4677 CASTLE HILL SERIES
Castle Hill
290 Argilla Road
Ipswich, MA 01938
Phone: 978-356-4351
Fax: 978-356-2143

Management:
   Events Manager: Jennifer Kyte
Mission: To offer a range of performing arts events at the historic R.T. Crane Estate.
Founded: 1951
Specialized Field: Vocal Music; Instrumental Music; limited small scale performances with local artists
Status: Professional; Nonprofit
Performs At: Crane Memorial Reservation
Organization Type: Performing; Educational; Sponsoring

4678 TANGLEWOOD FESTIVAL
West Street
Lenox, MA 01240
Phone: 413-637-1565
Fax: 413-637-4623
Toll-free: 800-266-1200
Web Site: www.tanglewood.org
Management:
   Managing Director: Mark Volpe
Mission: To provide a summer home to the Boston Symphony Orchestra; to offer two stages for diverse pops and classical concerts; to maintain a world class music school in the summer.
Specialized Field: Vocal Music; Instrumental Music; Festivals; Orchestral
Status: Professional; Nonprofit
Income Sources: Ticket sales, contributions
Season: Summer
Performs At: Tanglewood
Organization Type: Performing; Educational
Comments: Information at Tanglewood for the disabled is available at the Access Services Center at the Main Gate. The Service Center has alternate format materials, medical equipment, and trained staff available to assist patrons on an as-needed b

4679 CAPE & ISLANDS CHAMBER MUSIC FESTIVAL
216 C Orleans Road
North Chatham, MA 02650
Phone: 508-945-8060
Fax: 508-945-8059
Toll-free: 800-229-5739
e-mail: cicmf@c4.net
Web Site: www.capecodchambermusic.org
Management:
   Executive Director: Pamela Patrick
   Director Development: Lynne Pleffner
Mission: To present the finest classical and contemporary chamber music by both world-class ensembles and exceptional young emerging artists to Cape Cod audiences; to develop new and younger audiences for chamber music.
Founded: 1979
Specialized Field: Chamber Music
Paid Staff: 2
Volunteer Staff: 30

4680 CAPE COD CHAMBER MUSIC FESTIVAL
216C Orleans Road
Nickerson Corners
North Chatham, MA 02650
Phone: 508-945-8060
Fax: 508-945-8059
Toll-free: 800-229-5739
e-mail: contact@capecodchambermusic.org
Web Site: www.capecodchambermusic.org
Officers:
   President: Lawrence M Handley
   Treasurer: Laura S Emmons
   Secretary: George Dillion
Management:
   Artistic Director: Nicholas Kitchen
   Executive Directoror: Pamela Patrick
   Director Development: Lynne Pleffner
Mission: To present the finest classical and contemporary chamber music by both world-class ensembles and exceptional young emerging artists to Cape Cod audiences; to develop new and younger audiences for chamber music; to commission new chamber works whenever possible; and to provide educational activities and programs which encourage, broaden and deepen appreciation of the chamber music art form.
Founded: 1979
Specialized Field: Festivals
Status: Professional; Nonprofit
Paid Staff: 3
Paid Artists: 30
Facility Category: Usually churches
Seating Capacity: 250 - 300
Organization Type: Performing; Educational

4681 MASSACHUSETTS INTERNATIONAL FESTIVAL OF THE ARTS
274 Main Street
Northampton, MA 01060
Phone: 413-584-4425
Fax: 413-586-5368
Toll-free: 800-224-6432
e-mail: mifafestival@rcn.com
Web Site: www.mifafestival.org
Management:
   Artistic/Executive Director: Donald T Sanders
   Managing Director: Marta Ostapink
   Administrative Assistant: Melissa Hays
Mission: To present the finest contemporary practice in opera, theatre, dance, music, film and the visual arts in three counties of the Pioneer Valley of Western Massachusetts.
Founded: 1993
Specialized Field: Multidisciplinary / International Arts Festival
Paid Staff: 4
Volunteer Staff: 5
Paid Artists: 150

4682 SOUTH MOUNTAIN CONCERT SERIES
PO Box 23
Pittsfield, MA 01202
Phone: 413-442-2106
Management:

Director: Lou R Steigler
Specialized Field: Chamber Music

4683 ROCKPORT CHAMBER MUSIC FESTIVAL
PO Box 312
Rockport, MA 01966
Phone: 978-546-7138
e-mail: rcmf@shore.net
Web Site: www.rcmf.org
Officers:
   President: Phillip D Cutter MD
   VP: Dianne Anderson
   VP: Barbara Sparks
   Treasurer: William Hausman
   Clerk/Secretary: Mollie Byrnes
Management:
   Artistic Director: David Deveau
Mission: The presentation of a 16-concert series in June, featuring chamber ensembles performing alone and in collaboration.
Specialized Field: Chamber
Status: Professional; Nonprofit
Performs At: Rockport Art Association
Organization Type: Presenting

4684 BERKSHIRE CHORAL FESTIVAL
245 N Undermountain Road
Sheffield, MA 01257
Phone: 413-229-8586
Fax: 413-229-0109
e-mail: bcf@choralfest.org
Web Site: www.choralfest.org
Management:
   Executive Director: Trudy Weaver Miller

4685 MOHAWK TRAIL CONCERTS/MUSIC IN DEERFIELD
PO Box 75
Shelburne, MA 01370
Phone: 413-625-9511
Fax: 413-625-0221
e-mail: info@mohawktrailconcerts.org
Web Site: www.mohawktrailconcerts.org/tickets.html
Management:
   Executive Director: Anna Bartoli
   Artistic Director-Mohawk Trail: Ruth Black
   Artistic Director-Deerfield: John Montanari
Mission: To offer professional chamber music in the fall and summer; to provide educational music programs.
Founded: 1969
Specialized Field: Vocal Music; Instrumental Music; Festivals
Status: Professional; Nonprofit
Paid Staff: 3
Budget: $200,000
Performs At: Federated Church
Annual Attendance: 5,500
Seating Capacity: 225-500
Organization Type: Performing; Touring; Resident; Educational; Sponsoring

4686 MUSICORDA SUMMER FESTIVAL
PO Box 557
South Hadley, MA 01075
Phone: 413-538-2590
Fax: 413-538-3021
e-mail: musicorda@aol.com
Web Site: www.musicorda.org
Management:
    Artistic Director: Leopold Teraspulsky

4687 AMERICAN INTERNATIONAL COLLEGE SERIES
Sprague/Griswold Cultural Arts Center
1000 State Street
Springfield, MA 01109
Phone: 413-747-6393
Fax: 413-737-2803
Management:
    Visual/Performing Arts Director: Alvin Paige
Performs At: Auditorium

4688 SPRINGFIELD PERFORMING ARTS DEVELOPMENT CORPORATION
1 Columbus Center
Springfield, MA 01103
Phone: 413-788-7646
Fax: 413-737-9991
e-mail: tdagostino@citystage.symphonyhall.com
Web Site: www.citystage.symphonyhall.com
Management:
    General Manager: Cynthia Anzalotti
    Marketing Director: Tina D'Agostino
    Technical Director: Chad LaBombard
    Box Office Manager: Tara Garvey
Mission: Professional presenting theatres.
Founded: 1998
Paid Staff: 8
Volunteer Staff: 50

4689 BERKSHIRE THEATRE FESTIVAL
PO Box 797
Stockbridge, MA 01262
Phone: 413-298-5536
Fax: 413-298-3368
e-mail: info@berkshiretheatre.org
Web Site: www.berkshiretheatre.org
Management:
    Producing Director: Kate Maguire
    Artistic Associate: John Rando
Mission: To offer thought-provoking entertainment each summer.
Founded: 1928
Specialized Field: Theater; Festivals
Status: Professional; Nonprofit
Paid Staff: 12
Income Sources: Actors' Equity Association; Council of Resident Summer Theatres
Season: June - September
Performs At: Playhouse, Unicorn Theatre
Type of Stage: Proscenium, Thrust
Seating Capacity: 415, 122
Organization Type: Performing; Resident; Educational; Sponsoring

4690 BENTLEY COLLEGE BOWLES PREFORMANCE SERIES
LCC 225, 175 Forest Street
Waltham, MA 02154
Phone: 781-891-3424
Fax: 781-891-2839
e-mail: jmorris@bentley.edu
Management:
    Performing Arts Coordinato: Jim Morris
Performs At: Lindsay Auditorium

4691 BRANDEIS SYMPHONY ORCHESTRA
Slosberg Musical Building MS 051
Waltham, MA 02454
Phone: 781-736-3328
Fax: 781-736-3320
e-mail: brocksym@email.msn.com
Web Site: www.brandeis.edu/departments/music
Management:
    Music Director: Neal Hampton

4692 BRANDEIS UNIVERSITY SPINGOLD THEATER CENTER SERIES
PO Box 9100 MS072
Spingold Theater Center, Brandeis University
Waltham, MA 02454-9110
Phone: 781-736-3400
Fax: 781-736-3389
Management:
    General Manager: John-Edward Hill
Seating Capacity: 744

4693 LYDIAN STRING QUARTET CHAMBER MUSIC FESTIVAL
PO Box 549110, MS085
Brandies University, Summer School Office
Waltham, MA 02454-9110
Phone: 781-736-3424
Fax: 781-736-8124
e-mail: summerschool@brandeis.edu
Web Site: www.brandeis.edu/sumsch
Officers:
    Administrative Assistant: Heidi Foster
Management:
    Director: Rhonda Rider
    Director Summer Program: Gwenn Smaxwill
Mission: To provide chamber music performances, master classes, guest lecturers for serious amateurs, preprofessionals, and professional musicians.
Founded: 1989
Specialized Field: Instrumental Music
Status: Professional; Non-Professional
Performs At: Slosberg Hall; Brandeis University
Annual Attendance: 30
Facility Category: Slosberg Recital Hall
Organization Type: Performing; Resident; Educational
Resident Groups: Lydian String Quartet

4694 WALTHAM COMMUNITY CONCERT SERIES
124 Felton Street
Suite 2
Waltham, MA 02453-4119
Phone: 781-891-3740
Fax: 781-891-3740
e-mail: sbkilgore@mediaone.net
Management:
    Director: Stephen Kilgore
Performs At: Waltham Public Library

4695 ALL NEWTON MUSIC SCHOOL, THE ANDREW WOLF CONCERT SERIES
321 Chesnut Street
West Newton, MA 02465
Phone: 617-527-4553
Fax: 617-527-7710
e-mail: anms@mediaone.net
Management:
    Director: Paulette Bowes
Founded: 1911
Paid Staff: 5
Volunteer Staff: 49
Non-paid Artists: 20
Budget: $1,000,000
Income Sources: Tuition; Grants; Donations
Performs At: Auditorium
Annual Attendance: 3,000
Facility Category: Mansion
Type of Stage: Salon in the Round
Seating Capacity: 200
Year Built: 1900

4696 WESTFIELD STATE COLLEGE MUSIC & MORE PERFORMING ARTS SERIES
Western Avenue
Westfield, MA 01086
Phone: 413-572-5438

4697 CONCERTS-AT-THE-COMMON
Harvard Unitarian Chruch
Bernard J Fine
32 Coburn Road
Weston, MA 02193
Phone: 978-456-8752
Officers:
    Concert Series Director: Bernard J Fine
Mission: To present community concerts.
Founded: 1979
Specialized Field: Vocal Music; Instrumental Music
Status: Nonprofit
Organization Type: Sponsoring

4698 WILLIAMS COLLEGE SERIES
Bernhard Music Center
54 Chapin Hill Drive
Williamstown, MA 01267
Phone: 413-597-2736
Fax: 413-597-3100
e-mail: ernest.m.clark@williams.edu
Web Site: www.williams.edu/Music/

Officers:
    Music Department Chairman: David Kechley
Management:
    Concert Manager: Ernest Clark

4699 WILLIAMSTOWN THEATRE FESTIVAL
PO Box 517
Williamstown, MA 01267
Phone: 413-458-3200
Fax: 413-458-3147
Web Site: wtfestival.org
Officers:
    President: Dr. Ira Lapidus
    VP: William S Reed
    Secretary: Fred A Windover
    Treasurer: Jid Sprague
Management:
    Producer: Michael Ritchie
    General Manager: Deborah Fehr
    Associate Producer: Jenny Gersten
Mission: To present outstanding productions of modern classics on our main stage; to develop new acting, writing and musical talent.
Founded: 1955
Specialized Field: Theatrical Group
Status: Professional; Nonprofit
Paid Staff: 75
Volunteer Staff: 150
Paid Artists: 100
Non-paid Artists: 40
Budget: $2,500,000
Season: June - August
Performs At: Adams Memorial Theater; Nikos Stage
Annual Attendance: 50,000
Seating Capacity: 520
Organization Type: Performing

4700 WORCESTER MUSIC FESTIVAL
323 Main Street
Worcester, MA 01608
Phone: 508-754-3231
Fax: 508-754-8698
e-mail: music@musicworcester.org
Web Site: www.musicworcester.org
Management:
    Executive Director: Stasia B Hovenesian
    Marketing Assistant: Avril K Waye
    Marketing Coordinator: Cynthia Wood
Mission: To present performances of the highest quality through Worcester Music Festival, International Artist Series, Mass Jazz Festival and Music for Children; to educate all ages about music composers, history, etc.
Founded: 1858
Specialized Field: Classical Orchestras; Soloist; Chamber Ensembles; Jazz Groups; Dance Ensembles
Status: Nonprofit; Cultural Organization
Paid Staff: 5
Performs At: Mechanics Hall; Tuckerman Hall
Annual Attendance: 26,000
Facility Category: Concert Halls
Seating Capacity: 1,550 & 550 (2 stages)

Michigan

4701 ADRIAN COLLEGE EVENTS SERIES
Pellowe Hall
110 S Madison Street
Adrian, MI 49221
Phone: 517-264-3156
Fax: 517-264-3156
e-mail: awilson@adrian.edu
Management:
  Conference/Campus Programs Director: Jim Campbell
Performs At: Dawson Auditorium

4702 ALBION PERFORMING ARTIST & LECTURE SERIES
Albion College
4680 Kellogg Center
Albion, MI 49224
Phone: 517-629-0433
Fax: 517-629-0509
Web Site: www.albion.edu
Performs At: Goodrich Chapel

4703 GRAND VALLEY STATE UNIVERSITY ARTS AT NOON SERIES
Grand Valley State University
Allendale, MI 49401
Phone: 616-895-3484
Fax: 616-895-3100
e-mail: vandenwj@gvsu.edu
Management:
  Arts At Noon Coordinator: Julianne Vanden Wyngaard
Performs At: Louis Armstrong Theatre

4704 ALMA COLLEGE PERFORMING ARTS SERIES
Heritage Center
614 W Superior
Alma, MI 48801
Phone: 517-463-7256
Fax: 517-463-7277
e-mail: jamartin@alma.edu
Web Site: www.alma.edu
Management:
  Building Coordinator: Judy Deegan
Performs At: Heritage Center for the Performing Arts

4705 THUNDER BAY ARTS COUNCIL
313 1/2 N 2nd Avenue
Alpena, MI 49707-2805
Phone: 517-356-6678
e-mail: hoarts@freeway.net
Officers:
  President: Duane Beyer
Mission: The promotion of cultural arts through the coordination of events and the sponsoring of various performances.
Founded: 1971
Specialized Field: Dance; Vocal Music; Instrumental Music; Theater; Lyric Opera
Status: Professional; Nonprofit

Organization Type: Educational; Sponsoring

4706 ANN ARBOR BLUES & JAZZ FESTIVAL
PO Box 7456
Ann Arbor, MI 48107
Phone: 734-747-9955
e-mail: info@jazzfest.org
Web Site: www.a2.blues.jazzfest.org

4707 ANN ARBOR SUMMER FESTIVAL
400 4th Street
Room 150
Ann Arbor, MI 48103
Phone: 734-647-2278
Fax: 734-936-3393
e-mail: Evyw@umich.edu
Web Site: www.mlive.com/AASF
Officers:
  Business Manager: Jeanne Rowlette
  Marketing Director: Colleen Murdock
  President: John C Clark
  Chairman: Anne K. Rubin
Management:
  Festival Director: Evy Warshawski
  Production Manager: Henry Reynolds
Mission: To offer both ticketed and free of charge performing arts events to Ann Arbor area residents.
Founded: 1978
Specialized Field: Dance; Theater; Festivals
Status: Professional; Nonprofit
Paid Staff: 5
Volunteer Staff: 100
Paid Artists: 75
Budget: $1,000,000
Income Sources: Donations from Businesses & Individuals; Grants
Performs At: Power Center; Lydia Mendelssohn; Top of the Park
Affiliations: University of Michigan; City of Ann Arbor
Annual Attendance: 50,000
Type of Stage: Thrust, Proscenium
Stage Dimensions: 40x60
Seating Capacity: 1,300
Organization Type: Performing; Sponsoring

4708 MICHIGAN ASSOCIATION OF COMMUNITY ARTS AGENCIES
107 Miller Avenue
Ann Arbor, MI 48104
Phone: 734-996-2500
Fax: 734-996-3317
Toll-free: 800-203-9633
e-mail: demikula@macaa.com
Web Site: www.macaa.com
Officers:
  President: Oliver Ragsdale, Jr
Management:
  Executive Director: Deborah E Mikula
Mission: Exists to support, strengthen, and unite community arts and organizations in Michigan.
Founded: 1977
Specialized Field: Arts Service Organization
Paid Staff: 7

4709 MUSICAL SOCIETY OF THE UNIVERSITY SERIES
Burton Memorial Tower
881 N University
Ann Arbor, MI 48109-1011
Phone: 734-764-2538
Fax: 734-647-1171
Toll-free: 800-221-1239
e-mail: umstix@umich.edu
Web Site: www.ums.org
Officers:
Chairperson: Beverley Geltner
Vice Chair: Lester Monts
Secretary: Pruuueu Rosentnal
Treasurer: David Featherman
President: Kenneth C. Fischer
Management:
Director Programming: Michael Kondziolka
Director Administation: John Kennard
Director Development: Christina Thoburn
Director Marketing/Promotion: Sara Billmann
Director Education: Ben Johnson
Mission: To provide professional theatre, dance and music for Southeastern Michigan students and residents.
Founded: 1879
Specialized Field: Dance; Vocal Music; Instrumental Music; Theater; Festivals; Grand Opera
Status: Professional; Nonprofit
Paid Staff: 30
Budget: $6,000,000
Income Sources: Ticket Sales; Fundraising
Performs At: Hill Auditorium; Power Center; Rackham Auditorium
Annual Attendance: 150,000
Organization Type: Performing; Educational

4710 BAY ARTS COUNCIL
901 N Water Street
Bay City, MI 48708
Phone: 989-893-0343
Fax: 989-893-6443
Management:
Executive Director: Tom Niemann
Administrative Assistant: Carolyn White
Paid Staff: 2
Volunteer Staff: 50
Paid Artists: 25
Non-paid Artists: 10

4711 BAY VIEW MUSIC FESTIVAL
Box 1596
Bay View, MI 49770
Phone: 231-347-4210
Web Site: www.bayviewassoc.net
Management:
Director: Gary Glaze

4712 FERRIS STATE UNIVERSITY-ARTS & LECTURES SERIES
1201 S State
CSS 208A
Big Rapids, MI 49307
Phone: 231-591-3626
Fax: 231-591-3067
e-mail: hadley-p@ferris.edu
Officers:
Chairman: Daniel Cronk
Chairman: J Randall Groves
Management:
Auditorium Manager: Michael Terry
Paid Staff: 2
Budget: $40,000
Income Sources: Ticket Sales; Donations; Grants
Performs At: Williams Auditorium
Affiliations: Michigan Nonprofit Presenters Network
Type of Stage: Proscenium
Seating Capacity: 1,800

4713 AMERICAN ARTISTS SERIES
435 Goodhue Road
Bloomfield Hills, MI 48304
Phone: 313-547-2230
Fax: 313-547-1525
Management:
Artistic Director: Joann Freeman
Executive Director: Leonard Mazern
Business Manager: Morton Malitz
Mission: Sponsoring diverse performing arts programs, which include guest artists and native musicians.
Founded: 1970
Specialized Field: Instrumental Music; Theater; Chamber Music
Status: Professional; Nonprofit
Performs At: Kingswood Auditorium
Organization Type: Performing; Touring; Sponsoring

4714 CRANBROOK MUSIC GUILD CONCERT SERIES
PO Box 402
Bloomfield Hills, MI 48303
Phone: 248-645-0097
Officers:
Program Chairman: Anita Demarco Goor
President: William R Brashear
Performs At: Cranbrook House Library

4715 GOPHERWOOD CONCERT SERIES
119 Marble
Cadillac, MI 49601
Phone: 231-775-7084
e-mail: pbrown@michweb.net
Web Site: www.users.michweb.net/~pbrown/gopherwood.htm
Performs At: Auditorium

4716 VILLAGE BACH FESTIVAL
PO Box 27
Cass City, MI 48726
Phone: 517-872-3465
Fax: 517-872-2301
Mission: Promoting professional musical events in Michigan's Thumb Area.
Founded: 1979
Specialized Field: Vocal Music; Instrumental Music; Festivals

Status: Professional; Nonprofit
Organization Type: Performing

4717 CHEBOYGAN AREA ARTS COUNCIL CONCERT SERIES

PO Box 95
403 N Huron Street
Cheboygan, MI 49721
Phone: 231-627-5432
Fax: 231-627-2643
e-mail: jpl@nmo.net
Web Site: www.theoperahouse.org
Officers:
    President: Jeff Swadling
    VP: Ron Berg
    Treasurer: Alice Barron
    Secretary: Gussie Williams
Management:
    Executive Director: Joann Leal
    Education Coordinator/Secretary: Glad Remaly
    Technician: Jerry Bronson
    Box Office Manager: Millie Podgorski
Mission: To promote and encourage cultural and educational activites within the Straits Area and Northern Michigan; to provide services that stimulate and encourage participation and appreciation of the arts within all segments of the community.
Founded: 1972
Specialized Field: Multidisciplinary
Paid Staff: 4
Volunteer Staff: 150

4718 CASA DE UNIDAS SERIES

1920 Scotten
Detroit, MI 48209
Phone: 313-843-9598
Fax: 313-843-7307
Management:
    Program Coordinator: Marta Lagos
Mission: Providing community-based, performing arts presentations for Detroit's Hispanic communities.
Founded: 1981
Specialized Field: Dance; Vocal Music; Instrumental Music; Theater
Status: Nonprofit
Paid Staff: 10
Performs At: Clark Park Theatre
Organization Type: Performing; Touring; Educational; Sponsoring

4719 DETROIT FESTIVAL OF THE ARTS

4735 Cass Avenue
Detroit, MI 48202
Phone: 313-577-5088
Fax: 313-577-3332
e-mail: Maureen.Riley@wayne.edu
Web Site: www.detroitfestival.com
Officers:
    President: Susan Mosey
Management:
    Performing Arts Director: Njia Kai
Mission: To encourage use of the University Cultural Center of Detroit, and introduce the resources of the area to the metropoliton community.

Founded: 1915
Specialized Field: International, Arts & Music, outdoor festival
Paid Staff: 7
Volunteer Staff: 400
Paid Artists: 60
Non-paid Artists: 150
Budget: 1,300,000
Income Sources: Corporate; Private; State
Performs At: Outdoors; 20 Blocks
Affiliations: Wayne State University and University Cultural Center Association
Annual Attendance: 300,000
Facility Category: Various Outdoor Venues
Type of Stage: 3 Main, 1 Childrens, 2 Coffeehouses

4720 FORD DETROIT INTERNATIONAL JAZZ FESTIVAL

350 Madison Avenue
Detroit, MI 48226
Phone: 313-963-7622
Fax: 313-963-2462
Web Site: www.detroitjazzfest.com
Management:
    Director Operations: Eric R Dueweke
    Artistic Director: Frank Malfitano
    Director Media Relations: Michael Vigilant
Mission: Preserving, promoting and maintaining the understanding and appreciation of jazz music.
Founded: 1980
Specialized Field: Vocal Music; Instrumental Music; Festivals
Status: Nonprofit
Annual Attendance: 770,000
Facility Category: Outdoor Festival
Organization Type: Performing; Sponsoring

4721 SYRACUSE JAZZ FESTIVAL

655 Brush Street
#2815
Detroit, MI 48226
Phone: 313-961-2166
Fax: 313-961-2177
e-mail: info@syracusejazzfest.com
Web Site: www.syracusejazzfest.com

4722 UNITED BLACK ARTISTS: USA SERIES

7661 LaSalle Boulevard
Detroit, MI 48206
Phone: 313-898-5574
Fax: 313-895-8942
Management:
    Management Staff: Dr. Daphne W Ntiri
Mission: Encouraging cultural opportunities and education among Detroit's black communities.
Founded: 1987
Specialized Field: Instrumental Music; Theater
Status: Nonprofit
Paid Staff: 20
Income Sources: Harmony Park Playhouse
Organization Type: Educational; Sponsoring

4723 FLINT INSTITUTE OF MUSIC

1025 E Kearsley Street
Flint, MI 48503
Phone: 810-238-1350
Fax: 810-238-6385
Toll-free: 800-395-4849
e-mail: fim@thefim.com
Web Site: www.thefim.com
Officers:
   President: Paul Torre
Management:
   Marketing Director: Christina Ferris
   Director Flint School Performing: Davin Pierson Torre
   Manager Flint Symphony: Tom Glasscok
   Music Director: Enrique Diemecke
   Director Ticket: Linda Tomlinson
   Director Development: Carol Hartley
Mission: Providing a lifelong continuum of music and dance.
Founded: 1917
Status: Nonprofit
Performs At: Whiting Auditorium
Annual Attendance: 3,500

4724 MUSIC IN THE PARKS

Flint Symphony Orchestra
1025 E Kearsley Street
Flint, MI 48509
Phone: 810-238-1350
Fax: 810-238-6385
e-mail: fim@flint.org
Management:
   Manager: Tom Glasscock

4725 GAYLORD AREA COUNCIL FOR THE ARTS

PO Box 249
Gaylord, MI 49734
Phone: 517-732-3242
e-mail: nordeen@avci.net
Management:
   Manager: Kate Nordeen
Performs At: Auditorium

4726 FESTIVAL OF THE ARTS

300 Waters Building
161 Ottawa NW #300
Grand Rapids, MI 49503
Phone: 616-459-2787
Fax: 616-459-7160
Management:
   Executive Director: Tammy Ramaker
Mission: To support the arts and artists of the Greater Grand Rapids Community; to promote and support the arts financially and through technical assistance to organizations or individuals; to promote experiences for participants and observers from within the general public.
Founded: 1970
Specialized Field: Dance; Vocal Music; Instrumental Music; Theater; Festivals
Status: Professional; Nonprofit
Paid Staff: 3000
Budget: $300,000

Performs At: Calder Plaza
Annual Attendance: 300,000
Organization Type: Sponsoring
Resident Groups: Regional artists only

4727 REIF ARTS COUNCIL

720 Conifer Drive
Grand Rapids, MI 55744
Phone: 218-327-5780
Fax: 218-327-5798
e-mail: dmarty@reifcenter.org
Web Site: www.reifcenter.org
Management:
   Executive Director: David Marty
Mission: Stimulating arts in Northern Minnesota.
Founded: 1981
Specialized Field: Multi-Disciplinary
Paid Staff: 15
Paid Artists: 100
Budget: $620,000
Income Sources: Sales; Grants; Tuition
Annual Attendance: 18,000
Type of Stage: Proscenium; Modified Thrust
Seating Capacity: 642
Rental Contact: John Miller

4728 GROSSE POINTE WAR MEMORIAL

32 Lake Shore Drive
Grosse Pointe Farms, MI 48236
Phone: 313-881-7511
Fax: 313-884-6638
e-mail: laflanangan-wattrick@warmemorial.org
Web Site: www.warmemorial.org
Management:
   Director Lifelong Learning: Lou Anne Wattrick
Mission: To offer outdoor performances in the summer via Summer Music Festival and other events during the year.
Founded: 1957
Specialized Field: Vocal Music; Instrumental Music; Theater; Festivals; Lyric Opera
Status: Professional; Nonprofit
Performs At: Terrace of Alger House
Organization Type: Performing; Touring; Resident

4729 PINE MOUNTAIN MUSIC FESTIVAL

PO Box 406
Hancock, MI 49930
Phone: 906-482-1542
Fax: 906-487-3511
Toll-free: 888-309-7861
e-mail: Festival@pmmf.org
Web Site: www.pmmf.org
Officers:
   President: Virginia Feleppe
   VP: Alice Boyce
   Secretary: Darlene Strand
   Treasurer: Howard Zollinger
Management:
   Executive Director: Kathy Tompkins
   Artistic Director: Christopher Mattaliano
   Operations Manager: Nathan Barber
   Marketing Manager: Jane LeBouef

Mission: Serve upper Midwest with opera, symphony, and chamber music during June and July.
Founded: 1991
Specialized Field: Classical Music
Paid Staff: 6
Volunteer Staff: 200
Paid Artists: 150
Non-paid Artists: 20
Budget: 500,000
Income Sources: Grants; Box Office; Gifts
Performs At: Rented Theaters
Affiliations: Opera America
Annual Attendance: 8,000
Facility Category: Various

4730 HOLLAND AREA ARTS COUNCIL

150 E 8th Street
Holland, MI 49423
Phone: 616-396-3278
Fax: 616-396-6298
Management:
  Executive Director: Brenda S Nienhouse

4731 HOPE COLLEGE GREAT PERFORMANCE SERIES

Hope College
PO Box 9000
Holland, MI 49422-9000
Phone: 616-395-7893
Fax: 616-395-7191
e-mail: emerson@hope.edu
Web Site: www.hope.edu/arts
Management:
  Arts Coordinator: Derek Emerson
Paid Artists: 6
Performs At: DeWitt Center
Annual Attendance: 4000
Facility Category: 3 different venues

4732 MICHIGAN RENAISSANCE FESTIVAL

12600 Dixie Highway
Holly, MI 48442
Phone: 248-634-5552
Fax: 248-634-7590
Toll-free: 800-601-4848
e-mail: renfestmi@aol.com
Web Site: www.michaenfest.com
Management:
  General Manager: Christine Daye
  Site Operations/Special Events: Kathy Parker
Mission: Promoting Renaissance traditions in the area of Southeastern Michigan.
Founded: 1980
Specialized Field: Dance; Vocal Music; Instrumental Music; Theater; Festivals
Status: Professional; Commercial
Paid Staff: 30
Volunteer Staff: 200
Paid Artists: 100
Non-paid Artists: 100
Performs At: Hollygrove; Holly
Organization Type: Performing

4733 MTU/GREAT EVENTS SERIES

1400 Townsend Drive
Center Room 106
Houghton, MI 49931
Phone: 906-487-2844
Fax: 906-487-3552
e-mail: vepegg@mtu.edu
Web Site: www.greatevents.mtu.edu
Management:
  Director Great Events: Valerie Pegg
Specialized Field: Performing; Educational
Paid Staff: 7
Volunteer Staff: 60
Budget: $130,000
Income Sources: Box Office; Grants; Private Donations
Performs At: Performing Arts Theatre; Concert Hall
Facility Category: Performing Arts Center
Seating Capacity: 1,101
Year Built: 2000
Rental Contact: Kelly Thomas

4734 INTERLOCHEN ARTS FESTIVAL

PO Box 199
Interlochen, MI 49643-0199
Phone: 231-276-4455
Fax: 231-276-4417
e-mail: paulsontm@interlochen.org
Web Site: www.interlochen.org
Officers:
  Radio/Presentations VP: Thom Paulson
Mission: To offer an eight-week extension of the National Music Camp.
Founded: 1928
Specialized Field: Dance; Vocal Music; Instrumental Music; Theater
Status: Semi-Professional; Nonprofit
Performs At: Kresge Auditorium; Corson Auditorium
Organization Type: Performing; Educational

4735 MICHIGAN SHAKESPEARE FESTIVAL

Box 323
Jackson, MI 49204
Phone: 517-788-5032
Fax: 517-788-5254
e-mail: thebard@michshakefest.org
Web Site: www.michshakefest.org
Officers:
  President: Ann Green
  VP: Tom Mitchell
  Secertary: Rick Davies
  Treasurer: Margaret Musser
Management:
  Managing Director: Vicki TrudellIseler
  Artistic Director: John Neville-Andrews
  Marketing Director: Tonyaa Redding
Mission: Quality outdoor Shakespeare.
Founded: 1995
Status: Non-Equity; Nonprofit
Paid Staff: 8
Volunteer Staff: 6
Paid Artists: 60
Season: July - August
Type of Stage: Thrust
Stage Dimensions: 40' x 30'

Seating Capacity: 350

4736 BACH FESTIVAL SOCIETY OF KALAMAZOO

Kalamazoo College
1200 Academy Street
Kalamazoo, MI 49006
Phone: 616-337-7407
Fax: 616-337-7067
e-mail: jturner@kzoo.edu -or- bach@kzoo.edu
Management:
 Artistic Director/Conductor: James Turner

4737 FONTANA FESTIVAL OF MUSIC & ART

Fontana Concert Society
821 W South Street
Kalamazoo, MI 49007
Phone: 616-382-0826
Fax: 616-382-0812
e-mail: fontana@iserv.net
Web Site: www.fontanafestival.org
Management:
 Executive Director: Janet Karpus

4738 IRVING S GILMORE INTERNATIONAL KEYBOARD FESTIVAL

Epic Center
359 S Burdick
Kalamazoo, MI 49007
Phone: 616-342-1166
Fax: 616-342-0968
e-mail: gilmore@gilmore.org
Web Site: www.gilmore.org
Officers:
 President: Patti Huiskamp
Management:
 Director: Dan Gustin
 Operations Director: Juanita Nash
 Director Public Relations/Marketing: Carol Janowicz
 Box Office Manager/Secretary: Diane Gill
Mission: Identifying and supporting concert pianists; producing a biennial festival.
Founded: 1989
Specialized Field: Festivals
Status: Nonprofit
Paid Staff: 10
Income Sources: Association of Performing Arts Presenters
Performs At: Miller Auditorium; Dalton Center Recital Hall; others
Annual Attendance: Biennial Festival
Resident Groups: Gilmore Artist; Gilmore Young Artists

4739 NEW YEAR'S FEST

364 W Michigan Avenue
Kalamazoo, MI 49007
Phone: 616-388-3083
Fax: 616-388-2830
Officers:
 President: Chuck Wray
 Entertainment Chair: David Overton
Mission: To offer an alcohol-free celebration of New Year's Eve featuring performing arts to Kalamazoo.

Founded: 1986
Specialized Field: Dance; Vocal Music; Instrumental Music; Theater; Festivals; Lyric Opera
Status: Nonprofit
Organization Type: Festival

4740 MATRIX: MIDLAND FESTIVAL-CELEBRATION OF THE ARTS, SCIENCES & HUMANITIES

1801 W St Andrews Drive
Midland, MI 48640
Phone: 989-631-5930
Fax: 989-631-7890
Toll-free: 800-523-7649
e-mail: sabin@mcfta.org
Web Site: www.mcfta.org
Management:
 General Manager: Phyllis B Sabin
Mission: To encourage creativity of the highest level in the arts, sciences, humanties and all aspects of their interelationships.
Founded: 1978
Paid Staff: 1
Budget: $250,000
Income Sources: Corporate Sponsorships
Annual Attendance: 12,000

4741 MIDLAND COMMUNITY CONCERT SOCIETY

1801 W St. Andrews Road
Midland, MI 48640
Phone: 517-631-5930
Fax: 517-631-7890
e-mail: logan@mcfta.org
Officers:
 Chairman: Dr. Alice Ralston
Management:
 Operations Manager: Patricia E Logan
Mission: Encouraging concert audiences; Providing students with opportunities to experience professional performances.
Specialized Field: Vocal Music; Instrumental Music
Status: Nonprofit
Organization Type: Educational; Sponsoring

4742 MUSIC SOCIETY OF THE MIDLAND CENTER FOR THE ARTS

1801 W St. Andrews Road
Midland, MI 48640
Phone: 517-631-5931
Fax: 517-631-7890
e-mail: hohmeyer@mcfta.org
Web Site: www.mcfta.org
Management:
 Artistic Director: James Hohmeyer
Seating Capacity: 1492

4743 INTERMEDIA ARTS

2822 Lyndale Avenue S
Minneapolis, MI 55408-2108

Phone: 612-871-4444
Fax: 612-871-6927
e-mail: info@intermediaarts.org
Web Site: www.intermediaarts.org
Officers:
   Chair of the Board: Richard Ammmen
Management:
   Executive Director: Tom Borrup
   Associate Director: Sandy Agustin
Mission: Intermedia Arts is a catalyst that builds understanding among people through art.
Founded: 1973

4744   CROOKED TREE ARTS COUNCIL
461 E Mitchell Street
Petoskey, MI 49770
Phone: 231-347-4337
Fax: 231-347-5414
e-mail: liz@crookedtree.org
Web Site: www.crookedtree.org
Officers:
   President: Phoebea Wietzke
   VP: Stephen Palmer
   Treasurer: Richard Lent
   Secretary: Jane Miller
Management:
   Executive Director: Dale Hull
   Marketing Director: Elizabeth Ahrens
Mission: To sponsor and encourage cultural and educational activities in the fine arts for Charlevoix and Emmet Counties.
Founded: 1972
Specialized Field: Dance; Vocal Music; Instrumental Music; Festivals
Status: Nonprofit
Paid Staff: 10
Income Sources: National Guild of Community Schools of the Arts; Michigan Association of Community Arts Agencies; Michigan Council on the Arts
Performs At: Crooked Tree Arts Center
Annual Attendance: 50,000
Year Remodeled: 2002
Organization Type: Performing; Educational; Sponsoring

4745   TEMPLE THEATRE ORGAN CLUB
315 Court Street
Saginaw, MI 48602
Phone: 517-754-2575
Fax: 517-793-7225
Management:
   General Manager: Ken Wuepper
Mission: Restoring the Temple Theatre and reestablishing it as a prominent performing arts center.
Founded: 1960
Status: Nonprofit
Organization Type: Educational; Sponsoring; Historic Preservation

4746   LAKE SUPERIOR STATE UNIVERSITY CULTURAL EVENTS SERIES
Lake Superior State Univesity
Sault Sainte Marie, MI 49783
Phone: 906-635-2265
Fax: 906-635-6674
e-mail: jwilkinson@gw.lssu.edu
Officers:
   Cultural Events Chairman: John Wilkinson
Performs At: Auditoriums

4747   WEST SHORE COMMUNITY COLLEGE CULTURAL SERIES
3000 N Stiles Road
Scottville, MI 49454
Phone: 231-845-6211
Fax: 231-843-2680
Toll-free: 800-848-9722
e-mail: rjplummer@westshore.cc.mi.us
Web Site: www.westshore.cc.mi.us
Management:
   Theater/Cultural Arts Director: Dr. Rick Plummer
Volunteer Staff: 2
Paid Artists: 19
Non-paid Artists: 35
Performs At: Media Center Auditorium
Annual Attendance: 12,000+
Type of Stage: Thrust
Seating Capacity: 279
Year Built: 1971
Year Remodeled: 1999

4748   GREAT LAKES CHAMBER MUSIC FESTIVAL
17348 W Twelve Mile Road
Suite 102
Southfield, MI 48076
Phone: 248-559-2097
Fax: 248-559-2098
e-mail: chambermusic@juno.com
Web Site: www.greatlakeschambermusic.com
Management:
   Executive Director: Maury Okun

4749   DOWNRIVER COUNCIL FOR THE ARTS
20904 Northline Road
Taylor, MI 48180
Phone: 734-287-6103
Fax: 734-287-6151
e-mail: DC4arts@cs-net.net
Web Site: www.downriverarts.org
Management:
   Executive Director: Richard Green
Mission: Promoting a range of the fine and performing arts in Downriver communities.
Founded: 1978
Specialized Field: Dance; Vocal Music; Instrumental Music; Theater; Festivals
Status: Professional; Nonprofit
Paid Staff: 35
Income Sources: Grants, Donations, Membership
Organization Type: Educational; Sponsoring

4750 SAGINAW VALLEY STATE UNIVERSITY CONCERT: LECTURE SERIES
Campus Life
7400 Bay Road
University Center, MI 48710
Phone: 517-790-4170
Fax: 517-249-1695
e-mail: ebusch@tardis.svsu.edu
Management:
   Director: Eric Buschlen
Seating Capacity: 400

4751 WATERFORD CULTURAL COUNCIL
5860 Andersonville Road
Waterford, MI 48329-1510
Phone: 248-623-9389
Fax: 248-623-7907
e-mail: waterfordcc@earthlink.net
Web Site: www.waterford.wb.mi.us/win/ncc
Management:
   Executive Director: Tony Marha
   Program Director: Debra Berry
Mission: To strenthen, enrich and unite the community through the arts.
Founded: 1994
Specialized Field: Performing & Visual
Status: Nonprofit
Paid Staff: 4
Volunteer Staff: 120
Budget: $260,000
Income Sources: United Way; Waterford Township; Waterford Schools
Performs At: Waterford Mott High School Auditorium
Annual Attendance: 16,000
Facility Category: Performance Arena
Seating Capacity: 650

Minnesota

4752 ALEXANDRIA FESTIVAL OF THE LAKES
PO Box 863
Alexandria, MN 56308
Phone: 320-762-5666
Fax: 320-762-8246
e-mail: Alexfest@aol.com
Web Site: www.AlexFest.org
Management:
   Artistic Director: Nina Tobias
Founded: 1993
Specialized Field: Chamber Music

4753 HOBSON UNION PROGRAMING BOARD PERFORMING ARTISTS SERIES
Bemidji State University
15th & Birchmont Drive
Bemidji, MN 56601
Phone: 218-755-3760
Fax: 218-755-3757
Management:
   Director: Linda Blanchard
   (Student) Chair Cultural Arts: LaShawna Peterson

Paid Staff: 1
Paid Artists: 1
Performs At: Various Auditoriums

4754 COLLEGE OF ST. SCHOLASTICA MITCHELL AUDITORIUM
1200 Kenwood Avenue
Duluth, MN 55811-4199
Phone: 218-723-5908
Fax: 218-723-6290
Toll-free: 800-447-5444
e-mail: ngawinsk@css.edu
Web Site: www.css.edu
Management:
   Director: Neil A Gawinski
   Office Assistant: LeAnn Jopke
Founded: 1912
Paid Staff: 12
Performs At: Mitchell Auditorium
Annual Attendance: 38,000
Facility Category: Orchestra Hall/Arts Center
Type of Stage: Sprung Wood Maple Dance Floor
Stage Dimensions: 30 deep X 60 wide
Seating Capacity: 585
Year Built: 1993
Cost: $4.6 million
Rental Contact: Director Neil A. Gawinski

4755 REIF GREENWAY SERIES
720 Conifer Drive
Grand Rapids, MN 55744
Phone: 218-327-5780
Fax: 218-327-5798
e-mail: dmarty@reifcenter.org
Web Site: www.reifcenter.org
Management:
   Executive Director: David Marty
Mission: Stimulating arts in Northern Minnesota.
Founded: 1980
Budget: $520,000
Income Sources: Box Office; Grants; Foundations
Annual Attendance: 12,500
Facility Category: Auditorium
Type of Stage: Modified Thrust
Stage Dimensions: 45 x 46 (curtain lines)
Seating Capacity: 645
Year Built: 1980
Year Remodeled: 1999
Rental Contact: John Miller
Organization Type: Presenting

4756 BETHANY LUTHERAN COLLEGE CONCERTS & LECTURES
700 Luther Drive
Mankato, MN 56001-6163
Phone: 507-344-7365
Fax: 507-344-7380
e-mail: ljaeger@blc.edu
Management:
   Fine Arts Director: Lois Jaeger
Performs At: Theatre

4757 MINNEAPOLIS PARK & RECREATION BOARD-SUMMER MUSIC IN THE PARKS
200 Grain Exchange
400 S 4th Street
Minneapolis, MN 55415-1400
Phone: 612-661-4890
Fax: 612-661-4780
e-mail: linda.m.larson@ci.minneapolis.mn.us
Management:
Concert Coordinator: Linda Larson

4758 PLYMOUTH MUSIC SERIES OF MINNESOTA
1900 Nicollet Avenue
Minneapolis, MN 55403
Phone: 612-547-1451
Fax: 612-547-1484
e-mail: info@plymouthmusic.org
Web Site: www.plymouthmusic.org
Management:
Executive Director: Philip Brunelle
General Manager: Frank Stubbs
Mission: The presentation of newly commissioned choral and orchestral works.
Founded: 1969
Specialized Field: Choral Music
Status: Professional; Nonprofit
Paid Staff: 9
Paid Artists: 24
Non-paid Artists: 75
Budget: 1.2 million
Affiliations: Chorus America; IFCM
Organization Type: Performing; Educational; Sponsoring
Resident Groups: Ensamble Singers

4759 UNIVERSITY OF MINNESOTA AT MINNEAPOLIS SERIES
84 Church Street SE
Minneapolis, MN 55455
Phone: 612-625-9878
Fax: 612-626-1750
e-mail: schat001@axus.umn.edu
Web Site: www.northrop.umn.edu
Management:
Director: Dale Schatzlein
Performs At: Northrop Memorial Auditorium

4760 ALLIED CONCERT SERVICES
12450 Wayzata Boulevard
#200
Minnetonka, MN 55305
Phone: 952-542-8019
Fax: 952-542-8398
Officers:
President: Paul Folin

4761 CONCORDIA COLLEGE CULTURAL EVENTS SERIES
901 8th Street S
Moorhead, MN 56562
Phone: 218-299-4366
Fax: 218-299-3191

4762 MINNESOTA STATE UNIVERSITY MOOREHEAD SERIES
250D Bridges Hall
1104 7th Avenue S
Moorhead, MN 56563
Phone: 218-287-5031
Fax: 218-287-5037
e-mail: wigtil@mnstate.edu
Web Site: www.mnstate.edu/perform
Management:
Performing Arts Series Coordinator: Laurie Wigtil
Mission: To provide cultural programming of the highest calibre to the community and campus audiences.
Founded: 1930
Specialized Field: Dance; Vocal Music; Instrumental Music; Theater
Status: Professional; Nonprofit
Budget: $80,000
Performs At: Center for the Arts
Annual Attendance: 5,000
Facility Category: Center for the Arts
Type of Stage: Proscenium
Stage Dimensions: 41'x22'x33'
Seating Capacity: 850
Year Built: 1963
Organization Type: Performing; Educational; Sponsoring

4763 UNIVERSITY OF MINNESOTA MORRIS CAC PERFORMING ARTS SERIES
Office of Student Activities, UMM
600 E 4th Street
Morris, MN 56267-2134
Phone: 320-589-6080
Fax: 320-589-6084
e-mail: haugensj@mrs.umn.edu
Performs At: Edson Auditorium

4764 CARLETON COLLEGE CONCERT SERIES
One N College Street
Northfield, MN 55057
Phone: 507-646-4347
Fax: 507-633-4347
Management:
Concert Manager: Harry Nordstrom
Mission: Providing excellently performed music; offering an educational program.
Founded: 1945
Specialized Field: Vocal Music; Instrumental Music
Status: Professional; Nonprofit
Performs At: Carleton Concert Hall; Skinner Chapel
Organization Type: Educational; Sponsoring

4765 ST. OLAF COLLEGE ARTIST SERIES
Music Department
St. Olaf College
Northfield, MN 55057
Phone: 507-646-3179
Management:

Music Organizations Manager: BJ Johnson
Performs At: Skoglund Auditorium

4766 ROCHESTER CIVIC MUSIC

201 4th Street SE
Suite 170
Rochester, MN 55904
Phone: 507-281-6005
Fax: 507-281-6055
e-mail: sschmidt@ci.rochester.mn.us
Web Site: www.ci.rochester.mn.us/music/
Management:
  General Manager: Steven J Schmidt
Specialized Field: Concert Band; Choir Music; Presenter; Producer
Performs At: Mayo Civic Center

4767 SCHUBERT CLUB INTERNATIONAL ARTIST SERIES

302 Landmark Center
75 W 5th Street
Saint Paul, MN 55102
Phone: 651-292-3267
Fax: 651-292-4317
e-mail: schubert@schubert.org
Web Site: www.schubert.org
Management:
  Executive Director: Bruce Carlson
Mission: To promote the art of music, particularly recital music through education, performance, and museum programs and to maintain a high standard of artistic excellence.
Founded: 1982
Specialized Field: Performing Music Series and Museum.
Paid Staff: 10
Performs At: Ordway Music Theatre

4768 GUSTAVUS ADOLPHUS COLLEGE ARTIST SERIES

Gustavus Adolphus College
800 W College Avenue
Saint Peter, MN 56082
Phone: 507-933-7363
e-mail: al@gustavus.edu
Management:
  Fine Arts Programs Director: Alan Behrends
Performs At: Bjorling Concert Hall

4769 ST. CLOUD STATE UNIVERSITY PROGRAM BOARD PERFORMING ARTS SERIES

118 Atwood Memorial Center, SCSU
720 4th Avenue S
St. Cloud, MN 56301
Phone: 320-255-2205
Fax: 320-529-1669
Management:
  Programming Director: Jessica Ostman
  Assistant Director: Janice Courtney
Performs At: Atwood Center Ballroom

4770 PACIFIC COMPOSERS FORUM

332 Minnesota Street
Suite E145
St. Paul, MN 55101-1300
Phone: 651-228-1407
Fax: 651-291-7978
e-mail: info@composersforum.com
Web Site: www.composersforum.com

Mississippi

4771 JAZZ IN THE GROVE

PO Box 409
Bay Springs, MS 39422
Phone: 601-764-2121
Fax: 601-764-6866
Toll-free: 800-898-2782
e-mail: joeyg@tec.com
Web Site: www.bayspringstel.net
Management:
  Director: Emily Mixon
Specialized Field: Performing Series - Jazz Festival

4772 UNIVERSITY OF SOUTHERN MISSISSIPPI COLLEGE OF THE ARTS

Hardy Street
Box 5031
Hattiesburg, MS 39406-5031
Phone: 601-266-4984
Fax: 601-266-4127
Web Site: www.arts.usm.edu
Management:
  Interim Dean: Dr. Mary Ann Stringer
Specialized Field: Music, Dance, Theatre, Visual Arts
Budget: $35,000-60,000
Income Sources: State Funded

4773 BELHAVEN COLLEGE PRESTON MEMORIAL SERIES

Belhaven College
Jackson, MS 39202-1789
Phone: 601-968-8707
Fax: 601-968-9998
e-mail: cshelt@belhaven.edu
Web Site: www.belhaven.edu
Officers:
  Music Department Chairman: Christopher Shelt
Performs At: Girault Auditorium

4774 MISSISSIPPI ARTS COMMISSION

239 N Lamar Street
Suite 207
Jackson, MS 39201
Phone: 601-359-6030
Fax: 601-359-6008
e-mail: hedgepet@arts.state.ms.us
Management:
  Program Administrator: Tim Hedgepeth

4775 WORLD PERFORMANCE SERIES: THALIA MARA FOUNDATION
1440 N State Street
Jackson, MS 39202
Phone: 601-968-0090
Fax: 601-354-2781
e-mail: mail@thaliamara.org
Web Site: www.thaliamara.org
Management:
Executive Director: Leanne Mahoney
Budget: $400,000-1,000,000

4776 MISSISSIPPI STATE UNIVERSITY LYCEUM SERIES
PO Drawer HY
Mississippi State, MS 39762
Phone: 662-325-4201
Fax: 662-325-7456
Management:
Series Coordinator: Brenda Neubauer
Budget: $20,000-35,000
Performs At: Humphery Coliseum

4777 NATCHEZ OPERA FESTIVAL
64 Homochitto
Natchez, MS 39120
Mailing Address: PO Box 2207, Natchez, MS. 39121
Phone: 601-442-7464
Fax: 601-442-9686
Toll-free: 800-647-6724
e-mail: opera@bkbank.com
Web Site: www2.bkbank.com/opera/index.html
Management:
General/Artistic Director: David Blackburn
Performs At: Margaret Martin Performing Arts Center

4778 UNIVERSITY OF MISSISSIPPI ARTIST SERIES
University of Mississippi Artists Series
University, MS 38677
Phone: 662-232-7429
Fax: 662-232-7830
Web Site: www.olemiss.edu/depts/music/artist.html
Officers:
Chairman: Dr. Robert Riggs
Budget: $35,000-60,000
Performs At: Fulton Chapel

Missouri

4779 FRIENDS OF HISTORIC BOONVILLE PERFORMING ARTS
614 E Morgan
PO Box 1776
Boonville, MO 65233-1776
Phone: 660-882-7977
Fax: 660-882-9194
Toll-free: 888-588-1477
e-mail: friendsart@mid-mo.net
Web Site: mid-mo.net/friendsart
Officers:

President: Ron Lenz
Second VP: Barbara Holtzclaw
First VP: Gary Campbell
Secretary: Debby Koerner
Management:
Administrator: Maryellen McVicker
Mission: To provide a community arts program in our historic theatre, Thespian Hall.
Founded: 1971
Specialized Field: Dance; Vocal Music; Instrumental Music; Theater; Festivals; Lyric Opera; Grand Opera
Status: Nonprofit
Paid Staff: 4
Budget: $60,000-150,000
Income Sources: Donations; earned income
Performs At: Thespian Hall
Annual Attendance: 7,500
Facility Category: Theatre; Performing Arts Center
Type of Stage: Proscenium
Stage Dimensions: 80x100
Seating Capacity: 600
Year Built: 1857
Year Remodeled: 1980
Organization Type: Performing; Educational; Sponsoring

4780 MISSOURI RIVER FESTIVAL OF THE ARTS
PO Box 1776
614 E Morgan
Boonville, MO 65233
Phone: 660-882-7977
Fax: 660-882-9194
Toll-free: 888-588-1477
e-mail: friendsart@mid-mo.net
Web Site: www.mid-mo/friendsart
Management:
Administrator: Maryellen H McVicker
Founded: 1975
Seating Capacity: 600
Year Built: 1855
Year Remodeled: 2002

4781 SOUTHEAST MISSOURI STATE UNIVERSITY: CULTURAL SERIES
Southeast Missouri State University
Cape Girardeau, MO 63701
Phone: 573-651-2000
Fax: 573-651-2893
Management:
Dean College of Humanities: Dr. Martin Jones
Chairperson/Speech Communications: Dr. Ray G Ewing
Mission: To attract professional quality performing arts to the Southeast Missouri area; to offer professional workshops.
Founded: 1873
Specialized Field: Dance; Vocal Music; Instrumental Music; Theater
Status: Nonprofit
Income Sources: Missouri Council on the Arts
Performs At: Academic Hall Auditorium
Organization Type: Educational; Sponsoring

4782 UNIVERSITY OF MISSOURI: COLUMBIA CONCERT SERIES
409 Jesse Hall, MU
Columbia, MO 65211
Phone: 573-882-3875
Fax: 573-882-2636
Toll-free: 800-292-9136
e-mail: dunnm@missouri.edu
Web Site: www.concertseries.org
Management:
    Executive Director: Dr. Michael W Dunn
    Assistant Director: Julie Graff
Paid Staff: 20
Volunteer Staff: 50
Paid Artists: 42
Budget: $400,000-1,000,000
Annual Attendance: 65,000
Seating Capacity: 1,800

4783 CENTRAL METHODIST COLLEGE CONVOCATIONS
Central Methodist College
Fayette, MO 65248-1198
Phone: 660-248-6304
Fax: 660-248-2622
e-mail: jgeist@coin.org
Officers:
    Chairman: Dr. Joseph Geist
Budget: $20,000-35,000
Performs At: Little Theater; Lynn Memorial Chapel; Field House

4784 WILLIAM WOODS UNIVERSITY CONCERT & LECTURE SERIES
William Woods University
One University Avenue
Fulton, MO 65251
Phone: 573-592-4281
Fax: 573-592-1623
e-mail: jpotter@william-woods.edu
Web Site: www.williamwoods.edu
Management:
    Performing/Community: Paul Clervi
    Artistic Director of Theatre: Joe Potter
Founded: 1870
Budget: $10,000
Performs At: Cutlip Auditorium; Dulany Auditorium

4785 HANNIBAL CONCERT ASSOCIATION
22 Hamlin Heights
Hannibal, MO 63401
Phone: 573-221-3139
Fax: 573-221-6545
e-mail: debpriest@hotmail.com
Management:
    Booking Manager: Deb Priest
Budget: $10,000-20,000

4786 CAPITAL CITY COUNCIL ON THE ARTS
PO Box 1311
Jefferson City, MO 65102
Phone: 573-635-8355
Fax: 573-634-3805

Budget: $10,000

4787 PRO MUSICA
2700 E 15th Street
Joplin, MO 64804
Phone: 417-623-8865
Fax: 417-623-0402
e-mail: athena@ipa.net
Web Site: www.promusicajoplin.org
Management:
    Executive Director: Cynthia H Schwab
Paid Staff: 2
Volunteer Staff: 1
Budget: $35,000-60,000

4788 HEART OF AMERICA SHAKESPEARE FESTIVAL
4800 Main Street
Suite 302
Kansas City, MO 64112
Phone: 816-531-7728
Fax: 816-531-1911
e-mail: info@kcshakes.org
Web Site: www.kcshakes.org
Management:
    Executive Director: Tom Banks
Founded: 1991
Status: Nonprofit
Paid Staff: 3
Volunteer Staff: 700
Paid Artists: 35
Budget: $500,000-600,000
Income Sources: Foundations; Individuals; Corporations
Season: June - July
Annual Attendance: 25-35,000
Facility Category: Outdoor Park Setting
Stage Dimensions: 45'x 30'
Seating Capacity: 3000

4789 KANSAS CITY BLUES & JAZZ FESTIVAL
4200 Pennsylvania Avenue
Suite 230
Kansas City, MO 64111
Fax: 816-531-2583
Toll-free: 800-530-5266
e-mail: kcbluesjazz@kcbluesjazz.org
Web Site: www.kcbluesjazz.org
Management:
    Director: Greg Patterson
    Assistant Director: Connie Hemiston
Founded: 1991
Specialized Field: Music Festival
Paid Staff: 2
Volunteer Staff: 500
Paid Artists: 50

4790 KANSAS CITY RENAISSANCE FESTIVAL
207 Westport Road
Suite 206
Kansas City, MO 64111

Phone: 816-561-8005
Fax: 816-561-6493
Toll-free: 800-373-0357
e-mail: renfest@kcrenfest.com
Web Site: www.kcrenfest.com
Management:
    Executive Director: Carrie Shoptaw
Mission: To entertain and educate using a Renaissance theme.
Founded: 1977
Paid Staff: 15
Volunteer Staff: 2
Income Sources: Ticket sales; sponsorships
Annual Attendance: 180,000
Facility Category: 12 Outdoor Stages
Type of Stage: 4 Proscenium; 1 Jousting Field
Year Built: 1977

4791 KANSAS CITY YOUNG AUDIENCES SERIES

4601 Madison Avenue
Kansas City, MO 64112
Phone: 816-531-4022
Fax: 816-531-2787
e-mail: dwindham@crn.org
Management:
    President/CEO: Daniel Windham

4792 SUMMERFEST CONCERTS

PO Box 22697
Kansas City, MO 64113-0697
Phone: 913-262-2543
Management:
    Artistic Advisor: Nancy Beckmann

4793 UNIVERSITY OF MISSOURI-KANSAS CITY CONSERVATORY SERIES

4949 Cherry Street
Kansas City, MO 64110-2229
Phone: 816-235-2949
Fax: 816-235-5265
e-mail: urbana@umkc.edu
Web Site: www.umkc.edu/performance
Management:
    Marketing Director: Al Urban
    Concert Activities Manager: Stephen Steigman
Budget: $35,000-60,000
Performs At: White Recital Hall; Center for the Performing Arts

4794 TRUMAN STATE UNIVERSITY LYCEUM SERIES

Truman State University
Kirksville, MO 63501
Phone: 660-785-7423
Fax: 660-785-7424
e-mail: tlinares@truman.edu
Officers:
    Lyceum Committee Chairman: Thomas Linares
Budget: $60,000-150,000
Performs At: Baldwin Hall Auditorium

4795 HARRIMAN ARTS PROGRAM OF WILLIAM JEWELL COLLEGE

William Jewell College
500 College Hill, PO Box 1015
Liberty, MO 64068
Phone: 816-415-5025
Fax: 816-415-5035
e-mail: info@harrimanarts.org
Web Site: www.harrimanarts.org
Management:
    Director: Richard Harriman
    Associate Director: Clark Morris
Mission: To bring the best of the performing arts to the communities of William Jewell College and greater Kansas City.
Founded: 1965
Specialized Field: Music, Dance and Theatre Performance
Paid Staff: 6

4796 NORTHWEST MISSOURI STATE UNIVERSITY PERFORMING ARTS SERIES

800 University Drive
Maryville, MO 64468
Phone: 660-562-1562
Fax: 660-562-1121
Toll-free: 800-633-1175
e-mail: desser@mail.nwmissouri.edu
Web Site: www.nwmissouri.edu
Management:
    Chairman: Bayo Oludaja
Mission: Providing a range of lectures and performing arts for the University and area residents.
Specialized Field: Vocal Music; Instrumental Music; Theater
Status: Nonprofit
Budget: $60,000-150,000
Income Sources: Missouri Arts Council
Performs At: Charles Johnson Theatre; Mary Linn Performing Arts
Organization Type: Educational; Sponsoring

4797 MOBERLY AREA COUNCIL ON THE ARTS

Moberly Area Community College
Moberly, MO 65270
Phone: 660-263-4110
Fax: 660-263-6448
Budget: $20,000-35,000

4798 COTTEY LECTURERS & ARTISTS SUPER SERIES

Cottey College
Nevada, MO 64772
Phone: 417-667-8181
Web Site: www.cottry.edu
Management:
    Campus Activities Coordinator: Kristi L Korb
Budget: $20,000-35,000
Performs At: Center for the Arts

4799 THERON C BENNET RAGTIME & EARLY JAZZ FESTIVAL
21554 Lawrence 1032
Pierce City, MO 65723
Phone: 417-476-5408
Web Site: www.sound.net/~gary/theron/theron.htm
Management:
   Festival Organizer: Murray Bishoff

4800 PERFORMING ARTS ASSOCIATION OF SAINT JOSEPH
719 Edmond Street
Saint Joseph, MO 64501
Phone: 816-279-1225
Fax: 816-233-6704
e-mail: toihunt@paastjo.org
Web Site: www.paastjo.org
Management:
   Executive Director: Teresa Fankhauser
Budget: $60,000-150,000
Performs At: Missouri Theatre

4801 CITICORP SUMMERFEST
Powell Symphony Hall
718 N Grand Boulevard
Saint Louis, MO 63103
Phone: 314-533-2500
Fax: 314-286-4188
Web Site: www.slso.org
Management:
   Music Director/Conductor: Hans Vonk
Founded: 1966
Specialized Field: Instrumental Music
Status: Professional; Nonprofit
Performs At: Powell Symphony Hall At Grand Center
Affiliations: Saint Louis Symphony Orchestra
Organization Type: Performing

4802 FOX ASSOCIATES
527 N Grand
Saint Louis, MO 63103
Phone: 314-534-1678
Fax: 314-534-8702
e-mail: webmaster@mtix.com
Web Site: www.fabouousfox.com
Management:
   Executive Director: Richard Baker
Mission: Present live entertainment.
Founded: 1982
Budget: $1,000,000+

4803 NEW MUSIC CIRCLE SERIES
142 Willow Brook Road
Saint Louis, MO 63146
Phone: 314-432-6073
Fax: 314-567-5384
e-mail: alumrod@aol.com
Web Site: www.newmusiccircle.org
Management:
   Music Department: Rich O'Donnell
Founded: 1959
Paid Staff: 2
Volunteer Staff: 5

Paid Artists: 30
Budget: $34,000
Income Sources: St. Louis Regional Arts Commission, Missouri Arts Council
Annual Attendance: 1,000
Facility Category: Venues

4804 SAINT LOUIS CATHEDRAL CONCERTS
4431 Lindell Boulevard
Saint Louis, MO 63108
Phone: 314-533-7662
Fax: 314-533-2844
e-mail: concerts@cathedralstl.org
Web Site: www.cathedralstl.org
Budget: $60,000-150,000

4805 SAINT LOUIS HILLS ARTS COUNCIL
4924 Hampton Avenue
Saint Louis, MO 63109-3109
Phone: 314-352-1838
Fax: 314-352-3049
e-mail: Johnpwalsh@aol.com
Officers:
   President: John Powel Walsh
Budget: $10,000-20,000
Performs At: Powell Symphony Hall

4806 UNIVERSITY OF MISSOURI: SAINT LOUIS PREMIER PERFORMANCES
8001 Natural Bridge Road
Saint Louis, MO 63121-4499
Phone: 314-516-5818
Fax: 314-516-5881
e-mail: klbmezzo@umsl.edu
Web Site: www.umsl.edu/~premier/
Management:
   Director: Katharine Lawton Brown
   Production Associate: Gloria Kohn
Founded: 1986
Specialized Field: Chamber Music
Paid Staff: 3
Volunteer Staff: 2
Non-paid Artists: 50
Budget: $35,000-60,000
Income Sources: Public, Private and Grants
Performs At: Sheldon Concert Hall; Ethical Society Auditorium
Seating Capacity: 700/419

4807 SCOTT JOPLIN RAGTIME FESTIVAL
113 E 4th Street
Sedalia, MO 65301
Phone: 660-826-2271
Web Site: www.scottjoplin.org
Management:
   Festival Coordinator: John Moore
   Executive Secretary: Julie Renberg
Mission: To expose a greater variety of people to the historical and aesthetic value of Scott Joplin and ragtime music; to enrich our understanding.
Founded: 1974
Specialized Field: Orchestra; Ensemble; Instrumental Group; Electronic & Live Electronic; Band

Status: Nonprofit
Organization Type: Performing; Educational

4808 **EVANGEL UNIVERSITY ARTISTS & LECTURESHIP SERIES**
1111 N Glenstone
Springfield, MO 65802
Phone: 417-865-2811
Fax: 417-865-9599
e-mail: bernetg@evangel.edu
Management:
　Dean: Glenn Bernet
　Music Department: Dr. Linda Ligateng
Budget: $10,000-20,000

4809 **LINDENWOOD COLLEGE MAINSTAGE SEASON**
209 S Kings Highway
St. Charles, MO 63301
Phone: 636-949-4966
e-mail: breeder@lindenwood.edu
Management:
　Manager: Bryan Reeder

4810 **JUNETEENTH HERITAGE & JAZZ FESTIVAL**
625 N Euclid
Suite 225
St. Louis, MO 63108
Phone: 314-367-0100
Fax: 314-367-0200
Toll-free: 877-586-8684
e-mail: juntnthjaz@aol.com
Web Site: www.juneteenthjazz.org
Management:
　Executive Producer: Curtis Faulkner

4811 **SAINT LOUIS SYMPHONY: CLASSICS IN THE LOOP FESTIVAL**
Saint Louis Symphony Orchestra
718 N Grand Boulevard
St. Louis, MO 63103
Phone: 314-533-2500
Fax: 314-286-4140
e-mail: Symph@admiral.umsl.edu
Web Site: www.slso.org
Management:
　Conductor: David Loebel

4812 **ROYAL ARTS COUNCIL**
PO Box 273
Versailles, MO 65084
Phone: 573-378-6226
Management:
　Executive Director: Marilyn L Dimond
Budget: $10,000-20,000

4813 **CENTRAL MISSOURI STATE UNIVERSITY PERFORMING ARTS SERIES**
Office of Student Life
Union Building 307
Warrensburg, MO 64093
Phone: 660-543-8607
Fax: 660-543-4181
e-mail: hailey@cmsu1.cmsu.edu
Web Site: www.cmsu.edu/pas
Management:
　Special Activities Director: Thomas H Hailey
Budget: $60,000-150,000
Performs At: Hendricks Hall

Montana

4814 **RED LODGE MUSIC FESTIVAL**
2235 Saint Andrews Drive
Billings, MT 59105
Phone: 406-652-8146
e-mail: rlmf@mcn.net
Web Site: www.mcn.net/~rlmf/redldg.html
Officers:
　President: Kenneth Gilstrap

4815 **ASSOCIATED STUDENTS OF MONTANA STATE UNIVERSITY**
Strand Union Building
Room 282-B
Bozeman, MT 59717
Phone: 406-994-5828
Fax: 406-994-6911
Budget: $20,000-35,000
Performs At: Wilson Auditorium; Reynolds Recital Hall; Northwest Lounge

4816 **DILLON COMMUNITY CONCERT ASSOCIATION**
102 Legget
Dillon, MT 59725
Phone: 406-683-2285
Officers:
　Drive Chairman: Ingrid Joy Kaushagen
Budget: $10,000-20,000

4817 **MONTANA TRADITIONAL JAZZ FESTIVAL**
PO Box 956
Great Falls, MT 59403
Phone: 406-771-1642
Fax: 406-727-5869
e-mail: jazzfeset@montana.com
Web Site: www.montanatradjazz.com
Management:
　Director: Don West

4818 HAVRE COMMUNITY CONCERT ASSOCIATION
44 Saddle Butte Drive
Havre, MT 59501
Phone: 406-265-5254
Officers:
   President: Dan Heltne
Budget: $10,000-20,000

4819 MONTANA STATE UNIVERSITY NORTHERN SHOWCASE
MSU-Northern
PO Box 7751
Havre, MT 59501
Phone: 406-265-3732
Fax: 406-265-3555
e-mail: brewer@msun.edu
Management:
   Showcase Coordinator: Denise Brewer
Mission: To provide fine arts/culture to the Havre community and MSU Northern students.
Founded: 1932
Specialized Field: Havre and the Hiline community
Paid Staff: 1
Volunteer Staff: 20
Paid Artists: 4
Budget: $10,000-20,000

4820 FLATHEAD VALLEY FESTIVAL
545 Second Avenue E
Kalispell, MT 59901
Phone: 406-257-1065
Fax: 406-257-1065
e-mail: festival@cyberport.net
Web Site: www.cyberport.net/festival
Officers:
   VP: Bob Kieser
   Treasurer: Kris Fuehrer

4821 UNIVERSITY OF MONTANA PERFORMING ARTS SERIES
University of Montana
University Center #104
Missoula, MT 59812
Phone: 406-243-6661
Fax: 406-243-4905
e-mail: specialevents@umproductions.org
Web Site: www.umproductions.org
Management:
   Director: Ally Ruvolo
   Advisor: Marlene Hendckson
   Special Events Coordinator: Burke Jam
Founded: 1918
Paid Staff: 9
Income Sources: Student Funded
Performs At: Fieldhouse; Wilma Theatre; University Theater; UC Ballroom; Arena; Theaters
Facility Category: Theater
Type of Stage: Built In
Seating Capacity: 1,000
Year Remodeled: 1998
Rental Contact: Tom Webster

4822 YOUNG AUDIENCES OF WESTERN MONTANA SERIES
PO Box 9096
111 N Higgins #212
Missoula, MT 59807
Phone: 406-721-5924
Fax: 406-829-6432
e-mail: alaynusa@montana.com
Officers:
   President: John Engen
   Past President: John Bohyer
   Secretary: Jack Sturgis
   Treasurer: Dan Chisholm
Management:
   Executive Director: Alayne Dolson
Mission: To introduce elementary school children to various performing arts.
Founded: 1964
Specialized Field: Dance; Vocal Music; Instrumental Music; Theater; Story telling
Status: Professional; Nonprofit
Paid Staff: 1
Paid Artists: 36
Budget: $43,000
Income Sources: Grants, School Fees, Individual and business donors.
Performs At: Schools
Affiliations: Young Audience, New York, NY
Organization Type: Performing; Touting; Educational

4823 OLD TIMERS CONCERT SERIES
Sheridan High School
Sheridan, MT 59749
Phone: 406-842-5226
Management:
   Manager: Sue Nottingham
Mission: To encourage community talent; to raise money for scholarships and school music programs.
Founded: 1974
Specialized Field: Dance; Vocal Music; Instrumental Music; Theater; Festivals
Status: Semi-Professional; Non-Professional
Paid Staff: 50
Performs At: Sheridan School Gym
Organization Type: Performing; Resident

4824 FLATHEAD FESTIVAL OF THE ARTS
PO Box 1780
Whitefish, MT 59937
Phone: 406-862-1780
Management:
   Executive Director: Charles Buchwalter
   Artistic Director: Gordon Johnson
   Administrative Director: Rebecca Grouse
Founded: 1986
Specialized Field: Vocal Music Instrumental Music; Festivals; Lyric Opera
Status: Nonprofit
Organization Type: Performing; Touring; Educational; Sponsoring

Nebraska

4825 HARLAN COUNTY ARTS COUNCIL
PO Box 166
Alma, NE 68920
Phone: 308-234-4949
Officers:
President: Cindy Kauk
Budget: $10,000-20,000

4826 BASSETT ARTS COUNCIL
Box 429
Bassett, NE 68714
Phone: 402-684-3355
Fax: 402-684-2546
Officers:
President: Linda May
VP: Kathy Jorgenser
Treasurer: Betty Hall
Secretary: Mary M. Schelkopf
Management:
Secretary/ Contact Person: Mary M Schelkopf
Paid Staff: 50
Budget: $20,000-35,000

4827 COLUMBUS FRIENDS OF MUSIC ASSOCIATION
3485 18th Avenue
Columbus, NE 68601

4828 MIDLAND LUTHERAN COLLEGE CONCERT: LECTURE SERIES
900 N Clarkson
Fremont, NE 68025
Phone: 402-721-5480
Officers:
VP Institutional Advancement: Fred Pyle

4829 ABENDMUSIK SERIES
2000 D Street
Lincoln, NE 68502-1698
Phone: 402-476-9933
Fax: 402-476-8402
e-mail: sue@abendmusik.org
Web Site: www.abendmusik.org / www.firstplymouth.org
Management:
Executive Director: Sue J Buss
Founded: 1972
Budget: $60,000-150,000
Performs At: First-Plymouth Church
Facility Category: Church
Seating Capacity: 670-750
Rental Contact: Louise Bremers

4830 UNIVERSITY OF NEBRASKA AT LINCOLN LIED CENTER SEASON
Lied Center for Performing Arts
301 N 12th, PO Box 880151
Lincoln, NE 68588-0151
Phone: 402-472-4700
Fax: 402-472-2725
e-mail: cbethea2@unl.edu
Web Site: www.liedcenter.org
Management:
Executive Director: Charles Henry Bethea
Founded: 1989
Specialized Field: State of Nebraska
Paid Staff: 30
Volunteer Staff: 300

4831 HERITAGE DAYS FESTIVAL
PO Box 337
McCook, NE 69001
Phone: 308-345-3200
Fax: 308-345-3201
e-mail: info@aboutmecook.com
Web Site: www.aboutmecook.com
Management:
Director: Moris Owen
Assistant Director: Joan Parsons
Founded: 1969
Specialized Field: Dance; Vocal Music; Instrumental Music; Arts and Crafts
Status: Non-Professional; Nonprofit
Organization Type: Sponsoring

4832 BROWNVILLE CONCERT SERIES
740 S 75th Streer
Omaha, NE 68114
Phone: 402-346-1102
Fax: 402-346-1355
Officers:
Program Chairman: James Keene
Budget: $20,000-35,000

4833 CATHEDRAL ARTS PROJECT SERIES
100 N 62 Street
Omaha, NE 68132
Phone: 402-558-3800
Fax: 402-558-3026
e-mail: dorthy@tuma.net
Web Site: www.cathedralartsproject.org
Management:
Executive Director: William Woeger
Adminstrative Assistant: Dorothy Tuma
Founded: 1986
Specialized Field: Visual/Performing
Paid Staff: 2
Volunteer Staff: 50
Budget: $10,000-20,000
Performs At: St. Cecelia Cathedral

4834 NEBRASKA SHAKESPEARE FESTIVAL
Department of Fine Arts
Creighton University
Omaha, NE 68178
Phone: 402-280-2391
Management:
Artistic Director: Cindy Melby Phaneuf
Managing Director: Michael Markey

4835 TUESDAY MUSICAL CONCERT SERIES
8543 Hickory Street
Omaha, NE 68124
Phone: 402-391-4661
Fax: 402-397-9510
e-mail: barbarataxman@aol.com
Management:
    Program Chairman: Barbara Taxman
Mission: Offering an annual professional concert series.
Founded: 1892
Specialized Field: Present Classical Recitals
Status: Non-Professional; Nonprofit
Volunteer Staff: 30
Budget: $35,000-60,000
Income Sources: Ticket sales; Donations; Grants
Performs At: Joslyn Art Museum
Annual Attendance: 600
Facility Category: Art Museum/Concert Hall
Seating Capacity: 1,000
Organization Type: Sponsoring

4836 UNIVERSITY OF NEBRASKA AT OMAHA MUSIC SERIES
Music Department
60 and Dodge Street
Omaha, NE 68182
Phone: 402-554-3427
Fax: 402-554-2252
e-mail: amerit@mail.unomaha.edu
Web Site: www.unomaha.edu/~finearts/music/events.htm
Officers:
    Chairman Department of Music: James R Saker
Management:
    Events Coordinator: Adrienne Merit
    Coordinator/Performace Series: Roger Foltz
Founded: 1918
Paid Staff: 10
Paid Artists: 25
Non-paid Artists: 50
Budget: $25,000
Income Sources: University Funds, Foundation Support, Grants, Ticket Sales
Performs At: Strauss Performing Arts Center
Annual Attendance: 50,000+
Facility Category: Concert Hall
Type of Stage: Concert Only
Seating Capacity: 500
Year Built: 1975
Cost: $23 million
Rental Contact: Events Coordinator T. Heil

4837 CONCORDIA UNIVERSITY CONCERT SERIES
800 N Columbia Avenue
Seward, NE 68434
Phone: 402-643-7405
Fax: 402-643-4073
Budget: $10,000

4838 WAYNE STATE COLLEGE SPECIAL PROGRAMS BLACK & GOLD SERIES
Wayne State College
Wayne, NE 68787

Phone: 402-375-7359
Fax: 402-375-7204
Management:
    Dean: James O'Donnell
Budget: $35,000-60,000
Performs At: Ramsey Theatre; Ley Theatre

Nevada

4839 BOULDER CITY ARTS COUNCIL
PO Box 61314
Boulder City, NV 89006
Phone: 702-294-1499
Fax: 702-293-7743
Budget: $10,000

4840 NEVADA ARTS COUNCIL
602 N Curry Street
Carson City, NV 89703
Phone: 702-687-6680
Fax: 702-687-6688
e-mail: schannel@clan.lib.nv.us
Web Site: dmia.clan.lib.nv.us
Management:
    Community Development: Suzanne Channel

4841 CHURCHILL ARTS COUNCIL
PO Box 2204
Fallon, NV 89407
Phone: 775-423-1440
Fax: 775-423-0779
e-mail: charts@phonewave.net
Web Site: www.churchillarts.org
Management:
    Director: Valerie J Serpa
Founded: 1986
Specialized Field: Multi
Paid Staff: 2
Volunteer Staff: 20
Paid Artists: 35

4842 REED WHIPPLE CULTURAL ARTS CENTER
821 Las Vegas Boulevard N
Las Vegas, NV 89101
Phone: 702-229-6211
Fax: 702-382-5199
Web Site: www.ci.Las-Vegas.nv.us
Management:
    Center Coordinator: Ellis Rice
    Supervisor: Patricia Harris
Mission: Developing the arts community via programming, community involvement and education.
Founded: 1961
Specialized Field: Dance; Theatre; Concerts
Status: Nonprofit
Paid Staff: 100
Income Sources: American Council for the Arts; Nevada Recreation & Parks Society; Nevada Presenters Network
Affiliations: Las Vegas Civic Center; Las Vegas Woodwing Quintet
Type of Stage: Proscenium

Stage Dimensions: 18'x45'x24'
Seating Capacity: 300
Rental Contact: Patricia Harris
Organization Type: Performing; Touring; Educational; Sponsoring
Resident Groups: Rainbow Theatre Company

4843 UNIVERSITY OF NEVADA: LAS VEGAS MASTER SERIES
4505 Maryland Parkway
Box 455005
Las Vegas, NV 89154-5005
Phone: 702-895-3535
Fax: 702-895-4714
Web Site: www.pac.nevada.edu
Management:
  UNLV Performance Arts Director: Myron Martin

4844 UNIVERSITY OF NEVADA: RENO PERFORMING ARTS SERIES
UNR Division of Continuing Ed/048
Reno, NV 89557
Phone: 775-784-4046
Fax: 775-784-4801
e-mail: cjc@unr.edu
Web Site: www.dce.unr.edu/arts
Budget: $20,000-35,000
Annual Attendance: 3000
Facility Category: recital
Type of Stage: Proscenium
Year Built: 1989

4845 NEVADA SHAKESPEARE FESTIVAL
Box 871
Virginia City, NV 89440
Phone: 775-324-4198
e-mail: information@nevada-shakespeare.org
Web Site: www.nevada-shakespeare.org
Management:
  Communications Director: Martha Quarkziz
Founded: 1996

New Hampshire

4846 KEISER CONCERT SERIES
Saint Paul's School
325 Pleasant Street
Concord, NH 03301-2591
Phone: 603-229-4681
Fax: 603-229-5695
e-mail: dseaton@sps.edu
Management:
  Director: David D Seaton
Founded: 1978
Specialized Field: Music
Budget: 24,000
Seating Capacity: 125-150

4847 WILLIAM H GILE TRUST FUND CONCERT SERIES
17 Pleasant View Avenue
Concord, NH 03301-2555
Phone: 603-224-1217
Fax: 603-228-3901
e-mail: jiffi6s@aol.com
Officers:
  Committee Chairman: Dr. Robert C Rainie
  Advisor: MT Mennino
Budget: $85,000
Income Sources: Trust Fund
Performs At: Chubb Theatre; Capitol Center for the Arts
Annual Attendance: 1,400/performance
Facility Category: Capiyol Center for the Arts
Stage Dimensions: 40' wide/24 1/2' deep/4 1/2' apron
Seating Capacity: 1,425
Rental Contact: CEO M.T. Mennino

4848 NEW HAMPSHIRE SHAKESPEARE FESTIVAL
PO Box 191
Deerfield, NH 03037
Phone: 603-666-9088
e-mail: nhsf@nhsf.org
Web Site: www.nhsf.org
Management:
  Executive Director: Gail Mills
Founded: 1993
Status: Non-Equity; Nonprofit
Season: July - August

4849 UNIVERSITY OF NEW HAMPSHIRE CELEBRITY SERIES
Paul Creative Arts Center, M202
30 College Road
Durham, NH 03824-3538
Phone: 603-862-3242
Fax: 603-862-3155
Web Site: www.unh.edu/mub
Budget: $60,000-150,00
Performs At: Johnson Theatre
Type of Stage: proscenium
Stage Dimensions: 20x40
Seating Capacity: 688a
Year Built: 1963
Rental Contact: Theatre & Dance Dept. Michael Woood

4850 DARTMOUTH COLLEGE HOPKINS CENTER PERFORMING SERIES
Hopkins Center
6041 Lower Level Wilson Hall
Hanover, NH 03755-3543
Phone: 603-646-3453
Fax: 603-646-3911
Web Site: www.hop.dartmouth.edu
Management:
  Programming Director: Margaret Lawrence
Budget: $400,000-1,000,000
Performs At: The Moore Theatre; Rollins Chapel

4851 NEW ENGLAND COLLEGE CULTURAL EVENTS SERIES
24 Bridge Street
Henniker, NH 03242-0793
Phone: 603-428-2303
Budget: $10,000

4852 BELKNAP MILL SOCIETY
The Mill Plaza
Laconia, NH 03246
Phone: 603-524-8813
Management:
Executive Director: Mary Boswell
Budget: $10,000

4853 NORTH COUNTRY CHAMBER PLAYERS SUMMER FESTIVAL: MUSIC IN THE WHITE MOUNTAINS
PO Box 904
Littleton, NH 03561
Phone: 603-444-0309
Fax: 603-444-0309
e-mail: nccp@ncia.net
Web Site: www.newww.com/org/nccp
Officers:
President, Board of Directors: Len Reed
Management:
Executive Director: Stephen Dignazio
Artistic Director: Ronnie Bauch
Mission: Culturally enrich New Hamphire through chamber music performance and music education
Founded: 1978
Status: Nonprofit
Paid Staff: 1
Paid Artists: 12
Budget: $400,000-500,000
Income Sources: Earned Revenues by Government; Foundation; Corporate and Individual Donors

4854 SAINT ANSELM COLLEGE PERFORMING ARTS SERIES
Dana Humanities Center
100 Saint Anselm Drive
Manchester, NH 03104-1310
Phone: 603-641-7710
Fax: 603-641-7332
Web Site: www.anselm.edu
Management:
Campus Events Director: Robert Shea
Budget: $150,000-400,000
Performs At: Koonz Theatre

4855 AMERICAN STAGE FESTIVAL
14 Court Street
Nashua, NH 03060-3478
Phone: 603-889-2330
Fax: 603-889-2336
Web Site: www.americanstagefestival.org
Management:
Production Artistic Director: Robert Walsh
Founded: 1974
Status: Nonprofit

Season: June - August
Type of Stage: Proscenium
Stage Dimensions: 40' x 38'
Seating Capacity: 497

4856 NASHUA COMMUNITY CONCERT ASSOCIATION
31 Cushing Avenue
Nashua, NH 03064
Phone: 603-882-6840
Officers:
President: Ernest D Berube
Budget: $35,000-60,000

4857 COLBY-SAWYER COLLEGE
Ware Campus Center
100 Maint Street
New London, NH 03257
Phone: 603-526-3759
Fax: 603-526-2135
Web Site: www.colby-sawyer.edu
Management:
Campus Activities Director: Sharon Williamson
Budget: $10,000-20,000

4858 SUMMER MUSIC SERIES
PO Box 603
New London, NH 03257
Phone: 603-927-4647
Management:
Program Committee Chairman: Robert Fraley
Mission: Presenter of four summer concerts.
Founded: 1974
Specialized Field: Vocal Music; Instrumental Music
Status: Nonprofit
Budget: $45,000
Income Sources: Contributions; ticket sales
Performs At: College/high schoool/church/town hall facilities
Annual Attendance: 1500
Seating Capacity: 700
Organization Type: Sponsoring

4859 MONADNOCK MUSIC
PO Box 255
Peterborough, NH 03458
Phone: 603-924-7610
Fax: 603-924-9403
e-mail: mm@monadrockmusic.mv.com
Web Site: www.monadrockmusic.org
Officers:
President: Roger Sweet
Treasurer: Vance Finch
Secretary: Faith Hanson
Management:
Music Director: James Bolle
Executive Director: Gregory Pierre Cox
Mission: To present first-rate, professional performances of music representing as wide a repertory as possible; to maintain an atmosphere which is conducive to a close audience-performer relationship; to make these performances truly accessible to people in the Monadnock Region.

Founded: 1966
Specialized Field: Vocal Music; Instrumental Music;
Festivals; Lyric Opera
Status: Professional; Nonprofit
Paid Staff: 6
Paid Artists: 100
Budget: $400,000
Income Sources: Contributions, Grants, Tickets
Performs At: Peterborough Town House
Organization Type: Performing; Educational

4860 PLYMOUTH FRIENDS OF THE ARTS SERIES

Box 386
Plymouth, NH 03264-0386
Phone: 603-536-1182
Fax: 603-536-1182
Management:
   Executive Director: Jane Hamor
Budget: $20,000-35,000
Performs At: Silver Hall

4861 PLYMOUTH STATE COLLEGE SILVER CULTURAL ARTS CENTER SILVER SERIES

Silver Cultural Arts Center
Plymouth State College
Plymouth, NH 03264
Phone: 603-535-2801
Fax: 603-535-2917
e-mail: djeffery@plymouth.edu
Web Site: www.plymouth.edu
Management:
   Director: Diane Jeffery
Specialized Field: Central NH
Paid Staff: 7
Paid Artists: 14
Budget: $35,000-60,000
Income Sources: Ticket Revenue, Sponserships, Grants,
and Donations.
Performs At: Hanaway Theatre; Smith Recital Hall;
Studio Theatre
Facility Category: Performing Arts Center
Type of Stage: Proscenium
Stage Dimensions: 90' x 36'
Seating Capacity: 650
Year Built: 1992
Year Remodeled: 1992
Rental Contact: Director Diane Jeffery

4862 FRIENDS OF THE MUSIC HALL CONCERT SERIES

104 Congress Street
Suite 203
Portsmouth, NH 03801
Phone: 603-433-3100
Fax: 603-431-4103
e-mail: jforde@themusichall.org
Web Site: www.themusichall.org
Management:
   Artistic Director: Jane Forde
Budget: $150,000-400,000

4863 HARBOR ARTS JAZZ NIGHT: PORTSMOUTH JAZZ FESTIVAL

401 The Hill
Portsmouth, NH 03801
Phone: 603-436-8596
Fax: 603-433-2787
e-mail: events@cuzinrichard.com
Web Site: www.jazznightportsmouthnh.com
Management:
   Chairman Jazz Festival: Richard Smith
   Media Management: Joe Kelly
   Museum VP: Bob Marchewka
Mission: Raise funds for Harbor Arts Museum and for
school music art departments/music schools
Founded: 1991
Specialized Field: Performing Arts
Status: Nonprofit
Volunteer Staff: 25

4864 PRESCOTT PARK ARTS FESTIVAL

PO Box 4370
105 Marcy Street
Portsmouth, NH 03802
Phone: 603-436-2748
Management:
   Executive Director: Michael Greenblatt
   Festival Coordinator: Sue Bolduc
   Program Director: Mark Vadney
Mission: To provide a professional wide-ranging arts
festival for a diverse audience combining ticketed and free
access.
Founded: 1974
Specialized Field: Dance; Vocal Music; Theater;
Festivals
Status: Nonprofit
Season: July - August
Performs At: Prescott Park
Organization Type: Performing; Touring; Resident;
Educational; Sponsoring

4865 FRANKLIN PIERCE COLLEGE CRIMSON-GREY CULTURAL SERIES

Franklin Pierce College
Rindge, NH 03461
Phone: 603-899-4152
Fax: 603-899-6448
Management:
   Student Activities Director: Jacqueline Weeks
Budget: $10,000-20,000
Performs At: Fieldhouse; Ravencroft Theater

4866 WATERVILLE VALLEY FOUNDATION SUMMER FESTIVAL

Town Square
Waterville Valley, NH 03215
Phone: 603-236-8311
Fax: 603-236-4344
Web Site: www.waterville.com
Management:
   Town Square Manager: April Smith
Mission: To present a summer festival of the arts.
Founded: 1985

Specialized Field: Vocal Music; Instrumental Music;
Festivals; Concerts
Status: Nonprofit
Performs At: Town Square Concert Pavillion
Organization Type: Performing; Educational

4867 GREAT WATERS MUSIC FESTIVAL

PO Box 488
56 N Main Street
Wolfeboro, NH 03894
Phone: 603-569-7710
Fax: 603-569-7715
e-mail: info@greatwaters.org
Web Site: www.greatwaters.org
Management:
   Executive Director: Ben Anderson
Mission: To present a diversified summer concert series.
Founded: 1985
Facility Category: Acoustic Tent

New Jersey

4868 ASBURY PARK JAZZ FESTIVAL

1 Municipal Plaza
Asbury Park, NJ 07712
Phone: 732-502-5728
Fax: 732-502-5738

4869 GREAT GEORGE FESTIVAL

11 Elmwood Avenue
Belleville, NJ 07109
Phone: 973-759-3819
e-mail: dquinn711@aol.com
Management:
   Producer: Daniel P Quinn

4870 CAPE MAY JAZZ FESTIVAL

PO Box 2065
Cape May, NJ 08204
Phone: 609-884-7277
Fax: 609-884-7248
Web Site: www.capemayjazz.org
Officers:
   President: Carol Stone
Management:
   Artistic Director: Carol Stone
   Executive Director: Jane Henderson Hale
Mission: To hold 2 jazz festivals per year, education
programs and promote jazz to region
Founded: 1994
Specialized Field: Music
Paid Staff: 3
Volunteer Staff: 200
Annual Attendance: 15,000

4871 CAPE MAY MUSIC FESTIVAL

1048 Washington Street
PO Box 340
Cape May, NJ 08204

Phone: 609-884-5404
Fax: 609-884-0574
Toll-free: 800-275-4278
e-mail: mstewart@capemaymac.org
Web Site: www.capemaymac.org
Management:
   Artistic Director: Stephen Rogers Radcliffe
   Deputy Dirctor: Mary E Stewart
Founded: 1990
Specialized Field: Music; Instrumental
Paid Staff: 20
Volunteer Staff: 61
Paid Artists: 111

4872 EDISON ARTS SOCIETY

1729 Woodland Avenue
Edison, NJ 08820
Phone: 908-753-2787
Web Site: www.edisonnj.org
Officers:
   President: Angelo A Orlando
   Vice President: Denise Persico
   Treasurer: Denise Sirna
   Secretary: Karen McNamara
Management:
   Executive Director: Denise Farco

4873 APPEL FARM ARTS AND MUSIC CENTER

PO Box 888
Elmer, NJ 08318
Phone: 856-358-2472
Fax: 856-358-6513
Toll-free: 800-394-1211
e-mail: appelarts@aol.com
Web Site: appelfarm.org
Management:
   Executive Director: Mark E Packer
   Artistic Director: Trudy Hansen
Founded: 1960
Specialized Field: Dance; Vocal Music; Instrumental
Music; Theater; Festivals
Status: Professional; Nonprofit
Paid Staff: 18
Volunteer Staff: 500
Paid Artists: 21
Budget: $2.3 million
Affiliations: ArtPRIDE, NJSCA, SJCA, ABP
Facility Category: Regional Performing Arts Center
Type of Stage: Indoor/Outdoor
Stage Dimensions: 40'x50'
Seating Capacity: 250/12,000
Year Built: 1965
Rental Contact: Conference Center Director Walt Sibley
Organization Type: Performing; Resident; Educational

4874 JOHN HARMS CENTER FOR THE ARTS

30 N Van Brunt Street
Englewood, NJ 07631
Phone: 201-567-5797
Fax: 201-567-7357
e-mail: info@johnharms.org
Web Site: www.johnharms.org
Management:

All listings are in alphabetical order by state, then city, then organization within the city.

Executive Director: Jessica Finkelberg
Business Manager: Steve Nemiroff
Director Education: Cathy Roy
Communications/Marketing: Ed Kirchdoerffer
Founded: 1976
Status: Nonprofit
Paid Staff: 14
Volunteer Staff: 150
Paid Artists: 250
Budget: $3,000,000
Income Sources: Foundations, Grants, Corporate
Support, Individuals, Earned
Annual Attendance: 300,000
Facility Category: Theater
Type of Stage: Proscenium
Stage Dimensions: 33 x 30
Seating Capacity: 1322
Year Built: 1926

**4875 COLLEGE OF NEW JERSEY:
CELEBRATION OF THE ARTS**
Box 7718
Ewing, NJ 08628-0718
Phone: 609-771-2519
Fax: 609-637-5198
e-mail: hill@tcnj.edu
Web Site: www.tcnj.edu
Management:
    Performing Arts Director: Michael A Pedretti
Mission: To present high quality performing arts events
that enhance the cultural life of students, staff and
community.
Specialized Field: Presenting
Paid Staff: 1
Volunteer Staff: 20
Paid Artists: 3

4876 FAIR LAWN SUMMER FESTIVAL
Federated Arts Council
185 Prospect Avenue, Apartment 12M
Hackensack, NJ 07601
Phone: 201-646-1061
Fax: 201-796-5667
Management:
    Director: Isadore Freeman
Budget: $10,000
Annual Attendance: 1,000
Facility Category: Band Shell
Year Built: 1992

**4877 SOUNDFEST CHAMBER MUSIC
FESTIVAL, COLORADO QUARTET**
225 Prospect Avenue
Suite B
Hackensack, NJ 07601
Phone: 508-548-2290
Fax: 201-498-0019
e-mail: soundfest@coloradoquartet.com
Web Site: www.coloradoquartet.com
Management:
    Director: Diane Chaplin

**4878 CENTENARY COLLEGE PERFORMING
ARTS GUILD**
400 Jefferson Street
Hackettstown, NJ 07840
Phone: 908-979-0900
Fax: 908-979-4297
e-mail: rustc@centenarycollege.edu
Web Site: www.centenarystageco.org
Management:
    Producing Director: Carl Wallnau
    Associate Producer: Catherine Rust
    Education/Outreach Director: Maria Brodeur Ludwig
Founded: 1920
Paid Staff: 5
Volunteer Staff: 25
Paid Artists: 30
Non-paid Artists: 3

**4879 COMMUNITY ARTS PARTNERSHIP
SERIES WITH PEDDIE SCHOOL**
The Peddie School
Box A, S Main Street
Highstown, NJ 08520
Phone: 609-490-7550
Fax: 609-426-9019
e-mail: rrund@peddie.org
Web Site: www.peddie.org
Management:
    Executive Director: Robert Rund
Mission: Performing and Visual Arts Presenter and
Producer
Budget: $250,000
Performs At: William Mount-Burke Theatre; Masland
Room
Type of Stage: Proscenium
Seating Capacity: 535

4880 AM PRODUCTIONS SERIES
2 Woodland Road
Holmdel, NJ 07733
Phone: 732-264-2111
Fax: 732-264-0081
Toll-free: 800-995-8085
e-mail: amprod@aol.com
Officers:
    President: Stanley Andrucyk
Management:
    Marketing: Terry y McDermott
    Operations: Steven Katz
Founded: 1979
Paid Staff: 28
Volunteer Staff: 30

4881 NEW JERSEY REPERTORY COMPANY
179 Broadway
Long Branch, NJ 07740
Phone: 732-229-3166
Fax: 732-229-3167
e-mail: info@njrep.org
Web Site: www.njrep.org
Officers:
    Director Marketing: Debbie Mura
Management:

Artistic Director: SuzAnne Barabas
Executive Director: Gabor Barabas
Mission: The primary mission of the theater is to develop and produce new plays with diverse themes. It is also devoted to creating an atmosphere where classics can take on a fresh look and forgotten plays can find a home.
Founded: 1997
Status: Professional
Income Sources: Donation, Grants
Facility Category: Theater
Type of Stage: Black Box
Year Remodeled: 1998

4882 ARTS COUNCIL OF THE MORRIS AREA

PO Box 370
Madison, NJ 07940
Phone: 973-377-6622
Fax: 973-301-2040
e-mail: info@morrisarts.org
Web Site: www.morrisarts.org
Management:
Executive Director: Carolyn T Ward
Budget: $60,000-150,000

4883 NEW JERSEY SHAKESPEARE FESTIVAL

36 Madison Avenue (at Lancaster Road)
Madison, NJ 07940
Phone: 973-408-3278
Fax: 973-408-3361
e-mail: njsf@njshakespeare.org
Web Site: www.njshakespeare.org
Officers:
Board President: Jeanne Barrett
Management:
Artistic Director: Bonnie J Monte
Managing Director: Frank Mack
Chairman of the Board: S Dillard Kirby
Mission: The Festival strives to illuminate the universal and lasting relevance of the classics for contemporary audiences, and its mission places an equal emphasis on education, for young artists and audiences alike.
Founded: 1962
Specialized Field: Theatrical Group
Status: Professional; Nonprofit
Paid Staff: 35
Paid Artists: 120
Budget: 2.6 million
Income Sources: Actors' Equity Association; Society for Stage Directors and Choreographers; New Jersey State Council on the Arts; Corporations; Foundations, Businesses; Individuals
Season: May - December
Performs At: F.M. Kirby Shakespeare Theatre
Affiliations: New Jersey Theatre Group; Theatre Communications Group; Shakespeare Association of America; ArtPride; Artsweb NJ/NY
Annual Attendance: 100,000
Stage Dimensions: 28' wide x 33' deep
Seating Capacity: 308
Year Built: 1998
Organization Type: Performing; Educational; Sponsoring; Touring

4884 ALGONQUIN ARTS

171 Main Street, Suite 202
PO Box Q
Manasquan, NJ 08736
Phone: 732-528-9211
Fax: 732-528-3881
Web Site: www.manasquan-nj.org/algonquin
Officers:
President: John Drew
Treasurer: Frances Drew
Secretary: Marguerite Zschiegner
Management:
Executive Director: Frances Drew
Assistant Executive Director: Thomas Stephens
Founded: 1992
Specialized Field: Facility; Performing; multi-discipline
Paid Staff: 4
Volunteer Staff: 2
Paid Artists: 120
Non-paid Artists: 25

4885 ACADEMY OF SAINT ELIZABETH PERFORMING ARTS SERIES

Saint Elizabeth
2 Convent Road
Morristown, NJ 07960-6989
Phone: 973-290-0045
Management:
Artist in Residence: Dr. Teresa Walters
Budget: $10,000
Performs At: Founders Hall; McGuire Lounge

4886 RUTGERS UNIVERSITY CONCERT SERIES

106 Walters Hall
New Brunswick, NJ 08907
Phone: 732-932-7591
Fax: 732-932-6973
Management:
Assistant Dean Arts Programming: Lance Olson
Marketing Director: Charles Fessenden
Publicity Director: Ellen Saxon
Operations Manager: Kevin Coleman
Box Office Manager: Jeanne Salzman
Mission: To offer performances by contemporary musicians.
Founded: 1917
Specialized Field: Instrumental Music
Status: Professional
Performs At: Rutgers Arts Center
Organization Type: Presenting

4887 STATE THEATRE/NEW BRUNSWICK CULTURAL CENTER

11 Livingston Avenue
New Brunswick, NJ 08901
Phone: 732-247-7200
Fax: 732-247-4005
Toll-free: 877-782-8311
e-mail: info@statetheatrenj.org
Web Site: www.StateTheatreNJ.org
Officers:
President: Chris Butler

Management:
    Marketing/Public Relations Director: Marc Fleming
    Education Director: Lian Farer
    General Manager: David Hartkern
Mission: To present the finest of the performing arts.
Specialized Field: Presenting
Status: Nonprofit
Budget: $2,000,000
Performs At: State Theatre
Seating Capacity: 1800
Year Built: 1921
Year Remodeled: 1987
Organization Type: Performing; Educational;
Sponsoring

4888 NEW JERSEY SYMPHONY ORCHESTRA AMADEUS FESTIVAL

2 Central Avenue
Newark, NJ 07102
Phone: 973-624-3713
Fax: 973-624-2115
e-mail: kswanson@njsymphony.org
Web Site: www.njsymphony.org
Management:
    Music Director: Zdenek Macal

4889 NEWARK MUSEUM ASSOCIATION

49 Washington Street
PO Box 540
Newark, NJ 07101-0540
Phone: 973-596-6550
Fax: 973-642-0459
Toll-free: 800-768-7386
e-mail: pubblicrelations@newarkmusium.org
Web Site: www.newarkmuseum.org
Mission: The americas and the Pacific, Ancient Egypt,
Greece and Rome, Decorative Arts, Science, Planetarium,
Mini Zoo, Natural Sciences, Newark Black Film Festival,
Jazz in the Garden, Family, Adult and children's
programing
Founded: 1909
Specialized Field: American, Fold, Tibetan, Asian,
Africe
Budget: $20,000-35,000
Performs At: Billy Johnson Auditorium

4890 ANNUAL OCEAN GROVE CHOIR FESTIVAL

PO Box 126
Ocean Grove, NJ 07756
Phone: 732-775-0035
Fax: 732-775-5689
e-mail: info@oceangrove.org
Web Site: www.oceangrove.org
Management:
    Music Director: Lewis A Daniels

4891 RARITAN RIVER CONCERT SERIES

Box 454
Oldwick, NJ 08858-0454
Phone: 908-213-1100
Management:
    Music Co-Director: Michael Newman

Budget: $10,000

4892 RARITAN RIVER MUSIC FESTIVAL

PO Box 454
Oldwick, NJ 08858-0454
Phone: 908-213-1100
Management:
    Co-Music Director: Thomas Gallant

4893 JULIUS FORSTMANN LIBRARY SECOND SUNDAY SERIES

195 Gregory Avenue
Passaic, NJ 07055
Phone: 973-779-0474
Fax: 973-779-0889
Management:
    Music Director: Laurie Sansone

4894 PASSAIC COUNTY COMMUNITY COLLEGE SERIES

1 College Boulevard
Paterson, NJ 07505-1179
Phone: 973-684-6555
Fax: 973-684-5843
Web Site: www.pccc.cc.nj.us
Management:
    Cultural Affairs Director: Maria M Gillan
Mission: To serve poets and poetry, bring performing arts
to elementary schools and enjoy the arts as a community.
Founded: 1968
Specialized Field: Poetry; Childrens Theater; Art
Galleries
Paid Staff: 7
Paid Artists: 45
Budget: $35,000-60,000
Income Sources: Nassaic County College; NJ State
Council of the Arts; Geraldine K. Dodge Foundation
Performs At: Theater; Reading Rooms
Type of Stage: Proscenium
Seating Capacity: 300
Year Built: 1968
Year Remodeled: 1999
Rental Contact: Edna Ortiz

4895 CRESCENT CONCERTS

71 Watchung Avenue
Plainfield, NJ 07060
Phone: 908-756-2468
Fax: 908-756-3158
Web Site: www.capc.org
Officers:
    President: Alan Ganun
Management:
    Director: Ronald Thayer
Mission: Classical concert series, one per month from
October to May, all performances at Cresceent Avenue
Presbyterian Chruch.
Founded: 1981
Specialized Field: Vocal and Instrumental Music
Status: Active
Paid Staff: 1
Volunteer Staff: 12
Paid Artists: 50

Non-paid Artists: 125

4896 PRINCETON SHAKESPEARE FESTIVAL
44 Nassau Street
Suite 350
Princeton, NJ 08542
Phone: 609-921-3682
Web Site: www.princetonrep.org
Management:
  Artistic Director: Victoria Liberatori
  Executive Producer: Anne Reiss
  Press Contact: Carol Fineman
Founded: 1995
Status: Professional; Not-for-Profit

4897 PRINCETON UNIVERSITY CONCERTS
Woolworth Center
Princeton, NJ 08544
Phone: 609-258-4239
Fax: 609-258-1179
Management:
  Concert Manager: Nathan A Randall
Budget: $60,000-150,000
Performs At: Richardson Auditorium

4898 YOUNG AUDIENCES OF NEW JERSEY
12 Rpszel Road
Suite B102
Princeton, NJ 08540
Phone: 609-243-9000
Fax: 609-243-5999
e-mail: info@yanj.org
Web Site: www.yanj.org
Mission: To provide arts in education programs and
services to schools and other community settings.
Founded: 1973
Budget: $400,000-1,000,000

4899 RINGWOOD FRIENDS OF MUSIC SERIES
17 Kraft Place
Ringwood, NJ 07456
Phone: 973-962-6118
Officers:
  President: Donaldo Garcia
Budget: $10,000
Performs At: Ringwood Community Church

4900 WILLIAMS CENTER FOR THE ARTS
One Williams Plaza
Rutherford, NJ 07070
Phone: 201-939-6969
Fax: 201-939-0843
Web Site: www.williamscenter.org
Officers:
  President: Richard Theryoung
  Vice President: Carolyn Spann-Swallwood
  Secretary: Dr. Joseph DeFazi
  Treasurer: Evelyn Spath-Mercado
Management:
  Executive Director: GW McLuckey
Mission: To provide programs of artistic excellence at
affordable prices.

Founded: 1978
Paid Staff: 22
Budget: $650,000
Income Sources: Ticket Sales; grants; sponsorships;
rentals
Performs At: Newman Theatre
Annual Attendance: 50,000
Facility Category: Performing Arts Center
Type of Stage: Black Box; Proscenium Arch
Seating Capacity: 200; 642
Year Built: 1922
Year Remodeled: 1992
Rental Contact: G.W. McLuckey

4901 WATERLOO FOUNDATION FOR THE ARTS SERIES
525 Waterloo Road
Stanhope, NJ 07874
Phone: 973-347-0900
Fax: 973-347-3573
e-mail: info@waterloovillage.org
Web Site: www.waterloovillage.org
Officers:
  Controller: Cule Jorden
Management:
  Executive Director: Geoffery Opertner
  Director Museum Operations: John Kraft
Mission: To combine history, music, art and architecture;
to educate all persons in the state of New Jersey in
appreciation of these arts forms.
Founded: 1967
Specialized Field: Vocal Music; Instrumental Music;
Theater; Festivals; Historic Programs
Status: Professional; Nonprofit
Paid Staff: 10
Volunteer Staff: 40
Budget: $ 2.5 Million
Income Sources: Gate Admissions; New Jersey State
Council of the Arts; New Jersey Tourism Council;
Business/Corporate Donations
Season: April - November
Performs At: Waterloo Music Festival Tent; Waterloo
Concert Field
Affiliations: New Jersey Tourism Council
Annual Attendance: 150,000
Facility Category: Seasonal
Seating Capacity: 2,200-15,000
Year Built: 1964
Year Remodeled: 1997
Organization Type: Performing; Sponsoring

4902 CENTRAL PRESBYTERIAN CHURCH BROWN BAG CONCERT SERIES
70 Maple Street
Summit, NJ 07901
Phone: 908-273-0441
Fax: 908-273-0444
Management:
  Music Director: Noel Werner

4903 OCEAN COUNTY COLLEGE FINE & PERFORMING ARTS SELECT-A-SERIES
Ocean County College
College Drive
Toms River, NJ 08754
Phone: 732-255-0500
Fax: 732-255-0444
Management:
Fine Arts Center Director: Roberta F Krantz
Paid Staff: 3
Budget: $35,000-60,000
Income Sources: Ticket Sales
Facility Category: Fine Arts Center
Type of Stage: Proscenium
Seating Capacity: 564
Year Built: 1972
Rental Contact: Ronnie Mahoney

4904 JETTE PERFORMANCE COMPANY
10 Raymond Terrace
Vauxhall, NJ 07088
Phone: 212-459-4210
Fax: 212-840-0344
e-mail: JetteJazz@excite.com
Web Site: www.jettejazz.org
Management:
Artistic Director: JT Jenkins
Mission: Creates a fusion of classical and commersials styles of dance and brings them to the concert stage.
Founded: 1996
Specialized Field: Dance

4905 JAZZ IT UP FESTIVAL
William Paterson University
300 Pompton Road
Wayne, NJ 07470
Phone: 973-720-2371
Web Site: www.wpunj.edu

4906 WILLIAM PATERSON COLLEGE: THE JAZZ ROOM SERIES
300 Pompton Road
Wayne, NJ 07470
Phone: 973-720-2268
Fax: 973-720-2217
Management:
Producer: Martin Krivin
Artistic Advisor: Rufus Reid
Mission: Presenting a complete range of jazz music.
Founded: 1978
Specialized Field: Instrumental Music
Status: Professional
Performs At: Shea Center for the Performing Arts
Organization Type: Performing

4907 WILLOWBROOK JAZZ FESTIVAL
William Paterson College
300 Pompton Road
Wayne, NJ 07470
Phone: 201-595-2268
Fax: 201-595-2460
Management:
Special Projects Assistant: Dr. Martin Krivin

Director Jazz Program at William: Rufus Reid
Mission: Making jazz accessible by offering free concerts at convenient times and places.
Specialized Field: Jazz
Status: Professional; Nonprofit
Performs At: Willowbrook Mall
Organization Type: Performing

4908 YM-YWHA OF NORTH JERSEY CULTURAL ARTS SERIES
1 Pike Drive
Wayne, NJ 07470-2497
Phone: 973-595-0100
Fax: 973-595-5234
Management:
Cultural Arts Director: Sheila Hellman
Budget: $60,000-150,000
Performs At: Rosen Auditorium

New Mexico

4909 CHAMBER MUSIC ALBUQUERQUE PRESENTS THE JUNE MUSIC FESTIVAL
2400 Louisiana Boulevard NE
#3-215
Albuquerque, NM 87110
Phone: 505-268-1990
Fax: 505-268-6288
e-mail: cma@cma-abq.org
Web Site: www.cma-abq.org
Officers:
President: Heidi Frost Heard
VP: Calla Ann Pepmueller
Secretary: Geoffrey M Kalmu
Management:
Administrative Director: Judith O Smith
Mission: To present the world's finest chamber musicians in live performance, sharing the power of great music with the community.
Founded: 1942
Affiliations: June Music Festival; Chamber Music at the Simms

4910 NEW MEXICO JAZZ WORKSHOP
PO Box 40330
Albuquerque, NM 87103
Phone: 505-255-9798
Fax: 505-232-8420
e-mail: nmjw@flash.net
Web Site: www.flash.net/mmjw
Officers:
President: Paul Mansfield
Management:
Executive Director: Ed Uhlman
Education Coordinator: Sara Hutchinson
Mission: To present major jazz artists January-May for performing and educational activities.
Specialized Field: Jazz
Status: Professional; Nonprofit
Paid Staff: 2
Volunteer Staff: 50
Paid Artists: 30

Performs At: Hiland Theater; Kimo Theater
Facility Category: Various local venues
Organization Type: Performing; Touring

4911 CARLSBAD COMMUNITY CONCERT ASSOCIATION
611 N 4th Street
Carlsbad, NM 88220
Phone: 505-885-8255
Management:
   Manager: Jed Howard
Budget: $20,000-35,000

4912 DONA ANA ARTS COUNCIL
224 N Campo
Las Cruces, NM 88001
Phone: 505-523-6403
Budget: $20,000-35,000

4913 PAN AMERICAN CENTER
MSC 35E
PO Box 30001, Dept 3SE
New Mexico State University
Las Cruces, NM 88003
Phone: 505-646-4413
Fax: 505-646-3605
e-mail: wlofdahl@nmsu.edu
Web Site: panam.nmsu.edu
Management:
   Director Special Events: Will Lofdahl
Mission: Special events facilities, 13,000 seat arena, 500 seat Performing Arts Center
Paid Staff: 14

4914 LOS ALAMOS CONCERT ASSOCIATION
Box 572
Los Alamos, NM 87544
Phone: 505-662-9000
Web Site: www.losalamos.org/laca
Management:
   Artistic Director: Rosalie Heller
Founded: 1946
Volunteer Staff: 20
Paid Artists: 5
Budget: $35,000-60,000
Performs At: Duane Smith Auditorium

4915 PLACITAS ARTISTS SERIES
PO Box 944
Placitas, NM 87043
Phone: 505-867-2471
e-mail: Scoro9451@aol.com
Management:
   Artistic Director: Sally Curro
Budget: $20,000-35,000

4916 EASTERN NEW MEXICO UNIVERSITY
Station 17
Portales, NM 88130
Phone: 505-562-2153
Fax: 505-562-2822
Web Site: www.enmu.edu/athletics.html

Management:
   Athletic Director: Michael Maguire

4917 SANTA FE CHAMBER MUSIC FESTIVAL
PO Box 853
Santa Fe, NM 87504-0853
Phone: 505-983-2075
Fax: 505-986-0251
e-mail: evollmer@santafechambermusic.org
Web Site: www.santafechambermusic.org
Officers:
   President: Quarrier Cook
Management:
   Artistic Director: Marc Neikrug
   Executive Director: Robert Glick
Mission: To produce innovative chamber music concerts and related educational programs of exceptional artistic quality; to serve as a chamber music center attracting American musicians, composers and audiences whose combined influence, stimulation and energy will benefit American culture.
Founded: 1973
Specialized Field: Chamber Music, Jazz, World Music
Status: Professional; Nonprofit
Paid Staff: 12
Budget: 1.6 k
Performs At: Saint Francis Auditorium; Museum of Fine Arts
Annual Attendance: 11,000
Organization Type: Performing; Touring; Resident; Educational

4918 SANTA FE CONCERT ASSOCIATION
210 E Marcy Street
Santa Fe, NM 87501
Mailing Address: PO Box 4626, Santa Fe, NM. 87502
Phone: 505-984-8759
Fax: 505-984-8759
e-mail: sfca@gateway.net
Web Site: www.musicone.org
Officers:
   President: Clifford Vernick
Management:
   Managing Director: William Mullen
Budget: $60,000-150,000
Performs At: St. Francis Auditorium; James A. Little Theatre

4919 TWENTIETH CENTURY UNLIMITED SERIES
PO Box 2631
Santa Fe, NM 87504-2631
Phone: 505-820-6401
Fax: 505-995-0941
Management:
   Director: Eleanor C Eisenmenger

4920 TAOS ART ASSOCIATION
133 N Pueblo Road
Taos, NM 87571

Phone: 505-758-2052
Fax: 505-751-3305
e-mail: taa@taos.newmex.xom
Web Site: www.taosnet.com/taa
Management:
    Interim Executive Director: Bruce Ross

4921 TAOS SCHOOL CHAMBER MUSIC FESTIVAL

PO Box 1879
Taos, NM 87571
Phone: 505-776-2388
e-mail: tsofm@newmex.com
Web Site: www.taosschoolofmusic.com
Officers:
    President/Treasurer: Chilton Anderson
    VP: R Jamesson Burns
    Secretary: Grace M Parr
Management:
    Director: Chilton Anderson
Mission: Study and performance of chamber music.
Founded: 1963
Specialized Field: Instrumental Music; Festivals
Status: Nonprofit
Paid Artists: 6
Budget: $100,000
Income Sources: Contributions; Grants; Tuition
Performs At: Taos Community Auditorium; Hotel St. Bernard
Facility Category: Auditorium
Type of Stage: Platform
Seating Capacity: 290; 150
Organization Type: Performing; Educational
Resident Groups: Chicago String Quartet

New York

4922 AMERICAN MUSIC FESTIVAL

19 Clinton Avenue
Albany, NY 12207
Phone: 518-465-4755
Fax: 518-465-3711
e-mail: aso@global2000.net
Web Site: www.global2000.net/aso
Management:
    Manager: Sharon Walsh

4923 L'ENSEMBLE CHAMBER MUSIC

PO Box 38024
Albany, NY 12203-8024
Phone: 518-436-5321
Fax: 518-436-5322
Management:
    Executive/Artistic Director: Ida Faiella

4924 ALFRED UNIVERSITY ARTIST SERIES

Performing Arts Division
Alfred, NY 14802

Mailing Address: PO Box 781
Phone: 607-871-2562
Fax: 607-871-2587
e-mail: forsky@Alfred.edu
Web Site: www.alfred.edu
Management:
    Performing Arts Head: S Crosby
    Admissions Director: Scott Hooker
    Acting Professor: Becky Prophet
    Tech Theater: Michael Duprey
Mission: To provide professional performing artists for the area.
Founded: 1836
Specialized Field: Dance; Instrumental Music; Theater
Paid Staff: 1
Organization Type: Performing; Educational; Sponsoring

4925 MUSIC FESTIVAL OF THE HAMPTONS

PO Box 1525
Amagansett, NY 11930
Toll-free: 800-644-4418
Web Site: www.thehamptons.com/music_festival
Management:
    Artistic Director: Lukas Foss

4926 AMSTERDAM AREA COMMUNITY CONCERT ASSOCIATION

31 Young Avenue
Amsterdam, NY 12010
Phone: 518-843-3247
Budget: $10,000-20,000

4927 BARD MUSIC FESTIVAL

Bard College
Annandale-on-Hudson, NY 12504
Phone: 845-758-7410
Fax: 845-758-8043
e-mail: loftin@bard.edu
Web Site: www.bard.edu/bmf
Management:
    Executive Director: Mark Loftin

4928 LORRAINE PRODUCTIONS: EAST/WEST

28-04 33th Street
Suite 8
Astoria, NY 11102
Phone: 718-721-9785
Management:
    Executive Director: Scott Douglas Morrow
Budget: $150,000-400,000

4929 GENESEE COMMUNITY COLLEGE FINE ARTS COMMITTEE SERIES

1 College Road
Batavia, NY 14020
Phone: 716-345-6814
Fax: 716-345-6815
e-mail: mkmorrison@sunygenesee.suny-edu
Web Site: www.sunygenesee.cc.ny.us
Management:

Fine/Performing Arts Director: Marcia K Morrison
Box Office Manager: Patricia A Hawley

4930 PROFESSIONAL PERFORMING ARTS SERIES
Queensborough Community College/Cuny
222-05 56 Avenue
Bayside, NY 11364-1497
Phone: 718-631-6321
Fax: 718-631-6033
e-mail: acarobine@qcc.cuny.edu
Web Site: www.qcc.cuny.edu/boxoffice
Management:
 Executive Director: Sophia Fogliane
 Director Performing Arts: Anthony Carobine
Budget: $60,000-150,000
Annual Attendance: 12,000-15,000
Facility Category: Conventional Theatre
Type of Stage: Proscenium
Stage Dimensions: 40x40
Seating Capacity: 875
Year Built: 1970
Rental Contact: Terry Doria

4931 BINGHAMTON SUMMER MUSIC FESTIVAL
PO Box 112
Binghamton, NY 13903
Phone: 607-777-4777
Fax: 607-777-4000
e-mail: bsmf1@yahoo.com
Web Site: www.summermusic.binghamtom.edu
Officers:
 President: Jim Reyer
 VP: Karl Hirshman
 Secretary: Jim Gacioch
 Treasurer: Larry Deminster
Management:
 Executive Director: Kelly Wakeman
Mission: To provide an annual summer performing arts program for audiences in New York's Southern Tier.
Founded: 1985
Specialized Field: Dance; Vocal Music; Instrumental Music; Festivals
Status: Nonprofit
Paid Staff: 1
Volunteer Staff: 24
Paid Artists: 9
Performs At: Anderson Center for Performing Arts
Organization Type: Performing; Educational

4932 STATE UNIVERSITY OF NEW YORK AT BINGHAMTON PERFORMING ARTS SERIES
Binghamton University
Anderson Center for the Arts, PO Box 6000
Binghamton, NY 13902-6000
Phone: 607-777-6802
Fax: 607-777-6771
Web Site: www.anderson.binghamton.edu
Management:
 Director: Floyd R Herzog
Budget: $60,000-150,000

Performs At: Cmaber Hall; Watters Theater

4933 BAY SHORE-BRIGHTWATERS LIBRARY PERFORMING ARTS SERIES
1 S Country Road
Brightwaters, NY 11718
Phone: 631-665-4350
Fax: 631-665-4958
e-mail: jcreilly@suffolk.lib.ny.us
Management:
 Executive Director: John Clark
 Director: Judith Reilly
Budget: $35,000-60,000
Performs At: Suffolk Community College

4934 651 ARTS
651 Fulton Street
Brooklyn, NY 11217
Phone: 718-636-4181
Fax: 718-636-4166
e-mail: ionfo@651ARTS.org
Web Site: www.651ARTS.org
Management:
 Executive Director: Maurine Knighton

4935 ARTS AT ST. ANN'S
70 Washington Street
Brooklyn, NY 11201
Phone: 718-834-8794
Fax: 718-522-2470
e-mail: info@artsatstanns.org
Web Site: www.artsatstanns.org
Management:
 Artistic Director: Susan Feldman
Founded: 1979
Paid Staff: 8
Volunteer Staff: 10
Budget: $1,500,000
Income Sources: Foundation; Corporate; Government; Individual; Earned Income

4936 BROOKLYN ACADEMY OF MUSIC
30 Lafayette Avenue
Brooklyn, NY 11217
Phone: 718-636-4100
Fax: 718-857-2021
Officers:
 Chairman: Neil Chrisman
 Vice Chairman: Rita Hillman
 Vice Chairman: Franklin Weissberg
 Vice Chairman: I. Stanley Kriegel
 VP: David Kleiser
 Executive VP: Judith E. Daykin
 Treasurer: Richard Balzano
 President: Karen Brooks Hopkins
Management:
 Executive Producer: Joseph V Melilo
 Managing Director: Judith E Daykin
 Finance: Richard Balzano
 Promotion/Marketing: Doug Allan

Mission: Programming policy involves a commitment to provide our audiences with quality performing arts, new and innovative theatre, and dance and music, both foreign and domestic, as well as diversified choices in all areas at affordable and accessible prices.
Founded: 1861
Specialized Field: Dance; Vocal Music; Instrumental Music; Theater; Festivals
Status: Professional; Nonprofit
Income Sources: New York Department of Cultural Affairs
Performs At: Brooklyn Academy of Music
Organization Type: Performing; Touring; Educational; Sponsoring

4937 CELEBRATE BROOKLYN FESTIVAL

647 Fulton Street
Brooklyn, NY 11217
Phone: 718-855-7882
Fax: 718-802-9095
e-mail: celebrate@brooklyn.org
Web Site: www.brooklyn.org
Officers:
President: Nanette Rainone
Management:
Director: Jack Walsh
Mission: Supporting Brooklyn's international community through the presentation of original and professional performing arts.
Founded: 1979
Specialized Field: Dance; Vocal Music; Instrumental Music; Theater; Festivals
Status: Professional; Nonprofit
Performs At: Prospect Park Bandshell and Picnic House
Annual Attendance: 200,000
Facility Category: Ampitheatre
Type of Stage: Sprung Wood
Stage Dimensions: 70x40
Seating Capacity: 10,000
Year Built: 1939
Year Remodeled: 1999
Cost: $3.4 million
Rental Contact: Director Jack Walsh
Organization Type: Performing

4938 CW POST CHAMBER MUSIC FESTIVAL

Long Island University, CW Post Campus
720 Northern Boulevard
Brookville, NY 11548
Phone: 516-299-2103
Fax: 516-299-2884
Web Site: www.liu.edu/svpa/music/festival
Management:
Co-Director: Susan Deaver
Co-Director: Maureen Hynes
Mission: To study and perform of standard chamber music repertoire.
Founded: 1981
Paid Staff: 2
Volunteer Staff: 2
Paid Artists: 15
Performs At: Long Island And New York Metropolitan Area.

4939 AFRICAN-AMERICAN CULTURAL CENTER

350 Masten Avenue
Buffalo, NY 14209
Phone: 716-884-2013
Fax: 716-885-2590
e-mail: aacc@pcom.net
Web Site: www.paulrobesontheatre.com
Officers:
Chairman: Darlene Badgett
Vice Chairman: Emma Bassett
Secretary: Gwendolyn Neal
Treasurer: Paulett S. Counts
Management:
Executive Director: Agnes M Bain
Artistic Director: Paulette D Harris
Mission: Developing appreciation for African traditions through cultural events and the arts.
Founded: 1958
Specialized Field: Dance; Theater
Status: Nonprofit
Paid Staff: 35
Performs At: Paul Robeson Theatre
Type of Stage: proscenium
Stage Dimensions: 40x18
Seating Capacity: 130
Organization Type: Performing; Sponsoring

4940 JUNE IN BUFFALO

SUNY at Buffalo
222 Haird Hall
Buffalo, NY 14260
Phone: 716-645-2765
Fax: 716-645-3824
e-mail: mbg2@acsu.buffalo.edu
Web Site: www.music.buffalo.edu/jib
Officers:
Administrative Associate: Mara Gibson
Management:
Artistic Director: David Felder
Assistant Director: Amy Williams
Director Music Technology: David Boyle
Internet Design: Sam Hamm
Mission: To sponsor festival and conference dedicated to emerging composers, and the opportunity to work with outstanding professional musicians and distinguished composition faculty.
Founded: 1975
Status: Professional

4941 VIVA VIVALDI FESTIVAL XXIII

Ars Nova Musicians Chamber Orchestra
136 Goethe Street
Buffalo, NY 14206
Phone: 716-662-3598
Fax: 716-894-2456
e-mail: arsnovamusicians@aol.com
Management:
Music Director/Conductor: Marylouise Nanna
Executive/Managing Director: Susan Willet
Mission: ARS Nova Musicians is dedicated to performing a varied repertoire that extends from early Baroque through contemporary music, including frequent premiers.

Constantly aspire through creative and innovative means to attract new audiences to this wonderful medium of the musical art, called Chamber Music.
Founded: 1974
Specialized Field: Buffalo, Western New York, Southern Ontario, Northeastern Pennsylvania, Northern Ohio

4942 CHAUTAUQUA INSTITUTION

PO Box 28
Chautauqua, NY 14722
Phone: 716-357-6200
Fax: 716-357-9014
Toll-free: 800-836-2787
e-mail: info@chautauqua-inst.org
Web Site: www.chautaugua-inst.org
Management:
    Program Director: Marty Merkley
Mission: Combining the arts, religion, recreation and education in a Victorian community.
Founded: 1874
Specialized Field: Dance; Vocal Music; Instrumental Music; Theater; Grand Opera
Status: Professional; Semi-Professional; Non-Professional; Nonprofit
Paid Staff: 300
Income Sources: Opera America; American Symphony Orchestra League; Association for Performing Arts Presenters; Music Educators National Conference; American Arts Alliance
Performs At: Amphitheater; Norton Hall
Organization Type: Performing; Resident; Educational; Sponsoring

4943 PERFORMING ARTS AT HAMILTON

Performing Arts
Hamilton College
Clinton, NY 13323
Phone: 315-859-4350
Fax: 315-859-4632
e-mail: performingarts@hamilton.edu
Management:
    Performing Arts Director: Michelle Reiser-Memmer
Budget: $60,000-150,000
Performs At: Wellin Hall; Schambach Center

4944 HUDSON VALLEY SHAKESPEARE FESTIVAL

155 Main Street
Cold Spring, NY 10516
Phone: 845-265-7858
Fax: 845-265-7865
e-mail: info@shakespeare.org
Web Site: www.hvshakespeare.org
Officers:
    President: Sarah Geer
    Vice President: Betsy Simons
    Treasurer: Jerrold Gretzinger
Management:
    Executive Director: Susan Landstreet
    Artistic Director: Terrence O'Brien
    Director Marketing: Abigail Adams
Founded: 1987
Specialized Field: Summer Theater
Status: Nonprofit

Volunteer Staff: 250
Paid Artists: 24
Non-paid Artists: 11
Budget: $735,000
Income Sources: Ticket Sales and Fundraising
Season: June, July, August
Performs At: Tent Theater
Annual Attendance: 24,000
Type of Stage: Thrust
Seating Capacity: 450

4945 COOPERSTOWN CONCERT SERIES

PO Box 624
Cooperstown, NY 13326
Phone: 607-547-2918
Fax: 617-547-2918
Officers:
    Co-Director: Jane Johngren
    Co-Director: Donna Thomson
    Treasurer: Lois Hopper
    Secretary: Dottie Leslie
Management:
    Co-Director: Richard Brown
    Co-Director: Pamela Huntsman
Mission: To promote the cultural growth of our community by presenting live performances of high quality.
Founded: 1970
Specialized Field: Dance; Vocal Music; Instrumental Music; Theater
Status: Nonprofit
Budget: $10,000-20,000
Performs At: Sterling Auditorium
Organization Type: Sponsoring

4946 COOPERSTOWN THEATRE & MUSIC FESTIVAL

PO Box 851
Cooperstown, NY 13326
Phone: 607-547-2335
Management:
    Producer: Margarita Malinova

4947 CLARION CONCERTS IN COLUMBIA COUNTY

Box 43
Copake, NY 12516
Phone: 518-325-3815
Management:
    Music Director: Sanford Allen

4948 A FESTIVAL OF ART

1 Baron Steuben Place
Suite 8, Market Street
Corning, NY 14830
Phone: 607-962-5871
Fax: 607-936-2235
e-mail: thearts@stny.lrun.com
Web Site: www.eARTS.org
Management:
    Executive Director: Janet Newcomb

4949 CORNING-PAINTED POST CIVIC MUSIC ASSOCIATION
PO Box 1402
Corning, NY 14830
Phone: 607-936-9493
Fax: 607-974-7522
Web Site: www.pennynet.org/civicmus.htm
Mission: To provide professional performers at the lowest possible cost.
Founded: 1928
Specialized Field: Dance; Vocal Music; Instrumental Music; Jazz; Classical Presentation
Status: Professional
Budget: $60,000-150,000
Performs At: Corning Glass Center Auditorium
Organization Type: Performing

4950 STATE UNIVERSITY OF NEW YORK AT CORTLAND: CAMPUS ARTIST & LECTURE SERIES
Corey Union, Room 401
PO Box 2000
Cortland, NY 13045
Phone: 607-753-2321
Fax: 607-753-2808
e-mail: cals@snycorva.cortland.edu
Web Site: www.cortland.edu/cals
Management:
Coordinator Performing Arts Program: Judy Kopf
Mission: To enhance the cultural awareness of the Cortland College and general community.
Founded: 1984
Specialized Field: Dance; Instrumental Music; Theater; Festivals
Status: Professional; Nonprofit
Budget: $35,000-60,000
Income Sources: Association of Performing Arts Presenters; Upstate New York Presenters
Performs At: Dowd Fine Arts Theatre
Organization Type: Presenting

4951 GREAT PERFORMERS IN WESTCHESTER SERIES
5 Joseph Wallace Drive
Croton-on-Hudson, NY 10520
Phone: 914-271-2595
Management:
Executive Director: Beth Jennings Eggar
Budget: $10,000

4952 SEVENARS CONCERTS-SEVENARS MUSIC FESTIVAL
30 E End Avenue
Suite 3A-3D
Director, NY 10028
Phone: 212-288-4261
Fax: 212-288-4261
e-mail: sevenars@aol.com
Officers:
President/Artistic Director: Robert W Schrade
VP/Executive Director: Rolande Y Schrade
Director: David F James
Director: Robelyn Schrade-James

Director: Randolph RA Schrade
Director: Rorianne C Schrade
Executive Director: Rolande Young Schrade
Management:
Executive Director: Rolande Young Schrade
Artistic Director: Robert Schrade
Mission: To present music of the highest quality to the widest possible audience in an atmosphere of family warmth, acoustical perfection and serene beauty.
Founded: 1968
Specialized Field: Instrumental Music
Status: Professional; Nonprofit
Budget: $70,000-$80,000
Income Sources: Individual contributions; foundations; corporations & local cultural councils
Season: May to October in Worthington, Massachusetts
Performs At: Historic Academy/Concert Hall
Affiliations: Conservatories, universities, independent schools
Annual Attendance: 250+ at 7-8 events
Type of Stage: Raised; Acoustic
Seating Capacity: 250 - 350
Year Built: 1800
Year Remodeled: 1976
Organization Type: Performing; Educational
Resident Groups: Schrade and James family pianists
Comments: May-October: c/o Schrade, Worthington, Massachusetts, 01098, phone (413-338-5854)

4953 ROYCROFT CHAMBER MUSIC FESTIVAL
PO Box 281
East Aurora, NY 14052
Phone: 716-457-3565
Fax: 716-457-4119

4954 PIANOFEST
110 Pantigo Road
East Hampton, NY 11937
Mailing Address: PO Box 574, Wainscott, NY. 11975
Phone: 631-329-9115
Fax: 631-329-9115
e-mail: PSchenly@aol.com
Web Site: www.pianofest.org
Management:
Director: Paul Schenly

4955 ISLIP ARTS COUNCIL CHAMBER MUSIC SERIES
50 Irish Lane
East Islip, NY 11730
Phone: 631-224-5420
Fax: 631-224-5440
e-mail: iacouncil@aol.com
Web Site: www.isliparts.org
Officers:
President: Helene Katz
VP: Nicholas Wartella
Secretary: Jean Lipshie
Treasurer: Edward E. Wankel
Management:
Executive Director: Lillian Barbash
Co-Directror: Jodi Gianni
Artist Administrator: Dorothy Kalson

All listings are in alphabetical order by state, then city, then organization within the city.

Clerk Typist: Angela Wallace
Mission: To present a variety of disciplines ranging from fine classical music to young persons' programs to avant garde performance art; to enable and emerging art organizations to gain information and assistance from the Arts Council library and staff in applying for not-for-profit status, funding, computer services, publicity, mailing lists, etc.
Founded: 1974
Specialized Field: Vocal Music; Instrumental Music
Status: Professional; Nonprofit
Budget: $250,000
Income Sources: Town of Islip; Suffolk County
Performs At: Sayville Schools; Dowling College
Type of Stage: Semi-Thurst
Organization Type: Performing

4956 COLDEN CENTER PERFORMANCES

Colden Center for the Performing Arts
Queens College
Flushing, NY 11367-1597
Phone: 718-544-2996
Fax: 718-261-7063
e-mail: V.Charlop@coldcenter.org
Web Site: www.coldencenter.org
Management:
Director: Vivian Charlop
Budget: $150,000-400,000
Performs At: Irving & Susan Wallack Goldstein Theatre

4957 FLUSHING COUNCIL ON CULTURE & THE ARTS

Flushing Town Hall
137-35 Northern Boulevard
Flushing, NY 11354
Phone: 718-463-7700
Fax: 718-445-1920
e-mail: info@flushingtownhall.org
Web Site: www.flushingtownhall.org
Management:
Creative/Executive Director: Jo-Ann Jones
Mission: To make the arts a central part of life, to be a creative and revitalizing force for developing the arts in the community and to be a national and international destination for tourism.
Founded: 1979
Specialized Field: Greater New York metro area
Paid Staff: 16
Volunteer Staff: 900
Paid Artists: 160
Seating Capacity: 340
Rental Contact: Susan Agin

4958 MERANOFEST

6911 Yellowstone Boulevard
Suite B-5
Forest Hills, NY 11375
Phone: 718-575-8998
Fax: 718-575-2132
e-mail: info@meranofest.com -or- levnatofest@cs.com
Web Site: www.meranofest.com
Management:
Artistic Director: Professor Lev Natochenny

4959 SPECIALIST TO THE ARTS

5 Yorktown Place
Fort Salonga, NY 11768
Phone: 631-261-1576
Fax: 631-754-4616
e-mail: reabsld@aol.com
Officers:
President: Rea Jacobs

4960 SUFFOLK Y JCC INTERNATIONAL JEWISH ARTS FESTIVAL & THE CELEBRATION SERIES

5 Yorktown Place
Fort Salonga, NY 11768
Phone: 516-261-1576
Toll-free: 516-754-4616
e-mail: www.jewishartsfest.comsw
Management:
Specialist to the Arts: Rea Jacobs

4961 NASSAU COMMUNITY COLLEGE CULTURAL PROGRAM

Nassau Community College
1 Education Drive
Garden City, NY 11530
Phone: 516-572-7153
Fax: 516-222-2962
Management:
Student Activities Counselor: Phyllis Kurland
Mission: On campus presentations for student body.
Founded: 1970
Budget: $10,000-20,000
Performs At: College Center-Multipurpose Room
Type of Stage: Resess
Stage Dimensions: 16 x 24
Seating Capacity: 300

4962 HUDSON HIGHLANDS MUSIC FESTIVAL

PO Box 164
Garrison, NY 10516
Phone: 845-265-4273
e-mail: HHMF@highlands.com
Web Site: www.highlands.com/MusicFestival
Management:
Artistic Director: Heidi Stubner

4963 SUNY COLLEGE AT GENESEO LIMELIGHT ARTIST SERIES

College Union, SUNY College at Geneseo
1 College Circle
Geneseo, NY 14454
Phone: 585-245-5855
Fax: 585-245-5400
e-mail: rodgers@geneseo.edu
Management:
Campus Activities Director: Thomas Rodgers
Budget: $60,000-150,000
Income Sources: Student Feed; Ticket Revenue
Performs At: Wadsworth Auditorium
Affiliations: Arts Presenters National Association for Campus Activities

Facility Category: Auditorium
Type of Stage: Proscenium

4964 GENEVA CONCERTS

PO Box 709
Geneva, NY 14456
Phone: 315-781-3619
Fax: 315-781-3660
e-mail: mitchell@hws.edu
Web Site: www.hws.edu/genevaconcerts/
Officers:
   President: Kevin Mitchell
Mission: To promote the arts in Geneva and the
surrounding Finger Lakes community by presenting
music, dance and vocal performances.
Founded: 1938
Specialized Field: Dance; Vocal Music; Instrumental
Music; Lyric Opera; Grand Opera
Status: Professional; Nonprofit
Volunteer Staff: 22
Paid Artists: 290
Budget: $60,000-150,000
Performs At: Smith Opera House
Annual Attendance: 3,000
Facility Category: Opera House
Type of Stage: Proscenium Arts; Thrust Stage
Seating Capacity: 1,500
Year Built: 1894
Year Remodeled: 2000
Rental Contact: Kevin Mitchell
Organization Type: Educational; Sponsoring

4965 ADIRONDACK THEATRE FESTIVAL

PO Box 3203
Glens Falls, NY 12801
Phone: 518-798-7479
Fax: 518-793-1334
e-mail: atf@atfestival.org
Web Site: www.atfestival.org
Management:
   Artistic Director: Martha Banta
   Producing Director: David Turner
Mission: To present a season of new and contemporary
theater.
Founded: 1994
Specialized Field: Summer Theater
Status: Nonprofit
Paid Staff: 10
Volunteer Staff: 10
Paid Artists: 24
Budget: $150,000
Season: June - July
Performs At: Temporary theater in an old Woolworths
Store
Annual Attendance: 5,000
Type of Stage: Black Box
Seating Capacity: 150

4966 LOWER ADIRONDACK REGIONAL ARTS COUNCIL

7 Lapham Place
Glens Falls, NY 12801
Phone: 518-798-1144
Web Site: www.laracarts.org

Mission: To lead in the improvement of the quality of life
for the people of the lower Adirondack region by
supporting the arts and culture.
Founded: 1972
Status: Nonprofit
Affiliations: New York State Council on the Arts

4967 GLYDE RECITALS: NEW YORK VIOLA SOCIETY

26 Green Hill Road
Golden's Bridge, NY 10526
Mailing Address: New York Viola Society, PO Box 61,
New York, NY. 10019
Phone: 914-232-8159
Fax: 914-232-0521
e-mail: wsalchow@computer.net
Web Site: www.viola.com/nyvs
Budget: $10,000

4968 FESTIVAL OF BAROQUE MUSIC

Foundation for Baroque Music
165 Wilton Road
Greenfield Center, NY 12833
Phone: 518-893-7527
Fax: 518-893-2351
e-mail: baroque@global2000.net
Web Site: www.global2000.net/baroque
Management:
   Artistic Director/President: Robert Conant

4969 LONG ISLAND UNIVERSITY SERIES

Long Island University
CW Post Campus
Greenvale, NY 11548-0570
Phone: 516-299-2752
Fax: 516-299-2520
e-mail: elliott@tilles.liu.edu
Web Site: www.tillescenter.org
Management:
   Executive Director: Elliot Sroka
Budget: $1,000,000+
Performs At: Hillwood Recital Hall

4970 COLGATE UNIVERSITY CONCERT SERIES

Colgate University, Music Department
13 Oak Drive
Hamilton, NY 13346-1398
Phone: 315-228-7642
Fax: 315-228-7557
e-mail: shealey@mail.colgate.edu
Web Site: www.colgate.edu
Officers:
   Chairperson: Mariette Cheng
   Director, Chenango Summer Mus. Fest: Laura
   Klugherz
Management:
   Concert Manager: Roberta Healey
Mission: To provide music concerts for Colgate students
and the surrounding community.
Specialized Field: Vocal Music and Instrumental Music
Status: Non-Professional; Nonprofit
Budget: $20,000-35,000

Income Sources: Private
Performs At: Colgate Memorial Chapel
Facility Category: chapel
Type of Stage: wooden
Seating Capacity: 750
Organization Type: Educational; Sponsoring
Resident Groups: University Orchestra, Chamber Players, Chorus, Jazz Ensemble

---

4971 JOSEPH G ASTMAN INTERNATIONAL CONCERT SERIES
200 Hofstra University
Student Center, Room 107
Hempstead, NY 11549
Phone: 516-463-5042
Fax: 516-463-4793
e-mail: culrts@hofstra.edu
Management:
   Associate Director: Bob Spiotto MFA
Performs At: Monroe Lecture Center Theater

4972 BELLEAYRE MUSIC FESTIVAL
Belleayre Conservatory
PO Box 198
Highmount, NY 12441
Phone: 845-254-5600
Fax: 845-254-5608
Toll-free: 800-942-6904
e-mail: festival@catskill.net
Web Site: www.belleayremusic.org -or- www.belleayre.com
Management:
   Co-Artistic Director: Mel Litoff
   Co-Artistic Director: Phyllis Litoff
   Administrative Manager: Don L Myers
Founded: 1992
Specialized Field: A variety of live music from Folk, Rock, Chamber, Philharmonic to Opera, Jazz, and Broadway
Paid Staff: 8
Volunteer Staff: 100
Paid Artists: 14
Non-paid Artists: 3

4973 HORNELL AREA ARTS COUNCIL
PO Box 298
20 Broadway
Hornell, NY 14843
Phone: 607-324-3822
Fax: 607-324-3822
Management:
   Executive Director: Rene, Coombs
Budget: $10,000-20,000

4974 HOUGHTON COLLEGE ARTIST SERIES
Houghton College
Houghton, NY 14744
Phone: 716-567-9403
Fax: 716-567-9517
e-mail: BBrown@houghton.edu
Management:
   Director: Dr. Bruce Brown
Mission: To offer the finest music concerts.

Founded: 1930
Specialized Field: Vocal Music; Instrumental Music; Theater; Grand Opera
Status: Nonprofit
Budget: $20,000-35,000
Income Sources: Association of Performing Arts Presenters
Performs At: Wesley Chapel
Organization Type: Performing; Educational; Sponsoring

4975 HUNTINGTON ARTS COUNCIL
213 Main Street
Huntington, NY 11743
Phone: 631-271-8423
Fax: 631-271-8428
e-mail: info@huntingtonarts.org
Web Site: www.huntingtonarts.org
Management:
   Executive Director: Diana Cherryholmes
   Program Director: Dan Forte
Mission: The Huntington Arts Council supports and fosters the arts to enhance the lives of the citizens of Huntington Township and their visitors.
Founded: 1963
Specialized Field: Presenting, Education, Re-grants, Technical Assistance
Paid Staff: 8
Volunteer Staff: 27
Paid Artists: 57
Income Sources: Grants; Sponsorchip; Town and County Funding; Membership Dues
Annual Attendance: 90,000
Seating Capacity: 5,500
Year Built: 1979
Rental Contact: Dan Forte

4976 HUNTINGTON SUMMER ARTS FESTIVAL
Huntington Arts Council
213 Main Street
Huntington, NY 11743
Phone: 631-271-8423
Fax: 631-271-8428
e-mail: hsaf@huntingtonarts.org
Web Site: www.huntingtonarts.org
Management:
   Executive Director: Diana J Cherryholmes

4977 HUDSON VALLEY MUSIC CLUB SERIES
10 Riverview Terrace
Irvington, NY 10533
Phone: 914-591-6434
Fax: 914-591-7226
e-mail: wsalisbury@sasmedia.com
Officers:
   Artist Selection Chairman: Meredith P Salisbury
Budget: $10,000
Performs At: Dobbs Ferry Woman's Club; Dobbs Ferry

4978 CORNELL CONCERT SERIES
Cornell University
Lincoln Hall
Ithaca, NY 14853
Phone: 607-255-4363
Fax: 607-254-2877
Web Site: www.arts.cornell.edu/ccs
Management:
   Concert Manager: Richard Riley
Mission: Concert events per academic year, from solo recitals to orchestras presents; musicians of international renown.
Founded: 1903
Specialized Field: Classical Music, Jazz, World Music
Paid Staff: 2
Volunteer Staff: 80
Paid Artists: 10

4979 ITHACA COLLEGE CONCERTS
Ithaca College, School of Music
4201 Whalen Center
Ithaca, NY 14850-7240
Phone: 607-274-3169
Fax: 607-274-1727
e-mail: DVialet@ithaca.edu
Web Site: www.ithaca.edu/music
Management:
   Concert Manager: Debra L Vialet
Founded: 1892
Specialized Field: Classical Music7
Budget: $20,000-35,000
Income Sources: Ticket Revenue
Performs At: Ford Hall
Facility Category: Concert Hall
Type of Stage: Proscenium
Seating Capacity: 737
Year Built: 1960

4980 NEW DIRECTIONS CELLO FESTIVAL
501 Linn Street
Ithaca, NY 14850
Phone: 607-277-1686
Fax: 607-277-1686
Toll-free: 877-665-5815
e-mail: info@newdirectionscello.com
Web Site: www.newdirectionscello.com
Management:
   Director: Chris White
   Education Director: Sera Surslen
Mission: To bring together cellists and others interested in nonclassical uses of cello (jazz, blues, folk, rock, etc.). Workshops, jams, concerts.
Founded: 1995
Specialized Field: Music
Paid Staff: 2
Volunteer Staff: 10
Paid Artists: 12
Budget: Under $10,000
Income Sources: Sponsors, Participants, Donations
Season: July 11 - 13, 1999
Performs At: University of Connecticut, Storrs [Festival Site]
Annual Attendance: 100
Facility Category: Mehden Auditorium/Recital Hall

Stage Dimensions: 50x25
Seating Capacity: 500
Year Built: 1985
Cost: $150 - 3 day

4981 ARTS COUNCIL FOR CHAUTAUGUA COUNTY
116 E Third Street
Jamestown, NY 14701
Phone: 716-664-2465
Fax: 716-661-3829
Web Site: www.artscouncil.com
Management:
   Acting Executive Director: Keith Schmitt
Budget: $60,000-150,000
Performs At: Reg Lenna Civic Center

4982 JAMESTOWN CONCERT ASSOCIATION
315 N Main Street
Suite 200
Jamestown, NY 14701-5124
Phone: 716-487-1522
Fax: 716-483-5051
e-mail: icamusic@excite.com
Officers:
   President: R Richard Corbin
   VP: Sally Ulrich
   Treasurer: F John Fuchs
   Secretary: Mary Weeden
Management:
   Programming: Sally Ulrich
Mission: Purpose of presenting live classical performances in the Jamestown area.
Founded: 1934
Volunteer Staff: 16
Budget: $20,000-35,000
Income Sources: NYSCA; Local Foundations; PENNPAT

4983 CARAMOOR CENTER FOR MUSIC AND THE ARTS
Katonah, NY 10536
Phone: 914-232-1252
Fax: 914-232-5521
Web Site: www.caramoor.org
Officers:
   President/CEO: Erich Vollmer
Management:
   Executive Director: Howard Herring
   Managing Director: Paul Rosenblum
   Director Development: Susan Shine
   Director Operations: Melissa Montera
   Box Office Manager: Sal Vaccaro
Mission: To offer a performing arts venue in Bedford and New York State.
Founded: 1945
Specialized Field: Vocal Music; Instrumental Music; Festivals
Status: Professional; Nonprofit
Performs At: Museum Music Room Venetian Theatre
Organization Type: Performing; Educational; Sponsoring

4984 CARAMOOR INTERNATIONAL MUSIC FESTIVAL

PO Box 816
Katonah, NY 10536
Phone: 914-232-5035
Fax: 914-232-5521
Web Site: www.caramoor.com
Management:
Executive Director: Howard Herring

4985 LAKE GEORGE JAZZ WEEKEND

Lake George Arts Project
Canada Street
Lake George, NY 12845
Phone: 518-668-2616
Fax: 518-668-3050
Officers:
President: Ed Ostberg
Management:
Executive Director: John Strong
Music Director: Paul Pines
Mission: Sponsoring a two-day jazz festival every September featuring nationally acclaimed as well as emerging jazz artists.
Specialized Field: Instrumental Music; Jazz
Status: Professional; Nonprofit
Performs At: Shepard Park Bandstand
Organization Type: Performing; Touring

4986 LUZERNE CHAMBER MUSIC FESTIVAL

PO Box 35
Lake Luzerne, NY 12846
Phone: 518-696-2771

4987 ARTPARK

150 S 4th Street
Box 28
Lewiston, NY 14092
Phone: 716-754-9000
Fax: 716-754-2741
e-mail: gosborne@artpark.net
Web Site: www.artpark.net
Officers:
President: George D Osborn
Director Finance: Jean Stopa
Productions Manager: Susan Stimson
Mission: To provide arts education and programming to nuture and develop the talents of visual and performing artists; to provide quality volunteer experiences in the arts; to produce and present a series of theatre productions and concert events that will entertain and enrich the residents of Western New York, southeastern Canada, and area tourists.
Founded: 1974
Specialized Field: Dance; Vocal Music; Instrumental Music; Festivals; Grand Opera
Status: Professional; Nonprofit
Paid Staff: 15
Volunteer Staff: 500
Paid Artists: 150
Non-paid Artists: 60
Budget: $2,500,000
Income Sources: State Parks; Ticket Sales; Fees

Season: June - September
Affiliations: Actors' Equity Association; International Association of Theatrical Stage Employees; American Guild of Musical Artists
Annual Attendance: 120,000
Facility Category: Theatre; Concert Hall; Visual Arts; Musicals
Type of Stage: Proscenium
Stage Dimensions: 60' x 90'
Seating Capacity: 2,324
Year Built: 1973
Cost: $7,200,000
Rental Contact: Executive Director George Osborne
Organization Type: Performing; Resident; Sponsoring

4988 BEETHOVEN FESTIVAL

Friends of the Arts
PO Box 702
Locust Valley, NY 11560
Phone: 516-922-0061
Fax: 516-922-0770
Management:
Executive Director: Theodora Bookman
Mission: Presenting Beethoven's lifetime body of work during one spectacular weekend.
Specialized Field: Instrumental Music
Status: Professional; Nonprofit
Performs At: Planting Fields Arboretum
Organization Type: Performing

4989 EMELIN THEATRE FOR THE PERFORMING ARTS

153 Library Lane
Mamaroneck, NY 10543
Phone: 914-698-3045
Fax: 914-698-1404
e-mail: emelin98@aol.com
Web Site: www.emelin.org
Management:
Managing Director: John Raymond
Founded: 1973
Budget: $150,000-400,000
Performs At: Emelin Theatre
Type of Stage: Proscenium
Seating Capacity: 280

4990 OYSTER BAY ARTS COUNCIL DISTINGUISHED ARTISTS CONCERTS

977 Hicksville Road
Massapequa, NY 11758-1281
Phone: 516-797-7926
Fax: 516-797-7919
Management:
Executive Director: Dorothy Blumstein
Budget: $10,000

4991 INTERNATIONAL PIANO FESTIVAL AT WILLIAMS

The Taubman Institute
245 Route 351
Medusa, NY 12120

Fax: 518-239-6822
Toll-free: 800-826-3720
e-mail: es@taubman-institute.com
Web Site: www.taubman-institute.com
Management:
   Festival Director: Enid Stettner
Paid Artists: 13

4992 CHAMBER MUSIC FESTIVAL OF THE EAST

PO Box 1346
Melville, NY 11747-0422
Phone: 201-242-1277
e-mail: chmusic@tiac.net
Management:
   Music Director: Shem Guibbory

4993 MOUNT KISCO CONCERT ASSOCIATION

34 Lakeside Road, RD 4
Mount Kisco, NY 10549
Phone: 914-666-2242
Fax: 914-241-0034
Officers:
   Artist Selection Chairperson: Michael G Rothenberg
Budget: $20,000-35,000

4994 PIANO SUMMER AT NEW PALTZ

SUNY at New Paltz, Music Department
75 S Manheim Boulevard, Suite 9
New Paltz, NY 12561-2443
Phone: 845-257-2700
Fax: 845-257-3121
Web Site: www.newpaltz.edu/piano
Management:
   Artistic Director: Vladimir Feltsman

4995 92ND STREET Y

1395 Lexington Avenue
New York, NY 10128
Phone: 212-415-5500
Fax: 212-415-5788
e-mail: webmaster@92ndsty.org
Web Site: www.92ndsty.org
Officers:
   President: Matthew Bronfman
   Chairman: Philip L Milgrein
   VP: Claire B Benenson
   VP: Lini Lipton
   Treasurer: Martin J. Rabinpwitz
   Secretary: Lori A. Kasowitx
Management:
   Executive Director: Sol Adler
   Executive Assistant: Catherine Marino
   Director: Tamar C Podell
   Production Manager: Zoe Markwalter
Mission: Promotes individual and family development and participation in civic life within the context of Jewish values and American pluralism; creates, provides and disseminates programs of distinction that foster physical and mental health.
Founded: 1874
Status: Nonprofit

4996 AMERICAN FESTIVAL OF MICROTONAL MUSIC

318 E 70th Street
#5FW
New York, NY 10021
Phone: 212-517-3550
Fax: 212-517-5495
e-mail: Afmmjr@aol.com
Web Site: www.wchonyc.com/~jhhl/AFMM
Management:
   Director: Johnny Reinhard

4997 AMERICAN INDIAN COMMUNITY HOUSE SERIES

708 Broadway
8th Floor
New York, NY 10003
Phone: 212-598-0100
Fax: 212-598-4909
e-mail: akwesasne@aol.com
Web Site: www.oich.org
Management:
   Executive Director: Rosemary Richmond
   Performing Arts Director: Jim Cyrus
Founded: 1969
Status: Nonprofit; Equity; Non-Equity
Budget: $10,000-20,000
Season: September - June

4998 AMERICAN LANDMARK FESTIVALS

685 W End Avenue
Suite 1AF
New York, NY 10025
Phone: 212-866-2086
Fax: 212-825-6874
e-mail: AmLandmarKFstvls@aol.com
Officers:
   President: Francis L Heilbut
Mission: To present cultural performances in various historic settings.
Founded: 1973
Specialized Field: Dance; Vocal Music; Instrumental Music; Theater; Festivals; Lyric Opera; Grand Opera
Status: Professional
Organization Type: Performing

4999 ARTS INTERNATIONAL

251 Park Avenue S
5th Floor
New York, NY 10010
Phone: 212-674-9744
Fax: 212-674-9092
e-mail: info@artsinternational.org
Web Site: www.artsinternational.org
Officers:
   President: Noreen Tomassi

5000 ASIA SOCIETY

725 Park Avenue
New York, NY 10021-5025

Phone: 212-327-9249
Fax: 212-517-7246
e-mail: rachelc@asiasoc.org
Web Site: www.asiasociety.org
Management:
　　Associate Director Performing Arts: Rachel Cooper

5001　BANG ON A CAN
222 E 5th Street
#12
New York, NY 10003
Phone: 212-777-8442
Fax: 212-388-1727
e-mail: info@bangonacan.org
Web Site: www.bangonacan.org
Management:
　　Managing Director: Kenny Savelson
　　Artistic Director: Michael Gordon
　　Artistic Director: David Lang
　　Artistic Director: Julia Wolfe
Mission: To present contemporary musical works by emerging and young composers.
Founded: 1987
Specialized Field: Music Festivals
Status: Professional; Nonprofit
Income Sources: Public; Private Funding; Earned Income
Organization Type: Performing

5002　BASKETBALL CITY
Pier 63 W 23rd Street
New York, NY 10011
Phone: 212-924-4040
Fax: 212-924-5550
e-mail: bruce@basketballcity.com
Web Site: www.basketballcity.com
Management:
　　Director: Bruce Radler
Founded: 1997

5003　BELL ATLANTIC JAZZ FESTIVAL
74 Leonard Street
New York, NY 10013
Phone: 212-219-3006
Fax: 212-219-3401
Web Site: www.jazfest.com

5004　BLOOMINGDALE SCHOOL OF MUSIC CONCERT SERIES
323 W 108th Street
New York, NY 10025
Phone: 212-663-6021
Fax: 212-932-9429
e-mail: Mary_Hastings@Bloomingdalemusic.org
Web Site: www.bloomingdalemusic.org
Management:
　　Director: Mary Hastings
Budget: $10,000
Performs At: David Greer Recital Hall

5005　BOPI'S BLACK SHEEP/DANCE BY KRAIG PATTERSON
Jaf Station
PO Box 372
New York, NY 10116
Phone: 212-262-9499
Fax: 212-399-1349
e-mail: dancebopi@aol.com
Web Site: www.bopi.org
Management:
　　Artistic Director: Kraig Patterson
　　Booking Agent: Micocci Productions
Mission: Performance, touring and creation of works.
Specialized Field: Modern Dance
Paid Staff: 2
Paid Artists: 12

5006　BRIDGEHAMPTON CHAMBER MUSIC FESTIVAL
305 7th Avenue
16th Floor
New York, NY 10001
Phone: 212-741-9073
Fax: 212-691-9225
e-mail: bcmainc@aol.com
Web Site: www.bcmf.org
Management:
　　Artistic Director: Marya Martint

5007　CATHEDRAL ARTS
1047 Amsterdam Avenue
New York, NY 10025
Phone: 212-316-7563
Fax: 212-316-7445
Web Site: www.stjohndivine.org
Management:
　　Director: Karen De Francis
Budget: $10,000-20,000

5008　CENTRAL PARK SUMMERSTAGE
830 5th Avenue
New York, NY 10021
Phone: 212-360-2756
Fax: 212-360-2754
e-mail: info@SummerStage.org
Web Site: www.SummerStage.org
Management:
　　Director Arts/Cultural Programs: Alexa Birdsong
　　Associate Producer: Gayle Horio
　　Program Director: Walter Durkacz
　　Development/Outreach Manager: James Burke
Founded: 1986
Specialized Field: Music; Dance; Spokin Word; Opera
Status: Nonprofit
Paid Staff: 76
Volunteer Staff: 300
Paid Artists: 90
Budget: $800,000
Income Sources: Ticket Sales; State Local Grants; Memberships; Endowment Funds
Performs At: Rumsey Playfield
Annual Attendance: 350,000
Stage Dimensions: 36'x42'

Seating Capacity: 4,000-6,000
Year Built: 1986
Year Remodeled: 2000

5009   CLARION MUSIC SOCIETY
Kaye Playhouse
695 Park Avenue
New York, NY 10021
Phone: 212-463-7201
Fax: 212-463-7201
Web Site: www.kayeplayhouse.org
Management:
   Executive Director: Sandra Davis
Budget: $35,000-60,000
Performs At: Kaye Playhouse

**5010   CONCERT ARTISTS GUILD NEW YORK
RECITAL SERIES**
850 7th Avenue
Suite 1205
New York, NY 10019
Phone: 212-333-5200
Fax: 212-977-7149
e-mail: caguild@concertartists.org
Web Site: www.concertartists.org
Officers:
   President: Richard S Weinert
   Executive VP: Amy Roberts Frawley
   Senior VP: Brian D Bumby
Founded: 1951
Specialized Field: Classical Music
Performs At: Weill Recital Hall at Carnegie Hall

5011   CONCERT SOCIALS
110 W 96th Street
Suite 9D
New York, NY 10025
Phone: 212-749-5464
Management:
   Executive Director/President: Rae Metzgar
Performs At: Weill Recital Hall at Carnegie Hall

5012   CONCERTS AT THE CLOISTERS
The Cloisters
Fort Tryon Park
New York, NY 10040
Phone: 212-650-2290
Fax: 212-795-3640
Web Site: www.metmuseum.org
Management:
   Concert Manager: Nancy Wu
Budget: $50,000-100,000
Performs At: Fuentiduena Chapel; Metropolitan Museum
of Art

5013   CREATIVE TIME SERIES
307 7th Avenue
Suite 1904
New York, NY 10001
Phone: 212-206-6674
Fax: 212-255-8467
e-mail: staff@creativetime.org
Web Site: www.creativetime.org

Management:
   Office/Production Manager: Carol Stakenas
   Administrative/Outreach: Sarah Bacon
Budget: $10,000-20,000

5014   DIA CENTER FOR THE ARTS
548 W 22nd Street
New York, NY 10011
Phone: 212-989-5566
Fax: 212-989-4055
e-mail: info@diacenter.org
Web Site: www.diacenter.org
Management:
   Director: Michael Govan
   Administrator Art Programs: John Bowsher
   Development Associate: Katherine Carl
   Assistant Director: Stephen Dewhurst
Founded: 1974
Specialized Field: Contemporary Art
Status: Tax-exempt
Income Sources: Foundations; Corporations;
Affiliations: 1

**5015   ELAINE KAUFMAN CULTURAL
CENTER PRESENTATIONS**
129 W 67th Street
New York, NY 10023
Phone: 212-501-3386
Fax: 212-501-3317
e-mail: lhat@ekcc.org
Web Site: www.ekcc.org
Management:
   Merkin Concert Hall Director: Vicki Margulies
   Communications Director: Lizanne Hart
Budget: $60,000-150,000
Performs At: Ann Goodman Recital Hall

5016   FESTIVAL OF NEW MUSIC
30 Seaman Avenue
#4M
New York, NY 10034
Phone: 212-567-1493
Fax: 212-544-0738
e-mail: info@threetwo.org
Web Site: www.threetwo.org
Management:
   Co-Director: Taimur Sullivan

5017   FOOLS COMPANY
356 W 44th Street
New York, NY 10036
Phone: 212-307-6000
Fax: 212-307-6003
e-mail: foolsco@att.net
Web Site: www.foolsco.org
Officers:
   President: James Wertheim
   VP: Marcus Bicknell
   Secretary/Treasurer: Joseph Benitez
Management:
   Executive Director: Jill Russell
   Artistic Director: Martin Russell
   Executive Administrator: Susan Cline

All listings are in alphabetical order by state, then city, then organization within the city.

Mission: To produce a theatre arts festival and other works and workshops in the performing arts.
Founded: 1970
Specialized Field: Theater; Festivals
Status: Professional; Nonprofit
Budget: $10,000
Performs At: John Houseman Theatre Studio
Organization Type: Performing; Educational

5018 FRENCH INSTITUTE ALLIANCE FRANCAISE

22 E 60th Street
New York, NY 10022
Phone: 212-355-6100
Fax: 212-935-4119
e-mail: reception@fiaf.org
Web Site: www.fiaf.org
Management:
 Artistic Director: Jacqueline Chambord
 Client Relations Manager: Kin Hernandez
Founded: 1898
Budget: $150,000-400,000
Performs At: Theater, Dance, Music, Lecture and Film
Facility Category: Cultural Organization
Type of Stage: Proscenium
Stage Dimensions: 35'x22'
Seating Capacity: 400
Year Built: 1989
Rental Contact: Client Relations Manager Kin Hernandez

5019 FRICK COLLECTION CONCERT SERIES

1 E 70th Street
New York, NY 10021
Phone: 212-288-0700
Fax: 212-628-4417
e-mail: bodig@frick.org
Web Site: www.frick.org
Management:
 Concerts Coordinator: Joyce Bodig
Budget: $60,000-150,000

5020 GOTHAM EARLY MUSIC FOUNDATION SERIES

PO Box 231300
Ansonia Station
New York, NY 10023
Phone: 212-595-4036
Fax: 212-875-8503
e-mail: admin@gothamemf.com
Officers:
 President: Douglas K Dunn
Budget: $150,000-400,000
Performs At: Weill Recital Hall at Carnegie Hall; Ethical Culture Society

5021 GREENWICH HOUSE ARTS: NORTH RIVER MUSIC

46 Barrow Street
New York, NY 10014

Phone: 212-242-4770
Fax: 212-366-9621
e-mail: gharts@gharts.org
Web Site: www.gharts.org
Management:
 Concert Manager: Scott Taylor
Founded: 1902
Specialized Field: Music; Theatre
Budget: $10,000-20,000
Performs At: Renee Weiler Concert Hall

5022 HELICON FOUNDATION

27 W 67th Street
New York, NY 10023-6258
Phone: 212-874-6438
Fax: 212-874-6438
e-mail: helicon@dti.net
Management:
 Executive Director: James Roe
 Artistic Director: Albert Fuller
Budget: $10,000-20,000

5023 HENSON INTERNATIONAL FESTIVAL OF PUPPET THEATRE

117 E 69th Street
New York, NY 10021
Phone: 212-794-2400
Fax: 212-439-6036
e-mail: info@hensonfestival.org
Web Site: www.hensonfestival.org
Management:
 Executive Producer: Cherly Henson
 Generla Manager: Heidi Wilenius
 Development Officer: Meg Daniel
Mission: To provide some of the finest international puppetry performers for American audiences; to present the finest international puppet artists to American audiences.
Specialized Field: Puppet theatre
Status: Nonprofit
Performs At: Joseph Papp Public Theater
Organization Type: Sponsoring

5024 HISTORIC BRASS SOCIETY - EARLY BRASS FESTIVAL

148 W 23rd Street
Suite 2A
New York, NY 10011
Phone: 212-627-3820
Fax: 212-627-3820
e-mail: president@historicbrass.org
Web Site: www.historicbrass.org
Management:
 President: Jeff Nussbaum
Mission: To promote the study and performance of brass music.
Founded: 1988
Specialized Field: Brass Music
Volunteer Staff: 20

5025 HUDSON RIVER FESTIVAL

200 Liberty Street
New York, NY 10281

Phone: 212-945-0505
Fax: 212-945-3392
e-mail: wfcae@wfprop.com
Web Site: www.worldfinancialcenter.com
Management:
Director: Melissa Coley

5026 INTERNATIONAL OFFESTIVAL

Fools Company
423 W 46th Street
New York, NY 10036
Phone: 212-307-6000
Fax: 212-307-6003
e-mail: foolsco@att.net
Web Site: www.foolsco.org
Management:
Executive Director: Jill Russell
Artistic Director: Martin Russell

5027 JAPAN SOCIETY PERFORMING ARTS SERIES

333 E 47th Street
New York, NY 10017
Phone: 212-832-1155
Fax: 212-715-1262
e-mail: plawrence@japansociety.org
Web Site: www.japansociety.org
Management:
Director: Paula Lawrence
Senior Program Officer: Michiko Hirzano
Founded: 1907
Paid Staff: 4
Budget: $60,000-150,000
Performs At: Lila Acheson Wallace Auditorium
Annual Attendance: 6,000
Seating Capacity: 278
Year Built: 1971

5028 JAZZ AT LINCOLN CENTER'S ESSENTIALLY ELLINGTON JAZZ FESTIVAL

33 W 60th Street
New York, NY 10023-7999
Phone: 212-258-9800
Fax: 212-258-9900
e-mail: mfuss@jazzatlincolncenter.org
Web Site: www.jazzatlincolncenter.org
Management:
Executive Producer/Director: Rob Gibson
Artistic Director: Wynton Marsalis

5029 JAZZ IN JULY

92nd Street Y
1395 Lexington Avenue
New York, NY 10128
Phone: 212-415-5740
Fax: 212-415-5738
e-mail: tischctr@92ndsty.org
Web Site: www.92ndsty.org
Management:
Artistic Director: Dick Hyman

5030 JVC JAZZ FESTIVAL NEW YORK

PO Box 1169, Ansonia Station
311 W 74th Street
New York, NY 10023
Phone: 212-501-1390
Fax: 212-877-9916
Web Site: www.festivalproductions.net/jvc/ny
Management:
Producer: George T Wein

5031 LEAGUE OF COMPOSERS-ISCM NEW YORK SEASON

PO Box 250281
New York, NY 10025
Phone: 718-442-5225
e-mail: lqc5590@is9.nyu.edu
Web Site: www.unix.temple.edu/~mrimple/iscm.html
Officers:
President: Dan Wanner
Management:
Executive Director: Louis Conti
Budget: $10,000-20,000

5032 LOTUS FINE ARTS PRODUCTIONS

109 W 27th Street
8th Floor
New York, NY 10001
Phone: 212-627-1076
Fax: 212-675-7191
e-mail: info@lotusarts.com
Web Site: www.lotusarts.com
Management:
Artistic Director: Kamala Cesar

5033 MANNES COLLEGE OF MUSIC INTERNATIONAL KEYBOARD INSTITUTE AND FESTIVAL

150 W 85th Street
New York, NY 10024
Phone: 212-580-0210
Fax: 212-580-1738
e-mail: IKI@newschool.edu
Web Site: www.mannes.edu/IKI
Management:
Director: Jerome Rose

5034 MELLON JAZZ IN PHILADELPHIA

PO Box 1169
New York, NY 10023
Phone: 212-496-9000
Fax: 212-877-9916
e-mail: dan.melnick@fpiny.com
Web Site: www.festivalproductions.net
Management:
Senior Producer: Dan Melnick

5035 METROPOLITAN MUSEUM CONCERTS AND LECTURES

1000 5th Avenue and 82nd Street
New York, NY 10028

Phone: 212-570-3717
Fax: 212-570-3973
Web Site: www.metmuseum.org
Management:
    General Manager: Hilde Annik Limondjian
    Director: Philippe de Montebello
Mission: As one of the major presenting organizations in New York City to reflect the museum's charter in promoting education and cultural events which reflect the museum's holdings.
Founded: 1954
Specialized Field: Vocal Music; Instrumental Music; Festivals
Status: Professional
Income Sources: American Association of Museums
Performs At: Grace Rainey Rogers Auditorium
Seating Capacity: 705
Organization Type: Sponsoring

5036 MIDAMERICA PRODUCTIONS

70 W 36th Street
Suite 305
New York, NY 10018
Phone: 212-239-0205
Fax: 212-563-5587
e-mail: tiboris@midamerica-music.com
Web Site: www.midamerica-music.com
Management:
    General/Music Director: Peter Tiboris
    Executive Director: Norman Dunfee
    Public Relations Director: Dale Zeidman
Budget: $1,000,000+
Performs At: Avery Fisher Hall; Lincoln Center; Lakka Open Theatre

5037 MOSTLY MOZART FESTIVAL

70 Lincoln Center Plaza
New York, NY 10023
Phone: 212-875-5135
Fax: 212-875-5145
Web Site: www.lincolncenter.org
Management:
    Music Director: Gerard Schwarz

5038 MUSIC BEFORE 1800

529 W 121st Street
New York, NY 10027
Phone: 212-666-0675
Fax: 212-666-9266
e-mail: MB1800@aol.com
Management:
    Executive Director: Louise Basbas
Budget: $60,000-150,000
Performs At: Corpus Christi Church

5039 MUSIC FROM JAPAN

7 E 20th Street
#6F
New York, NY 10003-1106
Phone: 212-674-4587
Fax: 212-529-7855
e-mail: mfjrc@aol.com
Web Site: www.musicfromjapan.org
Management:

Artistic Director: Naoyuki Miura
Budget: $200,000
Income Sources: ANSCA; Japanese Government; Corporations; Foundations
Performs At: Merkin Concert Hall

5040 MUSIC IN ABE LEBEWOHL PARK

235 E 11th Street
New York, NY 10003
Phone: 212-777-3240
Fax: 212-477-1808
Management:
    Community Affairs/Concerts Director: Beth Flusser
Budget: $10,000
Performs At: Abe Lebewohl Park
Facility Category: Outdoor

5041 NEW YORK'S ENSEMBLE FOR EARLY MUSIC

217 W 71st Street
New York, NY 10023
Phone: 212-749-6600
Fax: 212-932-7348
Management:
    Managing Director: Carl K Steffes
Budget: $20,000-35,000
Performs At: Cathedral of Saint John the Divine

5042 NOONDAY CONCERTS

74 Trinity Place
New York, NY 10006-2088
Phone: 212-602-0768
Fax: 212-602-9630
e-mail: etucker@trinitywallstreet.org
Web Site: www.trinitywallstreet.org
Management:
    Trinity Concerts Director: Earl Tucker
Budget: $35,000-60,000
Performs At: St. Paul's Chapel & Trinity Church

5043 PLURAL ARTS INTERNATIONAL

22 E 67th Street
New York, NY 10021
Phone: 212-439-9800
e-mail: info@pluralarts.org
Web Site: www.pluralarts.org
Management:
    Executive Director: Todd J Fletcher

5044 PRO PIANO NEW YORK RECITAL SERIES

Pro Piano
85 Jane Street
New York, NY 10014
Phone: 212-206-8794
Fax: 212-633-1207
e-mail: ricard@propiano.com
Web Site: www.propiano.com
Management:
    Founder/Executive Director: Ricard de La Rosa
    Artistic Director: Chitose Okashiro
Mission: Present pianists to perform at Weill Hall NYC annually.

Budget: $60,000-150,000
Performs At: Weill Recital Hall at Carnegie Hall

5045 SCHNEIDER CONCERTS AT THE NEW SCHOOL

66 W 12th Street
New York, NY 10011
Phone: 212-243-9937
Fax: 212-243-9958
e-mail: nsconcerts@earthlink.net
Web Site: home.earthlink.net/~nsconcerts
Management:
   Administrative Director: Rohana Keninll
   Administrator: Frank Salomon
Mission: To offer young profesional classical musicians
performance opportunities and exposure at a vital stage of
career development and to present chamber music
concerts of the highest quality at modest ticket prices.
Founded: 1957
Specialized Field: Chamber Music
Paid Staff: 2
Volunteer Staff: 2
Paid Artists: 31
Non-paid Artists: 4
Budget: $30,000-45,000
Income Sources: Box Office; NYSCA; Private Donors;
Foundations
Annual Attendance: 4,000
Facility Category: Auditorium
Type of Stage: Proscenium
Seating Capacity: 510

5046 SHANDELEE MUSIC FESTIVAL

36 E 74th Street
New York, NY 10021
Phone: 212-288-4152
Fax: 212-879-2462
e-mail: shanfest@aol.com
Web Site: shandelee.org
Officers:
   Founding President: Daniel Stroup
   VP: Stephen Johnson
Management:
   Artistic Director: Lana Ivanov
Founded: 1993
Specialized Field: Classical Music Festival
Performs At: Concert Hall; Sunset Concert Pavilion
Seating Capacity: 200
Year Built: 2001

5047 ST. PATRICK'S CATHEDRAL CHAMBER MUSIC SERIES

St. Patrick's Cathedral
460 Madison Avenue
New York, NY 10022
Phone: 212-753-2261
Fax: 212-753-3925
e-mail: mlchamber@aol.com
Management:
   Manager: Monica Avitsur
Budget: $10,000

5048 SUMMERGARDEN

The Museum of Modern Art
11 W 53rd Street
New York, NY 10019
Phone: 212-708-9400
Fax: 212-333-1246
Web Site: www.moma.org
Management:
   Director: Joel Sachs

5049 SYMPHONY SPACE

2537 Broadway
New York, NY 10025-6947
Phone: 212-864-1414
Fax: 212-932-3228
e-mail: info@symphonyspace.org
Web Site: www.symphonyspace.org
Officers:
   Executive VP: Joanne Cossa
Management:
   Artistic Director: Ismiah Sheffer
   Managing Director: Peggy Wreen
   Director Marketing: Elizabeth Vilmik
   Director Development: Peter Shavitz
   Producer Music/Dance Program: Maren Bethelsen
Founded: 1978
Specialized Field: Music; dance; theatre; educational
Status: Nonprofit
Facility Category: Theater
Rental Contact: Patricia Sinnott

5050 THIRD STREET MUSIC SCHOOL SETTLEMENT FACULTY ARTISTS SERIES

235 E 11th Street
New York, NY 10003
Phone: 212-777-3240
Fax: 212-477-1808
Management:
   Community Affairs/Concerts Director: Beth Flusser
Budget: $10,000
Performs At: Mark's Park

5051 TRIBECA PERFORMING ARTS CENTER

199 Chambers Street
New York, NY 10007-1006
Phone: 212-346-8500
Fax: 212-732-2482
e-mail: boxoffice@tribecapac.org
Web Site: www.tribecapac.org
Management:
   Operations Director: Carol Cleveland
Budget: $60,000-150,000

5052 USDAN CENTER FOR THE CREATIVE & PERFORMING ARTS: FESTIVAL CONCERTS

420 E 79th Street
New York, NY 10021
Phone: 212-772-6060
Web Site: www.usdan.com
Management:

Executive Director: Dale Lewis

5053 WASHINGTON SQUARE MUSIC FESTIVAL

PO Box 1066, Village Station
New York, NY 10014-0706
Phone: 917-855-4205
e-mail: pacrasia@aol.com
Officers:
    Chairman: Liama Hood
Management:
    Executive Director: Peggy Friedman
    Festival Manager: Jean Lyman Geotz
    Music Director: Lutz Rath
Mission: To present free classical and classical jazz and salsa concerts in Washington Square Park in the summer, for the largest possible audiences. Outreach activities announce the series to as large and diverse asegment of the metropolitan population as possible.
Founded: 1953
Specialized Field: Music
Paid Staff: 3
Volunteer Staff: 15
Paid Artists: 50
Budget: $55,000
Income Sources: Public and Private Funds; NYSCA; NYC Cultural Affairs; Trust Fund through 802
Affiliations: Whashington Square Association
Annual Attendance: 6,000
Facility Category: Park

5054 WASHINGTON SQUARE CONTEMPORARY MUSIC SERIES

NYU Music Department FAS
268 Waverly Building
New York, NY 10003-6789
Phone: 212-998-8300
Fax: 212-995-4147
e-mail: FennellyBL@aol.com
Management:
    Co-Director: Brian Fennelly
Budget: $10,000-20,000
Performs At: Merkin Hall

5055 WORLD FINANCIAL CENTER ARTS & EVENTS PROGRAM

200 Liberty Street
New York, NY 10281
Phone: 212-945-0505
Fax: 212-945-3392
e-mail: wfcae@wfprop.com
Web Site: www.worldfinancialcenter.com
Management:
    Artistic Director/Vice-President: Melissa Coley
Budget: $150,000-400,000
Performs At: World Financial Center Winter Garden & Plaza

5056 WORLD MUSIC INSTITUTE

49 W 27th Street
#930
New York, NY 10001-6396

Phone: 212-545-7536
Fax: 212-889-2771
e-mail: WMI@HearTheWorld.org
Web Site: www.HearTheWorld.org
Management:
    Executive Director: Robert Browning
Budget: $150,000-400,000
Performs At: Washington Square Church; Sylvia & Danny Kaye Playhouse

5057 YOUNG CONCERT ARTISTS SERIES

250 W 57th Street
New York, NY 10019
Phone: 212-307-6655
Fax: 212-581-8894
e-mail: yca@yca.org
Web Site: www.yca.org
Management:
    Director: Susan Wadsworth
Budget: $60,000-150,000
Performs At: Kaufmann Concert Hall; Terrace Theatre; Kennedy Center

5058 GREECE PERFORMING ARTS SOCIETY SERIES

PO Box 300
North Greece, NY 14515
Phone: 716-227-2619
Officers:
    President: Rick Stein
    Treasurer: William Coons
    Secretary: Carol Coons
Management:
    Program Coordinator: William Coons
Mission: To foster the development, in the community of Greece, of an appreciation for artistic and cultural activities, GPAS sponsors the Greece Symphony Orchestra, Greece Community Orchestra and Greece Choral Society & GPAS Summer Theatre.
Founded: 1972
Specialized Field: Vocal Music; Instrumental Music; Theater
Status: Nonprofit
Organization Type: Sponsoring

5059 CHENANGO COUNTY COUNCIL FOR THE ARTS

27 W Main Street
Norwich, NY 13815
Phone: 607-336-2787
Fax: 607-336-1893
e-mail: artscoun@norwich.net
Web Site: www.norwich.net/~artscoun
Management:
    Manager: Victoria Kappel
Budget: $10,000-20,000

5060 NYACK COLLEGE PROGRAM OF CULTURAL EVENTS

Nyack College
1 S Boulevard
Nyack, NY 10960

Phone: 845-358-1710
Fax: 845-358-1718
Budget: $10,000
Performs At: Pardington Hall; Olson Auditorium

5061 OGDENSBURG COMMAND PERFORMANCES

1100 State Street
Ogdensburg, NY 13669
Phone: 315-393-2625
Fax: 315-393-2625
e-mail: manny@gisco.net
Management:
    Administrative Coordinator: Sally Palao

5062 ARTS CENTER/OLD FORGE

Route 28
PO Box 1144
Old Forge, NY 13420
Phone: 315-369-6411
Fax: 315-369-2431
e-mail: arts@telenet.net
Management:
    Executive Director: Pamela Pratt
    Program Coordinator: Julie Tabbitas
Founded: 1952
Specialized Field: Multi Arts
Paid Staff: 6
Volunteer Staff: 6
Budget: $250,000-300,000
Income Sources: Private Donations; Membership; State & Local Government
Annual Attendance: 30,000
Facility Category: Community Arts Center
Stage Dimensions: varies
Seating Capacity: 150

5063 FRIENDS OF GOOD MUSIC

PO Box 222
Olean, NY 14760
Phone: 716-373-1776
Fax: 716-373-2662
Budget: $35,000-60,000

5064 FESTIVAL OF THE ARTS

248 Main Street
Upper Catskill Community Council of the Arts
Oneonta, NY 13820
Phone: 607-432-2070
Fax: 607-431-9319
Management:
    Director: Pamela Cooley
Founded: 1969
Specialized Field: Dance; Vocal Music; Instrumental Music; Theater; Festivals
Status: Professional; Nonprofit
Income Sources: State University of New York-Oneonta
Performs At: Slade Auditorium; Anderson Theater
Organization Type: Educational; Sponsoring

5065 HARTWICK COLLEGE FOREMAN CREATIVE & PERFORMING ARTS SERIES

Office of Events Planning
Shineman Chapel
Oneonta, NY 13820
Phone: 607-431-4034
Fax: 607-431-4043
e-mail: markusonc@hartwick.edu
Web Site: www.hartwick.edu
Management:
    Event Planning/Stewardship Director: Cira P Markuson
Budget: $20,000-35,000
Performs At: Slade Theatre

5066 UPPER CATSKILL COMMUNITY COUNCIL OF THE ARTS

248 Main Street
Oneonta, NY 13820
Phone: 607-432-2070
Fax: 607-431-9319
Management:
    Executive Director: Pamela Cooley
    Associate Director: Elissa Kane
Mission: Sponsoring community performances and coordinating secondary and elementary school performances.
Founded: 1970
Specialized Field: Dance; Vocal Music; Theater
Status: Professional; Non-Professional; Nonprofit
Organization Type: Educational; Sponsoring

5067 OSWEGO HARBOR FESTIVALS

41 Lake Street
Oswego, NY 13126
Phone: 315-343-3733
Fax: 315-343-7390
Management:
    Program Administrator: Laurel Braun

5068 PAWLING CONCERT SERIES

700 Route 22
Pawling, NY 12564
Phone: 845-855-3100
Fax: 845-855-3816
e-mail: nreade@trinitypawling.org
Web Site: www.pawlingconcertseries.org
Management:
    Manager: Ned Reade
    Artistic Director: Keir Donaldson
Mission: To provide high-quality live performances of folk, jazz and classical music for the area.
Founded: 1973
Specialized Field: Vocal Music; Instrumental Music
Status: Nonprofit
Volunteer Staff: 13
Non-paid Artists: 24
Budget: $20,000-35,000
Income Sources: Subscriptions; Business; Sponsor Grants
Annual Attendance: 1,200
Facility Category: Gothic Chapel

Seating Capacity: 250; 400
Year Built: 1924
Organization Type: Sponsoring; Presenting

5069 CLASSICAL FRONTIERS
446 Pelhamdale Avenue
Pelham, NY 10803
Phone: 914-738-6537
Budget: $10,000

5070 YATES PERFORMING ARTS SERIES
PO Box 503
Penn Yan, NY 14527
Phone: 315-536-2095
Mission: To provide entertainment for Yates County residents.
Founded: 1972
Specialized Field: Dance; Vocal Music; Instrumental Music; Festivals; Lyric Opera
Status: Professional; Non-Professional; Nonprofit
Performs At: Penn Yan Academy
Organization Type: Performing; Touring

5071 MUSICAL CONCERTS AT THE BURLINGHAM INN
29 Vinegar Hill Road
Pine Bush, NY 12566
Phone: 845-744-8499
Fax: 845-744-8936
e-mail: BIConcerts@aol.com
Web Site: www.burlinghaminn.com/concerts
Management:
    Director: Jonathan Bley
Budget: $10,000
Performs At: Burlingham Inn Hall

5072 MUSIC AT PORT MILFORD
288 Washington Avenue
Pleasantville, NY 10570
Phone: 914-769-9046
e-mail: director@mpmcamp.org
Web Site: www.mpmcamp.org
Management:
    Director: Meg Hill

5073 SUMMIT MUSIC FESTIVAL
192 Edgewood Avenue
Pleasantville, NY 10570
Phone: 914-769-4111
Fax: 914-769-4111
e-mail: summitmusic2000@aol.com
Management:
    Executive Director: David Krieger
    Artistic Director: Efrem Breskin
    Administrator: Miriam Derivan
Mission: To provide an enriching musical experience for area students and exposure to the finest in solo, chamber, and orchestra performances.
Founded: 1991
Specialized Field: Classical Instrumental music instruction and performance for pre - professional high school and college age students
Paid Staff: 7

Paid Artists: 20

5074 COMMUNITY PERFORMANCE SERIES
Snell Music Theatre
Bishop Hall, SUNY
Potsdam, NY 13676
Phone: 315-267-2411
Fax: 315-267-2869
e-mail: olsenka@potsdam.edu
Web Site: www.potsdam.edu/cps
Management:
    Executive Director: Kathy Olsen
Paid Staff: 3
Paid Artists: 50
Non-paid Artists: 20
Budget: $300,000
Performs At: Hosmer Concert Hall; Snell Music Theater; MaxcyHall
Annual Attendance: 7,000
Facility Category: Concert Hall
Stage Dimensions: 40 x 40
Seating Capacity: 1,200
Year Built: 1971
Year Remodeled: 2000

5075 CRANE SCHOOL OF MUSIC ANNUAL SPRING FESTIVAL OF THE ARTS
State University of NY at Potsdam
Potsdam, NY 13676
Phone: 315-267-2412
Fax: 315-267-2413
e-mail: olsenka@potsdam.edu
Web Site: www.potsdam.edu/crane
Management:
    Executive Director: Kathleen Olsen

5076 CLEARWATER'S GREAT HUDSON RIVER REVIVAL
112 Market Street
Poughkeepsie, NY 12601
Phone: 845-454-7953
e-mail: revival@mail.clearwater.org
Web Site: www.clearwater.org

5077 EASTMAN SCHOOL OF MUSIC
26 Gibbs Street
Rochester, NY 14604
Phone: 585-274-1110
Fax: 585-274-1073
e-mail: agreen@esm.rochester.edu
Management:
    Director of Concert Operations: Andrew Green
Budget: $60,000-150,000
Performs At: Kilbourn Hall; Eastman Theatre

5078 NAZARETH COLLEGE ARTS CENTER SERIES
4245 E Avenue
Rochester, NY 14618-3090
Phone: 716-389-2175
Fax: 716-389-2182
e-mail: nlpeet@naz.edu

Officers:
Chairman: Fred E Strauss
President of the College: Dr. Rose Marie Beston
Management:
School Program Coordinator: Nancy Peet
Director: Dr David M Ferrell
Assistant Director: Terry Meyer
Mission: To present a subscription series of professional performing artists and organizations for the benefit of Nazareth students and the community of Rochester.
Founded: 1967
Specialized Field: Dance; Vocal Music; Instrumental Music; Theater
Status: Professional; Nonprofit
Budget: $150,000-400,000
Income Sources: Association of Performing Arts Presenters
Performs At: Nazareth College Arts Center
Organization Type: Performing; Sponsoring

5079 ROBERTS WESLEYAN COLLEGE
Roberts Cultural Life Center
2301 Westside Drive
Rochester, NY 14624-1997
Phone: 716-594-6026
Fax: 716-594-6812
e-mail: DunnDR@roberts.edu
Web Site: www.rwc.edu/clc
Management:
Director: David R Dunn
Technical Director: James R Price
Founded: 1866
Paid Staff: 6
Volunteer Staff: 45
Paid Artists: 7
Non-paid Artists: 155
Budget: $35,000-60,000
Income Sources: Ticket Sales
Performs At: Hale Auditorium
Annual Attendance: 45,000
Facility Category: Performing Arts
Type of Stage: Proscenium
Stage Dimensions: 50'x30'x25'
Seating Capacity: 1000
Year Built: 1996
Cost: $8 Million
Rental Contact: David Dunn

5080 RPO SUMMERMUSIC
Rochester Philharmonic Orchestra
108 East Avenue
Rochester, NY 14604
Phone: 716-454-2620
Fax: 716-423-2256
e-mail: rpo@rpo.org
Web Site: www.rpo.org
Management:
Operations Director: Randy Kemp

5081 MUSIC FROM SALEM
PO Box 631
Salem, NY 12865

Phone: 518-854-7232
e-mail: cmfs@sover.net
Web Site: www.musicfromsalem.org
Management:
Artistic Director: Lila Brown
Mission: To provide a summer home to international chamber musicians.
Founded: 1986
Specialized Field: Vocal Music; Instrumental Music
Status: Professional
Performs At: Hubbard Hall
Organization Type: Performing; Resident

5082 HILL & HOLLOW MUSIC
Weatherwatch Farm
550 #37 Road
Saranac, NY 12981
Phone: 518-293-7613
Fax: 518-293-7634
Management:
Co-Director: Angela Brown
Co-Director: Kellum Smith
Mission: To promote and present classical chamber music in a rural area.
Founded: 1995
Specialized Field: Chamber Music
Volunteer Staff: 2
Budget: $100,000
Income Sources: Box office, Grants, Private contributions
Performs At: Church in the Hollow; Highschool Auditorium
Affiliations: Chamber Music America; Country Dance & Song Society
Facility Category: Rural Venues
Seating Capacity: 220
Year Built: 1862

5083 ADIRONDACK FESTIVAL OF AMERICAN MUSIC
Gregg Smith Singers
PO Box 562
Saranac Lake, NY 12983
Phone: 518-891-1057
Fax: 518-891-1057
Management:
Artistic Director: Gregg Smith
Director Vocal Workshop: Linda Ferriera
Mission: To offer a program including American music of the present and past, and some traditional repertoire.
Specialized Field: Vocal Music; Instrumental Music; Choral
Status: Professional; Nonprofit
Performs At: Town Hall
Organization Type: Performing; Educational

5084 FREIHOFER'S JAZZ FESTIVAL AT THE SARATOGA PERFORMING ARTS CENTER
Saratoga Performing Arts Center
Saratoga Springs, NY 12866

Phone: 518-584-9330
e-mail: info@spac.org
Web Site: www.spac.org

5085 SKIDMORE MUSIC DEPARTMENT SERIES

Skidmore College
815 N Broadway
Saratoga Springs, NY 12866
Phone: 518-580-5320
Fax: 518-580-5799
e-mail: rhihn@skidmore.edu
Web Site: www.skidmore.edu
Officers:
   Music Department Chairman: Richard R Hihn
Budget: $35,000-60,000
Performs At: Filene Recital Hall

5086 SCHENECTADY MUSEUM: UNION COLLEGE CONCERT SERIES

857 Northumberland Drive
Schenectady, NY 12309
Phone: 518-372-3651
Officers:
   Chairman: Dr. Daniel Berkenblit
Budget: $35,000-60,000
Performs At: Union College Memorial Chapel

5087 SKANEATELES FESTIVAL

28 Hannum Street
Skaneateles, NY 13152
Phone: 315-685-7418
Fax: 315-685-4802
e-mail: music@scanfest.org
Web Site: www.skanfest.org
Management:
   Executive Director: Susan Mark
   Music Director: Robert Weirich
   Artistic Director: Diane Walsh
Mission: Bringing world-class musicians to this lakeside community for five weeks of chamber music, chamber orchestra and children's concerts in the late summer.
Founded: 1980
Specialized Field: Festivals
Status: Professional; Nonprofit
Organization Type: Performing; Educational

5088 SPENCERTOWN ACADEMY PERFORMING SERIES

790 Route 203
Box 80
Spencertown, NY 12165
Phone: 518-392-3693
Fax: 518-392-6521
e-mail: spencertown@taconic.net
Web Site: www.spencertown.org
Officers:
   President: Roberta Reynes
   Vice President: Ben Puccio
   Secretary: Claire Verenezi
   Treasurer: Jan Steinbrenner
Management:
   Director: Judy Staber

Associate Director: Susan Davis
Mission: To preserve the historic building and provide a welcoming space for all the arts.
Founded: 1970
Paid Staff: 3
Volunteer Staff: 10+
Paid Artists: 40
Non-paid Artists: 5
Budget: $100,000
Income Sources: Private Funds; Ticket Sales; Art Sales
Annual Attendance: 5,000
Facility Category: Performance & Visual Arts Center
Type of Stage: Proscenium
Seating Capacity: 130
Year Built: 1867
Year Remodeled: 1999

5089 STERLING RENAISSANCE FESTIVAL

15385 Farden Road
Sterling, NY 13156
Phone: 315-947-5783
Fax: 315-947-6905
Toll-free: 800-879-4446
e-mail: office@sterlingfestival.com
Web Site: www.sterlingfestival.com
Officers:
   President: Alisa Cook
   VP: John Kissler
   Secretary: Phil Holding
   Treasurer: Marylee Pangman
Management:
   Office Manager/Sales Director: Kelli Raymond
Mission: To present interactive and staged performances.
Paid Staff: 10
Paid Artists: 80
Season: June - August
Annual Attendance: 100,000
Facility Category: Outdoor
Type of Stage: 8 Stages
Year Built: 1977

5090 STATE UNIVERSITY OF NEW YORK AT STONY BROOK CONCERT SERIES

SUNY at Stony Brook
Stony Brook, NY 11794-5425
Phone: 516-632-7235
Fax: 516-632-7354
e-mail: ainkles@notes.cc.sunysb.edu
Web Site: www.stallercenter.com
Management:
   Director: Alan Inkles
Budget: $150,000-400,000
Performs At: Staller Center for the Arts; Three Black Box Theatres

5091 CIVIC MORNING MUSICALS

301 Apple Street
Syracuse, NY 13204-2107
Phone: 315-422-0553
Management:
   Public Relations Coordinator: Irene Boheme
Budget: $10,000
Performs At: Hosmer Auditorium; Everson Museum of Art

5092   CULTURAL RESOURCES COUNCIL OF SYRACUSE
411 Montgomery Street
Syracuse, NY 13202
Phone: 315-435-2155
Fax: 315-435-2160
Web Site: www.cspot.org
Management:
    Executive Director: Leo Crandace
Mission: Promote cultural development in Central NY; identify, coordinate, promote, and present performing arts for a 10-county area in Cedntral New York. Education and trainging; technical assistance.
Founded: 1968
Specialized Field: Dance; Theater; Festivals; Music; Visual Advocacy, Training, Education
Status: Professional; Nonprofit
Paid Staff: 9
Income Sources: International Society of Performing Arts Administrators
Performs At: Civic Center of Onondaga County
Organization Type: Performing

5093   SYRACUSE SOCIETY FOR NEW MUSIC
312 Crawford Avenue
Syracuse, NY 13224
Phone: 315-446-5733
Web Site: www.societyfornewmusic.org
Management:
    Program Advisor: Neva Pilgrim
Founded: 1971
Budget: $20,000-35,000
Performs At: Everson Museum; Carrier Theatre
Annual Attendance: 13,000

5094   TICONDEROGA FESTIVAL GUILD
124 Montclaim Street
PO Box 125
Ticonderoga, NY 12883
Phone: 518-585-6716
Fax: 518-543-6654
e-mail: tfguild@capital.net
Management:
    Executive Director: Cathie Burdick
Mission: To provide cultural events for a rural area.
Founded: 1980
Specialized Field: Festivals
Status: Nonprofit
Budget: $40,000
Income Sources: Grants; Donations; Tickets
Annual Attendance: 3500
Type of Stage: Wood
Stage Dimensions: 20'x30'
Seating Capacity: 200
Organization Type: Performing

5095   HUDSON VALLEY COMMUNITY COLLEGE CULTURAL AFFAIRS PROGRAM
80 Vandenburgh Avenue
Troy, NY 12180
Phone: 518-629-8073
e-mail: boggesar@hvcc.edu

Management:
    Community Relations Director: Sarah Boggess
Budget: $10,000
Performs At: Maureen Stapleton Theatre

5096   TROY CHROMATIC CONCERTS
PO Box 1574
Troy, NY 12181
Phone: 518-273-0038
e-mail: killeent@crisny.org
Web Site: www.crisny.org/not-for-profit/trychrom
Officers:
    President: Bernice Bornt-Ledeboer
    Artist Selection Committee Chair: Tracy Killeen
Budget: $35,000-60,000
Performs At: Troy Savings Bank Music Hall

5097   A GOOD OLD SUMMER TIME'S GENESEE STREET FESTIVAL
520 Seneca Street
Utica, NY 13502
Phone: 315-733-6976
Fax: 315-724-3177
Web Site: www.goodoldsummertime.org
Officers:
    President: Mark Minasi

5098   MOHAWK VALLEY COMMUNITY COLLEGE CULTURAL EVENTS SERIES
1101 Sherman Drive
Utica, NY 13501
Phone: 315-792-5439
Fax: 315-793-5666
e-mail: jgifford@mvcc.edu
Web Site: www.mvcc.edu
Management:
    Manager: James Gifford
Budget: $10,000

5099   MUNSON-WILLIAMS-PROCTOR ARTS INSTITUTE
310 Genesee Street
Utica, NY 13502-4799
Phone: 315-797-0000
Fax: 315-797-5608
Toll-free: 800-754-0797
e-mail: gtrudeau@mwpi.edu
Web Site: www.mwpi.edu
Management:
    Director Performing Arts: George Trudeau
Mission: To provide exemplary programs and educational opportunites in the performing and cinematic arts, setting a national standard for artistic achievement.
Founded: 1932
Specialized Field: Dance; Vocal Music; Instrumental Music; Theater; Festivals; Lyric Opera; Grand Opera; Jazz; Folk; Children's; Film
Status: Professional; Nonprofit
Paid Staff: 10
Volunteer Staff: 30
Paid Artists: 270
Budget: $919,000 (performing arts)

Income Sources: Ticket sales; grants; sponsorships; program advertising; endowment
Performs At: Stanley Performing Arts Center
Affiliations: International Society of Performing Arts Administrators, INTIX, American Symphony Orchestra League, Wellinhall/Hamilton Colletge
Annual Attendance: 45,550
Facility Category: Arts center
Type of Stage: Proscenium, thrust,museum courtyad
Seating Capacity: 2,960, 271, 500
Year Built: 1960
Cost: 10 Million
Organization Type: Performing; Educational; Sponsoring

5100 WESTBURY MUSIC FAIR

960 Brush Hollow Road
Westbury, NY 11590
Phone: 516-333-7228
Fax: 516-333-7991
Web Site: www.musicfair.com
Management:
Executive Vice President: Jason Stone
Theatre Manager: John Blenn
Marketing Director: Dan Kellachan
Publicist: Laura Nuzzolo
Group Sales Manager: Ed Denning
Mission: To offer the best entertainment of all kinds to metropolitan New York.
Founded: 1956
Specialized Field: Dance; Vocal Music; Instrumental Music; Theater
Status: Professional; Commercial
Season: year-round
Facility Category: Year-round Indoor
Type of Stage: In the round
Seating Capacity: 2,742
Year Built: 1956
Year Remodeled: 1998
Rental Contact: 516-333-2101 Ed Denning
Organization Type: Performing

5101 ARTS COUNCIL FOR THE NORTHERN ADIRONDACKS

PO Box 187
Westport, NY 12993
Phone: 518-962-8778
Fax: 518-962-8797
e-mail: artsco@westelcom.com
Web Site: www.artsnorth.org
Management:
Executive Director: Caroline Rubino
Budget: $10,000-20,000

5102 MAVERICK CONCERTS

Maverick Road
PO Box 102
Woodstock, NY 12498
Phone: 914-338-3074
Fax: 914-338-3074
e-mail: musicmavrk@aol.com
Web Site: www.beekman.net/maverickconcerts
Management:
Music Director: Vincent Wagner

Mission: To provide Sunday afternoon chamber music concerts in summer.
Budget: $60,000-150,000

North Carolina

5103 ASHEVILLE CHAMBER MUSIC SERIES

25 Brook Forest Drive
Arden, NC 28704
Phone: 828-684-5976
Web Site: www.main.nc.us/ashevillechambermusic/
Officers:
President: Dr. Harold Rotman
VP: Philip Walker
Secretary: Perien Gray
Treasurer: J. H. Wynn
Management:
Program Director: Bill van der Hoeven
Mission: To provide chamber music concerts.
Founded: 1952
Specialized Field: Instrumental Music
Status: Non-Professional; Nonprofit
Budget: $10,000-20,000
Income Sources: Chamber Music America
Organization Type: Performing

5104 UNIVERSITY OF NORTH CAROLINA AT ASHEVILLE CULTURAL & SPECIAL EVENTS

Highsmith Center
1 University Heights
Asheville, NC 28804
Phone: 828-232-5000
Fax: 828-232-2988
e-mail: bhalton@unca.edu
Web Site: www.unca.edu/student_activities
Management:
Assistant Director Student Life: Barbara Halton
Budget: $60,000-150,000
Performs At: Lipinsky Auditorium; Thomas Wolfe Auditorium; Pack Place
Annual Attendance: 7,000+
Facility Category: Campus Auditorium
Type of Stage: Proscenium
Seating Capacity: 600

5105 BEAUFORT COUNTY COMMUNITY CONCERTS ASSOCIATION

1117 Whealton Point Road
Aurora, NC 27806
Phone: 252-322-5259
Officers:
President: Helen Sommerkamp
Budget: $20,000-35,000

5106 LEES-MCRAE COLLEGE FORUM

PO Box 649
Banner Elk, NC 28604

All listings are in alphabetical order by state, then city, then organization within the city.

Phone: 828-898-8748
Fax: 828-898-8814
Toll-free: 800-280-4562
e-mail: ramsey@lmc.edu
Web Site: www.lmc.edu
Officers:
   President: Ed Hardin
   Vice President: Dick Collins
   Treasurer: Paul Weber
Management:
   Special Events Coordinator: Sandy M Ramsey
Mission: To bring a stimulating series of cultural events to the area.
Founded: 1979
Specialized Field: Performing
Paid Staff: 2
Volunteer Staff: 4
Budget: $40,000-45,000
Income Sources: Donations
Performs At: Hayes Auditorium
Annual Attendance: 6500
Facility Category: Concert hall/performance center
Seating Capacity: 750

5107 GARDNER-WEBB UNIVERSITY DISTINGUISHED ARTIST SERIES

Box 7298
Fine Arts Department
Boiling Springs, NC 28017
Phone: 704-406-3937
Fax: 704-406-3920
e-mail: tfern@gardner-webb.edu
Officers:
   Fine Arts Department Chairman: Dr. Terry Fern
Budget: $10,000-20,000
Performs At: Hamrick Hall Auditorium; Dover theatre

5108 AN APPALACHIAN SUMMER FESTIVAL

Appalachian State University
Office of Cultural Affairs, PO Box 32045
Boone, NC 28608-2045
Phone: 828-262-6084
Fax: 828-262-2848
Toll-free: 800-841-2787
e-mail: weissberg@appstate.edu
Web Site: www.appsummer.appstate.edu
Management:
   Artistic Director: Gil Morgenstern
   Marketing Director: Denise Rigler
Mission: To build new audiences for the fine arts; to enrich as well as to entertain.
Founded: 1983
Specialized Field: Multi-Disciplinary (Music, Dance, Theatre

5109 APPALACHIAN STATE UNIVERSITY PERFORMING ARTS & FORUM SERIES

Appalachian State University
PO Box 32045
Boone, NC 28608-2045
Phone: 828-262-4010
Fax: 828-262-2556
e-mail: mixterhp@appstate.edu
Web Site: www.oca.appstate.edu

Management:
   Director: Rachel Laney
Budget: $150,000-400,000
Performs At: Farthing Auditorium; Rosen Concert Hall; Valborg Theatre

5110 HORN IN THE WEST

PO Box 295
Boone, NC 28607
Phone: 828-264-2120
Fax: 828-264-4529
e-mail: smalling@boone.net
Web Site: www.boonenc.org/saha
Management:
   General Manager/Museum Director: Curtis Smalling
   Assistant General Manager: Debbie Grant
Mission: To bring the past to life, with emphasis on the Revolutionary War and the struggle between settlers and Native Americans.
Founded: 1952
Specialized Field: Dance; Vocal Music; Theater; Festivals
Status: Professional; Nonprofit
Income Sources: Southern Appalachian Historical Association
Season: June - Ausust
Performs At: Horn In The West
Organization Type: Performing; Educational

5111 BREVARD MUSIC FESTIVAL

1000 Probart Street
PO Box 312
Brevard, NC 28712
Phone: 828-862-2100
Fax: 828-884-2036
e-mail: brevardmusic@citcom.net
Web Site: www.brevardmusic.org
Management:
   Artistic Director: David Effron
Founded: 1936
Specialized Field: Music
Income Sources: Ticket Sales; Tuition; Donation
Performs At: Concert Hall
Annual Attendance: 70,000
Facility Category: Covered, Open-Sided Auditorium
Seating Capacity: 1,800
Year Built: 1965
Year Remodeled: 1998

5112 CAMPBELL UNIVERSITY COMMUNITY CONCERT SERIES

Music Department
PO Box 70, Campbell University
Buies Creek, NC 27506
Phone: 910-893-1495
Fax: 910-893-1515
Toll-free: 800-334-4111
e-mail: wilson@mailcenter.cambell.edu
Management:
   Director: Charles D Wilson
Budget: $10,000-20,000
Performs At: Scott Concert Hall

5113 CAROLINA UNION PERFORMING ARTS SERIES
Carolina Union
201 Student Union Building
Chapel Hill, NC 27599-5210
Phone: 919-966-3120
Fax: 919-962-3719
e-mail: lused@email.unc.edu
Web Site: carolinaunion.unc.edu
Management:
    Director: Don Luse
    Production Services Ass't Director: Michael Johnson
Budget: $150,000-400,000
Performs At: Memorial Hall university of North Carolina
Annual Attendance: 10,000

5114 CAROLINAS CONCERT ASSOCIATION
PO Box 11356
Charlotte, NC 28220
Phone: 704-527-6680
Fax: 704-527-1846
e-mail: bratton@carolinasconcert.com
Web Site: carolinasconcertassoc.com
Management:
    Booking Director: John Whitaker
    Executive Director: Shelley Bratton
Founded: 1930
Budget: $150,000-400,000
Performs At: North Carolina Blumenthal Performing Arts Center

5115 CHARLOTTE CENTER CITY PARTNERS
128 S Tyron Street
Suite 1960
Charlotte, NC 28202
Phone: 704-332-2227
Fax: 704-342-1233
e-mail: rkrumbine@charlottecentercity.org
Web Site: www.charlottecentercity.org
Management:
    VP Events: Rovbert Krumbine

5116 WESTERN CAROLINA UNIVERSITY LECTURES, CONCERTS & EXHIBITIONS
Western Carolina University
University Center
Cullowhee, NC 28723
Phone: 828-227-7234
Fax: 828-227-7250
Management:
    LCE Series: Beth Johnson
Paid Staff: 1
Budget: $35,000-60,000
Performs At: Ramsey Activities Center; Hoey Auditorium

5117 AMERICAN DANCE FESTIVAL
PO Box 90772
Durham, NC 27708-0772
Phone: 919-684-6402
Fax: 919-684-5459
e-mail: adf@americandancefestival.org
Web Site: www.americandancefestival.org
Management:
    Co-Director: Charles Reinhart
    Co-Director: Stephanie Reinhart
    Dean: Donna Faye Burchfield
    Director ADF Humanities: Dr. Gerald E Myers
    Dean Emeritus: Martha Myers
    Director Administration: Cynthia Wyse
    Director Community Activites: Martha Zeadler
    Director Press/Marketing: Anne Shoemake
Mission: Committed to encouraging and supporting the creation of our dance heritage by established and emerging choreographers; to offer a solid professional education.
Founded: 1934
Specialized Field: Modern Dance
Status: Professional; Nonprofit
Paid Staff: 18
Budget: $2,000,000
Performs At: Page Auditorium; Reynolds Industries Theatre; others
Annual Attendance: 32,000
Stage Dimensions: 30'x 37',48'x 35'
Seating Capacity: 1232; 589
Organization Type: Educational; Sponsoring

5118 BULL DURHAM BLUES FESTIVAL
Hayti Historic Center
801 Old Fayetteville Street
Durham, NC 27702
Phone: 919-683-1709
Fax: 919-682-5869

5119 DUKE UNIVERSITY ARTISTS SERIES
Box 90834
Duke University
Durham, NC 27708
Phone: 919-684-3227
Fax: 919-684-8395
e-mail: susan.coon@duke.edu
Management:
    Office of University Life Dean: Susan L Coon
Budget: $60,000-150,000
Performs At: Page Auditorium
Seating Capacity: 1232

5120 DUKE UNIVERSITY UNION BROADWAY COMMITTEE / ON STAGE COMMITTEE
Box 90834
Duke University
Durham, NC 27708-0834
Phone: 919-684-4682
Fax: 919-684-8395
e-mail: pcoyle@acpub.duke.edu
Management:
    Associate Dean: Peter Coyle
Budget: $35,000-60,000
Performs At: Page Auditorium
Seating Capacity: 1232

5121 SUMMER FESTIVAL OF CHAMBER MUSIC AT DUKE UNIVERSITY
Box 90834
Duke University
Durham, NC 27708
Phone: 919-684-3227
Fax: 919-684-8395
Management:
Office of University Life Dean: Susan Coon

5122 TRIANGLE THEATRE FESTIVAL
100 Timber Ridge Drive
Durham, NC 27713-9330
Phone: 919-490-8603
Fax: 919-401-3565
e-mail: info@theatrefestival.org
Web Site: www.theatrefestival.org
Management:
Director: Anthony C Caporale

5123 COA COMMUNITY CENTER AUDITORIUM
PO Box 2327
Elizabeth City, NC 27906-2327
Fax: 252-337-6622
Toll-free: 800-335-9050
e-mail: aswain@albemarle.edu
Web Site: www.albemarle.cc.nc.us/acadaff/finearts
Management:
Community Center Manager: Sam Johnson
Events Coordinator: Sandra Boyce
Box Office Manager: Angela Swain
Paid Staff: 4
Volunteer Staff: 20
Budget: $60,000-150,000
Performs At: Proscenium House Auditorium
Seating Capacity: 1,000
Rental Contact: Sam Johnson

5124 ELIZABETH CITY STATE UNIVERSITY LYCEUM SERIES
Campus Box 891
1704 Weeksville Road
Elizabeth City, NC 27909
Phone: 252-335-3345
Fax: 252-335-3482
e-mail: arjoyner@mail.ecsu.edu
Web Site: www.ecsu.edu
Management:
Art Department: Alexis Joyner

5125 ELON UNIVERSITY LYCEUM COMMITTEE
2800 Campus Box
Elon, NC 27244-2010
Phone: 336-278-5607
Fax: 336-278-5609
e-mail: troxlerg@elon.edu
Management:
Dean of Cultural/Special Programs: George Troxler
Paid Staff: 4
Budget: $35,000-60,000

Income Sources: University Funds
Performs At: McCrary Theatre; Whitley Auditorium
Seating Capacity: 572/370

5126 FARMVILLE COMMUNITY ARTS COUNCIL
PO Box 305
Farmville, NC 27828
Phone: 252-753-3832
Fax: 252-753-6910
e-mail: fcac@greenvillenc.com
Web Site: www.reflector.com
Management:
Executive Director: Barbara D Owens
Budget: $10,000
Performs At: Stage-Theater-Arts Center

5127 ARTS COUNCIL OF FAYETTEVILLE/CUMBERLAND COUNTY
301 Hay Street
Fayetteville, NC 28301
Mailing Address: PO Box 318, Fayetteville, NC 28302
Phone: 910-323-1776
Fax: 910-323-1727
e-mail: admin@theartscouncil.com
Web Site: www.theartscouncil.com
Officers:
President: Libby Seymour
Budget: $10,000

5128 ARTS COUNCIL OF MACON COUNTY
PO Box 726
Franklin, NC 28744
Phone: 828-524-7683
Fax: 828-524-7683
Management:
Executive Director: Bobbie Contino
Budget: $10,000
Performs At: Franklin Fine Arts Center; Highlands Civic Center

5129 EASTERN MUSIC FESTIVAL
200 N Davie Street
PO Box 22026
Greensboro, NC 27420
Phone: 336-333-7450
Fax: 336-333-7454
Toll-free: 877-833-6753
e-mail: easternmusicfestival@worldnet.att.net
Web Site: www.easternmusicfestival.com
Management:
President & CEO: Thomas Philion
Music Director: Sheldon Morgenstern
Development/Marketing: Juanita Lawson-Haith
Business Manager: Dianne Lyle
Admissions Director: Janis Nilsen
Artistic Administrator: Renee Ward
Artistic Director: Andre-Michel Schrub
Mission: To offer a six-week intensive study program for 200 talented young national and international musicians; to provide a quality music series to the Southeast.
Founded: 1961

All listings are in alphabetical order by state, then city, then organization within the city.

Specialized Field: Symphony; Orchestra; Chamber
Status: Professional; Nonprofit
Income Sources: Broadcast Music Incorporated;
American Society of Composers, Authors and Publishers
Organization Type: Performing; Educational

5130 GUILFORD COLLEGE ARTS

5800 W Friendly Avenue
Greensboro, NC 27410
Phone: 336-316-2388
Fax: 336-316-2949
e-mail: watkinsda@rascalguilford.edu
Web Site: www.guilford.edu
Management:
   Activities & Events Director: Dawn Watkins
Budget: $35,000-60,000
Performs At: Dana Auditorium; Sternberger Auditorium

5131 NORTH CAROLINA A&T STATE UNIVERSITY LYCEUM SERIES

North Carolina A&T State University
Greensboro, NC 27411
Phone: 336-334-7500
Fax: 336-334-7770
e-mail: jhgarner@ncat.edu
Officers:
   Chairman: Dr. Olen Cole, Jr.
   Student Affairs Vice-Chancellor: Dr. Sullivan
   Wellbourne, Jr
Status: Nonprofit
Budget: $35,000-60,000

5132 UNITED ARTS COUNCIL OF GREENSBORO

200 N Davie Street
PO Box 877
Greensboro, NC 27402
Phone: 336-373-7523
Fax: 336-373-7553
Web Site: www.uacgreensboro.org
Management:
   Community Events Director: Tina Foxx
   Marketing Director: Liz Summers

5133 UNIVERSITY OF NORTH CAROLINA AT GREENSBORO CONCERT/LECTURE SERIES

Aycock Auditorium, PO Box 26170
Spring Garden at Tate Street
Greensboro, NC 27402-6170
Phone: 336-334-5800
Fax: 336-334-3008
e-mail: ucls@uncg.edu
Web Site: ucls.uncg.edu
Management:
   UC/LS Director: Dawn Mays-Floyd
Paid Staff: 2
Budget: $150,000-400,000
Income Sources: Ticket Revenue
Performs At: Aycock Auditorium
Affiliations: NCPC; APAP
Type of Stage: Black Pine
Stage Dimensions: 39'8"

Seating Capacity: 2300
Year Built: 1926
Year Remodeled: 1970
Rental Contact: 336-334-5118 Jan Hullihan

5134 EAST CAROLINA UNIVERSITY S. RUDOLPH ALEXANDER PERFORMING ART SERIES

207 Mendenhall Student Center
East Carolina University
Greenville, NC 27858-4353
Phone: 252-328-4702
Fax: 252-328-4778
e-mail: clutterw@mail.ecu.edu
Web Site: www.ecu.edu
Management:
   Asst VC for Student Experiences: William B Clutter
Founded: 1907
Paid Staff: 2
Budget: $150,000-400,000
Performs At: Wright Auditorium
Annual Attendance: 14,000
Type of Stage: Proscenium
Seating Capacity: 1,500
Year Remodeled: 1985

5135 PITT COUNTY ARTS COUNCIL

PO Box 8191
Greenville, NC 27835
Phone: 252-757-1785
e-mail: pcac@greenville.com
Budget: $35,000-60,000

5136 NORTH CAROLINA SHAKESPEARE FESTIVAL

220 E Commerce Avenue
PO Box 6066
High Point, NC 27262
Phone: 336-841-2273
Fax: 336-841-8627
e-mail: bjatncsf@nr.infi.net
Web Site: www.ncshakes.org
Officers:
   Chairman: Christine Green
Management:
   Artistic Director: Louis Rackoff
   Marketing/Public Relations Director: Laura Ward
   Managing Director: Thomas G Gaffney
Mission: Seeks to serve the cultural and educational
needs of North Carolina audiences through traditional and
nontraditional staging of the plays of Shakespeare and
other classic playwrights.
Founded: 1977
Specialized Field: Theater
Status: Professional; Nonprofit
Paid Staff: 10
Paid Artists: 55
Budget: $1,400,000
Income Sources: Ticket sales; Touring fees; Contributors
Season: Late August - December
Performs At: High Point Theatre
Organization Type: Performing; Touring; Resident;
Educational

5137 HIGHLANDS CASHIERS CHAMBER MUSIC FESTIVAL

PO Box 1702
Highlands, NC 28741
Phone: 828-526-9060
Fax: 828-526-1865
e-mail: hccmf@aol.com
Web Site: www.h-cmusicfestival.org
Officers:
President/CEO: Sanford Cohen
Management:
Festival Manager: Thom Corrigan
Artistic Director: William Ransom
Mission: To promote the performance and appreciation of chamber music.
Founded: 1982
Specialized Field: Instrumental Chamber Music; Festivals
Status: Professional
Paid Staff: 2
Volunteer Staff: 5
Paid Artists: 35
Budget: $180,000
Income Sources: Contributions; Ticket Sales; Fund Raising
Performs At: Cashiers Carlton Public Library
Affiliations: Chamber Music America
Annual Attendance: 3500
Facility Category: Performing Arts Center
Seating Capacity: 200
Year Remodeled: 2001
Organization Type: Performing; Touring; Resident; Educational; Sponsoring

5138 COASTAL CAROLINA COMMUNITY COLLEGE

444 Western Boulevard
Jacksonville, NC 28546-6877
Phone: 910-455-1221
Fax: 910-455-7027
Management:
Concert Manager/Artist Director: Dr. Michael Daughtey
Budget: $10,000-20,000
Performs At: CCCC Fine Arts Auditorium
Seating Capacity: 182

5139 CALDWELL ARTS COUNCIL

PO Box 1613
601 College Avenue
Lenoir, NC 28645-1613
Phone: 828-754-2486
Fax: 828-754-2440
e-mail: caldart@conninc.com
Web Site: www.conninc.com/caldart/
Mission: To bring arts to the community.
Status: Nonprofit
Budget: $100,000
Income Sources: Grants; Private Donations
Performs At: J.E. Broyhill Civic Center
Annual Attendance: 2,500
Facility Category: Gallery
Type of Stage: None
Seating Capacity: 50

Year Built: 1900
Year Remodeled: 1973
Cost: Rental: $150.00
Rental Contact: Administrative Assistant Caron Banks

5140 LINCOLN ART COUNCIL

PO Box 45
Lincolnton, NC 28093
Phone: 704-732-9044
Fax: 704-732-9057
Officers:
President: Madeline Elmore
First VP: Kenneth Brown
Second VP: Beverly McAdams
Management:
Director: Lea Evelyn Tatich
Office Asssistant: Amy Crump
Mission: To develop, promote and foster all forms of creative and performing arts by arranging and offering exhibits, lectures, demonstrations, classes and performances, etc.
Founded: 1973
Specialized Field: Instrumental Music; Festivals
Status: Nonprofit
Income Sources: North Carolina Association of Arts Councils; North Carolina Arts Council
Performs At: Lincoln Citizens Center; Lincoln Cultural Center
Organization Type: Performing; Educational; Sponsoring

5141 LOUISBURG COLLEGE CONCERT SERIES

Louisburg College
501 N Main Street, Box 3125
Louisburg, NC 27549
Phone: 919-497-3251
Fax: 919-496-7141
Web Site: www.louisburg.edu
Management:
Concert and Auditorium Manager: Robert Poole
Founded: 1987
Paid Staff: 1
Budget: $35,000-60,000
Performs At: Louisburg College Performing Arts Center
Annual Attendance: 5,000
Facility Category: Auditorium
Type of Stage: Proscenium
Stage Dimensions: 56' wide x 16' high x 47' deep
Seating Capacity: 1,189
Year Built: 1987
Rental Contact: Robert Poole

5142 ROANOKE ISLAND HISTORICAL ASSOCIATION

1409 National Park Road
Manteo, NC 27954
Phone: 252-473-2127
Fax: 252-473-6000
e-mail: info@thecolony.org
Web Site: www.thecolony.org
Officers:
Chairman: Rick Gray
Vice-Chairman: Norma Mills

Secretary: Julie Daniels Nowells
Treasurer: Stuart Bell
Management:
    Executive Production Coordinator: Rhoda Dresken
    Marketing/PR Associate: Joshua M Gilliam
    Membership/Development Associate: Bette Self
    Office Manager: Terry Fowler
Mission: To celebrate the history of the first English colonies on Roanoke Island NC; to honor the founders of The Last Colony, to promote awareness of the historical value of this event; to educate through drama and literature.
Founded: 1937
Specialized Field: Dance; Theater
Status: Non-Equity; Nonprofit
Paid Staff: 30
Paid Artists: 145
Budget: $1.5 million
Income Sources: Ticket Sales; Grants; Donations
Performs At: Waterside Theatre
Affiliations: Professional Theatre Workshop (in-house)
Annual Attendance: 60,000-70,000
Facility Category: Outdoor
Type of Stage: Amphitheatre
Stage Dimensions: 80' x 40'
Seating Capacity: 1534
Year Built: 1937
Year Remodeled: 1998
Organization Type: Performing

5143 PFEIFFER UNIVERSITY ARTIST SERIES

Pfeiffer University
Misenheimer, NC 28109
Phone: 704-463-1360
Fax: 704-463-1363
e-mail: sharrill@pfeiffer.edu
Management:
    Manager: Stephen Harrill
Budget: $10,000
Performs At: Henry Pfeiffer Chapel

5144 SURRY ARTS COUNCIL

PO Box 141
Mount Airy, NC 27030
Phone: 336-786-7998
Fax: 336-786-9822
e-mail: surryarts@advi.net
Management:
    Executive Director: Tanya Rees
Mission: To give direction and encouragement in the arts via performances, workshops and classroom instruction to residents of all ages in Surry County.
Founded: 1968
Specialized Field: Musical
Status: Nonprofit
Budget: $60,000-150,000
Performs At: Andy Griffith Playhouse; Mount Airy Fine Arts Center
Organization Type: Educational; Sponsoring

5145 ARTS NCSTATE

NC State University
Box 7306
Raleigh, NC 27695-7306
Phone: 919-515-3503
Fax: 919-515-6163
e-mail: gallery@ncsu.edu
Web Site: www.fis.ncsu.edu/visualarts/

5146 ARTSPLOSURE: 2003 SPRING JAZZ & ART FESTIVAL

336 Fayetteville Street
Mall Suite 405
Raleigh, NC 27601
Phone: 919-832-8699
Fax: 919-832-0890
e-mail: info@artsplosure.org
Web Site: www.atsplosure.org
Management:
    Director: Michael Lowder
    Entry Coordinator: Christa Misenheiner
    Program Director: Terri Dollar
Founded: 1979
Specialized Field: Visual Arts, Music
Status: Nonprofit
Income Sources: Sposors; Grnats; Donations
Annual Attendance: 75,000
Facility Category: Outdoor Stages

5147 FIRST NIGHT RALEIGH

336 Fayetteville Street Mall
Suite 405
Raleigh, NC 27601
Phone: 919-832-8699
Fax: 919-832-0890
e-mail: info@artsplosure.org
Web Site: www.firstnightraleigh.com
Management:
    Program Director: Terri Dollar
Mission: To offer annual arts festivals to enhance cultural life in the communities of Raleigh and Walce.
Founded: 1991
Specialized Field: Dance; Vocal Music; Instrumental Music; Theater; Festivals
Status: Nonprofit
Paid Staff: 4
Annual Attendance: 50,000
Organization Type: Performing; Festivals

5148 NORTH CAROLINA ARTS COUNCIL

Mail Service Center 4632
Raleigh, NC 27699-4632
Phone: 919-733-2111
Fax: 919-733-4834
e-mail: ncarts@ncmail.net
Web Site: www.ncarts.org
Management:
    Executive Director: Mary Regan
Founded: 1967
Specialized Field: State Arts Agency for North Carolina
Paid Staff: 25

5149 PINE CONE-PIEDMONT COUNCIL OF TRADITIONAL MUSIC

PO Box 28534
Raleigh, NC 27611

Phone: 919-664-8333
Fax: 919-664-8301
e-mail: pinecone1@mindspring.com
Web Site: www.pinecone.org
Management:
   Executive Director: Susan Newberry
   Program Associate: Sarah Beth Woodruff
Mission: Pine Cone is dedicated to preserving, promoting, and presenting traditonal forms of music and dance and other folk performing arts in North Carolina.
Founded: 1984
Specialized Field: Traditional Music and Dance.
Paid Staff: 2

5150 UNITED ARTS COUNCIL OF RALEIGH AND WAKE COUNTY
336 Fayetteville Street Mall
Suite 440
Raleigh, NC 27601-1743
Phone: 919-839-1498
Fax: 919-839-6002
e-mail: gzehr@unitedarts.org
Web Site: www.unitedarts.org
Officers:
   President/CEO: Eleonor Jordan
   VP Education/Community Programs: Virginia Zehr
   Campaign Director: Yvette Holmes
   Community Arts/Grants Manager: Angela Carter
   Chair: V R Ramanan
   Chair-Elect: Brad Phillips
   Vice Chair Administration: David Otteni
   Vice Chair Grants: Priscilla Tyree
Mission: Builds better communities through support and advocacy of true arts.
Founded: 1962
Status: Nonprofit
Volunteer Staff: 1
Budget: 1.5 million
Organization Type: Educational; Sponsoring

5151 JOHNSTON COMMUNITY COLLEGE ON STAGE CONCERT SERIES
245 College Road
PO Box 2350
Smithfield, NC 27577
Phone: 919-209-2099
Fax: 919-209-2133
e-mail: mitchellken@johnstoncc.edu
Web Site: www.johnstoncc.edu
Management:
   Executive Director: Ken Mitchell
Paid Staff: 3
Budget: $60,000-150,000
Performs At: Paul A. Johnston Auditorium
Type of Stage: Proscenium
Seating Capacity: 1,000
Rental Contact: Ken Mitchell

5152 ARTS COUNCIL OF MOORE COUNTY
PO Box 405
Southern Pines, NC 28388
Phone: 910-692-4356
Fax: 910-693-1217
e-mail: acmc@pinehurst.net

Management:
   Assistant Director: Chris Dunn
Budget: $20,000-35,000

5153 SWANNANOA CHAMBER MUSIC FESTIVAL
WWC 6062
701 Warren Wilson Road
Swannanoa, NC 28778
Phone: 828-771-3035
Fax: 828-254-1733
e-mail: festival1@juno.com
Management:
   Director: Frank Ell
   Administrator: Margaret Gormley-Chapman
Mission: Five weeks of chamber music featuring compositions of traditional and contempory composers.
Founded: 1969
Specialized Field: Asheville, Hendersonville, Waynesville, North Carolina
Paid Staff: 1
Volunteer Staff: 15
Paid Artists: 9

5154 EDGECOMBE COUNTY ARTS COUNCIL
130 Bridgers Street
Tarboro, NC 27886
Phone: 252-823-4159
Fax: 252-823-6190
e-mail: edgecombearts@earthlink.net
Management:
   Executive Director: Meade Horne
Mission: Promote and preserve cultural heritage of the county.
Founded: 1985
Specialized Field: Visual Arts In School, Festival
Paid Staff: 4
Volunteer Staff: 12
Paid Artists: 1
Budget: $10,000
Income Sources: Private Donations; State and Local Government
Facility Category: Outdoor Stage; Intimate Gallery

5155 MESSIAH 2000
PO Box 502
Troy, NC 27371
Phone: 910-576-8742
e-mail: tmusic@mc-online.net
Officers:
   President: Dr. Paul Chandley

5156 TRYON CONCERT ASSOCIATION SUBSCRIPTION SERIES
PO Box 32
34 Melrose Avenue
Tryon, NC 28782
Phone: 828-859-8322
Fax: 828-859-0271
e-mail: tfac@alltel.net
Officers:
   President: Philip Cooper
Budget: $20,000-35,000

Performs At: Tryon Fine Arts Center

**5157 SOUTHEASTERN COMMUNITY
COLLEGE PERFORMING ARTS SERIES**
PO Box 151
4564 Chadbourn Highway
Whiteville, NC 28472
Phone: 910-642-7141
Fax: 910-642-5658
e-mail: rburkhardt@mail.southeast.cc.nc.us
Management:
    Director: Richard Burkhardt
Budget: $20,000-35,000
Performs At: College Auditorium; Bowers Auditorium

5158 CAPE FEAR BLUES FESTIVAL
PO Box 1487
Wilmington, NC 28402
Phone: 910-350-8822
e-mail: bluesociety@capefearblues.com
Web Site: www.capefearblues.com
Management:
    Director: Lan Nichols

**5159 UNIVERSITY OF NORTH CAROLINA AT
WILMINGTON**
UNCW-Kenan Auditorium
601 S College Road
Wilmington, NC 28403-3297
Phone: 910-962-3442
Fax: 910-962-3661
e-mail: bemelmansn@uncwil.edu
Web Site: www.uncwil.edu/kenan
Management:
    Kenan Auditorium Manager: Norman Bemelmans
Founded: 1970
Specialized Field: Variety
Paid Staff: 7
Budget: $60,000-150,000
Income Sources: University Support, Ticket Sales
Performs At: Kenan Auditorium
Facility Category: Auditorium/Concert Hall
Seating Capacity: 953
Rental Contact: Norman Bemelmans

**5160 BARTON COLLEGE CONCERT,
LECTURE & CONVOCATION
COMMITTEE SERIES**
Barton College
Wilson, NC 27896
Phone: 252-399-6368
Fax: 252-399-0893
Management:
    Chaplain: R Morgan Daughety
Budget: $10,000
Performs At: Howard Chapel

**5161 NOEL MUSICAL ARTIST SERIES, JESSE
BALL DUPONT FUND**
Campus Box 3017
Wingate University
Wingate, NC 28174

Phone: 704-233-8303
Fax: 704-233-8309
e-mail: santuccio@wingate.edu
Web Site: www.wingate.edu
Management:
    Director: Barbara Jenkins Williamson
    Fine Arts Center: George A Battle, Jr
Performs At: Hannah Covington McGee Theatre

**5162 NORTH CAROLINA SCHOOL OF THE
ARTS: SCHOOL OF MUSIC
PERFORMANCE SERIES**
1533 S Main
Winston-Salem, NC 27127
Mailing Address: PO Box 12189, Winston-Salem, NC.
27117-2189
Phone: 336-770-3255
Fax: 336-770-3248
e-mail: yekovb@ncarts.edu
Web Site: www.ncarts.edu
Management:
    School of Music Dean: Robert Yekovich
Budget: $10,000
Performs At: Crawford Hall; Stevens Center

5163 SALEM COLLEGE CONCERT SERIES
PO Box 10548
Winston-Salem, NC 27108-0548
Phone: 336-721-2636
Fax: 336-721-2683
e-mail: stegall@salem.eduu
Web Site: www.salem.edu
Management:
    Interim School of Music Dean: Joel Stegall
Budget: $10,000
Performs At: Hanes Auditorium; Shirley Recital Hall

**5164 WAKE FOREST UNIVERSITY SECREST
ARTISTS SERIES**
Reynolda Station
PO Box 7411
Winston-Salem, NC 27109
Phone: 336-758-5757
Fax: 336-758-4935
e-mail: sheltolb@wfu.edu
Web Site: www.wfu.edu/secrestartists
Management:
    Director: Lillian Britt Shelton
Budget: $60,000-150,000
Performs At: Wait Chapel; Brendle Hall

5165 CASWELL PERFORMING ARTS SERIES
536 Main Street E
PO Box 609
Yanceyville, NC 27379-0609
Phone: 336-694-4591
Fax: 336-694-5675
e-mail: ccfta@vnet.net
Management:
    Director: H Lee Fowlkes
Founded: 1979
Paid Staff: 5
Volunteer Staff: 30

Budget: $150,000
Annual Attendance: 7,000
Facility Category: civic center
Type of Stage: proscenium
Stage Dimensions: 45 x 30
Seating Capacity: 912
Year Built: 1979
Rental Contact: Hilce Fowlfes

North Dakota

5166 NORTH DAKOTA STATE UNIVERSITY LIVELY ARTS SERIES

PO Box 5476
360 Memorial Union, North Dakata State Univ.
Fargo, ND 58105-5476
Phone: 701-231-7350
Fax: 701-231-8043
e-mail: lee.hoedl@ndsu.nodak.edu
Web Site: www.ndsu.nodak.edu/memorial_union/las
Management:
   Associate Director: Lee Hoedl
Mission: To provide a quality performing arts program for all members of the university community including students, faculty, staff, alumni, guests, parents and Fargo-Moorhead community members. Performing arts provided by the Lively Arts Series must challenge and stimulate creativity and positive regard for a multicultural perspective and provide students with opportunities for experiential learning and involvement related to performing arts.
Founded: 1910
Paid Staff: 1
Budget: $30,000-50,000
Income Sources: Grants; Community Support
Affiliations: Lake Agassiz Arts Council
Annual Attendance: 2,000-3,000
Facility Category: Fully Functional Concert Hall
Seating Capacity: 1,000

5167 NORTH DAKOTA MUSEUM OF ART CONCERT SERIES

Box 7305
Grand Forks, ND 58202
Phone: 701-777-4195
Fax: 701-777-4425
e-mail: ndmuseum@gfherald.infi.net
Web Site: www.ndmoa.com
Management:
   Director: Laurel Reuter
Founded: 1972
Paid Staff: 15
Volunteer Staff: 70
Budget: $20,000-30,000
Performs At: museum gallery
Facility Category: Art Museum
Seating Capacity: 300

5168 MAYVILLE STATE UNIVERSITY (ND) FINE ARTS SERIES

Mayville State University
330 Third Street NE
Mayville, ND 58257
Mailing Address: 400 Groveland Avenue Minneapolis MN, 55403
Phone: 612-874-9238
Fax: 701-786-4748
e-mail: apthien@msn.com
Management:
   Series Director: Dr. Anthony Thein
Income Sources: Student Activity Fee, Concert Tickets, Contributions
Annual Attendance: 15-200
Facility Category: Fieldhouse
Type of Stage: Concrete
Seating Capacity: 400
Year Built: 1969

Ohio

5169 OHIO NORTHERN UNIVERSITY ARTIST SERIES

Fred Center for the Performing Arts
525 S Main Street
Ada, OH 45810
Phone: 419-772-2049
Fax: 419-772-1856
e-mail: e-williams@onu.edu/c-mcqhie.edu
Web Site: www.onu.edu/
Officers:
   Chairman Music Department: Dr. Edwin Williams
Management:
   Managing Director/Development: Catriena MacQhie
Founded: 1871
Specialized Field: Music; Dance; Theater
Paid Staff: 10
Budget: $35,000-60,000
Performs At: Freed Center for the Performing Arts
Facility Category: Concert Hall
Type of Stage: Moveable Proscenium/Black Box
Seating Capacity: 550/136
Year Built: 1990
Cost: $7,000,000
Rental Contact: Andrea Lawson

5170 CHILDREN'S CONCERT SOCIETY OF AKRON

Edwin J Thomas Performing Arts Hall
198 Hill Street
Akron, OH 44325-0501
Phone: 330-972-2504
Fax: 330-972-6571
Management:
   Administrative Director: Elizabeth Butler
Budget: $60,000-150,000
Seating Capacity: 2800

5171 GREATER AKRON MUSICAL ASSOCIATION
17 N Broadway
Akron, OH 44308
Phone: 330-535-8131
Fax: 330-535-7302
Officers:
President: Wayne Knabel
Executive Vice President: Ellen Otto
Management:
Music Director/Conductor: Alan Balter
Conductor/Youth Symphony: Eric Benjamin
General Manager: Connie F Linsler
Mission: To provide the Greater Akron Area with the finest quality symphonic and choral music and related fine arts; to educate the local public with respect to classical and contemporary music.
Founded: 1950
Specialized Field: Vocal Music; Instrumental Music
Status: Professional; Nonprofit
Performs At: E.J. Thomas Hall
Organization Type: Performing; Educational

5172 MUSIC FROM STAN HYWET
714 N Portage Path
Akron, OH 44303
Phone: 330-836-5533
Fax: 330-688-4839
Officers:
Concert Chairman: Lola Rothmann
Budget: $10,000
Seating Capacity: 160

5173 TUESDAY MUSICAL
198 Hill Street
Akron, OH 44325-0501
Phone: 330-972-2342
Fax: 330-972-6571
e-mail: tmc@uakron.edu
Management:
Concert Manager: Barbara Feld
Budget: $60,000-150,000
Performs At: Edwin J. Thomas Performing Arts Hall

5174 UNIVERSITY OF AKRON: EJ THOMAS HALL SERIES
198 Hill Street
Akron, OH 44325-0501
Phone: 330-972-7595
Fax: 330-972-6571
Management:
Executive Director: Dan Dahl
Assistant Director: Cynthia Hollis
Budget: $400,000-1,000,000
Seating Capacity: 2,956

5175 OHIO UNIVERSITY PERFORMING ARTS SERIES
Office of Public Occasions
Templeton-Blackburn Alumni Memorial Aud.
Athens, OH 45701
Phone: 740-593-1761
Fax: 740-593-1763
e-mail: gstephensl@ohiou.edu
Management:
Public Occassions Director: Grethen L Stephens
Budget: $60,000-150,000
Seating Capacity: 2,000

5176 LOGAN COUNTY COMMUNITY CONCERTS
PO Box 442
1200 Milligan Road
Bellefontaine, OH 43311
Phone: 937-592-5863
e-mail: barnwell@loganrec.com
Officers:
Treasurer: Robert J Barnell
Budget: $20,000-35,000

5177 BALDWIN-WALLACE BACH FESTIVAL
Baldwin-Wallace College Conservatory of Music
96 Front Street
Berea, OH 44017
Phone: 440-826-2369
Fax: 440-826-3239
Management:
Music Director: Dwight Oltman

5178 BALDWIN-WALLACE COLLEGE ACADEMIC & CULTURAL EVENTS SERIES
275 Eastland Road
Berea, OH 44017
Phone: 440-826-2157
Fax: 440-826-3020
e-mail: jhairsto@bw.edu
Management:
ACES Director: Jay Hairston
Budget: $10,000
Performs At: John Patrick Theatre; Kulas Musical Arts Building

5179 BLUFFTON COLLEGE ARTIST SERIES
Bluffton College
280 W College Avenue
Bluffton, OH 45817-1196
Phone: 419-358-3349
Fax: 419-358-3323
e-mail: schatta@bluffton.edu
Officers:
Artists Series Committee Chair: Dr. Adam J Schattschneider
Budget: $10,000-20,000
Performs At: Yoder Recital Hall; Founders Hall; Mosiman Hall

5180 BOWLING GREEN STATE UNIVERSITY: NEW MUSIC & ART FESTIVAL
BGSU
MidAmerican Center for Contemporary Music
Bowling Green, OH 43403

Phone: 419-372-2836
Fax: 419-372-2938
e-mail: bbeerma@bgnet.bgsu.edu
Web Site: www.bgsu.edu/colleges/music/maccm
Management:
    Director: Burton Beerman

5181 BOWLING GREEN STATE UNIVERSITY FESTIVAL SERIES
Moore Musical Arts Center
Bowling Green State University
Bowling Green, OH 43403-0290
Phone: 419-372-8654
Fax: 419-372-2938
e-mail: dfleitz@bgnet.bgsu.edu
Web Site: www.bgsu.edu/colleges/music
Management:
    Public Events Director: Deborah L Fleitz
Budget: $60,000-150,000
Performs At: Kobacker Hall; Bryan Hall

5182 CRAWFORD COUNTY COMMUNITY CONCERT ASSOCIATION
PO Box 469
Bucyrus, OH 44820
Phone: 419-562-3719
Fax: 416-562-9098
e-mail: slater@cybrtown.com
Web Site: www.slatertours.com
Officers:
    President: Robert A Slater
Budget: $35,000-60,000
Performs At: Bucyrus Middle School Auditorium

5183 LITHOPOLIS PERFORMING ARTISTS SERIES
3825 Cedar Hill Road
Canal Winchester, OH 43110-8929
Phone: 614-837-8925
Fax: 614-837-4765
Management:
    Series Director: Virginia E Heffner
Budget: $10,000-20,000
Performs At: Wagnalss Memorial Auditorium

5184 CEDARVILLE UNIVERSITY ARTIST SERIES
251 N Main Street
Box 601
Cedarville, OH 45314
Phone: 937-766-7956
Fax: 937-766-7581
Management:
    Ass't Campus Activities Director: Jeff Beste
    Director: Scott Van Loo
Budget: $20,000-35,000
Performs At: James T. Jeremiah Chapel

5185 COLLEGE-COMMUNITY ARTS COUNCIL
7600 State Route 703E
Celina, OH 45822

Phone: 419-678-2950
Fax: 419-678-2950
e-mail: eeweber@bright.net
Officers:
    President: Eugene Weber
Budget: $10,000-20,000
Seating Capacity: 150-470

5186 CINCINNATI ARTS ASSOCIATION: ARONOFF CENTER FOR THE ARTS
650 Walnut Street
Cincinnati, OH 45202
Phone: 513-977-4123
Fax: 513-977-4150
Web Site: www.cincinnatiarts.org
Officers:
    President/Executive Director: Stephen A Loftin
    VP/General Manager: Janet L Taylor
Founded: 1992
Budget: 10,000,000
Performs At: Proctor & Gamble Hall; Jarson-Kaplin Theater; Fifth Third Bank Trust
Annual Attendance: 1,100,000
Seating Capacity: 2,719; 437; 150

5187 CINCINNATI FOLK LIFE SERIES
PO Box 9008
Cincinnati, OH 45209
Phone: 513-533-4822
Fax: 513-533-4828
e-mail: cfl@fuse.net
Web Site: www.home.fuse.net/cfl
Management:
    Administrator: JoAnn Buck
Budget: $20,000-35,000
Seating Capacity: 150-500

5188 CINCINNATI GARDENS
2250 Seymour Avenue
Cincinnati, OH 45212
Phone: 513-631-7793
Fax: 513-631-2666
Management:
    Director: Joseph F Jagoditz

5189 CINCINNATI MAY FESTIVAL
Music Hall
1241 Elm Street
Cincinnati, OH 45210
Phone: 513-621-1919
Fax: 513-744-3535
e-mail: information@mayfestival.com
Web Site: www.mayfestival.com
Officers:
    Chairman: Mary Margret Rochford
    Vice Chairman: Alice Sweet
    Secretary: Ruthy Korelitz
Management:
    Music Director: James Conlon
    Chorus Director: Robert Porco
    Executive Director: Steven Monder
    Manager: Jeffrey Alexander
    Director Marketing/Development: Vera Menner

Mission: Cincinnati May Festival presents an exciting repertoire of choral and orchestral music featuring the May Festival Chorus, world-renowned guest soloists and conductors and the Cincinnati Symphony Orchestra.
Founded: 1873
Specialized Field: Vocal Music; Instrumental Music; Festivals
Status: Professional; Nonprofit
Paid Staff: 200
Income Sources: Cincinnati Symphony Orchestra
Performs At: Music Hall; Cathedral Basillica of the Assumption
Organization Type: Performing; Resident; Sponsoring

5190 CINCINNATI OPERA ASSOCIATION SUMMER FESTIVAL
1241 Elm Street
Cincinnati, OH 45210
Phone: 513-621-1919
Fax: 513-744-3520
e-mail: info@cincinnatiopera.com
Web Site: www.cincinnatiopera.com
Management:
    Artistic Director: Nicholas Muni

5191 CINCINNATI SHAKESPEARE FESTIVAL
717 Race Street
Cincinnati, OH 45202-4304
Phone: 513-381-2288
Fax: 513-381-2298
e-mail: info@cincyshakes.com
Web Site: www.cincyshakes.com
Officers:
    President: Richard Westheimer
    Treasurer: Mark Rubin
Management:
    Production Artistic Director: Jasson Minadakis
    Company Manager: Jason Bruffy
    Head of Production: Will Turbyne
    Technical Director: Todd Edwards
    Marketing Director: Andrea Reynolds
Founded: 1994
Status: Nonprofit; Equity
Volunteer Staff: 5
Season: August - June
Type of Stage: 3/4 Thrust
Stage Dimensions: 24' x 32'
Seating Capacity: 185

5192 CLASSICAL GUITAR SERIES
Xavier University
3800 Victoria Parkway
Cincinnati, OH 45207-2717
Phone: 513-745-3161
Fax: 513-745-2083
e-mail: heim@admin.xu.edu
Web Site: www.xu.edu
Management:
    Director: Father Jack Heim
Budget: $20,000-35,000
Performs At: University Center Theatre
Seating Capacity: 395

5193 CLASSICAL PIANO SERIES
Xavier University
3800 Victoria Parkway
Cincinnati, OH 45207-2717
Phone: 513-745-3161
Fax: 513-745-2083
e-mail: heim@admin.xu.edu
Web Site: www.xu.edu
Management:
    Director: Father Jack Heim
Budget: $20,000-35,000
Performs At: University Center Theatre
Seating Capacity: 395

5194 FALL ARTS FESTIVAL/JEWISH FOLK FESTIVAL
2615 Clifton Avenue
Cincinnati, OH 45220
Phone: 513-221-6728
Fax: 513-221-7134
e-mail: email@hillelcincinnati.orgf
Management:
    Executive Director: Rabbi Abie Ingber
Mission: Folkmusic, Theatre and World Music especially Jewish artists.
Founded: 1977
Specialized Field: Music, Theatre (Small Production, One Person Show)
Paid Staff: 6
Volunteer Staff: 35
Paid Artists: 3
Non-paid Artists: 3

5195 JAZZ GUITAR SERIES
Xavier University
3800 Victoria Parkway
Cincinnati, OH 45207-2717
Phone: 513-745-3161
Fax: 513-745-2083
e-mail: heim@admin.xu.edu
Web Site: www.xu.edu
Management:
    Director: Father Jack Heim
Budget: $20,000-35,000
Performs At: University Center Theatre
Seating Capacity: 395

5196 JAZZ PIANO SERIES
Xavier University
3800 Victoria Parkway
Cincinnati, OH 45207-2717
Phone: 513-745-3161
Fax: 513-745-2083
e-mail: heim@admin.xu.edu
Web Site: www.xu.edu
Management:
    Director: Father Jack Heim
Budget: $20,000-35,000
Performs At: University Center Theatre
Seating Capacity: 395

5197 LINTON CHAMBER MUSIC SERIES/ENCORE!
1223 Central Parkway
Cincinnati, OH 45214
Phone: 513-381-6868
Fax: 513-381-6888
e-mail: lintoninc@aol.com
Web Site: www.wguc.org/linton
Management:
Artistic Director: Richard Waller
Executive Director: Anne Black
Budget: $20,000-35,000
Performs At: First Unitarian Church; Cinicinnati City Council Chambers

5198 LINTON'S PEANUT BUTTER & JAM SESSIONS
4 W 4th Street
Cincinnati, OH 45202
Phone: 513-381-6868
Fax: 513-381-6888
e-mail: lintoninc@aol.com
Management:
Artistic Director: Richard Waller
Executive Director: Anne Black
Budget: $20,000-35,000
Performs At: First Unitarian Church; Cinicinnati City Council Chambers

5199 ART SONG FESTIVAL
11021 E Boulevard
Cleveland, OH 44106
Phone: 216-791-5000
Fax: 216-791-3063
e-mail: jxu3@po.cwru.edu
Web Site: www.cim.edu
Management:
Executive Coordinator: Dr. Joanne Uniatowski
Founded: 1985

5200 CHINA MUSIC PROJECT
334 Claymore Boulevard
Cleveland, OH 44143-1730
Phone: 216-531-2188
Management:
Director: Marjorie Ann Ciarillo

5201 CLEVELAND MUSEUM OF ART CONCERTS SERIES
11150 E Boulevard
Cleveland, OH 44106
Phone: 216-421-7340
Fax: 216-421-0921
e-mail: cox@cma-oh.org
Web Site: www.clemusart.com
Management:
Curator Musical Arts: Karel Paukert
Associate Curator Musical Arts: Paul Cox
Founded: 1920
Specialized Field: Vocal Music; Instrumental Music
Status: Nonprofit
Paid Staff: 3
Budget: $35,000-60,000
Performs At: Gartner Auditorium
Organization Type: Educational; Sponsoring

5202 CLEVELAND MUSIC SCHOOL SETTLEMENT ARTISTS CONCERT SERIES
11125 Magnolia Drive
Cleveland, OH 44106
Phone: 216-421-5806
Fax: 216-421-5813
e-mail: cmsselee@aol.com
Management:
Performing Arts Director: Ella W Lee
Budget: $10,000
Seating Capacity: 200

5203 CLEVELAND SHAKESPEARE FESTIVAL
PO Box 606272
Cleveland, OH 44106
Phone: 216-732-3311
e-mail: info@cleveshakes.org
Web Site: www.cleveshakes.org
Officers:
Business Manager: Elisabeth Madden
Management:
Managing Director: Joshua Brown
Co-Artistic Director: Kelly Elliot
Co-Artistic Director: Larry Nehring
Mission: Committed to producing the plays of Shakespeare in the way that the author intended—fun, at the speed of thought, and in the midst of a vibrant community. Committed to free admission, a festive atmosphere, and an earned attention to the work of the play.

5204 DARIUS MILHAUD SOCIETY
15715 Chadbourne Road
Cleveland, OH 44120
Phone: 216-921-4548
Fax: 216-921-4548
Officers:
President: Katherine M Warne
Budget: $10,000-20,000
Seating Capacity: 500

5205 GREAT LAKES THEATER FESTIVAL
1501 Euclid Avenue
Suite 423
Cleveland, OH 44115
Phone: 216-241-5490
Fax: 216-241-6315
e-mail: mail@greatlakestheater.org
Web Site: www.greatlakestheater.org
Officers:
President: David Porter
Co-Chairman: John Katzenmeyer
Co-Chairman: Joseph Lopresti
Management:
Producing Artistic Director: Charlie Fee
Marketing Director: Pam Mehenett
Education Director: Daniel Hahn

Mission: To produce theater emphasizing world classics, particularly Shakespeare and important nonclassical works of American theater.
Founded: 1962
Specialized Field: Classic Theater
Status: Professional; Nonprofit
Income Sources: League of Resident Theatres; American Arts Alliance
Performs At: Ohio Theatre Playhouse Square Center
Affiliations: LORT
Year Built: 1921
Organization Type: Performing; Educational

5206 TRI-C JAZZFEST

2900 Community College Avenue
Theatre 11
Cleveland, OH 44115
Phone: 216-987-4444
Fax: 216-987-4422
e-mail: terri.pontremoli@tri-c.cc.oh.us
Web Site: www.tri-c.cc.oh.us/jazz
Management:
    Director: Terri Pontremoli
    Education Events Coordinator: Susan Stone
    Booking Coordinator: Willard Jenkins
    Office Manager: Cliffie Jones
Mission: To provide an educational opportunity for students and people of all ages and backgrounds to further their abilities, understanding and appreciation for jazz. To increase public awareness and appreciation for jazz as an American art form. To preserve the history and foster the development of this unique music. To bring world class performers and educators to greater Cleveland audiences.
Founded: 1980
Specialized Field: Big Band; World Music; All Jazz Related
Status: Nonprofit
Paid Staff: 6
Volunteer Staff: 20
Paid Artists: 80
Budget: 500,000
Income Sources: Foundations; Corporate; Government; Private
Performs At: College Campus Auditorium; Severance Hall; Metro Campus
Affiliations: Cuyahoga Community College; International Association of Jazz Educators
Annual Attendance: 30,000-40,000
Type of Stage: Proscenium
Seating Capacity: 360-3,000
Organization Type: Performing; Educational
Resident Groups: Swing City; Tri-C Jazz Fest; High School All-Stars

5207 SHALHAVET FESTIVAL

2140 Lee Road
Suite 218
Cleveland Heights, OH 44118
Phone: 216-932-3455
Management:
    Executive Director: Clara Amster

5208 COLUMBIANA SUMMER CONCERT ASSOCIATION

2905 Middleton Road
Columbiana, OH 44408-9550
Phone: 330-482-2978
Officers:
    Chairman: Fred A Lynn
Budget: $10,000-20,000
Performs At: Firestone Park Gazebo Entertainment Center

5209 COLUMBUS ARTS FESTIVAL

55 E Broad Street
Suite 2250
Columbus, OH 43215
Phone: 614-224-2606
Fax: 614-224-7461
e-mail: festival@gcac.org
Web Site: www.gcac.org
Management:
    Director: Katie Lucas
Mission: To offer an annual festival of the arts.
Founded: 1961
Specialized Field: Dance; Vocal Music; Instrumental Music; Festivals
Status: Professional; Non-Professional; Nonprofit
Volunteer Staff: 300
Income Sources: Greater Columbus Arts Council
Annual Attendance: 550,000
Facility Category: Outdoor Stage
Organization Type: Performing; Festival

5210 COLUMBUS ASSOCIATION FOR THE PERFORMING ARTS: SIGNATURE SERIES

55 E State Street
Columbus, OH 43215-4264
Phone: 614-469-1045
Fax: 614-461-0429
e-mail: meilley@capa.com
Web Site: www.capa.com
Officers:
    VP: Michael Rilley
    President: Bill Conner
Management:
    Executive Director: Douglas F Kridler
Mission: To utilize entertainment to enliven and enrich metropolitan life through its work in all its venues, enhance a continuing downtown renaissance and install appreciation for diverse forms of entertainment.
Founded: 1969
Budget: $15,000,000+
Income Sources: 90 per cent Ticket Sales; Rentals; Grants;Contributions
Performs At: Ohio Theatre; Palace Theatre; Southern Theatre; Riffe Center Theatre; Chicago Theatre; Shubert Theater
Annual Attendance: 1,000,000+

5211 COLUMBUS SYMPHONY ORCHESTRA: PICNIC WITH THE POPS
Columbus Symphony Orchestra
55 E State Street
Columbus, OH 43215
Phone: 614-228-9600
Fax: 614-224-7273
Management:
Executive Director/President: Daniel Hart
V Chairman: Lynn Crawford
Past Chair: Bernie Woreman
Paid Staff: 35
Volunteer Staff: 750
Paid Artists: 8

5212 COOPER STADIUM
1155 W Mound Street
Columbus, OH 43223
Phone: 614-462-5250
Fax: 614-462-3271
e-mail: colsclipper@earthlink.com
Web Site: www.clippersbaseball.com
Management:
General Manager: Ken Schnake
Seating Capacity: 15,000

5213 EARLY MUSIC IN COLUMBUS
Capital University
2199 E Main Street
Columbus, OH 43209
Phone: 614-861-4569
Fax: 614-861-4569
e-mail: mkwole@insight.rr.com
Web Site:
www.capital.edu/acad/cons/erly/earlymusic.htm
Management:
Program Director: Katherine Wolfe
Paid Staff: 1
Volunteer Staff: 20
Paid Artists: 30
Budget: $20,000-35,000
Performs At: Mees Hall; Capital University; Huntington Recital Hall

5214 JEFFERSON ACADEMY OF MUSIC
OSU School of Music
1866 College Road
Columbus, OH 43210
Phone: 614-292-2693
Fax: 614-292-1102
e-mail: jeffacad@osu.edu
Management:
Executive Director: Ruth Triplett Haddock
Budget: $10,000-20,000
Performs At: Battle Fine Arts Center; Children's Hospital Auditorium

5215 MUSIC IN THE AIR
549 Franklin Avenue
Columbus, OH 43215
Phone: 614-645-7995
Fax: 614-645-6278
e-mail: klwiser@cmhmetro.net
Web Site: www.musicintheair.org
Management:
Managing Director: Karen Wiser
Contact: Ed Myers
Mission: Presents a variety of musicians and performers with four summer music series and Festival Latino. All performances are free.
Founded: 1973
Specialized Field: Performing Arts Presenter
Paid Staff: 5
Paid Artists: 300
Budget: 450,000
Performs At: Outdoor Amphitheater; Mobile Stage Van
Annual Attendance: 200,000
Seating Capacity: 5,000
Rental Contact: Karen Wiser

5216 SHORT NORTH PERFORMING ARTS ASSOCIATION
PO Box 8414
Columbus, OH 43201
Phone: 614-291-5854
Fax: 614-291-5854
e-mail: strosen@excite.com
Officers:
President: Toba Feldman
Secretary: Cathy Huston
Treasurer: Anita St. John
Management:
Artistic Director: Steve Rosenberg
Mission: To present the finest chamber and folk music and to provide after school programs in music to inner city children.
Founded: 1983
Specialized Field: Instrumental Music
Status: Nonprofit
Paid Staff: 2
Volunteer Staff: 1
Budget: $50,000-70,000
Income Sources: Ticket sales, grants, sponsorships, contributions
Performs At: Short North Tavern; Little Brothers; Greek Orthodox Church

5217 TRIUNE CONCERT SERIES
St. John's Evangelical Church
59 E Mound Street
Columbus, OH 43215
Phone: 614-224-8634
Fax: 614-224-6375
Management:
Minister of Music: Mary Schwarz
Budget: $10,000
Seating Capacity: 1,000

5218 WOMEN IN MUSIC: COLUMBUS
PO Box 14722
Columbus, OH 43214
Phone: 614-470-0098
Fax: 614-430-3144
e-mail: WmcCols@cs.com

All listings are in alphabetical order by state, then city, then organization within the city.

Performs At: Mees Hall; Huntington Recital Hall

5219 DAYTON'S JAZZ AT THE BEND FESTIVAL
City of Dayton
216 N Main Street
Dayton, OH 45402
Phone: 937-223-2489
Fax: 937-223-0795
Management:
   Festival Director: Walter Williams

5220 ERVIN J NUTTER CENTER
3640 Colonel Glenn Highway
Suite 430
Dayton, OH 45435
Phone: 937-775-3498
Fax: 937-775-2060
Web Site: www.nuttercenter.com
Management:
   Executive Director: John Siehl
Founded: 1990
Paid Staff: 24

5221 SOIREES MUSICALES PIANO SERIES
834 Riverview Terrace
Dayton, OH 45407-2433
Phone: 937-228-5802
Fax: 937-228-2380
e-mail: hagpia@interaxs.net
Management:
   Series Director: Donald C Hageman
Budget: $10,000-20,000
Performs At: Shiloh Church

5222 UNIVERSITY OF DAYTON ARTS SERIES
University of Dayton
Dayton, OH 45469-0290
Phone: 937-229-2787
Fax: 937-229-3916
e-mail: arts-series@udayton.edu
Web Site: www.udayton.edu/inarts-series
Management:
   Manager: Barbra Lupp
Mission: To present an annual performing arts series to campus and community.
Founded: 1961
Specialized Field: Dance; Vocal Music; Instrumental Music; Theater
Status: Professional; Nonprofit
Paid Staff: 1
Budget: $60,000
Income Sources: Ohio Arts Council; Box Office; Montgomery County; University Subsidy
Performs At: Boll Theatre
Annual Attendance: 2,000
Facility Category: Theater
Seating Capacity: 378
Organization Type: Performing; Sponsoring

5223 VANGUARD CONCERTS
5335 Far Hills Avenue
Suite 304
Dayton, OH 45429
Phone: 937-434-6902
Fax: 937-434-6903
Management:
   Manager: Elana Bolling
Budget: $20,000-35,000
Performs At: Dayton Art Institute

5224 WRIGHT STATE UNIVERSITY ARTIST SERIES
Music Department
Wright State University
Dayton, OH 45435
Phone: 937-775-2787
Fax: 937-775-3786
e-mail: alison.schray@wright.edu
Web Site: www.wright.edu/academics/music
Management:
   Manager: Alison Y Schray
Budget: $20,000-35,000
Performs At: Creative Arts Center Concert Hall

5225 MIDAMERICA CHAMBER MUSIC FESTIVAL
Ohio Wesleyan University
Music Department
Delaware, OH 43015
Phone: 740-368-3704
Fax: 740-368-3723
e-mail: machmi@owu.edu
Web Site: www.owu.edu/~machmi
Management:
   Director: Dr. Cameron Bennett
   Director: Charles Wetherber
Founded: 1995
Specialized Field: Music
Paid Staff: 2
Paid Artists: 8

5226 OHIO WESLEYAN UNIVERSITY PERFORMING ARTS/LECTURE SERIES
Sanborn Hall
Delaware, OH 43015
Phone: 740-368-3719
Fax: 740-368-3723
e-mail: cdbennet@cc.owu.edu
Officers:
   Concert Chairman: Cameron Bennett
Budget: $20,000-35,000
Performs At: Gray Chapel

5227 LORAIN COUNTY COMMUNITY COLLEGE: STOCKER ARTS CENTER PROGRAMMING
1005 N Abbe Road
Elyria, OH 44035
Phone: 440-366-4140
Fax: 440-366-4101
e-mail: kcrooker@lorainccc.edu

Management:
Director: Kasson E Crooker
Budget: $150,000-400,000
Performs At: Stocker Arts Center

5228 ARTS PARTNERSHIP OF GREATER HANCOCK COUNTY
112 W Front Street
Suite A
Findlay, OH 45840
Phone: 419-422-3412
Fax: 419-422-2765
e-mail: communication@artspartnership.com
Web Site: www.artspartnership.com
Officers:
President: Bill Hoffman
Management:
Program Coordinator: Alissa Simpson
Communication Coordinator: Angela McCracken
Education Coordinator: Shari Hellman
Operations Coordinator: Denise Traxler
Box Office Coordinator: Brenda Kaukonen
Executive Director: Carolyn Copos
Mission: To offer a variety of professional programs, as well arts and education programs for all ages.
Specialized Field: Performing, Educational
Budget: $500,000
Income Sources: Box office, grants, private and corporate donations
Performs At: Several Facilities
Seating Capacity: 1418

5229 DENISON UNIVERSITY VAIL SERIES
Colwell House
Granville, OH 43023
Phone: 614-587-0525
Fax: 614-587-6602
e-mail: wales@denison.edu
Management:
Director: Lorraine Wales

5230 ARTISTS SERIES & ARTS-IN-EDUCATION
Drake County Center for the Arts
Box 718
Greenville, OH 45331-0718
Phone: 937-547-0908
Web Site: decarts.org
Management:
Executive Director: Marilyn Delk
Founded: 1978
Paid Staff: 3
Budget: $60,000-150,000
Performs At: Henry St. Clair Memorial Hall
Annual Attendance: 15,000
Type of Stage: Proscenium
Stage Dimensions: 30'x24'x28'
Seating Capacity: 632
Year Built: 1912

5231 MIAMI UNIVERSITY: HAMILTON ARTIST SERIES
1601 Peck Boulevard
Hamilton, OH 45011
Phone: 513-785-3264
Fax: 513-785-3145
e-mail: epsteihr@muohio.edu
Management:
Series Director: Howard Epstein
Budget: $20,000-35,000
Performs At: Parrish Auditorium

5232 HIRAM COLLEGE CONCERT & ARTIST SERIES
Hiram College
Hiram, OH 44234
Phone: 330-569-5181
Fax: 330-569-5479
Management:
Chair of Special Events: Helen Wood
Budget: $10,000-20,000
Performs At: Hayden Auditorium

5233 FOOTHILLS ART FESTIVAL, SOUTHERN HILLS ARTS COUNCIL
Box 149
Jackson, OH 45640
Phone: 740-286-6355
Management:
Executive Director: Barbara Summers

5234 KENT/BLOSSOM MUSIC
E101 M&S, PO Box 5192
Kent State University
Kent, OH 44242
Phone: 330-672-2613
Fax: 330-672-7837
e-mail: jlacorte@kent.edu
Web Site: www.kent.edu/blossom
Management:
Director: Jerome LaCorte
Mission: The intensive study of chamber music under the guidance of renowned master artists, including more than two dozen performances before a wide public audience.
Founded: 1968
Specialized Field: Chamber Music

5235 KENTFEST
PO Box 248
Kent, OH 44240-0237
Phone: 330-673-1599
Officers:
Chairman: Mary Drongowski

5236 LAKESIDE ASSOCIATION
236 Walnut Avenue
Lakeside, OH 43440
Phone: 419-798-4461
Fax: 419-798-5033
e-mail: schedule@lakesideohio.com
Web Site: www.alkesideohio.com
Management:

Director Programs: G Keith Aody
Mission: To establish and maintain schools, conferences, institutes, lecture courses and other means of aesthetic culture.
Founded: 1873
Specialized Field: Dance; Vocal Music; Instrumental Music; Theater
Status: Professional; Nonprofit; Commercial
Performs At: Auditorium
Type of Stage: Proscenium
Seating Capacity: 2,900
Year Built: 1929
Organization Type: Sponsoring

5237 LANCASTER FESTIVAL

127 W Wheeling Street
Lancaster, OH 43130
Phone: 740-687-4808
Fax: 740-687-1980
e-mail: lanfest@lanfest.org
Web Site: www.lanfest.org
Officers:
   General Manager: Eleanor Hood
   General Manager: Barbara Hunzicker
Management:
   Production Manager: Carol Abbott
Founded: 1985
Specialized Field: Visual Arts; Performing Arts
Paid Staff: 4
Volunteer Staff: 600
Paid Artists: 180
Budget: $800,000
Income Sources: Ticket Sales, Private/Corporate Donations, Grants
Annual Attendance: 45,000
Stage Dimensions: 40'x60'

5238 COUNCIL FOR THE ARTS OF GREATER LIMA

130 W Elm Street
PO Box 1124
Lima, OH 45801
Phone: 419-222-1096
Fax: 419-222-3871
Web Site: www.limaartscouncil.org
Officers:
   President: Greg Phipps
   VP: Mike Hoffman
   Financial Officer: Terry Webb
   Secretary: Brenda Ellis
Management:
   Executive Director: Bart Mills
   Education Director: Sally Windle
   Operations Manager: Chris Craft
Mission: To enrich the quality of life in the Greater Lima community, the Council for the Arts will promote and encourage appreciation, respect and understanding of the arts through advocacy, education and programming.
Founded: 1966
Specialized Field: Dance; Vocal Music; Instrumental Music; Theater; Festivals; Lyric Opera
Status: Nonprofit
Performs At: Civic Center
Organization Type: Educational; Sponsoring

5239 LIVELY ARTS SERIES: PALACE CULTURAL ARTS ASSOCIATION

276 W Center Street
Marion, OH 43302
Phone: 740-383-2101
Fax: 740-387-3425
e-mail: marionpalace@marion.net
Web Site: www.marion.net/palace
Management:
   Managing Director: Elaine Merchant

5240 MENTOR PERFORMING ARTISTS CONCERT SERIES

6477 Center Street
Mentor, OH 44060
Phone: 440-205-3333
Fax: 440-974-5216
Web Site: www.mentorconcertseries.com
Management:
   Director: Theodore Hieronymus
Budget: $150,000-400,000
Performs At: Mentor Schools Fine Arts Center

5241 MOUNT VERNON NAZARENE COLLEGE: LECTURE ARTIST SERIES

800 Martinsburg Road
Mount Vernon, OH 43050
Phone: 740-397-6862
Fax: 740-392-1689
e-mail: bcochran@mvnu.edu
Web Site: www.mvnc.edu
Management:
   Chair Lecture Artist Committee: B Barnett Cochran
Founded: 1970
Volunteer Staff: 10
Budget: $10,000-20,000
Income Sources: Institutional budget
Performs At: R.R. Hodges Chapel-Auditorium; Recital Hall-Theater
Annual Attendance: 3,225
Facility Category: 2 Theatres
Seating Capacity: 2,000; 300
Year Built: 1990

5242 OHIO OUTDOOR HISTORICAL DRAMA ASSOCIATION

PO Box 450
New Philadelphia, OH 44633
Phone: 330-364-5111
Fax: 330-339-8140
e-mail: trumpet@tusco.net
Management:
   General Manager: Margaret M Bonamico
   Director: Joseph Bonamico
Mission: To produce Trumpet in the Land, an original outdoor drama by Paul Green.
Founded: 1967
Specialized Field: Musical
Status: Nonprofit
Income Sources: Actors' Equity Association
Performs At: Schoenbrunn Amphitheatre
Facility Category: Outdoor amphitheatre
Seating Capacity: 1200

Organization Type: Educational; Sponsoring

5243 CENTRAL OHIO TECHNICAL COLLEGE
1179 University Drive
Newark, OH 43055-1767
Phone: 740-364-9580
Fax: 740-364-9646
e-mail: irmscher.1@osu.edu
Management:
Assistant Director/Student Affairs: Krista Irmscher
Budget: $10,000-20,000
Performs At: Founders Hall

5244 OBERLIN BAROQUE PERFORMANCE INSTITUTE & FESTIVAL
Oberlin College Conservatory of Music
77 W College Street
Oberlin, OH 44074-1588
Phone: 440-775-8044
Fax: 440-775-6840
e-mail: OCBPI@oberlin.edu

5245 OBERLIN COLLEGE CONSERVATORY OF MUSIC ARTIST: RECITAL SERIES
Oberlin College
Conservatory of Music
Oberlin, OH 44074
Phone: 440-775-8293
Fax: 440-775-8942
e-mail: marci.alegant@oberlin.edu
Web Site: www.oberlin.edu
Management:
Assistant Dean: Marci Alegant
Budget: $60,000-150,000
Performs At: Finney Memorial Chapel

5246 MIAMI UNIVERSITY PERFORMING ARTS SERIES
102 Hall Auditorium
Oxford, OH 45056
Phone: 513-529-6333
Fax: 513-529-5482
e-mail: swoffoph@muohio.edu
Web Site: www.muohio.edu/performingartsseries
Management:
Executive Director: Patti Hannan Swofford
Budget: $150,000-400,000
Performs At: Millett Hall; Gates-Abegglen Theater; Art Museum; Hall Auditorium
Seating Capacity: 730

5247 VALLEY ARTISTS SERIES
University of Rio Grande
Fine & Performing Arts Center
Rio Grande, OH 45674
Phone: 740-245-7360
Fax: 740-245-7101
Management:
Fine & Performing Arts Coordinator: Dr. Greg Miller
Budget: $20,000-35,000

Performs At: Fine Arts Theater

5248 LANGE TRUST
1402 Columbus Avenue
Sandusky, OH 44870
Phone: 419-625-8312
Fax: 419-625-8380
Officers:
Chairman: Diane Ernst
Mission: To bring events of good quality and variety to the people of our county at no charge.
Founded: 1928
Volunteer Staff: 24
Budget: $50,000-60,000
Income Sources: Interest income from the Lange Trust
Performs At: State Theatre
Affiliations: Ohio Arts Presenter Network, Association of Performing Arts Presenters
Annual Attendance: 9,000
Facility Category: Renovated Vaudovillle House
Type of Stage: Proscenium
Stage Dimensions: 25x40
Seating Capacity: 1,570
Year Built: 1924
Rental Contact: Rob Dippel

5249 SANDUSKY CONCERT ASSOCIATION
1402 Columbus Avenue
Sandusky, OH 44870-3521
Phone: 419-625-8312
Fax: 419-625-8380
Management:
Talent Coordinator: Diane Ernst
Specialized Field: Classical Music
Budget: $35,000- $50,000
Income Sources: Tickets sales, local support
Performs At: Sandusky State Theatre
Affiliations: AOR Hearthland

5250 SPRINGFIELD ARTS COUNCIL BROADWAY & POPS ON TOUR & SEASON EXTRAS
PO Box 745
Springfield, OH 45501-0745
Phone: 937-324-2712
Fax: 937-324-3170
e-mail: sac4arts@aol.com
Web Site: www.springfieldartscouncil.org
Management:
Manager: J Chris Moore
Budget: $60,000-150,000
Performs At: Kuss Auditorium; Clark State Performing Arts Center

5251 SPRINGFIELD SUMMER ARTS FESTIVAL
PO Box 745
Springfield, OH 45501-0745
Phone: 937-324-2712
Fax: 937-324-3170
e-mail: sac4arts@aol.com
Web Site: www.springfieldartscouncil.org
Management:

Executive Director: J Chris Moore

5252 ARTS COUNCIL LAKE ERIE WEST
1700 N Reynolds Road
Toledo, OH 43615
Phone: 419-531-2046
Fax: 419-531-5049
Toll-free: 888-297-6645
e-mail: martinnagy@aol.com
Web Site: www.artscouncillew.org
Management:
  Executive Director: Martin W Nagy
  Program Director: Danette Olson
Mission: To support, nourish, and provide for a quality environment for the arts to flourish in our region.
Founded: 1983
Specialized Field: All
Budget: $10,000-20,000
Income Sources: Admission; grants; donations; sales
Affiliations: Americans for the Arts
Facility Category: Auditorium
Type of Stage: Proscenium
Stage Dimensions: 16 x 44
Seating Capacity: 800
Year Built: 1920
Year Remodeled: 2001

5253 UPPER ARLINGTON CULTURAL ARTS COMMISSION
3600 Tremont Road
Upper Arlington, OH 43221
Phone: 614-583-5310
Fax: 614-442-3208
Toll-free: 888-722-5845
Web Site: www.ua.ohio.net
Management:
  Arts Manager: Diane Deane
  Arts Coordinator: Lynette Santoro-Au
Mission: Encouraging, promoting and providing cultural opportunities for community enrichment.
Founded: 1972
Specialized Field: Dance; Vocal Music; Instrumental Music; Facility; Theater; Festivals
Status: Nonprofit
Paid Staff: 2
Volunteer Staff: 78
Budget: $82,000
Income Sources: OAC; Ohio Humanities Donations; In Kind
Performs At: Upper Arlington Municipal Center
Annual Attendance: 200-30,000
Facility Category: Schools; City Buildings
Organization Type: Sponsoring

5254 FINE ARTS COUNCIL OF TRUMBULL COUNTY
PO Box 48
Warren, OH 44482
Phone: 330-399-1212
Fax: 330-399-7710
e-mail: bbrown@trumbullarts.org
Web Site: www.trumbullarts.org
Management:
  Executive Director: Bobbie Brown

Founded: 1971
Paid Staff: 1
Budget: $80,000

5255 WARREN CIVIC MUSIC ASSOCIATION
PO Box 8731
Warren, OH 44484
Phone: 330-652-1118
Fax: 330-393-5348
Officers:
  Talet Chairperson: Jeannine Morris
Mission: Building and maintaining a permanent audience for concerts in Warren and the surrounding areas; cultivating interest in music; encouraging performance by skilled artists.
Founded: 1937
Specialized Field: Dance; Vocal Music; Instrumental Music; Theater; Lyric Opera; Grand Opera
Status: Professional; Semi-Professional; Nonprofit
Budget: $60,000-150,000
Income Sources: Ohio Arts Council
Performs At: W.D. Packard Music Hall and Convention Center
Organization Type: Performing; Educational; Sponsoring

5256 OTTERBEIN COLLEGE ARTIST SERIES
Cellar House
141 W Park Street
Westerville, OH 43081
Phone: 614-823-1600
Fax: 614-823-1360
e-mail: pkessler@otterbein.edu
Web Site: www.otterbein.edu
Management:
  Executive Director: Patricia Kessler
Budget: $35,000-60,000
Performs At: Cowan Hall

5257 CHAMBER MUSIC CONNECTION
242 N Sinsbury Drive
Worthington, OH 43085
Phone: 614-848-3312
e-mail: artsdir@cmconnection.org
Web Site: www.cmconnection.org
Management:
  Artistic Director: Deborah B Price

5258 WORTHINGTON ARTS COUNCIL
777 High Street
2nd Floor
Worthington, OH 43085
Phone: 614-431-0329
Fax: 614-431-2491
e-mail: info@worthingtonarts.org
Web Site: www.worthingtonarts.org
Management:
  Executive Director: Sean Cooper
Mission: To encourage arts appreciation, awareness and participation in Worthington.
Founded: 1977
Specialized Field: Community
Paid Staff: 4
Volunteer Staff: 15

Paid Artists: 4
Budget: $200,000
Income Sources: Grants; Sponsorships; Ticket Sales
Performs At: Theaters
Annual Attendance: 4,000
Seating Capacity: 1,174

5259 MONDAY MUSICAL CLUB OF YOUNGSTOWN, OHIO

1000 5th Avenue
Suite 3
Youngstown, OH 44504-1603
Phone: 330-743-2717
Fax: 330-743-3745
e-mail: tickets@mondaymusical.com
Web Site: www.mondaymusical.com
Management:
    Manager: Kathy Doyle
Paid Staff: 2
Volunteer Staff: 30
Budget: $60,000-150,000
Performs At: Stambaugh Auditorium
Seating Capacity: 2,535
Year Built: 1926

5260 YOUNGSTOWN STATE UNIVERSITY: DANA CONCERT SERIES

Dana School of Music, Youngstown University
1 University Plaza
Youngstown, OH 44555
Phone: 330-742-3640
Fax: 330-742-1490
e-mail: mgelfand@cc.ysu.edu
Management:
    Coordinator: Michael D Gelfand
Budget: $20,000-35,000
Performs At: Bliss Recital Hall

5261 ZANESVILLE CONCERT ASSOCIATION

3450 S River Road
Zanesville, OH 43701
Phone: 740-452-4325
Fax: 740-453-3103
Management:
    Booking Agent: Carol Boyse
Seating Capacity: 35,000-60,000

Oklahoma

5262 COMMUNITY CONCERTS OF BARTLESVILLE

PO Box 651
Bartlesville, OK 74005
Phone: 918-333-4599
e-mail: Cjswango@aol.com
Officers:
    President: Carol Swango
Budget: $20,000-35,000

5263 OKLAHOMA MOZART INTERNATIONAL FESTIVAL

500 SE Dewey, Suite A
PO Box 2344
Bartlesville, OK 74005
Phone: 918-333-9900
Fax: 918-336-9525
e-mail: jmswindell@okmozart.com
Web Site: www.okmozart.com
Management:
    Executive Director: Peggy Ball
    Artistic Director: Ransom Wilson
    Development Director: Linda Cubbage
    Public Relations Director: Jeanette Swindell
Founded: 1985
Specialized Field: Dance; Vocal Music; Instrumental Music; Festivals; Grand Opera
Status: Professional; Nonprofit
Paid Staff: 8
Volunteer Staff: 800
Paid Artists: 50
Non-paid Artists: 0
Budget: $890,000
Income Sources: Oklahoma State Arts Council; National Endowment for the Arts; Individuals; Businesses
Performs At: Bartlesville Community Center
Annual Attendance: 30,000
Facility Category: Concert Hall, Community Center
Seating Capacity: 1700
Year Built: 1982
Organization Type: Sponsoring
Resident Groups: New York Orchestra

5264 CHISHOLM TRAIL ARTS COUNCIL

717 W Willow
Suite 6
Duncan, OK 73533
Phone: 580-252-4160
Fax: 580-252-1631
e-mail: ctac@texhoma.net
Officers:
    President: Gina Flesher
Management:
    Executive Director: Patrick Brown
Mission: To promote the arts in all discipline in the community.
Founded: 1976
Paid Staff: 1
Volunteer Staff: 50
Budget: $60,000-150,000
Income Sources: Public and private support
Performs At: Jack A. Mauer Convention Center
Seating Capacity: 750
Year Built: 1990

5265 CENTRAL OKLAHOMA CONCERT SERIES

PO Box 5272
Edmond, OK 73083
Phone: 405-340-3500
Fax: 405-844-8795
e-mail: JanStan@swbell.net
Web Site: www.chopinsociety.com
Management:

Executive Director: Jan Steele
Founded: 1986
Specialized Field: Concert
Budget: $20,000-35,000
Performs At: Mitchell Hall UCO Campus

5266 PHILADELPHIA FOUNDATION

PO Box 3700
Edmond, OK 73083
Phone: 405-285-1010
Fax: 405-359-6280
e-mail: info@pfconcerts.org
Web Site: www.pfconcerts.org
Management:
   Concert Series Director: Ryan Malone
Founded: 1998
Status: Nonprofit
Stage Dimensions: 21x56
Seating Capacity: 900
Year Built: 2001

5267 TRI-STATE MUSIC FESTIVAL

PO Box 5908
Enid, OK 73702
Phone: 580-237-4964
Management:
   Managing Director: Dr. Margaret S Buvinger

5268 CAMERON UNIVERSITY: LECTURE & CONCERT SERIES

2800 W Gore Boulevard
Lawton, OK 73505
Phone: 580-581-2211
e-mail: thescoop@cameron.edu
Web Site: www.cameron.edu
Budget: $10,000
Seating Capacity: 500

5269 LAWTON ARTS & HUMANITIES DIVISION

801 NW Ferris
Lawton, OK 73507
Mailing Address: PO Box 1054, Lawton, OK. 73502
Phone: 580-581-3470
Fax: 580-581-3473
Management:
   Administrator: Margaret Chalfant
   Auditorium Coordinator: Jim McCarthy
Budget: $10,000-20,000
Performs At: McMahon Memorial Auditorium

5270 JAZZ IN JUNE

PO Box 2405
Norman, OK 73070
Phone: 405-325-3388
e-mail: dkritten@swbell.net
Management:
   Executive Director of the Norman Ar: Phoebe Morales
Mission: To offer Oklahoma residents a jazz festival.
Founded: 1985
Specialized Field: Vocal Music; Instrumental Music
Status: Professional; Semi-Professional

Income Sources: American Federation of Musicians
Organization Type: Performing

5271 ARTS COUNCIL OF OKLAHOMA CITY

400 W California
Oklahoma City, OK 73102
Phone: 405-270-4848
Fax: 405-270-4888
e-mail: info@artscounciloke.com
Web Site: www.artscouncilokc.com
Management:
   Stage Center Director: Ron Martin
Founded: 1967
Specialized Field: Dedicated to bringing art of all types to everyone. From oil painting to folk dancing, events are presented bringing visual and performing arts.
Paid Staff: 17
Income Sources: Grants; Corporate Sponsors; Ticket Sales
Performs At: Stage Center; 400 West Sheridan
Annual Attendance: 44,700
Facility Category: Theatre
Type of Stage: 3/4 Round; Full Round
Seating Capacity: 580; 210
Year Built: 1970
Year Remodeled: 1987
Rental Contact: Kevin Lesley

5272 DEEP DEUCE JAZZ FESTIVAL

PO Box 11014
Oklahoma City, OK 73136
Phone: 405-524-3800
Fax: 405-524-3800
Management:
   Executive Director: Anita G Arnold
   Office Manager: Elwreta Parker
Paid Staff: 2
Volunteer Staff: 3
Paid Artists: 10

5273 DUSK TILL DAWN BLUES FESTIVAL

701 DC Minner Street
Rentiesville, OK 74459
Phone: 918-473-2411
Fax: 918-473-0033
e-mail: dcminner@lakewebs.net
Web Site: www.okblues.org
Management:
   Director: DC Minner
   Manager: Selby Minner
Mission: To showcase the Oklahoma blues tradition, music strong on electric guitars and full bands.
Founded: 1988
Paid Staff: 2
Volunteer Staff: 60
Paid Artists: 200

5274 OKLAHOMA BAPTIST UNIVERSITY ARTIST SERIES

College of Fine Arts
Box 61276
Shawnee, OK 74804

All listings are in alphabetical order by state, then city, then organization within the city.

Phone: 405-878-2305
Fax: 405-878-2328
e-mail: paul.hammond@okbu.edu
Web Site: www.okbu.edu
Management:
Dean: Paul Hammond
Budget: 20,000
Performs At: Yarborough Auditorium
Facility Category: Potter Auditorium/Yarboroagh
Auditorium
Seating Capacity: 2,000/400
Year Built: 1963
Year Remodeled: 2000

5275 OKLAHOMA STATE UNIVERSITY ALLIED ARTS

Oklahoma State University
060 Student Union
Stillwater, OK 74078
Phone: 405-744-7509
Fax: 405-744-2680
e-mail: rayjc@okstate.edu
Web Site: www.osunet.okstate.edu
Management:
Coordinator: Joe Ray
Mission: To provide OSU students, faculty, and staff and
Stillwater residents with world class cultural presentations
which they would not otherwise have the opportunity to
experience.
Founded: 1922
Paid Staff: 2
Budget: $60,000-82,000
Income Sources: Student Fees; Ticket Sales; Grants
Performs At: MB Seretean Center Concert Hall
Affiliations: APAP; SWPAP
Facility Category: Concert Hall
Type of Stage: Proscenium
Stage Dimensions: 38x44
Seating Capacity: 801

5276 NORTHEASTERN OKLAHOMA STATE UNIVERSITY ALLIED ARTS SERIES

College of Arts & Letters
Tahlequah, OK 74464
Phone: 918-456-5511
Fax: 918-458-2348
e-mail: storerz@nsuok.edu
Web Site: www.nsuok.edu
Officers:
Series Chairperson: Dr. Kathryn Robinson
Budget: $10,000-20,000

5277 BOK/WILLIAMS JAZZ ON GREENWOOD

PO Box 52111
Tulsa, OK 74152
Phone: 918-584-3378
Fax: 918-699-3560
e-mail: traceway@aol.com
Management:
Director: Barbara Swiggart
Founded: 1988
Specialized Field: Music

Volunteer Staff: 9
Paid Artists: 250

5278 CONCERTIME

11317 E 4th Street
Tulsa, OK 74128-2006
Phone: 918-438-2582
Fax: 918-437-1848
e-mail: organist@mciworld.com
Web Site: www.webtek.com/concertime
Management:
Manager: Alta Selvey
Budget: $20,000-35,000
Performs At: Patti Johnson Wilson Hall; Philbrook
Museum

5279 LIGHT OPERA OKLAHOMA - LOOK

Harwelden
2210 S Main
Tulsa, OK 74114
Phone: 918-583-4267
Fax: 918-583-1780
e-mail: eric@lightoperaok.org
Web Site: www.lightoperaok.org
Management:
Artistic Director: Eric Gibson
Artistic Director Emeritus/Founder: John Everitt
Mission: To preserve and create awareness of the musical
comedy/operetta art form by producing a festival of such
every summer in Tulsa, OK.
Founded: 1984
Specialized Field: Music Comedy; Operetta; Plays
Paid Staff: 3
Volunteer Staff: 10
Paid Artists: 100
Non-paid Artists: 10
Budget: $300,000-350,000
Income Sources: Foundations; Corporations
Performs At: University of Tulsa School of Theatre
Annual Attendance: 6000-7500
Seating Capacity: 375

5280 TULSA PERFORMING ARTS CENTER TRUST

110 E 2nd Street
Tulsa, OK 74103-3212
Phone: 918-596-7122
Fax: 918-596-7144
Toll-free: 800-364-7111
e-mail: tgrufik@ci.tulsa.ok.us
Web Site: www.tulsapac.com
Management:
Program Director: Terry Grufik
Budget: $150,000-400,000
Performs At: Chapman Music Hall; Williams Theatre;
Doenges Theatre

Oregon

5281 CHILDREN'S PERFORMING ARTS SERIES
Albany Parks & Recreation
333 Broadalbin Street SW
Albany, OR 97321-2247
Phone: 541-917-7772
Fax: 541-917-7776
Management:
    Recreation Coordinator: Jan Taylor
Budget: $10,000
Performs At: Linn Benton Community College Forum

5282 CITY OF ALBANY PARKS AND RECREATION DEPARTMENT
433 SW 4th Avenue
Albany, OR 97321
Phone: 541-917-7777
Fax: 514-917-7776
Management:
    Director: Dave Clark
    Program Coordinator: Sherry Halligan
Mission: To offer an outdoor concert series in summer at no cost, as well as a concert series for children.
Founded: 1983
Specialized Field: Vocal Music; Instrumental Music; Festivals
Status: Nonprofit
Organization Type: Sponsoring

5283 RIVER RHYTHMS
Albany Parks & Recreation
333 Broadalbin Street Southwest
Albany, OR 97321-2247
Phone: 541-917-7772
Fax: 541-917-7776
Web Site: www.ci.albany.or.us
Management:
    Recreation Coordinator: Jan Taylor
Mission: To build community.
Founded: 1983
Paid Staff: 16
Volunteer Staff: 12
Paid Artists: 7

5284 ASHLAND FOLK MUSIC CLUB
PO Box 63
Ashland, OR 97520
Phone: 541-488-0679
Fax: 541-552-6693
e-mail: ashlandfolk@iname.com
Officers:
    President: Jay Michalson
    VP: Gordon Enns
Mission: Supporting traditional music and dance.
Founded: 1984
Specialized Field: Dance; Vocal Music; Instrumental Music
Status: Nonprofit
Volunteer Staff: 8
Performs At: Carpenter Hall
Organization Type: Performing; Sponsoring

5285 OREGON SHAKESPEAREAN FESTIVAL ASSOCIATION
15 S Pioneer
PO Box 158
Ashland, OR 97520
Phone: 541-482-4331
Fax: 541-482-0446
Web Site: www.osfashland.org
Management:
    Artistic Director: Libby Appel
    Executive Director: Paul Nicholson
    Director Marketing/Communications: Janeen Olsen
Mission: To create bold new interpretations of contemporary and classic plays in repertory, influenced by American diversity and inspired by the high standard of Shakespeare.
Founded: 1935
Status: Professional; Nonprofit
Paid Staff: 450
Volunteer Staff: 750
Budget: $17.1 million
Season: June - August
Performs At: Angus Bowmer Theatre; Black Swan; Elizabethan Theatre
Affiliations: Actors' Equity Association; ATA; University/Resident Theatre Association; Theatre Communications Group
Annual Attendance: 375,000+
Type of Stage: Thrust Stage; Black Box; Outdoors
Seating Capacity: 601; 250; 1188
Organization Type: Performing; Touring; Resident; Educational

5286 CASCADE FESTIVAL OF MUSIC
842 NW Wall Street
Suite 6
Bend, OR 97701
Phone: 541-382-8381
Fax: 541-388-2814
e-mail: musicinfo@cascademusic.org
Web Site: www.cascademusic.org
Management:
    Executive Director: Sally Russenberger
    Business Manager: Cindy Sundquist
    Executive Assistant: Coleen Shearer
Mission: Classical music event in Central Oregon as an eight day festival in late August
Founded: 1981
Paid Staff: 4
Volunteer Staff: 200
Paid Artists: 90
Performs At: Tent
Annual Attendance: 7,000 - 8,000

5287 OREGON COAST MUSIC FESTIVAL
PO Box 663
Coos Bay, OR 97420
Phone: 541-267-0938
Fax: 541-267-0938
Toll-free: 877-897-9350
e-mail: ocma@coosnet.com
Web Site: www.coosnet.com/music
Management:
    Music Director: James Paul

Administrative Assistant: Cory Smith
Mission: To present an annual Classical Music festival of the highest professional caliber and to support a wide range of year-round musical performances and educational activities.
Founded: 1979
Specialized Field: Music

5288 COQUILLE PERFORMING ARTS
PO Box 53
Coquille, OR 97423
Phone: 541-396-5131
e-mail: rwiese@ucinet.com
Officers:
President: Rochelle Wiese
Budget: $10,000
Performs At: Sawdust Theatre

5289 CORVALLIS-OREGON STATE UNIVERSITY MUSIC ASSOCIATION
3328 NW Firwood Drive
Corvallis, OR 97330
Phone: 541-737-1879
Fax: 541-346-5764
e-mail: mcclintt@ucs.orst.edu
Officers:
Chairman Program Committee: Thomas C McClintock
President: Larry Blus
Treasurer: Len Webber
Secretary: Midge Mueller
Founded: 1948
Specialized Field: Classical Music, No Chamber Groups Except Orchestra
Volunteer Staff: 15
Budget: $20,000-35,000
Income Sources: Ticket Sales, Member and Corporate Donations, Foundation Grants
Performs At: Austin Auditorium; LaSells Stewart Center
Annual Attendance: 20,000
Facility Category: Auditorium in Conference Center
Type of Stage: Proscenium
Seating Capacity: 1,200
Year Built: 1981

5290 OREGON BACH FESTIVAL
1257 University of Oregon
Eugene, OR 97403
Phone: 541-346-5666
Fax: 541-346-5669
Toll-free: 800-457-1486
e-mail: saltzman@oregon.ugregon.edu
Web Site: www.bachfest.uoregon.edu
Management:
Artistic Director: Helmuth Rilling
Executive Director: H Royce Saltzman
Marketing Director: George Evano
Mission: To offer high quality performances that elevate the spirits of both performers and audiences.
Founded: 1970
Specialized Field: Choral-Orchestral
Status: Professional; Nonprofit
Paid Staff: 8
Budget: 1.3 Million

Income Sources: Box office, grants, private donqtions
Performs At: University of Oregon School of Music; Beall Concert
Affiliations: University of Oregon School of Music
Annual Attendance: 33,000
Facility Category: Concert Hall
Type of Stage: Proscenium
Seating Capacity: 2500/550
Organization Type: Performing; Resident; Educational

5291 OREGON FESTIVAL OF AMERICAN MUSIC
The Shedd
868 High Street
Eugene, OR 97401
Mailing Address: PO Box 1497, Eugene, OR. 97440
Phone: 541-687-6526
Fax: 541-687-1589
e-mail: info@ofam.org
Web Site: www.ofam.org
Management:
Executive Director: James Ralph
Mission: Year-round production and presenting of American music genres.
Founded: 1991
Specialized Field: Music Performance; Education

5292 UNIVERSITY OF OREGON CHAMBER MUSIC SERIES
School of Music
1225 University of Oregon
Eugene, OR 97403-1225
Phone: 541-346-5679
Fax: 541-346-0723
e-mail: jjs@oregon.uoregon.edu
Web Site: www.music1.oregon.edu/cms/cmshomepage.html
Management:
Director: Janet J Stewart
Budget: $20,000-35,000
Performs At: Beall Concert Hall

5293 MT. HOOD COMMUNITY COLLEGE
26000 SE Stark Street
Gresham, OR 97030
Phone: 503-491-7260
Fax: 503-491-6077
Budget: $10,000

5294 COMMUNITY CONCERT ASSOCIATION
PO Box 1214
Klamath Falls, OR 97601
Phone: 541-882-6041
e-mail: jd4chunjn@aol.com
Officers:
President: Susan Fortune
Budget: $20,000-35,000
Performs At: Ross Ragland Theater

5295 EASTERN OREGON STATE COLLEGE PERFORMING ARTS PROGRAM
Student Activities Office
1 University Blvd, Hoke Center, Suite 321
La Grande, OR 97850-2899
Phone: 541-962-3704
Fax: 541-962-1849
e-mail: jkreider@eou.edu
Management:
   Student Activities Director: Jim Kreider
Budget: $10,000
Performs At: Inlow Hall; Loso Hall

5296 LAKE OSWEGO FESTIVAL OF THE ARTS
PO Box 385
368 S State Street
Lake Oswego, OR 97034
Phone: 503-636-1060
Fax: 503-635-2002
Web Site: www.lakewood-center.org
Management:
   Director: Dean Denton
   Director: Malcolm Mathes
Founded: 1962
Paid Staff: 1
Volunteer Staff: 22
Budget: $150,000
Income Sources: Gifts; Grants; Commisions
Annual Attendance: 22,000
Facility Category: Arts Center and Park
Type of Stage: Outdoor
Seating Capacity: 500-1,000

5297 CASCADE HEAD MUSIC FESTIVAL
PO Box 605
Lincoln City, OR 97367
Web Site: www.cascadeheadmusic.com
Management:
   Music Director: Sergiu Luca

5298 MARYLHURST MUSIC SERIES
Marylhurst University
17600 Pacific Highway
Marylhurst, OR 97036
Mailing Address: PO Box 261, Marylhurst, PA. 97036
Phone: 503-636-8141
Fax: 503-636-9526
Toll-free: 800-634-9982
e-mail: music@marylhurst.edu
Web Site: www.marylhurst.edu
Officers:
   Chair: John Paul
Paid Staff: 1
Performs At: St. Anne's Chapel; Wiegand Recital Hall
Annual Attendance: 1,000
Facility Category: Chapel
Seating Capacity: 325
Cost: $690/day

5299 BRITT FESTIVALS
PO Box 1124
Medford, OR 97501

Phone: 541-779-0847
Fax: 541-776-3712
e-mail: info@brittfest.org
Web Site: www.brittfest.org
Management:
   Executive Director: Ron McUne
   Music Director: Peter Bay
   Marketing/Public Relations Director: Kelly Gonzales
   Development Director: Ed Foss
   Booking/Production Director: Mike Sturgill
   Education Director: David MacKenzie
Mission: To present and sponsor, in Southern Oregon, performing arts of the highest quality for the education, enrichment and enjoyment of all.
Founded: 1963
Specialized Field: Classical; Jazz; Blues; Pop/Rock; Country; Folk; Bluegrass; World Music; Dance; Musical Theater; Comedy
Status: Professional; Nonprofit
Paid Staff: 12
Volunteer Staff: 600
Performs At: The Britt Gardens
Annual Attendance: 70,000
Facility Category: Outdoor Amphitheatre
Seating Capacity: 2200
Year Built: 1963
Year Remodeled: 1992
Organization Type: Performing; Touring; Resident; Educational; Sponsoring

5300 WESTERN OREGON UNIVERSITY EDGAR H SMITH FINE ARTS SERIES
Western Oregon University
345 N Monmouth Avenue
Monmouth, OR 97361
Phone: 503-838-8333
Fax: 503-838-1864
e-mail: fineart@fsa.wou.edu
Management:
   Series Director: Carole Orloff
Founded: 1976
Paid Staff: 1
Volunteer Staff: 16
Paid Artists: 4
Budget: $35,000-60,000
Performs At: Rice Auditorium
Facility Category: College Auditorium
Type of Stage: Proscenium
Stage Dimensions: 30 X 55
Seating Capacity: 617

5301 ERNEST BLOCH MUSIC FESTIVAL AT NEWPORT
PO Box 1617
Newport, OR 97365
Phone: 541-265-2787
Fax: 541-265-5008
Web Site: www.baymusic.org
Management:
   Music Director/Conductor: Sylvain Fremaux

5302 CHAMBER MUSIC NORTHWEST
522 SW 5th Avenue
Suite 725
Portland, OR 97204
Phone: 503-233-3202
Fax: 503-294-1690
e-mail: info@cmnw.org
Web Site: www.cmnw.org
Management:
  Executive Director: Linda Magee
  Artistic Director: David Shifrin
  Operations Director: Franck Avril
  Finance Director: Katherine King
  Marketing Manager: Garen Horgend
Mission: To present an annual summer music festival
(five weeks/25 concerts) with world renowned performers
in residence; to present concerts and educational activities
on a year-round basis.
Founded: 1971
Specialized Field: Chamber; Ensemble
Status: Professional; Nonprofit
Paid Staff: 6
Paid Artists: 75
Budget: One Million
Performs At: Reed College
Affiliations: Kaul Auditorium at Reed College; Cabell
Theatre at Catlin Gabel Schhool
Annual Attendance: 19,000
Facility Category: Concert Hall (private college)
Seating Capacity: 550
Year Built: 1998
Organization Type: Performing
Notes: Wheelchair seating available

5303 MOUNT HOOD FESTIVAL OF JAZZ: THE GOVERNOR BUILDING
408 SW 2nd Avenue
Portland, OR 97204
Phone: 503-232-3000
Fax: 503-232-2336
e-mail: billroyston@pocketmail.com
Web Site: www.mthoodjazz.com
Management:
  Director: Bill Royston

5304 PORTLAND UNIVERSITY PORTLAND INTERNATIONAL: PERFORMANCE FESTIVAL
PO Box 1491
Portland, OR 97207
Phone: 503-725-5389
Fax: 503-725-4840
e-mail: griggsm@ses.pdx.edu
Web Site: www.extended.pdx.edu/pipf/index.html
Management:
  Artistic Director: Michael Griggs

5305 PORTLAND STATE UNIVERSITY PIANO RECITAL SERIES
PO Box 751
Portland, OR 97207
Phone: 503-725-5400
Fax: 503-725-8215
e-mail: zagelop@mail.pdx.edu
Web Site: www.fpa.pdx.edu/prs/
Management:
  Executive Director: Pat Zagelow
Mission: The piano recital series is dedicated to
presenting the finest pianists in the world in recital
settings and outreach for the purpose of enriching and
educating our community.
Budget: $200,000
Income Sources: Tickets; Contributions
Performs At: Lincoln Hall Auditorium
Annual Attendance: 6,000
Type of Stage: Proscenium
Seating Capacity: 476

5306 TRIANGLE PRODUCTIONS
3430 SE Belmont
Portland, OR 97214
Phone: 503-239-5919
Fax: 503-239-5928
e-mail: trianglepro@juno.com
Web Site: www.tripro.org/general.html
Officers:
  Triangle Productions Board: Lennky Borer
  Board: Dennis Dohtery
  Board: Larry Esau
  Board: Sherman Tam
  Board: Edd Scott
  Board: Donald I Horn
  Past President: Sharon Knorr
  Honorary Member: Gus Van Sant
  Honorary Member: Dan Reed
Management:
  Managing Director/Founder: Donald I Horn
Founded: 1989
Status: Not-for-profit

5307 UNIVERSITY OF PORTLAND MUSIC AT MIDWEEK
5000 N Williamette Boulevard
Portland, OR 97203
Phone: 503-943-7382
Fax: 503-943-7399
e-mail: doyle@up.edu
Management:
  Manager: Roger Doyle
Budget: $10,000
Performs At: Hunt Center Recital Hall

5308 ABBEY BACH FESTIVAL
Mount Angel Abbey
One Abbey Drive
Saint Benedict, OR 97373
Phone: 503-845-3321
Fax: 503-845-3202
e-mail: bach@mtangel.edu
Web Site: www.mtangel.edu
Officers:
  President: Nathan Zodrow OSB
  Executive Director: Father Paschal Cheline OSB
Management:
  Administrative Assistant: Father Bruno Becker, OSB

Founded: 1972
Specialized Field: Vocal Music; Instrumental Music
Status: Professional; Semi-Professional
Performs At: Damian Center
Annual Attendance: 1500
Type of Stage: Proscenium
Seating Capacity: 500
Year Built: 1936
Year Remodeled: 1983
Organization Type: Performing

5309 SUNRIVER MUSIC FESTIVAL CHAMBER ORCHESTRA

PO Box 4308
Sunriver, OR 97707
Phone: 541-593-1084
Fax: 541-593-6959
e-mail: srmusic@coinet.com
Web Site: www.sunrivermusic.org
Officers:
   President: Bergen Bull
Management:
   Executive Director: Lori Noack
   Office Manager: Joan Fields
Mission: Present quality performances of classical music and educational programs for the youth of Central Oregon.
Founded: 1971
Specialized Field: Central Oregon
Paid Staff: 3
Volunteer Staff: 200
Budget: $250,000
Income Sources: Private; Business; Grants
Performs At: Great Hall
Annual Attendance: 3,500

5310 YACHATS MUSIC FESTIVAL

PO Box 566
Yachats, OR 97498
Mailing Address: Four Season Concerts, PO Box 507, Berkeley, CA. 94701
Phone: 510-451-0775
Fax: 510-549-3504
e-mail: fourseasonsconcerts@juno.com
Web Site: www.fourseasonsconcerts.com
Officers:
   President: Jesse W Anthony

Pennsylvania

5311 ALLENTOWN COMMUNITY CONCERTS

905 S Cedar Crest Boulevard
Allentown, PA 18103
Phone: 610-432-9143
Officers:
   President: William Lazenberg
Mission: To present four annual concerts with varied programs; membership is open to the public during the annual campaign.
Founded: 1927

Specialized Field: Dance; Vocal Music; Instrumental Music
Status: Nonprofit
Budget: $20,000-35,000
Income Sources: Community Concerts
Organization Type: Educational; Sponsoring

5312 MUHLENBERG COLLEGE CONCERT SERIES

2400 Chew Street
Allentown, PA 18104
Phone: 484-664-3363
Fax: 484-664-3633
Budget: $10,000-20,000
Season: June - August

5313 BLAIR COUNTY CIVIC MUSIC ASSOCIATION

PO Box 69
Altoona, PA 16603
Phone: 814-943-9951
Fax: 814-944-9811
Officers:
   President: Patricia Gildea
   First Vice President: Charlotte Morris
   Second VP: Richard Russell
   Third VP: Estrida McLocham
   Recording Secretary: Pauline Hoover
   Membership Secretary: Jane Gable
Mission: To provide the finest in performing arts for Blair County at reasonable cost to our subscribers.
Founded: 1944
Specialized Field: Dance; Vocal Music; Instrumental Music; Theater; Grand Opera
Status: Professional; Nonprofit
Budget: $60,000-150,000
Performs At: Roosevelt Junior High School Auditorium
Organization Type: Presenting

5314 BEAVER VALLEY COMMUNITY CONCERT ASSOCIATION

153 Oak Drive
Beaver Falls, PA 15010
Phone: 724-846-6814
Officers:
   President: EE Bass
Budget: $20,000-35,000

5315 BETHLEHEM BACH FESTIVAL

423 Heckewelder Place
Bethlehem, PA 18018
Phone: 610-866-4382
Fax: 610-866-6232
Toll-free: 888-743-3100
e-mail: office@bach.org
Web Site: www.bach.org
Management:
   Artistic Director/Conductor: Greg Funfgeld

5316 BETHLEHEM MUSIKFEST ASSOCIATION

25 W 3rd Street
Bethlehem, PA 18015
Phone: 610-861-0678
Fax: 610-861-2644
e-mail: jparks@fest.org
Web Site: www.musikfest.org
Officers:
   President: Jeffrey A Parks

5317 MORAVIAN COLLEGE ARTS & LECTURES SERIES

1200 Main Street
Bethlehem, PA 18018
Phone: 610-861-1686
Fax: 610-861-1657
e-mail: mecat01@moravian.edu
Officers:
   Chairperson: Carol Traupman-Carr
Budget: $20,000-35,000
Seating Capacity: 400

5318 BLOOMSBURG UNIVERSITY ARTIST-CELEBRITY SERIES

Bloomsburg University
400 E 2nd Street
Bloomsburg, PA 17815
Phone: 570-389-4201
Fax: 570-389-4201
e-mail: jmulka@bloomu.edu
Web Site: www.bloomu.edu
Management:
   Executive Director: Nancy Vought
   Special Assistant to VP: Dr. John S Mulka
Budget: $60,000-150,000
Performs At: Mitrani Hall; Haas Center for the Arts; Gross Auditorium

5319 MONTGOMERY COUNTY COMMUNITY COLLEGE LIVELY ARTS SERIES

340 DeKalb Pike
Box 400
Blue Bell, PA 19422-0796
Phone: 215-641-6505
Fax: 215-641-6645
e-mail: livarts@mc3.edu
Web Site: www.mc3.edu
Management:
   Director Cultural Affairs: Helen Haynes
   Assistant Director Cultural Affairs: Jennifer Merritt
Paid Staff: 2
Budget: $35,000-60,000
Performs At: Science Center Theater

5320 BRADFORD CREATIVE & PERFORMING ARTS CENTER

PO Box 153
Bradford, PA 16701

Phone: 814-362-1025
Fax: 814-368-7040
e-mail: jdg1@charter.net
Web Site: www.bcpac.com
Officers:
   President: James D Guelfi
Founded: 1984
Paid Staff: 1
Volunteer Staff: 15
Paid Artists: 5
Budget: $60,000-150,000
Income Sources: Sales; Grants; Patrons
Annual Attendance: 5,000
Seating Capacity: 1410

5321 CRS NATIONAL FESTIVAL FOR THE PERFORMING ARTS

724 Winchester Road
Broomall, PA 19008
Phone: 215-544-5920
Fax: 215-544-5921
e-mail: crsnews@erols.com
Web Site: www.erols.com/crsnews
Management:
   Artistic Advisor: Milton Babbitt
Mission: To offer performers, composers, teachers, libraries, educational institutions, amateurs, devotees of music and prosepective sponsors cultural enrichment through vast musical sources.
Founded: 1981
Specialized Field: Dance; Vocal Music; Instrumental Music; Festivals
Status: Professional; Semi-Professional; Nonprofit
Income Sources: Contemporary Record Society
Organization Type: Performing; Touring; Resident; Educational

5322 BRYN MAWR COLLEGE PERFORMING ARTS SERIES

Office for the Arts
101 N Merion Avenue
Bryn Mawr, PA 19010
Phone: 610-526-5210
Fax: 610-526-5205
e-mail: ngreaves@brynmawr.edu
Web Site: www.brynmawr.edu
Management:
   Coordinator: Nicole Greaves
Specialized Field: Dance; Theater; Chamber Music
Volunteer Staff: 2
Budget: $42,000
Seating Capacity: 800

5323 PENNSYLVANIA SHAKESPEARE FESTIVAL

2755 Station Avenue
Center Valley, PA 18034
Phone: 610-282-9455
Fax: 610-282-2084
e-mail: Kathryn.Cousar@desales.edu
Web Site: www.pashakespeare.org
Management:
   Artistic Director: Jack Young

All listings are in alphabetical order by state, then city, then organization within the city.

Managing Director: Kathryn Cousar
Managing Associate: Robyn Brady
Director Educational Outreach: Sandy Marino
Endowment Director: Gerard J Schubert, OSFS
Business Manager: Janice Hein
Founded: 1991
Status: Nonprofit; Equity
Paid Staff: 6
Volunteer Staff: 200
Paid Artists: 100
Season: May - August
Type of Stage: Thrust
Stage Dimensions: 38' x 40'
Seating Capacity: 473

5324   WILSON COLLEGE LECTURES & CONCERTS

1015 Philadelphia Avenue
Chamebrsburg, PA 17201
Phone: 717-262-2003
Fax: 717-264-2038
e-mail: klehman@wilson.edu
Web Site: www.wilson.edu
Management:
    Cultural Events Director: Kathy Lehman
Mission: To provide a series of artistic performances that enrich the educational and social lives of students, faculty, and staff. It is also our mission to enhance Wilson College's reputation as a cultural resource serving the Cumberland Valley c
Paid Staff: 3
Budget: $10,000-15,000
Income Sources: Grants, Foundation Funding, Gifts, Ticket sales
Performs At: Laird Hall; Thompson Hall
Facility Category: Auditorium
Stage Dimensions: 30'x30'
Seating Capacity: 800

5325   CLARION UNIVERSITY ACTIVITIES BOARD ARTS

273 Gemmell Student Center
Clarion, PA 16214
Phone: 814-393-2312
Management:
    Advisor: Jamie Bero-Johnson
Budget: $10,000-20,000
Performs At: Marwick - Boyd Auditorium

5326   LEHIGH VALLEY BLUES & JAZZ FESTIVAL

PO Box G
Coplay, PA 18037
Web Site: www.lvbluesfest.org

5327   MOUNT ALOYSIUS COLLEGE PERFORMING ARTS SERIES

7373 Admiral Peary Highway
Cresson, PA 16630
Phone: 814-886-6407
Fax: 814-886-2978
e-mail: jniebauer@mtaloy.edu
Management:

Director of Student Activities: Joyce Niebauer
Budget: $10,000-20,000

5328   DELAWARE WATER GAP CELEBRATION OF THE ARTS

PO Box 249
Delaware Water Gap, PA 18327
Phone: 717-424-2210
Web Site: www.welcome.to/cotajazz
Management:
    Director: Richard C Chamberlain

5329   ALLAN KURBY SPORTS CENTER

Lafayette College
Easton, PA 18042
Phone: 610-250-5470
Fax: 610-250-7651
Web Site: www.lafayette/sports.edu
Management:
    Director: Eve Atkinson

5330   LAFAYETTE COLLEGE CONCERT SERIES

Williams Center for the Arts
Easton, PA 18042
Phone: 610-250-5010
Fax: 610-250-8728
Management:
    Executive Director: Dr. Ellis Finger
Budget: $60,000-150,000
Seating Capacity: 400

5331   EDINBORO UNIVERSITY OF PENNSYLVANIA PERFORMING ARTS SERIES

Music Department
Room 109
Edinboro, PA 16444
Phone: 814-732-2518
Fax: 814-732-2518
e-mail: Barbaro@Edinboro.edu
Management:
    Executive Director: Dr. Cosmo A Barbaro
Budget: $35,000-60,000
Performs At: Memorial Auditorium

5332   MUSIC AT GRETNA

1 Alpha Drive
Elizabethtown, PA 17022
Phone: 717-361-1508
Fax: 717-361-1512
e-mail: music@mtgretna.com
Web Site: www.mtgretna.com/music
Officers:
    Founder: Carl Ellenberger, Jr
    President: Henry Kenderdine
Management:
    Executive Director: Douglas Blackstone
    Development Director: Suzanne Lieto
Founded: 1975
Specialized Field: Festivals
Status: Professional; Nonprofit

Budget: $60,000-150,000
Income Sources: Mt. Greten Playhouse; Clyde & Perk Center
Performs At: Leffler Chapel Performance Center
Organization Type: Educational; Sponsoring; Producing

5333 ERIE CIVIC CENTER/ WARNER THEATRE
809 French Street
Erie, PA 16512
Phone: 814-453-7117
Fax: 814-455-9931
Web Site: www.erieciviccenter.com
Management:
Managing Director: John Wells

5334 ERIE CIVIC MUSIC ASSOCIATION
1833 W 33 Street
Erie, PA 16508
Phone: 814-864-5681
Fax: 814-459-1509
e-mail: butchvick@aol.com
Web Site: www.eriecivicmusic.com
Officers:
President: Garlan Newcomb
Assistant Treasurer: Nora Fickle
VP: Joe Luckey
Executive Secretary: Bea Hansen
Treasurer: Chris Moser
Management:
Director: Joe Allen
Director: Alice Couchin
Mission: We present the greatest international talent available at the most reasonable costs.
Founded: 1928
Specialized Field: Vocal Music; Instrumental Music
Status: Nonprofit
Volunteer Staff: 35
Budget: $50,000-90,000
Income Sources: Erie Area Fund for the Arts; Season & Single Tickets Sales
Performs At: Warner Theatre
Annual Attendance: 7,500-9,000
Organization Type: Sponsoring

5335 MESSIAH COLLEGE CULTURAL SERIES
Messiah College
One College Avenue, PO Box 3020
Grantham, PA 17027
Phone: 717-691-6027
Fax: 717-796-5371
e-mail: ehager@messiah.edu
Web Site: www.messiah.edu
Management:
Performing Arts Coodinator: Eunice Hager
Paid Staff: 6
Budget: $20,000-35,000
Performs At: Miller Auditorium

5336 CENTRAL PENNSYLVANIA MELLON JAZZ FESTIVAL
PO Box 10738
Harrisburg, PA 17105
Phone: 717-540-1010
Fax: 717-540-7735
e-mail: pajazz@epix.net
Web Site: www.pa.jazz.org
Management:
Executive Director: David Lazorcik

5337 HARRISBURG AREA COMMUNITY COLLEGE
1 HACC Drive
Harrisburg, PA 17110-2999
Phone: 717-780-2545
Fax: 717-780-3281
Web Site: www.hacc.edu/rose
Management:
Performing Artist Series Director: Teri Guerrisi
Paid Staff: 6
Volunteer Staff: 30
Budget: $35,000-60,000
Performs At: Rose Lehrman Auditorium
Facility Category: Proscenium
Type of Stage: Hardwood, Spring Floor
Stage Dimensions: 36'x40'
Seating Capacity: 374
Year Built: 1975
Year Remodeled: 1993
Rental Contact: Teri Guerrsi

5338 MARKET SQUARE CONCERTS
301 Market Street
6th Floor
Harrisburg, PA 17101
Mailing Address: PO Box 1292, Harrisburg, PA. 17108
Phone: 717-221-9599
Fax: 717-221-9588
e-mail: lucy-miller@worldnet.att.net
Officers:
President: David Lehman
Management:
Executive Director: Lucy Miller
Mission: Presenting a wide range of chamber and solo music presentations by distinguished artists.
Specialized Field: Chamber Music
Status: Professional; Nonprofit
Budget: $60,000-150,000
Performs At: Market Square Church; Rose Lehrman Art Center; Whitaker Ctr.
Organization Type: Educational; Presenting

5339 NEXT GENERATION FESTIVAL
WITF-FM
1982 Locust Land
Harrisburg, PA 17105
Web Site: www.nextgenerationfestival.org

5340 HERSHEYPARK ARENA/STADIUM
100 W Hersherpark Drive
Hershey, PA 17033

Phone: 717-534-8966
Fax: 717-534-3113
Web Site: www.hersheypa.com
Management:
    General Manager: Matthew Ford

5341 JUNIATA COLLEGE ARTIST SERIES
1700 Moore Street
Huntingdon, PA 16652
Phone: 814-641-3471
e-mail: bargied@juniata.edu
Web Site: www.juniata.edu
Management:
    Artist Series Director: Diane Bargiel
Budget: $35,000-60,000

5342 INDIANA UNIVERSITY OF PENNSYLVANIA ONSTAGE: ARTS AND ENTERTAINMENT
102 Pratt Hall
Indiana, PA 15705
Phone: 724-357-2315
Fax: 724-357-2593
e-mail: destefan@iup.edu
Web Site: www.iup.edu/sao/artist.htmlx
Management:
    Assoc. Dir. Ctr. for Student Life: Frank DeStefano
Budget: $400,000
Performs At: Fisher Auditorium
Type of Stage: Proscenium
Seating Capacity: 1600

5343 LAUREL FESTIVAL OF THE ARTS
PO Box 206
Jim Thorpe, PA 18229
Phone: 570-325-4439
Fax: 570-325-4439
Management:
    Artistic Director: Marc Mostaroy
    Weeknight Concerts: Randall Perry
    Publicity: Herbert Thompson
    Marketing: Barbara Loeffler
Mission: To unite the finest performers in working together to present events for the public.
Founded: 1990
Specialized Field: Dance; Vocal Music; Instrumental Music; Festivals; Poetry
Status: Professional; Nonprofit
Performs At: Manch Chunk Opera House
Organization Type: Performing; Resident; Educational

5344 CAMBRIA COUNTY WAR MEMORIAL ARENA
326 Napoleon
Johnstown, PA 15901
Phone: 814-536-5156
Fax: 814-536-3670
Web Site: www.warmemorialarena.com
Management:
    General Manager: James L Vautar
Mission: Sports and entertainment
Founded: 1950
Paid Staff: 9

Budget: 1.5 million
Income Sources: Rental Events
Annual Attendance: 275,000
Facility Category: Arena
Type of Stage: Portable
Seating Capacity: 5,000
Year Built: 1950
Year Remodeled: 2003
Cost: $85 million
Rental Contact: Jim Vautar

5345 UNIVERSITY OF PITTSBURGH AT JAMESTOWN
450 Schoolhouse Road
Johnstown, PA 15904
Phone: 814-269-7200
Fax: 814-269-7240
Management:
    Executive Director: Patricia Carnevali

5346 CHRYSANTHEMUM FESTIVAL / CHRISTMAS FESTIVAL / SUMMER FESTIVAL OF FOUNTAINS
PO Box 501
Longwood Gardens
Kennett Square, PA 19348
Phone: 610-388-1000
Fax: 610-388-3833
Web Site: www.longwoodgardens.org
Management:
    Performing Arts Coordinator: Priscilla Johnson
    Performing Arts Assistant: Nancy Bleakley
    Production Coordinator: Ken Homer
    Performing Arts Associate: Sue Johnson
Founded: 1906
Paid Staff: 35
Paid Artists: 400
Non-paid Artists: 23

5347 LONGWOOD GARDENS PERFORMING ARTS
PO Box 501
Kennett Square, PA 19348
Phone: 610-388-1000
Fax: 610-388-3833
Web Site: www.longwoodgardens.org
Management:
    Performing Arts Coordinator: Priscilla Johnson
Mission: To enhance the gardens and follow tradition of founder Pierre S duPont.
Founded: 1929
Specialized Field: Instrumental Music; Theater; Festivals
Status: Nonprofit
Paid Staff: 50
Budget: $60,000-150,000
Income Sources: Ticket Sales
Annual Attendance: 1 Million to Gardens
Facility Category: Outdoor Historic Theatre
Stage Dimensions: 73 x 36
Seating Capacity: 2000
Year Built: 1920
Organization Type: Performing; Educational

5348 KUTZTOWN UNIVERSITY PERFORMING ARTISTS SERIES
Office of Cultural Affairs
Kutztown University
Kutztown, PA 19530
Phone: 610-683-4510
Fax: 610-683-4010
Management:
   Cultural Affairs Director: Ellen Finks
Budget: $60,000-150,000
Performs At: Schaeffer Auditorium

5349 NEW ARTS PROGRAM
173 W Main Street
PO Box 82
Kutztown, PA 19530
Phone: 610-683-6440
Fax: 610-683-6440
e-mail: napconn@aol.com
Web Site: www.napconnection.com
Officers:
   President: James FL Carroll
   VP: Michael Kessler
   Treasurer: James FL Carroll
   Secretary: Joanne P. Carroll
Management:
   Director: James FL Carroll
Mission: To present artists from the performing, visual and literary arts in one-to-one consultations; to offer a presentation/performance style collective consultation.
Founded: 1974
Specialized Field: Dance; Literary; Visual; Performing
Status: Professional; Nonprofit
Paid Staff: 1
Volunteer Staff: 2
Budget: $60,000
Income Sources: PCA, Foundations, Corporations, Individuals
Performs At: Saint Johns UCC
Annual Attendance: 3000
Facility Category: Gallery
Seating Capacity: 76 - 350
Organization Type: Performing; Resident

5350 FRANKLIN & MARSHALL COLLEGE SOUND HORIZONS CONCERT SERIES
PO Box 3003
Lancaster, PA 17604-3003
Phone: 717-291-4346
Fax: 717-358-7168
e-mail: D_Miller@admin.fandm.edu
Web Site: www.fandm.edu
Officers:
   Chairman Concert Committee: Bruce Gustafson
Management:
   Concert Coordinator: Deb Miller
   Performance Manager/Asst.Technical: Mark Miskinis
Founded: 1935
Paid Staff: 6
Volunteer Staff: 6
Budget: $35,000-50,000
Performs At: The Ann & Richard Barshinger Center; Miller Recital Hall

Facility Category: Concert Hall
Seating Capacity: 500
Year Built: 1925
Year Remodeled: 2000

5351 PHILADELPHIA COLLEGE OF BIBLE ARTIST LECTURE SERIES
Philadelphia Biblical University
200manor Avenue
Langhorne, PA 19047-2990
Phone: 215-702-4329
Fax: 215-702-4342
e-mail: music@pbu.edu
Web Site: www.pbu.edu
Officers:
   Dean: Dr. Paul R Isensee
Budget: $10,000
Affiliations: NASM
Facility Category: Chapel
Seating Capacity: 750

5352 BUCKNELL UNIVERSITY: WEIS CENTER PERFORMANCE SERIES
Weis Center for the Performing Arts
Bucknell University
Lewisburg, PA 17837-2005
Phone: 570-577-3700
Fax: 570-577-3701
e-mail: boswell@bucknell.edu
Web Site: http://www.departments.bucknell.edu
Management:
   Director Cultural Events: William Boswell
Mission: To provide the campus and region with opportunity for exposure to the essential cultural and educational values inherent in the great historical an radical traditions of the performing arts.
Founded: 1846
Budget: $150,000-400,000
Affiliations: APAP, CMA, PA Presenters, Others
Annual Attendance: 9000
Facility Category: Concert Hall
Type of Stage: Sprung Wood Floor
Seating Capacity: 1,200+
Year Built: 1988

5353 MIFFLIN-JUNIATA CONCERT ASSOCIATION
PO Box 870
Lewiston, PA 17044-0870
Phone: 717-248-4971
Fax: 717-248-2672
Management:
   Director Emeritus: Allen J Levin
Budget: $20,000-35,000

5354 MANSFIELD UNIVERSITY FINE ARTS SERIES
Music Department
Mansfield, PA 16933
Phone: 570-662-4710
Fax: 570-662-4114
Management:
   Manager: Kenneth Sarch

Budget: $10,000-20,000
Performs At: Steadman Theatre

5355 MUSIC AT FISHS EDDY

875 Welsh Road
Maple Glen, PA 19002
Mailing Address: PO Box 191, Fishs Eddy, NY. 13774
Phone: 607-637-3413
Fax: 607-637-3413
e-mail: fishsmusic@aol.com
Management:
   Artistic Director: Joyce Lindorff

5356 ALLEGHENY COLLEGE PUBLIC EVENTS SERIES

Allegheny College
520 N Main Street, Box 40
Meadville, PA 16335
Phone: 814-332-3101
Fax: 814-333-8180
Web Site: www.alleg.edu
Management:
   Events Director: Deb Baker
Budget: $35,000-60,000
Type of Stage: Proscenium
Seating Capacity: 1,700

5357 BRODHEAD CULTURAL CENTER SUMMER SERIES

Penn State Beaver
100 University Drive
Monaca, PA 15061-2799
Phone: 724-773-3817
Fax: 724-773-3557
e-mail: amk6@psu.edu
Web Site: www.br.psu.edu/bcc
Management:
   Director: Amy K Krebs
Mission: The Brodhead Cultural Center is operated through the Penn State Beaver Offices of University Relations to provide free and low-cost programs for the public.
Founded: 1977
Specialized Field: Various
Status: Nonprofit
Paid Staff: 1
Budget: $10,000-20,000
Affiliations: Pennsylvania State
Annual Attendance: 10,000
Facility Category: Outdoor Amphitheater
Type of Stage: Concrete
Seating Capacity: 750
Year Built: 1997

5358 ALLEGHENY VALLEY CONCERT ASSOCIATION

67 River Avenue
Natrona, PA 15065
Phone: 724-226-2155
Officers:
   President: Nora Ann Pastrick
Budget: $20,000-35,000

5359 WESTMINSTER COLLEGE CELEBRITY SERIES

Westminster College
New Wilmington, PA 16172-0001
Phone: 724-946-7371
Fax: 724-946-6243
Management:
   Celebrity Series Director: Gene DeCaprio
Budget: $150,000-400,000

5360 PCCA FESTIVAL AT LITTLE BUFFALO

PO Box 354
Newport, PA 17074
Phone: 717-567-7023
Fax: 717-567-7429
e-mail: pcca@perrycountyarts.org
Web Site: www.perrycountyarts.org
Management:
   Executive Director: Joni Williamson
Founded: 1983
Specialized Field: all mediums - music, dance, drams, literary, visual
Paid Staff: 4
Volunteer Staff: 500
Paid Artists: 100
Facility Category: Multi-Cultural

5361 BUCKS COUNTY COMMUNITY COLLEGE CULTURAL PROGRAMMING

Bucks County Community College
Swamp Road
Newtown, PA 18940
Phone: 215-968-8132
e-mail: mengersk@storm.bucks.edu
Management:
   Cultural Programming Director: Kay Mengers
Budget: $10,000-20,000
Seating Capacity: 345

5362 AMERICAN MUSIC THEATER FESTIVAL/PRINCE MUSIC THEATER

100 S Broad Street
Suite 650
Philadelphia, PA 19110
Phone: 215-972-1000
Fax: 215-972-1020
Web Site: www.amtf.org
Management:
   Artistic Director: Ben Levit
Founded: 1984
Performs At: Prince Music Theater
Facility Category: Theater
Type of Stage: Proscenium
Seating Capacity: 450

5363 BACH FESTIVAL OF PHILADELPHIA

8419 Germantown Avenue
Philadelphia, PA 19118
Phone: 215-247-2224
Fax: 215-247-4070
e-mail: bach@bach-fest.org
Web Site: www.bach-fest.org
Officers:

President: Toni Carey
Treasurer: Emilio Bonelli
VP: Samuel Swansen
Seceretary: Jeanette Cord
Management:
　Executive Director: Sharon R Derstine
Mission: The Bach Festival of Philadelphia is dedicated to enriching the community through concerts and educational programs presented by some of the best Baroque interpreters in the world.
Founded: 1976
Specialized Field: Vocal Music; Instrumental Music; Festivals
Status: Professional; Nonprofit
Paid Staff: 2
Volunteer Staff: 8
Income Sources: Government; Corporate and private foundations; Donations; Ticketsales; Advertising books
Performs At: Churches, Performance halls
Annual Attendance: 2,000-3,000
Organization Type: Educational; Presenting

5364　COMMUNITY EDUCATION CENTER

3500 Lancaster Avenue
Philadelphia, PA 19104-2434
Phone: 215-387-1911
Fax: 215-387-3701
Budget: $10,000-20,000
Seating Capacity: 100

5365　FIRST UNION CENTER

3601 S Broad Street
Philadelphia, PA 19148
Phone: 215-336-3600
Fax: 215-389-9403
Web Site: www.comcast-spectator.com
Management:
　President: Peter Luukko
　VP Event Producer: John Page
Specialized Field: Home of the Philadelphia 76ers (NBA), Philadelphia Flyers (NFHL) and the Philadelphia Wings (NLL)
Seating Capacity: 21,000, 19,500
Year Built: 1996

5366　FOLKLIFE CENTER OF INTERNATIONAL HOUSE

3701 Chestnut Street
Philadelphia, PA 19104
Phone: 215-895-6537
Fax: 215-895-6562
e-mail: helen@ihphilly.org
Web Site: www.ihousephilly.org
Management:
　Program Director: Helen Henry
Mission: Too present the highest caliber of traditional arts.
Founded: 1977
Specialized Field: Traditional Arts (ethnic)
Paid Artists: 50
Budget: $60,000-150,000
Performs At: Hopkinson Hall
Annual Attendance: 2500
Facility Category: Multi-use

Type of Stage: Thrust
Stage Dimensions: 14 x 40
Seating Capacity: 480
Year Built: 1970
Year Remodeled: 1987
Rental Contact: Helen Henry

5367　GERMAN SOCIETY OF PENNSYLVANIA

611 Spring Garden Street
Philadelphia, PA 19123
Phone: 215-627-2332
Fax: 215-627-5297
e-mail: contact@germansociety.org
Web Site: www.germansociety.org
Management:
　Executive Director: Annke Farago
Mission: Serve members and the community, espeially those who share our intrest in German and German-American culture.
Founded: 1764
Status: Nonprofit
Paid Staff: 5
Volunteer Staff: 40
Paid Artists: 10
Budget: $460,000
Facility Category: Historic Landmark Building
Seating Capacity: 370
Year Built: 1888
Year Remodeled: 1997
Organization Type: Educational; Language classes; Lectures; Concerts

5368　MARLBORO MUSIC FESTIVAL

135 S 18th Street
Philadelphia, PA 19103
Phone: 215-569-4690
Fax: 215-569-9497
e-mail: info@marlboromusic.org
Web Site: www.marlboromusic.org
Officers:
　Administrator: Anthony P Checchia
Management:
　Manager: Philip Maneval
　Box Office Manager: Beth Gaynor LaPat
　Projects Administrator: Derek Delaney
Mission: Artistic development of younger musicians with older, more experienced musicians.
Founded: 1951
Specialized Field: Instrumental Music
Status: Professional; Nonprofit
Paid Staff: 15
Volunteer Staff: 10
Season: August-June
Performs At: Persons Auditorium
Organization Type: Performing; Touring; Resident; Educational; Sponsoring

5369　MIDATLANTIC ARTS FOUNDATION PENNSYLVANIA PERFORMING ARTS ON TOUR

1811 Chestnut Street, 301
Philadelphia, PA 19103

Phone: 215-496-9424
Fax: 215-496-9585
e-mail: pennpat@erols.com
Web Site: www.libertynet.org/pennpat
Management:
   Director: Katie West

5370 NORTHEAST PHILADELPHIA CULTURAL COUNCIL

Jardel Recreation Center
Penny & Cottman Avenue
Philadelphia, PA 19111
Phone: 215-686-0592
Management:
   Coordinator: James Robb
Budget: $35,000-60,000
Performs At: Small Hall

5371 PENN PRESENTS

3680 Walnut Street
Philadelphia, PA 19104
Phone: 215-898-3900
Fax: 215-573-9568
e-mail: boxoffice@ac.upenn.edu
Web Site: www.pennpresents.org
Management:
   Managing Director: Michael Rose
   Director Marketing: Roy Wilbur
   Box Office Manager: David Sullivan
   Facilities and Events Manager: Marie Gallagher
Founded: 1971
Annual Attendance: 100000+
Facility Category: 5 theaters throughout Univ. of Pennsylvania
Type of Stage: Proscenium, Black Box
Seating Capacity: 120-1270
Year Built: 1971
Rental Contact: Marie Gallagher

5372 PHILADELPHIA ALL STAR-FORUM SERIES

PO Box 42276
Philadelphia, PA 19101-2276
Phone: 215-735-7506
Fax: 215-735-4129
Officers:
   Treasurer: Roy A Shubert
Budget: $400,000-1,000,000
Performs At: Academy of Music

5373 SETTLEMENT MUSIC SCHOOL WEXLER CONTEMPORARY

PO Box 25120
416 Queen Street
Philadelphia, PA 19147-3094
Phone: 215-336-0400
Fax: 215-551-0483
e-mail: smsmlc@smsmusic.org
Web Site: www.smsmusic.org
Management:
   Branch Director: Eric Anderson
Performs At: PNC Bank-Presser Recital Hall

5374 ST. STEPHEN'S

19 S 10 Street
Philadelphia, PA 19107
Phone: 215-922-3807
Fax: 215-829-4561
e-mail: ststevepa@email.msn.com
Management:
   Program Director: Mark Yurkanin
Performs At: St. Stephen's Sanctuary

5375 TONY WILLIAMS LABOR DAY JAZZ FEST

PO Box 27116
Philadelphia, PA 19118
Phone: 215-848-3677
Fax: 215-848-0297
e-mail: vwedwards@worldnet.att.net
Web Site: www.maccjazz.org
Officers:
   President: Donald Clark Ph.D
   Ambassador At Large: Thelma Anderson
   Secretary: Joseph Stevenson
Management:
   Director/Founder/President "Mall": Tony Williams
Mission: To increase community involvement with our youth. A commitment to helping the youth develop the proper attitude necessary in becoming a productive adult through the expressive arts with special emphasis on jazz, our only American art form
Founded: 1977
Specialized Field: Jazz
Status: Nonprofit
Volunteer Staff: 20
Non-paid Artists: 20

5376 ALLEGHENY COUNTY SUMMER CONCERT SERIES

515B COB, Office of Special Events
542 Forbes Avenue
Pittsburg, PA 15219-2904
Phone: 412-594-4823
Fax: 412-350-3280
e-mail: lkuzmanko@county.allegheny.pa.us
Web Site: www.county.allegheny.pa.us
Management:
   Director: J Larry Kuzmanko
Mission: Enhance quality of life for the people.
Paid Staff: 3
Volunteer Staff: 20
Paid Artists: 500

5377 THREE RIVERS ARTS FESTIVAL

707 Penn Avenue
Pittsburg, PA 15222
Phone: 412-281-8723
Fax: 412-281-7822
e-mail: pearlman@sgi.net
Web Site: www.artsfestival.net
Management:
   Executive Director: Jeanne Pearlman

5378 CARNEGIE-MELLON CONCERTS
CMU School of Music
Pittsburgh, PA 15213-3890
Phone: 412-268-2383
Fax: 412-268-1431
e-mail: musicschool@andrew.cmu.edu
Web Site: www.cmu.edu/cfa/music
Management:
    Manager: Amy Stabenow
Budget: $20,000-35,000
Performs At: Carnegie Music Hall; Lecture Hall;
Exhibition Hall
Seating Capacity: 450

5379 FIRST FRIDAY AT THE FRICK CONCERT SERIES
7227 Reynolds Street
Pittsburgh, PA 15208
Phone: 412-371-0600
Fax: 412-371-6030
e-mail: smartin@frickart.org
Web Site: www.frickart.org
Officers:
    Director Visitor Services: Sue Martin
Founded: 1995
Specialized Field: Music
Paid Staff: 50
Budget: $20,000
Annual Attendance: 10,000
Facility Category: Outdoor Stage
Type of Stage: Platform
Stage Dimensions: 24x40
Seating Capacity: 3,000

5380 FIRST FRIDAYS AT THE FRICK CONCERT SERIES
7227 Reynolds Street
Pittsburgh, PA 15208-2923
Phone: 412-371-0600
Fax: 412-371-6030
e-mail: smartin@frickart.org
Web Site: www.frickart.org
Management:
    Visitor Services Director: Sue N Martin
    Assistant Manager Visitors Services: Caito Amarose
    Services Assistant: Peggy McLean
Mission: Community cultural event sposored by our
museum complex.
Founded: 1995
Specialized Field: Electric Mix
Budget: $10,000-20,000
Performs At: Frick Art & Historical Center
Annual Attendance: 3,000 per concert
Facility Category: Outdoor
Type of Stage: Transtage
Stage Dimensions: 20x30
Organization Type: outdoor

5381 MANCHESTER CRAFTSMEN'S GUILD
Manchester Craftsmen's Guild
1815 Metropolitan Street
Pittsburgh, PA 15233

Phone: 412-322-1773
Fax: 412-321-2120
e-mail: mashby@mcg-btc.org
Web Site: www.mcjazz.org
Management:
    Executive Producer: Marty Ashby
    Producer: Jay Ashby
    Associate Producer: Georgina Gutierrez
    Associate Producer: Renee Govanucci
Mission: To present jazz performances as well as
community and educational activities.
Founded: 1987
Specialized Field: Jazz
Paid Staff: 11
Volunteer Staff: 6
Performs At: Manchester Craftmen's Guild Music Hall
Annual Attendance: 15,000
Facility Category: Concert Hall
Type of Stage: Concert stage
Stage Dimensions: 24x26
Seating Capacity: 350
Year Built: 1987
Organization Type: Educational; Presenting

5382 MUSIC FOR MT. LEBANON
2016 Worcester Drive
Pittsburgh, PA 15243-1542
Phone: 412-531-8588
Fax: 412-344-9054
Management:
    Artistic Director: Carl Apone
Budget: $60,000-150,000
Seating Capacity: 1,500

5383 POINT PARK COLLEGE GUEST ARTISTS SERIES
485 Wood Street & Boulevard of Allies
Pittsburgh, PA 15222
Phone: 412-621-4445
Fax: 412-621-4762
Performs At: John Hopkins Auditorium & Library
Center

5384 UNIVERSITY OF PITTSBURGH CONCERT SERIES
Music Building
Room 110
Pittsburgh, PA 15260
Phone: 412-624-4125
Fax: 412-624-4186
e-mail: musicdpt+@pitt.edu
Web Site: www.pitt.edu/~musicdpt/index.html
Budget: $10,000
Performs At: Frick Fine Arts Auditorium; William Pitt
Union Ballroom

5385 Y MUSIC SOCIETY OF THE JEWISH COMMUNITY CENTER
5738 Forbes Avenue
Pittsburgh, PA 15217

Phone: 412-421-6771
Fax: 412-208-9107
e-mail: mroth@jccpgh.org
Web Site: www.trfn.clpgh.org/yms
Management:
   Director: Mayda Roth
Budget: $60,000-150,000
Performs At: Carnegie Music Hall

5386 HILL SCHOOL CENTER FOR THE ARTS LIVELY ARTS SERIES
717 E High Street
Pottstown, PA 19464-5791
Phone: 610-326-1000
Fax: 610-326-0348
e-mail: bmerriam@thehill.org
Web Site: www.thehill.org
Budget: $20,000-35,000
Performs At: The Center Theatre

5387 CABRINI COLLEGE
610 King of Prussia Road
Radnor, PA 19087
Phone: 610-902-8380
Fax: 610-902-8285
Officers:
   Fine Arts Chairperson: Dr. Adeline Bethany
Budget: $10,000
Performs At: Lecture Hall; Mansion Grand Foyer

5388 ALBRIGHT COLLEGE CONCERT SERIES
PO Box 15234
13th & Bern Streets
Reading, PA 19612-5234
Phone: 610-921-7871
Fax: 610-921-7768
e-mail: beckyb@alb.edu
Management:
   Concert Series Director: Rebecca Butler
Budget: $10,000
Performs At: Memorial Chapel; Roop Hall

5389 BERKS JAZZ FESTIVAL
PO Box 854
The Pagoda
Reading, PA 19603-0854
Phone: 610-655-6374
Fax: 610-655-6378
Toll-free: 800-523-3781
e-mail: mikand@ptdprolog.net
Web Site: www.berksjazzfest.com
Management:
   Executive Director: Connie Leinbach
Paid Staff: 9
Volunteer Staff: 200
Paid Artists: 100

5390 STAR SERIES ASSOCIATION
147 N 5th Street
Reading, PA 19601

Phone: 610-373-0141
Fax: 610-376-3336
e-mail: cbreaux@redrose.net
Web Site: www.berks.net
Management:
   Manager: Chip Breaux
Performs At: Rajah Theatre; Albright Coll. Theatre; Albright Coll. Chapel

5391 SCRANTON COMMUNITY CONCERTS
404 N Washington Avenue
Scranton, PA 18503
Phone: 570-342-4137
Fax: 570-342-4856
e-mail: commconcerts@aol.com
Web Site: www.scrantonconcerts.org
Management:
   Director: Bridget Fitzpatrick
Mission: To present world-class performing arts in classical, jazz, opera and dance.
Founded: 1928
Specialized Field: Classical; Jazz
Status: Non-Profit
Paid Staff: 3
Budget: $170,000
Income Sources: Grants; Donations
Performs At: Scranton Cultural Center; Mellow Theater

5392 SUSQUEHANNA UNIVERSITY ARTIST SERIES
514 University Avenue
Selinsgrove, PA 17870
Phone: 570-372-4299
Fax: 570-372-2832
e-mail: artistseries@susqu.edu
Web Site: www.susqu.edu/artists
Management:
   Manager: Laura de Abruna
Budget: $35,000-60,000
Performs At: Weber Chapel Auditorium and Dogenstein Center Theatre

5393 CENTRAL COMMUNITY CONCERTS
52 E Independence Street
Shamokin, PA 17872
Phone: 570-648-3931
Officers:
   President: Irvin R Liachowitz
Budget: $20,000-35,000

5394 SLIPPERY ROCK UNIVERSITY - PERFORMING ARTS SERIES
105 University Union
Slippery Rock, PA 16057
Phone: 724-738-2092
Fax: 724-738-2624
e-mail: cheryl.knoch@sru.edu
Web Site: www.sru.edu
Management:
   Director of Student Life: Cherly Knoch
Performs At: Miller Auditorium; Swope Music hall

5395 CENTRAL PENNSYLVANIA FESTIVAL OF THE ARTS
PO Box 1023
State College, PA 16804
Phone: 814-237-3682
Fax: 814-237-0708
e-mail: office@arts-festival.com
Management:
   Executive Director: Philip L Walz
   Performing Arts Director: Doris Mack
Mission: To offer an annual festival which celebrates all the arts.
Founded: 1967
Specialized Field: Festivals
Status: Nonprofit
Paid Staff: 4
Budget: $490,000
Income Sources: Sponsorship; ticket sales; entry fees
Performs At: Indoor; Auditorium; Outdoor stages
Affiliations: PA Presenters
Annual Attendance: 100,000
Facility Category: Festival
Organization Type: Performing

5396 MUSIC AT PENN'S WOODS
Pennsylvania State University
254 Music Building
University Park, PA 16802
Phone: 814-863-1118
Fax: 814-865-6785
e-mail: pennswoods@psu.edu
Web Site: www.music.psu.edu/mpw
Management:
   Music Director: Gerardo Edelstein
   Manager: Russell Bloom
Mission: Orchestra and chamber music festival
Founded: 1985
Specialized Field: Orchestra; chamber music
Paid Staff: 3
Paid Artists: 45
Budget: $100,000
Performs At: Eisenhower Auditorium
Facility Category: Performing Arts Facility
Seating Capacity: 2500
Year Built: 1972

5397 MUSIC AT PENN'S WOODS
254 Music Building
Penn State University
University Park, PA 16802-1901
Phone: 814-863-1118
Fax: 814-865-6785
e-mail: pennswoods@psu.edu
Web Site: www.music.psu.edu/mpw
Management:
   Music Director: Gerardo Edelstein
   Manager: Russell Bloom
Founded: 1985
Specialized Field: Orchestra; Chamber Music
Paid Staff: 3
Paid Artists: 45
Budget: $100,000
Performs At: Eisenhower Auditorium
Facility Category: Performing Arts Facility

Seating Capacity: 2500
Year Built: 1972

5398 VILLANOVA UNIVERSITY CHAMBER SERIES
Office of Musical Activities
Villanova University
Villanova, PA 19085
Phone: 610-519-7214
Fax: 610-519-7596
Management:
   Manager: Peter Marino
Budget: $20,000-35,000
Performs At: St. Mary's Hall

5399 WILDFLOWER MUSIC FESTIVAL
PO Box 356
White Mills, PA 18473
Phone: 570-253-5500
Fax: 570-253-5196
e-mail: dglassmus@aol.com
Web Site: www.ibcco.com/dorflinger
Management:
   Artistic Director: Jane F Ables

5400 KING'S COLLEGE EXPERIENCING THE ARTS SERIES
133 N River Street
Wilkes-Barre, PA 18711-0801
Phone: 570-208-5900
Fax: 570-208-6013
e-mail: jfplumme@kings.edu
Web Site: www.kings.edu
Management:
   Co-Curricular Program Director: Judith F Plummer
Budget: $10,000-20,000
Performs At: Campus Ministry Center; Sheeny-Farmer Campus Center

5401 WILLIAMSPORT COMMUNITY CONCERT ASSOCIATION
1401 Washington Boulevard
Williamsport, PA 17701-5424
Phone: 570-322-7004
Officers:
   President: Terry L Ziegler
Budget: $35,000-60,000
Performs At: Scottish Rite Auditorium

5402 ARCADIA PERFORMING ARTS
1418 Graham Avenue
Windber, PA 15963
Phone: 814-467-9070
Fax: 814-467-5646
Web Site: www.arcadiatheater.net
Officers:
   Chairman of Board: Frank Consolo
Management:
   Artistic Director: Gerald Ledney
   Public Relations/Development Dir.: Denise Mihalick
Founded: 1998
Budget: $60,000-150,000

All listings are in alphabetical order by state, then city, then organization within the city.

Seating Capacity: 710
Year Built: 1921
Year Remodeled: 1998

5403 LOWER MAKEFIELD SOCIETY FOR THE PERFORMING ARTS

696 Briarwood Court
Yardley, PA 19067
Phone: 215-493-3010
Fax: 215-493-0754
e-mail: lmpspa.maryb@verizon.net
Web Site: www.lmt.org
Management:
    Executive Director: Mary Borkovitz
Founded: 1978
Volunteer Staff: 10
Budget: $24,000
Performs At: Township Community Room
Annual Attendance: 1050
Seating Capacity: 175
Year Built: 1976

5404 STRAND-CAPITOL PERFORMING ARTS CENTER SERIES

50 N George Street
York, PA 17401
Phone: 717-846-1155
Fax: 717-843-1208
e-mail: boxoffice@strandcapitol.org
Web Site: www.strandcapitol.org
Management:
    Director: Clyde Lindsley
    Interim Executive Director: Judy Simpson
    Director Marketing: Laura L Sullivan
Budget: $150,000-400,000

Rhode Island

5405 CONCERTS BY THE BAY

101 Ferry Road
Route 114
Bristol, RI 02809
Phone: 401-253-2707
Fax: 401-253-0412
e-mail: info@blitheworld.org
Web Site: www.blitheworld.org
Management:
    Site Administrator: Constance Coar

5406 CULTURAL ORGANIZATION OF THE ARTS

PO Box 258
111 Pierce Street
East Greenwich, RI 02818
Phone: 401-886-4530
Management:
    COA Director: Kate Leach
Budget: $10,000

5407 KINGSTON CHAMBER MUSIC FESTIVAL AT URI

PO Box 1733
Kingston, RI 02881
Phone: 401-874-2060
Fax: 401-874-2380
e-mail: sadd@egr.uri.edu
Web Site: www.mce.uri.edu
Management:
    Artistic Director Violin: David Kim
Mission: To provide outstanding classical music programs in New England. Offers both summer and winter concerts, and also outreach programs at local area schools.
Founded: 1989
Specialized Field: Classical music
Volunteer Staff: 15
Paid Artists: 1045
Budget: $60,000
Income Sources: Donations; Ticket sales
Affiliations: University of Rhode Island
Annual Attendance: 2800

5408 NEW ENGLAND PRESENTERS: UNIVERSITY OF RHODE ISLAND GREAT PERFORMANCES

105 Upper College Road
URI
Kingston, RI 02881
Phone: 401-874-2627
Fax: 401-874-2772
e-mail: rto9302u@postoffice.uri.edu
Management:
    Director: Roxana Tourigny
Budget: $35,000-60,000
Performs At: Veterans Memorial Auditorium; Edwards Hall; Will Theatre

5409 NEWPORT MUSIC FESTIVAL

PO Box 3300
Newport, RI 02840
Phone: 401-846-1133
Fax: 401-849-1857
e-mail: staff@newportmusic.org
Web Site: www.newportmusic.org
Officers:
    President: Mrs. Herbert B. Swope, Jr
    President Emeritus: Mrs. Robert Horne Charles
    VP Emeritus: Mrs. William Wood-Price
Management:
    General Director: Dr. Mark P Malkovich, III
    Marketing Director: Mark Malkovich, IV
Mission: To present little-known music from the Romantic era; to sponsor international artists making their North American debuts.
Founded: 1969
Specialized Field: Vocal Music; Instrumental Music; Chamber Music
Status: Nonprofit
Paid Staff: 21
Volunteer Staff: 250
Paid Artists: 71
Budget: $1,000,000

Income Sources: Box Office; Donations; Corporate & Foundation Support
Season: July
Performs At: Fabled Mansions of Newport; Churches; Tents
Affiliations: Yamaha Corporation of America; Roederer Champagne; Time, Inc.; Lufthansa
Annual Attendance: 28,000
Facility Category: Various Mansions; Churches; Tents
Seating Capacity: 250 - 500
Organization Type: Performing; Sponsoring
Comments: The Newport Music Festival is listed by Cadogen Press in their Ultimate List of 1000 Best Things in America.

5410 CAPITOLARTS PROVIDENCE CULTURAL AFFAIRS
Providence Parks Department
65 Waybosset Street, Mailbox 39
Providence, RI 02903
Phone: 401-621-1992
Fax: 401-621-1883
e-mail: festival@lds.net
Web Site: www.caparts.org
Management:
   Director: Bob Rizzo
   Programming Coordinator: Lynne McCormack
   Web Site Development: Remo Campopiano
Mission: Dedicated to producing arts events that enliven the cityscape of Providence, Rhode Island; working together with the City of Providence, Parks Department, Office of Cultural Affairs, CapitolArts Providence produces events, both large and small, that appeal to the region's diverse community.
Specialized Field: Producing arts events
Status: Nonprofit

5411 CONVERGENCE 2000 ARTS FESTIVAL: WORKSHOP WITH TS THOMAS
Providence Parks Department
400 Westminister Street 4th Floor
Providence, RI 02903
Phone: 401-621-1992
Fax: 401-621-1883
Web Site: www.vac.igs.net
Specialized Field: Two-day workshop - poetry of Walt Whitman

5412 FIRST NIGHT PROVIDENCE
10 Dorrance Street
Suite 920
Providence, RI 02903
Phone: 401-521-1166
Fax: 401-273-5630
e-mail: firstnight@firstnightprovidence.org
Web Site: www.firstnightprovidence.org
Management:
   Director: Doris Stephens
   Assistant Director: Annette Robinson
   Artistic Director: Kathleen Fletcher
   Business Director: Carolyn Tick
Mission: Nonalcoholic family celebration of the arts on New Year's Eve.
Founded: 1985

Specialized Field: Dance; Vocal Music; Instrumental Music; Theater
Status: Nonprofit
Paid Staff: 4
Budget: $550,000
Income Sources: Admission Sales; Corporate Sponsors; Individual Contributions
Performs At: Theaters; Performance Halls; Churches
Annual Attendance: 50,000
Facility Category: Arts festival
Type of Stage: Multi-Purpose
Organization Type: Performing; Educational; Sponsoring

5413 PROVIDENCE DIVISION OF PUBLIC PROGRAMMING DEPARTMENTS
Providence Parks Department
400 Westminster Street 4th Floor
Providence, RI 02903-3222
Phone: 401-621-1992
Fax: 401-621-1883
e-mail: info@caparts.org
Web Site: www.caparts.org
Management:
   Public Programming Director: Bob Rizzo
Budget: $60,000-150,000

5414 RHODE ISLAND COLLEGE: PERFORMING ARTS SERIES
301 Roberts Hall
Providence, RI 02908-1991
Phone: 401-456-8194
Fax: 401-456-8269
e-mail: jcuster@ric.edu
Management:
   Director: John Custer
Paid Staff: 9
Volunteer Staff: 24
Paid Artists: 80
Budget: $60,000-$150,000
Performs At: Roberts Auditorium; Sapinrey Hall; Forman Theatre

South Carolina

5415 UNIVERSITY OF SOUTH CAROLINA: AIKEN ETHERREDGE CENTER
471 University Parkway
Aiken, SC 29801
Phone: 803-641-3328
Fax: 803-641-3691
e-mail: janes@aiken.sc.edu
Web Site: www.usca.sc.edu/ec
Management:
   Executive Director: Jane Schumacher
Budget: $60,000-150,000
Affiliations: University of Saint Gerdina
Facility Category: Theater Complex
Type of Stage: Thrust Proscenium
Stage Dimensions: 38 by 24
Seating Capacity: 687
Year Built: 1986

Rental Contact: Jane Schumacher

5416 ANDERSON COLLEGE: RAINEY FINE ARTS CENTER

316 Boulevard
Anderson, SC 29621
Phone: 864-231-2002
Fax: 864-231-2083
Web Site: www.ac.edu
Management:
  Division Head Fine Arts: Dr. David Larson
Founded: 1911
Paid Staff: 3
Volunteer Staff: 20
Budget: $10,000-20,000
Seating Capacity: 1100; 200; 100

5417 CIVIC CENTER OF ANDERSON

3027 Mall Road
Anderson, SC 29625
Phone: 864-260-4800
Fax: 864-260-4847
Management:
  Director: Charles Wyatt

5418 UNIVERSITY OF SOUTH CAROLINA-BEAUFORT

801 Carteret Street
Beaufort, SC 29902
Phone: 843-521-4144
Fax: 843-521-4145
e-mail: info@beauforarts.com
Web Site: www.beaufortarts.com
Management:
  Executive Director: Eric Holowacz
Budget: $60,000-150,000
Performs At: Beaufort Waterfront Park

5419 CHARLESTON CONCERT ASSOCIATION

207 E Bay Street, Suite 213
PO Box 743
Charleston, SC 29401
Phone: 843-722-7667
Fax: 843-577-5173
Management:
  Director: Jason Nichols
  Executive Assistant: Toni Franklin
Budget: $150,000-400,000
Performs At: Gaillard Municipal Auditorium

5420 CITADEL FINE ARTS SERIES

The Citadel
Charleston, SC 29409
Phone: 843-953-5065
Fax: 843-953-6797
e-mail: Grant.Staley@citadel.edu
Officers:
  Chairman: Dr. Grant B Staley
Budget: $10,000-20,000
Performs At: Mark Clark Hall Auditorium

5421 PICCOLO SPOLETO FESTIVAL

Office of Cultural Affairs
133 Church Street
Charleston, SC 29401
Phone: 843-724-7305
Fax: 843-720-3967
e-mail: cultural_affairs@ci.charleston.sc
Web Site: www.charleston.net/charlestoncity/piccolo.htm
Management:
  Executive Director: Ellen Dressler Moryl

5422 SPOLETO FESTIVAL USA

478 E Bay Street
Suite 200
Charleston, SC 29403
Mailing Address: PO Box 157 Charleston, SC 29402
Phone: 843-579-3100
Fax: 843-723-6383
e-mail: receptionist@spoletousa.org
Web Site: www.spoletousa.org
Officers:
  Director Finance: Tasha Gandy
  Chairman of the Board: William B Hewitt
  President: Eric G Friberg
Management:
  Artistic Director: Joseph Flummerfelt
  Music Director: Emmanuel Villaume
  General Manager: Nigel Redden
  Producer: Nunally Kersh
Mission: To present opera, dance, theater, symphonic, choral and chamber music, jazz and visual arts exhibits of the highest quality; to serve as an educational environment for young artists and audiences alike.
Founded: 1977
Specialized Field: Opera; Chamber; Choral & Symphonic Music; Jazz; Theater; Dance
Status: Professional; Semi-Professional; Nonprofit
Paid Staff: 21
Income Sources: Opera America; Dance USA; Theatre Communications Group; National Institute for Music Theater; American Arts Alliance
Performs At: Gaillard Municipal Auditorium; Dock Street Theater; Garden Theater; Sottile Theatre; Grace Episcopal Church
Annual Attendance: 60,000
Organization Type: Performing; Educational; Sponsoring

5423 PRESBYTERIAN COLLEGE

503 S Broad Street
Clinton, SC 29325
Phone: 864-833-8923
Fax: 864-833-8600
e-mail: lwshealy@presby.edu
Web Site: www.presby.edu
Management:
  Cultural Events Director: Laura Shealy
Paid Staff: 3
Paid Artists: 10
Non-paid Artists: 30
Budget: $35,000-60,000
Annual Attendance: 25,000
Facility Category: Concert Hall/Recital Hall
Type of Stage: Proscenium

Stage Dimensions: 39'x24'/23'x49'
Seating Capacity: 1,100/335
Rental Contact: Not Available for Rental

5424 CAROLINA PRODUCTIONS, PERFORMING ARTS COMMISSION

Russell House University Union
Room 235
Columbia, SC 29208
Phone: 803-777-7130
Fax: 803-777-7132
Web Site: www.sa.sc.edu/cp
Officers:
　　President: Krista Wingard
Management:
　　Director Student Activities: Mike Duncan
Performs At: Koger Center for the Arts; Carolina Coliseum

5425 COLUMBIA COLLEGE SOSOHO PERFORMANCE SERIES

1301 Columbia College Drive
Columbia College Dance Department
Columbia, SC 29203
Phone: 803-786-3825
Fax: 803-786-3868
e-mail: mbrim@colacoll.edu
Web Site: www.columbiacollegesc.edu
Officers:
　　Dance Department Chair: Susan Haigler-Robles
Management:
　　Professional SoHo Director: Martha Brim
Founded: 1987
Specialized Field: Dance
Paid Staff: 2
Volunteer Staff: 45
Paid Artists: 5
Budget: $10,000
Performs At: Cottingham Theater, Columbia College
Affiliations: The Power Company; South Carolina Center for Dance Education
Annual Attendance: 12,000
Facility Category: Theater
Type of Stage: Proscenium
Stage Dimensions: 30 X 40
Seating Capacity: 385
Year Built: 1960
Rental Contact: Patrick Faulds

5426 KOGER CENTER FOR THE ARTS

Koger Center of the Arts
Columbia, SC 29208
Phone: 803-777-7500
Fax: 803-777-9774
Web Site: www.koger.sc.edu
Management:
　　Director: Ron Pearson
　　Assistant Director: Michael Taylor
Budget: $1,000,000+

5427 ERSKINARTS (THE FINE & PERFORMING ARTS AT ERSKINE COLLEGE)

Erskine College
Due West, SC 29639
Phone: 864-379-8831
Fax: 864-379-2167
e-mail: mattman@erskine.edu
Web Site: www.erskine.edu
Officers:
　　Chairman Music Department: Matthew Manwarren
Budget: $20,000-35,000
Performs At: Memorial Hall

5428 FRANCIS MARION UNIVERSITY ARTISTS SERIES

PO Box 100547
Florence, SC 29501-0547
Phone: 843-661-1385
Fax: 843-661-1219
Officers:
　　Fine Arts Department Chairman: Lawrence P Anderson
Budget: $10,000-20,000
Performs At: McNair Auditorium

5429 METROPOLITAN ARTS COUNCIL

123 W Broad Street
Greenville, SC 29601
Phone: 864-467-3132
Fax: 864-467-3133
e-mail: macsc@mindspring.com
Web Site: www.greenvillearts.com
Management:
　　Executive Director: Julie Richard
Mission: To stimulate and support artistic expression and its appreciation and enjoyment in ways that enrich all citizens, artsits, cultural organizations, and communities of the Metropolitan area.
Founded: 1973
Paid Staff: 3
Budget: $450,000
Income Sources: City, State and Federal grants, private donations

5430 GREENWOOD-LANDER PERFORMING ARTS

CPO Box 6044
Lander University
Greenwood, SC 29649
Phone: 864-388-8326
Fax: 864-388-8036
e-mail: lcone@lander.edu
Management:
　　Executive Director: Laurie Cone
Founded: 1946
Specialized Field: All Arts Areas
Paid Staff: 1
Budget: $70,000-80,000
Annual Attendance: 3,500- 4,000
Facility Category: Concert Hall
Seating Capacity: 700

5431 HARTSVILLE COMMUNITY CONCERT ASSOCIATION
PO Box 2283
Hartsville, SC 29551
Phone: 843-383-8145
e-mail: gsawyer@coker.edu
Officers:
  President: David M Tavernier
Founded: 1945
Budget: $20,000-35,000

5432 ARTS CENTER OF COASTAL CAROLINA
14 Shelter Cove Lane
Hilton Head Island, SC 29928
Phone: 843-686-3945
Fax: 843-842-7877
e-mail: artscenter@hargray.com
Web Site: www.artscenter-hhi.org
Officers:
  President/CEO: Kathleen P Bateson
Management:
  General Manager: Richard Feldman
Mission: Theatre and presenting.
Founded: 1996
Specialized Field: Performing, Visual Gallery
Status: Nonprofit
Paid Staff: 35
Paid Artists: 15
Budget: $3.2 million
Performs At: Elizabeth Wallace Theatre
Type of Stage: Proscenium
Seating Capacity: 350
Year Built: 1996
Rental Contact: Richard Feldman

5433 COASTAL CONCERT ASSOCIATION
1107 48 Avenue N
Suite 211-L
Myrtle Beach, SC 29577
Phone: 843-449-7546
Fax: 843-449-9391
e-mail: coastcon@sunnews.infi.net
Web Site: www.coastalconcert.com
Officers:
  President: John Trugdeau
  Treasurer: Kelli Shana Felt
  President: B Matt Morris
Management:
  Executive Director: Shirley Cope
Specialized Field: Arts Presenter
Paid Staff: 1
Volunteer Staff: 20
Paid Artists: 50
Budget: $35,000-60,000
Performs At: Performing Arts Center
Annual Attendance: 6,000
Seating Capacity: 1900

5434 ARTS ETC
PO Box 2692 CRS
Rock Hill, SC 29732

Phone: 803-324-8803
Fax: 803-324-8200
e-mail: karenb@infoave.net
Web Site: www.artsetc.org
Management:
  Executive Director: Karen Blankenship
Paid Staff: 5
Budget: $35,000-60,000
Performs At: Byrnes Auditorium
Type of Stage: Proscenium
Seating Capacity: 3,540
Year Built: 1938

5435 WINTHROP UNIVERSITY COLLEGE OF VISUAL & PERFORMING ARTS
College of Visual & Performing Arts
Winthrop University
Rock Hill, SC 29733
Phone: 803-328-2323
Fax: 803-323-2333
e-mail: svedlowa@winthrop.edu
Web Site: www.winthrop.edu
Management:
  Dean: Dr. Andrew J Svedlow
Budget: $35,000-60,000

5436 ARTS PARTNERSHIP OF GREATER SPARTANBURG
385 S Spring Street
Spartanburg, SC 29306-3350
Phone: 864-542-2787
Fax: 864-948-5353
e-mail: ahughes@teleplex.net
Management:
  Arts Education Director: Ava J Hughes
Budget: $35,000-60,000

5437 MUSIC FOUNDATION OF SPARTANBURG CONCERT SERIES
385 S Spring Street
Spartanburg, SC 29306
Mailing Address: Box 1274, Spartanburg, SC. 29304
Phone: 864-948-9020
Fax: 864-948-5353
e-mail: music@teleplex.net
Web Site: www.spartanarts.org
Management:
  Executive Director: Sarah Gunn
Budget: $60,000-150,000
Performs At: Twichell Auditorium

5438 FINE ARTS COUNCIL OF SUMTER PERFORMING ARTS SERIES
10 Mood Avenue
Sumter, SC 29150
Phone: 803-775-5580
Fax: 803-778-9664
e-mail: finearts@ftc-i.net
Web Site: www.angelfire.com/sc/finearts
Management:
  Executive Director: Ann Wilson Floyd

Mission: To enrich the cultural atmosphere of our area by presenting a Performing Arts Series; to reward students of the performing arts by sponsoring a school competition.
Founded: 1986
Paid Staff: 1
Volunteer Staff: 25
Budget: $100,000
Income Sources: Grants; ticket sales
Performs At: Patriot Hall
Facility Category: Auditorium
Type of Stage: Proscenium
Stage Dimensions: 47x21
Seating Capacity: 1,017
Year Remodeled: 1988

5439 NORTH GREENVILLE COLLEGE: FINE ARTS SERIES
Fine Arts
Tigerville, SC 29688
Phone: 864-977-7085
Fax: 864-977-7021
e-mail: orobertson@ngc.edu
Web Site: www.ngc.edu
Management:
 Manager: Owen Robertson
Budget: $10,000

South Dakota

5440 ABERDEEN COMMUNITY CONCERT ASSOCIATION
1312 3rd Avenue SE
Aberdeen, SD 57401
Phone: 605-226-3143
Officers:
 Secretary: Stacy Braun
Budget: $10,000-20,000
Performs At: Johnson Fine Arts Center

5441 SOUTH DAKOTA STATE UNIVERSITY STUDENT ACTIVITIES
PO Box 2815-USU065
Brookings, SD 57007-1599
Phone: 605-688-6129
Fax: 605-688-4973
Management:
 Program Advisor: Adam Karnopp
Budget: $20,000-35,000
Performs At: David B. Doner Auditorium

5442 LAURA INGALLS WILDER PAGEANT SOCIETY
PO Box 154
De Smet, SD 57231
Phone: 605-692-2108
Management:
 Managing Director: Portia Potvin
Mission: To present an outdoor pageant depicting The Little House on the Prairie books of Laura Ingalls Wilder. The pageant takes place across from the site of the Ingalls homestead.

Founded: 1971
Specialized Field: Theater
Status: Nonprofit
Organization Type: Performing

5443 HURON ARENA
150 5th Street SW
Huron, SD 57350
Phone: 605-353-6970
Fax: 605-353-6973
Management:
 Manager: Glen Ulvested

5444 MADISON AREA ARTS COUNCIL
PO Box 147
Madison, SD 57042
Phone: 605-256-5051
Management:
 Arts Coordinator: Eve Fisher
Mission: To promote arts appreciation; to sponsor arts activities; to offer opportunities for arts education to community members.
Founded: 1968
Specialized Field: Dance; Vocal Music; Instrumental Music; Theater; Festivals
Status: Nonprofit
Income Sources: South Dakota Arts Council; Community Arts Council Network; South Dakota Alliance
Performs At: Dakota Prairie Playhouse
Organization Type: Educational; Sponsoring

5445 PIERRE COMMUNITY CONCERTS ASSOCIATION
PO Box 519
808 W Pleasant
Pierre, SD 57501
Phone: 605-224-5803
Budget: $10,000-20,000

Tennessee

5446 ATHENS AREA COUNCIL FOR THE ARTS
PO Box 95
Athens, TN 37371-0095
Phone: 423-745-8781
Fax: 423-745-8635
e-mail: aaca@bellsouth.net
Management:
 Executive Director: Ellen Kimball
Budget: $10,000-20,000

5447 RIVERBEND FESTIVAL
1001 Market Street
Chattanooga, TN 37402
Phone: 423-756-2212
Fax: 423-756-2719
e-mail: Office@FriendsoftheFestival.com
Web Site: www.riverbendfestival.com

5448 UNIVERSITY OF TENNESSEE AT CHATTANOOGA
Fine Arts Center, Department 1351
615 McCallie Avenue
Chattanooga, TN 37403
Phone: 423-755-4379
Fax: 423-755-5249
e-mail: Kim-Renz@utc.edu
Web Site: www.utc.edu/finearts
Management:
Fine Arts Center Manager: Kim Edward Renz
Mission: Patten performances provides the Southeast
Tennessee area with a professional showcase of national
and international artists who perform and conduct
residency activities in music, theatre and dance.
Paid Staff: 3
Paid Artists: 12
Budget: $60,000-150,000
Performs At: Roland Hayes Concert Hall
Annual Attendance: 4,000-5,000
Facility Category: Fine Arts Center
Type of Stage: Modified Proscenium
Seating Capacity: 505
Year Built: 1979
Rental Contact: Sue Carroll

5449 AUSTIN PEAY STATE UNIVERSITY
Center of Excellence for the Creative Arts
PO Box 4666
Clarksville, TN 37044
Phone: 931-221-7034
Fax: 931-221-7149
e-mail: crown@apsu.edu
Management:
Associate Director: Marlon Crow
Founded: 1985
Specialized Field: Art; Creative Writing; Music; Theatre
Budget: $700,000
Income Sources: State
Performs At: Mass Communication Building
Type of Stage: Proscenium
Seating Capacity: 600

5450 LEE UNIVERSITY PRESIDENTIAL CONCERT SERIES
Lee University
Cleveland, TN 37311
Phone: 423-614-8240
Fax: 423-614-8242
e-mail: wmauldin@leeuniversity.edu
Web Site: www.leeuniversity.edu
Officers:
Dean: Stephen W Plate
Management:
Dean: Dr. Walt Mauldin
Specialized Field: Classical Theater
Status: Professioanl; Nonprofit
Budget: $20,000-35,000
Performs At: Dixon Center
Annual Attendance: 4,000+
Facility Category: Music/Drama Performing Hall
Type of Stage: Full

5451 SOUTHERN ADVENTIST UNIVERSITY
PO Box 370
Collegedale, TN 37315
Phone: 423-238-2813
Fax: 423-238-2441
e-mail: wohlers@southern.edu
Officers:
Student Services VP: William R Wohlers
Budget: $20,000-35,000
Performs At: Physical Education Center; Ackerman
Auditorium

5452 BRYAN COLLEGE DEPARTMENT OF MUSIC
PO Box 7000
Bryan College
Dayton, TN 37321
Phone: 423-775-2041
Fax: 423-775-7317
e-mail: Wilhoime@Bryan.edu
Web Site: www.Bryan.edu
Officers:
Chair Music Department: Mel R Wilhoit
Founded: 1930
Budget: $10,000
Performs At: Rudd Auditorium

5453 ETOWAH ARTS COMMISSION
PO Box 193
Etowah, TN 37331
Phone: 423-263-7608
Fax: 423-263-1670
Management:
Director: Charles Munn
Budget: $10,000
Performs At: Gem Theater

5454 GERMANTOWN PERFORMING ARTS CENTRE
1801 Exeter Road
Germantown, TN 38138
Phone: 901-751-7506
Fax: 901-751-7514
e-mail: info@GPACweb.com
Web Site: www.gpacweb.com
Management:
Executive Director: Albert Pertalion
Assistant Director: Paul Chandler
Principal Conductor: Michael Stern
Budget: $400,000-1,000,000
Income Sources: Box Office; Member Support

5455 JACKSON ARTS COUNCIL
314 E Main Street
Jackson, TN 38301
Mailing Address: PO Box 7534, Jackson, TN.
38302-7534
Phone: 901-423-2787
Fax: 901-424-2040
e-mail: jac@aeneas.net
Management:
Executive Director: Judy Truex

**5456 CARSON-NEWMAN COLLEGE
CONCERT-LECTURE SERIES**
Box 71987
Carson-Newman College
Jefferson City, TN 37760
Phone: 865-471-3409
Fax: 865-471-4849
e-mail: tteague@cn.edu
Web Site: www.cn.edu
Officers:
   Chairman: Thomas S Teague
Founded: 1917
Budget: $20,000-35,000
Performs At: Henderson Humanities Building

**5457 EAST TENNESSEE STATE UNIVERSITY
PERFORMING ARTS**
Box 70691, ETSU
Johnson City, TN 37614-0691
Phone: 423-439-6828
Fax: 423-439-4386
Web Site: www.estu.east-tenn-st.edu
Performs At: Brooks Gym

5458 JOHNSON CITY AREA ARTS COUNCIL
214 E Main Street
Johnson City, TN 37604
Mailing Address: Box 1033, Johnson City, TN. 37605
Phone: 423-928-8229
Fax: 423-928-4511
e-mail: jcarts@mounet.com
Web Site: www.arts.org
Management:
   Executive Director: Sarah K Davis
   Administrative Assistant: Susan Thomas
   Media Director: Christine Murdock
Mission: Dedicated to preserving the cultural communities in our area.
Paid Staff: 3
Volunteer Staff: 1
Budget: $10,000
Performs At: Small gallery space

5459 JUBILEE COMMUNITY ARTS
Laurel Theater
1538 Laurel Avenue
Knoxville, TN 37916
Phone: 865-522-5851
Fax: 865-522-5386
e-mail: info@jubileearts.org
Web Site: www.jubileearts.org
Management:
   Executive Director: Brent Cantrell
Budget: $35,000-60,000

**5460 UNIVERSITY OF TENNESSEE AT
KNOXVILLE: CULTURAL ARTS**
305 University Center
Knoxville, TN 37996-4800
Phone: 865-974-5455
Fax: 865-974-9252
e-mail: ronl@utk.edu
Management:

   Student Activities Director: Ron Laffitte
Budget: $150,000-400,000
Performs At: Clarence Brown Theatre

**5461 UNIVERSITY OF TENNESSEE AT
MARTIN ARTS COUNCIL**
102 Fine Arts Building
Martin, TN 38238
Phone: 901-587-7400
Fax: 901-587-7415
e-mail: dcook@utm.edu
Management:
   Director: Douglas Cook
Budget: $20,000-35,000
Performs At: Harriet Fulton Performing Arts Theater

5462 CONCERTS INTERNATIONAL
PO Box 770522
Memphis, TN 38177-0522
Phone: 901-527-3067
Fax: 901-682-1928
e-mail: barnbeca@mindspring.com
Web Site: Http://home.midsouth.rr.com
Officers:
   President: Barry White
   VP: Jeff Kass
   Secretary: Kacky Walton
   Treasurer: Dennis Norton
Management:
   Executive Director: Carol Barnett
   Artistic Director: Ralph Lake
Specialized Field: Chamber Music
Paid Staff: 1
Budget: $35,000-60,000
Performs At: Harris Concert Hall; University of Memphis
Seating Capacity: 385
Year Remodeled: 1999

**5463 MEMPHIS IN MAY INTERNATIONAL
FESTIVAL**
245 Wagner Place
Suite 220
Memphis, TN 38103
Phone: 901-525-4611
Fax: 901-525-4686
e-mail: mim@memphisinmay.org
Web Site: www.memphisinmay.org
Management:
   Executive Director: James L Holt
   Director of Programming: John Doyle
Mission: To promote and celebrate Memphis culture, foster economic growth and enhance international awareness.
Founded: 1976
Specialized Field: Dance; Vocal Music; Instrumental Music; Exhibits; Therater; Festivals
Status: Nonprofit
Paid Staff: 15
Volunteer Staff: 999
Performs At: Tom Lee Park in downtown Memphis, Tennessee and various venues throughout town
Annual Attendance: 300,000+
Organization Type: Educational; Sponsoring

5464 RHODES COLLEGE: MCCOY VISITING ARTIST SERIES
2000 N Parkway
Memphis, TN 38112
Phone: 901-843-3875
Fax: 901-843-3553
e-mail: templeton@rhodes.edu
Web Site: www.rhodes.edu
Budget: $10,000

5465 MIDDLE TENNESSEE STATE UNIVERSITY
Music Department
Murfreesboro, TN 37132
Phone: 615-898-2476
Fax: 615-898-5037
e-mail: jperkins@frank.mtsu.edu
Management:
    Music Professor: Jerry R Perkins
Budget: $10,000-20,000

5466 DAVID LIPSCOMB UNIVERSITY: MUSIC DEPARTMENT
David Lipscomb University
Nashville, TN 37204
Phone: 615-269-1000
Fax: 615-386-7620
e-mail: reedja@dlu.edu
Budget: $10,000-20,000
Performs At: Ward Lecture Auditorium; Alumni Auditorium

5467 FRIENDS OF MUSIC
PO Box 23593
Nashville, TN 37202-3593
Phone: 931-254-0469
Fax: 931-254-0469
Officers:
    President: Joseph S Johnson, Jr
Budget: $20,000-35,000
Performs At: James K. Polk Theater; Tennessee Performing Arts Center

5468 HOWARD C GENTRY COMPLEX
Tennessee State University
3500 John Merrit Boulevard
Nashville, TN 37209
Phone: 615-963-5000
Fax: 615-963-5911
Management:
    Athletic Director: Bill Thomas

5469 NASHVILLE SHAKESPEARE FESTIVAL
615 5th Avenue S
Nashville, TN 37203
Phone: 615-255-2273
Web Site: www.brotherswest.com/nsf
Officers:
    Chairman: Donald Capparella
    Secretary/Treasurer: Denah Shabal
Management:
    Artistic Director: Denice Hickes

    Managing Director: Denah Shabal
Mission: Dedicated to community enrichment and arts in education through innovative and relevant presentations of the works of William Shakespeare and other curriculum-based programming. We focus our work to stimulate imagination and inspire conversation, which are essential elements to a healthy society.
Founded: 1988
Specialized Field: Central Park
Status: Professional
Season: august
Performs At: Centennial Park Bandshell
Affiliations: Shakespeare Theatre Association of America
Annual Attendance: 14,000
Organization Type: Performing; Resident; Touring; Educational
Comments: Productions are free of charge or at a cost that makes them accesible regardless of socio-economic circumstances; Barrier free and multiculturally cast.

5470 VANDERBILT UNIVERSITY: GREAT PERFORMANCES
207 Sarratt Center
Student Center
Nashville, TN 37240
Phone: 615-322-2471
Fax: 615-343-8081
Web Site: www.vanderbilt.edu/sarratt/great.htm
Management:
    Assistant Director: Bridgette Sudbrink
Budget: $150,000-400,000

5471 OAK RIDGE CIVIC MUSIC ASSOCIATION
PO Box 4271
Oak Ridge, TN 37831
Phone: 865-483-5569
Fax: 865-483-5569
Management:
    Music Director: Serge Fourtier
Mission: To provide the community with quality music; to encourage community youth to enjoy good music.
Founded: 1944
Specialized Field: Vocal Music; Instrumental Music; Chamber Series
Status: Professional; Non-Professional; Nonprofit
Paid Staff: 50
Performs At: Oak Ridge High School Auditorium
Organization Type: Performing; Educational; Sponsoring

5472 SEWANEE SUMMER MUSIC FESTIVAL
735 University Avenue
Sewanee, TN 37383-1000
Phone: 931-598-1225
Fax: 931-598-1706
e-mail: ssmf@sewanee.edu
Web Site: www.sewanee.edu/ssmf
Management:
    Festival Coordinator: Kory Vrieze
Mission: To provide a comprehensive training program emphasizing performance experience.
Founded: 1957

Specialized Field: Symphony; Chamber Music; Composition; Conducting; Piano
Paid Staff: 4
Paid Artists: 50+
Facility Category: Concert Hall
Seating Capacity: 1,000

5473 UNIVERSITY OF THE SOUTH: PERFORMING ARTS SERIES
735 University Avenue
Sewanee, TN 37402
Phone: 615-598-1484
Fax: 615-598-1145
e-mail: sshrader@sewanee.edu
Management:
    Chairman: Steven Shrader

5474 WATERTOWN JAZZ FESTIVAL
Watertown Bed & Breakfast
116 Depot Avenue
Watertown, TN 37184
Phone: 615-237-9999
e-mail: mccomb28@earthlink.net
Web Site: www.bbonline.com/watertown/jazz.html
Management:
    Festival Director: Sharon McComb

Texas

5475 UNIVERSITY OF TEXAS AT ARLINGTON
EXCEL Campus Activities
300 W First Street, Uta Box 19348
Arlington, TX 76019-0348
Phone: 817-272-2963
Fax: 817-272-2962
e-mail: excell@uta.edu
Web Site: www.uta.edu/stuact
Management:
    Student Activities Director: Susan English
Specialized Field: University Center Art Gallery, Performing Arts, Childrens' Theatre, Touring Artists and Vendor Sales (in the arts)
Paid Staff: 15
Volunteer Staff: 50
Paid Artists: 20
Non-paid Artists: 6
Budget: $20,000-35,000
Performs At: Texas Hall; Rosebud Theatre; Blubonnet Ballroom

5476 AUSTIN CHAMBER MUSIC FESTIVAL
4930 Bornet Road
Suite 203
Austin, TX 78756
Phone: 512-454-7562
Fax: 512-454-0029
e-mail: info@austinchambermusic.org
Web Site: www.austinchambermusic.org
Officers:
    President: Barbara Grove
    VP: Bryce Williams

    Secretary: Dee Ann Kincke
    Treasurer: Diane Post
Management:
    Executive Director: Felicity Coltman
    Business Manager: Ira Shay
    Education Coordinator: Lisa Link Edwards
    Arts Administration Apprentice: Erin Hill
Mission: To enhance the quality of community life by nurturing and expanding knowledge, understanding, and appreciation of chamber music through education, community outreach and performance.
Founded: 1981
Specialized Field: Chamber Music
Paid Staff: 4
Paid Artists: 60
Budget: 265,000
Income Sources: Grants; Membership; Corporate Support; Government Funds; Individuals
Facility Category: Varies
Type of Stage: Varies

5477 AUSTIN SHAKESPEARE FESTIVAL
PO Box 683
Austin, TX 78767-0683
Phone: 512-454-2273
e-mail: asf@austinshakespeare.org
Web Site: www.austinshakespeare.org
Officers:
    President: Daniel B Wilson
    VP: Susan Threadgill
    Treasurer: Jill K Sawnson
    Secretary: Sylvester L. Ruffin
Mission: To produce professional quality productions of Classical theatre with an emphasis on the plays of William Shakespeare and to entertain and enrich the theatre-going public by presenting productions that are accessible, imaginative, and stimulating, while remaining true to the integrity of the plays and the author.
Founded: 1984
Status: Non-Equity; Nonprofit
Season: September - October
Type of Stage: Outdoor
Stage Dimensions: 50' x 40'
Seating Capacity: 3000

5478 FRANK ERWIN CENTER/ UNIVERSITY OF TEXAS-AUSTIN
1701 Red River
PO Box 2929
Austin, TX 78768-2929
Phone: 512-471-7744
Fax: 512-471-9652
e-mail: erwin.center@erwin.utexas.edu
Web Site: www.utexas.edu/admin/erwin/
Management:
    Director: John M Graham
    Associate Director: Jimmy Earl
Seating Capacity: 17,800, 16,500
Year Built: 1977

5479 NEW TEXAS MUSIC WORKS
2832 E Martin Luther King Jr Boulevard
Suite 103
Austin, TX 78702-1544

Phone: 512-476-5775
Fax: 512-481-1676
Founded: 1993
Affiliations: New Texas Music Works

5480 SALON CONCERTS
PO Box 163501
Austin, TX 78716-3501
Phone: 512-327-0004
Fax: 512-327-0046
e-mail: kmishell@aol.com
Management:
  Music Director: Robert Rudie
Budget: $10,000

5481 BAY CITY FESTIVAL ARTS ASSOCIATION
PO Box 111
Bay City, TX 77404-0111
Phone: 409-245-9062
Fax: 409-245-1622
e-mail: melvine@sat.net
Officers:
  Chairman Selection Committee: Melvin Epstein
Budget: $20,000-35,000
Performs At: Keye Ingram Auditorium

5482 FESTIVAL ARTS ASSOCIATION
PO Box 1794
Bay City, TX 77404-1794
Phone: 409-245-2727
Fax: 409-245-6966
e-mail: mseaman@alphainternet.net
Web Site: www.festarts.org
Management:
  Artistic Director: Mark Seaman

5483 BEAUMONT MUSIC COMMISSION
5640 North Circuit Drive
Beaumont, TX 77706
Phone: 409-898-1634
Fax: 409-833-7822
e-mail: emc@exp.net
Web Site: www.beaumontmusic.org
Officers:
  President: Matthew White
  VP/Chairman: Naaman J Woodland, Jr
  Second VP: David Hitt
  Third VP: J. Robert Madden
  Fourth VP: Virginia Christopher
  Recording Secretary: Gwenn Mercer
Mission: To offer instrumental and vocal artists in small ensembles, recitals/concerts, opera, musicals, dance groups and small orchestras.
Founded: 1923
Specialized Field: Dance; Vocal Music; Instrumental Music
Status: Nonprofit
Volunteer Staff: 60
Budget: $128,000
Performs At: Julie Rogers Theatre for the Performing Arts
Annual Attendance: 8,000

Organization Type: Educational; Sponsoring

5484 YOUNG AUDIENCES OF SOUTHEAST TEXAS
595 Orleans
Suite 414
Beaumont, TX 77701
Phone: 409-835-3884
Fax: 409-835-5504
e-mail: yasetx@aol.com
Web Site: www.geocities.com
Officers:
  President: Douglas E Fierce
Management:
  Executive Director: Sally Sessions
  Program Director/Business Manager: Mindy Wheeler
Mission: To provide students with an opportunity to experience live performances featuring professional artists; to further arts education.
Founded: 1973
Specialized Field: Dance; Instrumental Music; Theater; Drama
Status: Nonprofit
Paid Staff: 3
Paid Artists: 45
Budget: $155,598
Income Sources: Individual, Corporate, Grants/Foundations
Organization Type: Performing; Educational

5485 UNIVERSITY OF MARY HARDIN: BAYLOR LYCEUM
900 College Street
Box 8012, UMHB Station
Belton, TX 76513
Phone: 254-295-4678
Fax: 254-295-4535
e-mail: glayne@umbh.edu
Web Site: www.umbh.edu
Management:
  Dean School Fine Arts: George W Stansbury
Budget: $10,000
Performs At: Hughes Recital Hall

5486 BIG SPRING CULTURAL AFFAIRS COUNCIL
Box 1391
Big Spring, TX 79721
Phone: 915-263-7641
Fax: 915-264-9111
Management:
  Director: Marae Brooks
Mission: To offer balanced cultural activities to the community; to enhance natural cultural resources.
Specialized Field: Dance; Vocal Music; Instrumental Music; Theater
Status: Nonprofit
Budget: $10,000
Organization Type: Touring

5487 ARTS COUNCIL OF WASHINGTON COUNTY
701 Milroy Drive
Brenham, TX 77833
Phone: 979-836-3120
Fax: 979-830-4030
Mission: To advance local arts in our community; to bring events to our community that are not locally available.
Founded: 1981
Specialized Field: Vocal Music; Instrumental Music; Theater
Status: Professional; Semi-Professional; Non-Professional; Nonprofit
Income Sources: TCA
Organization Type: Touring; Resident; Educational; Sponsoring

5488 UNIVERSITY OF TEXAS AT BROWNSVILLE
80 Fort Brown
Brownsville, TX 78520
Phone: 956-544-8247
Fax: 956-982-0163
e-mail: surbis@utb1.utb.edu
Web Site: www.utb.edu/finearts
Management:
   Contact: Richard Urbis
   Contact: Sue Zanne Williamson Urbis
Budget: $10,000

5489 CITY OF BRYAN PARKS AND RECREATION
201 E 29th
PO Box 1000
Bryan, TX 77805
Phone: 979-209-5200
Fax: 979-209-5209
e-mail: cmessina@ci.bryan.tx.us
Management:
   Speical Events Coordinator: Linda Giffen
Mission: To provide area residents with quality entertainment.
Specialized Field: Dance; Vocal Music; Theater; Festivals
Status: Nonprofit
Paid Staff: 60
Performs At: Lake Byrant
Type of Stage: Amphitheatre; Outdoors
Organization Type: Performing; Touring; Resident; Educational; Sponsoring

5490 MONTGOMERY COUNTY PERFORMING ARTS SERIES
PO Box 1714
Conroe, TX 77305
Phone: 936-856-6243
Web Site: www.mcpas.org
Officers:
   President: Peggy Miller
Budget: $20,000-35,000

5491 CATHEDRAL CONCERT SERIES
505 N Upper Broadway
Corpus Christi, TX 78401
Phone: 361-888-6520
Fax: 361-888-6128
e-mail: lgccso@intercomm.com
Web Site: www.goccn.org/ccs/
Management:
   Executive Director: Lee Gwozdz
   Administrative Assistant: Fran Seagrave
Founded: 1985
Specialized Field: Vocal Music; Instrumental Music; Festivals
Status: Professional; Semi-Professional; Non-Professional; Nonprofit
Budget: $35,000-60,000
Income Sources: Donors; Grants; Foundations; Benefits
Annual Attendance: 6,000
Facility Category: Cathedral
Type of Stage: Portable
Seating Capacity: 900
Organization Type: Performing; Touring; Resident

5492 CORPUS CHRISTI COMMUNITY CONCERT
446 Troy
Corpus Christi, TX 78412
Phone: 361-992-9220
Fax: 361-992-9220
e-mail: pat@testx.net
Officers:
   President: Pat Townsend
Founded: 1935
Volunteer Staff: 20
Budget: $60,000-150,000
Income Sources: Subscriptions
Performs At: Bayfront Plaza Auditorium
Seating Capacity: 2,500

5493 DEL MAR COLLEGE STUDENT CULTURAL PROGRAMS
Del Mar College Music
Music & Drama Department, East Campus
Corpus Christi, TX 78404-3897
Phone: 361-886-1211
Budget: $10,000-20,000
Performs At: Nell Bartlett Theater

5494 TEXAS A&M UNIVERSITY: CORPUS CHRISTI, COLLEGE OF ARTS & HUMANITIES
6300 Ocean Drive
Corpus Christi, TX 78412
Phone: 361-825-2372
Fax: 361-825-6097
Officers:
   Visual/Performing Arts Dept. Chair: Carey Rote
Budget: $10,000-20,000
Performs At: Warren Theatre

5495 TEXAS JAZZ FESTIVAL SOCIETY

403 N Shoreline Boulevard
Corpus Christi, TX 78403
Phone: 361-883-4500
Fax: 361-883-4500
e-mail: james@microtek-sales.com
Web Site: www.texasjazz-fest.org/
Management:
Festival Originator: Al Beto Garcia
Mission: Producing the Texas Jazz Festival to the public annually, free of charge; promoting and preserving American jazz.
Founded: 1969
Specialized Field: Vocal Music; Instrumental Music; Festivals
Status: Professional; Nonprofit
Performs At: Bayfront Plaza Convention Center
Organization Type: Performing

5496 PINEY WOODS FINE ARTS ASSOCIATION

603 E Goliad, Suite 203
PO Box 1213
Crockett, TX 75835
Phone: 936-544-4276
Fax: 936-546-0927
e-mail: pwfaa@sat.net
Web Site: www.pwfaa.org
Management:
Executive Director: J Bryan Lake
Founded: 1991
Specialized Field: Performing/Visual
Paid Staff: 2
Volunteer Staff: 80
Paid Artists: 4
Non-paid Artists: 1
Performs At: General Purpose

5497 DALLAS FESTIVAL OF ARTS & JAZZ

MEI Festivals
2200 North Lamar #104
Dallas, TX 75202
Phone: 214-885-1881
Fax: 214-885-1882
e-mail: mei@meifestivals.com
Web Site: www.meifestivals.com/dalfest.html
Management:
Director: Stephen Millard

5498 DALLAS SUMMER MUSICALS

Music Hall at Fair Park
909 1st Avenue Parry
Dallas, TX 75210
Phone: 214-565-1116
Fax: 214-565-0071
Web Site: www.dallassummermusicals.org
Officers:
VP/General Manager: Nancy J Marshall
Management:
Staff Accountant: Linda White
Event Booking: Jayne Basse
Facilities Services Manager: Ben Perrin
Mission: To promote the performing arts.
Specialized Field: Musical

Paid Staff: 10
Season: June - August
Annual Attendance: 400,000+
Facility Category: Performance; Concert Hall
Type of Stage: Proscenium
Stage Dimensions: 100'x39'10'
Seating Capacity: 3,420
Year Built: 1925
Rental Contact: Jayne Basse
Organization Type: Performing

5499 DSO CLASSICAL SUMMER SAMPLER

2301 Flora Street
Suite 300
Dallas, TX 75201-2497
Phone: 214-692-0203
Fax: 214-953-1218
Web Site: www.dallassymphony.com
Officers:
President: Dr. Eugene Bonelli

5500 FAIR PARK

PO Box 159090
Dallas, TX 75315
Phone: 214-670-8400
Fax: 214-670-8907
e-mail: cls2nd@aol.com
Web Site: www.fairparkdallas.com
Management:
Executive General Manager: Eddie Hueston
Assistant General Manager: JB Gassaway
Events Manager: Les Studdard
Mission: Offers a 277 acre cultural and exhibition park including; Cotton Bowl Stadium; eight museums; the Old Mill Inn Restaurant; five indoor performance halls.
Specialized Field: 277 aacre cultural and exhibition park including: the Cotton Bowl Stadium, 8 museums, the Old Mill Inn Restaurant, 5 indoor performance halls
Seating Capacity: 72,500 (Cotton Bowl)
Year Built: 1936

5501 JUNIOR BLACK ACADEMY OF ARTS AND LETTERS

650 S Griffin
Dallas, TX 75202
Phone: 214-743-2440
Fax: 214-658-7163
Management:
Founder/President: Curtis King
Facility Operations Manager: Gwen Hargrove
Developmental Manager: Ken Rowe
Membership Developer: Gail Johnson
Publicist: Marilyn Clark
Mission: Promoting, fostering, cultivating, perpetuating and preserving Black Americans' arts and letters.
Founded: 1977
Specialized Field: Dance; Vocal Music; Instrumental Music; Theater; Festivals
Status: Professional; Nonprofit
Paid Staff: 100
Organization Type: Performing; Educational

All listings are in alphabetical order by state, then city, then organization within the city.

5502 SHAKESPEARE FESTIVAL OF DALLAS
3630 Harry Hine Boulevard
4th Floor
Dallas, TX 75219
Phone: 214-559-2778
Fax: 214-559-2782
e-mail: crivasfl@swbell.net
Web Site: www.shakespearedallas.org
Management:
Managing Director: Sandra L Greenway
Founded: 1972
Status: Professional; Nonprofit
Paid Staff: 3
Performs At: Fair Park Band Shell
Organization Type: Performing; Educational

5503 DEL RIO COUNCIL FOR THE ARTS
120 E Garfield
Del Rio, TX 78840
Phone: 830-775-0888
Fax: 830-774-0803
e-mail: drcarts@delrio.com
Web Site: firehousearts.org
Management:
Executive Director: Ann Stool
Founded: 1977
Specialized Field: Southwest Texas
Paid Staff: 5
Volunteer Staff: 21
Paid Artists: 105
Non-paid Artists: 15
Budget: $250,000
Income Sources: Grants; Ticket Sales; Fundraisers;
Corporate Sponsors; City; County; State; Foundation;
Performs At: Theatre, Schools, Fairgrounds,
Ampitheaters
Affiliations: Southwest Performing Arts Presenters;
Mid-America Arts Alliance, Heartland Fund
Annual Attendance: 16,000
Facility Category: Proscenium
Type of Stage: Wooden floor
Stage Dimensions: 25x27
Seating Capacity: 700
Year Built: 1930
Year Remodeled: 1980

5504 GRAYSON COUNTY COLLEGE HUMANITIES
6101 Grayson Drive
Denison, TX 75020
Phone: 903-465-6030
Web Site: www.grayson.edu
Management:
Manager: Joe Hick
Budget: $35,000-60,000

5505 DENTON ARTS & JAZZ FESTIVAL
PO Box 2104
Denton, TX 76202
Phone: 940-565-0931
Fax: 940-566-7007
Web Site: www.dentonjazzfest.com
Officers:
Board President: Murray Ricks

Management:
Festival Director: Carol Short
Artistic Manager: Ray Hair
Mission: Showcase visual and performing artists, both professional and amateur; free admission; 6 stages; children's art tent, food, games, etc.
Founded: 1980
Specialized Field: Denton Civic Center Park
Paid Staff: 2
Volunteer Staff: 300
Paid Artists: 250
Non-paid Artists: 900
Budget: $330,000
Income Sources: Sponsors; Booth Space Fees;
Concessions; Memberships
Performs At: Park
Annual Attendance: 100,000
Facility Category: Civic Center Park

5506 GREATER DENTON ARTS COUNCIL
207 S Bell Avenue
Denton, TX 76201-4259
Phone: 940-382-2787
Fax: 940-566-1486
Web Site: www.dentonarts.com
Budget: $10,000

5507 EASTLAND FINE ARTS ASSOCIATION
PO Box 705
108 N Lamar
Eastland, TX 76448
Phone: 254-629-2102
Fax: 254-629-2247
e-mail: majestic@txol.net
Management:
Manager: Ed Allcorn
Budget: $10,000
Performs At: Majestic Theatre

5508 EL PASO ARTS RESOURCES DEPARTMENT
2 Civic Center Plaza
6th Floor
El Paso, TX 79901
Phone: 915-541-4481
Fax: 915-541-4902
e-mail: drewaj@ci.el-paso.tx.us
Web Site: wwww.artsresources.org
Management:
Director: Alejandrina Drew
Budget: $150,000-400,000
Performs At: Chamizal National Memorial

5509 EL PASO ASSOCIATION FOR THE PERFORMING ARTS
PO Box 31340
El Paso, TX 79931
Phone: 915-565-6900
Fax: 915-565-6999
Web Site: www.viva-ep.org
Management:
Executive Director: David D Mills
Artistic Director: Hector M Serrano

Mission: An outdoor drama emphasizing dance, which celebrates the Western American, Native American, Mexican and Spanish cultures that have influenced El Paso's history. Shakespeare-on-the-Rocks presents four plays in repertory each September.
Founded: 1978
Specialized Field: Dance; Vocal Music; Theater; Ballet; Folkdance
Status: Professional; Nonprofit
Paid Staff: 15
Paid Artists: 100
Income Sources: Institute of Outdoor Drama
Season: June - August
Performs At: McKelligon Canyon Amphitheater
Organization Type: Performing; Resident

5510 EL PASO CHAMBER MUSIC FESTIVAL

PO Box 13328
El Paso, TX 79913
Phone: 915-833-9400
Fax: 915-833-9425
e-mail: info@elpasopromusica.org
Web Site: www.elpasopromusica.org
Management:
   Director: Kwang-Wu Kim

5511 EL PASO PRO-MUSICA

PO Box 13328
El Paso, TX 79913
Phone: 915-833-9400
Fax: 915-833-9425
e-mail: info@elpasopromusica.org
Web Site: www.elpasopromusica.org
Management:
   Artistic/Administrative Director: Kwang-Wu Kim
Budget: $60,000-150,000

5512 IMPACT: PROGRAMS OF EXCELLENCE

2626 N Stanton
El Paso, TX 79902
Phone: 915-545-5073
Fax: 915-545-5076
Management:
   Executive Director: Sally Gilbert

5513 BROOKHAVEN COLLEGE CENTER FOR THE ARTS

3939 Valley View Lane
Farmers Branch, TX 75244
Phone: 972-860-4730
Fax: 972-860-4385
e-mail: rpbfape@dcccd.edu
Web Site: www.dcccd.edu/bmc/centerforarts
Management:
   Dean Fine Arts: Rodger Bennett
Founded: 1978
Paid Staff: 3
Budget: $35,000-60,000
Income Sources: City Grants; Tickets
Annual Attendance: 7,000
Facility Category: Performance Center
Type of Stage: Proscenium
Seating Capacity: 680

Year Built: 1978
Rental Contact: Roger Bennett

5514 FORT HOOD COMMUNITY MUSIC AND THEATER

Building 2803
Fort Hood, TX 76544
Phone: 254-287-1110
Management:
   Mucsical Director/Theater: Jean Zavoina
   Music Director: Roland Gagne
   Technical Director: Fred Baker
   Costumer: Tom Ross
Mission: To provide opportunities for military personnel, their families and other area residents to participate in talent competitions, musicals and shows.
Founded: 1950
Specialized Field: Dance; Vocal Music; Instrumental Music; Theater; Festivals
Status: Non-Professional
Organization Type: Performing; Touring

5515 CHILDREN'S UNIVERSAL MUSIC FESTIVAL

4449 Camp Bowie Boulevard
Fort Worth, TX 76107-3834
Phone: 817-732-8161
Fax: 817-732-4774
e-mail: TGC@texasgirlschois.org
Web Site: www.Texasgirlschoir.org
Management:
   TX Girls' Choir/Executive Director: Shirley Carter
   Administrative Assistant: Debi Weir
Mission: To bring together childrens choirs from all over the world to share their music in performance.
Founded: 1998
Specialized Field: Children's choral music
Paid Staff: 10
Volunteer Staff: 55

5516 CLIBURN CONCERTS

Van Cliburn Foundation
2525 Ridgmar Boulevard, Suite 307
Fort Worth, TX 76116
Phone: 817-738-6536
Fax: 817-738-6534
e-mail: clistaff@cliburn.org
Web Site: www.cliburn.org
Officers:
   President: Richard Rodzinski
Management:
   General Manager: Maria Guralnik
Mission: To produce the Cilburn Piano Series.
Founded: 1962
Status: Professional; Nonprofit
Budget: $150,000-400,000
Performs At: Nancy Lee & Perry R. Bass Performance Hall

5517 COWTOWN COLISEUM

121 E Exchange Avenue
Fort Worth, TX 76106

Phone: 817-625-1025
Fax: 817-625-1148
e-mail: billy@cowtowncoliseum.com
Web Site: www.cowtowncoliseum.com
Management:
 General Manager: Hub Baker

5518 PERFORMING ARTS FORT WORTH
330 E 4th Street
#300
Fort Worth, TX 76102
Phone: 817-212-4200
Fax: 817-810-9294
e-mail: pbeard@basshall.com
Web Site: www.basshall.com
Management:
 Managing Director: Paul S Beard
 Director Operations: Don Fearing
 Director Communications: Carl Davis
 Special Events: Kelly Whitmarsh
 Box Office Manager: Patti Edwards
 Technical Director: Steve Truitt
Founded: 1992
Paid Staff: 35
Volunteer Staff: 750
Budget: $1,000,000+
Income Sources: Ticket Sales; Facility Rental; Donations
Performs At: One 2,056 seat multi-purpose theatre
Annual Attendance: 500,000 - 600,000
Facility Category: Multi-purpose theater
Type of Stage: Proscenium
Stage Dimensions: see www.basshall.com
Seating Capacity: 2,056
Year Built: 1998
Cost: 67 Million
Rental Contact: Managing Director Paul Beard
Resident Groups: Five local resident companies

5519 FREDERICKSBURG MUSIC CLUB
PO Box 1214
Fredericksburg, TX 78624
Phone: 830-997-5413
Fax: 830-997-2980
Officers:
 President: Patsy Hejl
 VP: Frances Gibson
Management:
 Artistic Director: Frances Gibson
Founded: 1937
Specialized Field: Classical Music Concerts
Budget: $10,000-20,000
Facility Category: Church; High School Auditorium

5520 GRAND 1894 OPERA HOUSE
2020 Post Office Street
Galveston, TX 77550
Phone: 409-763-7173
Fax: 409-763-1068
Toll-free: 800-821-1894
e-mail: mpatton@thegrand.com
Web Site: www.thegrand.com
Management:
 Executive Director: Maureen M Patton

Mission: To present professional performing arts in a restored, historic structure and to maintain that structure; to serve the Galveston and the Greater Houston areas.
Founded: 1974
Specialized Field: Dance; Vocal Music; Instrumental Music; Theater; Lyric Opera; Grand Opera; Meetings; Parties; Workshops
Status: Professional; Non-Professional; Nonprofit
Paid Staff: 12
Volunteer Staff: 300
Budget: $2.5 million
Income Sources: Earned and Contributed Revenue; Association of Performing Arts Presenters; League of Historic American Theatres; Southwest Performing Arts Presenters
Performs At: The Grand 1894 Opera House
Affiliations: APAP; ISPA; SWPAP; LHAT
Annual Attendance: 100,000+
Facility Category: Historic Theatre
Type of Stage: Proscenium
Stage Dimensions: 38x36
Seating Capacity: 1,040
Year Built: 1894
Year Remodeled: 1985
Rental Contact: Maureen Patton
Organization Type: Performing; Touring; Resident; Educational; Sponsoring; Presenting
Resident Groups: Galveston Symphony Orchestra

5521 GARLAND SUMMER MUSICALS
PO Box 462049
Garland, TX 75046
Phone: 972-205-2780
Fax: 972-205-2775
Management:
 Producer: Patty Granville
 Director: Buff Shurr
Mission: To bring to the community productions of the highest quality; to continue to provide excellent family entertainment.
Founded: 1983
Specialized Field: Dance; Vocal Music; Instrumental Music
Status: Semi-Professional; Nonprofit
Income Sources: Actors' Equity Association
Performs At: Garland Center for the Performing Arts
Organization Type: Sponsoring

5522 SOUTHWESTERN UNIVERSITY ARTIST SERIES
Southwestern University
The Sarofim School of Fine Arts
Georgetown, TX 78626
Phone: 512-863-1379
Fax: 512-863-1422
Web Site: www.southwestern.edu
Management:
 The Sarofim School of Fine Arts: Carole A Lee, Dean
Budget: $10,000-20,000
Performs At: Alma Thomas Theater

5523 HARLINGEN COMMUNITY CONCERT ASSOCIATION
PO Box 707
Harlingen, TX 78551
Phone: 956-748-3020
Fax: 956-425-3870
Officers:
President: James Hough
Management:
Publicity: Joyce Davis-Tucker
Mission: To entertain and influence community adults and students in culture and cultural events.
Founded: 1930
Specialized Field: a variety of cultural programs

5524 RIOFEST: A BLENDING OF THE ARTS AND ENTERTAINMENT
305 E Jackson, Suite 214
PO Box 531105
Harlingen, TX 78550
Phone: 956-425-2705
Fax: 956-440-0476
Toll-free: 800-746-3378
e-mail: RioFest@aol.com
Web Site: www.RioFest.com
Management:
Festival Director: Kathy Preddy
Mission: To develop new audiences for the arts and provide access to the arts for all citizens.
Founded: 1982
Specialized Field: Fine Arts & Crafts - Jueied; Unique Merchandise & Crafts - Jueied
Paid Staff: 1
Non-paid Artists: 100
Budget: $305,000
Income Sources: Gate; Sale of food & drink; Sponsors
Performs At: 40 Acre Park, One 1800 Seat Theatre & One 300 Seat Theatre
Affiliations: TFEA; TCA; City of Harlingen
Annual Attendance: 30,000
Facility Category: Multi-Venue; Indoor & Outdoor Theaters

5525 HILL COLLEGE
Box 619
Hillsboro, TX 76645
Phone: 254-582-2555
Fax: 254-582-7591
Management:
Music Coordinator: Philip Lowe
Budget: $10,000

5526 DA CAMERA OF HOUSTON
1427 Branard
Houston, TX 77006
Phone: 713-524-7601
Fax: 713-524-4148
Toll-free: 800-233-2226
e-mail: mlaleskie@decamara.com
Web Site: www.dacamera.com
Management:
Artistic Director: Sarah Rothenberg
Executive Director: Mary Lou Aleskie

Founded: 1987
Specialized Field: Chamber Music/Jazz
Paid Staff: 10
Paid Artists: 100
Budget: $1,200,000
Performs At: Cullen Theater; Wortham Center

5527 HOUSTON INTERNATIONAL FESTIVAL
7413-B Westview Drive
Houston, TX 77055
Phone: 713-654-8808
Fax: 713-654-1719
e-mail: info@hif.org
Web Site: ifest.org
Officers:
President/COO: Dr. James Austin
Mission: To sponsor a 10-day cultural celebration in an urban setting, focusing on a different country every year.
Founded: 1966
Specialized Field: Dance; Vocal Music; Instrumental Music; Festivals
Status: Professional; Nonprofit
Income Sources: Cultural Arts Council of Houston; Houston Convention & Visitors Center
Organization Type: Educational; Sponsoring

5528 HOUSTON INTERNATIONAL JAZZ FESTIVAL
PO Box 8031
Houston, TX 77288-8031
Phone: 713-839-7000
Fax: 713-839-8266
e-mail: jazzed@jazzeducation.org
Web Site: www.jazzeducation.org
Management:
Festival Director: Richard Dabon
Founded: 1990
Specialized Field: Performing Series
Paid Staff: 4
Volunteer Staff: 125
Paid Artists: 19

5529 HOUSTON SHAKESPEARE FESTIVAL
School of Theatre
University of Houston
Houston, TX 77204-5071
Phone: 713-743-3003
Fax: 713-749-1420
Web Site: www.hfac.uh.edu/theatre/hsf.htm
Management:
Producing Director: Sidney L Berger
Secretary: Sandy Judice
Business Administrator: Jerry Aven
Academic Advisor: Molly Dean
Lighting Designer: John Gow
Scene Shop Forman: Drew Hoovler
Costume Production Supervisor: Toni Lovaglia
Technical Director: Mo Tuttle
Mission: To provide classical theater at no cost to citizens of Houston and surrounding areas.
Founded: 1975
Specialized Field: Theater; Festivals
Status: Professional; Nonprofit
Income Sources: University of Houston

All listings are in alphabetical order by state, then city, then organization within the city.

Performs At: Miller Outdoor Theatre
Organization Type: Performing

5530 HOUSTON'S ANNUAL ASIAN-AMERICAN FESTIVAL

1714 Tannehill Drive
Houston, TX 77008
Phone: 713-861-8273
Fax: 713-861-3450
Management:
    Festival Director: Glenda Joe
Mission: Promote, preserve, present Asian cultural arts.
Founded: 1980
Specialized Field: Music, Dance, Hteatre, Puppetry
Paid Staff: 1
Volunteer Staff: 50
Paid Artists: 1600

5531 IMMANUEL & HELEN OLSHAN TEXAS MUSIC FESTIVAL

120 Scholl of Music Building
Houston, TX 77204-4017
Phone: 713-743-3167
Fax: 713-743-3391
e-mail: tmf@uh.edu
Web Site: www.uh.edu/music/tmf
Management:
    Executive Director: Alan Austin
Mission: The Texas Music Festival is an orchestral training program for talented young musicians ages 16-30. Performs four orchestral programs under internationally recognized conductors.
Founded: 1990
Specialized Field: Classical Music
Performs At: Cythia Woods Mitchell Pavilion
Annual Attendance: 7,000

5532 JEWISH COMMUNITY CENTER OF HOUSTON

5601 S Braeswood
Houston, TX 77096
Phone: 713-729-3200
Fax: 713-551-7223
Web Site: www.jcchouston.org
Management:
    Executive VP: Jerry Wische
Mission: To offer education, leisure activities and recreation to Southwest Houston; to promote the appreciation of theatre.
Founded: 1935
Specialized Field: Dance; Vocal Music; Instrumental Music; Theater; Festivals
Status: Nonprofit
Paid Staff: 50
Income Sources: Texas Nonprofit Theatre; National Council of Jewish Theatres
Performs At: Jewish Community Center; Kaplan Theatre; IW Marks Theatre Center; Joe Frank Theatre
Facility Category: Proscenium Theatre; Black Box Theatre
Type of Stage: Proscenium; Thrust
Seating Capacity: 330; 130

Organization Type: Performing; Educational; Sponsoring

5533 JONES HALL FOR THE PERFORMING ARTS

615 Louisiana Avenue
Houston, TX 77002
Phone: 713-227-3974
Web Site: www.ci.houston.tx.us/cef/jones.html
Management:
    Manager: Vivian Montejano
    Director: Gerald J Tollett
Opened: 1966

5534 SHEPHERD SCHOOL OF MUSIC CONCERT SERIES

Rice University
6100 Main Street
Houston, TX 77005
Phone: 713-348-4933
Fax: 713-348-5317
e-mail: littman@rice.edu
Web Site: www.rice.edu/music
Management:
    Concert Manager: Tom Littman
Founded: 1975
Performs At: Stude Concert Hall
Seating Capacity: 1000
Year Built: 1991
Rental Contact: Tom Littman

5535 SOCIETY FOR THE PERFORMING ARTS

615 Louisiana
Suite 100
Houston, TX 77002
Phone: 713-227-5134
Fax: 713-223-8301
e-mail: mattox@spahouston.org
Web Site: www.spahouston.org
Officers:
    Executive Director: Hoyt T Mattox
    Director Development: Chree Boydstun
    Director Marketing: Lynda Sanders
    Director Operations: June Christensen
    Chairman: Charles Davidson
    President: Stephen Trauber
Management:
    Executive Director: Sally Tyler
    Director Development: Priscilla Larson
    Director Marketing: Lynda Sanders
    Director Operations: June Christensen
    Director Ticketing Services: Greg Brown
Mission: To present the world's best in performing arts, whether dance, music or theatre.
Opened: 1966
Specialized Field: Modern; Mime; Ballet; Jazz; Ethnic; Folk
Status: Professional; Nonprofit
Budget: $2,500,000 - $4,000,000
Income Sources: Sales; Contributions
Performs At: Jones Hall; Wortham Theatre Center
Affiliations: ISPA; Arts Presenters; Dance USA

Annual Attendance: 50,000-60,0000
Type of Stage: Sprung Wood
Seating Capacity: 2912
Year Built: 1966
Year Remodeled: 1996
Cost: $9,000,000
Organization Type: Sponsoring

5536 UNIVERSITY OF ST. THOMAS GUEST RECITALS
3800 Montrose
Houston, TX 77006
Phone: 713-525-3560
Fax: 713-942-5912
Management:
   Department Coordinator: Sue Young
Mission: Enrichment for students, faculty and community.
Founded: 1947
Paid Staff: 1
Paid Artists: 30
Budget: $10,000-20,000

5537 HILL COUNTRY ARTS FOUNDATION
Highway 39
PO Box 176
Ingram, TX 78025
Phone: 830-367-5120
Fax: 830-367-5725
Management:
   Executive Director: Lane Tait
   Theatre Director: Susan Balentine
Mission: Promoting the performing and visual arts.
Founded: 1958
Specialized Field: Dance; Vocal Music; Instrumental Music; Theater
Status: Nonprofit
Paid Staff: 75
Income Sources: American Association of Community Theatres; Texas Nonprofit Theatre
Performs At: Outdoor Amphitheatre
Organization Type: Performing; Educational

5538 IRVING COMMUNITY CONCERT ASSOCIATION
3333 N Macarthur Boulevard
Suite 300
Irving, TX 75062
Phone: 972-252-7558
Fax: 972-570-4962
Web Site: www.ci.irving.tx.us
Officers:
   Chairman: Kim Dennis
   Vice-Chairman: Vanessa Bell
   Secretary: Laura Sanner
Management:
   Executive Director: Richard Huff
   Assistant Director: Rosie Meng
   Technical Theater Coordinator: Ross Moroney
   Box Office Manager: Andy Pate
   Director Marketing/Publications: Jo Trizila
Founded: 1956
Specialized Field: Dance; Vocal Music; Instrumental Music; Theater

Status: Nonprofit
Income Sources: Community Concerts
Organization Type: Sponsoring

5539 KERRVILLE FESTIVALS
Quiet Valley Ranch
PO Box 291466
Kerrville, TX 78029
Phone: 830-257-3600
Fax: 830-257-8680
e-mail: info@kerrville-music.com
Web Site: www.kerrvillefolkfestival.com
Management:
   Producer: Dalis Allen
Mission: To offer recordings, workshops and music festivals, featuring regional national and international artists and emphasizing acoustic musicians and songwriters.
Founded: 1972
Specialized Field: Songwriters Festival
Status: Professional; Commercial
Paid Staff: 3
Volunteer Staff: 600
Paid Artists: 100
Income Sources: Texas Festivals Association; Texas Music Association
Performs At: Festival Outdoor Theater
Organization Type: Performing

5540 KERRVILLE FOLK FESTIVAL
PO Box 291466
Kerrville, TX 78029
Phone: 830-257-3600
Fax: 830-257-8680
Toll-free: 800-435-8429
e-mail: staff@kerrville-music.com
Web Site: www.kerrville-music.com
Management:
   Producer: Rod Kennedy
Founded: 1972
Specialized Field: Songwriters Festival

5541 KILGORE COMMUNITY CONCERT ASSOCIATION
PO Box 47
Kilgore, TX 75663-0047
Phone: 903-984-4433
Fax: 903-984-1101
Officers:
   President: WS Morris
Budget: $20,000-35,000

5542 TEXAS SHAKESPEARE FESTIVAL
Kilgore College
1100 Broadway
Kilgore, TX 75662
Mailing Address: PO Box 2788, Kilgore, TX. 75663
Phone: 903-983-8117
Fax: 903-983-8124
e-mail: info@texasshakespeare.co
Web Site: www.texasshakespeare.com
Management:
   Artistic Director: Raymond Caldwell

Managing Director: John Dodd
Founded: 1986
Status: Non-Equity; Nonprofit
Season: June - July
Type of Stage: Flexible
Stage Dimensions: 30' x 30'
Seating Capacity: 240

5543 LUBBOCK ARTS ALLIANCE

2109 Broadway
Lubbock, TX 79401
Phone: 806-744-2787
Fax: 806-744-2790
e-mail: arts@nts-online.net
Web Site: www.lubbockarts.org
Officers:
President: Robby Vestal
Festival Chairman: Meredith McAlister
Management:
Executive Director: Libby Camp
Project Director: Brooke Witcher
Paid Staff: 2
Volunteer Staff: 250
Non-paid Artists: 300
Budget: $10,000-20,000
Income Sources: Grants; Corporate Sponsors
Performs At: Lubbock Memorial Civic Center

5544 LUBBOCK CHRISTIAN UNIVERSITY

5601 W 19th Street
Lubbock, TX 79407-2099
Phone: 806-720-7726
Fax: 806-720-7255
Web Site: lcu.edu
Management:
Dean Hancock College: Dr. E Don Williams
Chairman/Communication/Fine Arts: Dr. Michelle Kraff
Assistant Professor of Music: Laurie Doyle
Assistant Professor Music: Philip Camp
Professor Music: Dr. Ruth Holmes
Founded: 1957
Specialized Field: Music, Art, Theatre
Paid Staff: 6
Budget: $10,000
Type of Stage: Proscenium
Stage Dimensions: 35x20
Seating Capacity: 1,200
Year Built: 1967

5545 TEXAS TECH UNIVERSITY ARTISTS & SPEAKERS

PO Box 42031
TTU
Lubbock, TX 79409-2031
Phone: 806-742-3621
Fax: 806-742-0655
e-mail: campusactivitiesinvolvement@ttu.edu
Web Site: www.uc.ttu.edu
Management:
Activities/Involvement Coordinator: Nicole Kelly

5546 MARSHALL REGIONAL ARTS COUNCIL

2501 E End Boulevard
PO Box C
Marshall, TX 75671-3003
Phone: 903-935-4484
Fax: 903-927-2132
e-mail: arts@marshallartscouncil.org
Web Site: www.marshallartscouncil.org
Management:
Interim Executive Director: Geraldine Mautha n
Administrative Assistant: Joyce Weekly
Mission: Encouraging and supporting the performing arts in the East Texas area.
Founded: 1979
Specialized Field: Dance; Vocal Music; Instrumental Music; Theater; Festivals; Grand Opera
Status: Professional; Nonprofit
Paid Staff: 2
Volunteer Staff: 5
Budget: $100,000
Income Sources: Association of Performing Arts Presenters; National Association of Local Arts Agencies; Texas Arts Council; Country Music Association
Performs At: Marshall Theater at the Civic Center
Type of Stage: Proscenium
Stage Dimensions: 78 x 57
Seating Capacity: 1600
Year Built: 1984
Year Remodeled: 2001
Cost: 1.5 Million
Organization Type: Educational; Sponsoring

5547 MCALLEN PERFORMING ARTS

PO Box 790
McAllen, TX 78505
Phone: 956-631-2545
Fax: 956-631-8571
Management:
Executive Director: Genevia Crow
Mission: To provide the public with professional touring theatre productions and entertainment not available through local agencies.
Specialized Field: Vocal Music; Theater; Broadway Musicals
Status: Professional; Nonprofit
Performs At: McAllen Civic Center
Organization Type: Performing; Touring

5548 RIO GRANDE VALLEY INTERNATIONAL MUSIC FESTIVAL

PO Box 2315
McAllen, TX 78502
Phone: 956-618-6085
Officers:
Chairman: Dean R PhD Canty
Vice Chairman: Joy Judin
Secretary/Treasurer: Carol Edrington
Financial Secretary: Mildred Erhart
Mission: To present a major symphony orchestra annually, in varied concerts for students and adults, with emphasis on education of young listeners.
Founded: 1960

Specialized Field: Dance; Vocal Music; Instrumental Music; Festivals; Grand Opera
Status: Nonprofit
Paid Staff: 14
Performs At: McAllen International Civic Center
Organization Type: Performing; Touring; Educational; Presenting

5549 STEPHEN F AUSTIN UNIVERSITY VISUAL & PERFORMING ARTS

Box 13022 SFA
Nacogdoches, TX 75962
Phone: 409-468-2801
Fax: 409-468-1168
e-mail: rberry@sfasu.edu
Web Site: www.finearts.sfasu.edu
Budget: $60,000-150,000

5550 ADVENTURES WITH THE ARTS

602 Motley Drive
Overton, TX 75684-1021
Phone: 903-834-6234
Fax: 903-834-3574
e-mail: awamwc@aol.com
Budget: $35,000-60,000

5551 PITTSBURG/CAMP COUNTY ARTS COUNCIL

Box 72
Pittsburg, TX 75686
Phone: 903-856-6653
Budget: $35,000-60,000

5552 INTERNATIONAL FESTIVAL INSTITUTE AT ROUND TOP

PO Box 89
Round Top, TX 78954-0089
Phone: 979-249-3129
Fax: 979-249-5078
e-mail: alaind@festivalhill.org
Web Site: www.festivalhill.org
Management:
  Artistic Director: James Dick
  Managing Director: Richard Royall
  Program Director: Alain Declert
Performs At: Festival Concert Hall
Seating Capacity: 1,100

5553 ANGELO STATE UNIVERSITY

PO Box 11027
San Angelo, TX 76909
Phone: 915-942-2062
Fax: 915-942-2354
e-mail: program@angelo.edu
Web Site: www.angelo.edu/org/ucpc/
Management:
  Assistant Director Programming: Rick E Greig
  Assistant Program Director: Amy Horridge
Mission: The Arts Committee of the University Center Program Council presents performing and visual arts to the ASU and San Angelo communities.
Budget: $20,000-35,000

5554 CACTUS JAZZ & BLUES FESTIVAL

PO Box 2477
San Angelo, TX 76902
Phone: 915-653-6793
Fax: 915-658-6036
e-mail: sacac@wcc.net
Web Site: www.sanangeloarts.com

5555 ALAMO CITY PERFORMING ARTS ASSOCIATION

12915 Jones Maltsberger
Suite 200
San Antonio, TX 78247
Phone: 210-495-2787
Fax: 210-495-0872
e-mail: saspa@aol.com
Management:
  Executive Director: Nancy Grossenbacher
  Artistic Director: Scott Conway
Mission: To offer the best in music, both national and international, as well as theatre, dance and music to San Antonio year-round.
Founded: 1978
Specialized Field: Dance; Vocal Music; Instrumental Music; Theater; Festivals
Status: Nonprofit
Budget: $50,000
Income Sources: TCA; National Endowment for the Arts; City of San Antonio; Private Donations
Performs At: Theaters
Annual Attendance: 10,000
Organization Type: Sponsoring
Resident Groups: Alamo City Dance Company

5556 ARTS SAN ANTONIO

222 E Houston
Suite 630
San Antonio, TX 78205
Phone: 210-226-2891
Fax: 210-226-1981
e-mail: Frank@ArtsSanAntonio.com
Web Site: www.artsSanAntonio.com
Officers:
  Chairman: Tony Novoa
  President: Frank Villani
Mission: To offer theatre, music, ethnic dance, opera, ballet and family performances; to provide outreach programs.
Founded: 1992
Specialized Field: Multi-disciplinary
Paid Staff: 4
Paid Artists: 50
Budget: One million
Income Sources: Ticket sales - concession sales - in school workshops and grants
Performs At: Multiple
Affiliations: SWPAP; ISPA; Association of Performing Arts Presenters
Annual Attendance: 40,000
Seating Capacity: 400 - 5,000

5557 CARVER CULTURAL CENTER

226 N Hackberry
San Antonio, TX 78202

Phone: 210-207-7211
Fax: 210-207-4412
Web Site: www.thecarver.org
Officers:
   Chairperson: Prenza Woods
Management:
   Director: Desiree K Jordan
   Corporate Managere/Foundation Rel: Annalisa Peace
   Education Director: Roland Mazuca
   Public Information Officer: Sten Spence
Specialized Field: African American Visual and Performing Arts
Paid Staff: 20
Volunteer Staff: 50
Paid Artists: 15
Budget: $400,000-1,000,000
Annual Attendance: 50,000
Facility Category: Theatre and Arts School
Type of Stage: Proscenium
Seating Capacity: 640
Year Built: 1929
Year Remodeled: 2000
Rental Contact: 210-207-7215 Leticia Velazquez

5558 JAZZ'SALIVE

950 E Hildebrand
San Antonio, TX 78212
Phone: 210-207-3000
Fax: 210-207-3045
e-mail: kirvin@ci.sat.tx.us
Web Site: www.ci.sat.tx.us/sapar
Management:
   Director: Lila Cockrell
   Stage Manager: Bill Drain
Founded: 1984

5559 TUESDAY MUSICAL CLUB ARTIST SERIES

5410 Pawtucket Drive
San Antonio, TX 78230
Phone: 210-366-2464
Fax: 210-342-7748
Officers:
   Booking Chairman: Mrs. Harold Cockburn
Budget: $20,000-35,000
Income Sources: Tickets
Annual Attendance: 1,000
Facility Category: Chruch

5560 SOUTHWEST TEXAS STATE UNIVERSITY ARTS SERIES

Dance Department
San Marcos, TX 78666
Phone: 512-245-2194
Fax: 512-245-8181
e-mail: jwli@swt.edu
Officers:
   Artist Series Committee Chair: LeAnne Smith-Stedman
   Assistan Chair: Cary Michaels
Budget: $60,000-150,000

5561 TEXAS LUTHERAN UNIVERSITY CULTURAL ARTS EVENTS

1000 W Court
Seguin, TX 78155
Phone: 830-372-8180
Fax: 830-372-8096
Management:
   Jackson Auditorium Director: Susan Rinn
Budget: $20,000-35,000

5562 AUSTIN COLLEGE COMMUNITY SERIES

900 N Grand
Suite 61602
Sherman, TX 75090-4440
Phone: 903-813-2251
Fax: 903-813-2273
e-mail: jhicks@austinc.edu
Management:
   Manager: Joe Hicks
Founded: 1966
Paid Staff: 2
Volunteer Staff: 12
Budget: $35,000-60,000
Performs At: Wynne Chapel
Affiliations: AAAP
Annual Attendance: 7,000

5563 CROSS TIMBERS FINE ARTS COUNCIL

PO Box 1172
378 W Long Street
Stephenville, TX 76401
Phone: 254-965-6190
Fax: 254-965-6186
e-mail: ctfac@our-town.com
Web Site: www.our-town.com/ctfac/
Management:
   Executive Director: Debbie Reynolds
Budget: $60,000-150,000
Performs At: Clyde H. Wells Fine Arts Center

5564 TARLETON STATE UNIVERSITY STUDENT PROGRAMMING

Tarleton Station
Box T-0670
Stephenville, TX 76402
Phone: 254-968-9490
Fax: 254-968-9492
e-mail: spa@tarelton.edu
Management:
   Student Activities Coordinator: Donna Strohmeyer

5565 TEXARKANA REGIONAL ARTS & HUMANITIES COUNCIL

PO Box 1711
221 Main Street
Texarkana, TX 75504
Phone: 903-792-8681
Fax: 903-793-8510
e-mail: artsinfo@trahc.org
Web Site: www.trahc.org
Management:

Executive Director: Ruth Ellen Whitt
Budget: $60,000-150,000
Performs At: Perot theatre
Year Built: 1924
Year Remodeled: 1980

5566 TOMBALL REGIONAL ARTS COUNCIL

PO Box 1321
Tomball, TX 77377-1321
Phone: 713-351-2787
Officers:
President: Kathi Truex
Management:
Executive Director: Harriet Fether

5567 TYLER COMMUNITY CONCERT ASSOCIATION

PO Box 131673
Tyler, TX 75713-1673
Phone: 903-592-6266
Officers:
President: Gini Rainey
Budget: $35,000-60,000

5568 UNIVERSITY OF TEXAS AT TYLER

3900 University Boulevard
Tyler, TX 75701
Phone: 903-566-7250
Fax: 903-566-7287
e-mail: tallen@mail.uttyl.edu
Management:
Chairman Music Department: Dr. John Webb
Assistant: Gail Andrews
Budget: $35,000-60,000
Performs At: Fine & Performing Arts Center

5569 UVALDE ARTS COUNCIL

104 W North Street
Uvalde, TX 78801
Phone: 830-278-4184
Fax: 830-278-1658
e-mail: Esther@peppersnet.com
Officers:
President: Carol Kirlcham
VP: Michael Box
Treasurer: Esther Trevino
Management:
Managing Director: Esther Trevino
Founded: 1981
Paid Staff: 3
Volunteer Staff: 15
Budget: $20,000 - $30,000
Income Sources: memberships, ticket sales
Performs At: Grand Opera House
Annual Attendance: 14,000
Facility Category: Performing Arts & Presenter
Seating Capacity: 370
Year Built: 1891
Year Remodeled: 1981
Cost: 650,000

5570 CULTURAL COUNCIL OF VICTORIA

PO Box 1758
Victoria, TX 77902-1758
Phone: 361-572-2787
Fax: 361-572-6739
e-mail: leee@icsi.net
Web Site: www.ccvtx.org
Management:
Executive Director: LeOlive Rogge
Founded: 1981
Paid Staff: 3
Volunteer Staff: 200
Budget: $10,000
Facility Category: Victoria College Auditorium

5571 VICTORIA FINE ARTS ASSOCIATION

PO Box 1393
Victoria, TX 77902
Phone: 361-578-4564
Management:
Artistic Director: Carol Baker
Budget: $35,000-60,000

5572 BAYLOR UNIVERSITY DISTINGUISHED ARTIST SERIES

Box 97408
Baylor University, School of Music
Waco, TX 76798
Phone: 254-710-1162
Fax: 254-710-1191
e-mail: Music_School@baylor.edu
Web Site: www.baylor.edu
Management:
Distinguished Artist Series Manager: Kathy Johnson
Budget: $20,000-35,000
Performs At: Jones Concert Hall; Roxy Grove Hall

5573 WHARTON COUNTY JUNIOR COLLEGE FINE ARTS SERIES

911 Boling Highway
Wharton, TX 77488
Phone: 979-532-4560
Web Site: www.wcjc.cc.tx.us
Management:
Head Music Department: Phil Hart
Budget: $10,000
Performs At: Horton Foote Theatre

5574 MIDWESTERN STATE UNIVERSITY: ARTIST LECTURE SERIES

3410 Taft Boulevard
CSC Room 104
Wichita Falls, TX 76308
Phone: 940-397-4291
Fax: 940-397-4938
e-mail: jane.leishner@mwsu.edu
Management:
Associate VP for Student Affairs: Jane Leishner
Budget: $10,000-20,000

Utah

**5575 SOUTHERN UTAH UNIVERSITY
SUMMER EVENING CONCERTS**
Hunter Conference Center
Southern Utah University
Cedar City, UT 84720
Phone: 435-586-5483
Fax: 435-865-8087
e-mail: bingham@suu.edu
Web Site: www.suu.edu/ced/specialprojects/
Management:
   Manager: Marla Bingham
Budget: $10,000-20,000
Performs At: Randall Jones Performing Arts Theatre

5576 UTAH SHAKESPEAREAN FESTIVAL
351 W Center Street
Cedar City, UT 84720
Phone: 435-586-7880
Fax: 435-865-8003
Toll-free: 800-752-9849
e-mail: bahr@suu.edu
Web Site: www.bard.org
Officers:
   Development Director: Jyl Shuler
   Marketing Director: Donna Law
   Education Director: Michael Bahr
   Publications Director: Bruce Lee
Management:
   Executive Producer: Fred C Adams
   Managing Director: R Scott Phillips
   Producing Artistic Director: Cameron Harvey
   Associate Artistic Director: J R Sullivan
   Marketing Director: Donna Law
   Production Manager: Ran Inkel
   Director Plays-in-Progress: George Judy
   Education Director: Michael Don Bahr
   Publications Director: Bruce Lee
Mission: To present six classic and Shakespearean works
in repertory each summer.
Founded: 1961
Specialized Field: Theater
Status: Professional; Nonprofit
Paid Staff: 25
Volunteer Staff: 250
Paid Artists: 200
Budget: $5 Million
Income Sources: Box Office Sales; Contributed Income;
Endowment Income; Merchandise Sales
Season: June - August
Performs At: Adams Memorial Stage; Randall L. Jones
Theatre; University Stage
Affiliations: USA; SSD&C; Actors' Equity Association;
LORT; TCG
Annual Attendance: 155,000
Facility Category: Outdoor/Indoor
Type of Stage: Thrust; Proscenium
Stage Dimensions: 50Wx30D; 22Hx42Wx25D;
18Hx44Wx39D
Seating Capacity: 887; 769; 981
Year Remodeled: 1989
Rental Contact: Production Manager Ray Inkel
Organization Type: Performing; Resident; Educational

**5577 CACHE VALLEY CENTER FOR THE
ARTS**
43 S Main Street
Logan, UT 84321-4535
Phone: 435-753-6518
Fax: 435-753-1232
e-mail: lmiles@cache.net
Management:
   Executive Director: Lisette Miles
Founded: 1989
Paid Staff: 15
Volunteer Staff: 120
Budget: $900,000
Income Sources: City and County; Foundations;
Corporations and Individuals
Facility Category: Proscenium Theatre
Stage Dimensions: 36'x32'
Seating Capacity: 1,100
Year Built: 1923
Year Remodeled: 1993
Rental Contact: Mary Shope
Resident Groups: Utah Festival Opera, Alliance for the
Varied Arts, Paint Utah

**5578 UTAH STATE UNIVERSITY
PERFORMING ARTS SERIES**
Taggart Student Center, UMC-01
Logan, UT 84322-0105
Phone: 435-797-1732
Fax: 435-797-2571
Management:
   Student Activities Director: Randy Jensen
Budget: $150,000-400,000
Performs At: Chase Fine Arts Center

5579 WASSERMANN PIANO FESTIVAL
Utah State University, Music Department
4015 Old Main Hill
Logan, UT 84322-4015
Phone: 435-797-3257
Fax: 435-797-1862
e-mail: dhirst@hass.usu.edu
Management:
   Director: R Dennis Hirst

5580 MORMON MIRACLE PAGEANT
PO Box O
Manti, UT 84642
Phone: 435-835-3000
Management:
   Artistic Director: Macksene Rux
Mission: Portraying the religious history of the
Latter-Day Saints and relating it to national events.
Founded: 1967
Specialized Field: Theater
Status: Non-Professional; Nonprofit
Performs At: Manti Temple Grounds Amphitheatre
Organization Type: Performing; Resident

5581 CANYONLANDS ARTS COUNCIL
59 S Main Street
#236
Moab, UT 84532

Phone: 435-259-2742
Fax: 435-259-2418
Management:
   Director: Theresa King
Budget: $10,000-20,000

5582   MOAB MUSIC FESTIVAL

59 S Main
#3
Moab, UT 84532
Phone: 435-259-7003
Fax: 435-259-2418
e-mail: info@moabmusicfest.org
Web Site: www.moabmusicfest.org
Management:
   Music Director: Michael Barrett
   Director Artistic: Leslie Tomkins
   Admnistrative Director: Theresa King
Mission: Produce music festival and provide education outreach program to community schools.
Founded: 1991
Specialized Field: Classical Chamber Music
Paid Staff: 8
Volunteer Staff: 1

5583   WEBER STATE UNIVERSITY CULTURAL AFFAIRS

1904 University Circle
Ogden, UT 84408-1904
Phone: 801-626-6570
Fax: 801-626-7422
e-mail: dstern@weber.eduu
Management:
   Office Cultural Affairs Director: Diane Stern
Budget: $60,000-150,000
Seating Capacity: 1800

5584   FIDELITY INVESTMENTS PARK CITY JAZZ FESTIVAL

PO Box 680720
Park City, UT 84068-0720
Phone: 435-940-1362
Fax: 435-940-1464
Toll-free: 800-453-1360
e-mail: info@parkcityjazz.com
Web Site: www.parkcityjazz.com
Officers:
   Founder: Lew Fine
   Founder: Arlene Fine
   Interim Chairman: Martin Marmor
Management:
   Interim Executive Festival Director: Mike Andrews
   Assistant to Director: Janell James
Mission: Is committed to promoting jazz music through an annual showcase of national, regional, and local jazz musicians.
Founded: 1998
Specialized Field: Jazz Music; Education
Status: Nonprofit
Paid Staff: 2
Volunteer Staff: 186
Paid Artists: 11
Annual Attendance: 15,00
Seating Capacity: 5000

5585   PARK CITY INTERNATIONAL MUSIC FESTIVAL

1420 W Meadowloop Road
Park City, UT 84098
Phone: 435-649-5309
Fax: 435-615-1719
e-mail: lharlow@pcmusicfestival.com
Web Site: ww.pcmusicfestival.com

5586   BRIGHAM YOUNG UNIVERSITY PERFORMING ARTS SERIES

F-315 Harris Fine Arts Center
Provo, UT 84602
Phone: 801-378-5203
Fax: 801-378-8008
Officers:
   Director: Jon Hollsman
Management:
   Director: Jon Hollsman
Mission: A varied production and concert season in support of academic programs in music, dance and theatre.
Founded: 1875
Specialized Field: Dance; Vocal Music; Instrumental Music; Theater; Grand Opera
Status: Professional; Semi-Professional; Nonprofit
Paid Staff: 11
Budget: $60,000-150,000
Income Sources: Association of Performing Arts Presenters; Western Alliance of Arts Administrators
Performs At: Harris Fine Arts Center; Brigham Young University
Facility Category: Concert hall
Type of Stage: Proscenium w/hydralic pit
Stage Dimensions: 60 x 45
Seating Capacity: 1960
Year Built: 1963
Organization Type: Performing; Touring; Educational; Sponsoring

5587   DIXIE COLLEGE CELEBRITY CONCERT SERIES

225 S 700 E
Saint George, UT 84770
Phone: 435-652-7994
Fax: 435-656-4026
e-mail: gbunker@dixie.edu
Web Site: www.dixie.edu
Management:
   Director: Gail Bunker
Founded: 1958
Specialized Field: Multi-discipline Performance Arts
Paid Staff: 1
Volunteer Staff: 12
Paid Artists: 125
Budget: $150,000-200,000
Income Sources: Season Memberships; Ticket Sales; Grants; Donations; Endowment Income
Performs At: Avenna Center Cox Auditorium
Annual Attendance: 10,800
Facility Category: Theatre
Type of Stage: Proscenium
Seating Capacity: 1,200
Year Built: 1980

5588 DELTA CENTER
301 W South Temple
Salt Lake City, UT 84101
Phone: 801-325-2000
Fax: 801-325-2516
Web Site: www.deltacenter.com
Management:
   General Manager: Scott Williams
   VP Marketing: Jay Francis
   VP Event Services: Brent Allenbach
Specialized Field: Home of the Utah Jazz (NBA) and the
Utah Starzz (WNBA).
Seating Capacity: 19,911
Year Built: 1991

**5589 EASTERN ARTS INTERNATIONAL
DANCE THEATER**
PO Box 526362
Salt Lake City, UT 84152
Phone: 801-485-5824
e-mail: kstjohn@burgoyne.com
Web Site: www.easternartists.com
Officers:
   Dance Director: Katherine St John
   Music Director: Lloyd Miller
Management:
   Director: Katherine St. John
Mission: To promote time-honored traditions by offering
concerts, lectures, and workshops of cultures from Asia
and Eastern Europe.
Founded: 1960
Specialized Field: Ethnic
Status: Professional; Nonprofit
Paid Staff: 10
Income Sources: Western Alliance of Arts
Administrators; Society for Ethno-Musicology; Middle
East Studies Association; Society for Dance Ethnology
Organization Type: Performing; Educational;
Sponsoring

**5590 GINA BACHAUER INTERNATIONAL
PIANO COMPETITION & FESTIVAL**
138 W Broadway
Suite 220
Salt Lake City, UT 84101
Phone: 801-521-9200
Fax: 801-521-9202
e-mail: gina@bachauer.com
Web Site: www.bachauer.com
Management:
   Director: Dr. Paul C Pollei

5591 TEMPLE SQUARE CONCERT SERIES
LDS Church Office Building, 20th Floor
50 E North Temple
Salt Lake City, UT 84150
Phone: 801-240-3323
Fax: 801-240-1994
Management:
   Director: Iain B McKay
Performs At: Assembly Hall; Tabernacle at Temple
Square
Seating Capacity: 1200; 5500

5592 WESTMINSTER COLLEGE
1840 S 1300 E
Salt Lake City, UT 84105
Phone: 801-832-2435
Fax: 801-484-5579
e-mail: wccconcerts@rider.edu
Web Site: www.wcslc.edu/per_pages/
Management:
   Concert Series Director: Dr. Karlyn Bard
Budget: $10,000
Performs At: Jewett Center for the Performing Arts
Seating Capacity: 300

**5593 WORLD ARTS/NOON CONCERTS
SERIES**
PO Box 526362
Salt Lake City, UT 84152
Phone: 801-485-5824
Management:
   Contact: Lloyd Miller
Budget: $10,000

**5594 UTAH'S FESTIVAL OF THE AMERICAN
WEST**
4025 S Highway 89-91
Wellsville, UT 84339
Phone: 435-245-6050
Fax: 435-245-6052
Toll-free: 800-225-3378
e-mail: AWHC@cc.usu.edu
Web Site: www.americanwestcenter.org
Management:
   Executive Assistant: JoAnn Poulsen
Mission: Educate, entertain, and enlighten guests about
life from 1820-1920.
Founded: 1972
Paid Staff: 15
Volunteer Staff: 100
Paid Artists: 20
Non-paid Artists: 15

Vermont

5595 NEW ENGLAND BACH FESTIVAL
38 Walnut Street
Brattleboro, VT 05301
Phone: 802-257-4523
Fax: 802-254-7355
e-mail: info@bmcvi.org
Web Site: www.bmcvi.org
Management:
   Artistic Director: Blanche Honegger Moyse
   Managing Director: Zon Eastes
   Festival Coordinator: Beth Ann Betz
Founded: 1952

**5596 BURLINGTON DISCOVER JAZZ
FESTIVAL**
230 College Street
Burlington, VT 05401

Phone: 802-863-7992
Fax: 802-864-3927
e-mail: info@discoverjazz.com
Web Site: www.discoverjazz.com
Officers:
    Director Performing Arts: Andrea Rogers
Management:
    Director: Michael Bandelato
    Director Marketing/Development: Tara Perkins
    Chief Programming Officer: Arnie Malina
Mission: Offering the widest possible range of jazz and music educational programs; ticketed and free events.
Founded: 1984
Specialized Field: Vocal Music; Instrumental Music; Festivals
Status: Nonprofit
Paid Staff: 2
Volunteer Staff: 350
Budget: $300,000
Income Sources: Burlington City Arts; Flynn Center
Performs At: Multi-disciplinary
Annual Attendance: 45,000
Facility Category: city-wide (Burlington)
Organization Type: Performing; Educational; Sponsoring

5597 VERMONT MOZART FESTIVAL

110 Main Street
Burlington, VT 05401
Phone: 802-862-7352
Fax: 802-862-2201
Toll-free: 800-639-9097
Web Site: www.vtmozart.com/
Management:
    Executive Director: Laura Cole
    Associate Director: Regina Gonzales
Mission: To create opportunities for young people to appreciate and pursue excellence in music.
Founded: 1973
Specialized Field: Vocal Music; Instrumental Music; Festivals
Status: Professional; Nonprofit
Income Sources: Ticket sales, sponsorship, membership
Organization Type: Performing

5598 CASTLETON STATE COLLEGE PERFORMING ARTS SERIES

Castleton State College
Castleton, VT 05735
Phone: 802-468-5611
Fax: 802-468-1440
e-mail: mariko.hancock@castleton.edu
Web Site: www.csc.vsc.edu
Management:
    Fine Arts Center Coordinator: Mariko Hancock
Budget: $10,000-20,000

5599 GREEN MOUNTAIN FESTIVAL SERIES

PO Box 561
Chester, VT 05143
Phone: 802-875-4473
Fax: 802-875-3989
Management:
    Manager: Ann C. DiBernardo

Budget: $20,000-35,000

5600 MUSIC IN A GREAT SPACE

Saint Michael's College
Winooski Park
Colchester, VT 05439
Phone: 802-654-2508
Fax: 802-655-3680
Management:
    Music Director: Dr. William Tortolano

5601 ST. MICHAEL'S COLLEGE CONCERTS

St. Michael's College
Winooski Park
Colchester, VT 05439
Phone: 802-654-2508
Fax: 802-655-3680
Management:
    Music Director: Dr. William Tortolano
Budget: $10,000-20,000

5602 UNIVERSITY OF VERMONT: GEORGE BISHOP LANE SERIES

245 S Park Drive
Colchester, VT 05446-2501
Phone: 802-656-4455
Fax: 802-656-3891
e-mail: jambrose@zoo.uvm.edu
Web Site: www.uvm.edu/laneseries
Management:
    Director: Jane Ambrose
    Manager: Natalie Neuert
Founded: 1954
Specialized Field: Presenter
Volunteer Staff: 20
Budget: $500,000
Income Sources: Endowment; Ticket Sales; Fundraising
Performs At: Flynn Theatre

5603 DORSET THEATRE FESTIVAL

PO Box 510 Dorset
Dorset, VT 05251
Phone: 802-867-2223
Fax: 802-867-0144
e-mail: theatre@sover.net
Web Site: www.theatredirectories.com
Management:
    General Manager: Barbara Ax
    Artistic Director: John Nassicera
Founded: 1976
Specialized Field: Theater
Status: Professional; Nonprofit
Income Sources: Theatre Communications Group
Season: June-September
Performs At: Dorset Playhouse
Type of Stage: Proscenium
Seating Capacity: 218
Organization Type: Performing

5604 WAREBROOK CONTEMPORARY MUSIC FESTIVAL

276 Hillandale Road
Irasburg, VT 05845

Phone: 802-754-6631
Fax: 802-754-2562
e-mail: wcmf@sover.net
Web Site: www.warebrook.org
Management:
   Director: Sara Doncaster

5605 FESTIVAL OF THE ARTS
Southern Vermont Arts Center/West Coast
Manchester, VT 05254
Phone: 802-362-1405
Fax: 802-362-3274
Management:
   Executive Director: Christopher Madkour
Founded: 1929
Specialized Field: Vocal Music; Instrumental Music;
Festivals
Status: Professional; Nonprofit
Performs At: Southern Vermont Arts Center
Organization Type: Sponsoring

5606 MANCHESTER MUSIC FESTIVAL
PO Box 1165
58 Bonnet Street
Manchester, VT 05255
Phone: 802-362-1956
Fax: 802-362-0711
Toll-free: 800-639-5868
e-mail: mmf@vermontel.net
Web Site: www.mmfvt.org
Management:
   Managing Director: Diane Langevin
   Artistic Director: Michael Rudiakov
Mission: Educating young artists for a professional
career.
Founded: 1974
Specialized Field: Instrumental Music; Grand Opera;
Classical; Chamber
Status: Non-Professional; Nonprofit
Paid Staff: 2
Paid Artists: 15
Budget: $385,000
Income Sources: Ticket sales; contributions
Performs At: The Louise Arkell Pavilion
Annual Attendance: 4,000
Organization Type: Performing; Touring; Educational

5607 MANCHESTER MUSIC FESTIVAL
PO Box 1165
Manchester Center, VT 05255
Fax: 802-362-0711
Toll-free: 800-639-5868
Web Site: mmfvt.org
Management:
   Managing Director: Robyn Pruett
   Director: Ariel Rudiakov
Mission: To maintain a school for gifted instrumental
musicians; to offer festival concerts.
Founded: 1974
Specialized Field: Instrumental Music; Festivals
Status: Nonprofit
Paid Staff: 2
Volunteer Staff: 10
Paid Artists: 20

Non-paid Artists: 0
Performs At: Southern Vermont Arts Center
Seating Capacity: 460
Organization Type: Performing; Educational

5608 MIDDLEBURY COLLEGE CONCERT
SERIES
Middlebury College
Middlebury, VT 05753
Phone: 802-443-5307
Fax: 802-443-2084
Management:
   Director: Paul Nelson
Budget: $60,000-150,000
Performs At: Wright Theatre; Dance Performance Hall

5609 ONION RIVER ARTS COUNCIL:
CELEBRATION SERIES
41 Elm Street
Montpelier, VT 05602
Phone: 802-229-9408
Fax: 802-229-9408
e-mail: orac@together.net
Web Site: www.onionriverarts.org
Management:
   Executive Director: Diane Manion
Budget: $35,000-60,000

5610 YELLOW BARN MUSIC FESTIVAL
91 Old Route 5
Putney, VT 05346
Phone: 802-387-6637
Fax: 802-387-6637
Toll-free: 800-639-3819
e-mail: ybarn@sover.net
Web Site: www.yellowbarn.org
Officers:
   President: Douglas Cox
Management:
   Executive Director: Tova Malin
   Artistic Director: Seth Knopp
   Administrator: Maury McNaughton
Mission: To offer professional training and a performance
festival to talented young chamber artists.
Founded: 1969
Specialized Field: Chamber music
Status: Nonprofit
Paid Staff: 50
Volunteer Staff: 50+
Paid Artists: 22
Budget: $350,000
Income Sources: Private donations; Grants
Performs At: Concert Hall and touring events
Organization Type: Performing; Educational

5611 CHANDLER CENTER FOR THE ARTS
71-73 Main Street
Randolph, VT 05060
Phone: 802-728-9878
Fax: 802-728-4612
e-mail: chandler@innevi.com
Web Site: www.randolphvt.com
Officers:

President: Janet Watton
Management:
    Program Director: Rebecca B McMeekin
Mission: Providing opportunities to the community at large for artistic expression and educational pursuit by sponsoring and producing programs in the creative and performing arts in and for Chandler Music Hall.
Founded: 1978
Paid Staff: 2
Volunteer Staff: 50
Budget: $200,000
Income Sources: Individual and corporate donations; Grants; and Ticket sales
Annual Attendance: 13,000
Facility Category: Music hall and art gallery
Type of Stage: Proscenium
Stage Dimensions: 31'W x 20'H x 21'D
Seating Capacity: 589
Year Built: 1907
Rental Contact: Becky McMeekin

5612 CROSSROADS ARTS COUNCIL

39 E Center Street
Suite 3
Rutland, VT 05701
Phone: 802-775-5413
Fax: 802-747-3592
e-mail: CrossrdsW@aol.com
Web Site: www.crossroadsarts.com
Officers:
    President: Al Wakefield
    VP: Nina Keck Combs
    Secretary: Robert Rogan
    Treasurer: Kenneth McEwan
Management:
    Executive Director: Lequita P Vance-Watkins
    Executive Assistant: Lorraine M Record
    Office Assistant: Rebecca Combs-Ballard
Mission: To bring performing artists to the Rutland Region.
Paid Staff: 3
Budget: $225,000
Annual Attendance: 5,000+

5613 KILLINGTON MUSIC FESTIVAL

39 E Center Street
Rutland, VT 05701
Mailing Address: PO Box 386, Rutland, VT. 05702
Phone: 802-773-4003
Fax: 802-773-1168
e-mail: kmfest@sover.net
Web Site: www.killingtonmusicfestival.org
Management:
    Executive Director: Maria Fish
Mission: To present a series of summer chamber music concerts; To maintain a summer school to train aspiring musicians.
Founded: 1982
Specialized Field: Instrumental Music
Status: Nonprofit
Organization Type: Performing; Educational

5614 STOWE PERFORMING ARTS

1250 Waterbury Road
Stowe, VT 05672
Phone: 802-253-7792
Fax: 802-253-7140
e-mail: spa@stowearts.com
Web Site: www.stowearts.com
Management:
    Managing Director: Lynn Paparella
Mission: Stowe Performing Arts is a non-profit community organization with a volunteer Board of Directors dedicated to bringing high quality performances and opportunities for cultural enrichment through the Performing Arts to the community and surrounding areas.
Founded: 1976
Status: Nonprofit
Paid Staff: 1
Volunteer Staff: 15
Paid Artists: 10
Budget: $100,000
Income Sources: Donations and Ticket Sales
Performs At: Outdoor venue, Church, Ice Arena
Facility Category: Open Stage
Type of Stage: Wooden Platform
Stage Dimensions: 30'x40'
Seating Capacity: 2,200

5615 PENTANGLE COUNCIL ON THE ARTS AND THE WOODSTOCK TOWN HALL THEATRE

31 the Green
PO Box 172
Woodstock, VT 05091
Phone: 802-457-3981
Fax: 802-457-4972
e-mail: Pentarts@sover.net
Web Site: www.Pentangle Arts.org
Management:
    Executive Director: Sabrina Brown
Mission: To maintain an arts program of high quality for the enrichment of our community and schools.
Founded: 1973
Specialized Field: Mid Vermont and the Windsor Supervisory Union School District
Paid Staff: 3
Paid Artists: 35
Budget: $275,000
Income Sources: Annual Appeal; Membership; Endowment; Ticket Sales; Grants
Performs At: Town Hall Theatre; Little Theatre
Annual Attendance: 12,000
Facility Category: Theatre
Type of Stage: Proscenium
Seating Capacity: 400
Year Built: 1901
Year Remodeled: 1979
Rental Contact: Sabrina Brown

Virginia

5616 ALEXANDRIA RECITAL SERIES

5917 Berkshire Court
Alexandria, VA 22303-1632
Phone: 703-960-0616
Fax: 703-960-6691
e-mail: RecitalSeries@aol.com
Management:
    Program Director: Willis Bennett
Budget: $10,000
Performs At: The Lyceum

5617 INTERNATIONAL CHILDREN'S FESTIVAL

Arts Council of Fairfax
4022 Hummer Road
Annandale, VA 22003
Phone: 703-642-0862
Fax: 703-642-1773
e-mail: truemahon@artsfairfax.org
Web Site: www.artsfairfax.org
Officers:
    President/CEO: Toni Winters McMahon
Management:
    Performing Arts Director: Scott Fridy
Founded: 1971
Specialized Field: Dance; Vocal Music; Instrumental
Music; Theater; Festivals
Status: Professional; Nonprofit
Income Sources: Arts Council of Fairfax County, Inc.
Performs At: Wolf Trap Farm Park for the Performing
Arts
Annual Attendance: 30,000
Facility Category: Amphitheatre in a park
Seating Capacity: 4,000
Year Built: 1971
Organization Type: Performing; Resident; Sponsoring

5618 ARLINGTON CULTURAL AFFAIRS DIVISION

2700 S Lang Street
Arlington, VA 22206-3106
Phone: 703-228-6962
Fax: 703-228-6968
e-mail: jclari@co.arlington.va.us
Web Site: www.arlingtonarts.org
Management:
    Performing Arts Director: Jon Palmer Claridge
Budget: $60,000-150,000

5619 ARLINGTON'S ARTS AL FRESCO & THE INNOVATORS

2700 S Lang Street
Arlington, VA 22206
Phone: 703-228-6960
Fax: 703-228-6968
Management:
    Executive Director: Norma Kaplan
    Performing Arts Director: Jon Palmer Claridge
Budget: $60,000-150,000
Performs At: Thomas Jefferson Theatre; Ellipse Art
Center

5620 VIRGINIA TECH UNION LIVELY ARTS SEASON

Virginia Tech
325 Squires Student Center (0138)
Blacksburg, VA 24061
Phone: 540-231-5661
Fax: 540-231-7028
e-mail: pase@vt.edu
Web Site: www.vtu.org
Management:
    Student Activities Program Director: Jennifer
    MacDonald
Founded: 1969
Paid Staff: 1
Volunteer Staff: 20
Budget: $150,000-400,000
Income Sources: Ticket Sales; Student Activity Fees
Annual Attendance: 14,000
Facility Category: Auditorium
Type of Stage: Proscenium
Stage Dimensions: 58x34x32
Seating Capacity: 2,950
Year Built: 1935

5621 BRIDGEWATER COLLEGE LYCEUM SERIES

E College Street
Bridgewater, VA 22181
Phone: 540-828-5303
Fax: 540-828-5637
e-mail: jhopkins@bridgewater.edu
Web Site: www.bridgewater.edu
Management:
    Director: Jesse E Hopkins
Budget: $20,000-35,000
Performs At: Cole Hall

5622 ASHLAWN-HIGHLAND SUMMER FESTIVAL

1941 James Monroe Parkway
Charlottesville, VA 22902
Phone: 804-293-4500
Fax: 804-293-0736
e-mail: summerfestival@avenue.gen.va.us
Web Site: www.avenue.org/summerfestival
Management:
    General Director: Judith H Walker
Founded: 1978
Status: Non-Equity; Nonprofit
Paid Staff: 4
Volunteer Staff: 100
Paid Artists: 80
Non-paid Artists: 25
Season: June - August
Stage Dimensions: 24' x 16'
Seating Capacity: 450

5623 TUESDAY EVENING CONCERT SERIES

108 5th Street SE
Suite 205
Charlottesville, VA 22902

Phone: 434-244-9505
Fax: 434-244-9510
e-mail: kpellon@virginia.edu
Web Site: www.tecs.org
Management:
   Executive Director: Karen Pellon
Mission: Chamber music series with artists from around the world.
Founded: 1948
Specialized Field: Music
Status: Professional; Nonprofit
Paid Staff: 2
Paid Artists: 30
Budget: $100000+
Income Sources: Tickets; Advertising; Grants; Donations
Performs At: Concert Hall
Annual Attendance: 5,000
Facility Category: Concert Hall
Seating Capacity: 850
Year Built: 1896
Year Remodeled: 1995
Organization Type: Sponsoring

5624 JOHN TYLER COMMUNITY COLLEGE

John Tyler Community College
Chester, VA 23831
Phone: 804-594-1516
Fax: 804-796-4365
e-mail: cschofield@jt.cc.va.us
Management:
   Student Activities Specialist: Christine Schofield
Budget: $10,000

5625 ALLEGHANY HIGHLANDS ARTS COUNCIL/PERFORMING ARTS

PO Box 261
Covington, VA 24426
Phone: 540-962-6220
Fax: 540-962-4911
e-mail: ArtsCo@aol.com
Web Site: www.alleghanyhighlands.com/arts4all.html
Management:
   Executive Director: Tammy S Scruggs
Budget: $35,000-60,000
Performs At: Curfman Hall

5626 AVERETT UNIVERSITY CONCERT-LECTURE SERIES

420 W Main
Danville, VA 24541
Phone: 804-791-5621
Fax: 804-791-5819
e-mail: paul.bryant@averett.edu
Management:
   Dean of Students: Paul A Bryant
Budget: $10,000-20,000

5627 DANVILLE AREA ASSOCIATION FOR THE ARTS & HUMANITIES

435 Main Street
Danville, VA 24541

Mailing Address: PO Box 3581, Danville, VA. 24543-3581
Phone: 804-792-6965
Fax: 804-792-1307
e-mail: dwooten@mindspring.com
Web Site: www.danriverartalliance.com
Officers:
   President: John W Collins
Management:
   Executive Director: Alice Wooten
Founded: 1981
Paid Staff: 1
Budget: $35,000-60,000
Income Sources: Box office; Grants; Private donations
Annual Attendance: 5,500
Type of Stage: Proscenium
Stage Dimensions: 40x27
Seating Capacity: 1,119
Year Built: 1955

5628 EMORY & HENRY COLLEGE CONCERT SERIES

PO Box 947
Emory, VA 24327
Phone: 540-944-6846
Fax: 540-944-6259
e-mail: atcoulth@ehc.edu
Web Site: www.ehc.edu/inweb
Management:
   Arts Coordinator: Anita Coulthard
Mission: To provide cultural events that support the curriculum of the college.
Specialized Field: College arts organ
Paid Staff: 1
Paid Artists: 20
Non-paid Artists: 5
Budget: $20,000-35,000
Income Sources: College budget and grants
Performs At: Chapel, auditorium
Annual Attendance: 5,000
Facility Category: College campus, chapel and auditorium
Type of Stage: Proscenium
Seating Capacity: Chapel 500; auditorium - 300

5629 COLLEGE OF VISUAL AND PERFORMING ARTS

George Mason University
4400 University Drive, MSN 4C1
Fairfax, VA 22030-4444
Phone: 703-993-8877
Fax: 703-993-8883
e-mail: rdavi4@gmu.edu
Web Site: www.gmu.edu/cfa
Management:
   Dean: William Reeder
   Assistant Dean: Rick Davis
Budget: $400,000-1,000,000
Performs At: Harris Theatre
Facility Category: Performing Arts Hall
Type of Stage: Proscenium
Seating Capacity: 1,935

5630 GEORGE MASON UNIVERSITY PATRIOT CENTER
4400 University Drive
Fairfax, VA 22030
Phone: 703-993-3000
Fax: 703-993-3059
Web Site: www.sports-gmu.edu
Management:
Director: Jim Larsen

5631 FREDERICKSBURG MUSIC FESTIVAL
PO Box 7816
Fredericksburg, VA 22404
Phone: 540-374-5040
Fax: 540-368-1098
e-mail: fredfest@fls.infi.net
Web Site: www.fredfest.org
Management:
Executive Director: Susan Mullane
Mission: To foster excellence and diversity in the arts in Virginia and to bring world class arts events to the residents of the greater Fredericksburg area.
Founded: 1988
Specialized Field: Chamber Music; Pops; Big Band; Ethnic; Dance
Status: Nonprofit
Paid Staff: 3
Income Sources: Corporate & Individual Donations; Grants
Annual Attendance: 2,500+

5632 HAMPDEN-SYDNEY MUSIC FESTIVAL
Hampden-Sydney College
Box 25
Hampden-Sydney, VA 23943
Phone: 804-223-6304
Fax: 804-223-6399
Management:
Executive Director: James Kidd

5633 HAMPTON ARTS COMMISSION
4205 Victoria Boulevard
Hampton, VA 23669
Phone: 757-722-2787
Fax: 757-727-1621
Web Site: www.theamericantheatre.com
Management:
Director: Michael P Curry
Mission: Presenting and promoting the finest visual and performing arts.
Founded: 1987
Specialized Field: Dance; Vocal Music; Instrumental Music; Theater
Status: Professional
Income Sources: Association of Performing Arts Presenters
Performs At: American Theatre
Annual Attendance: 30,000
Facility Category: Theatre
Type of Stage: Procenium
Seating Capacity: 400
Year Built: 1908
Year Remodeled: 2000
Cost: $2.8 million

Organization Type: Performing; Educational; Sponsoring

5634 HAMPTON JAZZ FESTIVAL
PO Box 7309
Coliseum Drive
Hampton, VA 23666
Phone: 757-838-5650
Fax: 757-838-2595
Web Site: www.hamptonjazzfestival.com

5635 JAMES MADISON UNIVERSITY ENCORE SERIES
Harrison Hall A-104/MISC 2105
Harrisonburg, VA 22807
Phone: 540-568-6358
Fax: 540-568-3330
Toll-free: 877-201-7543
e-mail: weaverje@jmu.edu
Management:
Director: Jerry Weaver
Budget: $60,000-150,000
Affiliations: Association of Performing Arts Performers
Type of Stage: Proscenium
Stage Dimensions: 34 x 33
Seating Capacity: 1300

5636 SHENANDOAH VALLEY BACH FESTIVAL
Bach, EMU
1200 Park Road
Harrisonburg, VA 22802
Phone: 540-432-4367
Fax: 540-432-4622
e-mail: arancenab@emu.edu
Web Site: www.emu.edu/bach
Management:
Music Director/Conductor: Kenneth Nafziger
Bach Festival Coordinator: Beth Aracena
Mission: One week festival celebrating the music of Bach and another composer or geographical area.
Founded: 1993
Specialized Field: Performing Series

5637 MASTERWORKS FESTIVAL
PO Box 800
Haymarket, VA 22168
Fax: 703-753-0336
Toll-free: 888-836-2723
e-mail: cpaf@erols.com
Web Site: www.christianperformingart.org
Management:
Artistic Director: Dr. Patrick Kavanaugh
Music Director: Dr. James Kraft
Administrator: Dr. Richard Lambert
Dance Director: Robert Sturm
Mission: To train the next generation of Christian performing artists.
Founded: 1997
Specialized Field: Classical music (theater, dance, ballet)
Status: Professional; Nonprofit; Educational; Religious
Paid Staff: 5
Paid Artists: 52

Budget: $300,000 - $500,000
Income Sources: Donations, Tuition, Foundations
Performs At: Houghton College
Annual Attendance: 3,500 - 4,500
Facility Category: Professional; Non-profit-educational; Religious
Type of Stage: 3 stages; concert, recital, hall
Stage Dimensions: 60 x 45; 30 x 25, 45 x 38
Seating Capacity: 1200, 243, 210
Year Built: 1999

5638 TOWN OF HERNDON

PO Box 427
Herndon, VA 20170
Phone: 703-435-6868
Fax: 703-318-8652
e-mail: holly.popple@town.herndon.va.us
Management:
    Special Events Supervisor: Holly Popple
Mission: Functions as a talent buyer and events director.
Specialized Field: All Performing Arts; Festivals
Paid Artists: 80
Performs At: Industrial Strength Theatre; Worldgate Theatre

5639 BLUEMONT CONCERT SERIES

PO Box 208
Leesburg, VA 20178
Phone: 703-777-6306
Fax: 703-777-0574
e-mail: bluemontcs@aol.com
Web Site: www.bluemont.org
Management:
    Artistic Director: Dr. Peter Dunning
Mission: To offer a wide range of quality arts programs to the community.
Specialized Field: Festivals; Traditional; Variety
Status: Nonprofit
Budget: $60,000-400,000
Organization Type: Educational; Sponsoring

5640 WASHINGTON & LEE UNIVERSITY LENFEST SERIES

Lenfest Center, 100 Glasgow Street
Washington & Lee University
Lexington, VA 24450
Phone: 540-463-8001
Fax: 540-463-8041
e-mail: mgorman@wlu.edu
Management:
    Managing Director: Michael Gorman
Mission: Home of Theatre/Music/Dance Departments. Presenter of a few touring attractions.
Founded: 1991
Specialized Field: Theatre/Dance/Music
Budget: $35,000-60,000
Income Sources: Endowment/Ticket Sales
Performs At: Keller Theatre
Facility Category: Performing Arts Center
Type of Stage: Proscenium
Seating Capacity: 415
Year Built: 1991

5641 LYNCHBURG COMMUNITY CONCERT ASSOCIATION

PO Box 1332
Lynchburg, VA 24505
Phone: 804-845-3563
Fax: 804-845-3536
Management:
    Manager: Betty Sue Moehlenkamp
Budget: $35,000-60,000
Performs At: E.C. Glass High School Auditorium

5642 TOURING CONCERT OPERA COMPANY: MARTINSVILLE-HENRY COUNTY FESTIVAL OF OPERA

730 Craig Street
Martinsville, VA 24112
Phone: 540-632-5861
Fax: 518-851-6778
e-mail: tcoc@mhonline.com
Officers:
    President: Alberto Figols
    VP: Glenn Wilder
    Secretary/Treasurer: Anne de Figols
Management:
    Manager-Bookings: Priscilla Gordon
    Managing Director: Alberto Figols
    Public Relations: Ruth Johnson
    Bookkeeper: Alberto Fijolo
Mission: To bring live opera performances to audiences, internationally making it accessible to all.
Founded: 1977
Specialized Field: Dance, Vocal Music, Instrumental Music, Theater, Lyric Opera, Grand Opera
Annual Attendance: 5,000 - 10,000

5643 SWIFT CREEK ACADEMY OF THE PERFORMING ARTS

2808 Fox Chase Lane
Midlothian, VA 23112
Phone: 804-744-2801
Management:
    Director: Cassandra Lacey
Budget: $10,000

5644 CHRISTOPHER NEWPORT UNIVERSITY

1 University Place
Newport News, VA 23606
Phone: 757-594-7526
Fax: 757-594-7577
Management:
    Manager: Lawrence B Wood, Jr
Budget: $20,000-35,000
Performs At: John W. Gaines Theatre

5645 TIDEWATER PERFORMING ARTS SOCIETY

PO Box 1140
Norfolk, VA 23501-1140

Phone: 757-627-2314
Fax: 757-622-2803
e-mail: tpas@tpas.org
Web Site: www.tpas.org
Management:
    Executive Director: Karen E Levy
Budget: $35,000-60,000
Performs At: Pavilion Theatre; Wells Theatre; Harrison Opera House

---

5646 TOWN POINT JAZZ & BLUES FESTIVAL
Norfolk Festevents
120 W Main Street
Norfolk, VA 23501
Phone: 757-441-2345
Fax: 757-441-5098
Web Site: www.festeventsva.org

5647 VIRGINIA ARTS FESTIVAL
220 Boush Street
Norfolk, VA 23510
Mailing Address: PO Box 3595, Norfolk, VA 23514
Phone: 757-282-2800
Fax: 757-282-2787
Toll-free: 877-741-2787
e-mail: Lori@virginiaartsfest.com
Web Site: www.virginiaartsfest.com
Management:
    Director: Robert W Cross
    Marketing Manager: Lori Gubala
    Director Operations: Renae Adrian
Mission: Brings an imaginative and eclectic line-up of world-renowned performers, complemented by the region's own cultural stars, to the Virginia waterfront. Stages events in seven cities within a 60 mile radius. More than 80 performances in dance, theatre, classical, chamber, jazz and vocalmusic each season.
Founded: 1997
Specialized Field: Hampton Roads (Williamsburg to Virginia Beach)
Paid Staff: 22
Volunteer Staff: 300
Paid Artists: 700

5648 RADFORD UNIVERSITY PERFORMING ARTS SERIES
Box 6980
Radford University
Radford, VA 24142
Phone: 540-831-5265
Fax: 540-831-6313
e-mail: jscartel@radford.edu
Officers:
    Dean College/Visual/Performing: Dr. Joe Scartelli
Management:
    Technical Director: Doug Mead
Mission: Provide high end cultural artistic experiences for the campus and surrounding communities.
Founded: 1975
Specialized Field: Music, Dance, Theatre
Paid Staff: 2
Volunteer Staff: 8
Paid Artists: 5
Non-paid Artists: 20

Budget: $60,000-150,000
Income Sources: Student activities fees; Ticket revenues
Annual Attendance: 10,000
Facility Category: Auditorium
Type of Stage: Proscenium
Stage Dimensions: 40 x 25
Seating Capacity: 1500
Year Built: 1960

5649 CENTERSTAGE
2310 Colt Neck Road
Reston, VA 22090
Phone: 703-476-4500
Fax: 703-476-8617
e-mail: gordo@co.fairfax.va.us
Web Site: www.restoncommunitycenter.org
Management:
    Performing Arts Director: Leila Gordon
Founded: 1979
Specialized Field: Performing, Visual, Literary
Budget: $60,000-150,000
Income Sources: Government agency
Affiliations: Assoc. of Performing Arts Presenters
Annual Attendance: 25,000 +
Facility Category: Cultural and recreational
Type of Stage: Proscenium
Stage Dimensions: 32 W 18 H 25 Deep
Seating Capacity: 300
Year Built: 1979
Cost: $ 2 MM

5650 BIG GIG: RICHMOND'S SUMMER MUSICFEST
Downtown Presents
550 E Marshall Street, Suite 202
Richmond, VA 23219
Phone: 804-643-2826
Fax: 804-648-6834
e-mail: info@downtownpresents.org
Web Site: www.downtownpresents.org
Management:
    Booking Manager: Desiree Roots
Founded: 1988

5651 MODLIN CENTER FOR THE ARTS
University of Richmond
Richmond, VA 23173
Phone: 804-287-6632
Fax: 804-287-6681
e-mail: modlinarts@richmond.edu
Web Site: www.oncampus.richmond.edu
Management:
    Executive Director: Kathleen Panoff
Founded: 1996
Paid Staff: 7
Paid Artists: 30
Non-paid Artists: 15
Budget: $60,000-150,000

5652 RICHMOND SHAKESPEARE FESTIVAL
PO Box 27543
Richmond, VA 23261-7543

Phone: 804-270-3310
Toll-free: 888-373-2628
e-mail: cliffick@richmondshakespeare.com
Web Site: www.richmondshakespeare.com
Management:
 Managing Director: Cynde Liffick

5653 THEATREVIRGINIA

2800 Groove Avenue
Richmond, VA 23221
Phone: 804-353-6100
Fax: 804-353-8799
Web Site: www.theatreva.com
Management:
 Programming Artistic Director: Benny Ambush
 Assistant Director: Karen Brown
 Managing Director: Barbara Wells
Budget: $150,000-400,000

5654 VIRGINIA COMMONWEALTH UNIVERSITY COMMONS COLLEGE

907 Floyd Avenue
Box 842032
Richmond, VA 23284
Phone: 804-828-6500
Fax: 804-828-6182
e-mail: mhorvath@vcu.edu
Web Site: www.students.vcu.edu/commons
Management:
 Activities Coordinator: Mary Beth Horvath
Budget: $10,000-20,000
Performs At: University Student Commons
Commonwealth Ballroom

5655 HOLLINS UNIVERSITY PERFORMING ARTS SERIES

PO Box 9643
Presser Hall, 8226 Tinker Lane Northeast
Roanoke, VA 24020
Phone: 540-362-6511
Fax: 540-362-6648
e-mail: jcline@hollins.edu
Web Site: www.hollins.edu/academ/depts/music
Management:
 Manager: Judith Cline
Budget: $10,000

5656 ROANOKE COLLEGE PERFORMING ARTS SERIES

Roanoke College
221 College Lane
Salem, VA 24153
Phone: 540-375-2223
Fax: 540-375-2559
e-mail: weinstein@roanoke.edu
Management:
 Administrator: Alan Weinstein
Budget: $10,000-20,000
Performs At: Olin Hall
Seating Capacity: 404

5657 CARL BROMAN CONCERTS

Box 1
Mary Baldwin College
Staunton, VA 24401
Phone: 540-887-7188
Fax: 540-885-7039
e-mail: rtallen@mbc.edu
Management:
 Manager: Dr. Robert T Allen, III
Budget: $10,000-20,000
Performs At: Francis Auditorium

5658 MIDDLE PENINSULA COMMUNITY CONCERT ASSOCIATION

PO Box 198
Topping, VA 23169
Phone: 804-758-4819
Officers:
 President: Carolyn Shank
Budget: $20,000-35,000

5659 WOLF TRAP FOUNDATION FOR THE PERFORMING ARTS

1624 Trap Road
Vienna, VA 22182
Phone: 703-255-1900
Fax: 703-255-1918
e-mail: wolftrap@wolf-trap.org
Web Site: www.wolftrap.org
Officers:
 VP/Finance Officer: Charles A Walters, Jr
 VP, Performing Arts/Education: Ann McPherson McKee
Management:
 Sr Director/Commun/Marketing: Lisa LaCamera
 Director Special Events: Suzanne Musgrave
 Director Media Relations: Danette A Wilis
Mission: To provide enrichment, education and enjoyment to diverse audiences through presentation, production and creation of a broad spectrum of performing arts activities.
Founded: 1971
Specialized Field: Dance; Vocal Music; Instrumental Music; Theater; Lyric Opera
Status: Professional; Nonprofit
Budget: $20,000,000
Performs At: Filene Center at America's National Park for the Performing Arts
Facility Category: Indoor/Outdoor Amphitheatre
Type of Stage: Proscenium
Seating Capacity: 7,023 with lawn seats
Year Built: 1971
Year Remodeled: 1984
Organization Type: Educational; Sponsoring

5660 FALL FOLIAGE

Garth Newel Music Center
PO Box 240
Warm Springs, VA 24484

Phone: 540-839-5018
Fax: 540-839-3154
Toll-free: 877-558-1689
e-mail: office@garthnewel.org
Web Site: www.garthnewel.org
Founded: 1973
Specialized Field: music classical
Season: October

5661 GARTH NEWEL MUSIC CENTER
PO Box 240
Warm Springs, VA 24484
Phone: 540-839-5018
Fax: 540-839-3154
e-mail: office@garthnewel.org
Web Site: www.garthnewel.org
Management:
 Artistic Director: Evelyn Grau
 Artistic Director: Teresa Ling
 Artistic Director: Tobias Werner
Mission: Promoting and performing chamber music.
Founded: 1973
Specialized Field: Vocal Music; Instrumental Music;
Festivals, Concert Series
Status: Professional; Nonprofit; Student Program
Performs At: Herter Hall
Organization Type: Performing; Touring; Resident;
Educational

5662 MUSIC HOLIDAY WEEKENDS
Garth Newel Music Center
PO Box 240
Warm Springs, VA 24484
Phone: 540-839-5018
Fax: 540-839-3154
Toll-free: 877-558-1689
e-mail: office@garthnewel.org
Web Site: www.garthnewel.org
Mission: Music Holiday of offers a total experience in
social civility.
Founded: 1973
Specialized Field: music classical
Season: Fall; Winter; Spring

5663 SPECIAL MUSIC HOLIDAYS
Garth Newel Music Center
PO Box 240
Warm Springs, VA 24484
Phone: 540-839-5018
Fax: 540-839-3154
Toll-free: 877-558-1689
e-mail: office@garthnewel.org
Web Site: www.garthnewel.org
Founded: 1973
Specialized Field: music classical
Season: November; December

5664 SPRING 2003
Garth Newel Music Center
PO Box 240
Warm Springs, VA 24484

Phone: 540-839-5018
Fax: 540-839-3154
Toll-free: 877-558-1689
e-mail: office@garthnewel.org
Web Site: www.garthnewel.org
Founded: 1973
Specialized Field: music classical
Season: Spring

5665 SUMMER CHAMBER MUSIC FESTIVAL
Garth Newel Music Center
PO Box 240
Warm Springs, VA 24484
Phone: 540-839-5018
Fax: 540-839-3154
Toll-free: 877-558-1689
e-mail: office@garthnewel.org
Web Site: www.garthnewel.org
Mission: A tradition since 1973, the Summer Chamber
Music Festival makes Garth Newel the place to be on
weekends afternoons. Each concert consist of a unique
program featuring members of the Garth Newel Piano
Quartet and guest artists. Performances take place in
Herter Hall.
Founded: 1973
Specialized Field: music classical

5666 VIRGINIA SHAKESPEARE FESTIVAL
College of William and Mary
PO Box 8795
Williamsburg, VA 23187
Phone: 757-221-4563
Management:
 Executive Director: Jerry H Bledsoe
Mission: To offer quality Shakespeare performed in the
classical manner.
Founded: 1978
Specialized Field: Theater; Festivals
Status: Professional; Nonprofit
Paid Staff: 20
Income Sources: The College of William & Mary
Season: July - August
Performs At: Phi Beta Kappa Memorial Hall; The
College of Williamsburg
Organization Type: Performing; Educational

5667 WILLIAM & MARY CONCERT SERIES
The Campus Center 203
PO Box 8795
Williamsburg, VA 23187-8795
Phone: 757-221-3300
Fax: 757-221-3451
e-mail: mxcons@wm.edu
Management:
 Asst VP Student Affairs: Mark Constantine
Budget: $60,000-150,000
Performs At: Phi Beta Kappa Memorial Hall
Seating Capacity: 763

5668 WINTERGREEN PERFORMING ARTS
Box 816
Wintergreen, VA 22958

Phone: 540-343-6221
Fax: 540-325-1464
e-mail: info@wparts.com
Web Site: www.wparts.com
Officers:
    President: Stuart C Harvey
Management:
    Artistic Director/Conductor: David Wiley
    Managing Director: Sarah McCracken

5669 WINTERGREEN SUMMER MUSIC FESTIVAL

Wintergreen Performing Arts
Box 816
Wintergreen, VA 22958
Phone: 804-325-8292
Fax: 804-325-1464
e-mail: info@wparts.com
Web Site: www.wintergreenmusic.org
Management:
    Managing Director: Sarah McCracken
Mission: Summer Orchestra Concerts.
Founded: 1996
Paid Staff: 2
Volunteer Staff: 40
Paid Artists: 70
Non-paid Artists: 10

5670 SHENANDOAH VALLEY MUSIC FESTIVAL

PO Box 528
Woodstock, VA 22664
Phone: 540-549-3396
Fax: 540-459-3730
e-mail: svmf@shentel.net
Web Site: www.musicfest.org
Officers:
    Executive Director: Dennis M Lynch
Mission: To foster, promote, and increase the musical knowledge of the public by organizing and presenting programs chosen primarily from the literature of symphonic music, and incidentally from folk, bog band, jazz and family programming.
Founded: 1963
Specialized Field: Instrumental Music; Festivals; Symphonic; Jazz; Folk; Family; Big Band
Status: Nonprofit
Paid Artists: 3
Budget: $7,500
Income Sources: Government & private grants
Performs At: Orkney Springs Pavilion
Annual Attendance: 10,000
Organization Type: Sponsoring

Washington

5671 AUBURN ARTS COMMISSION

Auburn City Hall
25 W Main Street
Auburn, WA 98001
Phone: 253-804-5057
Fax: 253-288-3132

Management:
    Cultural Programs Manager: Susan Sagawa
Budget: $60,000-150,000

5672 BELLINGHAM FESTIVAL OF MUSIC

1300 N State Street
Suite 101
Bellingham, WA 98225
Phone: 360-676-5997
Fax: 360-647-3521
Toll-free: 800-335-5550
e-mail: andrew@bellinghamfestival.org
Web Site: www.bellinghamfestival.org
Officers:
    Chairperson: Marty Haines
Management:
    Executive Director: Andrew Moquin
    Operations Coordinator: Dimity Hammoney
Mission: To provide the area with educational opportunities to experience live music performances at the highest artistic level by nationally and internationally renowned musicians in a concentrated festival format.
Founded: 1993
Specialized Field: Summer Music Festival Featuring Classical, Chamber, Jazz, and Ethnic Music
Paid Staff: 3
Volunteer Staff: 6
Paid Artists: 50
Budget: $500,000
Income Sources: Grants from City; County; Private Foundations; Local Fund Drive; Ticket Sales
Performs At: Bellwether on the Bay
Annual Attendance: 9,000
Facility Category: Outdoor

5673 WESTERN WASHINGTON UNIVERSITY: COLLEGE OF FINE & PERFORMING ARTS

PAC, PA-361
516 High Street
Bellingham, WA 98225-9109
Phone: 360-650-3866
Fax: 360-650-3028
e-mail: Tamara.Mcdonald@wwu.edu
Web Site: www.pacseries.wwu.edu
Management:
    Dean: Bert van Boer
    Performing Arts Series Coordinator: Tamara McDonald
Budget: $40,000-55,000
Performs At: PAC Mainstage Theatre, PAC Concert Hall

5674 OLYMPIC COLLEGE

Student Programs
1600 Chester Avenue
Bremerton, WA 98337-1699
Phone: 360-475-7441
Fax: 360-475-7454
e-mail: jgallagher@oc.ctc.edu
Management:
    Associate Director: Jean Gallagher
Paid Staff: 2
Budget: $10,000-20,000

5675   LAKE CHELAN BACH FESTIVAL
PO Box 554
Chelan, WA 98816
Phone: 509-664-0412
Fax: 509-663-4849
Web Site: www.bachfest.org/
Officers:
   President: Bob Meyers
   Executive Director: Beth Jensen
   Vice President: Steve Palmbush
   Secretary: Kerry Travers
   Treasurer: Tom Thomas
Management:
   Artistic & Music Director: Kenneth Nafziger
Mission: To nurture the classical arts.
Founded: 1982
Specialized Field: Vocal Music; Instrumental Music;
Lyric Opera
Status: Professional; Non-Professional; Nonprofit
Paid Staff: 40
Organization Type: Performing; Educational

**5676   ORCAS THEATER & COMMUNITY
CENTER**
917 Mount Baker Road
PO Box 567
East Sound, WA 98245-0567
Phone: 360-376-2281
Fax: 360-376-6822
e-mail: orcascenter@rockisland.com
Web Site: www.rockisland.com/~orcascenter
Management:
   Director: Malissa White
Budget: $35,000-60,000

5677   EDMONDS ARTS COMMISSION
700 Main Street
Edmonds, WA 98020
Phone: 425-771-0228
Fax: 425-771-0253
e-mail: chapin@ci.edmonds.wa.us
Management:
   Cultural Resources Coordinator: Frances White
   Chapin
Budget: $10,000-20,000

5678   JAZZ IN THE VALLEY
PO Box 214
Ellensburg, WA 98926
Phone: 509-925-6677
e-mail: jazzinfo@jazzinthevalley.com
Web Site: www.jazzinthevalley.com
Management:
   Director: Larry Sharpe

5679   ENUMCLAW ARTS COMMISSION
1339 Griffin
Enumclaw, WA 98022
Phone: 360-802-0232
Fax: 360-825-1429
Management:
   Cultural Programs Manager: DeNae McGee
Budget: $35,000-60,000

Performs At: City Hall Park (summer)

5680   SAN JUAN JAZZ
PO Box 1666
Friday Harbor, WA 98250
Phone: 360-378-5509
Fax: 360-378-7796
e-mail: jazz@sanjuanjazz.org
Web Site: www.sanjuanjazz.org
Management:
   Manager: Bud Rodewald

5681   KENT PARKS & RECREATION
220 4th Avenue S
Kent, WA 98032-5895
Phone: 253-856-5050
Fax: 253-856-6050
Web Site: www.ci.kent.wa.us/culturalprograms
Management:
   Cultural Programs Manager: Ronda Billerbeck
Budget: $35,000-60,000
Annual Attendance: 50,000
Facility Category: Performing Arts Center/Outdoor
Festival - various

5682   ABBEY CHURCH EVENTS
Saint Martin's Abbey
5300 Pacific Avenue SE
Lacey, WA 98503-1297
Phone: 360-438-4476
Fax: 360-438-4387
Management:
   Director: Boniface V Lazzari, OSB
Budget: $10,000-20,000

5683   ICICLE CREEK CHAMBER FESTIVAL
PO Box 2071
Leavenworth, WA 98826
Phone: 509-548-6347
Fax: 509-548-3128
Toll-free: 877-265-6026
e-mail: icicle@icicle.org
Web Site: www.icicle.org
Management:
   Executive Director: Scott Hosfeld
   Artistic Director: Marcia Kaufmann
   Operations Manager: Vicki White
Founded: 1995
Specialized Field: Music/Chamber Music
Paid Staff: 5
Volunteer Staff: 20
Paid Artists: 18

5684   LYNNWOOD JAZZ FESTIVAL
20000 68th Avenue W
Lynnwood, WA 98036
Phone: 425-640-1650
Fax: 425-640-1083
e-mail: kmarcy@edcc.edu
Management:
   Festival Director: Kirk Marcy

5685 MERCER ISLAND ARTS COUNCIL
8236 SE 24th Street
Mercer Island, WA 98040
Phone: 206-236-3545
Fax: 206-236-3631
e-mail: diane.dobler@ci.mercer-island.wa.us.
Web Site: www.ci.mercer-island.wa.us
Management:
  Recreation Coordinator: Diane Dobler
  Recreation Supervisor: Jennifer Berner
Mission: To present cultural arts programs to the citizens of Mercer Island and to advocate for the arts and Mercer Island artists.
Founded: 1985
Paid Staff: 2
Volunteer Staff: 12
Budget: $20,000-35,000

5686 EVERGREEN STATE COLLEGE EVERGREEN EXPRESSIONS
Communications Building
Room 301
Olympia, WA 98505
Phone: 360-866-6000
Fax: 360-866-6794
e-mail: yatesc@evergreen.edu
Web Site: www.evergreen.edu
Management:
  Performing/Media Arts Manager: Christopher Yates
Budget: $20,000-35,000

5687 JUAN DE FUCA FESTIVAL OF THE ARTS
PO Box 796
Port Angeles, WA 98362
Phone: 360-457-5411
Fax: 360-457-5411
e-mail: festarts@olympus.net
Management:
  Executive Director: Anna Manildi

5688 DANCE FESTIVAL: CENTRUM FESTIVAL
PO Box 1158
Port Townsend, WA 98368
Phone: 360-385-3102
Fax: 360-385-2470
Toll-free: 800-733-3608
e-mail: centrum@olympus.net
Web Site: www.centrum.org
Management:
  Director: Carol Shiffman
Mission: To assist those who seek creative and intellectual growth and to present visual, literary and performing arts to the public.
Founded: 1973
Specialized Field: Multi-disciplinary
Paid Staff: 18
Volunteer Staff: 60
Paid Artists: 200

5689 JAZZ PORT TOWNSEND: CENTRUM FESTIVAL
PO Box 1158
Port Townsend, WA 98368
Phone: 360-385-3102
Fax: 360-385-2470
Toll-free: 800-733-3608
e-mail: centrum@olympus.net
Web Site: www.centrum.org
Management:
  Director: Carol Shiffman
Mission: To assist those who seek creative and intellectual growth and to present visual, literary and performing arts to the public.
Founded: 1973
Specialized Field: Multi-disciplinary
Paid Staff: 18
Volunteer Staff: 60
Paid Artists: 200

5690 PORT TOWNSEND BLUES HERITAGE FESTIVAL: CENTRUM FESTIVAL
PO Box 1158
Port Townsend, WA 98368
Phone: 360-385-3102
Fax: 360-385-2470
Toll-free: 800-733-3608
e-mail: centrum@olympus.net
Web Site: www.centrum.org
Management:
  Director: Carol Shiffman
Mission: To assist those who seek creative and intellectual growth and to present visual, literary and performing arts to the public.
Founded: 1973
Specialized Field: Multi-disciplinary
Paid Staff: 18
Volunteer Staff: 60
Paid Artists: 200

5691 WASHINGTON STATE UNIVERSITY
Washington State University
Pullman, WA 99164-1710
Phone: 509-335-2241
Fax: 509-335-3853
e-mail: kerrjf@wsu.edu
Web Site: www.wsu.edu/bpac
Management:
  Performing Arts Coliseum Director: Joseph Kerr
Budget: $10,000
Performs At: Performing Arts Coliseum Theatre

5692 CORNISH COLLEGE: CORNISH SERIES
710 E Roy Street
Seattle, WA 98102
Phone: 206-726-5030
Fax: 206-720-5183
Toll-free: 800-726-2787
e-mail: lkaminsky@cornish.edu
Web Site: www.cornish.edu
Officers:
  Music Department Chairperson: Laura Kaminsky
Founded: 1914

Specialized Field: Music
Budget: $20,000-35,000
Performs At: Poncho Concert Hall
Seating Capacity: 200
Year Remodeled: 2000

**5693 EARLY MUSIC GUILD
INTERNATIONAL SERIES/RECITALS**
2366 Eastlake Avenue E
#335
Seattle, WA 98102
Phone: 206-325-7066
Fax: 206-860-9151
e-mail: emg@earlymusicguild.org
Web Site: www.earlymusicguild.org
Management:
   Executive Director: Gus Denhard
Founded: 1977
Paid Staff: 2
Volunteer Staff: 11
Paid Artists: 30
Budget: $35,000-60,000

5694 EARSHOT JAZZ FESTIVAL
3429 Fremont Place
#309
Seattle, WA 98103-8650
Phone: 206-547-6763
Fax: 206-547-6826
e-mail: jazz@earshot.org
Web Site: www.earshot.org
Management:
   Executive Director: John Gilbreath

**5695 GOVERNORS CHAMBER MUSIC
SERIES**
205 McGraw Street
Seattle, WA 98109
Phone: 206-281-8292
Fax: 206-285-7610
Management:
   Artistic Director: Judith Cohen
Specialized Field: Only use Pacific Northwest artists
Budget: $10,000-20,000
Performs At: State Theatre, Olympia, Washington and the Governor's

5696 LADIES MUSICAL CLUB
Cobb Building 1305 Fourth Avenue
Suite 500
Seattle, WA 98101
Phone: 206-622-6882
Fax: 206-622-0791
e-mail: lmc@wolfenet.com
Web Site: www.lmcseattle.org
Officers:
   Concert Committee Chairperson: Barbara Sand
   President: Doris Eckert
   Recording Secretary: Susan Buttram
   Corresponding Secretary: Iris Ewing
   Treasurer: Ruth Caswell

Mission: To grant scholarships to deserving music students; to sponsor a yearly International Artists Series; to foster music among its members and the community.
Founded: 1891
Specialized Field: Vocal Music; Instrumental Music
Status: Professional; Semi-Professional; Nonprofit
Performs At: Meany Hall; University of Washington
Organization Type: Performing; Resident; Educational; Sponsoring

5697 NORTHWEST FOLKLIFE FESTIVAL
305 Harrison Street
Seattle, WA 98109
Phone: 206-684-7300
Fax: 206-684-7190
e-mail: folklife@nwfolklife.org
Web Site: www.nwfolklife.org
Officers:
   President: Scott Scher
   Vice President: Craig Beles
   VP: Ed D'Alessandro
   Secretary: Chuck Kichner
Management:
   Executive Director: Michael Herschensohn, PhD
   Program Director: Jill Linzee
   Director Operations: Mea Fischelis
   Public Relations/Marketing Director: Diane Walder
Mission: Preserving and presenting traditional and ethnic arts; fostering cultural understanding.
Founded: 1971
Specialized Field: Festivals
Status: Professional; Semi-Professional; Non-Professional; Nonprofit
Paid Staff: 14
Budget: $2,200,000
Income Sources: Fees; Commissions; Donations; Grants
Performs At: Seattle Center
Annual Attendance: 200,000
Organization Type: Performing; Touring; Educational; Sponsoring

5698 OLYMPIC MUSIC FESTIVAL
PO Box 45776
Seattle, WA 98145-0776
Phone: 206-527-8839
Fax: 206-526-8621
e-mail: info@musicfest.net
Web Site: www.musicfest.net
Management:
   Executive Director: Alan Iglitzin

5699 ON THE BOARDS
100 W Roy Street
Seattle, WA 98119
Mailing Address: PO Box 19515 Seattle, WA 98109
Phone: 206-217-9886
Fax: 206-217-9887
e-mail: info@ontheboards.org
Web Site: www.ontheboards.org
Management:
   Managing Director: Diane Ragsdale
   Artistic Director: Lane Czaplinski

Mission: Presentation oragnization featuring contemporary performance artists in dance, theater, music, multimedia and visual arts from around the globe.
Founded: 1978
Specialized Field: Contemporary Avanta Grade Performance
Paid Staff: 12
Budget: $1,200,000
Type of Stage: Black Box; Proscenium
Rental Contact: Operations Manager Brett McDowell

5700 ONE REEL
PO Box 9750
Seattle, WA 98109-0750
Phone: 206-281-7799
Fax: 206-281-7788
e-mail: rduff@onereel.org
Web Site: www.onereel.org
Management:
   Program Director: Reenie Duff
Budget: $400,000-1,000,000

5701 SEATTLE CHAMBER MUSIC FESTIVAL
10 Harrison Street
Suite 306
Seattle, WA 98109
Phone: 206-283-8710
Fax: 206-283-8826
e-mail: scmfmail@scmf.org
Web Site: www.scmf.org
Officers:
   President: Betty Lou Treiger
Management:
   Artistic Director: Toby Saks
   Executive Director: Connie Cooper
Mission: To present a four-week summer series of twelve outstanding chamber-music concerts annually.
Founded: 1982
Specialized Field: Chamber Music
Status: Professional; Nonprofit
Budget: $500,000
Performs At: Lakeside School; Saint Nicholas Hall; Benareya Recital Hall
Organization Type: Performing

5702 SEATTLE INTERNATIONAL CHILDREN'S FESTIVAL
305 Harrison Street
Seattle, WA 98109
Phone: 206-684-7338
Fax: 206-233-3944
e-mail: info@seattleinternational.org
Web Site: www.seattleinternational.org
Management:
   Executive Director: Andrea Wagner
   Producing Director: Brian Faker
   Director Education: Cathy Palmer
Mission: To offer an international festival of performing arts for children.
Founded: 1987
Specialized Field: Festivals
Status: Professional; Nonprofit

Income Sources: Western Alliance of Arts Administrators; International Association of Theatre for Children and Youth
Performs At: Seattle Center
Organization Type: Performing; Educational

5703 SEATTLE SHAKESPEARE FESTIVAL
1219 Westlake Avenue North
Suite 109
Seattle, WA
Phone: 206-286-0736
Fax: 206-286-0843
e-mail: ssf@seattleshakes.org
Web Site: www.seanet.com/~ssf/
Management:
   Producing Artistic Director: Stephanie Shine
Mission: To serve the community by presenting plays essential to our common culture in stagings that are vital and accesible to all.

5704 SEATTLE YOUTH SYMPHONY ORCHESTRA'S MARROWSTONE MUSIC FESTIVAL
11065 5th NE
Seattle, WA 98125
Phone: 206-362-2300
Fax: 206-361-9254
e-mail: info@syso.org
Web Site: www.syso.org
Management:
   Festival Director: Jonathan Shames

5705 WATER MUSIC FESTIVAL
PO Box 524
Seaview, WA 98644-0524
Phone: 360-642-5812
Fax: 360-642-5812
Toll-free: 800-451-2542
e-mail: normand@willapabay.org
Web Site: www.watermusicfsetival.com
   Board VP: Pat Reither
   Board Secretary: Sandy Jacoby
   Board Treasurer: Jane Schience
   Grants Coordinator: Jayne Dash
Founded: 1984
Specialized Field: Chamber Music
Volunteer Staff: 50

5706 CONNOISSEUR CONCERTS ASSOCIATION
315 W Mission Avenue
#21
Spokane, WA 99201-2325
Phone: 509-326-4942
Management:
   Executive Director: Gertrude Harvey
   Artistic Director: Gunther Schuller
Budget: $35,000-60,000
Performs At: Metropolitan Performing Arts Center

5707 PINESONG/SPOKANE FALLS COMMUNITY COLLEGE
3410 W Fort George Wright Drive
MS 3020
Spokane, WA 99204
Phone: 509-533-3800
Fax: 509-533-3433
Management:
    Festival Manager: Nancy Lindberg
    Festival Director: John Thompson
Mission: To offer a multi-cultural arts festival featuring hands-on participation.
Founded: 1986
Specialized Field: Festivals
Status: Nonprofit
Organization Type: Sponsoring

5708 BROADWAY CENTER FOR THE PERFORMING ARTS
901 Broadway
Tacoma, WA 98407
Phone: 253-591-5890
Fax: 253-591-2013
e-mail: administration@broadwaycenter.org
Web Site: www.broadwaycenter.org
Management:
    Executive Director: Eli D. Ashley
Paid Staff: 25
Volunteer Staff: 100
Budget: $150,000-400,000
Performs At: Pantages Theater; Rialto Theater
Seating Capacity: 1182
Year Built: 1918
Year Remodeled: 1979
Cost: 6.3 Million
Rental Contact: Marilyn Mullenax
Resident Groups: Tacoma Actors Guild

5709 EVERGREEN MUSIC FESTIVAL: TACOMA YOUTH SYMPHONY ASSOCIATION
901 Broadway Plaza
Suite 500
Tacoma, WA 98402-4415
Phone: 253-627-2792
Fax: 253-627-1682
e-mail: tacomayouthsymphony@msn.com
Web Site: www.tacomayouthsymphony@nisn.com
Management:
    Festival Music Director: Dr. Paul-Elliot Cobbs
    Executive Director: Dr. Loma Mosley
    Marketing Manager: Kristina Thomas
Mission: To provide an intense musical experience for younger students at the first session, and pre-professionals at the second session.
Founded: 1984
Specialized Field: Music

5710 PACIFIC LUTHERAN UNIVERSITY PROGRAM BOARD
Pacific Lutheran University
Tacoma, WA 98447
Phone: 253-535-7602
Fax: 253-535-8669
Web Site: www.plu.edu
Budget: $10,000
Performs At: Lutheran Concert Hall

5711 UNIVERSITY OF PUGET SOUND CULTURAL EVENTS
1500 N Warner
Tacoma, WA 98416
Phone: 253-879-3555
Fax: 253-879-3149
e-mail: mthorndill@ups.edu
Management:
    Public Events Director: Margaret Throndill
    Student Activities Director: Serni Solidarios
Budget: $20,000-35,000

West Virginia

5712 BETHANY COLLEGE
Renner Union
PO Box 37
Bethany, WV 26032
Phone: 304-829-7901
Fax: 304-829-7434
e-mail: b.nadzadi@bethanywv.edu
Web Site: www.bethanywv.edu
Management:
    Student Activities Director: Rebecca Nadzadi
Founded: 1860
Budget: $10,000-20,000
Income Sources: Private
Performs At: Sstage; Steinman Hall of Fine Arts; Hummel Field House
Annual Attendance: 750
Facility Category: College

5713 BLUEFIELD STATE COLLEGE
219 Rock Street
Bluefield, WV 24701
Phone: 304-327-4186
Fax: 304-327-4188
Management:
    Campus Life Director: JD Carpenter
Budget: $10,000

5714 CHARLESTON CIVIC CENTER
200 Civic Center Drive
Charleston, WV 25301
Phone: 304-345-1500
Fax: 304-357-7432
Management:
    General Manager: John D Robertson

5715 JEWISH CULTURAL SERIES
3828 Virginai Avenue SE
Charleston, WV 25304
Phone: 304-925-5112
Officers:
    Chairman: Dr. Steve Jubelirer

Budget: $10,000-20,000
Performs At: Temple Israel; B'nai Jacob Synagogue

5716 GLENVILLE STATE COLLEGE CULTURAL AFFAIRS COMMISSION
Glenville State College
Glenville, WV 26351-1292
Phone: 304-462-7361
Fax: 304-462-4407
e-mail: McKinneyj@glenville.wvnet.edu
Officers:
   Chairman Fine Arts: John S McKinney
Budget: $10,000-20,000

5717 CAM HENDERSON CENTER
Marshall University
400 Hal Greer Boulevard
Huntington, WV 25755
Phone: 304-696-3170
Fax: 304-696-6448
Web Site: www.marshall.edu
Management:
   Athletic Director: Lance West

5718 HUNTINGTON CIVIC ARENA
Ogeden Entertainment
One Civic Center Plaza
Huntington, WV 25701
Phone: 304-696-5990
Fax: 305-696-4463
e-mail: mail@hcarena.com
Web Site: www.hcarena.com
Management:
   Executive Director: Steven J Haver

5719 MARSHALL ARTISTS SERIES
Marshall University, Smith Hall 160
400 Hal Greek Boulevard
Huntington, WV 25755
Phone: 304-696-6656
Fax: 304-696-6658
e-mail: watkins@marshall.edu
Web Site: www.marshall.edu/muartser/index.html
Officers:
   President: J Wade Gilley
Management:
   Executive Director: Penny Watkins
   Administrative Assistant: Anne S Moncer
Mission: To aid, promote and contribute to the educational and cultural life of Marshall University and the surrounding area.
Founded: 1936
Specialized Field: Dance; Vocal Music; Instrumental Music; Theater; Lyric Opera; Grand Opera
Status: Nonprofit
Budget: $150,000-400,000
Income Sources: Marshall University
Performs At: Keith-Albee Theatre
Organization Type: Educational; Sponsoring

5720 WEST VIRGINIA STATE COLLEGE
PO Box 1000
Campus Box 4
Institute, WV 25112-1000
Phone: 304-766-3194
Fax: 304-766-5100
e-mail: byersrc@mail.wvsc.edu
Officers:
   Music Department Chairperson: Charlotte Giles
Budget: $35,000-60,000

5721 CARNEGIE HALL
105 Church Street
Lewisburg, WV 24901
Phone: 304-645-7917
Fax: 304-645-5228
e-mail: webmaster@carnegiehallwv.com
Web Site: www.carnegie-hall.com
Officers:
   President/CEO: Bruce Loving
Management:
   Artistic Director: Mary Leb
   Community Relations Director: Susan Bell
   Education Director: Christy Clemons-Rodgers
Founded: 1983
Paid Staff: 12
Volunteer Staff: 150
Budget: $35,000-60,000

5722 FAIRMONT CHAMBER MUSIC SOCIETY
5267 Arbugast Lane
Morgantown, WV 26508-8801
Phone: 304-291-8277
Fax: 304-367-4248
e-mail: jhashton@labs.net
Web Site: www.fcma.hypermart.net
Officers:
   President: John Ashton
   Vice President: Alison Poland
   Treasurer: Ruth Brooks
   Secretary: Marcella Yarenhuk
Mission: To present the finest of classical chamber music in the North Central West Virginia area.
Founded: 1982
Specialized Field: Chamber Music, Classical
Volunteer Staff: 8
Budget: $10,000
Performs At: St. Peter's Church
Seating Capacity: 700

5723 LYELL B CLAY CONCERT THEATRE
College of Creative Arts
PO Box 6111
1 Evandale Drive
Morgantown, WV 26506-6111
Phone: 304-296-4841
Fax: 304-293-6896
e-mail: msoreskovich@mail.wvu.edu
Web Site: www.wvu.edu/nccarts/
Management:
   Dean/Director: J Bernard Schultz

Chairman/Division Theatre & Dance: Margaret McKowen
Chairman Division of Art: Sergio Soave
Chairman Division Music: David Bess
Associate Director/Finance: Linda Queen
Director Operations: Mark S Oresicovich
Mission: Educational facility.
Specialized Field: Visual art, music theatre and dance
Income Sources: Stage and private
Performs At: Concert Theatre
Affiliations: National Association of Schools of Theatre; National Association of Schools of Art and Design, NASM
Annual Attendance: 200,000
Facility Category: Educational
Type of Stage: Proscenium
Stage Dimensions: 58 x 42
Seating Capacity: 1441
Year Built: 1968

5724 WVU ARTS SERIES
PO Box 6017
Morgantown, WV 26506-6017
Phone: 304-293-4407
Fax: 304-293-7574
e-mail: andrews@events.wvu.edu
Web Site: www.events.wvu.edu
Budget: $150,000-400,000

5725 WEST VIRGINIA UNIVERSITY AT PARKERSBURG
W Virginia University at Parkersburg
300 Campus Drive
Parkersburg, WV 26101
Phone: 304-424-8248
Fax: 304-424-8354
e-mail: hgyoung@alpha.wvup.wvnet.edu
Web Site: www.wvup.wvnet.edu
Management:
  Artistic Director: HG Young, III
Budget: $35,000-60,000

5726 CONTEMPORARY AMERICAN THEATER FESTIVAL
Box 429
Shepherdstown, WV 25443
Phone: 304-876-3473
Fax: 304-876-0955
Web Site: www.catf.org
Management:
  Producing Director: Ed Herendeen
  Managing Director: Catherine Irwin
Founded: 1991
Specialized Field: Theater Festival
Performs At: Main Stage, Studio Theater
Type of Stage: Proscenium, Black Box
Seating Capacity: 350, 99

5727 PERFORMING ARTS SERIES AT SHEPHERD
Shepherd College
101 College Center
Shepherdstown, WV 25443
Phone: 304-876-5113
Fax: 304-876-5137
e-mail: rmeads@shepherd.wvnet.edu
Officers:
  Chairperson: Rachael Meads
Budget: $35,000-60,000

5728 CHARLESTON COMMUNITY MUSIC ASSOCIATION
PO Box 8008
South Charleston, WV 25303
Phone: 304-744-1400
Fax: 304-343-7058
Officers:
  President: JB Wollenberger
Mission: Presenter.
Founded: 1933
Specialized Field: Music; Dance
Volunteer Staff: 100
Budget: $150,000
Income Sources: Ticket Sales; Contributions
Performs At: Concert Hall
Annual Attendance: 2,800-3,100
Type of Stage: Procenium
Seating Capacity: 3,450
Year Built: 1939

5729 WEST LIBERTY COLLEGE CONCERT SERIES
W Liberty College
Hall of Fine Arts
West Liberty, WV 26074-0335
Phone: 304-336-8135
Fax: 304-336-8056
e-mail: guerrjim@wtsc.wvnet.edu
Officers:
  Concert Committee Chairman: James C Guerriero
Budget: $20,000-35,000

5730 OGLEBAY INSTITUTE
Oglebay Park
Wheeling, WV 26003
Phone: 304-242-4200
Founded: 1930
Specialized Field: Dance; Instrumental Music; Theater; Lyric Opera
Status: Professional; Nonprofit
Organization Type: Performing; Touring; Educational

Wisconsin

5731 PERFORMING ARTS AT LAWRENCE
PO Box 599
115 S Drew Street
Appleton, WI 54912-0599
Phone: 920-832-6589
Fax: 920-832-6783
e-mail: shana.shallue@lawrence.edu
Web Site: www.lawrence.edu
Management:
  Manager of Public Events: Shana Shallue
Founded: 1847

Specialized Field: Jazz and classical concerts
Paid Staff: 2
Paid Artists: 8
Budget: $60,000-150,000
Income Sources: Ticket Revenue; Sponsorship
Annual Attendance: 10,000

5732 AL RINGLING THEATRE: LIVELY ARTS SERIES

PO Box 381
136 4th Avenue
Baraboo, WI 53913
Phone: 608-356-8864
Fax: 608-356-0976
e-mail: ringling@baraboo.com
Web Site: www.alringling.com
Management:
   Managing Director: Larry McCoy

5733 BELOIT COLLEGE PERFORMING ARTS SERIES

700 College Street
Beloit, WI 53511-5595
Phone: 608-363-2242
Fax: 608-363-2870
e-mail: freym@beloit.edu
Web Site: www.beloit.edu/~pubaff/events/pas00.html
Management:
   Events Coordinator: William F Faust
   Special Events/Projects Director: Mary Frey
Specialized Field: Dance; Vocal Music; Instrumental Music; Theater; Jazz
Status: Professional; Nonprofit
Budget: $20,000-35,000
Income Sources: Beloit College
Performs At: Eaton Chapel

5734 ST. NORBERT COLLEGE PERFORMING ARTS

St. Norbert College
De Pere, WI 54115
Phone: 920-403-4023
Fax: 920-403-4092
e-mail: garrett.grenz@snc.edu
Web Site: www.snc.edu
Management:
   Advisor: Garrett Grenz
Budget: $10,000-20,000
Performs At: Abbot Pennings Hall of Fine Arts
Annual Attendance: 7,000
Facility Category: vantons

5735 HEADWATERS COUNCIL FOR THE PERFORMING ARTS

Box 1481
Eagle River, WI 54521
Phone: 715-477-6206
Fax: 715-477-1736
Officers:
   President: Bernie Hupperts
   VP: Linnea Ebann
   Secretary: Tim Niehaus
   Treasurer: David Hanselman

Management:
   Community Contact: Nancy Berg
Mission: To bring quality entertainment to our remote community.
Founded: 1982
Specialized Field: Dance; Vocal Music; Instrumental Music; Theater
Status: Nonprofit
Volunteer Staff: 15
Budget: $24,000
Income Sources: Ticket Sales; Donations; Grants
Performs At: Northland Pines High School
Facility Category: High School Auditorium
Seating Capacity: 450
Year Built: 1980
Organization Type: Performing

5736 EAU CLAIRE REGIONAL ARTS CENTER

316 Eau Claire Street
Eau Claire, WI 54701
Phone: 715-832-2787
Fax: 715-832-0828
e-mail: ecrac@charters.net
Web Site: www.eraclairearts.com
Management:
   Executive Director: Peter Provost
   Facility Manager: Ron Rude
   Office Manager: Pat Teft
Founded: 1984
Paid Staff: 7
Budget: $300,000-400,000
Income Sources: Grants; Membership; Ticket Sales; Rentals
Annual Attendance: 80,000+
Facility Category: State Theatre
Type of Stage: Prosenium Theatre
Stage Dimensions: 50x29 prosc.@39'
Seating Capacity: 1,117
Year Built: 1926
Year Remodeled: 1986
Rental Contact: Office Manager
Resident Groups: Chippewa Valley Symphony, Chippewa Valley Theatre Guild, Eau Claire Childrens Theatre

5737 UNIVERSITY OF WISCONSIN AT EAU CLAIRE ARTISTS SERIES

University of Wisconsin-Eau Claire
Activities & Programs
Eau Claire, WI 54702-4004
Phone: 715-836-2787
Fax: 715-836-2521
e-mail: sollba@uwec.edu
Management:
   Performing Arts Coordinator: Beverly Soll
   Technical Services Manager: Laurie F Gapko
   Asst. Performing Arts Coordinator: Jennifer Hinners
Budget: $60,000-150,000
Performs At: Zorn Arena; Gantner Concert Hall
Annual Attendance: varies
Facility Category: varies

**5738 BIRCH CREEK MUSIC PERFORMANCE
CENTER**
PO Box 230
3821 County E
Egg Harbor, WI 54209
Phone: 920-868-3763
Fax: 920-868-1643
e-mail: mainoffice@birchcreek.org
Web Site: www.birchcreek.org
Officers:
   President: Lolly Ratajczak
Management:
   Executive Director: Kaye Wagner
   Public Relations Coordinator: Michael Brickley
Mission: To present a summer concert series; to train
young professionals and music students.
Founded: 1976
Specialized Field: Instrumental Music; Festivals
Status: Professional; Non-Professional; Nonprofit
Paid Staff: 100
Volunteer Staff: 100
Paid Artists: 4
Budget: $600,000
Income Sources: Student Tuitions; Concert Income;
Contributions
Facility Category: Concert Hall; Performance Center
Type of Stage: Thrust
Stage Dimensions: 30'x30'
Seating Capacity: 500
Year Built: 1900
Year Remodeled: 1976
Organization Type: Performing; Resident; Educational

5739 PENINSULA MUSIC FESTIVAL
PO Box 340
3045 Cedar Street
Ephraim, WI 54211
Phone: 920-854-4060
Fax: 920-854-1950
e-mail: musicfestival@dcwis.com
Web Site: www.musicfestival.com
Officers:
   Chairman: Patricia Hickey
Management:
   Executive Director: Sharon Grutzmacher
   Music Director/Conductor: Victor Yampolsky
   Assistant Conductor: Stephen Alltop
Mission: To perform quality music in a casual atmosphere
and promote young, new artists.
Founded: 1953
Specialized Field: Instrumental Music; Festivals
Status: Professional; Nonprofit
Paid Staff: 3
Volunteer Staff: 115
Paid Artists: 75
Budget: $450,000
Income Sources: Ticket Sales; Contributions;
Endowments
Season: August 6 - August 26, 2000
Performs At: Door Community Auditorium
Annual Attendance: 7,000
Facility Category: Concert Hall
Organization Type: Performing; Educational

**5740 DOOR COMMUNITY AUDITORIUM
SERIES**
3925 Highway 42
PO Box 397
Fish Creek, WI 54212
Phone: 920-868-2728
Fax: 920-868-2590
e-mail: dca@dcwis.com
Web Site: www.dcauditorium.org
Management:
   Executive Director: Katherine Liden
Founded: 1991
Paid Staff: 8
Volunteer Staff: 100
Budget: $600,000
Year Built: 1991
Rental Contact: Pete Evans

**5741 BROWN COUNTY CIVIC MUSIC
ASSOCIATION**
2818 St Ann Drive
Green Bay, WI 54311-5828
Phone: 920-469-7999
Fax: 920-469-7950
e-mail: civicmusic@aol.com
Officers:
   President: Amy L Kocha
   Executive Secretary: Sandra Eberhardt
Founded: 1926
Paid Staff: 1
Volunteer Staff: 150
Paid Artists: 5
Budget: $60,000-150,000
Annual Attendance: 5,000
Facility Category: H.S. auditorium
Seating Capacity: 1,522

5742 GREEN LAKE FESTIVAL OF MUSIC
PO Box 569
Green Lake, WI 54941
Phone: 920-748-9398
Fax: 920-748-6918
Toll-free: 800-662-7097
e-mail: office@greenlakefestival.org
Web Site: www.greenlakefestival.org
Management:
   Executive Director: Jeannette Kreston
   Administrative Director: Maria Dietrich
   Marketing Assistant: Pamela Nelson
Mission: The Green Lake Festival of Music is a
non-profit corporation founded for cultural enrichment
through the creation, promotion and public performance
of the musical arts.
Founded: 1979
Specialized Field: Vocal Music; Instrumental Music;
Festivals
Status: Professional; Semi-Professional;
Non-Professional; Nonprofit
Paid Staff: 3
Organization Type: Performing; Touring; Resident;
Educational; Sponsoring

5743 JANESVILLE CONCERT ASSOCIATION
PO Box 679
Janesville, WI 53547-0679
Phone: 608-756-1376
Management:
    Executive Director: Laurel A Canan
Budget: $20,000-35,000

5744 COUNCIL FOR THE PERFORMING ARTS
700 W Milwaukee Street
Jefferson, WI 53549-1717
Phone: 920-674-2179
Fax: 920-674-5140
e-mail: cpa@jefnet.com
Web Site: www.gojefferson.com/cpa
Management:
    Executive Director: Pat Guttenberg
Mission: To provide culturally and socially valuable entertainment and educational opportunities for this area.
Founded: 1977
Paid Staff: 2
Volunteer Staff: 100
Paid Artists: 100
Non-paid Artists: 175
Budget: $250,000
Income Sources: Ticket Sales; Grants; Donations
Affiliations: Arts Midwest
Annual Attendance: 15,000
Facility Category: Auditorium
Type of Stage: Proscenium
Stage Dimensions: 66'x44'
Seating Capacity: 996
Year Built: 1977
Organization Type: Performing; Educational

5745 CARTHAGE CHAMBER MUSIC SERIES
2001 Alford Drive
Kenosha, WI 53140-1994
Phone: 262-551-8500
Fax: 262-551-6208
e-mail: sjoerd1@carthage.edu
Web Site:
www.carthage.edu/departments/music/chamser.ht
Officers:
    Chairman Music Department: Dr. RD Sjoerdsma
Budget: $20,000-35,000
Performs At: Siebert Chapel

5746 CARTHAGE COLLEGE ARTS & LECTURE SERIES
2001 Alford Park Drive
Kenosha, WI 53140
Phone: 262-551-5859
Officers:
    Music Department Chairman: Richard Sjoerdsma

5747 DISTINGUISHED GUEST SERIES
725X Woodlake Road
Kohler, WI 53044-1334
Phone: 920-458-1972
Fax: 920-458-4280
e-mail: nancy.luczak@kohler.com
Web Site: www.kohlerfdn.org
Management:
    Executive Director: Terri Yorto
    Office Manager: Nancy Luczak
Paid Staff: 2
Volunteer Staff: 44
Budget: $60,000-150,000
Annual Attendance: 4,000
Facility Category: High School Theatre
Type of Stage: Wood
Stage Dimensions: 37'x30'x30'
Seating Capacity: 1,100

5748 KOHLER FOUNDATION
725X Woodlake Road
Kohler, WI 53044
Phone: 920-458-1972
Fax: 920-458-4280
e-mail: nancy.luczak@koheler.com
Web Site: www.kohlerfoundation.org
Management:
    Executive Director: Terri Yoho
    Office Manager: Nancy Luczak
Mission: To provide cultural opportunities for the benefit of the community.
Founded: 1940
Specialized Field: Dance; Vocal Music; Instrumental Music; Theater
Status: Nonprofit
Paid Staff: 6
Income Sources: Ticket Sales
Performs At: Kohler Memorial Theater
Annual Attendance: 4,000
Type of Stage: Wood Sprung Floor
Year Built: 1968
Organization Type: Performing

5749 GREAT RIVER FESTIVAL OF ARTS
PO Box 1434
La Crosse, WI 54602-1434
Phone: 608-784-3033
e-mail: grff@juno.com
Management:
    Administrator: Kathy Fitchuk

5750 PUMP HOUSE REGIONAL ARTS
119 King Street
La Crosse, WI 54601
Phone: 608-785-1434
Fax: 608-785-1432
e-mail: info@thepumphouse.org
Web Site: www.thepumphouse.org
Management:
    Executive Director: David Wells
Founded: 1977
Specialized Field: Vocal Music; Instrumental Music; Festivals, Acoustic, Folk
Status: Professional; Nonprofit
Paid Staff: 4
Volunteer Staff: 3
Non-paid Artists: 350

Budget: $98,000
Performs At: Dayton Gallery
Annual Attendance: 12,000
Facility Category: Arts Center
Seating Capacity: 130
Year Built: 1880
Rental Contact: Jodi Bente

5751 UNIVERSITY OF WISCONSIN AT LA CROSSE LECTURES

212 Cartwright Center
La Crosse, WI 54601
Phone: 608-785-8866
Fax: 608-785-6575
e-mail: richter.jara@uwlax.edu
Web Site: www.uwlax.edu/StuServ/SAC/LandC/index.html
Management:
   Program Adviser: Jaralee Richter
Budget: $20,000-35,000

5752 VITERBO UNIVERSITY BRIGHT STAR SEASON

815 S 9th Street
La Crosse, WI 54601
Phone: 608-796-3737
Fax: 608-796-3736
e-mail: maranscht@mail.viterbo.edu
Web Site: www.viterbo.edu
Management:
   Manager: Michael Ranscht
Budget: $200,000 - 250,000
Performs At: Fine Arts Center
Annual Attendance: 65,000
Facility Category: Multi-Disciplinary Arts Center
Type of Stage: Proscenium
Stage Dimensions: 40x30
Seating Capacity: 1,090
Year Built: 1971
Rental Contact: Michael Ranscht

5753 GREAT RIVER JAZZ FEST

811 20th Street S
LaCrosse, WI 54601
Toll-free: 888-711-7574
e-mail: Strong-RO@worldnet.att.net
Web Site: www.centurytel.net/jazzfest
Officers:
   President: Terry Rochester

5754 FLAMBEAU VALLEY ARTS ASSOCIATION

PO Box 343
Ladysmith, WI 54848
Phone: 715-532-7119
e-mail: cjohnson@jrec.com
Officers:
   President: Charmaine Johnson
Management:
   President: Charmaine Johnson
Mission: To present a season of 6-7 performing arts events to public audiences in their rural county.
Founded: 1971

Specialized Field: Performing Arts
Volunteer Staff: 13
Budget: $10,000-20,000
Income Sources: Donations; Grant Monies; Admissions
Performs At: High School Auditorium
Annual Attendance: 1600-2800
Type of Stage: Multipurpose auditorium w/fly space
Stage Dimensions: 60'x40'
Seating Capacity: 450
Year Built: 1968

5755 CAPITAL CITY JAZZ FEST

PO Box 8866
Madison, WI 53708
Phone: 608-850-5400
Fax: 608-850-5401
e-mail: marsch@chorus.net
Web Site: www.madisonjazz.com
Management:
   Director: Linda Marty Schmitz

5756 MADISON BLUES FESTIVAL

PO Box 5363
Madison, WI 53705
Phone: 608-836-0020
Fax: 608-836-8555
e-mail: madisonblues@madisonblues.com
Web Site: www.madisonblues.com

5757 SILVER LAKE COLLEGE GUEST ARTIST SERIES

2406 S Alverno Road
Manitowoc, WI 54220
Phone: 920-686-6172
Fax: 920-684-7082
e-mail: cgriff@silver.sl.edu
Web Site: www.sl.edu
Officers:
   Music Department Chairperson: Dr. Candice Griffith
Budget: $10,000

5758 UNIVERSITY OF WISCONSIN LECTURES AND FINE ARTS

PO Box 150
2000 W 5th Street
Marshfield, WI 54449
Phone: 715-389-6500
Fax: 715-389-6517
e-mail: dleick@uwc.edu
Web Site: www.marshfield.uwc.edu
Management:
   Music Professor: Robert I Biederwolf
   Drama Director: Greg Rindfleisch
   Performance Arts Series Coordinator: Darla Leick
Mission: Provide performances and lectures for the University and the community.
Founded: 1962
Specialized Field: Dance; Vocal Music; Instrumental Music; Theater
Status: Nonprofit
Performs At: University of Wisconsin Marshfield/Wodd County Theater
Type of Stage: Black Box

Organization Type: Educational; Sponsoring

5759 UNIVERSITY OF WISCONSIN CENTER - FOX VALLEY

PO Box 8002
1478 Midway Road
Menasha, WI 54952-1297
Phone: 920-832-2671
Fax: 920-832-2674
e-mail: JKuepper@uwc.edu
Management:
 Student Activities Director: Jeff Kuepper
Specialized Field: Dance; Vocal Music; Instrumental Music; Theater
Status: Nonprofit
Budget: $10,000-20,000
Performs At: Fine Arts Theatre
Organization Type: Performing; Educational

5760 CONCORDIA UNIVERSITY WISCONSIN

12800 N Lake Shore Drive
Mequon, WI 53097
Phone: 262-243-5700
Fax: 262-243-4351
Officers:
 Music Department Chairperson: Louis A Menchaca
Budget: $10,000
Performs At: Chapel of Christ Triumphant

5761 MERRILL AREA CONCERT ASSOCIATION

1103 Pierce Street
Merrill, WI 54452-2946
Phone: 715-536-3740
Management:
 Manager: Chad P Premeau
Budget: $20,000-35,000

5762 ALVERNO COLLEGE

Pitman Theatre
3401 S 39th Street, PO Box 343922
Milwaukee, WI 53234
Phone: 414-382-6044
Fax: 414-382-6354
e-mail: boxoffice@alverno.edu
Web Site: www.alverno.edu
Management:
 Assistant Director: Jan Kellogg
Mission: Alverno Presents, the performing arts series of Alverno College has presented the finest artists of all disciplines since 1960. Emphasis is on contemporary dance and world music. Artists perform in one of three theatre spaces or various locations throughout Milwaukee. Mission is to engage our community in stimulating arts experiences with both established and emerging artists from a variety of perspectives and cultural backgrounds.
Founded: 1960
Specialized Field: Presenter
Paid Staff: 3
Annual Attendance: 5000
Facility Category: Performing Arts Venue
Type of Stage: Proscenium
Stage Dimensions: 40'x30'

Seating Capacity: 930
Year Built: 1951
Rental Contact: Jan Kellogg

5763 ARTIST SERIES AT THE PABST

330 E Kilbourn Avenue
Suite 900
Milwaukee, WI 53202
Phone: 414-291-6010
Fax: 414-291-7610
Toll-free: 800-291-7605
e-mail: olsenb@milwaukeesymphony.org
Web Site: www.milwaukeesymphony.org
Officers:
 Chairman: Stephen E Richman
 Immediate Past-Chairman: Stanton J Bluestone
 Treasurer/Secretary: Robert A Wermuth
 President/Executive Director: Steven A. Ovitsky
Management:
 Public Relations Associate: Ceciclia M Francis
 Project Manager: Barbara Olsen
Founded: 1959
Specialized Field: Symphony; Orchestra
Status: Professional; Nonprofit
Performs At: Performing Arts Center; Uihlein Hall
Organization Type: Performing; Touring; Educational; Recording

5764 BRADLEY CENTER

1001 N 4th Street
Milwaukee, WI 53203-1314
Phone: 414-227-0400
Fax: 414-227-0497
e-mail: email@bcsec.com
Web Site: www.bradleycenter.com
Management:
 General Manager: David L Skiles
 Assistant General Manager: Steve Costello
Seating Capacity: 20k,000
Year Built: 1988

5765 CARDINAL STRITCH UNIVERSITY SCHOOL OF VISUAL AND PERFORMING ARTS

6801 N Yates Road
Milwaukee, WI 532173965
Phone: 414-410-4100
Fax: 414-410-4111
e-mail: dking@stritch.edu
Web Site: stritch.edu
Officers:
 Music Department Chairman: Dr. Dennis King
 Chairman Art Department: Tim Abler
 Chairman Theatre Arts Department: David Oswald
Specialized Field: Art; Music; Theatre; Dance; Film; Photography
Facility Category: Art Gallery
Type of Stage: Proscenium Arch
Seating Capacity: 400
Year Built: 1997
Comments: Theatre is air conditioned, handicapped accessible, infra-red hearing enhanced.

5766 EARLY MUSIC NOW
1630 E Royall Place
Milwaukee, WI 53202-1810
Phone: 414-225-3113
Fax: 414-278-0335
e-mail: emn@execpc.com
Web Site: www.execpc.com/~emn
Officers:
   President: Ralph Bulenburg
Management:
   Executive Director: Trallis Hoyt Drake
Paid Staff: 1
Volunteer Staff: 1
Budget: $75,000-80,000
Income Sources: Ticket sales; donations; grants
Annual Attendance: 2,000-3,000
Facility Category: Various halls and churches
Seating Capacity: 300-1,000

5767 WISCONSIN CONSERVATORY OF MUSIC
1584 N Prospect Avenue
Milwaukee, WI 53202
Phone: 414-276-5760
Fax: 414-276-6076
e-mail: joycea@aol.com
Web Site: www.wcmusic.org
Management:
   Executive Assistant: Denise M Traub
Mission: Music education and performance opportunities.
Founded: 1899
Specialized Field: Music
Paid Staff: 16
Volunteer Staff: 50
Paid Artists: 84
Budget: $1,400,000
Performs At: Recital Hall
Affiliations: NASM; NGCSA
Annual Attendance: 5,000

5768 LAKELAND PERFORMING ARTS ASSOCIATION
PO Box 1279
Minocqua, WI 54548
Phone: 715-356-2480
Officers:
   President: Jack Erwin
Budget: $10,000

5769 UNIVERSITY OF WISCONSIN AT OSHKOSH CHAMBER ARTS SERIES
Music Department N105
N105 A-C
Oshkosh, WI 54901
Phone: 920-424-4224
Fax: 920-424-1266
e-mail: hassel@uwosh.edu
Web Site: www.uwosh.edu/music/
Management:
   Faculty Advisor: Beverly Hassel
Mission: To offer the highest quality series of four professional classical music performances each season.
Founded: 1967

Specialized Field: Chamber Music
Volunteer Staff: 10
Budget: $20,000-35,000
Income Sources: Student Allocations and Box Office
Affiliations: University of Wisconsin-Oshkosh
Annual Attendance: 2,000
Facility Category: University Recital Hall
Type of Stage: Open
Stage Dimensions: 43'x 23'
Seating Capacity: 500
Year Built: 1970

5770 UNIVERSITY OF WISCONSIN-PLATTEVILLE PERFORMING ARTS
Center for the Arts
Platteville, WI 53818
Phone: 608-342-1480
Fax: 608-342-1478
e-mail: swanonk@uwplatt.edu
Management:
   Business Manager for the Arts: Kris Swanson
Budget: $35,000-60,000
Performs At: Center for the Arts-Concert Hall

5771 PRAIRIE PERFORMING ARTS CENTER
4050 Lighthouse Drive
Racine, WI 53402
Phone: 262-260-3545
Fax: 262-260-3790
e-mail: mpaffrath@prairieschool.com
Web Site: www.prairieschool.com
Management:
   Series Managing Director: Mark Paffrath
Budget: $10,000

5772 NORTHWOODS CONCERT ASSOCIATION
1960 Larsen Director
Rhinelander, WI 54501
Phone: 715-362-4912
Officers:
   President: Meredith Pirazzini
Budget: $20,000-35,000

5773 RIPON COLLEGE: CAESTECKER FINE ARTS SERIES
300 Seward Street
PO Box 248
Ripon, WI 54971
Phone: 920-748-8112
Fax: 920-748-8707
Management:
   Director Student Activities: Eric Tammes
Mission: To present four to five performing and visual artists, representing diverse backgrounds and arts areas each season for the college and surrounding Ripon community.
Specialized Field: Dance; Vocal Music; Instrumental Music; Theater
Status: Nonprofit
Performs At: Memorial Hall Gym; Benstead Theater
Organization Type: Sponsoring

5774 UNIVERSITY OF WISCONSIN RIVER FALLS: WYMAN CONCERTS & LECTURES SERIES
River Falls 410 South 3rd Street
River Falls, WI 54022
Phone: 715-425-4911
Fax: 715-425-3296
e-mail: kaye.e.schendel@uwrf.edu
Web Site: www.uwrf.edu
Management:
 Assistant Director Of Leadership: Kaye Schendel

5775 JOHN MICHAEL KOHLER ARTS CENTER: FOOTLIGHTS
PO Box 489
608 New York Avenue
Sheboygan, WI 53082-0489
Phone: 920-458-6144
Fax: 920-448-4473
e-mail: kbonin@jmkac.com
Web Site: www.jmkac.com
Budget: $35,000-60,000

5776 LAKELAND COLLEGE KRUEGER FINE ARTS SERIES
Lakeland College
PO Box 359
Sheboygan, WI 53082-0359
Phone: 920-565-1000
Fax: 920-565-1206
Web Site: www.lakeland.edu
Officers:
 Fine Arts Series Co-Chair: Dr. Michael Gill
 Fine Arts Series Co-Chair: Dr. JC Crawford
Management:
 Kraeger Fine Arts Coordinator: Debra Fale
Paid Staff: 1
Volunteer Staff: 4
Paid Artists: 8
Budget: $20,000-35,000
Performs At: Bradley Building
Seating Capacity: 495

5777 INDIANHEAD ARTS & EDUCATION CENTER
802 1st Street
Shell Lake, WI 54871
Phone: 715-468-2414
Fax: 715-468-4570
e-mail: iaec@uwec.edu
Web Site: www.IndianheadArtsCenter.com
Officers:
 President of Board: William Taubman
 VP: Jeanne Chamberlain
 Director: Howard Lehman
 Assistant Director: Andrea Pelloquin
 Secretary: Gloria Carlson
 Treasurer: Dale Larson
Mission: To provide creative arts education and enrichment experiences for diverse populations of youth and adult learners.
Founded: 1968

Specialized Field: Instrumental & Chorus Music; Visual Arts; Arts Education
Paid Staff: 4
Volunteer Staff: 104
Paid Artists: 60
Affiliations: University of Wisconsin-Eau Claire Continuing Education

5778 LUCIUS WOODS PERFORMING ARTS CENTER: MUSIC IN THE PARK
PO Box 295
Solon Springs, WI 54873
Phone: 715-378-4272
Fax: 715-378-2354
e-mail: luciuswoods@lwmusic.org
Web Site: www.lwmusic.org
Management:
 General Manager: Mary Giesen

5779 UNIVERSITY OF WISCONSIN AT STEVENS POINT PERFORMING ARTS
Quandt Fieldhouse
Stevens Point, WI 54481
Phone: 715-346-3265
Fax: 715-346-4655
e-mail: cseefeld@uwsp.edu
Management:
 Manager: Chris Seefeldt
Budget: $35,000-60,000
Performs At: Michelsen Concert Hall; Sentry Theatre

5780 UNIVERSITY OF WISCONSIN: SUPERIOR UNIVERSITY
1800 Grand Avenue
Superior, WI 54880-2898
Phone: 715-394-8115
Fax: 715-394-8454
Management:
 URS Manager: Harris L Balko
Budget: $10,000

5781 WAUPACA FINE ARTS FESTIVAL
Box 55
Waupacu, WI 54981
Phone: 715-842-1676
Fax: 715-848-4314
Officers:
 Chairman: Gerald Knoepfel
 Co-Chairman: Charles Spanhauer
 Treasurer: Blanche Fanik
Mission: Encouragement of active participation of musicians, artists and listeners/viewers of all the fine arts.
Founded: 1962
Specialized Field: Dance; Vocal Music; Instrumental Music; Theater
Status: Nonprofit
Paid Staff: 300
Income Sources: Wisconsin Art Council
Performs At: High School Auditorium
Organization Type: Performing

5782 UNIVERSITY OF WISCONSIN MARATHON COUNTY
518 S 7th Avenue
Wausau, WI 54401
Phone: 715-261-6234
Fax: 715-261-6333
e-mail: jgreenwo@uwc.edu
Management:
    Program Coordinator: Jean Greenwood
Paid Staff: 1
Budget: $15,000-25,000
Income Sources: Grants, student fees
Annual Attendance: 2500
Facility Category: Proscenium Stage
Stage Dimensions: 26 x 36
Seating Capacity: 240

5783 WAUSAU PERFORMING ARTS FOUNDATION
401 4th Street
PO Box 1553
Wausau, WI 54402-1553
Phone: 715-842-0988
Fax: 715-842-8715
Toll-free: 888-239-0421
e-mail: joconnell@grandtheater.org
Web Site: www.grandtheater.org
Management:
    Executive Director: Jim O'Connell
Founded: 1972
Specialized Field: Multi-disciplinary
Paid Staff: 18
Volunteer Staff: 200
Paid Artists: 30
Budget: $150,000-400,000
Income Sources: Ticket Sales; Theater Rental; Annual United Arts Fund Drive
Performs At: Proscenium Theater; Multi-purpose Room
Affiliations: Arts Presenters; Wisconsin Presenter's Network; Wisconsin Assembly for Local Arts
Annual Attendance: 100,000+
Facility Category: Performing Arts Center
Type of Stage: Proscenium
Stage Dimensions: 42 x 42
Seating Capacity: 1200
Year Built: 1927
Year Remodeled: 1987

5784 UNIVERSITY OF WISCONSIN AT WHITEWATER
Irvin L Young Auditorium
University of Wiscocsin at Whitewater
Whitewater, WI 53190
Phone: 262-472-4444
Fax: 262-472-4400
e-mail: youngaud@mail.uww.edu
Web Site: www.u.ww.edu
Management:
    Program Director: Randy Mayes
    Technical Director: David Nees
    Audience Services Manager: Michael Morrissey
    Marketing Director: Leslie LaMuro

Mission: Performing arts series for community, on-school-time presentations for school children and academic facility for the university arts students.
Paid Staff: 7
Volunteer Staff: 200
Paid Artists: 50
Budget: $150,000-400,000
Facility Category: Multi-Purpose Auditorium
Type of Stage: Proscenium
Stage Dimensions: 48'x30'
Seating Capacity: 1,335
Year Built: 1993
Rental Contact: Malinda Hunter

5785 ARTS COUNCIL OF SOUTH WOOD COUNTY
240 Johnson Street
PO Box 818
Wisconsin Rapids, WI 54495-0818
Phone: 715-421-4552
Fax: 715-421-4245
e-mail: swcarts.wctc.net
Management:
    Administrator: Mary Beth Rokus
Founded: 1976
Budget: $10,000-20,000
Performs At: Library Fine Arts Center; Performing Arts Center
Annual Attendance: 10,000
Seating Capacity: 800

Wyoming

5786 ARTCORE
Box 874
Casper, WY 82602
Phone: 307-265-1564
e-mail: artcorewy@aol.com
Web Site: www.members.aol.com/wycasper/artcore
Management:
    Executive Director: Carolyn Deuel
Budget: $20,000-35,000

5787 WYOMING ARTS COUNCIL
2320 Capitol Avenue
Cheyenne, WY 82002
Phone: 307-777-7742
Fax: 307-777-5499
Web Site: www.wyoarts.com
Officers:
    Chairman: Jim Willms
Management:
    Director: John G Coe
    Community Services/Performing Arts: Rita Basom
    Literature Manager: Mike Shay
    Visual Arts Manager: Liliane Francuz
    Grants Data Manager: Donna French
    Fiscal Officer: Justine Morris
    Office Manager: Evangeline Bratton
Mission: Promoting performing and literary and visual arts in Wyoming.
Founded: 1967

All listings are in alphabetical order by state, then city, then organization within the city.

Specialized Field: Dance; Vocal Music; Instrumental Music; Theater; Festivals; Lyric Opera; Grand Opera
Status: Nonprofit
Paid Staff: 10
Income Sources: National Endowment for the Arts; National Association of State Arts Agencies; WESTAF; Americans for the Arts
Organization Type: Educational; Sponsoring

5788 UNIVERSITY OF WYOMING CULTURAL PROGRAMS
Box 3951 University Station
Fine Arts Buiding, Room 113
Laramie, WY 82071
Phone: 307-766-5139
Fax: 307-766-5139
e-mail: husker@uwyo.edu
Web Site: uwadmnweb.uwyo.edu/culturalprograms
Management:
   Director: Cedric D Reverand, II
   Coordinator: Wendy Fanning
   Administrative Assistant: Janelle A Fletcher-Kilmer
Paid Staff: 3
Volunteer Staff: 6
Paid Artists: 25+
Budget: $60,000-$150,000
Annual Attendance: 5,000 - 6,000
Facility Category: Concert Hall
Type of Stage: Concert Stage
Seating Capacity: 699
Year Built: 1974
Year Remodeled: 2001

5789 WESTERN ARTS MUSIC FESTIVAL
University of Wyoming Department of Music
PO Box 3037
Laramie, WY 82071
Phone: 307-766-5242
Management:
   Chairman Music Department: Fredrick Gersten
Mission: To offer quality music to audiences during the summer.
Founded: 1972
Specialized Field: Vocal Music; Instrumental Music; Festivals; Lyric Opera
Status: Professional; Nonprofit
Income Sources: Wyoming Council of the Arts
Performs At: The Fine Arts Council Hall; University of Wyoming
Organization Type: Performing; Touring; Resident; Educational

5790 NORTHWEST COLLEGE
Northwest College
231 W 6th Street
Powell, WY 82435
Phone: 307-754-6307
Fax: 307-754-6700
e-mail: hansenn@nwc.cc.wy.us
Web Site: www.northwestmusic.org
Management:
   Music Coordinator: Neil Hansen
Budget: $10,000-$20,000

5791 WESTERN WYOMING COLLEGE
PO Box 428
Rock Springs, WY 82902
Phone: 307-382-1729
Fax: 307-382-7665
Officers:
   Chairman Cultural Affairs: Billy Smith
Management:
   Theatre Director: Billy Smith
Budget: $20,000-$35,000

5792 GRAND TETON MUSIC FESTIVAL
4015 W Lake Creek Drive
#1
Wilson, WY 83014
Phone: 307-733-3050
Fax: 307-739-9043
e-mail: gtmf@gtmf.org
Web Site: www.gtmf.org
Officers:
   President: Allan Tessler
Management:
   Executive Director: Donald Reinhold
   Marketing Director: Heather Hawkins
   Artistic Administrator: Nick Johnson
Mission: To establish a resident ensemble of like-minded artists to perform in small ensembles in a superb symphony orchestra; to bring the musical resources of a great metropolis to the Northern Rocky Mountain region for the summer season.
Founded: 1962
Specialized Field: Vocal Music; Instrumental Music; Festivals
Status: Professional; Nonprofit
Paid Staff: 9
Volunteer Staff: 100
Paid Artists: 250
Budget: 1,900,00
Income Sources: Donations; Sales
Performs At: Walk Festival Hall
Affiliations: ASOL; Jackson Hole Chamber of Commerce
Annual Attendance: 50,000
Facility Category: Concert Hall
Stage Dimensions: 60'wx 40'd
Year Built: 1974
Organization Type: Performing; Sponsoring

Alabama

5793 DIXON CENTER FOR THE PERFORMING ARTS
PO Box 1418
Andalusia, AL 36420
Phone: 334-222-6591
Fax: 205-222-6567
e-mail: info@lbw.com
Web Site: www.lbw.edu

5794 ANNISTON MUSEUM OF NATURAL HISTORY
800 Museum Drive
P.O. Box 1587
Anniston, AL 36207
Mailing Address: PO Box 1587, Anniston, AL 36202-1587
Phone: 256-237-6766
Fax: 256-237-6776
e-mail: info@annistonmuseum.org
Web Site: www.annistonmuseum.org
Management:
Marketing Manager: Susan Robertson
Founded: 1929
Budget: $10,000
Annual Attendance: 85,000
Seating Capacity: 175-200

5795 BEARD EAVES MEMORIAL COLISEUM
Auburn University
Room 2047
Auburn, AL 36849
Phone: 334-844-4442
Fax: 334-844-2399
e-mail: sparrtw@auburn.edu
Web Site: www.auburn.edu
Management:
Director: Tom Sparrow
Founded: 1969
Annual Attendance: 173,249
Seating Capacity: 13,000

5796 JOEL H EAVES MEMORIAL COLISEUM
Auburn University
Coliseum Office, Room 2047
Auburn, AL 36849
Phone: 334-844-4750
Fax: 334-844-4750
Management:
Director: Thomas W Sparrow
Assistant Director: Keith Bagwell
Seating Capacity: 14,000

5797 ALYS ROBINSON STEPHENS PERFORMING ARTS CENTER
1200 Tenth Avenue South
Birmingham, AL 35294
Phone: 205-975-9540
Fax: 205-975-2341
e-mail: trevor.cox@vpuadv.uab.edu
Web Site: www.alysstephens.org
Founded: 1996

Seating Capacity: 1,330

5798 BIRMINGHAM-JEFFERSON CONVENTION COMPLEX: ARENA
2100 Richard Arrington Jr Boulevard N
PO Box 13347
Birmingham, AL 35203
Phone: 205-458-8400
Fax: 205-458-8437
Toll-free: 877-843-2522
e-mail: info@bjcc.org
Web Site: www.bjcc.org
Officers:
CEO: Frank Poe
Management:
Sales/Marketing: Susette Hunter
Founded: 1973
Facility Category: Arena
Type of Stage: Varies
Seating Capacity: 19,000
Year Built: 1973
Rental Contact: Safety/Marketing Director Susette Hunter

5799 BIRMINGHAM-JEFFERSON CONVENTION COMPLEX - CONCERT HALL
2100 Richard Arrington Jr Boulevard North
PO Box 13347
Birmingham, AL 35203
Phone: 205-458-8400
Fax: 205-458-8494
Toll-free: 877-843-2522
e-mail: info@bjcc.org
Web Site: www.bjcc.org
Officers:
CEO: Frank Pos
Management:
Executive Director: Frank Poe
Sales/Marketing Director: Susette Hunter
Founded: 1973
Facility Category: Concert Hall
Seating Capacity: 3,000
Rental Contact: Sales/Marketing Director Susette Hunter

5800 BIRMINGHAM-JEFFERSON CONVENTION COMPLEX - THEATRE
2100 Richard Arrington Jr Boulevard North
PO Box 13347
Birmingham, AL 35203
Phone: 205-458-8400
Fax: 205-458-8494
Toll-free: 877-843-2522
e-mail: info@bjcc.org
Web Site: www.bjcc.org
Management:
Executive Director: Frank Poe
Sales/Marketing Director: Susette Hunter
Founded: 1970
Annual Attendance: 2,000,000
Seating Capacity: 1,000
Rental Contact: Sales/Marketing Director Susette Hunter

5801 BIRMINGHAM-JEFFERSON CIVIC CENTER - THEATRE
1 Civic Center Plaza
PO Box 13347
Birmingham, AL 35203
Phone: 205-458-8400
Fax: 205-458-8437

5802 BIRMINGHAM-SOUTHERN COLLEGE THEATRE
900 Arkadelphia Road
Birmingham, AL 35254
Phone: 205-226-4782
Fax: 205-226-3044
Toll-free: 800-523-5793
Web Site: www.bsc.edu

5803 LEGION FIELD STADIUM
400 Graymont Avenue West
Birmingham, AL 35204
Phone: 205-254-2391
Fax: 205-254-2515
e-mail: wegarre@ci.birmingham.al.us
Web Site: www.ci.bham.al.us
Management:
　　Stadium Manager: Walter Garrett
　　Director: Melvin Miller
Founded: 1926
Seating Capacity: 80,673
Year Built: 1927
Year Remodeled: 1991

5804 SAMFORD UNIVERSITY
800 Lakeshore Drive
Birmingham, AL 35229
Phone: 205-726-2011
Fax: 205-726-2243
Toll-free: 800-888-7218
e-mail: web@samford.edu
Web Site: www.samford.edu
Management:
　　Wright Center Managing Director: David Hartley
Founded: 1841
Budget: $150,000-400,000
Performs At: Wright Center
Seating Capacity: 2,640

5805 UAB ARENA
University of Alabama at Birmingham
1530 3RD AVE S
Birmingham, AL 35294
Phone: 205-934-7296
Fax: 205-975-8015
Management:
　　Director: Steve Mitchell
Type of Stage: Concert Stage
Seating Capacity: 9,000

5806 BOUTWELL MUNICIPAL AUDITORIUM
1930 8th Avenue N
Birminham, AL 35203

Phone: 205-254-2820
Fax: 205-254-2921
Web Site: www.ci.bham.al.us
Management:
　　Director: Kevin Arrington

5807 PRINCESS THEATRE CENTER FOR THE PERFORMING ARTS
112 2nd Avenue NE
Decatur, AL 35601
Phone: 256-350-1745
Fax: 256-350-1712
e-mail: lindy@princesstheatre.org
Web Site: www.princesstheatre.org
Management:
　　Executive Director: Lindy Ashwander
Mission: City performing arts center; presenter and rental facility.
Founded: 1983
Paid Staff: 5
Volunteer Staff: 250
Budget: $500,000
Affiliations: SAF
Annual Attendance: 60,000
Facility Category: Proscenium
Year Built: 1919

5808 DOTHAN CIVIC CENTER
Room 214 Civic Center
126 N St. Andrews Street PO Box 2128
Dothan, AL 36303
Phone: 334-793-0126
Fax: 334-712-4264
e-mail: civiccenter@dothan.org
Web Site: www.dothan.org
Management:
　　Director: JC Fredeman
Founded: 1975
Paid Staff: 12
Budget: $1,600,000
Income Sources: Municipal
Performs At: Proscenium Stages
Annual Attendance: 296,000
Facility Category: Arena and Opera House
Type of Stage: Proscenium
Seating Capacity: 3,100

5809 VON BRAUN CENTER
700 Monroe Street
Huntscille, AL 35801
Phone: 256-533-1953
Fax: 256-551-2203
Web Site: www.vbcc.com
Management:
　　Execcutive Director: Ronald D Avans
　　Assistant Director: Steven Maples
Seating Capacity: 8,748

5810 MILTON FRANK STADIUM
2801 15th Ave
Huntsville, AL 35805
Phone: 256-532-3090
Management:

Director: Bill Matthews
Founded: 1949
Seating Capacity: 11,000

5811 VON BRAUN CIVIC CENTER

700 Monroe Street SW
Huntsville, AL 35801
Phone: 256-533-1953
Fax: 256-551-2203
e-mail: marketing@vanbrauncenter.com
Web Site: www.vonbrauncenter.com
Founded: 1965

5812 VON BRAUN CIVIC CENTER - ARENA

700 Monroe Street SW
Huntsville, AL 35801
Phone: 256-533-1953
Fax: 256-551-2203
e-mail: marketing@vanbrauncenter.com
Web Site: www.vonbrauncenter.com
Founded: 1965
Seating Capacity: 10,000

5813 VON BRAUN CIVIC CENTER - CONCERT HALL

700 Monroe Street SW
Huntsville, AL 35801
Phone: 256-533-1953
Fax: 256-551-2203
e-mail: marketing@vanbrauncenter.com
Web Site: www.vonbrauncenter.com
Founded: 1965
Seating Capacity: 2,153

5814 VON BRAUN CIVIC CENTER - EXHIBIT HALL

700 Monroe Street SW
Huntsville, AL 35801
Phone: 256-533-1953
Fax: 256-551-2203
e-mail: marketing@vanbrauncenter.com
Web Site: www.vonbrauncenter.com
Founded: 1965

5815 VON BRAUN CIVIC CENTER - PLAYHOUSE

700 Monroe Street SW
Huntsville, AL 35801
Phone: 256-533-1953
Fax: 256-551-2203
e-mail: marketing@vanbrauncenter.com
Web Site: www.vonbrauncenter.com
Founded: 1965
Seating Capacity: 502

5816 PAUL SNOW MEMORIAL STADIUM

Jacksonville State University
700 Pelham Road N
Jacksonville, AL 36265

Phone: 256-782-5368
Fax: 256-782-5666
e-mail: info@jsucc.jsu.edu
Web Site: www.jsu.edu
Management:
  Director: Tom Seitz
Founded: 1951
Seating Capacity: 14,000

5817 PETE MATHEWS COLISEUM

Jacksonville State University
700 Pelham Road N
Jacksonville, AL 36265
Phone: 256-782-5368
Fax: 256-782-5666
e-mail: info@jsucc.jsu.edu
Web Site: www.jsu.edu
Management:
  Director: Tom Seitz
Seating Capacity: 6,000

5818 MOBILE CIVIC CENTER

401 Civic Center Drive
Mobile, AL 36602
Phone: 251-208-7261
Fax: 334-208-7551
Web Site: www.mobilecivicctr.com
Management:
  General Manager: Jay Hagerman
  Marketing Manager: Francie Unger
  Director Operations: Peter Caruso
  Director Finance: Sharee Self
  Director Marketing: Bob Brazier
Seating Capacity: 1,940

5819 MOBILE CIVIC CENTER - ARENA

401 Civic Center Drive
Mobile, AL 36602
Phone: 251-208-7261
Fax: 334-208-7551
Web Site: www.mobilecivicctr.com
Seating Capacity: 10,112

5820 MOBILE THEATRE GUILD

14 N Lafayette Street
Mobile, AL 36607
Phone: 334-433-7513

5821 USA SAENGER THEATRE

6 Joachim Street S
Mobile, AL 36602
Phone: 334-438-5686
Fax: 334-433-2087

5822 ALABAMA SHAKESPEARE FESTIVAL - FESTIVAL STAGE

One Festival Drive
Montgomery, AL 36117
Phone: 334-271-5300
Fax: 334-271-5348
Toll-free: 800-841-4ASF
Web Site: www.asf.net

Founded: 1985
Annual Attendance: 300,000
Seating Capacity: 750

5823 ALABAMA SHAKESPEARE FESTIVAL - OCTAGON
One Festival Drive
Montgomery, AL 36117
Phone: 334-271-5300
Fax: 334-271-5348
Web Site: www.asf.net
Founded: 1985
Annual Attendance: 300,000
Seating Capacity: 225

5824 GARRET COLISEUM
1555 Federal Drive
Montgomery, AL 36107
Mailing Address: PO Box 70026
Phone: 334-242-5597
Fax: 334-240-3242
Management:
    Executive Director: William H Johnson
    Assistant Director: Ed Wesson
Founded: 1951
Paid Staff: 10

5825 JOE L REED ACADOME
Montgomery, AL 36101-0271
Phone: 334-229-4529
Fax: 334-229-4988
Management:
    Facility Director: Jim Parker

5826 MONTGOMERY CIVIC CENTER
300 Bibb Street
PO Box 4037
Montgomery, AL 36104
Phone: 334-241-2100
Fax: 334-241-2117
e-mail: bmclain@civic-center.ci.montgomery.al.us
Web Site: www.civic-center.ci.montgomery.al.us
Management:
    Director: Robert G McLain
    Assistant Director Marketing: Rebie Tylor-Morris
    Assistant Director: Lainey Jenkins
Founded: 1977
Paid Staff: 43
Annual Attendance: 510,000
Type of Stage: Sico
Seating Capacity: 4,800

5827 OZARK CIVIC CENTER
East College Street
City of Ozark
Ozark, AL 36360
Phone: 334-774-2618
Fax: 334-445-1623
Toll-free: 877-622-2322
e-mail: civic@ozarkalabama.org
Web Site: www.ozarkciviccenter.com
Management:
    Box Office Manager: Doris Walters

Type of Stage: Concert Stage
Seating Capacity: 4,000

5828 BAMA THEATRE PERFORMING ARTS CENTER
600 Greensboro Avenue
Tuscaloosa, AL 35401
Phone: 205-758-5195
Fax: 205-345-2787

5829 BRYANT DENNY STADIUM
University of Alabama
Athletic Development, Box 870343
Tuscaloosa, AL 35487
Phone: 205-348-9727
Fax: 205-348-0789
e-mail: crimsontraditionfund@ia.ua.edu
Web Site: www.roll.tide.ua.edu
Management:
    Athletic Director: Bob Bockrath
Founded: 1929
Seating Capacity: 83,818

5830 COLEMAN COLISEUM
University of Alabama
Athletic Development, Box 870343
Tuscaloosa, AL 35487
Phone: 205-348-9727
Fax: 205-348-0789
e-mail: crimsontraditionfund@ia.ua.edu
Web Site: www.roll.tide.ua.edu
Management:
    Director Facilities: Bobby Rice
Founded: 1968
Seating Capacity: 15,043

5831 UNIVERSITY OF ALABAMA - CONCERT HALL
Frank Moody Music Building
PO Box 870366
Tuscaloosa, AL 35487-0366
Phone: 205-348-7110
Fax: 205-348-1473
e-mail: mjohnson@music.ua.edu
Web Site: www.music.ua.edu
Founded: 1987
Seating Capacity: 1,000

5832 UNIVERSITY OF ALABAMA - GALLAWAY THEATRE
Department of Theatre & Dance
PO Box 870239
Tuscaloosa, AL 35487-0239
Phone: 205-348-5283
Fax: 205-348-9048
e-mail: pmccray@theatre.as.ua.edu
Web Site: www.as.ua.edu

5833 UNIVERSITY OF ALABAMA - HUEY RECITAL HALL
Frank Moody Music Building
PO Box 870366
Tuscaloosa, AL 35487-0366
Phone: 205-348-7110
Fax: 205-348-1473
e-mail: mjohnson@music.ua.edu
Web Site: www.music.ua.edu
Seating Capacity: 140

5834 UNIVERSITY OF ALABAMA - MORGAN AUDITORIUM
Department of Theater & Dance
PO Box 870239
Tuscaloosa, AL 35487-0239
Phone: 205-348-5283
Fax: 205-348-9048
e-mail: pmccray@theatre.as.ua.edu
Web Site: www.as.ua.edu

5835 LOGAN HALL
Tuskegee University
321 Chappie James Center Arena
Tuskeegee, AL 36088
Phone: 337-727-8849
Fax: 334-724-4233
Management:
Manager: Wayvle Lewis
Seating Capacity: 3,000

5836 ALUMNI BOWL STADIUM
Tuskegee University
321 Chappie James Center Arena
Tuskeegee, AL 36088
Phone: 334-727-8849
Fax: 334-724-4233
Web Site: www.tusk.ed
Management:
Manager: Wayvle Lewis

Alaska

5837 ALASKA CENTER FOR THE PERFORMING ARTS
621 West Sixth Avenue
Anchorage, AK 99501
Phone: 907-263-2900
Fax: 907-263-2927
e-mail: acpa@alaskapac.org
Web Site: www.alaskapac.org
Officers:
President/COO: Nancy M Harbour
Founded: 1988
Annual Attendance: 250,000
Type of Stage: Proscenium

5838 WILLIAM A EGAN CIVIC AND CONVENTION CENTER
555 West Fifth Avenue
Anchorage, AK 99501
Phone: 907-263-2800
Fax: 907-263-2858
Web Site: www.egancenter.com

5839 ALASKALAND CIVIC CENTER
Airport Way & Peger Road
Fairbanks, AK 99701
Phone: 907-452-4244

5840 UNIVERSITY OF ALASKA - CHARLES W. DAVIS CONCERT HALL
UAF Music Department
PO Box 755660
Fairbanks, AK 99775
Phone: 907-474-7555
Fax: 907-474-6420
e-mail: fymusic@uaf.edu
Web Site: www.vaf.edu/music/department
Stage Dimensions: 30x60
Seating Capacity: 950
Year Built: 1968

5841 CHILKAT CENTER FOR THE ARTS
P.O. Box 1004
Haines, AK 99827
Phone: 907-766-3573
Fax: 907-766-3574
e-mail: arts@ChilkatCenterfortheArts.com
Web Site: www.chilkatcenterforthearts.com
Type of Stage: Flexible

5842 PIER ONE THEATRE
PO Box 894
Homer, AK 99603
Phone: 907-235-7333
Fax: 907-235-7333
e-mail: lance@xyz.net
Web Site: www.pieronetheatre.org

5843 CENTENNIAL HALL CONVENTION CENTER
101 Egan Drive
Juneau, AK 99801
Phone: 907-586-5283
Fax: 907-586-1135
Toll-free: 800-587-2201
e-mail: doyle_tennison@mail.ci.juneale.ak.u
Web Site: www.traveljuneau.com
Founded: 1985
Seating Capacity: 3,106

5844 KODIAK ARTS COUNCIL
PO Box 1792
Kodiak, AK 99615
Phone: 907-486-5291
Fax: 907-486-5591
e-mail: kodiak-arts-council@gci.net
Management:

Executive Director: Nancy Kemp
Founded: 1963
Budget: $190,000
Income Sources: Grants; membership; ticket sales
Facility Category: Auditorium
Type of Stage: Proscenium
Stage Dimensions: 40'x35'
Seating Capacity: 750
Year Built: 1986
Cost: 10,000,000

5845 SITKA CENTENNIAL BUILDING
330 Harbor Drive
Sitka, AK 99835
Phone: 907-747-3225
Fax: 907-747-8495
Founded: 1967
Seating Capacity: 500

Arizona

5846 CHANDLER CENTER FOR THE ARTS
250 N Arizona Avenue
Chandler, AZ 85225
Phone: 480-782-2683
Fax: 480-782-2684
e-mail: katrinamueller@ci.chandler.az.us
Web Site: www.chandlercenter.org
Management:
   Manager: Katrina Mueller

5847 COCONINO CENTER FOR THE ARTS
2800 S Lone Tree Rd
PO Box 296
Flagstaff, AZ 86001
Phone: 928-527-1222
Fax: 928-226-4101
Toll-free: 800-350-7122
e-mail: ladams@coco.cc.az.us
Web Site: www.coco.cc.az.us/

5848 SUN ENTERTAINMENT
Northern Arizona University
PO Box 5670
Flagstaff, AZ 86011-5670
Phone: 520-523-4313
Fax: 520-523-9219
e-mail: sun-p@www.nau.edu
Web Site: www.nau.edu/sun-p
Management:
   Associate Director: James P Conley
   Coordinator: Niki Graham
Performs At: NAU Walkup Skydrome; Ardrey
Auditorium; Prochnow Auditorium
Seating Capacity: 20,000

5849 J LAWRENCE WALK-UP SKYDOME
Northern Arizona University
PO Box 15096
Flatgstaff, AZ 86011
Phone: 520-523-3440
Fax: 928-523-5847

Management:
   Director: Dave Brown

**5850 GLENDALE COMMUNITY COLLEGE
PERFORMING ARTS CENTER**
6000 W Olive Avenue
Glendale, AZ 85302
Phone: 623-845-3000
e-mail: phil.randolph@gcmail.maricopa.edu
Web Site: www.gc.maricopa.edu

5851 GLENDALE PUBLIC LIBRARY
5959 W Brown Street
Glendale, AZ 85302
Phone: 623-930-3558
Fax: 623-842-4209
e-mail: aowens@glenpub.lib.az.us
Web Site: www.glendalelibrary.org/ill.htm
Management:
   Adult Programming Librarian: Anne Owens
Budget: $10,000
Performs At: Glendale Public Library
Seating Capacity: 207

5852 MOHAVE COMMUNITY COLLEGE
1971 Jagerson Avenue
Kingman, AZ 86401
Phone: 520-757-0851
Fax: 520-757-0837
e-mail: MohaveInfo@mohave.edu
Web Site: www.mohave.cc.az.us
Founded: 1971

5853 BARTON COLISEUM
2600 Howard Street
Little Rock, AZ 72206
Phone: 501-372-8341
Fax: 501-372-4197
e-mail: booking@arkfairgrounds.com
Web Site: www.arkfairgrounds.com
Management:
   EVP: Jim Pledger
Type of Stage: Outside Stages
Seating Capacity: 10,195

**5854 MESA COMMUNITY CENTER -
AMPHITHEATRE**
201 N Center Street
Mesa, AZ 85201
Phone: 480-644-2178
Fax: 480-644-2617
e-mail: commcntr_rental_info@ci.meza.az.us
Web Site: www.ci.mesa.az.us/commcntr
Type of Stage: Outside Stages
Seating Capacity: 4,200

**5855 MESA COMMUNITY CENTER -
CENTENNIAL HALL**
201 N Center Street
Mesa, AZ 85201

Phone: 480-644-2178
Fax: 480-644-2617
e-mail: commcntr_rental_info@ci.meza.az.us
Web Site: www.ci.mesa.az.us/commcntr
Type of Stage: Outside Stages

5856 MESA COMMUNITY CENTER CONFERENCE CENTER

201 N Center Street
Mesa, AZ 85201
Phone: 480-644-2178
Fax: 480-644-2617
Web Site: www.ci.mesa.az.us/commcntr
Paid Staff: 23
Facility Category: Amphitheatre
Seating Capacity: 4,200
Year Built: 1978

5857 ALLTEL ARENA

One Alltel Arena Way
North Little Rock, AZ 72114
Phone: 501-340-5660
Fax: 501-340-5668
e-mail: arena@alltelarena.com
Web Site: www.alltelarena.com
Management:
   General Manager: Michael Marion
   Assistant General Manager: John McDonald
Founded: 1999
Paid Staff: 35
Seating Capacity: 18,000

5858 PEORIA SPORTS COMPLEX

16101 N 83rd Avenue
Peoria, AZ 85382
Phone: 623-412-4211
Fax: 623-412-4249
Toll-free: 800-409-1511
e-mail: SportsComplex@peoriaaz.com
Web Site: www.peoriaaz.com/sports.htm
Management:
   Operations Coordinator: Nathan Torree
   Community Promotions Manager: Jim K Brink
   Director Human Resources: Greg Eckamann
   Executive Director: Jon Richardson
Founded: 1994
Volunteer Staff: 486
Annual Attendance: 450,000
Seating Capacity: 20,000

5859 AMERICA WEST ARENA

201 E Jefferson Street
P.O.Box - 433
Phoenix, AZ 85004
Phone: 602-379-2000
Fax: 602-379-2002
Web Site: www.americawestarena.com
Management:
   General Manager: Paige Peterson
   Director Ticket Operations: John Walker
   Sales Manager: Chris Montgomery

5860 BANK ONE BALL PARK

401 E Jefferson Street
PO Box 433
Phoenix, AZ 85001
Phone: 602-514-8400
Fax: 602-514-8699
Web Site: www.azdiamondback.com
Management:
   General Manager: Paige Peterson
   VP Event Services: Russ Amaral
Specialized Field: Ballpark home of the Arizona Diamondbacks
Seating Capacity: 49,500
Year Built: 1998

5861 CELEBRITY THEATRE

440 N. 32nd
Phoenix, AZ 85008
Phone: 602-267-1600
Fax: 602-267-4882
e-mail: khansen@celebritytheatre.com
Web Site: www.celebritytheatre.com
Management:
   Owner: Bill Bachand
   Marketing & Advertising Director: Kathy Hansen
Founded: 1963
Type of Stage: Proscenium
Seating Capacity: 2,651
Year Built: 1963
Year Remodeled: 1997
Rental Contact: Reed Glick

5862 GRAND CANYON UNIVERSITY

3300 W Camelback Road
Phoenix, AZ 85017-1097
Phone: 602-589-2482
Fax: 602-589-2492
Toll-free: 800-800-9776
e-mail: musicdepartment@grand-canyon.edu
Management:
   Chairperson Music Department: Dr. Sheila Corley
   Piano Area Coordinator: Dr. Judy Lively
   Instrumental Area Coordinator: Joe Lloyd
   Choral Activities: Dr. Keith Whitlock
   Director Vocal Activities: Nathan Wight
Budget: $10,000
Performs At: Ethington Theatre
Seating Capacity: 300
Rental Contact: Nathan Wight

5863 ORPHEUM THEATRE FOUNDATION

203 W Adams Street
Phoenix, AZ 85003
Phone: 602-252-9678
Fax: 602-252-1223
e-mail: orpheumphx@aol.com
Web Site: www.orpheumtheatrefoundation.org
Management:
   Executive Director: Joan Weil
Founded: 1929
Paid Staff: 3

5864 PHOENIX CIVIC PLAZA
225 E Adams Street
Phoenix, AZ 85004
Phone: 602-262-6225
Fax: 602-495-3643
Toll-free: 800-282-4842
e-mail: kevin.hill@phoenix.gov
Management:
  General Manager: Jay Green
  Marketing Director: Kevin Hall
Paid Staff: 200
Volunteer Staff: 120
Seating Capacity: 8,210

**5865 PHOENIX CIVIC PLAZA -
CONVENTION CENTER AND STAGE**
225 E Adams Street
Phoenix, AZ 85004
Phone: 602-262-6225
Fax: 602-495-3608

**5866 PHOENIX CIVIC PLAZA - EXHIBITION
HALLS**
225 E Adams Street
Phoenix, AZ 85004
Phone: 602-262-6225
Fax: 602-495-3608

**5867 PHOENIX CIVIC PLAZA - GRAND
BALLROOM**
225 E Adams Street
Phoenix, AZ 85004
Phone: 602-262-6225
Fax: 602-495-3642

5868 PHOENIX STAGES
203 W Adams Street
Phoenix, AZ 85003
Phone: 602-534-4874
Fax: 602-534-5622
Web Site: www.phoenixstages.com
Management:
  Booking Coordinator: Donna McWalters
  Manager: Bob Allen
Mission: Division of the city of Phoenix which manages
the Orpherm Theatre and Symphony Hall.
Paid Staff: 50
Volunteer Staff: 500

**5869 GOLDEN LION STADIUM
University of Arkansas- Pine Bluff**
1200 N University Drive
Pine Bluff, AZ 71601
Phone: 870-575-8000
Fax: 870-543-8013
e-mail: whimper_c@vx4-500.uapb.edu
Web Site: www.uapb.edu
Management:
  Director Public Relations: Carl Whimper

5870 HESTAND STADIUM
420 N Blake
Pine Bluff, AZ 71601
Phone: 870-535-2900
Fax: 870-534-2864
e-mail: hollandl@seark.com
Web Site: www.pinebluffonline.com/hestand.htm
Management:
  Manager: Robert Tollson
Seating Capacity: 7,000

5871 YAVAPAI COLLEGE
1100 E Sheldon
Prescott, AZ 86301
Phone: 520-776-2034
Fax: 520-776-2032
e-mail: debbie_mccasland@yavapai.cc.az.us
Web Site: www.yavapai.edu
Management:
  Community Events Mamager: Debbie McCasland
Mission: To present a broad variety of music, dance and
theatre.
Founded: 1976
Paid Staff: 4
Paid Artists: 300
Income Sources: Ticket Sales; Grants
Performs At: Performance Hall
Annual Attendance: 30,000
Facility Category: Theater
Type of Stage: Proscenium; Thurst
Stage Dimensions: 40'x50'
Seating Capacity: 1100
Year Built: 1992
Cost: $6.5 Million
Rental Contact: Garry Charter

5872 RAWHIDE PAVILION & RODEO ARENA
23023 N Scottsdale Road
Scottsdale, AZ 85255
Phone: 480-502-1880
Fax: 480-502-1301
Toll-free: 800-527-1880
e-mail: info@rawhide.com
Web Site: www.rawhide.com
Management:
  Manager: Marc Lemer
Founded: 1971
Annual Attendance: 960,000
Seating Capacity: 4,500

5873 SCOTTSDALE CENTER FOR THE ARTS
7380 E 2nd Street
Scottsdale, AZ 85251
Phone: 480-994-2787
Fax: 480-874-4699
e-mail: info@sccarts.org
Web Site: www.scottsdalearts.org
Officers:
  President/CEO: Frank Jacbson
Management:
  Director/VP: Kathy Hotchner
  Director Marketing/VP: Matt Lehrman
  Education Director: Linda Jane Austen
Specialized Field: Performing Arts

Paid Staff: 60
Type of Stage: Proscenium/Thrust
Seating Capacity: 833

5874 SCOTTSDALE COMMUNITY COLLEGE

9000 E Chaparral
Scottsdale, AZ 85250
Phone: 480-423-6350
Fax: 480-423-6365
e-mail: admissions@scinfo.sc.maricopa.edu
Web Site: www.sc.maricopa.edu
Management:
    Coordinator Fine Arts: James P O'Brien
Founded: 1970
Budget: $20,000-35,000
Performs At: Theatre; Recital Hall; Outdoor
Amphitheatre
Seating Capacity: 349; 105; 1000

5875 COCHISE COLLEGE

901 Colombo
Sierra Vista, AZ 85635
Phone: 520-515-5440
Toll-free: 800-966-7943
Web Site: www.cochise.edu
Management:
    Manager: M David Meeker
Founded: 1961

5876 SIERRA VISTA PARKS AND LEISURE SERVICES

1011 N Coronado Drive
Sierra Vista, AZ 85635
Phone: 520-417-6980
Fax: 520-417-6992
e-mail: tadkins@ci.sierra-vista.az.us
Web Site: www.ci.sierra-vista.az.us/
Management:
    Cultural Lifestyles Supervisor: Tracey Adkins
Budget: $35,000-60,000
Performs At: Buena Performing Arts Center
Type of Stage: Flexible
Seating Capacity: 1,366

5877 ARIZONA STATE UNIVERSITY: SUNDOME CENTER

19403 RH Johnson Boulevard
Sun City West, AZ 85375
Phone: 623-584-3118
Fax: 623-584-7947
Web Site: www.asusundome.com
Management:
    Director: M Smokey Renehan
    Technical Director: Rob Neyman
    Event / Rental Coordinator: Melissa Schwartz
Paid Staff: 35
Volunteer Staff: 250
Paid Artists: 35
Non-paid Artists: 60
Affiliations: Arizona State University; APAP; WAA
Annual Attendance: 300,000
Facility Category: Performing Arts
Type of Stage: Proscenium

Seating Capacity: 7036
Year Built: 1978
Rental Contact: Melissa Schwartz

5878 ARIZONA STATE UNIVERSITY - GAMMAGE AUDITORIUM

Corner of Mill Ave. & Apache Blvd.
Tempe, AZ 85287
Phone: 480-965-5062
Fax: 480-965-3583
Web Site: www.asugammage.com/home.shtml
Founded: 1962
Type of Stage: Concert Stage; Flexible
Seating Capacity: 3,000

5879 ARIZONA STATE UNIVERSITY ACTIVITY CENTER

Tempe, AZ 85287
Phone: 480-965-5062
Fax: 480-965-7663

5880 SUN DEVIL STADIUM

500 E Stadium Drive
PO Box 872405
Tempe, AZ 85287
Phone: 480-965-3933
Fax: 480-965-8154
Toll-free: 888-786-3857
e-mail: linda.gorman@asu.edu
Web Site: www.thesundevils.com
Management:
    Director Stadium Management: Tom Sadler
    Marketing Director: Lyn Music
    Senior Program Coordinator: Heather Morris
    Concessions Manager: Chris Nations
Founded: 1968
Specialized Field: Facility
Seating Capacity: 74,000

5881 NAVAJO DINE COLLEGE

1 College Circle
Tsaile, AZ 86556
Phone: 928-724-6630
Fax: 928-724-3349
e-mail: wjensen@crystal.ncc.cc.nm.us
Web Site: www.crystal.ncc.cc.nm.us
Management:
    Student Programs Director: Walter Jensen

5882 TUBAC CENTER OF THE ARTS

9 Plaza Road
PO Box 1911
Tubac, AZ 85646
Phone: 520-398-2371
Fax: 520-398-9511
e-mail: artcntr@flash.net
Web Site: www.tubacarts.org
Management:
    Performing Arts Coordinator: Marty Spencer
Founded: 1972
Paid Staff: 4
Volunteer Staff: 200
Budget: $10,000

Performs At: Auditorium
Annual Attendance: 36,000
Facility Category: Regional Art Center
Type of Stage: Flexible
Seating Capacity: 175
Year Built: 1972
Year Remodeled: 1999

5883 ARIZONA STADIUM UNIVERSITY OF ARIZONA

University of Arizona
Tucson, AZ 85721
Phone: 520-621-2287
Fax: 520-621-2419
Toll-free: 800-452-2287
Web Site: www.arizcats.com
Management:
    Director Operations: Mark Harlan
Specialized Field: Sports Facility
Affiliations: NCAA, Home to University of Arizona athletics, football season games
Seating Capacity: 56,136
Year Built: 1979

5884 HI CORBETT FIELD

900 South Randolph Way
Tucson, AZ 85716
Phone: 520-327-2621
Toll-free: 520-327-2371
Management:
    Director: James Ronstadt

5885 MCKALE MEMORIAL CENTER

University of Arizona
1020 E University Boulevard
Tucson, AZ 85721
Phone: 520-621-2200
Fax: 520-621-9690
Management:
    Director: Larrry R Duffin
    Assistant Manager: Mary Jean Draper
Seating Capacity: 20,000

5886 TUCSON CONVENTION CENTER

260 S Church Avenue
Tucson, AZ 85701
Phone: 520-791-4101
Fax: 520-791-5572
e-mail: eaguirr1@ci.tucson.az.us
Web Site: www.ci.tucson.az.us/tcc
Management:
    Director: Hymie Gonzales
    Marketing Director: Clarence Boykins
    Finance Director: Juanita Williams
    Public Relations: Vikki Hibberd
Founded: 1971
Paid Staff: 100
Seating Capacity: 6,000
Rental Contact: Marketing Director Clarence Boykins

5887 TUCSON CONVENTION CENTER - ARENA

260 S Church Avenue
Tucson, AZ 85701
Phone: 520-791-4101
Fax: 520-791-5572
e-mail: eaguirr1@ci.tucson.az.us
Web Site: www.ci.tucson.az.us
Management:
    Director: Hymie Gonzales
    Marketing Director: Clarence Boykins
    Finance Director: Juanita Williams
    Public Relations: Vikki Hibberd
Founded: 1981
Paid Staff: 100
Facility Category: Arena
Type of Stage: Flexible
Seating Capacity: 9,278
Year Built: 1971
Rental Contact: Marketing Director Clarence Boykins

5888 TUCSON CONVENTION CENTER - EXHIBITION HALL

260 S Church Avenue
Tucson, AZ 85701
Phone: 520-791-4101
Fax: 520-791-5572
e-mail: eaguirr1@ci.tucson.az.us
Web Site: www.ci.tucson.az.us
Management:
    Director: Hymie Gonzales
    Marketing Director: Clarence Boykins
    Finance Director: Juanita Williams
    Public Relations: Vikki Hibberd
Founded: 1981
Paid Staff: 100
Facility Category: Exhibition Hall
Seating Capacity: 6,000
Year Built: 1981
Rental Contact: Marketing Director Clarence Boykins

5889 TUCSON CONVENTION CENTER - LEO RICH THEATRE

260 S Church Avenue
Tucson, AZ 85701
Phone: 520-791-4101
Fax: 520-791-5572
e-mail: eaguirr1@ci.tucson.az.us
Web Site: www.ci.tucson.az.us
Management:
    Director: Hymie Gonzales
    Marketing Director: Clarence Boykins
    Finance Director: Juanita Williams
    Public Relations: Vikki Hibberd
Founded: 1981
Paid Staff: 100
Type of Stage: Proscenium
Seating Capacity: 511
Rental Contact: Marketing Director Clarence Boykins

**5890   TUCSON CONVENTION CENTER -
MUSIC HALL**
260 S Church Avenue
Tucson, AZ 85701
Phone: 520-791-4101
Fax: 520-791-5572
e-mail: eaguirr1@ci.tucson.az.us
Web Site: www.ci.tucson.az.us
Management:
   Director: Hymie Gonzales
   Marketing Director: Clarence Boykins
   Finance Director: Juanita Williams
   Public Relations: Vikki Hibberd
Founded: 1981
Paid Staff: 100
Facility Category: Music Hall
Type of Stage: Concert Stage
Seating Capacity: 4,506
Rental Contact: Marketing Director Clarence Boykins

**5891   TUCSON CONVENTION CENTER -
THEATRE**
260 S Church Avenue
Tucson, AZ 85701
Phone: 520-791-4101
Fax: 520-791-5572
e-mail: eaguirr1@ci.tucson.az.us
Web Site: www.ci.tucson.az.us

**5892   UNIVERSITY OF ARIZONA -
CENTENNIAL HALL**
The University of Arizona
1020 East University Boulevard
Tucson, AZ 85721
Phone: 520-621-3341
Fax: 520-621-8991
e-mail: uapresents@arizona.edu
Web Site: www.uapresents.arizona.edu

**5893   UNIVERSITY OF ARIZONA - CROWDER
HALL**
College of Fine Arts, P.O. Box 210004
Music Bldg Rm. 111, Tucson
Tucson, AZ 85721
Phone: 520-621-1778
Fax: 520-621-1307
e-mail: sevigny@u.arizona.edu
Web Site:
www.web.cfa.arizona.edu/students/crowder.php
Management:
   Technical Director: Julie B Bunker
Mission: Faculty and student music and dance recitals
Founded: 1934
Paid Staff: 2
Performs At: Recital Hall
Seating Capacity: 544

5894   ARIZONA WESTERN COLLEGE
PO Box 929
9500 S Avenue 8 E
Yuma, AZ 85366

Phone: 520-317-6000
Fax: 520-344-7730
Toll-free: 888-293-0392
e-mail: aw_hawkey@awc.cc.az.us
Web Site: www.awc.cc.az.us
Management:
   Student Activities Coordinator: Christina Hawkey
Budget: $60,000-150,000
Performs At: Snider Auditorium; Post; Convention
Center;
Seating Capacity: 721; 1000; 1800

5895   RAY KROC BASEBALL COMPLEX
Yuma Civic & Convention Center
1440 Desert Hills Drive, Yuma
Yuma, AZ 85365
Phone: 928-344-3800
Fax: 928-344-9121
e-mail: yccc@deyocomplex.com
Web Site: www.deyocomplex.com
Management:
   Director: Anthony Guerrera
   Complex Supervisor: Joel Hubbard
   Marketing Rep: Mary Jane Chambers
   Booking Manager: Becky Franks
Seating Capacity: 6,590

**5896   YUMA CIVIC AND CONVENTION
CENTER - YUMA ROOM**
Yuma Civic & Convention Center
1441 Desert Hills Drive, Yuma
Yuma, AZ 85365
Phone: 928-344-3800
Fax: 928-344-9121
e-mail: yccc@deyocomplex.com
Web Site: www.deyocomplex.com
Management:
   Marketing Director: Mary Jane Chambers
   Facilities Director: Ben Velasquez
Founded: 1973
Paid Staff: 20
Budget: 1,200,000.00
Income Sources: earned revenue, hospitality tax
Affiliations: IAAM, MPI, SGMP
Type of Stage: portable
Stage Dimensions: 30x40
Seating Capacity: 2,000
Year Built: 1973
Cost: 550.00

Arkansas

5897   GEORGE M SULLIVAN SPORTS ARENA
1600 Gambell Street
Anchorage, AR 99501
Phone: 907-279-0618
Fax: 907-274-0676
Management:
   Marketing Director: Tanya Hoak

All listings are in alphabetical order by state, then city, then organization within the city.

5898 UAA SPORTS ARENA
UAA Athletics, Anchorage
3211 Providence Drive
Anchorage, AR 99508
Phone: 907-786-1250
Fax: 907-786-1142
e-mail: goseawolves@uaa.alaska.edu
Web Site: www.goseawolves.com
Management:
  Athletic Director: Steve Cobb
  Sports Information Director: Nate Sagan
  Associate Athletic Director: Tim McDriffett
Seating Capacity: 1,250

5899 OUACHITA BAPTIST UNIVERSITY: DEPARTMENT OF THE ARTS
410 Ouachita Street
Arkadelphia, AR 71998
Phone: 870-245-5000
Fax: 870-245-5500
e-mail: wrightc@obu.edu
Web Site: www.obu.edu
Seating Capacity: 1,500

5900 RITZ CIVIC CENTER
306 W Main Street
Blytheville
Blytheville, AR 72315
Phone: 501-762-1744
Fax: 501-763-1950
e-mail: artscouncil@arkansas.net
Web Site: www.arkansas.com
Management:
  Director: Rae Glidewell

5901 EL DORADO MUNICIPAL AUDITORIUM
100 W 8th Street
El Dorado, AR 71730
Phone: 870-862-1387

5902 SOUTH ARKANSAS ARTS CENTER
110 East 5th Street
Suite 206
El Dorado, AR 71730
Phone: 870-862-5474
Fax: 870-862-4921
e-mail: saac@cox-internet.com
Web Site: www.saac-arts.org
Officers:
  President: Paul Stuart
  Vice President: Dan Francis
  Secretary: Carol Wofsey
  Treasurer: John Niemann
Management:
  Manager: Virginia Matthews

5903 CARLSON CENTER
Ogden Entertainment
2010 2nd Avenue
Fairbanks
Fairbanks, AR 99701

Phone: 907-451-7800
Fax: 907-451-1195
e-mail: info@carlson-center.com
Web Site: www.carlson-center.com
Management:
  General Manager: Joyce White
  Operations Manager: Kirk Patton
  Catering Manager: Martha Stickler
Mission: Event Facility
Type of Stage: Concert Stage; Portable; Sico
Seating Capacity: 3,470; 6,539

5904 FINE ARTS CONCERT HALL
University of Arkansas
Fayetteville, AR 72701
Phone: 479-575-4701
Fax: 479-575-5409
e-mail: smitche@uark.edu
Web Site: www.uark.edu

5905 UNIVERSITY OF ARKANSAS BUD WALTON ARENA
PO Box 7777
Fayetteville
Fayetteville, AR 72701
Phone: 479-575-2000
Fax: 501-575-3716
e-mail: arkansas@comp.uark.edu
Web Site: www.uark.edu
Management:
  Arena Manager: Fred Vorsanger
  Concession Manager: Mike Holbrook
Specialized Field: Sports Arena
Seating Capacity: 19,500

5906 WALTON ARTS CENTER
229 North School Street, PO Box 3547
Fayetteville
Fayetteville, AR 72702
Phone: 479-443-9216
Fax: 479-443-6461
e-mail: jpburns@uark.edu
Web Site: www.waltonartscenter.org
Officers:
  President/CEO: Anita K Scism
  Senior VP: Jenni Taylor Swain
Management:
  VP/Communications: Terri Trotter
  Programs: Jenni Taylor Swain
Mission: Visual and performing arts center.
Founded: 1992
Paid Staff: 45
Volunteer Staff: 300
Non-paid Artists: 50
Budget: $4 million
Income Sources: Ticket Sales, Corporate Sponsors, Members, Grants
Performs At: 1200 Seat Hall; 200 Seat Black Box
Affiliations: APAP, Midwest Arts Alliance
Annual Attendance: 150,000+
Type of Stage: Proscenium
Stage Dimensions: 58 x 40
Seating Capacity: 1,200
Year Built: 1992

Cost: 9 Million

5907 FORT SMITH CIVIC CENTER - EXHIBITION HALL

55 S 7th Street
Fort Smith
Fort Smith, AR 72901
Phone: 479-788-8932
Fax: 479-788-8930
e-mail: bmurphy@fsark.com
Web Site: www.fsark.com

5908 FORT SMITH CIVIC CENTER - THEATER

55 S 7th Street
Fort Smith
Fort Smith, AR 72901
Phone: 479-788-8932
Fax: 479-788-8930
e-mail: bmurphy@fsark.com
Web Site: www.fsark.com

5909 FORT SMITH CONVENTION CENTER

55 S 7th Street
Fort Smith, AR 72901
Phone: 501-788-8932
Fax: 501-788-8930
e-mail: mjordin@fsark.com
Web Site: www.fsark.com
Management:
    Director Convention Center: Frankie Hamilton
    Entertainment Director: Melanie Jordin
    Operations Manager: Wesley Hooks
Mission: Multipurpose facility for conventions, tradeshows, banquets, meetings, PAC performances and 40,000 square feet Exhibit Hall with riser seating.
Founded: 1966
Status: Operational
Paid Staff: 12
Income Sources: Concerts; Tradeshows; Conventions; Banquets; Rental Facilities
Annual Attendance: 500,000
Facility Category: Convention Center
Type of Stage: Hardwood on plywood substrate
Stage Dimensions: 58 x 42
Seating Capacity: 1330; 4700
Year Built: 1966
Year Remodeled: 2000
Cost: $27 Million
Rental Contact: Melanie Jordin

5910 FORT SMITH LITTLE THEATRE

401 North 6th Street
Fort Smith
Fort Smith, AR 72913
Phone: 479-783-1295
e-mail: billcovey@worldnet.att.net
Web Site: www.fslt.20fr.com
Founded: 1948

5911 KAY ROGERS PARK

4317 N 50th Street
Fort Smith, AR 72904

Phone: 507-738-6176
Fax: 501-782-9944
Management:
    Director: Jim Berry
Seating Capacity: 13,000

5912 WESTARK COMMUNITY COLLEGE - BREEDLOVE AUDITORIUM

5210 Grand Avenue, PO Box 3649
Fort Smith
Fort Smith, AR 72913
Phone: 479-788-7000
Fax: 501-788-7308
e-mail: information@uafortsmith.edu
Web Site: www.uafortsmith.edu

5913 HOT SPRINGS CONVENTION AND VISITORS' BUREAU

134 Convention Boulevard, PO Box K
Hot Springs
Hot Springs, AR 71902
Phone: 501-321-2835
Fax: 501-321-2136
e-mail: hscvb@hotsprings.org
Web Site: www.hotsprings.org

5914 FORUM

115 East Monroe
Jonesboro, AR 72401
Phone: 870-935-2726
Fax: 870-933-9505
e-mail: foa@insolwwb.net
Web Site: www.clt.astate.edu
Founded: 1926

5915 FOUNDATION OF ARTS

115 East Monroe
PO Box 310
Jonesboro, AR 72403
Phone: 870-935-2726
Fax: 870-933-9505
e-mail: foa@jonesborofoa.com
Web Site: www.jonesborofoa.com
Management:
    Manager: Karen Tjaden
Performs At: Auditorium
Seating Capacity: 690

5916 RAY WINDER FIELD

War Memorial Park
PO Box 55066
Little Rock, AR 72215
Phone: 501-664-1555
Fax: 501-664-1834
e-mail: travs@travs.com
Web Site: www.travs.com
Management:
    Executive Vice President: Bill Valentine
    Assistant General Manager: Hap Seliga
    Assistant General Manager: John Evens
    Superintendant: Greg Johnson
    Director Stadium Operations: Scott Tyler
    Assistant Park Supervisor: Reggi Temple

Founded: 1932
Seating Capacity: 6,083

5917 ROBINSON CENTER MUSIC HALL
Markham and Broadway
P. O. Box 3232
Little Rock, AR 72203
Phone: 501-376-4781
Fax: 501-374-2255
Toll-free: 800-844-4781
e-mail: lrcvb@littlerock.com
Web Site: www.littlerock.com
Affiliations: Arkansas Symphony Orchestra Celebrity Attractions
Year Built: 1939
Year Remodeled: 1989
Rental Contact: Lisa Simmons

5918 UNIVERSITY OF ARKANSAS-LITTLE ROCK
2801 South University Avenue
Little Rock, AR 72204
Phone: 501-569-3000
Fax: 501-569-3181
e-mail: recoates@ualr.edu
Web Site: www.ualr.edu

5919 WAR MEMORIAL STADIUM
Markham - Van Buren Street
Little Rock
Little Rock, AR 72205
Phone: 501-663-6385
Fax: 501-663-6387
Web Site: www.state.ar.us/wms
Management:
  Manager: Charlie Staggs
  Assistant Manager: Wayne Dyer
Seating Capacity: 53,715

5920 WILDWOOD PARK FOR THE PERFORMING ARTS
20919 Denny Road
Little Rock, AR 72223
Phone: 501-821-7275
Fax: 501-821-7280
Toll-free: 888-821-7225
e-mail: achotard@wildwoodpark.org
Web Site: www.wildwoodpark.org
Officers:
  Chairman Emeritus: Lucy C Cabe
  Chairman: Bill Morton
  President: Ellen M Gary
  VP: Melissa Thoma
  Secretary: Dolores Bruce
  Treasurer: William Mortan, MD
Management:
  Founder/Artistic Director: Dr. Ann Chotard
  Director of Finance: Benny Cagle
  Diector Education: Mary Smith
  Conductor: Pioir SulKowski
Founded: 1991
Paid Staff: 4
Budget: $1.2 Million

Income Sources: Friends of Wildwood, Grants, City and State Fundings
Affiliations: Opera America
Annual Attendance: 3,750
Facility Category: Opera House
Type of Stage: Thrust
Seating Capacity: 625
Year Built: 1996
Cost: $6 Million

5921 WILKINS STADIUM
Southern Arkansas University
100 East University
Magnolia, AR 71753
Phone: 870-235-4000
Fax: 870-235-4988
e-mail: muleriders@saumag.edu
Web Site: www.saumag.edu
Management:
  Executive Assistant to President: Ronnie Birdsong
  Director Development: Sharon Eichenberger
  University Editor: Mark Trout
Seating Capacity: 6,000

5922 ARTS AND SCIENCE CENTER FOR SOUTHEAST ARKANSAS
701 S Main Street
Pine Bluff, AR 71601
Phone: 870-536-3375
Fax: 870-536-3380
e-mail: asc@seark.net
Management:
  Director Performing Arts: Philip Counts
Founded: 1968
Paid Staff: 2
Volunteer Staff: 300
Non-paid Artists: 80
Budget: $110,000
Income Sources: Ticket Sales; Sponsorship; Grants
Annual Attendance: 5,500
Facility Category: multi-use
Seating Capacity: 232
Year Built: 1994

5923 PINE BLUFF CONVENTION CENTER
One Convention Center Plaza
701, Main street
Pine Bluff, AR 71601
Phone: 870-536-3375
Fax: 870-536-3380
Toll-free: 800-536-7660
e-mail: pbinfo@pinebluff.com
Web Site: www.pinebluff.com
Management:
  Executive Director: Bob Purvis

5924 PINE BLUFF CONVENTION CENTER - ARENA
1 Convention Center Plaza
701, Main street
Pine Bluff, AR 71601

Phone: 870-536-3375
Fax: 870-536-3380
Toll-free: 800-536-7660
e-mail: pbinfo@pinebluff.com
Web Site: www.pinebluff.com
Management:
  Deputy Director: Steven Burnett
  Sales/Marketing Director: Pam Jones
  Events Manager: Auryo Smith
  Events Manager: Marion Anderson
  Sales Manager: Dena Warner
Paid Staff: 26

5925 PINE BLUFF CONVENTION CENTER - AUDITORIUM
500 E 8th Street
701, Main street
Pine Bluff, AR 71601
Phone: 870-536-3375
Fax: 870-536-3380
e-mail: pbinfo@pinebluff.com
Web Site: www.pinebluff.com

5926 ARKANSAS RIVER VALLEY ARTS CENTER
PO Box 2112
Russellville
Russellville, AR 72811
Phone: 479-968-2452
Fax: 479-968-5015
e-mail: artscenter@centurytel.net
Web Site:
www.museumsusa.org/data/museums/AR/116979.htm
Management:
  Executive Director: Christine Tracy
Founded: 1981
Annual Attendance: 5,000
Seating Capacity: 400

5927 ARKANSAS TECH UNIVERSITY - WITHERSPOON ARTS ARENA
1505 North Boulder Avenue
Russellville
Russellville, AR 72801
Phone: 479-968-0244
Fax: 501-964-0812
e-mail: donna.vocate@mail.atu.edu
Web Site: www.atu.edu

5928 JOHN E TUCKER COLISEUM
Arkansas Tech Athletic Department
Tucker Coliseum, 1604 Coliseum Drive
Russellville, AR 72801
Phone: 479-968-0345
Fax: 479-964-0829
e-mail: larry.smith@mail.atu.edu
Web Site: www.atu.edu
Management:
  Athletic Director: Earl Dowman
Founded: 1976
Seating Capacity: 3,500

5929 ARTS CENTER OF THE OZARKS
214 South Main street
P.O. Box 725, Springdale
Springdale, AR 72765
Phone: 479-751-5441
Fax: 479-927-0308
e-mail: acozarks@swbell.net
Web Site: www.artscenteroftheozarks.org

5930 CONVOCATION CENTER
Arkansas State University
217 Olympic Drive
PO Box 880
State University, AR 72467
Phone: 870-972-3870
Fax: 870-972-3825
e-mail: timd@astate.edu
Web Site: www.convo.astate.edu
Management:
  Director: Tim L Dean
Founded: 1987
Budget: $1 million
Annual Attendance: 350,000
Facility Category: Arena
Type of Stage: Sico
Stage Dimensions: 60'x40'
Seating Capacity: 10,500
Year Built: 1987
Year Remodeled: 2001
Cost: $18.6 million
Rental Contact: Tim Dean

California

5931 ANAHEIM CONVENTION CENTER
800 W Katella Avenue
Anaheim
Anaheim, CA 92802
Phone: 765-999-8950
Fax: 714-999-8965
Web Site: www.anaheimoc.org

5932 ANAHEIM CONVENTION CENTER - ARENA
800 W Katella Avenue
Anaheim
Anaheim, CA 92802
Phone: 765-999-8950
Fax: 714-999-8965
Web Site: www.anaheimoc.org

5933 EDISON INTERNATIONAL FIELD OF ANAHEIM
2000 Gene Autry Way
Anaheim
Anaheim, CA 92806
Phone: 714-634-2000
Fax: 714-940-2001
e-mail: pr@angels.mlb.com
Web Site: www.angelsbaseball.com
Management:

Director Ticket Sales, Disney: Steve Shiffman
General Manager ARA Services: Lonco Irvins
Specialized Field: Home to the Anaheim Angels (MLB) and many other events and consumer shows.
Seating Capacity: 45,050
Year Built: 1966
Year Remodeled: 1998

5934 CABRILLO COLLEGE THEATER

6500 Soquel Drive
Aptos
Aptos, CA 95003
Phone: 831-479-6429
Fax: 831-464-8382
e-mail: contactus@cabrillostage.com
Web Site: www.cabrillostage.com
Founded: 1981

5935 CENTERARTS
Humboldt State University

Humboldt State University, 1 Harpst Street
Arcata
Arcata, CA 95521
Phone: 707-826-4411
Fax: 707-826-5980
e-mail: 20srb1@humboldt.edu
Web Site: www.humboldt.edu
Management:
   Director: Roy Furshpan

5936 HUMBOLDT STATE UNIVERSITY - EAST GYMNASIUM

Humboldt State University, 1 Harpst Street
Arcata
Arcata, CA 95521
Phone: 707-826-4411
Fax: 707-826-5980
e-mail: 20srb1@humboldt.edu
Web Site: www.humboldt.edu
Seating Capacity: 1,400

5937 HUMBOLDT STATE UNIVERSITY - FULKERSON RECITAL HALL

Humboldt State University, 1 Harpst Street
Arcata
Arcata, CA 95521
Phone: 707-826-4411
Fax: 707-826-5980
e-mail: 20srb1@humboldt.edu
Web Site: www.humboldt.edu
Seating Capacity: 201

5938 HUMBOLDT STATE UNIVERSITY - JOHN VAN DUZER THEATRE

Humboldt State University, 1 Harpst Street
Arcata
Arcata, CA 95521
Phone: 707-826-4411
Fax: 707-826-5980
e-mail: 20srb1@humboldt.edu
Web Site: www.humboldt.edu
Seating Capacity: 862

5939 HUMBOLDT STATE UNIVERSITY - KATE BUCHANAN ROOM

Humboldt State University, 1 Harpst Street
Arcata
Arcata, CA 95521
Phone: 707-826-4411
Fax: 707-826-5980
e-mail: 20srb1@humboldt.edu
Web Site: www.humboldt.edu
Seating Capacity: 600

5940 BAKERSFIELD CIVIC AUDITORIUM

Bakersfield Convention Center
1001 Truxton Avenue
Bakersfield, CA 93301
Phone: 661-852-7300
Fax: 661-861-9904
Toll-free: 888-255-2200
e-mail:
BroadwayInBakersfield@BroadwayAcrossAmerica.c
Web Site: www.centennialgarden.com

5941 CALIFORNIA STATE UNIVERSITY: DORE THEATRE

9001 Stockdale Highway
Bakersfield, CA 93311
Phone: 805-664-2221
Fax: 661-665-6901

5942 BERKELEY COMMUNITY THEATRE

1930 Allston Way
Berkeley
Berkeley, CA 94710
Phone: 415-346-7222
Fax: 415-771-9710
Web Site: www.premiertickets.com/berkeley.htm

5943 JULIA MORGAN CENTER FOR THE ARTS

2640 College Avenue
Berkeley, CA 94704
Phone: 510-845-8542
Fax: 510-845-3133
e-mail: bridget@juliamorgan.org
Web Site: www.juliamorgan.org
Management:
   Production Coordinator: Bridget Frederick
   Executive Director: Sabrina Klein
   Producing Manager: Patrick Dooley
Mission: The Julia Morgan Center for the Arts is a home for artists, educators, learners and the community.
Founded: 1980
Specialized Field: Music, Dance, Visual Arts, Theatre
Status: Nonprofit
Paid Staff: 8
Budget: $700,000
Type of Stage: Proscenrum
Stage Dimensions: 39'4" x 31'6"
Seating Capacity: 400
Year Built: 1908
Year Remodeled: 1990
Cost: $650-$1250
Rental Contact: Bridget Frederick

5944 LA PENA CULTURAL CENTER
3105 Shattuck Avenue
Berkeley
Berkeley, CA 94705
Phone: 510-849-2568
Fax: 510-849-9397
e-mail: info@lapena.org
Web Site: www.lapena.org
Management:
   Contact: Paul B Chin
Mission: To present cultural educational programs that
increase understanding of different cultures and support
efforts to build a more just society based on respect for
human, social and economic rights for all people; to
operate a multi-use cultural center/community gathering
place where people of all races and cultures can share the
rich and diverse heritages of the Americas and learn about
conditions in the US, Latin American and the world.
Founded: 1975
Specialized Field: Latin American Music
Paid Staff: 7
Volunteer Staff: 20
Paid Artists: 4
Annual Attendance: 25,000
Facility Category: Black Box
Type of Stage: Raised Platform
Stage Dimensions: 24'x14'
Seating Capacity: 170
Year Built: 1932
Year Remodeled: 1990
Cost: $100,000
Rental Contact: Paul Chin

5945 UNIVERSITY OF CALIFORNIA-BERKELEY
Visitor Services, 101 University Hall
2200 University Avenue, Berkeley
Berkeley, CA 94720
Phone: 510-642-5215
Fax: 510-643-6707
e-mail: visitor_info@pa.urel.berkeley.edu
Web Site: www.berkeley.edu

5946 UNIVERSITY OF CALIFORNIA-BERKELEY, ZELLERBAC AUDITORIUM
Cal Performances, 101 Zellerbach Hall #4800
University of California, Berkeley
Berkeley, CA 94720
Phone: 510-642-5215
Fax: 510-643-6707
e-mail: lbaqir@calperfs@calperfs.berkeley.edu
Web Site: www.berkeley.edu
Type of Stage: Proscenium
Seating Capacity: 2,089

5947 CAL PERFORMANCES
University of CA Berkley
101 Zellerbach Hall
#480
Berkley, CA 94720-4800

Phone: 510-642-0212
Fax: 510-643-6707
e-mail: rcole@calperfs.berkley.edu
Web Site: www.calperfs.berkley.edu
Management:
   Director: Robert W Cole
   Associate Director: Hollis Ashby

5948 BEVERLY HILLS PLAYHOUSE
254 S Robertson Boulevard
Beverly Hills, CA 90212
Phone: 310-855-1556
e-mail: info@katselas.com
Web Site: www.katselas.com
Management:
   Rental Coordinator: Tom McCafferty
Season: Year Round
Type of Stage: Proscenium

5949 BIG BEAR LAKE PERFORMING ARTS CENTER
39707 Big Bear Boulevard
PO Box 10000
Big Bear Lake, CA 92315
Phone: 909-866-4970
Fax: 909-878-2183
e-mail: pac@bigbearpac.com
Web Site: www.bigbearpac.com
Volunteer Staff: 10
Annual Attendance: 18,000
Facility Category: Performing Arts Center
Type of Stage: Wood
Stage Dimensions: 40'x55'
Seating Capacity: 398
Year Built: 1988
Cost: $3 million
Rental Contact: Manager Don Gavitte

5950 CURTIS THEATRE
1 Civic Center Circle
Brea, CA 92821
Phone: 714-990-7722
Fax: 714-990-7635
e-mail: curtistheatre.ci@brea.ca.us
Web Site: www.ci.brea.ca.us
Management:
   Manager: Christian Wolf
   Technical Director: Kevin Clowes
   Box Office: Amber Jackson
Affiliations: Western Arts Alliance; California
Presenters; Association of Performing Arts
Facility Category: Theatre
Type of Stage: Procenium
Stage Dimensions: 42W X 36D
Seating Capacity: 199
Year Built: 1981
Rental Contact: Manager Christian Wolf

5951 AIA ACTOR'S STUDIO
1918 Magnola Boulevard
Suite 204
Burbank, CA 91506

Phone: 818-563-4142
Fax: 818-563-4042
e-mail: emily@aiastudios.com
Web Site: www.aiastudios.com
Officers:
   VP/Director: Emily Yost
Mission: Mission is help actors achieve professional excellence. Has sucessfully integrated the business of acting with formal training. Insructors from the firlds of casting, producing, directing, writing and acting teach a diverse array of classe
Facility Category: Actor's Studio
Rental Contact: VP/Director Emily Yost

5952 SUNSET CENTER
City of Carmel
PO Box 1950
Carmel, CA 93921
Phone: 831-624-3996
Fax: 831-624-0147
e-mail: bdonog@aol.com
Web Site: www.sunsetcenter.com
Management:
   Director: Brian Donoghue

5953 CALIFORNIA STATE UNIVERSITY-DOMINGUEZ HILLS
1000 E Victoria Street
Carson, CA 90747
Phone: 310-243-3696
Fax: 310-516-4268
e-mail: info@csudh.edu
Web Site: www.csudh.edu

5954 OLYMPIC VELODROME/CALIFORNIA STATE UNIVERSITY
Dominguez Hills
1000 E Victoria Street
Carson, CA 90747
Phone: 310-516-4000
Fax: 310-217-6848
e-mail: bhornet@earthlink.net
Management:
   General Manager: Brad House
Seating Capacity: 8,500

5955 CERRITOS CENTER
12700 Center Court Drive
Cerritos, CA 90703
Phone: 562-916-8510
Fax: 562-916-8514
Toll-free: 800-300-4345
Web Site: cerritoscenter.com
Management:
   Operations: Tom Hamilton
   Box Office Manager: Kate Ladd
   Performance Manager: Michael Wolfe
   Executive Director: Craig M Sprenger PhD
Founded: 1993
Specialized Field: Dance; Music; Theatre
Paid Staff: 100
Volunteer Staff: 500
Paid Artists: 100

Non-paid Artists: 0
Budget: $11,000,000
Income Sources: Ticket Sales; Rental Revenue
Affiliations: California Presenters; Western Arts Alliance; APAP; ISPA; IAAM; IATT
Annual Attendance: 200,000
Facility Category: Multi-configuration auditorium
Seating Capacity: 950-1800
Year Built: 1992
Cost: $105,000,000
Rental Contact: Cynthia Doss

5956 CALIFORNIA STATE UNIVERSITY, CHICO
400 West First Street
Chico, CA 95929
Phone: 530-898-4636
Fax: 530-898-4797
e-mail: kfernandes@csuchico.edu
Web Site: www.csuchico.edu
Management:
   Director: Dan De Wayne
Budget: $400,000-$1,000,000
Performs At: Laxson Auditorium; Adams Theatre
Facility Category: Pit Stage; Proscenium
Seating Capacity: 1300; 500

5957 CLAREMONT COLLEGES - GARRISON THEATRE
150 E. Eighth Street
Claremont, CA 91711
Phone: 909-621-8000
Web Site: www.cuc.claremont.edu

5958 CLAREMONT COLLEGES - MABEL SHAW BRIDGES AUDITORIUM
450 N College Way
Claremont, CA 91711
Phone: 909-621-8031
Fax: 909-621-8398
e-mail: sharon_kuhn@cucmail.claremont.edu
Management:
   Events Manager: Sharon L Kuhn

5959 CHRONICLE PAVILION
2000 Kirker Pass Road
Concord, CA 94521
Phone: 925-676-8742
Fax: 510-676-7262
e-mail: chroniclepavilion@clearchannel.com
Web Site: www.chroniclepavilion.com

5960 WILLOWS THEATRE
1425 Gasoline Alley
Concord, CA 94520
Phone: 925-798-1300
Fax: 925-676-5726
e-mail: info@willowstheatre.org
Web Site: www.willowstheatre.org
Management:
   Managing Director: Andrew Holtz
Founded: 1975

Status: Nonprofit
Season: January - December
Annual Attendance: 48,000
Type of Stage: Proscenium; Amphitheater
Stage Dimensions: 40' x 26'
Seating Capacity: 210; 1200

5961 ORANGE COUNTY PERFORMING ARTS CENTER

600 Town Center Drive
Costa Mesa, CA 92626
Phone: 714-556-2122
Fax: 714-556-0156
e-mail: info@ocpac.org
Web Site: www.ocpac.org
Officers:
   President/COO: Jerry E Mandel, PhD
Management:
   VP Programming: Judy Morr

5962 SOUTH COAST REPERTORY - SEGERSTROM AUDITORIUM

655 Town Center Drive
Costa Mesa, CA 92626
Phone: 714-957-2603
e-mail: theatre@scr.org.
Web Site: www.scr.org

5963 VETERAN'S MEMORIAL AUDITORIUM

4117 Overland Avenue
Culver City, CA 90230
Phone: 310-253-6625

5964 FLINT CENTER FOR THE PERFORMING ARTS

De Anza College
21250 Stevens Creek Boulevard
PO Box 1897
Cupertino, CA 95015
Phone: 408-864-8820
Fax: 408-864-8918
e-mail: flintgm@ix.netcom.com
Web Site: www.flintcenter.com
Management:
   General Manager: Paula J Davis
Founded: 1971
Annual Attendance: 265,000
Type of Stage: Proscenium
Seating Capacity: 2,300

5965 DAVIS ART CENTER

1919 F Street
PO Box 4340
Davis, CA 95617
Phone: 530-756-4100
Fax: 530-756-3041
e-mail: davisart@dcn.davis.ca.us
Web Site: www.davisartcenter.com
Founded: 1961
Annual Attendance: 50,000

5966 RECREATION HALL

University of California-Davis
Davis, CA 95616
Phone: 530-752-6071
Fax: 530-752-3055
e-mail: bcburns@ucdavis.edu
Web Site: www.rechall.ucdavis.edu
Management:
   Facility Director: James Dodems
   Assistant Manager: Brett Burns
   Assistant Manager: Dan Manfinger
Founded: 1977
Paid Staff: 130
Seating Capacity: 10,111

5967 VETERANS' MEMORIAL THEATRE

203 E 14th Street
Davis, CA 95616
Phone: 530-757-5665

5968 EVENT FACILITIES MANAGEMENT OFFICE

164 Pauley Pavilion
Drake Stadium, CA 90095-1552
Phone: 310-825-4546
Fax: 310-825-5775
Web Site: www.uclabruins.fansonly.com
Management:
   Assistant Director: Rich Mylin

5969 EAST COUNTY PERFORMING ARTS CENTER - THEATRE

210 E Main Street
El Cajon, CA 92020
Phone: 619-440-2277
Fax: 619-440-6429
e-mail: ecpac@ecpac.com
Web Site: www.ecpac.com
Officers:
   President/CEO: Dick Zellner
Management:
   Marketing: Sally Buckelew
   Director Operations/VP: Jennie Mayes
Mission: Perfroming arts presenter and rental house. We book nationally and internationally recognized performers, from the Dixie Chicks to Bob Newhart, from Alvin Ailey to Dave Kue.
Founded: 1977
Specialized Field: Concert presenter; Arts education; Visual arts, Touring theaters
Paid Staff: 8
Budget: $1,900,000
Income Sources: Ticket revenues; Corporate sponsors; Individual donors; Foundations
Performs At: East County Performing Arts Center
Affiliations: Western Alliance of Arts Admistrators, International Association ofAuditorium Managers
Annual Attendance: 100,000
Facility Category: Concert Hall
Type of Stage: Proscenium
Stage Dimensions: 40 x 70
Seating Capacity: 1,142
Year Built: 1977

Year Remodeled: 1998
Rental Contact: Director of Operations Jennie Mayes

5970 SOUTHWEST PERFORMING ARTS THEATRE
2001 Ocotillo Drive
El Centro, CA 92243
Phone: 760-336-4228
Fax: 760-353-2906
e-mail: mcferron@cuhsd.k12.ca.us
Management:
   Theatre Manager: Stephen McFerron

5971 CALIFORNIA CENTER FOR THE ARTS-ESCONDIDO
340 N Escondido Boulevard
Escondido, CA 92025
Phone: 760-839-4138
Fax: 760-739-0205
Toll-free: 800-988-4253
e-mail: ftracey@artcenter.org
Web Site: www.artcenter.org
Officers:
   VP/General Manager: Vicky Basehore
Management:
   Performing Arts Director: JoAnne Ewan-Kroeger
   Assistant Performing Arts Director: Fred Tracey

5972 FONTANA CIVIC AUDITORIUM
9460 Sierra Avenue
Fontana, CA 92335
Phone: 909-428-8360
Fax: 909-428-2546
Web Site: www.fontana.org

5973 FONTANA PERFORMING ARTS CENTER
9460 Sierra Avenue
Fontana, CA 92335
Phone: 909-428-8390
Fax: 909-428-2546
Management:
   Coordinator: Larry Watson

5974 SMITH CENTER FOR THE FINE AND PERFORMING ARTS
Ohlone College
43600 Mission Boulevard
Fremont, CA 94539
Phone: 510-659-6000
Fax: 510-659-6188
e-mail: amillican@ohlone.cc.ca.us
Web Site: www.ohlone.cc.ca.us
Management:
   Dean Fine Arts: R Michael Gros

5975 BULLDOGS STADIUM
California State University- Fresno
5305 N Campus Drive NG27
Fresno, CA 93740

Phone: 559-278-2643
Fax: 559-278-6611
e-mail: mail@gobulldogs.com
Management:
   Athletic Center: Tom Kane
Founded: 1981

5976 CALIFORNIA STATE UNIVERSITY-FRESNO
5241 N Maple
Fresno, CA 93740
Phone: 559-278-4240
Web Site: www.csufresno.edu
Founded: 1911

5977 CALIFORNIA STATE UNIVERSITY-FRESNO, WAHLBERG
2380 E Keats
Fresno, CA 93740
Phone: 559-278-4240
Web Site: www.csufresno.edu

5978 FRESNO CONVENTION CENTER
848 M Street
Fresno, CA 93721
Phone: 559-498-1511
Fax: 559-488-4634
e-mail: valdez@ci.fresno.ca.us
Web Site: www.fresnoconventioncenter.com
Management:
   Convention Center Director: Ernest Valdez
   Convention Manager: Mike Sweeney
   Operations Manager: Greg Eisner
   Marketing Coordinator: Bruce Bucz
Mission: To provide superior customer service to both patrons and clients through selectively booking quality events that enhance the entertainment, assembly and cultural offerings to the Fresno area.
Founded: 1966
Paid Staff: 60
Volunteer Staff: 150
Budget: $2 Million
Income Sources: Rentals
Performs At: Performing Arts Theater
Stage Dimensions: 52'50'
Seating Capacity: 11,300
Year Built: 1966
Year Remodeled: 1992
Cost: $ 3 Million
Rental Contact: Mercy Tritian

5979 RATCLIFFE STADIUM
1101 E University Avenue
Fresno, CA 93741
Phone: 559-442-4600
Fax: 559-485-5322
Toll-free: 866-245-3276
e-mail: kathleen.bonilla@scccd.com
Web Site: www.fcc.cc.ca.us
Management:
   Athletic Director: Ron Scott
Founded: 1910
Seating Capacity: 13,500

5980 TOWER THEATRE FOR THE PERFORMING ARTS
815 E Olive
Fresno, CA 93728
Phone: 559-485-9050
Fax: 209-485-3941

5981 WARNOR'S THEATER
1400 Fulton Street
Fresno, CA 93721
Phone: 559-264-2848
Founded: 1908

5982 MUCKENTHALER CULTURAL CENTER
1201 W Malvern Avenue
Fullerton, CA 92833
Phone: 714-738-6595
Fax: 714-738-6366
e-mail: info@muckenthaler.org
Web Site: www.muckenthaler.org
Management:
Executive Director: Patricia House
Member Services: Beverly Travers
Mission: Dedicated to the study, exhibition and collection of multicultural arts, as well as to the professional staging of performing arts. The center is a multi-disciplinary venue that celebrates the traditions of a variety of cultures and encourages appreciation and creative expression in art, music, dance, literature, drama, local history, landscaping and botanical gardening.
Founded: 1965
Specialized Field: Multi-Cultural/Multi Discipline
Paid Staff: 8

5983 PLUMMER AUDITORIUM
201 E Chapman Avenue
Fullerton, CA 92832
Phone: 714-738-6317
Fax: 714-870-3768
Founded: 1930
Seating Capacity: 1,300

5984 ALEX THEATRE
216 N Brand Boulevard
Glendale, CA 91203
Phone: 818-243-7700
Fax: 818-243-3622
Toll-free: 818-243-ALEX
e-mail: admin@alextheatre.org
Web Site: www.alextheatre.org
Management:
Executive Director: Ellen Ketchum
Founded: 1925

5985 CITRUS COLLEGE HAUGH PERFORMING ARTS CENTER
1000 W Foothill Boulevard
Glendora, CA 91741
Phone: 626-963-9411
Fax: 626-335-4715
e-mail: hpac@citruscollege.edu
Web Site: www.haughpac.com

Management:
Performing Arts Director: Greg Hinrichsen
Annual Attendance: 100,000
Type of Stage: Flexible; Proscenium
Seating Capacity: 1,400

5986 CALIFORNIA STATE UNIVERSITY-HAYWARD - MAIN THEATRE
Carlos Bee Boulevard
25800 Carlos Bee Boulevard
Hayward, CA 94542
Phone: 510-885-3000
e-mail: applycsh@csuhayward.edu
Web Site: www.csuhayward.edu

5987 CHABOT COLLEGE PERFORMING ARTS CENTER
25555 Hesperian Boulevard
1998, Chabot College.
25555 Hesperian Blvd.
Hayward, CA 94545
Phone: 510-723-6600
Fax: 510-723-7157
e-mail: rnoyes@clpccd.cc.ca.us
Web Site: www.chabot.cc.ca.us
Management:
Theatre Manager: Roger Noyes
Founded: 1967
Paid Staff: 3
Volunteer Staff: 6
Income Sources: Rentals
Annual Attendance: 100,000
Type of Stage: Flexible; Proscenium
Stage Dimensions: 46'x22'
Seating Capacity: 1,432 and 200
Year Built: 1967
Cost: $1.8 million

5988 RAMONA BOWL AMPHITHEATRE
27400 Ramona Bowl Road
Hemet, CA 92544
Phone: 909-658-3111
Fax: 909-658-2695
Toll-free: 800-645-4465
e-mail: ramona@ramonapageant.com
Web Site: www.ramonabowl.com
Management:
General Manager: Roger Vitaich
Business Manager: Kathy Long
Box Office Supervisor: Lori West
Marketing and Communications: Janine Mundiler
Mission: To promote and produce The Ramona Pageant, America's longest running outdoor drama; to promote the Ramona Bowl Amphitheatre for events.
Founded: 1923
Paid Staff: 8
Volunteer Staff: 2
Paid Artists: 2
Non-paid Artists: 2

5989 COMPLEX
6476 Santa Monica Boulevard
Hollywood, CA 90038
Phone: 323-465-0383
Fax: 323-465-0008
e-mail: info@complexhollywood.com
Web Site: www.complexhollywood.com

5990 HOLLYWOOD BOWL
2301 N Highland Avenue
Hollywood, CA 90078
Phone: 323-850-2000
e-mail: dborda@laphil.org
Web Site: www.hollywoodbowl.com
  Director Development: Emily Laskin
Founded: 1922
Seating Capacity: 18,000

5991 HOLLYWOOD PALLADIUM
6215 W Sunset Boulevard
Hollywood, CA 90028
Phone: 323-962-7600
Fax: 323-962-7502
Web Site: www.hollywoodpalladium.com
Mission: we are an all purpose revue that has music acts as well as conventions and dinner events.
Founded: 1940

5992 JAMES A DOOLITTLE THEATRE
1615 N Vine Street
Hollywood, CA 90028
Phone: 213-972-0700
Fax: 213-926-2936

5993 JOHN ANSON FORD THEATRES
2580 Cahauga Boulevard E
Hollywood, CA 90068
Phone: 323-461-3673
Fax: 323-464-1158
e-mail: dpiern@bos.co.la.ca.us
Web Site: www.fordamphitheatre.org
Management:
  Managing Director: David Pier
Founded: 1920
Status: Volunteer
Facility Category: Amphitheatre/ Black Box
Seating Capacity: 1245/87
Rental Contact: David Pier

5994 GOLDEN WEST COLLEGE COMMUNITY THEATRE
15744 Golden West Street
Huntington Beach, CA 92647
Phone: 714-892-7711
Fax: 714-895-8784
e-mail: slombard@.gwc.cccd.edu
Web Site: www.gwc.cccd.edu
Management:
  Theatre Director: David Anthony

5995 GOLDEN WEST COLLEGE - MAINSTAGE THEATRE
15744 Golden W Street
Huntington Beach, CA 92647
Phone: 714-892-7711
Fax: 714-895-8784
e-mail: slombard@.gwc.cccd.edu
Web Site: www.gwc.cccd.edu

5996 GREAT WESTERN FORUM
3900 W Manchester Boulevard
Inglewood, CA 90305
Phone: 310-419-3100
Fax: 310-679-2375
Web Site: www.gwforum.com
Management:
  Managing Director: Adam Larr
  Operations Director: Albert Galicia
Specialized Field: Home of the Los Angeles Sparks (WNBA)
Seating Capacity: 17,505, 16,005
Year Built: 1966

5997 BREN EVENTS CENTER
University of California
Irvine, CA 92717
Phone: 949-824-5050
Fax: 949-824-5097
e-mail: bmstrobe@uci.edu
Web Site: www.bren.uci.edu
Founded: 1987
Annual Attendance: 175,000
Type of Stage: Portable
Seating Capacity: 5,700

5998 IRVINE BARCLAY THEATRE
4242 Campus Drive
Irvine, CA 92612
Phone: 949-854-4607
Fax: 949-854-4999
e-mail: info@thebarclay.org
Web Site: www.thebarclay.org
Management:
  General Manager: Christopher Burrill
  President: Douglas C Rankin
  Communications/Program Development: Karen Drews
Type of Stage: Proscenium
Seating Capacity: 756

5999 UNIVERSITY OF CALIFORNIA-IRVINE - VILLAGE THEATRE
University of California
Irvine, CA 92697
Phone: 949-824-5011
Fax: 510-643-6707
Web Site: www.uci.edu
Type of Stage: Concerts

6000 ATHENAEUM MUSIC & ARTS LIBRARY
1008 Wall Street
La Jolla, CA 92037

Phone: 858-454-5872
Fax: 858-454-5835
e-mail: Athlib@pacbell.net
Management:
    Program Director: Geoffrey Brooks
    Executive Director: Erika Torri
Founded: 1898
Paid Staff: 20
Volunteer Staff: 150
Paid Artists: 80
Non-paid Artists: 20
Budget: $ 1.2 Million
Income Sources: Memberships; Donations
Performs At: Athenaem; Neurosciences Institute
Facility Category: Library
Seating Capacity: 140; 350
Rental Contact: Susan Dilts

6001 MANDELL WEISS PERFORMING ARTS CENTER
9500 Gilman Drive MC0344
La Jolla, CA 92037
Phone: 858-550-1010
Fax: 619-534-1080
Type of Stage: Proscenium
Seating Capacity: 500

6002 MUSEUM OF CONTEMPORARY ART, SAN DIEGO
700 Prospect Street
La Jolla, CA 92037
Phone: 858-454-3541
Fax: 858-454-6985
e-mail: info@mcasd.org
Web Site: www.mcasandiego.org
Management:
    Events/Visitor Services Manager: Jini Bernstein
Performs At: Sherwood Auditorium
Seating Capacity: 500

6003 SHERWOOD AUDITORIUM
Museum of Contemporary Art - San Diego
700 Prospect Street
La Jolla, CA 92037
Phone: 858-454-2594
e-mail: jsantuccio@sdco.org
Web Site: www.sdco.org

6004 UNIVERSITY OF CALIFORNIA-SAN DIEGO - MANDEVILLE
UCSD Department of Theatre and Dance
La Jolla, CA 92093
Phone: 858-534-3791
Fax: 858-534-1080
e-mail: lmontano@ucsd.edu
Web Site: www.ucsd.edu

6005 BIOLA UNIVERSITY
13800 Biola Avenue
La Mirada, CA 90639

Phone: 562-903-6000
Fax: 562-903-4746
e-mail: georgeboesflug@truth.biola.edu
Web Site: www.biola.edu
Management:
    Music Department Chairman: George Boespflug
Founded: 1908
Income Sources: Ticket sales
Performs At: Lansing Auditorium
Seating Capacity: 450

6006 LA MIRADA THEATRE FOR THE PERFORMING ARTS
14900 La Mirada Boulevard
La Mirada, CA 90638
Phone: 714-994-6310
Fax: 714-994-5796
Web Site: www.lamiradatheatre.com
Management:
    Executive Director: Jeff Brown
    Ticketing Services Manager: Debbie J Walker
    Production Manager: Bobby DeLuca
Annual Attendance: 200,000
Facility Category: Performing Arts
Type of Stage: Proscenium
Stage Dimensions: 46'x26'x40'
Seating Capacity: 1,264
Year Built: 1977
Year Remodeled: 1999

6007 LAGUNA PLAYHOUSE
606 Laguna Canyon Road
Laguna Beach, CA 92652
Phone: 949-494-8021
Fax: 949-376-8185
Toll-free: 800-946-5556
e-mail: rstein@lagunaplayhouse.com
Web Site: www.lagunaplayhouse.com
Founded: 1920
Annual Attendance: 100,000
Type of Stage: Open Proscenium
Seating Capacity: 420

6008 JORDAN THEATRE
6500 Atlantic Avenue
Long Beach, CA 90805
Phone: 562-423-1471

6009 LONG BEACH COMMUNITY PLAYHOUSE - STAGE
5021 East Anaheim Street
Long Beach, CA 90804
Phone: 562-494-1014
Web Site: www.longbeachplayhouse.com
Annual Attendance: 34,000
Type of Stage: Proscenium

6010 LONG BEACH CONVENTION AND ENTERTAINMENT CENTER
300 East Ocean Boulevard
Long Beach, CA 90802

Phone: 562-436-3636
Fax: 562-436-9491
e-mail: dspellens@longbeachcc.com
Web Site: www.longbeachcc.com
Management:
    Director Theaters/Entertainment: Dan Spellens
Facility Category: Performing Arts Center
Type of Stage: Permanent; Proscenium
Stage Dimensions: 66 x 35
Seating Capacity: 825
Year Built: 1928
Year Remodeled: 1999
Rental Contact: Director of Theaters Dan Spellens

**6011 LONG BEACH PLAYHOUSE:
MAINSTAGE AND STUDIO THEATRES**
5021 E Anaheim Street
Long Beach, CA 90804
Phone: 562-494-1014
Fax: 562-961-8616
e-mail: lbphmandir@earthlink.net
Web Site: www.longbeachplayhouse.com
Management:
    Managing Director: Gigi Fuscomeese
Founded: 1929
Specialized Field: Performance Art
Paid Staff: 12
Volunteer Staff: 300
Income Sources: Ticket Sales
Performs At: Mainstage, Studio
Annual Attendance: 40,000
Facility Category: Non Union Space/AEA 99-56
Type of Stage: Thrust/Proscenium
Seating Capacity: 200, 98
Year Built: 1949

**6012 LONG BEACH PLAYHOUSE - STUDIO
THEATRE**
5021 East Anaheim Street
Long Beach, CA 90804
Phone: 562-494-1014
Web Site: www.longbeachplayhouse.com
Annual Attendance: 34,000
Type of Stage: Proscenium

**6013 RICHARD & KAREN CARPENTER
PERFORMING ARTS CENTER**
6200 Atherton Street
Long Beach, CA 90815-4500
Phone: 562-985-2488
Fax: 562-985-7024
e-mail: plesnik@csulb.edu
Web Site: www.carpenterarts.org
Management:
    Executive Director: Peter Lesnik
    General Manager: Michele Roberge
Mission: Presenting organization. Also, home to 4
resident companies.
Founded: 1994
Paid Staff: 15
Paid Artists: 40
Budget: $1,800,000

Income Sources: Individual Donor; Corporations; Rental
Clients; Ticket Buyers
Performs At: Performing Arts Center with continental
seating.
Affiliations: CSALB
Annual Attendance: 150,000
Type of Stage: Proscenium
Stage Dimensions: 70'x70'
Seating Capacity: 1,065
Year Built: 1994
Rental Contact: 562-985-7047 Glennis Watceman

6014 WOODROW WILSON HIGH SCHOOL
4400 E 10th Street
Long Beach, CA 90804
Phone: 562-433-0481
Fax: 562-433-2731

6015 ROBERT C SMITHWICK THEATRE
12345 El Monte Road
Los Altos Hills, CA 94022
Phone: 650-941-2500
Fax: 415-949-7375

6016 AGENCY FOR THE PERFORMING ARTS
9200 Sunset Boulevard
Suite 900
Los Angeles, CA 90069
Phone: 310-273-0744
Fax: 310-275-9401
e-mail: jhumiston@apa-agency.com
Management:
    Agent: Josh Humiston

**6017 CALIFORNIA STATE UNIVERSITY-LOS
ANGELES - PLAYERS**
5151 State University Drive
Los Angeles, CA 90032
Phone: 323-343-3000
e-mail: cdunn@cslanet.calstatela.edu
Web Site: www.calstatela.edu
Founded: 1947

6018 CELEBRATION THEATRE
7051B Santa Monica Boulevard
Los Angeles, CA 90028
Phone: 323-957-1884
e-mail: celebrationthtr@earthlink.net
Web Site: www.celebrationtheatre.com
Founded: 1982

**6019 CITY OF LOS ANGELES CULTURAL
AFFAIRS DEPARTMENT-PERFORMING
ARTS DIVISION**
514 S Spring Street
Los Angeles, CA 90013
Mailing Address: 433 S Spring Street 10th Floor Los
Angeles, CA 90013
Phone: 213-473-0686
Fax: 213-473-0620
Web Site: www.culturela.org
Officers:

General Manager: Margie J Reese
Management:
  Performing Arts Director: Ernest Dillihay
  Business/Theatre Manager: Lee Sweet
  Theatre Manager: Joyce Maddox
  Theatre Manager: Anisa Humlan
Specialized Field: Theatre, Dance, Music, Variety
Volunteer Staff: 12
Budget: 13.2 million
Income Sources: Rentals, Ticket Sales, Municipal Fund
Performs At: Theatre, 1; 2; 3; 4; Madrid Theatre; Warner Grand Theatre
Affiliations: Theatre LA; CALAA
Annual Attendance: 80,000
Facility Category: Theatre Complex
Type of Stage: Trust; Proscenium
Seating Capacity: 500; 296; 323; 90; 471; 1500

6020 DODGER STADIUM

1000 Elysian Park Avenue
Los Angeles, CA 90012
Phone: 323-224-1448
Fax: 323-224-1833
Web Site: www.dodgers.com
Management:
  VP Stadium Operations: Doug Duennes
  Sr Executive VP Marketing: Kris Rone
Founded: 1962
Specialized Field: Home of the Los Angeles Dodgers (MLB). Available for rental and concerts.d
Seating Capacity: 56,000
Year Built: 1962

6021 GETTY CENTER

1200 Getty Center Drive
Los Angeles, CA 90049
Phone: 310-440-7300
Fax: 310-440-7751
e-mail: communications@getty.edu
Web Site: www.getty.edu
Founded: 1953

6022 GREEK THEATRE

2700 N Vermont Avenue
Los Angeles, CA 90027
Phone: 323-666-8202
e-mail: concerts@nederlander.com
Web Site: www.nederlander.com
Founded: 1930

6023 HARRIET & CHARLES LUCKMAN
Fine Arts Complex

5151 State University Drive
Los Angeles, CA 90032
Phone: 323-343-6611
Fax: 323-343-6423
e-mail: AField@cslanet.calstatela.edu
Web Site: www.luckmanfineartscomplex.org
Management:
  Executive Director: Clifford D Harper
Founded: 1994
Seating Capacity: 250

6024 JAPANESE AMERICAN CULTURAL & COMMUNITY CENTER

244 S San Pedro Street
Los Angeles, CA 90012
Phone: 213-628-2728
Fax: 213-617-8576
e-mail: info@jaccc.org
Web Site: www.jaccc.org
Management:
  Managing Director: Victor Wong
Founded: 1980
Performs At: Japan America Theatre; Plaza
Seating Capacity: 878; 2000

6025 L'ERMITAGE FOUNDATION

11724 Gwynne Lane
Los Angeles, CA 90077
Phone: 310-472-3330
Fax: 310-476-8003
Management:
  Chairman: Renee Cherniak
Income Sources: Member Donations
Performs At: Salon Setting
Annual Attendance: 100
Facility Category: Hotel Salon
Seating Capacity: 200-250

6026 LOS ANGELES MEMORIAL COLISEUM SPORTS ARENA

3939 South Figueroa Street
Los Angeles, CA 90037
Phone: 213-748-6136
Fax: 213-746-9346
e-mail: info@lacoliseum.com
Web Site: www.lacouiseuwm.com
Management:
  General Manager: Patrick J Lynch
  Assistant General Manager: Ron Lederkramer
  Marketing/Sales Director: Jonathan Lee
  Event Coordinator: Yrene Asalde
  Event Director: Todd Destefano
  Event Coordinator: Rob Joyner
Mission: spaorts/ enterainment.
Founded: 1959
Paid Staff: 32
Type of Stage: Proscenium
Seating Capacity: 16,500
Year Built: 1923
Year Remodeled: 1994

6027 LOS ANGELES TENNIS CENTER

UCLA, 164 Pauley Pavilion
Los Angeles, CA 90095
Phone: 310-825-4403
Fax: 310-825-5775
e-mail: jhenson@ucla.edu
Web Site: www.performingarts.ucla.edu
Management:
  Manager: Rich Mylin
Seating Capacity: 6,800

6028 LOS ANGELES THEATRE CENTER

514 S Spring Street
Los Angeles, CA 90013
Phone: 213-627-6500
Fax: 213-624-6096
Type of Stage: Black Box; Flexible

6029 LOS ANGELES THEATRE CENTER - THEATRE 2

514 S Spring Street
Los Angeles, CA 90013
Phone: 213-627-6500
Fax: 213-847-3169
Type of Stage: Black Box; Flexible

6030 LOS ANGELES THEATRE CENTER - THEATRE 3

514 S Spring Street
Los Angeles, CA 90013
Phone: 213-627-6500
Fax: 213-847-3169
Type of Stage: Black Box; Flexible

6031 LOS ANGELES THEATRE CENTER - THEATRE 4

514 S Spring Street
Los Angeles, CA 90013
Phone: 213-627-6500
Fax: 213-847-3169
Type of Stage: Black Box; Flexible

6032 LOS ANGELES THEATRE CENTER - TOM BRADLEY THEATRE

514 S Spring Street
Los Angeles, CA 90013
Phone: 213-627-6500
Fax: 213-847-3169
Type of Stage: Black Box; Flexible
Seating Capacity: 498

6033 MUNICIPAL ART GALLERY - GALLERY THEATER

Barnsdall Art Park
4800 Hollywood Boulevard
Los Angeles, CA 90027
Phone: 213-473-8432
Fax: 213-473-8527
e-mail: cadmag@earthlink.net
Web Site: www.culturela.org

6034 MUSIC CENTER OF LOS ANGELES COUNTY

717 W Temple Street
Suite 400
Los Angeles, CA 90012
Phone: 213-202-2220
Fax: 213-481-1176
e-mail: general@musiccenter.org
Web Site: www.musiccenter.org
Management:
   President/COO: Joanne Corday Kozberg

VP Education Division: Mark Slaukin
   Director Public Relations: Ann Bradley
Founded: 1964
Specialized Field: Los Angeles Philharmonic, Los Angeles Opera, Los Angeles Master Chorale, Center Theatre Group (Mark Taper & Ahmanson Theatre).

6035 OCCIDENTAL COLLEGE - THORNE HALL

1600 Campus Road
Los Angeles, CA 90041
Phone: 323-259-2604
Fax: 323-341-4868
e-mail: abart@oxy.edu
Web Site: www.oxy.edu

6036 PAULEY PAVILION

University California - Los Angeles/UCLA
164 Pauley Pavilion
Los Angeles, CA 90095
Phone: 310-825-4546
Fax: 310-825-5775
Web Site: www.performingarts.ucla.edu
Management:
   Manager: Rich Mylin
   Assistant Manager: Susan Brown
Seating Capacity: 128,193

6037 PERFORMING ARTS OF LOS ANGELES COUNTY

135 N Grand Avenue
Los Angeles, CA 90012
Phone: 213-972-7211
Fax: 213-687-8490
e-mail: lamc@lamc.orgera.com
Web Site: www.performingartsla.com
Founded: 1964

6038 PERFORMING ARTS CENTER OF LOS ANGELES COUNTY

135 N Grand Avenue
Los Angeles, CA 90012
Phone: 213-628-2772
Fax: 213-628-2796
e-mail: tickets@ctgla.com
Web Site: www.taperahmanson.com
Founded: 1964
Annual Attendance: 750,000

6039 PLAZE GRAND PERFORMANCES

350 South Grand Avenue
Los Angeles, CA 90071
Phone: 213-687-2159
Fax: 213-687-2191
e-mail: booking@grandperformances.org
Web Site: www.grandperformances.org
Founded: 1987
Specialized Field: Southern California
Paid Staff: 10
Volunteer Staff: 3
Paid Artists: 40
Annual Attendance: 70,000

Type of Stage: Amphitheater; Thrust-Style
Seating Capacity: 6,500

**6040 SHRINE AUDITORIUM AND
EXPOSITION CENTER**
649 W Jefferson Boulevard
Los Angeles, CA 90007
Phone: 213-749-5123
Fax: 213-742-9922
e-mail: shringaud@aol.com
Management:
   General Manager: Douglas Worthington
Founded: 1920
Specialized Field: Los Angeles
Paid Staff: 20
Facility Category: Auditorium with adjoining Expo
Center
Type of Stage: Concerts; Masonite; Wood
Stage Dimensions: 193'x73'
Seating Capacity: Auditorium 6,500; Expo Center 2,000
Year Built: 1926
Cost: $2,500,000
Rental Contact: Douglas Worthington

6041 SHUBERT THEATRE
2020 Avenue of the Stars
Century City
Los Angeles, CA 90067
Phone: 310-201-1500
Fax: 310-201-1585
Toll-free: 800-233-3123

6042 STAPLES CENTER
1111 S Fugueroa Street
Los Angeles, CA 90017
Phone: 213-742-7300
Fax: 213-624-3054
Web Site: www.staplescenter.com
Management:
   President: Tim Leiweke
   SVP/General Manager: Bobby Goldwater
Seating Capacity: 16,096

6043 UCLA PERFORMING ARTS
Royce Hall, B100
PO Box 951529
Los Angeles, CA 90095
Phone: 310-794-4046
Fax: 310-206-3843
e-mail: across@ucla.edu
Web Site: www.performingarts.ucla.edu
Management:
   Director: David Sefton
Founded: 1929
Annual Attendance: 200,000
Seating Capacity: 1,818

**6044 UNIVERSITY OF CALIFORNIA-LOS
ANGELES - WADSWORTH**
405 Hilgard Avenue
Los Angeles, CA 90024
Phone: 310-206-8745
Founded: 1919

**6045 UNIVERSITY OF SOUTHERN
CALIFORNIA**
STU B7
Los Angeles, CA 90089
Phone: 213-740-2311
Fax: 213-740-5293
Web Site: www.usc.edu
Management:
   Dean School of Theater: Robert Scales
Founded: 1880
Type of Stage: Concerts

**6046 PEPPERDINE UNIVERSITY CENTER
FOR THE ARTS**
24255 Pacific Coast Highway
Malibu, CA 90263
Phone: 310-506-4522
Fax: 310-506-4556
e-mail: rob.witt@pepperdine.edu
Web Site: www.pepperdine.edu
Management:
   Managing Director: Marnie Mitze
Facility Category: Smothers Theatre
Seating Capacity: 450
Year Built: 1980
Rental Contact: Managing Director Marnie Mitze

**6047 PEPPERDINE UNIVERSITY -
AMPHITHEATRE, FINE ARTS**
24255 Pacific Coast Highway
Malibu, CA 90263
Phone: 310-456-4264
Fax: 310-456-4327
e-mail: rob.witt@pepperdine.edu
Web Site: www.pepperdine.edu

**6048 PEPPERDINE UNIVERSITY -
MINI-THEATRE, FINE ARTS**
24255 Pacific Coast Highway
Malibu, CA 90263
Phone: 310-456-4462
Fax: 310-456-4077
e-mail: rob.witt@pepperdine.edu
Web Site: www.pepperdine.edu

**6049 PEPPERDINE UNIVERSITY -
SMOTHERS THEATRE**
24255 Pacific Coast Highway
Malibu, CA 90263
Phone: 310-456-4000
Fax: 310-456-4556
e-mail: rob.witt@pepperdine.edu
Web Site: www.pepperdine.edu

**6050 MENDOCINO ART CENTER - HELEN
SCHOENI THEATER**
45200 Little Lake Street
P.O. Box 765
Mendocino, CA 95460

Phone: 707-937-5818
e-mail: mendoart@mcn.org.
Web Site: www.mendocinoartcenter.org
Founded: 1959

6051 MODESTO JUNIOR COLLEGE
435 College Avenue
Modesto, CA 95350
Phone: 209-575-6020
Fax: 209-575-6745
e-mail: mjcinfo@mail.yosemite.cc.ca.us
Web Site: www.gomjc.org
Founded: 1967

6052 MONTCLAIR CIVIC CENTER - STARLITE PATIO THEATRE
Montclair Civic Center
Montclair, CA 91763
Phone: 909-625-9457
Fax: 909-399-9751

6053 MOUNTAIN VIEW CENTER FOR THE PERFORMING ARTS
PO Box 7540
500 Castro Street
Mountain View, CA 94039
Phone: 650-903-6565
Fax: 650-903-6560
e-mail: performingarts@mvcpa.com
Web Site: www.mvcpa.com
Management:
　Executive Director: Ellen Miner
　Marketing/Public Relations Manager: Michele Roberts
　Operations Manager: W Scott Whisler
　Business Manager: Cindy Miksa
Mission: Seeks to enrich Silicon Valley audiences through enjoyment, celebration and interaction with the arts.
Founded: 1991
Paid Staff: 50
Volunteer Staff: 300
Budget: 1.3 Million
Performs At: Theaters
Affiliations: United States Institute for Theater Technolgies Inc., International Assocation of Auditorium Managers
Annual Attendance: 170,000
Type of Stage: Black Box; Mainstage-proscenium
Seating Capacity: Mainstage 600, Black Box 200, Park 300
Year Built: 1991
Resident Groups: Theatre Works, Peninsula Youth Theatre

6054 NAPA VALLEY OPERA HOUSE
1030 Main Street
Suite 100
Napa, CA 94559
Phone: 707-226-7372
Fax: 707-226-5392
e-mail: office@operahousetheatre.org
Web Site: www.napavalleyoperahouse.org

Founded: 1879
Seating Capacity: 180

6055 BALBOA PERFORMING ARTS THEATER
PO Box 752
Newport Beach, CA 92661
Phone: 949-673-0895
Fax: 949-673-0938
e-mail: mmroberge@prodigy.net
Management:
　Executive Director: Michele Roberge
Seating Capacity: 350

6056 CALIFORNIA STATE UNIVERSITY-NORTHRIDGE
18111 Nordhoff Street
Northridge, CA 91330
Phone: 818-677-1200
e-mail: university.advancement@csun.edu
Web Site: www.csun.edu

6057 ARENA IN OAKLAND AND NETWORK ASSOCIATES COLISEUM
7000 Coliseum Way
Oakland, CA 94621
Phone: 510-569-2121
Fax: 510-569-4246
e-mail: networkassociates@stadianet.com
Web Site: www.stadianet.com
Management:
　General Manager: Sally Roach
Founded: 1966
Seating Capacity: 62,500

6058 HENRY J KAISER CONVENTION CENTER
10 10th Street
Oakland, CA 94607
Phone: 510-238-7765
Fax: 510-238-7767
Web Site: www.hjkevents.com
Management:
　Facility Manager: Jacque Birdsong-James
　Booking Coodinator: Barbara S Sheppard
　Technical Director: Eli Morgan
　Special Events Assistant: Sarah Backes
Mission: The Henery J Kaiser Convention Center is a sophisticated, diverse avenue which can accomodate all types of events from pefforming arts, to entertainment, sports and private receptions.
Founded: 1917
Specialized Field: multi - use facility with theatre and arena space

6059 MILLS COLLEGE CONCERT HALL
5000 MacArthur Boulevard
Oakland, CA 94613
Phone: 510-430-2255
Fax: 510-430-3314
e-mail: ramon@mills.edu
Web Site: www.mills.edu

Founded: 1852

6060 NETWORK ASSOCIATES COLISEUM
7000 Coliseum Way
Oakland, CA 94621
Phone: 510-569-2121
Fax: 510-569-4246
e-mail: networkassociates@stadianet.com
Web Site: www.stadianet.com
Founded: 1966
Seating Capacity: 62,500

6061 OAKLAND-ALAMEDA COUNTY ARENA & NETWORK ASSOCIATES COLISEUM
7000 Coliseum Way
Oakland, CA 94621
Phone: 510-569-2121
Fax: 510-569-4246
e-mail: networkassociates@stadianet.com
Web Site: www.stadianet.com
Management:
  General Manager: Sally Roach
  Marketing Manager: Allison Miller
Founded: 1966
Seating Capacity: 62,500

6062 PARAMOUNT THEATRE
2025 Broadway
Oakland, CA 94612
Phone: 510-893-2300
Web Site: www.paramounttheatre.com

6063 OROVILLE STATE THEATER
1735 Montgomery Street
Oroville, CA 95965
Phone: 916-538-2471
Fax: 916-538-2460
e-mail: vorinj@onemain.com
Web Site: www.cityoforoville.org

6064 OXNARD CIVIC AUDITORIUM
800 Hobson Way
Oxnard, CA 93030
Phone: 805-486-2424
e-mail: dale.belcher@ci.oxnard.ca.us
Web Site: www.oxnardpacc.com

6065 OXNARD PERFORMING ARTS AND CONVENTION CENTER
800 Hobson Way
Oxnard, CA 93030-6786
Phone: 805-385-8149
Fax: 805-483-7303
e-mail: bevera.skelton@ci.oxnard.ca.us
Web Site: www.oxnardpacc.com
Management:
  Executive Director: Robert W Holden

6066 MCCALLUM THEATRE FOR THE PERFORMING ARTS
73-000 Fred Waring Drive
Palm Desert, CA 92260
Phone: 760-346-6506
Fax: 760-341-9508
e-mail: info@mccallum-theatre.org
Web Site: www.mccallumtheatre.com
Officers:
  President/CEO: Ted Giatas
  Director Presentations/Theatre: Mitchell Gershenfeld
  Director Development: Steve Sharp
  Director Marketing/Communications: Walter Marlock
Founded: 1988
Paid Staff: 40
Volunteer Staff: 400
Budget: $7.5 Million
Income Sources: Earned; Contributed revenues
Performs At: Presenting Theatre
Annual Attendance: 250,000
Type of Stage: Proscenium
Stage Dimensions: 41'D x 84'W
Seating Capacity: 1,127

6067 PALM SPRINGS DESERT MUSEUM: ANNENBERG THEATER
101 Museum Drive
PO Box 2310
Palm Springs, CA 92263
Phone: 760-325-7186
Fax: 760-327-5069
e-mail: bwitte@psmuseum.org
Web Site: www.psmuseum.org
Management:
  Performing Arts Director: Bill Witte
Founded: 1976
Performs At: Annenberg Theatre
Affiliations: APAP
Stage Dimensions: 50x30
Seating Capacity: 440
Year Built: 1976
Year Remodeled: 1999
Rental Contact: Bill Witte

6068 SPANGENBURG THEATRE
780 Arastradero Road
Palo Alto, CA 94306
Phone: 650-354-8220
Fax: 650-354-8277
e-mail: spangenberg@earthlink.net
Web Site: www.spangenbergtheatre.com
Management:
  Theatre Manager: Jorgen Wedseltoft
Founded: 1965
Facility Category: Performance Center; Art House; Cinema
Type of Stage: Proscenium
Seating Capacity: 953
Year Remodeled: 2002

6069 CALIFORNIA INSTITUTE OF TECHNOLOGY
1200 East California Boulevard
Pasadena, CA 91125
Phone: 626-395-6811
Fax: 626-577-0130
Toll-free: 888-222-5832
e-mail: dnn@caltech.eduk
Web Site: www.caltech.edu
Management:
  Direcktor: Denise Nelson Nash
Mission: Provides a broad spectrum of high quality multi-disciplinary cultural, educational and information programs. These programs are designed to compliment the Caltech experience of Institutes, students, faculty and staff, as well as serving as cultural enhancement to the greater Pasadena community.
Founded: 1891
Paid Staff: 60
Paid Artists: 100

6070 PASADENA CIVIC AUDITORIUM
300 E Green Street
Pasadena, CA 91101
Phone: 626-449-7360
Fax: 818-793-8014
e-mail: bgarcia@pasadenacal.com
Web Site: www.pasadenacal.com/civic.htm
Founded: 1931
Seating Capacity: 3,029

6071 PASADENA PLAYHOUSE - MAINSTAGE THEATRE
39 S El Molino Avenue
Pasadena, CA 91101
Phone: 626-356-7529
Fax: 626-792-7343
e-mail: patroninfo@pasadenaplayhouse.org
Web Site: www.pasadenaplayhouse.org
Management:
  Artistic Director: Sheldon Epps
  Executive Director: Lyla L. White
  Producing Director: Thomas Ware
  General Manager: Brian Colburn
Founded: 1917
Seating Capacity: 682
Year Built: 1925
Rental Contact: Thomas Ware

6072 ROSE BOWL
1001 Rose Bown Drive
Pasadena, CA 91103
Phone: 626-577-3100
Fax: 626-405-0992
e-mail: rosebowlstadium@yahoo.com
Web Site: www.rosebowlstadium.com
Management:
  General Manager: Darryl Dunn
Founded: 1921
Seating Capacity: 92,542

6073 PICO RIVERA SPORTS ARENA
11003 Rooks Road
Pico Rivera, CA 90660
Phone: 562-699-1751
Fax: 562-699-0005
Web Site: www.hauser-ent.com
Management:
  Manager: Ralph Hauser
  Assistant Manager: Jacqueline Hauser
  Marketing Director: Malu Elizondo
  Concessions Manager: Anothony Hauser
  Sound Engineer: Daniel Esparza
Seating Capacity: 5,452

6074 CALIFORNIA POLYTECHNIC UNIVERSITY-POMONA
3801 W Temple Avenue
University Theatre, Technical Services
Pomona, CA 91768
Phone: 909-869-7659
Fax: 909-869-3185
e-mail: dlogan@csupomona.edu
Web Site: www.csupomona.edu
Management:
  Technical Services: Dennis Logan
Mission: University theatre with 515 continental seating - university theatre arts education, concerts, dance, on campus activities and outside lease.
Founded: 1938

6075 POWAY CENTER FOR THE PERFORMING ARTS
15498 Espola Road
Poway, CA 92064
Phone: 858-748-0505
Fax: 619-486-2701
e-mail: powayarts@aol.com
Web Site: www.powayarts.org
Management:
  Executive Director: Gary A Neiger
Performs At: Poway Center for the Performing Arts
Seating Capacity: 815

6076 REDDING CIVIC AUDITORIUM - TRADE AND CONVENTION CENTER
777 Auditorium Drive
Redding, CA 96099
Phone: 530-225-4100
Fax: 530-225-4354
e-mail: admin@ci.redding.ca.us
Web Site: www.ci.redding.ca.us

6077 SHASTA COLLEGE - FINE ARTS THEATRE
11555 Old Oregon Trail
PO Box 496006
Redding, CA 96049
Phone: 530-225-4769
e-mail: info@shastacollege.edu
Web Site: www.shastacollege.edu
Founded: 1948

6078 REDLANDS COMMUNITY MUSIC ASSOCIATION
PO Box 466
25 Grant Street
Redlands, CA 92373
Phone: 909-793-7316
Fax: 909-793-5086
e-mail: BowlProgDir@aol.com
Web Site: www.redlandsbowl.org
Founded: 1923
Seating Capacity: 6,000

6079 AVIATION PARK COMPLEX
1935 Manhattan Beach Boulevard
Redondo Beach, CA 90278
Phone: 310-318-0610
Fax: 310-643-0096
Management:
Manager: Steve Bonnell
Seating Capacity: 1,425

6080 MATEEL COMMUNITY CENTER
59 Rusk Lane
PO Box 1910
Redway, CA 95560
Phone: 707-923-3368
Fax: 707-923-3370
e-mail: mateel@mateel.org
Web Site: www.mateel.org
Management:
Executive Director: Kathryn Manspeaker
Founded: 1939
Annual Attendance: 45,000

6081 RICHMOND MEMORIAL CONVENTION CENTER
PO Box 4046
Richmond, CA 94804
Phone: 510-620-6789
Fax: 510-620-6583

6082 RIVERSIDE CONVENTION CENTER
3443 Orange Street
Riverside, CA 92501
Phone: 909-787-7950
Fax: 909-222-4706
e-mail: riversidecb@linkline.com
Web Site: www.riversidecb.com/rcc.htm
Management:
General Manager: Scott Megna
Facility Category: Convention Center
Seating Capacity: 2,000
Rental Contact: Pamela Sturrock

6083 RIVERSIDE MUNICIPAL AUDITORIUM
3485 Mission Inn Avenue
Riverside, CA 92501
Phone: 909-787-7678
Fax: 909-682-8464
e-mail: MuniBoxOffice@aol.com
Web Site: www.riversidemunicipalauditorium.com
Officers:

President: Robert Stein
Management:
General Manager: Carlosc Von Frankenceng
Box Office Assistant Manager: Ryan White
Operator: Robert Stein
Founded: 1927
Paid Staff: 8
Annual Attendance: 50,000
Type of Stage: Proscenium
Seating Capacity: 1,776

6084 UNIVERSITY OF CALIFORNIA AT RIVERSIDE, CULTURAL EVENTS
133 Costo Hall
Riverside, CA 92521
Phone: 909-787-4629
Fax: 909-787-2221
e-mail: todd.wingate@ucr.edu
Web Site: www.culturalevents.ucr.edu

6085 NORRIS CENTER FOR THE PERFORMING ARTS
27570 Crossfield Drive
Rolling Hills Estates, CA 90274
Phone: 310-544-0403
Fax: 310-377-2997
e-mail: jrossier@norristheatre.org
Web Site: www.norriscenter.com
Management:
Executive Director: Richard S Kordos
Marketing Director: Jennifer Rossler
Development Director: Bryna Alper
Mission: To offer performing arts and performing arts education to the Los Angeles South Bay community.
Founded: 1983
Specialized Field: All Performing Arts - Presenting House
Volunteer Staff: 80
Income Sources: Private donations and ticket sales
Performs At: 450 seats, all clean sight lines
Annual Attendance: 14,000
Facility Category: Presenting; Producing; Rental
Type of Stage: Proscenium
Seating Capacity: 450
Year Built: 1983
Rental Contact: Box Office Manager David Barr

6086 ARCO ARENA
1 Sports Parkway
Sacramento, CA 95834
Phone: 916-928-3650
Fax: 916-928-6936
e-mail: tickets@arcoarena.com
Web Site: www.arcoarena.com
Management:
President: John Thomas
VP Food/Beverage: Mark Stone
Chief Marketing Officer: Steve Wille
Public Relations: Troy Hanson
Specialized Field: Sports Facility alsohosts numerous concerts, ice shows, festivals and other family events.
Affiliations: Home of the Sacramento Kings, Sacramento Monarchs and Sacramento Knights.
Seating Capacity: 17,317

Year Built: 1985

6087 ARDEN PLAYHOUSE
2120 Royale Road
Sacramento, CA 95815
Phone: 916-927-1814
Fax: 916-782-1072

6088 CROCKER ART MUSEUM
216 O Street
Sacramento, CA 95814
Phone: 916-264-5423
Toll-free: 800-735-2929
e-mail: cam@cityofsacramento.org
Web Site: www.crockerartmuseum.org
Management:
   Museum Director: Barbara Gibbs
Mission: Providing performances in an intimate museum setting.
Founded: 1885
Specialized Field: Dance; Vocal Music; Instrumental Music; Theater
Status: Nonprofit
Performs At: Crocker Museum Ballroom
Annual Attendance: 140,000
Organization Type: Sponsoring

6089 SACRAMENTO COMMUNITY CENTER EXHIBITION HALL
1400 J Street
Sacramento, CA 95814
Phone: 916-264-5291
Fax: 916-264-7687
e-mail: mvoreyer@cityofsacramento.org
Web Site: www.sacamenities.com
Founded: 1926
Type of Stage: Proscenium Arch
Seating Capacity: 6,500

6090 SACRAMENTO COMMUNITY CENTER THEATRE
1301 L Street
Sacramento, CA 95814
Phone: 916-264-5291
Fax: 916-264-7687
e-mail: mvoreyer@cityofsacramento.org
Web Site: www.sacamenities.com
Founded: 1926
Type of Stage: Proscenium Arch
Seating Capacity: 2,452

6091 SACRAMENTO COMMUNITY CONVENTION CENTER
1030 15th Street
Suite 100
Sacramento, CA 95814
Phone: 916-449-5291
Fax: 916-264-7687
e-mail: mvoreyer@cityofsacramento.org
Web Site: www.sacamenities.com
Founded: 1926

6092 SACRAMENTO PERFORMING ARTS CENTER
1924 T Street
Sacramento, CA 95814
Phone: 916-452-7722
Fax: 916-452-0757
e-mail: sparcenter@aol.com
Web Site: www.sacperformingartscenter.homestead.com
Management:
   Producer: Lisa Caretto
Mission: To provide a place where artists and arts organizations can afford to work, rehearse and teach.
Founded: 2000
Specialized Field: Plays; Children's Musical Theatre Workshops; Children's Vocal Workshoops
Income Sources: Box Office; Rents; Registration Fees
Affiliations: League of Sacramento Theatres; Sacramento Area Regional Theatre Alliance; Sacramento Arts Advocate
Facility Category: Office and Rehearsal Space
Year Remodeled: 1999
Rental Contact: Lisa Caretto
Organization Type: Performing
Resident Groups: Cisneros Studios of Dance

6093 CALIFORNIA STATE UNIVERSITY - CREATIVE ARTS BUILDING
5500 University Parkway
San Bernardino, CA 92407
Phone: 909-887-7452

6094 CALIFORNIA THEATRE OF PERFORMING ARTS
562 W 4th Street
San Bernardino, CA 92402
Phone: 909-386-7361
Fax: 909-885-8672
e-mail: joseph@theatricalarts.com
Web Site: www.theatricalarts.com

6095 BLACKFRIARS THEATRE
1057 1st Avenue
San Diego, CA 92101
Phone: 619-232-4088

6096 CAFE DEL REY MORO
House of Hospitality
1549 El Prado
San Diego, CA 92101
Phone: 619-557-9441
Web Site: www.cohnrestaurants.com

6097 COPLEY SYMPHONY HALL
1245 7th Avenue
750 B Street
San Diego, CA 92101
Phone: 619-235-0800
Fax: 619-231-8178
e-mail: epapel@sandiegosymhpony.org
Web Site: www.sandiegosymphony.com
Founded: 1929

6098 COX ARENA AT AZTEC BOWL
5500 Canyon Crest Drive
San Diego, CA 92182
Phone: 619-594-0234
Fax: 619-594-6423
e-mail: jenna.mcfarland@sdsu.edu
Web Site: www.cox-arena.com
Management:
   Director Facilities: John Kolek
Mission: Facility - 12,000 seat multi-purpose area.
Founded: 1997
Seating Capacity: 12,000

6099 GASLAMP QUARTER THEATRE COMPANY
444 4th Avenue
San Diego, CA 92101
Phone: 619-234-9583

6100 HORTON GRAND THEATRE
444 Fourth Avenue
San Diego, CA 92101
Phone: 619-234-3588
Fax: 619-234-3587
e-mail: matt@tripleespresso.com
Web Site: www.tripleespresso.com
Management:
   General Manager: Matt Boden
Founded: 1985
Paid Staff: 20
Paid Artists: 20
Income Sources: Ticket Sales
Affiliations: San Diego Performing Arts League; San Diego Chamber of Commerce; San Diego Convention & Visitors Bureau
Annual Attendance: 50,000
Facility Category: Rental house
Type of Stage: Proscenium
Stage Dimensions: 29'9" x 18'x22'6"
Seating Capacity: 250
Year Built: 1983
Rental Contact: General Manager Matt Boden

6101 LYCEUM THEATRES COMPLEX
San Diego Repertory Theatre
79 Horton Plaza
San Diego, CA 92101
Phone: 619-231-3586
Fax: 619-235-0939
e-mail: jmcintyre@sandiegorep.com
Web Site: www.sandiegorep.com
Founded: 1976
Annual Attendance: 50,000
Seating Capacity: 545

6102 QUALCOMM STADIUM
9449 Friars Road
San Diego, CA 92108
Phone: 619-641-3100
Fax: 619-283-0460
e-mail: stadium@sandiego.gov
Web Site: www.sannet.gov/qualcomm
Management:

Stadium Manager: Bill Wilson
Assistant Manager/Concessions: Ken Wilson
VP Marketing: Don Johnson
Director Sales: Lynn Abramson
Founded: 1961
Seating Capacity: 71,500

6103 RECITAL HALL: BALBOA PARK
2130 Pan American Road W
San Diego, CA 92101
Phone: 619-235-1100

6104 SAN DIEGO CONCOURSE
202 C Street MS#57
San Diego, CA 92101
Phone: 619-615-4100
Fax: 619-615-4115
e-mail: gayle.falkenthal@sdccc.org
Web Site: www.sdccc.org

6105 SAN DIEGO MUSEUM OF ART
1450 El Prado
Balboa Park
San Diego, CA 92101
Mailing Address: PO Box 122107, San Diego, CA. 92112-2107
Phone: 619-232-7931
Fax: 619-232-9367
e-mail: sdmaprog@pacbell.net
Web Site: www.sdmart.org
Management:
   Program Director: Wesley O Brustad
Founded: 1926
Specialized Field: Visual
Budget: 9.0 Million
Performs At: Copley Auditorium
Annual Attendance: 400,000
Facility Category: Auditorium
Type of Stage: Proscenium
Seating Capacity: 425
Year Remodeled: 1999

6106 SAN DIEGO SPORTS ARENA
3500 Sports Arena Boulevard
San Diego, CA 92110
Phone: 619-224-4171
Fax: 619-224-3010
e-mail: ssaadch@sandiegoarena.com
Web Site: www.sandiegoarena.com
Management:
   General Manager: Ernie Hahn
   VP/Box Office: Bob Brown
   Director Booking: Sean Saadeh
   Director Public Relations: Stephanie Coolich
   VP/Operations: John Sanders
   Event Manager: Jason Lebdetter
   Director Group Sales: Ddkjennifer Darnell
   Programs/Novelties: Mike Kokun
   Director Sponsorship Marketing: Laurie Bianchi
Founded: 1967
Paid Staff: 60
Affiliations: Clear Channel Entertainment
Facility Category: Arena
Stage Dimensions: 60' x 40'

Seating Capacity: 14,000
Year Built: 1966
Year Remodeled: Cur.
Cost: 6.4 million
Rental Contact: Sean Saadeh

6107 SPRECKELS ORGAN PAVILION
Balboa Park Administration Building
2125 Park Boulevard
San Diego, CA 92101
Phone: 619-235-1100
Fax: 619-235-1112

6108 STARLIGHT THEATER
Balboa Park
PO Box 3519
San Diego, CA 92163
Phone: 619-544-7827
e-mail: artistic@starlighttheatre.org
Web Site: www.starlighttheatre.org
Founded: 1945

6109 ALCAZAR THEATRE
650 Geary Street
San Francisco, CA 94102
Phone: 415-441-4042
Fax: 415-441-9567
e-mail: AlcazarTheatre@aol.com
Management:
 Artistic Director: Steve Dobbins
 Administrative Director: Alan Ramos
 Casting Director: Kim Parolari
 House Manager: Bernadette Lopes
Founded: 1978
Status: Commercial
Volunteer Staff: 3
Budget: Varies
Season: Year Round
Performs At: Commercial, For Profit Theatre
Annual Attendance: 200,000
Type of Stage: Proscenium
Stage Dimensions: 45'x31'
Seating Capacity: 520
Year Built: 1917
Year Remodeled: 1991
Cost: $2.5 million
Rental Contact: Artistic Director Steve Dobbins

6110 BAYVIEW OPERA HOUSE
4705 3rd Street
San Francisco, CA 94124
Phone: 415-824-0386
Fax: 415-824-7124
Toll-free: 877-227-5544
e-mail: SBBPR@pacbell.net
Web Site: www.bayviewoperahouse.org
Officers:
 President: Gaylon Logan
Management:
 Associate Director: Ivory X Morton
 Program Director: Birta Leighton
 Events Coordinator: Eugene Steptoe
Founded: 1968
Seating Capacity: 300

6111 CENTER FOR AFRICAN AND AMERICAN ART
762 Fulton Street
Suite 300
San Francisco, CA 94102
Phone: 415-928-8546
Fax: 415-928-0466
e-mail: info@aaacc.org
Web Site: www.aaacc.org
Founded: 1989

6112 COMMUNITY MUSIC CENTER
544 Capp Street
San Francisco, CA 94110
Phone: 415-647-6015
Fax: 415-647-3890
e-mail: info@sfmusic.org
Web Site: www.sfmusic.org
Type of Stage: Proscenium
Seating Capacity: 90

6113 COW PALACE
PO Box 34206
Geneva Avenue and Santos Street
San Francisco, CA 94134
Phone: 415-404-4111
Fax: 415-469-6111
e-mail: info@cowpalace.com
Web Site: www.cowpalace.com
Management:
 CEO: Michael Wegher
 Director Operations: William Mendes
Specialized Field: Home of the Grand National Rodeo, Horse and Stock Show. Hosts ice events, basketball, motorcycle races.
Type of Stage: Proscenium
Seating Capacity: 8,849
Year Built: 1941

6114 CURRAN THEATRE
445 Geary Street
P O Box 7110
San Francisco, CA 94102
Phone: 415-512-7770
Fax: 415-431-5052
Web Site: www.bestofbroadway-sf.com
Officers:
 CEO: Greg Holland
Founded: 1922
Seating Capacity: 1,667

6115 FLORENCE GOULD THEATRE IN CALIFORNIA
Lincoln Park
34th Avenue and Clement Street
San Francisco, CA 94121
Phone: 415-750-3638

6116 FORT MASON CENTER - COWELL THEATRE
Fort Mason Center Building A
San Francisco, CA 94123

Phone: 415-441-3400
Fax: 415-441-3405
e-mail: wayne@fortmason.org
Web Site: www.fortmason.org
Founded: 1976
Annual Attendance: 1,500,000
Facility Category: Rental Theatre
Type of Stage: Proscenium
Stage Dimensions: 30'x40'
Seating Capacity: 437
Year Built: 1989
Rental Contact: Wayne Hazzard

6117 GOLDEN GATE THEATRE

1 Taylor Street at Market
San Francisco, CA 94102
Phone: 415-512-7770
Fax: 415-431-5052
Web Site: www.bestofbroadway-sf.com
Management:
  CEO: Greg Holland
Seating Capacity: 2,297

6118 NEW PERFORMANCE GALLERY OF SAN FRANCISCO

3153 17th Street
San Francisco, CA 94110
Phone: 415-626-6745
Fax: 415-863-9833

6119 NOB HILL MASONIC CENTER

1111 California Street
San Francisco, CA 94108
Phone: 415-776-4702
Fax: 415-776-3945
e-mail: erhall@sfmasoniccenter.com
Web Site: www.sfmasoniccenter.com
Facility Category: Event Center

6120 ORPHEUM THEATRE

1192 Market Street at Hyde
San Francisco, CA 94102
Phone: 415-512-7770
Fax: 415-431-5052
Web Site: www.bestofbroadway-sf.com
Officers:
  CEO: Greg Holland
Seating Capacity: 2,203

6121 PACIFIC BELL PARK

24 Willie Mays Plaza
San Francisco, CA 94107
Phone: 415-972-2000
Toll-free: 800-544-2687
Web Site: www.sfgiants.com
Management:
  Sr VP Ballpark Operations: Jorge Costa
  VP Community Affairs: Staci Slaughter
Founded: 1962
Seating Capacity: 40,930

6122 PALACE OF FINE ARTS THEATRE

3301 Lyon Street
San Francisco, CA 94123
Phone: 415-563-6504
Fax: 415-567-4062
e-mail: kevin@palaceoffinearts.org
Web Site: www.palaceoffinearts.com
Officers:
  President: Jerry Firedman
Management:
  Executive Director: Kevin J O'Brien
  Production Manager: Ursula D Smith
  House Manager: Viktoria Faktor
  House Manager: David Ypung
Founded: 1970
Specialized Field: Multidiscipliary, Multi-Use
Paid Staff: 15
Income Sources: Rental and concession fees
Performs At: Rental Theatre
Annual Attendance: 120,000
Facility Category: Theatre
Type of Stage: Proscenium
Stage Dimensions: 73'x54'
Seating Capacity: 1,000
Year Built: 1970
Rental Contact: Kevin O'Brien

6123 SAN FRANCISCO CIVIC AUDITORIUM

99 Grove Street
San Francisco, CA 94102
Phone: 415-974-4000
Fax: 415-974-4073
e-mail: mlendaro@billgrahamcivic.com
Web Site: www.billgrahamcivic.com
Officers:
  Director Sales: Melody Lendaro
  General Manager: Richard Shaff
  Building Manager: Thaddeus Watkins
Mission: Special events.
Founded: 1915
Paid Staff: 30
Affiliations: City of San Francisco
Annual Attendance: 300,000
Facility Category: Multi-Use Arena
Type of Stage: Flexible
Seating Capacity: 7,000
Year Built: 1918
Year Remodeled: 1986
Rental Contact: Melody Lendaro

6124 SAN FRANCISCO COUNTY FAIR BUILDING

Lincoln Way & 9th Avenue
Golden Gate Park
San Francisco, CA 94122
Phone: 415-666-7079
Web Site: www.sfgov.org

6125 HERBEST THEATRE

401 Van Ness Avenue
Suite 110
San Francisco, CA 94102
Phone: 415-621-6600
Fax: 415-621-5091

Founded: 1932
Affiliations: Owned and operated by the War Memorial, a department of the city of San Francisco
Annual Attendance: 127,000
Facility Category: theatre
Type of Stage: proscenium
Stage Dimensions: 33 x 40
Seating Capacity: 928
Year Built: 1937
Year Remodeled: 1979
Rental Contact: Jennifer Norris

6126 YERBA BUENA CENTER FOR THE ARTS

701 Mission Street
San Francisco, CA 94103
Phone: 415-978-2710
Fax: 415-978-9635
e-mail: info@yerbabuenaarts.org
Web Site: www.yerbabuenaarts.org
Management:
    Marketing/Communications Director: MaryBeth Smith
    Performing Arts Director: Nancy Martin
    Reservations Coordinator: Joan Curry
Founded: 1993
Paid Staff: 80
Volunteer Staff: 100
Budget: $7,300,000
Income Sources: Contributions; Rental Revenue; Ticket Revenue
Affiliations: LATSE
Annual Attendance: 205,000
Facility Category: Theater ; Multi-Use Forum
Type of Stage: Proscenium and Flexible
Stage Dimensions: 43'x93'
Seating Capacity: 750; 400
Year Built: 1993

6127 HP PAVILION AT SAN JOSE

525 W Santa Clara Street
San Jose, CA 95113
Phone: 408-287-7070
Fax: 408-999-5797
Web Site: www.hppavilion.com
Management:
    Director Booking/Events: Steve Kirsner
Founded: 1993
Performs At: Sports/Entertainment Arena
Affiliations: IAAM; Arena Network; MPI
Facility Category: Arena
Type of Stage: Portable
Seating Capacity: 4,500-18,000
Year Built: 1995
Rental Contact: Steve Kirsner

6128 MONTGOMERY THEATRE

408 Almaden Boulevard
San Jose, CA 95110
Phone: 408-277-5277
Fax: 408-277-3535
Web Site: www.sjcc.com
Management:
    Acting General Manager: Julie Mark

Founded: 1936
Seating Capacity: 537

6129 SAN JOSE CENTER FOR THE PERFORMING ARTS

408 Almaden Boulevard
San Jose, CA 95110
Phone: 408-277-5277
Fax: 408-277-3535
Web Site: www.sjcc.com
Officers:
    Chairman: Patrick J D'Angelo
    President/Executive Producer: Stewart Slater
    Immediate Past-Chairman: Frank S Greene, Jr
Management:
    Executive Producer: Stewart Slater
    Artistic Director: Dianna Shuster
    Associate Artistic Director: Marc Jacobs
    Technical Director: Nick Nichols
    Marketing Associate: Kari Henrichsen

6130 SAN JOSE CONVENTION & CULTURAL FACILITIES

Administrative Office
408 Almaden Boulevard
San Jose, CA 95110
Phone: 408-277-5277
Fax: 408-277-3535
Toll-free: 800-533-2345
e-mail: SJCC.Counseling@sjeccd.cc.ca.us
Web Site: www.sjcc.com

6131 SAN JOSE MUNICIPAL STADIUM

San Jose Giants Baseball
588 E Alma Avenue & Senter Road
San Jose, CA 95112
Phone: 408-297-1435
Fax: 408-297-1453
e-mail: sanjose_giants@mindspring.com
Web Site: www.sjgiants.com
Management:
    Stadium Manager: Rick Tracy
    General Manager: Mark Wilson
Founded: 1988
Annual Attendance: 154,324
Type of Stage: Baseball Stadium
Seating Capacity: 4,500

6132 SAN JOSE STATE UNIVERSITY - CONCERT HALL

Washington Square
San Jose, CA 95192
Phone: 408-924-4673
Fax: 408-924-4773
e-mail: bgottesm@email.sjsu.edu
Web Site: www.sjsu.edu

6133 SAN JOSE STATE UNIVERSITY THEATRE

One Washington Square
San Jose, CA 95192

Phone: 408-924-4530
Fax: 408-924-4574
e-mail: info@tvradiofilmtheatre.com
Web Site: www.tvradiofilmtheatre.com

6134 CUESTA COLLEGE AUDITORIUM

Cuesta College Campus
PO Box 8106
San Luis Obispo, CA 93403
Phone: 805-546-3100
Fax: 805-546-3904
Web Site: www.cuesta.cc.ca.us
Founded: 1973

6135 SAN MATEO PERFORMING ARTS CENTER

600 N Delaware
San Mateo, CA 94401
Phone: 650-579-5568
e-mail: info@bbbay.org
Web Site: www.pclo.org
Seating Capacity: 1,600

6136 ANGELS GATE CULTURAL CENTER

3601 S Gaffey Street
San Pedro, CA 90731
Phone: 310-519-0936
Fax: 310-519-8698
e-mail: artatgate@aol.com
Web Site: www.angelsgateart.org
Management:
    Executive Director: Robin Hinchliffe
Mission: Angels Gate Cultural Center, a nonprofit corporation, serves to develop an active environment mutually nourishing to the growth of artists, cultural arts and the community.
Founded: 1982
Paid Staff: 4
Volunteer Staff: 6
Paid Artists: 15

6137 WARNER GRAND THEATRE

478 West 6th Street
San Pedro, CA 90731
Phone: 310-548-2493
Fax: 310-548-2498
e-mail: WarnerGrand@earthlink.net
Web Site: www.warnergrand.org

6138 DOMINICAN COLLEGE - AUDITORIUM

50 Acacia
San Rafael, CA 94901
Phone: 415-457-4440
Fax: 415-485-3205
e-mail: publicrelations@dominican.edu
Web Site: www.dominican.edu
Founded: 1890

6139 MARIN CENTER - SHOWCASE THEATRE

10 Avenue of the Flags
San Rafael, CA 94903

Phone: 415-499-6400
Fax: 415-499-3700
e-mail: webmaster@co.marin.ca.us
Web Site: www.marincenter.org

6140 MARIN CENTER: SHOWCASE THEATRE

Avenue of the Flags
San Rafael, CA 94903
Phone: 415-472-3500
Fax: 415-499-3700

6141 MARIN CENTER: VETERANS MEMORIAL AUDITORIUM

Avenue of the Flags
San Rafael, CA 94903
Phone: 415-472-3500
Fax: 415-499-3700

6142 ARLINGTON CENTER FOR THE PERFORMING ARTS

1317 State Street
Santa Barbara, CA 93101
Phone: 805-963-4408
Fax: 805-966-4688
e-mail: karenkillingsworth_@hotmail.com
Founded: 1931
Facility Category: Theatre
Seating Capacity: 2,018
Year Built: 1931
Year Remodeled: 1977
Rental Contact: Karen Killingsworth

6143 HARDER STADIUM

University of California, Santa Barbara
Santa Barbara, CA 93106
Phone: 805-893-4156
Fax: 805-893-8640
e-mail: customer.service@pf.ucsb.edu
Web Site: www.facilities.ucsb.edu
Management:
    Manager: Joe Ballesteros

6144 LOBERO THEATRE FOUNDATION

33 E Canon Perdido Street
Santa Barbara, CA 93101
Phone: 805-966-4946
Fax: 805-963-8752
Toll-free: 888-456-2376
e-mail: agardner@lobero.com
Web Site: www.lobero.com
Management:
    Theatre Manager: David Asbell
Founded: 1873
Specialized Field: California Central Coast
Paid Staff: 15
Volunteer Staff: 100
Affiliations: APAP WAA Ca. Presenters
Annual Attendance: 100,000
Seating Capacity: 1,300
Year Built: 1924
Year Remodeled: 1996

Cost: 3 Million

6145 MUSIC THEATER OF SANTA BARBARA

1216 State Street
#200
Santa Barbara, CA 93101
Phone: 805-962-1922
Fax: 805-963-3510
e-mail: info@mtsb.org
Web Site: www.mtsb.org
Management:
   Executive Producer: Anthony Rhine
Mission: To enrich the community through musical theater.
Founded: 1989
Paid Staff: 15
Volunteer Staff: 20
Paid Artists: 100
Budget: $5 million
Income Sources: Tickets and Donations
Performs At: Granada Theater
Affiliations: National Association of Musical Theatre
Annual Attendance: 120,000
Facility Category: Theater
Type of Stage: Proscenium
Stage Dimensions: 60x40
Seating Capacity: 953
Year Built: 1908
Resident Groups: Santa Barbara Civic Light Opera

6146 SANTA BARBARA CONTEMPORARY ARTS FORUM

653 Paseo Nuevo
Santa Barbara, CA 93101
Phone: 805-966-5373
Fax: 805-962-1421
e-mail: sbcaf@sbcaf.org
Web Site: www.sbcaf.org
Management:
   Executive Director: Meg Linton
   Assistant Director: Rita Ferri
Mission: To provide an arena for the presentation, documentation and support of a broad variety of visual, media and performing arts representing a wide range of attitudes.
Founded: 1976
Specialized Field: Visual and Performing Arts Organization
Status: Nonprofit
Paid Staff: 7
Volunteer Staff: 30
Budget: $300,000
Income Sources: Membership; Business Sponsorship
Performs At: Center Stage Theater
Facility Category: Black Box
Year Built: 1990

6147 MUSIC AND ARTS INSTITUTE

2699 Maplewood Lane
Santa Clara, CA 95051
Phone: 408-296-7689

6148 KUUMBWA JAZZ CENTER

320-2 Cedar Street
Santa Cruz, CA 95060
Phone: 831-427-2227
Fax: 831-427-3342
e-mail: kuumbwa@kuumbwajazz.org
Web Site: www.kuumbwajazz.org
Management:
   Director: Tim Jackson
   Assistant Director: Kurt Brinkmeyer
   Education Development: Bobbi Todaro
Mission: To present jazz and educational opportunities to Santa Cruz County and surrounding areas.
Founded: 1975
Specialized Field: Jazz Music
Status: Nonprofit
Paid Staff: 7
Volunteer Staff: 50
Budget: $950,000
Income Sources: Membership; Grants
Performs At: Jazz Music
Stage Dimensions: 20'x14'6"
Seating Capacity: 200
Rental Contact: Kurt Brinkmeyer

6149 SANTA CRUZ CIVIC AUDITORIUM

307 Church Street
Santa Cruz, CA 95060
Phone: 831-420-5243
Fax: 831-420-5260
e-mail: info@santacruzcivic.com
Web Site: www.santacruzcivic.com
Management:
   Manager: Andrea Botsford
Founded: 1948
Annual Attendance: 87,000
Type of Stage: Proscenium
Seating Capacity: 1,957

6150 UNIVERSITY OF CALIFORNIA-SANTA CRUZ - PERFORMING ARTS

1156 High Street
Santa Cruz, CA 95064
Phone: 831-459-3500
Fax: 831-459-3502
e-mail: crede@cats.ucsc.edu
Web Site: www.ucsc.edu

6151 PACIFIC CONSERVATORY OF THE PERFORMING ARTS

800 S College Drive
PO Box 1700
Santa Maria, CA 93456-1700
Phone: 805-928-7731
Fax: 805-928-1142
e-mail: pcpa@pcpa.org
Web Site: www.pcpa.org
Management:
   Artistic Director: R Michael Gross
   Managing Director: Judy Frost6
   Associate Artistic Director: Mark Booher
   Marketing Director: Maria Centrella
Founded: 1964

Specialized Field: Professional Live Theatre;
Conservatory Training Program

6152 MORGAN-WIXSON THEATRE
2627 Pico Boulevard
Santa Monica, CA 90405
Phone: 310-828-7519

6153 SANTA MONICA CIVIC AUDITORIUM
1855 Main Street
Santa Monica, CA 90401
Phone: 310-393-9961

6154 LUTHER BURBANK CENTER FOR THE ARTS
50 Mark W Springs Road
Santa Rosa, CA 95403
Phone: 707-546-3600
Fax: 707-545-0518
e-mail: shekeynab@lbc.net
Web Site: www.lbc.net
Management:
    Scheduling Manager: Shekena Black
Mission: To enrich, educate and entertain in the North
Bay Community through outstanding artistic, cultural and
popular programming.
Founded: 1981
Annual Attendance: 500,000
Facility Category: Arts Center
Type of Stage: Thrust
Seating Capacity: 1,560
Year Remodeled: 2000

6155 LUTHER BURBANK CENTER FOR THE ARTS - CONCERT CHAMBER
50 Mark W Springs Road
Santa Rosa, CA 95403
Phone: 707-546-3600
Fax: 707-545-0518
e-mail: shekeynab@lbc.net
Web Site: www.lbc.net
Founded: 1981

6156 LUTHER BURBANK CENTER FOR THE ARTS - GOLD ROOM
50 Mark W Springs Road
Santa Rosa, CA 95403
Phone: 707-546-3600
Fax: 707-545-0518
e-mail: shekeynab@lbc.net
Web Site: www.lbc.net
Founded: 1981

6157 FALLON HOUSE THEATRE
Columbia State Historic Park
PO Box 3030
Sonora, CA 95370
Phone: 209-532-3120
Fax: 209-532-7270
e-mail: srt@mlode.com
Web Site: www.sierrarep.com
Management:

Managing Director: Sara Jones
Mission: To produce a year-round season of professional
theatre including musicals, drama and comedy.
Founded: 1980
Specialized Field: Theatre
Paid Staff: 25
Paid Artists: 200
Annual Attendance: 50,000
Type of Stage: Proscenium
Seating Capacity: 270

6158 STANFORD UNIVERSITY - ANNENBURG AUDITORIUM
Lasuen Mall Stanford University
Cummings Art Building
Stanford, CA 94305
Phone: 650-723-3404
Fax: 650-725-0140
Web Site: www.stanford.edu
Seating Capacity: 351

6159 STANFORD UNIVERSITY - BRAUN RECITAL HALL
Stanford University
Santa Theresa Street
Stanford, CA 94305
Phone: 650-723-3404
Fax: 650-725-0140
Web Site: www.stanford.edu

6160 STANFORD UNIVERSITY - CAMBLE RECITAL HALL
Santa Teresa Mall Stanford University
Braun Music Center
Stanford, CA 94305
Phone: 650-723-3404
Fax: 650-725-0140
Web Site: www.stanford.edu
Seating Capacity: 221

6161 STANFORD UNIVERSITY - COVERLY AUDITORIUM
Stanford University
Santa Theresa Street
Stanford, CA 94305
Phone: 650-723-3404
Fax: 650-725-0140
Web Site: www.stanford.edu

6162 STANFORD UNIVERSITY - DINKELSPIEL AUDITORIUM
Santa Teresa Mall Stanford University
Dinkelspiel
Stanford, CA 94305
Phone: 650-723-3404
Fax: 650-725-0140
Web Site: www.stanford.edu
Seating Capacity: 716

All listings are in alphabetical order by state, then city, then organization within the city.

6163 STANFORD UNIVERSITY - MEMORIAL AUDITORIUM
Stanford University
Memorial Hall
Stanford, CA 94305
Phone: 650-725-3335
Fax: 650-725-0140
Web Site: www.stanford.edu

6164 ATHERTON AUDITORIUM
5151 Pacific Avenue
Stockton, CA 95207
Phone: 209-474-5051
e-mail: questions@deltacollege.edu
Web Site: www.deltacollege.edu

6165 UNIVERSITY OF THE PACIFIC THEATRE ARTS DEPARTMENT
3601 Pacific Avenue
Stockton, CA 95211
Phone: 209-946-2116
Fax: 209-946-2118
e-mail: plach@uop.edu
Web Site: www.uop.edu
Management:
    Acting Chair: William Wolar
Founded: 1956
Paid Staff: 5
Non-paid Artists: 19
Budget: $82,900
Income Sources: Tickets, University
Annual Attendance: 1,800
Facility Category: Black Box
Type of Stage: Flexible
Stage Dimensions: 40 x 40
Seating Capacity: 80-120
Year Built: 1956

6166 UNIVERSITY OF THE PACIFIC - FAYE SPANOS CONCERTS
3601 Pacific Avenue
Stockton, CA 95211
Phone: 209-946-2415
e-mail: admissions@uop.edu
Web Site: www.uop.edu
Founded: 1987
Seating Capacity: 950

6167 UNIVERSITY OF THE PACIFIC - LONG THEATRE
3601 Pacific Avenue
Stockton, CA 95211
Phone: 209-946-2054
Fax: 209-946-2118
e-mail: plach@uop.edu
Web Site: www.uop.edu
Management:
    Theatre Manager: Jack Platt
Founded: 1976
Paid Staff: 1
Non-paid Artists: 19
Performs At: Proscenium

Annual Attendance: 8-10,000
Facility Category: Proscenium
Type of Stage: Proscenium
Stage Dimensions: 40 x 80
Seating Capacity: 400
Year Built: 1950
Year Remodeled: 1998

6168 UNIVERSITY OF THE PACIFIC - RECITAL HALL
3601 Pacific Avenue
Conservatory of Music
Stockton, CA 95211
Phone: 209-946-2415
e-mail: admissions@uop.edu
Web Site: www.uop.edu
Seating Capacity: 120

6169 WARREN ATHERTON AUDITORIUM
Delta College
5151 Pacific Avenue
San Joaquin County Delta Community College
Stockton, CA 95207
Phone: 209-954-5051
Fax: 209-954-5600
e-mail: timcox@sjddccT.cc.ca.us
Web Site: www.deltacollege.edu
Mission: Atherton Auditorium is one of the finest theater facilities in California. It maintains an independent staff of technical personnel who coordinate the productions presented on stage.
Specialized Field: Performing arts facility
Type of Stage: Proscenium
Stage Dimensions: 60 W x 26 L x 40 D
Seating Capacity: 1,456
Year Built: 1977
Rental Contact: Dr. Tim Cox

6170 THEATRE EAST
12655 Ventura Boulevard
Studio City, CA 91604
Phone: 818-760-4160
e-mail: theatreeast@yahoo.com
Founded: 1960

6171 CALIFORNIA LUTHERAN UNIVERSITY - PREUS-BRANDT FORUM
60 W Olsen Road
Thousand Oaks, CA 91360
Phone: 805-493-3195
Fax: 805-493-3513
e-mail: www@clunet.edu
Web Site: www.clunet.edu

6172 THOUSAND OAKS CIVIC ARTS PLAZA
2100 Thousand Oaks Boulevard
Thousand Oaks, CA 91362
Phone: 805-449-2787
Fax: 805-449-2750
e-mail: tmitze@toaks.org
Web Site: www.civicartsplaza.com
Management:

Technical Director: Gary Mintz
Box Office Supervisor: Sharon Lauritzen
Theatre House Supervisor: Nancy Loncto
Media Services Coordinator: Vanessa Greenberg
Founded: 1994
Performs At: Performing Arts Center
Affiliations: City of Thosand Oaks
Annual Attendance: 300,000+
Facility Category: Performing Arts Center
Type of Stage: Proscenium
Seating Capacity: 1800; 400
Year Built: 1994
Rental Contact: Tom Mitze
Resident Groups: Cabrillo Music Theatre and New West Symphony

6173 EL CAMINO COLLEGE/CENTER FOR THE ARTS
16007 S Crenshaw Boulevard
Torrance, CA 90506
Phone: 310-660-3748
Fax: 310-660-3734
e-mail: artstickets@elcamino.cc.ca.us
Web Site: www.elcamino.cc.ca.us
Management:
Center for the Arts Exec. Director: Tim Van Leer
Mission: To train college musicians; to provide community musicians with an opportunity to read and perform a greater variety of music than in other local groups.
Organization Type: Performing; Educational

6174 TORRANCE CULTURAL ARTS CENTER - JAMES R. ARMSTRONG THEATRE
3330 Civic Center Drive
Torrance, CA 90503
Phone: 310-781-7150
Fax: 310-781-7199
e-mail: jbotiller@tornet.com
Web Site: www.tcac.tornet.com
Management:
Theatre Booking Manager: Anita Molsen
Facility Booking Manager: Lisa Gomes
Paid Staff: 50
Volunteer Staff: 200
Income Sources: Facility rentals
Performs At: Theatre,, Visual & Performing Arts Studios(dance,crafts,etc)
Affiliations: City of Torrance, Torrance Cultural Arts Center Foundation
Facility Category: Multi-purpose complex (theater,art studios,rental)
Type of Stage: Proscenium
Stage Dimensions: 47 Feet Wide
Seating Capacity: 502
Year Built: 1991
Cost: $12 Million

6175 CALIFORNIA STATE UNIVERSITY-STANISLAUS
801 W Monte Vista Avenue
Turlock, CA 95382
Phone: 209-667-3451
Fax: 209-667-3782
e-mail: summerarts@calstate.edu
Web Site: www.calstate.edu/SummerArts
Mission: University degree.
Founded: 1986
Seating Capacity: 50-800

6176 HELENA PRODUCTIONS & MEDLEY SOCIETY THEATER
3069 Alamo Drive
Suite 319
Vacaville, CA 95687-6344
Phone: 707-477-9644
Fax: 707-447-9644

6177 VICTOR VALLEY COLLEGE PERFORMING ARTS CENTER
18422 Bear Valley Road
Victorville, CA 92392
Phone: 760-245-4271
Fax: 760-245-9744
e-mail: EPearson@victor.cc.ca.us
Web Site: www.victor.cc.ca.us
Founded: 1961
Seating Capacity: 493

6178 VISALIA CONVENTION CENTER - EXHIBIT HALL
303 E Acequia Street
Visalia, CA 93291
Phone: 559-713-4040
Fax: 209-738-3579
Toll-free: 800-225-2277
e-mail: vcc@ci.visalia.ca.us
Web Site: www.visalia.org
Seating Capacity: 2,000 to 4,000

6179 VISALIA CONVENTION CENTER
303 E Acequia Street
Visalia, CA 93291
Phone: 559-713-4040
Fax: 209-738-3574
e-mail: vcc@ci.visalia.ca.us
Web Site: www.visalia.org

6180 VISALIA CONVENTION CENTER - ROTARY THEATRE
330 S Dollner
Visalia, CA 93291
Phone: 559-730-7000
Fax: 209-738-3386
e-mail: vcc@ci.visalia.ca.us
Web Site: www.visalia.org

6181 MOONLIGHT AMPHITHEATRE
1200 Vale Terrance Drive
Vista, CA 92084
Phone: 760-639-6199
Fax: 760-941-9724
e-mail: moonlight@ci.vista.ca.us
Web Site: www.moonlightstage.com

Founded: 1976

**6182 DEAN LESHER REGIONAL CENTER
FOR THE ARTS**
1601 Civic Drive
Walnut Creek, CA 94596
Phone: 925-943-7469
Fax: 925-943-7222
e-mail: dlrca@dlrca.org
Web Site: www.dlrca.org
Management:
General Manager: Scott B Denison
Marketing Director: Lindsay Murray
Artistic Director: Lee Sankowich
Casting Director: Annie Stuart
Founded: 1966
Paid Staff: 11
Performs At: Dean Lesher Regional Center for the Arts,
Walnut Creek
Seating Capacity: 800
Year Built: 1991
Rental Contact: General Manager Scott B. Denison

**6183 COLLEGE OF THE SISKIYOUS -
THEATRE**
800 College Avenue
Weed, CA 96094
Phone: 530-938-5366
Fax: 916-938-5227
Toll-free: 888-397-4339
e-mail: ronge@siskiyous.edu
Web Site: www.siskiyous.edu
Seating Capacity: 584

**6184 RIO HONDO COLLEGE - MERTON
WRAY THEATRE**
3600 Workman Mill Road
Whittier, CA 90601
Phone: 562-692-0921
Fax: 562-908-3446
Web Site: www.riohondo.edu

6185 WOODLAND OPERA HOUSE
340 2nd Street
P.O. Box 1425
Woodland, CA 95776
Phone: 530-666-9617
Fax: 530-666-4783
e-mail: wohtheatre@afes.com
Web Site: www.wohtheatre.org
Founded: 1885

**6186 YREKA COMMUNITY THEATRE
CENTER**
810 N Oregon Street
Yreka, CA 96097
Phone: 916-842-2355
Fax: 916-842-4836

Colorado

**6187 ARVADA CENTER FOR THE ARTS AND
HUMANITIES**
6901 Wadsworth Boulevard
Arvada, CO 80003
Phone: 720-898-7285
Fax: 720-898-7204
e-mail: kathy-k@arvadacenter.org
Web Site: www.arvadacenter.org
Management:
Performing Arts Director: Kathy Kuehn
Executive Director: Deborah Jordy
Founded: 1976
Seating Capacity: 500

6188 MUSIC TENT
980 N 3rd Street
Aspen, CO 81611
Phone: 970-925-3254

6189 WHEELER OPERA HOUSE
320 E Hyman Avenue
Aspen, CO 81611
Phone: 970-920-5790
Fax: 970-920-5798
e-mail: nidat@ci.aspen.co.us
Web Site: www.wheeleroperahouse.com
Founded: 1889

6190 AURORA FOX ARTS CENTER
9900 E Colfax Avenue
PO Box 9
Aurora, CO 80010
Phone: 303-361-2910
Fax: 303-361-2909
e-mail: recreation@auroragov.org
Web Site: www.ci.aurora.co.us
Management:
Director: Robert Salisbury

6191 BICENTENNIAL ART CENTER
13655 E Alameda
Aurora, CO 80012
Phone: 303-344-1776
Fax: 303-341-7985

6192 BOULDER ART CENTER
1750 13th
Boulder, CO 80302
Phone: 303-443-2122
Fax: 303-447-1633

**6193 FOLDSOM FIELD
University of Colorado- Boulder**
Regent Drive & 28th Street
Boulder, CO 80309
Phone: 303-492-7930
Fax: 303-492-7753
e-mail: rose.hauber@colorado.edu
Web Site: www.cubuffs.ocsn.com
Management:

Director: John Krueger

6194 NAROPA INSTITUTE
2130 Arapahoe Avenue
Boulder, CO 80302
Phone: 303-444-0202
Fax: 303-444-0410
Web Site: www.naropa.edu

6195 NAROPA UNIVERSITY PERFORMING ARTS CENTER
2130 Araphoe Avenue
Boulder, CO 80302
Phone: 303-546-3538
Fax: 303-444-0410
e-mail: orotolano@naropa.edu
Web Site: www.naropa.edu
Management:
   Performing Arts Center Director: David Ortolano
   PAC Production Manager: Gary McCrumb
Performs At: Performing Arts Center

6196 UNIVERSITY OF COLORADO - MACKY AUDITORIUM
Box 285
Boulder, CO 80309
Phone: 303-492-8423
Fax: 303-492-5105
e-mail: macky@stripe.colorado.edu
Web Site: www.colorado.edu/Macky/contact.html
Founded: 1914
Type of Stage: Concert Hall
Seating Capacity: 2,047

6197 BACKSTAGE THEATRE
PO Box 297
Breckenridge, CO 80424
Phone: 970-453-0199
Fax: 970-453-4382
e-mail: backstagetheatre@hotmail.com
Web Site: www.backstagetheatre.org
Founded: 1974

6198 COORS EVENTS: CONFERENCE CENTER
Regent Drive & 28th Street
Colorado, CO 80309
Phone: 303-492-5316
Fax: 303-492-4801
Management:
   Director: Steve Wells

6199 ARNOLD HALL THEATER - UNITED STATES AIR FORCE
2302 Cadet Drive
Colorado Springs, CO 80840
Phone: 719-472-4497
Fax: 719-472-4597

6200 CITY AUDITORIUM
221 E Kiowa Street
Colorado Springs, CO 80903
Phone: 719-578-6652
Fax: 719-635-7806
e-mail: bwade@ci.colospgs.co.us
Web Site: www.springsgov.com
Management:
   Manager: Bob Wade
Founded: 1923
Paid Staff: 4
Volunteer Staff: 6
Annual Attendance: 125,000
Type of Stage: Raised Stage
Seating Capacity: 2,500

6201 COLORADO SPRINGS FINE ARTS CENTER THEATRE
30 W Dale Street
Colorado Springs, CO 80903
Phone: 719-634-5581
Fax: 719-634-0570
e-mail: info@csfineartscenter.org
Web Site: www.csfineartscenter.org/contact.htm
Management:
   Director Performing Arts: Robert T Geers
Founded: 1936

6202 PIKES PEAK CENTER
190 S Cascade
Colorado Springs, CO 80903
Phone: 719-520-7453
Fax: 719-520-7462
e-mail: ppcwes@pikespeakcenter.org
Web Site: www.pikespeakcenter.org
Management:
   Director: Steve Martin
   Booking Manager: Cindy Ballard
Founded: 1982
Paid Staff: 10
Annual Attendance: 200,000
Facility Category: Theat7e
Type of Stage: Proscenium
Seating Capacity: 2,061
Year Built: 1982
Cost: 13.2 Million
Rental Contact: Booking Manager Cindy Ballard

6203 SKY SOX STADIUM
4385 Tutt Boulevard
Colorado Springs, CO 80922
Phone: 719-597-1449
Fax: 719-597-2491
e-mail: info@skysox.com
Web Site: www.skysox.com
Management:
   Vice President/Operations: Dwight Hall
   EVP: Rai Henniger
Founded: 1988
Seating Capacity: 8,500

6204 CREEDE REPERTORY THEATRE
124 North Main Street
P. O. Box 269
Creede, CO 81130
Phone: 719-658-2343
Fax: 719-658-2343
e-mail: crt@creederep.com
Web Site: www.creederep.com
Founded: 1966
Type of Stage: Black Box; Proscenium
Seating Capacity: 313

6205 CRESTED BUTTE MOUNTAIN THEATRE
2nd and Elk
PO Box 611
Crested Butte, CO 81224
Phone: 970-349-0366
e-mail: mttheatre@crestedbutte.net
Web Site: www.visitcrestedbutte.com
Founded: 1972
Annual Attendance: 4,000
Type of Stage: Black Box
Seating Capacity: 100

6206 GOLD BAR ROOM THEATRE, IMPERIAL HOTEL
123 N 3rd Street
PO Box 1003
Cripple Creek, CO 80813
Phone: 719-689-7777
Fax: 719-689-1008

6207 AUDITORIUM THEATER - DENVER PERFORMING ARTS COMPLEX
14th and Curtis Streets
Denver, CO 80204
Phone: 303-832-4676
Fax: 303-640-2397
e-mail: info@denverbrass.org
Web Site: www.denverbrass.org
Management:
  General Manager: Rodney Smith
  Assistant General Manager: Elizabeth M Miller
  Event Coordinator: Dante Dunlap
Founded: 1908
Affiliations: Colorado Ballet, Colorado Symphony, Center Attractions
Annual Attendance: 1,500,000
Seating Capacity: 2,100
Year Built: 1908
Rental Contact: Bobbi McFarland

6208 AUGUSTANA ARTS
5000 E Alameda Avenue
Denver, CO 80246
Phone: 303-388-4678
Fax: 303-388-1338
e-mail: donald@augustanaarts.org
Web Site: www.augustanaarts.org
Officers:
  President: Cindy Linden Martin
  VP: Margaret Aarestad

Treasurer: Donald Fink
Secretary: Joel Haas
Management:
  Executive Director: Donald Tallman
  Education Director: Alfred Born
  Artistic Director: Michael Shasberger
Mission: To enhance the cultural life of the Denver Community: by supporting the efforts of local performing artists; by presenting performers of international renown; and performing arts outreach and educational programming.
Founded: 1997
Specialized Field: Music: Instrumental; Vocal; Opera
Budget: $250,000
Income Sources: Ticket Sales; Grants; Donations
Performs At: Primary - Church
Annual Attendance: 8,000
Seating Capacity: 700

6209 BOETTCHER CONCERT HALL - DENVER PERFORMING ARTS
950 13th Street
Denver, CO 80204
Phone: 303-640-2637
Fax: 303-640-2397
e-mail: smithr@ci.denver.co.us
Web Site: www.denvergov.org
Management:
  General Manager: Rodney Smith
  Assistant General Manager: Scott Rowitz
  Customer Services: Beth Miller
Founded: 1978
Facility Category: Concert Hall
Seating Capacity: 2,634
Year Built: 1978
Rental Contact: Bobbi McFarland

6210 CHANGING SCENE THEATER
1527 1/2 Champa Street
Denver, CO 80202
Phone: 303-893-5775

6211 COORS FIELD
2001 Blake Street
Denver, CO 80205
Phone: 800-388-ROCK
Fax: 303-312-2116
e-mail: tickets@rockies.mlb.com
Web Site: www.colorado.rockies.mlb.com
Management:
  Director Stadium Operations: Kevin Kahn
  Director Coors Field: Dave Moore
Founded: 1960
Annual Attendance: 7,701,861
Seating Capacity: 50,445
Year Built: 1995

6212 DENVER AUDITORIUM - ARENA
1323 Champa Street
Denver, CO 80204
Phone: 303-575-2637
Fax: 303-572-4709

6213 DENVER AUDITORIUM - CURRIGAN EXHIBITION HALL
1324 Champa Street
Denver, CO 80204
Phone: 303-640-3856
Fax: 303-572-4709

6214 DENVER AUDITORIUM - MCNICHOLS SPORTS ARENA
1635 Bryant Street
Denver, CO 80204
Phone: 303-640-7300
Fax: 303-572-4709

6215 DENVER AUDITORIUM - THEATRE
14th and Curtis
Denver, CO 80204
Phone: 303-575-2637
Fax: 303-572-4709

6216 DENVER BRONCOS STADIUM
Metropolitan Football Stadium District
1805 Bryant Street
Denver, CO 80204
Phone: 303-244-1002
Fax: 303-244-1003
e-mail: jbroz@mfsd.com
Web Site: www.mfsd.com
Management:
  Executive Director: Tim Romani
  Director Operations: Kelly Leid
  Director Events: Tua Bkakacj
Seating Capacity: 76,125

6217 DENVER CENTER FOR THE PERFORMING ARTS
1245 Champa Street
Denver, CO 80204-2104
Phone: 303-893-4000
e-mail: denvercenter@dcpa.org
Web Site: www.denvercenter.org
Founded: 1972
Status: Nonprofit; Professional
Seating Capacity: 1,577

6218 DENVER COLISEUM
4600 Humboldt Street
Denver, CO 80216
Phone: 303-295-4444
Fax: 303-572-4792
e-mail: gonzaam@ci.denver.co.us
Web Site: www.denvercoliseum.com
Management:
  Director: Fabbey Hillyard
Founded: 1947
Type of Stage: Concert Stage

6219 DENVER PERFORMING ARTS COMPLEX
950 13th Street
Denver, CO 80204

Phone: 303-640-7176
Fax: 303-640-2397
e-mail: diane.saslow@ci.denver.co.us
Web Site: www.denvergov.org/dpac
Management:
  General Manager: Rodney Smith
  Assistant General Manager: Scott Rowitz
  Customer Services: Beth Miller
Founded: 1908
Specialized Field: Broadway Shows
Affiliations: Center Attractions
Type of Stage: Proscenium
Year Built: 1991

6220 DENVER VICTORIAN PLAYHOUSE
4201 Hooker Street
Denver, CO 80211
Phone: 303-433-4343
Mission: Presenting a season of plays with five productions, including a variety of comedy and drama.
Founded: 1911
Specialized Field: Community; Theatrical Group
Status: Semi-Professional; Nonprofit; Commercial
Paid Staff: 30
Season: Year Round
Seating Capacity: 73
Organization Type: Performing; Sponsoring

6221 EL CENTRO SU TEATRO
4725 High Street
Denver, CO 80216
Phone: 303-296-0219
Fax: 303-296-4614
e-mail: elcentro@suteatro.org
Web Site: www.suteatro.org
Founded: 1971

6222 HISTORIC PARAMOUNT FOUNDATION/PARAMOUNT THEATRE
1631 Glenarm Place
Suite 200
Denver, CO 80202
Phone: 303-623-0106
Fax: 303-623-8062
e-mail: paramount@historicparamounttheatre.com
Web Site: www.historicparamounttheatre.netfirms.com
Management:
  Executive Director: Jim Sprinkle
Founded: 1930
Seating Capacity: 2,000

6223 HOUSTON FINE ARTS CENTER
Lamont School of Music
7111 Montview Boulevard
Denver, CO 80220
Phone: 303-871-6404
Fax: 303-871-3118
Web Site: www.du.edu/maps/houston.html
Rental Contact: Jennifer L. Olcott
Resident Groups: The Climb ((jazz), Davinici Quartet string ensemble)

6224 MAY BONFILS STANTON CENTER FOR THE PERFORMING ARTS
3001 S Federal Boulevard
Denver, CO 80110
Phone: 303-935-9110

6225 MILE HIGH STADIUM
2755 W 17th Avenue
Denver, CO 80204
Phone: 303-458-4848
Fax: 303-458-4861
Web Site: www.denverbroncos.com
Management:
   General Manager: Mac Freeman
   Director Operations: Gary Jones
Founded: 1970
Seating Capacity: 76,098

6226 MIZEL CENTER FOR ARTS AND CULTURE
350 S Dahlia Street
Denver, CO 80246-8102
Phone: 303-316-6360
Fax: 303-320-0042
e-mail: info@jccdenver.org
Web Site: www.mizelarts.org
Management:
   Artistic Director: Steve Wilson
   Technical Director: Cj Mosier
   Education Director: Roberta Bloom
   Arts Center Director: Joanne Kauvar
Budget: $300,000
Income Sources: Ticket Sales; Grants; City; State
Annual Attendance: 20,000
Type of Stage: Proscenium; Thrust
Seating Capacity: 300; 95
Year Built: 1970
Year Remodeled: 1995

6227 PEPSI CENTER
1000 Chopper Place
Denver, CO 80204
Phone: 303-405-1111
Fax: 303-893-6685
e-mail: webmaster@pepsicenter.com
Web Site: www.pepsicenter.com
Officers:
   President: Don Elliman
Management:
   Director Sponsorships/Ad Sales: Brian Jones
   SVP/Operations: Gene Feeling
   General Manager: Tim Romjani
Founded: 1999
Type of Stage: Concert Stage
Seating Capacity: 20,000

6228 RED ROCKS AMPHITHEATRE - MORRISON COLORADO
1380 Lawrence Street
Suite 790
Denver, CO 80204

Phone: 303-640-2637
Fax: 303-572-4792
Web Site: www.redrocksonline.com
Founded: 1941

6229 FORT LEWIS COLLEGE COMMUNITY CONCERT HALL
1000 Rim Drive
College Heights
Durango, CO 81301
Phone: 970-247-7162
Fax: 970-247-7058
e-mail: penington_g@fortlewis.edu
Web Site: www.durangoconcerts.com
Management:
   Manager: Gary Penington
Founded: 1997
Annual Attendance: 44,783
Type of Stage: Proscenium

6230 CITY OF FORT COLLINS: LINCOLN CENTER
417 W Magnolia
Fort Collins, CO 80521
Phone: 970-221-6735
Fax: 970-484-0424
Management:
   Director: David T Siever

6231 COLORADO STATE UNIVERSITY
McGraw Athletic Building
Fort Collins, CO 80523
Phone: 970-491-6211
Fax: 970-491-1348
Web Site: www.csurams.com
Management:
   Assistant Athletic Director: Doug Max
Founded: 1860
Specialized Field: Moby Arena, Hughes Stadium
Seating Capacity: 8,300

6232 COLORADO STATE UNIVERSITY - UNIVERSITY THEATRE
Fort Collins, CO 80523
Phone: 970-491-5116
Fax: 303-491-6423
Web Site: www.colostate.edu
Type of Stage: Black Box

6233 HUGHES STADIUM
Colorado State University
McGraw Athetic Building
Fort Collins, CO 80523
Phone: 970-491-6211
Fax: 970-491-1348
Web Site: www.csurams.com
Management:
   Assistant Athletic: Doug Max

6234 LINCOLN PARK STOCKER STADIUM
250 N 5th Street
Grand Junction, CO 81501

Phone: 970-244-1542
Fax: 970-242-1637
e-mail: cross@mesastate.edu
Web Site: www.mesastate.edu
Management:
  Director: Erik Joe Stevens
Seating Capacity: 6,600

6235 MESA COLLEGE: WALTER WALKER AUDITORIUM

PO Box 2647
Grand Junction, CO 81502
Phone: 970-248-1020
Fax: 970-248-1159

6236 UNION COLONY CIVIC CENTER

701 10th Avenue
Greeley, CO 80631
Phone: 970-350-9454
Fax: 970-350-9475
Toll-free: 800-315-2787
e-mail: uccc@ci.greeley.co.us
Web Site: www.ucstars.com
Management:
  Cultural Affairs Director: Jill Rosentrater
  UCCC Manager: Lonnie EJ Cooper
  Marketing Coordinator: Mary M Russell
  Event Coordinator: Julianne Givan
Founded: 1988
Paid Staff: 14
Volunteer Staff: 250
Budget: $1.5 Million
Income Sources: Ticket Sales; Rentals; Sponsorships;
City Subsidy
Annual Attendance: 110,000
Facility Category: Concert Hall; Auditorium;
Performance
Stage Dimensions: 50 x 60
Seating Capacity: 1660
Year Built: 1988
Cost: $9.2 Million
Rental Contact: Julie Givan

6237 UNIVERSITY OF NORTHERN COLORADO

Frazier Hall
501 20th Street
Greeley, CO 80639
Phone: 970-351-1890
Fax: 303-351-1923
e-mail: barbara.lowenbach@unco.edu
Web Site: www.unco.edu
Founded: 1954

6238 OTERO JUNIOR COLLEGE - HUMANITIES CENTER THEATRE

1802 Colorado
La Junta, CO 81050
Phone: 719-384-6831
Fax: 719-384-6880
e-mail: tim.walsh@ojc.edu
Web Site: www.ojc.edu
Founded: 1941

6239 PICKETWIRE PLAYERS AND COMMUNITY THEATRE

802 San Juan Ave.
La Junta, CO 81050
Phone: 719-384-8320
Founded: 1968
Seating Capacity: 350-394

6240 TOWN HALL ARTS CENTER

2450 W Main Street
Littleton, CO 80120
Phone: 303-794-2787
Fax: 303-794-6580
e-mail: bilroded@aol.com
Web Site: www.townhallartscenter.com
Management:
  Executive Director: Bill Rodgers
Mission: Offering live broadway musicals in an intimate
setting for families.
Specialized Field: Live Theater; Art Gallery

6241 DICKENS OPERA HOUSE

302 Main Street
Longmont, CO 80501
Phone: 303-651-7773
Fax: 303-651-7774

6242 LOVELAND CIVIC MUSIC ASSOCIATION

PO Box 952
Loveland, CO 80539
Phone: 970-633-9420

6243 SANGRE DE CRISTO ARTS AND CONFERENCE CENTER

210 N Santa Fe Avenue
Pueblo, CO 81003
Phone: 719-295-7222
Fax: 719-543-0134
e-mail: mail@sdc-arts.org
Web Site: www.sdc-arts.org
Founded: 1972

6244 NORTHEASTERN JUNIOR COLLEGE THEATRE

Northeastern Junior College
100 College Avenue
Sterling, CO 80751
Phone: 970-521-6600
Fax: 970-521-6703
e-mail: melissa.bornhoft@njc.edu
Web Site: www.njc.edu
Type of Stage: Proscenium
Seating Capacity: 566

Connecticut

6245 DOWNTOWN CABARET THEATRE

263 Golden Hill Street
Bridgeport, CT 6604

All listings are in alphabetical order by state, then city, then organization within the city.

Phone: 203-576-1634
Fax: 203-576-1444
e-mail: mail@dtcab.com
Web Site: www.dtcab.com
Management:
   Executive Producer Manager: Richard Hallinan
   Associate Producer: Hugh Hallinan
Founded: 1975
Status: Nonprofit
Paid Staff: 12
Season: Year Round
Annual Attendance: 80,000
Type of Stage: Proscenium
Seating Capacity: 276
Year Remodeled: 1995

6246 KLEIN MEMORIAL AUDITORIUM
910 Fairfield Avenue
Bridgeport, CT 6605
Phone: 203-576-8115

6247 UNIVERSITY OF BRIDGEPORT - BERNHARD CENTER
84 Iranistan Avenue
Bridgeport, CT 6601
Phone: 203-576-4000
Fax: 203-576-4051
e-mail: nas@bridgeport.edu
Web Site: www.bridgeport.edu
Founded: 1971

6248 CHARLES IVES CENTER - PAVILION
PO Box 2957
Danbury, CT 6813
Phone: 203-837-9226
Fax: 203-837-9230
e-mail: ivescenter@aol.com
Web Site: www.ivesconcertpark.com
Founded: 1974
Type of Stage: Concert Stage
Seating Capacity: 5,500

6249 O'NEILL CENTER
Western Connecticut State University
Lake Avenue & University Boulevard
Danbury, CT 6811
Phone: 203-837-8343
Fax: 203-837-8345
e-mail: dellaripav@wcsu.ctstate.edu
Web Site: www.vax.wcsu.edu
Management:
   Buiness Manager: Mike Palrea
   Excutive Director: Victor J Dellaripa, Jr
Founded: 1995
Paid Staff: 12
Seating Capacity: 3,500

6250 GOODSPEED OPERA HOUSE
Route 82
PO Box A
East Haddam, CT 06423

Phone: 860-873-8664
Fax: 860-873-2329
e-mail: info@goodspeed.org
Web Site: www.goodspeed.org
Management:
   Executive Director: Michael P Price
   Associate Producer: Sue Frost
Founded: 1963
Specialized Field: Opera House
Performs At: Goodspeed Opera House, Goodspeed-at-Chester
Type of Stage: Proscenium, Adaptable Proscenium
Seating Capacity: 400, 200

6251 QUICK CENTER FOR THE ARTS
Fairfield University
Fairfield, CT 06430-7524
Phone: 203-254-4242
Fax: 203-254-4113
Toll-free: 877-278-1396
e-mail: info@quickcenter.com
Web Site: www.quickcenter.com
Management:
   Director Programming: Deborah Sommers
   Executive Director: Thomas V Zingarelli
Mission: A year round Regional Arts Center that provides professional performances in all disciplines, outreach and educational programs and a 6'exhibit visual arts gallery.
Founded: 1990
Specialized Field: University owed; performing and visual educational
Paid Staff: 14
Volunteer Staff: 200
Budget: 2 Million
Income Sources: Ticket Revenue; Rentals; Sponsorships; Donations; Grants
Performs At: Kelley Theatre, Wien Experimental Theatre, Walsh Art Gallery
Affiliations: New England Presenters, National Association of Gallerys, Museums, Connecticut Dance Alliance, Association of Preforming Arts Presenters
Annual Attendance: 90,000
Facility Category: Two theatres
Type of Stage: Proscenium & Black Box
Seating Capacity: 741
Year Built: 1990
Rental Contact: House Manager T.J. Murphy

6252 ALBANO BALLET AND PERFORMING ARTS CENTER
15 Girard Avenue
Hartford, CT 6105
Phone: 860-232-8898

6253 BUSHNELL CENTER FOR THE PERFORMING ARTS
166 Capitol Avenue
Hartford, CT 06106
Phone: 860-987-6000
Fax: 860-987-6070
e-mail: info@bushnell.org
Web Site: www.bushnell.org
Management:
   Executive Director: David Fay

Associate Executive Director: Deidre Tavera
Founded: 1930
Paid Staff: 70
Volunteer Staff: 700
Annual Attendance: 350,000
Facility Category: Performing Arts Center
Type of Stage: Proscenium
Seating Capacity: 2,800
Year Built: 1929
Year Remodeled: 2001
Rental Contact: Jodi Arnmark

6254 CHARTER OAK CULTURAL CENTER

21 Charter Oak Avenue
Hartford, CT 06106
Phone: 860-249-1207
Fax: 860-524-8014
e-mail: cocc@hartnet.org
Officers:
President: Raymond Baker
Management:
Executive Director: Rabbi Donna Berman PhD
Specialized Field: Dance; Visual Arts; Music; Theatre; Exhibits; Film
Paid Staff: 2
Volunteer Staff: 1
Budget: $200,000
Income Sources: Private Foundations; Grants; Business and Individual Donations; Box Office; Government; Endowments
Affiliations: Greater Hartford Arts Council; Dance Connecticut
Annual Attendance: 2,500
Facility Category: Former Synagogue
Type of Stage: Stage and Dance Floor
Stage Dimensions: 40'x60'
Seating Capacity: 200
Year Built: 1876

6255 HARTFORD CIVIC CENTER

One Civic Center Plaza
Hartford, CT 6103
Phone: 860-249-6333
Fax: 860-727-8010
e-mail: nancy.gallagher@thegarden.com
Web Site: www.hartfordciviccenter.com
Management:
General Manager: Marty Brooks
Director Facility Booking: Nancy N Gallagher
Seating Capacity: 16,500
Year Built: 1978
Year Remodeled: 1998

6256 HARTFORD OFFICE OF CULTURAL AFFAIRS

2 Holcomb Street
Hartford, CT 06112
Phone: 860-543-8874
Fax: 860-722-6786
e-mail: yharris@ci.hartford.ct.us
Management:
Program Director: Yvonne Harris

Mission: To administer arts programs for city of Hartford residents and provide an exhibition space for all Connecitcut residents.
Founded: 1979
Specialized Field: Multi-Visual, Music, Poetry, Theater
Paid Staff: 150
Volunteer Staff: 25
Budget: $85,000
Income Sources: City Government

6257 HORACE BUSHNELL MEMORIAL HALL

166 Capitol Avenue
Hartford, CT 6106
Phone: 860-987-5900
Fax: 860-987-6080
Toll-free: 888-824-2874
e-mail: info@bushnell.org
Web Site: www.bushnell.org
Founded: 1929
Annual Attendance: 350,000
Type of Stage: Flexible; Proscenium

6258 TRINITY COLLEGE: AUSTIN ARTS CENTER

300 Summit Street
Hartford, CT 06106-3100
Phone: 860-297-2199
Fax: 860-297-5380
e-mail: jeffry.walker@mail.trincoll.edu
Web Site: www.austinarts.org
Management:
Austin Arts Center Director: Jeffry Walker
Mission: The Austin Arts Center (AAC) is Trinity College's premier venue for the performing and visual arts. Centrally-located on campus, it houses two performance spaces (Goodwin Theater and Garmany Hall) and the Widener Gallery. Annually presenting over 40 public events featuring guest artists, facility and students, programming can range from the creation of Tibetan mandalas to modern opera to political theater.
Paid Staff: 4
Facility Category: Performing; Visual Arts
Type of Stage: Proscenium; Black Box

6259 MASHANTUCKET PEQUOT MUSEUM & RESEARCH CENTER

110 Pequot Trail
PO Box 3180
Mashantucket, CT 06339-3180
Phone: 860-396-6835
Fax: 830-396-7013
e-mail: sdennin@mptn.org
Web Site: www.mashantucket.com
Management:
Marketing/Development Director: Steve Dennin
Founded: 1998
Annual Attendance: 300,000
Seating Capacity: 320

6260 CENTER FOR THE ARTS
Wesleyan University
283 Washington Terrace
Middletown, CT 06459-0442
Phone: 860-685-2695
Fax: 860-685-2061
e-mail: boxoffice@wesleyan.edu
Web Site: www.wesleyan.edu/CFA
Management:
  Director: Pamela Tatge
  Events Manager: Barbara Ally
Founded: 1973
Specialized Field: Music, dance, theatre, visual arts
Performs At: Crowell Concert Hall/Theater
Annual Attendance: 41,000
Facility Category: Concert Hall, Theatre
Type of Stage: Flexible
Seating Capacity: 1,799
Year Built: 1973

6261 INGALLS RINK
Yale University
Yale University
PO Box 208216
New Haven, CT 6520
Phone: 203-432-2489
Fax: 203-432-7772
e-mail: joseph.snecinski@yale.edu
Web Site: www.yale.edu/athletic
Management:
  Rink Manager: Joe Snecinski
Founded: 1958
Seating Capacity: 3,486

6262 LONG WHARF THEATRE
222 Sargent Drive
Exit 46 Off I-95
New Haven, CT 6511
Phone: 203-787-4282
Fax: 203-776-2287
Toll-free: 800-782-8497
e-mail: info@longwharf.org
Web Site: www.longwharf.org
Founded: 1965
Annual Attendance: 100,000
Type of Stage: Thrust
Seating Capacity: 487

6263 LONG WHARF THEATRE - STAGE II
222 Sargent Drive
Exit 46 Off I-95
New Haven, CT 6511
Phone: 203-787-4282
Fax: 203-776-2287
Toll-free: 800-782-8497
e-mail: info@longwharf.org
Web Site: www.longwharf.org
Founded: 1965
Annual Attendance: 100,000
Type of Stage: Proscenium
Seating Capacity: 204

6264 LYMAN CENTER
Southern Connecticut State University
501 Crescent Street
New Haven, CT 6515
Phone: 203-392-6161
Fax: 203-392-6158
e-mail: tomascak@southernct.edu
Web Site: www.southernct.edu/aboutscsu/lyman/
Management:
  Director: Dr. Cynthia DiSano
  Associate Director: Lawrence Tomascak
Type of Stage: Thrust
Seating Capacity: 1,568

6265 NEW HAVEN VETERANS MEMORIAL COLISEUM
275 South Orange Street
New Haven, CT 6510
Phone: 203-772-4200
Fax: 203-495-7745
Web Site: www.nhcoliseum.com
Management:
  Executive Director: James E Perillo
  Marketing: Jan Barese
  Assistant Director: Stephanie Panico
  Facility Coordinator: Jason Smith
Seating Capacity: 11,000

6266 PALACE THEATRE
248 College Street
New Haven, CT 6510
Phone: 203-789-2120
Fax: 203-773-0478

6267 SHUBERT THEATER
247 College Street
New Haven, CT 06510-2419
Phone: 203-562-5666
Fax: 203-789-2286
Toll-free: 800-228-6622
e-mail: shubert@shubert.com
Web Site: www.shubert.com
Officers:
  President/CEO: William Conner
Management:
  VP/Executive Director: John F Fisner
  Director Operations: Shari Kaplan
Facility Category: Theater
Type of Stage: Proscenium
Seating Capacity: 1,655
Year Built: 1914
Year Remodeled: 1997
Rental Contact: Debbi Rosenthal

6268 YALE BASEBALL STADIUM
Yale University
PO Box 208216
New Haven, CT 6520
Phone: 203-432-1420
Fax: 203-432-7772
e-mail: kenneth.place@yale.edu
Web Site: www.yale.edu/athletic/
Management:

All listings are in alphabetical order by state, then city, then organization within the city.

Assistant Athletic Director: Kenneth Place
Athletic Director: Tom Beckett
Founded: 1928
Seating Capacity: 6,200

6269 YALE BOWL

Yale University
PO Box 208216
New Haven, CT 6520
Phone: 203-432-1420
Fax: 203-432-7772
e-mail: kenneth.place@yale.edu
Web Site: www.yale.edu/athletic/
Management:
    Athletic Director: Tom Beckett
    Assistant Athletic Director: Kenneth Place
Founded: 1914
Seating Capacity: 64,269

6270 YALE REPERTORY THEATRE

1120 Chapel Street
P.O. Box 1257
New Haven, CT 6505
Phone: 203-432-1234
Fax: 203-432-6423
e-mail: yalerep@yale.edu
Web Site: www.yalerep.org
Founded: 1966
Seating Capacity: 487

6271 CONNECTICUT COLLEGE - PALMER AUDITORIUM

270 Mohegan Avenue
PO Box 5512
New London, CT 6320
Phone: 860-439-2605
Fax: 203-439-2700
Toll-free: 888-553-8760
e-mail: dthol@conncoll.edu
Web Site: www.conncoll.edu
Founded: 1911
Annual Attendance: 1,800
Type of Stage: Black Box; Concert Stage
Seating Capacity: 1,298

6272 GARDE ARTS CENTER

325 State Street
New London, CT 06320
Phone: 860-444-6766
Fax: 860-447-0503
Toll-free: 888-061-2033
e-mail: info@gardearts.org
Web Site: www.gardearts.org
Officers:
    Marketing Director: Jean Brown
    Director Finance: Edward Wozniak
Management:
    Production Manager: Lawrence Ryan
    Director Operations: George Dowker
    Executive Director: Steve Sigel
Founded: 1976
Paid Staff: 22
Volunteer Staff: 200

Budget: $2,000,000
Income Sources: Ticket Sales; Sponsorships
Affiliations: Easter Connecticut Symphony Orchestra; Summer Music
Annual Attendance: 72,000
Type of Stage: Proscenium
Stage Dimensions: 41'x 36'
Seating Capacity: 1,488
Year Built: 1926
Year Remodeled: 1999
Cost: $11,000,000
Organization Type: Proscenium Theatre

6273 RIDGEFIELD PLAYHOUSE FOR MOVIES & THE PERFORMING ARTS

80 East Ridge Avenue
Ridgefield, CT 6877
Phone: 203-438-6635
Fax: 203-438-1905
e-mail: info@ridgefieldplayhouse.org
Web Site: www.ridgefieldplayhouse.org
Management:
    Programing Director: Andrea Jabara
Founded: 1938
Seating Capacity: 509

6274 SHERMAN PLAYHOUSE

PO Box 471
Sherman, CT 6784
Phone: 860-354-3622
e-mail: ewscholze@aol.com
Web Site: www.geocities.com
Founded: 1926
Annual Attendance: 3,200
Type of Stage: Proscenium
Seating Capacity: 120

6275 SOUTHINGTON COMMUNITY THEATRE

1237 Marion Avenue, Marion
PO Box 411
Southington, CT 6444
Phone: 860-276-1961
e-mail: flozie18@aol.com
Web Site: www.southingtoncommunitytheatre.org
Founded: 1957

6276 RICH FORUM

307 Atlantic Street
Stamford, CT 6901
Phone: 203-358-2305
Fax: 203-358-2313
Web Site: www.onlyatsca.com
Management:
    Executive Director: George Moredock
Founded: 1992
Type of Stage: Proscenium
Seating Capacity: 757

6277 JORGENSEN CENTER FOR THE PERFORMING ARTS
University of Connecticut
2132 Hillside Road
Unit 3104
Storrs, CT 06269-3104
Phone: 860-486-1983
Fax: 860-486-6781
e-mail: rodney.rock@uconn.edu
Web Site: www.jorgensen.ct-arts.com
Management:
   Director: Rodney Rock
   Marketing/Publicity Director: Catherine Kalonia
   Operations Director: Gary Yakstis
   Box Office Director: Lucy Clarke
Mission: Through the presentation fo the performing arts, enlightens, entertains and inspires the intellectual curiosity in the university's students, faculty and staff, as well as the community at large.
Specialized Field: Multi-Disciplinary
Paid Staff: 13
Volunteer Staff: 8
Budget: $2 million
Income Sources: Sales; University Fees; Grants
Performs At: Jorgensen Center For The Performing Arts; Von Der Mehden Recital Hall
Affiliations: NEP, APAP
Annual Attendance: 70,000
Facility Category: Auditorium
Type of Stage: Proscenium
Seating Capacity: 2,630/500

6278 SPORTS COMPLEX, UNIVERSITY OF CONNECTICUT
2095 Hillside Road,U-78
Storrs, CT 6269
Phone: 860-486-2725
Fax: 860-486-1204
e-mail: kyle@maya.ath.uconn.edu
Web Site: www.uconn.edu
Management:
   Athletic Director: Lew Perkins
Seating Capacity: 10,027

6279 UNIVERSITY OF CONNECTICUT: SCHOOL OF FINE ARTS
Jorgensen Center for the Performing Arts
2132 Hillside Road, Unit 3104
Storrs, CT 06269-3104
Phone: 860-486-5225
Fax: 860-486-6781
e-mail: rodney.rock@uconn.edu
Web Site: www.jorgensen.ct-arts.com
Management:
   Director: Rodney Rock
   Director/Marketing-Publicity: Catherine Kalonia
   Director/Box Office: Lucy Clarke
   Director/Operations: Gary Yakstis
   Technical Director: Tom Meddick
Founded: 1955
Specialized Field: East of the River
Paid Staff: 14
Paid Artists: 45

6280 UNIVERSITY OF CONNECTICUT - HARRIET S. JORGEN CENTER
U-127
802 Bolton Road
Storrs, CT 6269
Phone: 860-486-4025
Fax: 860-486-3110
Web Site: www.uconn.edu

6281 COE PARK CIVIC CENTER
101 Litchfield Street
Torrington, CT 6790
Phone: 860-489-2274

6282 WARNER THEATRE
68 Main Street
PO Box 1012
Torrington, CT 6790
Phone: 860-489-7180
Fax: 860-482-4076
e-mail: warner@cttel.net
Web Site: www.warnertheatre.org
Management:
   Executive Director: Barry C Hughson
Founded: 1931
Annual Attendance: 10,000
Seating Capacity: 80

6283 OAKDALE THEATRE
95 S Turnpike Road
Wallingford, CT 06492
Phone: 203-269-8721
Fax: 203-294-6988
e-mail: reginashelton@clearchannel.com
Web Site: www.oakdale.com
Management:
   Booking: Anna Cappala
   Marketing: Jim Bozzi
Seating Capacity: 4,800

6284 PAUL MELLON ARTS CENTER
Choate Rosemary Hall
333 Christian Street
Wallingford, CT 6492
Phone: 203-697-2488
Fax: 203-697-2396
e-mail: rbrandt@choate.edu
Web Site: www.choate.edu
Management:
   Director: Paul J Tines
Founded: 1890
Annual Attendance: 45,000
Type of Stage: Proscenium
Seating Capacity: 750

6285 LINCOLN THEATER
200 Bloomfield Avenue
West Hartford, CT 6117
Phone: 860-768-4228

6286 SPORTS CENTER: UNIVERSITY OF HARTFORD
200 Bloomfield Avenue
West Hartford, CT 06117
Phone: 860-768-4536
Fax: 860-768-4229
Management:
    Director: Daivd Bell
Seating Capacity: 3,545

6287 LEVITT PAVILION FOR THE PERFORMING ARTS
260 South Compo Road
Westport, CT 6880
Phone: 203-226-7600
Fax: 203-226-2330
e-mail: levitt@ci.westport.ct.us
Web Site: www.levittpavilion.com
Management:
    Executive Director: Freda Walsh
Mission: The Pavilion provides over 50 nights of diverse, top-quality entertainment every summer, at no charge, plus 1-5 special ticketed events, to the residents of Connecticut and beyond.
Founded: 1973
Specialized Field: Performing Arts
Status: Nonprofit
Paid Staff: 6
Volunteer Staff: 20
Budget: $490,000
Income Sources: Fundraisingevents; Foundation Grants; Corporate Donations; Individual Donations
Affiliations: Friends of the Levitt Pavilion and the Town of Westport
Annual Attendance: 50,000
Facility Category: Outdoor
Type of Stage: Proscenium
Stage Dimensions: 26'x45'
Seating Capacity: 2,500
Year Built: 1973
Year Remodeled: 1990

6288 WESTPORT COMMUNITY THEATRE
110 Myrtle Avenue
Westport, CT 6880
Phone: 203-226-1983

6289 WESTPORT COUNTRY PLAYHOUSE
25 Powers Court
PO Box 629
Westport, CT 6881
Phone: 203-227-5137
Fax: 203-221-7482
e-mail: info@westportplayhouse.org
Web Site: www.westportplayhouse.org
Founded: 1931
Seating Capacity: 707

6290 SCHWARTZ CENTER FOR THE ARTS
Friends of the Capitol Theater
PO Box 1449
Dover, DE 19903
Phone: 302-678-3583
Fax: 302-678-1267
Toll-free: 800-778-5078
e-mail: thearts@schwartzcenter.com
Web Site: www.schwartzcenter.com
Management:
    Executive Director: Jeffery R Fulgham
    Adminastrative Director: Judy Rling
    Office Manager: JoAnn Glenn-Lewin
    Accociate Director: Mark Gallagher
Founded: 2001
Paid Staff: 4
Volunteer Staff: 50

6291 BOB CARPENTER CENTER
University of Delaware
631 S College Avenue
Newark, DE 19716
Phone: 302-831-4016
Fax: 302-831-4019
e-mail: dbs@udel.edu
Web Site: www.udel.edul/bcc
Management:
    Director: Domenick B Sicilia
    Events Coordinator: Karen Lofthouse
    Box Office Manager: Tammy Jackson-Harmon
Mission: To provide a venue for University of Deleware home basketball games, convocations, entertainment and special events.
Founded: 1992
Paid Staff: 25
Volunteer Staff: 5
Facility Category: Arena
Rental Contact: Domenick B Sicilia

6292 GRAND OPERA HOUSE
818 North Market Street
Wilmington, DE 19801-3080
Phone: 302-658-7897
Fax: 302-652-5346
e-mail: grandopera@grandopera.org
Web Site: www.grandopera.org
Founded: 1871
Type of Stage: Proscenium
Seating Capacity: 1,190

6293 PLAYHOUSE THEATRE
DuPont Building
10 & Market Streets
Wilmington, DE 19801
Phone: 302-656-4401
Fax: 302-594-1437
e-mail: Patricia.L.Dill@usa.dupont.com
Web Site: www.playhousetheatre.com
Management:
    General Manager: Patricia Dill

All listings are in alphabetical order by state, then city, then organization within the city.

District of Columbia

6294 AMERICAN UNIVERSITY - MCDONALD RECITAL HALL
4400 Massachusetts Avenue NW
Washington, DC 20016
Phone: 202-885-3420
Fax: 202-885-1092
e-mail: dpa_tech@american.edu
Web Site: www.american.edu

6295 AMERICAN UNIVERSITY - NEW LECTURE HALL
4400 Massachusetts Avenue NW
Washington, DC 20016
Phone: 202-885-3420
Fax: 202-885-1092
e-mail: dpa_tech@american.edu
Web Site: www.american.edu
Founded: 1968

6296 BENDER ARENA
American University
4400 Massachusetts Avenue NW
Washington, DC 20016
Phone: 202-885-3075
Fax: 202-885-3033
e-mail: sportsinfo@american.edu
Web Site: www.aueagles.com
Management:
   Athletic Director: Benjamin Ladner
   Assistant Athletic Director: Ed McLaughlin
Founded: 1988
Seating Capacity: 5,000 to 6,000

6297 CONSTITUTION HALL
18th and D Streets NW
Washington, DC 20006
Phone: 202-628-4780
Fax: 202-628-2570
e-mail: wwwfeedback@dar.org
Web Site: www.dar.org/conthall/
Founded: 1929

6298 DC ARMORY
2400 East Capitol Street, SE
Washington, DC 20003
Phone: 202-547-9077
Fax: 202-547-7460
e-mail: comments@dcarmory.com
Web Site: www.dcsportscommission.com
Management:
   Executive Director: James Dalrymple
Seating Capacity: 10,000

6299 FOLGER CONSORT
201 East Capitol Street, SE
Washington, DC 20003
Phone: 202-544-7077
Fax: 202-544-7520
e-mail: institute@folger.edu
Web Site: www.folger.edu

Management:
   Manager: Susanne Oldham
Founded: 1970

6300 GASTON HALL
37th and O Streets NW
Washington, DC 20057
Phone: 202-687-4081
Fax: 202-687-2191
e-mail: lignellr@georgetown.edu
Web Site: www.georgetown.edu
Founded: 1789
Annual Attendance: 15,000
Type of Stage: Black Box
Seating Capacity: 728

6301 GEORGETOWN UNIV. OFFICE OF PERFORMING ARTS
316 Leavey Center
Washington, DC 20057-1063
Phone: 202-687-3838
Fax: 202-687-8940
e-mail: lignellr@georgetown.edu
Web Site: www.georgetown.edu
Management:
   Director Performing Arts: Ron Lignelli

6302 HALL OF NATIONS BLACK BOX THEATRE
37th and O Streets NW
Washington, DC 20057
Phone: 202-687-4081
Fax: 202-687-2191
e-mail: lignellr@georgetown.edu
Web Site: www.georgetown.edu
Type of Stage: Black Box; Masonite
Seating Capacity: 200

6303 HOWARD UNIVERSITY CRAMTON AUDITORIUM
Howard University, Cramton Auditorium
2455 6th Street NW
Washington, DC 20059
Phone: 202-806-7194
Fax: 202-806-4862
e-mail: ddsaunders@howard.edu
Web Site: www.howard.edu
Management:
   Manager: Denise D Saunders
Performs At: Performing Arts; Educational Event; Keynote Speakers
Affiliations: Association of Performing Arts Presenters
Type of Stage: Proscenium
Seating Capacity: 1,500
Year Built: 1961
Rental Contact: Denise D Saunders

6304 JOHN F KENNEDY CENTER FOR THE PERFORMING ARTS
2700 F Street NW
Washington, DC 20566

Phone: 202-416-8000
Fax: 202-416-8018
Toll-free: 800-444-1324
Web Site: www.kennedy-center.org
Management:
   President: Lawrence J Wilker
   Program Director/National Programs: Kathi R Levin
   Program Director/ SR/Youth/Family: Kim Peter Kovac
   Program Manager/Performance Plus: Marlene Cooper

6305 LIBRARY OF CONGRESS
10, 1st Street SE
Washington, DC 20540
Phone: 202-707-5000

6306 GW'S LISNER AUDITORIUM
George Washington University
730 21st Street NW
Washington, DC 20052
Phone: 202-994-6800
Fax: 202-994-6906
e-mail: lisner@lisner.org
Web Site: www.lisner.org
Management:
   Director: Rosanna Ruscetti
Affiliations: George Washington University
Annual Attendance: 200,000
Facility Category: Auditorium
Seating Capacity: 1490
Year Built: 1942
Year Remodeled: 1990
Rental Contact: Rosanna Ruscetti

6307 MCI CENTER
601 F Street NW
Washington, DC 20001
Phone: 202-628-3200
Fax: 301-808-3002
Web Site: www.mcicenter.com
Officers:
   President: John Stranix
Management:
   VP/Executive Director: Nancy Lacy
   Booking Director: Patt Darr
   Assistant General Manager: Fritz Smith
   Director Excutive Seating: Bernie Deluca
Seating Capacity: 19,000

6308 SHAKESPEARE THEATRE
450 7th Street NW
Washington, DC 20004-2207
Phone: 202-547-3230
Fax: 202-547-0226
Toll-free: 877-487-8849
e-mail: webadmin@shakespearedc.org
Web Site: www.shakespearetheatre.org
Seating Capacity: 451

6309 SMITHSONIAN INSTITUTION - BAIRD AUDITORIUM
10th and Constitution Avenue NW
Washington, DC 20560
Phone: 202-357-1300
e-mail: ssmith@retail.si.edu
Web Site: www.mnh.si.edu

6310 SMITHSONIAN INSTITUTION - CARMICHAEL AUDITORIUM
14th and Constitution Avenue NW
Washington, DC 20560
Phone: 202-357-1300
e-mail: Info@info.si.edu.
Web Site: www.mnh.si.edu

6311 THEATER J
1529 16th Street NW
Washington, DC 20036
Phone: 202-518-9400
Fax: 202-518-9421
e-mail: theaterj@dcjcc.org
Web Site: www.theaterj.org
Management:
   Technical Director: Tim Getman
   Artistic Director: Joshua S Ford
   Managing Director: Caitlin Barile
   Artistic Director: Ari Roth
   Director Marketing/Communications: Jill Levin
Specialized Field: Theater
Season: October - May
Annual Attendance: 25,000
Facility Category: Theatre
Type of Stage: Thrust/Proscenium
Stage Dimensions: 20' x 20'
Seating Capacity: 258
Year Built: 1925
Year Remodeled: 1996
Rental Contact: Wanda ChiChester

6312 WARNER THEATRE
1299 Pennsylvania Avenue
NW Suite 111
Washington, DC 20004
Phone: 202-783-4000
Fax: 202-783-0204
Toll-free: 202-783-4000
e-mail: vradke@warnertheatre.com
Web Site: www.warnertheatre.com
Mission: Rental facility for local and touring presenters.
Founded: 1924
Performs At: Rental
Facility Category: Theater
Type of Stage: Proscenium
Seating Capacity: 1,847
Year Built: 1924
Year Remodeled: 1992
Rental Contact: 202-626-8250 B Newman

6313 CHARLES E SMITH CENTER
George Washinton University
600 22nd Street NW
Washington DC, DC 20052

Phone: 202-994-6650
Fax: 202-994-6818
e-mail: jahrens@gwu.edu
Web Site: www.gwu.edu
Management:
    Facilities Manager: Jason Wilson

Florida

6314 ISLAND PLAYERS THEATRE
Gulf Drive at Pine Avenue
PO Box 2059
Anna Maria, FL 34216
Phone: 941-778-5755

6315 DOLLY HANDS CULTURAL ARTS CENTER
Palm Beach Community College
M091920010ge Drive
Belle Glade, FL 33430
Phone: 561-992-6160
Fax: 407-992-6179
e-mail: woodhaml@pbcc.cc.fl.us
Web Site: www.pbcc.cc.fl.us
Management:
    Manager: Leigh Woodham

6316 PALM BEACH COMMUNITY COLLEGE, GLADES CAMPUS
1977 College Drive
Belle Glade, FL 33430
Phone: 561-992-6160
Fax: 561-992-6179
e-mail: woodhaml@pbc.cc.fl.us
Web Site: www.pbcc.cc.fl.us
Management:
    Manager: Leigh Woodham
Founded: 1982
Specialized Field: Performing
Paid Staff: 2
Volunteer Staff: 40
Budget: $350,000
Performs At: Dolly Hands Cultural Arts Center
Annual Attendance: 80,000
Type of Stage: Proscenium
Stage Dimensions: 40x40
Seating Capacity: 500
Year Built: 1982
Year Remodeled: 1996

6317 WT NEAL CIVIC CENTER
PO Box 40
Blountstown, FL 32424
Phone: 850-674-4500
Fax: 850-674-2459
e-mail: wtnealcc@gtcom.net

6318 CENTURY VILLAGE THEATRES
19296 Lyons Road
Boca Raton, FL 33434

Phone: 561-451-1227
Fax: 561-451-1218
e-mail: akoffler@cencec.com
Officers:
    VP: Abby Koffler
Management:
    Entertainment Director/VP: Abby C Koffler

6319 UNIVERSITY CENTER AUDITORIUM
500 NW 20th Street
Boca Raton, FL 33432
Phone: 561-297-3730
Fax: 561-297-3733
e-mail: dleland@fau.edu
Web Site: www.fau.edu
Founded: 1987

6320 FLAGLER AUDITORIUM
3265 E NHighway 100
PO Box 755
Bunnell, FL 32110
Phone: 386-437-7547
Toll-free: 866-352-4537
Web Site: www.flaglerauditorium.org
Founded: 1989
Type of Stage: Concert Stage
Seating Capacity: 1,000

6321 RUTH ECKERD HALL
1111 McMullen Booth Road
Clearwater, FL 33759
Phone: 727-791-7060
Fax: 727-724-5976
e-mail: lpoppens@rutheckerdhall.net
Web Site: www.rutheckerdhall.com
Officers:
    President/CEO: Robert Freedman
Management:
    Director Entertainment: Bob Rossi
    House Manager: Gregory Wright
    Director Marketing/Communication: Lex Poppens
Mission: To present major national and international artists and attractions year-round in a fine acoustic hall; to present educational programming, visual arts exhibits and senior citizen programs.
Founded: 1978
Specialized Field: Dance; Vocal Music; Instrumental Music; Theater
Status: Nonprofit
Paid Staff: 50
Paid Artists: 120
Budget: $9,000,000 million
Income Sources: Association of Performing Arts Presenters; International Society of Performing Arts Administrators; Florida Professional Presenters Association
Annual Attendance: 200,000
Facility Category: Performing Arts Center
Seating Capacity: 2,173
Year Built: 1982
Year Remodeled: 2002
Rental Contact: Gregory Wright
Organization Type: Performing; Educational; Sponsoring

6322 COCOA EXPO SPORTS CENTER
500 Friday Road
Cocoa, FL 32926
Phone: 321-639-3976
Fax: 321-639-0598
e-mail: gilesmalone@cocoaexpo.com
Web Site: www.cocoaexpo.com
Management:
    President/ General Manager: Giles Malone
Founded: 1985
Specialized Field: Brevard County/Space Coast
Performs At: 25,000 Square Foot Arena
Annual Attendance: 225,000
Facility Category: Multi-Purpose
Type of Stage: Concert Stage
Seating Capacity: 5000; 1500

6323 COCOA VILLAGE PLAYHOUSE
300 Brevard Avenue
Cocoa, FL 32922
Phone: 321-636-5050
Fax: 321-636-5050
e-mail: playhouse@cocoavillage.com
Web Site: www.playhouse.cocoavillage.com
Management:
    Executive Director: Staci Hawkins
Founded: 1924
Paid Staff: 20
Volunteer Staff: 250
Paid Artists: 35

6324 OMNI AUDITORIUM - BROWARD COMMUNITY COLLEGE
1000 Coconut Boulevard
Coconut Creek, FL 33066
Phone: 954-973-2233
Web Site: www.broward.cc.fl.us
Type of Stage: Flexible
Seating Capacity: 1900+

6325 WYNMOOR RECITAL HALL
1300 Avenue of the Stars
Coconut Creek, FL 33066
Phone: 954-978-2632
Fax: 954-978-2626
Officers:
    Chairman Fine Arts Committee: Murray Ross
Founded: 1974
Budget: $100,000
Income Sources: Ticket sales
Performs At: Recital Hall
Annual Attendance: 12,000
Facility Category: Concert Hall
Type of Stage: Double thrust
Stage Dimensions: 38' 10" x 21' 9'
Seating Capacity: 950
Year Built: 1979

6326 CORAL SPRINGS CITY CENTER
2855 Coral Springs Drive
Coral Springs, FL 33065

Phone: 954-344-5999
Fax: 954-344-5980
e-mail: info@coralspringscenterforthearts.com
Web Site: www.coralspringscenterforthearts.com
Management:
    General Manager: Kevin Barrett
Founded: 1989
Annual Attendance: 200,000
Type of Stage: Proscenium
Seating Capacity: 1,456

6327 DAYTONA BEACH COMMUNITY COLLEGE - THEATRE CENTER
1200 Volusia Avenue
Daytona Beach, FL 32115
Phone: 904-254-3000
Fax: 904-254-3044

6328 DAYTONA PLAYHOUSE
100 Jessamine Boulevard
Daytona Beach, FL 32118
Phone: 386-255-2431
Fax: 386-255-2432
e-mail: info@daytonaplayhouse.com
Web Site: www.daytonaplayhouse.com
Founded: 1945

6329 JACKIE ROBINSON BALL PARK
108 E Orange Avenue
Daytona Beach, FL 32114
Phone: 386-322-5133
Fax: 904-239-6550
Management:
    Manager: Hillary Rowley
Founded: 1946

6330 OCEAN CENTER
101 N Atlantic Avenue
Daytona Beach, FL 32118
Phone: 904-254-4500
Fax: 904-254-4512
Toll-free: 800-858-6444
e-mail: csmith@oceancenter.com
Web Site: www.oceancenter.com
Management:
    Director: Rick Hamiliton
    Assistant Director: Chad Smith
Founded: 1985
Annual Attendance: 525,000
Type of Stage: Sico
Seating Capacity: 10,000

6331 PEABODY AUDITORIUM
600 Auditorium Blvd
PO Box 551
Daytona Beach, FL 32118
Phone: 904-255-1318
Fax: 904-258-3169
Seating Capacity: 2,560

6332 DELRAY BEACH PLAYHOUSE
950 NW Ninth Street
PO Box 1056
Delray Beach, FL 33444
Phone: 561-272-1281
Fax: 561-272-5884
e-mail: eastons111@aol.com
Web Site: www.delraybeachplayhouse.com
Founded: 1947
Seating Capacity: 238

6333 MESA PARK
100 Mesa Park Boulevard
Fellsmere, FL 32948
Phone: 561-571-2000
Fax: 561-571-1008
e-mail: info@mesapark.com
Web Site: www.mesapark.com
Officers:
   President: Jefff Parsons
Management:
   Operations Manager/NASRA: Matt Graney

6334 BAILEY CONCERT HALL
3501 SW Davie Road
Fort Lauderdale, FL 33314
Phone: 954-475-6884
Fax: 954-424-3154
Toll-free: 888-475-6884
e-mail: tjones@broward.edu
Web Site: www.broward.cc.fl.us

6335 BROWARD CENTER FOR THE PERFORMING ARTS
201 SW Fifth Avenue
Fort Lauderdale, FL 33312
Phone: 954-462-0222
Fax: 954-468-3282
Toll-free: 800-564-9539
e-mail: mnerenhausen@curtianup.org
Web Site: www.curtainup.org
Management:
   President: Mark Nerenhausen
   General Manager: Kelley Shanley
Type of Stage: Concert Stage
Seating Capacity: 2,700

6336 FORT LAUDERDALE STADIUM
Lockhart Stadium
1401 N.W. 55th Street
Fort Lauderdale, FL 33309
Phone: 954-828-4980
Fax: 305-938-4979
Web Site: www.ci.ftlaud.fl.us
Management:
   Stadium Manager: Vincent Gizzi

6337 PARKER PLAYHOUSE
707 NE Eighth Street
PO Box 4603
Fort Lauderdale, FL 33304
Phone: 954-763-2444
Fax: 954-764-0708
Seating Capacity: 1,200

6338 BROWARD CENTER FOR THE PERFORMING ARTS
201 SW Fifth Avenue
Fort Lauderdale, FL 33312
Phone: 954-522-5334
Fax: 954-462-3541
e-mail: jjoseph@curtainup.org
Web Site: www.browardcenter.org
Management:
   Programming Coordinator: Judy Joseph
Performs At: The Performing Arts Center

6339 PTG-FLORIDA/PARKER PLAYHOUSE
707 NE Eighth Street
Fort Lauderdale, FL 33304
Phone: 954-763-2444
Fax: 954-764-0708

6340 WAR MEMORIAL AUDITORIUM
800 NE Eight Street
Fort Lauderdale, FL 33301
Phone: 954-761-5380
Fax: 954-761-5360
Web Site: www.ci.ftlaud.fl.us
Founded: 1949
Seating Capacity: 2,110

6341 BARBARA B MANN PERFORMING ARTS HALL
8099 College Parkway SW
Fort Myers, FL 33919
Phone: 941-489-3033
Fax: 941-481-4620
Toll-free: 800-440-7469
e-mail: genmgr@bbmannpah.com
Web Site: www.bbmannpah.com
Management:
   General Manager: Mary Bensel
   Director Marketing: Peg Welty
   Operations Manager: Eva Calhoun
   Technical Director: Robb McCoy
Mission: The Barbara B. Mann Performing Arts Hall countinues to improve the quality and accessiblity of touring broadway and star performing artists to the communities of Southwest Florida.
Founded: 1985
Specialized Field: Broadway; variety theatre
Paid Staff: 9
Volunteer Staff: 150
Paid Artists: 500
Affiliations: League of American Theatres & Producers; Florida Facility Managers; Southern Arts, APAP
Facility Category: Performing Arts Hall
Type of Stage: Non-Sprung
Stage Dimensions: 160'x47'
Seating Capacity: 1,753
Year Built: 1985
Year Remodeled: 1998

All listings are in alphabetical order by state, then city, then organization within the city.

6342 FORT MYERS HARBORSIDE
1375 Monroe Street
Fort Myers, FL 33902
Phone: 800-294-9516
Fax: 941-332-2242
e-mail: fmcc@fmharborside.com
Web Site: www.fmharborside.com

6343 WILLIAM H HAMMOND STADIUM
Lee County Parks & Recreation
3410 Palm Beach Boulevard
Fort Myers, FL 33916
Phone: 941-338-3300
Fax: 941-339-3333
e-mail: emc14@aol.com
Web Site: www.lee-county.com
Management:
   Director: John Yardbrough
   Manager: Ed McLntyre
Seating Capacity: 7,600

6344 WILLIAM R FRIZZELL CULTURAL CENTRE & CLAIBORNE & NED FOULDS THEATRE
10091 McGregor Boulevard
Fort Myers, FL 33919
Phone: 941-939-2787
Fax: 941-939-0794
e-mail: arts@artinlee.org
Management:
   Executive Director: Karl H Hollander

6345 SAINT LUCIE COUNTY CIVIC CENTER
2300 Virginia Avenue
Fort Pierce, FL 34982
Phone: 561-462-1530
Fax: 561-462-1526
e-mail: cappara@stlucieco.gov
Web Site: www.stlucieco.gov/leisure/civiccenter.htm
Seating Capacity: 4,000

6346 WAR MEMORIAL AUDITORIUM
800 NE 8th Street
Ft. Laudersale, FL 33301
Phone: 954-761-5380
Fax: 954-761-5361
Web Site: www.ci.ftlaud.fl.us/warmemorial.com
Management:
   Manager: Robert Stried
Seating Capacity: 2,110

6347 CURTIS M PHILLIPS CENTER FOR PERFORMING ARTS
315 Hull Road
PO BOX 112750
Gainesville, FL 32611
Phone: 352-392-1900
Fax: 352-392-3775
Toll-free: 800-905-2787
e-mail: bruce86@ufl.edu
Web Site: www.cpa.ufl.edu
Management:

Director: Michael Blachly
Annual Attendance: 6,800
Type of Stage: Black Box; Proscenium
Seating Capacity: 1,754

6348 HARN MUSEUM: UNIVERSITY OF FLORIDA
University of Florida
SW 34th Street & Hull Road, PO Box 112700
Gainesville, FL 32611-2700
Phone: 352-392-9826
Fax: 352-392-3892
e-mail: laurap@ufl.edu
Web Site: www.arts.ufl.edu/harn/
Management:
   Programs Director: Laura Pursley
   Dir Public Relations/Marketing: Karen Ilyse Wyman
Performs At: Harn Museum-Chandler Auditorium

6349 HIPPODROME STATE THEATRE
25 SE Second Place
Gainesville, FL 32601
Phone: 352-375-4477
Fax: 352-371-9130
e-mail: hipp@afn.org
Web Site: www.hipp.gator.net
Management:
   Producing Director: Mary Hausch
   Artistic Director: Lauren Caldwell
   General Manager: Mark Sexton
Mission: To explore the truth of human experience and the human spirit through the examination and presentation of dramatic work. Our purpose is to accomplish this through our commitment to create an artistic home.
Founded: 1973
Specialized Field: theatre
Status: Professional; Nonprofit
Paid Staff: 38
Volunteer Staff: 63
Budget: $243,074,800
Income Sources: Ticket sales; Concession sales; Corporate support, Federal, State and local grants
Season: Year round
Performs At: Hippodrome
Annual Attendance: 167,000
Facility Category: Live stage and movie theatre
Type of Stage: Thrust
Seating Capacity: 266
Year Built: 1911
Year Remodeled: 1980
Architect: $1.5 Million
Rental Contact: General Manager Mark Sexton
Organization Type: Performing; Touring; Resident; Educational; Sponsoring

6350 STEPHEN C O'CONNELL CENTER
University of Florida
Suite 1232, N-S Drive
Gainesville, FL 32611-5850
Mailing Address: PO Box 115850 Gainesville, FL 32611
Phone: 352-392-5500
Fax: 352-392-7106
e-mail: dariusd@ufl.edu
Web Site: www.oconnnellcenter.ufl.edu

Management:
Director: Lionel J Dubay
Assocaite Director: Darius Dunn
Business Manager: Renee Musson
Budget: $2.3 million
Performs At: Multi-Purpose Arena
Type of Stage: Portable
Seating Capacity: 12,000
Year Built: 1980
Year Remodeled: 1998
Cost: $16.5 million
Rental Contact: Associate Director Darius Dunn

6351 YOUNG CIRCLE PARK AND BANDSHELL
US Highway 1 and Hollywood Boulevard
Hollywood, FL 33020
Phone: 954-921-3404
Fax: 305-921-3233

6352 HOMESTEAD SPORTS COMPLEX
1601 SE 28th Avenue
Homestead, FL 33030
Phone: 305-247-1801
Fax: 305-246-3200
Management:
Director Parks/Recreation: Alan Ricke

6353 ALHAMBRA DINNER THEATRE
12000 Beach Boulevard
Jacksonville, FL 32246
Phone: 904-641-1212
Fax: 904-642-3505
Toll-free: 800-688-7469
e-mail: info@alhambradinnertheatre.com
Web Site: www.alhambradinnertheatre.com
Founded: 1967
Annual Attendance: 120,000
Type of Stage: Proscenium
Seating Capacity: 400

6354 ALLTEL STADIUM
One Alltel Stadium Place
Jacksonville, FL 32202
Phone: 904-633-6100
Fax: 904-633-6338
Web Site: www.jaguars.com/ALLTELStadium/
Management:
General Manager: Robert Downing
Marketing Assistant: Christina Mitalis
Founded: 1995
Seating Capacity: 80,000
Year Built: 1995
Resident Groups: Home to the Jacksonville Jaguars

6355 FLORIDA NATIONAL PAVILION
1410 E Adams Street
Jacksonville, FL 32202
Phone: 904-630-0837
Fax: 904-630-0538

6356 FLORIDA THEATRE
128 E 40th Street
Suite 300
Jacksonville, FL 32202
Phone: 904-355-2787
Fax: 904-353-3251
e-mail: info@floridatheatre.com
Web Site: www.floridatheatre.com
Management:
Executive Director: J Erik Hart
Founded: 1927
Annual Attendance: 250,000
Type of Stage: Flexible

6357 GATOR BOWL
1 Alltel Stadium Place
Jacksonville, FL 32202
Phone: 904-690-0335
Fax: 904-633-6113
Management:
Director Sports Complex: Doug Hall
Founded: 1945

6358 SAM WOLFSON BASEBALL PARK
1201 E Duval Street
Jacksonville, FL 32202
Phone: 904-358-2846
Fax: 904-358-2845
e-mail: jaxsuns@bellsouth.net
Web Site: www.jaxsuns.com
Officers:
President: Peter Bragan
Management:
Director Marketing: Kirk Goodman
Director Ticket Operations: Jamie Smith
Director Broadcasting: Dave Schultz
Director Stadium Operations: Russ Oliver
Office Manager: Cathy Wiggins
Community Affairs: Shannon Sharp
Administrative Assistant: Jen Adkison
Assistant To President: Jerry Lemoine
Founded: 1888
Annual Attendance: 1,500

6359 VETERANS MEMORIAL COLISEUM
SMG-Jacksonville
1145 E Adams Street
Jacksonville, FL 32202
Phone: 904-630-3900
Fax: 904-630-3913
e-mail: marketing@coj.net
Web Site: www.jaxevents.com
Management:
Director: Drew Armstrong
Marketing Manager: Nan Coyle Coyle
Seating Capacity: 10,276

6360 TENNIS CENTER AT CRANDON PARK
7300 Crandon Boulevard
Key Biscayne, FL 33149

All listings are in alphabetical order by state, then city, then organization within the city.

Phone: 305-365-2300
Fax: 305-365-2327
e-mail: parks@miamidade.gov
Web Site: www.co.miami-dade.fl.us
Seating Capacity: 14,000

6361 SOUTH FLORIDA CENTER FOR THE ARTS

29 Jolly Rodger Drive
PO Box 2540
Key Largo, FL 33037
Phone: 350-453-4224
Fax: 305-853-7122
e-mail: checker@terranova.net

6362 FLORIDA KEYS COMMUNITY COLLEGE

Tennessee Williams Fine Arts Center
5901 W College Road
Key West, FL 33040
Phone: 305-296-9081
Fax: 305-292-5155
e-mail: twfac@aol.com
Web Site: www.keywesttheater.org
Management:
    Production Director: Mike Boyer
Founded: 1977
Specialized Field: Dance; Symphony; Pops Symphony; Theatre; Community Choir; Musicals
Paid Staff: 3
Volunteer Staff: 3
Type of Stage: Flexible
Seating Capacity: 476

6363 RED BARN THEATRE

319 Duval Street
Rear Key West
Key West, FL 33041
Phone: 305-296-9911
Fax: 305-293-3035
Web Site: www.redbarntheatre.com
Seating Capacity: 88

6364 TENNESSEE WILLIAMS THEATRE

5901 Junior College Road
Key West, FL 33040
Phone: 305-296-9081
Fax: 305-292-3725
e-mail: info@twfac.com
Web Site: www.tennesseewilliamstheatre.com
Management:
    General Manager: Rebecca Tomlinson
    Technical Director: Michael Boyer
    Resident Lighting Designer: Kevin Shaw
Affiliations: Performing Arts Centers for Key West
Rental Contact: Rebecca Tomlinson

6365 OSCEOLA CENTER FOR THE ARTS

2411 E Bronson Highway
PO Box 451088
Kissimmee, FL 34745-1088

Phone: 407-846-6257
Fax: 407-846-7902
e-mail: ocfta@kua.net
Web Site: www.ocfta.com
Officers:
    Executive Director: Kip Watson
Mission: To promote, cultivate and foster interest and participation in the arts by providing affordable and accessible programs and facilities that encourage artistc expression in the diverse community we serve.
Founded: 1963
Specialized Field: Visual Arts; Music; Craft; Local Art Council
Paid Staff: 6
Volunteer Staff: 150
Paid Artists: 240
Non-paid Artists: 125
Budget: $580,000
Performs At: Theatre; Tours
Affiliations: Artexhibits
Facility Category: Art Center
Seating Capacity: 250
Year Built: 1913
Year Remodeled: 2002

6366 OSCELOA COUNTY STADIUM & SPORTS COMPLEX

1000 Bill Beck Boulevard
Florida Home of the Houston Astros, Kissimmee
Kissimmee, FL 34744
Phone: 407-933-5400
Fax: 407-847-6237
e-mail: osceolastadium@yahoo.com
Management:
    Director: Don Miers
Seating Capacity: 5,200

6367 WALT DISNEY WIDE WORLD OF SPORTS

3250 N Fort Wilderness Trail
Lake Buena Vista, FL 32830-1000
Phone: 407-939-7810
Fax: 407-938-3469
e-mail: wdw_golf_classic@wda.disney.com
Web Site: www.disneyworldsports.com
Management:
    Director/Event Programming: Mike Millay
    Manager/Sports Programming: Jeff Sturgeon
    Manager Sports Programming: John Bisignano
    Sports Special Events Manager: Sherri Noble
    CEO: Michael Eisner

6368 DUNCAN THEATRE
Palm Beach Community College

4200 South Congress Avenue
Lake Worth, MS15
Lake Worth, FL 33461
Phone: 561-868-3309
Fax: 561-439-8287
e-mail: gibsonbd@pbcc.edu
Web Site: www.pbcc.cc.fl.us
Management:
    Theatre Manager: Dawn Gibson-Brehon

6369 PALM BEACH COMMUNITY COLLEGE

4200 Congress Avenue
MS #58, Lake Worth
Lake Worth, FL 33461
Phone: 561-868-3350
Fax: 561-439-8287
e-mail: faocent@pbcc.edu
Web Site: www.pbcc.cc.fl.us
Paid Staff: 5
Annual Attendance: 48,000
Facility Category: Performing Arts Center
Type of Stage: Proscenium Opening
Stage Dimensions: 42'x36'
Seating Capacity: 720
Year Built: 1985

6370 BRANSCOMB MEMORIAL AUDITORIUM

Florida Southern College
111 Lake Hollingsworth Drive, Lakeland
Lakeland, FL 33801
Phone: 863-680-4296
Fax: 813-680-3758
e-mail: ltadlock@flsouthern.edu
Web Site: www.flsouthern.edu
Founded: 1959
Annual Attendance: 2,000
Type of Stage: Proscenium
Seating Capacity: 1,700

6371 FLORIDA SOUTHERN COLLEGE - BUCKNER THEATRE

111 Lake Hollings Worth Drive
Lakeland
Lakeland, FL 33801
Phone: 863-680-4296
Fax: 863-680-4120
e-mail: ltadlock@flsouthern.edu
Web Site: www.flsouthern.edu
Management:
   Office Manager: Kity Oelker
   Department Chair: James Beck
   Costumer/Faculty: Mary Albright
Status: Student Theater
Paid Staff: 3
Budget: $30,000
Income Sources: College/Academic Budget
Affiliations: Florida Southern College
Facility Category: Line Theatre Production
Year Built: 1971
Year Remodeled: 2000

6372 GENERAL MOTORS PLACE

Lakeland Center
700 West Lemon Street
Lakeland
Lakeland, FL 33815
Phone: 863-834-8100
Fax: 863-834-8101
e-mail: allison.jones@lakelandgov.net
Web Site: www.thelakelandcenter.com
Management:
   Director: Allen Johnson

6373 LAKELAND CENTER

701 West Lemon Street
Lakeland
Lakeland, FL 33815
Phone: 863-834-8100
Fax: 863-834-8101
e-mail: allison.jones@lakelandgov.net
Web Site: www.thelakelandcenter.com
Management:
   Director: Allen Johnson
   Assistant Director: Anthony Delgado
   Booking Manager: Tim Holloway
   Marketing Manager: Kevin Cook
   Operations Manager: Tom Prais
   Business Manager: Steven Collazo
Seating Capacity: 10,000

6374 KING CENTER FOR THE PERFORMING ARTS

Brevard Community College-Melbourne
3865 N Wickham Road
Melbourne
Melbourne, FL 32935
Phone: 321-632-1111
Fax: 321-634-3738
e-mail: sjanicki@kingcenter.com
Web Site: www.kingcenter.com
Management:
   Executive Director: Steven G Janicki
Founded: 1988
Paid Staff: 10
Volunteer Staff: 400
Type of Stage: Proscenium
Seating Capacity: 2,001

6375 MELBOURNE AUDITORIUM

625 Hibiscus Boulevard
Melbourne
Melbourne, FL 32903
Phone: 321-674-5700
Fax: 321-674-5736
e-mail: Auditorium@melbourneflorida.org

6376 AMERICAN AIRLINES ARENA

601 Biscayne Boulevard
Miami
Miami, FL 33132
Phone: 786-777-1000
Fax: 305-377-9716
e-mail: GuestServices@heat.com
Web Site: www.aaarena.com
Management:
   General Manager: Roger Newton
Founded: 1999
Seating Capacity: 20,000

6377 DADE COUNTY AUDITORIUM

2901 West Flagler Street
Miami
Miami, FL 33135
Phone: 305-547-5414
Fax: 305-541-7782
Seating Capacity: 2,498

6378 GOLDEN PANTHER SPORTSPLEX
Florida International University
RM 255/ University Park
Miami, FL 33199
Phone: 305-348-2756
Fax: 305-348-2963
Management:
   Athletic Director: Jose Sotolongo

6379 GUSMAN CENTER FOR THE PERFORMING ARTS
25 SE 2nd Avenue
Suite 415, Miami
Miami, FL 33131
Phone: 305-374-2444
Fax: 305-374-0303
e-mail: mwharton@gusmancenter.org
Web Site: www.gusmancenter.org
Management:
   Theater Operations Director: Jeannie Piazza-Zuniga
Founded: 1970
Seating Capacity: 1,700

6380 JAMES L KNIGHT CENTER
400 SE 2nd Avenue
Miami, FL 33131
Phone: 305-372-4633
Fax: 305-350-7910
Web Site: jlknightcenter.com
Founded: 1982
Specialized Field: Music, Theatre, Dance

6381 MIAMI ARENA
701 Arena Boulevard
Suite 415, Miami
Miami, FL 33136
Phone: 305-530-4400
Fax: 305-530-4429
Web Site: www.miamiarena.com
Management:
   General Manager: Betty Segul
   Assistant General Manager: Patrick McGrew
   Assistant Director Entertainment: Brenda Carter
Specialized Field: Concerts; Family Shows; Exhibitions
Facility Category: Arena
Seating Capacity: 15,500
Year Built: 1986
Rental Contact: Mike Carr

6382 ORANGE BOWL STADIUM
1501 NW 3rd Street
Suite 415, Miami
Miami, FL 33125
Phone: 305-643-7100
Fax: 305-643-7115
e-mail: igomez@ci.miami.fl.us
Management:
   Stadium Manager: Ileana Gomez
Founded: 1937
Seating Capacity: 82,000

6383 PERFORMING ARTS CENTER OF GREATER MIAMI
1444 Biscayne Boulevard
Suite 100, Miami
Miami, FL 33132
Phone: 305-377-1220
Fax: 305-377-1015
e-mail: tomt@pacmiami.com
Web Site: www.pacfmiami.org
Officers:
   Executive Director/CEO: Tom Tomlinson

6384 JACKIE GLEASON THEATER
1700 Washington Avenue
Miami Beach
Miami Beach, FL 33139
Phone: 305-673-7300
Fax: 305-588-6810
e-mail: jgtinfo@smgmb.com
Web Site: www.gleasontheater.com
Founded: 1950
Annual Attendance: 185,000
Type of Stage: Proscenium
Seating Capacity: 2,705

6385 MOBILE CIVIC CENTER - EXPOSITION HALL
401 Civic Center Drive
Mobile
Mobile, FL 33602
Phone: 251-208-7261
Fax: 334-208-7551
Web Site: www.mobilecivicctr.com
Type of Stage: Concert Stage; Portable
Seating Capacity: 3,000

6386 MOBILE CIVIC CENTER - THEATRE
401 Civic Center Drive
Mobile
Mobile, FL 33602
Phone: 251-208-7261
Fax: 334-208-7551
Web Site: www.mobilecivicctr.com
Seating Capacity: 1,940

6387 MONTICELLO OPERA HOUSE
Courthouse Square
PO Box 518
Monticello, FL 32345
Phone: 904-997-4242
Fax: 904-997-7142
e-mail: moperahouse@juno.com

6388 PHILHARMONIC CENTER FOR THE ARTS
5833 Pelican Bay Boulevard
Naples
Naples, FL 34108
Phone: 239-596-7575
Fax: 239-272-4674
e-mail: tbullis@thephil.org
Web Site: www.naplesphilcenter.org

All listings are in alphabetical order by state, then city, then organization within the city.

Officers:
Chairman/Presient/CEO: Myra Janco Daniels
Management:
Operations Director/Programing: Maureen Quilty Shallcross
Founded: 1989
Seating Capacity: 1,421

6389 CENTER FOR THE ARTS AT RIVER RIDGE
11646 Town Center Road
New Port Richey
New Port Richey, FL 34654
Phone: 727-774-7381
Fax: 727-774-7389
e-mail: pascocpa@pasco.k12.fl.us

6390 ATLANTIC CENTER FOR THE ARTS
1414 Art Center Avenue
New Smyrna Beach
New Smyrna Beach, FL 32168
Phone: 386-427-6975
Fax: 904-427-5669
Toll-free: 800-393-6975
e-mail: program@atlanticcenterforthearts.or
Web Site: www.atlanticcenterforthearts.org
Founded: 1982
Specialized Field: Florida; National; All disciplines
Paid Staff: 15
Volunteer Staff: 15
Budget: $1 million
Income Sources: Grants; Donations; Fundraisers
Annual Attendance: 250
Facility Category: 5 studios
Type of Stage: Black Box
Year Built: 1996
Rental Contact: Frankie Robert

6391 OKALOOSA-WALTON COMMUNITY COLLEGE, THE ARTS CENTER
100 College Boulevard
Niceville
Niceville, FL 32578
Phone: 850-729-5382
Fax: 850-729-5286
Toll-free: 888-838-2787
e-mail: arts@owcc.net
Web Site: www.owcc.cc.fl.us
Management:
Executive Director/Arts Center: Clifford Herron

6392 LEE CIVIC CENTER
11831 Bayshore Road
Fort Myers
Noah Fort Myers, FL 33917
Phone: 239-543-8368
Fax: 239-543-4110
e-mail: swffair@iline.com
Web Site: www.leeciviccenter.com
Management:
General Manager: Alta Mosley
Operations Manager: Simon Train
Conssesions Manager: Al Bertoni

Seating Capacity: 7,800

6393 LEE CIVIC CENTER - ARENA
11831 Bayshore Road
Fort Myers
North Fort Myers, FL 33917
Phone: 239-543-8368
Fax: 239-543-4110
e-mail: swffair@iline.com
Web Site: www.leeciviccenter.com

6394 LEE CIVIC CENTER - SMALL THEATER
11831 Bayshore Road
Fort Myers
North Fort Myers, FL 33917
Phone: 239-543-8368
Fax: 239-543-4110
e-mail: swffair@iline.com
Web Site: www.leeciviccenter.com

6395 VICTORY PARK AUDITORIUM
17011 NE 19th Avenue
North Miami Beach, FL 33162
Phone: 305-948-2957
Fax: 305-787-6037

6396 BOB CARR PERFORMING ARTS CENTER
401 West Livingston Street
Orlando
Orlando, FL 32801
Phone: 407-849-2577
Type of Stage: Proscenium
Seating Capacity: 2,518

6397 ORANGE COUNTY CONVENTION CENTER
9800 International Drive
Orlando
Orlando, FL 32819
Phone: 407-685-9800
Fax: 407-685-9884
Toll-free: 800-345-9845
e-mail: Info@occc.net
Web Site: www.orlandoconvention.com
Management:
Marketing Manager: Kathie Canning
Director Public Relations: Joe Boyd
Director Sales: Steve Bellas
Sales Assistant: Willie Nelson
Founded: 1996
Income Sources: Conventions, Tradeshows, Seminars/Workshops, Tourist Development Tax
Affiliations: Orange County Government
Facility Category: Performance Auditorium
Type of Stage: Performance Stage with Dock Access
Stage Dimensions: 26'x145'5"x49'6"
Seating Capacity: 2,643
Year Built: 1983
Year Remodeled: 1996
Rental Contact: Sales Assistant Willie Nelson

All listings are in alphabetical order by state, then city, then organization within the city.

6398 **ORLANDO CENTROPLEX**
600 West Amelia Street
Orlando
Orlando, FL 32801
Phone: 407-849-2000
Fax: 407-849-2329
Web Site: www.orlandocentroplex.com
Management:
   Arena Manager: Bill Becker
   Deputy Director: John Dorman
   Events Manager: Michael Thompson
   Convention Sales/Booking: Robin R Handlan
Seating Capacity: 17,500
Year Built: 1989

6399 **TD WATERHOUSE CENTRE**
Orlando Centroplex
600 West Amelia Street, Orlando
Orlando, FL 32801
Phone: 407-849-2000
Fax: 407-849-2329
Web Site: www.orlandocentroplex.com
Management:
   Director: William L Becker
   Marketing Director: Craig O'Niel
   Concessions Manager: Jim Breig
   Deputy Director: Jon Dorman
   Business Manager: Cindy Mitchum
Founded: 1989
Seating Capacity: 17,320

6400 **UCF ARENA**
PO Box 161500
Building 50 North Gemini Boulevard, Orlando
Orlando, FL 32816
Phone: 407-823-3070
Fax: 407-823-5154
e-mail: tgenoves@mail.ucf.edu
Web Site: www.arena.ucf.edu
Management:
   Director: Terry M Genovese
Founded: 1991
Seating Capacity: 5,322

6401 **VALENCIA COMMUNITY COLLEGE - BLACK BOX THEATRE**
East Campus, 701 N Econlockhatchee Trail
Orlando
Orlando, FL 32825
Phone: 407-299-5000
Fax: 407-277-0621
Web Site: www.valenciacc.edu

6402 **VALENCIA COMMUNITY COLLEGE - PERFORMING ARTS**
East Campus, 701 N Econlockhatchee Trail
Orlando
Orlando, FL 32825
Phone: 407-299-5000
Fax: 407-277-0621
Web Site: www.valenciacc.edu

6403 **PENSACOLA CIVIC CENTER**
201 East Gregory Street
Pensacola
Pensacola, FL 32501
Phone: 850-432-0800
Fax: 850-432-1707
e-mail: webmaster@pensacolaciviccenter.com
Web Site: www.pensacolaciviccenter.com
Management:
   Event Services Director: Cyndee Pennington
Founded: 1985
Facility Category: Arena
Seating Capacity: 10,000

6404 **PENSACOLA JUNIOR COLLEGE LYCEUM**
1000 College Boulevard
Pensacola
Pensacola, FL 32504
Phone: 850-484-1000
Fax: 850-484-1835
Toll-free: 888-897-3605
e-mail: sdean@pjc.cc.fl.us
Web Site: www.pjc.cc.fl.us
Management:
   Lyceum Director: Stan Dean
Founded: 1948
Performs At: Ashmore Fine Arts Auditorium
Annual Attendance: 7,000
Type of Stage: Proscenium
Seating Capacity: 314
Year Built: 1990

6405 **PENSACOLA JUNIOR COLLEGE, MUSIC AND DRAMA DEPARTMENT**
1000 College Boulevard
Pensacola
Pensacola, FL 32504
Phone: 850-484-1800
Fax: 850-484-1835
Toll-free: 888-897-3605
e-mail: dsnowden@pjc.cc.fl.us
Web Site: www.pjc.cc.fl.us
Annual Attendance: 2,000
Facility Category: Theatre
Type of Stage: Proscenium
Seating Capacity: 314
Year Built: 1958
Year Remodeled: 1990

6406 **SAENGER THEATRE**
118 South Palafox Place
Pensacola
Pensacola, FL 32501
Phone: 850-444-7699
Fax: 850-444-7684
e-mail: saengerweb@c:.pensacola.fl.us
Web Site: www.pensacolasaenger.com
Founded: 1925
Annual Attendance: 150,000
Facility Category: performing arts theatre
Type of Stage: Proscenium
Seating Capacity: 1,802

Year Built: 1925
Year Remodeled: 1981
Rental Contact: Douglas Lee

6407 UNIVERSITY OF WEST FLORIDA CENTER FOR FINE & PERFORMING ARTS

Music Department building 82
11000 University Parkway, Pensacola
Pensacola, FL 32514
Phone: 850-474-2147
Fax: 850-474-3247
e-mail: music@uwf.edu
Web Site: www.uwf.edu
Management:
   Assistant Director: Linda May
Mission: To support and educate the students and the community.
Founded: 1992
Paid Staff: 2
Volunteer Staff: 2
Paid Artists: 6
Budget: $40,000
Income Sources: SGA Funds; State and Private Donations
Performs At: Music Hall; Concert Hall
Annual Attendance: 33,000
Facility Category: Performance
Seating Capacity: 309
Year Built: 1992
Rental Contact: Assistant Director Linda May
Organization Type: Education

6408 CHARLOTTE COUNTY MEMORIAL AUDITORIUM

75 Taylor Street
Punta Gorda
Punta Gorda, FL 33950
Phone: 941-639-5833
Fax: 941-639-3814
Toll-free: 800-329-9988
e-mail: diana.finnegan@charlottefl.com
Web Site: www.charlottecountyfl.com
Founded: 1969
Annual Attendance: 250,000
Type of Stage: Proscenium
Seating Capacity: 2,230

6409 SEMINOLE COUNTY SPORTS TRAINING CENTER

Seminole County Government
845 Lake Markham Road
Sanford, FL 32703
Phone: 407-324-1217
Fax: 407-324-4317
e-mail: semcvb@ix.netcom.com
Web Site: www.co.seminole.fl.us
Management:
   Sports/Events Manager: John Giantonio

6410 ED SMITH STADIUM/ SPORTS COMPLEX

2700 12th Street
Sarasota, FL 34237
Phone: 941-954-4101
Fax: 941-365-1587
e-mail: ess@sarasotagov.com
Web Site: www.sarasotagov.com
Management:
   Sports Facility Manager: Patrick M Calhoon

6411 FLORIDA STUDIO THEATRE

1241 N Palm Avenue
Sarasota, FL 34236
Phone: 941-366-9017
Fax: 941-955-4137
e-mail: james@fst200.org
Web Site: www.fst2000.org
Management:
   Casting/Literary Coordinator: James Ashford
Founded: 1973
Paid Staff: 40
Volunteer Staff: 100
Paid Artists: 70

6412 THE PLAYERS THEATRE AND BOX OFFICE

838 North Tamiami Trail
US 41 at 9th Street
Sarasota, FL 34236
Phone: 941-365-2494
Fax: 941-954-0282
e-mail: info@theplayers.org
Web Site: www.theplayers.org
Founded: 1930
Annual Attendance: 80,000
Type of Stage: Proscenium
Seating Capacity: 497

6413 VAN WEZEL AUDITORIUM

777 N Tamiami Trail
Sarasota, FL 34236
Phone: 941-955-7676
Fax: 941-951-1449
Toll-free: 800-826-9303
e-mail: vanwezel@gte.net
Web Site: www.vanwezel.org
Founded: 1970
Annual Attendance: 200,000
Type of Stage: Proscenium
Seating Capacity: 1,736

6414 VAN WEZEL PERFORMING ARTS HALL

777 N Tamiami Trail
Sarasota, FL 34236
Phone: 941-955-7676
Fax: 941-951-1449
e-mail: vanwezel@verizon.net
Web Site: www.vanwezel.org
Management:
   Executive Director: John D Wildges
   Marketing Manager: Margaret Fuesy
   Events Coordinator: Charmaine McVicker

Facility Category: Performing Arts Hall
Type of Stage: Proscenium
Stage Dimensions: 60' wide x 30' high x 49' deep
Seating Capacity: 1736
Year Built: 1970
Year Remodeled: 2000
Rental Contact: Charmaine McVicker

6415 SPRINGSTEAD THEATRE

3300 Mariner Boulevard
Spring Hill, FL 34609
Phone: 352-797-7010
Fax: 352-797-7110

6416 TIMES/MAHAFFEY THEATRE FOR THE PERFORMING ARTS

400 1st Street S
St. Petersburg, FL 33701
Phone: 727-892-5024
Fax: 727-892-5858
e-mail: lauren.kleinfeld@stpete.org
Web Site: www.stpete.org/venues.htm
Management:
   Director Facilities: Michael R Barber
   Booking/Marketing Manager: Lauren Kleinfeld
Facility Category: Theatre/Arena

6417 TROPICANA FIELD

One Tropicana Drive
St. Petersburg, FL 33705
Phone: 888-326-7297
Fax: 727-825-3167
Web Site: www.devilrays.com
Management:
   VP/Operations/Facilities: Rick Nafe
   Event Manager: Tom Karac
   VP/sales/marketing: John Brown
Seating Capacity: 45,200

6418 RIVERSIDE THEATRE

3250 Riverside Park Drive
Vero Beach, FL 32963
Phone: 772-231-5860
Fax: 772-234-5298
Toll-free: 800-445-6745
e-mail: info@riversidetheatre.com
Web Site: www.riversidetheatre.com
Officers:
   President: Robert Bauchman
   VP: Gay Bain
   Secretary: Craig Marshall
   Treasurer: Robert Kingston
Management:
   Executive Director: Chuck Still
   Artistic Director: Allen D Cornell
   Education Director: Linda Downey
   Production Manager: Jon R Moses
Mission: Riverside Theatre is committed to providing a total theatre arts experience that entertains, challenges, and educates both adults and children.
Founded: 1973
Status: Letter of Agreement with Actors' Equity Association

Paid Staff: 35
Volunteer Staff: 150
Budget: $3 million
Income Sources: Corproate and Private Donations; Rentals; Grants; Fund-Raising Events; Ticket Sales
Season: October - May
Annual Attendance: 100,000
Type of Stage: Proscenium
Seating Capacity: 615 & 300 (2 stages)
Year Built: 1973
Cost: $1 Million
Rental Contact: Jon R Moses
Organization Type: Professional; Regional producing Theatre that occasionally serving as a presenter
Resident Groups: The Acting Company

6419 VERO BEACH CONCERT ASSOCIATION

PO Box 4024
Vero Beach, FL 32964
Phone: 561-231-6990
Fax: 561-231-2186
e-mail: CWITTEN@SUNET.com
Officers:
   President: Cora Witten

6420 KRAVIS CENTER FOR THE PERFORMING ARTS

701 Okeechobee Boulevard
West Palm Beach, FL 33401-6323
Phone: 561-833-8300
Fax: 561-833-3901
Toll-free: 800-572-8471
e-mail: kravis@kravis.org
Web Site: www.kravis.org
Officers:
   CEO: Judith Mitchell
Management:
   Senior Director of Programming: Lee Bell
Founded: 1992
Paid Staff: 75
Volunteer Staff: 800
Annual Attendance: 500,000
Facility Category: Performing Arts Center
Type of Stage: Proscenium
Seating Capacity: 2,200
Year Built: 1992
Cost: $68 million
Rental Contact: Shirnette Ball

6421 STEPHEN FOSTER STATE FOLK CULTURE CENTER

US 41 N
PO Drawer G
White Springs, FL 32096
Phone: 904-397-2733
Fax: 904-397-4262
Web Site: www.stephenfostercenter.com

6422 ROLLINS COLLEGE: ANNIE RUSSELL THEATRE

1000 Holt Avenue-2735
Winter Park, FL 32789-1199

Phone: 407-646-2501
Fax: 407-646-2257
e-mail: jnassif@rollins.edu
Management:
    Producing Director/Dept Chairman: Dr. S Joseph
    Nassif
Founded: 1932
Budget: $375,000
Income Sources: Ticket Sales; Donations
Performs At: Theatre Stages/Dance Studios
Annual Attendance: 15,000
Type of Stage: Proscenium/Thrust
Seating Capacity: 380/100
Year Built: 1932
Year Remodeled: 1978
Cost: $1,000,000

Georgia

6423 ALBANY JAMES H GRAY SR: CIVIC CENTER
100 W Oglethorpe Boulevard
Albany, GA 31701
Phone: 912-430-5200
Fax: 912-430-5163
Web Site: www.albanyciviccenter.com
Management:
    Director: Matty B Goddar

6424 ALBANY STATE UNIVERSITY DEPARTMENT OF FINE ARTS
Albany State University
504 College Dr.
Albany, GA 31705
Phone: 229-430-4849
Fax: 229-430-1617
e-mail: lbynum@asurams.edu
Web Site: www.argus.asurams.edu/asu
Officers:
    Chairman: Dr. Leroy E Bynum, Jr
Performs At: Albany Municipal Auditorium

6425 HUGH MILLS MEMORIAL STADIUM
PO Box 1470
Albany, GA 31703
Phone: 912-431-3308
Fax: 912-431-3309
Management:
    Athletic Director: Frank Orgel

6426 THEATRE ALBANY
514 Pine Avenue
Albany, GA 31702
Phone: 229-439-7141
Fax: 912-439-7193
Seating Capacity: 314

6427 SANFORD STADIUM
University of Georgia
PO Box 1472
Athens, GA 30602

Phone: 706-542-9094
Fax: 706-542-2980
Web Site: www.sports.uga.edu
Management:
    Athletic Director: Vince Dooley
Seating Capacity: 86,117

6428 UNIVERSITY OF GEORGIA OFFICE OF PERFORMING ARTS
Room 214 Performing Arts Center
230 River Road
Athens, GA 30602-7280
Phone: 706-542-1668
Fax: 706-542-8867
e-mail: ugaarts@arches.uga.edu
Web Site: www.uga.edu/pac/
Management:
    Director: Timothy Bartholow
Performs At: Hugh Hodgson Concert Hall; Ramsey
Concert Hall; Fine Arts Theatre; UGA Chapel; Franklin
College Chamber Music Series
Seating Capacity: 1100

6429 14TH STREET PLAYHOUSE
173 14th Street
Atlanta, GA 30309
Phone: 404-733-4754

6430 ACADEMY THEATRE: FIRST STAGE
PO Box 191306
Atlanta, GA 31119
Phone: 404-525-4111

6431 ACADEMY THEATRE: LAB
173 14th Street
PO Box 191306
Atlanta, GA 31119
Phone: 404-525-4111

6432 ACADEMY THEATRE: PHOEBE THEATRE
PO Box 191306
Atlanta, GA 31119
Phone: 404-525-4111

6433 ATLANTA CIVIC CENTER- THEATRE AUDITORIUM
395 Piedmont Avenue NE
Atlanta, GA 30308
Phone: 404-523-6275
Fax: 404-525-4634
e-mail: information@atlantaciviccenter.com
Web Site: www.atlantaciviccenter.com
Founded: 1968
Facility Category: procenium theatre
Type of Stage: Proscenium
Seating Capacity: 86,520
Year Built: 1968
Year Remodeled: 2001
Cost: 2 million
Rental Contact: Joyce Whisenant

All listings are in alphabetical order by state, then city, then organization within the city.

6434 FOX THEATRE
660 Peachtree Street NE
Atlanta, GA 30308
Phone: 404-881-2100
Fax: 404-872-2972
e-mail: information@foxtheatre.org
Web Site: www.thefoxtheatre.com
Management:
    General Manager: Edgar Neiss
Founded: 1920
Seating Capacity: 4,000

6435 GEORGIA DOME
285 Andrew Young International Blvd NW
Atlanta, GA 30313
Phone: 404-223-4000
Fax: 404-223-4011
e-mail: ContactUs@gwcc.com
Web Site: www.gadome.com
Management:
    Genaral Manager: Khalil Johnson
    Sales Manager: Greg Barckhoff
Mission: Cable-supported dome stadium. Home for
National Football League's Atlantic Falcons. Offers a
variety of events.
Seating Capacity: 71,500
Year Built: 1992

6436 GLENN MEMORIAL AUDITORIUM
1660 N Decatur Road NE
Atlanta, GA 30307
Phone: 404-634-3936
Fax: 404-634-1994
e-mail: bettyj@glennumc.org
Web Site: www.glennumc.org
Founded: 1920

6437 GRANT FIELD
Georgia Institute of Technology
225 N Avenue NW
Atlanta, GA 30332
Phone: 404-894-2000
Fax: 404-894-1300
Web Site: www.gatech.edu
Management:
    Director: Homer Rice

6438 PHILIPS ARENA
1 Philips Drive
Atlanta, GA 30303
Phone: 404-878-3000
Fax: 404-215-3878
e-mail: philipsarena-questions@philipsarena.com
Web Site: www.philipsarena.com
Management:
    President: Robert R Williams
    Sr Vice President: Mike Oshust
Founded: 1999
Seating Capacity: 20,000

6439 RIALTO CENTER FOR THE PERFORMING ARTS
George State University
University Plaza
Atlanta, GA 30303
Phone: 404-651-1234
Fax: 404-651-1573
e-mail: wbaites@gsu.edu
Web Site: www.rialtocenter.org
Management:
    Director: William Baites

6440 ROBERT FERST CENTER FOR THE ARTS AT GEORGIA TECH
349 Ferst Drive NW
Atlanta, GA 30332
Phone: 404-894-9600
Fax: 404-864-9864
e-mail: jay.constantz@ferstcenter.org
Web Site: www.Ferstcenter.gatech.edu
Management:
    Director: Andrea Hoffer
    Marketing Manager: Sharon Anmed
    Development Director: Alisa Smallwood
    Operations Manager: Brian Renkopf
    Technical Director: Brian Frey
    Box Office Manager: Chris Dreger
Founded: 1992
Performs At: 1,155 seat theatre
Annual Attendance: 60,000
Facility Category: Theatre & 2 galleries
Type of Stage: Proscenium
Stage Dimensions: 37x52
Seating Capacity: 1,155
Rental Contact: Tori Wallingford

6441 ROBERT W WOODRUFF ARTS CENTER: ALLIANCE THEATRE
1280 Peachtree Street
Atlanta, GA 30309
Phone: 404-733-4650
Fax: 404-733-4493

6442 ROBERT W WOODRUFF ARTS CENTER: SYMPHONY HALL
1280 Peachtree Street
Atlanta, GA 30309
Phone: 404-733-4900
Fax: 404-733-4493

6443 SEVEN STAGES
1105 Euclid Avenue
Atlanta, GA 30307
Phone: 404-522-0911
Fax: 404-522-0913
e-mail: boxoffice@7stages.org
Web Site: www.7stages.org
Officers:
    Board Chair: Ran Jan Dattagupta
    Borad Secretary: Tobie Kranitz
    Board Treasurer: Chris Ames
Management:

Artistic Director: Del Hamilton
Producing Director: Faye Allen
Managing Director: Raye Varney
Marketing Director: Joe Gfaller
Mission: Producing new works and international collaborations as well as contemporary theatre and reinterpretations of classics.
Founded: 1978
Specialized Field: Musical; Community; Theatrical Group
Status: Professional; Nonprofit
Paid Staff: 7
Volunteer Staff: 2
Paid Artists: 65
Budget: $850,000
Income Sources: Theatre Communications Group; National Endowment for the Arts; Georgia Council of the Arts; City of Atlanta Bureau of Cultural Affairs; Trust for Mutual Understanding; AT&T
Affiliations: Theatre Communications Group; Atlanta Coalition for the Performing Arts
Annual Attendance: 15,000
Facility Category: 2 Performing Arts Theatres
Type of Stage: Black Boxes
Seating Capacity: 99; 202
Year Built: 1928
Year Remodeled: 1994
Architect: $1.6 million
Rental Contact: Del Hamilton

6444 TURNER FIELD

755 Hank Aaron Drive
Atlanta, GA 30315
Phone: 404-522-7630
Fax: 404-614-1329
Management:
 Director Marketing: Wayna Long
Seating Capacity: 52,007

6445 AUGUSTA/RICHMOND COUNTY CIVIC CENTER COMPLEX

601 7th Street
PO Box 2306
Augusta, GA 30903
Phone: 706-722-3521
Fax: 706-724-7545
e-mail: info@arcc.com
Web Site: www.augustaciviccenter.com
Management:
 General Manager: Reggie Williams
 Assistant General Manager: Linda G Roberts
Mission: Complex with over 52,000 square feet of exhibit space. Arena floor 24,000 square feet, 65 foot ceiling. Sporting events, trade shows, meetings.
Type of Stage: Proscenium
Seating Capacity: 8500 Arena, 2690 Auditorium
Year Built: 1979
Rental Contact: Mike McGhee (713)623-4583

6446 IMPERIAL THEATRE

749 Broad Street
Augusta, GA 30901

Mailing Address: PO Box 31126, Augusta, GA. 30903
Phone: 706-722-8293
Fax: 706-722-8293
e-mail: greg@imperialtheatre.com
Web Site: www.imperialtheatre.com
Management:
 Business Manager: Elizabeth Swain Brownlee
Founded: 1918

6447 MAURICE K TOWNSEND CENTER FOR THE PERFORMING ARTS

State University of West Georgia
Carrollton, GA 30118-1400
Phone: 770-836-6694
Fax: 770-830-2346
e-mail: tcpa@westga.edu
Web Site: townsendcenter.org
Management:
 Director: Robert Jennings
Paid Staff: 4
Facility Category: Performing Arts
Type of Stage: Proscenium
Stage Dimensions: 42x74
Year Built: 1988
Cost: $3.5 Million
Acoustical Consultant: Jennings

6448 CEDARTOWN CIVIC AUDITORIUM

205 E Avenue
Cedartown, GA 30125
Phone: 770-748-4168
Fax: 770-748-8754
Toll-free: 800-830-8910
e-mail: director@ccauditorium.com
Web Site: www.ccauditorium.com
Management:
 Director: Wanda Cagle
 Assistant: Linda deGraauw
 Tech Director: Brian Keith
Founded: 1976
Paid Staff: 2
Income Sources: City of Cedartown; Ticket Sales; Donations; Grants
Affiliations: City of Cedartown; Georgia Council for the Arts; Southeast Arts Federation
Facility Category: Auditorium/Theater
Type of Stage: Proscenium
Seating Capacity: 976
Year Built: 1976
Rental Contact: Director Gary Redding

6449 COLUMBUS CIVIC CENTER

400 4th Street
Columbus, GA 31902
Phone: 706-653-4482
Fax: 706-653-4481
e-mail: info@columbusga.org
Web Site: www.columbusciviccenter.org
 Operations Manager: Dale Aester
Seating Capacity: 10,000

All listings are in alphabetical order by state, then city, then organization within the city.

6450 MEMORIAL STADIUM
S Commons Sports
Entertainment Complex
Columbus, GA 31902-1340
Phone: 706-653-4482
Fax: 706-653-4481
Management:
    General Manager: Anthony L Ford
    Project Analyst: Jim Jackson
    Operations Manager: Dale Hestter
    Marketing/Sales Manager: Valerie Edwards
Seating Capacity: 15,000

6451 RIVERCENTER FOR THE PERFORMING ARTS
900 Broadway
PO Box 2425
Columbus, GA 31902
Phone: 706-653-7993
Fax: 706-653-8664
e-mail: istreby@rivercenter.org
Web Site: www.rivercenter.org
Management:
    Executive Director: James Baudoin
Facility Category: Concert Hall; Recital Hall; Studio
Thaetre
Seating Capacity: 2,670

6452 THREE ARTS THEATRE
1020 Talbotton Road
Columbus, GA 31901
Phone: 706-653-4183

6453 AGNES SCOTT COLLEGE
141 E College Avenue
Decatur, GA 30030
Phone: 404-471-6285
Fax: 404-471-6298
Toll-free: 800-868-8602
e-mail: info@AgnesScott.edu
Web Site: www.AgnesScott.edu
Management:
    Cultural Programs Coordinator: James Boynton
    Special Events/Conferences Director: Demetrice
    Parks
Founded: 1889
Performs At: Gaines Chapel

6454 GWINNETT PERFORMING ARTS CENTER
6400 Sugarloaf Parkway
Building 100
Duluth, GA 30097
Phone: 770-623-4966
Fax: 770-623-4808
Toll-free: 800-224-6422
e-mail: info@gwinnettciviccenter.com
Web Site: www.gwinnettciviccenter.com
Type of Stage: Proscenium
Seating Capacity: 702

6455 JEKYLL ISLAND AMPHITHEATER
Stable Road
Jekyll Island, GA 31527
Phone: 912-635-4060

6456 JEKYLL ISLAND SOCCER COMPLEX
P.O. Box 13186
Jekyll Island, GA 31527
Phone: 877-453-5955
Fax: 912-635-4073
Toll-free: 877-4JE-KYLL
e-mail: meredithkid@cs.com
Web Site: www.jekyllisland.com
Management:
    Director Soccer Marketing: Jim Canter

6457 GRAND OPERA HOUSE
651 Mulberry Street
Macon, GA 31201
Phone: 912-749-6580

6458 GRAND OPERA HOUSE-A PERFORMING ARTS CENTER
Mercer University
1400 Coleman Avenue
Macon, GA 31207
Phone: 478-301-5460
Fax: 478-301-5469
e-mail: goss_km@mercer.edu
Management:
    Executive Director: Karen Goss

6459 WESLEYAN COLLEGE - PORTER AUDITORIUM
4760 Forsyth Road
Macon, GA 31210
Phone: 478-477-1110
Fax: 478-757-4030
Toll-free: 800-447-6610
e-mail: sallen@wesleyancollege.edu
Web Site: www.wesleyancollege.edu
Founded: 1836

6460 MADISON: MORGAN CULTURAL CENTER
434 S Main Street
Madison, GA 30650
Phone: 706-342-4743
Fax: 706-342-1154
Web Site: www.morgan.public.lib.ga.us/madmorg
Management:
    Executive Director: Cassandra E Baker

6461 COBB COUNTY CIVIC CENTER
548 S Marietta Parkway
Marietta, GA 30060
Phone: 770-528-8450
Fax: 770-528-8457

6462 COBB COUNTY CIVIC CENTER - JENNIE T. ANDERSON
548 S Marietta Parkway
Marietta, GA 30060
Phone: 770-528-8490
Fax: 770-528-8457

6463 COBB COUNTY CIVIC CENTER - ROMEO HUDGINS MEMORIAL CENTER
548 S Marietta Parkway
Marietta, GA 30060
Phone: 770-528-8450
Fax: 770-528-8457

6464 THEATRE IN THE SQUARE
11 Whitlock Avenue
Marietta, GA 30064
Phone: 770-422-8369
Fax: 770-424-2637
e-mail: boxoffice@theatreinthesquare.com
Web Site: www.theatreinthesquare.com
Management:
    Marketing Director: Monica Williamson
    Producer: Palmer Wells
Founded: 1982

6465 SPIVEY HALL
Clayton College & State University
5900 N Lee Street
Morrow, GA 30260
Phone: 770-961-3683
Fax: 770-961-3670
e-mail: spiveyhall@mail.clayton.edu
Web Site: www.spiveyhall.org
Founded: 1991

6466 COLQUITT COUNTY ARTS CENTER
401 7th Avenue SW
Moultrie, GA 31768
Phone: 229-985-1922
Fax: 229-890-6746
e-mail: artscenter@hotmail.com
Management:
    Director: Cary Carmichael

6467 ROME CITY AUDITORIUM
601 Broad Street
Rome, GA 30161
Mailing Address: PO Box 1433, Romega, GA. 30162
Phone: 706-236-4416
Fax: 706-236-4549
e-mail: joesmith@Romegacitygov.org
Facility Category: Auditorium
Type of Stage: Wood
Seating Capacity: 1,112

6468 ARMSTRONG STATE COLLEGE FINE ARTS AUDITORIUM
11935 Abercorn Street
Savannah, GA 31419-1997
Phone: 912-927-5325
Fax: 912-921-5472
e-mail: finearts@mail.armstrong.edu
Web Site: www.finearts.armstrong.edu/departments.htm
Seating Capacity: 1,000

6469 SAVANNAH CIVIC CENTER
301 W Ogelthorpe Avenue
PO Box 726
Savannah, GA 31402
Phone: 912-651-6550
Fax: 912-651-6552
Web Site: www.savannahcivic.com
Specialized Field: SE Coastal Area
Seating Capacity: 2524; 3,500 to 9,600

6470 SAVANNAH CIVIC CENTER - ARENA
301 W Ogelthorpe Avenue
PO Box 726
Savannah, GA 31402
Phone: 912-651-6550
Fax: 912-651-6552
Web Site: www.savannahcivic.com
Seating Capacity: 3,500 to 9,600

6471 SAVANNAH CIVIC CENTER - THEATRE
301 W Ogelthorpe Avenue
PO Box 726
Savannah, GA 31402
Phone: 912-651-6550
Fax: 912-651-6552
Web Site: www.savannahcivic.com
Seating Capacity: 2,524

6472 GEORGIA SOUTHERN UNIVERSITY - PUPPET THEATRE
PO Box 8124
Statesboro, GA 30460
Phone: 912-681-0336
Fax: 912-681-0822
e-mail: mikesull@gasou.edu
Web Site: www.gasou.edu

6473 THOMASVILLE CULTURAL CENTER AUDITORIUM
Thomasville Entertainment Foundation
600 East Washington Street
Thomasville, GA 31792
Phone: 229-226-0588
Web Site: www.tccarts.org
Founded: 1915

6474 VALDOSTA STATE COLLEGE - SAWYER THEATRE
Fine Arts Building
Valdosta, GA 31698
Phone: 912-333-5820
Fax: 912-245-3799
e-mail: ccates@valdosta.edu
Web Site: www.valdosta.edu
Founded: 1969
Seating Capacity: 225

6475 VALDOSTA STATE COLLEGE - WHITEHEAD AUDITORIUM
Fine Arts Building
Valdosta, GA 31698
Phone: 912-333-5816
Fax: 912-245-3799
e-mail: sarcher@valdosta.edu
Web Site: www.valdosta.edu
Type of Stage: Proscenium
Seating Capacity: 773

Hawaii

6476 ALOHA STADIUM
99-500 Salt Lake Boulevard
PO Box 30666
Honolulu, HI 96820
Phone: 808-486-9500
Fax: 808-486-9520
Web Site: www.hawaii.edu
Management:
    Stadium Manager: Edwin K Hayashi
Affiliations: NCAA; NFL Pro Bowl; Hawaii Bowl
Concerts
Seating Capacity: 50,419
Year Built: 1975
Rental Contact: Edwin K. Hayashi

6477 HONOLULU ACADEMY OF ARTS
900 S Beretania Street
Honolulu, HI 96814-1495
Phone: 808-532-8700
Web Site: www.honoluluacademy.org
Founded: 1927
Opened: 1927
Status: Nonprofit
Annual Attendance: 250,000

6478 HONOLULU DANCE THEATRE
3041 Manoa Road
Honolulu, HI 96822
Phone: 808-988-3202
Fax: 808-988-5199
e-mail: matthewwright@honoluludancetheatre.com
Web Site: www.honoluludancetheatre.com
Management:
    Executive Director: Matthew Wright
Mission: To develop, produce and present high quality
dance and or theatre works for the purposes of education
and entertainment and to promote the performing arts in
Hawaii.
Founded: 1993
Specialized Field: Dance
Paid Staff: 1
Volunteer Staff: 1
Non-paid Artists: 50
Annual Attendance: 13,200
Type of Stage: Concert
Seating Capacity: 1,400

6479 NEAL S BLAISDELL CENTER
777 Ward Avenue
Honolulu, HI 96814
Phone: 808-527-5400

6480 SAINT LOUIS CENTER FOR THE PERFORMING ARTS -
3142 Waialae Avenue
Honolulu, HI 96816-1579
Phone: 808-739-7777
Fax: 808-739-4853
e-mail: info@saintlouishawaii.org
Web Site: www.saintlouishawaii.org

6481 MAUI ARTS & CULTURAL CENTER
1 Cameron Way
Kahului, HI 96732
Phone: 808-242-2787
Fax: 808-242-4665
e-mail: info@mauiarts.org
Web Site: www.mauiarts.org
Management:
    President/CEO: Christina Cowan
    Managing Director: Karen Fisher
    General Manager: Art Vento
Mission: A gathering place where our community
celebrates creativity.
Founded: 1994
Specialized Field: Presenter
Annual Attendance: 250,000
Facility Category: Visual and performing arts
Type of Stage: Proscenium and open air
Seating Capacity: 5,000 + 1,200 + 300
Year Built: 1994
Cost: $32 million
Rental Contact: Candace Croteau

6482 KAHILU THEATRE
67 1186 Lindsey Road
PO Box 549
Kamuela, HI 96743
Phone: 808-885-6017
Fax: 808-885-0546
e-mail: renee@kahilutheatre.org
Web Site: www.kahilutheatre.org
Officers:
    President: Evarts Fox
    VP: Mike Luce
    Secretary: Barbara Campbell
    Treasurer: Lauri Ainslie
Management:
    Acting Director: Renee Mueller
Mission: To maintain performing arts center designed to
present high-quality national and international
artists/groups.
Founded: 1981
Status: Professional; Nonprofit
Paid Staff: 2
Volunteer Staff: 10
Income Sources: Western Alliance of Arts
Administrators; Association of Performing Arts
Presenters; International Society of Performing Arts
Administrators
Annual Attendance: 6,500

Facility Category: Theater
Type of Stage: Proscenium
Stage Dimensions: 35 x 65
Seating Capacity: 490
Year Built: 1981
Rental Contact: Acting Director Renee Mueller
Organization Type: Performing; Sponsoring

6483 MCKAY AUDITORIUM AT BRIGHAM YOUNG UNIVERSITY

Brigham Young University
55-220 Kulanui Street
Laie, HI 96762
Phone: 808-293-3903
Web Site: www.byuh.edu

Idaho

6484 BANK OF AMERICA CENTRE

233 S Capitol Boulevard
Boise, ID 83702
Phone: 208-424-2200
Fax: 208-424-2222
e-mail: sales@bofacentre.com
Web Site: www.bofacentre.com
Management:
  General Manager: John Cunningham
  Communications/Media Director: Jack Careefix
Mission: Capable of hosting a variety of events including
professional ice hockey and professional tennis, concerts,
and family shows, trade shows.
Seating Capacity: 5,100
Year Built: 1997

6485 MORRISON CENTER FOR THE PERFORMING ARTS

1910 University Drive
Boise, ID 83725
Phone: 208-426-1609
Fax: 208-426-3021
e-mail: mcpa@email.boisestate.edu
Web Site: www.boisestate.edu
Management:
  Executive Director: Frank Heise
Founded: 1984
Type of Stage: Proscenium
Seating Capacity: 2,000

6486 PAVILION AT BOISE STATE

Boise State University
1910 University Drive
Boise, ID 83725
Phone: 208-426-1900
Fax: 208-426-1998
e-mail: jgrimes@boisestate.edu
Web Site: www.boisestate.edu
Management:
  Executive Director: Dexter King
  Assistant Director: Greg Marchant
Founded: 1982
Seating Capacity: 2,500 to 13,265

6487 PALMER COLLEGE

1000 Brady Street
Davenport, ID 52803
Phone: 319-884-5856
Fax: 319-326-8414
e-mail: obrien_r@palmer.edu
Web Site: www.palmer.edu
Management:
  Manager: Ron O'Brien
Seating Capacity: 4,000

6488 CIVIC AUDITORIUM

501 S Holmes Avenue
Idaho Falls, ID 83401
Phone: 208-529-1396
Fax: 208-552-0476
Management:
  Manager: Roger T Ralphs
Seating Capacity: 1,892

6489 LEWIS - CLARK CENTER FOR ARTS AND HISTORY

415 Main Street
Lewiston, ID 83501
Phone: 208-792-2243
Fax: 208-792-2850
e-mail: coakes@lcsc.edu
Web Site: www.csc.edu/centerforarts

6490 LEWIS-CLARK STATE COLLEGE CENTER FOR ARTS AND HISTORY

415 Main Street
Lewiston, ID 83501
Phone: 208-792-2243
Fax: 208-792-2850
e-mail: kpacker@lcsc.edu
Web Site: www.artsandhistory.org
Management:
  Director: Carlton Oakes
Founded: 1884
Performs At: Lewiston High School Auditorium
Affiliations: Collaborations

6491 KIBBIE-AUSI ACTIVITY CENTER

University of Idaho
Moscow, ID 83844-2307
Phone: 208-885-7928
Fax: 208-885-0562
Web Site: www.uidaho.edu
Management:
  Manager: Thomas McGann
  Assistant Manager: Joy Farmer
Seating Capacity: 8,500

6492 MOUNTAIN HOME ARTS COUNCIL

PO Box 974
Mountain Home, ID 83647
Phone: 208-587-3706
e-mail: mharts@earthlink.net
Management:
  Executive Director: Rhonda Urquidi

6493 NAMPA CIVIC CENTER
311 3rd Street South
Nampa, ID 83651
Phone: 208-465-2252
Fax: 208-465-2255
e-mail: stephanb@ci.nampa.id.us
Web Site: www.nampaciviccenter.com
Management:
　Director: Bill Stephan
Founded: 1990
Seating Capacity: 640

6494 IDAHO STATE UNIVERSITY
921 South 8th Avenue
PO Box 8281
Pocatello, ID 83209
Phone: 208-282-0211
Fax: 208-282-4741
e-mail: kovarudo@isu.edu
Web Site: www.isu.edu

6495 IDAHO STATE UNIVERSITY: HOLT ARENA
550 Memorial Drive
Pocatello, ID 83209
Phone: 208-236-2831
Fax: 208-236-4089
Web Site: www.isu.edu
Management:
　Manager: John Novosel

6496 IDAHO STATE UNIVERSITY - GORANSON HALL
Department of Music
PO Box 8099
Pocatello, ID 83209
Phone: 208-282-3636
Fax: 208-282-4884
e-mail: music@isu.edu
Web Site: www.isu.edu/music/
Type of Stage: Proscenium
Seating Capacity: 446

6497 IDAHO STATE UNIVERSITY - POWELL LITTLE THEATRE
Campus Box 8115
Pocatello, ID 83209
Phone: 208-282-3695
Fax: 208-282-4598
e-mail: jeppkare@isu.edu
Web Site: www.isu.edu/commthea/

6498 ELIZA R SNOW PERFORMING ARTS CENTER
Rexburg, ID 83460-1210
Phone: 208-496-1260
Fax: 208-496-1249
e-mail: robertsl@byui.edu
Web Site: www.byui.edu/music
Annual Attendance: 2100
Facility Category: Concert Hall
Type of Stage: Raised

Stage Dimensions: 53'x 48'
Seating Capacity: 700
Year Built: 1981
Rental Contact: Karla Ricks

6499 RICKS COLLEGE
Rexburg, ID 83460-1661
Phone: 208-356-1152
Fax: 208-356-1184
e-mail: sparhawkd@ricks.edu
Web Site: www.ricks.edu

6500 SUN VALLEY CENTER FOR THE ARTS AND HUMANITIES
PO Box 656
Sun Valley, ID 83353
Phone: 208-726-9491
Fax: 208-726-2344
e-mail: information@sunvalleycenter.org
Web Site: www.sunvalleycenter.org
Management:
　Director Performing Arts: Amy Wigstrom
Mission: To offer performances in all varieties of theatre, music and dance.
Founded: 1971
Specialized Field: Dance; Vocal Music; Instrumental Music; Theater
Paid Staff: 12
Budget: $60,000-$150,000
Performs At: Sun Valley Center for the Arts and Humanities
Organization Type: Presenting

6501 INTERMOUNTAIN CULTURAL CENTER AND MUSEUM
2295 Paddock Avenue
P.O. Box 307
Weiser, ID 83672
Phone: 208-549-0205

6502 SNAKE RIVER HERITAGE CENTER MUSEUM
PO Box 307
2295 Paddock Avenue
Weiser, ID 83672
Phone: 208-549-0205
Fax: 208-549-2740
e-mail: rain/@ruralnework.net
Management:
　President/Board of Directors: Pat Harberd
Mission: To bring together and preserve the culture and heritage of all the peoples of the Snake River Country for the education of this and future generations.
Founded: 1979
Specialized Field: Regional Culture Plus All Other Area's Of Interest
Volunteer Staff: 45
Paid Artists: 3
Non-paid Artists: 15

Illinois

6503 METROPOLIS PERFORMING ARTS CENTRE
111 W Campbell Street
Arlington Heights, IL 60005
Phone: 847-577-5982
Fax: 847-577-5992
e-mail: metropolis@interaccess.com
Web Site: www.metropolisarts.com
Management:
   Executive Director: Tim Rater
Founded: 2000

6504 ILLINOIS WESLEYAN UNIVERSITY - WESTBROOK AUDITORIUM
303 E. University Avenue, Presser Hall
School of Music, PO Box 2900
Bloomington, IL 61702-2900
Phone: 309-556-3061
Fax: 309-556-3121
e-mail: ldolan@titan.iwu.edu
Web Site: www.iwu.edu
Seating Capacity: 600

6505 SIU ARENA
Southern Illinois University
Room 117
Carbondale, IL 62901-6619
Phone: 618-453-2321
Fax: 618-453-2602
Management:
   Arena Director: Gary Drake
   Assistant Director: Russell Driver
   Deputy Director: Michelle J Suarez
Seating Capacity: 10,014

6506 SOUTHERN ILLINOIS UNIVERSITY AT CARBONDALE-SHRYOCK AUDITORIUM EVENTS
Shryock Auditorium, SIUC
Mailcode 4326
Carbondale, IL 62901-4326
Phone: 618-453-3379
e-mail: shryock@siu.edu
Web Site: www.siu.edu/~shryock/
Management:
   Shryock Auditorium Director: Robert Cerchio
Founded: 1917
Seating Capacity: 1,249

6507 ASSEMBLY HALL
University of Illinois
1800 S 1st Street
Champaign, IL 61820
Phone: 217-333-2923
Fax: 217-244-8888
e-mail: WebComment@uofiassemblyhall.com
Web Site: www.uofiassemblyhall.com
Management:
   Director: Kevin Ullestard
Founded: 1963

Paid Staff: 42
Seating Capacity: 16,000 to 17,200

6508 EASTERN ILLINOIS UNIVERSITY: O' BRIAN STADIUM
Campus Scheduling, MLK University Union
Room 208
Charleston, IL 61920
Phone: 217-581-3861
Fax: 217-581-7064
e-mail: camsched@eiu.edu
Web Site: www.mlkunion.eiu.edu
Management:
   Assistant Director: Kathy Cartwright
Seating Capacity: 10,000

6509 EASTERN ILLINOIS UNIVERSITY: LANTZ GYM
Campus Scheduling MLK University Union
Room 2
Charleston, IL 61920
Phone: 217-581-3861
Fax: 217-581-7064
Web Site: www.eiu.edu
Management:
   Assistant Director: Kathy Cartwright
Seating Capacity: 5,200

6510 ARIE CROWN THEATRE
McCormick Place
2301 S. Lake Shore Drive
Chicago, IL 60616
Phone: 312-791-6190
Type of Stage: Proscenium

6511 ATHENAEUM THEATRE
2936 N Southport Avenue
Chicago, IL 60657
Phone: 773-935-6860
Fax: 773-935-6878
Toll-free: 800-433-7285
e-mail: cfoster29@surfbest.net
Web Site: www.athenaeum.livedomain.com
Founded: 1925
Annual Attendance: 20,000+
Type of Stage: Proscenium
Seating Capacity: 1,325

6512 AUDITORIUM THEATRE
50 E Congress Parkway
Chicago, IL 60605
Phone: 312-922-2110
Fax: 312-431-2360
e-mail: info@auditoriumtheatre.org
Web Site: www.auditoriumtheatre.org
Founded: 1889

6513 AUDITORIUM THEATRE
50 E Congress Parkway
Chicago, IL 60605

Phone: 312-431-2395
Fax: 312-431-9668
Web Site: www.auditoriumtheatre.org
Management:
    Executive Director: Jan Kallish

6514 BEVERLY ART CENTER
2407 West 111th Street
Chicago, IL 60655
Phone: 773-445-3838
Fax: 773-445-0386
e-mail: beverlyartcenter@ameritech.net
Web Site: www.beverlyartcenter.org
Founded: 1968
Seating Capacity: 422

6515 CIVIC STAGES CHICAGO
20 N Wacker Drive
Suite 452
Chicago, IL 60606
Phone: 312-346-4744
Fax: 312-704-6030

6516 CIVIC STAGES CHICAGO - CIVIC THEATRE
20 N Wacker Drive
Suite 452
Chicago, IL 60606
Phone: 312-332-2244
Fax: 312-419-8345

6517 CIVIC STAGES CHICAGO - OPERA HOUSE
20 N Wacker Drive
Suite 452
Chicago, IL 60606
Phone: 312-332-2244
Fax: 312-419-8345

6518 COMISKEY PARK
333 W 35th Street
Chicago, IL 60616
Phone: 312-674-1000
Fax: 312-674-5102
Web Site: www.whitesox.com
Management:
    Concessions Manager: Patrick Redden
    Sr VP Marketing: Robert Gallas
Specialized Field: Home of the Chicago White Sox
Seating Capacity: 44,321
Year Built: 1991

6519 CURTISS HALL
410 S Michigan Avenue
Chicago, IL 60603
Phone: 312-939-3380

6520 CURTISS HALL: FINE ARTS BUILDING
410 S Michigan Avenue
Chicago, IL 60605
Phone: 312-939-3380
Management:

Bookings Manager: Lee Newcomer
Performs At: Hall

6521 DE PAUL UNIVERSITY - BLACKSTONE THEATRE
1 E Jackson
Chicago, IL 60604
Phone: 312-362-8000
Toll-free: 800-4DE-PAUL
e-mail: admitdpu@depaul.edu
Web Site: www.depaul.edu
Founded: 1898

6522 DMITRI ROUDNEV
47 W Division Street
Chicago, IL 60610
Phone: 773-404-0417
Fax: 312-440-0301
e-mail: ballet@concentric.net
Web Site: www.balletrussianteachers.com
Officers:
    Associate Director: Mary Van Dyke Roudnev
    Director: Dmitri Roundnev
Management:
    Repetiteur/Teacher: Valery Dolgallo

6523 CHICAGO SYMPHONY ORCHESTRA - ORCHESTRA HALL
220 S Michigan Avenue
Chicago, IL 60604
Phone: 312-294-3333
Fax: 312-294-3329
Web Site: www.cso.org

6524 CHICAGO THEATRE COMPANY PARKWAY PLAYHOUSE
500 E 67th Street
Chicago, IL 60637
Phone: 773-493-0901
Fax: 773-493-5360
Toll-free: 773-493-0360
e-mail: info@chicagotheatrecompany.com
Web Site: www.chicagotheatrecompany.com
Founded: 1984

6525 PETRILLO MUSIC SHELL
425 E McFetridge Drive
Columbus Dr and Jackson Blvd
Chicago, IL 60603
Phone: 312-742-4763
Fax: 312-616-3719

6526 ROOSEVELT UNIVERSITY - PATRICK L. O'MALLEY THEATRE
430 S Michigan Avenue
Room 780
Chicago, IL 60605
Phone: 312-341-3500
Fax: 312-341-3814
e-mail: pbernade@roosevelt.edu
Web Site: www.roosevelt.edu

6527 BROADWAY IN CHICAGO SHUBERT THEATRE
22 W Monroe Street
Ste 700
Chicago, IL 60603
Phone: 312-977-1700
Fax: 312-977-1740
Web Site: www.broadwayinchicago.com
Founded: 1914

6528 SOLDIER FIELD
425 E. McFetridge Drive
Chicago, IL 60605
Phone: 312-747-1285
Fax: 312-747-6694
e-mail: kofinn@soldierfield.net
Web Site: www.soldierfield.net
Management:
    General Manager: Bob Glazebrook
Founded: 1924
Seating Capacity: 66,950

6529 THEATRE BUILDING CHICAGO
1225 W Belmont Avenue
Chicago, IL 60657-3205
Phone: 773-929-7367
Fax: 773-327-1404
e-mail: jaon@theatrebuildingchicago.org
Web Site: www.theatrebuildingchicago.org
Officers:
    Operations/Building Manager: Lorraine Townsend
Management:
    Artistic Director: John Sparks
    Executive Director: Joan Mazzonelli
Mission: To develop and produce new musicals.
Founded: 1969
Specialized Field: Theatre, Musical
Status: Nonprofit
Paid Staff: 10
Volunteer Staff: 800
Paid Artists: 200
Non-paid Artists: 107
Budget: $1,000,000
Annual Attendance: 35,000
Facility Category: multiplex
Type of Stage: 3 black box
Seating Capacity: 444
Year Built: 1962
Year Remodeled: 2002
Cost: 100,000
Rental Contact: Lorraine Townsend

6530 TRUMAN COLLEGE - O'ROURKE CENTER FOR THE PERFORMING ARTS
1145 W Wilson
Chicago, IL 60640
Phone: 773-878-9761
Fax: 773-907-4479

6531 UNITED CENTER
1901 W Madison Street
Chicago, IL 60612
Phone: 312-455-4500
Fax: 312-455-4511
e-mail: info@united-center.com
Web Site: www.unitedcenter.com
Management:
    Diretor Event Operations: Johnathan Zirin
    SVP/Marketing: Steve Schanwald
    SVP/Operations: Terry Savarise
    Director Concessions: Eric Delisle
    Director Premium Seating: Greg Hanrahan
    Director Building Operations: James Koehler
Seating Capacity: 20,500

6532 VICTORY GARDENS THEATER
2257 N Lincoln Avenue
Chicago, IL 60614
Phone: 773-871-3000
e-mail: information@victorygardens.org
Web Site: www.victorygardens.org
Founded: 1974
Annual Attendance: 60,000
Type of Stage: Black Box; Thrust
Seating Capacity: 195

6533 WRIGLEY FIELD
1060 W Addison Street
Chicago, IL 60613
Phone: 773-404-2827
Fax: 773-404-4129
Management:
    VP/Marketing/Broadcasting: John McDonough
Founded: 1914
Seating Capacity: 38,710

6534 EGYPTIAN THEATRE
135 N 2nd Street
De Kalb, IL 60115
Phone: 815-758-1215
e-mail: cltsb53@aol.com
Web Site: www.egyptiantheatre.org
Founded: 1929
Seating Capacity: 1,475

6535 DECATUR CIVIC CENTER
2010 W. U.S. 380
PO Box 894
Decatur, IL 76234
Phone: 940-627-2369
Fax: 940-267-6400
e-mail: info@decaturciviccenter.com
Web Site: www.decaturciviccenter.com
Founded: 1980

6536 DECATUR CIVIC CENTER - ARENA
2010 W. U.S. 380
PO Box 895
Decatur, IL 76234
Phone: 940-627-2369
Fax: 940-267-6400
e-mail: info@decaturciviccenter.com
Web Site: www.decaturciviccenter.com

6537 DECATUR CIVIC CENTER - THEATER

2010 W. U.S. 380
Decatur, IL 76234
Phone: 940-627-2369
Fax: 940-267-6400
e-mail: info@decaturciviccenter.com
Web Site: www.decaturciviccenter.com

6538 MILLIKIN UNIVERSITY KIRKLAND FINE ARTS CENTER

1360 W Main Street
Decatur, IL 62522
Phone: 217-424-6253
Fax: 217-362-6417
e-mail: bdiver@mail.millikin.edu
Web Site: www.millikin.edu/kirkland
Management:
   Scheduling/Events Coordinator: Lynn Kickle
   Technical Director: Bryan Diver
   Box Office Manager: Jan Traughber
   Assistant Technical Director: Mark Beal
   Marketing Manager: Ralf Pansch
Paid Staff: 6
Volunteer Staff: 12
Paid Artists: 20
Annual Attendance: 60,000
Facility Category: Fine Arts Center
Type of Stage: Proscenium
Seating Capacity: 1,907
Year Built: 1970
Rental Contact: Scheduling & Events Coordinator Lynne Kickle

6539 ELGIN COMMUNITY COLLEGE VISUAL & PERFORMING ARTS CENTER

1700 Spartan Drive
Elgin, IL 60123
Phone: 847-214-7421
Fax: 847-214-7757
e-mail: mhatch@mail.elgin.cc.il.us
Web Site: www.elgin.edu
Management:
   Director: Mary Hatch
   Technical Operations Director: Cindy Gaspardo
Founded: 1994
Specialized Field: Dance, Music, Theatre, Visual Arts
Paid Staff: 20
Volunteer Staff: 80
Paid Artists: 15
Annual Attendance: 40,000
Type of Stage: Proscenium
Seating Capacity: 662

6540 HEMMENS CULTURAL CENTER

150 Dexter Court
Elgin, IL 60120
Phone: 847-697-3616
Fax: 847-931-5940
e-mail: hemmens@cityofelgin.org
Web Site: www.cityofelgin.org
Management:
   Cultural Center Manager: Blythe Rainey-Cuyler

Technical Supervisor: Butch Wilhelmi
Front-of-House Supervisor: Bill Folk
Mission: To offer a 1,200-seat theatre that is both a presenting venue of high-quality entertainment and a rental facility.
Founded: 1969
Specialized Field: Presents general audience programs/concerts and youth programing for the Chicago region.
Paid Staff: 33
Volunteer Staff: 35
Type of Stage: Proscenium Arch
Seating Capacity: 1,200

6541 NATIONAL/LOUIS UNIVERSITY LIBRARY

2840 N Sheridan Road
Evanston, IL 60201
Phone: 847-256-5150
Fax: 847-256-1057
e-mail: nluinfo@wheeling1.nl.edu
Web Site: www.nl.edu
Founded: 1930

6542 NORTHWESTERN UNIVERSITY: DYCHE STADIUM

1501 Central Street
Evanston, IL 60208
Phone: 847-491-7887
Fax: 847-467-6915
Web Site: www.nusports.com
Management:
   Director: John A Freeman

6543 PICK-STAIGER CONCERT HALL

1977 Sheridan Road
Evanston, IL 60208
Phone: 847-491-5441
Fax: 708-467-1831

6544 KNOX COLLEGE: ELEANOR ABBOTT FORD CENTER FOR THE PERFORMING ARTS

2 E South Street
Galesburg, IL 61401
Phone: 309-343-0112
Fax: 309-341-7090

6545 COLLEGE OF DUPAGE ARTS CENTER

McAninch Arts Center
425 Fawell Boulevard
Glen Ellyn, IL 60137
Phone: 630-942-4000
Fax: 630-790-9806
e-mail: raffel@cdnet.cod.edu
Web Site: www.cod.edu/artscntr
Management:
   Performing Arts Director: Jane Oldfield
Founded: 1986

6546 COLLEGE OF DUPAGE ARTS CENTER - MAINSTAGE

McAninch Arts Center
425 Fawell Boulevard
Glen Ellyn, IL 60137
Phone: 630-942-4000
Fax: 630-790-9806
e-mail: raffel@cdnet.cod.edu
Web Site: www.cod.edu/artscntr
Founded: 1986
Seating Capacity: 793

6547 COLLEGE OF DUPAGE ARTS CENTER - STUDIO THEATRE

McAninch Arts Center
425 Fawell Boulevard
Glen Ellyn, IL 60137
Phone: 630-942-4000
Fax: 630-790-9806
e-mail: raffel@cdnet.cod.edu
Web Site: www.cod.edu/artscntr
Founded: 1986
Specialized Field: Theatre
Type of Stage: Black Box
Seating Capacity: 75
Resident Groups: Buffalo Theatre Ensemble

6548 COLLEGE OF DUPAGE ARTS CENTER - THEATRE 2

McAninch Arts Center
425 Fawell Boulevard
Glen Ellyn, IL 60137
Phone: 630-942-4000
Fax: 630-790-9806
e-mail: raffel@cdnet.cod.edu
Web Site: www.cod.edu/artscntr
Founded: 1986
Type of Stage: Thrust
Seating Capacity: 195

6549 SOUTHEASTERN ILLINOIS COLLEGE VISUAL & PERFORMING ARTS CENTER

3575 College Road
Harrisburg, IL 62946
Phone: 618-252-5400
Fax: 618-252-3156
Toll-free: 866-338-2742
e-mail: kellye@sic.cc.il.us
Web Site: www.sic.cc.il.us
Management:
  Visual/Performing Arts: Kellye Whitler

6550 RIALTO SQUARE THEATRE

15 E Van Buren Street
Joliet, IL 60432
Phone: 815-726-7171
Fax: 815-726-0352
e-mail: information@rialtosquare.com
Web Site: www.rialtosquare.com
Management:
  General Manager: Randy Green

Director Marketing/Sales: Annette Louch
Director Development: Martha Scheidler
Director Programming: Nancy Bertnik
Finance Manager: Dale Evans
Founded: 1926
Paid Staff: 11
Volunteer Staff: 300
Budget: $2,000,000
Income Sources: Corporate; Individual; Foundations
Facility Category: Performing Arts
Type of Stage: Proscenium
Stage Dimensions: 52' 0" wide x 23' 6" high
Seating Capacity: 1,000
Year Built: 1926
Year Remodeled: 1981
Cost: $7,000,000
Rental Contact: Mary Beth DeGrush

6551 DAVID ADLER CULTURAL CENTER

1700 N Milwaukee Avenue
Libertyville, IL 60048
Phone: 847-367-0707
Fax: 847-367-0804
e-mail: info@adlercenter.org
Web Site: www.adlercenter.org
Mission: Dedicated to promoting the cultural arts as an integral part of everyday life; designed to foster critical thinking and interpretation, participation, entertainment, and achievement in the arts for the people of Northern Illinois and Southern Wisconsin; maintains and interprets the historic home of architect David Adler, which is the base of its activities.
Founded: 1957
Organization Type: Performing; Edcuational

6552 WESTERN ILLINOIS UNIVERSITY - HAINLINE THEATRE

1 University Circle
Macomb, IL 61455
Phone: 309-298-1414
Fax: 309-298-2695
e-mail: info@wiu.edu
Web Site: www.wiu.edu/users/mithea/facilities.html
Type of Stage: Proscenium
Seating Capacity: 387

6553 MARION CULTURAL AND CIVIC CENTER

PO Box 51
Marion, IL 62959-0051
Phone: 618-997-4030
Fax: 618-997-2028
e-mail: marionccc@hcis.net
Web Site: www.marionccc.org
Management:
  Director: Mike Bennett
  Director/Asst Arts Coordinator: Bill Hamer
Founded: 1974
Specialized Field: Musicals; Plays; Concerts; Classical Dance
Paid Staff: 4
Budget: $200,000
Income Sources: Donations
Annual Attendance: 52,000

Type of Stage: Proscenium
Stage Dimensions: 45'x36'
Seating Capacity: 1,100
Year Built: 2004
Cost: $8 Million

6554 THE MARK OF QUAD CITIES
1201 River Drive
Moline, IL 61265
Phone: 309-764-2001
Fax: 309-764-2192
e-mail: meetingsandbanquets@themark.org
Web Site: www.themark.org
Management:
 Executive Director: Stephen R Hyman
 Director Finance: Rocky R Jones
 Marketing/Sales Director: Brett Cornish
 Director Operations: John Watts
Founded: 1993
Annual Attendance: 700,000
Seating Capacity: 12,000

6555 EWING COLISEUM
Northeast Louisiana University
Athletic Department, Malone Stadium
700 University Avenue
Monroe, IL 71209
Phone: 318-342-5360
Fax: 318-342-5367
Web Site: www.ulm.edu/tour/10/welcome.html
Management:
 Athletic Director: Warmer Alford
Founded: 1971
Type of Stage: Wood
Seating Capacity: 8,000

6556 HANCOCK STADIUM
7130 Horton Field House
Normal, IL 61790
Phone: 309-438-2000
Fax: 309-438-3513
Management:
 Athletic Director: Perk Weisenburger
Founded: 1969
Seating Capacity: 15,000

6557 ILLINOIS STATE UNIVERSITY:
REDBIRD ARENA
203 W College
Normal, IL 61790-2660
Phone: 309-438-2000
Fax: 309-438-3513
Management:
 Athletic Director: Perk Wesenburger
Seating Capacity: 10,500

6558 SHEELY CENTER FOR THE
PERFORMING ARTS
2300 Shermer Road
Northbrook, IL 60062
Phone: 708-272-6400
Fax: 708-272-4330

6559 MORAINE VALLEY COMMUNITY
COLLEGE FINE & PERFORMING ARTS
CENTER
10900 S 88th Avenue
Palos Hills, IL 60465
Phone: 708-974-4300
Fax: 708-974-5366
e-mail: nedza@morainevalley.edu
Web Site: www.moraine.cc.il.us
Management:
 Director Fine/Performing Arts: Susan Linn
Founded: 1967
Seating Capacity: 780

6560 FREEDOM HALL: NATHAN MANILOW
THEATRE
410 Lakewood Boulevard
Park Forest, IL 60466
Phone: 708-747-0580
Fax: 708-503-7737

6561 ILLINOIS THEATRE CENTER
400A Lakewood Boulevard
Park Forest, IL 60466
Phone: 708-481-3510
Fax: 708-481-3693

6562 RICHARD BURTON PERFORMING
ARTS CENTER
2000 5th Avenue
River Grove, IL 60171
Phone: 708-456-0300
Fax: 708-456-0049
e-mail: triton@triton.cc.il.us
Web Site: www.triton.cc.il.us

6563 TRITON COLLEGE PERFORMING
ARTS CENTER
2000 5th Avenue
River Grove, IL 60171
Phone: 708-456-0300
Fax: 708-583-3778
e-mail: triton@triton.cc.il.us
Web Site: www.triton.cc.il.us
Management:
 Manager/Tech Director: Marie Correa
Facility Category: Performing Arts Center
Type of Stage: Proscenium
Seating Capacity: 412
Rental Contact: Manager Maria Correa

6564 AUGUSTANA COLLEGE - CENTENNIAL
HALL
639 38th Street
Rock Island, IL 61201
Phone: 309-794-7000
Fax: 309-794-7678
Founded: 1860

6565 MIDWAY THEATRE
721 E State Street
Rockford, IL 61104
Phone: 815-965-5211
Fax: 815-964-8378

6566 LEWIS UNIVERSITY THEATRE
Institutional Advancement
Lewis University
Romeoville, IL 60446
Phone: 815-836-5471
Fax: 815-836-5641
Management:
   Theater Director: Jo Slowik
   Director Theatre: Keith White
   Technical Director of Theatre: Harold McCay
Founded: 1974
Budget: $6,000
Performs At: Philip Lynch Theatre
Facility Category: Educational Theatre
Type of Stage: 3/4 Thrust
Seating Capacity: 240
Year Built: 1976

6567 ALLSTATE ARENA
6920 N Mannheim Road
Rosemont, IL 60018
Phone: 847-635-6601
Fax: 847-635-6606
Web Site: www.allstatearena.com
Management:
   Director: Harry Pappas
Founded: 1979
Annual Attendance: 1,500,000
Seating Capacity: 18,500

6568 ARCH-OPERA HOUSE OF SANDWICH
140 E Railroad Street
Sandwich, IL 60548
Phone: 815-786-2555
Fax: 815-786-7012
e-mail: operahouse@sannauk.com
Web Site: www.sandwichoperahouse.com
Founded: 1878
Annual Attendance: 20,000
Type of Stage: Proscenium Arch
Seating Capacity: 310

6569 PRAIRIE CENTER FOR THE ARTS
201 Schuamburg Court
Schuamburg, IL 60193-1899
Phone: 847-895-3600
Fax: 847-895-1837
e-mail: earmistead@ci.schaumburg.il.us
Web Site: www.prairiecenter.org
Management:
   Director: Elizabeth Armistead
Founded: 1986
Paid Staff: 20
Volunteer Staff: 50
Budget: $1 million
Income Sources: Tickets; Rentals; Foundation Support
Annual Attendance: 75,000

Type of Stage: Proscenium
Year Built: 1986
Rental Contact: Pat DeBartolo

6570 NORTHSHORE CENTER FOR THE PERFORMING ARTS
9501 N Skokie Boulevard
Skokie, IL 60077
Phone: 847-679-9501
Fax: 847-679-7945
e-mail: pcowen@nscpas.org
Web Site: www.centreast.org
Management:
   Executive Director: Phyllis Cowen
   Office Manager: Pat Adams
Founded: 1979
Paid Staff: 3
Volunteer Staff: 8
Seating Capacity: 848
Year Built: 1996

6571 SPRINGFIELD COLLEGE - MUSIC HALL
1500 N 5th Street
Springfield, IL 62702
Phone: 217-525-1420
Fax: 217-525-0694

6572 NORRIS CULTURAL ARTS CENTER
1040 Dunham Road
PO Box 747
St. Charles, IL 60174
Phone: 630-584-7200
Fax: 630-584-7262
e-mail: mail@norristheatre.com
Web Site: www.norristheatre.com
Management:
   Managing Director: Robert Destocki
Seating Capacity: 1,052

6573 STERLING CENTENNIAL AUDITORIUM
202 E 5th
Sterling, IL 61081
Phone: 815-625-8200
Fax: 815-625-8363

6574 CENTER FOR THE PERFORMING ARTS
Governers State University
1 University Parkway
University Park, IL 60466
Phone: 708-235-2222
Fax: 708-235-2180
e-mail: tickets@govst.edu
Web Site: www.govst.edu/center
Officers:
   President: Karen Reid
Management:
   Executive Director: Burton Dikelsky
   Theater Manager: John McCall
   Development Officer: Jackie Small
   Box Office Manager: Diane Giles
Founded: 1995
Paid Staff: 7

Volunteer Staff: 50
Paid Artists: 40
Budget: $975,000
Income Sources: Tickets; Rentals; Donations; Sales
Annual Attendance: 60,000
Facility Category: Theater
Type of Stage: Proscenium
Stage Dimensions: 45'x35'
Seating Capacity: 1,171
Year Built: 1995
Cost: $8,000,000
Rental Contact: Les Alberts
Organization Type: Performing

6575 KRANNERT CENTER FOR THE PERFORMING ARTS

500 S Goodwin Avenue
Urbana, IL 61801
Phone: 217-333-6700
Fax: 217-244-0810
Toll-free: 800-527-2849
e-mail: webmaster@kcpa.uiuc.edu
Web Site: www.krannertcenter.com
Management:
   Director: Mike Ross
   Senior Associate Director/Marketing: Rebecca McBride
   Associate Director/Production: Susan McDonald
   Public Information Manager: Tammey Kikta
Mission: Auxiliary unit of the University of Illinois College of Fine and Applied Arts, Krannert Center offers about 350 performances each year by world renowned professional artists and university faculty and students, including classical music, jazz, dance, theatre, and family fare. The facility houses four theatres, a cafe and gift shop, and complete technical shops and rehearsal facilities.
Founded: 1969

6576 KRANNERT CENTER FOR THE PERFORMING ARTS - STUDIO

500 S Goodwin Avenue
Urbana, IL 61801
Phone: 217-333-6700
Fax: 217-244-0810
e-mail: webmaster@kcpa.uiuc.edu
Web Site: www.krannertcenter.com

6577 KRANNERT CENTER FOR THE PERFORMING ARTS - THEATRE 2

500 South Goodwin Avenue
Urbana, IL 61801
Phone: 217-333-6700
Fax: 217-244-0810
e-mail: webmaster@kcpa.uiuc.edu
Web Site: www.krannertcenter.com
Founded: 1969
Type of Stage: Proscenium
Seating Capacity: 4,000; (200 to 2,094)

6578 KRANNERT CENTER FOR THE PERFORMING ARTS - THEATRE 3

500 South Goodwin Avenue
Urbana, IL 61801
Phone: 217-333-6700
Fax: 217-244-0810
e-mail: webmaster@kcpa.uiuc.edu
Web Site: www.krannertcenter.com
Founded: 1969
Type of Stage: Proscenium
Seating Capacity: 4,000; (200 to 2,094)

6579 ODEUM SPORTS & EXPO CENTER

1033 North Villa Avenue
Villa Park, IL 60181
Phone: 630-941-9292
Fax: 630-831-9183
e-mail: mike@odeumexpo.com
Web Site: www.odeumexpo.com
   President/Owner: Philip Greco
Seating Capacity: 5,500

6580 GOODFELLOW HALL-THE JACK BENNY CENTER FOR THE ARTS

39 Jack Benny Drive
Waukegan, IL 60087
Phone: 847-360-4740
Fax: 847-662-0592
e-mail: cpetrusky@waukeganparks.org
Web Site: www.waukeganparks.org/jbc/
Founded: 1986
Seating Capacity: 100

6581 WHEATON COLLEGE - ARENA THEATER

501 College Avenue
Student Activities Office, Wheaton College
Wheaton, IL 60187
Phone: 630-752-5181
Fax: 630-752-5381
e-mail: studentactivities@wheaton.edu
Web Site: www.wheaton.edu
Officers:
   President: David Reifsnyder
Management:
   Associate Producer/Director: Michael Stauffer
   Assistant Producer: Mark Lewis
Founded: 1973

6582 WHEATON COLLEGE - EDMAN CHAPEL

501 College Avenue
Student Activities Office, Wheaton College
Wheaton, IL 60187
Phone: 630-752-5000
Fax: 630-752-5381
e-mail: studentactivities@wheaton.edu
Web Site: www.wheaton.edu

6583 DILLER STREET THEATER

310 Green Bay Road
Winnetka, IL 60093

Phone: 847-446-0674
Fax: 847-446-0675
e-mail: JAxelson@nscds.org
Web Site: www.nscds.pvt.k12.il.us/
Founded: 1919
Seating Capacity: 480

6584 CHRISTIAN ARTS AUDITORIUM
Dowie Memorial Drive
Zion, IL 60099
Phone: 708-746-2221
Fax: 847-548-5622
e-mail: padfield@ourzion.com
Web Site: www.ourzion.com
Founded: 1960
Seating Capacity: 522

Indiana

6585 REARDON AUDITORIUM
1100 East Fifth Street
Anderson, IN 46012
Phone: 765-649-9071
Fax: 765-641-3647
e-mail: clshark@anderson.edu
Web Site: www.anderson.edu
Management:
Director Conference: Cheryl L Jhank
Assistant Director Conference: Lisa D Crouse
Technical Director: Jeff Bates
Founded: 1983
Paid Staff: 4
Paid Artists: 4
Income Sources: University Administration; Facility Rental
Facility Category: Auditorium
Stage Dimensions: 52' x 75'
Seating Capacity: 23,000
Year Built: 1983
Cost: $5.1 million

6586 ASSEMBLY HALL
Indiana University
1001 E 17th Street
Bloomington, IN 47408-1590
Phone: 812-855-2127
Fax: 812-856-5155
e-mail: ccrabb@indiana.edu
Web Site: www.athletics.indiana.edu
Management:
Associated Director Events: Chuck Crabb

6587 INDIANA UNIVERSITY AUDITORIUM
1211 E 7th Street
Bloomington, IN 47405
Phone: 812-855-9528
Fax: 812-855-4244
Toll-free: 800-411-1512
e-mail: tickets@indiana.edu
Web Site: www.iuauditorium.com
Management:
General Manager: Bryan Rives

Founded: 1941
Annual Attendance: 88,390
Type of Stage: Proscenium Arch
Seating Capacity: 3,200

6588 INDIANA UNIVERSITY MUSICAL ARTS CENTER
Indiana University
School of Music
Bloomington, IN 47405
Phone: 812-855-7433
e-mail: cesbronv@indiana.edu
Web Site: www.music.indiana.edu

6589 INDIANA UNIVERSITY SCHOOL OF MUSIC
Indiana University
Bloomington, IN 47405
Phone: 812-855-1583
e-mail: musicadm@indiana.edu
Web Site: www.music.indiana.edu
Founded: 1820
Seating Capacity: The Musical Arts Center seats 1,460; Recital

6590 INDIANA UNIVERSITY THEATRE
Theatre 200, 275 North Jordan Avenue
Indiana University
Bloomington, IN 47405
Phone: 812-855-4502
Fax: 812-855-4704
e-mail: threatre@indiana.edu
Web Site: www.indiana.edu
Mission: Education, training, entertainment, scholarship, research.
Specialized Field: Theatre and drama

6591 BRONCO STADIUM
1910 University Drive
Boise, IN 83725
Phone: 208-426-1900
Fax: 208-426-1998
e-mail: jgrimes@boisestate.edu
Web Site: www.boisestate.edu
Management:
Executive Director: Joyce Grims
Founded: 1967
Seating Capacity: 30,000

6592 EVANSVILLE AUDITORIUM AND CONVENTION CENTRE
715 Locust Street
Evansville, IN 47708
Phone: 812-435-5770
Fax: 812-435-5500
Toll-free: 877-598-7603
e-mail: saaron@smgevansville.com
Web Site: www.smgevansville.com
Management:
Regional General Manager: Sandie Aaron
Assistant General Manager: Mick Conabi
Sales Manager: Marylinn Reinhart

Assistant General Manager: Kathy Lebarron

6593 ROBERTS MUNICIPAL STADIUM
2600 Division Street
Evansville, IN 47711
Phone: 812-476-1383
Fax: 812-476-1881
e-mail: saaron@smgevansville.com
Web Site: www.smgevansville.com
Management:
Regional General Manager: Sandie Aaron
Assistant General Manager: Mick Conati
Assistant General Manager: Kathy LeSarron
Operations Directoror: Kevin McAllister
Marketing Manager: JoNell Reich
Marketing Manager: Becky Pike
Seating Capacity: 12,500

6594 VETERANS MEMORIAL COLISEUM
300 Court Street
Evensville, IN 47736
Phone: 812-424-5879
Fax: 812-424-2798
Management:
Manager: Mark Acker
Seating Capacity: 4,055

6595 FOELLINGER THEATER IN FRANKE PARK
3411 Sherman Boulevard
Fort Wayne, IN 46805
Phone: 219-427-6715
Web Site: www.fortwayneparks.org
Founded: 1949
Annual Attendance: 52,000

6596 PERFORMING ARTS CENTER
303 E Main Street
Fort Wayne, IN 46802
Phone: 219-422-8641
Fax: 219-422-6699
e-mail: fwcvb@visitfortwayne.com
Web Site: www.fwcvb.org
Seating Capacity: 150

6597 SCOTTISH RITE CENTER
431 W Berry Street
Fort Wayne, IN 46802
Phone: 260-423-2593
Fax: 260-426-4126
Toll-free: 877-480-8020
e-mail: srcenter1@juno.com
Web Site: www.srcenter.org
Management:
Director Marketing/Events: Samantha Teter
Founded: 1925
Paid Staff: 8
Volunteer Staff: 20
Facility Category: Theater, Ballroom, Banquet Rooms
Type of Stage: Proscenium
Stage Dimensions: 90 w x 30 d
Seating Capacity: 50 to 2,086
Year Built: 1928

Year Remodeled: 2001
Rental Contact: Director of Marketing & Events
Samantha Teter

6598 ALLEN COUNTY WAR MEMORIAL COLISEUM
4000 Parnell Avenue
Ft. Wayne, IN 46805
Phone: 260-482-9502
Fax: 260-484-1637
e-mail: rbrown@memorialcoliseum.com
Web Site: www.memorialcoliseum.com
Management:
General Manager: Randy L Brown
Founded: 1952
Specialized Field: Concerts; Family Shows;
Trade/Consumer Shows; Private Meetings & Banquets
Paid Staff: 300
Seating Capacity: 13,000

6599 IUDONS
3400 Broadway
PO Box M622
Gary, IN 46408
Phone: 219-980-6500
Fax: 219-981-4208
e-mail: vesmith@iun.edu
Web Site: www.iun.edu
Officers:
President: Dr. Vernon G Smith
Founded: 1969
Budget: 5,000 - 10,000
Annual Attendance: 2,000
Facility Category: University Auditorium
Type of Stage: Professional
Seating Capacity: 2,000
Year Built: 1980

6600 GOSHEN COLLEGE - JOHN S. UMBLE CENTER
1700 S Main
Goshen, IN 46526
Phone: 219-535-7393
Fax: 219-535-7660
e-mail: douglc@goshen.edu
Web Site: www.goshen.edu
Founded: 1978
Type of Stage: Proscenium; Thrust
Seating Capacity: 495

6601 EASTERN HOWARD PERFORMING ARTS SOCIETY
120 South Green Street
Greentown, IN 46936
Phone: 765-628-4025
Fax: 765-628-5017
Toll-free: 888-649-2787
e-mail: info@ehpas.com
Web Site: www.ehpas.com
Management:
Executive Director: Kelli Austin

Mission: Be catalysts for the cultural enrichment of the community by presenting performing arts programs to entain and enrich all audiences: futhermore, the society hopes to foster intrest and development of the arts in the schools.
Founded: 2000
Paid Staff: 2
Volunteer Staff: 27
Type of Stage: Proscenium
Year Built: 1999

6602 BUTLER ATHLETIC STADIUM

510 W 49th Street
Indianapolis, IN 46208
Phone: 317-940-9375
Fax: 317-940-9808
e-mail: info@butler.edu
Web Site: www.butler.edu
Management:
   Athletic Director: John Parry

6603 BUTLER UNIVERSITY: HINKLE FIELDHOUSE

4602 Sunset Avenue
Indianapolis, IN 46208
Phone: 317-940-9375
Fax: 317-940-9734
Management:
   Director: Elise Kushigian

6604 CLOWES MEMORIAL HALL

Butler University
4600 Sunset Avenue
Indianapolis, IN 46208
Phone: 317-940-9697
Fax: 317-940-9820
Toll-free: 800-732-0804
e-mail: ekushigi@butler.edu
Web Site: www.cloweshall.org
Founded: 1963
Annual Attendance: 185,000
Type of Stage: Proscenium
Seating Capacity: 2,172

6605 EITELJORG MUSEUM

500 W Washington Street
Indianapolis, IN 46204
Phone: 317-636-9378
e-mail: museum@eiteljorg.org
Web Site: www.eiteljorg.org
Management:
   President/CEO: John Vanausdall
   VP/Chief Curator: James Nottage
   Director Education: Cathy Burton
Mission: To inspire an appreciation and understanding of the arts, history and cultures of the American West and the indigenous people of North America. The Eiteljorg Museum collects and preserves Western art and Native American art cultural objects of the highest quality, and serves the public through ongoing exhibitions, educational programs, cultural exchanges, and entertaining special events.

6606 INDIANAPOLIS ARTS GARDEN

Arts Council of Indianapolis
47 S Pennsylvania Street
Suite 303
Indianapolis, IN 46204
Phone: 317-631-3301
Fax: 317-624-2559
e-mail: indyarts@indyarts.org
Web Site: www.indyarts.org
Mission: To enable a large and diverse audience to see, understand and enjoy the best of the worlds visual arts; to this end, the Museum collects, preserves, exhibits and interprets original works of art.
Founded: 1995

6607 INDIANAPOLIS MUSEUM OF ART

4000 Michigan Road
Indianapolis, IN 46208
Phone: 317-920-2660
Fax: 317-931-1978
e-mail: ima@ima-art.org
Web Site: www.ima-art.org
Founded: 1883
Annual Attendance: 490,000
Type of Stage: Theater
Seating Capacity: 200

6608 PIKE PERFORMING ARTS CENTER

6701 Zionsville Road
Indianapolis, IN 46268
Phone: 317-387-2783
Fax: 317-216-5460
e-mail: MAbdulla@pike.k12.in.us
Web Site: www.pike.k12.in.us/
Management:
   Executive Director: Don Steffy
   Technical Director: David Bauer
   Box Office Manager: Lorna Startzman
   Bookkeeper: Sue Thatcher
Mission: To offer quality performances and educational activities for the enjoyment and enlightenment of its public.
Founded: 1996
Paid Staff: 5
Budget: $200,000+
Income Sources: Box Office, Grants, Sponsors
Affiliations: Association of Performing Arts Presenters; Indiana Presenters Network; League of Indianapolis Theatres
Annual Attendance: 7,800
Facility Category: Performance Center
Type of Stage: Proscenium
Stage Dimensions: 52'w x 24'h x 36'8"d
Seating Capacity: 1,449
Year Built: 1997

6609 VICTORY FIELD: INDIANAPOLIS BASEBALL CLUB

501 W Maryland Street
Indianapolis, IN 46225

Phone: 317-269-3542
Fax: 317-269-3541
e-mail: indyindians@indyindians.com
Web Site: www.indyindians.com
Management:
   Chairman/President: Max B Schumacher
   General Manager: D Cal Burleson
   Business Manager: Brad Morris
   Director Operations: Randy Lewandowski
   Office Manager: Scott Rubin
   Media Relations Director: Tim Harms
   Director Advertising: Daryle Keith
   Director Special Projects: Bruce Schumacher
   Director Ticket Operations: Mike Schneider
Seating Capacity: 15,500

6610 WARREN PERFORMING ARTS CENTER

9301 E 18th Street
Indianapolis, IN 46229
Phone: 317-532-6300
Fax: 317-352-6440
e-mail: sheminge@warren.k12.in.us
Performs At: Grand Stage Auditorium, Studio Theatre
Type of Stage: Flexible
Seating Capacity: 1000; 150

6611 WARREN PERFORMING ARTS CENTER - ESCH AUDITORIUM

9301 E 18th Street
Indianapolis, IN 46229
Phone: 317-532-6280
Fax: 317-532-6440

6612 WARREN PERFORMING ARTS CENTER - STUDIO THEATER

9301 E 18th Street
Indianapolis, IN 46229
Phone: 317-532-6280
Fax: 317-532-6440

6613 MARKEY SQUARE ARENA

Pacers Basketball Corporation
300 E Market Street
Indianapolos, IN 46204
Phone: 317-639-6411
Fax: 317-261-6299
Web Site: www.marketsquaresarena.com
Management:
   VP/General Manager: Rick Fuson
   Communications Manager: Jeff Johnson
   VP/Scheduling/Production Manager: Jeff Bowen
   Concessions Manager: Rich Kapp
Seating Capacity: 16,900

6614 RCA DOME

100 S Capitol Avenue
Indianpolis, IN 46225
Phone: 317-262-3403
Fax: 317-262-3455
e-mail: blevengood@iccrd.com
Web Site: www.iccrd.com
Management:
   Executive Director: Barney Levengood

Marketing Director: Linda Addaman
Stadium Director: Michael A Fox
Suites/Special Services Manager: Heidi Mallin
General Manager/Volume Service: Dennis Cullinane
Ticket Manager: Mary Dyer
Seating Capacity: 60,500

6615 JASPER ARTS CENTER

951 College Avenue
Jasper, IN 47546
Phone: 812-482-3070
Fax: 812-634-6997
e-mail: jasperarts@psci.net
Web Site: www.jasperarts.org
Founded: 1975
Type of Stage: Proscenium

6616 LONG CENTER FOR THE PERFORMING ARTS

111 N 6th Street
Lafayette, IN 47902
Phone: 765-742-5664
Fax: 765-742-2375
e-mail: info@longcentertheater.com
Web Site: www.longcentertheater.com
Officers:
   President: Mary Reece
Management:
   Manager: Judi Best
   Technical/Maintenance: Dick Emery
   Secretary/Ticket Sales: Connie Moore
   Accountant: Shelly McConnaughey
Mission: To provide quality facilities and supporting services for the performing arts community and community gatherings, an environment that facilitates and promotes performing arts in the Lafayette community.
Founded: 1921
Paid Staff: 5

6617 BALL STATE UNIVERSITY EMENS AUDITORIUM

Ball State University
Worthen Arena 140
Muncie, IN 47306
Phone: 765-285-1539
Fax: 765-285-3719
Web Site: www.bsu.edu
Management:
   General Manager: Dan P Bymes
   Assistant Manager: Julie Strider
   Stage Manager: Keven Byral
Mission: To provide cultural, fine arts and enterainment opportunties for East Central Indiana.
Founded: 1964
Paid Staff: 10
Performs At: Emens Auditorium
Type of Stage: Black Box
Seating Capacity: 3,581

6618 CENTER FOR VISUAL AND PERFORMING ARTS

1040 Ridge Road
Munster, IN 46321

Phone: 219-836-3255
Fax: 219-836-9073
e-mail: cvpa@surfnetinc.com
Web Site: www.cvpa.org
Management:
    President: Vick Russell
Mission: To touch, enrich and entertain human beings
with live professional theatre.
Founded: 1989
Type of Stage: Thrust
Seating Capacity: 450

**6619 PAUL W OGLE CULTURAL &
COMMUNITY CENTER**
Indiana University Southeast
4201 Grant Line Road
New Albany, IN 47150-6405
Phone: 812-941-2266
Fax: 812-941-2541
e-mail: kridout@ius.edu
Web Site: www.ius.indiana.edu
Management:
    Manager: Kyle Ridout
Performs At: Concert Hall

**6620 MANCHESTER COLLEGE - CORDIER
AUDITORIUM**
604 East College Avenue
North Manchester, IN 46962
Phone: 219-982-5247
Fax: 219-982-6868
Web Site: www.manchester.edu
Founded: 1889
Seating Capacity: 1,300
Year Built: 1978

**6621 JOYCE ATHLETIC & CONVOCATION
CENTER UNIVERSITY OF NOTRE
DAME**
Notre Dame University
112 Joyce Center
Notre Dame, IN 46556
Phone: 574-631-5000
Fax: 219-631-8596
e-mail: develop.1@nd.edu
Web Site: www.nd.edu
Management:
    Director Athletic Facilities: Michael J Danch
Founded: 1842
Seating Capacity: 11,400

6622 NOTRE DAME STADIUM
1100 Grace Hall, University of Notre Dame
Notre Dame, IN 46556
Phone: 574-631-7164
Fax: 574-631-8325
e-mail: develop.1@nd.edu
Web Site: www.und.com
Management:
    Director Athletic Facilities: Michael J Danch
Seating Capacity: 80,530

**6623 CIVIC HALL PERFORMING ARTS
CENTER**
380 Hub Etchison Parkway
Richmond, IN 47374
Phone: 765-973-3350
Fax: 765-973-3346
Toll-free: 888-248-4242
e-mail: boxoffice@civichall.com
Web Site: www.civichall.com
Management:
    Facilities Director: Stuart Secttor
Founded: 1993
Specialized Field: multi-discipline
Paid Staff: 5
Volunteer Staff: 150
Seating Capacity: 924

6624 RICHMOND CIVIC THEATRE
1003 E Main Street
Richmond, IN 47374
Phone: 765-962-1816
Fax: 765-939-2572
e-mail: BMyers1068@aol.com
Web Site: www.richmondcivictheatre.org
Management:
    Office Manager: Robert Hofmann
    Technical Director: Ron Church
    Dir. Stage One Children's Theatre: Becky Jewison
Mission: To produce high quality theatrical productions
that will engage, entertain, educate, and inspire the people
of Richmond and the surrounding community, participants
and audience alike.
Type of Stage: Concert Stage

6625 CENTURY CENTER - BENDIX THEATRE
120 S St. Joseph Street
South Bend, IN 46601
Phone: 574-235-9711
Fax: 574-235-9185
e-mail: info@centurycenter.org
Web Site: www.centurtcenter.org
Founded: 1977
Type of Stage: Thrust
Seating Capacity: 694

**6626 CENTURY CENTER - CONVENTION
HALL**
120 S St. Joseph Street
South Bend, IN 46601
Phone: 574-235-9711
Fax: 574-235-9185
e-mail: info@centurycenter.org
Web Site: www.centurycenter.com
Founded: 1977

6627 CENTURY CENTER: RECITAL HALL
120 S St. Joseph Street
South Bend, IN 46601
Phone: 219-235-9711
Fax: 219-235-9185
Web Site: www.centurycenter.com

6628 MORRIS PERFORMING ARTS CENTER

211 N Michigan Street
South Bend, IN 46601
Phone: 574-235-9198
Fax: 574-235-5604
Toll-free: 800-537-6415
e-mail: dandres@morriscenter.org
Web Site: www.morriscenter.org
Management:
Executive Director: Dennis J Andres
Assistant Director: Susan Halteman
Booking Associate: Denise Chambers
Box Office Manager: Wendy Garuer
Mission: To provide a performing arts venue to the community, as well as a for community resident users.
Founded: 1922
Specialized Field: Symphony; Dance; Theatre
Paid Staff: 10
Volunteer Staff: 150
Annual Attendance: 160,000
Type of Stage: Proscenium
Seating Capacity: 2,560

6629 COMMUNITY THEATRE OF TERRE HAUTE

1431 S 25th Street
Terre Haute, IN 47803
Phone: 360-373-5152
Fax: 360-373-6754
Web Site: www.mama.indstate.edy
Officers:
President: Sonni Crawford
VP: Tim Porter
Secretary: Marti Cornelius
Treasurer: Wayne Huston

6630 HULMAN CENTER INDIANA STATE UNIVERSITY

Indiana State University
200 N 8th Street
Terre Haute, IN 47809
Phone: 812-237-3770
Fax: 812-237-3741
e-mail: hcclori@isugw.indstate.edu
Web Site: www.indstate.edu/hctaf
Management:
Director: Cliff Lambert
Facility Marketing/Ticket Sales: Jennifer Cook
Operations/Event Services Manager: Judy Price
Technical Services Supervisor: Don Knott
Founded: 1973
Specialized Field: Multi Purpose Venue
Seating Capacity: 11,000
Year Built: 1973

6631 HONEYWELL CENTER

275 W Market Streeet
Wabash, IN 46992-3057
Phone: 219-563-1102
Fax: 219-563-0873
Toll-free: 800-626-6345
e-mail: honeywell@honeywell.org
Web Site: www.honeywell.org

Management:
Executive Director: Philip L Zimmerman
Scheduling Manager: Sharon Shrider
Technical Director: Mark Goff
Executive Assistant: Bonnie McKee
Mission: Serve the local and surrounding communities through cultural and educational programs.
Founded: 1952
Status: Nonprofit
Paid Staff: 24
Volunteer Staff: 150
Budget: $3,100,000
Income Sources: Earned
Annual Attendance: 30,000
Facility Category: cultural arts/ conference
Type of Stage: Proscenium
Stage Dimensions: 50' x 30' x45'
Seating Capacity: 1500
Year Built: 1994
Year Remodeled: 1994
Cost: $17,000,000
Rental Contact: Shannon Shrider

6632 ELLIOTT HALL OF MUSIC

Purdue University
West Lafayette, IN 47907
Phone: 765-494-3935
Fax: 317-494-6621
e-mail: sdhall@purdue.edu
Web Site: www.purdue.edu/hlmc/
Management:
Assistant to the Director: Jennifer Molden
Account Clerk: Janice Sigman
Director: Steve Hall
Assistant Director: Jim Chapman
Box Office Manager: Carolanne Robinson
Fiscal Administrator: Michael Smolen
Account Clerk: Kay Gohn
House Manager: Joyce Banta
Mission: To serve our customers in West Lafayette, IN by providing an environment which enhances their Purdue university expirence while supporting the University's overall objectives of "Education Research, and Service".
Founded: 1940
Type of Stage: Proscenium
Seating Capacity: 6,025

6633 MACKEY ARENA

Purdue University
1790 Mackey Arena
West Lafayette, IN 47907
Phone: 765-494-4600
Fax: 765-784-4497
e-mail: ofd.cc@purde.edu
Web Site: www.purdue.edu
Management:
Athletic Director: Morgan Burke
Seating Capacity: 14,121

6634 PURDUE UNIVERSITY: ROSS-AIDE STADIUM

SCAA/Big Ten Conference
Purdue University
West Lafayette, IN 47907

Phone: 765-494-3189
Fax: 765-496-1280
Web Site: www.purduesports.com
Management:
  Athletic Director: Morgan Burke
  Senior Associate Athletic Director: Glenn Tompkins
  Senior Associate Athletic Director: Nancy Cross
  Associate Athletic Director: Roger Blalock
Founded: 1869
Seating Capacity: 67,332

Iowa

6635 AMES CITY AUDITORIUM
515 Clark Avenue
P.O. Box 811
Ames, IA 50010
Phone: 515-239-5365
Fax: 515-239-5404
e-mail: auditorium@city.ames.ia.us
Web Site: www.city.ames.ia.us/
Management:
  Auditorium/Activities Supervisor: Mike King
Type of Stage: Concert Stage
Seating Capacity: 869

6636 IOWA STATE UNIVERSITY-IOWA STATE CENTER
Scheman Building
Suite 4
Ames, IA 50011
Phone: 515-294-3347
Fax: 515-294-3349
Toll-free: 877-843-2368
e-mail: center@center.iastate.edu
Web Site: www.center.iastate.edu
Management:
  Executive Director: Mark North
  Director of Business and Finance: Patrick Kennedy
  Director Marketing: Curt Miller
  Director Marketing: Sara Huber
  Director Operations: Randy Baumeister
  Director Programing: Mark E Ewalt
  Tech. Director/Sound Engineering: James B Ewalt Ewalt
Mission: To develop and support the programming facilities and services necessaryto establish the Iowa State Center as the premier university public assembly complex in the United States.
Type of Stage: Concert Stage; Flexible
Seating Capacity: 3,650
Year Built: 1971

6637 IOWA STATE UNIVERSITY-IOWA STATE CENTER - STEPHENS AUDITORIUM
Scheman Building
Suite 4
Ames, IA 50011

Phone: 515-294-8123
Fax: 515-294-8997
Toll-free: 877-843-2368
e-mail: slharder@center.iastate.edu
Web Site: www.center.iastate.edu
Seating Capacity: 2,750

6638 IOWA STATE UNIVERSITY-IOWA STATE CENTER - HILTON COLLISEUM
Scheman Building
Suite 4
Ames, IA 50011
Phone: 515-294-3347
Fax: 515-294-3349
Toll-free: 877-843-2368
e-mail: center@center.iastate.edu
Web Site: www.center.iastate.edu
Seating Capacity: 14,900

6639 IOWA STATE UNIVERSITY - IOWA STATE CENTER - FISHER THEATRE
Scheman Building
Suite 4
Ames, IA 50011-1112
Phone: 515-294-3347
Fax: 515-294-3349
Toll-free: 877-843-2368
e-mail: shuber@center.iastate.edu
Web Site: www.center.iastate.edu
Seating Capacity: 450

6640 UNI-DOME
University of Northern Iowa
Business Office NE, Lower NE Offices
Cedar Falls, IA 50613
Phone: 319-273-6307
Fax: 319-273-2913
e-mail: Gerald.Peterson@uni.edu
Web Site: www.uni.edu
Management:
  Facility Coodinator: Dave Kohrs
  Ticket Manager: Greg Davies
  Special Events Coordinator: Shandon Hoffmeier
  Associate AD/Internal Operations: Justin Sell
  Assistant Operations Coordinator: Ryan McKernan
Founded: 1976
Seating Capacity: 25,000
Rental Contact: Ryan McKernan

6641 UNIVERSITY OF NORTHERN IOWA - GALLAGHER BLUEDORN
Gallagher Bluedorn Performing Arts Center
University of Northern Iowa
Cedar Falls, IA 50614
Phone: 319-273-3660
Fax: 319-273-7470
Toll-free: 877-549-7469
e-mail: gbpac@uni.edu
Web Site: www.uni.edu/gbpac
Management:
  Executive Director: Steve Carignan
  Department Secretary: Carol Aswegan-Thornhill
  House/Events Manager: Kimberly Buchan

Technical Director: Shawn DuBois
Assistant Technical Director: Jennifer Gray
Outreach/Education Director: Beatrice Foley
Assistant House Manager: Joan Hovey
Audio Engineer: Sandy Norcdahl
Assistant Box Office Manager: Susan Trahan
Founded: 2000
Specialized Field: Present Arts
Paid Staff: 12
Volunteer Staff: 350
Type of Stage: Tongue-in-groove oak
Stage Dimensions: 55'W X 40'H

6642 UNIVERSITY OF NORTHERN IOWA: STRAYER-WOOD THEATRE

Department of Theatre
125 SWT
Cedar Falls, IA 50614-0371
Phone: 319-273-6307
Fax: 319-273-6390
e-mail: Steve.Taft@uni.edu
Web Site: www.uni.edu
Management:
   Department Head: Steve Taft
Mission: Education of future theatre artists.
Founded: 1976
Specialized Field: Theatre
Paid Staff: 3
Paid Artists: 11
Facility Category: Theater house
Type of Stage: Proscenium
Stage Dimensions: 22 x 84 x 39
Seating Capacity: 500
Year Built: 1978
Rental Contact: Eric Lange

6643 FIVE SEASONS CENTER

370 1st Avenue NE
Cedar Rapids, IA 52401
Phone: 319-398-5211
Fax: 319-362-2102
e-mail: s.cummins@5seasons.com
Web Site: www.5seasons.com
Management:
   Assistant Executive Director: Sharon Cummins
   Director Programs: Roy Nowers
   Director Marketing: Tammky Koolbeck
Founded: 1920
Specialized Field: Multi-purpose arena
Type of Stage: Wood
Seating Capacity: 1,901
Year Built: 1979

6644 PARAMOUNT THEATRE

123 3rd Avenue SE
Cedar Rapids, IA 52401
Mailing Address: 370 1st Avenue NE Cedar Rapids IA, 52401
Phone: 319-398-5211
Fax: 319-362-2102
e-mail: s.cummins@uscellularcenter.com
Web Site: www.uscellularcenter.com
Management:
   Executive Director: Sharon Cummins

   Director Programming: Roy Nowers
   Marketing Manager: Christy Frost
Affiliations: Homr of Cedar Rapids Symphony Orchestra, Cedar Rapids Area Theatre Organ Society, Community Concerts, Broadway Series, School Programming Series

6645 US CELLULAR CENTER

370 1st Avenue NE
Cedar Rapids, IA 52401
Phone: 319-398-5211
Fax: 319-362-2102
e-mail: s.cummins@uscellularcenter.com
Web Site: www.uscellularcenter.com
Management:
   Executive Director: Sharon Cummins
   Director Programming: Roy Nowers
   Marketing Manager: Christy Frost
Facility Category: Arena
Type of Stage: Stageright
Seating Capacity: 914
Year Built: 1978
Rental Contact: R Nowers

6646 RIVERVIEW STADIUM

PO Box 1295
Clinton, IA 52733
Phone: 563-242-0727
Fax: 563-242-1433
e-mail: lumberkings@lumberkings.com
Web Site: www.lumberkings.com/contact_us.htm
Management:
   General Manager: Ted Tornow
Founded: 1937
Seating Capacity: 3,600

6647 GALVIN FINE ARTS CENTER

518 W Locust Street
Davenport, IA 52803
Phone: 319-333-6251
Fax: 319-333-6243
e-mail: lsadlek@saunix.sau.edu
Web Site: www.sau.edu/administration/galvin/
Management:
   Director: Lance Sadlek
Founded: 1971
Performs At: Allaert Hall

6648 QUAD CITY RIVER BANDITS BASEBALL CLUB

PO Box 3496
209 S Gaines Street
Davenport, IA 52808
Phone: 563-324-3000
Fax: 319-324-3109
e-mail: bandit@riverbandits.com
Web Site: www.riverbandits.com
Management:
   Genaral Manager: Dave Ziedells
   Sales Director: Pete Cunico
   Marketing Director: Matt Beatty
Seating Capacity: 6,200

6649 SAINT AMBROSE COLLEGE - ALLAERT AUDITORIUM
Galvin Fine Arts Center
518 W Locust Street
Davenport, IA 52803
Phone: 319-333-6000
Fax: 319-336-6243
e-mail: webmaster@sau.edu
Web Site: www.sau.edu
Founded: 1882
Specialized Field: Art; Music; Theatre; Communication
Annual Attendance: 134,000
Facility Category: Auditorium
Type of Stage: Proscenium
Seating Capacity: 1,200

6650 SAINT AMBROSE COLLEGE - GALVIN FINE ARTS CENTER
518 W Locust Street
Davenport, IA 52803
Phone: 563-333-6427
e-mail: cjohnson@sau.edu
Web Site: www.web.sau.edu/theatre
Officers:
    Chairperson Theatre: Dr. Corinne Johnson
Founded: 1971

6651 CIVIC CENTER OF GREATER DES MOINES
221 Walnut Street
Des Moines, IA 50309
Phone: 515-246-2328
Fax: 515-246-2325
e-mail: info@civiccenter.org
Web Site: www.civiccenter.org
Management:
    General Manager: Jeffrey L Chelesvig
Founded: 1979
Opened: 1979
Status: Nonprofit
Annual Attendance: 275,000
Seating Capacity: 2,735
Rental Contact: General Manager Bill McElrath

6652 DES MOINES WOMEN'S CLUB
Hoyt Sherman Place
1501 Woodland
Des Moines, IA 50309
Phone: 515-244-0507
Fax: 515-237-3582
e-mail: barcus@hoytsherman.org
Web Site: www.hoytsherman.org/contact.html
Founded: 1995
Specialized Field: Theatre
Annual Attendance: 200,000
Type of Stage: Proscenium
Seating Capacity: 1,400

6653 DRAKE STADIUM
Drake University
2507 University Avenue
Des Moines, IA 50311

Phone: 515-271-2889
Fax: 515-271-3015
Web Site: www.drakebulldogs.org
Management:
    Athletic Director: Dave Blank
Founded: 1925
Seating Capacity: 18,000

6654 DRAKE UNIVERSITY - OLD MAIN AUDITORIUM
2507 University Avenue
Des Moines, IA 50311
Phone: 515-271-3939
Fax: 515-271-3977
e-mail: lisa.lacher@drake.edu
Web Site: www.drake.edu
Seating Capacity: 100-200

6655 DRAKE UNIVERSITY - HALL OF PERFORMING ARTS HARMON FINE ARTS CENTER
2508 University Avenue
Des Moines, IA 50311
Phone: 515-271-2018
Fax: 515-271-3977
e-mail: lisa.lacher@drake.edu
Web Site: www.drake.edu
Seating Capacity: 460

6656 VETERANS MEMORIAL AUDITORIUM
Regional Facilities, Polk County
833 5th Avenue
Des Moines, IA 50309
Phone: 515-323-5400
Fax: 515-323-5401
e-mail: eventscenterfriends@hotmail.com
Web Site: www.co.polk.ia.us
Management:
    Director: F Michael Grimaldi
    Marketing/Event Manager: Joy Giudicessi
Founded: 1954
Facility Category: Arena
Type of Stage: Concert
Seating Capacity: 7,200
Year Built: 1954
Year Remodeled: 1997

6657 DUBUQUE FIVE FLAGS CENTER
PO Box 628
Dubuque, IA 52001
Phone: 563-589-4254
Fax: 563-589-4351
e-mail: 5flags@cityofdubuque.org
Web Site: www.cityofdubuque.org
Management:
    Director: Carole Barry
Founded: 1971
Seating Capacity: 5,200

6658 FIVE FLAGS CENTER - ARENA
4th and Main Streets
PO Box 628
Dubuque, IA 52001
Phone: 563-589-4258
Fax: 563-589-4351
e-mail: 5flags@cityofdubuque.org
Web Site: www.cityofdubuque.org
Founded: 1971
Seating Capacity: 5,200

6659 FIVE FLAGS CENTER - THEATRE
4th and Main Streets
PO Box 628
Dubuque, IA 52001
Phone: 563-589-4258
Fax: 563-589-4351
e-mail: 5flags@cityofdubuque.org
Web Site: www.cityofdubuque.org

6660 MAHARISHI UNIVERSITY OF MANAGEMENT - STUDENT ACTIVITIES
1000 North Fourth Street
Maharishi University of Management, SU 361
Fairfield, IA 52557
Phone: 641-472-1104
Fax: 641-472-7000
e-mail: student_activities@mum.edu
Web Site: www.mum.edu

6661 OLD CREAMERY THEATRE
39 38th Avenue
Suite 200
Garrison, IA 52203
Phone: 319-622-6194
Toll-free: 800-352-6262
Web Site: www.oldcreamery.com
Officers:
   President-Amana: Bruce Eickhacker
   VP-Cedar Rapids: Richard Welch
   Secretary - Vinton: Ron Baldwin
   Treasurer-Amana: Vic Rathje
Management:
   Producing/Artistic Director: Thomas P Johnson
   Associate Artistic Director: Meg Merckens
   Associate Artistic Director: Sean McCall
   General Manager: Pat Wagner
Founded: 1971
Seating Capacity: 275

6662 KINNICK STADIUM/UNIVERSITY OF IOWA
University of Iowa
157 Carver-Hawkeye Arena
Iowa City, IA 52242
Phone: 319-335-9410
Fax: 319-335-9333
e-mail: gohawks@hawkeyesports.com
Web Site: www.hawkeyesports.com
Management:
   Facility Manager: Dilbert E Gehrke
Specialized Field: Home of University of Iowa athletics

Seating Capacity: 70,111

6663 UNIVERSITY OF IOWA - HANCHER AUDITORIUM
The University of Iowa Foundation
PO Box 4550
Iowa City, IA 52244
Phone: 319-335-3305
Toll-free: 800-648-6973
e-mail: margaret-reese@uiowa.edu
Web Site: www.uifoundation.org/hancher
Management:
   Associate Director of Development: Margaret Nothnagle Reese
   Assistant Director Development: Erik Thurman
Founded: 1972
Annual Attendance: 20,000+

6664 CHARLES H MACNIDER ART MUSEUM
303 2nd Street SE
Mason City, IA 50401
Phone: 641-421-3666
e-mail: macnider@macniderart.org
Web Site: www.macniderart.org
Management:
   Director: Richard Leet
   Education Coordinator: Linda Willeke
   Financial Secretary: Audrey Gabel

6665 NORTH IOWA COMMUNITY AUDITORIUM
500 College Drive
Mason City, IA 50401
Phone: 641-423-1264
Fax: 641-423-1711
e-mail: request@niacc.edu
Web Site: www.niacc.com

6666 NORTHWESTERN COLLEGE
101 7th Street SW
Orange City, IA 51041
Phone: 712-707-7000
Web Site: www.nwciowa.edu
Mission: To provide a distinctively Christian liberal arts education of recognized quality in a primarily undergraduate, co-educational, multicultural, residential environment.

6667 ROBERTS STADIUM
1491 S Paxton
PO Box 3183
Sioux City, IA 51102
Phone: 712-279-6651
Fax: 712-279-6651
e-mail: saaron@smgevansville.com
Web Site: www.robertstadium.com
Management:
   Manager Public Schools: Ray Rowe
Seating Capacity: 7,000

6668 HOPE MARTIN THEATRE
PO Box 433
Waterloo, IA 50704
Phone: 319-235-0367
Fax: 319-235-7489
e-mail: wcpbhct@cedarnet.org
Web Site: www.cedarnet.org/wcpbhct/
Officers:
 President: Bryan Molinaro-Blonigan
 VP Fund Developement: Stephen Saladrigas
 VP Marketing: Beverly McCusker
 Secretary: Linda Neese
 Treasurer: Chad Abbas
 Past President: Jerry Oberheu
Management:
 Artistic/Managing Director: Charles Stilwill
 Designer/Production Manager: Steve Stabenow
 Marketing/Development Director: Mary Beth
 O'Brien

6669 WATERLOO RIVERFRONT STADIUM
850 Park Road
Waterloo, IA 50704
Phone: 319-232-5633
Fax: 319-232-6140
Management:
 Manager: Eric Snider
Seating Capacity: 4,000

6670 WARTBURG COLLEGE - NEUMANN AUDITORIUM
PO Box 1003
100 Wartburg Blvd
Waverly, IA 50677
Phone: 319-352-8200
Fax: 319-352-8501
Toll-free: 800-772-2085
e-mail: webmaster@wartburg.edu
Web Site: www.wartburg.edu/tour/Neumann.html
Officers:
 Art Department Chairman: Thomas Payne
Seating Capacity: 1,400

Kansas

6671 MEMORIAL AUDITORIUM
101 S Lincoln
PO Box 907
Chanute, KS 66720
Phone: 316-431-5229
Fax: 316-431-5239
Toll-free: 800-735-5229
e-mail: tourism@chanute.org
Web Site: www.chanute.org
Founded: 1925
Paid Staff: 2
Seating Capacity: 1,243

6672 FLORAL HALL
PO Box 1629
Coffeyville, KS 67337
Phone: 316-251-9794

Stage Dimensions: 8x15 (meters)

6673 DODGE CITY CIVIC CENTER
PO Box 939
311 W Spruce
Dodge City, KS 67801
Phone: 620-227-9501
Fax: 620-338-8734
Toll-free: 800-381-3690
e-mail: dodgedev@pld.com
Web Site: www.dodgedev.org

6674 FORT HAYS STATE UNIVERSITY-FELTON CENTER
600 Park Street
Hays, KS 67601
Phone: 785-628-5801
Fax: 785-628-4007
e-mail: cbrock@fhsu.edu
Web Site: www.fhsu.edu
Management:
 Special Events Coordinator: Carol Brock

6675 KANSAS STATE FAIR - GRANDSTAND
2000 N Poplar Street
Hutchinson
Hutchinson, KS 67502
Phone: 620-669-3600
Fax: 620-669-3640
e-mail: info@kansasstatefair.com
Web Site: www.kansasstatefair.com

6676 BOWLUS FINE ARTS CENTER
205 E Madison
Iola, KS 66749
Phone: 316-365-4765
Web Site: www.bowluscenter.com
Management:
 Marketing/Finance Director: Tammu Porter
 Executive Director: Mary Martin
Mission: Attracts nationally-acclaimed performers to the area. Also houses a fine arts education center. The Bowlus provides display areas for local and visiting artists, while maintaining a permanent collection of distinctive paintings.

6677 ALLEN FIELDHOUSE
Athletics Department, University of Kansas
1651 Naismith Drive, Lawrence
Lawrence, KS 66045
Phone: 785-864-3143
Fax: 785-864-5517
e-mail: facilities@jayhawks.org
Web Site: www.jayhwks.edu
Management:
 Director Promotions: Rick Mullen
Founded: 1955
Seating Capacity: 16,300

6678 LIED CENTER OF KANSAS
University of Kansas
1600 Stewart Drive, Lawrence
Lawrence, KS 66045
Phone: 785-864-3469
Fax: 785-864-5450
e-mail: lied@ku.edu
Web Site: www.lied.ku.edu
Management:
  Executive Director: Tim Van Leer
  Associate Director: Karen Lane Christilles
Founded: 1993
Specialized Field: Presenting
Type of Stage: Proscenium
Seating Capacity: 2,018

6679 UNIVERSITY OF KANSAS: CRAFTON-PREYER THEATRE
Murphy Hall
1530 Naismith Drive
Lawrence, KS 66045
Phone: 785-864-3381
Fax: 785-864-5251
e-mail: cjenkins@ku.edu
Web Site: www.kutheatre.com
Management:
  Public Relations Director: Charla Jenkins
  Artistic Director: John Staniunas
Founded: 1923
Specialized Field: Theatre
Paid Staff: 10
Income Sources: State of Kansas and Box Office
Annual Attendance: 65,000
Facility Category: University Theatre
Type of Stage: Proscenium
Seating Capacity: 1,180
Year Built: 1957

6680 SAINT MARY COLLEGE - XAVIER HALL THEATRE
4100 S 4th Street
Leavenworth
Leavenworth, KS 66048
Phone: 913-682-5151
Fax: 914-758-6140
Toll-free: 800-752-7043
e-mail: enroll@hub.smcks.edu
Web Site: www.smcks.edu

6681 BETHANY COLLEGE - BURNETT CENTER
421 North First Street
Lindsborg
Lindsborg, KS 67456
Phone: 785-227-3311
Fax: 785-227-2004
Toll-free: 800-826-2281
e-mail: legault@bethanylb.edu
Web Site: www.bethanylb.edu

6682 FRED BRAMIAGE COLISEUM
Kansas State University
Bramlage Coliseum, 1800 College Avenue
Suite 133, Manhattan
Manhattan, KS 66502
Phone: 785-532-7600
Fax: 785-532-7655
e-mail: bramlage@ksu.edu
Web Site: www.ksu.edu
Management:
  Director: Charles E Thomas
Founded: 1988
Type of Stage: Concert Stage
Seating Capacity: 14,000

6683 KANSAS STATE UNIVERSITY - MCCAIN AUDITORIUM
Kansas State University
207 McCain Auditorium, Manhattan
Manhattan, KS 66506
Phone: 785-532-6428
Fax: 785-532-5870
e-mail: mcctxt@ksu.edu
Web Site: www.ksu.edu
Officers:
  President: Eugene Klingler
  President Elect: Katie Philip
  VP: Ann Murray
  Secretary: Nancy Ryan
  Treasurer: Eugene Laughlin
Management:
  Director: Richard P Martin
  Operations Officer: Kathleen Emig
  Marketing/Development Officer: Thomas E Jackson
  Public Programming/Performance Tech: Terri Lee
  Ticket Services Manager: Karen Kimbrough
Seating Capacity: 1,751

6684 MANHATTAN ARTS CENTER
1520 Poyntz Avenue
Manhattan
Manhattan, KS 66502
Phone: 785-537-4420
Fax: 785-539-3356
e-mail: boxoffice@manhattanarts.org
Web Site: www.manhattanarts.org
Officers:
  President: Jim Hamilton
Management:
  Executive Director: Penny Senftem
Mission: To make arts activities available to all.
Founded: 1996
Specialized Field: Galleries; Live Theatre; Concerts; Classes
Status: Nonprofit
Paid Staff: 3
Volunteer Staff: 75
Budget: $250,000
Income Sources: Kansas Arts Commission; City of Manhattan; Foundations; Private Donations
Performs At: Multi-use Arts Center
Annual Attendance: 4,500
Type of Stage: Black Box
Seating Capacity: 160

Year Remodeled: 1996
Organization Type: Educational; Sponsoring

6685 MCPHERSON COLLEGE - BROWN AUDITORIUM
1600 East Euclid
P.O. Box 1402, McPherson
McPherson, KS 67460
Phone: 316-241-0731
Fax: 316-241-8443
Toll-free: 800-365-7402
e-mail: admiss@mcpherson.edu
Web Site: www.mcpherson.edu
Management:
    Computer Services Director: David D Gitchell
    Business Manager: Shirley Reissig
    Library/Media Services Director: Rowena Olsen

6686 NEODESHA ARTS ASSOCIATION
PO Box 65
5th Street & Indiana
Neodesha, KS 66757
Phone: 316-325-3422
Fax: 316-325-3122
e-mail: neodeshaart@yahoo.com
Management:
    Executive: Teresa Railsback
Mission: The mission is to improve the quality of life in Neodesha and surrounding area through presentation of cultutral activities in which the arts fourish.
Founded: 1973
Paid Staff: 1
Volunteer Staff: 13
Paid Artists: 1
Non-paid Artists: 3

6687 OTTAWA MUNICIPAL AUDITORIUM
PO Box 452
301 South Hickory Street, Ottawa
Ottawa, KS 66067
Phone: 785-242-8810
Fax: 785-229-3760
Founded: 1890
Seating Capacity: 840

6688 JOHNSON COUNTY COMMUNITY COLLEGE, CARLSEN CENTER
12345 College Boulevard, CC 105
Overland Park, KS 66210
Phone: 913-469-8500
Fax: 913-469-4409
e-mail: webmaster@jccc.net
Web Site: www.jccc.net
Management:
    Carlsen Center Director: Charles Rogers
Performs At: Yardley Hall

6689 CARNIE SMITH STADIUM
1701 South Broadway
Pittsburg, KS 66762

Phone: 316-231-7000
Fax: 316-235-4661
e-mail: acad@pittstate.edu
Web Site: www.pittstate.edu
Management:
    Athletic Director: Chuck Broyles
Annual Attendance: 238,911
Seating Capacity: 8,343

6690 MEMORIAL AUDITORIUM AND CONVENTION CENTER
503 N Pine
Pittsburg, KS 66762
Phone: 316-231-7827
Fax: 316-231-5967
e-mail: judyc@pittks.org
Web Site: www.pittks.org
Management:
    Manager: Judy Collins
    Office Manager: Janice Arthur
    Technical Director: David Stubbs
Founded: 1925
Paid Staff: 5
Annual Attendance: 10,000
Facility Category: Concert Hall, Children's theater
Type of Stage: Proscenium
Stage Dimensions: 90 x 37
Seating Capacity: 1588
Year Built: 1923
Year Remodeled: 1984
Architect: Seidler, Owsley and Associates
Cost: $3.4 million
Rental Contact: Manager Judy Collins

6691 PITTSBURGH STATE UNIVERSITY: WEEDE ARENA
1701 S Broadway
Pittsburg, KS 66762
Phone: 316-235-4646
Fax: 316-235-4661
Web Site: www.oitstate.edu
Management:
    Athletic Director: Chuck Broyles
    Sports Information Director: Dan Wilkes
    Head Football Coach: Chuck Broyles
    Head Basketball Coach (M): Swede Trenkle
    Head Basketball Coach (W): Steve High
    Assistant Director Athletics: Steve Bever
    Marketing/Promotions Director: Tommy Riggs
Seating Capacity: 6,000

6692 SALINA BICENTENNIAL CENTER
PO Box 1727
800 The Midway
Salina, KS 67402
Phone: 785-826-7200
Fax: 785-826-7207
Toll-free: 888-826-7469
e-mail: info@bicentennial.org
Web Site: www.bicentennial.org
Seating Capacity: 2,000

All listings are in alphabetical order by state, then city, then organization within the city.

6693 KANSAS EXPOCENTRE
One Expocentre Drive
Topeka, KS 66612
Phone: 785-235-1986
Fax: 785-235-2967
e-mail: RoyM@ksexpo.com
Web Site: www.ksexpo.com
Management:
General Manager: HR Cook
Director Operations: Roy Mitchell
Director Marketing: Shannon Reilly
Founded: 1987
Specialized Field: Multi-purpose facility
Seating Capacity: 10,000
Year Built: 1987

6694 TOPEKA PERFORMING ARTS CENTER
214 E 8th Avenue
Topeka, KS 66603
Phone: 785-297-9000
Fax: 785-234-2307
e-mail: hhansen@tpactix.org
Web Site: www.tpactix.org
Management:
Executive Director: Harold Hansen
Founded: 1990
Seating Capacity: 4,200

6695 WASHBURN UNIVERSITY: LEE ARENA
1700 College Avenue
Topeka, KS 66621
Phone: 785-231-1010
Fax: 785-231-1091
Web Site: www.washburn.edu
Management:
Athletic Director: Loren Ferre
Facilities Manager: Gilbert Herrera
Seating Capacity: 4,500

6696 KANSAS COLISEUM
1229 E 85th Street N
Valley Center, KS 67147
Phone: 316-755-1243
Fax: 316-755-2869
e-mail: info@kansascoliseum.com
Web Site: www.kansascoliseum.com
Management:
Director: John W Nath
Assistant Director: David Rush
Specialized Field: Multi-purpose arena. Home of the
Wichita Thunder (CHL) and Wichita Stealth
Annual Attendance: 700,000
Seating Capacity: 9,600; 12,400
Year Built: 1978

6697 COLUMBIAN THEATRE: MUSEUM & ART CENTER
521 Lincoln Avenue
PO Box 72
Wamego, KS 66547

Phone: 785-456-2029
Fax: 785-456-9498
Toll-free: 800-899-1893
e-mail: ctheatre@wamego.net
Web Site: www.columbiantheatre.com
Founded: 1895
Annual Attendance: 12,000
Seating Capacity: 284

6698 WELLINGTON MEMORIAL AUDITORIUM
PO Box 564
Wellington, KS 67152
Phone: 316-326-3303
Fax: 316-326-8506
Management:
Manager: Ellen McCue

6699 CENTURY II CIVIC CENTER - CONVENTION HALL
225 W Douglas Avenue
Wichita, KS 67202
Phone: 316-264-9121
Fax: 316-268-9268
e-mail: kpearson@century2.org
Web Site: www.century2.org
Type of Stage: Proscenium
Seating Capacity: 5244 ; 4,100

6700 CENTURY II CIVIC CENTER - EXHIBITION HALL
225 W Douglas Avenue
Wichita, KS 67202
Phone: 316-264-9121
Fax: 316-268-9268
e-mail: kpearson@century2.org
Web Site: www.century2.org
Type of Stage: Proscenium
Seating Capacity: 2,000

6701 CENTURY II CIVIC CENTER - THEATRE
225 W Douglas Avenue
Wichita, KS 67202
Phone: 316-264-9121
Fax: 316-268-9268
e-mail: kpearson@century2.org
Web Site: www.century2.org
Type of Stage: Proscenium

6702 CENTURY II CONVENTION & PERFORMING ARTS CENTER
225 W Douglas Avenue
Wichita, KS 67202
Phone: 316-264-9121
Fax: 316-303-8688
e-mail: kpearson@century2.org
Web Site: www.century2.org
Facility Category: Convention & performing arts center
Type of Stage: Proscenium
Stage Dimensions: 60 W x 29 H x 33 D
Year Built: 1960

Rental Contact: Kathy Pearson

6703 CESSNA STADIUM
Wichita State University
1845 Fairmount Street
Wichita, KS 67260
Phone: 316-978-3023
Fax: 316-978-3336
e-mail: hicks@twsuvm.uc.twsu.edu
Web Site: www.wichita.edu
Management:
  Sports Information Director: Larry Rankin
Founded: 1969
Seating Capacity: 10,432

6704 WICHITA STATE UNIVERSITY: HENRY LEVITT ARENA
1845 Fairmount Street
Campus Box 12
Wichita, KS 67260
Phone: 316-978-STET
Fax: 316-978-3336
Web Site: www.twsu.edu
Management:
  Director Athletics: Jim Schalf

Kentucky

6705 PARAMOUNT ARTS CENTER
1300 Winchester Avenue
PO Box 1546
Ashland, KY 41105
Phone: 606-324-3175
Fax: 606-324-1233
e-mail: tysonc@paramountartscenter.com
Web Site: www.paramountartscenter.com
Management:
  Executive Director: Kathleen Timmons
  Marketing Director: Tyson Compton
Mission: The Paramount Theatre, originally designed and built to show motion pictures, has provided an intamite venue for a variety of performances since it opened in 1931.
Paid Staff: 10
Volunteer Staff: 100
Annual Attendance: 240,000
Facility Category: Performing Arts
Type of Stage: Proscenium
Seating Capacity: 1400
Year Built: 1931
Year Remodeled: 2001
Cost: $ 9 Million
Rental Contact: Cindy Collins

6706 J DAN TALBOTT AMPHITHEATRE
My Old Kentucky Home State Park
Bardstown, KY 40004
Phone: 502-348-5971
Toll-free: 800-626-1563
Web Site: www.stephenfoster.com/theatre.htm
Founded: 1959
Season: June - August

Seating Capacity: 1450
Year Built: 1959
Year Remodeled: 1997
Cost: $1.6 million

6707 PHELPS-STOKES AUDITORIUM AT BEREA COLLEGE
Berea College Campus
CPO 2220
Berea, KY 40404
Phone: 606-985-3000
Fax: 606-985-3512
Toll-free: 800-326-5948
e-mail: linda_avery@berea.edu
Web Site: www.berea.edu

6708 CAPITOL ARTS CENTER
416 E Main Street
Bowling Green, KY 42101
Phone: 270-782-2787
Fax: 270-782-2804
Toll-free: 877-694-2787
Web Site: www.capitolarts.com

6709 DIDDLE ARENA
Western Kentucky University
1 Big Red Way
Bowling Green, KY 42101
Phone: 502-745-3542
Fax: 502-745-6187
e-mail: western@wku.edu
Web Site: www.wku.edu/athletics
Management:
  Director: Wood Selid

6710 LT SMITH STADIUM/WESTERN KENTUCKY UNIVERSITY
1 Big Red Way
Bowling Green, KY 42101
Phone: 502-745-3542
Fax: 502-745-6187
Web Site: www.wku.edu/athletics
Management:
  Director: Wood Selid
  Associate Athletic Director: Pam Herriford
  Associate Athletic Director: Matt Pope
  Coordinator Marketing/Promotions: Wayne Orscheln
Seating Capacity: 17,000

6711 NORTON CENTER FOR THE ARTS
Centre College
600 W Walnut Street
Danville, KY 40422
Phone: 859-236-4692
Fax: 859-238-5448
Toll-free: 877-448-7469
e-mail: chafin@centre.edu
Web Site: www.centre.edu
Founded: 1973
Seating Capacity: Newlin Hall-1500; Weisiger Theatre-360

All listings are in alphabetical order by state, then city, then organization within the city.

Year Built: 1973
Year Remodeled: 1994

6712 HENDERSON FINE ARTS CENTER
Henderson Fine Arts Center
2660 S Green Street
Henderson, KY 42420
Phone: 270-827-1867
Fax: 270-830-5307
Toll-free: 800-696-9958
Web Site: www.hencc.kctcs.net
Management:
    Director: Rachael Baar

6713 COMMONWEALTH STADIUM
University of Kentucky
Memorial Coliseum
Room 23
Lexington, KY 40506
Phone: 859-257-3838
Fax: 859-323-4310
Web Site: www.ukathletics.com
Management:
    Athletic Director: CM Newton
    Facility Manager: Suzanne Truitt
Founded: 1973
Seating Capacity: 57,800
Year Built: 1973

6714 LEXINGTON CENTER COMPLEX
430 W Vine Street
Lexington, KY 40507
Phone: 606-233-4567
Fax: 606-253-2718
e-mail: comments@rupparena.com
Web Site: www.lexingtoncenter.com
Officers:
    President: William B Owen
Management:
    Director Sports/Entertainment: Rick Reno
Seating Capacity: 23,500

6715 LEXINGTON OPERA HOUSE
430 W Vine Street
Lexington, KY 40507
Phone: 606-233-4567
Fax: 606-253-2718
e-mail: rreno@rupparena.com
Web Site: www.lexingtonoperahouse.com
Founded: 1886
Seating Capacity: 1,000
Year Built: 1886
Year Remodeled: 1972

6716 SINGLETARY CENTER FOR THE ARTS
University of Kentucky
Lexington, KY 40506
Phone: 606-257-1706
Fax: 606-323-9991
Web Site: www.uky.edu/SCFA/
Founded: 1979
Paid Staff: 71
Volunteer Staff: 70

Annual Attendance: 115,000
Seating Capacity: Concert Hall-1500; Recital Hall-400

6717 TRANSYLVANIA UNIVERSITY
300 N Broadway
Lexington, KY 40508
Phone: 859-233-8300
Fax: 859-233-8797
e-mail: Admissions@transy.edu
Web Site: www.transy.edu
Founded: 1780

6718 UNIVERSITY OF KENTUCKY: MEMORIAL COLISEUM
UKAA Memorial Coliseum
Lexington, KY 40506
Phone: 606-257-8000
Fax: 606-257-6303
Web Site: www.ukathletics.com
Management:
    Athletic Director: CM Newton
    Senior Associate Director Athletics: Larry Ivy
    Associate Director Athletics: Kathleen DeBoer
    Associate Director: Bob Bradley
    Assistant Director Athletics: Sandy Bell
    Assistant Director Athletics: John Cropp
    Assistant Director Athletics: Alvis Johnson
    Assistant Director Athletics: Kyle Moats
    Assistant Director Athletics: Russ Pear
Seating Capacity: 11,500

6719 CARDINAL STADIUM
937 Phillips Lane
PO Box 37130
Louisville, KY 40209
Phone: 502-367-5000
Fax: 502-367-5139
e-mail: clark.bertloff@mail.state.ky.us
Web Site: www.kyfairexpo.org
Management:
    President/CEO: Harold Workman
    Operations Director: Larryy Faue
Specialized Field: Sports Stadium for baseball and NCAA.
Seating Capacity: 47,925
Year Built: 1956
Year Remodeled: 1981

6720 FREEDOM HALL ARENA
PO Box 37130
Louisville, KY 40233
Phone: 502-367-5000
Fax: 502-367-5139
e-mail: ellen.anderson@mail.state.ky.us
Web Site: www.kyfairexpo.org
Management:
    President/CEO: Harold Workman
    Operations Director: Larry Faue
Specialized Field: Home of University of Louisville athletics (NCAA)
Seating Capacity: 19,169
Year Built: 1956
Year Remodeled: 1984

6721 KENTUCKY CENTER FOR THE ARTS
501 W Main Street
Louisville, KY 40202
Phone: 502-562-0100
Fax: 502-562-0750
e-mail: info@kca.org
Web Site: www.kca.org
Management:
   Program Director: Ken Clay
Founded: 1980

**6722 KENTUCKY CENTER FOR THE ARTS -
BOMHARD THEATRE**
501 W Main Street
Louisville, KY 40202
Phone: 502-562-0100
Fax: 502-562-0150
e-mail: info@kca.org
Web Site: www.kca.org
Seating Capacity: 619

**6723 KENTUCKY CENTER FOR THE ARTS -
WHITNEY HALL**
501 W Main Street
Louisville, KY 40202
Phone: 502-562-0100
Fax: 502-562-0150
e-mail: info@kca.org
Web Site: www.kca.org
Seating Capacity: 2,406

**6724 LOUISVILLE MEMORIAL
AUDITORIUM**
970 S 4th Street
Louisville, KY 40202
Phone: 502-584-4911
Fax: 502-574-4318
Specialized Field: Gospel Shows; Stage Plays; Small
Concerts; Children's Shows; Dance and Talent
Competitions
Paid Staff: 4
Annual Attendance: 100,000
Facility Category: Auditorium
Stage Dimensions: 50' x 85'
Year Built: 1929
Rental Contact: Dale Royer

6725 MACAULEY THEATRE
315 W Broadway
Louisville, KY 40202
Phone: 502-562-0194
Fax: 502-562-0188

**6726 MADISONVILLE COMMUNITY
COLLEGE GLEMA MAHR CENTER FOR
THE ARTS**
2000 College Drive
Madisonville, KY 42431
Phone: 270-821-2250
Fax: 270-821-5555
e-mail: bradley.downall@kctcs.net
Web Site: www.madcc.kctcs.net

6727 JAYNE STADIUM
150 University Blvd.
Morehead, KY 40351
Phone: 606-783-2088
Fax: 606-783-5035
e-mail: s.mays@moreheadstate.edu
Web Site: www.morehead-st.edu
Management:
   VP/Director: Mike Mincey

**6728 MURRAY STATE UNIVERSITY: LOVETT
AUDITORIUM**
1401 State Route 121 N
Murray, KY 42071-3362
Phone: 270-762-5577
Fax: 270-762-5511
Web Site: www.murraystate.edu
Management:
   Facility Manager: Shelley Todd
Founded: 1926
Facility Category: Auditorium

**6729 RACER ARENA/MURRAY STATE
UNIVERSITY**
Murray State University
Athletic Department
Murray, KY 42071
Phone: 502-762-6800
Fax: 270-762-5498
e-mail: webmaster@murraystate.edu
Web Site: www.murraystate.edu
Management:
   Athletic Director: EW Dennison
Founded: 1997
Seating Capacity: 5,500

6730 REGIONAL SPECIAL EVENTS CENTER
1401 State Soute 121 N
Murray, KY 42071
Phone: 270-762-5577
Fax: 502-762-5511
e-mail: rsec@murraystate.edu
Web Site: www.murraystate.edu
Management:
   Director Sales/Marketing: Shelly Todd
   Operations Supervisor: Kenny Gibson
Seating Capacity: 8,538

**6731 OWENSBORO SPORTSCENTER CITY
OF OWENSBORO**
101 East 4th Street
PO Box 10003
Owensboro, KY 42302
Phone: 270-687-8600
Fax: 270-687-8787
e-mail: fred@owensboro.com
Web Site: www.owensboro.com
Management:
   Facility Manager: Hal L Mischel
Seating Capacity: 5,000

6732 RIVERPARK CENTER
PO Box 548
101 Daviess Street
Owensboro, KY 42303
Phone: 270-687-2770
Fax: 270-687-2775
e-mail: jbolt1@occ.uky.campus.mci.net
Web Site: www.riverparkcenter.org
Management:
    Executive Director: John Bolton

6733 FOUR RIVERS CENTER FOR THE PERFORMING ARTS
417 S 4th Street, Suite 1
PO Box 2194
Paducah, KY 42003
Phone: 270-443-9932
Fax: 270-443-9947
e-mail: dowen@fourrivercenter.org
Web Site: www.fourriverscenter.org
Officers:
    Chairman: Ted Borodofsky
    Vice Chairman: Mike Livingston
    Treasurer: Linda Miller
    Secretary: Anne Gwinn
Management:
    Executive Director: Desiree Owen Lyles
    Assistant Director: Suzanne Clinton
    Events Coordinator: Tara Camacho
Founded: 1996
Specialized Field: Performing
Paid Staff: 3
Seating Capacity: 1,800

6734 PADUCAH COMMUNITY COLLEGE FINE ARTS CENTER
PO Box 7380
4810 Alben Barkley Drive
Paducah, KY 42002-7380
Phone: 270-554-9290
Fax: 270-552-6310
e-mail: PCC.PR@kctcs.edu
Web Site: www.pccky.com
Officers:
    Chairman: Gail Robinson
Management:
    Fine Arts Center Director: Gail Robinson
Founded: 1983
Performs At: Auditorium
Type of Stage: Proscenium
Seating Capacity: 500

6735 ALUMNI COLISEUM
Eastern Kentucky University
521 Lancaster Avenue
Richmond, KY 40475
Phone: 859-622-2122
Fax: 859-622-5108
e-mail: tickets@eku.edu
Web Site: www.ekusports.com
Management:
    Business Manager: David Parke
Paid Staff: 2

Volunteer Staff: 4

Louisiana

6736 RAPIDES COLISEUM
5600 Coliseum Boulevard
Alexandria, LA 71303
Phone: 318-443-1110
Fax: 318-443-0611
e-mail: rapcol1@cricket.net
Web Site: www.louisianarangers.com
Management:
    Executive Director: Don Guillory
Seating Capacity: 6,000

6737 ALEX BOX STADIUM
Athletic Administrative Building
S Stadium Drive
Baton Rouge, LA 70803
Phone: 225-578-8266
Fax: 225-388-2430
e-mail: chan@lsu.edu
Web Site: www.lsu.edu
Management:
    Manager Facilities: Jeff Kershow
Annual Attendance: 7,460
Seating Capacity: 7,760

6738 LOUISIANA STATE UNIVERSITY: TIGER STADIUM
Athletic Department
PO Box 25095
Baton Rouge, LA 70894-5095
Phone: 225-334-4578
Fax: 225-388-2430
e-mail: jacksonv@alpha0.gram.edu
Web Site: www.lsu.edu
Management:
    Manager Athletic Facilites: Jeff Kershaw
    Athletic Director: Joe Dean
Seating Capacity: 79,940

6739 LSU UNION THEATER
Raphael Semmes Road
Louisiana State University
Baton Rouge, LA 70803
Phone: 225-578-5124
Fax: 225-578-4329
e-mail: union@lsu.edu
Web Site: www.lsu.edu
Mission: The generation, preservation, dissemination, and application of knowledge and cultivation of the arts for the benefit of the people of the state, the nation, and the global community.

6740 PETE MARAVICH ASSEMBLY CENTER
Louisiana State University
N Stadium Drive
Baton Rouge, LA 70803

Phone: 225-578-8205
Fax: 225-578-8437
e-mail: lsupmac@lsu.edu
Web Site: www.lsu.edu
Management:
Director: Eric Edwards
Assistant Director: Jeff Campbell
Operations Manager: Eddie Crawford
Assistant Operations Manager: Nathan Hanson
Founded: 1971
Seating Capacity: 4,500 to 15000

6741 RIVERSIDE CENTROPLEX
275 S River Road
Baton Rouge, LA 70810
Phone: 225-389-3030
Fax: 225-389-4954
e-mail: wwilton@brcentroplex.com
Web Site: www.brcentroplex.com
Seating Capacity: 2,000;12,000

6742 RIVERSIDE CENTROPLEX - ARENA
275 S River Road
Baton Rouge, LA 70810
Phone: 225-389-3030
Fax: 225-389-4954
e-mail: wwilton@brcentroplex.com
Web Site: www.brcentroplex.com
Seating Capacity: 12,000

6743 RIVERSIDE CENTROPLEX - EXHIBITION HALL
275 S River Road
Baton Rouge, LA 70810
Phone: 225-389-3030
Fax: 225-389-4954
e-mail: wwilton@brcentroplex.com
Web Site: www.brcentroplex.com

6744 RIVERSIDE CENTROPLEX - THEATRE FOR PERFORMING ARTS
275 S River Road
Baton Rouge, LA 70810
Phone: 225-389-3030
Fax: 225-389-4954
e-mail: wwilton@brcentroplex.com
Web Site: www.brcentroplex.com
Seating Capacity: 2,100

6745 EUNICE PLAYERS THEATRE
PO Box 306
Eunice, LA 70535
Phone: 337-546-0163
Fax: 337-457-3081

6746 GRAMBLING UNIVERSITY: MEMORIAL GYMNASIUM
403 Main Street
Grambling, LA 71245

Phone: 318-247-3811
Fax: 318-274-3265
e-mail: jacksonv@alpha0.gram.edu
Web Site: www.gram.edu
Management:
Director Facility: Mark Blake
Associate Director: Betty Jones
Human Resources Director: Karen Emmanuel
Seating Capacity: 2,200

6747 SOUTHEASTERN LOUISIANA UNIVERSITY
Hammond, LA 70402
Phone: 985-549-2000
Fax: 985-549-3595
e-mail: rmoffett@selu.edu
Web Site: www.selu.edu

6748 SOUTHEASTERN LOUISIANA UNIVERSITY: STRAWBERRY STADIUM
PO Box 309
Hammond, LA 70402
Phone: 504-549-2253
Fax: 504-549-2253
Management:
Director: Tom Douple
Seating Capacity: 9,300

6749 SOUTHEASTERN LOUISIANA UNIVERSITY: UNIVERSITY CENTER
Southeastern Louisiana University
Hammond, LA 70402
Phone: 985-549-3818
Fax: 985-549-5383
Web Site: www.selu.edu/athletics
Management:
Head Basketball Coach (M): Bill Kennedy
Director: Larry M Hymel
Athletic Director: Frank Pergolizzi
Head Basketball Coach (W): Lori Davis Jones
Seating Capacity: 7,500

6750 HOUMA TERREBONNE CIVIC CENTER
346 Civic Center Boulevard
Houma, LA 70360
Phone: 985-850-4657
Fax: 985-850-4663
Toll-free: 888-771-4822
e-mail: info@houmaciviccenter.com
Web Site: www.houmaciviccenter.com
Management:
Director: Linda McCarthy
Marketing Manager: Tammy Damangne
Business Manager: Chris Moore
Paid Staff: 15
Annual Attendance: 200,000+
Facility Category: Civic Center
Type of Stage: Portable
Stage Dimensions: 40x80x150
Seating Capacity: 5,000
Year Built: 1999
Cost: $20 million
Rental Contact: Linda McCarthy

6751 BLACKHAM COLISEUM
201 Reinhardt Drive
Lafayette, LA 70506
Phone: 337-482-2001
Fax: 337-482-5830
Management:
General Manager: Sheila Blanco
Seating Capacity: 9,800

6752 CAJUN STADIUM
University of South West Louisiana
University of Southwestern Louisiana
Lafayette, LA 70506
Phone: 318-482-6331
Fax: 734-482-5830
Management:
General Manager: Mike Broussard
Founded: 1971
Seating Capacity: 31,000

6753 CAJUNDOME
444 Cajundome Boulevard
Lafayette, LA 70506
Phone: 337-265-2100
Fax: 337-265-2311
e-mail: pdeville@cajundome.com
Web Site: www.cajundome.com
Management:
Director: Gregory A Davis
Assistant Director: Pam Deville
Seating Capacity: 13,232

6754 HEYMANN PERFORMING ARTS CENTER
PO Box 52979
1373 S College Road
Lafayette, LA 70503
Phone: 337-291-5540
Fax: 337-291-5580
e-mail: hpacc@eatel.net
Officers:
CFO: Frank Bradshaw
Management:
Executive Director: Jacqueline Lyle
General Manager: James Edmunds
Marketing Director: Jamie Pierce

6755 HEYMANN PERFORMING ARTS - CONVENTION CENTER
1373 S College Road
Lafayette, LA 70503
Phone: 337-291-5540
Fax: 337-291-5580
e-mail: hpacc@eatel.net

6756 LAFAYETTE COMMUNITY THEATRE
529 Jefferson Street
Lafayette, LA 70501
Phone: 318-235-1532

6757 ARTISTS CIVIC THEATRE AND STUDIO
One Reid Street
PO Box 278, Lake Charles
Lake Charles, LA 70602
Phone: 337-433-2287
Fax: 337-491-1534
e-mail: information@actstheatre.com
Web Site: www.actstheatre.com
Specialized Field: Community Theatre
Organization Type: Performing; Educational

6758 BURTON COLISEUM
McNeese State University
7001 Gulf Highway
Lake Charles
Lake Charles, LA 70607
Phone: 337-478-9010
Fax: 337-474-4413
e-mail: webmaster@mail.mcneese.edu
Web Site: www.mcneese.edu
Management:
Director: Johnny Suydam
Founded: 1976
Seating Capacity: 8,000

6759 COWBOY STADIUM
700 E McNeese
Lake Charles, LA 70607
Phone: 318-475-5200
Fax: 318-475-5202
Web Site: www.mcneese.edu
Management:
Director: John Suydam

6760 LAKE CHARLES CIVIC CENTER
900 Lakeshore Drive
PO Box 900, Lake Charles
Lake Charles, LA 70602
Phone: 337-491-1256
Fax: 337-491-1534
e-mail: civiccenter@mail.city-lakecharles.or
Web Site: www.lakecharlesciviccenter.bigstep.com

6761 LAKE CHARLES CIVIC CENTER - JAMES E SUDDUTH COLISEUM
900 Lakeshore Drive
PO Box 900, Lake Charles
Lake Charles, LA 70602
Phone: 337-491-1256
Fax: 337-491-1534
Web Site: www.lakecharlesciviccenter.bigstep.com
Seating Capacity: 7,450

6762 LAKE CHARLES CIVIC CENTER - EXHIBITION HALL
900 Lakeshore Drive
PO Box 900, Lake Charles
Lake Charles, LA 70602
Phone: 337-491-1256
Fax: 337-491-1534
e-mail: civiccenter@mail.city-lakecharles.o
Web Site: www.lakecharlesciviccenter.bigstep.com

Seating Capacity: 1,400

6763 LAKE CHARLES CIVIC CENTER - ROSA HART THEATRE
900 Lakeshore Drive
PO Box 900, Lake Charles
Lake Charles, LA 70602
Phone: 337-491-1256
Fax: 337-491-1534
e-mail: civiccenter@mail.city-lakecharles.o
Web Site: www.lakecharlesciviccenter.bigstep.com
Seating Capacity: 2,050

6764 MALONE STADIUM
The University of Louisiana at Monroe
700 University Avenue, Monroe
Monroe, LA 71209
Phone: 318-342-5360
Fax: 318-342-5367
e-mail: stark@ulm.edu
Web Site: www.nlu.edu
Management:
  Director: Warner Alford
  Associate Athletic Director: Diane Stark
  Assistant Athletic Director/Busines: Alisa Hale
  Assistant Athletic Director: Cory Rogers
Founded: 1978
Seating Capacity: 30,427

6765 MONROE CIVIC CENTER
401 Lea Joyner Memorial Expressway
Monroe
Monroe, LA 71201
Phone: 318-329-2225
Fax: 318-329-2548
e-mail: christine.walters@ci.monroe.la.us
Web Site: www.ci.monroe.la.us
Management:
  General Manager: Greg Gregory

6766 PRATHER COLISEUM
NSU Athletic Department
Natchitoches, LA 71497
Phone: 318-357-5251
Fax: 318-357-4221
e-mail: nsudemons@hotmail.com
Web Site: www.nsudemons.com
Management:
  Associate Athletic Director: Donnie Cox
  Assitant Athletic Director: Rob Zinkan
  Assistant Athletic Director: Rob Dill
  Business Manager: Roxanne Freeman
Seating Capacity: 3,500

6767 TURPIN STADIUM
Northweatern Stare University
NSU Athletic Field House
Natchitoches, LA 71497
Phone: 318-357-5251
Fax: 318-357-4221
e-mail: nsudemons@hotmail.com
Web Site: www.nsudemons.com
Management:

Manager: Chris Sampite
Seating Capacity: 16,000

6768 CONTEMPORARY ARTS CENTER
900 Camp Street
New Orleans
New Orleans, LA 70130
Phone: 504-528-3805
Fax: 504-528-3828
e-mail: jweigel@cacno.org
Web Site: www.cacno.org
Management:
  Executive Director: Jay Weigel
Founded: 1976
Status: Non-Equity; Nonprofit
Type of Stage: Concert Stage; Flexible
Seating Capacity: 200-3,500

6769 LE PETIT THEATRE DU VIEUX CARRE
616 St. Peter
New Orleans, LA 70116
Phone: 504-522-9958
Fax: 504-524-9027
e-mail: sborey@bellsouth.net
Web Site: www.lepetittheatre.com
Management:
  Executive Artistic Director: Sonny Borey
  Assistant Artistic Director: Derek Franklin
  Business Manager: Jim Word
  Development/Marketing Director: Brandt Blocker
  Technical Director: Bill Walker
  Box Office Manager: Jenny Richardson
  House Manager: Linda Wegmann
Founded: 1917
Specialized Field: Community/Regional Theatre
Paid Staff: 11
Seating Capacity: 325

6770 LOUISIANA SUPERDOME
SMG
Sugar Bowl Drive, New Orleans
New Orleans, LA 70112
Phone: 504-587-3663
Fax: 504-587-3848
Toll-free: 800-756-7074
e-mail: info@superdome.com
Web Site: www.superdome.com
Management:
  General Manager: Doug Thornton
  Director Public Relationsration: Bill Curl
  Director Sales/Events Coordinator: Mark Kaufaman
Founded: 1975
Type of Stage: Concert Stage
Seating Capacity: 87,500
Year Built: 1975
Year Remodeled: 1997

6771 LOYOLA UNIVERSITY - LOUIS J. ROUSSEL PERFORMANCE CENTER
College of Music Communications/Music Complex
6363 Street Charles Avenue
New Orleans, LA 70118

Phone: 504-865-3037
e-mail: music@loyno.edu
Web Site: www.loyno.edu
Seating Capacity: 600

6772 LOYOLA UNIVERSITY - MARQUETTE THEATRE
6364 Street Charles Avenue
Department of Drama and Speech
New Orleans, LA 70118
Phone: 504-865-3840
Fax: 504-865-2284
Toll-free: 800-456-9652
e-mail: drama@loyno.edu
Web Site: www.loyno.edu
Type of Stage: Proscenium
Seating Capacity: 150

6773 NEW ORLEANS ARENA
1501 Girod Street
New Orleans
New Orleans, LA 70113
Phone: 504-587-3663
Fax: 504-587-3848
e-mail: susan.ballard@superdome.com
Web Site: www.neworleansarena.com
Management:
    General Manager: Doug Thorton
    Assistant General Manager: Glenn Menard
Seating Capacity: 17,232

6774 NEW ORLEANS MUNICIPAL AUDITORIUM
1201 St. Peter Street
New Orleans
New Orleans, LA 70116
Phone: 504-565-7470
Fax: 504-565-7477

6775 ORPHEUM THEATRE
129 University Place
New Orleans
New Orleans, LA 70112
Phone: 504-524-3285
Fax: 504-524-3286
e-mail: jeff@orpheumneworleans.com
Web Site: www.orpheumneworleans.com
Seating Capacity: 1,780

6776 SAENGER THEATRE
142 N Rampart Street
New Orleans
New Orleans, LA 70112
Phone: 504-525-1052
Fax: 504-569-1533
e-mail: mail@saengertheatre.com
Web Site: www.saengertheatre.com
Founded: 1927
Seating Capacity: 2,794
Year Built: 1927
Year Remodeled: 1980

6777 TAD GORMLEY STADIUM
New Orleans City Park
Improvement Association, 1 Palm Drive
New Orleans, LA 70124
Phone: 504-483-9496
Fax: 504-593-7620
e-mail: rdoussan@tadgromley.com
Web Site: www.tadgormley.com
Management:
    Stadium Manager: Russell Soussan
    Assistant Manager: Scott Thurman
Seating Capacity: 25,600

6778 TULANE UNIVERSITY
Department of Theatre and Dance
6823 St. Charles Avenue, New Orleans
New Orleans, LA 70118
Phone: 504-865-5000
Fax: 504-865-6737
Toll-free: 800-873-9283
e-mail: website@tulane.edu
Web Site: www.tulane.edu
Founded: 1834
Performs At: Albert Lupin Experimental Theatre, Dixon Hall
Type of Stage: Black Box; Proscenium
Seating Capacity: Proscenium theatre seats 1,000

6779 TULANE UNIVERSITY
James Wilson Center, Athletic Department
6824 St. Charles Avenue, New Orleans
New Orleans, LA 70118
Phone: 504-865-5000
Fax: 504-865-5512
Toll-free: 800-873-9283
e-mail: website@tulane.edu
Web Site: www.tulane.edu
Management:
    Associate Director Athletics: Naurice L Lagrade
    Athletic Director: Scott Devine
    Sports Law Professor: Gary Roberts
Founded: 1834
Seating Capacity: 3,600

6780 UNIVERSITY OF NEW ORLEANS PERFORMING ARTS CENTER
Lakefront
New Orleans
New Orleans, LA 70148
Phone: 504-280-6317
Fax: 504-280-6318
e-mail: kgraves@uno.edu
Web Site: www.uno.edu

6781 AILLET STADIUM
1450 W Alabama
Ruston, LA 71272
Phone: 318-257-3144
Fax: 318-257-3456
Management:
    Director Athletic Facilities: Tommy Sisemore
Founded: 1968
Seating Capacity: 30,200

All listings are in alphabetical order by state, then city, then organization within the city.

6782 LOUISIANA TECH - HOWARD AUDITORIUM CENTER FOR PERFORMING ARTS
Corner of Arizona & Adams
PO Box 8608
Ruston, LA 71272
Phone: 318-257-2711
Fax: 318-257-4571
e-mail: krobbins@latech.edu
Web Site: www.performingarts.latech.edu
Founded: 1898
Paid Staff: 6
Annual Attendance: 2,000
Type of Stage: Proscenium
Seating Capacity: 150
Year Built: 1938
Year Remodeled: 2001

6783 THOMAS ASSEMBLY CENTER
Louisiana Tech University
PO Box 3042
Ruston, LA 71272
Phone: 318-257-4111
Fax: 318-257-4437
Management:
    Manager: Tommy Sisemore
Seating Capacity: 8,698

6784 CENTENARY COLLEGE - RECITAL HALL
Hurley School of Music
PO Box 41188
Shreveport, LA 71134
Phone: 318-869-5011
Fax: 318-869-5248
Web Site: www.centenary.edu

6785 HIRSCH MEMORIAL COLISEUM
State Fair of Louisiana
3701 Hudson Street
Shreveport, LA 71109
Phone: 318-635-1361
Fax: 318-631-4909
e-mail: info@statefairoflouisiana.com
Web Site: www.statefairoflouisiana.com
Officers:
    President/General Manager: Sam Giordano
    Assistant Manger: Chris Giordano
    Administrative Assistant: Mary M Gasper
    Chairman: Davis Means, III
    Vice Chairman: George McInnis
    Past Chairman: Ed Powell
    Secretary/Treasurer: James Elrod
Mission: To serve as the State Fair of Louisiana's prime facility; to host-year round events such as major concerts, circuses, rodeos, ice shows, sporting events and motor thrill shows.
Founded: 1954
Paid Staff: 10
Budget: $80,000
Income Sources: Concerts; Rodeos; Circuses
Annual Attendance: 300,000
Facility Category: Multi-Purpose

Type of Stage: Portable
Seating Capacity: 10,300
Year Built: 1954
Year Remodeled: 1994
Cost: $300,000
Rental Contact: Mary M Gasper

6786 SHREVEPORT CIVIC THEATRE
600 Clyde Fant Parkway
Shreveport, LA 71101
Phone: 318-673-5100
Fax: 318-673-5105
e-mail: spar@ci.shreveport.la.us
Specialized Field: Municipal Performance Theater
Type of Stage: Proscenium
Stage Dimensions: 49 x 41
Seating Capacity: 1,725
Year Built: 1965
Year Remodeled: 1997

6787 SHREVEPORT MUNICIPAL AUDITORIUM
705 Elvis Presley Avenue
Shreveport, LA 71101
Phone: 318-673-5100
Fax: 318-673-5105
e-mail: spar@ci.shreveport.la.us
Type of Stage: Proscenium
Stage Dimensions: 58' wide x 29' high x 37' deep
Seating Capacity: 3,007
Year Built: 1929

6788 STRAND THEATRE OF SHREVEPORT
619 Louisiana Avenue
PO Box 1547
Shreveport, LA 71165
Phone: 318-226-1481
Fax: 318-424-5434
Toll-free: 800-313-6373
e-mail: strand@thestrandtheatre.com
Web Site: www.thestrandtheatre.com
Management:
    Manager: Penne Mobley
Founded: 1925

6789 NICHOLLS STATE UNIVERSITY GYM
PO Box 2032
Thibodaux, LA 70310
Phone: 504-448-4794
Fax: 504-448-4814
e-mail: nichweb@nicholls.edu
Web Site: www.nicholls.edu
Management:
    Athletic Director: Robert J Bernardi
Seating Capacity: 15,500

Maine

6790 AUGUSTA CIVIC CENTER
76 Community Drive
Augusta, ME 4330

Phone: 207-626-2405
Fax: 207-626-5968
e-mail: acc@biddeford.com
Web Site: www.augustaciviccenter.org

6791 AUGUSTA CIVIC CENTER - ARENA
76 Community Drive
Augusta, ME 4330
Phone: 207-626-2405
Fax: 207-626-5968
e-mail: acc@biddeford.com
Web Site: www.augustaciviccenter.org

6792 AUGUSTA CIVIC CENTER - NORTH HALL
76 Community Drive
Augusta, ME 4330
Phone: 207-626-2405
Fax: 207-626-5968
e-mail: acc@biddeford.com
Web Site: www.augustaciviccenter.org

6793 BANGOR CIVIC CENTER & AUDITORIUM
100 Dutton Street
Bangor, ME 4401
Phone: 207-947-5555
Fax: 207-947-5105
e-mail: sally.bilancia@bgrme.org
Web Site: www.bangorciviccenter.com
Mission: To serve as Maine's premier multi-purpose convention, tradeshow, meeting and entertainment show place.
Founded: 1954
Type of Stage: Portable
Seating Capacity: 6,000

6794 PICKARD THEATRE
Memorial Hall
Bowdoin College
Brunswick, ME 4011
Phone: 207-725-3663
Fax: 207-725-3372
e-mail: theater-dance@bowdoin.edu
Web Site: www.bowdoin.edu
Founded: 1955
Type of Stage: Proscenium
Seating Capacity: 600

6795 WHITTIER FIELD
Bowdoin College
9000 College Station
Brunswick, ME 4011
Phone: 207-725-3326
Fax: 207-725-3019
e-mail: jcoyne@polar.bowdoin.edu
Web Site: www.bowdoin.edu
Management:
   Athletic Director: Jeff Ward
   Sports Information Director: Jac Coune
   Human Resources Director: Cathy Gubser
Seating Capacity: 4,500

6796 CAMDEN OPERA HOUSE
29 Elm Street
PO Box 1207
Camden, ME 04843
Phone: 207-236-7963
Fax: 207-236-7956
e-mail: khadley@town.camden.me.us
Web Site: www.camdenoperahouse.com
Officers:
   President: Chris Wolf
Management:
   Opera House: Kerry Hadley
   Artistic Director: Karen Elisen Hever
Mission: Providing an elegant, historic yet practical facility for performing arts serving the mid coast region; providing affordable space for local nonprofit groups to perform and meet; and state of the art conference facility hosting numerous annual international conferences.
Specialized Field: Regional
Paid Staff: 2
Volunteer Staff: 100
Performs At: Opera, Theatre, Concerts
Facility Category: Performing Arts
Type of Stage: Thrust
Stage Dimensions: 37'x34'
Seating Capacity: 500
Year Built: 1894
Year Remodeled: 1994
Resident Groups: The Maine Grand Opera

6797 BATES COLLEGE: CONCERT HALL
Olin Arts Center
Lewiston, ME 04240
Phone: 207-786-6135
Fax: 207-786-8335

6798 BATES COLLEGE: GARCELON FIELD
130 Central Avenue
Lewiston, ME 04240
Phone: 207-786-6345
Fax: 207-786-8232
Web Site: www.bates.edu
Management:
   Assistant Athletic Director: Dana Mulholland

6799 UNIVERSITY OF MAINE AT MACHIAS - PERFORMING ARTS CENTER
The Arts Downeast
#9 O'Brien Avenue
Machias, ME 4654
Phone: 207-255-1200
Fax: 207-255-4864
e-mail: ummadmissions@maine.edu
Web Site: www.umm.maine.edu
Mission: To host campus and community meetings, seminars, festivals and the performing arts.
Founded: 1985
Seating Capacity: 358
Organization Type: Amphitheater auditorium

All listings are in alphabetical order by state, then city, then organization within the city.

6800   CUMSTON HALL
Main Street
PO Box 239
Monmouth, ME 4259
Phone: 207-933-4788
Fax: 509-471-2100
e-mail: allstaff@cumston.lib.me.us
Web Site: www.cumston.lib.me.us
Officers:
   Chairman: Benjamin Lund
Founded: 1900

6801   OGUNQUIT PLAYHOUSE
PO Box 915
Ogunquit-by-the-Sea, ME 3907
Phone: 207-646-2402
Fax: 207-646-4732
e-mail: mail@ogunquitplayhouse.org
Web Site: www.ogunquitplayhouse.org
Founded: 1933

6802   ALFOND ARENA
University of Maine
5747 Memorial Gym
Orono, ME 4469
Phone: 207-581-1052
Fax: 207-581-3070
e-mail: john.gregory@umit.maine.edu
Web Site: www.umaine.edu
Management:
   Director: James Dyer
Founded: 1977
Type of Stage: Sports Arena
Seating Capacity: 5,641

6803   ALUMNI STADIUM
University of Maine Memorial Gym
Orono, ME 4469
Phone: 207-581-1110
Fax: 207-581-3070
e-mail: john.gregory@umit.maine.edu
Web Site: www.umaine.edu
Management:
   Athletic Director: Suzanne Tyler

6804   UNIVERSITY OF MAINE - MAINE CENTER FOR THE ARTS
5746 Maine Center For The Arts
Orono, ME 4469
Phone: 207-581-1755
Fax: 207-581-1837
e-mail: john.patches@umit.maine.edu
Web Site: www.umaine.edu
Management:
   Director: John I Patches
   Ticket Services Manager: Mary Addison
   Box Office Assistant: Sue Melvin
   Assistant Director/External Affairs: Adala Adkins
   Outreach/Education Coordinator: Stephen Wicks
   Manager Theatre Operations: Joe Cota
   Technical Director: Jeff Richards
   Assistant Technical Director: Scott Stiham
   Secretary: Deborah Seekins

Mission: Provides a cultural focus for the University of Maine campus, the communities of the region. and all the citizens of the State of Maine. The center coordinates the development of performances, exhibitions outreach programs, and conferences, and works with the related academic departments to unsure both diversity - that is, it serves as a resource to the State of Maine by providing oppotunities for talented people to share thie accomplishments.
Founded: 1986
Specialized Field: Performing Arts
Paid Staff: 10
Volunteer Staff: 60

6805   CENTER FOR CULTURAL EXCHANGE
1 Longfellow Square
Portland, ME 4101
Phone: 207-761-0591
Fax: 207-775-4254
e-mail: info@centerforculturalexchange.org
Web Site: www.artsandculture.org
Management:
   Director Marketing: Stew Cruernsey
   Finance Manager: Ben Dacey
Founded: 1998
Paid Staff: 12
Volunteer Staff: 20
Annual Attendance: 3,000
Facility Category: Small Concert hall
Type of Stage: Modular Platform
Stage Dimensions: 25' x 30'
Seating Capacity: 200
Year Built: 1999
Year Remodeled: 1999
Organization Type: Performing

6806   CUMBERLAND COUNTY CIVIC CENTER
1 Civic Center Square
Portland, ME 4101
Phone: 207-775-3481
Fax: 207-828-8344
Web Site: www.theciviccenter.com
Mission: Multi-purpose entertainment and sports facility that annually hosts a wide variety of family shows, concerts, sporting events, and trade shows.

6807   MERRILL AUDITORIUM
20 Mystic Street
Portland, ME 04101
Phone: 207-874-8200
Web Site: www.portlandevents.com
Management:
   Executive Director: Frank P Latorre
Facility Category: Upscale Arts Facility
Type of Stage: Proscenium
Seating Capacity: 1900
Year Built: 1912
Year Remodeled: 1996

6808   PORTLAND EXPO/HADLOCK FIELD
239 Park Avenue
Portland, ME 4102

Phone: 207-874-8200
Fax: 207-874-8130
e-mail: Frank@ci.portland.me.us
Web Site: www.portlandevents.com
Management:
   Executive Director: Frank P Latorre
   Assistant Director: Authur H Stephenson
Founded: 1994
Facility Category: Arena
Type of Stage: Sports Arena
Stage Dimensions: 60x40
Seating Capacity: 7,000
Year Built: 1915
Year Remodeled: 1990

6809 PORTLAND EXPOSITION BUILDING

239 Park Avenue
Portland, ME 4102
Phone: 207-874-8200
Fax: 207-874-8130
e-mail: andrea@ci.portland.me.us
Web Site: www.portlandevents.com
Officers:
   Division Director: Frank P LaTorre
Management:
   Booking Coordinator: Andrea Smith
Founded: 1915
Facility Category: Arena
Type of Stage: Portable
Stage Dimensions: 60' wide x 40' deep
Seating Capacity: 3,000
Year Built: 1914
Rental Contact: Andrea Smith

6810 PORTLAND PERFORMING ARTS CENTER

25A Forest Avenue
Portland, ME 4101
Phone: 207-761-0591
Fax: 207-775-4254

6811 ROCKPORT OPERA HOUSE

PO Box 10
Central Street
Rockport, ME 4856
Phone: 207-236-2823
Fax: 207-230-0454
e-mail: info@baychamberconcerts.org
Web Site: www.baychamberconcerts.org
Founded: 1891
Type of Stage: Flexible
Seating Capacity: Auditorium 400; Meeting room 100
Year Built: 1891
Year Remodeled: 1993
Cost: $1 million

6812 CELEBRATION BARN THEATER

190 Stock Farm Road
South Paris, ME 4281
Phone: 207-743-8452
Fax: 207-743-3889
e-mail: info@celebrationbarn.com
Web Site: www.celebrationbarn.com

Management:
   Executive Director/Owner: Carol Brett
   Artistic Director: Tony Montanaro
   Managing Director: Fritz Grobe
Founded: 1972

6813 COLBY COLLEGE: STRIDER THEATER

4520 Mayflower Hill
Waterville, ME 04901
Phone: 207-872-3388
Fax: 207-872-3803
e-mail: djward@culby.edu
Web Site: www.colby.edu/theater
Seating Capacity: 274
Cost: $850,000

6814 WATERVILLE OPERA HOUSE IMPROVEMENT ASSOCIATION

93 Main Street 3rd Floor
Waterville, ME 4901
Phone: 207-873-5381
Fax: 207-861-7096
e-mail: operainfo@operahouse.com
Web Site: www.operahouse.com
Officers:
   Chairman: Earle Bessey III
   Vice-Chair: Jim Lynch
   Treasurer: Kathleen Livollen
Management:
   Office Manager: Janis White
Founded: 1902
Annual Attendance: 80,000
Type of Stage: Proscenium
Seating Capacity: 918

Maryland

6815 ALUMNI HALL

675 Decatour Road
US Naval Academy
Annapolis, MD 21402
Phone: 410-293-2234
Fax: 410-293-3218
Management:
   Manager: Gregory B Zingler

6816 FRANCIS SCOTT KEY AUDITORIUM

60 College Avenue
St. John's College
Annapolis, MD 21401
Phone: 410-626-2547
Fax: 410-263-4828
e-mail: webmaster@mailhost.sjca.edu
Web Site: www.sjca.edu/college
Seating Capacity: 600
Year Built: 1958

6817 MARYLAND HALL FOR THE CREATIVE ARTS

801 Chase Street
Annapolis, MD 21401

Phone: 410-263-5544
Fax: 410-263-5114
e-mail: mdhall@annap.infi.net
Web Site: www.mdhallarts.org
Officers:
   President: Tom Marquardt
   First VP: Veronica Meneely
   Second VP: Mary G Petersen
   Third VP: Judi Herrmann
   Treasurer: Brian E. Lees
   Secretary: Aileen Carlucci
Management:
   Executive Director: Linnell R Bowen
   Technical Director: Sid Curl
   Education Director: Emily Garvin
   Registration Coordinator: Jennifer Alder
   Theatre/Rental Manager: Tom Fridrich
   Director Operations/Finance: Leslie Rose
Specialized Field: Visual, Performing, and Creative Arts
Status: Active; Nonprofit

6818 ARENA PLAYERS

801 McCulloh Street
Baltimore, MD 21201
Phone: 410-383-2691
Fax: 410-383-2692
e-mail: arena@fcsmd.org
Web Site: www.fcsmd.org/locations/baltimorecity/arena

6819 BALTIMORE ARENA

201 W Baltimore Street
Baltimore, MD 21201
Phone: 410-347-2020
Fax: 410-347-2042
Web Site: www.baltimorearena.com
Management:
   General Manager: Donna P Julian
   Contracts Coordinator: Trish Howerton
Performs At: Entertainment; Sports
Seating Capacity: 14,000
Year Built: 1962
Year Remodeled: 1984

6820 BALTIMORE MUSEUM OF ART

10 Art Museum Drive
Baltimore, MD 21218
Phone: 410-396-6342
Fax: 410-396-7153
Web Site: www.artbma.org
Management:
   Auditorium Technical Coordinator: Don Weiland
Mission: Visual arts institution with a 360 seat public auditorium which is available for rental to performing and cultural arts groups.

6821 CENTER STAGE

700 N Calvert Street
Baltimore, MD 21202-3686
Phone: 410-332-0033
Fax: 410-539-3912
e-mail: info@centerstage.org
Web Site: www.centerstage.org
Management:
   Managing Director: Thomas Pechar

Artistic Director: Irene Lewis
Director Development: Dawn Helsing
Production Manager: Katheryn Davis
Company Management: Katie Byrnes
Public Relations Manager: Richard Gorelick
Founded: 1963
Budget: $6.2 million
Affiliations: BACVA, Baltimore Tourism Association, Baltimore Theatre Alliance, TCG, AEA
Type of Stage: Semi-Thrust and Flexible
Stage Dimensions: 40'x36' and 67'x118'
Seating Capacity: 541 and 850
Year Remodeled: 2000
Rental Contact: Harry Delair

6822 DUNBAR PERFORMING ARTS CENTER

1400 Orleans Street
Baltimore, MD 21231
Phone: 410-534-6614

6823 JOHNS HOPKINS UNIVERSITY: THE MERRICK BARN

3400 N Charles Street
Baltimore, MD 21218
Phone: 410-516-7159
Fax: 410-516-8198
e-mail: thehop@jhu.edu

6824 JOHNS HOPKINS UNIVERSITY: HOMEWOOD FIELD

3400 N Charles Street
Baltimore, MD 21218
Phone: 410-516-7490
Fax: 410-516-7482
Web Site: www.hopkinssports.com
Management:
   Athletic Director: Tom Calder

6825 LOYOLA COLLEGE IN MARYLAND: MCMANUS THEATER/REITZ ARENA

4501 N Charles Street
Baltimore, MD 21210
Phone: 410-617-5077
Fax: 410-617-2211
Web Site: www.loyola.edu
Management:
   Director: Joan M Flynn
Founded: 1852
Seating Capacity: 3,000

6826 LYRIC OPERA HOUSE

140 W Mount Royal Avenue
Baltimore, MD 21201
Phone: 410-685-5086
Fax: 410-332-8234
e-mail: info@lyricoperahouse.com
Web Site: www.lyricoperahouse.com

6827 MORGAN STATE UNIVERSITY: HUGHES STADIUM

1700 E Cold Spring Lane
Baltimore, MD 21251

Phone: 443-885-3050
Fax: 410-319-3221
Web Site: www.morgan.edu
Management:
    Athletic Director: David Thomas

6828 ORIOLE PARK AT CAMDEN YARDS
State of Maryland
555 Russell Street, Suite A
Baltimore, MD 21230
Phone: 410-576-0300
Fax: 410-539-7640
Management:
    Director Facility Management: Sherman B Kerbel
    Deputy Director: Ed Cline
    Concessions Manager: Bernie Kloppenburg
    Private Suite Coordinator: Julie Wagner
    Director Marketing: Scott Nickle
Seating Capacity: 48,031

6829 PSINET STADIUM AT CAMDEN YARDS
1100 Russell Street
Baltimore, MD 21230
Phone: 410-333-1560
Fax: 410-333-1888
Toll-free: 877-637-8234
e-mail: msa@mdstad.com
Web Site: www.mdstad.com
Management:
    Executive Director: Bruce H Hoffman, PE
    Deputy Director: Edward E Cline
Founded: 1998
Seating Capacity: 69,400

6830 BOWIE STATE UNIVERSITY- MARTIN LUTHER KING JR. CENTER
14000 Jericho Park Road
Bowie, MD 20715-9465
Phone: 301-464-3441
Toll-free: 877-772-6943

6831 NATIONAL ORCHESTRAL INSTITUTE
2110 Clarice Smith Performing Arts Center
University Of Maryland
College Park, MD 20742-1620
Phone: 301-405-2317
Fax: 301-314-9504
e-mail: noi@accmail.umd.edu
Web Site: www.nationlaorchestralinstitute.com
Management:
    Assistant Manager: Phil Kancianic
    Manager: Richard Scerbo
    Aristic Director: James Ross
    Artistic Director: Christopher Kendall
Mission: The NOI offers an intensive three-week training experience in orchestral musicianship and professional development for musicians on the threshold of their careers.
Founded: 1987
Specialized Field: Music
Paid Staff: 2
Paid Artists: 41
Budget: $380,000

Income Sources: University Funds, Ticket Revenue
Performs At: University Performing Arts Facility
Annual Attendance: 3500
Facility Category: Concert Hall
Type of Stage: Open
Seating Capacity: 1100
Year Remodeled: 2001

6832 UNIVERSITY OF MARYLAND: CLARICE SMITH PERFORMING ARTS CENTER
Suite 3800
College Park, MD 20742-1625
Phone: 301-405-5974
Fax: 301-405-5977
e-mail: sfarr@deans.umd.edu
Web Site: claricesmithcenter.umd.edu
Management:
    Executive Director: Susie Farr
    Program Coordinator: Rose Ann Cleveland

6833 TOBY'S DINNER THEATRE
5900 Symphony Woods Road
PO Box 1003
Columbia, MD 21044
Phone: 410-730-8311
Fax: 410-730-8311
Toll-free: 800-888-6297
Web Site: www.tobysdinnertheatre.com
Founded: 1980

6834 JOHN ADDISON CONCERT HALL
10701 Livingston Road
Fort Washington, MD 20744
Phone: 301-203-6070
Fax: 301-203-6071
Web Site: www.pgparks.com
Management:
    Art Director: Dr. Lawrence J Knowles

6835 FROSTBURG STATE UNIVERSITY: BOBCAT STADIUM
101 Braddock Street
Frostburg, MD 21532
Phone: 301-687-4000
Fax: 301-689-6034
Management:
    Facilities Director: Ralph Brewer

6836 MARYLAND THEATRE
21 S Potomac Street
Hagerstown, MD 21740-5598
Phone: 301-790-3500
Fax: 301-791-6114
e-mail: pww@mdtheatre.org
Web Site: www.mdtheatre.org
Management:
    Director: Patricia Wolford

6837 COLLEGE OF SOUTHERN MARYLAND FINE ARTS CENTER
Box 910
Mitchell Road
La Plata, MD 20646-0910
Phone: 301-934-7863
Fax: 301-934-7682
e-mail: johnm@csm.cc.md.us
Web Site: www.csm.cc.md.us
Management:
   Executive Director: John Maerhofer
   Technical Director: Emmutt Woodey
   Box Office Manager: Cathy Brooks
Type of Stage: proscenium
Seating Capacity: 404
Year Built: 1983

6838 FEDEX FIELD
1600 Raljon Road
Landover, MD 20785-4236
Phone: 301-276-6000
Fax: 301-276-6002
Web Site: www.redskins.com
Management:
   Sr VP: Michael Dillow
Specialized Field: Home of the Washington Redskins (NFL)
Seating Capacity: 78,600
Year Built: 1997

6839 STRATHMORE HALL ARTS CENTER
10701 Rockville Pike
North Bethesda, MD 20852
Phone: 301-530-0540
Fax: 301-530-9050
e-mail: concerts@strathmore.org
Web Site: www.strathmore.org

6840 ROLAND E POWELL CONVENTION CENTER
4001 Coastal Highway
40th Street
Ocean City, MD 21842
Phone: 410-289-8311
Fax: 410-289-0058
Toll-free: 800-626-2326
e-mail: mnoah@ococean.com
Web Site: www.ocean-city.com/convention
Management:
   Director: Mike Noah

6841 GORDON CENTER FOR THE PERFORMING ARTS
3506 Gwynnbrook Avenue
Owings Mills, MD 21117
Phone: 410-356-7469
Fax: 410-356-7605
e-mail: gordoncenter@hotmail.com
Web Site: www.gordoncenter.com
Management:
   Executive Director: Nancy Goldberg
   Technical Director: Mark Quackenbush

Mission: To offer professional, high-quality performances in all genres to all ages.
Status: Nonprofit
Income Sources: Grants; Endowments
Annual Attendance: 35,000
Facility Category: Performing Arts Center
Type of Stage: Proscenium
Stage Dimensions: 70'x 40'
Seating Capacity: 550
Year Built: 1995
Rental Contact: Nancy Goldberg

6842 JEWISH COMMUNITY CENTER OF GREATER WASHINGTON
6125 Montrose Road
Rockville, MD 20852
Phone: 301-881-0100
Fax: 301-881-8802
Management:
   Cultural Arts Director: Maida Barron
Performs At: Gliddenhorn/Speisman Center for the Arts

6843 MONTGOMERY COLLEGE: ROBERT E PARILLA PERFORMING ARTS CENTER
51 Mannakee Street
Rockville, MD 20850
Phone: 301-251-7536
Fax: 301-251-7542
e-mail: dfyodoro@mc.cc.md.us
Management:
   Theatre Manager: Deborah Fyodorov

6844 WICOMICO YOUTH AND CIVIC CENTER
500 Glen Avenue
Salisbury, MD 21804
Phone: 410-548-4900
Fax: 410-546-0490
Web Site: www.wicomicociviccenter
Management:
   Manager: Charles R Rousseau
   Director Marketing/Public Relations: Tara Zaiser

6845 TOWSON STATE UNIVERSITY: FINE ARTS CENTER
Towson, MD 21204
Phone: 410-830-3289
Fax: 410-830-3914

6846 TOWSON STATE UNIVERSITY: STEPHENS AUDITORIUM
Towson, MD 21204
Phone: 410-830-3289
Fax: 410-830-3914

Massachusetts

6847 UNIVERSITY OF MASSACHUSETTS: FINE ARTS CENTER
2 Curry Hicks
100 Hicks Way
Amherst, MA 01003-9267
Phone: 413-545-0190
Fax: 413-545-0132
Toll-free: 800-999-8627
e-mail: jsmar@art.umass.edu
Web Site: www.fineartscenter.com
Specialized Field: Performing Series
Facility Category: Concert Hall and Bowker Auditorium
Type of Stage: Proscenium
Seating Capacity: 1980 Concert Hall, 700 Bowker Auditorium

6848 UNIVERSITY OF MASSACHUSETTS: CONCERT HALL
2 Curry-Hicks
Amherst, MA 01003
Phone: 413-545-0190
Fax: 413-545-0132

6849 WILLIAM D MULLINS MEMORIAL CENTER
University of Massachusetts
Amherst, MA 01003
Phone: 413-545-3001
Fax: 413-656-3005
Web Site: www.mullins.center.umass.edu
Management:
Executive Director: Paul Gould
Seating Capacity: 10,500

6850 BOSTON CENTER FOR THE ARTS: CYCLORAMA
539 Tremont Street
Boston, MA 02116
Phone: 617-426-5000
Fax: 617-426-5336
Web Site: www.bcaonline.org
Mission: Seeks to sustain artists seriously engaged in the advancement of an artistic discipline and to create an ever-changing array of meaningful opportuniities for people to encounter the work of living artists.
Status: Nonprofit

6851 BOSTON CENTER FOR THE ARTS: THE NATIONAL THEATRE
539 Tremont Street
Boston, MA 02116
Phone: 617-426-5000
Fax: 617-426-5336

6852 BOSTON OPERA HOUSE
539 Washington Street
Boston, MA 02111
Phone: 617-426-5300

6853 BOSTON UNIVERSITY: SCHOOL OF FINE ARTS
855 Commonwealth Avenue
Boston, MA 02215-1303
Phone: 617-353-3350
Fax: 617-353-5331
e-mail: esmuller@bu.edu
Web Site: www.bu.edu/ofa
Management:
Director Public Relations: Elly Muller
Specialized Field: Music; Visul Arts; Theatre

6854 BOSTON UNIVERSITY THEATRE
264 Huntington Avenue
Boston, MA 02115
Phone: 617-266-7900
Fax: 617-363-8300
Web Site: www.bu.edu/but
Management:
Production Management: Jeff Clark
Sound Design: Ben Emerson
Costume Production: Caroline Errington
Stage Management: Thom Kauffman
Technical Production: Stratton McGrady
Theatre Management: Michael Maso

6855 BOSTON UNIVERSITY THEATRE: MAIN STAGE
264 Huntington Avenue
Boston, MA 02115
Phone: 617-266-7900
Fax: 617-363-8300

6856 BOSTON UNIVERSITY: NICKERSON FIELD
285 Babcock Street
Boston, MA 02215
Phone: 617-353-4632
Fax: 617-353-6428
Management:
Athletic Director: Gary Strickler
Seating Capacity: 15,500

6857 EMERSON COLLEGE: EMERSON MAJESTIC THEATRE
219 Tremont Street
Boston, MA 02116-1809
Phone: 617-824-8000
Fax: 617-824-8725
e-mail: majestic@emerson.edu
Web Site: www.maj.org
Management:
Manager: Lance Olson
Technical Director: Michael Wilder
Assistant Manager/Business: Susan Roberts
Ticketing Manager: Donna Aitken
Mission: To provide a first class performance home for New England's finest non-profit performers and presenters.
Founded: 1984
Paid Staff: 40
Volunteer Staff: 40

Annual Attendance: 150,000
Facility Category: Opera/Dance Theatre
Type of Stage: Proscenium
Stage Dimensions: 40'x 40'
Seating Capacity: 1,000
Year Built: 1903
Year Remodeled: 2003
Rental Contact: Manager Lance Olson
Resident Groups: Dance Umbrella, World Music, BAM Opera, Celebrity Series, Jose Mateo's Ballet Theatre, The Revels...

6858 FENWAY PARK
4 Yawkey Way
Boston, MA 02215
Phone: 617-267-9440
Fax: 617-375-0944
Web Site: www.redsox.com
Management:
  CEO: John Harrington
  Executive VP Administrator: John Buckley
  VP Marketing/Sales: Larry Cancro
Seating Capacity: 33,871
Year Built: 1912
Year Remodeled: 1934

6859 FLEETCENTER
One Fleetcenter
Suite 200
Boston, MA 02114-1310
Phone: 617-624-1050
Fax: 617-624-1818
e-mail: courtney@fleetcenter.com
Web Site: www.fleetcenter.com
Management:
  President: Richard Krezwick
  Sr VP Finance: James Bednarek
  Director Marketing: Jim Delaney
Mission: The FleetCenter is a large multi-purpose sports entertainment facility with many opportunities to accommodate various types of events from full arena concerts to client lunches.
Founded: 1995
Specialized Field: New England/s largest sports and entertainment complex is home to the Boston Celtics(NBA) and the Boston Bruins(NHL).Hosts a wide variety of events.
Seating Capacity: 18,600, 17,200
Year Built: 1995

6860 HARVARD UNIVERSITY: HARVARD STADIUM/BRIGHT ARENA
Murr Center
65 N Harvard Street
Boston, MA 02163
Phone: 617-495-4848
Fax: 617-495-9950
Web Site: www.harvard.edu/~athletic/
Management:
  Assistant Athletic Director: Lauren Dougherty

6861 HUNTINGTON THEATRE COMPANY
264 Huntington Avenue
Boston, MA 02115
Phone: 617-266-0800
Fax: 617-353-8300
Web Site: www.huntingtontheatre.org
Management:
  MS Director: Michael Maso
  Artistic Director: Nicholas Martin
Founded: 1982

6862 ISABELLA STEWART GARDNER MUSEUM
280 The Fenway
2 Palace Road
Boston, MA 02115
Phone: 617-566-1401
Fax: 617-232-8039
e-mail: information@isgm.org
Web Site: www.gardnermuseum.org
Management:
  Director: Anne Hawley
  Director Operations/Finance: Peter Bryant
  Curator: Alan Chong
Mission: Providing a venue for contemporary and historical exhibitions, lectures, family programs and concerts.
Founded: 1903
Specialized Field: Vocal Music; Instrumental Music; Chamber Music; Recitals
Status: Nonprofit
Budget: $130,000
Performs At: Museum Gallery
Annual Attendance: 200,000
Facility Category: Museum
Seating Capacity: 250
Organization Type: Sponsoring

6863 JORDAN HALL AT NEW ENGLAND CONSERVATORY
30 Gainsboro Street
Boston, MA 02115
Phone: 617-262-1120
Fax: 617-262-0500
Web Site: www.newenglandconservatory.edu
Founded: 1903
Annual Attendance: 125,000
Facility Category: Performance Hall
Seating Capacity: 1013
Year Built: 1903
Year Remodeled: 1995
Architect: Ann Beha Associates
Cost: 8.2 Million

6864 MATTHEWS ARENA
238 Street Botoloph Street
Boston, MA 02115
Phone: 814-272-2261
Fax: 814-272-3775
Management:
  Manager: Mark Coates
  Operations Director: Mike Winson
Seating Capacity: 5,700

6865 NEW ENGLAND CONSERVATORY
290 Huntington Avenue
Boston, MA 02115
Phone: 617-585-1100
Fax: 617-585-1336
e-mail: rhoenich@newenglandconservatory.edu
Web Site: www.newenglandconservatory.edu
Management:
Music Director: Richard Hoenich
Mission: To serve society by training outstanding performers, composers, and teachers. With a diverse faculty of exceptional caliber and a flexible curriculum, we strive to develop these young artists individually and integrate them into the larger world of music.

6866 NORTHEASTERN UNIVERSITY CENTER FOR THE ARTS
118 Cushing Halll
102 The Fenway
Boston, MA 02115
Phone: 617-373-2249
Fax: 617-373-4488
Web Site: www.casctn.nev.edu/arten
Management:
Director: Del Lewis
Specialized Field: Performances in Dance, Theatre and Music.
Paid Staff: 6
Paid Artists: 810

6867 NORTHEASTERN UNIVERSITY: PARSONS FIELD STADIUM
360 Huntington Avenue
Boston, MA 02215
Phone: 617-566-5955
Fax: 617-373-5000
Management:
Assistant Director: Sue Ekizan
Seating Capacity: 7,000

6868 SYMPHONY HALL
301 Massachusetts Avenue
Boston, MA 02115
Phone: 617-266-1492
Fax: 617-637-9367

6869 WANG THEATRE
Wang Center for the Performing Arts
270 Tremont Street
Boston, MA 02116
Phone: 617-482-9393
Fax: 617-357-0804
e-mail: mszczepkowski@wangcenter.org
Web Site: www.wangcenter.org
Management:
Booking/Programming Manager: Michael Szczepkowski
Facility Category: Theatre
Type of Stage: Proscenium
Stage Dimensions: 80 x 60
Seating Capacity: 3561
Year Built: 1910
Year Remodeled: 1996

6870 LOEB DRAMA CENTER
64 Brattle Street
Cambridge, MA 02138
Phone: 617-495-2668
Fax: 617-495-1705
Founded: 1960
Type of Stage: Proscenium
Stage Dimensions: 26 x 60
Seating Capacity: 556 each configuration
Year Built: 1960
Architect: h
Cost: Hugh Stubins Associates

6871 RADCLIFFE COLLEGE: AGASSIZ THEATER
10 Garden Street
Cambridge, MA 02138
Phone: 617-495-8676
Fax: 617-495-8690
Web Site: www.fas.harvard.edu
Management:
Associate Technical Director: Adam Kibbe
Technical Director College Theatre: Alan Symonds
Mission: To integrate creative thinking and expression into the undergraduate educational experience. The Theatre serves as a try-out house for plays which students select, direct, produce, perform and occasionally write. Approximately 750 undergraduates are involved in Agassiz Theatre productions each year and thousands more attend its productions.
Founded: 1904

6872 RADCLIFFE COLLEGE: LYMAN COMMON ROOM
10 Garden Street
Cambridge, MA 02138
Phone: 617-495-8676
Fax: 617-495-8690

6873 BOSTON COLLEGE: ALUMNI FIELD STADIUM
140 Commonwealth Avenue
Chestnut Hill, MA 02467
Phone: 617-552-3004
Fax: 617-552-4903
e-mail: defilieu@bc.edu
Web Site: www.bceagles.com
Management:
Athletic Director: Gene Defillippo

6874 SILVIO O CONTE FORUM/BOSTON COLLEGE
140 Commonwealth Avenue
Chestnut Hill, MA 02467
Phone: 617-552-4681
Fax: 617-552-4903
e-mail: defilieu@bc.edu
Web Site: www.bceagles.com
Management:
Head Football Coach: Tom O'Brien
Athletic Director: Gene Difillppo
Senior Associate Athletic Director: John Kane

Senior Associate Athletic Director: Ed Carroll
Head Basketball Coach (M): Al Skinner
Head Basketball Coach (W): Cathy Inglese
Seating Capacity: 8,606

6875 CAPE PLAYHOUSE

820 Main Street
Route 6A
Dennis, MA 02638
Mailing Address: PO Box 2001 Dennis, MA 02638
Phone: 508-385-3838
Fax: 508-385-8162
Toll-free: 877-385-3911
Web Site: www.capeplayhouse.com
Officers:
President: James Wilson
VP: Avard Craig
Treasurer: Katherine Dorshimer
Secretary: Robert Oek
Management:
Managing Director: Kathleen A Fahle
Artistic Director: Evans Haile
Mission: Established by the Raymond Moore Foundation and chartered by the Commonwealth of Massachusetts in 1948, Cape Playhouse operates for educational and charitable purposes as well as presenting top summer entertainment with stars of stage, screen and television.
Founded: 1927
Specialized Field: Summer Stock
Status: Professional; Nonprofit

6876 M HARRIET MCCORMACK CENTER FOR THE PERFORMING ARTS/STRAND THEATER

543 Columbia Road
PO Box 255247
Dorchester, MA 02125
Phone: 617-282-5230
Fax: 617-282-5252
e-mail: info@strandtheatreboston.com
Web Site: www.strandtheatreboston.com
Officers:
President: Joyce Williams
Treasurer: Carla Sharpe
Management:
Executive Director: Victoria Jones
Marketing Director: Lisa Jones
Program Manager: Margie Shaheed
Mission: To continue to bring and produce innovative entertainment through productions, film series, music and our youth programs. The Strand is a cutting edge theatre that continues to cater to the community, nations and international audiences.
Founded: 1918
Specialized Field: Theatre/Entertainment
Income Sources: Grants; Productions
Affiliations: Uphams Corner Main Street Association
Type of Stage: Proscenium
Stage Dimensions: 39x29
Seating Capacity: 1400
Year Built: 1918
Year Remodeled: 1978

6877 FESTIVAL THEATRE

56 Centre Street
Dover, MA 02030
Phone: 508-785-0068

6878 ART COMPLEX AT DUXBURY

189 Alden Street
Box 2814
Duxbury, MA 02331
Phone: 781-934-6634
Fax: 781-934-5117
Web Site: www.artcomplex.org
Management:
Communications Coordinator: Laura Doherty
Founded: 1971
Specialized Field: Asian; American/European Prints; Paintings; Shaker
Paid Staff: 10
Volunteer Staff: 50
Performs At: Art; Music; Theater; Japanese Tea Ceremonies
Annual Attendance: 10,000+
Facility Category: Museum w/gallery space; tea house

6879 BRISTOL COMMUNITY COLLEGE ARTS CENTER

777 Elsbree Street
Fall River, MA 02720
Phone: 508-678-2811
Fax: 508-674-3117
Management:
Dean Administration: Richard Sobel

6880 HIGHFIELD THEATRE

PO Drawer F
Falmouth, MA 02541
Phone: 508-548-2211
Fax: 508-548-2211

6881 FOXBORO STADIUM

60 Washington Street
Foxboro, MA 02035
Phone: 508-543-8200
Fax: 508-543-0285
Web Site: www.patriots.com
Management:
General Manager: Dan Murphy
Director Marketing/Special Events: Lou Imbriano
Seating Capacity: 61,000
Year Built: 1971

6882 FOXBOROUGH REGIONAL CENTER FOR THE PERFORMING ARTS

PO Box 266
Foxborough, MA 02035
Phone: 508-543-4434
e-mail: frepa-info@frcpa.org
Web Site: www.orpheum.org
Mission: Dedicated to providing audiences with quality performing arts events, as well as providing an environment which will allow performing arts groups within the community to flourish.

Founded: 1993
Status: Nonprofit

6883 LAWRENCE ACADEMY THEATRE
Powderhouse Road
Groton, MA 01450
Phone: 508-448-6535
Fax: 508-448-6535
Web Site: www.lacademy.edu

6884 HINGHAM HIGH SCHOOL - AUDITORIUM
41 Pleasant Street
Hingham, MA 02043
Phone: 781-741-1500

6885 LOWELL MEMORIAL AUDITORIUM: MILL CITY MANAGEMENT
50 E Merrimack Street
Lowell, MA 01852-1205
Phone: 978-937-8688
Fax: 978-452-7342
e-mail: lowellauditorium.com
Web Site: www.lowellauditorium.com
Management:
Executive Director: Thomas F McKay

6886 UNIVERSITY OF MASSACHUSETTS AT LOWELL: CENTER FOR THE ARTS
One University Avenue
Lowell, MA 01854
Phone: 978-934-4000

6887 LYNN CITY HALL MEMORIAL AUDITORIUM
3 City Hall Square
Lynn, MA 01901
Phone: 617-598-4000
Fax: 617-592-9411

6888 TWEETER CENTER FOR THE PERFORMING ARTS
885 S Main Street
PO Box 810
Mansfield, MA 02048
Phone: 508-339-2331
Fax: 508-339-0550
Facility Category: Open Air Amphitheater
Seating Capacity: 19,900

6889 BOCH CENTER FOR THE PERFORMING ARTS
13 Steeple Street
Mashpee, MA 02649-1997
Phone: 508-477-2580
Fax: 508-477-2595
e-mail: bochctr@cape.com
Web Site: capecodtravel.com/boch
Management:
President/Executive Director: TK Thompson

6890 ZEITERION THEATRE
684 Purchase Street
PO Box 4084
New Bedford, MA 02741
Phone: 508-997-5664
Fax: 508-999-5956
e-mail: zeiterion@usa.net
Web Site: www.zeiterion.com
Management:
Executive Director: Christopher J Le Blanc
Technical Director: Tom Hanks

6891 FIREHOUSE CENTER FOR THE ARTS
One Market Square
Newburyport, MA 01950
Phone: 978-462-7336
Fax: 978-462-9911
e-mail: johnbudzyna@hotmail.com
Web Site: firehousecenter.com
Management:
Executive Director: Kathaleen Miller
Business Manager: John Budzyna
Paid Staff: 6
Volunteer Staff: 2
Seating Capacity: 195
Year Remodeled: 1991
Rental Contact: Kathleen Miller

6892 MASSACHUSETTS MUSEUM OF CONTEMPORARY ART
87 Marshall Street
1040 Mass Moca Way
North Adams, MA 01247
Phone: 413-664-4481
Fax: 413-663-8548
e-mail: jonathan@massmoca.org
Web Site: www.massmoca.org
Management:
Performing Arts Director: Jonathan Secor
Specialized Field: Contemporary visual arts and performing arts, Dance, Theatre, Live Music Film

6893 ACADEMY PLAYHOUSE
120 Main Street
PO Box 1843
Orleans, MA 02653
Phone: 508-255-1963
Fax: 508-255-8704
e-mail: apa@cape.com
Web Site: www.apal.org/playhouse
Management:
Executive Administrator: Ralph Basset
Artistic Director: Peter Earle
Mission: To enrich the life of the Cape Cod community through the performing arts. The APA carries out its mission through Playhouse, School, and Outreach programs.
Founded: 1975
Specialized Field: Theatre
Paid Staff: 10
Volunteer Staff: 150
Facility Category: Arena Theatre
Type of Stage: Arena
Seating Capacity: 164

6894 ROBERT BOLAND THEATRE - KOUSSEVITZKY PERFORMING ARTS CENTER
Berkshire Community College
1350 W Street
Pittsfield, MA 01201
Phone: 413-499-4660
e-mail: jjgardner@cc.berkshire.org
Management:
 Technical Director: Jeffrey L Gardner
Type of Stage: Proscenium
Stage Dimensions: 56'W x 46'D x 66'H
Seating Capacity: 510

6895 SPRAGUE - GRISWOLD CULTURAL ART CENTER
American International College
1000 State Street
Springfield, MA 01109
Phone: 413-747-6393
Fax: 413-737-2803

6896 SPRINGFIELD CIVIC CENTER
1277 Main Street
Springfield, MA 01103
Phone: 413-787-6610
Fax: 413-787-6645
e-mail: palumbo@javanet.com
Web Site: www.mccahome.com/staff
Management:
 General Manager: Stuart Hurwitz
 Advertising Manager: Adrianne Palumbo
 Director Operations/Technical: Scott Griffith
 Box Office Director: Anne DeWolf
 Administrative Assistant: Debbie Pafumi

6897 SPRINGFIELD SYMPHONY HALL
Court Square
Springfield, MA 01103
Phone: 413-787-6610
Fax: 413-787-6645

6898 KATHARINE CORNELL MEMORIAL THEATRE
21 Spring Street
PO Box 1239
Tisbury, MA 02568
Phone: 508-696-4200

6899 BRANDEIS UNIVERSITY: SPINGOLD THEATER CENTER
Waltham, MA 02254
Phone: 781-736-2000
Fax: 617-736-3389

6900 BRANDEIS UNIVERSITY: GOSMAN SPORTS & CONVOCATION CENTER
415 S Street
Waltham, MA 02254
Phone: 781-736-4300
Fax: 781-736-4305
Web Site: www.brandeis.edu
Management:
 Athletic Director: Jeff Cohen

6901 CAPE COD CONSERVATORY OF MUSIC, ART, DANCE & DRAMA
Route 132
West Barnstable, MA 02668
Phone: 508-362-2772
Fax: 508-362-4071
Management:
 Director: Robert Wyatt

6902 HORACE A MOSES BUILDING
1305 Memorial Avenue
West Springfield, MA 01089
Phone: 413-737-2443
Fax: 413-787-0127

6903 REGIS COLLEGE FINE ARTS CENTER
235 Wellesley Street
Weston, MA 02493
Phone: 781-768-7034
Fax: 781-768-7030
e-mail: rosemary.noon@regiscollege.edu
Web Site: www.regiscollege.edu
Management:
 Manager: Rosemary Noon

6904 PRISCILLA BEACH THEATER SCHOOL
Rocky Hill Road
Whitehorse Beach, MA 02381
Phone: 508-224-4888

6905 STERLING & FRANCINE CLARK ART INSTITUTE
Sterling & Francine Clark Institute
Box 8
Williamstown, MA 01267
Phone: 413-458-2303
Fax: 413-458-2318
e-mail: info@clarkart.edu
Web Site: www.clarkart.edu
Management:
 Consultant: Brian O'Grady
Founded: 1955
Specialized Field: Visual Arts with Supporting Performances
Performs At: Auditorium
Annual Attendance: 200,000
Seating Capacity: 320
Year Built: 1973

6906 WILLIAM COLLEGE: WESTON FIELD
Lasell Gymnasium, Spring Street
Williamstown, MA 01267
Phone: 413-597-2366
Fax: 413-594-4272
Web Site: www.wiliams.edu
Seating Capacity: 8,000

6907 WILLIAMS COLLEGE: CHAPIN HALL
Williamstown, MA 01267
Phone: 413-597-2127
Web Site: www,williams.edu

6908 MECHANICS HALL
321 Main Street
Worcester, MA 01608
Phone: 508-752-5608
Fax: 508-754-8442
Web Site: www.mechanicshall.com
Management:
  Executive Director: Norma J Sandison
  Sales/Marketing: Sharon Onorato
  Sales/Marketing: Rich Miller
  Business Manager: Steven Grasseschi
  Publicist: Kathleen Gagne
  Building Manager: Robert Blair
Mission: Performing arts center, recording venue,
social/civic function hall.
Founded: 1857
Specialized Field: 1500 Seat Concert Hall
Paid Staff: 12
Year Built: 1857

6909 PERFORMING ARTS SCHOOL OF WORCESTER
29 High Street
Worcester, MA 01608
Phone: 508-755-8246
Fax: 508-795-0640
e-mail: jrlene@performingartsworc.com
Web Site: www.performingartsworc.com
Officers:
  President: Susan Jacobs
  Chair: Chris Cuccaro
  Treasurer: Nigel Belgrave
  VP: Joe Sgro
Management:
  Music Director: Kallin Johnson
  Dance Director: Deidre Miles-Burger
Mission: To expand and anhance the cultural
opportunities of all people by providing diversified
individual and group instruction musci, dance and theatre
arts within and organizational environment that honors
every person. To provide outreach programs to
under-served population that reflect ourrich ethnic
cultures and to remove the socioeconomic barriers that
deny access to the performing arts.
Founded: 1966
Specialized Field: Music Dance Thatre

Michigan

6910 ADRIAN COLLEGE
110 S Madison
Rush Union
Adrian, MI 49221

Phone: 517-264-3156
Fax: 517-264-3331
Toll-free: 800-877-2246
e-mail: admissions@adrian.edu
Web Site: www.adrian.edu

6911 KERRYTOWN CONCERT HOUSE
415 N 4th Avenue
Ann Arbor, MI 48104
Phone: 734-769-2999
Fax: 734-994-0504
e-mail: kch@ic.net
Management:
  Executive Director: Deanna Relyea

6912 MICHIGAN STADIUM
University of Micgigan-Ann Arbor
530 S State Street
Ann Arbor, MI 48103
Phone: 734-936-9358
Fax: 734-936-9345
Web Site: www.umich.edu/~mgoblue/
Management:
  Director: Kevin Gilmartin
Seating Capacity: 101,701

6913 MICHIGAN THEATER
603 E Liberty
Ann Arbor, MI 48104
Phone: 734-668-8397
Fax: 734-668-7136
e-mail: rcollins@michtheater.com
Web Site: www.michtheater.com
Officers:
  President: Ruth Bardenstein
  VP: Albert Barriz
  Secretary: Russell Collins
Management:
  Executive Director: Russell Collins
  Director Operations: Nancy Doyle
Mission: To preserve, restore and operate the historic
Michigan Theater for the benefit of the community and
the arts.
Founded: 1928
Status: Nonprofit
Paid Staff: 12
Volunteer Staff: 300
Paid Artists: 3
Non-paid Artists: 4
Budget: $ 2 Million
Income Sources: 20% Memberiship; Contributions;
Grants
Affiliations: National Association of Theater Owners
Annual Attendance: 2,100,000
Facility Category: Historic Movie Palace
Type of Stage: Precenium
Stage Dimensions: 55x30
Seating Capacity: 1710
Year Built: 1928
Year Remodeled: 2000
Cost: 8.4 Million
Rental Contact: Director Operations Nancy Doyle

**6914 POWER CENTER FOR THE
PERFORMING ARTS**
12 Fletcher Street at E Huron
911 N University
Ann Arbor, MI 48109-1265
Phone: 734-763-3333
Fax: 734-647-2282
e-mail: blarue@umich.edu
Web Site: www.theatre.music.umich.edu/uprod/uprod
Management:
    Facilities Manager: Shannon Rice
Founded: 1971

**6915 UNIVERSITY OF MICHIGAN:
MENDELSSOHN THEATRE**
911 North University
Ann Arbor, MI 48109
Phone: 734-763-1085
Fax: 734-747-2282
Web Site: www.theatre.music.umich.edu
Management:
    Facilities Manager: Shannon Rice
Founded: 1929
Performs At: Intimate, shoe-box theatre with a
cyclorama.
Type of Stage: Proscenium
Stage Dimensions: 29'11" x 16'10"
Seating Capacity: 658
Year Built: 1929
Year Remodeled: 1995

**6916 UNIVERSITY OF MICHIGAN:
TRUEBLOOD THEATRE**
State Street at Washington
Ann Arbor, MI 48109
Phone: 734-763-5213
Fax: 734-647-2282
Web Site: threatre.music.umich.edu/uprod/uprod
Management:
    Facilities Manager: Shannon Rice
Affiliations: UM School of music
Type of Stage: black box
Seating Capacity: varies

6917 YOST ICE ARENA
University of Michigan
1000 S State Street
Ann Arbor, MI 48109-2201
Phone: 734-764-4600
Fax: 734-764-4597
e-mail: yostice@umich.edu
Web Site: www.umich.edu/yost
Management:
    Manager: Craig Wotta
    Assistant Manager: Steve Ponka
Mission: Hockey Games and Tournaments, Figure
skating shows, and general public seating.
Paid Staff: 20
Seating Capacity: 6,193

6918 PALACE AT AUBURN HILLS
2 Championship Drive
Auburn Hill, MI 48326

Phone: 248-377-8200
Fax: 248-377-4262
Web Site: www.palacenet.com
Officers:
    President: Tom Wilson
Management:
    Director Events: Bill Newton
    VP/Marketing: Dan Hauser
    Marketing Director: Marilyn Desjardins
    EVP: John Ciszewski
    Director Corporate Sales: Jon Dierkes
Seating Capacity: 21,454

6919 BATTLE CREEK CIVIC THEATRE
PO Box 519
Battle Creek, MI 49106
Phone: 616-441-2708
Web Site: www.bcarts.org/civictheatre

6920 CO BROWN STADIUM
1392 Capital Avenue NE
Battle Creek, MI 49017
Phone: 269-660-2287
Fax: 269-660-2288
Web Site: www.battlecatsbaseball.com
Management:
    General Manager: Jerry Burkot

6921 KELLOGG ARENA
1 McCamly Square
Battle Creek, MI 49017
Phone: 616-963-4800
Fax: 616-968-8840
e-mail: kschreibler@kelloggarena
Web Site: www.kelloggarena.com
Management:
    General Manager: Kevin Scheibler
    Director Operations: Martin R Whiting
Seating Capacity: 6,000

**6922 UNITED ARTS COUNCIL DISCOVERY
THEATRE**
51 W Michigan Avenue
Battle Creek, MI 49017
Mailing Address: PO Box 1079, Battle Creek, MI. 49016
Phone: 616-441-2700
Fax: 616-441-2707
e-mail: bcunitedartscouncil@prodigy.net
Web Site: www.unitedartscouncil.org
Management:
    Acting Executive Director: Kevin S Henning

**6923 LAKE MICHIGAN COLLEGE, MENDEL
CENTER FOR THE ARTS &
TECHNOLOGY**
2755 E Napier Avenue
Benton Harbor, MI 49022-1899
Phone: 616-927-8193
Fax: 616-927-6587
e-mail: schutze@raptor.lmc.cc.mi.us
Management:
    Mainstage Services Director: Cindy Shutze

6924 CHEBOYGAN OPERA HOUSE: CITY HALL
403 N Huron
Cheboygan, MI 49721
Phone: 231-627-5432
Fax: 231-627-2643
Toll-free: 800-357-9408
e-mail: jpl@nmo.net
Web Site: theoperahouse.org
Management:
    Executive Director/Arts Council: Joann P Leal
Mission: To promote and encourage cultural and educational activities within the Straits Area of Northern Michigan and to provide services that stimulate and encourage participation in the arts within all segments of the community.
Founded: 1877
Budget: $250,000
Income Sources: Ticket Sales; Contributions; Annual Campaigns; Grants
Affiliations: Association of Performing Arts Presenters
Type of Stage: Proscenium
Stage Dimensions: 34 x 23
Seating Capacity: 582
Year Built: 1877
Year Remodeled: 1982

6925 MACOMB CENTER FOR THE PERFORMING ARTS
44575 Garfield Road
Clinton Township, MI 48038-1139
Phone: 810-286-2141
Fax: 810-286-2272
e-mail: biddle@macomb.cc.mi.us
Web Site: www.macomb.cc.mi.us
Management:
    Executive Director: William Biddle

6926 COBO ARENA
600 Civic Center Drive
Detroit, MI 48226
Phone: 313-396-7600
Fax: 313-396-7998
Web Site: www.detroitwtewings.com
Management:
    VP/General Manager: Randy Lippe
    Director Events: Robert Baker
Seating Capacity: 12,200
Year Built: 1959

6927 COMERICA PARK
Detroit, MI 48216
Phone: 313-962-4000
Fax: 313-471-2099
Web Site: www.detroittigers.com
Management:
    President/CEO: John McHale
    VP Baseball Operations/Gen. Manager: Randyk Smith
Seating Capacity: 40,000
Year Built: 2000

6928 DETROIT SYMPHONY ORCHESTRA HALL
3711 Woodward
Detroit, MI 48201
Phone: 313-576-5111

6929 FISHER THEATRE
3011 W Grand Boulevard
Detroit, MI 48202
Phone: 313-872-1156
Fax: 313-872-0632
Web Site: www.nederlanderdetroit.com
Management:
    Manager: James Manduzzi
Mission: To offer the best in national stage and concert entertainment.
Founded: 1961
Status: Professional; Nonprofit
Income Sources: Box Office
Facility Category: Live Stage Theater
Type of Stage: Proscenium House
Stage Dimensions: 50' 0" x 32' 6"
Seating Capacity: 2,089
Year Remodeled: 2001
Architect: Rapp & Rapp of Chicago

6930 FOX THEATRE
2211 Woodward Avenue
Detroit, MI 48201
Phone: 313-965-7100
Fax: 313-471-3220
Web Site: www.olympiaentertainment.com
Founded: 1928

6931 JOE LOUIS ARENA
600 Civic Center Drive
Detroit, MI 48226
Phone: 313-396-7444
Fax: 313-396-7998
Web Site: www.detroitredwings.com
Management:
    VP Sports/Entertainment: Stuart Mayer
    Director Marketing: Bill Lee
    General Sales Manager: William A Ley
Seating Capacity: 19,965
Year Built: 1979

6932 MASONIC TEMPLE THEATRE
500 Temple Avenue
Detroit, MI 48201
Phone: 313-832-5900
Fax: 313-832-1047

6933 MUSIC HALL CENTER FOR THE PERFORMING ARTS
350 Madison Avenue
Detroit, MI 48226
Phone: 313-963-7622
Fax: 313-963-2462
Web Site: www.musichall.org
Officers:
    President: Cameron Duncan

Management:
  Marketing Manager: Andrea Saglimbene
  Marketing Director: Michael Vigilant
  Artistic Director: Frank Malfitano
  Events Director: Karen McBride
Mission: To present high-quality programming to a variety of audiences, while preserving and maintaining a nationally recognized historic building and remaining a financially viable institution.
Founded: 1928
Paid Staff: 20
Volunteer Staff: 200
Paid Artists: 600
Seating Capacity: 1701
Year Built: 1928
Year Remodeled: 1995
Organization Type: Performing

6934 UNIVERSITY OF DETROIT MERCY: CALIHAN HALL
University of Detroit Mercy
4001 W McNichols
Detroit, MI 48219
Phone: 313-993-1700
Fax: 313-993-2449
Web Site: www.udmercy.edu
Management:
  Athletic Director: Brad Kinsman

6935 WAYNE STATE UNIVERSITY: COLLEGE OF FINE, PERFORMING & COMMUNICATION ARTS
5104 Gullen Mall
Linsell House
Detroit, MI 48202
Phone: 313-577-5342
Fax: 313-577-5355
Web Site: www.cfpca.wayne.edu
Founded: 1868
Specialized Field: All

6936 SPARTAN STADIUM
Michigan State University
One Birch Road
East Kansing, MI 48824
Phone: 517-432-1989
Fax: 517-432-1510
Web Site: www.breslincenter.msu.edu
Management:
  Director: Scott Breckner
Seating Capacity: 72,027

6937 BRESLIN STUDENT EVENTS CENTER
1 Birch Road
East Landing, MI 48824-1004
Phone: 517-432-1989
Fax: 517-432-1510
Web Site: www.breslincenter.msu.edu
Management:
  Director: Scott H Breckner

6938 MICHIGAN STATE UNIVERSITY WHARTON CENTER PRESENTATIONS
Wharton Center
East Lansing, MI 48824-1318
Phone: 517-353-1982
Fax: 517-353-5329
e-mail: wrightw@pilot.msu.edu
Web Site: www.msu.edu/wharton
Management:
  Executive Director: William Wright
Founded: 1982
Paid Staff: 30
Budget: $8,000,000
Income Sources: Ticket Sales, Funding, Rentals
Performs At: Great Hall
Annual Attendance: 250,000
Facility Category: Theatre (5)
Type of Stage: Premium, Thrust
Seating Capacity: 2,500,000
Year Built: 1982

6939 1515 BROADWAY PERFORMANCE VENUE
29205 Greening Boulevard
Farmington Hills, MI 48334
Phone: 248-932-0090
Fax: 248-932-8763
Toll-free: 877-683-4452
e-mail: jsapub@aol.com
Web Site: www.the-feds.com
Management:
  Managing Director: Joseph S Ajlouny, Jr
  Marketing Director: Patte Miller
Mission: Urban performance venue.
Founded: 1990
Specialized Field: Music; Theatre
Status: Profit
Paid Staff: 6
Volunteer Staff: 10
Budget: $160,000
Income Sources: Tickets; Sponsorship
Performs At: Black Box Theater
Annual Attendance: 4,000
Facility Category: Independent Theater
Type of Stage: Proscenium; In-the-Round
Stage Dimensions: 18' x 16' with thrust
Seating Capacity: 120
Year Built: 1979
Year Remodeled: 1989

6940 COMMUNITY CENTER FARMINGTON
24705 Farmington
Farmington Hills, MI 48336
Phone: 313-477-8404

6941 ATWOOD STADIUM
1101 S Saginaw Street
Flint, MI 48502
Phone: 810-766-7463
Fax: 810-766-7468
Management:
  Director: Art Evans

6942 FLINT INSTITUTE OF MUSIC
1025 E Kearsley Street
Flint, MI 48503
Phone: 810-238-1350
Fax: 810-238-1350
Toll-free: 800-395-4849
e-mail: fim@thefim.com
Web Site: www.thefim.com
Officers:
   President: Paul Torre
Management:
   Marketing Director: Christina Ferris
   Director Flint School Performing: Davin Pierson
   Torre
   Manager Flint Symphony: Tom Glasscok
   Music Director: Enrique Diemecke
   Director Ticket: Linda Tomlinson
   Director Development: Carol Hartley
Mission: Providing a lifelong continuum of music and
dance.
Founded: 1917
Status: Nonprofit
Performs At: Whiting Auditorium
Annual Attendance: 3,500

6943 IMA SPORTS ARENA
3501 Lapeer Road
Flint, MI 48503
Phone: 810-744-0580
Fax: 810-744-2906
Management:
   General Manager: Tony Sertich

6944 MAPLEWOOD COMMUNITY CENTER
31735 Maplewood
Garden City, MI 48135
Phone: 734-525-8848
Fax: 734-261-7112
Web Site: www.ci.maplewood.mn.us

**6945 CITY OF GRAND HAVEN COMMUNITY
CENTER**
421 Columbus
Grand Haven, MI 49417
Phone: 616-842-2550
Fax: 616-842-5287
Web Site: www.grandhavenlive.com/ghee
Seating Capacity: 300-350

6946 CALVIN COLLEGE FINE ARTS CENTER
3201 Burton Street SE
Grand Rapids, MI 49546
Phone: 616-957-6280
Fax: 616-957-6469
Web Site: www.calvin.edu

**6947 DELTAPLEX ENTERTAINMENT & EXPO
CENTER**
2500 Turner NW
Grand Rapids, MI 49544

Phone: 616-364-9000
Fax: 616-559-8001
e-mail: robh@deltaplex.com
Web Site: www.deltaplex.com
Management:
   Director Sales/Marketing: Mike Vandervelde
   GM: Rob Harley
   Event Coordinator: Amy Dittweiler
Seating Capacity: 7,000

6948 FOUNTAIN STREET CHURCH
24 Fountain Street NE
Grand Rapids, MI 49503
Phone: 616-459-8386
Fax: 616-459-4809
Web Site: www.fountainstreet.org
Management:
   Interim Character School Director: Lydia Stubs
   Execuktive Minister: Dr. Don Hoekstra
   Senior Programming Director: Mary Thompson
Mission: To liberate and cultivate the human spirit. For
this liberation to take place, it is our goal to provide a
community where a person can unfold into their
individuality and become a fully functioning free
individual.

6949 GRAND CENTER: DEVOS HALL
245 Monroe Avenue NW
Grand Rapids, MI 49503
Phone: 616-742-6600
Fax: 616-742-6590
Web Site: www.grandcenter.com
Management:
   General Manager: Rich Mackeigan
   Director Events Services: Steve Miller
Performs At: Theater
Facility Category: theater
Type of Stage: Proscenium
Seating Capacity: 2446
Year Built: 1980
Rental Contact: Steve Miller

6950 GRAND CENTER: AUDITORIUM
245 Monroe Avenue NW
Grand Rapids, MI 49503
Phone: 616-742-6600
Fax: 616-742-6590
Web Site: www.grandcenter.com
Management:
   General Manager: Rich MacKeigan
   Assistant General Manager: Jim Watt
   Director Events Services: Steve Miller
   Stage Manager: Sandy Thomley
Founded: 1980
Paid Staff: 13
Performs At: DesVos Hall and Welsh Auditorium
Seating Capacity: 2446 and 4396

**6951 URBAN INSTITUTE FOR
CONTEMPORARY ARTS**
41 Sheldon Boulevard SE
Grand Rapids, MI 49503

Phone: 616-454-7000
Fax: 616-454-7013
e-mail: uica@iserv.net
Web Site: www.uica.org

6952 VAN ANDEL ARENA
130 Folton W
Grand Rapids, MI 49503
Phone: 616-742-6600
Fax: 616-742-6590
Management:
General Manager: Craig Liston
Seating Capacity: 12,048

6953 HOPE COLLEGE THEATRE DEPARTMENT
Holland, MI 49423
Phone: 616-392-5111
Fax: 616-395-7182
Web Site: www.hope.edu/academic/theatre
Management:
Theatre Director: John KV Tammi
Office Manager: Judyth Thomas
Producing Director: Mary Schakel
Production Manager: Anne de Velder

6954 INTERLOCHEN CENTER FOR THE ARTS - DENDRINOS CENTER
PO Box 199
Interlochen, MI 49643
Phone: 231-276-7200
Fax: 231-276-6321
Seating Capacity: 200
Year Built: 1991

6955 INTERLOCHEN CENTER FOR THE ARTS: KRESGE AUDITORIUM
PO Box 199
Interlochen, MI 49643
Phone: 231-276-7200
Fax: 231-276-6321

6956 IRONWOOD THEATRE
109 E Aurora Street
Ironwood, MI 49938
Phone: 906-932-0618
Fax: 906-932-0457
e-mail: office@ironwoodtheatre.org
Web Site: www.ironwoodtheatre.org
Officers:
President: Dale Ballone
VP: Tom Brown
Secretary: Lee Brown
Treasurer: David Sauter
Management:
Administrative Assistant: Andrea Soltis
Mission: To provide cultural entertainment of the highest possible quality to the greatest number of people in the western upper Peninsula of Michigan and Northern Wisconsin.
Founded: 1928
Budget: $125,000

Income Sources: Grants; State of Michigan; Fund Raisers
Performs At: Auditorium
Affiliations: Michigan Council for Arts-Cultural Affairs
Annual Attendance: 20,000
Facility Category: Performing Arts Center
Type of Stage: Proscenium
Stage Dimensions: 28'6wx23'l
Seating Capacity: 732
Year Built: 1928
Year Remodeled: 1983
Cost: $160,000

6957 JAMES W MILLER AUDITORIUM
1903 W Michigan Avenue
Kalamazoo, MI 19008
Phone: 269-387-2311
Fax: 269-387-2317
Toll-free: 800-228-9858
e-mail: William.Biddle@wmich.edu
Web Site: www.millerauditorium.com
Management:
Building Coordinator: Elaine Williams
Founded: 1968
Specialized Field: Symphonies; Broadway Musicals; Opera; Comedy; Concert
Facility Category: Auditorium
Seating Capacity: 3; 497

6958 KALAMAZOO CIVIC AUDITORIUM
329 S Park Street
Kalamazoo, MI 49006
Phone: 616-343-1313
Fax: 616-343-0532
Web Site: www.kazoocivic.com

6959 KALAMAZOO COLLEGE
1200 Academy Street
Kalamazoo, MI 49006
Phone: 616-337-7070
Web Site: www.kzoo.edu

6960 WESTERN MICHIGAN UNIVERSITY PATRONS
Department of Theatre
Kalamazoo, MI 49008-5029
Phone: 616-387-3224
Fax: 616-387-3222
e-mail: williamst@wimch.edu
Web Site: www.wmich.edu
Management:
Chairman: D Terry Williams PhD
Performs At: James W. Miller Auditorium

6961 WINGS STADIUM
3600 Van Rick Drive
Kalamazoo, MI 49001
Phone: 616-345-1125
Fax: 616-345-6452
e-mail: info@wingsstadium.com
Web Site: www.wingsstadium.com
Management:
CEO: RT Parfet

VP/General Manager: Paul L Pickard
Event Coordinator: Andrea Pluta
Seating Capacity: 5,113

6962 LANSING CIVIC ARENA

505 W Allegan Street
Lansing, MI 48933
Phone: 517-483-7425
Fax: 517-483-7400

6963 BERRY EVENTS CENTER

1401 Presquesolo
Marquette, MI 49855
Phone: 906-227-1150
Fax: 906-227-2855
Web Site: www.nmu.edu
Management:
   Facility Director: Steve Van Der Kamp

6964 LAKEVIEW ARENA

401 E Fair Avenue
Marquette, MI 49855-4763
Phone: 906-228-0493
Fax: 906-228-0493
Management:
   Event Coordinator: Victoria Snyder
   Park/Recreation Director: High Leslie
Seating Capacity: 3,500

6965 NORTHERN MICHIGAN UNIVERSITY: SUPERIOR HOME

Northern Michigan University Superior Dome
C-105
Marquette, MI
Phone: 906-227-2850
Fax: 906-227-2855
Management:
   Director/Manager: Carl Bammert
   Ticket Manager: Joan Mulder
Seating Capacity: 9,000

6966 MIDLAND CENTER FOR THE ARTS

1801 W St. Andrews Road
Midland, MI 48640-2695
Phone: 989-631-5930
Fax: 989-631-7890
e-mail: info@mcfta.org
Web Site: www.mcfta.org
Management:
   President/CEO: Michael Tiknis

6967 RIVER RAISIN CENTRE FOR THE ARTS

114 S Monroe Street
Monroe, MI 48161
Phone: 734-242-7722
Fax: 734-242-9238
e-mail: kreutzberg@riverraisincentre.org
Web Site: www.riverraisincentre.org
Management:
   Executive Director: James D Kreutzberg

6968 CENTRAL MICHIGAN UNIVERSITY

1303 W Campus Drive
Mount Pleasant, MI 48859
Phone: 517-774-3355
Fax: 517-774-7957
e-mail: Robert.J.Ebner@cmich.edu
Web Site: www.cmich.edu/events.html
Management:
   University Events Director: Robert Ebner

6969 ROSE ARENA: BASKETBALL ARENA

Central Michigan University
Rose Center
Mount. Pleasant, MI 48859
Phone: 517-774-3041
Fax: 517-774-5391
Web Site: www.smich.edu
Seating Capacity: 5,200

6970 KELLY/SHORTS STADIUM

Center Michigan University
306 Warriner Hall
Mt Pleasant, MI 48859
Phone: 517-774-3355
Fax: 517-774-7957
e-mail: keith.e.voeks@cmich.edu
Web Site: www.cmich.edu
Management:
   Assistant Director: Keith E Voeks
Seating Capacity: 30,000

6971 MACOMB CENTER FOR THE PERFORMING ARTS

44575 Garfield
Mt. Clemens, MI 48038
Phone: 810-286-2222
Fax: 313-286-2272
Management:
   Marketing Director: Tara Arnold
   Technical Director: George Hommowun
   Facility Rentals: Susan Hier
   Executive Director: Ron Koenig
   Operations Manager: Nancy Kramarcyzk
Mission: To enhance and enrich the cultural development and awareness of the community by offering a diversified selection of quality cultural experiences and to inspire and encourage artistic expression through education, performance and volunteer opportunities.
Type of Stage: Proscenium
Stage Dimensions: 48 x 29
Seating Capacity: 1271

6972 FRAUENTHAL CENTER FOR THE PERFORMING ARTS

425 W Western Avenue
Muskegon, MI 49440
Phone: 231-722-9750
Fax: 231-722-4616
e-mail: smogabry@cffmc.org
Web Site: www.frauenthal.org
Officers:
   President Community Foundation: Chris McGuigan
Management:

Executive Director: Kirk M Wahamaki
Interim Director: Susan Elliott McGarry
Operations Manager: Jennifer Witham
Technical Director: Bill Bodell
Mission: To increase appreciation of film and the performing arts in Western Michigan.
Founded: 1974
Specialized Field: Dance; Vocal Music; Instrumental Music; Theater
Status: Professional; Non-Professional; Nonprofit
Paid Staff: 7
Volunteer Staff: 385
Budget: $890,000
Income Sources: Ticket Sales; Endowments
Performs At: Frauenthal Theatre; Beardsley Theatre
Affiliations: League of Historic American Theatres; American Association of Arts Presenters
Annual Attendance: 185,000
Facility Category: Historic Theater
Type of Stage: Proscenium
Stage Dimensions: 41'6"x30H
Seating Capacity: 1,748
Year Built: 1930
Year Remodeled: 1998
Cost: $8,500,000
Rental Contact: Interim Director Susan Elliot McGarry
Organization Type: Performing; Resident; Educational; Sponsoring; Presenter
Resident Groups: Muskegon Community Concert Association, Muskegon Civic Theatre, Cherry County Playhouse, West Shore

6973 FRAUENTHAL FOUNDATION FINE ARTS CENTER
221 S Quarterline Road
Muskegon, MI 49442
Phone: 231-773-9131
Fax: 231-722-4616
Mission: The heart of the Frauenthal Fine Arts Center is the 344-seat Overbrook Theater and adjacent art gallery, where works by students, faculty, and guest artists are exhibited. The center also includes a large rehearsal room for band, orchestra, and chorus, practice rooms, and a listening library where students may enjoy recordings. The Center also has 12 electronic pianos for instruction and practice.
Specialized Field: Fine Arts Center
Performs At: Overbrook Theater
Seating Capacity: 344

6974 WALKER ARENA
955 4th Street
Muskegon, MI 49440
Phone: 231-726-3939
Fax: 231-726-4620
Management:
  Director: Neil Hawryliw
Seating Capacity: 6,400

6975 PONTIAC SILVERDOME
1200 Featherstone
Pontiac, MI 48342

Phone: 248-858-7358
Fax: 248-456-1691
e-mail: info@silverdome.com
Web Site: www.silverdome.com
Management:
  Executive Director: Eric Walker
  Director Marketing: Greg Roberts
Founded: 1975
Seating Capacity: 93,000

6976 MCMORRAN PLACE THEATRE
701 McMorran Boulevard
Port Huron, MI 48060
Phone: 810-985-6166
Fax: 810-985-3358
Toll-free: 800-858-6166
e-mail: webmaster@mcmorran.com
Web Site: www.mcmorran.com
Officers:
  President: Ernest Werth
  First VP: Denise Selby
  Second VP: John Shirky
  Secretary: Jo Lantz
Management:
  General Manager: Larry Krabach
  Administrative Director: Lynn Hines
  Technical Director/Webmaster: Scot W Kavanaugh
  Box Office Manager: Pat David
Mission: Bring the Arts and culture to the community. To provide public facilities to the community.
Founded: 1957
Specialized Field: Community; Theatrical Group
Status: Semi-Professional; Nonprofit
Paid Staff: 10
Income Sources: College
Facility Category: Performing Arts
Type of Stage: Procenium
Stage Dimensions: 50x30
Seating Capacity: 1159
Year Built: 1959

6977 KIRTLAND COMMUNITY COLLEGE: KIRTLAND CENTER FOR THE PERFORMING ARTS
10775 N St. Helen Road
Roscommon, MI 48653
Phone: 989-275-5000
Fax: 989-275-6757
e-mail: cartong@kirtland.cc.mi.us
Web Site: www.kirtland.cc.mi.us/~kcpahome
Management:
  Director: Gary Carton
  Director Kirtland Youth Theatre: Shirley Carton
  Ticket Office Manager: Beth Petrik
  Technical Director: Jeani Vermillion
Mission: Arts Center for four county area
Founded: 1966
Paid Staff: 4
Volunteer Staff: 30
Budget: 300,000
Income Sources: Ticket Sal;es; Donations; College Funding
Affiliations: Arts Midwest; APAP; USITT; MACAA
Annual Attendance: 30,000

Facility Category: Theatre
Type of Stage: Modified Thrust
Seating Capacity: 846
Year Built: 1966
Rental Contact: Director Gary Carlton

6978 COUNTY EVENT CENTER: HERITAGE THEATER

303 Johnson Street
Saginaw, MI 48607
Phone: 989-759-1320
Fax: 989-759-1322
Founded: 1970
Facility Category: Theatre
Year Remodeled: 2002
Rental Contact: Allan C. Vella

6979 PARAMOUNT THEATRE

913 W Saint Germain Street
Saint Cloud, MI 56301-3460
Phone: 320-259-5463
Fax: 320-257-3111
e-mail: lolson@paramountarts.org
Web Site: www.paramountarts.org
Management:
   Executive Director: Lori Olsen

6980 TECUMSEH CIVIC AUDITORIUM

400 N Maumee
Tecumseh, MI 49286-0056
Phone: 517-423-6617
Fax: 517-423-3610
e-mail: CivicDir@tecumseh.mi.us
Web Site: www.Tecumseh.mi.us/TheCivic
Management:
   Executive Director: Paul H Sullivan

6981 DENNOS MUSEUM CENTER

Northwestern Michigan College
1701 E Front Street
Traverse City, MI 49686
Phone: 231-995-1055
Fax: 231-995-1597
e-mail: dmc@nmc.edu
Web Site: www.dennosmuseum.org
Management:
   Museum Center Director: Eugene A Jenneman
   Performing Art Manager: Robert Weiler
Mission: Seeks to engage, entertain and enlighten its
audiences through the collection of art; and through the
presentation of exhibitions and programs in the visual
arts, sciences and performing arts.
Founded: 1991

6982 DENNOS MUSEUM CENTER: MILLIKEN AUDITORIUM

1701 E Front Street
Traverse City, MI 49686
Phone: 231-995-1055
Fax: 231-995-1597
Toll-free: 800-748-0566
e-mail: dmc@rmc.edu
Web Site: www.dennosmuseum.org

Management:
   Museum Director: Eugene Jenneman
   Assistant to the Director: Judith Albers
   Curator: Kathleen Buday
   Auditorium Coordinator: Martha Griggs
Paid Staff: 9
Volunteer Staff: 160
Budget: $900,000
Annual Attendance: 600,000
Facility Category: Art Museum/ Performance Center
Stage Dimensions: 30' X 50'
Seating Capacity: 367
Year Built: 1991
Rental Contact: Assistant to the Director Judith Albers

6983 PARK PLACE HOTEL

300 E State Street
Traverse City, MI 49684
Phone: 231-946-5000
Fax: 231-941-9812
Toll-free: 800-748-0133
e-mail: hotel@park-place-hotel.com
Web Site: www.park-place-hotel.com

6984 JAMES E O'NEILL JR ARENA
Saginaw Valley State University

7400 Bay Road
University Center, MI 48710
Phone: 517-791-7333
Fax: 517-790-0545
e-mail: waske@svsu.edu
Web Site: www.svsu.edu
Management:
   Manager: Joe Vogl

6985 JEWISH COMMUNITY CENTER OF METROPOLITAN DETROIT

D. Dan & Betty Kahn Building
6600 W Maple Road
West Bloomfield, MI 48322-3002
Phone: 248-661-1000
Fax: 248-432-5540
Web Site: www.jccdet.org
Management:
   President: Sharon Hart
   Executive Director: David H Sorkin
   Marketing Director: Heidi Press
Mission: To support Jewish unity, ensure Jewish
continuity and enrich Jewish life while conveying the
importance of well-being within the Jewish and general
community and the people of Israel.
Founded: 1926
Paid Staff: 491
Volunteer Staff: 999

6986 CRILSER ARENA

260 Lakeview Drive
Whitmore, MI 48189
Phone: 734-998-7236
Fax: 734-615-0224
Management:
   Facility Director: Lisa Panettalalt

6987 YACK ARENA
246 Sycamore Street
Wyandotte, MI 48192
Phone: 734-324-7290
Fax: 734-324-7296
e-mail: lupo2390@cs.com
Web Site: www.wyandotte.net
Management:
   Festival Manager: Lelsie Lupo
   Arena Manager: James Knopp
Seating Capacity: 3,800

6988 BOWEN FIELDHOUSE
Easter Michigan University
200 Bowen Fieldhouse
Ypsilanti, MI 48197
Phone: 734-487-1050
Fax: 734-487-6898
Management:
   Athletic Director: Dave Diles

6989 EASTERN MICHIGAN UNIVERSITY OFFICE OF CULTURAL LIFE
11 McKenny Union
Ypsilanti, MI 48197
Phone: 734-487-3045
Fax: 734-480-1927

6990 RYNEARSON STADIUM
Eastern Michigan University
200 Bowen Fieldhouse
Ypsilanti, MI 48197
Phone: 734-487-1050
Fax: 734-487-6898
Web Site: www.emich.edu
Management:
   Manager Facilities/Events: Brett Roach
   Sports Information Director: Jim Streeter
   Head Football Coach: Rick Rasnick
   Head Basketball Coach (M): Milton Barnes
   Head Basketball Coach (W): Paulette Stein
Seating Capacity: 30,200

Minnesota

6991 ALBERT LEA CITY ARENA
Lake Chapeau Drive
Albert, MN 56007
Phone: 507-377-4374
Fax: 507-377-4336
Management:
   Director: Bob Furland

6992 ALBERT LEA CIVIC THEATER
147 N Broadway
Albert Lea, MN 56007
Phone: 507-377-4372
Fax: 507-377-4336
Management:
   Theatre Manager: Patrick Rasmussen
Paid Staff: 1

Facility Category: Theatre
Type of Stage: Proscenium
Stage Dimensions: 29' 6" x 23' x 28'
Seating Capacity: 255
Year Remodeled: 1989
Rental Contact: Patrick Rasmussen

6993 RIVERSIDE ARENA
501 2nd Avenue NE
Austin, MN 55912
Phone: 507-437-8315
Fax: 507-433-9078
Management:
   Manager: Dennis Maschka
Facility Category: Arena
Type of Stage: Portable
Seating Capacity: 4,200

6994 BEMIDJI STATE UNIVERSITY: BANGSBERG FINE ART BUILDING
1500 Birchmont Drive NE
Bemidji, MN 56601
Phone: 218-755-3990
Fax: 218-755-4369
Web Site: www.bemidji.msus.edu/
Mission: Faculty and departmental/program offices for theatre and speech communication, music and mass communication; studios; classrooms; Thompson Recital Hall; main stage and black box theatres; rehearsal rooms; KAWE public television offices. Facilities are utilized by both the campus and the community.
Specialized Field: Fine Arts Complex
Performs At: Thompson Recital Hall
Facility Category: Main Stage and Black Box

6995 NATIONAL SPORTS CENTER
1700 105th Avenue N
Blaine, MN 55449
Phone: 612-785-5600
Fax: 612-785-5699
Web Site: www.nscsports.com
Management:
   Marketing Director: Dave Christie
Founded: 1990
Seating Capacity: 12,000

6996 ARTS IN THE PARKS: PORTABLE STAGE
2215 W Old Shakopee Road
Bloomington, MN 55431
Phone: 952-948-3925
Fax: 612-887-9695

6997 TORO COMPANY
81111 Lyndale Avenue S
Bloomington, MN 55420
Phone: 612-887-8960
Fax: 612-887-8258
Web Site: www.toro.com
Management:
   Director Public Relations: Don Dennis
   Contractor Sales Manager: Mark Roberts

All listings are in alphabetical order by state, then city, then organization within the city.

6998 BROOKLYN CENTER
6301 Shingle Creek Parkway
Brooklyn Center, MN 55430-2199
Phone: 763-569-3300
Fax: 763-569-3494
e-mail: info@ci.brooklyn-center.mn.us
Web Site: www.ci.brooklyn-center.mn.us/

6999 NORTH HENNEPIN COMMUNITY COLLEGE
7411 85th Avenue N
Brooklyn Park, MN 55445
Phone: 763-493-0505
Fax: 763-493-0542

7000 DEPOT ST. LOUIS CO. HERITAGE AND ARTS CENTER
506 W Michigan Street
Duluth, MN 55802
Phone: 218-727-8025
Fax: 218-733-7506
Web Site: www.duluthdepot.org/
Management:
 Executive Director: Paula Davidson
 Administrative Coordinator: Rose Case
 Technical Services: Tim Klande
 Finance Director: Bob Larkin

7001 DULUTH ENTERTAINMENT CONVENTION CENTER
350 Harbor Drive
Duluth, MN 55802
Phone: 218-722-5573
Fax: 218-722-4247
Toll-free: 800-628-8385
e-mail: decc@decc.org
Web Site: www.decc.org/
Management:
 Director Sales: Anna Schnell
 Director Event Planning: Annette Eberhart
 Human Resources Manager: Bryan French
 Director of Entertainment: Craig Samborski

7002 FAIRMONT OPERA HOUSE
45 Downtown Plaza
PO Box 226
Fairmont, MN 56031
Phone: 507-238-4900
Web Site: www.fairmont.org/foh/home.htm
Management:
 Managing Director: Michael Burgraff

7003 GRAND RAPIDS COMMUNITY COLLEGE: FORD FIELDHOUSE
11 Lyon Street NE
Grand Rapids, MN 49503
Phone: 616-771-4261
Fax: 616-771-4262
Web Site: www.grcc.cc.mi.us
Management:
 Head Football Coach: Fred Julian

7004 PRAIRIE ARTS CENTER
PO Box 94
310 1st Avenue Norther
Long Prairie, MN 56347
Phone: 320-732-6080
Officers:
 President: Linda Kielty

7005 MIDWEST WIRELESS CIVIC CENTER
One Civic Center Plaza
Mankato, MN 56001-7797
Phone: 507-389-3000
Fax: 507-345-1627
Web Site: www.midwestwirelessciviccenter.com
Management:
 General Manager: Marshall Madsen
 Executive Director: Burt Lyman
 Marketing Manager: Eric Jones
 Operations Manager: Dave Randalls
 Food/Beverage Director: Scott Schonike
Seating Capacity: 7,310

7006 MINNESOTA STATE UNIVERSITY: ELIAS J HALLING RECITAL HALL
202 Performing Arts Center
Mankato, MN 56001
Phone: 507-389-2118
Fax: 507-389-2922
e-mail: music@mnsu.edu
Web Site: www.intech.mnsu.edu
Management:
 Events Coordinator/Music: Dale Haefner
Paid Staff: 5
Budget: $55,000
Income Sources: Gate Receipts; Grants; Advertising; Corporate Contributions
Annual Attendance: 14,000
Facility Category: Performing Arts Center
Type of Stage: Proscenium
Stage Dimensions: 80'x40'
Seating Capacity: 350
Year Built: 1968
Rental Contact: 507-398-5549 Dale Haefner

7007 GUTHRIE THEATER
725 Vineland Place
Minneapolis, MN 55403
Phone: 612-347-1100
Fax: 612-347-1188
Toll-free: 877-447-8243
Web Site: www.guthrietheater.org
Seating Capacity: 1,293
Year Built: 1963

7008 HENNEPIN CENTER FOR THE ARTS
528 Hennepin Avenue
Minneapolis, MN 55403
Phone: 612-332-4478
Fax: 612-340-1255
Web Site: www.artspaceprojects.org
Founded: 1888

7009 HISTORIC ORPHEUM THEATRE
910 Hennepin Avenue
Minneapolis, MN 55403
Phone: 612-339-0075
Fax: 612-339-5917
Web Site: www.state-orpheum.com

7010 HISTORIC STATE THEATRE
805 Hennepin Avenue
Minneapolis, MN 55403
Phone: 612-339-0075
Fax: 612-339-0601
Web Site: www.state-orpheum.com

7011 HUBERT H HUMPHREY METRODOME
900 S 5th Street
Minneapolis, MN 55415
Phone: 612-332-0386
Fax: 612-332-8334
e-mail: alftond@msfc.com
Web Site: www.msfc.com
Management:
   Executive Director: William Lester
   Director Operations/Marketing: Dennis Alfton
Founded: 1982
Seating Capacity: 65,000 (football), 55,500 (basketball)
Year Built: 1982

7012 MACPHAIL CENTER FOR THE ARTS
1128 LaSalle Avenue
Minneapolis, MN 55403
Phone: 612-321-0100
Management:
   Assistant Director: Joanna Cortright
Mission: Lessons and classes in music to both adults and children.
Founded: 1907
Specialized Field: Vocal Music; Instrumental Music
Status: Semi-Professional; Nonprofit
Income Sources: University of Minnesota; National Guild of Community Schools of Music
Organization Type: Educational

7013 MARIUCCI ARENA
University of Minnesota
1901 4th Street SE, Room 137
Minneapolis, MN 55455
Phone: 612-625-5804
Fax: 612-624-5887
Management:
   Program Director: Scott P Ellison
   Asssistant Program Director: Craig Flor
Seating Capacity: 16,900

7014 ORCHESTRA HALL
1111 Nicollet Mall
Minneapolis, MN 55403
Phone: 612-371-5600
e-mail: info@mnorch.com
Web Site: www.minnesotaorchestra.org
Officers:
   President: David H Hyslop
   VP: E Benton Gill

Mission: To enrich lives with great music.
Founded: 1903
Paid Staff: 150
Paid Artists: 100
Budget: $28,000,000
Annual Attendance: 400,000
Facility Category: Concert Hall
Type of Stage: Proscenium
Seating Capacity: 2,450
Year Built: 1974

7015 TARGET CENTER
600 1st Avenue
Minneapolis, MN 55403
Phone: 612-673-1300
Fax: 612-673-1370
e-mail: mail@tagretcenter.com
Web Site: www.targetcenter.com
Management:
   VP/Basketball Operations: Kevin McHale
   Marketing Director: Sandy Sweetser
   Executive Director: Dane Warg
   Concessions Manager: Ajay Sekhran
Seating Capacity: 19,006

7016 THEATRE IN THE ROUND PLAYERS
245 Cedar Avenue
Minneapolis, MN 55454-1054
Phone: 612-333-2919
Web Site: www.theatreintheround.org

7017 UNIVERSITY OF MINNESOTA: SPORTS PAVILLION
1923 University Avenue SE
Minneapolis, MN 55455
Phone: 612-625-5804
Fax: 612-624-5887
Management:
   Director/Athletic Facilities: Scott P Ellison
   Assistant Program Director: Leon Freese
Seating Capacity: 5,700

7018 WALKER ART CENTER
Vineland Place
Minneapolis, MN 55403
Phone: 612-375-7600
Fax: 612-375-7618
e-mail: diane.anderson@walkerart.org
Web Site: www.walkerart.org

7019 NEW HOPE OUTDOOR THEATRE
4401 Xylon Avenue N
New Hope, MN 55428
Phone: 763-531-5151
Fax: 763-531-5136
Web Site: www.ci.new-hope.mn.us

7020 MARTIN LUTHER COLLEGE LYCEUM
1995 Luther Court
New Ulm, MN 56073
Fax: 507-354-8225

All listings are in alphabetical order by state, then city, then organization within the city.

7021 MAYO CIVIC CENTER
30 Civic Center Drive SE
Rochester, MN 55904
Phone: 507-281-6184
Fax: 507-281-6277
Web Site: www.mayociviccenter.com

7022 MAYO CIVIC CENTER: ARENA
30 2nd Avenue SE
Rochester, MN 55904
Phone: 507-281-6184
Fax: 507-281-6277

7023 MAYO CIVIC CENTER: AUDITORIUM
30 Civic Center Drive SE
Rochester, MN 55904
Phone: 507-281-6184
Fax: 507-281-6277

7024 MAYO CIVIC CENTER: THEATRE
30 Civic Center Drive SE
Rochester, MN 55904
Phone: 507-281-6184

**7025 COLLEGE OF SAINT BENEDICT -
BENEDICTA ARTS CENTER**
37 S College Avenue
Saint Joseph, MN 56374
Phone: 320-363-5777
Fax: 320-363-6097
e-mail: amthompson@csbsju.edu
Web Site: www.csbsju.edu/finearts
Management:
    Executive Director: Anna M Thompson
Paid Staff: 13
Volunteer Staff: 20
Paid Artists: 9
Non-paid Artists: 400
Income Sources: NEA, MSAB, Heartland Arts Fund,
Target Stores, local corporations, fees and tickets
Annual Attendance: 15,000
Facility Category: Performing Arts Center
Type of Stage: Proscenium
Stage Dimensions: 59' X 38
Seating Capacity: 1,084
Year Built: 1963
Cost: 2.5 million
Rental Contact: Mary Darnall

7026 FITZGERALD THEATER
10 E Exchange Street
Saint Paul, MN 55101
Phone: 651-290-1200
Fax: 651-290-1195
e-mail: fitzgerald@mpr.org
Web Site: www.fitzgeraldtheater.org
Management:
    General Manager: Brian Sanderson
    Production Manager: Thomas Campbell
    Event Service Manager: Katie Burger
    Box Office Manager: Shane Wethers
Founded: 1980

Specialized Field: Concerts; Theater; Broadcasting;
Dance
Paid Staff: 15
Volunteer Staff: 15
Budget: 350,000
Income Sources: Box Office; Rent; Concession; Grant
from Parent Company
Facility Category: Rental-Performing Arts
Type of Stage: Sprung Floor
Stage Dimensions: 36'x30'
Year Built: 1910
Year Remodeled: 1986
Rental Contact: General Manager Brian Sanderson

**7027 ORDWAY CENTER FOR THE
PERFORMING ARTS**
345 Washington Street
Saint Paul, MN 55102
Phone: 651-282-3000
Fax: 651-224-5319
Web Site: www.ordway.org
Officers:
    President/CEO: David Galligan
Management:
    Associate Producer: Lynn Von Eschen
    Director Marketing/Sales: Ron Smith
Founded: 1985
Paid Staff: 80
Volunteer Staff: 100

**7028 ORDWAY MUSIC THEATRE:
MCKNIGHT THEATRE**
345 Washington Street
Saint Paul, MN 55102
Phone: 651-224-4222
Fax: 651-282-3160

7029 ORDWAY MUSIC THEATRE
345 Washington Street
Saint Paul, MN 55102
Phone: 651-282-3000
Fax: 651-224-5319
Web Site: www.ordway.org

**7030 ROY WILKINS AUDITORIUM AT RIVER
CENTRE**
175 W Kellogg Boulevard
Saint Paul, MN 55102
Phone: 651-265-4800
Fax: 651-265-4899
e-mail: info@rivercentre.org
Web Site: www.rivercentre.org
Management:
    Director: Susan Hubbard
    Vice President: Jim Iblister
    Director Marketing: Mary Sienko
Founded: 1930
Facility Category: Auditorium with flat floor and
blacony setting
Type of Stage: portable
Stage Dimensions: 6' x 8'x 8' sections
Seating Capacity: 5,500
Year Built: 1931

Year Remodeled: 1984

7031 GUSTAVUS ADOLPHUS COLLEGE: SCHAEFFER FINE ARTS CENTER
800 W College Avenue
Saint Peter, MN 56082
Phone: 507-933-7363
Fax: 507-933-6253

7032 MIDWAY STADIUM
1771 Energy Park
Sait Paul, MN 55108
Phone: 615-646-1679
Management:
    Director: Bob Klepperich
Seating Capacity: 6,329

7033 COLLEGE OF ST. CATHERINE: O'SHAUGHNESSY AUDITORIUM
2004 Randolph Avenue
Mail F-24
St. Paul, MN 55105
Phone: 651-690-6925
Fax: 651-690-6769
Management:
    Managing Director: Jamie Ryan

7034 RIVERCENTER
175 W Kellogg Boulevard
St. Paul, MN 55102-1299
Phone: 651-465-4800
Fax: 651-265-4899
Web Site: www.rivercentre.org
Management:
    Managing Director: Barbara Chandler
    Interim Director: Erich Mische
Seating Capacity: 16,000

7035 XCEL ENERGY CENTER
7th Street
St. Paul, MN 55102
Phone: 651-222-9453
Web Site: www.wild.com
Management:
    Director Marketing: Peter Johns
    General Manager: Chris Hansen
    Arena Project Director: Ray Chandler
Seating Capacity: 18,600

7036 LAKESHORE PLAYHOUSE
4820 Steward Avenue
PO Box 10562
White Bear Lake, MN 55110
Phone: 651-426-3275

Mississippi

7037 DEPOT THEATRE
110 Magnolia Street
Belzoni, MS 39038

Phone: 662-247-4838
Season: June - September

7038 MISSISSIPPI COAST COLISEUM
2350 Beach Boulevard
Biloxi, MS 39531
Phone: 228-594-3700
Fax: 228-594-3812
Toll-free: 800-726-2781
e-mail: mail@mscoastcoliseum.com
Web Site: www.mscoastcoliseum.com
Management:
    Executive Director: Williams F Holmes
    Assistant Executive Director: Matt McDonnell
    Director Marketing: Paula April
Seating Capacity: 11,500

7039 SAENGER THEATRE OF THE PERFORMING ARTS
170 Reynoir Street
PO Box 775
Biloxi, MS 39530
Phone: 228-435-6291
Web Site: www.biloxi.ms.us/saenger/
Management:
    Theatre Manager: Lee Hood
    Technical Director: Bob Montgomery

7040 DELTA STATE UNIVERSITY BOLOGNA PERFORMING ARTS CENTER
PO Box 3213
Cleveland, MS 38733
Phone: 662-846-4625
Fax: 662-846-4627
e-mail: spapian@dsu.deltast.edu
Web Site: www.deltast.edu/perf-arts
Management:
    Director: Sharon Papian
Performs At: Delta & Pine Land Theatre

7041 WHISTLE STOP PLAYHOUSE
Cleveland Community Theatre
PO Box 44
Cleveland, MS 38732
Phone: 601-843-3096

7042 COLUMBUS CONVENTION AND CIVIC CENTER
2n Avenue N
Columbus, MS 39701
Phone: 601-328-4164

7043 PRINCESS THEATRE
5th Street S
Columbus, MS 39701
Phone: 662-328-7860

7044 COLISEUM CIVIC CENTER
404 Taylor Street
PO Box 723
Corinth, MS 38834

All listings are in alphabetical order by state, then city, then organization within the city.

Phone: 662-287-6079
Fax: 662-286-0903

7045 LEFLORE COUNTY CIVIC CENTER
Highway 7 N
PO Box 1659
Greenwood, MS 38930
Phone: 662-453-4065
Fax: 662-453-4067
e-mail: mcqueen@msdelta.com
Management:
   Director: Andrew McQeen
   Booking: Flo Long
Paid Staff: 5
Budget: $350,000
Income Sources: Lefrore County
Facility Category: Arena/Meeting Rooms
Type of Stage: Proscenium
Seating Capacity: 3000
Year Built: 1980

7046 MANNONI PERFORMING ARTS CENTER
Southern Station
PO Box 5052
Hattiesburg, MS 39406
Phone: 601-266-4988

7047 SAENGER THEATRE
Forrest/Front Streets
PO Box 1898
Hattiesburg, MS 39403-1898
Phone: 601-545-4944
Fax: 850-444-7684
e-mail: asanders@hattiesburgms.com
Web Site: hattiesburgms.com
Paid Staff: 13
Volunteer Staff: 10
Paid Artists: 10
Budget: $100,000
Income Sources: Revenue Taxes
Annual Attendance: 100,000+
Facility Category: Theatre
Seating Capacity: 1000
Year Built: 1929
Year Remodeled: 2000
Cost: 3.75 Million
Rental Contact: H. Allen Sanders

7048 UNIVERSITY OF SOUTHERN MISSISSIPPI: MM ROBERTS STADIUM
Fairchild Fieldhouse, Universal Boulevard
Hattiesburg, MS 39406-5017
Phone: 601-266-5017
Fax: 601-266-4044
Web Site: www.athletics.usm.edu
Management:
   Athletic Director: Richard Giannini
Seating Capacity: 33,000

7049 UNIVERSITY OF SOUTHERN MISSISSIPPI: PETE TAYLOR BASEBALL PARK
University of Southern Mississippi
W 4th Street
Hattiesburg, MS 39406
Phone: 601-266-5017
Fax: 601-226-6595
Web Site: www.athletics.usm.edu
Management:
   Athletic Director: Richard C Giannini
Seating Capacity: 3,678

7050 UNIVERSITY OF SOUTHER MISSISSIPPI: REED GREEN COLISEUM
PO Box 5017
Hattiesburg, MS 39406-5017
Phone: 601-226-5017
Fax: 601-266-6690
Web Site: www.athletics.usm.edu
Management:
   Athletic Director: Richard Giannini
Seating Capacity: 8,095

7051 INDIANOLA LITTLE THEATRE
Main and Sunflower Avenue
Indianola, MS 38751
Phone: 662-887-9920

7052 MISSISSIPPI VALLY STATE UNIVERSITY
14000 Highway 82 W
Itta Bena, MS 38941
Phone: 601-254-3550
Fax: 601-254-3639
Web Site: www.mvsu.edu
Management:
   Athletic Director: Charles Prophet
   Head Football Coach: Latal Jones
   Head Basketball Coach (Mens): Lafayette Stribling
   Head Basketball Coach (Womens): Jessie L Haris
Seating Capacity: 6,000

7053 BELHAVEN COLLEGE: GIRAULT AUDITORIUM
Belhaven College
1500 Peachtree Street
Jackson, MS 39202
Phone: 601-968-8707

7054 JACKSON MUNICIPAL AUDITORIUM: THALIA MARA HALL
255 E Pacagoula Street
Jackson, MS 39205
Mailing Address: PO Box 288
Phone: 601-960-1537
Fax: 601-960-1583
Management:
   Coordinator/Booking: Vicki Green
   Manager: Maxine Dilday

All listings are in alphabetical order by state, then city, then organization within the city.

Mission: Theatre style venue for operas, ballet, symphony plays, small seminars and some musical performances.
Founded: 1968
Paid Staff: 4
Affiliations: City of Jackson
Annual Attendance: 160,000
Facility Category: Theatre
Seating Capacity: 2,350
Year Built: 1968
Rental Contact: Vicki Green

7055 MISSISSIPPI VETERANS MEMORIAL STADIUM

2531 N State Street
Jackson, MS 39296
Phone: 601-354-6021
Fax: 601-354-6019
Web Site: www.mveteransstadium.com
Management:
   Director: Matt Watley
Seating Capacity: 60,492

7056 ALCORN STATE UNIVERSITY ATHLETIC COMPLEX

1000 Asu Drive
Highway 552, Whitney Complex
Lorman, MS 39096
Phone: 601-877-6500
Fax: 601-877-3821
e-mail: peter@loman.edu
Web Site: www.alcorn.edu
Management:
   Athletic Director: Lloyd N Hill

7057 MISSISSIPPI STATE UNIVERSITY: DUDY NOBLE STADIUM

Mississippi State University
Collegeview Drive
MS State, MS 39762
Phone: 601-325-2808
Fax: 601-325-7904
Web Site: www.msstate.edu
Management:
   Athletic Director: Larry Templeton

7058 WOOD COLLEGE: THEATRE

Wood College Road
PO Box 289
Mathiston, MS 39752
Phone: 662-263-5352
Fax: 662-263-4964

7059 STATE THEATRE

220 State Street
PO Box 1141
McComb, MS 39648
Phone: 601-684-5229

7060 MERIDIAN COMMUNITY COLLEGE-THEATRE

5500 Highway 19 N
Meridian, MS 39301

Phone: 601-483-8241
Fax: 601-482-3936
Management:
   Chair/Fine Arts: Ronnie Miller
Founded: 1937
Specialized Field: Visual Arts, Music, Theatre
Paid Staff: 5

7061 MISSISSIPPI STATE UNIVERSITY: SCOTT FIELD

Lee Boulevard, PO Box HY
Mississippi State, MS 39762
Phone: 662-325-2970
Fax: 662-325-3850

7062 SCOTT FIELD

Mississippi State University
PO Box 5327
Mississippi State, MS 39762
Phone: 601-325-2808
Fax: 804-982-5213
Web Site: www.msstae.edu
Management:
   Athloetic Director: Larry Templeton
Seating Capacity: 40,656

7063 UNIVERSITY OF MISSISSIPPI: MEEK AUDITORIUM

Oxford, MS 38677
Phone: 662-232-7268
Fax: 662-915-7443
e-mail: music@olemiss.edu

7064 UNIVERSITY OF MISSISSIPPI: FULTON CHAPEL

Oxford, MS 38677
Phone: 662-232-7411
Fax: 662-232-5082
Web Site: www.olemiss.edu
Founded: 1927
Seating Capacity: 915
Year Built: 1927

7065 UNIVERSITY OF MISSISSIPPI: STUDIO THEATRE

Oxford, MS 38677
Phone: 662-232-7411
Fax: 662-232-5082
Web Site: www.olemiss.edu

7066 PANOLA PLAYHOUSE

212 S Main Street
Sardis, MS 38666
Mailing Address: PO Box 43, Sandis, MS 38666-0043
Phone: 662-487-3975
Fax: 662-487-1421
e-mail: lee@panola.com
Officers:
   President: Carla Mettetal
   VP: Matthew Domas
   Secretary: Melissa Baker
   Treasurer: Lee Dixon

Management:
    Treasurer: Lee Dixon
Mission: To provide an outlet for entertainment and performance for the mostly rural area of Panola County and the surrounding area of North Mississippi.
Founded: 1963
Specialized Field: Community Theatre
Status: Active
Volunteer Staff: 15
Budget: $20,000
Income Sources: Membership; Donations; Box Office; Fundraising
Affiliations: Mississippi Arts Commission
Annual Attendance: 1,200
Seating Capacity: 163
Year Built: 1946
Year Remodeled: 1970
Rental Contact: Lee Dixon

7067 TUPELO COLISEUM
PO Box 7288
Tupelo, MS 38802
Phone: 601-841-6573
Fax: 601-841-6413
e-mail: toddhunt@ebicome.net
Web Site: www.tupelociliseum.com
Management:
    Manager: Todd Hunt
Seating Capacity: 10,000

7068 UNIVERSITY OF MISSISSIPPI: CM TAD SMITGH COLISEUM
University of Mississippi
Department of Athletics
All American Drive
University, MS 38677
Phone: 662-232-7241
Fax: 662-915-7683
Management:
    Athletic Director: John Shafer

7069 UNIVERSITY OF MISSISSIPPI: VAUGH-HEMINGWAY STADIUM
Department of Athletics
University, MS 38677
Phone: 601-232-7241
Fax: 601-232-7683
Web Site: www.olemisssports.com
Management:
    Athletic Director: John Shafer
Seating Capacity: 42,577

7070 TRIANGLE CULTURAL CENTER
322 N Main
Yazoo City, MS 39194
Phone: 662-746-2273
Toll-free: 800-381-0662

7071 LYCEUM THEATRE
Main Street
Arrow Rock, MO 65320
Phone: 660-837-3311
Fax: 660-837-3112
e-mail: boxoffice@lyceum.ork.uk
Web Site: www.lyceumorg.uk/
Management:
    Artistic Director: Michael Bollinger

7072 CULVER-STOCKTON COLLEGE PERFORMING ARTS HALL
Culver-Stockton College
One College Hill
Canton, MO 63435
Phone: 217-231-6352
Fax: 217-231-6614
Toll-free: 800-537-1883
e-mail: jdieker@culver.edu
Web Site: www.culver.edu
Officers:
    Fine Arts Department Chair: Joseph Deiker
Mission: Private liberal Arts college with a strong progam in Art, Theatre and Music.
Founded: 1853
Specialized Field: Art; Music; Theatre
Status: Nonprofit
Paid Staff: 10
Paid Artists: 8
Budget: $10,000-20,000
Performs At: Alexander Campbell Auditorium; Meriallat Recital Hall
Annual Attendance: 5,000
Facility Category: College Campus
Type of Stage: Recital Hall; Proscenium; Black Box
Stage Dimensions: 60'x40'
Seating Capacity: 200; 969; 150
Year Built: 1966
Year Remodeled: 1990
Rental Contact: 217-231-6346 Judy Garkie

7073 SHOW ME CENTER
Number 1 University Plaza
SE Missouri State
Cape Girardeau, MO 63701
Phone: 573-651-2297
Fax: 573-651-5054
e-mail: smc@semo.edu
Web Site: www2.semo.edu/showmecenter
Management:
    Marketing Director: Brad Gentry
    Business Manager: Greg Talbut
    Director: David Ross
    Event Supervisor: Jack Davis
Seating Capacity: 7,000

7074 SOUTHEAST MISSOURI STATE UNIVERSITY
1 University Plaza
Cape Girardeau, MO 63701

Phone: 573-651-2000
Fax: 573-651-2893
Web Site: www.semo.edu

7075 MISSOURI THEATRE
203 S 9th Street
Columbia, MO 65205
Phone: 573-882-7529
e-mail: wbloss@stjoearts.org

7076 OKOBOJI SUMMER THEATRE
Stephens College
Columbia, MO 65215
Mailing Address: Box 341, Spirit Lake, IA. 51360
Phone: 573-876-7194
Web Site: www.okoboji.com/summertheatre/
Founded: 1958

7077 UNIVERSITY OF MISSOURI: COLUMBIA/JESSE AUDITORIUM
311 Jesse Hall
Columbia, MO 65211
Phone: 573-882-3753
Fax: 573-884-5411
Web Site: www.missouri.edu

7078 UNIVERSITY OF MISSOURI: FAUROT FIELD
University of Missouri
600 Stadium Boulevard
Room 260
Columbia, MO 65211
Phone: 573-882-2056
Fax: 573-882-4298
e-mail: hickmantl@missouri.edu
Web Site: www.mutigers.com
Management:
   Director: Timothy L Hickman
Facility Category: Stadium

7079 UNIVERSITY OF MISSOURI: HEARNES CENTER
600 Stadium Boulevard
Room 260
Columbia, MO 65211
Phone: 573-882-2056
Fax: 573-882-4298
e-mail: hickmanti@missouri.edu
Web Site: www.hearnescenter.com
Management:
   Director: Timothy L Hickman
   Operations Manager: Jeff Roberts
Seating Capacity: 13,500
Year Built: 1972

7080 UNIVERSITY OF MISSOURI: MEMORIAL STADIUM
University of Missouri-Columbia
600 Stadium Boulevard
Columbia, MO 65211

Phone: 573-882-6501
Fax: 573-882-4298
e-mail: hickmantl@missouri.edu
Web Site: www.missouri.edu/~hearnes
Management:
   Director: Tim Hickman
   Event Manager: Roger Crumpton
Founded: 1969

7081 WESTMINSTER COLLEGE: WESTMINSTER CHAMP AUDITORIUM
Fulton, MO 65251
Phone: 573-642-3361
e-mail: webmaster@jaynet.wcmo.edu
Management:
   President: Dr. Fletcher M Lamkin
Founded: 1851

7082 WESTMINSTER COLLEGE: WINSTON CHURCHILL MEMORIAL HALL
7th and Westminster
Fulton, MO 65251
Phone: 314-642-3361

7083 WILLIAM WOODS COLLEGE: CAMPUS CENTER
200 W 12th Street
Fulton, MO 65251
Phone: 573-642-2251
Fax: 612-690-3279
Web Site: www.williamwoods.edu

7084 WILLIAM WOODS COLLEGE: DULANY AUDITORIUM
200 W 12th Street
Fulton, MO 65251
Phone: 612-690-8112
Fax: 612-690-3279

7085 ARROWHEAD STADIUM
One Arrowhead Drive
Kansas City, MO 64129
Phone: 816-920-9300
Fax: 816-920-4287
Management:
   VP Administratoring/Sales: Dennise Watley
   Director Stadium Operations: Steve Schneider
   Director Ticket Operations: Doug Hopkins
Specialized Field: Sports Facility, home of the Kansas City Chiefs and the Kansas City Wizards
Seating Capacity: 79,451
Year Built: 1972
Rental Contact: 816-921-3600 John Friedmann

7086 AVILA COLLEGE: GOPPERT THEATRE
11901 Wornall Road
Kansas City, MO 64145
Phone: 816-501-2411
Fax: 816-501-2442
Toll-free: 800-462-8452
e-mail: gouidcj@mail.avila.edu
Web Site: www.avila.edu

Officers:
  Theatre Director: Dr. Charlene Gould
Founded: 1973
Specialized Field: Goppert Theatre
Budget: $10,000
Performs At: Goppert Theater

7087 FOLLY THEATER
300 W 12th Street
PO Box 26505
Kansas City, MO 64196
Phone: 816-842-5500
Fax: 816-842-8709
e-mail: follytheater@aol.com

7088 KANSAS CITY MUNICIPAL AUDITORIUM: MUSIC HALL
301 W 13th Street
Suite 100
Kansas City, MO 64105
Phone: 816-513-5000
Fax: 816-513-5001
Toll-free: 800-821-7060
e-mail: sue_hodes@kcmo.org
Web Site: www.kcconvention.com
Management:
  Sales Associate: Sue Hides
  Sales Associate: Felecia Fremont
  Marketing Manager: Liz Bouman
  Executive Director: William H LaMette
  Deputy Director: Bill Langley
  Director Sales/Marketing: Kathleen Lee
  Assistant Director Sales/Marketing: Alan Schmelzle
Founded: 1936
Paid Staff: 120
Income Sources: Rental and User Fees
Performs At: Performance Hall
Facility Category: Fine Arts Performing Arts
Type of Stage: Proscenium
Stage Dimensions: 85'6"wx35'lx46'h
Seating Capacity: 2,400
Year Built: 1936
Year Remodeled: 1981
Architect: $1,200,000
Rental Contact: Sales Associate Sue Hodes

7089 KANSAS CITY MUNICIPAL AUDITORIUM: ARENA
Convention & Entertainment Centers
301 W 13th Street
Suite 100
Kansas City, MO 64105
Phone: 816-513-5000
Fax: 816-513-5001
Toll-free: 800-821-7060
Web Site: www.kcconvention.com
Management:
  Sales Manager: Larry Joneshill
  Contract Administrator: Felicia Fremont-Alexiou
  Marketing Manager: Liz Bowman
Seating Capacity: 10,700

7090 KAUFFMAN STADIUM
1 Royal Way
PO Box 419969
Kansas City, MO 64129
Phone: 816-921-8000
Fax: 816-921-1366
Web Site: www.kcroyals.com
Management:
  Sr VP Business Operations: Art Chaudry
  Vp/Marketing/Communications: Mike Levy
  VP Administration/Development: Jay Hinrichs
  Director Marketing/Sales: Tonya Mangels
Specialized Field: Home of the Kansas City Royals (MLB)
Seating Capacity: 40,625
Year Built: 1973

7091 KEMPER ARENA/AMERICAN ROYAL CENTER
1800 Genessee Street
Suite 100
Kansas City, MO 64102
Phone: 816-513-4000
Fax: 816-513-4001
Toll-free: 800-634-3942
Web Site: www.kcconvention.com
Officers:
  Media/Public Relations Manager: Ken Gies
  Executive Director: William Lamette
Management:
  General Manager: Deb Churchill
  Director Sales/Marketing: Kathleen Lee
  Event Coordinator: Todd Mitchell
  Event Coordinator: Michael Young
Founded: 1973
Specialized Field: Sports and entertainment arena. Home of the Kansa City Comets (Misl)
Paid Staff: 60
Seating Capacity: 19,500
Year Built: 1974
Year Remodeled: 1997

7092 MUNICIPAL AUDITORIUM
301 W 13th Street
Suite 100
Kansas City, MO 64105
Phone: 816-871-3700
Fax: 816-871-3710
Toll-free: 800-821-7060
Web Site: www.kcconvention.com
Management:
  Direector: Bill Lamette
  Director Operations: Dean Barrett
Seating Capacity: 8,189

7093 PARK COLLEGE: GRAHAM TYLER MEMORIAL CHAPEL
8700 River Park Drive
Kansas City, MO 64152
Phone: 816-741-2000

7094 UNICORN THEATRE
3820 Main Street
Kansas City, MO 64111
Phone: 816-531-0421

7095 LIBERTY PERFORMING ARTS THEATRE
1600 S Withers Road
Liberty, MO 64068-4604
Phone: 816-792-6130
Fax: 816-792-6148
e-mail: info@libertytheatre.org
Web Site: www.libertytheatre.org
Management:
  Mayor: Steven Hawkins
  Recreation Director: Chris Deal
  Theatre Coordinator: Paul Miler
  Technical Director: Hunter Burgess
Mission: A rental venue hosting a wide range of dance, music, drama, ceremonial, and other special events — striving to provide the best in personnel, services, and equipment. The Theatre also serves as a co-presenter of high quality, family-oriented art events.
Founded: 1992
Specialized Field: All performing Arts Disciplines
Paid Staff: 10
Budget: $110,000
Income Sources: Rental venue, Ticket revenue, Private donations
Performs At: Liberty Performing Arts Theatre
Affiliations: Kansas City Jazz Ambassadors, Plain Presenters Consortium, local Chamber of Commerce
Annual Attendance: 80,000
Facility Category: Multi-discipline theatrical space
Type of Stage: Proscenium
Stage Dimensions: 85x41
Seating Capacity: 725 (700 permanent)
Year Built: 1992
Cost: $1.5 milion
Rental Contact: Theatre Coordinator Paul Miller

7096 NORTHWEST MISSOURI STATE UNIVERSITY
800 University Drive
Department of Music
Maryville, MO 64468
Phone: 660-562-1317
Fax: 660-562-1346
e-mail: music@mail.nwmissouri.edu
Web Site: www.nwmissouri.edu
Management:
  Department Chair/Music: Dr. Ernest Woodruff
Mission: Educational
Founded: 1905
Specialized Field: Instrumental music, vocal music
Performs At: Mary Linn Performing Arts Center
Affiliations: National Association of Schools of Music

7097 MISSISSIPPI STATE UNIVERSITY: HUMPHREY COLISEUM
PO Box 5327
Mississippi State, MO 39762
Phone: 601-325-2532
Fax: 662-325-7456
Web Site: www.msstae.edu
Management:
  Director Support Services: Walter G Hunt

7098 PARK COLLEGE: ALUMNI HALL THEATRE
Park College
Parkville, MO 64152
Phone: 816-741-2000

7099 COLLEGE OF THE OZARKS: JONES AUDITORIUM
PO Box 17
Point Lookout, MO 65726
Phone: 417-334-6411
Fax: 417-335-2618
Web Site: www.coso.edu

7100 UNIVERSITY OF MISSOURI-ROLLA
College of Arts & Sciences
121 Fulton
Rolla, MO 65409-1130
Phone: 573-341-4141
Fax: 573-341-6127
Web Site: web.umr.edu/~upas/
Officers:
  Den/Chair Campus Performing Arts: Paula M Lutz
Management:
  Administrative Assistant: Barbara Palmer
  House Manager: Barbara Griffin
Budget: $60,000-150,000
Income Sources: Box Office; Subscriptions; Grants
Performs At: Leach Theatre; Castleman Hall
Affiliations: Plains Presenters
Annual Attendance: 3,900
Facility Category: Theater/Concert Hall
Type of Stage: Proscenium
Stage Dimensions: 45'x21'
Seating Capacity: 656
Year Built: 1991
Rental Contact: House Manager Barbara Griffen

7101 MISSOURI THEATER
717 Edmond Street
Saint Joseph, MO 64501
Phone: 816-271-4717
Fax: 816-232-9213
Toll-free: 800-821-5052
e-mail: kbrock@ci.st-joseph.om.us
Management:
  Manager: Kathy Brock
  Maintenance/Operations: Steve O'Neal
  Assistant: Carolyn Hitchings
Founded: 1980
Specialized Field: Performing Art Association
Paid Staff: 5
Income Sources: City Owned Facility
Facility Category: Performing Arts Facility
Type of Stage: Permanent
Seating Capacity: 1,200
Year Built: 1927

Year Remodeled: 1995
Resident Groups: Robidouk Resident Theatre

7102 MISSOURI WESTERN STATE COLLEGE
Music Department
Saint Joseph, MO 64507
Phone: 816-271-4420
Fax: 816-271-5974
Officers:
   Music Department Chairman: Matt Gilmour
Budget: $10,000
Performs At: Fine Arts Theatre

7103 SAINT JOSEPH CIVIC ARENA
100 N 4th Street
Saint Joseph, MO 64501
Phone: 816-271-4717
Fax: 816-232-9213
Toll-free: 800-821-5052
e-mail: kbrock@ci.st-joseph.mo.us
Web Site: ci.st-joseph.mo.us
Management:
   Manager: Kathy Brock
   Assistant: Carolyn Hitchings
   Operations Supervisor: John Whitmore
Paid Staff: 4
Income Sources: City Owned Facility/Arena
Facility Category: multi-use facility/arena
Type of Stage: Portable
Stage Dimensions: 36'x48'
Seating Capacity: 5000
Year Built: 1980
Year Remodeled: 1997

7104 AMERICAN THEATRE
1401 S Brentwood Boulevard
Suite 700
Saint Louis, MO 63144
Phone: 314-962-4000
Fax: 314-436-0483

7105 CATHEDRAL OF SAINT LOUIS
4431 Lindell Boulevard
Saint Louis, MO 63108-2496
Phone: 314-533-7662
Fax: 314-533-2844
e-mail: music@cathedralstl.org
Web Site: www.cathedralstl.org

7106 CENTER OF CONTEMPORARY ARTS
524 Trinity Avenue
Saint Louis, MO 63130
Phone: 314-725-1834
Fax: 314-725-6222
e-mail: coca@cocastl.org
Web Site: www.cocastl.org

7107 FABULOUS FOX THEATRE
Grand Center
527 N Grand Boulevard
Saint Louis, MO 63103
Phone: 314-534-1111
Fax: 314-534-8702

7108 GRAND CENTER
634 N Grand
#10A
Saint Louis, MO 63103-1025
Phone: 314-533-1884
Fax: 314-533-3345
e-mail: mconcannon@grandcenter.org
Web Site: www.grandcenter.org
Management:
   Marketing/Programming Director: Merrell Wiegraffe
Budget: $60,000-150,000

7109 JEWISH COMMUNITY CENTER OF SAINT LOUIS
Cultural Arts Department
2 Millstone Campus Drive
Saint Louis, MO 63146
Phone: 314-432-5700
Fax: 314-432-5825
Management:
   Theatre Coordinator: Kathleen Sitzer

7110 MISSOURI BOTANICAL GARDEN
PO Box 299
Saint Louis, MO 63166-0299
Phone: 314-577-9598
Toll-free: 800-642-8842
Web Site: www.mobot.org
Management:
   Public Events Manager: Jim Kalkbrenner
   Public Relations Manager: Anne Shepherd
   Director of Marketing: Brenda Jones
Mission: To discover and share knowledge about plants and their environment, in order to preserve and enrich life.
Founded: 1859
Paid Staff: 385
Volunteer Staff: 99+
Income Sources: Admission charges; Membership fees; Grants; Private donations
Annual Attendance: 750,000
Facility Category: Auditorium; Outdoor Ampitheatre
Type of Stage: Proscenium
Seating Capacity: 300

7111 MUNY
Forest Park
Saint Louis, MO 63112
Phone: 314-361-1900
Fax: 314-361-0009
e-mail: munyinfo@muny.com
Web Site: www.muny.com
Management:
   Marketing Director: Laura Peters Reilly
Mission: Broadway-style musical theatre productions
Founded: 1919
Specialized Field: Theatre
Paid Staff: 550
Paid Artists: 200
Non-paid Artists: 200
Season: June - August
Annual Attendance: 400,000
Facility Category: Outdoor Amphitheatre
Type of Stage: Traditional
Seating Capacity: 11,000

Year Built: 1919
Year Remodeled: 2000

7112 POWELL SYMPHONY HALL AT GRAND CENTER

718 N Grand Boulevard
Saint Louis, MO 63103
Phone: 314-533-2500
Fax: 314-286-4142

7113 SARRIS CENTER

1401 Clark Avenue
Saint Louis, MO 63102
Phone: 618-222-2900
Fax: 314-466-4660

7114 SHELDON CONCERT HALL AND BALLROOM

3648 Washington Avenue
Saint Louis, MO 63108
Phone: 314-533-9900
Fax: 314-533-2958
Web Site: www.sheldonconcerthall.org
Management:
   Executive Director: Paul Reuter
   Director Events (Rentals): Laurie Hasty
Mission: To present concerts of jazz, folk and classical music, art exhibits in the Sheldon Galleries and community events in 500 and 250 seat rental spaces.
Founded: 1912
Budget: $2.4 million
Income Sources: Subscriptions, rentals and contributions
Annual Attendance: 100,000
Facility Category: Concert Hall
Type of Stage: Flexible; platform
Stage Dimensions: 17 x 24
Seating Capacity: 702
Year Built: 1912
Year Remodeled: 1998
Rental Contact: Director of Events (Rentals) Laurie Hasty

7115 UNION AVENUE OPERA THEATRE/ARTS GROUP

733 N Union Boulevard
Saint Louis, MO 63108
Phone: 314-361-8844
Fax: 314-361-3036
e-mail: uaccstl@swbell.net

7116 WASHINGTON UNIVERSITY: EDISON THEATRE

Mallinckrodt Center
Campus Box 1119
Saint Louis, MO 63130
Phone: 314-935-6543
Fax: 314-935-7362
e-mail: edison@artsci.wustl.edu
Web Site: www.wustl.edu/edison

7117 WEBSTER UNIVERSITY-LORETTO: HILTON CENTER FOR THE ARTS

130 Edgar Road
Saint Louis, MO 63119
Phone: 314-968-6933
Fax: 314-963-6102
Management:
   Executive Director: Dean Peter Sargent

7118 HAMMONS STUDENT CENTER

661 S John Q Hammons Parkway
Springfield, MO 65807
Phone: 417-836-5240
Fax: 417-836-6344
Management:
   Athletic Director: Bill Rowe

7119 LANDERS THEATRE

311 E Walnut Street
Springfield, MO 65806
Phone: 417-869-3869
Fax: 417-869-4047
e-mail: aabryce@hotmail.com
Web Site: www.landerstheatre.org
Officers:
   President: Todd Smith
   Senior VP: Richard Ollis
Management:
   Executive Director: Alan Bryce
   Finance Director: Chris Volkmen
   Technical Director: Matt Young
Founded: 1936
Specialized Field: Southwest Missouri
Paid Staff: 9
Budget: $750,000
Income Sources: Tickets; Underwriting; Grants
Annual Attendance: 35,000
Facility Category: Theatre
Type of Stage: Proscenium

7120 PLASTER SPORTS COMPLEX

Southwest Missouri State University
901 S National Avenue
Springfield, MO 65804
Phone: 417-836-4640
Fax: 417-736-7660
Management:
   Director: Randall Blackwood
   Associate Director: Chris W Bowser
   Assistant Director: Lance M Kettering
   Manager: Beverly Nickols
Seating Capacity: 16,000

7121 SOUTHWEST MISSOURI STSTE UNIVERSITY: JUANITA K HAMMON HALL FOR THE PERFORMING ARTS

901 S National
Springfield, MO 65804
Phone: 417-836-6776
Fax: 417-836-6891
e-mail: emorris@smsu.edu
Web Site: www.hammonhall.com
Management:

Executive Director: Enoch Morris
Founded: 1992
Paid Staff: 15
Volunteer Staff: 250
Budget: $400,000-1,000,000
Annual Attendance: 125,000
Facility Category: Performing Arts Center
Type of Stage: Proscenium
Seating Capacity: 2,220
Year Built: 1992
Cost: $17.3 million
Rental Contact: Jack Wheeler

7122 BUSCH STADIUM

St. Louis Cardinals
250 Stadium Plaza
St Louis, MO 63102
Phone: 314-421-3060
Fax: 314-425-0640
Web Site: www.stlcardinals.com
Management:
   Director: Marian Rhodes
   VP Stadium Operations: Joe Abernathky
   Senior VP Corporate Sales: Dan Farrell
Specialized Field: Operated bhy St. Louis Cardinals
Seating Capacity: 49,625
Year Built: 1966
Year Remodeled: 1997

7123 FAMILY ARENA

2002 Arena Parkway
St. Charles, MO 63303
Phone: 636-896-4200
Fax: 636-896-4205
Web Site: www.familyarena.com
Management:
   Director: Matt Hacker
Founded: 1999
Specialized Field: Arena/Facility
Income Sources: Tickets; Concessions; Suites;
Advertising
Affiliations: St. Charles County Government
Annual Attendance: 750,000
Facility Category: Arena
Type of Stage: Stageright
Seating Capacity: 11,000
Year Built: 1999
Cost: $32 million

7124 SAINT JOSEPH CIVIC ARENA

100 N 4th Street
St. Joseph, MO 64501
Phone: 816-271-4717
Fax: 816-232-9213
e-mail: civicfac@ci.st-joseph.mo.us
Management:
   Assistant/Recreation Department: Bill France
   Manager Civic Facilities: Kathy Brock
Seating Capacity: 5,000

7125 GRAND CENTER / GRANDEL THEATRE

634 N Grand
#10A
St. Louis, MO 63103-1025

Phone: 314-533-1884
Fax: 314-533-3345
e-mail: mwiefgraffe@grandcenter.org
Web Site: www.grandcenter.org
Management:
   Facilities Manager: Merrill Wiegraffe

7126 SAVIS CENTER

1401 Clarke Avenue
St. Louis, MO 63103
Phone: 314-622-5400
Fax: 314-589-5981
e-mail: webmastr@gw.kiel.com
Web Site: www.saviscenter.net
Management:
   Sr VP/General Manager Savis Center: Dennis
   Petrullo
   Sr VP Marketing: Jim Woodcockne
   Food/Beverage Director: Skip Aurell
   VP/Operations: Fred Corsi
   Box Office Director: Carol Chilton
   Boc Offive Manager: Debra Freking
   Publicity/Special Events Manager: Cindy Underwood
   Director Manager: Gayle Leonard
   Marketing Manager: Michele Peck
Seating Capacity: 20,000 basketball, 19,267 hockey
Year Built: 1994

7127 TRANSWORLD DOME AT AMERICAS' CENTER

701 Convention Plaza
St. Louis, MO 63101
Phone: 314-342-5036
Fax: 314-342-5040
Management:
   Director: Bruce Sommer
   Director Sports Entertainment: Jack Croghan
   General Manager/Sports Service: Tom Schlaker
   Executive Suites Director/Catering: Gregory Lee
Seating Capacity: 65,600

7128 MULE BARN THEATRE

224 Main
Tarkio, MO 64491
Phone: 660-736-4430

7129 CENTER OF CONTEMPORARY ARTS

524 Trinity Avenue
University City, MO 63130
Phone: 314-725-6555
Fax: 314-725-6222
e-mail: coca@cocastl.org
Web Site: www.cocastl.org
Management:
   Executive Director: Stephanie Riven
Founded: 1986
Specialized Field: isual, Performing Arts

7130 CENTRAL MISSOURI STATE UNIVERSITY: VERNON KENNEDY STADIUM
Central Missouri State University
203 Multipurpose Building
Warrensburg, MO 64093
Phone: 660-543-4250
Fax: 660-543-8034
Web Site: www.cmsu.edu
Management:
    Athletic Director: Jerry Hughes
Seating Capacity: 12,000

7131 SOUTHWEST MISSOURI STATE UNIVERSITY
128 Garfield
West Plains, MO 65775
Phone: 417-257-3310
Fax: 417-257-7682
e-mail: kmorrissey@wp.smsu.edu
Web Site: www.users.townsqr.com/arts
Management:
    Theater/Events Coordinator: Kahtleen Morrissey
Budget: $20,000-35,000

Montana

7132 BIGFORK CENTER FOR THE PERFORMING ARTS
PO Box 1230
Bigfork, MT 59911
Phone: 406-837-4885

7133 ALBERTA BAIR THEATRE FOR THE PERFORMING ARTS
PO Box 1556
Billings, MT 59103
Phone: 406-256-8915
Fax: 406-256-5060
Toll-free: 877-321-2074
e-mail: bfisher@albertabairtheater.org
Web Site: www.albertabairtheater.org
Management:
    Executive Director: Bill Fisher
    Program/Marketing Director: Corby Skinner
    Technical Director: Tom Lund
Founded: 1983
Paid Staff: 15
Volunteer Staff: 200
Budget: $1.2 million
Income Sources: Ticket income
Annual Attendance: 123,000
Facility Category: Performing Arts
Type of Stage: Proscenium
Stage Dimensions: 54 x 30
Seating Capacity: 1416
Year Remodeled: 1987
Cost: 5-6 million
Rental Contact: Bill Fisher

7134 METRAPARK
308 6th Avenue N
Billings, MT 59101
Phone: 406-256-2400
Fax: 406-254-2479
Web Site: www.metrapark.com
Management:
    Manager: Bill Chiesa
Seating Capacity: 12,000

7135 MONTANA STATE UNIVERSITY SPORTS FACILITITES: BREENDEN FIELD HOUSE
Bozeman, MT 59717
Phone: 406-994-7117
Fax: 406-994-4400
e-mail: mstocks@monatan.edu
Web Site: www.montana.edu/wwwsfac
Management:
    Director Sports Facilities: Melanie J Stocks

7136 RENO H SALES STADIUM/MONTANA STATE UNIVERSITY
Sports Facilities
#1 Bobcat Circle
Bozeman, MT 59717
Phone: 406-994-4221
Fax: 406-994-2278
e-mail: mstock@montana.edu
Web Site: www.montana.edu/wwwsfac
Management:
    Director Sports Facilities: Melanie Stocks
    Operations Manager: Brad Murphy
    Marketing: Duane Morris
    Sports Information Director: Tom Schulz
Seating Capacity: 12,500

7137 FOUR SEASONS ARENA
400 3rd Street NW
Great Falls, MT 59404
Phone: 406-727-8900
Fax: 406-452-8955
e-mail: expopark@ci.great-falls.mt.us
Web Site: www.ci.great-falls.mt.us
Management:
    General Manager: Patty Gumberg

7138 GREAT FALLS CIVIC CENTER THEATER
PO Box 5021
Great Falls, MT 59403
Phone: 406-454-3915
Fax: 406-454-3468

7139 MONTANA STATE FAIR & FOUR SEASONS ARENA
400 3rd Street NW
PO Box 1888
Great Falls, MT 59404

All listings are in alphabetical order by state, then city, then organization within the city.

Phone: 406-727-8900
Fax: 406-452-8955
e-mail: expopark@city-of-great-falls.com
Web Site: www.city-of-great-falls.com
Management:
    Interim Director: Patty Gumenberg
    Concession Manager: Karen Rossberg
Seating Capacity: 6,134

7140 CARROLL COLLEGE: THEATRE
North Benton Avenue
Helena, MT 59625
Phone: 406-442-3450
Fax: 406-447-4533
Toll-free: 800-942-3648

7141 HELENA CIVIC CENTER: AUDITORIUM
340 Neill Avenue
Helena, MT 59601
Phone: 406-447-8481
Fax: 406-447-8480
Management:
    Manager: Diane Stavnes
    Director Comm Facility/Tech Direct: Gery Carpenter
    Administrative Assistant: Barb Olsen
Paid Staff: 7
Income Sources: City of Helena; ticket sales; rental income.
Performs At: Auditorium
Facility Category: City owned and managed for rental.
Stage Dimensions: 45'x38'x17'6"
Seating Capacity: 2,000
Year Built: 1920
Year Remodeled: 1995
Rental Contact: Manager Diane Stavnes

7142 HELENA CIVIC CENTER: BALLROOM
340 Neill Avenue
Helena, MT 59601
Phone: 406-447-8481
Fax: 406-447-8480
Management:
    Manager: Diane Stavnes
    Director Comm Facility/Tech Direct: Gery Carpenter
    Administrative Assistant: Barb Olsen
Paid Staff: 7
Facility Category: Ballroom
Stage Dimensions: 25'x15'x12'
Seating Capacity: 1,500
Year Built: 1920
Year Remodeled: 1995
Rental Contact: Manager Diane Stavnes

7143 MYRNA LOY CENTER
15 N Ewing
Helena, MT 59601
Phone: 406-443-0287
Fax: 406-443-6620
e-mail: moonared@aol.com
Officers:
    Chairman: Bob Anderson
    VP: Jim Nys
    VP: Hattie Jo Lehmann
    Secretary: Al Sheppard

    Treasurer: Melanie White
Management:
    Executive Director: Ed Noonan
Mission: To provide programs in the visual and performing arts; to provide educational programs.
Founded: 1976
Specialized Field: Dance; Vocal Music; Instrumental Music; Theater; Festivals; Lyric Opera
Status: Nonprofit
Paid Staff: 12
Budget: $400,000
Income Sources: Business, grants, fundraising
Performs At: Myrna Loy Center; Helena Middle School, Civic Center
Affiliations: NPN
Annual Attendance: 8000
Facility Category: Media and performance center
Type of Stage: Proscenium
Seating Capacity: 250
Year Built: 1875
Year Remodeled: 1990
Cost: 1.6 Million
Rental Contact: Rental Coordinator Christy Stile
Organization Type: Performing; Touring; Resident; Educational; Sponsoring

7144 ADAMS EVENT CENTER
University of Montana-Missoula
Adams Center 103
Missoula, MT 59812
Phone: 406-243-5355
Fax: 406-243-4265
e-mail: musem@mso.umf.edu
Web Site: www.adamseventcenter.com
Management:
    Executive Director: Mary Muse
    Assistant Director Business Affairs: Jan Pierce
    Operations Supervisor: Janet White
    Executive Assistant: Betty Jo Miller
Mission: Venue for staging performing and nonperforming arts and sports.
Founded: 1955
Specialized Field: Sports; Concerts; Flatshows; Special Events
Paid Staff: 10
Budget: $1,000,000
Income Sources: Rent; Contracted Services
Facility Category: Sports Arena; Concert Hall
Seating Capacity: 7,500
Year Built: 1955
Year Remodeled: 1999
Cost: $15,000,000
Rental Contact: Director Mary Muse

7145 UNIVERSITY OF MONATANA-MISSOULA: GRIZZILI STADIUM
University of Monatana- Missoula
Missoula, MT 59812
Phone: 406-243-4051
Fax: 406-243-6859
Web Site: www.umn.edu
Management:
    Facilities Manager: Gary Hughes

7146 UNIVERSITY OF MONTANA: MONTANA THEATRE
Department of Drama and Dance
Missoula, MT 59812-8736
Phone: 406-243-4481
Fax: 406-243-5726
e-mail: drama@selway.umt.edu
Web Site: www.umt.edu/drama

Nebraska

7147 COMMUNITY PLAYERS
412 Ella Street
Beatrice, NE 68310
Phone: 402-228-1801

7148 BELLEVUE LITTLE THEATRE
203 W Mission
Bellevue, NE 68005
Phone: 402-291-1554

7149 BLADEN OPERA HOUSE
Main Street
Bladen, NE 68928

7150 CHADRON STATE COLLEGE: MEMORIAL HALL
10th and Main
Chadron, NE 69337
Toll-free: 800-242-3766

7151 GOTHENBURG COMMUNITY PLAYHOUSE: SUN THEATRE
10th and D Street
PO Box 15
Gothenburg, NE 69138
Phone: 308-537-3235

7152 KEARNEY COMMUNITY THEATRE
83 Plaza Boulevard
Kearney, NE 68847
Phone: 308-234-1529

7153 UNIVERSITY OF NEBRASKA: UNIVERSITY THEATRE
905 W 25th Street
Kearney, NE 68849
Phone: 308-865-8441

7154 UNK SPORTS CENTER
University of Nebraska at Kearney
Health and Sports Center
Kearney, NE 68849
Phone: 308-865-8514
Fax: 308-865-8832
Web Site: www.unk.edu
Management:
  Athletic Director: Micheal Sumtter

Seating Capacity: 5,842

7155 LIED CENTER FOR PERFORMING ARTS
301 N 12th
PO Box 880151
Lincoln, NE 68588-0151
Phone: 402-472-4700
Fax: 402-472-4730
e-mail: mmoorel@unl.edu
Web Site: www.liedcenter.org

7156 PERSHING CENTER
226 Centennial Mall S
Lincoln, NE 68508
Phone: 402-441-7500
Fax: 402-441-7913
e-mail: info@pershingauditorium.com
Web Site: pershirgauditorium.com
Management:
  Manager: Tom Lorenz
  Marketing Director: Derek Andersen
  Event Director: Phil Potter
  Operations Director: Fred McCoy
  Assistant General Manager: Howard Feldman
Performs At: Multi-purpose arena and exhibit hall
Stage Dimensions: 42'x105'
Seating Capacity: 6,818
Year Built: 1956
Rental Contact: Manager Tom Lorenz

7157 UNIVERSITY OF NEBRASKA-LINCOLN: LINCOLN MEMORIAL STADIUM
118 S Stadium
Lincoln, NE 68588-0119
Phone: 402-472-1960
Fax: 402-472-4662
Web Site: www.huskerwebcast.com
Management:
  Director Athlettic Facilities: John M Ingram
  Director Athletics Events: Butch Hug
Seating Capacity: 73,650

7158 UNIVERSITY OF NEBRASKA-LINCOLN: BOB DEVANEY SPORTS CENTER
University of Nebraska-Lincoln
103 S Stadium
Lincoln, NE 68588-0119
Phone: 402-472-4224
Fax: 402-472-9675
Web Site: www.huskerwebcast.com
Management:
  Director Athletic Facilities: John M Ingram

7159 UNIVERSITY OF NEBRASKA-LINCOLN: KIMBALL RECITAL HALL
321 Canfield Administration Building
PO Box 880424
Lincoln, NE 68588-0424

Phone: 402-472-8518
Fax: 402-472-7825
e-mail: scarlet@unl.edu
Web Site: www.unl.edu/scarlet/
Management:
  Editor: Kim Hachiya
  Editorial Assistant: Diane Taurins

7160 OMAHA CIVIC AUDITORIUM
City of Omaha
1804 Capitol Avenue
Ohaha, NE 68101
Phone: 402-444-4750
Fax: 402-444-4739
Web Site: www.ci.omaha.ne.us
Management:
  Manager: Lawrence Lahaie
Seating Capacity: 10,950

7161 AK-SAR-BEN FUTURE TRUST
7800 Mercy Road
Suite 100
Omaha, NE 68106
Phone: 402-561-7000
Fax: 402-561-7012
Toll-free: 800-228-6601
e-mail: marketing@aksarbenomaha.com
Web Site: www.aksarbenomaha.com
Management:
  General Manager: Leslie Douglas
  Director Marketing/Sales: Kay Telford
  Manager Plant Operations: Leonard Larson
Specialized Field: Sports Facility
Seating Capacity: 7200
Year Built: 1965
Resident Groups: Omaha Lancers, Hosts Hoop It Up, WCW Wrestling, US Hockey League

7162 AKSARBEN COLISEUM
6800 Mercy Road
Suite 100
Omaha, NE 68106
Phone: 402-561-7000
Fax: 402-561-7012
e-mail: marketing@aksarbenomaha.com
Web Site: www.aksarbenomaha.com
Management:
  General Manager: Leslie Douglas

7163 JEWISH COMMUNITY CENTER OF OMAHA
333 S 132nd Street
Omaha, NE 68154
Phone: 402-334-6403
Fax: 402-334-6466
Web Site: www.jewishomaha.org
Management:
  Program Director: Rachel Shkolnick
Budget: $10,000

7164 OMAHA CIVIC AUDITORIUM: MUSIC HALL
1804 Capitol Avenue
Omaha, NE 68134
Phone: 402-444-4750
Fax: 402-444-4739

7165 ORPHEUM THEATRE
409 S 16th Street
Omaha, NE 68102
Phone: 402-444-4750
Fax: 402-444-4739

7166 UNIVERSITY OF NEBRASKA AT OMAHA
6001 Dodge
Omaha, NE 68182
Phone: 402-554-2305
Fax: 402-554-3694
Web Site: www.cidunomaha.edu/cyberman/
Management:
  Sports Information Director: Gary Anderson
  Athletic Director: Bob Danenhauer
  Head Football Coach: Pat Behrns
  Head Basketball Coach (M): Kevin McKenna
Seating Capacity: 3,800

7167 WEST NEBRASKA ARTS CENTER
PO Box 62
106 E 18th Street
Scottsbluff, NE 69363-0062
Phone: 308-632-2226
Fax: 308-632-2226
e-mail: wnearts@prairieweb.com
Management:
  Executive Director: Susan Selvey
Budget: $10,000-20,000

7168 WAYNE STATE COLLEGE/ATHLETIC DEPARTMENT
1111 Main Street
Wayne, NE 68787
Phone: 402-375-7520
Fax: 402-375-7271
Web Site: www.wsc.edu
Management:
  Athletic Director: Pete Chapman
  Assistnat Athletic Director: Mike Barry
  Head Football Coach: Kevin Haslam
  Head Basketball Coach (W): Ryun Williams
  Head Basketball Coach (M): Greg McDermott
Seating Capacity: 6,000

Nevada

7169 BREWERY ARTS CENTER
449 W King Street
Carson City, NV 89703

Phone: 775-883-1976
Fax: 775-883-1922
e-mail: ann@breweryarts.org
Web Site: www.breweryarts.org
Management:
    Executive Director: Joe McCarthy
Budget: $10,000
Performs At: Carson City Community Center

7170 CAESARS PALACE
3570 Las Vegas Boulevard S
Las Vegas, NV 89109
Phone: 702-731-7320
Fax: 702-731-7328
Web Site: www.caesarspalace.com
Management:
    Director: Charry Kennedy

7171 CHARLESTON HEIGHTS ARTS CENTER
800 S Brush
Las Vegas, NV 89107
Phone: 702-229-6383
Fax: 702-258-8286
Management:
    Center Coordinator: Joanne Lentino
Budget: $35,000-60,000
Performs At: Ballroom , Theatre
Seating Capacity: 365
Year Built: 1979
Year Remodeled: 1989
Rental Contact: phone 702-229-5256 Roy Ramirez

**7172 LAS VEGAS CONVENTION AND
VISITORS AUTHORITY**
850 Las Vegas Boulevard N
Las Vegas, NV 89101
Phone: 702-386-7100
Fax: 702-386-7126
Web Site: www.vegasfreedom.com
Management:
    Director/Facilities Cashman Center: Vel Jones

7173 MGM GRAND GARDEN
3799 Las Vegas Boulevard S
Las Vegas, NV 89109
Phone: 702-891-7824
Fax: 702-891-7831
e-mail: prowsm@aol.com
Web Site: www.mgmgrand.com
Officers:
    Assistant VP: Rich Baccellieri
Management:
    VP/Convention: Mark W Prows
    Assistant VP Arena/Convention: John Huska
    Executive Director/Arena/Convention: Karen Prescia
    Senior Event Manager: Dick Hill
Seating Capacity: 15,200

**7174 REED WHIPPLE CULTURAL ARTS
CENTER**
821 Las Vegas Boulevard N
Las Vegas, NV 89101

Phone: 702-229-6211
Fax: 702-382-5199
Web Site: www.ci.Las-Vegas.nv.us

7175 THOMAS & MACK CENTER
4505 Maryland Parkway
Las Vegas, NV 89154-0003
Phone: 702-895-3761
Fax: 702-895-1099
Web Site: www.thomasandmack.com
Management:
    Director: Daren Libonati
    Assistant Director: Joseph Santiago
    Associate Director Operations: Rick Picone
    Public Relations: Windy Lawson-Whitney
Founded: 1983
Paid Staff: 100
Seating Capacity: 18,500

**7176 UNIVERSITY OF NEVADA-LAS VEGAS:
ARTEMUS HAM**
4505 Maryland Parkway
Box 45-5005
Las Vegas, NV 89154
Phone: 702-865-3011
Fax: 702-895-1940

**7177 UNIVERSITY OF NEVADA-LAS VEGAS:
PERFORMING ARTS CENTER**
4505 Maryland Parkway
Box 455005
Las Vegas, NV 89154-5005
Phone: 702-895-3535
Fax: 702-895-4714
e-mail: henley@communitynevada.edu
Web Site: pac.nevada.edu
Management:
    Director Artistic Programming: Larry Henley
    Director Huest Relations: Lori James
    Technical Director: Trent Downing
Mission: To be the cultural heart of Southern Nevada and
provide quality performances.
Founded: 1996
Specialized Field: Present world's greatest talent
Budget: $400,000-1,000,000
Income Sources: Box office, sponsorships, rentals
Performs At: Artemus W. Ham Concert Hall, Judy
Bayley Theater
Affiliations: Western Alliance of Arts Administrators,
Association of Performing Arts Administrators,
International Society of Performing Arts Administrators
Facility Category: Concert hall, theatre, black box
Seating Capacity: 1870/550/200
Year Built: 1976
Rental Contact: Facilities Manager Larry Henley

7178 SAM BOYD STADIUM
4505 Maryland Parkway
Los Vegas, NV 89145-0003
Phone: 702-895-3716
Fax: 702-895-1099
Web Site: www.thomasandmackcenter.com
Management:

Director: Patrick J Christenson
Assistant Director: Robert P Anderson
Assistant Director/Booking: Daren Libonati
Assistant Director/Sports Marketing: Steve Stallworth
Assistant Director Operations: Rick Picone
Promotions/Public Relations Manager: Cliff Clinger
Seating Capacity: 42,500

7179 CENTENNIAL COLISEUM: RENO SPARKS CONVENTION
4590 S Virginia
Reno, NV 89502
Phone: 775-825-2627

7180 LAWLOR EVENTS CENTER
University of Nevada Athletic Department
Legacy Hall/232
Reno, NV 89557
Phone: 775-784-4659
Fax: 775-784-4428
Web Site: www.unr.edu
Management:
   Athletic Director: Chris Ault
Seating Capacity: 12,400

7181 MACKEY STADIUM
University of Nevada
Legacy Hall 232
Reno, NV 98557
Phone: 775-784-6900
Fax: 775-784-4497
Web Site: www.nevadawolfpack.com
Management:
   Athletic Director: Chris Ault
Seating Capacity: 30,000

7182 PIONEER CENTER FOR THE PERFORMING ARTS
100 S Virginia Street
Reno, NV 89501
Phone: 702-686-6010
Fax: 702-686-6630

7183 RENO LITTLE THEATER
690 N Sierra
PO Box 2088
Reno, NV 89505
Phone: 775-329-0661

7184 UNIVERSITY OF NEVADA-RENO: CHURCH FINE ARTS
Reno, NV 89557
Phone: 775-784-6847

7185 UNIVERSITY OF NEVADA-RENO: LAWLOR EVENTS CENTER
Virginia Street
Reno, NV 89557
Phone: 775-784-4700
Fax: 775-784-1025

7186 PIPER'S OPERA HOUSE
PO Box J
12 N B Street
Virginia City, NV 89440
Phone: 775-847-0433
Fax: 775-847-9668
e-mail: pipers@vcnevada.com
Web Site: www.pipers opera.org
Founded: 1878

New Hampshire

7187 CLAREMONT OPERA HOUSE
City Hall on Tremont Square
PO Box 664
Claremont, NH 03743
Phone: 603-542-0064
Fax: 603-542-7014
e-mail: twincloud@pobox.com
Web Site: www.claremontoperahouse.com
Management:
   Executive Artistic Director: Thom Wolke
Mission: Multi-use performing arts center.
Opened: 1977
Specialized Field: Upper Connecticut Valley
Budget: $150,000
Income Sources: Tickets; Membership; Sponsers
Affiliations: APAP; APNNE
Annual Attendance: 15,000
Facility Category: Theatre
Type of Stage: Proscenium
Seating Capacity: 780
Year Built: 1897
Year Remodeled: 1975

7188 CAPITOL CENTER FOR THE ARTS
44 S Main Street
Concord, NH 03301
Phone: 603-225-1111
Fax: 603-224-3408
e-mail: mtmennino@ccanh.com
Web Site: www.ccanh.com
Management:
   Executive Director: Mary-Therese Mennino
Mission: To inspire, educate and entertain audiences by providing both the finest venue for the performing arts and a wide range of professioanlly excellent and artistically significant presentations.
Founded: 1995
Status: Nonprofit
Paid Staff: 15
Budget: $1.8 Million
Annual Attendance: 100,000
Seating Capacity: 1300
Year Built: 1927
Year Remodeled: 1995

7189 FRIENDS OF THE CONCORD CITY AUDITORIUM
Prince Street
Concord, NH 03302-0652

Mailing Address: PO Box 652
Phone: 603-225-2164
Fax: 603-224-1036
e-mail: carolbagan@mediaone.net
Web Site: concordcityauditorium.org
Officers:
President: Merwyn Bagan
VP: Esther Crowley
Mission: To restore and renovate our historic theatre and to foster its use for the benefit of all the people in our community. We will assist all presenters who wish to book the City Auditorium.
Founded: 1991
Specialized Field: Theatre; Music; Dance; Series; Community Based A&E
Performs At: Auditorium; Adjoining Reception Lobby
Annual Attendance: 100,000
Facility Category: Municipal Theatre
Type of Stage: Proscenium
Stage Dimensions: 25'x 25'
Seating Capacity: 850
Year Built: 1904
Year Remodeled: 1991
Rental Contact: DJ Sartwell

7190 UNIVERSITY OF NEW HAMPSHIRE
Paul Creative Arts Center
4 Ballard Street
Durham, NH 03824-2303
Phone: 603-862-3322
Fax: 603-868-8992
e-mail: durhamnhmainst@ttlc.net
Management:
Executive Director: Pati Frew-Waters

7191 UNIVERSITY OF NEW HAMPSHIRE-DURHAM: BRATTON RECITAL HALL
Paul Creative Arts Center
Durham, NH 03824
Phone: 603-862-3038
Fax: 603-862-3038

7192 UNIVERSITY OF NEW HAMPSHIRE-DURHAM - HENNESSY CENTER
Paul Creative Arts Center
Durham, NH 03824
Phone: 603-862-3038
Fax: 603-862-3038

7193 WHITTEMORE CENTER
University of New Hampshire
Main Street
Durham, NH 03824
Phone: 603-862-1850
Fax: 603-862-4069
Web Site: www,unh.edu/athletics
Management:
Athletic Director: Judith Ray
Marketing Director: Dan Raposa
Media Relations Director: Scott Stapin
Seating Capacity: 6,000

7194 HAMPTON PLAYHOUSE THEATRE ARTS WORKSHOP
357 Winnacunnet Road
Hampton, NH 03842
Phone: 603-926-3073

7195 MEMORIAL STADIUM/DARTMOUTH COLLEGE
Athletic Department
6083 Alumni Gym
Hanover, NH 03755
Phone: 603-646-3654
Fax: 603-646-3348
e-mail: jennifer.coleman@darthmouth.edu
Web Site: www.dartmouth.edu
Management:
Facilities Manager: Jennifer Coleman
Seating Capacity: 20,416

7196 THOMPSON ARENA
Dartmouth College
Athletic Department
Hanover, NH 03755-3512
Phone: 603-646-2673
Fax: 603-646-3348
e-mail: jennifer.coleman@darthmouth@edu
Web Site: www.darthmouth.edu
Management:
Athletic Facilities Manager: Jennifer Coleman
Seating Capacity: 3,500

7197 COLONIAL THEATRE
PO Box 77
95 Main Street
Keene, NH 03431
Phone: 603-357-1233
Fax: 603-357-7817
e-mail: info@thecolonial.org
Web Site: www.thecolonial.org
Management:
Executive Director: Ken Kohberger
Season: year round

7198 REDFERN ARTS CENTER ON BRICKYARD POND
Keene State College
229 Main Street
Keene, NH 03435-2401
Phone: 603-358-2167
Fax: 603-358-2145
e-mail: bmenezes@keene.edu
Web Site: www.keene.edu/racbp/
Management:
Director: Bill Menezes
Mission: Educational
Founded: 1979
Specialized Field: theatre, dance, music
Paid Staff: 4
Budget: $250,000
Income Sources: tickets sales, college subs, corparate sponsors, private donations
Affiliations: Green Mountain Consortium; New England Presenters; Assoc. Performing Arts Presenters

Annual Attendance: 15,000
Facility Category: Multipurpose
Type of Stage: proscenium
Stage Dimensions: 36'x 30'x 56'
Seating Capacity: 572
Year Built: 1979
Rental Contact: B. Denehy

7199 NCCA PAPERMILL THEATRE

PO Box 1060
Lincoln, NH 03251
Phone: 603-745-6032
Fax: 603-745-2564
Web Site: www.papermilltheatre.org
Officers:
    President: Bill Hollager
    VP: John Hettinger
Management:
    Business Director: Tony Ferrelli
    Administrative Assistant: Ellen Ferrelli
Mission: To provide theatre, cultural programming and theatre education for children and adults.
Founded: 1986
Specialized Field: Theater; Festivals; Touring Children's Theatre; Art Gallery
Status: Professional; Nonprofit
Paid Staff: 3
Volunteer Staff: 50
Paid Artists: 60
Non-paid Artists: 20
Organization Type: Performing; Touring; Educational

7200 NEW LONDON BARN PLAYHOUSE

209 Main Street
PO Box 285
New London, NH 03257
Phone: 603-526-6710
Fax: 603-526-2849
e-mail: nlbarn@juno.com
Season: June - August

7201 EASTERN SLOPE INN PLAYHOUSE

Main Street
PO Box 265
North Conway, NH 03860
Phone: 603-356-5776
Fax: 603-356-8357
Mission: To keep the tradition of line performance, especially musical.

7202 MUSIC HALL

28 Chestnut Street
104 Congress Street
Portsmouth, NH 03801-4078
Phone: 603-433-3100
Fax: 603-431-4103
e-mail: info@themusichall.com
Web Site: www.themusichall.org
Management:
    Artistic Director: Jane Forde
Specialized Field: Seacoast, NH
Paid Staff: 12
Volunteer Staff: 274

New Jersey

7203 BAYONNE VETERANS MEMORIAL STADIUM

W 26th Street
Bayonne, NJ 07002
Phone: 201-858-6164
Fax: 201-858-6092
Management:
    Director: Steve Gallo

7204 BLAIR ACADEMY

PO Box 600
2 Park Street
Blairstown, NJ 07825
Phone: 908-362-6121
Fax: 908-362-2029
e-mail: habers@blair.edu
Web Site: www.blair.edu
Management:
    Special Events/Performing Arts Dir.: Susan K Habermann
    Director Bartow Series: Chris Eanes
Mission: Educational insititution.
Founded: 1848
Specialized Field: Armstrong-Hepkins Center for the Arts

7205 CALDWELL COLLEGE: STUDENT UNION BUILDING

9 Ryerson Avenue
Caldwell, NJ 07006
Phone: 973-618-3000
Fax: 201-228-3851

7206 RUTGERS-CAMDEN CENTER FOR THE ARTS

3rd and Pearl Streets
Fine Arts Building/Gordon Theater
Camden, NJ 08102-1403
Phone: 856-225-6676
Fax: 856-225-6597
e-mail: cjgrimes@camden.rutgers.edu
Management:
    Theater Program Manager: Capucine Jackson-Grimes

7207 WALT WHITMAN CULTURAL ARTS CENTER

2nd and Cooper Streets
Camden, NJ 08102
Phone: 856-964-8300
Fax: 856-964-2953
Management:
    Executive Director: Pamela Bridgeforth
Budget: $60,000-150,000

7208 MID-ATLANTIC CENTER FOR THE ARTS

PO Box 340
1048 Washington Street
Cape May, NJ 08204

Phone: 609-884-5404
Fax: 609-884-0574
Toll-free: 800-275-4278
e-mail: mstewart@capemaymac.org
Web Site: www.capemaymac.org
Officers:
  President: Tom Carroll
  First VP: Niels Favre
  Second VP: Ed Henry
  Deputy Director External Affair: Mary Stewart
  Deputy Director Operations: Bill Ten Eyck
  Treasurer: Richard Juliano
  Secretary: Joan Wells
Management:
  Festival Artistic Director: Stephen Rogers Radcliffe
  Director: B Michael Zuckerman
  Deputy Director: Mary Stewart
Mission: Dedicated to promoting preservation, awareness and interpretation of the Victorian era and its customs, heritage and architecture, as well as striving to promote the performing arts.
Founded: 1970
Specialized Field: Instrumental Music; Special Events
Status: Professional; Nonprofit
Performs At: Cape May Convention Hall
Organization Type: Sponsoring

7209 MIDDLE TOWNSHIP PERFORMING ARTS CENTER

1 Penkethman Way
Cape May, NJ 08210
Phone: 609-463-1924
Fax: 609-463-1928
e-mail: mtpac@bellatlantic.net
Management:
  Theater Manager: Richard Ludwig
Budget: $60,000-150,000

7210 CRANFORD DRAMATIC CLUB THEATRE

78 Winans Avenue
PO Box 511
Cranford, NJ 07016
Phone: 908-276-7611

7211 DOVER LITTLE THEATRE

Elliott Street
PO Box 82
Dover, NJ 07801
Phone: 973-328-9202

7212 GIANTS STADIUM

50 Route 120
E. Rutherford, NJ 07073
Phone: 201-935-8500
Fax: 201-460-4294
e-mail: webmaster@meadowlands.com
Web Site: www.meadowlands.com
Management:
  Senior Executive VP: Robert Castronovo
  VP Marketing: Eric Krasnoo
Mission: Home of the New York Giants and the New York Jets, The Metro Stars, College football and concerts.

Seating Capacity: 79,469, 60,000
Year Built: 1976

7213 MEADOWLANDS/NEW JERSEY SPORTS & EXPOSITION AUTHORITY

Executive Offices
50 St Route 120
E. Rutherford, NJ 07073-0700
Phone: 201-240-4038
Fax: 201-507-8130
Web Site: www.meadowlands.com
Officers:
  President: James A Dieleuterio
Management:
  Chairman: Ray H Batemen
  Assistant General Manager: Rober E Carney
  COO: Robdert Castronovo
Seating Capacity: 7,200

7214 CONTINENTAL AIRLINES ARENA

50 Route 120
East Rutherford, NJ 07073
Phone: 201-460-4374
Fax: 201-507-8122
Web Site: www.meadowlands.com
Officers:
  Sr VP: Tim Hassett
Management:
  VP Event Booking: Ron VanDeVeen
Budget: $3 million
Facility Category: Arena
Seating Capacity: 20,029
Year Built: 1981
Rental Contact: Ron VanDeVeen

7215 APPEL FARM ARTS AND MUSIC CENTER

PO Box 888
Elmer, NJ 08318
Phone: 609-358-2472
Fax: 609-358-6513

7216 JOHN HARMS CENTER FOR THE ARTS

30 N Van Brunt Street
Englewood, NJ 07631
Phone: 201-567-5797
Fax: 201-567-7357
e-mail: info@johnharms.org
Web Site: www.johnharms.org
Management:
  Executive Director: Jessica Finkelberg
  Business Manager: Steve Nemiroff
  Director Education: Cathy Roy
  Communications/Marketing: Ed Kirchdoerffer
Founded: 1976
Status: Nonprofit
Paid Staff: 14
Volunteer Staff: 150
Paid Artists: 250
Budget: $3,000,000
Income Sources: Foundations, Grants, Corporate Support, Individuals, Earned
Annual Attendance: 300,000

Facility Category: Theater
Type of Stage: Proscenium
Stage Dimensions: 33 x 30
Seating Capacity: 1322
Year Built: 1926

7217 ROWAN UNIVERSITY: GLASSBORO CENTER FOR THE ARTS
Rowan University
Wilson Hall, Room 211
Glassboro, NJ 08028
Phone: 856-256-4548
Fax: 856-256-4919
e-mail: centerarts@rowan.edu
Web Site: www.rowan.edu/centerarts
Management:
    Marketing Director: Amy Lebo
    Director: Mark Fields
Mission: To provide several different professional cultural events for the Southern New Jersey area.
Founded: 1989
Specialized Field: Dance; Vocal Music; Instrumental Music; Theater; Lyric Opera; Grand Opera; Jazz
Status: Professional
Budget: $950,000
Income Sources: New Jersey State Council on the Arts; Bergen Foundation; PSEG;
Performs At: Wilson Concert Hall
Annual Attendance: 35,000
Facility Category: Auditorium
Type of Stage: Proscenium
Stage Dimensions: 50' X 35'
Seating Capacity: 895
Year Built: 1971
Rental Contact: Stu McKee
Organization Type: Performing; Touring; Resident; Educational; Sponsoring

7218 ORRIE DE NOOYER AUDITORIUM
Bergen County Technical School
200 Hackensack Avenue
Hackensack, NJ 07601
Phone: 201-343-6000

7219 RICHARD L SWIG ARTS CENTER
The Peddie School
Box A, S Main Street
Highstown, NJ 08520
Phone: 609-490-7550
Fax: 609-426-9019
e-mail: rrund@peddie.org
Web Site: www.peddie.org
Management:
    Director: Robert Rund

7220 LIBERTY SCIENCE CENTER
Liberty State Park
Jersey City, NJ 07305-4699
Phone: 201-451-0006
Fax: 201-451-6383
e-mail: webleam@lsc.org
Web Site: www.lsc.org
Management:

Arts/Sciences Coordinator: Christine Bodwitch

7221 STRAND THEATRE
400 Clifton Avenue
Lakewood, NJ 08701
Phone: 732-367-7789
Fax: 732-367-7819
Management:
    Executive Director: Theresa Beaugard
    Event Manager: Patti Curtis
    Technical Director: Chris Staton
    Office Manager: Linda Hassa
    House Manager: Jose Pastrana
Paid Staff: 35
Volunteer Staff: 30
Non-paid Artists: 80
Income Sources: Rentals; Grants; Ticket Sales
Facility Category: Theatre
Seating Capacity: 1,042
Year Built: 1922
Year Remodeled: 2001
Cost: $5,000,000
Rental Contact: Linda Hassa

7222 RIDER UNIVERSITY: THE YVONNE THEATER
Rider University
2083 Lawrenceville Road
Lawrenceville, NJ 08648
Phone: 609-896-5168
Fax: 609-896-5232
e-mail: chmel@rider.edu
Web Site: www.theatre.rider.edu
Seating Capacity: 450
Year Remodeled: 2000
Rental Contact: Tharyle Prather

7223 DREW UNIVERSITY: BOWNE THEATRE
36 Madison Avenue
Madison, NJ 07940
Phone: 908-272-0100
Fax: 908-272-3949
e-mail: info@dgdco.com

7224 RAMAPO COLLEGE OF NEW JERSEY: BERRIE CENTER FOR PERFORMING AND VISUAL ARTS
Ramapo College of New Jersey
505 Ramapo Valley Road
Mahwah, NJ 07430
Phone: 201-684-7844
Fax: 201-684-7979

7225 CULTURE HALL OF MEDFORD NEW JERSEY
2 Friends Avenue
Medford, NJ 08055
Phone: 609-654-7587
Web Site: www.medfordstation.com
Specialized Field: Performing Arts Center; Banquet Facility

7226 PAPER MILL PLAYHOUSE
Brookside Drive
Millburn, NJ 07041
Phone: 973-379-3636
Fax: 973-376-2359
Web Site: www.papermill.org

7227 COMMUNITY THEATRE
100 S Street
Morristown, NJ 07960
Phone: 973-539-0345
Fax: 973-455-1607
e-mail: lksmith2@bellatlantic.net
Web Site: www.communitytheatrenj.com
Management:
   Producing Manager: Linda Smith

7228 MORRIS MUSEUM
6 Normandy Heights Road
Morristown, NJ 07960
Phone: 973-971-3700
Fax: 973-538-0154
Web Site: www.morrismuseum.org
Founded: 1913
Specialized Field: Theatre/Performing Arts
Paid Staff: 20
Type of Stage: Proscenium
Stage Dimensions: 40x80
Seating Capacity: 300
Year Built: 1975
Year Remodeled: 1987
Resident Groups: The Bickford Theatre

7229 WILLIAM G MENNEN SPORTS ARENA
161 E Hanover Avenue
Morristown, NJ 07962
Phone: 973-326-7651
Fax: 973-829-8698
Seating Capacity: 3,500

7230 RUTGERS ARTS CENTER
George Street and Route 18
New Brunswick, NJ 08903
Phone: 732-932-4636
e-mail: info-update@cis.rutgers.edu

7231 STATE THEATRE
15 Livingston Avenue
New Brunswick, NJ 08901-1903
Mailing Address: 11 Livingston Avenue
Phone: 732-246-7469
Fax: 732-745-5653
Toll-free: 877-782-8311
e-mail: info@statetheatrenj.org
Web Site: www.statetheatrenj.org
Management:
   Communications Manager: Paul Fantini
   VP Programming/Operations: Chris Butler
   President/CEO: Mark Hough
Founded: 1921
Specialized Field: Music, Dance & Live Performing Arts
Paid Staff: 45
Volunteer Staff: 20

Paid Artists: 100
Budget: $5 million
Income Sources: Individuals, Government, Corporations
Performs At: Presenting House Theatre
Affiliations: League Of Historic Theatres New Brunswick Cultural Center, Others
Annual Attendance: 275,000
Facility Category: Performing Arts Center
Type of Stage: Procenium
Stage Dimensions: 45'x28'
Seating Capacity: 1,800
Year Built: 1921
Year Remodeled: 1988
Rental Contact: David Hartkern

7232 NEW JERSEY PERFORMING ARTS CENTER
1 Center Street
Newark, NJ 07102
Phone: 973-642-8989
Fax: 973-642-0654
Toll-free: 888-466-5722
e-mail: ldenmark@njpac.org
Web Site: www.njpac.org
Officers:
   President/CEO: Lawrence P Goldman
   COO: M John Richard
   Treasurer: Leonard Lieberman
   Assistant Treasurer: Marc E. Berson
   Secretary: Clive S. Cummis
   Co-Chairman: Raymond G. Chambers
   Co-Chairman: Arthur E. Ryan
Management:
   Vice President Programming: Leon Denmark
   VP Development: Diane Nixa
   VP Finance: Bobbie Arbesfeld
   VP Arts Education: Philip S Thomas
   VP Operations: Audrey Winkler
   Vice President Public Affairs: Jeffrey Norman
Mission: To be a world class cultural complex and center stage for New Jersey's best performing artists; to aid in providing economic revitalization in Newark.
Founded: 1988
Paid Staff: 146
Budget: $22 million
Income Sources: Earned revenue: Ticket sales, Fees, Parking, Restaurant Commission and Philanthropy
Performs At: New Jersey Performing Arts Center
Annual Attendance: 550,000
Type of Stage: Proscenium
Stage Dimensions: 37'x 39'4'x 3'2'/116' x 49'x 3'6'
Seating Capacity: 514/2,750
Year Built: 1997
Year Remodeled: N/A
Cost: $187 million
Organization Type: Performing, Resident, Educational, Sponsoring, Touring

7233 NEWARK SYMPHONY HALL
1030 Broad Street
Newark, NJ 07102
Phone: 973-643-8009

7234 LOUIS BROWN ATHLETIC CENTER
Rutgers University
83 Rockafeller Road
Piscataway, NJ 08853
Phone: 732-445-4220
Fax: 732-445-2752
Management:
    Athletic Director: Bob Mulcahy
Seating Capacity: 8,4000

7235 RUTGERS UNIVERSITY: RUTGERS ATHLETIC CENTER
Rutgers University
83 Rockefeller Road
Piscataway, NJ 08854
Phone: 732-445-4223
Fax: 732-445-2990
Management:
    Assistant Athletic Director: Douglas S Kokoskie
Seating Capacity: 9,000

7236 RUTGERS UNIVERSITY: RUTGERS STADIUM
Rutgers University
PO Box 1149
Piscataway, NJ 08855-1149
Phone: 732-445-4223
Fax: 732-445-2990
Management:
    Assistant Athletic Director: Douglas S Kokoskie
Seating Capacity: 42,000

7237 SILVER CULTURAL ARTS CENTER
Plymouth State College
Plymouth, NJ 03264
Phone: 603-535-2874
Fax: 603-535-2917
Toll-free: 800-799-3869
e-mail: djeffrey@mail.plymouth.edu
Web Site: www.plymouth.edu/psc/cac
Management:
    Director: Diane Jeffrey

7238 STOCKTON PERFORMING ARTS CENTER
PO Box 195
Jim Leeds Road
Pomona, NJ 08240-0195
Phone: 609-652-9000
Fax: 609-748-5523
e-mail: pac@loki.stockton.edu
Web Site: www.stockton.edu/~pac
Management:
    Director: Michael Cool
Budget: $150,000-400,000
Performs At: Main House Theatre

7239 JADWIN GYMNASIUM
Princeton University
Princeton, NJ 08544

Phone: 609-258-3000
Fax: 609-258-4477
Web Site: www.nj.com/princeton/basketball/stadium
Management:
    Athletic Director: Gary D Walters

7240 MCCARTER THEATRE
91 University Place
Princeton, NJ 08540
Phone: 609-258-6500
Fax: 609-497-0369
e-mail: admin@mccarter.org
Web Site: www.mccarter.org

7241 PRINCETON UNIVERSITY: RICHARDSON AUDITORIUM IN ALEXANDER HALL
Princeton University
Princeton, NJ 08544
Phone: 609-258-4239
Fax: 609-258-6793

7242 UNION COUNTY ARTS CENTER
1601 Irving Street
Rahway, NJ 07065
Phone: 732-499-0441
Fax: 732-499-8227
Web Site: www.ucac.org
Management:
    Theatre Manager: Sharon Surber
Paid Staff: 8
Volunteer Staff: 50
Budget: 1.5 million
Performs At: Arts Center

7243 COUNT BASIE THEATRE
99 Monmouth Street
Red Bank, NJ 07701
Phone: 732-842-9000
Fax: 732-842-9323
e-mail: info@countbasietheatre.org
Web Site: www.countbasietheatre.org
Management:
    CEO: Numa Saisselin
    Marketing Director: Regina Paleau
    Education Director: Yvonne Lamb Scudiery
    Technical Directpr: Mike Jacoby
Specialized Field: Dance; Theatre; Vocal Music; Instrumental Music
Seating Capacity: 1,400
Year Built: 1926
Rental Contact: Annette Bartolomeo

7244 WILLIAMS CENTER FOR THE ARTS
One Williams Plaza
Rutherford, NJ 07070
Phone: 201-939-6969
Fax: 201-939-0843
Web Site: www.williamscenter.org
Officers:
    President: Richard Theryoung
    Vice President: Carolyn Spann-Swallwood
    Secretary: Dr. Joseph DeFazi

Treasurer: Evelyn Spath-Mercado
Management:
 Executive Director: GW McLuckey
Mission: To provide programs of artistic excellence at affordable prices.
Founded: 1978
Paid Staff: 22
Budget: $650,000
Income Sources: Ticket Sales; grants; sponsorships; rentals
Performs At: Newman Theatre
Annual Attendance: 50,000
Facility Category: Performing Arts Center
Type of Stage: Black Box; Proscenium Arch
Seating Capacity: 200; 642
Year Built: 1922
Year Remodeled: 1992
Rental Contact: G.W. McLuckey

7245 RARITAN VALLEY COMMUNITY COLLEGE: NASH THEATREY

Route 28 and Lamington Road
PO Box 3300
Somerville, NJ 08876-1265
Phone: 908-218-8867
Fax: 908-526-7890
e-mail: theatre@raritanval.edu
Web Site: www.raritanval.edu/theatre
Management:
 Founding RVCC Trustee/President: Edward Nash
Mission: To pleease audience.
Seating Capacity: 1,000

7246 JCC ON THE PALISADES

411 E Clington Avenue
Tenafly, NJ 07670
Phone: 201-569-7900
Fax: 201-569-2765
e-mail: olistokin@jcconthepalisades,org
Management:
 Cultural Arts Director: Ophrah Listokin

7247 NEW JERSEY STATE MUSEUM AUDITORIUM

205 W State Street
PO Box 530
Trenton, NJ 08625-0530
Phone: 609-292-6464
Fax: 609-599-4098
e-mail: feedback@sos.state.nj.us
Web Site: www.state.nj.us/state/museum/
Officers:
 President: Kenneth Newcomb
 Vice President Board of Directors: Doug Setzer
 Treasurer: Charles Moseley
 Secretary: Louise Barrett
Management:
 Acting Director: Lorraine E Williams
Mission: To produce the historical outdoor drama From This Day Forward annually; to produce Dickens' A Christmas Carol annually; to produce other dramas, engage in outreach activities, and sponsor workshops and cultural events.
Founded: 1895

7248 PATRIOTS THEATER AT THE WAR MEMORIAL

Memorial Drive
Trenton, NJ 08608
Mailing Address: PO Box 232 Treton, NJ 08625
Phone: 609-984-8400
Fax: 609-777-0581
Toll-free: 800-955-5566
e-mail: thewarmemorial@sos.state.nj.us
Web Site: www.thewarmemorial.com
Management:
 Executive Director: Molly S McDonough
 Production Corrdinator: Bill Nutter
 Director Ticketing/Sales: Andrew Burkett
 Director Ticketing/Sales: Rebecca Jensen
Founded: 1932
Paid Staff: 20
Volunteer Staff: 100
Income Sources: State of New Jersey
Performs At: 1800 seat concert hall, 12,000 square feet of facilities
Affiliations: State of New Jersey, Department of State Division of War Memorial
Facility Category: Theater
Type of Stage: Proscenium
Stage Dimensions: 50 x 30
Seating Capacity: 1800
Year Built: 1932
Year Remodeled: 1998
Cost: 34.5 Million
Rental Contact: Executive Director Molly S. McDonough
Resident Groups: New Jersey Symphony, Greater Trenton Sympony, Boheme Opera, American Repertory Ball

7249 SOVEREIGN BANK ARENA

81 Hamilton Avenue
Trenton, NJ 08611
Phone: 609-656-3200
Fax: 609-656-3201
e-mail: mail@soverignbankarena.com
Web Site: www.sovereignbankarena.com
Management:
 General Manager: Michael Scanlon
 Assistant General Manager: Rick Hontz
 Operations Manager: Jason Robertson
 Event Coordinator: Chad Jeffrey
 Event Coordinator: Kris Brassil
Mission: Theatre events, concerts, sports, family shows and community events.
Founded: 1999
Seating Capacity: 8,600
Year Built: 1999

7250 KEAN COLLEGE OF NEW JERSEY: WILKENS THEATRE

1000 Morris Avenue
Union, NJ 07083
Phone: 908-527-2000
Fax: 908-527-8345
Web Site: www.kean.edu

Mission: To offer theatre to all citizens in our county, primarily through the schools, providing one selected offering annually.

7251 PARK THEATRE PERFORMING ARTS CENTRE
560 32nd Street
Union City, NJ 07087
Phone: 201-865-5301
Fax: 201-865-5339
e-mail: passnplay@aol.com
Web Site: www.passionplayusa.org
Management:
    Director: Kevin Ashe
Founded: 1983
Budget: $400,000
Income Sources: Earned Income; State Grants; Private Funds
Stage Dimensions: 70x40
Seating Capacity: 1400
Year Built: 1933

7252 MONTCLAIR STATE COLLEGE: MEMORIAL AUDITORIUM
1 Normal Avenue
Upper Montclair, NJ 07043
Phone: 973-655-4000
Toll-free: 800-624-7780
e-mail: webmaster@montclair.edu
Web Site: www.montclair.edu
Mission: Producing and promoting high quality, accessible, professional theatre; training and developing the talents of musicians, actors and technicians.

7253 WILLIAM PATTERSON UNIVERSITY
300 Pompton Road
Wayne, NJ 07470
Phone: 973-720-2000
Officers:
    Preisdent: Mary Harper
    President: Libby Noah
    Treasurer: Leslie Madigan
    Treasurer-Elect: Ernestine Worley
    Immediate Past President: Janet Bondurant
Mission: Children's Theatre Board provides opportunities for students, educators and families to experience and participate in the perforrming arts. CTB offers multidisciplinary, culturally diverse programs to foster sensitivity and acceptance.

7254 JCC METROWEST
760 Northfield Avenue
West Orange, NJ 07052
Phone: 201-736-3200
Fax: 201-736-6871
Management:
    Director/Arts/Education: Isabel Margolin

7255 JEWISH COMMUNITY CENTER OF METROPOLITAN NEW JERSEY
760 Northfield Avenue
West Orange, NJ 07052
Phone: 201-736-3200
Fax: 201-736-6871
Management:
    Programming Supervisor: Jo Goldstien
    Program Assistant: Marsha Fleisch
Founded: 1877
Specialized Field: Vocal Music; Instrumental Music; Theater; Festivals; Film Series
Status: Professional; Non-Professional; Nonprofit
Performs At: Maurice Levin Theater
Organization Type: Performing; Educational; Sponsoring

7256 MAURICE LEVIN THEATER
760 Northfield Avenue
West Orange, NJ 07052
Phone: 201-736-3200
Fax: 201-736-6871
Management:
    President of the Board: Eva Wu
Mission: To provide for all within the community an avenue for education and development in all aspects of theatrical arts and to provide entertainment for the community by offering a series of well-staged performances of live theatre.

7257 BARRON ARTS CENTER
582 Rahway Avenue
Woodbridge, NJ 07095
Phone: 732-634-0413
Management:
    Director: Stephen J Kager
Mission: To offer professional productions of musicals and plays including original and renowned works with universal as well as ethnic (African-American) themes.

New Mexico

7258 FLICKINGER CENTER FOR PERFORMING ARTS
1110 New York Avenue
PO Box 1214
Alamogordo, NM 88311
Phone: 505-437-2202
Fax: 505-434-0067
e-mail: fcinalamo@wayfarer1.com
Web Site: www.flickinger.org
Founded: 1988
Paid Staff: 5
Volunteer Staff: 60
Non-paid Artists: 200
Facility Category: Performing arts center
Type of Stage: Proscenium
Stage Dimensions: 30 x 40
Seating Capacity: 675
Year Built: 1954
Year Remodeled: 1991
Rental Contact: Ron Geisheimer

7259 TINGLEY COLISEUM/NEW MEXICO STATE FAIR

300 San Pedro NE
PO Box 8546
Albuqerque, NM 87108
Phone: 505-265-1791
Fax: 505-268-6753
Web Site: www.nmstatefair.com
Management:
  General Manager: Kay Shollenbarger
  Deputy General Manager: Staci Brown
  Media Director: Veronica Valencia
Founded: 1942
Performs At: Multi-Purpose
Facility Category: Arena
Type of Stage: Standard
Stage Dimensions: 40' x 60'
Seating Capacity: 12,000
Year Remodeled: 2000
Cost: $3,500
Rental Contact: Booking Manager Peggy Durkin

7260 ALBUQUERQUE CONVENTION CENTER

401 Second Street NW
Albuquerque, NM 87103
Phone: 505-768-4575
Fax: 505-768-3239
e-mail: cchavez@cabq.gov@cabq.gov
Paid Staff: 56
Facility Category: Convention Center; Ballroom; Auditorium
Type of Stage: Flexible, Platform/Proscenium
Seating Capacity: 3000
Year Built: 1972
Year Remodeled: 1990
Rental Contact: Scheduling Manager Carol Chavez

7261 ALBUQUERQUE SPORTS STADIUM

1340 University SE
Albuquerque, NM 87102
Phone: 505-848-1359
Fax: 505-857-8641
Web Site: www.dukes.com
Management:
  Director: Pleas Gleen

7262 NATIONAL HISPANIC CULTURAL CENTER OF NEW MEXICO

Quickel Building
600 Central SW
Suite 201
Albuquerque, NM 87102-3194
Phone: 505-246-2261
Fax: 505-246-2613
e-mail: rlove@state.nm.us
Management:
  Director Performing Arts: Reve Love

7263 SOUTH BROADWAY CULTURAL CENTER

1025 Broadway SE
Albuquerque, NM 87102
Phone: 505-848-1320
Fax: 505-848-1329
e-mail: lulibarri@cabq.gov
Web Site: www.cabq.gov/sbec
Management:
  Director: Linda Ulibarri
  Technical Director: Antonio Aragon
  Gallery Curator: John Peterson
Mission: To produce theatrical productions reflecting a high degree of professionalism; to develop artists in the theatre as well as responsive audiences.
Founded: 1970
Paid Staff: 8

7264 UNIVERSITY OF NEW MEXICO: UNIVERSITY ARENA

1414 University Boulevard SE
Albuquerque, NM 87131
Phone: 505-925-5500
Fax: 505-925-5559
Web Site: www.unm.edu/lobo
Management:
  Athletic Director: Rudy Davalos
  Sports Information Director: Greg Remington
  Head Football Coach: Rocky Long
  Head Basketball Coach (M): Fran Fraschilla
  Head Basketball Coach (W): Don Douple
Seating Capacity: 18,018

7265 UNIVERSITY OF NEW MEXICO: POPEJOY HALL

Center for the Arts
University of New Mexico
Albuquerque, NM 87131-3176
Phone: 505-277-3824
Fax: 505-277-7353
e-mail: psuozzi@unm.edu
Web Site: www.popejoyhall.com
Officers:
  President: Carol Leevers
  VP: Jane Traynor
  Treasurer/Secretary: Dean Petska
Management:
  Director: Tom Tkach
  Public Relations Manager: Terry Davis
  Technical Director: Billy Tubb
  Artistic Director: Judy Ryan
Mission: To present Touring Broadway, plus national as well as international music and dance.
Paid Staff: 12
Volunteer Staff: 200
Budget: $2,000,000
Income Sources: State legislature; Event revenue
Affiliations: University of New Mexico-Center for the Arts
Annual Attendance: 100,000
Seating Capacity: 2044
Year Built: 1966
Year Remodeled: 1996
Rental Contact: Thomas Tkach

Resident Groups: Musical Theatre Southwest & New Mexico Symphony Orchestra

7266 UNIVERSITY OF NEW MEXICO: UNIVERSITY STADIUM
1414 University Boulevard SE
Albuquerque, NM 87131
Phone: 505-925-5500
Fax: 505-925-5559
Web Site: www.enm.edu/lobo
Management:
   Sports Information: Greg Remington
   Head Football Coach: Rocky Long
   Head Basketball Coach: Fran Fraschilla
   Head Basketball Coach (M): Don Flanahan
   Athletic Director: Rudy Davalos
Seating Capacity: 30,000

7267 SPENCER THEATER FOR THE PERFORMING ARTS
PO Box 140
Alto, NM 88312
Phone: 505-336-0010
Fax: 505-336-4001
Toll-free: 886-818-7872
e-mail: centilli@spencertheater.com
Web Site: www.spencertheater.com
Management:
   Executive Director: Theta Smith
Founded: 1997
Paid Staff: 13
Volunteer Staff: 30
Income Sources: Private, Contributions
Annual Attendance: 5,000
Facility Category: Tjeater
Stage Dimensions: 50 x 80
Seating Capacity: 514
Year Built: 1979
Cost: $22 Million
Rental Contact: Charles Centilli

7268 FARMINGTON CIVIC CENTER
200 W Arrington
Farmington, NM 87401
Phone: 505-599-1150
Fax: 505-599-1146
e-mail: lparks@fmtn.org
Web Site: www.farmington.nm.us
Officers:
   President Civic Center Foundation: Melissa Sharpe
Management:
   Civic Center Supervisor: Loretta J Parks
Mission: To further promote the cultural enrichment of the citizens of the City of Farmington and surrounding area.
Founded: 1976
Specialized Field: Performing and Visual
Paid Staff: 14
Budget: $571,000
Income Sources: Diuvision of City of Farmington supported by tax revenue. Government Municipality.
Performs At: Broadway Musicals, SJ Community Concert & Symphony Leage
Affiliations: WAA and IAAM

Annual Attendance: 150,000
Facility Category: Performing Arts Theatre & Convention Center
Type of Stage: Proscenium
Stage Dimensions: 52 w x 72 deep
Seating Capacity: 1200
Year Built: 1976

7269 NEW MEXICO STATE UNIVERSITY: AMERICAN SOUTHWEST CENTER
PO Box 3072
Las Cruces, NM 88003
Phone: 505-646-4517
Fax: 505-646-5767
Mission: The state's land grant university, serving the educational needs of New Mexico's diverse population through comprehensive programs of education, research, extension education, and public service.

7270 PAN AMERICAN CENTER
Department 3 SE
Corner of Payne & Univ, PO Box 30001
Las Cruces, NM 88003
Phone: 505-646-4413
Fax: 505-646-3605
Management:
   Director Special Events: Will Lofdahl
   Assistant Director Special Events: Gary Rachele
   Box Office Manager: Barbara Welch
Seating Capacity: 13,007

7271 DUANE SMITH AUDITORIUM
1300 Diamond Drive
Los Alamos, NM 87544
Phone: 505-662-9000
Web Site: www.losalamos.org/laca
Management:
   Artistic Director: Rosalie Heller
Founded: 1946
Volunteer Staff: 30
Paid Artists: 5

7272 NEW MEXICO MILITARY INSTITUTE
101 W College Boulevard
Roswell, NM 88201-5173
Phone: 505-624-8011
Fax: 505-624-8025
Toll-free: 800-421-5376
e-mail: miller@nmmi.edu
Web Site: www.nmmi.edu
Management:
   Secretary to the Commandant: Stacy Garrett
Mission: To make available theatre arts (acting, directing and so forth) to the people of a rural community.
Paid Staff: 3
Income Sources: State Education Funds
Annual Attendance: 20,000 -
Facility Category: Auditorium
Seating Capacity: 1,100

7273 NEW MEXICO MILITARY INSTITUTE: PEARSON AUDITORIUM
New Mexico Military Institute
College of Main
Roswell, NM 88201
Phone: 505-622-6250
Fax: 505-624-8459
Web Site: www.nmmi.cc.nm.us
Officers:
  President: Ken Haarstad
  VP: Shirley Olson
  Secretary: Lori Garnes
  Treasurer: Jerry Jorgenson
Mission: Community theatre to promote adult education and provide theatre arts to surroundings communities children's educational performing arts.

7274 COLLEGE OF SANTA FE: GREER GARSON THEATRE CENTER
1600 St. Michael's Drive
Santa Fe, NM 87505
Phone: 505-473-6439
Fax: 505-473-6016
Toll-free: 800-456-2673
e-mail: jkilbourn@csf.edu
Web Site: www.csf.edu
Management:
  Assistant Director: Jennifer Kilbourn
  Chair: John Weckesser
Mission: Provide undergraduate degrees, BA and BFA in Theatre, Acting, Music Theatre, Design Tech and Theatre Management.
Founded: 1936
Specialized Field: Acting; Musical Theatre; Technical Theatre; Theatre Management; Stage Management
Paid Staff: 25

7275 GUADALUPE HISTORIC FOUNDATION (SANTUARIO DE GUADALUPE)
100 S Guadalupe Street
Santa Fe, NM 87501
Phone: 505-988-2027
Management:
  preident/Owner/Executive Producer: Prescott F Griffith
Mission: Elegant Dinner Theatre featuring live Broadway musical productions.

7276 SANTA FE CONVENTION AND VISITORS BUREAU: SWEENEY CENTER
201 W Marcy
PO Box 909
Santa Fe, NM 87501
Phone: 505-955-6200
Fax: 505-955-6222
Toll-free: 800-777-2489
Web Site: www.santafe.org

7277 SANTA FE STAGES
100 N Guadalu Place
Santa Fe, NM 87501
Phone: 505-982-6680
Fax: 505-982-6682
e-mail: info@santafestages.org
Web Site: www.santafestages.org
Management:
  Performing Director: Craig Strong
  General Manager: Suzanne Mannard

7278 WECKESSER STUDIO THEATRE
Greer Garson Theatre Center
1600 St. Michael's Drive
Santa Fe, NM 87505
Phone: 505-473-6270
Fax: 505-473-6286

New York

7279 ARTS IN EDUCATION: CAPITAL REGION CENTER
SUNY at Albany
Ten Broeck 107, Dutch Quad
Albany, NY 12222
Phone: 518-442-4240
Fax: 518-442-3239
Management:
  Director: Marlinda Menashe
Budget: $10,000

7280 CAPITAL REPERTORY THEATRE
111 N Pearl Street
Albany, NY 12207
Phone: 518-462-4531
Fax: 518-465-0213
e-mail: info@capitalrep.org
Web Site: www.capitalrep.org
Management:
  Artistic Director: Margaret Mancinelli-Cahill
  Managing Director: Jeff Dannick
  Marketing/Public Relations Director: Nancy Laribee
  Production Manager: Robin MacDuffil
Founded: 1981
Status: Nonprofit
Budget: 2,100,000
Income Sources: Corporate Sponsors; Individual Donors; Subscriptions; Ticket Sales
Season: July - May
Performs At: Producing Theatre
Affiliations: LORT
Annual Attendance: 63,000+
Facility Category: LORT Theatre
Type of Stage: Thrust
Seating Capacity: 285

7281 EGG
PO Box 2065
Empire State Plaza
Albany, NY 12220
Phone: 518-473-1061
Fax: 518-473-1848
e-mail: info@theecg.com
Web Site: www.theecg.com
Management:

Executive Director: Peter Lesser
Founded: 1978

7282 EMPIRE CENTER AT THE EGG

Empire State Plaza
PO Box 2065
Albany, NY 12220
Phone: 518-473-1061
Fax: 518-473-1848
e-mail: info@theegg.org
Web Site: www.theegg.org
Organization Type: Performing

7283 EMPIRE STATE PERFORMING ARTS CENTER: KITTY CARLISLE HART

PO Box 2065
Albany, NY 12220
Phone: 518-473-1061
Fax: 518-473-1848

7284 EMPIRE STATE PERFORMING ARTS CENTER: LEW

PO Box 2065
Albany, NY 12220
Phone: 518-473-1061
Fax: 518-473-1848

7285 PALACE PERFORMING ARTS CENTER

19 Clinton Avenue
Albany, NY 12207
Phone: 518-465-0681
Fax: 518-427-0151
e-mail: palaceth@aol.com
Management:
    Executive Director: Robert C Goepfert
Founded: 1931
Specialized Field: Albany, Capital District

7286 PEPSI ARENA

51 S Pearl Street
Albany, NY 12207
Phone: 518-487-2000
Fax: 518-487-2020
e-mail: info@pepsiarena.com
Web Site: www.pepsiarena.com
Management:
    General Manager: Robert Belber
Seating Capacity: 17,000

7287 STATE UNIVERSITY OF NEW YORK-ALBANY: ARENA

Albany Performing Arts Center
1400 Washington Avenue
Albany, NY 12222
Phone: 518-442-3995
Fax: 518-442-4206

7288 STATE UNIVERSITY OF NEW YORK-ALBANY: MAIN THEATRE

Albany Performing Arts Center
1400 Washington Avenue
Albany, NY 12222
Phone: 518-442-3995
Fax: 518-442-4206

7289 STATE UNIVERSITY OF NEW YORK-ALBANY: RECITAL HALL

Albany Performing Arts Center
1400 Washington Avenue
Albany, NY 12222
Phone: 518-442-3995
Fax: 518-442-4206

7290 ALFRED UNIVERSITY: MERRILL FIELD

Alfred University Saxon Drive
Office of Conferences Carnegie Hall
Alfred, NY 14802-1205
Phone: 607-871-2183
Fax: 607-871-2293
e-mail: emrick@alfred.edu
Web Site: www.alfred.edu
Management:
    Director: William T Emrick
Founded: 1836
Seating Capacity: 3,000

7291 DAEMEN COLLEGE: DAEMEN THEATRE

4380 Main Street
Amherst, NY 14226
Phone: 716-839-8540

7292 US MILITARY ACADEMY

Wells College
Student Activities
Aurora, NY 13026
Phone: 315-364-3330
Fax: 315-364-3325

7293 JUNE COMPANY

28 Coolidge Way
Averil Park, NY 12018
Phone: 518-447-5414
Fax: 518-447-5446
e-mail: edward_j_hackney@fleet.com

7294 QUEENSBOROUGH COMMUNITY COLLEGE THEATER

222-05 56th Avenue
Bayside, NY 11364-1497
Phone: 718-631-6311
Fax: 718-631-6033
e-mail: boxoffice@qcc.cuny.edu
Web Site: www.qcc.cuny.edu
Management:
    Director Room Reservations: Anthony Carobine
Founded: 1970

Annual Attendance: 15,000+
Facility Category: Conventional Theatre
Type of Stage: Proscenium
Stage Dimensions: 40x40
Seating Capacity: 875
Year Built: 1970

7295 BROOME COUNTY VETERANS MEMORIAL ARENA

1 Stuart Street
Binghamton, NY 13901
Phone: 607-778-1528
Fax: 607-778-6041
e-mail: mmarinaccio@co.broome.ny.us
Web Site: www.gobroomecounty.com
Management:
   General Manager: Mike Marinaccio
Founded: 1972
Paid Staff: 30
Budget: 800,000
Income Sources: Sports; Concerts, Government; State; County; Concessions; Trade Shows

7296 STATE UNIVERSITY OF NEW YORK-BINGHAMPTON: ANDERSON CENTER FOR THE ARTS

PO Box 6000
Binghamton, NY 13902
Phone: 607-777-6802
Fax: 607-777-6771

7297 ADIRONDACK LAKES CENTER FOR THE ARTS

Route 28
PO Box 205
Blue Mountain Lake, NY 12812
Phone: 518-352-7715
Fax: 518-352-7333
e-mail: alca@telenet.net
Web Site: www.telenet.net/~alca
Officers:
   President: Roland B Stearns
   Vice President: Cathleen Collins
   Treasurer: Polly Fagan
   Secretary: Jamie Nile
Management:
   Executive Director: Ellen C Butz
   Program Coordinator: Darren Miller
Mission: To promote visual and performing arts through programs and services in our region, to serve established professional and aspiring artists.
Founded: 1967
Paid Staff: 5
Income Sources: Membership; grants; admission fees
Annual Attendance: 3,500
Facility Category: Concert Hall; Performance Center; Theatre
Type of Stage: Platform
Stage Dimensions: varible
Seating Capacity: 170
Year Remodeled: 1991

7298 SPECIAL OLYMPICS STADIUM

State University of New York, College at
Brockport, 350 New Campus Drive
Brockport, NY 14420-2989
Phone: 716-395-2218
Fax: 716-395-2160
e-mail: mandriat@brockport.edu
Web Site: www.brockport.edu
Management:
   Sports Information Director: Eric McDowell
Seating Capacity: 10,000

7299 STATE UNIVERITY OF NEW YORK COLLEGE AT BROCKPORT: TOWER FINE ARTS CENTER AND HARTWELL HALL

350 New Campus Drive
Brockport, NY 14420-2983
Phone: 716-395-2797
Fax: 716-395-5872
e-mail: sbixler@brockport.edu
Web Site: www.brockport.edu
Type of Stage: procenium/dance stage/black box
Stage Dimensions: 45'x30'
Seating Capacity: 400; 270; 100
Year Built: 1968
Year Remodeled: 1999

7300 STATE UNIVERSITY OF NEW YORK COLLEGE-BROCKPORT

Department of Dance
Brockport, NY 14420
Phone: 716-395-2153
Fax: 716-395-5134

7301 LEHMAN CENTER FOR THE PERFORMING ARTS

250 Bedford Park Boulevard W
Bronx, NY 10468
Phone: 718-960-8232
Fax: 718-960-8233
Web Site: lehman.cuny.edu
Management:
   Managing Director: Jack Globenfelt
Founded: 1980
Budget: $400,000-1,000,000
Facility Category: Concert Hall
Type of Stage: Proscenium
Seating Capacity: 2,310
Year Built: 1979

7302 YANKEE STADIUM

800 Ruppert
Bronx, NY 10451
Phone: 718-293-4300
Fax: 718-293-7431
Web Site: www.yankees.com
Management:
   General Manager: Bob Cashman
   Director Marketing: Beborah Tymon
   Director/Hospitality: Joel White
   Director Stadium Operations: Kirk Randazzo

Seating Capacity: 55,545

7303 BROOKLYN ACADEMY OF MUSIC
30 Lafayette Avenue
Brooklyn, NY 11217
Phone: 718-636-4100
Fax: 718-857-2021

7304 BROOKLYN ACADEMY OF MUSIC: CAREY PLAYHOUSE
30 Lafayette Avenue
Brooklyn, NY 11217
Phone: 718-636-4100
Fax: 718-857-2021

7305 BROOKLYN ACADEMY OF MUSIC: OPERA HOUSE
30 Lafayette Avenue
Brooklyn, NY 11217
Phone: 718-636-4100
Fax: 718-857-2021

7306 BROOKLYN CENTER FOR THE PERFORMING ARTS AT BROOKLYN COLLEGE
Campus Road & Hillel Place
PO Box 100163
Brooklyn, NY 11210
Phone: 718-951-4600
Fax: 718-951-4437
e-mail: richardg@brooklyn.cuny.edu
Web Site: www.brooklyncenter.com
Management:
    Director/General Manager: Richard Grossberg
    Producing Director: Julie Pareles
Budget: $400,000-1,000,000
Performs At: Walt Whitman Hall
Seating Capacity: 2,400
Rental Contact: Director/General Manager Richard Grossberg

7307 BROOKLYN CONSERVATORY OF MUSIC
58 7th Avenue
Brooklyn, NY 11217
Phone: 718-622-3300
Fax: 718-622-3957
Web Site: www.brooklynconservatory.com
Officers:
    President: David Rivel
Founded: 1898

7308 PRATT INSTITUTE: AUDITORIUM
200 Willoughby Avenue
Brooklyn, NY 11205
Phone: 718-636-3422
Fax: 718-636-3497

7309 SAINT JOSEPH'S COLLEGE
245 Clinton Avenue
Brooklyn, NY 11205

Phone: 718-636-6880
Fax: 718-636-6830
e-mail: rdavis@sjcny.edu
Web Site: www.sjcny.edu
Officers:
    Council for the Arts Co-Chair: Ruth Davis

7310 CW POST CAMPUS: HICKOX FIELD
CW Post Campus
Brookville, NY 11548
Phone: 516-299-2289
Fax: 516-299-3155
Management:
    Athletic Director: Vincent Salamone

7311 AFRICAN-AMERICAN CULTURAL CENTER: PAUL ROBESON HALL
350 Masten Avenue
Buffalo, NY 14209
Phone: 716-884-2013
Fax: 716-885-2590

7312 BUFFALO STATE COLLEGE-PERFORMING ARTS CENTER
1300 Elmwood Avenue
Rockwell Hall 210
Buffalo, NY 14222
Phone: 716-878-3032
Fax: 716-878-4234
e-mail: rhpac@bscmail.buffalostate.edu
Web Site: www.buffalostate.edu
Management:
    Director Of Operations: Jeff Marsha
    Technical Director: Thomas Kostusiak
Mission: To provide a first class professional performing arts facility that enhances the quality of life for the campus and the citizens of Western New York.
Founded: 1987
Specialized Field: Music.Dance.Theatre
Paid Staff: 5

7313 DUNN TIRE PARK
275 Washington Street
Buffalo, NY 14203
Phone: 716-846-2000
Fax: 716-852-6530
Web Site: www.bisons.com
Management:
    VP/Sales/Marketing: Marta Hiczewski

7314 HSBC ARENA
1 Seymore H Knox III Plaza
Buffalo, NY 14203
Phone: 716-855-4100
Fax: 716-855-4110
Web Site: www.hsbcarena.com
Management:
    Director Event Booking: Jennifer Van Rysdam

7315 KLEINHANS MUSIC HALL

Symphony Circle
Buffalo, NY 14201
Phone: 716-883-3560
Fax: 716-883-7430
Management:
   Manager: Kirsten R Carlon
Founded: 1941
Facility Category: Music Hall/Theater
Seating Capacity: 2,839
Rental Contact: Kristen R Carlsen

7316 MARINE MIDLAND ARENA

1 Seymour H Knox III Plaza
Buffalo, NY 14203-3007
Phone: 716-855-4100
Fax: 716-855-4110
Web Site: wwww.marinemidlandarena.com
Management:
   Director Building Operations: Stan Makowski
   Director Arena Booking: Jennifer Stich

7317 SHEA'S PERFORMING ARTS CENTER

646 Main Street
Buffalo, NY 14202
Phone: 716-847-1410
Fax: 716-847-1644
e-mail: pfagan@sheas.org
Web Site: www.sheas.org
Management:
   President/COO: Patrick Fagan

7318 STATE UNIVERSITY OF NEW YORK AT BUFFALO: DEPARTMENT OF THEATRE & DANCE

285 Alumni Arena
Buffalo, NY 14260
Phone: 716-645-6898
Fax: 716-645-6992
e-mail: clwhelan@acsu.buffalo.edu
Management:
   Secretary: Christine Whelan
Affiliations: Irish Classical Theatre Company;
Shakespeare in Delaware Park; Kavinoky; Musical Fare;
Art Park
Type of Stage: Proscenium; Black Box
Seating Capacity: 120; 388
Year Built: 1995
Cost: $500,000,000
Rental Contact: Center for the Arts S. Fazekas

7319 UNIVERSITY AT BUFFALO: SLEE CONCERT HALL

105 Slee Hall Department of Music
University at Buffalo
Buffalo, NY 14260
Phone: 716-645-2921
Web Site: www.slee.buffalo.edu/

7320 UNIVERSITY OF BUFFALO: CENTER FOR THE ARTS

103 Center for the Arts
University of Buffalo
Buffalo, NY 14260-6000
Phone: 716-645-6259
Fax: 716-645-6973
e-mail: fazekas@acsu.buffalo.edu
Web Site: www.arts.buffalo.edu
Management:
   Director: Thomas Burrows
   Assistant Director: Sandra Fazekas
   Assistant Director: Rob Falgiano
Mission: Mission is to create an environment for the
visual and performing arts to flourish through education,
exploration, collaboration, and presentation, while
enriching cultural opportunities for the surrounding
community.
Founded: 1994
Paid Staff: 30
Volunteer Staff: 300
Budget: $2 million
Income Sources: Rental, ticket sales, 60% salaries.
Affiliations: State University of New York at Buffalo
Annual Attendance: 130,000
Facility Category: Performing and Visual Arts
Type of Stage: Proscenium
Stage Dimensions: 42' X 102'
Seating Capacity: 1,748
Year Built: 1994
Cost: $2,500 commercial & labor
Rental Contact: Associate Director Sandra Fazekas
Organization Type: Mainstage 1748; Drama Theatre
388; Screening Room 210; Black Box 185.

7321 ST. LAWRENCE UNIVERSITY: AUGSBURY CENTER

Park Street
Canton, NY 13617
Phone: 315-229-5423
Fax: 315-229-5589
Web Site: www.stlawu.edu
Management:
   Associate Director Athletics: Randolph W LaBrake
   Athletic Director: Margie Strait
   Sports Information Director: Walter Johnson
   Head Football Coach: Chris Phelps
   Head Basketball Coach (M): Chris Downs
   Head Basketball Coach (W): GP Bromacki
Seating Capacity: 3,500

7322 CHAUTAUQUA INSTITUTION: AMPHITHEATER

PO Box 28
Chautauqua, NY 14722
Phone: 716-357-6200
Fax: 716-357-9014
Toll-free: 800-836-2787
e-mail: info@chautanqua-inst.org
Web Site: www.ciweb.org

7323 CHAUTAUQUA INSTITUTION: NORTON HALL
Chautauqua, NY 14722
Phone: 716-357-6000
Fax: 716-357-4175

7324 HAMILTON COLLEGE: MINOR THEATRE
198 College Hill Road
Clinton, NY 13323
Phone: 315-859-4205

7325 KIRKLAND ART CENTER
PO Box 213
E Park Row
Clinton, NY 13323-0213
Phone: 315-853-8871
Fax: 425-889-2963
e-mail: kacinc@dreamscape.com

7326 171 CEDAR ARTS CENTER
171 Cedar Street
Corning, NY 14830
Phone: 607-936-4647
Fax: 607-936-2081
e-mail: welkl@171cedararts.com
Web Site: www.171cedararts.com
Management:
    Executive Director: Lois Welk
Budget: $60,000-150,000

7327 MERCY COLLEGE: LECTURE HALL
555 Broadway
Dobbs Ferry, NY 10566
Phone: 914-693-9455

7328 EARLVILLE OPERA HOUSE
6-22 West Main Street
Earlville, NY 13332
Phone: 315-691-3550
Fax: 315-691-4111
e-mail: earlopra@dreamscape.com
Web Site: www.earlvilleopenhouse.com
Management:
    Executive Director: P Lockwood Blais
Mission: To promote the arts in a rural region of Central
New York State by offering programs of cultural,
educational and historical significance.
Status: Nonprofit
Paid Staff: 2
Facility Category: Theater
Type of Stage: Racked; Proscenium Arch
Seating Capacity: 300
Year Built: 1892

7329 CLEMENS CENTER
207 Clemens Center Parkway and Gray Street
PO Box 1046
Elmira, NY 14902

Phone: 607-733-5639
Fax: 607-737-1162
Toll-free: 800-724-0159
e-mail: info@clemenscenter.com
Web Site: www.clemenscenter.com
Management:
    Executive Director: Tom Weidemann
    Associate Executive Director: Julie Kriston
    Director Facility: Michael Kenna
    Stage Manager: Scott Tolbert
    Marketing Director: Jensen Monroe
Mission: To enhance the performing arts and the
entertainment experiences for the people of our region by
providing superior facilities and programs.
Founded: 1977
Specialized Field: Year-round presenter 10, 5 canty
region, resident companies and rentals
Paid Staff: 17
Volunteer Staff: 200

7330 ELMIRA COLLEGE
1 Park Place
Elmira, NY 14901
Phone: 607-735-1814
Fax: 607-735-1757
e-mail: manderson@elmira.edu
Web Site: www.elmira.edu
Management:
    Performing Arts Program Coordinator: Marjorie
    Anderson
Mission: Performing Arts program established as a
graduation requirement for freshmen and sohomores. We
want to keep the arts alive through making them a
necessary part of their college education. Community
patrons may purchase tickets also.
Founded: 1855
Status: Educational Institution
Income Sources: Course Fees; Ticket Sales
Type of Stage: Proscenium
Stage Dimensions: 28'x30'x15'
Seating Capacity: 448
Year Remodeled: 1995

7331 WESTCHESTER BROADWAY THEATRE
1 Broadway Plaza
Elmsford, NY 10523
Phone: 914-592-2222
Fax: 914-592-6917

7332 ARTHUR ASHE STADIUM
USTA National Tennis Center
Flushing Meadow, Corona Park
Flushing, NY 11368
Phone: 718-760-6200
Fax: 718-592-9488
Web Site: www.usta.com
Management:
    Facility Director: David Meehan

7333 BROOKLYN-QUEENS CONSERVATORY OF MUSIC
42-76 Main Street
Flushing, NY 11355

Phone: 718-461-8910
Fax: 718-886-2450
Web Site: www.brooklynconservatory.com
Officers:
　President: David Rivel

7334 COLDEN CENTER FOR THE PERFORMING ARTS

Queens College
Kissena Boulevard
Flushing, NY 11367
Phone: 718-544-2996
Fax: 718-261-7063
e-mail: PattyPrice@aol.com
Web Site: www.coldencenter.org
Management:
　Director: Vivian Charlop
　General Manager: Stephen Mallalieu
　Public Relations Director: Patty Price
　Box Office Manager: Stephanie McWoods
Founded: 1961
Paid Staff: 9
Performs At: Auditorium w/permanent acoustical shell
Facility Category: Performing Arts
Seating Capacity: 2143
Year Built: 1961
Rental Contact: Stephen Mallalieu

7335 SHEA STADIUM

123-01 Roosevelt Avenue
Flushing, NY 11368
Phone: 718-507-6387
Fax: 718-507-6395
Web Site: www.mets.com
Management:
　VP/Operations: Robert Mandt
　SVP/Marketing/Broadcasting: Mark Bingham
　SVP/Business/Legal Affairs: Dave Howard
　SVP/Treasurer: Harry O'Shaughnessy
　VP/Ticket Sales/Service: Bill Lannicielle
　Director Media Relations: Jay Horowitz
　Director Stadium Operations: Kevin McCarthy
　Director Ptom: James Plummer
　Director Community Outreach: Bill Knee
Seating Capacity: 55,000

7336 USTA NATIONAL TENNIS CENTER

Flushing Meadow-Corona Park
Flushing, NY 11368
Phone: 718-760-6200
Fax: 718-592-9488
Web Site: www.usta.com
Management:
　Facility Manager: Daivd Meehan

7337 STATE UNIVERSITY OF NEW YORK-FREDONIA: MICHAEL C ROCKEFELLER ARTS CENTER

Michael C Rockefeller Arts Center
Fredonia, NY 14063
Phone: 716-673-3217
Fax: 716-673-3617
e-mail: arts.center@fredonia.edu
Web Site: www.fredonia.edu/rac
Founded: 1969
Annual Attendance: 58,000
Facility Category: Multi-Vennue
Seating Capacity: 1,145/400/200

7338 WADSWORTH AUDITORIUM

State University of New York-Geneseo
1 College Circle
Geneseo, NY 14454
Phone: 716-245-5855
Fax: 716-245-4500
Web Site: www.geneseo.edu~sopa

7339 SMITH OPERA HOUSE

82 Seneca Street
Geneva, NY 14456
Phone: 315-789-2221
Fax: 315-789-6360
e-mail: thesmith1@capital.net
Web Site: www.thesmith.org
Management:
　Executive Director: Kevin Schoonover
Mission: A 107-year-old, fully restored, acoustically perfect performing arts venue and movie theatre catering to college students, senior citizens, families, and children.
Founded: 1894
Specialized Field: Music, Theatre, Dance, Film, Childrens Programing
Paid Staff: 4
Paid Artists: 80

7340 GLENS FALLS CIVIC CIENTER

1 Civic Center Plaza
Glens Falls, NY 12801
Phone: 518-798-0366
Fax: 518-793-7750
e-mail: oei@superior.ent
Management:
　Executive Director: Don M Ostrom

7341 ANDY KERR STADIUM

Colgate University
Hamilton, NY 13346
Phone: 315-228-7611
Fax: 315-228-7008
Web Site: www.athletics.colgate.edu
Management:
　Athletic Director: Mark Murphy

7342 COLGATE UNIVERSITY: BREHMER THEATER

Dana Arts Center
13 Oak Drive
Hamilton, NY 13346
Phone: 315-228-1000

7343 COLGATE UNIVERSITY: UNIVERSITY THEATER
Dana Arts Center
13 Oak Drive
Hamilton, NY 13346
Phone: 315-228-1000

7344 HOFSTRA UNIVERSITY STADIUM & ARENA
200 Hofstra University
Room 112
Hempstead, NY 11549
Phone: 516-463-6625
Fax: 516-463-6520
Web Site: www.hofstra.edu
Management:
    Associated Director: Ann Baller

7345 DOME CENTER
2695 E Henrietta Road
Henrietta, NY 14467
Phone: 716-334-4000
Fax: 716-334-3005
e-mail: fairlady@frontiernet.net
Web Site: www.domecenter.com
Management:
    Executive Director: Frances Tepper
Mission: Exhibition Hall, Concert Venue, County Fair
Founded: 1823
Paid Staff: 11
Budget: $1,000,000
Income Sources: Rentals
Affiliations: IAMM, SAFE, ORBA, NYSAAP
Annual Attendance: 80,000
Seating Capacity: 1200
Year Built: 1973
Rental Contact: Executive Director Fran Tepper

7346 HOUGHTON COLLEGE: WESLEY CHAPEL
Houghton College
Houghton, NY 14744
Phone: 716-567-2211
Fax: 716-567-9517
Web Site: www.houghton.edu

7347 INTER-MEDIA ART CENTER
370 New York Avenue
Huntington, NY 11713
Phone: 516-549-9666
e-mail: imac@ix.netcom.com
Web Site: www.imactheater.org
Management:
    Executive Director: Michael Rothbard

7348 ALICE STATLER HALL
Statler School of Hotel Administration
Cornell University
Ithaca, NY 14853-6902
Phone: 607-254-2604
Fax: 607-257-6432

7349 HANGAR THEATRE
Cass Park
PO Box 205
Ithaca, NY 14851
Phone: 607-273-8588
Fax: 607-273-4516
Web Site: www.hangartheatre.org

7350 ITHACA COLLEGE: DILLINGHAM CENTER FOR THE PERFORMING ARTS
Department of Theatre Arts
201 Dillingham Center
Ithaca, NY 14850
Phone: 607-274-3345
Fax: 607-274-3672
e-mail: theatrearts@ithaca.edu
Web Site: www.ithaca.edu/theatre
Management:
    Chairman/Director Theatre: Lee Byron
Specialized Field: Theatre Education
Paid Staff: 25

7351 JIM BUTTERFIELD STADIUM
201 Ceracchie Athletic Center
Ithaca College
Ithaca, NY 14850-7198
Phone: 607-274-3209
Fax: 607-274-1667
Web Site: www.ithaca.edu
Management:
    Director Athletics: Kristen Ford

7352 JAMAICA CENTER FOR THE PERFORMING & VISUAL ARTS
161-04 Jamaica Avenue
Jamaica, NY 11432
Phone: 718-658-7400
Fax: 718-658-7922
Management:
    Presenting Program Manager: JD Rose

7353 ST. JOHN'S UNIVERSITY
8000 Utopia Parkway
Jamaica, NY 11439
Phone: 718-990-6217
Fax: 718-969-8213
Management:
    Director: Edward J Manetta
    Sr Associate Director: Kathleen Meehan
    Associate Director: Charlie Elwood
    Sports Information Director: Dominic Scianna
Seating Capacity: 6,008

7354 LUCILLE BALL LITTLE THEATRE BUILDING
18-24 East Second Street
Jamestown, NY 14701
Phone: 716-483-1095
Fax: 716-483-1099
Officers:
    President: Marvin Anderson
Management:

Business Manager: Marshall Dahlin
Mission: Produce five plays and musicals from September through May.
Founded: 1936
Paid Staff: 3
Volunteer Staff: 2
Non-paid Artists: 100
Budget: $150,000
Income Sources: Ticket sales, grants
Annual Attendance: 12,000
Facility Category: Auditorium theatre house
Type of Stage: Proscenium
Stage Dimensions: 80 x 40 x 24
Seating Capacity: 400
Year Built: 1925
Year Remodeled: 1968

7355 CARAMOOR CENTER FOR MUSIC AND THE ARTS

149 Girdle Ridge Road
Katonah, NY 10536
Phone: 914-232-5035
Fax: 914-232-5521
Web Site: www.caramoor.org
Officers:
  President/CEO: Erich Vollmer
Management:
  Executive Director: Howard Herring
  Managing Director: Paul Rosenblum
  Director Development: Susan Shine
  Director Operations: Melissa Montera
  Box Office Manager: Sal Vaccaro
Mission: To offer a performing arts venue in Bedford and New York State.
Founded: 1945
Specialized Field: Vocal Music; Instrumental Music; Festivals
Status: Professional; Nonprofit
Performs At: Museum Music Room Venetian Theatre
Organization Type: Performing; Educational; Sponsoring

7356 VENETIAN THEATRE

Caramoor
Girdle Ridge Road
Katonah, NY 10536
Phone: 914-232-5035
Fax: 914-232-5521

7357 ULSTER PERFORMING ARTS CENTER

601 Broadway
Kingston, NY 12401
Phone: 845-331-1613
Fax: 845-339-3814
e-mail: director@upac.org
Web Site: www.upac.org
Year Remodeled: 2001
Rental Contact: Jodi Longto

7358 LAKE GEORGE DINNER THEATRE

2223 Route 9
PO Box 266
Lake George, NY 12845

Phone: 518-668-5781
Fax: 518-668-9213
Web Site: www.lakegeorgedinnertheatre.com
Management:
  Producer: Victoria Eastwood
Founded: 1968

7359 LAKE PLACID CENTER FOR THE ARTS-THEATER

91 Saranac Avenue
Lake Placid, NY 12946
Phone: 518-523-2512
Fax: 518-523-2521
e-mail: lpca@northnet.org
Web Site: www.lpartscenter.org
Management:
  Director: Nadine Duhaime
Mission: Dedicated to presenting and fostering quality arts which inspire, enrich, educate and entertain people of all ages.
Founded: 1972
Specialized Field: multi- purpose arts center
Paid Staff: 8
Volunteer Staff: 50
Budget: $600,000
Income Sources: Grants; Rentals
Annual Attendance: 35,000
Facility Category: Theatre/Gallery/Studio
Type of Stage: Proscenium
Seating Capacity: 355
Year Built: 1971
Rental Contact: Nadine Danaime

7360 OLYMPIC CENTER

Olympic Regional Development Authority
218 Main Street
Lake Placid, NY 12946
Phone: 518-523-1655
Fax: 518-523-9275
Web Site: www.orda.org
Management:
  General Manager: Dennis R Allen
Seating Capacity: 11,100

7361 LANCASTER NEW YORK OPERA HOUSE

21 Central Avenue
Lancaster, NY 14086
Phone: 716-683-1776
Fax: 716-683-8220
Web Site: www.lancopera.org

7362 STUDIO THEATRE

141 S Wellwood Avenue
Lindenhurst, NY 11757
Phone: 631-226-1833

7363 MOHAWK VALLEY CENTER FOR THE ARTS

401 S Ann Street
Little Falls, NY 13365
Phone: 315-823-0808

7364 KENAN CENTER
433 Locust Street
Lockport, NY 14094
Phone: 716-433-2617
Fax: 716-433-6645
Management:
   Executive Director: Susan Przybyl

7365 LAGUARDIA PERFORMING ARTS CENTER
31-10 Thomson Avenue
Room E-241
Long Island City, NY 11101
Phone: 718-482-5151
Fax: 718-482-5155
Management:
   Producing Director: Zuri McKie
Budget: $60,-150,000
Performs At: Little Theatre

7366 EMELIN THEATRE FOR THE PERFORMING ARTS
Library Lane
Mamaroneck, NY 10543
Phone: 914-698-3045
Fax: 914-698-1404

7367 AARON DAVIS HALL
W 135th Street & Convent Avenue
New York, NY 10031
Phone: 212-650-6900
Fax: 212-862-4600
e-mail: adh@interport.net
Management:
   General Manager: James King
Performs At: Marian Anderson Theater

7368 AMBASSADOR THEATRE
215 W 49th Street
New York, NY 10019
Phone: 212-239-6200

7369 AMERICAN PLACE THEATRE
111 W 46th Street
New York, NY 10036
Phone: 212-840-2960
Fax: 212-391-4019
e-mail: apt@americanplacetheatre.org
Web Site: www.americanplacetheatre.org
Management:
   Artistic Director: Wynn Handman
   General Manager: Carl H Jeynes
Paid Staff: 75
Annual Attendance: 90,000
Facility Category: Three Theatres; Cabaret; Black Box
Seating Capacity: 74/74/350
Year Built: 1971

7370 APOLLO THEATRE
253 W 125th Street
New York, NY 10027

Phone: 212-531-5300
Fax: 212-749-2743

7371 ASCAP
One Lincoln Plaza
New York, NY 10023
Phone: 212-621-6407
Fax: 212-873-3133
Toll-free: 800-652-7227
e-mail: aalexander@ascap.com
Web Site: www.ascap.com
Management:
   Director, Symphonic Educational: Allen Alexander
   Account Services Manager: Krystal Jones

7372 BAKER FIELD
Columbia University
533 W 218th Street
New York, NY 10027
Phone: 212-942-0431
Fax: 212-854-2988
e-mail: jar14@columbia.edu
Web Site: www.columbia.edu

7373 BMI (BROADCAST MUSIC)
320 W 57th Street
New York, NY 10019
Phone: 212-586-2000
Fax: 212-262-2824
e-mail: classical@bmi.com
Web Site: www.bmi.com
Officers:
   President/CEO: Frances W Preston
   Senior VP Performing Rights: Del R Bryant
   VP Corporate Relations: Robbin Ahrold
   President BMI Foundation: Ralph N Jackson
Management:
   Assistant VP Classical Music: Barbara A Petersen
   VP Writer Publisher Relations: Charles Feldman
   Senior Director Jazz & Musical Thea: Jean Banks
   General Licensing Executive: William Grothe
Mission: BMI is a performing rights licensing organization representing composers, songwriters and publishers with a repertory of more than 4.5 million musical works.
Founded: 1940
Specialized Field: Music

7374 BOOTH THEATRE
222 W 45th Street
New York, NY 10036
Phone: 212-239-6200

7375 BROADHURST THEATRE
235 W 44th Street
New York, NY 10035
Phone: 212-239-6200

7376 BROADWAY THEATRE
1681 Broadway
New York, NY 10019
Phone: 212-239-6200

7377 BROOKS ATKINSON THEATRE
256 W 47th Street
New York, NY 10036
Phone: 212-719-4099

7378 CARNEGIE HALL CORPORATION
881 7th Avenue
New York, NY 10019
Phone: 212-903-9600
Fax: 212-581-6539
Web Site: www.carnegiehall.org
Management:
Executive/Artistic Director: Robert Harth
Mission: To continue to be one of the world's leading institutions in presenting great music and in promoting music education, music creation and music enjoyment in landmark concert hall.
Founded: 1891
Paid Staff: 250
Volunteer Staff: 150

7379 CENTER FOR TRADITIONAL MUSIC & DANCE
200 Church Street
Room 303
New York, NY 10013-3831
Phone: 212-571-1555
Fax: 212-571-9052
e-mail: jschlefer@ctmd.org
Web Site: www.ctmd.org
Management:
Director Artist Management: James R Schlefer
Mission: to identify and present artists of traditional global cultures who now make their home in New York City. To develop and provide educational programming and material that fosters cross-cultural dialouge and understanding through the perform
Founded: 1976
Specialized Field: World Music; Dance
Paid Staff: 8
Volunteer Staff: 2

7380 CIRCLE IN THE SQUARE
Broadway & 50th Street
New York, NY 10019
Phone: 212-307-0388
Web Site: www.circlesquare.org
Officers:
President: Paul Libin
Management:
Artistic Director: Theodore Mann
Executive Director: E Colin O'Leary
Associate Director: Dr. Rhonda R Dodd
Development & Arts Education: Jonathan Mann
Development Associate: Holly Ricciuti
Mission: School of training.
Status: Nonprofit

7381 CITY CENTER
130 W 56th Street
New York, NY 10019

Phone: 212-247-0430
Fax: 212-246-9778
e-mail: elowery@citycenter.org
Web Site: www.citycenter.org
Officers:
President/Executive Director: Judith E Daykin
Senior VP/ Managing Director: Mrk G Litvin
Management:
Senior Director Theatre Operations: Eugene Lowery
Senior Manager Operations: Ann Tuomey
Founded: 1943
Status: Nonprofit
Paid Staff: 32
Budget: $1,000,000+
Income Sources: Ticket Sales; Donations
Annual Attendance: 200,000
Facility Category: Theater
Type of Stage: Proscenium
Stage Dimensions: 43'x45'
Seating Capacity: 2,684
Year Built: 1923
Rental Contact: Eugene Lowery

7382 CITY CENTER OF MUSIC AND DRAMA
70 Lincoln Central Plaza
4th Floor
New York, NY 10023
Phone: 212-870-4266
Fax: 212-870-4286
Management:
Director: Michael Edwards
Mission: To provide ballet, theatre and opera for the community at low cost or no charge.
Founded: 1943
Specialized Field: Dance; Vocal Music; Instrumental Music; Theater
Status: Professional; Nonprofit
Performs At: New York State Theater
Organization Type: Performing; Touring; Educational

7383 COLUMBIA UNIVERSITY: WIEN STADIUM
Columbia University, Dodge Fitness Center
3030 Broadway, Mail Code 1902
New York, NY 10027
Phone: 212-854-2538
Fax: 212-854-2988
Management:
Athletic Director: John Reeves
Seating Capacity: 3,405

7384 CORT THEATRE
138 W 48th Street
New York, NY 10036
Phone: 212-239-6200
Fax: 212-239-5134

7385 DANCE THEATER WORKSHOP
219 W 19th Street
New York, NY 10011

Phone: 212-691-6500
Fax: 212-633-1974
e-mail: dtw@dtw.org
Web Site: www.dtw.org
Management:
   Executive Director/Producer: David R White
   Senior Producer: Craig T Peterson

7386 DELACORTE THEATER IN CENTRAL PARK
81st Street at Central Park W
New York, NY 10003
Phone: 212-539-8750
Fax: 212-839-8505
Web Site: www.publictheater.org
Officers:
   Producer: George C Wolfe
   Managing Director: Mark Litvin
Management:
   General Manager: Michael Hurst
Founded: 1954
Season: June - September
Facility Category: Ampitheatre (open air)
Type of Stage: Thrust
Seating Capacity: 1900
Year Built: 1962
Year Remodeled: 1999
Rental Contact: General Manager Michael Hurst
Comments: The Delacorte Theater is operated by the Joseph Papp Public Theater/New York Shakespeare Festival Shakespeare productions. Free tickets are distributed starting at 1 PM on days of performances.

7387 EDEN'S EXPRESSWAY
537 Broadway
New York, NY 10012
Phone: 212-226-8988

7388 ENSEMBLE STUDIO THEATRE
549 W 52nd Street
New York, NY 10019
Phone: 212-247-3405
Fax: 212-664-0041

7389 ETHEL BARRYMORE THEATRE
243 W 47th Street
New York, NY 10036
Phone: 212-239-6200

7390 GERSHWIN THEATRE
222 W 51st Street
New York, NY 10019
Phone: 212-586-6510
Web Site: www.gershwintheatre.com

7391 GOETHE-INSITUT/INTER NATIONES GERMAN CULTURAL CENTER
1014 5th Avenue
New York, NY 10028

Phone: 212-439-8700
Fax: 212-439-8705
e-mail: director@goethe-newyork.org
Web Site: www.goethe.de/newyork
Management:
   Director: Stephan Nobbe, PhD
Budget: $10,000

7392 HB PLAYWRIGHTS FOUNDATION THEATRE HOUSE
124 S Bank Street
New York, NY 10014
Phone: 212-989-6540
Fax: 212-627-4288

7393 IMPERIAL THEATRE
249 W 45th Street
New York, NY 10036
Phone: 212-944-3700

7394 JEWISH MUSEUM
1109 5th Avenue
New York, NY 10128
Phone: 212-423-3224
Fax: 212-423-3232
Web Site: www.thejewishmuseum.org
Management:
   Media/Public Programs Director: Aviva Weintraub

7395 JOHN GOLDEN THEATRE
252 W 45th Street
New York, NY 10036
Phone: 212-944-4136

7396 JOSEPH PAPP PUBLIC THEATER
425 Lafayette Street
New York, NY 10003
Phone: 212-539-8530
Fax: 212-539-8505
Web Site: www.publictheater.org
Management:
   Director: George C Wolfe
   Literary Director: John Eiqw
   Associate Producer Musicals: Wiley Hausam
Mission: Historical landmark and former site of the Astor Library, the Public Theater was saved from the wrecking ball by the legendary Joseph Papp to become home to six theaters, producing the best of original drama and comedy as well as new productions of timeless classics.
Founded: 1954
Specialized Field: Public theater
Performs At: Newman Theater, Anspacher Theater, Martinson Hall, LuEsther Hall, Shiva Theater
Type of Stage: Proscenium, Thrust, Flexible
Seating Capacity: 299, 275, 200, 150, 100

7397 JOYCE THEATER
175 8th Avenue
New York, NY 10011

Phone: 212-691-9740
Fax: 212-727-3658
e-mail: staff@joyce.org
Web Site: www.joyce.org
Management:
  Director Programming: Martin Wechsler
  Executive Director: Linda Shelton
Mission: Mission is to serve and support the art of dance and choreography, to promote the richness and variety of the art form in its fullest expression.
Founded: 1981
Specialized Field: Dance
Annual Attendance: 136,000
Facility Category: Theater
Type of Stage: Proscenium
Stage Dimensions: 64x35
Seating Capacity: 472
Year Built: 1930
Year Remodeled: 1982

7398 KAYE PLAYHOUSE AT HUNTER COLLEGE
695 Park Avenue
New York, NY 10021
Phone: 212-772-5207
Fax: 212-650-3919
Web Site: www.kayeplayhouse.org
Management:
  General Manager: Nancy B Dodds

7399 KAZUKO HIRABAYASHI DANCE THEATRE
330 Broome Street
New York, NY 10002
Phone: 212-966-6414

7400 KITCHEN
512 W 19th Street
New York, NY 10011
Phone: 212-255-5793
Fax: 212-645-4258
e-mail: info@thekitchen.org
Web Site: www.thekitchen.com
Management:
  Executive Director: Elise Bernhardt
  New Media Director: Christina Yang
  Education/Outreach Curator: Treba Offutt
Founded: 1971
Specialized Field: Dance, Music, Performance, Literature, Film & Video, New Media Arts
Paid Staff: 20
Volunteer Staff: 10
Paid Artists: 40

7401 LAMB'S THEATRE
130 W 44th Street
New York, NY 10036
Phone: 212-997-1780
Fax: 212-997-1082

7402 LEHMAN CENTER FOR THE PERFORMING ARTS
Bedford Park Boulevard W
New York, NY 10468
Phone: 718-960-8881
Fax: 212-960-8935

7403 LONGACRE THEATRE
220 W 48th Street
New York, NY 10036
Phone: 212-239-6200

7404 LUCILLE LORTEL THEATRE
121 Christopher Street
New York, NY 10014
Phone: 212-924-2817
Fax: 212-939-0036

7405 LUNT-FONTANNE THEATRE
205 W 46th Street
New York, NY 10036
Phone: 212-575-9200
Mission: To promote and increase awareness and interest in the theatre and performing arts locally, nationally and globally.

7406 LYCEUM THEATRE
149 W 45th Street
New York, NY 10036
Phone: 212-239-6200

7407 MADISON SQUARE GARDEN
4 Pennsylvania Plaza
New York, NY 10001
Phone: 212-456-6000
Fax: 212-465-6029
Web Site: www.thegarden.com
Officers:
  President: James Dolan
  Chairman: Charles Dolan
  Vice Chairman: Robert Lemle
Management:
  President/CEO: David W Checketts
  Executive VP/General Manager: Robert Russo
Mission: Madison Square Garden is part of Madison Square Garden, L.P. Cablevision Systems Corporation owns a majority interest in MSG.

7408 MAJESTIC THEATRE
245 W 44th Street
New York, NY 10036
Phone: 212-239-6200

7409 MANHATTAN THEATRE CLUB
453 W 16th Street
New York, NY 10011
Phone: 212-399-3030
Fax: 212-691-9106
e-mail: questions@mtc-nyc.org
Web Site: www.mtc-nyc.org

7410 MARQUIS
211 W 45th Street
New York, NY 10036
Phone: 212-382-0100

7411 MARTIN BECK THEATER
302 W 45th Street
New York, NY 10036
Phone: 212-239-6200

7412 MARYMOUNT MANHATTAN COLLEGE
221 E 71st Street
New York, NY 10021
Phone: 212-517-0475
Fax: 212-517-0541

7413 MERKIN CONCERT HALL AT KAUFMAN CENTER
Goodman House
129 W 67th Street
New York, NY 10023-5976
Phone: 212-501-3340
Fax: 212-501-3317
e-mail: lhart@ekcc.org
Web Site: www.ekcc.org
Officers:
    Honorary Chairman: Leonard Goodman
    Chairman: Elaine Kaufman
    President: Phyllis Feder
    VP: R. Devon
Management:
    Executive Director: Lydia Kontos
    Director Concert Division: Vicki Margulies
    Director Communications: Lizanne Hart
    Director Development: Judy Ringer
Mission: To awaken and enhance appreciation of and participation in music and other arts; seeks to further this mission as an independent concert hall. Merkin Hall's programming reflects a diverse society and encompasses a breath of musical styles, periods, and traditions, with emphasis on new work, new artists, events and programs which draw on our rich Jewish cultural heritage.
Founded: 1952
Specialized Field: Concert Hall
Status: Professional; Nonprofit
Paid Staff: 19
Paid Artists: 500
Budget: $720,000
Income Sources: Earned and Contributed; Foundation; Individual; Government Support
Performs At: Merkin Concert Hall
Affiliations: Chamber Music America
Annual Attendance: 60,000
Facility Category: Professional Concert Hall
Type of Stage: Fixed Proscenium
Stage Dimensions: 35'x57'x20'
Seating Capacity: 457
Year Built: 1978
Rental Contact: Booking/Operations Manager Kelly Ransell
Resident Groups: Poppyseed Players

7414 MICHAEL SCHIMMEL CENTER FOR THE ARTS
3 Spruce Street
Pace University, 1 Pace Plaza
New York, NY 10038
Phone: 212-346-1398
Fax: 212-346-1645
e-mail: culture@pace.edu
Web Site: www.pace.edu
Management:
    Managing Director: Jillian C Panfel
Founded: 1970
Specialized Field: Dance, Jazz, Theatrical Student Productions, Location for Film and TV

7415 MINETTA LANE THEATRE
18 Minetta Lane
New York, NY 10012
Phone: 212-420-8000
Fax: 212-420-8214

7416 MINSKOFF THEATRE
200 W 45th Street
New York, NY 10036
Phone: 212-869-0550
Fax: 212-944-8644
Seating Capacity: 1685

7417 MUSIC BOX
239 W 45th Street
New York, NY 10036
Phone: 212-239-6200

7418 NEDERLANDER THEATRE
208 W 41st Street
New York, NY 10036
Phone: 212-921-8000
Web Site: www.siteforrent.com

7419 NEIL SIMON THEATRE
250 W 52nd Street
New York, NY 10019
Phone: 212-757-8646
Fax: 212-262-2400
Seating Capacity: 1334

7420 NEW DRAMATISTS
424 W 44th Street
New York, NY 10036
Phone: 212-757-6960
Fax: 212-265-4738

7421 OPEN EYE: NEW STAGINGS
270 W 89th Street
New York, NY 10024
Phone: 212-226-8435
Fax: 212-343-1065

7422 ORPHEUM THEATRE
126 2nd Avenue
New York, NY 10003

Phone: 212-477-2477

7423 PALACE THEATRE

1564 Broadway
New York, NY 10036
Phone: 212-730-8200
Fax: 212-730-7932

7424 PAN AMERICAN MUSICAL ART RESEARCH

198 Broadway
Room 807
New York, NY 10038
Phone: 212-267-8723
Fax: 212-267-8723
e-mail: panmarj@aol.com
Web Site: www.pamar.org
Management:
    Executive Director: Jan Michael Hanvik

7425 PERFORMANCE SPACE

150 1st Avenue
New York, NY 10009
Phone: 212-477-5829
Fax: 212-353-1315
e-mail: ps122@ps122.org
Web Site: www.ps122.org
Management:
    Executive Director: Mark Russell

7426 PLYMOUTH THEATRE

236 W 45th Street
New York, NY 10036
Phone: 212-239-6200

7427 PROMENADE THEATRE

2162 Broadway
New York, NY 10023
Phone: 212-707-8270
Fax: 212-707-8775

7428 QUEBEC GOVERNMENT HOUSE

1 Rockefeller Plaza
26th Floor
New York, NY 10020
Phone: 212-843-0985
Fax: 212-376-8984
e-mail: renee.ovellet@mri.gouv.qc.ca
Web Site: www.quebecusa.org
Management:
    Director Cultural Services: Renee Ovellet

7429 RADIO CITY MUSIC HALL

1260 Avenue of the Americas
New York, NY 10020
Phone: 212-632-4000
Web Site: www.radiocity.com
Mission: Since 1932, Radio City Hall has been synonymous with the very in entertainment.
Founded: 1932
Resident Groups: Radio City Rockettes

7430 RICHARD ROGERS THEATRE

226 W 46th Street
New York, NY 10036
Phone: 212-221-1211

7431 ROYALE THEATRE

242 W 45th Street
New York, NY 10036
Phone: 212-239-6200
Seating Capacity: 1,068

7432 SAINT CLEMENT'S CHURCH

423 W 46th Street
New York, NY 10036
Phone: 212-246-7277
Fax: 212-307-1447

7433 SAINT JAMES THEATER

246 W 44th Street
New York, NY 10036
Phone: 212-239-6200

7434 SHUBERT THEATRE

225 W 45th Street
New York, NY 10036
Phone: 212-239-6200
Seating Capacity: 1,513

7435 SOHO REP

46 Walker Street
New York, NY 10013
Phone: 212-941-8632
Fax: 212-941-7148
Web Site: www.sohorep.org
Management:
    Managing Director: Alexandra Conley
Founded: 1974
Status: Nonprofit
Season: March - August
Stage Dimensions: 25' x 35'
Seating Capacity: 99

7436 SULLIVAN STREET PLAYHOUSE

181 Sullivan Street
New York, NY 10012
Phone: 212-674-3838
Fax: 212-674-4706
Seating Capacity: 153

7437 SUPPER CLUB

240 W 47th Street
New York, NY 10036
Phone: 212-921-1940
Fax: 212-391-3982

7438 SURDNA FOUNDATION

330 Madison Avenue
30th Floor
New York, NY 10017
Phone: 212-557-0010

7439 TISCH CENTER FOR THE ARTS OF THE 92ND STREET Y
1395 Lexington Avenue
New York, NY 10128
Phone: 212-415-5739
Fax: 212-415-5738
e-mail: tischctr@92ndsty.org
Web Site: www.92ndsty.org
Management:
Director: Hanna Arie-Gaifman
Budget: $400,000-1,000,000
Performs At: Theresa L. Kaufmann Concert Hall

7440 TOWN HALL
123 W 43rd Street
New York, NY 10036
Phone: 212-997-1003
Fax: 212-997-1929
e-mail: info@the-townhall-nyc.org
Web Site: www.the-townhall-nyc.org
Management:
Executive Director: Lawrence C Zucker
Director Public Relations: Kerrie L Smith
Director Marketing: Ellen A Katnolos
Mission: To offer affordable entertainment to all ages.
Annual Attendance: 500,000
Facility Category: Concert Hall
Type of Stage: Proscenium
Seating Capacity: 1,495
Year Built: 1921
Year Remodeled: 1985

7441 TRIBECA PERFORMING ARTS CENTER
199 Chambers Street
New York, NY 10007-1006
Phone: 212-346-8500
Fax: 212-732-2482
e-mail: boxoffice@tribecapac.org
Web Site: www.tribecapac.org
Management:
Operations Director: Carol Cleveland
Executive Director: Linda Herring
Marketing Director: Donald Briggs
Mission: Producing and presenting theatre, dance and music for diverse audiences of all ages.
Founded: 1983
Specialized Field: Performing Arts
Paid Staff: 14
Paid Artists: 5
Budget: $600,000
Income Sources: Earned Income; Rental Income; Charitable Contributions
Affiliations: TCG; ART New York
Annual Attendance: 40,000
Facility Category: Multi-theatre Performing Arts
Type of Stage: Proscenium; Thrust
Seating Capacity: 913/262
Year Built: 1983
Rental Contact: Carol Cleveland

7442 UNION SQUARE THEATRE
126 2nd Avenue
New York, NY 10003

Phone: 212-505-0700
Fax: 212-477-7732

7443 UNIVERSITY SETTLEMENT
184 Eldridge Street
New York, NY 10002
Phone: 212-674-9120
Fax: 212-475-3278

7444 VIRGINIA THEATER
245 W 52nd Street
New York, NY 10019
Phone: 212-840-8181

7445 WALTER KERR THEATRE
219 W 48th Street
New York, NY 10036

7446 WEB CONCERT HALL
2565 Broadway
Suite 316
New York, NY 10025
Phone: 212-280-8187
Fax: 212-280-8187
e-mail: info2@musicalonline.com
Web Site: www.webconcerthall.com
Management:
Music Director: Mi Jung Im
Budget: $10,000

7447 WESTBETH THEATRE CENTER
151 Bank Street
New York, NY 10014
Phone: 212-691-2272
Fax: 212-924-7185
e-mail: WbethTC@aol.com
Web Site: www.westbeththeatre.com
Management:
Producing Director: Arnold Engelman
Associate Producer: Kirsten Ames
Founded: 1977
Status: Nonprofit
Season: Year-Round
Type of Stage: Thrust and Arena
Seating Capacity: 60-300

7448 WESTBETH THEATRE CENTER: BIG ROOM
151 Bank Street
New York, NY 10014
Phone: 212-691-2272
Fax: 212-924-7185
Web Site: www.westbeththeatre.com

7449 WESTBETH THEATRE CENTER: SECOND FLOOR THEATRE
151 Bank Street
New York, NY 10014
Phone: 212-691-2272
Fax: 212-924-7185
Web Site: www.westbeththeatre.com

7450 WESTBETH THEATRE CENTER: STUDIO THEATRE
151 Bank Street
New York, NY 10014
Phone: 212-691-2272
Fax: 212-924-7185
Web Site: www.westbeththeatre.com

7451 WESTSIDE THEATRE
407 W 43rd Street
New York, NY 10036
Phone: 212-315-2302
Fax: 212-315-2307
Type of Stage: proscenium/ thrust
Stage Dimensions: 40'x 26' 6"/ 40'x 18'3"
Seating Capacity: 299/ 250
Organization Type: Theatre Complex; Performance Center; Commercial Rental Theatre

7452 WHITNEY MUSEUM OF ART
120 Park Avenue at 42 Street
New York, NY 10017
Phone: 212-878-2475
Fax: 212-907-5770

7453 WINTER GARDEN THEATRE
1634 Broadway
New York, NY 10019
Phone: 212-239-6200

7454 HERSHELL CARROUSEL FACTORY MUSEUM
180 Thompson Street
PO Box 672
North Tonawanda, NY 14120
Phone: 716-693-1885
Fax: 716-743-9018
e-mail: hcfm@carrouselmuseum.org
Web Site: www.carrouselmuseum.org

7455 HELEN HAYES PERFORMING ARTS CENTER
PO Box 229
Nyack, NY 10960
Phone: 914-358-2847
Management:
    Managing Director: Joel Warren
    Artistic Director: Rod Kaats
Founded: 1996
Status: Nonprofit
Season: October - July
Type of Stage: Proscenium
Stage Dimensions: 60' x 28'
Seating Capacity: 600

7456 RALPH WILSON STADIUM
One Bills Drive
Orchard Park, NY 14127
Phone: 716-648-1800
Fax: 716-649-6446
Web Site: www.buffalobills.com
Management:
VP Operations: William G Munson
Director Stadium Operations: Joe Frandina
Seating Capacity: 79,902

7457 PARAMOUNT CENTER FOR THE ARTS
1008 Brown Street
Peekskill, NY 10990
Phone: 914-739-2333
Fax: 914-736-4674
Web Site: www.paramountcenter.org
Management:
    Executive Director: Alice Jane Bryant
    Manager: Anthony Corcoran
Mission: To provide quality programming in live perfromance and the visual arts. Serving the interest of the Hudson Valley and raising the level of cultural enrichment of all who enter this unique theater.
Founded: 1981
Seating Capacity: 1024
Year Built: 1930

7458 THEATRE THREE PRODUCTIONS: MAINSTAGE
412 Main Street
PO Box 512
Port Jefferson, NY 11777
Phone: 631-928-9202
Fax: 631-928-9120
Facility Category: Theatre House
Rental Contact: Vivian Koutrakas

7459 THEATRE THREE PRODUCTIONS: SECOND STAGE
412 Main Street
PO Box 512
Port Jefferson, NY 11777
Phone: 631-928-9202
Fax: 631-928-9120

7460 BARDAVON 1869 OPERA HOUSE
35 Market Street
Poughkeepsie, NY 12601-9990
Phone: 845-473-5288
Fax: 845-473-4259
e-mail: slamarca@bardavon.org
Web Site: www.bardavon.org
Management:
    Managing Director Production: Stephen LaMarca
    Executive Director: Chris Silva
    Music Director: Randall Craig Fleischer
Founded: 1869
Paid Staff: 17
Volunteer Staff: 80
Seating Capacity: 944
Year Built: 1869

7461 MID-HUDSON CIVIC CENTER
14 Civic Center Plaza
Poughkeepsie, NY 12601
Phone: 845-454-9800
Fax: 845-454-5877
e-mail: Dumoulins@netstep.net
Web Site: www.midhudsonciviccenter.com

Management:
Executive Director: Susan DuMoulin

7462 PURCHASE COLLEGE, SUNY: THE PERFORMING ARTS CENTER
The Performing Arts Center, SUNY Purchase
735 Anderson Hill Road, Box 140
Purchase, NY 10577-0140
Phone: 914-251-6222
Fax: 914-251-6171
e-mail: center@purchase.edu
Web Site: www.artscenter.org
Management:
Director: Christopher Beach

7463 BLUE CROSS ARENA
1 War Memorial Square
Rochester, NY 14614
Phone: 716-546-3020
Fax: 716-758-5327
Web Site: www.bluecrossarena.com
Management:
General Manager: Jeffrey E Calkins

7464 EASTMAN SCHOOL OF MUSIC KILBOURN HALL
26 Gibbs Street
Rochester, NY 14604
Phone: 716-274-1110

7465 EASTMAN SCHOOL OF MUSIC
26 Gibbs Street
Rochester, NY 14604
Phone: 716-274-1110
Fax: 716-274-1073
e-mail: agrn@mail.rochester.edu
Management:
Director Concert Operations: Andrew Green
Budget: $60,000-150,000
Performs At: Kilbourn Hall; Eastman Theatre

7466 FRONTIER FIELD
333 N Plymounth Avenue
Rochester, NY 14608
Phone: 716-262-2009
Fax: 716-232-3453
Management:
Director: Jim Lebeau
Seating Capacity: 10,500

7467 NAZARETH COLLEGE: NAZARETH ARTS CENTER
4245 E Avenue
Rochester, NY 14618
Phone: 716-586-2483

7468 PYRAMID ARTS CENTER
PO Box 30330
Rochester, NY 14603

Phone: 716-461-2222
Fax: 716-461-2223
e-mail: pyramid1@frontiernet.net
Web Site: www.pyramidarts.org
Management:
Executive Director: Elizabeth McDade

7469 UNIVERSITY OF ROCHESTER-RIVER CAMPUS: STRONG THEATRE
Rochester, NY 14627
Phone: 716-275-2330
Fax: 716-273-5306

7470 CAPITOL CIVIC CENTER
220 W Dominick Street
Rome, NY 13440
Phone: 315-337-6277
Fax: 315-337-6277

7471 RYE ARTS CENTER
51 Milton Road
Rye, NY 10580
Phone: 914-967-0700

7472 SARATOGA PERFORMING ARTS CENTER
Saratoga Spa State Park
Hall of Springs
Saratoga Springs, NY 12866
Phone: 518-584-9330
Fax: 518-584-0809
Web Site: www.spac.org
Officers:
Vice Chairman: Wallace A Graham
Chairman: Charles E Matter
President: Herbert A Chesbrough
Secretary/Treasurer: Edward P. Swyer
Vice Chairman: John Breyo
Mission: To host performing arts events.
Founded: 1966
Specialized Field: Dance; Vocal Music; Instrumental Music; Theater; Opera
Status: Professional; Nonprofit
Paid Staff: 11
Budget: $11 Million
Income Sources: International Association of Auditorium Managers; New York Performing Arts Association; Membership ticket sales
Affiliations: Summer home of New York City Ballet, Philadelphia Orchestra and Saratoga Chamber Music Festival
Annual Attendance: 350,000
Facility Category: Ampitheatre
Type of Stage: Proscenium
Stage Dimensions: 80 W x 60 D
Seating Capacity: 5100
Year Built: 1966
Organization Type: Performing; Educational; Sponsoring

7473 PROCTOR'S THEATRE
432 State Street
Schenectady, NY 12305

Phone: 518-382-3884
Fax: 518-346-2468
e-mail: info@proctors.org
Web Site: www.proctors.org

7474 SCHENECTADY CIVIC PLAYERS
12 S Church Street
Schenectady, NY 12305
Phone: 518-382-2081

7475 SUFFOLK COUNTY COMMUNITY COLLEGE: SHEA THEATRE
533 College Road
Selden, NY 11784
Phone: 631-451-4163
Fax: 631-451-4601
Management:
  Theatre Director: Charles Wittreich

7476 LONG ISLAND UNIVERSITY: FINE ARTS THEATRE
Southampton Campus
Montauk Highway
Southampton, NY 11968
Phone: 516-283-4000

7477 REILLY CENTER ARENA
St. Bonaventure University
PO Box BZ
St. Bonaventure, NY 14778
Phone: 716-375-2514
Fax: 716-375-3583
Management:
  Director: Steve Pleasec
Seating Capacity: 6,500

7478 CENTER FOR THE ARTS AT THE COLLEGE OF STATEN ISLAND
2800 Victory Boulevard
Building 1P-116
Staten Island, NY 10314
Phone: 718-982-2787
Fax: 718-982-2251
e-mail: boxoffice@postbox.csi.cuny.edu
Web Site: www.csi.cuny.edu/arts
Management:
  Manager/Artistic Director: Lisa Reilly
  Theatre Operations Manager: John Jankowski
  Contracts/Reservations: Rita Balsamo
  Contracts/Reservations: Dorothy Zarilla
  Marketing/Development: Barbara Caldwell
Mission: To bring artists and audiences together on Staten Island.
Founded: 1996
Paid Staff: 10
Budget: $850,000
Income Sources: Ticket sales; other earned revenue; grants and contributions
Affiliations: Association of Performing Arts Presenters, onsortium of Eastern Regional Theatres
Annual Attendance: 100,000
Facility Category: Performing Arts Center

Type of Stage: Theatre
Seating Capacity: 440
Year Built: 1996
Cost: $35 million
Resident Groups: Staten Island Symphony; Staten Island Ballet, NeverLand Theatre Company; Enrichment Through the Arts

7479 CENTER FOR THE ARTS AT THE COLLEGE OF STATEN ISLAND: LECTURE HALL
2800 Victory Boulevard
Building 1P-116
Staten Island, NY 10314
Phone: 718-982-2787
Fax: 718-982-2251
e-mail: boxoffice@postbox.csi.cuny.edu
Web Site: www.csi.cuny.edu/arts
Management:
  Manager/Artistic Director: Numa C Saisselin
  Theatre Operations Manager: Chris Van Alstyne
  Contracts/Reservations: Rita Balsamo
  Contracts/Reservations: Dorothy Zarilla
Mission: To bring artists and audiences together on Staten Island.
Founded: 1996
Paid Staff: 10
Budget: $850,000
Income Sources: Ticket sales; other earned revenue; grants and contributions
Affiliations: Association of Performing Arts Presenters, onsortium of Eastern Regional Theatres
Annual Attendance: 100,000
Facility Category: Performing Arts Center
Type of Stage: Lecture Hall
Seating Capacity: 150
Year Built: 1996
Cost: $35 million
Resident Groups: Staten Island Symphony; Staten Island Ballet, NeverLand Theatre Company; Enrichment Through the Arts

7480 CENTER FOR THE ARTS AT THE COLLEGE OF STATEN ISLAND: RECITAL HALL
2800 Victory Boulevard
Building 1P-116
Staten Island, NY 10314
Phone: 718-982-2787
Fax: 718-982-2251
e-mail: boxoffice@postbox.csi.cuny.edu
Web Site: www.csi.cuny.edu/arts
Management:
  Manager/Artistic Director: Numa C Saisselin
  Theatre Operations Manager: Chris Van Alstyne
  Contracts/Reservations: Rita Balsamo
  Contracts/Reservations: Dorothy Zarilla
Mission: To bring artists and audiences together on Staten Island.
Founded: 1996
Paid Staff: 10
Budget: $850,000
Income Sources: Ticket sales; other earned revenue; grants and contributions

Affiliations: Association of Performing Arts Presenters, onsortium of Eastern Regional Theatres
Annual Attendance: 100,000
Facility Category: Performing Arts Center
Type of Stage: Recital Hall
Seating Capacity: 150
Year Built: 1996
Cost: $35 million
Resident Groups: Staten Island Symphony; Staten Island Ballet, NeverLand Theatre Company; Enrichment Through the Arts

7481 SNUG HARBOR CULTURAL CENTER

1000 Richmond Terrace
Staten Island, NY 10301-1116
Phone: 718-448-2500
Fax: 718-442-8534
Management:
   Presentations Director: Ellen Kodadek
   Presentations Associate: Elizabeth LaCause
Budget: $60,000-150,000
Performs At: Veterans Memorial Hall; Performance Meadow; Cabaret

7482 VETERANS MEMORIAL HALL

1000 Richmond Terrace
Staten Island, NY 10301
Phone: 718-448-2500
Fax: 718-442-8534

7483 SPORTS COMPLEX

Stony Brook University
Stony Brook, NY 11794-3500
Phone: 516-632-7174
Fax: 516-632-7122
Management:
   Managing Director: Kay Don
Seating Capacity: 5,000

7484 CIVIC CENTER OF ONONDAGA COUNTY

411 Montgomery Street
Syracuse, NY 13202
Phone: 315-435-2121
Fax: 315-435-8099

7485 CIVIC CENTER OF ONONDAGA COUNTY: CARRIER THEATRE

411 Montgomery Street
Syracuse, NY 13202
Phone: 315-435-2121
Fax: 315-435-8099

7486 CIVIC CENTER OF ONONDAGA COUNTY: CROUSE-HIND HALL

411 Montgomery Street
Syracuse, NY 13202
Phone: 315-435-2121
Fax: 315-435-8099

7487 MULROY CIVIC CENTER AT ONCENTER

800 S State Street
Syracuse, NY 13202
Phone: 315-435-8000
Fax: 315-435-8099
e-mail: sales@oncenter.org
Web Site: www.oncenter.org
Officers:
   President/CEO: Jerry Gallagher
Founded: 1976
Specialized Field: Onondage County / Central New York
Status: Rental Houses / Not A Presentor
Paid Staff: 300
Volunteer Staff: 300
Paid Artists: 200
Non-paid Artists: 250

7488 P&C STADIUM

One Tex Simone Drive
Syracuse, NY 13208
Phone: 315-474-7833
Fax: 315-474-2658
e-mail: baseball@skychiefs.com
Web Site: www.skyshiefs.com
Management:
   Executive VP/COO: Tex Simone
   General Manager: John Simone
   Assistant General Manager: Tom Van Schaack
Founded: 1961
Specialized Field: Professional Baseball Club
Paid Staff: 12
Seating Capacity: 11,071

7489 SYRACUSE AREA LANDMARK THEATRE

362 S Salina Street
Syracuse, NY 13202
Phone: 315-475-7979
Fax: 315-473-7993

7490 SYRACUSE UNIVERSITY: CARRIER DOME

Syracuse University
900 Irving Avenue
Syracuse, NY 13244
Phone: 315-443-4634
Fax: 315-443-5203
e-mail: boxoffice@carrierdome.syr.edu
Web Site: carrierdome.syr.edu
Management:
   Managing Director: Patrick M Campbell
Seating Capacity: 50,000 Football, 32,000 Basketball
Year Built: 1980

7491 KNICKERBACKER RECREATIONAL FACILITY AND ICE ARENA

191 103rd Street
Troy, NY 12180
Phone: 518-235-7761
Fax: 518-235-0219
Web Site: www.troynet.net

Officers:
President: Bruce Arnold
VP: Steven Angle
Management:
Facility Manager: Irma A Magee
Mission: To provide the public with recreation and special events in a healthy atmosphere.
Founded: 1990
Specialized Field: Figure Skating, Speed Skaters, Hockey
Paid Staff: 10
Income Sources: City of Troy
Season: Year Round
Affiliations: City of Troy
Facility Category: Ice arena, baseball field, softball fields
Rental Contact: Facility Manager Irma Magee
Organization Type: Ice arena, baseball and softball fields, tennis courts, pool, basketball courts, 400 meter oval, out-door rink, street hockey suface, sand volleyball courts, children's playground
Resident Groups: Predominantly Figure Skaters

7492 RENSSELAER POLYTECHNIC INSTITUTE: HOUSTON FIELD HOUSE
1900 Peoples Avenue
Troy, NY 12180
Phone: 518-276-6262
Fax: 518-276-2833
Management:
Manager: Norris A Pearson
Box Office Manager: Dorthy Conroy
Supervisor: Brian Darby
Department Specialist: Kim M Forette
Seating Capacity: 6,900

7493 RENSSELAER NEWMAN FOUNDATION CHAPEL AND CULTURAL CENTER
2125 Burden Avenue
Troy, NY 12180
Phone: 518-274-7793

7494 TROY SAVINGS BANK MUSIC HALL
7 State Street
Troy, NY 12180-3920
Phone: 518-273-0038
Fax: 518-273-1564
e-mail: info@troymusichall.org
Web Site: www.troymusichall.org
Management:
Manager: Peter Clough

7495 NASSAU VETERANS MEMORIAL COLISEUM
SMG Facilities Management
1255 Hempstead Turnpike
Uniondale, NY 11553
Phone: 516-794-9303
Fax: 516-794-9389
e-mail: nassauco@aol.com
Web Site: www.nassaucoliseum.com
Management:
General Manager: David Reuss
Seating Capacity: 16,285

7496 STANLEY PERFORMING ARTS CENTER
259 Genesee Street
Utica, NY 13501
Phone: 315-724-5919
Fax: 315-724-3854

7497 UTICA MEMORIAL AUDITORIUM
400 Oriskany Street W
Utica, NY 13502
Phone: 315-738-0164
Fax: 315-738-9597
e-mail: UticaAud@aol.com
Management:
General Manager: Will Berkeiser
Arena Administrator: Betsy Woish
Director Operations: Frank LaBella
Paid Staff: 79
Facility Category: Arena
Type of Stage: Wenger
Stage Dimensions: 56x44
Year Built: 1959
Rental Contact: Will Berkheiser/Gen.Mgr.

7498 EUGENE O'NEILL THEATER CENTER
305 Great Neck Road
Waterford, NY 06385
Phone: 860-443-5378
Fax: 860-443-9653
Management:
Executive Director: Howard Sherman

7499 JEFFERSON COMMUNITY COLLEGE
Jefferson Community College
Watertown, NY 13601
Phone: 315-786-2289
Fax: 315-788-0716
Web Site: www.sunyjefferson.edu
Management:
Ass't Student Activities Director: Mary Kinne
Budget: $35,000-60,000
Performs At: McVean Student Center Theater

7500 US MILITARY ACADEMY: EISENHOWER HALL THEATRE
655 Ruger Road
West Point, NY 10996-1593
Phone: 845-938-2782
Fax: 845-446-5302
e-mail: vw0304@exmail.usma.edu
Web Site: www.eisenhowerhall.com
Management:
Cultural Arts Director: William A Yost
Budget: $400,000-1,000,000
Seating Capacity: 4,400

7501 US MILITARY ACADEMY: MISHIE STADIUM
United States Military Academy
Michie Stadium Odia Building 639, Usma
West Point, NY 10996

Phone: 914-938-3002
Fax: 914-938-2210
Web Site: www.usma.com
Management:
    Director: Ben Russell
Seating Capacity: 41,000

7502 KLEINERT/JAMES ARTS CENTER

34 Tinker Street
Woodstock, NY 12498
Phone: 845-679-2079
Fax: 845-679-4529
e-mail: wguild@ulster.net
Web Site: www.woodstockguild.org
Management:
    Executive Director: Carla T Smith
Founded: 1957
Paid Staff: 5
Budget: $25,000
Income Sources: Concerts; Rentals
Annual Attendance: 1,500
Facility Category: Indoor
Seating Capacity: 135
Year Built: 1957
Year Remodeled: 1994
Rental Contact: Carla Smith

7503 MAVERICK CONCERT HALL

PO Box 102
Woodstock, NY 12498
Phone: 845-679-8217

7504 HUDSON RIVER MUSEUM

511 Warburton Avenue
Yonkers, NY 10701-1899
Phone: 914-963-4550
Fax: 914-963-8558
Web Site: www.hrm.org
Management:
    Director: Michael Botwinick
    Curator Public Programs: Barbara Davis
Founded: 1919
Paid Staff: 55
Volunteer Staff: 100
Paid Artists: 200
Season: Seasonal

North Carolina

7505 STANLY COUNTY AGRI-CIVIC CENTER

26032-B Newt Road
Albemarle, NC 28001
Phone: 704-986-3666
Fax: 704-986-3817
e-mail: tharris@co.stanly.nc.us
Web Site: www.stanlyciviccenter.com
Management:
    Director: Tim K Harris
Specialized Field: Music; Theater; Dance; Meetings
Paid Staff: 5
Performs At: Performing Arts Theatre
Facility Category: Performing Arts Theatre

Type of Stage: Pine
Stage Dimensions: 53 x 38
Seating Capacity: 1200
Year Built: 1988
Rental Contact: Tim Harris

7506 ASHEVILLE CIVIC CENTER

87 Haywood Street
Asheville, NC 28801
Phone: 828-259-5736
Fax: 828-259-5777
e-mail: DavidP@mail.ci.asheville.nc.us
Web Site: www.ci.ashville.mc.us/ashville/civic.intern
Management:
    Director: David Pisha

7507 LEES MCRAE COLLEGE: HAYES AUDITORIUM

Main Street
Banner Elk, NC 28604
Phone: 828-898-5241
Fax: 704-898-8711

7508 APPALACHIAN STATE U DEPARTMENT OF ATHLETICS: KIDD BREWER STADIUM

Appalachian State U Department of Athletics
Boone, NC 28608
Phone: 828-262-4010
Fax: 828-651-2556
Management:
    Director: Roachel Laney
Seating Capacity: 18,000

7509 FARTHING AUDITORIUM

Rivers Street
ASU
Boone, NC 28608
Phone: 704-262-6372
Fax: 704-262-2848

7510 BREVARD MUSIC CENTER: STRAUS AUDITORIUM

Probart Street
PO Box 592
Brevard, NC 28712
Phone: 704-884-2011
Fax: 704-884-2036

7511 BREVARD MUSIC CENTER: WHITTINGTON-PFOHL AUDITORIUM

Probart Street
PO Box 592
Brevard, NC 28712
Phone: 704-884-2011
Fax: 704-884-2036

7512 PORTER CENTER FOR PERFORMING ARTS

400 N Broad Street
Brevard, NC 28712

Phone: 828-884-8330
Fax: 828-884-8353
e-mail: ccalabrese@brevard.edu
Web Site: www.brevard.edu/portercenter
Management:
    Concerts Division: Lynn Wood Bertrand
    Managaing Director: Cynthia Calabrese
Budget: $20,000-35,000
Performs At: The Concert Hall; Porter Center for
Performing Arts

7513 CAMP THEATER
Building 19
Camp Lejeune, NC 28542
Phone: 919-451-1759
Fax: 919-451-1879

7514 TOWN OF CARY CULTURAL ARTS DIVISION
PO Box 8005
Cary, NC 27512-8005
Phone: 919-469-4061
Fax: 919-469-4344
e-mail: lcollins@ci.cary.nc.us
Web Site: www.townofcary.org
Management:
    Cultural Arts Supervisor: Lyman Collins
    Cultural Arts Program Coordinator: Joy Cox
Mission: Present high quality cultural arts events musical
and theatrical in the Town of Cary.
Founded: 1994
Specialized Field: Music, Classical, Jazz, Pop
Paid Staff: 6

7515 UNIVERSITY OF NORTH CAROLINA: DEANE E SMITH CENTER
Chapel Hill
Chapel Hill, NC 27515
Phone: 919-962-7777
Fax: 919-966-3173
Web Site: www.smithcenter.unc.edu
Management:
    Managing Director: Angelyn S Bitting

7516 UNIVERSITY OF NORTH CAROLINA: KENAN STADIUM
Carolina Football
PO Box 2126
Chapel Hill, NC 27515-2126
Phone: 919-966-2575
Fax: 919-962-0393
Web Site: www.tarheelblue.com
Management:
    Athletic Director Game Operations: William Scroggs
    Associate Athletic Director: Bob Savod
    Ticket Manager: Darren Lucas
Specialized Field: Home of University of North Carolina
football (NCAA)
Seating Capacity: 60,000
Year Built: 1927
Year Remodeled: 1997

7517 AFRO-AMERICAN CULTURAL CENTER
401 N Myers Street
Charlotte, NC 28202-2910
Phone: 704-374-1565
Fax: 704-374-9273
Web Site: www.aacc-charlotte.org
Officers:
    President: Michael Vaughn
    VP: Angeline Clinton
    Second VP: Dee Merrill
    Treasurer: Chris Carter
Management:
    Executive Director: John Moore
    Director External Affairs: June Saunders Grayson
    Director Performing Arts Programs: Sidney Horton
    Director Development: Alecia Bracy
Mission: To preserve, promote and present
African-American art, history and culture.
Founded: 1976
Specialized Field: Multi-disciplinary
Paid Staff: 6
Paid Artists: 50
Budget: $35,000-60,000

7518 BELK THEATER
345 N College Street
Charlotte, NC 28202
Phone: 704-348-5793
Fax: 704-348-5794

7519 CENTRAL PIEDMONT COMMUNITY COLLEGE: SUMMER THEATRE
Box 35009
Charlotte, NC 28235
Phone: 704-330-6016

7520 CHARLOTTE COLISEUM
100 Paul Buck Boulevard
Charlotte, NC 28266-9247
Phone: 704-357-4701
Fax: 704-357-4757
e-mail: sjeralds@charlottecoliseum.com
Web Site: www.charlottecoliseum.com
Management:
    Managing Director: Michael E Crum
    Director Marketing: Ereka Crawford
Mission: Home of the Charlotte Hornets and the Charlotte
Sting. Also hosts family shows, motorsports and concert
events.
Seating Capacity: 23,698

7521 CRICKET ARENA
2700 E Independent Boulevard
Charlotte, NC 28205
Phone: 704-372-3600
Fax: 704-335-3118
Web Site: cricketarenacharlotte.com
Management:
    Managing Director: Michael E Crum
    Cricket Arena Manager: George Height
    Director Marketing: Ereka Cranford
Founded: 1955

7522 ERICSSON STADIUM
Carolinas Stadium Corporation
800 S Mint Street
Charlotte, NC 28202
Phone: 704-358-7407
Fax: 704-358-7619
e-mail: pauls@panthers.nfl.com
Web Site: www.panthers.com
Management:
    President Carolinas Stadium Corp: Jon Richardson
    Stadium Operations Mamager: Scott Pul
    Director Tickets: Phil Youtsey
Specialized Field: Home of the Carolina Panthers (NFL).
Seating Capacity: 73,250
Year Built: 1996

7523 NORTH CAROLINA BLUMENTHAL PERFORMING ARTS CENTER
130 N Tryon Street
Founders Hall, 2nd Floor
Charlotte, NC 28202
Phone: 704-379-1279
Fax: 704-444-2111
e-mail: Jallen@ncbpac.org
Web Site: www.performingartsctr.org
Officers:
    President: Judith Allen

7524 OVENS AUDITORIUM
2700 E Independence Boulevard
Charlotte, NC 28205
Phone: 704-372-3600
Fax: 704-372-3620

7525 SPIRIT SQUARE CENTER FOR THE ARTS
345 N College Street
Charlotte, NC 28202
Phone: 704-372-1000
Fax: 704-377-9808

7526 RAMSEY REGIONAL ACTIVITY CENTER
Western Carolina University
Cullowhee, NC 28723
Phone: 828-227-7677
Fax: 828-227-7680
e-mail: clarke@emcit.wcu.edu
Web Site: www.ramsey.wcu.edu
Management:
    Director of University Events: Bill Clarke
    Operations Manager: Jim Irvin
    Ticket Office Manager: Laura Sellers
Founded: 1986
Budget: $35,000-60,000
Annual Attendance: 100,000
Facility Category: Multipurpose
Seating Capacity: 8000
Year Built: 1986

7527 ST. JOSEPH'S HISTORIC FOUNDATION/HAYTI HERITAGE CENTER
804 Old Fayetteville Street
Durham, NC 27701
Mailing Address: PO Box 543, Durham, NC. 27702
Phone: 919-683-1709
Fax: 919-682-5869
e-mail: hayti@hayti.org
Web Site: www.hayti.org
Officers:
    President/CEO: V Dianne Pledger
    Programs Director: Darrell Stover
Founded: 1975
Budget: 1.2 Million
Seating Capacity: 450

7528 CUMBERLAND COUNTY COLISEUM COMPLEX
1960 Coliseum Drive
PO Drawer 64549
Fayetteville, NC 28306
Phone: 910-323-5088
Fax: 919-323-0489
e-mail: comments@crowncoliseum.com
Web Site: www.fayetville.com/cccc
Management:
    President/General Manager: Kendall B Wall
    Director Sales: Patricia Fields
Seating Capacity: 13,500
Year Built: 1997

7529 AYCOCK AUDITORIUM
University of North Carolina at Greensboro
Greensboro, NC 27412
Phone: 919-334-5800
Fax: 919-334-3008

7530 CAROLINA THEATRE
310 S Greene Street
Greensboro, NC 27401
Phone: 336-333-2600
Fax: 336-333-2604
e-mail: comments@carolinatheatre.com
Web Site: www.carolinatheatre.com
Management:
    Executive Director: Brian Gray

7531 GREENSBORO COLISEUM COMPLEX
1921 W Lee Street
PO Box 5447
Greensboro, NC 27403
Phone: 336-373-7400
Fax: 336-373-2170
e-mail: scott.johnson@ci.greensboro.nc.us
Web Site: www.greenborocoliseum.com
Management:
    Director Booking/Event Service: Scott E Johnson
    Booking Assistant: Robin Welborn
Founded: 1959
Specialized Field: Greensboro/High Point/Winston-Salem
Seating Capacity: 23,500

Year Built: 1959
Year Remodeled: 1994

7532 GREENSBORO COLISEUM: WAR MEMORIAL AUDITORIUM
1921 W Lee Street
PO Box 5447
Greensboro, NC 27403
Phone: 336-373-7400
Fax: 336-373-2170
Web Site: www,greensborocoliseum.com

7533 HENDRIX THEATRE
Mendenhall Student Center
Greenville, NC 27858
Phone: 919-757-4702
Fax: 919-757-4778

7534 WRIGHT AUDITORIUM
E Carolina University
Campus Circle
Greenville, NC 27858
Phone: 919-757-6269
Fax: 919-757-4778

7535 LENOIR - RHYNE COLLEGE FACILITIES
7th Avenue and 8th NE
Hickory, NC 28601
Phone: 828-328-7254
Fax: 828-328-7329
e-mail: helpdesk@lrc.edu
Web Site: www.irc.edu
Management:
    Director: Caroline Cauthen
    Athletic Facilities Coordinator: Joe Fisher
Seating Capacity: 3,000

7536 HIGH POINT THEATRE AND EXHIBITION CENTER
220 E Commerce Street
High Point, NC 27260
Phone: 336-883-3401
Fax: 336-883-3533
Web Site: www.ci.high-point.nc.us
Annual Attendance: 60,000+
Facility Category: Theatre and Exhibition Center
Seating Capacity: 967
Year Built: 1975
Rental Contact: Louisa Hart

7537 HIGHLANDS PLAYHOUSE
PO Box 896
Highlands, NC 28741
Phone: 828-526-9443
Season: June - August

7538 GRAINER STADIUM
400 E Grainer Avenue
Kinston, NC 28501

Phone: 252-527-9111
Fax: 919-527-2328
Web Site: www.kinstinindians.com
Management:
    Director/Manager: North Johnson

7539 CALDWELL COMMUNITY COLLEGE: JE BROYHILL CIVIC CENTER
1913 Hickory Boulevard SE
PO Box 600
Lenoir, NC 28645
Phone: 828-726-2401
Fax: 828-726-2405
e-mail: dbriggs@caldwell.cc.nc.us
Web Site: www.broyhillcenter.com
Management:
    Director: David Briggs
    Program Assistant: Cheryl Bolt
    Technical Director: Jeff Bentley
Founded: 1993
Paid Staff: 7
Budget: $350,000
Income Sources: Tickets, local and state support, sponsors and advertising.
Annual Attendance: 80,000
Facility Category: Performing Arts/ Meeting Center
Type of Stage: Procenium
Stage Dimensions: 42W X 45D X 22H
Seating Capacity: 999
Year Built: 1993
Cost: 6.1 million
Rental Contact: Jean Rondeau

7540 LINCOLN CULTURAL CENTER
403 E Main Street
Lincolnton, NC 28092
Phone: 704-732-9055
Fax: 704-732-9057
e-mail: lcc@vnet.net
Management:
    Director: Lyle Back

7541 MOORE AUDITORIUM
Mars Hill College
Marshall Highway
Mars Hill, NC 28754
Phone: 704-689-1260
Fax: 704-689-1474

7542 CITY OF MORGANTON MUNICIPAL AUDITORIUM
401 S College Street
PO Box 3448
Morganton, NC 28680
Phone: 828-438-5294
Fax: 828-438-5246
e-mail: wilsonbcomma@hci.net
Web Site: www.ci.morganton.nc.us
Management:
    Director: John W Wilson, III

**7543 MOUNT AIRY FINE ARTS CENTER
ANDY GRIFFITH PLAYHOUSE**
218 Rockford Street
Mount Airy, NC 27030
Phone: 336-786-7998
Fax: 919-986-9822

**7544 CHOWAN COLLEGE: MCDOWELL
COLUMNS AUDITORIUM**
Jones Drive
Murfreesboro, NC 27855
Phone: 919-398-4101
Fax: 919-398-1190

**7545 UNIVERSITY OF NORTH CAROLINA AT
PEMBROKE: GIVENS PERFORMING
ARTS CENTER**
PO Box 1510
Pembroke, NC 28372-1510
Phone: 910-521-6287
Fax: 910-521-6552
e-mail: thaggard@sassette.uncp.edu
Web Site: www.uncp.edu/gpac
Management:
Director: David P Thaggard

**7546 BTI CENTER FOR THE PERFORMING
ARTS: AJ FLETCHER OPERA THEATER**
2 S Street
500 Payette Street Mall
Raleigh, NC 27601
Phone: 919-831-6011
Fax: 919-831-6013
e-mail: hollyj@raleighconvention.com
Web Site: www.raleighconvention.com

**7547 BTI CENTER FOR THE PERFORMING
ARTS: MEYMANDI CONCERT HALL**
500 Fayetteville Street Mall
Raleigh, NC 27601
Phone: 919-831-6011
Fax: 919-831-6013
e-mail: hollyj@raleighconvention.com
Web Site: www.raleighconvention.com

7548 JS DORTIN ARENA
1025 Blue Ridge Boulevard
Raleigh, NC 27607
Phone: 919-733-2626
Fax: 919-733-5079
Web Site: www.arg.state.nc.us/fair
Management:
Manager: Wesley Rowley

7549 NCSU CENTER STAGE
Campus Box 7306
Raleigh, NC 27695-7306
Phone: 919-515-3030
Fax: 919-515-1406
e-mail: sharon_moore@ncsu.edu
Web Site: www.ncsu.edu/arts

Management:
Director: Sharon Moore

7550 NORTH CAROLINA MUSEUM OF ART
2110 Blue Ridge Road
Raleigh, NC 27607
Mailing Address: 4630 Mail Service Center, Raleigh,
NC. 27699-4630
Phone: 919-839-6262
Fax: 919-733-2309
e-mail: gholt@ncmamail.dcr.state.nc.us
Web Site: www.ncartmuseum.org
Management:
Public Programs Director: George Holt
Production Manager: Suzanne Gorden
Founded: 1997
Specialized Field: Raleigh/Durham, NC.
Paid Staff: 2
Volunteer Staff: 50
Paid Artists: 40
Budget: $275,000
Income Sources: Ticket; Sponsorships
Performs At: Outdoor Theatre
Affiliations: NC Museum of Art
Annual Attendance: 40,000+
Facility Category: Outdoor Theatre/cinema
Type of Stage: Open Air/Concert
Seating Capacity: $3,000
Year Built: 1997
Cost: 3,000,000

**7551 NORTH CAROLINA STATE
UNIVERSITY: CARTER FINLEY
STADIUM**
103 Dunn Avenue
Raleigh, NC 27695
Phone: 919-515-3050
Fax: 919-515-1161
Web Site: www.athletics.ncsu.edu

**7552 NORTH CAROLINA STATE
UNIVERSITY CENTER STAGE**
Campus Box 7306
Raleigh, NC 27695-7306
Phone: 919-513-3030
Fax: 919-515-1406
e-mail: sharon_moore@ncsu.edu
Web Site: www.ncsu.edu/arts
Management:
NCSU Center Stage Director: Sharon Herr Moore
Specialized Field: Multi-disciplinary
Budget: $60,000-150,000
Income Sources: Student fees, Ticket sales, Grants
Performs At: Stewart Theatre; Thompson Theatre
Annual Attendance: 8,500
Facility Category: Theatre
Type of Stage: Thrust
Stage Dimensions: 40'
Seating Capacity: 802
Year Built: 1972

All listings are in alphabetical order by state, then city, then organization within the city.

7553 NORTH CAROLINA STATE UNIVERSITY: REYNOLDS COLISEUM
103 Dunn Avenue
Raleigh, NC 27695
Phone: 919-515-3050
Fax: 919-515-1161
e-mail: les_robinson@ncsu.edu
Web Site: www.ecsu.edu
Management:
    Athletic Director: Les Robinson
Seating Capacity: 11,400

7554 RALEIGH CIVIC CENTER COMPLEX
500 Fayetteville Street Mall
Raleigh, NC 27601
Phone: 919-831-6011
Fax: 919-831-6013
Management:
    Executive Director: Roger Krupa
    Marketing/Promotions Director: James G Lavery
Seating Capacity: 3,800

7555 RALEIGH ENTERTAINMENT & SPORTS ARENA
1400 Edward Mill Road
Raleigh, NC 27607
Phone: 919-467-7825
Fax: 919-462-7030
Toll-free: 888-645-8494
Web Site: www.caneshockey.com
Management:
    VP Arena Management: Sims Hinds
Seating Capacity: 19,000

7556 RALEIGH LITTLE THEATRE
301 Pogue Street
PO Box 5637
Raleigh, NC 27650
Phone: 919-821-4579
Fax: 919-821-7961
e-mail: rallittletheatre@mindspring.com
Web Site: www.raleighlittletheatre.com
Management:
    Office Manager: Sarah Corrie
Mission: A community theatre that enriches, educates and entertains our community.
Founded: 1936
Specialized Field: Performing Arts - Theatre
Paid Staff: 14
Volunteer Staff: 200
Paid Artists: 50
Non-paid Artists: 300

7557 THEATRE IN THE PARK
107 Pullen Road
Raleigh, NC 27605
Phone: 919-831-6936
Fax: 919-831-9475
Web Site: tip.dreamhost.com/davidwood/davidpage.htm

7558 CATAWBA COLLEGE: COLLEGE COMMUNITY CENTER
2300 W Inves Street
Salisbury, NC 28144
Phone: 704-637-4200
Fax: 704-637-4211
Toll-free: 800-228-2922
e-mail: ccurrent@catawba.edu
Web Site: www.catawba.edu
Founded: 1851
Paid Staff: 5
Annual Attendance: 20,000+
Facility Category: Theatre
Type of Stage: Proscenium
Stage Dimensions: 48'x35'
Seating Capacity: 1,451
Year Built: 1963
Year Remodeled: 1998
Rental Contact: Clark Current

7559 TEMPLE THEATRE COMPANY
PO Box 1391
120 Carthage Street
Sanford, NC 27331-1391
Phone: 919-774-4512
Fax: 919-774-7531
Toll-free: 800-752-2765
Web Site: www.transoftinc.com/temple/frmain.htm

7560 ISOTHERMAL COMMUNITY COLLEGE PERFORMING ARTS CENTER
PO Box 804
286 ICC Loop Road
Spindale, NC 28160
Phone: 828-286-3636
Fax: 828-287-8090
e-mail: pacc@isothermal.cc.nc.us
Management:
    Director: Russell J Wicker

7561 TRYON FINE ARTS CENTER
208 Melrose Avenue
Tryon, NC 28782
Phone: 828-859-8322

7562 WALKER EVENTS
PO Box 120
Wilkesboro, NC 28697-0120
Phone: 336-838-6133
Fax: 336-838-6277
e-mail: grayk@wikes.cc.nc.us
Web Site: wilkes.cc.nc.us
Officers:
    President: Arnold Lakey
Management:
    Special Projects Coordinator: Kathy T Gray
Mission: To provide an entertainment facility, and banquet & meeting facility.
Founded: 1985
Specialized Field: Dance; Vocal Music; Instrumental Music; Theater; Festivals
Status: Nonprofit
Budget: $150,000-400,000

Income Sources: Association of Performing Arts Presenters; North Carolina Arts Council
Performs At: John A. Walker Community Center
Organization Type: Performing; Touring; Resident; Educational; Sponsoring

7563 LEGION STADIUM
PO Box 1810
Wilmington, NC 28402
Phone: 910-341-7855
Fax: 910-341-7854
Management:
   Manager: Gary Shell
Seating Capacity: 6,500

7564 THALIAN HALL CENTER FOR THE PERFORMING ARTS
PO Box 371
310 Chestnut Street
Wilmington, NC 28402
Phone: 910-343-3660
Fax: 910-343-3662
e-mail: rivenbark@thalianhall.com
Web Site: www.thalianhall.com
Management:
   Executive Director: Tony Rivenbark

7565 WAKE FOREST UNIVERSITY: GROVES STADIUM
499 Deacon Boulevard
Winston- Salem, NC 27105
Phone: 336-759-5000
Fax: 336-759-6090
e-mail: wellman@wfu.edu
Management:
   Athletic Director: Ron Wellman

7566 BOWMAN GRAY STADIUM
Coliseum Complex
Winston-Salem, NC 27102
Phone: 336-723-4267
Fax: 336-727-2922
e-mail: cwebster@ljum.com
Web Site: www.wjum.com
Management:
   Coliseum Director: Benjamin B Dame
Founded: 1937
Performs At: Football; Racing
Seating Capacity: 17,000

7567 LAWRENCE JOEL VETERANS MEMORIAL COLISEUM
Coliseum Complex
2825 University Parkway
Winston-Salem, NC 27105
Phone: 336-727-5635
Fax: 336-727-2922
e-mail: info@wscvb.com
Web Site: www.ljvm.com
Management:
   Coliseum Director: Benjamin B Dame
   Coliseum Operations Supervisor: Charlie R Vestal

Booking/Marketinng Director: Brian A Scott
Seating Capacity: 15,290

7568 NORTH CAROLINA SCHOOL OF THE ARTS - ROGER
405 W 4th Street
Winston-Salem, NC 27101
Phone: 336-723-6320
Fax: 336-722-7240
Web Site: www.ncarts.edu/stevens_center
Annual Attendance: 175,000
Facility Category: Theatre
Seating Capacity: 1,380
Year Built: 1979
Year Remodeled: 1983
Rental Contact: Scott Spencer

7569 REYNOLDS MEMORIAL AUDITORIUM
301 N Hawthorne Road
Winston-Salem, NC 27104
Phone: 336-727-2061
Fax: 336-727-2053

7570 WINSTON-SALEM STATE UNIVERSITY
601 Martin Luther King Jr Drive
PO Box 19402
Winston-Salem, NC 27110
Phone: 336-750-3350
Fax: 336-750-3355
e-mail: cumbow@wssumits.wssu.edu
Management:
   Thompson Center Director: Willie A Cumbo
Budget: $20,000-35,000
Performs At: K.R. Williams Auditorium

7571 WINSTON-SALEM UNIVERSITY: CE GAINES COMPLEX
Winston-Salem State University
601 Martin Luther King Drive
CB 19529
Winston-Salem, NC 27110
Phone: 336-750-2000
Fax: 336-750-2144
Web Site: www.wssu.edu
Management:
   Athletic Director: Anne Little

7572 CASWELL COUNTY CIVIC CENTER
Intersection of Highway 158 & Highway 62
PO Box 609
Yanceyville, NC 27379
Phone: 910-694-4591
Fax: 910-694-5675

North Dakota

7573 BISMARCK CIVIC CENTER: ARENA
201 N 6th Street
PO Box 1075
Bismarck, ND 58502

Phone: 701-222-6487
Fax: 701-222-6599
e-mail: dpelton@state.nd.us
Web Site: www.bismarckciviccenter.com
Management:
   General Manager: Richard Petersen
   Marketing Director: Ross Horner
   Operations Director: Ron Staiger
Facility Category: Arena
Type of Stage: portable slogerignt
Stage Dimensions: various
Seating Capacity: 9,000
Year Built: 1969
Year Remodeled: 1999
Cost: $10 million

7574 BISMARCK CIVIC CENTER: CITY AUDITORIUM

201 N 6th Street
Bismarck, ND 58502
Phone: 701-222-6487
Fax: 701-222-6599
e-mail: dpelton@state.nd.us
Web Site: www.bismarckciviccenter.com
Management:
   Events Coordinator: Darla Pelton
Facility Category: Theatre
Type of Stage: sprung/wood
Seating Capacity: 600
Year Built: 1929
Year Remodeled: 1990

7575 BISMARK CIVIC CENTER

601 E Sweet Avenue
PO Box 1075
Bismark, ND 58504-1075
Phone: 701-222-6487
Fax: 701-222-6599
e-mail: bccdp@btigate.com
Web Site: www.bismarckciviccenter.com
Management:
   General Manager: Richard L Petersen
   Marketing Director: Ross Horner
Founded: 1969
Paid Staff: 20

7576 FARGODOME

1800 N University Drive
Fargo, ND 58102
Phone: 701-241-9100
Fax: 701-237-0987
Web Site: www.fargodome.com
Management:
   Executive Director: Paul A Johnson

7577 UNIVERSITY OF NORTH DAKOTA: FESTIVAL CONCERT HALL

1241 N University Drive
Fargo, ND 58105
Phone: 701-231-8011
Fax: 701-237-8043

7578 HYSLOP SPORTS CENTER

University Sports Center
PO Box 9013
Grand Forks, ND 58202
Phone: 701-777-2234
Fax: 701-777-4352
Web Site: www.und.nodak.edu/dept/athletics/
Management:
   Director: Roger Thomas

7579 UNIVERSITY OF NORTH DAKOTA: CHESTER FRITZ AUDITORIUM

PO Box 9028
University Station
Grand Forks, ND 58202-9028
Phone: 701-777-3076
Fax: 701-777-4710
Web Site: www.cfa.und.edu
Management:
   Director: Wallace Bloom
   Events: Betty Allan
   Box Office Manager: Tom Swanglier
   Technical Director: Patrick Hill
Founded: 1972

7580 UNIVERSITY OF NORTH DAKOTA

Columbia Road and Second Avenue
Grand Forks, ND 58202
Phone: 701-777-2236
Fax: 701-777-4352
Web Site: www.und.edu
Management:
   Athletic Director: Roger Thomas
Seating Capacity: 10,000

7581 JAMESTOWN CIVIC CENTER

212 3rd Avenue NE
PO Box 389
Jamestown, ND 58402
Phone: 701-252-8088
Fax: 701-252-8089
e-mail: jmstnd@daktel.com
Web Site: www.jamestown.com
Management:
   Manager: Charlie Jeske
   Marketing/Sales Manager: Fred Walker
Seating Capacity: 5,500
Year Built: 1973

Ohio

7582 AKRON CIVIC THEATRE

182 S Main Street
Akron, OH 44308
Phone: 216-535-3179

7583 EJ THOMAS PERFORMING ARTS HALL

University Avenue and Hill Streets
The University of Akron
Akron, OH 44325

Phone: 330-972-7595
Fax: 216-972-6571

7584 JAMES A RHODES ARENA
University of Akron
373 Carrol Street, MH69
Akron, OH 44325-5104
Phone: 330-972-6849
Fax: 330-972-5847
e-mail: athfac@uakron.edu
Web Site: www.gozips.com
Management:
Assistant Athletic: Riku Chung

7585 UNIVERSITY OF AKRON: AKRON RUBBER BOWL
800 George Washington Boulevard
Akron, OH 44312
Phone: 330-972-6849
Fax: 330-972-5847
e-mail: athfac@uakron.edu
Web Site: www.gozips.com
Management:
Assistant Athletic: Paul Hammond
Founded: 1941
Budget: $250,000

7586 ASHTABULA ARTS CENTER
2928 W 13th Street
Ashtabula, OH 44004
Phone: 440-964-3396
Management:
Music Coordinator: Lyn Savarise

7587 DAIRY BARN CULTURAL ARTS CENTER
8000 Dairy Lane
PO Box 747
Athens, OH 45701-0747
Phone: 740-592-4981
Fax: 740-592-5090
e-mail: info@dairybarn.org
Web Site: www.dairybarn.org
Management:
Executive Director: Krista Campbell
Program Director: Julie Clark
Education Director: Lisa Quinn
Mission: To present the arts, crafts, and cultural heritage of Southeast Ohio. The Dairy Barn achieves its mission through offering programs that are creative, unique, high quality, educational and family oriented.
Founded: 1978
Specialized Field: Arts, crafts and cultural
Paid Staff: 6
Paid Artists: 24
Budget: $320,000
Income Sources: Grants, membership, private donations
Annual Attendance: 15,000
Facility Category: Cultural Arts Center
Type of Stage: wood/rented
Seating Capacity: 200
Year Built: 1914
Year Remodeled: 2000

Rental Contact: Mark Rice

7588 OHIO UNIVERSITY: PATIO THEATER
307 Kantner Hall
School of Theater
Athens, OH 45701
Phone: 740-593-2845

7589 OHIO UNIVERSITY: SCHOOL OF MUSIC
Athens, OH 45701
Phone: 740-593-2845

7590 MAGICAL THEATRE COMPANY
565 W Tuscarawas Avenue
Barberton, OH 44203
Phone: 216-848-3708

7591 UC CLERMONT COLLEGE: CALICO THEATRE
4200 Clermont College Drive
Batavia, OH 45103
Phone: 513-732-5281
Fax: 513-732-5329
e-mail: communityarts@uc.edu
Web Site: www.ucclermont.com
Management:
Community Arts Coordinator: Summer Tyler
Specialized Field: Children's and Family Entertainment; Musical; Theatre; Dance
Paid Staff: 1
Income Sources: Grants; Ticket Sales
Facility Category: Auditorium
Type of Stage: procenium
Stage Dimensions: 20x30
Seating Capacity: 400
Rental Contact: Katie Turning

7592 HUNTINGTON PLAYHOUSE
28601 Lake Road
Bay Village, OH 44140
Phone: 440-871-8333
Fax: 216-221-9495
e-mail: huntingtonplayhouse@huntingtonplauhouse.com
Web Site: www.huntingtonplayhouse.com
Management:
Managing Director: Tom Meyrose

7593 BALDWIN WALLACE COLLEGE: KULAS MUSICAL ARTS
96 Front Street
Berea, OH 44017
Phone: 440-826-2369
Fax: 440-826-3239
Toll-free: 866-296-2148
e-mail: thecon@bw.edu
Web Site: www.bw.edu/con
Management:
Director/Conservatory Music: Catherine Jarjisian
Assistan Director/Conserv of Music: Nanette Canfield
Outreach Director/Conserv of Music: Bryan Bowser

Mission: To educate and train undergraduate musicians.
Founded: 1899
Specialized Field: Music
Paid Staff: 4
Performs At: Recital Hall
Affiliations: United Methodist Church
Facility Category: Conservatory of Music
Type of Stage: Concert
Stage Dimensions: 35x41
Seating Capacity: 650
Year Built: 1913
Year Remodeled: 1988
Rental Contact: Ellen Hansen-Ellis

7594 BOWLING GREEN STATE UNIVERSITY: ANDERSON ARENA

Bowling Green State University
BGSU Athletic Department
Bowling Green, OH 43403
Phone: 419-372-2401
Fax: 419-372-6015
Web Site: www.bgsu.edu
Management:
   Athletic Director: Paul Krebs

7595 BOWLING GREEN STATE UNIVERSITY: DOYT L PERRY FIELD

Bowling Green University
Bowling Green, OH 43403
Phone: 419-372-2401
Fax: 419-372-6015
Web Site: www.bgsu.edu/athletics
Management:
   Athletic Director: Paul Krebs

7596 BRECKSVILLE LITTLE THEATRE

49 Public Square
Brecksville, OH 44141
Phone: 216-526-4477

7597 CANTON MEMORIAL CIVIC CENTER

1101 Market Avenue N
Canton, OH 44702
Phone: 330-489-3090
Fax: 330-471-8840
Management:
   Manager: Robert D Patt
Seating Capacity: 4500

7598 PLAYERS GUILD OF CANTON

1001 North Market Street
Canton, OH 44702
Phone: 216-453-7619

7599 ARTS CONSORTIUM STUDIO THEATRE

1515 Linn Street
Cincinnati, OH 45214
Phone: 513-381-0645
Fax: 513-345-3743

7600 CINCINNATI JEWISH COMMUNITY CENTER

1580 Summit Road
Cincinnati, OH 45237
Phone: 513-761-7500
Fax: 513-761-0084

7601 CINCINNATI MUSIC HALL ASSOCIATION

1243 Elm Street
Cincinnati, OH 45210
Phone: 513-621-1919
Fax: 513-744-3345
Mission: To maintain a performance and concert hall.
Organization Type: Performing; Touring; Resident; Educational

7602 CINCINNATI PLAYHOUSE: ROBERT S MARX THEATRE

962 Mount Adams Circle
Eden Park
Cincinnati, OH 45202
Phone: 513-345-2242
Fax: 513-345-2254

7603 CINCINNATI PLAYHOUSE: THOMPSON SHELTERHOUSE

962 Mount Adams Circle
Eden Park
Cincinnati, OH 45202
Phone: 513-345-2242
Fax: 513-345-2254

7604 CINERGY FIELD

201 E Pete Rose Way
Cincinnati, OH 45202-3596
Phone: 513-946-8000
Fax: 513-946-8006
Web Site: www.cinergy-field.com
Management:
   Operations Manager: Rick Portmann
   Administrative Manager: Jackie Kordenbrock
Mission: Home of the Cincinnati Reds and the Cincinnati Bengals.
Seating Capacity: 60,311
Year Built: 1970

7605 NIPPERT STADIUM

University of Cincinnati
One Stadium Drive
Cincinnati, OH 45221
Phone: 513-556-2170
Fax: 513-556-5059
Web Site: www.ucbearcats.com
Management:
   Athletic Director: Bob Goin
   Associate Athletic Director: Paul Klaczak
   Operations/Maintenance Director: Bob Bauer
Seating Capacity: 30,000

7606 PAUL BROWN STADIUM
Two Paul Brown Way
Cincinnati, OH 45202
Phone: 513-455-4800
Fax: 513-455-4801
Web Site: www.paulbrownstadium.com
Management:
 Managing Director: Eric J Brown
Seating Capacity: 65,600

7607 RIVERBEND MUSIC CENTER
6295 Kellogg Avenue
Cincinnati, OH 45230
Phone: 513-232-5882
Fax: 513-232-7577

7608 UNIVERSITY OF CINCINNATI: CORBETT AUDITORIUM
Corbett Center for the Performing Arts
College Conservatory of Music
Cincinnati, OH 45221-0003
Phone: 513-556-9430
Fax: 513-556-9988
e-mail: brian.anderson@uc.edu
Web Site: www.ccm.uc.edu

7609 UNIVERSITY OF CINCINNATI: ROBERT J WERNER RICITAL HALL
Robert J Werner Recital Hall
PO Box 210003
Cincinnati, OH 45221-0003
Phone: 513-556-9430
Fax: 513-556-9988
e-mail: brian.anderson@uc.edu
Web Site: www.ccm.uc.edu

7610 UNIVERSITY OF CINCINNATI: WATSON HALL
Corbett Center for the Performing Arts
College Conservatory of Music
Cincinnati, OH 45221
Phone: 513-556-9430
Fax: 513-556-9988
e-mail: brian.anderson@uc.edu
Web Site: www.ccm.uc.edu
Seating Capacity: 143
Year Built: 1967
Rental Contact: Brian Anderson

7611 UNIVERSITY OF CINCINNATI: MYRL L SHOEMAKER CENTER
University Of Cincinnati
ML 021, Room 327, Stadium Drive
Cincinnati, OH 45221-0021
Phone: 513-556-2170
Fax: 513-556-5059
e-mail: Bob.Goin@uc.edu
Web Site: www.ucbearcats.com
Officers:
 Band Director: Dr. Terren Frenz
Management:
 Athletic Director: Bob Goin

Associate Athletic Director: Paul Klaczak
Operations/Maintenance Director: Bob Bauer
Dance Team Coach: Lisa Spears
Assistant Director Marketing: Joe Roberts
Senior Associate Athletic Director: John Sheffield
Cheerleading Coach: Tabby Fagan
Paid Staff: 150
Seating Capacity: 13,176

7612 US BANK ARENA
100 Broadway
Cincinnati, OH 45202
Phone: 513-421-4111
Fax: 513-333-3040
e-mail: info@usbankarena.com
Web Site: www.usbankarena.com
Management:
 General Manager: Jim Moehring
 Director Markting/Public Relations: Morrello Raleigh
 Director Operations: Kristin Poluha
 Director Programming/Bus. Develop.: Matt Dunne
Founded: 1975
Performs At: Arena
Seating Capacity: 17,566
Year Built: 1975
Year Remodeled: 1997
Rental Contact: Matt Dunne

7613 WESTWOOD TOWN HALL
3017 Harrison Avenue
Cincinnati, OH 45213
Phone: 513-662-9109

7614 CASE WESTERN RESERVE UNIVERSITY: ELDRED HALL
10900 Euclid Avenue
Cleveland, OH 44106
Phone: 216-368-4868
Fax: 216-368-5184
e-mail: ksg@po.cwru.edu
Web Site:
www.cwru.edu/artsci/thtr/website/theahome.htm
Management:
 Chairman Department Theater Arts: Ron Wilson
Status: Nonprofit
Paid Staff: 3
Performs At: College Theater
Type of Stage: PProscenium
Seating Capacity: 152
Year Built: 1898
Year Remodeled: 1997

7615 CLEVELAND BROWNS STADIUM
1085 W 3rd Street
Cleveland, OH 44114
Phone: 440-891-5000
Fax: 440-891-5009
Web Site: www.clevelandbrowns.com
Management:
 VP/Director Stadium Operations: Lew Merletti
 Stadium Operations Manager: Diane Downing
Specialized Field: Home of the Cleveland Browns

All listings are in alphabetical order by state, then city, then organization within the city.

Seating Capacity: 62m799
Year Built: 1999

**7616 CLEVELAND MUSEUM OF ART:
GARTNER AUDITOR**
11150 E Boulevard
Cleveland, OH 44106
Phone: 216-421-7340
Fax: 216-421-0411

7617 CLEVELAND PLAY HOUSE
8500 Euclid Avenue
Cleveland, OH 44106
Phone: 216-795-7000
Fax: 216-795-7005
Web Site: www.cleveplayhouse.org

**7618 CLEVELAND PLAY HOUSE: BOLTON
THEATRE**
8500 Euclid Avenue
PO Box 1989
Cleveland, OH 44106
Phone: 216-795-7010
Fax: 216-795-7005
Management:
  Artistic Director: Peter Hackett
  Managing Director: Dean Gladden

**7619 CLEVELAND PLAY HOUSE: BROOKS
THEATRE**
8500 Euclid Avenue
Cleveland, OH 44106
Phone: 216-795-7010
Fax: 216-795-7005

**7620 CLEVELAND PLAY HOUSE: DRURY
THEATRE**
8500 Euclid Avenue
Cleveland, OH 44106
Phone: 216-795-7010
Fax: 216-795-7005

7621 CLEVELAND PUBLIC THEATRE
6415 Detroit Avenue
Cleveland, OH 44102
Phone: 216-631-2727
Fax: 216-631-2575
e-mail: cpt@clevelandartists.net
Web Site: www.clevelandartists.net/cpt

**7622 CLEVELAND STATE UNIVERSITY:
CONVOCATION CENTER**
2000 Prospect Avenue
Cleveland, OH 44115-2318
Phone: 216-687-9292
Fax: 216-687-5450
Web Site: www.csuohio.edu/convo
Management:
  General Manager: Joe Mazur
  Director Food/Beverage: Sean Sullivan

Mission: Arena located on the campus of Cleveland State
University. Home of the Cleveland Crunch and CSU
Vikings Men's and Women's basketball teams.
Seating Capacity: 15,000+
Year Built: 1991

**7623 CSU CONVOCATION CENTER
Cleveland State University**
2000 Prospect Avenue
Cleveland, OH 44115
Phone: 216-687-5119
Fax: 216-687-7257
Web Site: www.csuohio.edu/convo
Management:
  Athletic Director: Ronald A Willner

7624 GUND ARENA
1 Center Court
Cleveland, OH 44115
Phone: 216-420-2000
Fax: 216-420-2260
Web Site: www.gunarena.com
Management:
  Executive VP/General Manager: Roy Jones
  Sr VP Sales/Marketing: Jim Kahler
Mission: Home of the Cleveland Cavaliers and the
Cleveland Lumberjacks.
Seating Capacity: 20,600
Year Built: 1994

**7625 JACOBS FIELD
Cleveland Indians**
2401 Ontario Street
Cleveland, OH 44115-4003
Phone: 216-420-4200
Fax: 216-420-4430
Web Site: www.indian.com
Management:
  Director Ballpark Operations: Jim Folk
  Sr Director Corp Mktg/Brdcst: Jon Starrett
  Concession General Manager: Charlie Henningsen
Mission: Home of the Cleveland Indians. Offers ballpark
signage and branded products opportunities.
Seating Capacity: 43,368
Year Built: 1994

**7626 KARAMU HOUSE PERFORMING ARTS
THEATRE**
2355 E 89th Street
Cleveland, OH 44106
Phone: 216-795-7070
Fax: 216-795-7073

**7627 KARAMU HOUSE PERFORMING ARTS
THEATRE: AMPHITHEATRE**
2355 E 89th Street
Cleveland, OH 44106
Phone: 216-795-7070
Fax: 216-795-7073

All listings are in alphabetical order by state, then city, then organization within the city.

7628 KARAMU HOUSE PERFORMING ARTS THEATRE: ARENA
2355 E 89th Street
Cleveland, OH 44106
Phone: 216-795-7070
Fax: 216-795-7073

7629 KARAMU HOUSE PERFORMING ARTS THEATRE: PROSCE HALL
2355 E 89th Street
Cleveland, OH 44106
Phone: 216-795-7070
Fax: 216-795-7073

7630 PLAYHOUSE SQUARE CENTER
1501 Euclid Avenue
Cleveland, OH 44115
Phone: 216-771-4444
Fax: 216-771-0217

7631 PLAYHOUSE SQUARE CENTER: OHIO THEATRE
1519 Euclid Avenue
Cleveland, OH 44115
Phone: 216-771-4444
Fax: 216-771-0217

7632 PLAYHOUSE SQUARE CENTER: PALACE THEATRE
1519 Euclid Avenue
Cleveland, OH 44115
Phone: 216-771-4444
Fax: 216-771-0217

7633 PLAYHOUSE SQUARE CENTER: STATE THEATRE
1519 Euclid Avenue
Cleveland, OH 44115
Phone: 216-771-4444
Fax: 216-771-0217

7634 SAINT SAVA SERBIAN ORTHODOX CATHEDRAL
6306 Broadview
Cleveland, OH 44134
Phone: 216-741-3002
Management:
   Director: Dragica Zamiska
Mission: To encourage and perpetuate Serbian music, dance, language, culture and heritage.
Founded: 1982
Specialized Field: Ethnic; Folk
Status: Non-Professional; Nonprofit
Income Sources: Saint Sava Free Serbian Orthodox Church; School Congregation; Cleveland Area Arts Council
Organization Type: Performing; Touring; Resident; Educational

7635 SEVERANCE HALL
11001 Euclid
Cleveland, OH 44106
Phone: 216-231-7300
Fax: 216-231-0202

7636 CAIN PARK THEATRE
Lee and Superior Roads
40 Severance Circle
Cleveland Heights, OH 44118
Phone: 216-291-5796
Fax: 216-291-3705
e-mail: cainpark@clvhts.com
Web Site: www.cainpark.com
Officers:
   City Manager: Robert C Downey
Management:
   General Manager: Janet Herman-Barlow
   Operations Manager: William D Thomas
   Public Relations: Ksenia Roshchakovsky
   Development Office: Jennifer Kuzma
Founded: 1938
Specialized Field: Dance; Vocal Music; Instrumental Musical Theater; Arts Festival; Visual Arts Gallery
Status: Professional; Nonprofit
Paid Staff: 60
Paid Artists: 700
Budget: $630,000
Income Sources: Ticket sales; Grants; City of Cleveland Heights
Performs At: Evans Amphitheater; Alma Theater
Affiliations: Ohio Arts Council; Arts Midwest; Association of Performing Arts Presenters; Ohio Arts Presenters Network
Annual Attendance: 125,000+
Facility Category: Summer outdoor, covered open-air theatres
Type of Stage: Proscenium, Thrust
Seating Capacity: 1,222 + lawn; 262
Year Built: 1938
Year Remodeled: 1989
Organization Type: Sponsoring

7637 CAIN PARK: CITY OF CLEVELAND HEIGHTS
Cain Park, Lee & Superior Roads
40 Severance Circle
Cleveland Heights, OH 44118-1576
Phone: 216-291-5796
Fax: 216-291-3705
e-mail: cainpark@clvhts.com
Web Site: www.clevelandheights.com
Management:
   General Manager: Janet Herman Barlow
Mission: Presents local, regional and national acts during an 11 week summer season, in addition to producing 2-musical theatre productions, art gallery show, and a major weekend-long arts festival.
Founded: 1938
Status: municipally ownes and operated summer arts park.
Volunteer Staff: 300
Paid Artists: 100
Non-paid Artists: 40

7638 DOBAMA THEATRE
1846 Coventry Road
Cleveland Heights, OH 44118
Phone: 216-932-6838
Fax: 216-932-3259

7639 EUGENE S BLANCHE AND R HALLE THEATRE
Mayfield JCC
3505 Mayfield Road
Cleveland Heights, OH 44118
Phone: 216-382-4000
Fax: 216-382-5401
e-mail: halltheatre@clevejcc.org
Web Site: www.clevejcc.org
Management:
   Administrative Director: Amy Kenerup
   Technical Director: Tony Kovacic
   Playmakers Youth Theatre Director: Sheri Gross
Mission: To provide opportunities through the arts for persons of all ages to explore and strengthen Jewish identity, arts expertise, and human-relation skills.
Founded: 1949
Specialized Field: Dance; Theater; Visual Arts
Status: Professional; Non-Professional; Nonprofit
Paid Staff: 10
Volunteer Staff: 50
Paid Artists: 90
Budget: $300,000
Income Sources: Jewish Community Center; Ohio Arts Council
Performs At: Eugene S. & Blanche R. Halle Theatre
Annual Attendance: 10,000
Facility Category: Theatre; Community Theatre
Type of Stage: Proscenium
Stage Dimensions: 29x35
Seating Capacity: 270
Year Built: 1960
Rental Contact: Administrative Director Amy Kenerup
Organization Type: Performing; Resident; Educational

7640 CREW STADIUM
2121 Velma Avenue
Columbus, OH
Phone: 614-447-4100
Web Site: www.thecrew.com
Management:
   Stadium Manager: Mark McCullers

7641 DAVIS DISCOVERY CENTER: AGNES JEFFREY SHEDD
549 Franklin Avenue
Columbus, OH 43215
Phone: 614-645-7469
Fax: 614-645-6278

7642 DAVIS DISCOVERY CENTER: HENRY VAN FLEET THEATRE
549 Franklin Avenue
Columbus, OH 43215
Phone: 614-645-7469
Fax: 614-645-6278

7643 FRANKLIN COUNTY VETERANS MEMORIAL
300 W Broad Street
Columbus, OH 43215
Phone: 614-221-4341
Fax: 614-221-8422
e-mail: info@fvcm.com
Web Site: www.fcvm.com
Management:
   General Manager: Richard P Nolan
   Assistant Manager: Melody A Stevens
Mission: Veterans Memorial is a non profit multi-purpose facility providing rental spaces for concerts
Founded: 1955
Paid Staff: 25
Volunteer Staff: 50
Budget: $1.6 million
Income Sources: Self Generator Revenue
Facility Category: Auditorium and Exhibition Facility
Type of Stage: Proscenium
Stage Dimensions: 32'x26'
Seating Capacity: 3916
Year Built: 1955
Year Remodeled: 2000
Cost: $11.5 million
Rental Contact: Richard Nolan

7644 JEROME SCHOTTENSTEIN CENTER AT OHIO STATE UNIVERSITY
555 Borror Drive
Suite 1030
Columbus, OH 43210
Phone: 614-688-8400
Fax: 614-292-5067
e-mail: osuarena@osu.edu
Web Site: www.schottensteincenter.com
Management:
   Director Booking: Sharon Rone
Founded: 1998
Annual Attendance: 1,000,000
Facility Category: Arena
Type of Stage: Portable
Stage Dimensions: 60x80
Seating Capacity: 20,000
Year Built: 1998
Rental Contact: Sharon Rone

7645 JEWISH COMMUNITY CENTER OF CLEVELAND: BLANCH HALL
3505 Mayfield Road
Columbus, OH 44118
Phone: 216-382-4000

7646 MARTIN LUTHER KING JR. PERFORMING AND CULTURAL ARTS COMPLEX
867 Mt. Vernon Avenue
Columbus, OH 43203
Phone: 614-645-5464
Fax: 614-645-0672
Management:
   Executive Director: Dr. Barbara Nicholson
   Assistant Executive Director: Zoraba Q Ross

Mission: To enrich and improve our community and society by preserving, presenting, and fostering the contributions of African-Americans through the arts and education.
Founded: 1987
Paid Staff: 16
Budget: $1.4 million
Income Sources: Box office, grants, private donations
Performs At: 1 Multi Purpose, 1 Theatre; 1 Ballroom
Seating Capacity: 444
Year Remodeled: 2000
Rental Contact: Howard Newman

7647 OHIO STATE UNIVERSITY: STADIUM II THEATRE

1089 Drake Union
1849 Cannon Drive
Columbus, OH 43210
Phone: 614-292-5821
Fax: 614-292-3222

7648 OHIO STATE UNIVERSITY: THURBER THEATRE

1089 Drake Union
1849 Cannon Drive
Columbus, OH 43210
Phone: 614-292-5821
Fax: 614-292-3222

7649 OHIO STATE UNIVERSITY WEXNER CENTER FOR THE ARTS

1871 N High Street
Columbus, OH 43210-1393
Phone: 614-292-5821
Fax: 614-292-7824
e-mail: helm.9@osu.edu
Web Site: www.wexarts.org
Management:
   Performing Arts Director: Charles Helm
   Assistant Director: Mychaelyn Michalec
   Technical Director: John Smith
Specialized Field: Contemporary
Budget: $150,000-400,000
Performs At: Mershon Auditorium; Weigel Hall Auditorium
Type of Stage: Black Box
Rental Contact: Claudia Bonham

7650 OHIO STATE UNIVESRITY: OHIO STADIUM

411 Woody Hayes Drive, Room 155
Ohio Stadium Rotunda
Columbus, OH 43210
Phone: 614-292-5821
Management:
   Director: Elizabeth Conlisk
   Assistant Director: Amy Murray
   Assistant Director: Lesley D Deaderick
   Media Relations Coordinator: Reginald Anglen
   Media Relations Coordinator: Karissa Shivley
Founded: 1922
Seating Capacity: 98,000

7651 PLAYERS THEATRE COLUMBUS

Verm Rifle Center for Government & the Arts
77 High Street South
Columbus, OH 43215
Phone: 614-470-4809

7652 VETERANS MEMORIAL

300 W Broad Street
Columbus, OH 43215
Phone: 614-221-4341
Fax: 614-221-8422
e-mail: info@fcum.com
Web Site: www.fcum.com
Facility Category: Multi-purpose facility
Type of Stage: Proscenium
Stage Dimensions: 73x31
Seating Capacity: 3,916
Year Built: 1955
Year Remodeled: 2000
Cost: $11.5 million
Rental Contact: Richard Nolan

7653 WEXNER CENTER FOR THE ARTS: MERSHON AUDITORIUM

30 W 15th Avenue
Columbus, OH 43210
Phone: 614-292-5785
Fax: 614-292-7824
Web Site: www.wexarts.org

7654 POMERENE CENTER FOR THE ARTS

317 Mulberry Street
Coshocton, OH 43812
Phone: 740-622-0326
e-mail: Kricor@coshocton.com
Management:
   Director: Anne Cornell
Budget: $10,000
Seating Capacity: 75-900

7655 BLOSSOM MUSIC CENTER

1145 W Steels Corners Road
Cuyahoga Falls, OH 44223
Phone: 216-566-8184
Fax: 216-920-0968
e-mail: blossommusic@umusic.com
Web Site: www.blossommusic.com -or- clevelandorch.com
Management:
   General Manager: David E Carlucci

7656 DAYTON CONVENTION AND EXHIBITION CENTER

22 E 5th Street
Dayton, OH 45402
Phone: 937-333-4711
Fax: 937-333-4700
Toll-free: 800-822-3498

7657 DAYTON HARA ARENA

1001 Shiloh Springs Road
Dayton, OH 454415

Phone: 937-278-4776
Fax: 937-278-4633
e-mail: harapr@haracomplex.com
Web Site: www.haracomplex.com
Management:
  Owner: Ralph M Wampler
  Community Affairs Director: Karen Wanpler
Founded: 1964
Facility Category: Arena; Exhibtion Centers
Seating Capacity: 7,000
Year Built: 1964
Year Remodeled: 1997
Rental Contact: Corey Rose

7658 DAYTON HARA COMPLEX
1001 Shiloh Springs Road
Dayton, OH 45415
Phone: 973-278-9776
Fax: 973-278-4633
e-mail: harapr@coax.net
Web Site: www.coax.net/hara
Management:
  President: Johnny Walker
  Sales Director: Larry Neace
  Promotion Director: James Reynolds
Specialized Field: Full-service sports, entertainment and family show facility.
Seating Capacity: 5,900, 7,000
Year Built: 1964
Year Remodeled: 1987

7659 DAYTON PLAYHOUSE
1301 E Siebenthaler Avenue
Dayton, OH 45414
Phone: 937-333-7469
Fax: 937-277-9539

7660 UNIVERSITY OF DAYTON ARENA
PO Box 8806
Dayton, OH 45401-4461
Phone: 937-229-2100
Fax: 937-229-4461
e-mail: sid@udayton.edu
Web Site: www.udayton.edu
Management:
  Athletic Director: Ted Kissell
  Sports Information Director: Doug Hauschild
  Head Football Coach: Mike Kelly
  Head Basketball Coach (M): Oliver Purneil
  Head Basketbal Coach: Jaci Clark
  Director: Timothy J O'Connell
  Operations Coordinator: Norm Dupler
  Ticket Office Manager: Joe Granito
  Office Supervisor: Tina Wheelock
Founded: 1850
Seating Capacity: 14,000

7661 VICTORIA THEATRE
138 N Main Street
Dayton, OH 45402
Phone: 937-228-7591
Fax: 937-449-5068
Web Site: www.victoriatheatre.com
Officers:

President: Mark Light
  Executive Director: Dione Kennedy
Specialized Field: Theatre
Paid Staff: 80
Volunteer Staff: 999
Budget: $1,000,000+
Annual Attendance: 300,000
Facility Category: Theatre
Type of Stage: Proscenium
Seating Capacity: 1,139
Year Built: 1868
Year Remodeled: 1990
Rental Contact: JoAnn Brown

7662 WRIGHT STATE UNIVERSITY: ERVIN J NUTTER CENTER
Wright State University
3640 Colonel Glenn Highway
Dayton, OH 45435
Phone: 937-775-3498
Fax: 937-775-2060
e-mail: john.siehl@wright.edu
Web Site: www.nuttercenter.com
Management:
  Executive Director: John Siehl
  Associate Director: Jim Brown
  Events Coordinator: Dan Bago
Specialized Field: Home of Wright State University athletics (NCAA) and Dayton Bombers East Coast Hockey League team.
Seating Capacity: 12,000
Year Built: 1990

7663 DELAWARE COUNTY CULTURAL ARTS CENTER
190 W Winter Street
Delaware, OH 43015
Phone: 740-369-2787
Fax: 740-363-2733
Management:
  Executive Director: Krista Campbell
Budget: $10,000
Seating Capacity: 2,000

7664 SELBY STADIUM
Ohio Weslyan University
Delaware, OH 43015
Phone: 740-368-3725
Fax: 740-368-3751
Management:
  Athletic Director: John Martin
Seating Capacity: 9,300

7665 FOSTORIA FOOTLIGHTERS
PO Box 542
Fostoria, OH 44830
Phone: 419-435-7501

7666 ARIEL THEATRE
426 2nd Avenue
Gallipolis, OH 45631
Phone: 740-446-2787
Management:

Artistic Director: Lora Snow

**7667 MEMORIAL ATHLETIC &
CONVOCATION CENTER**
150 Momorial Gym
Kent, OH 44242
Phone: 330-672-3120
Fax: 330-672-2112
Web Site: www.kent.edu/athletics
Management:
    General Manager: Kenny Long
Seating Capacity: 6,327

**7668 FRAZE PAVILION FOR THE
PERFORMING ARTS**
Lincoln Park Center
695 Lincoln Park Boulevard
Kettering, OH 45429
Phone: 937-296-3300
Fax: 937-296-3302
e-mail: fraze@ketteringoh.org
Web Site: www.fraze.com
Management:
    General Manager: Karen Durham
Founded: 1991
Budget: $400,000-1,000,000
Income Sources: Ticket sales
Annual Attendance: 200,000
Facility Category: Amphitheatre
Seating Capacity: 4,300
Year Built: 1991

**7669 KENNETH C BECK CENTER FOR THE
PERFORMING ARTS**
17801 Detroit Avenue
Lakewood, OH 44107
Phone: 216-521-2540
Fax: 216-228-6050
e-mail: grumio85@aol.com
Web Site: www.beckcenter.org

**7670 VETERANS MEMORIAL CIVIC AND
CONVENTION CENTER**
7 Town Square
Lima, OH 45801
Phone: 419-224-5222
Fax: 419-224-6964
Toll-free: 888-377-0674
e-mail: vmccc@wcoil.com
Web Site: www.vmccc.com
Officers:
    President: Frank Wellmann
    VP: James Bourk
    Treasurer: Cecil Baylor
Management:
    Director: Brian Keegan
    Booking Coordinator: Joe Shaffner
Founded: 1984
Specialized Field: Performing Arts
Paid Staff: 20
Volunteer Staff: 40
Income Sources: 50% earned; 50% subsidy
Affiliations: I.A.A.M.

Annual Attendance: $250,000
Facility Category: Multi-Purpose
Type of Stage: Proscenium
Stage Dimensions: 60'x40'
Seating Capacity: 1792
Year Built: 1984
Cost: $9 Million
Rental Contact: Joe Shaffnerr
Resident Groups: Lima Symphony Orchestra

7671 PALACE CIVIC CENTER
Broadway at 6th Street
Lorain, OH 44052
Phone: 440-245-2323
Fax: 440-246-6076

7672 CENTRAL PARK BANDSHELL
Mansfield City Square
Mansfield, OH 44902
Phone: 419-755-9819
Fax: 419-522-9841

7673 PALACE THEATRE
276 W Center Street
Marion, OH 43302
Phone: 740-383-2101
Fax: 740-387-3425
e-mail: marionpalace@marion.net
Web Site: www.marion.net/palace

7674 NATIONWIDE ARENA
77 E Nationwide Boulevard
Nationwide Arena, OH 43215
Phone: 614-677-9000
Fax: 614-232-5910
Toll-free: 800-645-2657
Web Site: www.columbusbluejackets.com
Management:
    President/General Manager: Doug McLean
    Assistant General Manager: Jim Clark
Founded: 2000
Seating Capacity: 18,500

**7675 KENT STATE UNIVERSITY:
TUSCARAWAS**
330 University Drive
New Philadelphia, OH 44663
Phone: 330-339-3391
Fax: 330-339-3321
Management:
    Public Relations Coordinator: Pam Patacca
Specialized Field: Allarew

7676 SCHOENBRUNN AMPHITHEATRE
PO Box 450
New Philadelphia, OH 44663
Phone: 330-364-5111

7677 TRUMBULL NEW THEATRE
5883 Youngstown-Warren Road
Niles, OH 44446
Phone: 330-652-1103

7678 TOWNE AND COUNTRY PLAYERS
55 E Main Street
PO Box 551
Norwalk, OH 44857
Phone: 419-668-1641

7679 FAIRMOUNT FINE ARTS CENTER
8400 Fairmount Road
PO Box 80
Novelty, OH 44072
Phone: 440-338-3171
Fax: 440-338-4218

7680 MIAMI UNIVERSITY: MILLET HALL
Millett Hall
Room 218
Oxford, OH 45056
Phone: 513-529-3355
Fax: 513-529-6729
Management:
    Manager Special Events: John T Walker
Seating Capacity: 10,000

7681 CUYAHOGA COMMUNITY COLLEGE: WESTERN CAMPUS THEATRE
11000 Pleasant Valley
Parma Heights, OH 44130
Phone: 216-987-5538

7682 SHAWNEE STATE UNIVERSITY: VERN RIFFE CENTER FOR THE ARTS
940 2nd Street
Portsmouth, OH 45662
Phone: 740-351-3622
Fax: 740-351-3414
e-mail: info@vrcfa.org
Web Site: www.vrcfa.org
Management:
    Executive Director: Carl Daehler
    Technical Director: Leo Schiosser
Specialized Field: Broadway; Theatre; Orchestra; Pop; Dance; Folk
Paid Staff: 4
Volunteer Staff: 120
Performs At: Kahl Studio Theater; Howland Recital Hall
Affiliations: AAPA, OAPN
Annual Attendance: 75,000
Type of Stage: Proscenium and Concert Hall
Stage Dimensions: 58'x 30'
Seating Capacity: 1,139
Year Built: 1995
Cost: $16,000,000
Rental Contact: Gloria Horsley

7683 SOUTHERN OHIO MUSEUM & CULTURAL CENTER
PO Box 990
825 Gallia Street
Portsmouth, OH 45662
Phone: 740-354-5629
Fax: 740-354-4090
e-mail: museum826falcon1.com

Management:
    Curator Performing Arts: Pegi Wilkes
Mission: To educate, enlighten, entertain and enrich the regional community through quality exhibitions of art and artifacts; through conversation and promotion in the permanent collection; and through satellite interpretive events and performances designed to interpret, reinforce and enhance access to exhibition concepts.
Founded: 1979
Specialized Field: Visual Arts; Performing Arts
Paid Staff: 8
Paid Artists: 5

7684 CLARK STATE PERFORMING ARTS CENTER
300 S Fountain Avenue
PO Box 570
Springfield, OH 45501-0570
Phone: 937-328-3857
Fax: 937-328-3879
e-mail: eckstrandk@clark.cc.oh.us
Web Site: www.clark.cc.oh.us/pac
Management:
    Director: Katherine L Eckstrand
    Operations Manager: Karen Clark
    Technical Director: Dan Hunt
    Box Office Manager: Mary Lu Shobe
    Administrative Assistant: Lori Common
    Education/Outreach Director: Tim Rowe
Mission: To present quality and diverse performing arts events to a wide regional audience.
Specialized Field: Dayton/Springfield
Paid Staff: 8
Volunteer Staff: 280
Paid Artists: 80
Budget: $660,000
Income Sources: Box Office, Rentals, Grants, Sponsorships, Donations
Performs At: Kuss Auditorium; Turner Studio Theatre
Affiliations: Association of Performing Arts Presenters; Ohio Arts Performers Network
Annual Attendance: 90,000
Facility Category: Auditorium Studio Theatre
Type of Stage: Proscenium/ Studio Theatre
Stage Dimensions: 55'x 40'
Seating Capacity: 1,500/200
Year Built: 1993
Cost: $15.1 million
Rental Contact: Operations Manager Karen Clark
Organization Type: Arts Center

7685 FRANCISCAN CENTER
6832 Convent Boulevard
Sylvania, OH 43560-2896
Phone: 419-885-1547
Fax: 419-882-2981
e-mail: director@franciscancenter.org
Web Site: www.francisancenter.org
Management:
    OSF Director: Sheila Shea

7686 COLLINGWOOD ARTS CENTER
2413 Collingwood Boulevard
Toledo, OH 43626-1153

Phone: 419-244-2787
Fax: 419-244-2820
Officers:
   President: Ed Hoffman

7687 GLASS BOWL STADIUM
2801 W Bancroft
Toledo, OH 43606
Phone: 419-530-4226
Fax: 419-530-4428
Web Site: www.utoledo.edu/athletics/nonframe
Management:
   Asst. Athletic Dir./Ext. Affairs: Mike Karabin
   Athletic Facilities Coordinator: Tim Warga

7688 OHIO THEATRE
3114 Lagrange Street
Toledo, OH 43608
Phone: 419-241-6785

7689 SEAGATE CENTRE
401 Jefferson Avenue
Toledo, OH 43604
Phone: 419-255-3300
Fax: 419-255-7731
e-mail: jdonnelly@toledo~seagate.com
Web Site: www.toledo~seagate.com
Officers:
   President: James E Donnelly
Management:
   Director Operations: Jim Thielman
   Director Sales/Marketing/Booking: Carol Dupuis
Seating Capacity: 7,500

7690 TOLEDO MASONIC AUDITORIUM
4645 Heather Downs Boulevard
Toledo, OH 43614
Phone: 419-381-8851
Fax: 419-381-9525
Web Site: stranahantheater.org
Management:
   Box Office Manager: Cherie Gime
   Facility Category: Performing Arts
   Stage Dimensions: 100 x 106
   Seating Capacity: 2424
   Year Built: 1968
   Year Remodeled: 2000
   Cost: $1,900
   Rental Contact: General Manager Ward Whiting

7691 TOLEDO MUSEUM OF ART
2445 Monroe Street
PO Box 1013
Toledo, OH 43697
Phone: 419-255-8000
Fax: 419-255-5638
Toll-free: 800-644-6862
e-mail: information@toledomuseum.org
Web Site: www.toledomuseum.org
Management:
   Marketing Manager: Holly Taylor
   Advertising/Promotions Coordinator: Chris Peiffer
   Marketing Director: Barbara Stahl

Mission: The power of art to ignite the imagination, stimulate thought, and provide enjoyment. Through our collection and programs, we strive to integrate art into the lives of people.
Founded: 1901
Specialized Field: Fine Arts - Ancient through Contemporary
Status: Nonprofit
Paid Staff: 150
Volunteer Staff: 500
Paid Artists: 20

7692 TOLEDO SPORTS ARENA
1 Mail Street
Toledo, OH 43605
Phone: 419-698-1598
Fax: 419-693-3299
Management:
   General Manager: Gary Wyse
Seating Capacity: 7,500

7693 UNIVERSITY OF TOLEDO: JOHN F SAVAGE HALL
University of Toledo
2801 W Bancroft Street
Toledo, OH 43606
Phone: 419-530-4226
Fax: 419-530-2096
Web Site: www.utoledo.edu
Management:
   Athletic Director: Pete Liske
Seating Capacity: 9,600

7694 HOBART SPORTS ARENA
255 Adams Street
Troy, OH 45373
Phone: 937-339-2911
Fax: 937-335-0046
Management:
   Manager: Charles R Sharrett

7695 TROY-HAYNER CULTURAL CENTER
301 W Main Street
Troy, OH 45373
Phone: 937-339-0457
Fax: 937-335-6373
e-mail: hayner@tdnpublishing.com
Web Site: www.tdn-net.com/hayner
Management:
   Director: Linda Lee Jolly

7696 COWAN HALL
30 Grove Street
Westerville, OH 43081
Phone: 614-823-1557
Fax: 614-823-1998

7697 MURPHY THEATRE
50 W Main
Wilmington, OH 45177

Phone: 937-382-3643
Fax: 937-382-6364
e-mail: members.aol.com/murphytheatre
Management:
Theatre Director: Doug Lynn
Paid Staff: 7
Volunteer Staff: 20
Paid Artists: 14
Budget: $175,000 - 225,000
Income Sources: Donations, ticket sales; and rentals
Facility Category: Renovated theatre
Type of Stage: Original style
Seating Capacity: 795
Year Built: 1918
Year Remodeled: 1992

7698 BEEGHLY GYM
Youngstown State University
Youngstown, OH 44555
Phone: 330-742-3717
Fax: 330-742-3191
Web Site: www.ysu.edu
Management:
Human Resiurces Director: Jeanne Wainio

7699 STAMBAUGH AUDITORIUM
Monday Musical Club
1000 5th Avenue
Youngstown, OH 44504
Phone: 330-743-2617

7700 STAMBAUGH STADIUM
Youngstown State University
Youngstown, OH 44555
Phone: 330-742-3717
Fax: 330-742-3191
Web Site: www.ysu.edu
Management:
Athletic Director: Jim Tressel
Associate Athletic Director: Pauline Saternow
Associate Athletic Director: Daniel O'Connell
Associate Athletic Director: Judy Richards
Seating Capacity: 16,000

7701 YOUNGSTOWN PLAYHOUSE
600 Playhouse Lane
Youngstown, OH 44511
Phone: 330-788-8739
Fax: 330-788-1208

7702 YOUNGSTOWN STATE UNIVERSITY: BLISS RECITAL HALL
410 Wick Avenue
Youngstown, OH 44555
Phone: 330-742-3636
Fax: 330-742-1496

7703 YOUNGSTOWN STATE UNIVERSITY: FORD THEATRE
410 Wick Avenue
Youngstown, OH 44555

Phone: 330-742-3625
Fax: 330-742-2341

7704 YOUNGSTOWN STATE UNIVERSITY: SPOTLIGHT ARENA
410 Wick Avenue
Youngstown, OH 44555
Phone: 330-742-3625
Fax: 330-742-2341

7705 YOUNGSTOWN SYMPHONY CENTER: POWERS AUDITORIUM
260 Federal Plaza W
Youngstown, OH 44503
Phone: 330-744-4269
Fax: 330-742-2341

7706 SECREST AUDITORIUM
334 Shinnick Street
Zanesville, OH 43701
Phone: 740-454-6851
Fax: 740-454-6852
e-mail: auditorium@coz.org
Management:
Manager: John P Kunkel, III

7707 ZANESVILLE ART CENTER
620 Military Road
Zanesville, OH 43701
Phone: 740-452-0741
Fax: 740-452-0797
Management:
Director: Philip A LaDouceur
Founded: 1936
Paid Staff: 7
Volunteer Staff: 50
Paid Artists: 5
Budget: $300,000
Income Sources: Multiple Sources
Annual Attendance: 15,000
Facility Category: Auditorium
Stage Dimensions: 30'x
Seating Capacity: 80
Year Built: 1984
Rental Contact: Debbie Lowe

Oklahoma

7708 EAST CENTRAL UNIVERSITY: D0ROTHY I SUMMERS
Ada, OK 74820
Phone: 580-332-8000
Fax: 580-436-3329
Management:
Ass't Professor of Speech/Drama: Bret Jones
Technical Director: Theo Peshehonoff
Annual Attendance: 1200 - 1500
Seating Capacity: 430

7709 ALVA PUBLIC LIBRARY AUDITORIUM
504 7th
Alva, OK 73717
Phone: 580-327-1833
Fax: 580-327-5329

7710 BARTLESVILLE COMMUNITY CENTER
300 SE Adams Boulevard
Bartlesville, OK 74003
Mailing Address: PO Box 1027, Bartlesville, OK. 74005
Phone: 918-337-2787
Fax: 918-337-3783
Toll-free: 800-618-2787
e-mail: bartcent@onenet.net
Web Site: www.bartlesvilleok.com/ee/cc
Officers:
    Chairman: Edd Grigsby
Management:
    Managing Director: Patricia Dickerson
    Facility Manager: Pat Patterson
    Office Manager: Bonnie Williams
    Events Coordinator: Shallan John
Founded: 1982
Specialized Field: Performing Arts Hall and Rental Facility
Paid Staff: 15
Volunteer Staff: 400
Budget: $860,000
Income Sources: Interest Income; Endowment; Rental Income; Hotel/Motel Tax Revenue; Donations; Admissions; Rentals
Affiliations: City of Bartlesville
Annual Attendance: 130,000
Facility Category: Performing Arts Hall; Rental Facility
Type of Stage: Proscenium
Stage Dimensions: 40-60wx30d
Seating Capacity: 1,702
Year Built: 1982
Cost: $13,000,000
Rental Contact: Events Coordinator Shallan John

7711 AMERICAN LEGION
121 W 8th Street
Bristow, OK 74010

7712 KLINGENSMITH PARK AMPHITHEATRE
110 W 7th Street
Bristow, OK 74010
Phone: 918-367-2237
Fax: 918-367-2237

7713 OKLAHOMA PANHANDLE STATE COLLEGE: CARL WOOTEN STADIUM
Oklahoma Panhandle State College
600 S College
Goodwell, OK 73939
Phone: 580-349-2611
Fax: 405-346-2302
Web Site: www.opsu.edu
Management:
    Director: Kevin Emerick

7714 GREAT PLAINS COLISEUM
920 Sheridan Road
Lawton, OK 73502
Phone: 580-357-1483
Fax: 580-357-1192
e-mail: gpc@ionet.net
Web Site: www.gpcoliseum.com
Management:
    Executive Director: Richard Pool

7715 MCMAHON MEMORIAL AUDITORIUM
801 Ferris
PO Box 522
Lawton, OK 73502
Phone: 580-581-3470
Fax: 580-581-3473
Web Site: www.lawtonok.com/mcmahon.shtml
Founded: 1954
Affiliations: Lawton Philharmonic Society
Type of Stage: Proscenium
Stage Dimensions: 92'Wx40'D
Orchestra Pit: 1
Architect: Paul Harris
Rental Contact: Jim McCarthy

7716 MUSKOGEE LITTLE THEATRE
Box 1974
Muskogee, OK 74402
Phone: 918-683-5332

7717 LLYOD NOBLE CENTER
2900 Jenkins Avenue
Norman, OK 73019
Phone: 405-646-1935
Fax: 864-656-0299
e-mail: Inc@ou.edu
Web Site: www.ou.eud
Management:
    Director: James C Dunn
Seating Capacity: 12,000

7718 UNIVERSITY OF OKLAHOMA THEATRE
563 Elm Street
#209
Norman, OK 73019-0310
Phone: 405-325-4021
Fax: 405-325-0400
Management:
    Director: Steven W Wallace
Mission: We seek to educate and train theatrical artists, craftpeoples and audiences.
Budget: $8,000; $1,500
Seating Capacity: 600; 144

7719 BLACK LIBERATED ARTS CENTER
PO Box 11014
Oklahoma City, OK 73136
Phone: 405-524-3800
Fax: 405-524-3800
Management:
    Director: Anita G Arnold
Budget: $35,000-60,000

Performs At: Civic Center Music Hall

7720 CIVIC CENTER MUSIC HALL
201 Channing Square
Suite 100
Oklahoma City, OK 73102
Phone: 405-297-2584
Fax: 405-297-3896

7721 MYRIAD CONVENTION CENTER
One Myriad Gardens
Oklahoma City, OK 73102
Phone: 405-297-3300
Fax: 405-297-1683
e-mail: gray@ionet.net
Web Site: www.myriadevents.com
Management:
General Manager: John Zeigler
Marketing Director: Kim Jones
Founded: 1972
Seating Capacity: 14,380

7722 OKLAHOMA CITY UNIVERSITY
2501 N Blackwelder
Oklahoma City, OK 73106
Phone: 405-521-5315

7723 OKLAHOMA CITY UNIVERSITY: BURG THEATRE
2501 N Blackwelder
Oklahoma City, OK 73106
Phone: 405-521-5315

7724 OKLAHOMA CITY UNIVERSITY: KIRKPATRICK AUDITORIUM
2501 N Blackwelder
Oklahoma City, OK 73106
Phone: 405-521-5315

7725 OKLAHOMA CITY ZOO AMPHITHEATRE
2101 NE 50th
Oklahoma City, OK 73111
Phone: 405-297-3300
Fax: 405-297-1683

7726 OKLAHOMA SUMMER ARTS INSTITUTE
105 N Hudson
Suite 101
Oklahoma City, OK 73102
Phone: 405-319-9099
Fax: 405-319-9019
e-mail: okarts@telepath.com
Web Site: www.okartinst.org
Management:
Artistic/Managing Director: Lee Warren

7727 PONCA PLAYHOUSE
516 E Grand
Ponca City, OK 74601

Phone: 580-465-5360

7728 STILLWATER COMMUNITY CENTER
PO Box 1449
Eighth & Duck Streets
Stillwater, OK 74076
Phone: 405-747-8003
Fax: 405-747-8022
e-mail: communitycenter@stillwater.org
Management:
Manager: Stephanie Nicholas
Budget: $10,000
Performs At: Continental Auditorium

7729 CHEROKEE HERITAGE CENTER AMPHITHEATER
Willis Road
PO Box 515
Tahlequah, OK 74465
Phone: 918-456-6007
Fax: 918-456-6165

7730 BRADY THEATRE/LARRY SHAEFFER PRESENTS
105 W Brady
Tulsa, OK 74103
Phone: 918-582-7239
Fax: 918-587-9531
e-mail: larryshaffer@hotmail.com
Web Site: www.bradytheatre.com
Management:
President: Larry Shaffer
Publicity Director/Marketing: Matt Alcott

7731 MABEE CENTER ARENA
Oral Roberts University
7777 S Lewis Avenue
Tulsa, OK 74136
Phone: 918-495-6444
Fax: 918-495-6478
e-mail: vbarker@oru.edu
Web Site: www.mabeecenter.com
Management:
Building Manager: Vick Barker
Operations Director: Tony Winters
Founded: 1972
Paid Staff: 25
Seating Capacity: 11,763

7732 SKELLY STADIUM
University of Tulsa
600 S College Avenue
Tulsa, OK 74104-3189
Phone: 918-631-5223
Fax: 918-631-5220
Web Site: www.tulsahurriccane.com
Management:
Director/Facilities: Terry Hossack
Athletic Director: Judy Macleod
Director Marketing: Cam Pepper
Sports Information Director: Don Tomkalski
Seating Capacity: 40,235

7733 TULSA PERFORMING ARTS CENTER
110 E 2nd Street
Tulsa, OK 74103
Phone: 918-596-7122
Fax: 918-596-7144
e-mail: jscott@ci.tulsa.ok.us
Web Site: www.webtek.com/pastrust
Management:
    Director: John E Scott

7734 TULSA PERFORMING ARTS CENTER: CHAPMAN MUSIC
110 E 2nd Street
Tulsa, OK 74103
Phone: 918-596-7122
Fax: 918-596-7144

7735 TULSA PERFORMING ARTS CENTER: JOHN H WILLIAM HALL
110 E 2nd Street
Tulsa, OK 74103
Phone: 918-596-7122
Fax: 918-596-7144

7736 TULSA PERFORMING ARTS CENTER: DOENGES THEATER
110 E 2nd Street
Tulsa, OK 74103
Phone: 918-596-7122
Fax: 918-596-7144

7737 TULSA PERFORMING ARTS CENTER: STUDIO II
110 E 2nd Street
Tulsa, OK 74103
Phone: 918-596-7122
Fax: 918-596-7144

7738 UNIVERSITY OF TULSA: KENDALL HALL
600 S College
Tulsa, OK 74104
Phone: 918-631-2000

7739 UNIVERSITY OF TULSA: TYRRELL HALL
600 S College
Tulsa, OK 74114
Phone: 918-631-2000
Fax: 918-631-3589

7740 WALTER ARTS CENTER
Holland Hall
5666 E 81 Street
Tulsa, OK 74137-2099
Phone: 918-481-1111
Fax: 918-481-1193
e-mail: bandoe@hollandhall.org
Web Site: hollandhall.org
Management:

Director: Bill Andoe
Founded: 1992
Specialized Field: Performing and Visual
Budget: $10,000
Performs At: Branch Theatre
Facility Category: Arts Education
Type of Stage: Proscenium
Seating Capacity: 1,119
Year Built: 1992
Rental Contact: Jackie Hewitt

7741 TULSA COMMUNITY COLLEGE PERFORMING ARTS CENTER FOR EDUCATION
10300 E 81st Street
Tusla, OK 74133-4513
Phone: 918-595-7752
Fax: 918-595-7778
e-mail: kclark@vm.tulsa.cc.ok.us
Management:
    Director: Kelly Clark

7742 SOUTHWESTERN OKLAHOMA STATE UNIVERSITY: FINE ARTS CENTER
Department of Music
100 Campus Drive
Weatherford, OK 73096
Phone: 580-774-3708
Fax: 405-774-3795

7743 SOUTHWESTERN OKLAHOMA: MILAN STADIUM
Southweatern Oklahoma State University
100 Campus Drive
Weatherford, OK 73096
Phone: 404-774-3068
Fax: 405-774-7106
Web Site: www.swosu.edu
Management:
    Athletic Director: Cecil Perkins
    Sports Information Director: Chris Doyle
Seating Capacity: 9,000

Oregon

7744 OREGON SHAKESPEARE FESTIVAL: ANGUS BOWMER THEATRE
15 S Pioneer
Ashland, OR 97520
Phone: 541-482-4331
Fax: 541-482-8045
e-mail: info@osfashland.org
Web Site: www.osfashland.org
Founded: 1935
Specialized Field: Performing Arts; diama
Paid Staff: 300
Volunteer Staff: 500
Paid Artists: 75

7745 OREGON SHAKESPEARE FESTIVAL: BLACK SWAN THEATER
15 S Pioneer
Ashland, OR 97520
Phone: 541-482-2111
Fax: 541-482-8045
Web Site: www.orshakes.org

7746 OREGON SHAKESPEARE FESTIVAL: ELIZABETH STATION
15 S Pioneer
Ashland, OR 97520
Phone: 541-482-2111
Fax: 541-482-8045
Web Site: www.orshakes.org

7747 SOUTHERN OREGON UNIVERSITY
1250 Siskiyou Boulevard
Ashland, OR 97520
Phone: 541-552-6456
Fax: 541-552-6440
e-mail: olbrich@sou.edu

7748 CLATSOP COMMUNITY COLLEGE/ARTS & IDEAS
1653 Jerome Street
Astoria, OR 97103
Phone: 503-338-2473
Fax: 503-338-2333
e-mail: kmace@clatsop.cc.or.us.us
Web Site: www.clatsopcollege.com/Arts&Ideas
Management:
 Community Arts Coordinator: Katherine Mace
Mission: Presented in a setting of artistry and education, the program provides opportunities for creativity and learning to both artists and audience.
Specialized Field: Visual; Performing; Lectures
Facility Category: Theatre
Type of Stage: Plywood
Seating Capacity: 255
Year Built: 1920

7749 COASTER THEATER
108 N Hemlock
PO Box 643
Cannon Beach, OR 97110
Phone: 503-436-1242

7750 LASELLS STEWART CENTER
Oregon State University
100 LaSells Stewart Center
Corvallis, OR 97331
Phone: 541-737-2402
Fax: 541-737-3187
e-mail: shawn.tucker@orst.edu
Web Site: oregonstate.edu/dept/lasells/index
Founded: 1981
Income Sources: Rental And Fees
Performs At: Concert Hall
Facility Category: Auditorium
Type of Stage: Hardwood Concert
Stage Dimensions: 53x42

Seating Capacity: 1200
Year Built: 1981
Rental Contact: Vi Anderson

7751 OREGON STATE UNIVERSITY: GILL COLISEUM
Oregon State University
103 Gill Coliseum
Corvallis, OR 97331
Phone: 541-737-7371
Fax: 541-737-1790
e-mail: mike.corwin@orst.edu
Management:
 Associate: Mike Corwin

7752 RESER STADIUM
Oregon State University
201 Cill Coliseum
Corvallis, OR 97331
Phone: 541-737-2785
Fax: 541-737-3570
Web Site: www.osubeavers.com
Management:
 Director: Mitch Barnhart
Seating Capacity: 35,000

7753 COMMUNITY CENTER FOR THE PERFORMING ARTS
WOW Hall
291 West Eighth
Eugene, OR 97401
Phone: 541-687-2746
Fax: 541-687-1664
e-mail: wowhall@efn.org
Web Site: www.efn.org/~wowhall
Officers:
 Board Chair: John Mathison
Management:
 Booking Coordinator: Abe Nielson
 Publicity: Bob Fennessey
Paid Staff: 10
Volunteer Staff: 100

7754 HULT CENTER FOR THE PERFORMING ARTS
One Eugene Center
Eugene, OR 97401
Phone: 541-682-5087
Fax: 541-682-5426
Web Site: www.hultcenter.org
Management:
 Executive Director: Richard A Schuland
 Programming Manager: Darrel Kane
Founded: 1982
Income Sources: City of Eugene
Seating Capacity: 2,500; 1,500

7755 JOHN C SHEDD INSTITUTE FOR THE ARTS
The Shedd
868 High Street
Eugene, OR 97401

Phone: 541-687-6526
Fax: 541-687-1589
Mission: Multi-venue performance space and educational facilities.
Facility Category: Concert Hall; Recital Hall; Gymnasium
Seating Capacity: 750; 175; 300
Year Built: 1926
Year Remodeled: 02/3
Rental Contact: Erik Martin

7756 UNIVERSITY OF OREGON: BEALL CONCERT HALL
Eugene, OR 97403
Phone: 541-696-5678

7757 UNIVERSITY OF OREGON: AUTZEN STADIUM
University of Oregon
2727 Leo Harris Parkway
Eugene, OR 97401
Phone: 541-346-5860
Fax: 541-346-5031
Web Site: www.goducks.com
Management:
    Events Manager: Vicky Strand

7758 FLORENCE EVENTS CENTER
715 Quince Street
Florence, OR 97439
Phone: 541-997-1994
Fax: 541-902-0991
e-mail: gmgr@eventcenter.org
Web Site: www.eventscenter.org
Management:
    Director: Kevin Rhodes
    Community Outreach Manager: Lis Farm
Mission: The mission is to provide multi cultural enrichment to the community; to provide a welcoming, accessible facility for residents and visitors; and to promote events and conventions of the benefit of the greater Florence areas economy
Founded: 1996
Paid Staff: 3
Seating Capacity: 457
Year Built: 1996

7759 FLORENCE PERFORMING ARTS
PO Box 3287
Florence, OR 97439
Phone: 541-997-2128
e-mail: jrincon@harbourside.com

7760 PACIFIC UNIVERSITY
2043 College Way
Forest Grove, OR 97116
Phone: 503-359-2925
Fax: 503-359-2252
e-mail: thatchep@pacificu.edu

7761 PACIFIC UNIVERSITY: TOM MILES THEATRE
2043 College Way
Forest Grove, OR 97116
Phone: 503-359-2200
Fax: 503-359-2242

7762 THEATRE IN THE GROVE
2028 Pacific Avenue
PO Box 263
Forest Grove, OR 97116
Phone: 503-359-5349

7763 LAKE OSWEGO PARKS & REC
PO Box 369
Lake Oswego, OR 97304
Phone: 503-636-9673
Fax: 503-697-6579
e-mail: cic@ci.oswego.or.us
Web Site: www.ci.oswego.or.us

7764 LAKEWOOD CENTER FOR THE ARTS
368 S State Street
PO Box 274
Lake Oswego, OR 97034
Phone: 503-635-6338
Fax: 503-635-2002
e-mail: center.info@lakewood-center.org
Web Site: www.lakewood-center.org
Management:
    Executive Director: Andrew Edwards

7765 YAMHILL COUNTY FAIRGROUNDS
2070 Lafayette Avenue
McMinville, OR 97128
Phone: 503-434-7524
Fax: 503-435-1860
e-mail: ycec@onlinemac.com
Web Site: www.yamhillcountyfair.com
Officers:
    Board Member: Bruce Distler
    Fair Board Chairman: Larry Collver
    Secretary: Gary Wetz
    Fair Board Vice Chairman: Russ Christensen
Management:
    Fairgrounds Manager: Darcie Vanderyacht
    Maintenance Foreman: Kevin Rose
Mission: Yamhill County Fair and Rodeo, horse Shows, Weddings, Wedding Receptions, Horse Boarding, Concerts, Canine Training, Master Gardeners Test Garden, Saturday Market, Talent Contests during Yamhill County Fair, Flea Maret and Rodeo.
Founded: 1854
Paid Staff: 2
Volunteer Staff: 6
Income Sources: Horseshows; Horseboarding; Fairs & Rodeos; USDA or Lottery; Receptions; Weddings; Banquets
Performs At: Fairgrounds
Seating Capacity: 4,000
Rental Contact: Darcie Vanderyacht

7766 CRATERIAN GINGER ROGERS THEATER
23 S Central Avenue
Medford, OR 97501
Phone: 541-779-8195
Fax: 541-779-8175
e-mail: stephen@craterian.org
Web Site: www.craterian.org
Mission: To present national, international and local performing artists to foster the development of the performing arts, to serve as a multi-purpose community center.
Founded: 1991
Specialized Field: Performing arts presentation and rental venue
Paid Staff: 7
Volunteer Staff: 120

7767 MCARTHUR SPORTS FIELD
Western Oregon University
345 N Monmouth
Monmouth, OR 97631
Phone: 503-838-8000
Fax: 503-838-8370
Web Site: www.wou.edu
Management:
   Athletic Director: Jon Carey
   Sports Information Director: Russ Blunck
Seating Capacity: 2,500

7768 WESTERN OREGON UNIVERSITY
345 Monmouth Avenue
Monmouth, OR 97361
Phone: 503-838-8462
Fax: 503-838-8995

7769 NEWPORT PERFORMING ARTS CENTER
777 W Olive Street
PO Box 1315
Newport, OR 97365
Phone: 541-265-9231
Fax: 541-265-9464
Toll-free: 888-701-7123
e-mail: occa@coastarts.org
Web Site: coastarts.org
Specialized Field: Theatre, Music, Dance, Film, Literary
Facility Category: Live performance venue
Type of Stage: Proscenium
Stage Dimensions: 23 x 42
Seating Capacity: 393
Year Built: 1988
Year Remodeled: 2000
Rental Contact: Jan Eastman
Resident Groups: 8 major resident presenting organizations

7770 PENDLETON CONVENTION CENTER
1601 Westgate
Pendleton, OR 97801
Phone: 541-276-6569
Fax: 541-278-1317
Toll-free: 800-863-9358
e-mail: pkennendy@oregontrail.net
Web Site: www.pendleton.or.us/pcc.htm
Management:
   Director: Pat Kennedy
Founded: 1991
Specialized Field: Columbia River Basin
Paid Staff: 4
Seating Capacity: 128,193

7771 COMMUNITY MUSIC CENTER: DAVID CAMPBELL RECITAL HALL
3350 SE Francis
Portland, OR 97202
Phone: 530-823-3177
Fax: 530-823-3178

7772 EARLE A CHILES CENTER
5000 N Willamette Boulevard
Portland, OR 97203
Phone: 503-943-7523
Fax: 503-943-7451
Toll-free: 800-227-4568
e-mail: reed@up.edu
Web Site: www.up.edu
Management:
   University Events: Bill Reed
   Chiles Center Building Manager: Bill Reed
Founded: 1901

7773 KELLER AUDITORIUM
1111 SW Broadway
Portland, OR 97205
Phone: 503-248-4335
Fax: 503-274-7490
e-mail: lori@pcpa.com
Web Site: www.pcpa.com
Management:
   Booking Manager: Lori Kramer
   Operations Manager: Don Scorby
   Events Manager: Patricia Iron
   Box Office Manager: Ron Sanders
   Director: Robyn Williams
   Booking Coordinator: Judy Siemssen
Paid Staff: 150
Volunteer Staff: 600
Annual Attendance: 400,000
Facility Category: Theatre
Type of Stage: Proscenium
Seating Capacity: 2,992
Year Built: 1952
Year Remodeled: 1968
Rental Contact: Booking Manager Lori Kramer

7774 LEWIS AND CLARK COLLEGE
MSC 37
Portland, OR 97219
Phone: 503-768-7216
Fax: 503-768-7205
e-mail: mford@lclark.edu

7775 MEMORIAL COLISEUM
1 Center Court
Suite 20
Portland, OR 97227
Phone: 503-235-8771
Fax: 507-736-2187
e-mail: facilitymarketing@rosequarters.com
Web Site: www.rosequarter.com
Management:
   SVP: J Isaac
   VP/Facility Sales/Marketing: Jim McCue
   General Manager: Ron Woodbridge
Seating Capacity: 12,500

7776 NEW ROSE THEATRE
904 SW Main Street
Portland, OR 97205
Phone: 503-781-2061

7777 PGE PARK
1844 SW Madison Street
Portland, OR 97205
Phone: 503-248-4345
Fax: 503-221-3983
Web Site: www.civicstadium.com
Management:
   General Manager: Barry Strasacci
Seating Capacity: 30,500

7778 PORTLAND CENTER FOR THE PERFORMING ARTS
222 SW Clay Street
Portland, OR 97201
Phone: 503-248-4335
Fax: 503-247-7490

7779 PORTLAND CIVIC STADIUM
1844 SW Morrison
Portland, OR 97205
Phone: 503-244-8434
Fax: 503-221-3983
Web Site: www.civicstadium.org
Management:
   Operations Manager: Eric Eriksen
   Interim Stadium Manager: Barry J Strafacci
Founded: 1923
Seating Capacity: 13,000

7780 PORTLAND INSTITUTE FOR CONTEMPORARY ART
219 NW 12th Avenue
#100
Portland, OR 97209
Phone: 503-242-1419
Web Site: www.pica.org

7781 REED COLLEGE: REED THEATRE
3203 Southeast Woodstock
Portland, OR 97202
Phone: 503-771-1112
Fax: 503-777-7769
Web Site: http://web.reed.edu

Paid Staff: 4

7782 ROSE GARDEN
1 Center Court
Suite 200
Portland, OR 97227
e-mail: facilitymarketing@rosequarter.com
Officers:
   Supervisor Business Affairs: J Isaac
   CFO: Jim Kotchik
   Executive VP: Erin Hubert
   VP Sales/Marketing: Jim McCue
Seating Capacity: 20,300

7783 ROSE QUARTER
1 Center Court
Suite 200
Portland, OR 97227
Phone: 503-235-8771
Fax: 503-736-2187
Web Site: www.rosequarter.com
Management:
   VP/General Manager: Ron Woodbridge
   SVP/Business Affairs: J Isaac
   SVP/Marketing: Harry Holt
   Sr VP/CFO: Jim Kotchik
   VP/Cutting Edge Concepts: Mark Lewis
   VP/General Counsel: Mike Fennel
   VP/Facility Sales/Marketing: Jim McCue
   VP/Marketing/Communications: Marta Monetti
   VP/Sponsorship Sales: Erin Hubert
Seating Capacity: 12,000

7784 WILSON CENTER FOR THE PERFORMING ARTS
1111 SW 10th
Portland, OR 97205
Phone: 503-746-9293

7785 SEASIDE CIVIC AND CONVENTION CENTER
415 1st Avenue
Seaside, OR 97138
Phone: 503-738-8585
Fax: 503-738-0197
e-mail: gretchen@theoregonshore.com
Web Site: www.datsop.com/convention
Management:
   Manager: Karen Wilson

Pennsylvania

7786 J BIRNEY CRUM STADIUM
31 S Penn Street
Allentown, PA 18105
Phone: 610-821-2604
Fax: 610-821-2628

7787 SYMPHONY HALL
23 N 6th Street
Allentown, PA 18103

Phone: 610-432-6715
Fax: 610-432-6009

7788 MISHLER THEATRE
1208 12th Avenue
Altoona, PA 16601
Phone: 814-942-4728

7789 NEUMANN COLLEGE
1 Neumann Drive
Aston, PA 19014-1298
Phone: 610-558-5626
Fax: 610-558-5644
e-mail: rrobinso@smtpgate.neumann.edu
Web Site: www.neumann.edu
Management:
    Cultural Programming Coordinator: Lisa Cadorette
Performs At: Meagher Theatre

7790 MORAVIAN COLLEGE: MUSIC INSTITUTE
1200 Main Street
Bethlehem, PA 18018
Phone: 610-861-1650
Fax: 610-861-1657
e-mail: menec01@moravian.edu
Web Site: www.moravian.edu
Management:
    Assistant Dean: Nancy Clark

7791 STABLER ARENA
Lehigh University
124 Goodman Drive
Bethlehem, PA 18015
Phone: 610-758-3770
Fax: 610-866-8070
Web Site: www.stablerarena.com
Management:
    Director: Richard Fritz
    Event Coodinator: Darius Dunn
Seating Capacity: 6,700

7792 TOUCHSTONE THEATRE
321-323 E 4th Street
Bethlehem, PA 18015
Phone: 610-867-1689
Fax: 610-867-0561

7793 LEHIGH UNIVERSITY: ZOELLNER ARTS CENTER
420 E Packer Avenue
Bethlehem, PA 18015
Phone: 610-758-5323
Fax: 610-758-6537
e-mail: els7@lehigh.edu
Web Site: www.lehigh.edu/zoellner
Management:
    Managing Director: Elizabeth Scofield
    Programming Director: Deborah Sacarahs
    Production Manager: Joshua Kovar
    Audience Services Director: Sandra Anderson

Mission: Performing arts venue presents guest artists and academic groups.
Founded: 1997
Specialized Field: Performing
Paid Staff: 20
Volunteer Staff: 150
Paid Artists: 18
Non-paid Artists: 500
Budget: $400,000
Income Sources: Ticket Revenues; Grants; Development; Rentals
Performs At: Baker Hall; Diamond Theater; Black Box Theatre; Presenting Series
Annual Attendance: 43,000
Type of Stage: Proscenium
Stage Dimensions: 37x25
Seating Capacity: 1,000
Year Built: 1997
Architect: 33,000,000
Rental Contact: Annette Stolte

7794 BRADFORD CREATIVE & PERFORMING ARTS CENTER
PO Box 153
Bradford, PA 16701f
Phone: 814-362-2522
Fax: 814-368-7040
e-mail: jjg@penn.com
Web Site: www.bcpac.com
Management:
    President: James D Guelfi

7795 WIDENER UNIVERSITY: ALUMNI AUDITORIUM/BERT AUDITORIUM
1 University Place
Chester, PA 19013
Phone: 610-499-1102
Fax: 610-499-1155

7796 MARWICK-BOYD AUDITORIUM
Clarion University
Clarion, PA 16214
Phone: 814-226-2000
Fax: 814-393-1623

7797 UPPER DARBY PERFORMING ARTS CENTER
4820 Drexelbrook Drive
Drexel Hill, PA 19026-5305
Phone: 610-284-5861
Fax: 610-394-9502
e-mail: harryd1@bellatlantic.net
Management:
    Director: Harry Dietzler

7798 STATE THEATRE CENTER FOR THE ARTS
27 E Main Street
Easton, PA 15401

Phone: 610-258-7766
Fax: 610-258-2570
e-mail: stcfta@hhs.net
Web Site: www.statetheatrecenter.org
Management:
  Executive Director: Christine Wagner
  Administrative Assistant: Kathleen Loomis
  Box Office Manager: Suzanne Baron
  Accounts Coordinator: Debra Grimm
  Stage Manager: Erica Miller
  Technical Director: Leonard Baron
Founded: 1989
Annual Attendance: 10,000
Facility Category: Performing Arts Theatre
Seating Capacity: 1,400
Year Built: 1922
Year Remodeled: 2000

7799 ERIE COUNTY CONVENTION CENTER AUTHORITY: WARNER THEATRE

811 State Street
PO Box 6140
Erie, PA 16512
Phone: 814-452-4857
Fax: 814-455-9931
e-mail: ecccasey@erie.net
Web Site: www.erieciviccenter.com
Management:
  Executive Director: John Casey Wells
Founded: 1931
Budget: $600,000
Annual Attendance: 140,000
Facility Category: Historic Performing Arts Center
Type of Stage: Proscenium
Stage Dimensions: 60x32
Seating Capacity: 2506
Year Built: 1931
Cost: $ 1.5 Milion

7800 ERIE CIVIC CENTER: LJ TULLIO CONVENTION HALL

811 State Street
PO Box 6140
Erie, PA 16512
Phone: 814-452-4857
Fax: 814-455-9931

7801 MERCYHURST COLLEGE: D'ANGELO PERFORMING ARTS CENTER

501 E 38th Street
Erie, PA 16546
Phone: 814-824-3000
Fax: 814-824-3098
e-mail: mfuhrman@mercyhurst.edu
Web Site: www.mercyhurst.edu
Management:
  Manager: Michael J Fuhrman

7802 TOTEM POLE PLAYHOUSE

PO Box 603
Fayetteville, PA 17222-0603

Phone: 717-352-2164
Fax: 717-352-8870
Toll-free: 888-805-7056
e-mail: boxoffice@totempoleplayhouse.org
Web Site: www.totemplayhouse.org

7803 MUSSELMAN STADIUM

Gettysburg College
300 N Washington Street
Gettysburg, PA 17325
Phone: 717-337-6000
Fax: 717-337-6528
Web Site: www.gettysburg.edu
Management:
  Athletic Director: Chuck Winters
Seating Capacity: 6,000

7804 PALACE THEATRE

Center for the Performing Arts
21 W Otterman Street
Greensburg, PA 15601
Phone: 724-836-8000

7805 FARM SHOW ARENA

2301 N Cameron Street
Harrisburg, PA 17110
Phone: 717-787-5373
Fax: 717-783-8710
Web Site: www.pda.state.pa.us
Management:
  Director: Dennis L Grumbine
  Soccer Manager: Gregg Cook
  American Rodeo Association Manager: Chris Sciabica
Specialized Field: Home of the Harrrisburg Heat (NPSL)
Seating Capacity: 7,400
Year Built: 1938

7806 STATE MUSEUM OF PENNSYLVANIA

The State Museum of Pennsylvania
300 N Street
Harrisburg, PA 17120-0024
Phone: 717-787-4979
Fax: 717-783-7842
e-mail: museum@statemuseumpa.org
Web Site: www.statemuseumpa.org
Management:
  Director: Anita Blackaby
  Community Relations: Gina McLean-Linton
Mission: To collect and preserve artifacts illustrating the Commonwealth's history and to interpret our heritage through exhibits and programs; to highlight Pennsylvania artists and performers.
Facility Category: Auditorium

7807 WHITAKER CENTER FOR SCIENCE AND THE ARTS

222 Market Street
Harrisburg, PA 17101
Mailing Address: 301 Market Street Harrisburg PA 17101
Phone: 717-221-8201

Fax: 717-221-8208
e-mail: skrempasky@whitakercenter.org
Web Site: www.whitaker center.org
Officers:
  VP Theater Operations: Stephen F Krempasky
Paid Staff: 12
Volunteer Staff: 75
Facility Category: Theater
Type of Stage: Proscenium
Stage Dimensions: 45 x 80
Seating Capacity: 636
Year Built: 1997

7808 HERSHEY THEATRE
15 E Caracas Avenue
Hershey, PA 17033
Phone: 717-534-3411

7809 MOUNTAIN PLAYHOUSE
PO Box 205
Jennerstown, PA 15547
Phone: 814-629-9201
Fax: 814-629-6221
e-mail: boxoffice@mountainplayhouse.com
Web Site: www.mountainplayhouse.com

7810 POINT STADIUM
City Hall Recreation Department
401 Main Street
Johnstown, PA 15901
Phone: 814-533-2104
Fax: 814-833-2111
Management:
  Manager: Karl Kilduff
Volunteer Staff: +
Seating Capacity: 10,500

**7811 UNIVERSITY OF PITTSBURGH AT
JOHNSTOWN: PASQUERILLA
PERFORMING ARTS CENTER**
450 Schoolhouse Road
Johnstown, PA 15904
Phone: 814-269-7200
Fax: 814-269-7240
Toll-free: 800-846-2787
e-mail: upjarts@pitt.edu
Web Site: www.arts-center.upj.pitt.edu
Management:
  Executive Director: Patricia Carnevali

7812 OPEN AIR THEATRE
Longwood Gardens
PO Box 501
Kennett Square, PA 19348
Phone: 610-388-1000

**7813 KUTZTOWN UNIVERSITY: SCHAEFFER
AUDITORIUM**
College Hill
Kutztown, PA 19530
Phone: 610-683-4060
Fax: 215-683-4671

**7814 BUCKNELL UNIVERSITY: WEIS
CENTER PERFORMANCE SERIES**
Weis Center for the Performing Arts
Bucknell University
Lewisburg, PA 17837-2005
Phone: 570-577-3700
Fax: 570-577-3701
e-mail: boswell@bucknell.edu
Web Site: http://www.departments.bucknell.edu
Management:
  Director Cultural Events: William Boswell
Mission: To provide the campus and region with
opportunity for exposure to the essential cultural and
educational values inherent in the great historical and
radical traditions of the performing arts.
Founded: 1846
Budget: $150,000-400,000
Affiliations: APAP, CMA, PA Presenters, Others
Annual Attendance: 9000
Facility Category: Concert Hall
Type of Stage: Sprung Wood Floor
Seating Capacity: 1,200+
Year Built: 1988

7815 MILLBROOK PLAYHOUSE
Country Club Lane
PO Box 161
Mill Hall, PA 17751
Phone: 570-748-8083
Web Site: www.millbrookplayhouse.org
Season: May - August

7816 LACKAWANNA COUNTY STADIUM
235 Montage Mountain Road
Moosic, PA 18507
Phone: 570-969-2255
Fax: 570-963-6564
Web Site: www.redbarons.com
Management:
  Director: Rick Muntean
Founded: 1989
Seating Capacity: 10,800

7817 POCONO PLAYHOUSE
Playhouse Lane
Mountainhome, PA 18342
Phone: 570-595-7456
Fax: 570-595-7465

7818 BUCKS COUNTY PLAYHOUSE
70 S Main
PO Box 313
New Hope, PA 18938
Phone: 215-862-2041
Fax: 215-862-0220

**7819 WESTMINSTER COLLEGE: BEEGHLY
THEATER**
New Wilmington, PA 16172
Phone: 724-946-8761

7820 WESTMINSTER COLLEGE: WILL W ORR AUDITORIUM
Market Street
New Wilmington, PA 16172
Phone: 724-946-8761

7821 MCCARTHY STADIUM
Lasalle Iniversity
1900 W Oleny Avenue, PO Box 805
Philadelohia, PA 19141-1199
Phone: 215-951-1694
Fax: 215-951-1694
e-mail: athletics@lasalle.edu
Web Site: www.lasalle.edu
Management:
   Director Athletics: Tom Brennan
Seating Capacity: 7,500

7822 ACADEMY OF MUSIC
Broad and Locust Streets
Philadelphia, PA 19102
Phone: 215-893-1935
Fax: 215-545-4588

7823 ACADEMY OF MUSIC: HALL
Broad and Locust Streets
Philadelphia, PA 19102
Phone: 215-893-1935
Fax: 215-545-4588

7824 ACADEMY OF MUSIC: MAIN AUDITORIUM
Broad and Locust Streets
Philadelphia, PA 19102
Phone: 215-893-1935
Fax: 215-545-4588

7825 CURTIS INSTITUTE OF MUSIC
1724 Locust Street
Philadelphia, PA 19103
Phone: 215-893-5252
Fax: 215-839-0537

7826 FIRST UNION SPECTRUM
3601 S Broad Street
Philadelphia, PA 19148
Phone: 215-336-3600
Fax: 215-389-9506
Web Site: www.comcast-spectator.com
Management:
   President: Peter Luukko
   VP Marketingducer: Bob Schwartz
Seating Capacity: 18,000
Year Built: 1965

7827 FORREST THEATRE
1114 Walnut Street
Philadelphia, PA 19107
Phone: 215-923-1515

7828 MANN CENTER FOR THE PERFORMING ARTS
123 S Broad Street
Suite 1930
Philadelphia, PA 19109
Phone: 215-546-7900
Fax: 215-546-9524
Web Site: www.manncenter.org
Management:
   President: Peter B Lane
   General Manager: Jerry W Grasey
   Director Marketing/Performance: Rosie Vergilio
   Director Development: Nancy Newman
Founded: 1925
Specialized Field: Presenter, venue address: 52nd and Parkside
Status: Nonprofit
Paid Staff: 7
Budget: $4.2 Million
Income Sources: Ticket sales, grants, sponsorships
Annual Attendance: 275,000
Facility Category: Amphitheatre
Type of Stage: Proscenium
Stage Dimensions: 263 x 200 x 107
Year Remodeled: 1975
Rental Contact: Director Marketing & Dprogramming Rosie Vergilio

7829 MERRIAM THEATER
250 S Broad Street
Philadelphia, PA 19102
Phone: 215-732-5446
Fax: 215-732-1396
Toll-free: 888-451-5761
e-mail: merriumtheater@juno.com
Web Site: www.broadwayseries.com
Management:
   General Manager: DeVida Jenkins
   Marketing Director: Collie Andrew
Founded: 1987
Paid Staff: 35
Income Sources: Ticket Sales
Performs At: Procenium Theater
Annual Attendance: 301,847
Facility Category: Road House
Type of Stage: Proscenium
Stage Dimensions: 45'x25',44'x85'
Seating Capacity: 1870
Year Built: 1910
Year Remodeled: 1986
Rental Contact: General Manager DeVida Jenkins

7830 PAINTED BRIDE
230 Vine Street
Philadelphia, PA 19104
Phone: 215-925-9914
Fax: 215-925-7402
Web Site: www.paintedbride.org
Management:
   Executive Director: Laurel Raczka
   Director Programs: Ellen Rosenholtz
   Communications Director: Lisa Nelson

Mission: The Painted Bride Art Center works with artists to create and present programs that affirm the intrinsic values of all cultures, the inspirational and healing powers of the arts, and their ability to effect social change.
Founded: 1969
Specialized Field: Multi-Disciplinary
Paid Staff: 15

7831 REGIONAL PERFORMING ARTS CENTER

260 S Broad Street
Suite 901
Philadelphia, PA 19102
Phone: 215-790-5800
Fax: 215-790-5801
e-mail: lschwartz@rpac.org
Web Site: www.kimmelcenter.org
Management:
    Booking Manager: Lilly Schwartz
    Assistant Director Marketing: Tiffany Madden
Mission: The Regional Performing Arts Center manages The Kimmel Center for the Performing Arts Academy of Music in Philadelphia, and presents a wide variety of programming including jazz, dance, theatre, classical and world music.
Specialized Field: Facility/Presenter

7832 SOCIETY HILL PLAYHOUSE

507 S 8th Street
Philadelphia, PA 19147
Phone: 215-923-0210
Fax: 215-923-1789
e-mail: SHP@erols.com
Web Site: www.societyhillplayhouse.com

7833 SPECTRUM

Pattison Place
Philadelphia, PA 19148
Phone: 215-336-3600

7834 TEMPLE UNIVERSITY

Esther Boyer College of Music
Philadelphia, PA 19122
Phone: 215-204-8301
Fax: 215-204-4957
Officers:
    Associate Dean: Steven Kreinberg

7835 UNIVERSITY OF PENNSYLVANIA: THE PALESTRA

233 S 33rd Street
Philadelphia, PA 19104
Phone: 215-898-6121
Fax: 215-898-6117
Web Site: www.upenn.edu/athletics
Management:
    Athletic Director: Steve Bilsky
Seating Capacity: 8,700

7836 UNIVERSITY OF PENNSYLVANIA: FRANKLIN FIELD

University of Pennsylvania
235 S 33rd Street
Philadelphia, PA 19104
Phone: 215-898-9231
Fax: 215-573-2161
e-mail: kowalski@pobox.upenn.edu
Web Site: www.pennathletics.com
Management:
    Director: Dave Bryan
    Associate Director: Peggy Kowalski
Specialized Field: Home of University of Pennsylvania athletics (NCAA). Site of the Penn Relays, one of the largest track and field events in the country.
Seating Capacity: 52,593
Year Built: 1996

7837 VETERANS STADIUM

3501 S Broad Street
Philadelphia, PA 19148
Phone: 215-463-2500
Fax: 215-393-5464
Management:
    Director Sales: Rory McNeil
    Ogden Entertainment Services: Brian Hastings
    VP/Sales: Vic Gregovitz
    Director Penthouse Operations: Christy Noyalas
Seating Capacity: 62,382

7838 WALNUT STREET THEATRE

825 Walnut
Philadelphia, PA 19107
Phone: 215-574-3550
Fax: 215-574-3598
e-mail: wstpc@erols.com
Web Site: www.wstonline.org

7839 WALNUT STREET THEATRE: MAINSTAGE

825 Walnut
Philadelphia, PA 19107
Phone: 215-574-3550
Fax: 215-574-3598
e-mail: wstpc@erols.com
Web Site: www.wstonline.org

7840 WALNUT STREET THEATRE: STUDIO 3

825 Walnut
Philadelphia, PA 19107
Phone: 215-574-3550
Fax: 215-574-3598
e-mail: wstpc@erols.com
Web Site: www.wstonline.org

7841 WALNUT STREET THEATRE: STUDIO 5

825 Walnut
Philadelphia, PA 19107
Phone: 215-574-3550
Fax: 215-574-3598
e-mail: wstpc@erols.com
Web Site: www.wstonline.org

7842 BENEDUM CENTER
719 Liberty Avenue
Pittsburgh, PA 15222
Phone: 412-456-2600
Fax: 412-456-2645
e-mail: ciavarra@pgharts.org
Web Site: www.pgharts.org
Specialized Field: Performing Arts
Paid Staff: 18
Volunteer Staff: 550
Facility Category: Proscenium theater
Type of Stage: FIR
Stage Dimensions: 75x142
Seating Capacity: 2,889
Year Built: 1927
Year Remodeled: 1987
Cost: $42 million
Rental Contact: Gene Ciavarra

7843 CARNEGIE: LECTURE HALL
4400 Forbes Avenue
Pittsburgh, PA 15213
Phone: 412-622-3360
Fax: 412-688-8664

7844 CARNEGIE: MUSEUM OF ART THEATRE
4400 Forbes Avenue
Pittsburgh, PA 15213
Phone: 412-622-3360
Fax: 412-688-8664

7845 CARNEGIE: MUSIC HALL
4400 Forbes Avenue
Pittsburgh, PA 15213
Phone: 412-622-3360
Fax: 412-688-8664

7846 DUQUESNE UNIVERSITY TAMBURITZANS
1801 Boulevard of the Allies
Pittsburgh, PA 15219
Phone: 412-396-5185
Fax: 412-396-5583
e-mail: stafura@duq.edu
Web Site: www.tamburitzans.duq.edu
Management:
    Director: Paul Stafura

7847 FITZGERALD FIELDHOUSE
University of Pittsburgh
Pittsburgh, PA 15213
Phone: 412-648-8200
Fax: 412-648-8306
Management:
    Athletic Director: Steve Pederson

7848 HEINZ HALL FOR THE PERFORMING ARTS
600 Penn Avenue
Pittsburgh, PA 15222
Phone: 412-392-4800
Fax: 412-392-4909

7849 MANCHESTER CRAFTSMEN'S GUILD
1815 Metropolitan Street
Pittsburgh, PA 15233
Phone: 412-322-1773
Web Site: www.artsnet.org/mcg/

7850 MELLON ARENA
300 Auditorium Place
Pittsburgh, PA 15219
Phone: 412-642-2062
Fax: 412-562-9913
Web Site: www.civiccenter.com
Management:
    Directir: Rich Engler
Seating Capacity: 18,000

7851 PITTSBURGH CIVIC ARENA
Gate Number 9
66 Mariolemieux Place
Pittsburgh, PA 15219
Phone: 412-642-1800
Fax: 412-642-1925
Web Site: www.civicarena.com
Management:
    General Manager: Hank Abate
    Director Operations: Jay Roberts
    Comcessions Manager: Rob Sunday
Seating Capacity: 17,500

7852 PNC PARK
600 Stadium Circle
Pittsburgh, PA 15212
Phone: 412-323-5000
Fax: 412-323-5009
Web Site: www.pirateball.com
Management:
    VP New Ballpark Development: Steve Greenberg
Seating Capacity: 38,127

7853 UNIVERSITY OF PITTSBURGH: PITT STADIUM
University of Pittsburgh
PO Box 7436
Pittsburgh, PA 15213-0436
Phone: 412-648-8200
Fax: 412-648-8306
Management:
    Athletic Director: Steve Pederson
    Excutive Athletic Director: Marc Boehm
    Senior Associate Athletic Director: Carol Sprague
    Associate Athletics for Business: Jim Earle
Seating Capacity: 56,500

7854 RAJAH THEATRE
136 North Sixth Street
Reading, PA 19601
Phone: 610-371-8820
Fax: 610-371-8691

7855 SCRANTON CULTURAL CENTER AT THE MASONIC TEMPLE
420 North Washington Avenue
Scranton, PA 18503
Phone: 570-346-7369
Fax: 717-346-7365
Management:
    Executive Director: Jo Ann Freriotti
    Facility/Technical Director: John Cardoni
    Programming Director: Patricia Rosetti
Founded: 1996
Specialized Field: Mid Atlantic
Paid Staff: 12
Volunteer Staff: 100
Paid Artists: 50
Annual Attendance: 140,000+
Facility Category: Theatre
Stage Dimensions: 48x32x64
Seating Capacity: 2500
Year Built: 1927

7856 LAUREL ARTS/THE PHILIP DRESSLER CENTER
PO Box 414
214 S Harrison Avenue
Somerset, PA 15501-0414
Phone: 814-443-2433
Fax: 814-443-3870
e-mail: arts@laurelarts.org
Web Site: www.laurelarts.org
Management:
    Executive Director: George Fattman

7857 BRYCE JORDAN CENTER
Penn State University
127 Bryce Jordan Center
University Park, PA 16802
Phone: 814-865-5555
Fax: 814-863-5705
e-mail: jordancenter@psu.edu
Web Site: www.bjc.psu.edu

7858 PENN STATE UNIVERSITY BEAVER STADIUM
103 Bryce Jordan Center
University Park, PA 16802
Phone: 814-863-5500
Fax: 814-863-8569
Web Site: www.psu.edu
Management:
    Director Food & Beverage: Toby Scott
Specialized Field: Home of Penn State University athletics.
Seating Capacity: 93,500

7859 PENN STATE UNIVERSITY: CENTER FOR THE PERFORMING ARTS
Eisenhower Auditorium
University Park, PA 16802
Phone: 814-863-0388
Fax: 814-863-7218
e-mail: se523@psu.edu
Web Site: www.cpa.psu.edu
Mission: To enhance the community experience through the presentation of a diverse program of professional, high quality performing arts events; to support other University programs, productions and activities; to complement and supplement the academic programs of the College of Arts and Architecture; to provide cultural experiences that augment and enrich general education.
Organization Type: Performing; Presenting

7860 PENNSYLVANIA CENTRE STAGE
106 Arts Building
University Park, PA 16802
Phone: 814-863-0381
Fax: 814-863-7327
e-mail: wtdz@psm.edu
Season: June - August

7861 FARREL STADIUM
West Chester University
West Chester, PA 19383
Phone: 610-436-1000
Fax: 610-436-3275
Web Site: www.wecpa.edu
Management:
    Director Facility: Stephen Quigley

7862 FM KIRBY CENTER FOR THE PERFORMING ARTS
71 Public Square
Wilkes-Barre, PA 18701
Mailing Address: PO Box 486, Wilkes-Barre, PA. 18703
Phone: 570-823-4599
Fax: 570-823-4890
e-mail: kirby@tl.infi.net
Web Site: www.kirbycenter.org
Officers:
    Board Chairman: Robert Cioruttoli
    Vice Chairman: Denise Ceasare
    Treasurer: Dr. Wallace Steitler
Management:
    Executive Director: Marilyn Santarelli
    Program Manager: Bob Nocek
    Technical Director: Fran McMullen
    Director Operations: John Domzalski
Mission: To promote and present the performing arts in our region.
Founded: 1986
Budget: $400,000-$1,000,000
Performs At: Film, concerts, broadway
Type of Stage: Proscenium
Stage Dimensions: 47'3" x 30' x 30' deep30'
Seating Capacity: 1800
Year Built: 1936
Year Remodeled: 1986
Rental Contact: Director of Operations John Domzalski

7863 WILKES UNIVERSITY: DOROTHY DICKSON DARTE CENTER
S Street
Wilkes-Barre, PA 18766
Phone: 717-824-4651
Fax: 717-408-7842

7864 STRAND-CAPITOL PERFORMING ARTS CENTER
50 N George Street
York, PA 17401
Phone: 717-846-1155
Fax: 717-843-1208

Rhode Island

7865 UNIVERSITY OF RHODE ISLAND FINE ARTS CENTER
105 Upper College Road
Fine Arts Center
Kingston, RI 02881
Phone: 401-874-5921
Fax: 401-874-5618
Management:
   Chairman: Paula McGlasson
   Administrative Assistant: Bonnie Bosworth
Founded: 1950
Paid Staff: 4
Volunteer Staff: 20
Paid Artists: 10
Non-paid Artists: 10
Type of Stage: Proscenium; Black Box
Rental Contact: Bonnie Besworth

7866 AS220
115 Empire Street
Providence, RI 02903
Phone: 401-831-9327
Fax: 401-454-7445
e-mail: info@as220.org

7867 BROWN STADIUM
235 Hope Street
Providence, RI 02912
Phone: 401-863-2295
Fax: 401-863-1436
e-mail: tom_bold@brown.edu
Management:
   Athletic Director: David Roach

7868 PERISHABLE THEATRE
95 Empire Street
PO Box 23132
Providence, RI 02903
Phone: 401-331-2695
Fax: 401-331-7811
e-mail: info@perishable.org
Web Site: www.perishable.org
Management:
   Office Manager: Lauryn Sasso
   Artistic Director: Mark Lerman
Managing Director: Claudia Traub
PR Director: Marilyn Dubois
Mission: Perishable Theatre brings together artists from all media and provides them with the opportunity to perform and develop their craft. The theatre offers a mainstage season of new plays, a theatre arts school, and touring children's theatre.
Founded: 1982
Paid Staff: 12
Volunteer Staff: 4
Paid Artists: 20
Budget: $500,000
Performs At: Theatre Arts Center
Affiliations: TCG
Annual Attendance: 3,000
Facility Category: Performing Arts Center
Type of Stage: Black Box
Seating Capacity: 75

7869 PROVIDENCE CIVIC CENTER
1 LaSalle Square
Providence, RI 02903
Phone: 401-331-0700
Fax: 401-751-6792
Web Site: www.pov.cc.com
Management:
   CEO: Ed Anderson
Seating Capacity: 14,500

7870 PROVIDENCE PERFORMING ARTS CENTER
220 Weybosset Street
Providence, RI 02903
Phone: 401-421-2997
Fax: 401-421-5767
e-mail: info@ppacri.org
Web Site: www.ppari.org
Officers:
   President: JL Singleton
Management:
   General Manager: Alan Chille
Specialized Field: Touring Broadway, Concerts, Film

7871 TRINITY ARTS CENTER
55 Locust Street
Providence, RI 02906
Phone: 401-272-1595

7872 VETERANS MEMORIAL AUDITORIUM
Brownell Street and Park Streets
Providence, RI 02903
Phone: 401-831-3123
Fax: 401-277-1466

7873 STADIUM THEATRE PERFORMING ARTS CENTER
PO Box 665
28 Monument Square
Woonsocket, RI 02895
Phone: 401-762-4545
Fax: 401-765-4949
e-mail: stadiumpac@aol.com
Web Site: www.stadiumtheatre.com

Officers:
  Marketing Director: Jeffrey Polucha
  President: Robert P Picards
  Events Chairman/First VP: Jean Rondeau
  Second VP: Joan Gahan
  Secretary: Donna Palreiro
Founded: 1996
Paid Staff: 2
Volunteer Staff: 200
Income Sources: Rentals; Donations; Grants; Box Office
Performs At: Live theatre, classic films, local & national entertainment
Affiliations: Encore Repertory Company
Annual Attendance: 60,000-100,000
Facility Category: Performing arts center
Seating Capacity: 1100
Year Built: 1926
Year Remodeled: 2000
Cost: $2.5 Million
Rental Contact: Jean Rondeau
Resident Groups: Encore Reportory Company

South Carolina

7874 ABBEVILLE OPERA HOUSE
Court Square
PO Box 247
Abbeville, SC 29620
Phone: 864-459-8118
Fax: 803-459-9266

7875 FINE ARTS CENTER OF KERSHAW COUNTY
PO Box 1498
Camden, SC 29020
Phone: 803-425-7676
Fax: 803-425-7679
Web Site: www.fineartscenter.org
Management:
  Manager: Susan DuPlessis

7876 DOCK STREET THEATRE
135 Church Street
Charleston, SC 29401
Phone: 843-720-3968
Fax: 843-720-3967

7877 FOOTLIGHT PLAYERS THEATRE
20 Queen Street
PO Box 62
Charleston, SC 29401
Phone: 843-722-7521
Fax: 843-722-3777
e-mail: footlightplayers.aol.com
Web Site: www.footlightplayers.com
Officers:
  President: Hope Grayson
Management:
  Artistic Director: Sheri Grace Wenger
  Business Manager: Gail Pike
Founded: 1931
Specialized Field: Theatre

7878 GAILLARD MUNICIPAL AUDITORIUM
77 Calhoun Street
Charleston, SC 29403
Phone: 843-577-7400
Fax: 843-724-7389

7879 JOHNSON HAGOOD STADIUM
The Citadel Athletic Department
171 Moultrie Street
Charleston, SC 29409
Phone: 843-953-5030
Fax: 843-953-5058
Web Site: www.citadel.edu
Management:
  Assoociate Athletic Director: Ray Whiteman
Seating Capacity: 22,500

7880 MCALISTER FIELDHOUSE
The Citadel Athletic Department
171 Moultrie Street
Charleston, SC 29409
Phone: 843-503-0
Fax: 843-953-6727
Web Site: www.thecitadel.edu
Management:
  Assocaite Athletic Director: Robert Bennett
Seating Capacity: 6,000

7881 CLEMSON UNIVERSITY: BROOKS CENTER FOR THE PERFORMING ARTS
Clemson University
Box 340526
Clemson, SC 29634-0526
Phone: 864-656-3043
Fax: 864-656-1013
e-mail: harderl@clemson.edu
Web Site: www.clemson.edu/Brooks
Management:
  Director: Lillian U Harder

7882 CLEMSON UNIVERSITY: CLEMSON MEMORIAL STADIUM
602 University Union
PO Box 344056
Clemson, SC 29634
Phone: 864-656-5827
Fax: 864-656-1858
e-mail: mkern@clemson.edu
Web Site: www.clemson.edu
Management:
  Director: Marty Kern
Mission: Successfully produce area shows with capacity of 20,000-70,000

7883 CLEMSON UNIVERSITY: LITTLEJOHN COLISEUM
Jarvey Athletic Center
PO Box 31
Clemson, SC 29633
Phone: 864-646-1935
Fax: 864-646-0299
Management:

Director Programs/Services: Michael Arnold
Seating Capacity: 10,820

7884 KOGER CENTER FOR THE ARTS
University of South Carolina
Columbia, SC 29208
Phone: 803-777-7500
Fax: 803-777-5774

7885 UNIVERSITY OF SOUTH CAROLINA: LONGSTREET THEATRE
Green and Sumter Streets
Columbia, SC 29208
Phone: 803-777-4288

7886 UNIVERSITY OF SOUTH CAROLINA: CAROLINA COLISEUM
701 Assembly Street
Columbia, SC 29201
Phone: 803-777-5113
Fax: 803-777-5114
e-mail: jbolin@sc.edu
Web Site: www.coliseum.sc.edu
Management:
   Director: John Bolin
   Business Manager: Dick Marks
Specialized Field: Home to USC basketball.
Seating Capacity: 12,500
Year Built: 1969

7887 UNIVERSITY OF SOUTH CAROLINA: DRAYTON HALL
Green and Sumter Streets
Columbia, SC 29208
Phone: 803-777-4288

7888 WILLIAMS-BRICE STADIUM/UNIVERSITY OF SOUTH CAROLINA
701 Assembly Street
Couumbia, SC 29201
Phone: 704-223-8193
Fax: 704-233-8170
Web Site: www.wingate.edu
Management:
   Head Basketball Coach (W): Johnny Jacumin
   Managing Director/CEO: John C Bondi
   Director Marketing: Connie O Scrivens
   Athletic Director: Beth Lawrence
   Sports Information Director: David Sherwood
   Head Football Coach: Doug Malone
   Head Basketball Coach (M): Jeff Reynolds
Seating Capacity: 72,000

7889 FLORENCE CIVIC CENTER
3300 W Radio Drive
Floremce, SC 29501-7802
Phone: 843-679-9417
Fax: 843-679-9429
Web Site: www.florenceciviccenter.com
Management:
   General Manager: Mark Lavaway

7890 CHARLOTTE KNIGHTS BASEBALL STADIUM
2280 Deerfield Drive
Ft. Hill, SC 29716
Phone: 803-548-8050
Fax: 513-548-8055
e-mail: percival@aaaknights.com
Web Site: www.aaaknights.com
Management:
   Assistant General Manager/Facility: Jon Percival
   Assistant General Manager: Mark Viniard
Seating Capacity: 10,000
Year Built: 1990

7891 BI-LO CENTER
650 N Academy Street
Greenville, SC 29601
Phone: 864-241-3800
Fax: 864-250-4939
e-mail: erubinstein@biloctr.com
Web Site: www.bilocenter.com
Management:
   Executive Director: Ed Rubenstein
   Director Operations: Steve Chastain
   Marketing Director: Jill Weninger
Founded: 1998
Specialized Field: Sports and entertainment arena in upstate South Carolina.
Seating Capacity: 16,,d000
Year Built: 1998

7892 FURMAN UNIVERSITY: MCALISTER AUDITORIUM
Greenville, SC 29613
Phone: 864-294-2000
Fax: 864-294-3035

7893 GREENVILLE MUNICIPAL STADIUM
One Braves Avenue
Greenville, SC 29607
Phone: 864-299-3456
Fax: 864-277-7369
Web Site: www.gbraves.com
Management:
   General Manager: Steve Desalvo

7894 PEACE CENTER FOR THE PERFORMING ARTS
101 W Broad Street
Greenville, SC 29601
Phone: 864-467-3030
Fax: 864-467-3040
e-mail: MRiegel@peacecenter.org
Web Site: www.peacecenter.org
Officers:
   President: Megan Riegel
Mission: Providing a world-class home for Resident Companies
Founded: 1985
Specialized Field: Performing
Paid Staff: 130
Volunteer Staff: 57
Budget: $400,000

Income Sources: Board, Edowment, Patrons
Annual Attendance: 97,000
Facility Category: Performing Arts7
Type of Stage: Proscenium
Stage Dimensions: 34' x 58'
Seating Capacity: 2089
Year Built: 1985
Year Remodeled: 2002
Cost: 4 million
Rental Contact: Tom Bugg

7895 GREENWOOD CIVIC CENTER
PO Box 3008
Greenwood, SC 29648
Phone: 864-942-8606

7896 CENTER THEATER
212 N 5th Street
Hartsville, SC 29550
Phone: 843-332-5721

7897 NORTH CHARLESTON PERFORMING ARTS CENTER
5001 Coliseum Drive
North Charleston, SC 29418
Phone: 843-529-5050
Fax: 843-529-5020
e-mail: dholsher@knology.com
Web Site: www.coliseumpac.com
Officers:
    General Manager: Dave Holscher
Founded: 1999
Type of Stage: Proscenium
Seating Capacity: 2254
Year Built: 1999
Rental Contact: Dave Holscher

7898 SOUTH CAROLINA STATE UNIVERSITY
300 College Avenue
Orangeburg, SC 29115
Phone: 803-536-8998
Fax: 803-533-3661
Web Site: www.scsu.edu
Management:
    Athletics Director: Timothy Autry
Seating Capacity: 2,500

7899 WINTHROP COLLEGE: JAMES F BYRNES AUDITORIUM
Rock Hill, SC 29733
Phone: 803-323-2196
Fax: 803-323-3438

7900 SPARTANBURG MEMORIAL AUDITORIUM: ARENA
385 N Church Road
PO Box 1410
Spartanburg, SC 29304
Phone: 803-582-8107
Fax: 803-583-9850

7901 SPARTANBURG MEMORIAL AUDITORIUM: THEATRE
385 N Church Street
PO Box 1410
Spartanburg, SC 29304
Phone: 803-582-8107
Fax: 803-583-9850

7902 SUMTER COUNTY CULTURAL CENTER
135 Haynsworth
Sumter, SC 29150
Phone: 803-436-2260
Fax: 803-436-2258
e-mail: patriot_hall@sumtercountysc.org
Paid Staff: 4
Income Sources: Sumter County Government
Facility Category: Auditorium
Type of Stage: Proscenium
Stage Dimensions: 47wx21hx26-38l
Seating Capacity: 1,013
Year Built: 1935
Year Remodeled: 1986
Cost: $4 million
Rental Contact: Martha Greenway

7903 MCCELVEY CENTER OF YORK
PO Box 457
212 E Jefferson Street
York, SC 29745
Phone: 803-684-3948
Fax: 803-684-3599
e-mail: mccelvey@cetlink.net
Management:
    Director: Liz Funderburk

South Dakota

7904 COUGHLIN ALUMNI STADIUM
16th Avenue and 11th Street
Brookings, SD 57007
Phone: 605-688-5625
Fax: 605-688-5999
Management:
    Athletic Director: Fred Oien

7905 SOUTH DAKOTA ART MUSEUM
PO Box 2250
Brookings, SD 57007
Phone: 605-688-5423
Fax: 605-688-4445

7906 CORN PALACE
604 N Main Street
Mitchell, SD 57301
Phone: 605-996-5031
Fax: 605-996-8273
Web Site: www.compalace.org
Management:
    Director Sales: Dale Odegard

7907 RUSHMORE PLAZA CIVIC CENTER

444 Mount Rushmore Road N
Rapid City, SD 57701
Phone: 605-394-4115
Fax: 605-394-4119
e-mail: civicctr@rapidnet.com
Web Site: www.got.mine.com
Management:
    General Mmanager: Jim Walczak
Seating Capacity: 11,000

7908 SIOUX FALLS ARENA

Odgen Entertainment
1201 W Avenue N
Sioux Falls, SD 57104
Phone: 605-367-7288
Fax: 605-338-1463
Web Site: www.sfarena.com
Management:
    Executive Director: Russ Decurtins
    Assistant Director: Debra D Esche
Seating Capacity: 8,000

7909 SIOUX FALLS COLISEUM

600 E 7th Street
Sioux Falls, SD 57102
Phone: 605-367-7288
Fax: 605-338-1463

7910 SIOUX FALLS COMMUNITY PLAYHOUSE

315 N Phillips
PO Box 600
Sioux Falls, SD 57101
Phone: 605-336-7418
Fax: 605-336-2243

7911 WASHINGTON PAVILION OF ARTS & SCIENCE

301 S Main Avenue
Sioux Falls, SD 57104
Mailing Address: PO Box 984, Sioux Falls, SD.
57101-0984
Phone: 605-367-7397
Fax: 605-367-7399
Toll-free: 877-927-4728
e-mail: shoffman@washingtonpavilion.org
Web Site: www.washingtonpavilion.org
Management:
    Executive Director: Steven A Hoffman
    Director Marketing: Christen Rennich
    Sr Events Coordinator: Jeff Venekamp
    Director Operations: Jon Loos
Mission: To provide residents, students and visitors with a distinguished array of cultural, scientific and artistic experiences drawn from within and beyond the greater Sioux Falls area. The Washington Pavilion challenges, involves and educates audiences and motivates them to incorporate the arts, humanities and sciences into their daily lives.
Founded: 1999
Specialized Field: South Dakota, Northwest Iowa, Southwest Minnesota, Northeast Nebraska

Paid Staff: 150
Volunteer Staff: 230

7912 AMERICA'S SHRINE TO MUSIC MUSEUM

414 E Clark Street
Vermillion, SD 57069-2390
Phone: 605-677-5306
Fax: 605-677-5073
e-mail: smm@usd.edu
Web Site: www.usd.edu/smm
Management:
    Director: Andr, Larson

7913 UNIVERSITY OF SOUTH DAKOTA: SLAGLE AUDITORIUM

414 E Clark
Vermillion, SD 57069
Phone: 605-677-5481
Fax: 605-677-5988

7914 UNIVERSITY OF SOUTH DAKOTA: WARREN M LEE CENTER

414 E Clark
Vermillion, SD 57069
Phone: 605-677-5481
Fax: 605-677-5988

7915 UNIVERSITY OF SOUTH DAKOTA: DAKOTA DOME

Dakota Dome #205
414 E Clark
Vermillion, SD 57069
Phone: 605-677-5309
Fax: 605-677-5618
Web Site: www.usd.edu
Management:
    Athletic Director: Kelly Higgins

Tennessee

7916 VIKING HALL CIVIC CENTER

1100 Edgemont Avenue
Bristol, TN 37625
Phone: 423-764-4171
Fax: 423-765-3299
Web Site: www.vikinghal.com
Management:
    Director: Terrie Smith
    Box Office Manager: Tommy Baker
Seating Capacity: 6,200

7917 ROLAND HAYES CONCERT HALL

University of Tennessee
615 McCallie Avenue/FAC #324
Chattanooga, TN 37403
Phone: 423-755-4269
Fax: 615-755-5249

7918 TIVOLI THEATRE
709 Broad Street
Chattanooga, TN 37402
Phone: 423-757-5457
Fax: 615-757-5326

**7919 UNIVERSITY OF
TENNESSEE-CHATTANOOGA: UTC
MCKENZIE ARENA**
615 McCallie Avenue
Department 3403
Chattanooga, TN 37403
Phone: 423-755-4706
Fax: 423-755-4783
e-mail: ken-kapelinski@utc.edu
Web Site: www.utc.edu/utcarena
Management:
    Acting Director Arena: Ken Kapelinski
    Assistant Director: Obie Webster
Founded: 1982
Paid Staff: 15
Volunteer Staff: 30
Budget: $1.2 Million
Income Sources: Rental, Concessions, Services
Affiliations: University of Tennessee, Chatanooga
Annual Attendance: 240,000
Facility Category: Arena
Type of Stage: Flexible
Stage Dimensions: 64x48
Seating Capacity: 12,000
Year Built: 1982
Rental Contact: Ken Kapelinski

7920 DUNN CENTER
PO Box 4515
Clarksville, TN 37044
Phone: 931-221-7011
Fax: 931-221-7830
Web Site: www.apsu.edu
Management:
    Director: Roy Gregory

**7921 TENNESSEE TECH UNIVERSITY:
HOOPER EBLEN CENTER**
PO Box 5057
Cookeville, TN 38505
Phone: 931-372-3940
Fax: 931-372-3114
Management:
    Athletic Director: David Larimore

7922 TULANE UNIVERSITY
Tennessee Tech University
PO Box 5057
Cookeville, TN 38505
Phone: 931-372-3940
Fax: 931-372-3114
Management:
    Director: David Lorimore
Seating Capacity: 16,500

7923 JACKSON CIVIC CENTER
400 South Highland Avenue
Jackson, TN 38301
Phone: 901-425-8580
Fax: 901-425-8385

**7924 LAMBUTH COLLEGE: LAMBUTH
THEATRE**
Department of Theatre
705 Lamburth Boulevard
Jackson, TN 38301
Phone: 901-425-2500
Fax: 901-423-3493

7925 AMAN ARENA
City of Jackson
179 Lane Avenue
Jackson, TN 38301
Phone: 901-425-8390
Fax: 701-425-8390
Web Site: www.cj.jacksoin.tn.us
Management:
    Manager: Martha A Pope
Seating Capacity: 5,612

7926 FREEDOM HALL CIVIC CENTER
Liberty Bell Boulevard
Johnson City, TN 37604
Phone: 423-461-4855
Fax: 423-461-4867
e-mail: director@freedomhall-tn.com
Web Site: www.freedomhall-tn.com
Management:
    Director: Lisa Chamness
    Box Office Manager: Bobbie Shirley
Founded: 1974
Paid Staff: 7
Volunteer Staff: 100
Paid Artists: 125
Seating Capacity: 6,215

**7927 MILLIGAN COLLEGE: DERTHICK
THEATRE**
Johnson City, TN 37682
Phone: 423-461-8782
Fax: 423-461-8755

**7928 MILLIGAN COLLEGE: SEEGER
CHAPEL CONCERT HALL**
Johnson City, TN 37682
Phone: 423-461-8782
Fax: 423-461-8755

7929 MINI DOME
E Tennessee State University
Johnson City, TN 37614
Phone: 423-439-4343
Fax: 423-439-5294
Management:
    Director: Bill Toohey
Seating Capacity: 16,000

7930 BIJOU THEATRE CENTER
803 S Gay Street
Knoxville, TN 37901
Phone: 865-522-0832
Fax: 615-524-0821

7931 KNOXVILLE CIVIC AUDITORIUM AND COLISEUM-AUDITORIUM
500 East Howard Baker Jr. Avenue
PO Box 2603
Knoxville, TN 37915
Phone: 865-544-5399
Fax: 865-544-5386
Management:
   Event Services Coordinator: Robbie Sandoval
   General Manager: Dale Dunn
   Stage Manager: David Scruggs
Facility Category: Auditorium and Arena
Stage Dimensions: Auditorium 57x57x27, Arena 60x40
Seating Capacity: Auditorium- 2,500 Arena- 6,000
Year Built: 1961
Year Remodeled: 1987
Rental Contact: Robbie Sandoval

7932 NEYLAND STADIUM
University of Tennessee
1600 Stadium Drive
Knoxville, TN 37996
Phone: 723-974-0953
Fax: 423-974-2800
Management:
   Manager: Tim Reese
   Associtae Director Athletics: Robert J Dobell
Seating Capacity: 103,000

7933 TENNESSEE THEATER
604 S Gay Street
Knoxville, TN 37902
Phone: 865-522-1174
Fax: 615-523-3954

7934 THOMPSON-BOLING ARENA
University of Tennessee
1600 Stadium Drive, Suite 202
Knoxville, TN 37996
Phone: 423-974-0953
Fax: 423-974-2800
Web Site: www.knoxvilletickets.com
Management:
   Manager: Timothy L Reese
Seating Capacity: 24,451

7935 UNIVERSITY OF TENNESSEE MUSIC HALL
1741 Volunteer Boulevard
Knoxville, TN 37996
Phone: 865-974-5110

7936 CUMBERLAND UNIVERSITY AUDITORIUM
S Greenwood Street
Lebanon, TN 37087
Phone: 615-444-2562
Fax: 615-444-2569

7937 UNIVERSITY OF TENNESSEE-MARTIN: SKYHAWK ARENA
University of Tennessee-Martin
1020 Elam Center
Martin, TN 38238
Phone: 901-587-7745
Fax: 901-587-7725
Web Site: www.utm.edu
Management:
   Interim Director Campus Recreation: Gina Warren
Seating Capacity: 6,600

7938 MARYVILLE COLLEGE
Maryville, TN 37801
Phone: 865-981-8000
Fax: 865-981-8001
Toll-free: 800-597-2687

7939 EWING CHILDREN'S THEATRE
2599 Avery Avenue
Memphis, TN 38112
Phone: 901-452-3968
Fax: 901-452-3805
e-mail: ewingct1949@aol.com
Founded: 1949
Income Sources: Memphis Park Services
Annual Attendance: 10,000
Facility Category: Theatre
Type of Stage: Proscenium
Seating Capacity: 193
Year Built: 1982
Rental Contact: Kay Lightfoot

7940 LIBERTY BOWL MEMORIAL STADIUM
335 S Hollywood
Memphis, TN 38104
Phone: 901-729-4344
Fax: 901-276-2756
Web Site: www.libertybowl.org
Management:
   Managerr: Johnny Sowell
Seating Capacity: 64,000
Year Built: 1963
Year Remodeled: 1965

7941 MEMPHIS COOK CONVENTION CENTER COMPLEX
Cannon Center for the Performing Arts
255 N Main Street
Memphis, TN 38103
Phone: 901-576-1200
Fax: 901-576-1212
Toll-free: 800-726-0915
Web Site: www.memphisconvention.com
Management:
   Sales/Marketing Director: Debbi Forshee
Mission: They are a full service convention center with a performing arts center.
Founded: 1974

Seating Capacity: 2,100
Year Built: 2002

7942 MID-SOUTH COLISEUM
996 Early Maxwell Boulevard
Memphis, TN 38104
Phone: 901-274-3982
Fax: 901-276-8653
e-mail: fox@midsouthcoliseum.com
Web Site: www.midsouthcoliseum.com
Management:
  Managing Director: Alan Freemarl
  Assistant Director: Steve Fox
  Food/Beverage Manager: Jim Orcholski
Seating Capacity: 12,000

7943 ORPHEUM THEATRE
203 S Main Street
PO Box 3370
Memphis, TN 38173
Phone: 901-525-7800
Fax: 901-526-0829
e-mail: orpheumnt@aol.com
Web Site: www.orpheum-memphis.com
Officers:
  Chief Administrative Officer: Donna Darwin
Management:
  Director Education/Programs: Alica Donohoe
  Technical Director: Richard Reinach

7944 PYRAMID ARENA
One Auction Avenue
Memphis, TN 38105
Phone: 901-521-9675
Fax: 901-528-0153
Web Site: www.pyramidarena.com
Management:
  General Manager: Alan Freeman
  Assistant General Manager: Chuck Jabbour
  Office Manager/Booking Coordinator: Terri Knight
  Director Sales/Marketing: Greg Lowry
  Director Finance: Mary Burd
  Director Operations: Denise Brown
  Director Event Services: Eric Granger
  Box Office Manager: Anita Biles
Founded: 1991
Seating Capacity: 22,000

7945 THEATRE MEMPHIS
PO Box 240117
Memphis, TN 38124-0117
Phone: 901-682-8601
Fax: 901-763-4096
Web Site: www.theatrememphis.org
Management:
  Business Manager: David Allen
  Executive Producer: Ted Strickland
Founded: 1920
Status: Nonprofit
Paid Staff: 13
Paid Artists: 4
Budget: $1,100,000
Income Sources: Ticket sales, Contributions, Foundation
Season: Year-Round

Annual Attendance: 2,000
Type of Stage: Proscenium; Flexible
Seating Capacity: 424; 100
Year Built: 1975
Rental Contact: Administrative Asst.

7946 THEATRE GUILD
314 S Hill Street
Morristown, TN 37814
Phone: 423-586-9260

7947 TENNESSEE STATE UNIVERSITY: CHARLES M MURPHY ATHLETIC CENTER
Tennesse Boulevard
Box 203
Murfreesboro, TN 37132
Phone: 615-898-2873
Fax: 615-898-2873
Management:
  Director Activities: Harold Smith

7948 ADELPHIA STADIUM
1 Tittans Way
Nashville, TN 37213
Phone: 615-565-4000
Fax: 615-673-1524
Management:
  Director: Jerry Tuggle

7949 CHAFFIN'S BARN
8204 Highway 100
Nashville, TN 37221
Phone: 615-646-9977
Fax: 615-662-5439
Toll-free: 800-282-2276
e-mail: info@dinnertheatre.com
Web Site: www.dinnertheatre.com
Management:
  Managing Director: Angela Burnett
  Producer/Owner: John Chaffin
  Marketing Director: Martha Wilkinson
Facility Category: Dinner Theatre
Type of Stage: In the Round
Stage Dimensions: 16'x16'
Seating Capacity: 300
Year Built: 1967
Rental Contact: Regina Brock

7950 GAYLORD ENTERTAINMENT CENTER
501 Broadway
Nashville, TN 37203
Phone: 615-770-2000
Fax: 615-770-2010
e-mail: info@gaylordcenter.com
Web Site: www.gaylordentertainmentcenter.com
Management:
  Sr VP/General Manager: Russ Simons
  Assistant General Manager: Jeff Gaines
Specialized Field: Home of the Nashville Predators (NHL) and the Nashville Kats (AFL)
Seating Capacity: 17,298, 20,000
Year Built: 1996

7951 GRAND OLE OPRY HOUSE
2804 Opryland Drive
Nashville, TN 37214
Phone: 615-871-6612
Fax: 615-871-5719
e-mail: swilliams@opry.com
Web Site: www.opry.com
Management:
    Events Manager: Sally Williams
Founded: 1974
Facility Category: Threatre
Type of Stage: Procenium
Stage Dimensions: 80w x 60d
Seating Capacity: 4400
Year Built: 1974
Cost: 4,500 vs 12% gbr

7952 GREER STADIUM
534 Chestnut Street
Nashville, TN 37203
Phone: 615-242-4371
Fax: 615-256-5684
e-mail: chrissnyder@nashvillesounds.com
Web Site: www.nashvillesounds.com
Management:
    Manager: Chris Snyder
Founded: 1978
Paid Staff: 20

7953 LANGFORD AUDITORIUM
Garland Avenue
Nashville, TN 37232
Phone: 615-322-2170

7954 NASHVILLE CONVENTION CENTER
601 Commerce Street
Nashville, TN 37203
Phone: 615-742-2000
Fax: 615-742-2014
e-mail: conventionceter@metro.nashville.org
Web Site: www.nashvilleconventioncenter.com
Founded: 1987

7955 NASHVILLE JEWISH COMMUNITY CENTER
801 Percy Warner Boulevard
Nashville, TN 37205
Phone: 615-356-7170
Fax: 931-352-0056

7956 NASHVILLE MUNICIPAL AUDITORIUM
417 4th Avenue N
Nashville, TN 37201
Phone: 615-862-6392
Fax: 615-862-6394
e-mail: sharon.hill@metro.nashville.org
Web Site: www.nashville.org/ma
Management:
    Auditorium Manager: Robert C Skoney
    Sales Manager: Sharon Hill
    Operations Manager: Jim Raver
    Box Office Manager: Bill Williams
    Marketing Manager: Steve West
Founded: 1962
Paid Staff: 11
Annual Attendance: 500,000
Type of Stage: Portable
Stage Dimensions: 60' x 40'
Seating Capacity: 9,654
Year Built: 1962
Year Remodeled: 1995
Cost: $5 million
Rental Contact: Sharon Hill

7957 RYMAN AUDITORIUM
116 5th Avenue N
Nashville, TN 37219
Phone: 615-889-3060
Fax: 615-458-8701
e-mail: rymaninfo@oprylandusa.com
Web Site: www.ryman.com
Founded: 1892
Specialized Field: Museum; Concert Hall
Year Built: 1892
Year Remodeled: 1994
Rental Contact: Brian Gavron

7958 TENNESSEE PERFORMING ARTS CENTER
505 Deaderick Street
PO Box 190660
Nashville, TN 37219
Phone: 615-782-4000
Fax: 615-782-4001
e-mail: sgreil@tpac.org
Web Site: www.tpac.org
Officers:
    President/CEO: Steven J Greil
    Executive VP/Manager: Ted DeDee
Management:
    Executive VP: Ted DeDee
    President/CEO: Steven J Greil

7959 TENNESSEE PERFORMING ARTS CENTER: ANDREW JACKSON HALL
505 Deaderick Street
Nashville, TN 37219
Phone: 615-741-7975
Fax: 615-741-1266

7960 VANDERBILT STADIUM
M091920010 University
25th & Kensington Place
Nashville, TN 37212
Phone: 615-322-4727
Fax: 615-343-8126
Management:
    Stadium Director: Mike Leary
    Athletic Director: Todd Turner
Seating Capacity: 41,203

7961 VANDERBILT UNIVERSITY: MEMORIAL GYM
2601 Jess Neely Drive
Nashville, TN 37212

Phone: 615-322-4727
Fax: 615-343-8738
Web Site: www.vanderbilt.edu
Management:
    Athletic Director: Todd Turner
Seating Capacity: 15,626

7962   W.J. HALE STADIUM
Tennessee State University
3500 John Merrit Boulevard
Nashville, TN 37209
Phone: 615-320-3598
Management:
    Athletic Director: Bill Thomas
Seating Capacity: 16,500

7963   SOUTH JACKSON CIVIC CENTER
Corner of S Jackson and Decherd Streets
Tullahoma, TN 37388
Phone: 931-455-7239

Texas

7964   ABILENE CIVIC CENTER
1100 N 6th Street
PO Box 60
Abilene, TX 79604
Phone: 915-676-6211
Fax: 915-676-6343

7965   ABILENE CIVIC CENTER: EXHIBIT HALL
1100 N 6th Street
PO Box 60
Abilene, TX 79604
Phone: 915-676-6211
Fax: 915-676-6343

7966   ABILENE CIVIC CENTER: THEATER
1100 N 6th Street
PO Box 60
Abilene, TX 79604
Phone: 915-676-6211
Fax: 915-676-6343

7967   AZTEC
Albany Chamber of Commerce
PO Box 185
Albany, TX 76430
Phone: 915-762-3838
Fax: 915-762-3125

7968   FORT GRIFFIN FANDANGLE OUTDOOR THEATRE
PO Box 155
#1 Railroad Street
Albany, TX 76430
Phone: 915-762-3838
Fax: 915-762-3125

7969   OLD JAIL ART CENTER
201 S 2nd Street
Albany, TX 76430
Phone: 915-762-2269
Fax: 915-762-2260
e-mail: ojac@camalott.com
Web Site: www.albanytexas.com
Management:
    Education Assistant: Kathryn Mitchell
Mission: To serve as an educational and cultural center focused on the visual arts through collections, interpretation, programs and regional history resources to enhance the education of the audience.
Founded: 1980
Specialized Field: Art Meseum
Paid Staff: 8
Volunteer Staff: 89
Paid Artists: 28
Non-paid Artists: 20

7970   AMARILLO CIVIC CENTER
401 S Buchanan
PO Box 1971
Amarillo, TX 79105
Phone: 806-378-4297
Fax: 806-378-4234
e-mail: civama@ci.amarillo.tx.us
Web Site: www.civicamarillo.com
Management:
    Manager: Kris J Miller
    Assistant Manager: Sherman Bass
Specialized Field: Multi-purpose public assembly facility including convention space, coliseum and theatre. Meeting and conventions, professional ice hockey and shows.
Affiliations: Western Professional Hockey League
Seating Capacity: 4900 Sporting Events, 7000 Concerts
Year Built: 1968

7971   AMARILLO CIVIC CENTER: ARENA
401 S Buchanan
Amarillo, TX 79101
Phone: 806-378-4297
Fax: 806-378-4234

7972   AMARILLO CIVIC CENTER: MUSIC HALL
401 S Buchanan
Amarillo, TX 79101
Phone: 806-378-4297
Fax: 806-378-4234

7973   BALLPARK IN ARLINGTON
1000 Ballpark Way
Suite 400
Arlington, TX 76011
Phone: 817-273-5222
Fax: 817-273-5174
Web Site: www.texasrangers.com
Management:
    VP Event Services: Tim Murphy
    Director Facility Event Operations: Kevin Jimison

Specialized Field: Sports Facility, home of the Texas Rangers. Also includes a baseball museum, youth baseball park, amphitheatre and an office building.
Seating Capacity: 49,166
Year Built: 1994

7974 THEATRE ARLINGTON
305 W Main Street
Arlington, TX 76010
Phone: 817-275-7661

7975 UNIVERSITY OF TEXAS AT ARLINGTON: THEATRE ARTS
PO Box 19103
502 South Cooper
Arlington, TX 76019
Phone: 817-272-2650
Fax: 817-272-2697
e-mail: inman@uta.edu
Web Site: www.uta.edu
Management:
    Director: Kim LaFontaine
    Head of Theatre Recruitment: Angela Inman
Mission: Pre-professional training program for Theatre
Specialized Field: Theatre Performance and Designs
Paid Staff: 13
Affiliations: University of Texas system
Facility Category: Mainstage Theater; Black Box Theater
Type of Stage: Proscenium; Black Box
Seating Capacity: 425; 150

7976 UNIVERSITY OF TEXAS AT ARLINGTON: MAVERICK STADIUM
University of Texas at Arlington
1409 W Mitchell Street
Arlington, TX 76013
Phone: 817-272-2261
Fax: 817-272-5037
Web Site: www.uta.edu/athletics
Management:
    Athletic Director: Pete Carlon
    Director: Kathryn Beeler
Seating Capacity: 12,800

7977 FRANK C ERWIN JR SPECIAL EVENTS CENTER
1701 Red River
PO Box 2929
Austin, TX 78701
Phone: 512-471-7744
Fax: 512-471-9652
e-mail: j.earl@mail.utexas.edu
Web Site: www.utexas.edu/admin/erwin

7978 ONE WORLD THEATRE
7701 Bee Caves Road
Austin, TX 78746
Phone: 512-330-9500
Fax: 512-330-9600
e-mail: info@oneworldtheatre.org
Web Site: oneworldtheatre.org

7979 PARAMOUNT THEATER FOR THE PERFORMING ARTS
713 Congress Avenue
Austin, TX 78701
Mailing Address: PO Box 1566 Austin, TX 78767
Phone: 512-472-2901
Fax: 512-472-5824
Web Site: www.austintheatrealliance.org
Management:
    Director Programming: Paul Bewtel
Mission: Presting performing arts and film.
Founded: 1975
Paid Staff: 25
Volunteer Staff: 200
Performs At: Proscenium Theatre
Affiliations: APAP; LHAT
Type of Stage: Proscenium
Seating Capacity: 1,300
Year Built: 1915
Year Remodeled: 1980
Rental Contact: Paul Bentel

7980 UNIVERSITY OF TEXAS AT AUSTIN PERFORMING ARTS CENTER
PO Box 7818
Austin, TX 78713-7818
Phone: 512-471-1194
Fax: 512-471-3636
e-mail: nbarclay@mail.utexas.edu
Web Site: www.utpac.org
    Associate Director: Neil Barclay
    Assistant /Associate Director: JB Tuttle
    Assistant Director: Suzanne Cooper
    Production Manager: Charles Leslie
    Programmer: Neil Barclay
    Events Manager: Peter Melnick
Management:
    Director: Pebbles Wadsworth
    Associate Director: Neil Barclay
Mission: The University of Texas at Austin Performing Arts Center is a fully professional presenter of the performing arts. The PAC also seeks to educate, enlighten and entertain residents of the state with diverse and innovative programs that reflect the tradtional and evolving culture of the United States and of the world.
Budget: $1,000,000+
Performs At: Bass Concert Hall; Bates Recital Hall; McCullough Theatre
Facility Category: Performance Center; Opera House
Type of Stage: Proscenium
Stage Dimensions: 30'Wx36'D; 30'Wx18'H
Rental Contact: Pebbles Wadsworth

7981 UNIVERSITY OF TEXAS AT AUSTIN: DARRELL K ROYAL-TEXAS MEMORIAL STADIUM
PO Box 7399
Austin, TX 78713-7399
Phone: 512-471-9405
Fax: 512-471-+130
Web Site: www.texassports.com
Management:
    Facility Director: Doug Wilson

All listings are in alphabetical order by state, then city, then organization within the city.

Assistant Director: Larry Falk
Assistant Director: Mike Korth
Specialized Field: Home of University of Texas athletics (NCAA).
Seating Capacity: 79,450
Year Built: 1924
Year Remodeled: 1998

7982 UNIVERSITY OF TEXAS AT AUSTIN: THEATRE ROOM

Winship Drama Building
Austin, TX 78712
Phone: 512-471-5793
Fax: 512-471-0824

7983 UNIVERSITY OF TEXAS AT AUSTIN: TEXAS MEMORIAL STADIUM

University of Texas At Austin
1701 Red River
Austin, TX 78704
Phone: 512-471-3333
Management:
  Director: John M Graham
Seating Capacity: 75,524

7984 OLD BASTROP OPERA HOUSE

711 Spring
PO Box 691
Bastrop, TX 78602
Phone: 512-321-6283

7985 BEAUMONT CIVIC CENTER COMPLEX: EXHIBIT HALL

701 Main Street
Beaumont, TX 77701
Phone: 409-838-3435
Fax: 409-838-3715
Toll-free: 800-782-3081
e-mail: info@beaumont-tx-complex.com
Web Site: www.beaumont-tx-complex.com

7986 BEAUMONT CIVIC CENTER COMPLEX: JULIE ROGERS THEATRE

765 Pearl Street
Beaumont, TX 77701
Phone: 409-838-3435
Fax: 409-838-3715
Toll-free: 800-782-3081
e-mail: info@beaumont-tx-complex.com
Web Site: www.beaumont-tx-complex.com

7987 CIVIC CENTER COMPLEX

PO Box 3827
Beaumont, TX 77704-3827
Phone: 409-838-3435
Fax: 409-838-3715
e-mail: bookings@beaumont-tx-complex.com
Web Site: www.beaumont-tx-complex.com
Management:
  Director: Claudie D Hawkins
Paid Staff: 21

7988 LAMAR UNIVERSITY PROSCENIUM

Beaumont, TX 77710
Phone: 409-880-7011
Fax: 409-880-2286

7989 LAMAR UNIVERSITY STUDIO THEATRE

Beaumont, TX 77710
Phone: 409-880-7011
Fax: 409-880-2286

7990 LAMAR UNIVERSITY: CARDINAL STADIUM

4400 MLK Parkway
Beaumont, TX 77710
Phone: 409-880-2329
Fax: 409-880-1814
Web Site: www.athletics.lamar.edu
Management:
  Athletic Director: Dean Billick

7991 MONTAGNE CENTER

Lamar University
4400 MLK Parkway
Beaumont, TX 77710
Phone: 409-880-2329
Fax: 409-880-8990
Management:
  Athletic Director: Dean Billick
Seating Capacity: 10,080

7992 COASTAL BEND COLLEGE

3800 Charco Road
Beeville, TX 78102
Phone: 361-354-2300
Fax: 361-358-3971
e-mail: jimlee@cbc.cc.tx.us
Web Site: www.cbc.cc.tx.us
Officers:
  Performing Arts Division Chair: James L Lee

7993 CAMILLE LIGHTNER PLAYHOUSE

1 Dean Porter Park
Brownsville, TX 78520
Phone: 956-542-8900
Fax: 956-986-0639
e-mail: camillight@aol.com
Web Site: camilleplayhouse.vtl.com
Officers:
  President: John Kinch
  First VP: Robert Torres
  Second VP: Laura Partridge
  Treasurer: Dan Anderson
  Secretary: Pat Crow
Management:
  Executive Director: Joel Humphries
  Business Manager: Clara Reynolds
Mission: To stimulate an interest in the performing arts through the presentation of live theatre, utilizing the talents of the entire Valley community.
Founded: 1963
Specialized Field: Live theatre

Paid Staff: 2
Volunteer Staff: 3
Facility Category: Theatre house
Type of Stage: Thrust, proscenium
Stage Dimensions: 20 x 48 x 28
Seating Capacity: 301
Year Built: 1964
Rental Contact: Executive Director Joel Humphries

7994 BROWNWOOD COLISEUM
500 E Baker
Brownwood, TX 76801
Phone: 915-646-3586
Fax: 915-646-0938
Management:
General Manager: David Withers
Facility Manager: Kevin Dearling
Facility Category: Arena; Multy- Purpose
Type of Stage: flexible
Stage Dimensions: 60 4'x 8' stage segments
Seating Capacity: 3,000
Year Built: 1963
Rental Contact: David Withers

7995 KIMBROUGH MEMORIAL STADIUM
West Texas A&M University
PO Box 60049
Canyon, TX 79016
Phone: 806-651-2069
Fax: 806-651-2688
Management:
Athletic Director: Ed Harris
Seating Capacity: 20,000

7996 PIONEER AMPHITHEATRE
Palo Duro Canyon State Park
PO Box 268
Canyon, TX 79015
Phone: 806-488-2421
Fax: 806-655-7425

7997 WEST TEXAS STATE UNIVERSITY: BRANDING IRON THEATRE
Canyon, TX 79016
Phone: 806-651-2799
Fax: 806-651-2818
e-mail: wcrafton@mail.utamu.edu
Seating Capacity: 305
Year Built: 1959
Rental Contact: Perry Crafton

7998 G ROLLIE WHITE COLISEUM
Texas A&M University
Athletic Department
College Station, TX 77843-1128
Phone: 409-845-2313
Fax: 409-845-6825
Web Site: sports.tamu.edu
Management:
Athletic Director: Wally Groff

7999 KYLE FIELD
Texas A&M Athletic Department
161 Wellborn Road
College Station, TX 77843
Phone: 979-845-5725
Fax: 979-845-0564
e-mail: dsouth@athletics.tamu.edu
Web Site: www.sports.tamu.edu
Management:
Associate Athletic Director: Dave South
Sr Assoc Athletic Director: Billy Pickard
Specialized Field: Home of Texas A&M University athletics NCAA
Seating Capacity: 58,000
Year Built: 1927
Year Remodeled: 1998

8000 UNIVERSITY CENTER THEATRE COMPLEX AND CONFERENCE CENTER
Texas A&M University
College Station, TX 77840
Phone: 979-845-8903
Fax: 979-845-7312

8001 BAYFRONT PLAZA CONVENTION CENTER: AUDITORIUM
1901 N Shoreline Drive
Corpus Christi, TX 78401
Phone: 361-883-8543
Fax: 512-883-0788

8002 RICHARDSON AUDITORIUM
101 Baldwin Avenue
Corpus Christi, TX 78404
Phone: 512-855-0264
Fax: 512-886-1276

8003 WAREHOUSE LIVING ARTS CENTER
119 W 6th
Corsicana, TX 75110
Phone: 903-872-5421
Fax: 903-874-2923

8004 DISCOVER HOUSTON COUNTY VISITORS CENTER: MUSEUM
303 S 5st
Crockett, TX 75835
Phone: 936-544-9520

8005 BATH HOUSE CULTURAL CENTER
521 E Lawther Drive
Dallas, TX 75218
Phone: 214-670-8749
Fax: 214-670-8751
e-mail: bathhousecultural@hotmail.com
Web Site: www.bathhousecultural.com
Management:
Manager: David Fisher
Paid Staff: 3
Facility Category: Art/Cultural Center

Type of Stage: Thrust
Stage Dimensions: 13' x 20'
Seating Capacity: 120
Year Built: 1930
Year Remodeled: 1997
Rental Contact: Manager David Fisher

8006 BIBLICAL ARTS CENTER
7500 Park Lane
Dallas, TX 75225
Phone: 214-691-4661
Fax: 214-691-4752

8007 BRONCO ARENA
2600 Ft. Worth Avenue
Dallas, TX 75211
Phone: 214-943-1777
Fax: 214-943-2014
Web Site: www.broncobull.com
Management:
 Director: Susan Palmer

8008 COTTON BOWL/FAIR PARK
3809 Tower Building
PO Box 159090
Dallas, TX 75315
Phone: 214-670-8400
Fax: 214-670-8907
Web Site: www.tgimaps.com
Management:
 General Manager: Eddie Hueston
 Sales/Event Manager: Leslie Studard
Seating Capacity: 22,528 Soccer, 67,000 Football
Year Built: 1935

8009 DALLAS CONVENTION CENTER: ARENA
650 S Griffin
Dallas, TX 75202
Phone: 214-939-2700
Fax: 214-939-2795

8010 DALLAS CONVENTION CENTER: THEATER
650 S Griffin
Dallas, TX 75202
Phone: 214-939-2700
Fax: 214-939-2795

8011 DALLAS THEATER CENTER: ARTS DISTRICT
2401 Flora Street
Dallas, TX 75204
Phone: 214-922-0422
Fax: 214-521-7666

8012 DALLAS THEATER CENTER: KALITA HUMPHREYS THEATRE
3636 Turtle Creek Boulevard
Dallas, TX 75219

Phone: 214-526-8210
Fax: 214-521-7666

8013 MAJESTIC THEATRE
1925 Elm Street
Dallas, TX 75201
Phone: 214-880-0137
Fax: 214-880-0097
e-mail: jwilborn@dallassummermusicals.org
Web Site: www.dallassummermusicals.org

8014 MOODY COLISEUM
Southern Methodist University
6405 Boaz Lane, Suite 101
Dallas, TX 75275
Phone: 214-768-2864
Fax: 214-768-2044
Management:
 Assistant Manager: Kevin Diggs
Seating Capacity: 9,500

8015 MORTON H MEYERSON SYMPHONY CENTER
2301 Flora Street
PO Box 26207
Dallas, TX 75201
Phone: 214-670-3737
Fax: 214-670-4334
Web Site: www.dallassymphony.com

8016 MUSIC HALL AT FAIR PARK
909 Frist Avenue Parry
Dallas, TX 75315
Phone: 214-565-1116
Fax: 214-428-4526
Web Site: www.dallassummermusicals.org
Paid Staff: 10

8017 REUNION ARENA
777 Sports Street
Dallas, TX 75207
Phone: 214-939-2770
Fax: 214-800-3040
Management:
 General Manager: David R Brown
 Director Events/Booking: Ken Kurl
 Director Operations: Bob Jordan
 Concessions Manager: David Jenkins
 Director Marketing: Vicki Huxel
 Box Office Manager: Mike Chilers
 EVP/CFO: Graig Courson
 Group Sales Assistant: Melissa Mezger
Seating Capacity: 18,042

8018 SOUTH DALLAS CULTURAL CENTER
3400 S Fitzhugh
Dallas, TX 75210
Phone: 214-939-2787
Fax: 214-939-2787
Web Site: www.dallasblack.com

8019 SOUTHERN METHODIST UNIVERSITY
Owen Fine Arts Center
Dallas, TX 75275
Phone: 214-692-3383
Fax: 214-692-4138

8020 SOUTHERN METHODIST UNIVERSITY: BOB HOPE THEATRE
Owen Fine Arts Center
Dallas, TX 75275
Phone: 214-692-3383
Fax: 214-692-4138

8021 SOUTHERN METHODIST UNIVERSITY: CARUTH AUDITORIUM
Owen Fine Arts Center
Dallas, TX 75275
Phone: 214-692-2713
Fax: 214-692-4138

8022 SOUTHERN METHODIST UNIVERSITY: MCFARLIN MEMORIAL
6400 Hillcrest Avenue
PO Box 152
Dallas, TX 75275
Phone: 214-692-3129
Fax: 214-692-4138

8023 THANKSGIVING SQUARE: CHAPEL OF THANKSGIVING
Intersection of Bryan, Pacific and Ervay
PO Box 131770
Dallas, TX 75221
Phone: 214-969-1977
Fax: 214-754-0152
e-mail: info@thanksgiving.org
Web Site: www.thanksgiving.org

8024 THANKSGIVING SQUARE: COURTYARD AT THANKSGIVING
Intersection of Bryan, Pacific and Ervay
PO Box 131770
Dallas, TX 75313-1770
Phone: 214-969-1977
Fax: 214-754-0152
e-mail: info@thanksgiving.org
Web Site: www.thanksgiving.org

8025 TEXAS WOMAN'S UNIVERSITY: REDBUD THEATRE
PO Box 23865
TWU Station
Denton, TX 76204
Phone: 817-898-2500
Fax: 817-898-3198

8026 UNIVERSITY OF NORTH TEXAS: CONCERT HALL
College of Music
Denton, TX 76203

Phone: 817-565-2791
Fax: 817-565-4919

8027 UNIVERSITY OF NORTH TEXAS: DEPARTMENT OF DANCE
PO Box 13126
Denton, TX 76203
Phone: 817-565-2211
Fax: 817-565-4919

8028 UNIVERSITY OF NORTH TEXAS FINE ARTS SERIES
PO Box 310710
Denton, TX 76203-0710
Phone: 940-565-3815
Fax: 940-565-3773
e-mail: Keffer@unt.edu
Web Site: www-lan.unt.edu/usl/home/www
Officers:
  Chairman: Lindsay Keffer
Management:
  Chairman: J Lindsay Keffer
Founded: 1924
Specialized Field: Performing, Visual, Literary
Paid Staff: 1
Volunteer Staff: 9
Budget: $60,000-150,000
Income Sources: Grants; Ticket Sales; Underwriting; Student Service Fees
Affiliations: A.A; APA
Type of Stage: Thrust; Proscenium
Seating Capacity: 200/8,000

8029 UNIVERSITY OF TEXAS-PAN AMERICAN: FINE ARTS
Pan American University
Edinburg, TX 78539
Phone: 956-381-3471
Fax: 956-381-3472

8030 UNIVERSITY OF TEXAS-PAN AMERICAN: THEATER
1201 W University Drive
Edinburg, TX 78539
Phone: 512-381-3581
Fax: 956-381-3472

8031 CHAMIZAL NATIONAL MEMORIAL: THEATER
800 S San Marcial
PO Box 722
El Paso, TX 79905
Phone: 915-532-7273
Fax: 915-532-7240

8032 COHEN STADIUM
9700 Gateway North Boulevard
El Paso, TX 79924
Phone: 915-755-2000
Fax: 915-757-0671
Web Site: www.diablos.com
Management:

President: Rick Parr

8033 DON HASKINS CENTER
Baltimore & Mesa STS
500 W University Avenue
El Paso, TX 79968-0557
Phone: 915-747-5265
Fax: 915-747-5228
e-mail: dhc@utep.edu
Web Site: www.utep.edu/venues
Management:
   Director: Mike Spence
   Program Coordinator: Lucretia Boucher
   Technical Staff Assistant IV: Fernie Mabini
Paid Staff: 9
Affiliations: University of Texas at El Paso
Facility Category: SICO
Seating Capacity: 12,000
Year Remodeled: 2001
Rental Contact: (915)747-5481 Carol Roberts-Spence

8034 DUDLEY FIELD
PO Box 4797
El Paso, TX 79914
Phone: 915-544-1950
Management:
   Owner: Jim Paul

8035 EL PASO CIVIC CENTER: EXHIBITION HALL
1 Civic Center Plaza
El Paso, TX 79901
Phone: 915-534-0600
Fax: 915-534-0686
Web Site: www.elpaso.com

8036 EL PASO CIVIC CENTER: THEATRE
1 Civic Center Plaza
El Paso, TX 79901
Phone: 915-541-4920
Fax: 915-534-0686

8037 EL PASO CONVENTION & PERFORMING ARTS CENTER
One Civic Center Plaza
El Paso, TX 79901
Phone: 915-534-0609
Fax: 915-532-2963
Toll-free: 800-351-6024
e-mail: eportillo@elpasocvb.com
Web Site: www.elpasocvb.com
Management:
   Facility Sales Manager: Esther Portillo

8038 EL PASO COUNTY COLISEUM
4100 Paisano
El Paso, TX 79997
Phone: 915-534-4229
Fax: 915-532-4048
Management:
   Director: Joyce Trujillo

8039 SUN BOWL
500 W University Avenue
El Paso, TX 79968-0557
Phone: 915-747-5265
Fax: 915-747-5228
e-mail: events@utep.edu
Web Site: www.utep.edu-events
Management:
   Director Facility: Mike Spence
   Spence Director Special Events: Carol Roberts
Seating Capacity: 52,000

8040 UNIVERSITY OF TEXAS AT EL PASO: MAIN PLAYHOUSE
500 W University
El Paso, TX 79968
Phone: 915-747-5146
Fax: 915-747-5134
Web Site: www.utap.org/utph/theatre

8041 CARAVAN OF DREAMS
312 Houston Street
Fort Worth, TX 76102
Phone: 817-877-3000
Fax: 817-877-3752

8042 CASA MANANA THEATRE
3101 W Lancaster
Fort Worth, TX 76107
Phone: 817-332-9319
Fax: 817-332-5711
Season: june - august

8043 OAK ACRES AMPHITHEATRE
1620 Las Vegas Trail N
at Loop 820 N
Fort Worth, TX 76108
Phone: 817-246-9775

8044 SOUTHWESTERN BAPTIST THEOLOGICAL SEMINARY
190 W Broadus Street
PO Box 22390
Fort Worth, TX 76122-0390
Phone: 817-923-1921
Fax: 817-921-8762
e-mail: scmusic@swbts.edu
Web Site: www.swbts.edu
Performs At: Graduate School Recital Hall
Facility Category: Concert Halls, Auditorium, studio
Seating Capacity: 500
Year Built: 1933
Year Remodeled: 1960
Rental Contact: Ext 3160 Joseph King

8045 TEXAS CHRISTIAN UNIVERSITY: ED LANDRETH AUDITORIUM
School of Fine Arts
PO Box 32928
Fort Worth, TX 76129
Phone: 817-921-7625
Fax: 817-921-7333

8046 TEXAS WESLEYAN COLLEGE: FINE ARTS
Rosedale and Wesleyan
PO Box 50010
Fort Worth, TX 76105
Phone: 817-531-4443
Fax: 817-531-6583

8047 WILLIAM EDRINGTON SCOTT THEATRE
3505 W Lancaster
Fort Worth, TX 76107
Phone: 817-738-1938
Fax: 817-731-0835
e-mail: wescotttheatre@prodigy.net

8048 DANIEL-MEYER COLISEUM
Texas Chsitioan University
PO Box 297600
Ft Worth, TX 76129
Phone: 817-257-7965
Fax: 817-257-7656
Web Site: www.tcu.edu
Management:
    Associated Director: Brian Florko

8049 TEXAS CHRISTIAN UNIVERSITY: AMOIN G CARTER STADIUM
3500 Bellaire Drive N
Ft. Worth, TX 76129
Phone: 817-257-7965
Fax: 817-257-7656
Web Site: www.gofrogs.com
Management:
    Athletic Director: Eric Hyman

8050 GRAND 1894 OPERA HOUSE
2020 Postoffice Street
Galveston, TX 77550
Phone: 409-763-7173
Fax: 409-763-1068
Toll-free: 800-821-1894
e-mail: m.patton@thegrand.com
Web Site: www.thegrand.com

8051 MOODY CIVIC CENTER: EXHIBITION HALL
2100 Seawall Boulevard
Galveston, TX 77550
Phone: 409-762-8626
Fax: 406-762-8911

8052 GARLAND CENTER FOR THE PERFORMING ARTS
PO Box 469002
Garland, TX 75046
Phone: 972-205-2780
Fax: 972-205-2775
Web Site: www.cagarland.tx.us/tac

8053 GARLAND CENTER FOR THE PERFORMING ARTS: THEATRE
PO Box 469002
Garland, TX 75046
Phone: 972-205-2780
Fax: 972-205-2775

8054 GRANBURY OPERA HOUSE
116 E Pearl Street
PO Box 297
Granbury, TX 76048
Phone: 817-573-9191
Fax: 817-579-5529

8055 CAPITAL BASEBALL STADIUM
Harlingen Municipal Auditorium Complex
1204 Fair Park Boulevard
Harlingen, TX 78550
Phone: 956-430-6690
Fax: 956-364-2975
e-mail: harlingnarts@xanadu2.net
Management:
    Director: Susan Thomae-Morphew

8056 HARLINGEN CULTURAL ARTS CENTER: AUDITORIUM
576'76 Drive
PO Box 609
Harlingen, TX 78551
Phone: 210-423-9736

8057 ALLEY THEATRE
615 Texas Avenue
Houston, TX 77002
Phone: 713-228-9341
Fax: 713-222-6542
Management:
    Artistic Director: Gregory Boyd
    Managing Director: Paul Tetreault
    Direction Production: Sean Skeeman

8058 ALLEY THEATRE: LARGE STAGE
615 Texas Avenue
Houston, TX 77002
Phone: 713-228-9341
Fax: 713-222-6542
Web Site: www.alleytheatre.org or teatroalley.org

8059 ASTRODOME
8400 Kirby Lane
PO Box 288
Houston, TX 77054-0288
Phone: 713-799-9500
Fax: 713-799-9722
e-mail: twinspin@astros.com
Web Site: www.astros.com
Management:
    President/CEO: Mike Puryear
    VP Marketing/Sales: George Coenig
Seating Capacity: 53,000 (Stadium, 6,000 (Arena)
Year Built: 1963
Year Remodeled: 1988

8060 COMMUNITY MUSIC CENTER

3100 Cleburne
Houston, TX 77004
Phone: 713-523-9710
Fax: 713-523-0507
Management:
Executive Director: Gary Wilkins
Music Director: Anne Lundy

8061 COMPAQ CENTER

10 Greenway Plaza
Houston, TX 77046
Phone: 713-843-3900
Fax: 713-843-3986
e-mail: info@compaqcenter.com
Web Site: www.compaqcenter.com
Management:
General Manager: Gerald McDonald
Assistant General Manager: Bryan Blaum
Seating Capacity: 17,000
Year Built: 1975
Year Remodeled: 1994

8062 DELMAR STADIUM COMPLEX

2020 Magnum
Houston, TX 77092
Phone: 713-957-7700
Fax: 713-957-7704
Management:
Director: Mike Truelove

8063 DIVERSEWORKS

1117 E Freeway
Houston, TX 77002
Phone: 713-223-8346
Fax: 713-223-4608
e-mail: info@diverseworks.org
Web Site: www.diverseworks.org
Management:
Performing Arts Director: Sixto Wagan
Mission: Dedicated to presenting new visual, performing, and literary art. A place where the process of creating art is valued and where artists can test new ideas in the public arena. By encouraging the investigation of current artistic, cultural and social issues, they build, educate, and sustain audiences for contemporary art.
Founded: 1982
Specialized Field: Multidisciplinary Performance and Visual
Status: Nonprofit

8064 ENRON FIELD

PO Box 288
Houston, TX 77001-0288
Phone: 713-799-9500
Fax: 713-799-9881
Web Site: www.astros.com
Management:
Facility Manager: Don Collins
Sr VP Marketing Advertising: Pam Gardner
Specialized Field: Home of the Houston Astros (MLB).
Seating Capacity: 42,000
Year Built: 2000

8065 HOFHEINZ PAVILION

3100 Cullen Boulevard
Houston, TX 77204-6742
Phone: 713-743-9370
Fax: 713-743-9375
Web Site: www.uhcougars.com
Management:
Athletic Director: Chet Gladchuk

8066 HOUSTON CIVIC CENTER

PO Box 61649
Houston, TX 77208
Phone: 713-247-1000
Fax: 713-583-8090

8067 HOUSTON CIVIC CENTER: JESSE H JONES HALL FOR THE PERFORMING ARTS

615 Louisiana
PO Box 61469
Houston, TX 77208
Phone: 713-227-3974
Fax: 713-228-9629

8068 HOUSTON CIVIC CENTER: GEORGE R BROWN CONVENTION CENTER

1001 Convention Center Boulevard
Houston, TX 77010
Phone: 713-853-8000
Fax: 713-583-8011

8069 HOUSTON CIVIC CENTER: GUS WORTHAM THEATER

510 Preston 4th Floor
Houston, TX 77002
Phone: 713-237-1439
Fax: 713-237-9313

8070 ALLEY THEATRE: HUGO V NEUHAUS ARENA STAGE

615 Texas Avenue
Houston, TX 77002
Phone: 713-228-9341
Fax: 713-222-6542
Web Site: www.alleytheatre.org or www.teatroalley.org
Year Remodeled: 2001

8071 MILLER OUTDOOR THEATRE

Hermann Park
PO Box 1562
Houston, TX 77251
Phone: 713-284-8358

8072 RICE STADIUM

Rice University
6100 S Main Street
Houston, TX 77005
Phone: 713-527-4077
Fax: 713-527-6019
Web Site: www.riceowls.com
Management:

Athletic Director: Bobby May
Seating Capacity: 70,000

8073 RICE UNIVERSITY: HAMMAN HALL
PO Box 1892
Houston, TX 77251
Phone: 713-348-4027

8074 ROBERTSON STADIUM
University of Huston
3100 Cullen Boulevard
Houston, TX 77204-6742
Phone: 713-743-9370
Fax: 713-743-9375
Web Site: www.uhcougars.com
Management:
    Athletic Director: Chet Gladchuk
    Sports Information Director: Chris Burkholter
    Head Football Coach: Kim Helton
    Head Basketball Coach (M): Claude Drexler
    Head Basketball Coach (W): Joe Curl
Seating Capacity: 22,000

8075 STAGES REPERTORY THEATRE
3201 Allen Parkway
 # 101
Houston, TX 77019
Phone: 713-527-0240
Web Site: www.stagestheatre.com

8076 THEATRE SUBURBIA
1410 W 43rd
Houston, TX 77018
Phone: 713-682-3525

8077 BERNARD G JOHNSON COLISEUM
Sam Houston State University
Avenue H & Bowers Boulevard
Huntsville, TX 77341
Phone: 936-294-1740
Fax: 936-294-1913
e-mail: rca_elc@shsu.edu
Web Site: www.shsu.edu
Management:
    Director: Ed Chatal

8078 SAM HOUSTON STATE UNIVERSITY THEATRE & DANCE
Theatre & Dance Department
Avenue H at 17th Street, PO Box 2297
Huntsville, TX 77341
Phone: 936-294-1329
Fax: 936-294-3898
e-mail: drm_jrm@shsu.edu
Web Site: shsu.edu/ndrm.www
Management:
    Chairman: Dr. James Miller
Type of Stage: Proscenium and Thrust
Seating Capacity: 396, 96
Year Built: 1976
Year Remodeled: 2001

8079 IRVING ARTS CENTER
3333 N MacArthur Boulevard
Suite 300
Irving, TX 75062
Phone: 972-252-7558
Fax: 972-570-4962
e-mail: jtrizila@ci.irving.tx.us
Web Site: www.ci.irving.tx.us/arts
Management:
    Director Marketing/Publication: Jo Trizila
    Executive Director: Richard E Huff
    Facilities Director: Kass Price
Mission: To serve the citizens of Irving through the support and development of artistic opportunities.
Founded: 1986
Paid Staff: 25
Volunteer Staff: 800
Affiliations: City of Irving
Annual Attendance: 100,000
Type of Stage: Proscenium; Black Box
Seating Capacity: 700; 450; 500
Year Built: 1990

8080 TEXAS STADIUM
2401 E Airport Freeway
Irving, TX 75062
Phone: 972-438-7676
Fax: 975-785-4709
Management:
    VP/General Manager: Bruce Hardy
    Concessions Manager: Amy Bersen
Seating Capacity: 63,855

8081 FESTIVAL OUTDOOR THEATER
Quiet Valley Ranch
PO Box 291466
Kerrville, TX 78029-1466
Phone: 830-257-3600
Fax: 830-257-8680
Toll-free: 800-435-8429
e-mail: rad@karrville/music.com
Web Site: www.festival/music.com

8082 JONES STADIUM/TEXAS TECH UNIVERSITY OF ATHLETICS
Texas Tech Athletics Department
6 & Red Raider Avenue
Lubbock, TX 79409
Phone: 806-742-3355
Fax: 806-742-1970
e-mail: sportsinfo@ttu.edu
Web Site: www.texastech.edu
Management:
    Athletic Director: Gerald Myers
    Senior Associate Athletic Director: Steve Locke
    Associate Athletics: Judi Henry
    Senior Associate Athletic Director: Bobby Gleason
    Assistant Athletic Director: Richard Kilwien
    Assistant Athletic Director: Byron Waters
    Associate Athletic Director: Ron Famrom
    Assistant Athletic Director: Russell Warren
    Associate Athletic Director: Steve Uryasz
Seating Capacity: 50,500

8083 LUBBOCK MEMORIAL CIVIC CENTER
1501 6th Street
Lubbock, TX 79401
Phone: 806-770-2000
Fax: 806-775-3240

8084 LUBBOCK MEMORIAL CIVIC CENTER BANQUET HALL
1501 6th Street
Lubbock, TX 79401
Phone: 806-770-2000

8085 LUBBOCK MEMORIAL CIVIC CENTER COLISEUM
4th and Boston
Lubbock, TX 79457
Phone: 806-770-2000
Fax: 806-765-5803

8086 LUBBOCK MEMORIAL CIVIC CENTER EXHIBIT HALL
1501 6th Street
Lubbock, TX 79457
Phone: 806-770-2000
Fax: 806-765-5803

8087 LUBBOCK MEMORIAL CIVIC CENTER MUNICIPAL AUDITORIUM
4th and Boston
Lubbock, TX 79457
Phone: 806-770-2000
Fax: 806-765-5803

8088 LUBBOCK MEMORIAL CIVIC CENTER THEATER
1501 6th Street
Lubbock, TX 79457
Phone: 806-770-2000
Fax: 806-765-5803

8089 TEXAS TECH UNIVERSITY CENTER: ALLEN THEATRE
15th and Boston Avenue
PO Box 42031
Lubbock, TX 79409
Phone: 806-742-3636
Fax: 806-742-0655
e-mail: felix.moore@ttu.edu
Web Site: www.uc.ttu.edu
Paid Staff: 10
Facility Category: rental
Type of Stage: proeswien
Stage Dimensions: 60 x 20
Seating Capacity: 928
Year Built: 1976

8090 TEXAS TECH UNIVERSITY SCHOOL OF MUSIC
18th and Boston
Box 42033
Lubbock, TX 79409-2033
Phone: 806-742-2270
Fax: 806-742-2294
e-mail: garry.owens@ttu.edu
Web Site: www.ttu.edu/~music

8091 MARSHALL CIVIC CENTER
2501 E End Boulevard S
Marshall, TX 75670
Phone: 903-935-4472
Fax: 903-935-0538
e-mail: awright@marshalltexas.net
Management:
    Event Facilites Director: Ardis Wright
Founded: 1976
Paid Staff: 5

8092 MARSHALL THEATER AT THE CIVIC CENTER
2501 E End Boulevard S
Marshall, TX 75670
Phone: 903-935-4472
Fax: 903-935-0538

8093 RESISTOL ARENA/RODEO CENTER EXHIBIT HALL
SW Sports Group
1818 Rodeo Drive
Mesquiet, TX 75149
Phone: 972-285-8777
Fax: 972-289-2999
e-mail: eddie@mesquietroedo.com
Web Site: www.mesquietroedo.com
Officers:
    President: Jack B Beckman
Management:
    Director: Chris Beckman
Seating Capacity: 5,300

8094 CHAPARRAL CENTER
Midland College
3600 N Garfield
Midland, TX 79705
Phone: 915-685-4584
Fax: 915-685-4740
e-mail: mstevens@midland.edu
Management:
    Director: Michael J Stevens
Founded: 1978
Affiliations: Midland College
Facility Category: Small arena with curtain system
Type of Stage: Stageright Portable
Stage Dimensions: 60' x 40'
Seating Capacity: 1800; 2400; 5000
Year Built: 1978

8095 STEPHEN F AUSTIN STATE UNIVERSITY: HOMER BRYCE STADIUM
Stephen F. Austin State University
PO Box 13010, SFA Station
Nacogdoches, TX 75962
Phone: 409-468-3501
Web Site: www.athletics.sfasu.edu
Management:
Athletic Director: Steve McCarty

8096 WILLIAM R JOHNSON COLISEUM
Stephen F Austin State University
PO Box 13010-SFA Station
Nacogdoches, TX 75962
Phone: 936-468-3501
Fax: 936-468-4070
Web Site: fajacks.com
Management:
Athletic Operations Director: John Branch
Seating Capacity: 7,200

8097 LUTCHER THEATER
707 W Main Street
Orange, TX 77630
Phone: 409-886-5535
Fax: 409-886-5537
Toll-free: 800-828-5535
e-mail: lutcher@exp.net
Web Site: www.lutcher.org

8098 PALESTINE CIVIC CENTER COMPLEX
Highway 287-19N
Palestine, TX 75801
Phone: 903-723-3014
Fax: 903-729-6067
Toll-free: 800-659-3484
e-mail: avapcvb@flash.net

8099 MK BROWN AUDITORIUM
1100 W Coronado Drive
Pampa, TX 79065
Phone: 806-669-5790
Fax: 806-669-5842
e-mail: mkb@pan-tex.net
Management:
Auditorium Manager: Jackie Harper
Stage Dimensions: 3,150 square feet
Seating Capacity: 1,500

8100 PARIS JUNIOR COLLEGE
2400 Clarksville
Paris, TX 75460
Phone: 903-785-7661
Fax: 903-784-9370

8101 SAN JACINTO COLLEGE CENTRAL
8060 Spencer Highway
PO Box 2007
Pasadena, TX 77501-2007
Phone: 281-476-1829
Fax: 281-476-1892

Management:
Theater Manager: Jerry Ford
Budget: $10,000

8102 SLOCOMB AUDITORIUM
8060 Spencer Highway
Pasadena, TX 77501
Phone: 713-476-1829

8103 RICHARDSON PERFORMING ARTS & CORPORATE PRESENTATION CENTER
959 E Lookout Drive
Richardson, TX 75081
Phone: 972-907-8205
Fax: 972-276-3
e-mail: bruce_macpherson@cor.gov
Management:
Managing Director: Bruce MacPherson

8104 INTERNATIONAL FESTIVAL-INSTITUTE AT ROUND TOP
State Highway 237 at Jaster Road
Round Top, TX 78954
Phone: 979-249-3129
Fax: 979-249-5078
e-mail: festinst@fai.net
Web Site: www.festivalhill.org
Management:
Founder/Artistic Director: James Dick
Program Director: Alain G Declert
Managing Director: Richard R Royall
Director Operations: David Bowman
Director Library/Museum: Lamar Lentz
Mission: Educational project.
Founded: 1971
Specialized Field: Classical Music
Status: Not-for-profit educational
Budget: 1.6 Million
Income Sources: Individual gifts, foundations, grants, box office, gift shop
Performs At: Orchestral and chamber music concerts.
Affiliations: Chamber Music of America, America Orchestra Symphony League
Facility Category: Concert Hall, Auditorium
Type of Stage: Proscenium
Stage Dimensions: 70 x 50
Seating Capacity: 1100
Rental Contact: Program Director Alain G. Declert

8105 ANGELO STATE UNIVERSITY AUDITORIUM
2601 W Avenue N
San Angelo, TX 76909
Phone: 915-942-2021
Fax: 915-942-2229
e-mail: greg.pecina@angelo.edu
Web Site: www.angelo.edu

8106 HOUSTON HARTE UNIVERSITY CENTER
1910 Rosemont
San Angelo, TX 76909

Phone: 915-942-2021
Fax: 915-942-2229
e-mail: greg.pacina@angelo.edu

8107 SAN ANGELO CITY AUDITORIUM

500 Rio Concho Drive
72 West College
San Angelo, TX 76903
Phone: 915-653-9577
Fax: 915-659-0900
e-mail: sacc@wcc.net
Web Site: www.sanangelotexas.org

8108 ALAMODOME

100 Montana
San Antonio, TX 78203
Phone: 210-207-3663
Fax: 210-207-3646
Toll-free: 800-884-3663
e-mail: dmarketing@alamodome.com
Web Site: www.alamodome.com
Management:
  Director: Michael Abington
  Operations Manager: Jim Mery
  Booking Manager: Kyle Kirousis
Founded: 1993
Paid Staff: 50
Type of Stage: Stadium
Seating Capacity: 65,000

8109 ARNESON RIVER THEATRE

418 Villita Street
San Antonio, TX 78205
Phone: 210-212-6771
Fax: 210-299-8444

8110 BEETHOVEN HALL: SAN JOSE CONVENTION CENTER

200 E Market
San Antonio, TX 78205
Phone: 210-299-8500
Fax: 210-223-1495

8111 CARVER COMMUNITY CULTURAL CENTER

226 N Hackberry
San Antonio, TX 78202
Phone: 210-207-7211
Fax: 210-207-4412
e-mail: kjordan@ci.sat.tx.us
Web Site: www.thecarver.org
Management:
  Interim Manager: Kim Jordan
Mission: To celebrate the diverse cultures of our world, nation and community, with emphasis on its African American heritage by providing challenging artistic presentations, community outreach activities and educational programs.
Founded: 1976
Specialized Field: Multi-ethnic and multi-cultural performing and visual arts center
Paid Staff: 18
Paid Artists: 10

8112 CARVER COMPLEX

226 N Hackberry
San Antonio, TX 78202
Phone: 210-207-7211
Fax: 210-207-4412
Web Site: www.thecarver.org

8113 FREEMAN COLISEUM

3201 E Houston
PO Box 200283
San Antonio, TX 78220
Phone: 210-226-1177
Fax: 210-226-5081
e-mail: lynettec@freemancoliseum.com
Web Site: www.freemancoliseum.com
Management:
  Marketing Director: Lynette Crisp
  General Manager: JC Hrubetz
Mission: Multi-purpose concert and performance facility
Founded: 1949
Specialized Field: Dance, Music, Facility

8114 MUNICIPAL AUDITORIUM

100 Auditorium Circle
San Antonio, TX 78205
Phone: 210-207-8511
Fax: 210-223-1495

8115 NELSON W WOLFF MUNICIPAL STADIUM

5757 New Highway 90 W
San Antonio, TX 78227
Phone: 210-207-3750
Fax: 210-670-8251
Management:
  Stadium Manager: James G Mery
Seating Capacity: 6,100

8116 SAN ANTONIO CONVENTION CENTER

200 E Market Street
San Antonio, TX 78205
Phone: 210-731-6611
Fax: 210-223-1495

8117 SAN ANTONIO CONVENTION CENTER LILA COCKRELL HALL

200 E Market Street
San Antonio, TX 78205
Phone: 210-731-6611
Fax: 210-223-1495

8118 TRINITY UNIVERSITY: DEPARTMENT OF SPEECH AND THEATRE

715 Stadium Drive
San Antonio, TX 78284
Phone: 210-736-8511
Fax: 210-736-7305

8119 TRINITY UNIVERSITY: LAURIE AUDITORIUM

San Antonio, TX 78212

Phone: 210-736-8119
Fax: 210-736-8100

8120 SOUTHWEST TEXAS STATE UNIVERSITY: STRAHAN COLISEUM

174 Jowers Center
San Marcos, TX 78666
Phone: 512-245-2023
Fax: 512-245-2967
Management:
    Director Facility/Game Operations: Timothy Atkinson
    Director Facility: Adam Alonzo
Seating Capacity: 7,739

8121 SOUTHWEST TEXAS STATE UNIVERSITY: BOBCAT STADIUM

176 Jowers Center
San Marcos, TX 78666
Phone: 512-245-2023
Fax: 512-245-2967
Management:
    Director Athletic Facilities: Timothy Atkinson

8122 JACKSON AUDITORIUM

1000 W Court
Seguin, TX 78155
Phone: 210-372-8180
Fax: 210-372-8096

8123 CULTURAL ACTIVITIES CENTER

3011 N 3rd Street
Temple, TX 76501
Phone: 254-773-9926
Fax: 254-773-9929
e-mail: cac@cacarts.org
Web Site: www.cacarts.org
Management:
    Visual Arts Director: Marilyn Ritchie
    Executive Director: David Pennington
Mission: Provide area residents, especially children, with opportunities to expirence visual and performing arts.
Founded: 1958
Specialized Field: Visual Arts; Performing Arts
Status: Professional; Semi-Professional; Non-Professional; Nonprofit
Paid Staff: 8
Budget: $500,000
Income Sources: Heartland Fund; Texas Commission on the Arts; Foundations; Grants; Memberships
Affiliations: Southwest Performing Arts Presenters; Texas Association of Museums; Texas Alliance for Education & The Arts
Annual Attendance: 80,000
Facility Category: Auditorium
Type of Stage: Proscenium
Stage Dimensions: 38Wx30D
Seating Capacity: 487
Year Built: 1978
Rental Contact: Aileen Snyder
Organization Type: Performing; Touring; Resident; Educational; Sponsoring

8124 TEMPLE CIVIC THEATRE

2413 S 13th Street
Temple, TX 76504
Phone: 254-778-4751
Fax: 254-778-4980
Web Site: www.artstemple.com

8125 PEROT THEATRE

221 Main Street
PO Box 1171
Texarkana, TX 75501
Phone: 903-792-8681
Fax: 903-793-8510
e-mail: mstarrett@trahc.org
Web Site: www.trahc.org
Officers:
    Executive Director: Ruth Ellen
    Administrative Director: Mary Starrett
    Director Marketing/Development: Nita Fran Hutcheson
    Operations Director: Randal Conry
Mission: To enrich the human experience in the region by increasing public awareness of, exposure to and participation in the arts and humanities in their many diverse forms.
Founded: 1981
Paid Staff: 14
Volunteer Staff: 114

8126 CYNTHIA WOODS MITCHELL PAVILION

2005 Lake Robbins Drive
The Woodlands, TX 77380
Phone: 281-363-3300
Fax: 713-364-3011
Web Site: www.pavillion.woodlandcenter.org

8127 REGIONAL ARTS CENTER

PO Box 1321
500 Malone, Suite B
Tomball, TX 77377-1321
Phone: 281-351-2787
Fax: 281-351-2702
e-mail: harriet@regional-arts.org
Web Site: www.regional-arts.org
Management:
    Executive Director: Harriet Fether

8128 ROSE STADIUM

PO Box 2035
Tyler, TX 75710
Phone: 903-531-3602
Fax: 765-496-1280
Management:
    Athletic Director: Billy Hall
Seating Capacity: 12,018

8129 FERREL CENTER

Baylor University
150 Bear Run
Waco, TX 76711

Phone: 254-710-1011
Fax: 254-710-1968
Web Site: www.baylor.edu
Management:
Director: Jim Trego

8130 WACO CONVENTION CENTER
100 Washington Avenue
PO Box 2570
Waco, TX 76703
Phone: 254-299-0630
Fax: 817-750-5801

8131 WACO CONVENTION CENTER CHISHOLM HALL
100 Washington Avenue
PO Box 2570
Waco, TX 76703
Phone: 254-299-0630
Fax: 817-750-5801

8132 WACO HIPPODROME
724 Austin Avenue
Waco, TX 76701
Phone: 254-752-7745
Fax: 254-752-9806
Toll-free: 800-701-2787
e-mail: boxofficewpac@texnet.net
Web Site: www.wacohippodrome.com
Management:
Technical Director/Facilities Man.: Len Howard
Mission: To preserve the historic Waco Hippodrome, originally a vaudeville show house; to provide quality Broadway entertainment and nationally known children's shows based on children's literature at an affordable price.
Founded: 1913
Paid Staff: 4
Volunteer Staff: 60
Budget: $150,000-400,000
Annual Attendance: 21,000-35,000
Facility Category: Performing Arts Center
Seating Capacity: 943
Rental Contact: Facilities Manager Len Howard

8133 MEMORIAL AUDITORIUM
1300 7th Street
Wichita Falls, TX 76307
Phone: 940-716-5500
Fax: 940-716-5509
Management:
Manager: George Casper

Utah

8134 ECCLES COLISEUM/SOUTHERN UTAH UNIVERSITY
351 W Center Street
Cedar City, UT 84720
Phone: 435-586-1937
Fax: 435-586-5444
Management:

Athletic Director: Tom Douple

8135 LAGOON ENTERTAINMENT DIVISION
375 N Lagoon Drive
Farmington, UT 84025
Phone: 801-451-8059
Fax: 801-451-8015
Toll-free: 800-748-5246

8136 UTAH STATE UNIVERSITY: D GLEN SMITH SPECTRUM
Athletic Department
7400 Old Main Hill
Logan, UT 84322-7400
Phone: 435-797-1850
Fax: 435-797-2615
Web Site: www.utahstateuniversity.edu
Management:
Director: Rance Pugmire
Marketing Director: Michelle Wilson
Seating Capacity: 10,270

8137 UTAH STATE UNIVERSITY: CHASE FINE ARTS CENTER
Logan, UT 84322
Phone: 435-797-1094

8138 UTAH STATE UNIVERSITY: KENT CONCERT HALL
Chase Fine Arts Center
Logan, UT 84322
Phone: 435-797-1094

8139 UTAH STATE UNIVERSITY: MORGAN THEATRE
Chase Fine Arts Center
Logan, UT 84322
Phone: 435-797-1094

8140 MANTI TEMPLE GROUNDS AMPHITHEATRE
Manti, UT 84642
Phone: 435-835-3000

8141 ECCLES COMMUNITY ART CENTER
2580 Jefferson Avenue
Ogden, UT 84401
Phone: 801-392-6935
e-mail: eccles@ogden4arts.org
Web Site: www.ogden4arts.org

8142 VAL A BROWNING CENTER FOR THE PERFORMING ARTS
Weber State University
Ogden, UT 84408
Phone: 801-626-7000
Fax: 801-626-6811

8143 WEBER STATE UNIVERSITY: DEE EVENTS CENTER
4400 Harrison Boulevard
Box 3401
Ogden, UT 84408-3401
Phone: 801-626-6665
Fax: 801-626-7190
e-mail: jlake@weber.edu
Management:
Manager: Jody G Lake

8144 BRIGHAM YOUNG UNIVERSITY: MARRIOTT CENTER
Marriot Center/Cougar Stadium
Brigham Young Univ, PO Box 20530
Provo, UT 84602-0530
Phone: 801-378-6022
Fax: 801-378-2042
Web Site: www.byu.edu
Management:
Director: Larry R Duffin
Assistant Manager: Mary Jean Draper
Seating Capacity: 23,000

8145 BRIGHAM YOUNG UNIVERSITY COUGAR STADIUM
PO Box 20530
Provo, UT 84602-2042
Phone: 801-378-6022
Fax: 801-378-2042
Web Site: www.byucougars.com
Management:
Director: Larry D Duffin
Assistant Manager: Mary Jean Draper
Seating Capacity: 65,524
Year Built: 1982

8146 BRIGHAM YOUNG UNIVERSITY HARRIS FINE ARTS CENTER
Harris Fine Arts Center
Provo, UT 84602
Phone: 801-412-2819
Fax: 801-422-0253
e-mail: hfac@byu.edu
Web Site: www.byu.edu/cfac
Officers:
Dean College Fine Arts/Commun.: K Newell Dayley
Year Built: 1965
Rental Contact: Russell Richins

8147 DIXIE COLLEGE: FINE ARTS CENTER
225 S 700th E
Saint George, UT 84770
Phone: 435-652-7790
Fax: 435-656-4021

8148 DIXIE COLLEGE FINE ARTS CENTER ARENA THEATRE
225 S 700th E
Saint George, UT 84770
Phone: 435-652-7790
Fax: 435-656-4021

8149 DIXIE COLLEGE FINE ARTS CENTER PROSCENIUM THEATRE
225 S 700th E
Saint George, UT 84770
Phone: 435-652-7790
Fax: 435-656-4021

8150 CAPITOL THEATRE
48 W Second S
Salt Lake City, UT 84101
Phone: 888-451-2787
Fax: 801-538-2272

8151 SYMPHONY HALL
123 W South Temple
Salt Lake City, UT 84101
Phone: 801-323-6800

8152 UNIVERSITY OF UTAH: KINGSBURY HALL
1395 E Presidents Circle
Room 190
Salt Lake City, UT 84112-0040
Phone: 801-581-6261
Fax: 801-585-5464
e-mail: lchristensen@kingsbury.utah.edu
Web Site: www.kingsburyhall.org
Management:
Director: Greg Gailmann
Manager Events/Operations: Lynda Christensen
Development Director: Kathleen Harmon Gardner
Technical Director: Randy Rasmussen
Founded: 1930
Specialized Field: Performing Arts Center
Paid Staff: 20
Income Sources: Rentals
Affiliations: University of Utah Music Department
Annual Attendance: 200,000
Facility Category: Auditorium
Type of Stage: Proscenium
Stage Dimensions: 120 x 48 x 72
Seating Capacity: 1,913
Year Built: 1930
Year Remodeled: 1996
Rental Contact: Manager of Events & Operations Lynda Christensen
Resident Groups: University of Utah Associated Students (Ballet, Organization theaters, operat, etc.)

8153 UNIVERSITY OF UTAH: JON M HUNTSMAN CENTER
1825 East South Campus Drive, Front
Salt Lake City, UT 84112
Phone: 801-581-5155
Fax: 801-581-6670
e-mail: rljames@huntsman.utah.edu
Management:
Director: Richard L James
Box Office Supervisor: Jon Jabobsen
Seating Capacity: 15,000

Vermont

8154 BARRE OPERA HOUSE
6 N Main Street
PO Box 583
Barre, VT 05641
Phone: 802-476-8188
Fax: 802-476-5648
e-mail: staff@barreoperahouse.org
Web Site: www.barreoperahouse.org
Management:
Executive Director: Carol Dawes
Paid Staff: 2
Annual Attendance: 22,000
Facility Category: Performance Hall
Type of Stage: Proscenium
Stage Dimensions: 32x30
Seating Capacity: 645
Year Built: 1899
Year Remodeled: 1993
Rental Contact: Carol Dawes

8155 BURLINGTON MEMORIAL AUDITORIUM
250 Main Street
Burlington, VT 05401
Phone: 802-864-6044
Fax: 802-863-4322

8156 FLYNN CENTER FOR THE PERFORMING ARTS
153 Main Street
Burlington, VT 05401
Phone: 802-652-4500
Fax: 802-863-8788
e-mail: amalina@flynncenter.org
Web Site: www.flynncenter.org
Management:
Programming Director: Arnie Malina
Founded: 1981
Paid Staff: 35
Volunteer Staff: 300
Annual Attendance: 100,000+
Facility Category: 150 Seat Modular Black Box
Type of Stage: Proscenium
Seating Capacity: 1,450; 150
Year Built: 1930
Year Remodeled: 2000
Rental Contact: Aimee Petrin

8157 FLYNN THEATRE FOR THE PERFORMING ARTS
153 Main Street
Burlington, VT 05401
Phone: 802-652-4500
Fax: 802-863-8788
e-mail: amalina@flynntheatre.org
Web Site: www.flynntheatre.org
Management:
Chief Programming Officer: Arnie Malina

8158 UNIVERSITY OF VERMONT: RECITAL HALL
Music Building
Redstone Campus - S Prospect Street
Burlington, VT 05405
Phone: 802-656-3040

8159 MIDDLEBURY COLLEGE: THEATRE PROGRAM
Seelek Studio Theatre
Wright Theatre Center for the Arts
Middlebury, VT 05753
Phone: 802-443-6433
Fax: 802-443-2137
Mission: Education

8160 YELLOW BARN
Rural Delivery 2
Box 371
Putney, VT 05346
Phone: 802-387-6637
Fax: 802-387-6637

8161 CHANDLER MUSIC HALL AND CULTURAL CENTER
71-73 Main Street
Randolph, VT 05060
Phone: 802-728-9878

Virginia

8162 BARTER PLAYHOUSE/THEATRE HOUSE
Main Street
PO Box 867
Abingdon, VA 24210
Phone: 540-628-3991
Fax: 540-676-6064

8163 VIRGINIA TECH UNIVERSITY: LANE STADIUM
Lane Stadium/Virgina Tech Athletics
Jamerson Center
Blacksburg, VA 24061-0502
Phone: 540-231-6796
Fax: 540-231-3060
Web Site: www.hokiesports.com
Management:
Director Athletics: Jim Weaver
Senior Associate Director Athletics: Sharon McCloskey
Associate Director Athletics: Tom Gabhard
Associate Director Athletics: Jon Jaudon
Director Fiance Affairs: Randy Butt
Assistant Dorector Athletics: Tim East
Director Sports Pronmotions: Tim East
Seating Capacity: 50,000

All listings are in alphabetical order by state, then city, then organization within the city.

8164 **VIRGINIA TECH UNIVERSITY: BURRUSS AUDITORIUM**
Virginia Technical Campus
225 Squires Center
Blacksburg, VA 24061
Phone: 703-231-5431
Fax: 703-231-5430

8165 **VIRGINIA TECH UNIVERSITY: CASELL COLISEUM**
Virginia Tech University
Washington Street
Blacksburg, VA 24061
Phone: 540-231-9963
Fax: 540-231-3060
Web Site: www.hokiesports.com
Management:
 Athletic Diretor: Jim Weaver

8166 **SAINT ANNE'S-BELFIELD SCHOOL SUMMER MUSIC ACADEMY**
1503 Wilton Farm Road
Charlottesville, VA 22911
Phone: 804-295-5499
Fax: 804-963-9964
Management:
 Executive Director: Susan Black

8167 **SCOTT STADIUM**
University of Virginia
PO Box 3785
Charlottesville, VA 22903
Phone: 804-982-5100
Fax: 804-982-5213
Management:
 Athletic Director: M Terry Holland
Seating Capacity: 40,000

8168 **UNIVERSITY OF VIRGINIA: UNIVERSITY HALL**
University of Virginia
PO Box 400846
Charolottsville, VA 22904-4846
Phone: 804-924-3791
Fax: 804-982-5212
Web Site: www.virginiasports.com
Management:
 Associate Athletic Director: Mark Fletcher
 Associate Athletic Director: Barry Parkhill
 Athletic Director: Craig Littlepage
 Sports Information Director: Rich Murray
 Head Football Coach: George Welsh
 Head Men's Basketball Coach: Pete Gillen
 Head Women's Basketball Coach: Debbie Ryan
 Associate Athletic Director: Mike Thomas
 Ticket Manager: Dick Mathias
Seating Capacity: 8,450

8169 **GEORGE MASON UNIVERSITY: PATRIOT CENTER**
George Mason University
4400 University Drive
Fairfax, VA 22030-4444
Phone: 703-993-3009
Fax: 703-993-3079
e-mail: bgeisler@gmu.edu
Web Site: www.patroitcenter.com
Management:
 General Manager: Barry H Geisler
 Director Arena Administration: John Besanko
 Director Operations: John Gabbert
Seating Capacity: 10,200

8170 **GEORGE MASON UNIVERSITY CENTER FOR THE ARTS**
4400 University Drive
Fairfax, VA 22030
Phone: 703-993-8877
Fax: 703-993-8883
e-mail: bbrining@gmu.edu
Web Site: www.gmu.edu/cfa
Management:
 Center for the Arts Director: Betsy Brininger

8171 **FORT EUSTIS MUSIC AND VIDEO CENTER**
ATZF-PRC-MT BUILDING 224
Fort Eustis, VA 23604
Phone: 757-878-3436

8172 **FORT EUSTIS MUSIC AND VIDEO CENTER - JACOBS THEATRE**
ATZF-PRC-MT BUILDING 224
Fort Eustis, VA 23604
Phone: 757-878-3436

8173 **RIVERSIDE CENTER DINNER THEATER AND CONFERENCE FACILITY**
95 Riverside Parkway
Fredericksburg, VA 22406
Phone: 540-370-4300
Fax: 540-370-4304
Web Site: www.riversidedt.com

8174 **HAMPTON COLISEUM**
1000 Coliseum Drive
PO Box 7309
Hampton, VA 23666
Phone: 757-838-5650
Fax: 757-838-2595
e-mail: jtsao@city.hampton.va.us
Web Site: www.hampton.va.us/coliseum
Management:
 Director: Joe Tsao

8175 HAMPTON UNIVERSITY: ARMSTRONG STADIUM
Hampton University
121 Holland Hall
Hampton, VA 23668
Phone: 757-727-5641
Fax: 757-728-6995
Management:
Athletic Director: Dennis E Thomas

8176 BRIDGEFORTH STADIUM
Godwin Hall, MSC 2301
Harrisonburg, VA 22807
Phone: 540-568-6164
Fax: 540-568-3489
Management:
Athletic Director: Jeff Boume

8177 JAMES MADISON UNIVERSITY: WILSON HALL AUDITORIUM
James Madison University
Harrisonburg, VA 22807
Phone: 540-568-6211
Fax: 540-568-6598

8178 VIRGINIA MILITARY INSTITUTE: CAMERON HALL
Virginia Military Institute
North Main Street
Lexington, VA 24450
Phone: 540-464-7529
Fax: 540-646-7622
Web Site: www.vmi.edu
Management:
Director: Donny White

8179 VIRGINIA UNIVERSITY: ALUMNI FIELD STADIUM
North Main Street
Lexington, VA 24450
Phone: 540-464-7251
Fax: 540-464-7622
Web Site: www.vmi.edu
Management:
Athletic Director: Donny White

8180 LIBERTY UNIVERSITY: WILLIAM STADIUM
Liberty University
1971 University Boulevard
Lynchburg, VA 24502
Phone: 804-582-2100
Fax: 804-582-2076
Management:
Director: Woody Galbreath
Seating Capacity: 12,000

8181 LIBERTY UNIVERSITY: VINES CENTER
Liberty University
1971 University Boulevard
Lynchburg, VA 24502

Phone: 804-582-2000
Fax: 804-582-2076
Web Site: www.liberty.edu
Management:
Director: Woody Galbreath
Seating Capacity: 9,000

8182 LYNCHBURG FINE ARTS CENTER
1815 Thomson Drive
Lynchburg, VA 24501
Phone: 434-846-8451
Fax: 434-846-3806
e-mail: finearts@lynchburg.net
Web Site: www.lynchburgbiz.com/fac
Officers:
Chairman: Michael Gillette
Interim Executive Director: Judy Wynne
Management:
Executive Director: Mary Brumbaugh
Founded: 1962
Paid Staff: 12
Paid Artists: 100
Budget: $640,000
Income Sources: contributions, rentals, classes, performances
Annual Attendance: 50,000
Facility Category: arts center
Type of Stage: proscenium
Stage Dimensions: 20x40x30
Seating Capacity: 501
Year Built: 1962
Rental Contact: Fred Saheib

8183 PRINCE WILLIAM COUNTY STADIUM
14420 Bristow Road
Manassas, VA 22191
Phone: 703-792-7060
Fax: 703-792-4219
Management:
Director: Rich Artenian
Sports Marketing Coordinator: Marvin Vann
Seating Capacity: 6,000

8184 TULTEX CORPORATION
101 Commonwealth Boulevard
Martinsville, VA 24112
Phone: 540-632-2961
Fax: 510-632-9123

8185 MCLEAN COMMUNITY CENTER: ALDEN THEATRE
1234 Ingleside Avenue
McLean, VA 22101
Phone: 703-790-0123
Fax: 703-556-0547
e-mail: clare.kiley@co.fairfax.va.us
Web Site: www.mcleancenter.org
Management:
Performing Arts Director: Clare Kiley

8186 GENERIC THEATER
912 W 21st Street
PO Box 11071
Norfolk, VA 23517
Phone: 757-441-2729
Fax: 757-441-2729
e-mail: generic@whro.net
Web Site: www.generictheater.org/

8187 LITTLE THEATRE OF NORFOLK
801 Claremont Avenue
Norfolk, VA 23508
Phone: 757-627-8551

8188 NORFOLK SCOPE CULTURAL AND CONVENTION CENTER
Scope Plaza
201 E Brambleton Avenue
Norfolk, VA 23510
Phone: 757-664-6464
Fax: 757-664-6990
Web Site: www.norfolk.gov
Management:
   Media/Promotions Manager: Cynthia Carter-West
   Event Coordinator: Beth Spangler
   Productions Manager: Brock Jones
   Assistant Director: Bob Wagoner
Mission: To present the best in sports, family and cultural entertainment.
Founded: 1971
Specialized Field: Instrumental music, vocal music, theater, performing series, sports, concerts
Paid Staff: 56

8189 WELLS THEATRE
Monticello Avenue and Tazewell Street
Norfolk, VA 23514
Phone: 757-627-6988
Fax: 757-628-5958

8190 ROGERS STADIUM
Virginia State University
PO Box 9058
Petersburg, VA
Phone: 804-524-5030
Fax: 804-524-5763
Web Site: www.vsu.edu
Management:
   Interim Athletic Director: Edward Cooper
Seating Capacity: 13,500

8191 RADFORD UNIVERSITY THEATRE
Norwood Street
PO Box 6969
Radford, VA 24142
Phone: 540-831-5207
Fax: 540-831-6313

8192 CENTER STAGE
2310 Colts Neck Road
Reston, VA 22091

Phone: 703-476-4500
Fax: 703-476-8617

8193 CARPENTER CENTER FOR THE PERFORMING ARTS
600 E Grace Street
Richmond, VA 23219
Phone: 804-225-9000
Fax: 804-649-7402
e-mail: info@carpentercenter.org
Web Site: www.carpentercenter.com
Management:
   Executive Director: Joel Katz
   Administrative Manager/Group Sales: Carolyn Barefoot
   Business Manager: Maria Donaldson
   Director Marketing: Kristen Berrier
   Facility Manager: Joe Yarborough
Founded: 1983
Annual Attendance: 180,000
Type of Stage: proscenium
Stage Dimensions: width 76'6", depth 26'6"
Seating Capacity: 2,041
Year Built: 1928
Year Remodeled: 1983
Rental Contact: Joel Katz

8194 EMPIRE THEATRE COMPLEX
114 W Broad Street
Richmond, VA 23220
Phone: 804-344-8040
Fax: 804-643-2671

8195 EMPIRE THEATRE COMPLEX EMPIRE STAGE
118 W Broad Street
Richmond, VA 23220
Phone: 804-344-8040
Fax: 804-643-2671

8196 EMPIRE THEATRE COMPLEX: LITTLE THEATRE
114 W Broad Street
Richmond, VA 23220
Phone: 804-783-1688
Fax: 804-775-2325

8197 RICHMOND COLISEUM
City of Richmond
601 E Leigh Street
Richmond, VA 23219
Phone: 804-780-4970
Fax: 804-780-4606
Web Site: www.richmondcoliseum.org
Management:
   General Manager: Kathleen Turner
   Interim Manager: Tim Murphy
Seating Capacity: 15,523

8198 RICHMOND STADIUM
University of Richmond
Richmond, VA 23173

Phone: 804-289-8371
Fax: 804-289-8820
e-mail: athletic@richmond.edu
Web Site: www.richmond.edu/~athletic
Management:
    Athletic Director: Charles S Boone
Seating Capacity: 22,319

8199 ROBINS CENTER
University of Richmond
Richmond, VA 23173
Phone: 804-289-8371
Fax: 804-289-8820
Web Site: www.richmond.edu
Management:
    Athletic Director: Charles S Boone
    Sports Information Director: Phil Stantoon
    Head Football Coach: Jim Reid
    Head Basketball Coach (M): John Beilein
    Head Basketball Coach (W): Bob Foley
Seating Capacity: 9,171

8200 UNIVERSITY OF RICHMOND: JAMES L CAMP MEMORIAL
Richmond, VA 23173
Phone: 804-289-8263
Fax: 804-287-6006

8201 ROANOKE CIVIC CENTER
PO Box 13005
710 Williamson Road Northeast
Roanoke, VA 24016
Phone: 540-853-2241
Fax: 540-853-2748
e-mail: info@roanokeciviccenter.com
Web Site:
www.roanokeciviccenter.com/html/contact.html
Management:
    Interim Civic Facilities Director: Chip Snead
    Civic Facilities Manager: Chris Powell
    Booking Manager: Tricia Downie
    Marketing Director: Robyn Schon
    Business Manager: Mae Huff
    Event Services Manager: Lisa Moorman
    Catering Manager: Jed McCracken
    Box Office Manager: Judy Jennings
    Operations Superintendent: Gary Hannabass
Founded: 1971
Paid Staff: 35
Annual Attendance: 500,000
Facility Category: Public Assembly - Coliseum, Auditorium, Ex. Hall
Seating Capacity: 11,000
Year Built: 1971
Cost: $14 million
Rental Contact: Booking Manager Tricia Downie

8202 SALEM CIVIC CENTER
1001 Boulevard
Salem, VA 24153

Mailing Address: PO Box 886
Phone: 540-375-3004
Fax: 540-375-4011
Web Site: www.salenciviccenter.com
Management:
    Director Civic Center: Carey Harveycutter
    Assistant Director Civic Facilities: John Saunders
    Civic Center Supervisor: Paul Bowles
Mission: Multi purpose entertainment facility with Arena, Ballroom and parlors.
Founded: 1967

8203 SWEET BRIAR COLLEGE: BABCOCK AUDITORIUM
Box AU
Sweet Briar College
Sweet Briar, VA 24595
Phone: 804-381-6123
Fax: 804-381-6173
e-mail: Whittman@sbc.edu
Management:
    Manager: Loretta Whittman

8204 WOLF TRAP FARM PARK FOR THE PERFORMING ARTS
1624 Trap Road
Vienna, VA 22180
Phone: 703-255-1900
Fax: 703-255-1918

8205 VIRGINIA BEACH PAVILION CONVENTION CENTER
1000 19th Street
Virginia Beach, VA 23458
Phone: 804-428-8000
Fax: 804-422-8860

8206 WILLIAM & MARY HALL
College of Williams & Mary
PO Box HC
Williamsburg, VA 23187
Phone: 804-221-3355
Fax: 413-545-3005
Management:
    Director: Bettie S Adams
Seating Capacity: 11,300

8207 WILLIAM AND MARY COLLEGE: CARY FIELD
PO Box 399
Williamsburg, VA 23187
Phone: 804-221-3400
Fax: 413-545-3412
Web Site: www.wm.edu

Washington

8208 BISHOP CENTER FOR PERFORMING ARTS
1610 EP Smith Drive
Aberdeen, WA 98520
Phone: 206-533-0177
Fax: 206-532-6716

8209 GRAYS HARBOR COLLEGE: BISHOP CENTER FOR PERFORMING ARTS
1620 Edward P Smith Drive
Aberdeen, WA 98520
Phone: 360-538-4066
Fax: 360-538-4293
Management:
VP for Student Services: Arlene Torgerson
Coordinator of Student Programs: Morgan Brown
Volunteer Staff: 5
Budget: $60,000
Annual Attendance: 7,000
Type of Stage: Proscenium
Seating Capacity: 440
Year Built: 1975
Rental Contact: Maureen Espedal

8210 INTERURBAN CENTER FOR THE ARTS
12401 SE 320th Street
Auburn, WA 98092-3699
Phone: 253-833-9111
Fax: 253-288-3481
e-mail: pthomas@grcc.ctc.edu
Web Site: www.greenriver.ctc.edu
Management:
Program Manager: Patricia Thomas
Budget: $10,000

8211 CITY OF BELLINGHAM FACILITIES
2221 Pacific Street
Bellingham, WA 98226
Phone: 360-676-6854
Fax: 360-647-6367
Web Site: www.cob.org
Management:
Director: Jack Gamer

8212 MOUNT BAKER THEATRE
106 N Commercial
Bellingham, WA 98225
Phone: 360-733-5793
Fax: 360-671-0114
Web Site: www.mtbakertheatre.com

8213 WESTERN WASHINGTON UNIVERSITY PERFORMING ARTS CENTER
WWU College of Fine & Performing Arts
MS-9109
Bellingham, WA 98225
Phone: 360-650-2829
Fax: 360-650-3028
e-mail: cfpa@wwu.edu
Web Site: www.wwu.edu/~cfpa

Management:
Dean: Bertil van Boer

8214 WESTERN WASHINGTON UNIVERSITY EXPERIMENTAL
Performing Arts Center
Bellingham, WA 98225
Phone: 360-650-3000

8215 WESTERN WASHINGTON UNIVERSITY MAIN STAGE
Performing Arts Center
Bellingham, WA 98225
Phone: 360-650-3000
Fax: 206-676-3028

8216 WESTERN WASHINGTON UNIVERSITY OLD MAIN THEATRE
High Street
Bellingham, WA 98225
Phone: 360-650-3000

8217 COMMUNITY THEATRE
599 Lebo Boulevard
Bremerton, WA 98310
Phone: 360-373-5152
Fax: 360-373-6754
Toll-free: 800-865-1706
e-mail: bet@silverlink.net
Web Site: www.silverlink.net/bet

8218 CENTRALIA COLLEGE: CORBET THEATRE
600 W Locust
Centralia, WA 98531
Phone: 360-736-9391
Fax: 206-753-3404

8219 EVERETT CIVIC AUDITORIUM
2415 Colby Avenue
Everett, WA 98201
Phone: 425-388-4746
Fax: 425-339-4675

8220 EVERETT PARKS AND RECREATION DEPT.
1507 Wall Street
Everett, WA 98201
Phone: 425-257-8300
Fax: 425-257-8389
e-mail: wbecker@ci.everett.wa.us

8221 7TH STREET THEATRE
313 7th Street
Hoquiam, WA 98550
Phone: 360-532-0302

8222 KENT CIVIC AND PERFORMING ARTS CENTER
PO Box 1617
Kent, WA 98035
Phone: 253-520-2525
Fax: 253-520-2424
e-mail: cmiller@ci.kent.wa.us
Web Site: www.kcpac.org
Management:
   Executive Director: Christopher Miller

8223 KIRKLAND PERFORMANCE CENTER
350 Kirkland Avenue
Kirkland, WA 98033-6504
Phone: 425-828-0422
Fax: 425-889-9827
e-mail: slerian@kpcenter.org
Web Site: www.kpcenter.org
Management:
   Executive Director: Steve Lerian
   Marketing Director: Frank Stilwagner
   Development Director: Joe McAlwain
   Technical Director: Anthony Hughes
Mission: Responsive to the cultural needs of the community, Kirkland Performance Center opened in 1998 to provide a home for the presentation, support and promotion of the performing arts.
Founded: 1998
Specialized Field: Theatre; Dance; Music
Status: Nonprofit
Seating Capacity: 402

8224 MCCLELLAND ARTS CENTER
951 Delaware
Longview, WA 98632
Phone: 360-577-3345
Fax: 360-577-4002

8225 LINCOLN THEATRE CENTER
712 S 1st Street
PO Box 2312
Mt. Vernon, WA 98273
Phone: 360-336-2408
Fax: 360-336-2408
e-mail: ltheatre@sos.net
Web Site: www.lincolntheatre.org

8226 WHIDBEY PLAYHOUSE
1094 Midway Boulevard
Oak Harbor, WA 98277
Phone: 360-679-2237
e-mail: playhous@whidbey.net

8227 SOUTH PUGET SOUND COMMUNITY COLLEGE
2011 Mottman Road SE
Olympia, WA 98512
Phone: 360-754-7711
e-mail: director@spscc.ctc.edu

8228 WASHINGTON CENTER FOR THE PERFORMING ARTS
512 Washington Street SE
Olympia, WA 98501
Phone: 360-753-8585
Fax: 360-754-1177
e-mail: tiovanne@washingtoncenter.org
Web Site: www.washingtoncenter.org
Management:
   Executive Director: Thomas Iovanne

8229 A CONTEMPORARY THEATRE
700 Union Street
Seattle, WA 98101
Phone: 206-292-7660
Fax: 206-292-7676
Web Site: www.tickets.com/venue_info

8230 BATHHOUSE THEATRE
7312 W Greenlake Drive N
Seattle, WA 98103
Phone: 206-524-3608
Fax: 206-527-1942

8231 KEYARENA AT SEATTLE CENTER
305 Harrison Street
Seattle, WA 98109
Phone: 206-684-7200
Fax: 206-684-7366
e-mail: eventsales.seattlecenter@ciseattle.wa.us
Web Site: www.seattlecenter.com
Management:
   Director: Virginia Anderson
   Director Event Producer: John Rhamstine
   Associate Director: Margaret Wetter
Mission: Home to Seattle Supersonics (NBA) and Seattle Thunderbirds (WHL).
Seating Capacity: 15,000, 6000
Year Built: 1995

8232 MARION OLIVER MCCAW HALL
Seattle Center
305 Harrison Street
Seattle, WA 98109
Phone: 206-684-7202
Fax: 206-684-7366
e-mail: SCBooking@ci.seattle.wa.us
Web Site: www.seattlecenter.com
Management:
   Director: Virginia Anderson
   Marketing Manager: Barbara Bryant
   McCaw Hall Manager: Shelley Singh
   Director Human Resources: John Cunningham
   Booking Representative: Allison McGuire
Mission: Marion Oliver McCaw Hall is a renovation of the Opera House at Seattle Center. McCaw Hall will be completed and available for booking in the fall of 2003. Contact Alison McGuire, for your booking questions.
Seating Capacity: 2,890 Auditorium; 388 Racked Seat Lecture Hal
Organization Type: Grand Lobby available for special events

Resident Groups: Seattle Opera and Pacific Northwest Ballet

8233 MERCER ARENA AT SEATTLE CENTER
305 Harrison Street
Seattle, WA 98109
Phone: 206-684-7200
Fax: 206-684-7342
e-mail: eventsales.seattlecenter@ci.seattle.wa.us
Web Site: www.seattlecenter.com
Management:
    Director: Virginia Anderson
    Associate Director: Margaret Wetter

8234 SAFECO FIELD
PO Box 4100
Seattle, WA 98104-4100
Phone: 206-346-4000
Fax: 206-346-4400
Management:
    Manager Suite Services: Tad Richardson
    Manager Ballpark Events: Gus Peterson
    Manager Events Services: Kameron Durham
    Director Guest Relations: Alexi Kelly
    Director Safeco Field Operations: Tony Pereira
    VP/Ballpark Planning: John Palmer
    VP/Ballpark Operations: Neil Campbell
Seating Capacity: 47,000

8235 SEATTLE CENTER
305 Harrison Street
Seattle, WA 98109
Phone: 206-684-7202
Fax: 206-684-7366
e-mail: eventsales.seattlecenter@ci.seattle.wa.us
Web Site: www.seattlecenter.com
Management:
    Director: Virginia Anderson
    Director Event Production: John Rhamstine
    Director Human Resources: John Cunningham
Seating Capacity: 17,000

8236 SEATTLE CENTER OPERA HOUSE
321 Mercer Street
Seattle, WA 98109
Phone: 206-684-7200
Fax: 206-615-0306

8237 SEATTLE REPERTORY THEATRE
155 Mercer Street
Seattle, WA 98109-9982
Phone: 206-443-2222
Fax: 206-443-2379
Toll-free: 877-900-9285
e-mail: info@seattlerep.org
Web Site: www.seattlerep.org

8238 UNIVERSITY OF WASHINGTON: HUSKY STADIUM
University of Washington
208 Graves Building, Room 207
Box 354070
Seattle, WA 98195-4070
Phone: 206-543-2246
Fax: 206-616-1523
Web Site: www.gohuskies.com
Management:
    Asst Athletics: Chip Lydum
    Event Manager: Steve Harper
Mission: Home of the University of Washington athletics (NCAA).
Seating Capacity: 72,484
Year Built: 1920

8239 UNIVERSITY OF WASHINGTON: HEC EDMUNDSON PAVILION
University of Washington
208 Graves Building
Box 354070
Seattle, WA 98195
Phone: 206-543-7373
Fax: 206-616-1523
Web Site: www.gohuskies.com
Management:
    Assistant Athletic Director: Chip Lydum
Founded: 1927
Year Built: 1927
Year Remodeled: 1999

8240 UNIVERSITY OF WASHINGTON: MEANY HALL FOR THE PERFORMING ARTS
Box 351150
Meany Hall
Seattle, WA 98195-1150
Phone: 206-543-4882
Fax: 206-685-2759
e-mail: krashan@u.washington.edu
Web Site: www.meany.org
Management:
    Director: Matthew Krashan

8241 AVISTA STADIUM
602 N Havana
Spokane, WA 99202
Phone: 509-535-2922
Fax: 509-534-5368
Management:
    Manager: Dolly Hughes

8242 GONZAGA UNIVERSITY: GENE RUSSELL THEATRE
Spokane, WA 99258
Phone: 509-328-4220

8243 JOE ALBI STADIUM
W 334 Spokane Falls Boulevard
Spokane, WA 99201

Phone: 509-353-6500
Fax: 509-353-6511
Web Site: www.spokanecenter.com
Management:
   Events Manager: Maxey D. Adams

8244 METROPOLITAN PERFORMING ARTS CENTER
901 W Sprague
Spokane, WA 99204
Phone: 509-835-2638

8245 SPOKANE ARENA
City of Spokane Arena
W 720 Mallon Avenue
Spokane, WA 99201
Phone: 509-324-7000
Fax: 509-324-7050
e-mail: abb@spokanearena.com
Web Site: www.spokanearena.com
Management:
   General Manager: Kevin J Twohig
   Marketing Manager: Amy B Brown
Seating Capacity: 12,500

8246 SPOKANE CONVENTION CENTER
334 W Spokane Falls Boulevard
Spokane, WA 99201
Phone: 509-353-6500
Fax: 509-353-6511
Web Site: spokanecenter.com

8247 SPOKANE OPERA HOUSE
334 W Spokane Falls Boulevard
Spokane, WA 99201
Phone: 509-353-6500
Fax: 509-353-6511
Web Site: spokanecenter.com
Management:
   Director: Johnna Boxley
   Events Manager: Maxey Adams
Performs At: Performing Arts
Annual Attendance: 315,000
Facility Category: Performing Arts
Type of Stage: Wood
Stage Dimensions: 149.5'x59'
Seating Capacity: 2,700
Year Built: 1974
Rental Contact: Events Manager Maxey Adams

8248 CHENEY STADIUM
Tacoma Rainiers Baseball Club
2502 South Tyler Street
Tacoma, WA 98405
Phone: 253-752-7700
Fax: 253-752-7135
Web Site: www.tacomarainiers.com
Management:
   Asst. GM of Stadium Operations: Phil Cowan
Mission: The rental of the stadium, parking area and/or meeting rooms for as many outside events as possible. Includes concerts, car shows, travelling performers, etc.
Facility Category: Baseball Stadium

Rental Contact: Philip Cowan

8249 TACOMA DOME
2727 East D Street
Tacoma, WA 98421
Phone: 253-272-3663
Fax: 253-593-7620
e-mail: bbeard@tacomadome.org
Web Site: www.tacomadome.org
Management:
   Assistant Director: Jody Hodgson
   Director: Mike Combs
   Marketing Manager: Beth Beard
Founded: 1983
Seating Capacity: 20,200

8250 WHITMAN COLLEGE: CORDINER HALL
Walla Walla, WA 99362
Phone: 509-527-5111

8251 CAPITAL THEATRE
19 S 3rd Street
PO Box 102
Yakima, WA 98907
Phone: 509-575-6267
Fax: 509-575-6251

8252 YAKIMA VALLEY SUNDOME
1301 S Fair Avenue
Yakima, WA 98901
Phone: 509-248-7160
Fax: 509-248-8093
Web Site: www.fairfund.com
Management:
   General Manager: Greg Stewart
   Assistant General Manager: Greg Lybeck
   Events Manager: Ray Mata
Seating Capacity: 8,000

West Virginia

8253 WEST VIRGINIA WESLEYAN COLLEGE ATKINSON AUDITORIUM
59 College Avenue
Buckhannon, WV 26201
Phone: 304-473-8000
Fax: 304-472-2571

8254 OLD OPERA HOUSE COMPANY
204 N George Street
Charles Town, WV 25414
Phone: 304-725-4420
Fax: 304-725-4420

8255 CHARLESTON CIVIC CENTER
200 Civic Center Drive
Charleston, WV 25301
Phone: 304-345-1500
Fax: 304-357-7432

Management:
   General Manager: John D Robertson

8256   GEARY AUDITORIUM
2300 MacCorkle Avenue SE
Charleston, WV 25304
Phone: 304-357-4807
Fax: 304-357-4915

**8257   LAIDLEY FIELD ATHLETIC
RECREATIONAL CENTER**
200 Elizabeth Street
Charleston, WV 25311
Phone: 304-348-1134
Fax: 304-348-6559
Management:
   Facility Director: Lou Ann Lanham
Seating Capacity: 22,000

8258   WATT POWELL STADIUM
35th Street & Mac Corkle Avenue
Charleston, WV 25304
Phone: 304-925-8222
Fax: 304-344-0083
Web Site: www.charlestonallycats.com
Management:
   General Manager: Tim Bordein
Seating Capacity: 7,500

**8259   WEST VIRGINIA STATE COLLEGE
CAPITOL CENTER**
123 Summers Street
Charleston, WV 25301
Phone: 304-342-6522

8260   HUNTINGTON CIVIC ARENA
1 Civic Center Plaza
Huntington, WV 25701
Phone: 304-696-5990
Fax: 304-696-4463
Web Site: www.hcarena.com
Management:
   General Manager: Pete Wenzel
   Director Marketing: Hearth Brown
   Director Of Operations: Steve Kessick
   Ticket Director: Martha Lunsford
Facility Category: civic arena\ conference center
Year Built: 1977
Year Remodeled: 1999
Rental Contact: Pete Wenzel

**8261   HUNTINGTON MUSEUM OF ART
AMPHITHEATRE**
2033 McCoy Road
Huntington, WV 25701
Phone: 304-529-2701
Fax: 304-529-7447
Web Site: www.hmoa.org
Management:
   Executive Director: Margaret Mary Lane
   Director of Marketing/PR: John Gillispie
   Senior Curator: Janine Culligan

Director of Education: Katharine Cox
Mission: To provide services and education in the fine and performing arts.
Founded: 1952
Specialized Field: Visual
Paid Staff: 24
Volunteer Staff: 400
Budget: $1.9 million
Income Sources: Endowment; Gifts; Grants
Affiliations: AAM Accredited
Annual Attendance: 60,000
Facility Category: Museum with 300-Seat Auditorium
Type of Stage: Proscenium
Seating Capacity: 300
Year Built: 1970
Cost: $1 million
Rental Contact: Larry Mullins

**8262   HUNTINGTON MUSEUM OF ART
AUDITORIUM**
Park Hills
Huntington, WV 25701
Phone: 304-529-2701
Fax: 304-529-7447

8263   KEITH-ALBEE THEATRE
925 4th Avenue
Huntington, WV 25720
Phone: 304-525-4440

8264   MARSHALL ATHLETICS
2001 3rd Avenue
Huntington, WV 25703
Phone: 304-696-6448
Fax: 304-676-6448
Web Site: www.herdzone.com
Management:
   Athletic Director: Lance A West
Seating Capacity: 30,000

**8265   MARSHALL UNIVERSITY: JOAN C
EDWARDS PLAYHOUSE**
400 Halgreer Boulevard
Huntington, WV 25755
Phone: 304-696-2787

**8266   MARSHALL UNIVERSITY: SMITH
RECITAL HALL**
400 Halgreer Boulevard
Huntington, WV 25755
Phone: 304-696-3117
Fax: 304-696-4379
Web Site: marshall.edu/music

8267   VETERANS MEMORIAL FIELD HOUSE
PO Boox 5455
Huntington, WV 25703
Phone: 304-528-5173
Fax: 304-528-5185
Management:
   Manager: Donald S Ewanus
Seating Capacity: 6,800

8268 WEST VIRGINIA STATE COLLEGE THEATRE

Fine Arts Building
Institute, WV 25112
Phone: 304-766-3186
Fax: 304-766-5100

8269 CARNEGIE HALL

105 Church Street
Lewisburg, WV 24901
Phone: 304-645-7917
Fax: 304-645-5228

8270 COLLEGE OF CREATIVE ARTS: CHORAL RECITAL HALL

PO Box 6111
1 Evandale Drive
Morgantown, WV 26506-6111
Phone: 304-296-4841
Fax: 304-293-6896
e-mail: mark.oresovich@mail.wvu.edu
Web Site: www.wvu.edu/nccarts/
Management:
   Facilities Manager: Mark Oreskovick
   Interim Chairman Division Music: David Bess
   Associate Director/Finance: Linda Queen
   Director Operations: Mark S Oresicovich
Mission: Educational facility
Specialized Field: Visual art, music theatre and dance
Income Sources: Stage and private
Performs At: Choral Recital Hall
Affiliations: NASM - National Association of Schools of Theatre - NASAD
Annual Attendance: 22,500
Facility Category: Educational
Type of Stage: Indoor ampitheatre
Stage Dimensions: 18 x 56
Seating Capacity: 180
Year Built: 1968
Year Remodeled: 2000
Cost: $500,000

8271 LYELL B CLAY CONCERT THEATRE

College of Creative Arts
PO Box 6111
1 Evandale Drive
Morgantown, WV 26506-6111
Phone: 304-296-4841
Fax: 304-293-6896
e-mail: msoreskovich@mail.wvu.edu
Web Site: www.wvu.edu/nccarts/
Management:
   Dean/Director: J Bernard Schultz
   Chairman Division Theatre/Dance: Margaret McKowen
   Chairman Division of Art: Sergio Soave
   Chairman Division Music: David Bess
   Associate Director/Finance: Linda Queen
   Director Operations: Mark S Oresicovich
Mission: Educational facility
Specialized Field: Visual art, music theatre and dance
Income Sources: Stage and private
Performs At: Concert Theatre

Affiliations: National Association of Schools of Theatre; National Association of Schools of Art and Design, NASM
Annual Attendance: 200,000
Facility Category: Educational
Type of Stage: Proscenium
Stage Dimensions: 58 x 42
Seating Capacity: 1441
Year Built: 1968

8272 MONTAINEER FIELD

W Virginia University
Room 107
Morgantown, WV 26507-0877
Phone: 307-293-5621
Fax: 717-337-6528
Web Site: www.msnsportsnet.com
Management:
   Athletic Director: Ed Pastilong
Seating Capacity: 63,500

8273 WEST VIRGINIA UNIVERSITY COLISEUM

W Virginia University
PO Box 6017
Morgantown, WV 26506-6017
Phone: 304-293-4407
Fax: 304-293-7574
e-mail: andrews@events.wvu.edu
Web Site: www.events.wvu.edu
Management:
   Program Manager: Eric Andrews
Seating Capacity: 15,000

8274 WEST VIRGINIA UNIVERSITY CREATIVE ARTS CENTER

PO Box 6111
Morgantown, WV 26506-6111
Phone: 304-293-4841
Fax: 304-293-6896
e-mail: mark.oreskovich@mail.wvu.edu
Web Site: www.wvu.edu
Management:
   Assistant Director: Mark Oreskovich
Founded: 1969
Specialized Field: Visual; Music; Theatre; Dance
Annual Attendance: 300,000
Facility Category: Performing and Educational Arts Center
Year Built: 1965
Year Remodeled: 2002

8275 CAPITOL MUSIC HALL

1015 Main Street
Wheeling, WV 26003
Phone: 304-232-1170
Fax: 304-234-0067
Toll-free: 800-624-5456
e-mail: jamboree@jamboreeusa.com
Web Site: www.jamboreeusa.com
Officers:
   VP/General Manager: Larry Anderson
Management:

Theatre Manager: Paula Anderson
Promotions/Marketing Director: Terri A Phillips
Stage Manager: Tom Beck
Mission: Entertainment from country music artists, Broadway productions, comedy acts, Las Vegas-style acts and pop groups.
Founded: 1933
Budget: $400,000-1,000,000

8276 WHEELING CIVIC CENTER
Two 14th Street
Wheeling, WV 26003
Phone: 304-223-7000
Fax: 304-233-7001
Web Site: www.wheelingciviccenter.com
Seating Capacity: 8,000

8277 WHEELING ISLAND STADIUM
S Front Street
Wheeling, WV 26003
Phone: 304-243-0431
Fax: 304-243-0328
Web Site: www.wphs.ohio.k12.wv.us
Management:
   Manager: Robert Conaway
Seating Capacity: 10,000

Wisconsin

8278 LAWRENCE UNIVERSITY: MUSIC-DRAMA CENTER
420 E College Avenue
Appleton, WI 54912
Phone: 920-832-7000
Fax: 920-832-6633

8279 CEDARBURG PERFORMING ARTS CENTER
W 68 N 611 Evergreen Boulevard
Cedarburg, WI 53012
Phone: 262-376-6160
Fax: 262-376-6163
e-mail: jweninger@cedarburg.k12.wi.us
Management:
   Box Office Manager: Kathleen Pier
   Managing Director: John W Weninger
   Technical Director: Paul Thur
Founded: 1999
Paid Staff: 3
Volunteer Staff: 20
Income Sources: Ticket Revenue; District Funding
Performs At: School District Functions; Tear 1 &2 Arts; Local Talent
Annual Attendance: 50,000
Facility Category: Performing Arts Center
Stage Dimensions: 50x22x34
Seating Capacity: 580
Year Built: 1998
Cost: 1.5 million
Rental Contact: Managing Director John Weninger

8280 NORTHLAND PINES HIGH SCHOOL
Eagle River
PO Box 1269
Eagle River, WI 54521
Phone: 715-479-4473
Fax: 715-479-5808

8281 WL ZORN ARENA
University of Wisconsin: Eau Claire
105 Garfield Avenue
Eau Claire, WI 54701
Phone: 715-836-3881
Fax: 715-836-4268
Web Site: www.uwec.edu
Management:
   Conference Manager: Karen Stuber
Seating Capacity: 3,200

8282 BIRCH CREEK MUSIC CENTER
PO Box 230
Egg Harbor, WI 54209
Phone: 920-868-3763
Fax: 920-868-1643

8283 LAMBEAU FIELD
Green Bay Packers
1265 Lombardi Avenue
Green Bay, WI 54304
Phone: 920-496-5700
Fax: 920-496-5712
Web Site: www.packers.com
Management:
   President: Robert Harland
   Public Relations Executive Director: Lee Remmel
   Stadium Manager: Ted Eisenreich
   Marketing Director: Jeff Cieply
Specialized Field: Home of the Green Bay Packers
Seating Capacity: 60,790
Year Built: 1957
Year Remodeled: 1990

8284 UNIVERSITY OF WISCONSIN:P BROWN COUNTY ARENA
2420 Nicolet Drive
Green Bay, WI 54311-7001
Phone: 920-494-6868
Fax: 920-465-2178
Management:
   Director: Les Raduenz

8285 UNIVERSITY OF WISCONSIN: WEINDER CENTER FOR THE PERFORMING ARTS
University of Wisconsin-Green Bay
Green Bay, WI 54311
Phone: 920-465-2691
Fax: 920-465-2619
e-mail: erwinl@uwgb.edu
Web Site: www.weidnercenter.com
Management:
   Managing Director: Linda Erwin

Mission: To present cultural entertaining and educational programs to Northeast Wisconsin and serve as home for university and local performing arts organizations.
Organization Type: Performing

8286 PHIPPS CENTER FOR THE ARTS

109 Locust Street
Hudson, WI 54016
Phone: 715-386-2305
Fax: 715-381-2177
e-mail: info@thephipps.org
Web Site: www.thephipps.org
Officers:
  President: Sarah J Andersen
  VP: Mark J Gherty
  Secretary: Roberta Pominville
  Treasurer: James Steel
Management:
  Executive Director: John H Potter
Mission: To celebrate the creative spirit.
Founded: 1981
Specialized Field: Multi-Disciplinary
Paid Staff: 7
Volunteer Staff: 500
Paid Artists: 100
Non-paid Artists: 200
Budget: $900,000
Income Sources: Earned and Contributed
Affiliations: Wisconsin Presenters Network
Annual Attendance: 22,500
Facility Category: Arts Center
Type of Stage: Proscenium
Stage Dimensions: 36' x 34'/247
Year Built: 1983
Year Remodeled: 1992
Cost: $7 million
Rental Contact: Executive Director John H Potter

8287 UNIVERSITY OF WISCONSIN AT PARKSIDE

900 Wood Road
Box 2000
Kenosha, WI 53141-2000
Phone: 262-595-3339
Fax: 262-595-2202
Management:
  Activities Assistant Director: Stephanie Sirovatka
Budget: $35,000-60,000
Performs At: Communication Arts Theatre

8288 MITCHELL HALL GYMNASIUM

University of Wisconsin-Lacrosse
1725 State Street
La Cross, WI 54601
Phone: 608-785-8679
Fax: 608-785-8674
Web Site: www.uwlax.edu
Management:
  Facilities Director: Mark Guthrie
Seating Capacity: 3,400

8289 CAMP RANDALL STADIUM

1440 Monroe Street
Madison, WI 53711
Phone: 608-262-1866
Fax: 608-265-3036
e-mail: arn@athletics.wisc.edu
Web Site: www.uwbadgers.com
Management:
  Interim Athletic Director: Andrea Nilsen
  Facility Director: Barry Fox
Specialized Field: Home of University of Wisconsin athletics.
Seating Capacity: 77,745
Year Built: 1917
Year Remodeled: 1968

8290 KOHL CENTER

601 W Dayton Street
Madison, WI 53715-1233
Phone: 608-263-5645
Fax: 608-265-4700
e-mail: arn@athletics.wisc.edu
Web Site: www.uwbadgers.com
Management:
  Associate Athletic Director: Jamie Pollard
  Interim Assistant Athletic Director: Andrea Nilsen
  Facility Director: Barry Fox
Seating Capacity: 17,142
Year Built: 1998

8291 MADISON AREA TECHNICAL COLLEGE, MITBY THEATER

3550 Anderson Road
Madison, WI 53704-2599
Phone: 608-246-6529
Fax: 608-246-6880
e-mail: dhesler@madison.tec.wi.us
Web Site: www.mitbytheater.madison.tec.wi.us
Management:
  Managing Director: D Corey Hesler
Budget: $20,000-35,000
Performs At: Norman Mitby Theater

8292 MADISON CIVIC CENTER

211 State Street
Madison, WI 53703
Phone: 608-258-4177
Fax: 608-258-4971
e-mail: civiccenter@ci.madison.wi.us
Web Site: www.madcivic.org
Management:
  Director: Robert B D'Angelo
  Associate Director: Reynold Peterson
  Events Manager: Rudy Lienau
  Marketing Director: Anna Hahn
  Ticket Office Manager: Bob Palmer
Mission: Multi-venue regional Performing Arts Center.
Founded: 1980
Specialized Field: Community Facility, all types
Paid Staff: 45
Volunteer Staff: 250
Budget: 3.5 - 4.5 Million
Income Sources: Operations; Government
Performs At: Oscar Mayer Theatre

Affiliations: Madison Cultural Arts District
Annual Attendance: 250,000
Facility Category: Theater
Type of Stage: Proscenium
Year Built: 1928
Year Remodeled: 1980
Rental Contact: Rudy Lienau

8293 UNIVERSITY OF WISCONSIN: SPORTS CENTER

1440 Monroe Street
Madison, WI 53711
Phone: 608-262-7974
Fax: 608-265-3036
e-mail: firstname.lastname@ccmail.adp.wisc.edu
Web Site: www.wisc.edu/ath/
Management:
   Athletic Director: Pat Richter
Seating Capacity: 3,000

8294 UNIVERSITY OF WISCONSIN: UNIVERSITY FIELDHOUSE

University of Wisconsin
1440 Monroe Street
Madison, WI 53711
Phone: 608-262-1866
Fax: 608-265-3036
Web Site: www.wisc.ed/ath/
Management:
   Sports Information Director: Tam Flarup
   Athletic Director: Pat Richter
   Head Football Coach: Barry Alvarez
   Head Basketball Coach (M): Dick Bennett
   Head Basketball Coach (W): Jane Albright/Dieterl
Seating Capacity: 11,500

8295 CAPITOL CIVIC CENTRE

913 S 8th Street
PO Box 399
Manitowoc, WI 54221-0399
Phone: 920-683-1937
Fax: 920-683-0272
e-mail: ccc@cccshows.org
Web Site: www.cccshows.org
Management:
   Executive Director: Joseph A Ferlo
   Assistant Director: Peggy Krey
Budget: $60,000-150,000
Seating Capacity: 1,150
Year Built: 1921
Year Remodeled: 1987

8296 SILVER LAKE COLLEGE

2406 S Alverno Road
Manitowoc, WI 54220
Phone: 920-684-6691

8297 MUSIC LIBRARY ASSOCIATION

8551 Research Way
Suite 180
Middletown, WI 53562

Phone: 608-836-5825
Fax: 608-831-8200
e-mail: mla@areditions.com
Web Site: www.musiclibraryassoc.org
Officers:
   President: James P Cassaro
   Past-President: Paula D Matthews
   Treasurer/Executive Secretary: Laura Gayle Green
   Recording Secretary: Lynn Gullickson
Founded: 1931

8298 ALVERNO COLLEGE

Pitman Theatre
3401 S 39th Street, PO Box 343922
Milwaukee, WI 53234
Phone: 414-382-6044
Fax: 414-382-6354
e-mail: boxoffice@alverno.edu
Web Site: www.alverno.edu
Management:
   Assistant Director: Jan Kellogg
   Director: Amanda Lang
Paid Staff: 3
Annual Attendance: 5000
Facility Category: Performing Arts Venue
Type of Stage: Proscenium
Stage Dimensions: 40' x 30'
Seating Capacity: 930
Year Built: 1951
Rental Contact: Jan Kellogg

8299 MARCUS CENTER FOR THE PERFORMING ARTS

929 N Water Street
Milwaukee, WI 53202-3122
Phone: 414-273-7121
Fax: 414-273-5480
Toll-free: 800-612-3500
e-mail: hlofy@marcuscenter.org
Web Site: www.marcuscenter.org
Officers:
   President: Paul Mathews
   Executive VP: Tom Gergerich
   Finance/Human Resource VP: Carol Hayden
   Director Marketing/Public Relations: Heidi Lofy
Management:
   Service Director: Mark Barnes
   Technical Director: Eric Zaun
   Facilities Director: Dick Hecht
Mission: To serve the community, offer facilities and services of the highest quality, also makes a wide range of performing arts available.
Income Sources: Technical income; County grants
Affiliations: Milwaukee Ballet Company; Florentine Opera Company; First Stage Children's Theatre; Milwaukee Youth Symphony Orchestra
Resident Groups: Milwaukee Ballet Co.; Florentine Opera Co.; Milwaukee Symphony Orch.; First Stage Children's Theater

8300 MILLER PARK

1135 S 70th Street
Suite 500
Milwaukee, WI 53214

Phone: 414-607-4040
Fax: 414-607-4044
Web Site: www.millerpark.org
Management:
   COB: Robert Trunzo
   Executive Direector: Michael Duckett

8301 MILWAUKEE AREA TECHNICAL COLLEGE: COOLEY AUDITORIUM
700 W State Street
Milwaukee, WI 53233
Phone: 414-297-6600
Fax: 414-271-2195

8302 MILWAUKEE COUNTY STADIUM
201 W 46th Street
Milwaukee, WI 53214
Phone: 414-933-4114
Fax: 414-933-2604
Web Site: www.milwaukeebrewery.com
Management:
   Director Operations: Steve Ethier
   Marketing Director: Dean Rennick
   Suites Director: Geoff Campion
   Concessions Manager: Tom Olsen
Seating Capacity: 55,000

8303 MILWAUKEE THEATRE
Wisconsin Center District
400 West Wisconsin Avenue
Milwaukee, WI 53203
Phone: 414-908-6000
Fax: 414-908-6010
e-mail: slange@wcd.org
Web Site: www.wcd.org
Officers:
   President: Richard A Geyer
Management:
   Director Marketing/Sales: Sandra A Lange
   Director Event Services: David Anderson
   Box Office Manager: Donna Piotrowski
   Director Business Development: Richard Freiberg
Facility Category: Theatre
Type of Stage: Proscenium
Seating Capacity: 4,200
Year Built: 1905
Year Remodeled: 2002
Cost: $34 million
Rental Contact: Director Marketing/Sales Sandra Lange

8304 PABST THEATRE
144 E Wells Street
Milwaukee, WI 53202
Phone: 414-286-3665
Fax: 414-278-2154
e-mail: psbstth@execpc.com
Management:
   Executive Director: Philip Procter

8305 US CELLULAR ARENA
Wisconsin Center District
400 W Winconsin Avenue
Milwaukee, WI 53203

Phone: 414-908-6000
Fax: 414-908-6010
e-mail: rfreiber@wed.org
Web Site: www.wed.org
Officers:
   President: Richards A Geyer
Management:
   Box Office Manager: Donna Piotrowski
   Director Marketing/Sales: Sandra A Lange
   Director Event Services: David Anderson
   Director Business Development: Richard Freiberg
Seating Capacity: 12,600

8306 MONROE ARTS CENTER
PO Box 472
Monroe, WI 53566
Phone: 608-325-5700
Fax: 608-329-4004
e-mail: mac@cppweb.com
Management:
   Executive Director: Sandra Brown
   Assistant Director: Lori Grinnell

8307 GRAND OPERA HOUSE
100 High Avenue
PO Box 1004
Oshkosh, WI 54903
Phone: 414-424-2355
Fax: 920-424-2357
e-mail: bobi@grandoperahouse.org
Web Site: www.grandoperahouse.org
Officers:
   Chairman: Betty Adams
Management:
   Executive Director: Robert Destocki
   Business Manager: Meery Little
   Tech Director: Tom Hanson
Founded: 1883
Specialized Field: All
Paid Staff: 7
Volunteer Staff: 100
Paid Artists: 20
Non-paid Artists: 20
Budget: $500,000
Income Sources: Public; Private
Affiliations: City of Oshkosh
Stage Dimensions: 30'x30'
Seating Capacity: 660
Year Built: 1883
Year Remodeled: 1986
Rental Contact: Merry Little

8308 PIONEER FIELD
University of Wisconsin
One University Plaza
Platteville, WI 53818
Phone: 608-342-1567
Fax: 608-342-1567
Web Site: www.uwplatt.edu
Management:
   Athletic Director: Mark Wolesworth
Seating Capacity: 10,000

All listings are in alphabetical order by state, then city, then organization within the city.

8309 UNIVERSITY OF WISCONSIN: CENTER FOR THE ARTS
One University Plaza
Platteville, WI 53818
Phone: 608-342-1298
Fax: 608-342-1478
e-mail: hassig@nwplatt.edu
Web Site: www.uwplat.edu/ncfa
Officers:
    Reservationist: Giner Zielke
    Chair, Fine Arts Department: Dan Fairchild
Management:
    Program Coordinator: John Hassig
Founded: 1866
Paid Staff: 1
Income Sources: Box office, grants, student support
Facility Category: Concert Hall, Theatre House
Type of Stage: Flexible; Proscenium
Stage Dimensions: 55 x 48
Seating Capacity: 578
Year Built: 1981
Cost: 5.2 Million
Rental Contact: Reservationist Ginger Zielke

8310 RIPON COLLEGE: DEMMER RECITAL HALL
Rodman Arts Center
300 Seward Street, Box 248
Ripon, WI 54971
Phone: 414-748-8120
Fax: 414-748-9262

8311 FINE ARTS THEATRE
One University Drive
Sheboygan, WI 53081
Phone: 414-459-6600
Fax: 920-459-6602

8312 JOHN MICHAEL KOHLER ARTS CENTER
608 New York Avenue
Sheboygan, WI 53081
Phone: 920-458-6144
Fax: 920-458-4473

8313 LUCILLE TACK CENTER FOR THE ARTS
PO Box 337
300 School Street
Spencer, WI 54479
Phone: 715-659-4499
Fax: 715-659-5470
Web Site: www.spencer.kiz.wi.us/ltca
Management:
    Executive Director: Deborah Janz
Mission: To provide an environment that encourage a variety of opportunities to enlighten, enrich and develop acttitud growth for community members of all ages.
Paid Staff: 1
Volunteer Staff: 50
Seating Capacity: 500

8314 UNIVERSITY OF WISCONSIN-SUPERIOR
Superior, WI 54880
Phone: 715-394-8369

8315 WAUKESHA CIVIC THEATRE
Margaret Brate Bryant Civic Theatre
264 W Main Street
Waukesha, WI 53186
Phone: 262-547-4911
Fax: 262-547-8454
e-mail: planious@waukeshacivictheatre.com
Web Site: ww.waukeshacivictheatre.com
Founded: 1957

8316 WARHAWK STADIUM
University of Wisconsin
800 W Main Street
Whitewater, WI 53190
Phone: 414-472-1234
Fax: 414-472-2791
e-mail: myersw.wwwvax.uww.edu
Web Site: www.uww.edu
Management:
    Athletic Director: Willie Myers
    Athletic Director/Women's: Dianne Jones
Seating Capacity: 11,500

Wyoming

8317 CASPER COLLEGE: DURHAM HALL
125 College Drive
Casper, WY 82601
Phone: 307-268-2110

8318 CASPER EVENTS CENTER
1 Events Center Drive
PO Box 128
Casper, WY 82602
Phone: 307-235-8441
Fax: 307-235-8445
e-mail: bobbit@trib.com
Web Site: www.caspereventscenter.com
Management:
    Director: Max L Torbert
Seating Capacity: 10,452

8319 CHEYENNE CIVIC CENTER
2101 O'Neil Avenue
Cheyenne, WY 82001
Phone: 307-637-6364
Fax: 307-637-6365
e-mail: drohla@cheyennecity.org
Management:
    Director: Dru A Rohla

8320 CAM-PLEX HERITAGE CENTER
1635 Reata Drive
Gillette, WY 82718

Phone: 307-682-0552
Fax: 307-682-8418
Toll-free: 800-358-1897
e-mail: camplex@ccg.co.campbell.wy.us
Web Site: www.cam-plex.com
Management:
   Theatre Manager: Phyllis Colpitts

8321 UNIVERSITY OF WYOMING: ARENA AUDITORIUM
University of Wyoming
University Station
Laramie, WY 82071
Phone: 307-766-2292
Fax: 307-766-5414
e-mail: wyosid@uwyo.edu
Web Site: www.uwyo.edu/om/ath/inercol/index.htm
Management:
   Head Football Coach: Vick Koenning
   Head Basketball Coach (M): Steve McClain
   Head Basketball Coach (W): Cindy Fisher
   Athletic Director: Lee Moon
   Associate Ath/Etic Director: Keener Fry
   Sports Information Director: Kevin McKinney
   Senior Women's Adminstrator: Barbara Burke
   Executive Director: Randy Woliniak
Seating Capacity: 15,028

8322 UNIVERSITY OF WYOMING: ARTS AND SCIENCES AUDITORIUM
PO Box 3254
Laramie, WY 82071
Phone: 307-766-5242
Fax: 307-766-5326

8323 UNIVERSITY OF WYOMING: FINE ARTS CONCERT HALL
PO Box 3037
Laramie, WY 82071
Phone: 307-766-5242

8324 WAR MEMORIAL STADIUM (WY)
University of Wyoming
PO Box 3414
Laramie, WY 82071
Phone: 307-766-2293
Fax: 307-766-2346
e-mail: wyosid@uwyo
Web Site: www.uwyo.edu
Management:
   Athletic Director: Lee Moon
   Associate Athletic Director: Randy Welniak
   Sports Informations Director: Kevin McKinney
Seating Capacity: 33,500

8325 COMMUNITY FINE ARTS CENTER
400 C Street
Rock Springs, WY 82901
Phone: 307-362-6212
Fax: 307-382-4101
e-mail: cfac@rock.sw1.k12.wy.us
Web Site: www.cfac4art.com

Management:
   Director: Gregory Gaylor

8326 WYO THEATER
PO Box 528
42 N Main Street
Sheridan, WY 82801
Phone: 307-672-9083
Fax: 307-672-8074
e-mail: wyotheater@wavecom.net
Web Site: www.wyotheater.com
Management:
   Executive Director: Marcia F Dunsmore

Arizona

8327 PATRICIA ALBERTI PERFORMING ARTISTS MANAGEMENT
11250 N Pinto Drive
Fountain Hills, AZ 85268
Phone: 480-816-8462
Fax: 480-816-8464
e-mail: palberti@earthlink.net
Web Site: www.performingarts.net
Officers:
    President/Owner: Patricia Alberti
Mission: To offer our eclectic roster of artists including Jazz, Classical, and Children's Programming to arts personnel with quality and efficient service.
Founded: 1989
Specialized Field: Music; Opera; Music Theater; Theater
Paid Staff: 1

8328 ENCORE ATTRACTIONS
9580 E Ranch Gate Road
Scottsdale, AZ 85255
Phone: 480-502-9779
Fax: 480-502-9363
Web Site: www.encoreattractions.com
Management:
    Producer: Jerry Lonn
    Sales/Marketing: Anna Vogel
    Contracts/Publicity: Ginny Lonn
Mission: Specializes in producing and touring theatrical productions for mid-sized and smaller markets and theaters.
Founded: 1994

California

8329 BERKELEY AGENCY
2608 9th Street
Suite 301
Berkeley, CA 94710
Phone: 510-843-4902
Fax: 510-843-7271
Web Site: www.berkeleyagency.com
Officers:
    Owner: Jim Cassell
Specialized Field: Music

8330 CHL ARTISTS
269 S Beverly Drive #466
Beverly Hills, CA 90212
Phone: 310-247-2248
Fax: 310-247-2254
e-mail: chlartists@aol.com
Web Site: www.chlartists.com
Officers:
    President/CEO: Christopher H Ling
Mission: CHL Artists is the preeminent classical artist management company on the west coast of the United States, representing some of the most exciting, individual and dynamic soloists and conductors throughout North America today.
Founded: 1992

8331 WILLIAM MORRIS AGENCY
One William Morris Place
Beverly Hills, CA 90212
Phone: 310-859-4000
Fax: 310-859-4462
Web Site: www.wma.com

8332 NANCY CARLIN ASSOCIATES
Concord, CA
Mailing Address: PO Box 6499 Concord, CA 94524
Phone: 925-686-5800
Fax: 925-680-2582
e-mail: nancy@nancycarlinassociates.com
Web Site: www.nancycarlinassociates.com
Mission: Nancy Carlin Associates currently books North America tours for folk, ethnic and world musicians. Our focus is on Celtic music - Irish, Scottish and especially the Welsh.
Founded: 1976

8333 PRINCE/SF PRODUCTIONS
1450 Southgate Avenue
Suite 206
Daly City, CA 94015-4021
Phone: 650-550-0005
Fax: 650-550-0006
e-mail: ACappella@PrinceSF.com
Web Site: www.princesf.com
Mission: Worldwide booking source for vocal-only groups.

8334 SPOTOMA
17027 Tennyson Place
Granada Hills, CA 91423
Phone: 818-366-3637
Fax: 818-363-3258
e-mail: bralston@bobralston.com
Web Site: www.bobralston.com
Management:
    Music Director: Bob Ralston

8335 ISLAND HEART ARTISTS
PO Box 1354
Hoboken, CA 07030
Phone: 201-868-2246
Fax: 201-868-3964

8336 CADENCE ARTS NETWORK
10516 Clarkson Road
Los Angeles, CA 90064
Phone: 310-838-0849
Fax: 310-838-1922
e-mail: cadencearts@aol.com
Web Site: www.dance90210.com/Cadence.html
Management:
    Director: Rachel Cohen
    Associate: Lori Perkovich
Mission: Cadence Arts Network is a development, booking, resource and referral network specializing in Dance, New Performance, World Music and Jazz.
Founded: 1989
Specialized Field: Dance; Cirque; World Music; Jazz

8337 CHAMJO GROUP
PO Box 491160
Los Angeles, CA 90049
Phone: 310-535-5609
Fax: 636-230-0001
Web Site: www.chamjo.com
Mission: ChAmJo concentrates on four basic yet specific areas of concentration of our efforts: Management; Entertainment; Investments; Publishing.
Founded: 1990

8338 HARMORY ARTISTS
8455 Beverly Boulevard
Suite 400
Los Angeles, CA 90048
Phone: 323-655-5007
Fax: 323-655-5154
e-mail: contact-us@harmoryartists.com
Web Site: www.harmonyartists.com

8339 PARADISE ARTISTS
108 E Matilija Street
Ojai, CA 93023
Phone: 805-646-8433
Fax: 805-646-3367
Web Site: www.paradiseartists.com

8340 OPEN DOOR MANAGEMENT
865 Via de la Paz
Suite 365
Pacific Palisades, CA 90272
Phone: 310-459-2559
Fax: 310-454-7803
e-mail: bill@opendoormanagement.com
Web Site: www.opendoormanagement.com
Mission: Personal management company specializing in jazz artists.

8341 STEVEN BARCLAY AGENCY
12 Western Avenue
Petaluma, CA 94952
Phone: 707-773-0654
Fax: 707-778-1868
Web Site: www.braclayagency.com
Officers:
  Director: Steven Barclay

8342 SACRAMENTO ARTS ADVOCATE
Sacramento, CA 95814
Phone: 916-452-7722
Fax: 916-452-0757
e-mail: info@sacramentoartsadvocate.org
Web Site: www.sacramentoartsadvocate .org
Management:
  Choreographer/Director: Ron Cisneros
  Director: Lisa Caretto
Mission: To raise public awareness about the vital, cultural, educational and economic role of the arts in our communities and to engage residents of the Sacramento region in advocating of the arts.
Founded: 2001

8343 CSTAR
89 Melville Avenue
San Anselmo, CA 94960
Phone: 415-458-2882
Fax: 415-458-2992
e-mail: greg@cstartists.com
Web Site: www.cstartists.com

8344 CALIFORNIA ARTISTS MANAGEMENT
41 Sutter Street
Suite 420
San Francisco, CA 94104-4903
Phone: 415-362-2787
Fax: 415-362-2838
e-mail: don@calartists.com
Web Site: www.calartists.com
Officers:
  Founder: Susan Endrizzi
Management:
  Director: Donald E Osborne
Mission: California Artists Management is a professional booking agency representing an international roster of early, classical and world music, theater and performance art.
Founded: 1978
Specialized Field: Classical Music
Paid Staff: 2

8345 CIRCUM ARTS
2940 16th Street
Suite 110
San Francisco, CA 94103
Phone: 415-565-0725
Fax: 415-565-0731
Web Site: www.circum.org
Management:
  Executive Director: Richard Biles
  Membership Coordinator: Doris Caravaglia
Mission: Circum-Arts is a not-for-profit arts service organization with the mission to assist, advocate and encourage performing artists and visual arts projects. Our goal is to provide a complete service structure of administrative, technical and educational resources that are accessible and affordable to individual artists and emerging companies in the performing arts.
Status: Not-For-Profit

8346 CORBETT ARTS MANAGEMENT LTD.
41 Sutter Street
Suite 518
San Francisco, CA 94104-4903
Phone: 415-982-2505
Fax: 415-982-5295
e-mail: info@corbettarts.com
Web Site: www.corbettarts.com
Officers:
  President: Joanne Corbett-Barnes
Management:
  Artists' Administrative Associate: Erika Johnson
  Office Manager/Artists' Service: Brandon Adams
  Booking Services: David J Dieni
Mission: The agency is a culmination of a lifetime of performance, teaching, management and artistic administration experience by the founder.

Founded: 1991

8347 GARY LINDSEY ARTIST SERVICES
2700 15th Avenue
San Francisco, CA 94127
Phone: 415-759-6410
Fax: 415-681-9801
Toll-free: 800-947-9274
e-mail: LindseyArtists@aol/com
Web Site: www.napama.org/lindsey
Management:
   Director: Gary Lindsey
   Associated Director: Whitney Trilling
   Sales Representative: Sandra J Calvin

8348 MARIEDI ANDERS ARTISTS MANAGEMENT
535 El Camino del Mar
San Francisco, CA 94121-1099
Phone: 415-752-4404
Fax: 415-752-7451
e-mail: maaminc@aol.com
Web Site: www.andersmanagement.com
Founded: 1960

8349 MATTHIAS VOGT ARTISTS' MANAGEMENT
211 Gough Street
Suite 112
San Francisco, CA 94102
Phone: 415-788-8073
Fax: 530-684-5535
e-mail: matthias.vogt@usa.net
Web Site: www.matthiasvogt.com

8350 ROBERT FRIEDMAN PRESENTS
1353 4th Avenue
San Francisco, CA 94122
Phone: 415-759-1992
Fax: 415-759-6663
Toll-free: 800-706-2787
e-mail: info@rfpresents.com
Web Site: www.rfpresents.com
Officers:
   President: Robert Friedman
Founded: 1973

8351 ROSEBUD AGENCY
PO Box 170429
San Francisco, CA 94117
Phone: 415-386-3456
Fax: 415-386-0599
e-mail: info@rosebuds.com
Web Site: www.rosebuds.com
Founded: 1976

8352 FOLKLORE PRODUCTIONS
1671 Appian Way
Santa Monica, CA 90401
Phone: 310-451-0767
Fax: 310-458-6005
e-mail: info@folkloreproductions.com
Web Site: www.folkloreproductions.com
Officers:
   Founder: Manuel Greenhill
   President: Mitchell Greenhill
   VP: Matthew Greenhill
Mission: Folklore Productions has represented artists in the folk, traditional and roots music worlds for many years.
Founded: 1950

8353 SCOTT STANDER & ASSOCIATES
13701 Riverside Drive
Suite 201
Sherman Oaks, CA 91423
Phone: 818-905-7000
Fax: 818-990-0582
Web Site: www.scottstander.com

8354 UNDERGROUND SOUND DJ BOOKINGS & MANAGEMENT COMPANY
PO Box 341746
West Los Angeles, CA 90064-6746
Phone: 310-479-7339
Fax: 310-861-9061
e-mail: ruth@ugsoundmgmt.com
Web Site: www.ugsoundmgmt.com
Management:
   Booking Manager: Ruth Nakada
Mission: Artist management and promotions, event promotions and music production. Our goal is to promote the music of established recording artists and up and coming recording artists through our own event promotions, booking and music production on our own record label.
Founded: 1994

Colorado

8355 IZNALOA GUITAR WORKS
PO Box 462072
Aurora, CO 80046
Phone: 303-693-6267
Fax: 303-766-9332
e-mail: vbrandys@iznaolaguitarworks.com
Web Site: www.iznaolaguitarworks.com
Management:
   General Manager: Victoria Brandys
Mission: An independent publishing and recording company, as well as an Artist Managing and Booking Agency to promote classical Guitarist Ricardo Iznaola's publications, recordings and performing international career.
Founded: 1990
Specialized Field: Classical Guitar
Status: Limited Liability
Paid Artists: 1
Non-paid Artists: 1

Connecticut

8356 GAMI/SIMONDS
24 Church Hill Road
Washington Depot, CT 06794
Phone: 860-354-5295
Fax: 860-354-5298
e-mail: gamisim@worldnet.att.net
Web Site: www.gamisim.com
Mission: Gami/Simonds is a full service performing arts management company offering personal management and booking for internationally acclaimed artists from North and South America.
Founded: 1991
Type of Stage: Proscenium
Stage Dimensions: 28'x30,
Seating Capacity: 222
Year Built: 1964
Year Remodeled: 2001

8357 PHILLIP TRUCKENBROD CONCERT ARTISTS
97 S Street, Suite 100
PO Box 331060
West Hartford, CT 06133-1060
Phone: 860-560-7800
Fax: 860-560-7788
e-mail: email@concertartists.com
Web Site: www.concertartists.com
Officers:
   President: Phillip Truckenbrod
   VP: Raymond Albright
   Operations: Victoria Burns
   Booking: James Rogers
Founded: 1967
Paid Staff: 5

District of Columbia

8358 LOIS HOWARD & ASSOCIATES
4834 W Street NW
Washington, DC 20007-1518
Phone: 202-342-1655
Fax: 202-342-5192
e-mail: lois@loishoward.com
Web Site: www.loishoward.com
Officers:
   President: Lois Howard
Mission: To provide highly personalized services to artists and clients in the classical music field. In addition to artist representation, we offer a broad range of consulting services to cassical artists as well as performing arts organizations.
Founded: 1995
Specialized Field: Classical Music

Florida

8359 BLADE AGENCY
203 SW 3rd Avenue
Gainesville, FL 32601
Mailing Address: PO Box 1556 Gainesville, FL 32602-1556
Phone: 352-372-8158
Fax: 352-372-1700
Toll-free: 800-367-1700
e-mail: info@bladeagency.com
Web Site: www.bladeagency.com
Officers:
   Owner/Manager: Charles Steadham
Mission: Blade Agency is an international full-service agency representing a variety of performers whose primary interest is providing their audiences with the best possible entertainment.
Founded: 1974

8360 PEYTON & DAY ENTERTAINMNET
PO Box 617289
Orlando, FL 32861
Phone: 407-299-0996
Fax: 407-299-5606
e-mail: lee@peytonday.com
Web Site: www.peytonday.com
Management:
   Agent: Lee Peyton
Mission: Full service entertainment bureau providing a wide range of highest quality performers for every conceivable event.

8361 NEW CENTURY ARTISTS
67 Sugar Mill Drive
Osprey, FL 34229
Phone: 941-966-9700
Fax: 941-966-9702
e-mail: sgeorge@newcentury.nu
Web Site: www.newcentury.nu
Officers:
   President: Scott George

8362 SIEGEL ARTIST MANAGEMENT
1220 Kirby Street
Palatka, FL 32177-0528
Phone: 368-325-8080
Fax: 368-325-8080
Web Site: www.siegelartist.com
Management:
   Contact: Jeanie Thompson

8363 ARTS GROUP
4957 Peregrine Point Way
Sarasota, FL 34231-3244
Phone: 941-927-1155
Fax: 941-925-2470
e-mail: aajupin@aol.com
Officers:
   President: A Alexandra Jupin

8364 SIEGEL ARTIST MANAGEMENT
283 W Lake Elbert Drive NE
Winter Haven, FL 33881-4736
Phone: 863-294-1586
Fax: 863-293-1415
Web Site: www.siegelartist.com
Management:

All listings are in alphabetical order by state, then city, then organization within the city.

Contact: Jane Lawrence Curtis

Georgia

8365 ALKAHEST AGENCY
Atlanta, GA 30359
Mailing Address: PO Box 49571
Phone: 404-315-0709
Fax: 404-636-0844
e-mail: alkagency@aol.com
Web Site: www.alkahest.net
Officers:
   President: Scott A Bridges
Founded: 1896
Specialized Field: Musci; Opera; Music Theater; Theater

8366 EASTCOAST ENTERTAINMENT
296 14th Street NW
Atlanta, GA 30318
Phone: 404-351-2263
Fax: 404-351-1558
Toll-free: 800-876-0016
Web Site: www.eastcoastentertainment.com
Mission: Worldwide booking agency, supplying talent
throughout this country and overseas for a wide range of
situations, including conventions and concerts, presidents
and royalty, movies and television, bar mitzvahs and
weddings.
Founded: 1976

8367 WORLD ARTISTS
3126 Bolero Drive
Atlanta, GA 30341
Phone: 770-939-4343
Fax: 770-908-1231
e-mail: lynnmc@mindspring.com
Web Site: www.lynnmcconnell.com

Illinois

8368 ARTRA-ARTISTS MANAGEMENT
555 W Madison Street
Suite 2110
Chicago, IL 60661
Phone: 312-648-4100
Fax: 312-648-0600
Toll-free: 800-354-1645
e-mail: artra@aol.com
Web Site: www.artra.com
Officers:
   President: Robert Bauchens
   VP: Terry Jares
Mission: ARTRA Artists Management is well known in
the music industry for the personalized service they give
to their artists and presenters.
Founded: 1984
Specialized Field: Music

8369 EARWIG MUSIC COMPANY
1818 W Pratt Boulevard
Chicago, IL 60626-3120
Phone: 773-262-0278
Fax: 773-626-0285
e-mail: info@earwigmusic.com
Web Site: www.earwigmusic.com
Officers:
   Founder/President/CEO: Michael Frank

8370 OVATION MANAGEMENT
6161 N Hamilton
Chicago, IL 60659
Phone: 773-338-4182
Fax: 773-338-8331
e-mail: ovationmgmt@aol.com
Web Site: www.ovationmanagement.org
Officers:
   President: Blanche Lewis
Mission: International concert agency representing
talented and unique classical artists.
Founded: 1989
Paid Artists: 7

8371 SIEGEL ARTIST MANAGEMENT
1416 Hinman Avenue
Evanston, IL 60201-5310
Phone: 847-475-4224
Fax: 847-475-0440
Web Site: www.siegelartist.com

**8372 CAPITOL INTERNATIONAL
PRODUCTIONS**
44 Fox Trail
Lincolshire, IL 60069
Toll-free: 800-770-0030
Web Site: www.capitolint.com/index.htm
Mission: Supplying acts for every type of events for over
four decades — fairs, festivals, theme parks, performing
arts centers, private functions or corporate fund raisers.

Indiana

8373 JEJ ARTISTS
2450 Rock Creek Drive
Bloomington, IN 47401-6822
Phone: 812-323-0427
Fax: 812-323-1453
e-mail: janet@jejartists.com
Web Site: www.jejartists.com
Management:
   Personal Representative: Janet Jarriel
Mission: Provides personal representation for some of the
finest musicians performing today. From opera singers to
concert organists to conductors, each artist holds a
reputation of outstanding musicianship and proven talent.
Founded: 1996
Specialized Field: Music Management
Paid Staff: 2
Paid Artists: 10

Iowa

8374 JECKLIN ASSOCIATES
2717 Nichols Lane
Davenport, IA 52803
Phone: 563-359-0866
Fax: 563-359-1266
e-mail: jecklin@webtv.net
Web Site: www.jecklinassociates.com
Officers:
   President: Lois Jecklin
Mission: Limits its roster to carefully chosen group of the most gifted artists with worldwide performing and recording credits. Their diverse repertoires encompass the classical, as well as less performed works, in keeping with our devotion to broadening musical understanding.
Founded: 1988
Specialized Field: Composers; Instrumentalists
Paid Staff: 2

Massachusetts

8375 ANNIE TIBERIO AGENCY
PO Box 2058
Amherts, MA 01004-2058
Phone: 413-256-0036
Fax: 413-256-0035
e-mail: annie@a-tiberio.com
Web Site: www.a-tiberio.com
Mission: A national arts booking agency, representing exclusively a small number of performing companies whose focus is music and theater celebrating the Earth and World Cultures. The agency and its artists maintain the highest standards of efficient service to clients and unique artistry and creativity to their audiences. Can fulfill programming needs for preforming arts series, festivals, arts councils, colleges, museums, special events, conferences.
Founded: 1983

8376 MARGE GUILLARDUCCI AGENCY
724 Berkley Street
Berkley, MA 02779
Phone: 508-822-3735
Fax: 508-880-6214
e-mail: margecris@mail.com
Web Site: www.welcome.to/ghilarducci
Founded: 1986

8377 ED KEANE ASSOCIATES
32 St. Edward Road
Boston, MA 02128
Phone: 617-567-6300
Fax: 617-569-5949
e-mail: info@edkeane.com
Web Site: www.edkeane.com

8378 KURLAND ASSOCIATES
173 Brighton Avenue
Boston, MA 02134
Phone: 617-254-0007
Web Site: www.tedkurland.com

Officers:
   President: Ted Kurland
   VP/Director Management Division: David Sholemson

8379 LORDLY & DAME
51 Church Street
Boston, MA 02116
Phone: 617-482-3593
Fax: 617-426-8029
e-mail: lordly@lordly.com
Web Site: www.lordly.com
Mission: Provide the finest speakers and programs pertaining to the most significant issues and defining moments of the times.
Founded: 1954

8380 MUSIC AMADOR
199 Pemberton Street
Cambridge, MA 02140
Phone: 617-492-1515
Fax: 617-492-1515
e-mail: mail@musicamador.com
Web Site: www.musicamador.com
Management:
   Director: Rosi Amador
Mission: Represents some of the foremost Latin music ensembles. The variety offered expands the very definition of the term Latin music.
Specialized Field: Music

8381 SIEGEL ARTIST MANAGEMENT
PO Box 67116
Chestnut Hill, MA 02467-0001
Phone: 617-232-2219
Fax: 617-232-2219
Web Site: www.siegelartist.com
Management:
   Contact: Jennifer Morris

8382 INTERNATIONAL MUSIC NETWORK
278 Main Street
Gloucester, MA 01930
Phone: 978-283-2883
Fax: 978-283-2330
Web Site: www.imnworld.com
Management:
   International Agent: Scott Southard
   European Agent: Katherine McVicker
   International Coordinator: Kristen Teixeira
   West Coast Agent: AnneMarie Southard
   West Coast Coordinator: Betty Bonney
   Northeast Agent: Todd Walker
   Midwest Asgent: David Lloyd
   South & MidAtlantic Agent: Jeanna Disney
   Administrative Coordinator: Susan Day
Mission: National and international booking agency exclusively representing more than forty musicians in a variety of genres including jazz, roots and other progressive musical styles.

8383 BERKSHIRE ARTISTS GROUP

PO Box 781
Lee, MA 01238
Phone: 413-243-6662
Fax: 208-988-1325
Web Site: www.berkshuireartistsgroup.com
Officers:
  Artistic Director: Ericka Wilcox
Specialized Field: Music; Opera; Music Theatre; Theatre

8384 CONCERTED EFFORTS

PO Box 600099
Newtonville, MA 02460
Phone: 617-969-0810
Fax: 617-969-6761
e-mail: concerted@concertedefforts.com
Web Site: www.concertedefforts.com
Management:
  Director/Artist Representative: Paul Kahn
  Artist Representative: Mike Leahy
  Artist Representative: Chris Colbourn
  Artist Representative: Dan Peraino
Mission: Concerted Efforts is proud to represent the finest in world music, zydeco, blues, folk, soul, rock, jazz, gospel, and singer/songwriters.

8385 JOAN SHERMAN ARTIST MANAGEMENT

106 Winona Street
Peabody, MA 01960-4637
Phone: 978-535-1358
Fax: 978-535-1378
Web Site: www.joansherman.com
Management:
  Eastern Representative: Joan Sherman
Mission: Represents the top names in the world of folk and world music, and spoken word artistry.

Michigan

8386 GREAT LAKES PERFORMING ARTIST ASSOCIATES

1969 W Stadium Boulevard
Suite 211
Ann Arbor, MI 48103
Phone: 734-665-4029
Fax: 734-769-9297
e-mail: info@greatlakespaa.org
Web Site: www.greatlakespaa.org
Officers:
  President: Robert F Whitman
  VP: Stephen T Bemis
  Treasurer: Peter Darrow
  Secretary: Jo-Ann M Featherman
Management:
  Executive Director: Matthew Ardizzone
  Administrative Associate: Corinne Nair
  Development Director: Ann Edwards
Mission: To encourage and promote the cultural and artistic development of Great Lake region by supporting the performance careers of execptional regional artists.

8387 ZAJONC/VALENTI

PO Box 7023
Ann Arbor, MI 48103
Toll-free: 800-650-8742
e-mail: ZVGMT@aol.com
Web Site: www.napama.org/Zajonc.htm

Minnesota

8388 BIG SKY ARTISTS MANAGEMENT

3812 Thomas Avenue S
Minneapolis, MN 55410
Phone: 612-926-2135
Fax: 612-926-2135
e-mail: bigsky@bsam.net
Web Site: www.bsam.net
Mission: Management, programming, and producing career development grant/competition search and coordination contract negotiation.
Founded: 1993

8389 NED KANTAR PRODUCTIONS

3430 St. Paul Avenue
Minneapolis, MN 55416
Phone: 612-926-5655
Fax: 612-920-8482
e-mail: ned@nedkantar.com
Web Site: www.nedkantar.com
Officers:
  President: Ned Kantar
Founded: 1975
Specialized Field: Jazz; Kelzmer Music

Missouri

8390 CHAMJO GROUP

167 Lamp & Lantern Village #142
Chesterfield, MO 63017
Phone: 636-230-0252
Fax: 636-230-0001
Web Site: www.chamjo.com
Mission: ChAmJo concentrates on four basic yet specific areas of concentration for our efforts: Management; Entertainment; Investments; Publishing.

8391 MAINSTAGE ARTIST MANAGEMENT

8144A Big Bend Boulevard
St. Louis, MO 63119-3205
Phone: 314-962-4478
Fax: 314-962-6960
e-mail: main@mainstage-mgmt.com
Web Site: www.mainstage-mgmet.com
Officers:
  President: Terry Kippenberger
Management:
  Director Sales: Deborah Sharn
  Contract Administrator/Publicity: Beverly Thomas
  Sales Associate: Patti Walley
Mission: Booking agency and producer in the Broadway and performing arts touring market.

Paid Staff: 4

Nebraska

8392 NORTHERN LIGHTS MANAGEMENT
437 Live Oak Loop NE
Albuquerque, NE 87122-1406
Phone: 505-856-7100
e-mail: nlightmgt@aol.com
Web Site: www.northenlightsmgt.com

Nevada

8393 NATIONWIDE ENTERTAINMENT SERVICES
2756 N Green Valley Parkway
Suite 449
Las Vegas, NV 89014-2100
Phone: 702-451-8090
Fax: 561-362-0079
e-mail: info@entertainmentservices.com
Web Site: www.entertainmentservices.com
Mission: A full service entertainment production company producing shows and supplying entertainers worldwide.

New Hampshire

8394 SKYLINE MUSIC AGENCY
PO Box 31
Lancaster, NH 03583
Phone: 603-586-7171
Fax: 603-586-7068
e-mail: bruce@skylineonline.com
Web Site: www.skylineonline.com
Management:
    Arts, East and Midwest: Andrea Sabota
    Arts, West Coast and Mountain: Tracy Tingley
Founded: 1983
Specialized Field: Music
Paid Staff: 10
Paid Artists: 35

New Jersey

8395 LOIS SCOTT MANAGEMENT
PO Box 140
Closter, NJ 07624
Phone: 201-768-6970
Fax: 201-768-7257
e-mail: lsminc@aol.com
Web Site: www.LoisScottMansgement.com

8396 AVIV PRODUCTIONS
4-23 Second Street
Fair Lawn, NJ 07410
Phone: 201-791-8414
Fax: 201-791-7283
e-mail: itzik@aviv2.com
Web Site: www.aviv2.com
Mission: Aviv Productions is a management booking producing agency located in the United States.

8397 STANLEY WEINSTEIN
Arts Management
408 Charlestown Road
Suite 3
Hampton, NJ 08827
Phone: 908-537-6832
Fax: 908-537-6832
e-mail: stainweinstein@sprintmail.com
Officers:
    President: Stanley Weinstein
Mission: Manager Agent; Arts Consultant; Grants Writer
Founded: 1984
Specialized Field: Various
Paid Staff: 2
Paid Artists: 25

8398 ARTSPOWER NATIONAL TOURING THEATRE
39 S Fullerton Avenue
Montclair, NJ 07042-3354
Phone: 973-744-0909
Fax: 973-744-3609
e-mail: info@artspower.org
Web Site: www.artspower.org
Officers:
    Founding Co-Director: Gary W Blackman
    Founding Co-Director: Mark A Blackman
    Director Operations: Caitlin Evans-Jones
Management:
    Artistic Director: Greg Gunning
Mission: ArtsPower has emerged as one of America's largest, and most active producers of Actors' Equity Association theatre for young and family audiences presented in theatres, cultural centers, and schools throughout 40 states.
Founded: 1985

8399 SUPREME TALENT INTERNATIONAL
210 Summit Avenue
Montvale, NJ 07645
Phone: 201-307-0604
Fax: 201-307-5656
Toll-free: 800-677-2731
e-mail: supremetal@aol.com
Web Site: www.supremetalent.com
Management:
    Contact: Larry Carter
    Contact: Mary Lynam
Mission: One-stop resource for event and meeting planners and entertainment buyers, Supreme Talent International has more than twenty years of experience in the special events industry, ranging from conceptual design to full-service production mana

8400 ARTISTS INTERNATIONAL MANAGEMENT

Morristown, NJ 07962-2146
Mailing Address: PO Box 2146
Phone: 973-538-0302
Fax: 973-734-1737
e-mail: aimartists@aol.com
Web Site: www.artistsinternational.com
Officers:
   Marketing: Norbert Schmid
Management:
   Executive Director: Birgit Schmid-Salm
   Program Coordinator: Georg von Hochstetter
Mission: AIM consists of young dynamic management
team that draws on previous experience in music and art,
marketing and international media. It has also assisted
young musicians to accomplish their goal of international
appearances. AIM represents chamber ensembles, choirs,
orchestras, conductors, pianists, string soloists and
vocalists.

8401 SAIL PRODUCTIONS

PO Box 134
Readington, NJ 08870
Phone: 908-788-6871
Fax: 908-788-1815
e-mail: info@sailproductions.com
Web Site: www.sailproductions.com
Founded: 1983

8402 GENEVIEVE SPIELBERG

12 Princeton Street
Summit, NJ 07901
Phone: 908-608-1325
Fax: 908-608-1326
e-mail: genevieve@gsiartists.com
Web Site: www.gsiartists.com
Officers:
   President: Genevieve Spielberg
   Associate Manager: Ann Rosenblum
Mission: A full service Performing Arts consultancy
established to meet the needs of today's concert artirts.

8403 DRAKE & ASSOCIATES/TAM

177 Woodland Avenue
Westwood, NJ 07675
Phone: 201-263-9200
Fax: 201-358-8784
e-mail: info@draketam.com
Web Site: www.draketam.com
Management:
   Agent: David Tamulevich
   Agent: Tim Drake
   Agent: Mike June
Mission: Representing artists across genres and cultures,
Drake is exclusive with its clients, working with clubs,
festivals, performing arts centers and some private events.
Founded: 1994
Paid Staff: 6
Paid Artists: 15

New York

8404 STANTON MANAGEMENT

45-05 Newtown Road
Astoria, NY 11103
Phone: 718-956-6092
Fax: 718-956-5385
e-mail: TDStanton@aol.com
Web Site: www.stantonmgt.com
Mission: Dedicated to providing personalized artist
management services to a select group of international
artists.
Founded: 1986

8405 BERNSTEIN ARTISTS

282 Flatbush Avenue
Suite 101
Brooklyn, NY 11217
Phone: 718-623-1214
Fax: 718-638-6110
e-mail: BernsArts@aol.com
Web Site: www.bernsarts.com
Officers:
   President: Sue Renee Bernstein
   Associate: Nancy Kushner
Mission: Dedicated to the development and advancement
of artists seeking to extend the boundaries of their given
genres, our roster embraces a broad spectrum of arts, from
new music to contemporary music theater, early music,
theater and jazz. We aim to develop new audiences, and
believe that these innovative artists speak to new
generation.
Founded: 1994

8406 HORIZON MANAGEMENT

PO Box 8770
Endwell, NY 13762
Phone: 607-785-9120
Fax: 607-785-4516
e-mail: HMI67@aol.com
Officers:
   President: Tom Varano
Mission: Live entertainment events such as concerts,
fairs, festivals, etc.
Founded: 1967
Paid Staff: 50
Volunteer Staff: 4
Paid Artists: 600

8407 NOVO ARTISTS

14 Townsend Avenue
Hartsdale, NY 10530
Phone: 914-948-4581
Fax: 914-761-3382
e-mail: novoarts@aol.com
Web Site: www.novoartists.com
Officers:
   President: Celia Novo
Mission: Management and career-counseling firm.
Founded: 1995

8408 AI ARTISTS

356 Pine Valley Road
Hoosick Falls, NY 12090
Phone: 518-686-0972
Fax: 518-686-1960
e-mail: cynthia@aiartists.com
Web Site: www.aiartists.com
Management:
    Director: Cynthia B Herbst
Mission: AIA is an artist management firm devoted to the career development of its composers and jazz and classical performers, and to the development and coordination of special projects.
Founded: 1978

8409 JEFFREY JAMES ARTS CONSULTING

316 Pacific Street
Massapequa Park, NY 11762
Phone: 516-797-9166
Fax: 516-797-9166
e-mail: jamesarts@worldnet.att.net
Web Site: www.jamesarts.com
Officers:
    President: Jaffrey James
    VP: Tristan Willems
Mission: Full service arts agency dedicated to management and public relations. Representing composers, ensembles, instrumentalists and special attractions, with a very special interest in the music of the 20th century

8410 JONATHAN WENTWORTH ASSOCIATES LIMITED

10 Fiske Place
Suite 5330
Mt. Vernon, NY 10550
Phone: 914-667-0707
Fax: 914-667-0784
e-mail: office@jwentworth.com
Web Site: www.jwentworth.com
Officers:
    President: Kenneth Wentworth
    VP: Martha Woods
Management:
    Artist Liaison: Kathryn Cardy
Mission: Respected resource for world-class chamber music, chamber orchestra, Irish & Scotish music, early music, percussive dance, orchestral soloists, conductors and recitals. The agency serves the performing arts presenting field including college and university series, festivals, orchestras, chamber music series and other presenters.

8411 AARON CONCERT ARTISTS

331 W 57th Street
New York, NY 10019
Mailing Address: Box 334
Phone: 212-665-0313
e-mail: info@aaronconcert.com
Web Site: www.aaronconcert.com
Management:
    Managing Director: Jon Aaron

Mission: ACA was created to provide management services, tour management and production support for variety of artists and special projects.
Founded: 2000

8412 ABACA PRODUCTIONS

711 W End Avenue
New York, NY 10025
Phone: 212-316-6372
e-mail: abacaprd@panix.com
Web Site: www.abacaproductions.com

8413 ABC ASSOCIATED BOOKING CORPORATION

1995 Broadway
New York, NY 10023
Phone: 212-874-2400
Fax: 212-769-3649
Web Site: www.abcbooking.com

8414 AEOLIAN ARTISTS INTERNATIONAL MANAGEMENT

244 5th Avenue
2nd Floor J234
New York, NY 10001
Phone: 212-252-2648
Fax: 212-591-6158
e-mail: aeolinartists@aol.com
Web Site: www.aeolianartists.com
Officers:
    President: Catherine Marchese Sidoti
Founded: 2001
Specialized Field: Classical Music; Opera
Paid Staff: 2
Volunteer Staff: 1
Paid Artists: 5

8415 AGENCY GROUP

1775 Broadway
New York, NY 10019
Phone: 212-581-3100
Fax: 212-581-0015
Web Site: www.theagency group.com

8416 ALBERT KAY ASSOCIATES

58 W 58th Street
Tower 58, Suite 31E
New York, NY 10019-2510
Phone: 212-593-1640
Fax: 212-759-7329
e-mail: jay-yoo@msn.com
Web Site: www.albertkay-jayyoo.com
Officers:
    President: Jay S Yoo
    VP: W Douglas Ryno
Management:
    Associate: Kenneth Leedom
Mission: Represents performers appearing worldwide in various opera houses, concert halls, theaters and institutions of learning.
Founded: 1963
Paid Staff: 4
Volunteer Staff: 2

Paid Artists: 25
Non-paid Artists: 35
Budget: $150,000-400,000
Performs At: Alice Tully Hall; Carnegie Hall; Weill Recital Hall

8417 ANTHONY GEORGE ARTIST MANAGEMENT
250 W 77th Street
New York, NY 10024
Phone: 212-580-1306
Fax: 212-721-9144
e-mail: operaag@aol.com
Web Site: www.ageorge.dezines.com

8418 ARDANI ARTISTS MANAGEMENT
130 W 56th Street
Floor 5M
New York, NY 10019
Phone: 212-399-0002
Fax: 212-399-9889
e-mail: SDanilian@aol.com
Web Site: www.ardani.com
Management:
   Producer: Sergei Danilian
Founded: 1990

8419 ARTHUR SHAFMAN INTERNATIONAL
163 Amsterdam Avenue
Suite 121
New York, NY 10023-5001
Phone: 212-799-4814
Fax: 212-874-3613
e-mail: ashafman@aol.com
Web Site: arthurshafman.com
Officers:
   President: Arthur Shafman
Mission: Concert producer
Founded: 1969

8420 ARTIST MANAGEMENT
300 W 55th Street
Suite 5L
New York, NY 10019-5138
Phone: 212-581-8479
e-mail: rwam@mcimail.com
Web Site: www.concentric.net/~Rwam/
Mission: For more than a quarter century RWAM has been engaged in representing some of the world's finest instrumental soloists and ensembles. It has especially sought out major talent from overseas, making them available to US sponsors.

8421 ARTS MANAGEMENT GROUP
1133 Broadway
Suite 1025
New York, NY 10010
Phone: 212-337-0838
Fax: 212-924-0382
e-mail: info@artsmg.com
Web Site: www.artsmg.com
Management:
   Associate: Arlene Paskalian

Associate: Alisa L Herrington
Managing Director: Vincent J Ryan
Managing Director: William J Capone

8422 ARTS4ALL
2 W 45th Street
Suite 500
New York, NY 10036
Phone: 212-391-4007
Fax: 212-391-4024
e-mail: mekernagham@arts4all.com
Web Site: www.arts4all.com
Officers:
   Director Content: Maryellen Kernaghan
Specialized Field: Dance

8423 ASSOCIATED BOOKING CORPORATION
1995 Broadway
Suite 501
New York, NY 10023-5877
Phone: 212-874-2400
Fax: 212-769-3649
e-mail: info@abcbooking.com
Web Site: www.abcbooking.com
Officers:
   President: Oscar Cohen

8424 BERNARD SCHMIDT PRODUCTIONS
461 W 49th Street
E Office
New York, NY 10019
Phone: 212-307-5046
Fax: 212-397-2459
e-mail: bschmidtpd@aol.com
Web Site: www.bernardschmidtproductions.com
Mission: An international performing arts agency promoting cultural exchange between the United States and countries around the world.

8425 BESENARTS
80 Varick Street
Suite 9D
New York, NY 10013
Phone: 212-226-7570
Fax: 212-343-8867
e-mail: contact@besenarts.com
Web Site: www.besenarts.com
Officers:
   Director: Robert Besen
Founded: 1999

8426 BIG LEAGUE THEATRICALS
1501 Broadway
Suite 2015
New York, NY 10036
Phone: 212-575-1601
Fax: 212-575-9817
e-mail: generalinfo@bigleague.org
Web Site: www.bigleague.org
Management:
   General Manager: Carolyn Clark Smith
   Director Publicity: Marni Kuhn

Mission: Big League Theatricals produces, general manages and represents Broadway and Off-Broadway shows as well as international attractions for touring worldwide. Big League Theatricals is dedicated to providing diverse, high quality theatrical a

8427 BOOKING GROUP

145 West 45th Street
8th Floor
New York, NY 10036
Phone: 212-869-9280
Fax: 212-869-3028
e-mail: kgebhart@tbgsuites.com
Web Site: www.thebookinggroup.com
Officers:
President: Meredith Blair
Specialized Field: Opera, Music Theatre; Theatre

8428 BRAD SIMON ORGANIZATION

122 E 57th Street
New York, NY 10022
Phone: 212-980-5920
Fax: 212-980-3193
e-mail: brad@bsoinc.com
Web Site: www.bsoinc.com
Officers:
President: Brad Simon
President: Barbara Simon
Management:
Agent: Keith Ghion
Office Manager: Larry Lees
Mission: Management and booking agency specializing in family entertainment, theatrical entertainment and music.
Founded: 1980

8429 CIRCUM ARTS

151 W 30th Street
Suite 200
New York, NY 10001
Phone: 212-904-1422
Fax: 212-904-1426
Web Site: www.circum.org
Management:
Executive Director: Richard Biles
Membership Coordinator: Doris Caravaglia
Mission: Circum-Arts is a not-for-profit arts service organization with the mission to assist, advocate and encourage performing artists and visual arts projects. Our goal is to provide a complete service structure of administrative, technical and educational resources that are accessible and affordable to individual artists and emerging companies in the performing arts.
Status: Not-For-Profit

8430 COLUMBIA ARTISTS MANAGEMENT

165 57th Street
New York, NY 10019-2276
Phone: 212-841-9500
Fax: 212-841-9744
e-mail: info@cami.com
Web Site: www.cami.com
Officers:
Chairman/CEO: Ronald A Wilford

Mission: Columbia Artists Management is an international leader in managing the touring activities of instrumental soloists, opera singers, conductors, classical music ensembles, orchestras, dance companies, popular and theatrical attractions, and fine arts media productions.
Founded: 1930

8431 DCA PRODUCTIONS

330 W 38th Street
Suite 303
New York, NY 10018
Phone: 212-245-2063
Fax: 212-245-2367
e-mail: info@dcaproductions.com
Web Site: www.dcaproductions.com
Officers:
President: Daniel Abrahamsen
VP: Gerri Abrahamsen
Office Manager: Lauren Pellegrino
Management:
Juggling Champion: Mark Nizer
Ventriloquist: Lynn Trefzger
Mission: Entertainment management company providing acts to theatre venues, colleges, clubs, TV performances, festivals and more.
Founded: 1983
Specialized Field: Comedy, Music, Variety Acts
Paid Staff: 3
Volunteer Staff: 1
Paid Artists: 20
Facility Category: Theatre, College, Festival, TV Studio; Indoor/Outdoor

8432 DODGER TOURING LIMITED

230 W 41st Street
Suite 2015
New York, NY 10036
Phone: 212-575-1120
Fax: 212-575-0520
e-mail: info@d-tours.com
Web Site: www.d-tours.com
Officers:
President: L Glenn Poppleton
Director Operations: Barbara Haven
Marketing: Dana Vokolek
Management:
Booking Agent: Michael Sinder
Booking Assistant: David Carpenter
Mission: Dodger Touring also known as D-Tours, is an independent booking and marketing company providing the touring industry with the highest quality talent and theatrical entertainment.
Founded: 1995

8433 ENTOURAGE TALENT ASSOCIATES

133 W 25th Street
New York, NY 10001
Phone: 212-633-2600
Fax: 212-633-1818
e-mail: administration@entouragetalent.com
Web Site: www.entouragetalent.com

8434 EXTREMETASTE LIMITED

307 W 38th Street
New York, NY 10018
Phone: 646-473-1414
Fax: 646-473-1415
e-mail: wheeler@extremetaste.com
Web Site: www.extremetaste.com
Management:
    Manager/Producer: Jedediah Wheeler
Mission: Manager and producer working in the creative performing arts. Wheeler has produced and toured work in dance, music, theater, opera and perfomance art across the United States and throughout the world.

8435 FINE ARTS MANAGEMENT CORPORATION

201 W 54th Street
Suite 1C
New York, NY 10019
Phone: 212-974-2470
Fax: 212-974-2743
Web Site: www.fineartsmanagement.com
Management:
    Managing Director: Steven Sobol
    Management Director: Amy Rhodes
Mission: The Fine Arts Management Corporation represents a new, multi-disciplinary approach to the performing arts field. Fine Arts Management offers a unique combination of artist management, and technology consultation and software solutions for Orchestras, Music Schools, Performing Arts Centers and Artist Managers.
Founded: 1994

8436 FRANK SALOMON ASSOCIATES

201 W 54th Street
1C
New York, NY 10019
Phone: 212-581-5197
Fax: 212-581-4029
e-mail: frank@franksalomon.com
Web Site: www.franksalomon.com
Officers:
    Founder/President: Frank Salomon
Management:
    Director: Barrie Steinberg
    Booking Associate: Jenna Grein
Mission: Commited to generating new audiences through a variety of imaginative and educational and educational outreach activities for students and audiences of all ages.
Type of Stage: Proscenium

8437 GARDNER ARTS NETWORK

155 W 72nd Street
Suite 605
New York, NY 10023
Phone: 212-496-9121
Fax: 212-496-9123
e-mail: gardnerart@aol.com
Web Site: www.napama.org
Officers:
    President: Jeannette Gardner
Management:
    Administrative Assistant: Juliay Barker
    Administrative Assistant: Lisa Bouley

    Consultant: Donalee Katz
Mission: Booking management which specializes in Dance and a wide variety of programming for family/young audiences.
Founded: 1988
Volunteer Staff: 3

8438 GLOBAL TALENT ASSOCIATES

120 W 44th Street
Suite 603
New York, NY 10036
Phone: 212-921-8500
Fax: 212-921-8599
e-mail: info@globaltalentassoc.com
Web Site: www.globaltalentassoc.com

8439 GURTMAN AND MURTHA ARTIST MANAGEMENT

450 7th Avenue
Suite 603
New York, NY 10123
Phone: 212-967-7350
Fax: 212-967-7341
Toll-free: 800-666-8742
e-mail: JMurtha457@aol.com
Mission: Public relations organization, representing many of the world's great artists, attractions and cultural institutions. They act as tour impresarios, concert promoters and booking agents.

8440 HANS SPENGLER ARTISTS MANAGEMENT

30 Beekman Place
New York, NY 10022
Phone: 212-355-2219
Fax: 212-421-6689
e-mail: hans@hans-splenger.com
Web Site: www.hans-spengler.com

8441 HARWOOD MANAGEMENT GROUP

5090 W 110th Street
New York, NY 10025
Phone: 212-864-0773
Fax: 212-663-1129
e-mail: jim@harwood-management.com
Web Site: harwood-management.com
Mission: Innovative arts management organization manages the carees of classical singers in opera, orchestra/choral works, recitals, concerts; cross-over/musical theater performers in Broadway, off-Broadway, touring productions, pops concerts; as well as conductors and stage directors for these venues. Also serves as artists consultants, artistic administrators and producers.
Founded: 1982
Specialized Field: Classical; Broadway
Paid Staff: 4

8442 IMG ARTISTS

825 7th Avenue
8th Floor
New York, NY 10019

Phone: 212-489-8300
Fax: 212-246-1596
e-mail: artistsny@imgworld.com
Web Site: www.imgartists.com
Management:
Managing Director: Edna Landau
Associate Director: Elizabeth Sobol
Director/Vocal Division: Alec C Treuhaft
Director/Dance Division: Nancy Gabriel
Director/Attractions: Mark S Maluso
Mission: Recognized as one of the world's foremost companies specializing in classical music management, as well as touring and special events, with offices in London, New york, Paris and Kuala Lumpur and affiliated branches in Tokyo, Hong Kong and Australia. IMG Artists combines the highest standards of presonal management with an unparalleled range of services to all its clients.

8443   J CHRISS & COMPANY

300 Mercer Street
Suite 3J
New York, NY 10003
Phone: 212-353-0855
Fax: 212-353-0094
e-mail: info@jchriss.com
Web Site: www.jchriss.com
Mission: Books, manages, consults and produces major music projects worldwide, and our client roster gives presenters the opportunity to choose from the greatest talents the world of jazz has to offer.
Founded: 1986

8444   JANICE MAYER & ASSOCIATES, LLC

250 W 57th Street
Suite 2214
New York, NY 10107
Phone: 212-541-5511
Fax: 212-541-7303
Web Site: www.janicemayer.com
Officers:
Persident: Janice Mayer
VP: Gloria Narramore Moody
Mission: An international artist management company dedicated to advancing and serving the vocal arts. The organization represents classical vocalists in the areas of concert and opera.

8445   JOHN GINGRICH MANAGEMENT

PO Box 1515
New York, NY 10023
Phone: 212-799-5080
Fax: 212-874-7652
e-mail: gingarts@erols.com
Web Site: www.gingarts.com
Mission: Represents an exclusive list of chamber music ensembles, conductors and instrumental and vocal soloist both in the United States and abroad.

8446   KAYLOR MANAGEMENT

130 W 57th Street
Suite 8G
New York, NY 10019

Phone: 212-977-6779
Fax: 212-977-6856
e-mail: hughkaylor@msn.com
Officers:
President: Kaylor Kaylor

8447   KIRSHBAUM DEMLER & ASSOCIATES

711 W End Avenue
Suite 5KN
New York, NY 10025
Phone: 212-222-4843
Fax: 212-222-7321
Web Site: www.skassoc.com
Officers:
Director: Shirley Kirshbaum
Director: Susan Demler
Artist Services Associate: Peri Stedman
Booking Associate: Jason M Belz
Sr Public Relations Associate: Austin S Wrubel
Public Relations Associte: Helane Anderson

8448   LISA BOOTH MANAGEMENT

145 W 45th Street
Suite 602
New York, NY 10036
Phone: 212-921-2114
Fax: 212-921-2504
e-mail: artslbmi@msn.com
Officers:
President: Lisa Booth
Specialized Field: Dance; Theatre

8449   MARK KAPPEL

252 W 76th Street
Suite 6E
New York, NY 10023
Phone: 212-724-3889
Fax: 212-874-5039
e-mail: markkapl1@aol.com
Web Site:
members.aol.com/MARKKAPL1/MARKKAPL1.htm
Officers:
President: Mark Kappel
Specialized Field: Ballet; Modern Dance

8450   MATTHEW LAIFER ARTISTS MANAGEMENT

410 W 24th Street
Suite 2i
New York, NY 10011
Phone: 212-929-7429
Fax: 212-633-2628
e-mail: laiferart@aol.com
Web Site: www.laiferart.com
Officers:
President: Matthew Laifer
Executive Assistant: Antje Hobner
Mission: The goal is to bring the finest artists to the finest theaters worldwide, with careful attention given to establishing and maintaining professional careers. The Laifer roster is divided among Americans and Europeans, stars and emerging tal

8451 MICOCCI PRODUCTIONS, LLC
253 W Street
Suite 8G
New York, NY 10023
Phone: 212-874-2030
Fax: 212-874-1175
e-mail: tony@micocci.com
Web Site: micocci.com
Mission: Performing arts, events and tour producer and management company, associated with performances in the major venues of New York City such as Carnegie Hall and Lincoln Center, as well as throughout the United States and internationally.

8452 MULTIARTS PROJECTS & PRODUCTIONS
140 2nd Avenue
Suite 502
New York, NY 10003
Phone: 646-602-9390
Fax: 646-602-9395
Web Site: www.multiprojects.com
Management:
   Executive Director: Ann Rosenthal
   Co-Director: Cathy Zimmerman
   Projects Manager: Jordana Phokompe
   Director Booking: Thomas O. Kriegsmann
Mission: Dedicated to producing and sustaining performing artists as they develop multidisciplinary projects that raise questions about the complexities of our time. Works in close collaboration with artists, arts organizations and other arts professionals to provide a holistic set of production services tailored to the specific nature and needs of each project.

8453 PARADISE ARTISTS
888 7th Avenue
New York, NY 10106
Phone: 212-397-7888
Fax: 212-397-6953
Web Site: www.paradiseartists.com

8454 PENTACLE
246 W 38th Street
8th Floor
New York, NY 10018
Phone: 212-278-8111
Fax: 212-278-8555
Web Site: www.pentacle.org
Mission: Provide some of the country's most exciting performing artists with essential administrative services and serve the broader performing arts community with innovative projects of local and national impact.

8455 PERFORMING ARTSERVICES
260 W Broadway
New York, NY 10013
Phone: 212-941-8911
Fax: 212-334-5149
e-mail: artservice@aol.com
Web Site: www.lovely.com/artservices
Mission: Non-profit organization whose mission is to produce, present and facilitate the endeavors of artists working in contemporary forms of music, theater and dance.
Founded: 1972

8456 RANDMASN ARTISTS' MANAGEMENT
400 W 43rd Street
Suite 18E
New York, NY 10036
Phone: 213-290-2281
Fax: 213-290-2284
e-mail: info@randsman.com
Web Site: www.randsman.com

8457 RICHARD REALMUTO ARTIST MANAGEMENT
PO Box 760
New York, NY 10033
Phone: 212-932-6131
Fax: 212-923-6132
e-mail: richard@realmutoartists.com
Web Site: www.rram.com
Officers:
   President: Richard Realmuto

8458 ROAD COMPANY
165 W 46th Street
Suite 1101
New York, NY 10036
Phone: 212-302-5200
Fax: 212-302-5374
e-mail: tours@theroadcompany.com
Web Site: www.theroadcompany.com
Management:
   Co-Founder: Stephen Lindsay
   Co-Founder: Brett Sirota
Mission: Theatrical booking agency, distributing musicals, plays and attractions internationally.
Founded: 1997

8459 ROBERT LOMBARDO & ASSOCIATES
61 W 62nd Street
Suite 6F
New York, NY 10023
Phone: 212-586-4453
Fax: 212-581-5771
e-mail: office@RobertLombardo.com
Web Site: www.rlombardo.com
Officers:
   Associate: Michael Rosen
   Associate: Lewis Ehlers
   Office Manager: Mark Lameier
   Assistant: Annamaria Pace
   Accounts Manager: Steve Sherling
Management:
   Accounts Manager: Steven Sherling
Founded: 1974
Specialized Field: Opera

8460 TIMOTHY GILLIGAN ARTIST MANAGEMENT
2475 Braodway
Suite 155
New York, NY 10025
Phone: 212-874-6360
Fax: 212-874-6376
e-mail: Gillartsny@aol.com
Web Site: www.gilliganartists.com

8461 TRAWICK ARTISTS MANAGEMENT
250 W 57th Street
Suite 901
New York, NY 10107
Phone: 212-581-6181
Fax: 212-581-4002
e-mail: info@trawickartists.net
Web Site: www.trawickartists.net
Management:
   Director Association Services: Sheila Gallagher
Mission: Organization focusing on management, concert presentation and the development of exciting new projects in the arts and entertainment industry. Community Concerts continues to bring the highest quality artists to an organized audience network of close to 400 concert presenters across the United States.

8462 WASHINGTON SQUARE ARTS
310 Bowery
2nd Floor
New York, NY 10012
Phone: 212-253-0333
Fax: 212-253-0330
Web Site: www.washingtonsquarearts.com
Mission: Booking and management company dedicated to artists who are unique, challenging, powerful and fun: artists whose work is designed for diverse and wide ranging audiences.

8463 WILLIAM MORRIS AGENCY
1325 Avenue of the Americas
New York, NY 10019
Phone: 212-586-5100
Fax: 212-246-2463
Web Site: www.wma.com

8464 WINDWOOD THEATRICALS
1504 Broadway
Suite 309
New York, NY 10036-5501
Phone: 211-239-8317
Web Site: www.windwoodtheatricals.com
Management:
   Agent: Paul Bartz
Mission: An agency headed by veteran agent Paul Bartz that concentrates on developing, producing and touring new and established productions from and for Broadway, Off-Broadway and regional theaters, along with a roster of special attractions.

8465 WORLDSTAGE ENTERTAINMENT, LLC
160 W End Avenue
Suite 18-A
New York, NY 10023
Phone: 212-769-1969
Fax: 212-769-2113
e-mail: wse@wstage.com
Web Site: www.wstage.com

8466 YOUNG CONCERT ARTISTS
250 W 57th Street
Suite 1222
New York, NY 10107
Phone: 212-307-6655
Fax: 212-581-8894
e-mail: yca@yca.org
Web Site: www.yca.com
Management:
   Director: Susan Wadsworth
   Director Development/Finance: Sara Sill
   Associate Director: Mark Hayman
   Director Artists Management: Monica J Felkel
   Far East Representative: Rong-Hong Ma
   Artist Manager: Vicki Marguiles
   Operations Manager: Rachel Zucker
   Development Manager: Jacqueline Fanelli
   Development Assistant: Lauren E Bennett
Mission: Non-profit organization dedicated to discovering and launching the careers of extraordinary young musicians. The artists are chosen through the Young Concerts Artists International Auditions, whose sole criteria are musicianship, vistuosity, communicative power and readiness for a concert career.
Founded: 1961

8467 ANTONIA ARTS MANAGEMENT
23 North Division Street
Peekskill, NY 10566
Phone: 914-788-0059
Fax: 914-788-0058
e-mail: AntiniArts@aol.com

8468 IRELAND ON STAGE
150 Main Street
Port Washington, NY 11050
Phone: 516-944-7393
Fax: 516-883-9487
e-mail: vmitchell@irelandonstage.com
Web Site: www.irelandonstage.com
Mission: Based on Long Island, we have national reputation and presence in the world of Irish Music. Ready to bring your organization talented and creative artists. Our mission is to bring the American public the finest in Irish entertainment.

8469 ON QUEUE PERFORMING ARTISTS
517 County Highway 27
Richfield Springs, NY 13439
Phone: 315-858-1434
Fax: 315-858-1431
e-mail: info@onqueueartists.com
Web Site: www.onqueueartists.com

Mission: Dedicated to promoting interest in traditional and world arts, featuring oustanding artists who not only preserve, but stretch beyond their traditions.
Founded: 1997

8470 POETRY IN MOTION
1445 S Fitzhugh Street
Suite 3
Rochester, NY 14608-2274
Toll-free: 888-860-2780
e-mail: poetinmo@aol.com
Web Site: www.poetinmo.com

8471 PRESTIGE AGENCY
109 S Warren Street, State Tower Building
Suite 911
Syracuse, NY 13202
Phone: 315-472-7637
Fax: 315-472-2693
e-mail: prestige@aol.com
Web Site: www.prestigeagency.com

8472 BENNETT MORGAN & ASSOCIATES LIMITED
1022 Route 376
Wappingers Falls, NY 12590
Phone: 845-227-6065
Fax: 845-227-4002
e-mail: ben@bennettmorgan.com
Web Site: www.bennettmorgan.com
Mission: Artist representative for the top stars of Jazz.

8473 MONICA ROBINSON LIMITED
2431 Pinetree Place
Yorktown Heights, NY 10598
Phone: 914-962-6062
Fax: 914-962-6068
e-mail: mrltd6062@aol.com
Web Site: www.monicarobinsonltd.com

North Carolina

8474 ARTSOURCE MANAGEMENT
104 Reton Court
Cary, NC 27513-9274
Phone: 919-319-9274
Fax: 919-319-9274
Web Site: www.artsourcemanagement.com
Officers:
    President: Art Waber
Specialized Field: Dance; Music

8475 RACHEL NARULA MANAGEMENT
408 Fairoaks Circle
Chapel Hill, NC 27516
Phone: 919-932-9045
Toll-free: 877-932-9045
e-mail: RNarula@bellsouth.net
Web Site: www.rachelnarulamanagement.com

8476 EASTCOAST ENTERTAINMENT
8910 Lenox Pointe Drive
Suite E
Charlotte, NC 28273
Phone: 704-339-0100
Fax: 704-372-9436
Toll-free: 800-950-2263
Web Site: www.eastcoastentertainment.com
Mission: Worldwide booking agency, supplying talent throughout this country and overseas for a wide range of situations, including conventions and concerts, presidents and royalty, movies and television, bar mitzvahs and weddings.
Founded: 1976

8477 HORTON SMITH MANAGEMENT
PO Box 51007
Durham, NC 27717-1007
Phone: 919-982-1395
e-mail: hortonsmith@aol.com
Web Site: www.hortonsmithmanagement.com
Mission: International performing artist management company with a proven track record of high quality, fairness and creativity
Founded: 1992

8478 INDIA ARTIST MANAGEMENT
PMB 44
2007 Yanceyville Street #3312
Greensboro, NC 27405
Phone: 336-275-2994
Fax: 336-274-1761
e-mail: lori@indiaartist.com
Web Site: www.indiaartist.com
Officers:
    President/Owner: Lori Jarrett
Mission: Mission is to promote India music and dance international venues.
Founded: 1999
Specialized Field: World Music
Paid Staff: 1
Volunteer Staff: 1
Paid Artists: 6
Budget: $50,000
Income Sources: Booking Fees

8479 EASTCOAST ENTERTAINMENT
Building F
Suite 102
Raleigh, NC 27609
Phone: 919-875-1800
Toll-free: 800-242-1243
Web Site: www.eastcoastentertainment.com
Mission: Worldwide booking agency, supplying talent throughout this country and overseas for a wide range of situations, including conventions and concerts, presidents and royalty, movies and television, bar mitzvahs and weddings.
Founded: 1976

Ohio

8480 KAREN MCFARLANE ARTISTS
2385 Fenwood Road
Cleveland, OH 44118
Fax: 216-397-7716
Toll-free: 866-721-9095
Web Site: www.concertorganists.com
Officers:
  President: John McElliot
Mission: Manages the performing careers of more than
thirty concert organists from the United States and
Europe, in addition to offering only the finest British and
American Choirs in the English Choral tradition. Artists
are available for dedicatory or series recitals, concerts
with orchestra, master classes, lectures and workshops.

8481 WESTWATER ARTS
105 N Merkle
Columbus, OH 43209
Phone: 614-234-2004
Fax: 614-231-5540
e-mail: westwater@westwaterarts.com
Web Site: www.westwaterarts.com
Management:
  Contact: James Westwater
Mission: Dedicated to live performance of great works of
classical music, artfully blended with giant-screen
multi-image photography that honors the music.
Founded: 1973

Oklahoma

8482 INTERNATIONAL ARTISTS
3126 S Boulevard
PO Box 138
Edmond, OK 73013
Phone: 405-341-0442
Fax: 405-349-9880
e-mail: hammons@bigplanet.com
Web Site: www.interartinc.com

8483 SOUTHWEST CONCERT ARTISTS
1601 S Madison Boulevard
Oklahoma, OK 74006
Phone: 914-333-8288
e-mail: swca@swbell.com
Web Site: www.concertart.com
Mission: Full-service arts management firm representing
a select group of hand-picked attractions.
Founded: 1992

Pennsylvania

8484 ELSIE MANAGEMENT
132 Prospect Place
#2R
Brooklyn, PA 11217

Phone: 718-638-9862
Fax: 718-638-0241
Web Site: www.elsieman.org
Management:
  Director: Laura Colby
  Artists Representative: Tessa Chandler
  Artists Representative: Meghan Dunne
Mission: Represents touring contemporary, modern and
world dance companies, artists and projects ranging in
size from chamber groups to large scale spectacles with
live music. All artists offer extensive outreach and
educational activities.
Founded: 1995
Specialized Field: Dance, Contemporary, Modern

8485 BAYLIN ARTISTS MANAGEMENT
18 West State Street
Suite 203
Doylestown, PA 18901
Phone: 267-880-3750
Fax: 267-880-3757
e-mail: mbaylin@baylinartists.com
Web Site: www.baylinartists.com
Officers:
  President: Marc J Baylin
  Director Operations: Kristen Lee
  Contracts Manager: Kara Ruiz
  Administrative Assistant: Jill Dulany
Management:
  Management Associate: Christopher Joy
Mission: Baylin Artists Management has earned a
reputation for superb servicing, innovative roster
management, and unique special projects.
Founded: 1993

8486 JOANNE RILE ARTISTS MANAGEMENT
801 Old York Road, Noble Plaza
Suite 212
Jenkintown, PA 19046-1611
Phone: 215-885-6400
Fax: 215-885-9929
Web Site: www.rilearts.com
Officers:
  President: Joanne Rile
  Executive VP: John R Rile
Management:
  Co-Director: Joanne Rile
  Co-Director: Jonh R Rile
Founded: 1972

8487 ENTERTAINMENT BUSINESS
2075 Leedoma Drive
Newtown, PA 18940-9420
Mailing Address: PO Box 32 Newtown, PA 18940-0032
Phone: 215-493-2500
Fax: 215-493-2507
e-mail: infp@theentertainmentbusiness.com
Web Site: www.theentertainmentbusiness.com

8488 BRITTON MANAGEMENT
28 E Willow Grove Avenue
Philadelphiall, PA 19118

Phone: 610-828-7537
Fax: 215-242-4953
e-mail: brittonmgt@aol.com
Web Site: www.gobritton.com
Officers:
    Founder/Chairman of the Board: Charlotte Britton
    President: Brian Patrone
Management:
    VP Marketing: Edward N Patrone
    VP Performing Arts: Carlos da Costa
    VP Contemporary Arts: Mary Collins
Mission: Britton Management has built a reputation of excellence in arts presenting with a focus on multi-cultural performing arts.
Founded: 1953
Specialized Field: Music, Dance, Theatre
Paid Staff: 5
Paid Artists: 50

8489 DAN KAMIN

366 Avon Drive
Pittsburgh, PA 15228
Phone: 412-563-0468
Fax: 412-563-4706
e-mail: dan@dankamin.com
Web Site: www.dankamin.com
Mission: Dan Kamin performs worldwide for theatres, colleges and symphony orchestras. On film, he created the physical comedy sequences for Chaplin and Benny and Joon, and trained Robert Downey Jr. and Johnny Depp for the acclaimed starring performances. He also created Martian movement for Tim Burton's Mars Attacks and played the wooden Indian come to life in the cult classic Creepshow 2.

8490 GEORGE BALDEROS

1414 Pennsylvania Avenue
Pittsburgh, PA 15233-1419
Phone: 412-323-2707
Fax: 412-323-1817
e-mail: info@music-tree.com
Web Site: www.music-tree.com

8491 JOAN SHERMAN ARTIST MANAGEMENT

3604 Bandera Street
Pittsburgh, PA 15201-1816
Phone: 412-621-9449
Fax: 412-291-1081
Web Site: www.joansherman.com
Management:
    Western Representative: Les Getchell
Mission: Represents the top names in the world of folk and world music ans spoken word artistry

8492 MUSIC TREE ARTIST MANAGEMENT

1414 Pennsylvania Avenue
Pittsburgh, PA 15233-1419
Phone: 412-323-2707
Fax: 412-323-1817
e-mail: info@music-tree.com
Web Site: www.music-tree.com
Management:

Managing Director: George Balderose
Associate Director: Leslie Clark
Founded: 1984
Specialized Field: Traditional Folk; Contemporary Folk
Paid Staff: 3

South Carolina

8493 MAGICMUSIC PRODUCTIONS

PO Box 26088
Greenville, SC
Phone: 864-676-9314
Fax: 864-676-0434
Toll-free: 888-273-3925
e-mail: magicmusic@infoave.net
Web Site: www.emilepandolfi.com
Management:
    General Manager: Judy Pandolfi
    Booking Manager: Kelley King
Mission: Record label and artist management for pianist Emile Pandolfi.
Founded: 1990
Status: Artist-Owned Corporation

8494 EASTCOAST ENTERTAINMENT

100 Harmon Street
Suite 204
Lexington, SC 29072
Phone: 803-957-7744
Fax: 803-957-7801
Toll-free: 800-323-3599
Web Site: www.eastcoastentertainment.com
Mission: Worldwide booking agency, supplying talent throughout this country and overseas for a wide range of situations, including conventions and concerts, presidents and royalty, movies and television, bar mitzvahs and weddings.
Founded: 1976

8495 EASTCOAST ENTERTAINMENT

1039 D Anna Knapp Boulevard
Mt. Pleasant, SC 29464
Phone: 843-856-9922
Fax: 843-846-8522
Toll-free: 800-521-2007
Web Site: www.eastcoastentertainment.com
Mission: Worldwide booking agency, supplying talent throughout this country and overseas for a wide range of situations, including conventions and concerts, presidents and royalty, movies and television, bar mitzvahs and weddings.
Founded: 1976

8496 GROUP H ENTERTAINMENT

10517 Ocean Highway
PMB 333
Pawleys Island, SC 29585
Phone: 843-235-3040
Fax: 843-235-3043
e-mail: grouph@aol.com
Web Site: www.grouph.com

Mission: Supplying entertainers and speakers for many of the nation's most respected concert halls, as well as colleges and universities, fairs, festivals and corporate events.

Tennessee

8497 HERSCHEL FREEMAN AGENCY
7684 Apahon Lane
Germantown, TN 38138
Phone: 901-757-4567
Fax: 901-757-5424
e-mail: hfreeman@herschelfreemanagency.com
Web Site: www.herschelfreemanagency.com
Mission: Herschel Freeman Agency manages North American tours for Ethnic, Folk and World Musicians. We have represented musicians from Eastern and Western Europe, Africa, Asia, and the indigenous cultures of the Americas and Canada.
Founded: 1980

8498 WILLIAM MORRIS AGENCY
2100 W End Avenue
#1000
Nashville, TN 37203
Phone: 615-963-3000
Fax: 615-963-3090
Web Site: www.wma.com

8499 CLASS ACT ENTERTAINMENT
107 Music City Circle
Suite 112
Nasville, TN 37214
Mailing Address: PO Box 160236 Nashville, TN 37216
Phone: 615-262-6886
Fax: 615-262-6881
e-mail: mail@classactentertainment.com
Web Site: www.classactentertainment.com
Officers:
   Founder: Mike Drudge
Mission: Class Act Entertainment was created to offer professional representation to the brightest talent in acoustic country, bluegrass and folk music today. The agency specializes in giving personalized attention to the artist and buyer alike.

Texas

8500 MELISSA J EDDY PRO ARTS MANAGEMENT
8506 Cima Oak Lane
Suite B
TX 78759
Phone: 512-342-2785
Fax: 512-342-0515
Web Site: www.hometown.aol.com/proartsmgt
Management:
   Owner/Principal: Melissa J Eddy

Mission: To provide a range of administrative services to performing arts organizations and individual artists. Offers administration, bookkeeping, marketing, production, resources development planning, grant writting and general operations management on a contract or consulting basis.
Founded: 2000

8501 HOLDEN & ARTS ASSOCIATES
PO Box 50120
Austin, TX 78763
Phone: 512-477-1859
Fax: 512-477-3908
e-mail: mh4arts@aol.com
Web Site: www.holdenarts.org
Mission: Booking and management company serving performing artist and performing arts presenters
Founded: 1983

8502 ARTISTS MANAGEMENT & ARTS CONSULTANT
6310 Turner Way
Dallas, TX 75230-1839
Phone: 972-661-9074
Fax: 972-661-9514
e-mail: friends@mec-sing.com
Web Site: www.mec-sing.com
Mission: Our select roster of singers include those with international and major national experiences, as well as some of the brightest emerging stars. We also offer lectures, workshops, consultations for artists, and arts consultant services.
Founded: 1985

Vermont

8503 DAVIS ROWE ARTISTS
303 Harlan Road
Bennington, VT 05257
Phone: 510-482-8903
Fax: 510-482-9923
e-mail: DavidRowe@aol.com
Web Site: www.davidroweartists.com

8504 MELVIN KAPLAN
115 College Street
Burlington, VT 05401
Phone: 802-658-2592
Fax: 802-658-6089
e-mail: music@melkap.com
Web Site: www.melkap.com
Officers:
   President: Melvin Kaplan
   Bookeeper: Tracy Cotnoir
   Office Manager: Karey Young
Management:
   Associate: Cynthia Seybolt
   Agent: Jessica Kuhlman
   Agent: Matthew Kulas
   Operations Director: Sharon Riley

Mission: To provide representation for chamber music groups; recital soloists; and attractions who possess the highest artistic integrity and seek to broaden the scope of classical music.
Specialized Field: Chamber Music

8505 ABBEY MUSIC MANAGEMENT
106 Brown Lane
Orwell, VT 05760-9779
Phone: 802-948-2848
Fax: 809-948-2856
e-mail: pax4arts@aol.com
Web Site: www.abbeymusic.net
Mission: Abbey Music Management was founded in 1997 as an early music booking agency handling instrumental and vocal ensembles and soloists performing music written before 1800 and played on original instruments exclusively.
Founded: 1997

Virginia

8506 FEUCHTENBERGER MANAGEMENT
804 Fincastle Drive
Bluefield, VA 24605
Phone: 276-326-1491
Fax: 276-326-1491
e-mail: pfeuch@netscope.net
Web Site: www.feucharts.com
Management:
    Director: Pat Feuchtenberger
Mission: Represent distinguished performing artists worldwide and remain dedicated to their career advancement, to promote, appreciate and enjoy classical music.
Founded: 1983
Specialized Field: Classical Performing Artists

8507 MARSJAZZ BOOKING AGENCY
1006 Ashby Place
Charlottesville, VA 22901-4006
Phone: 434-979-6374
Fax: 434-970-2270
e-mail: reggie@marsjazz.com
Web Site: www.marsjazz.com
Mission: To secure work for our roster of artists.
Founded: 1997
Specialized Field: Jazz Music

8508 WINDWOOD THEATRICALS
575 Windwood Lane
Paris, VA 20130-3003
Phone: 540-592-9576
Fax: 540-592-9574
e-mail: paul@aindwoodtheatricals.com
Web Site: www.windwoodtheatricals.com
Officers:
    President: Paul Bartz

Mission: An agency headed by veteran agent Paul Bartz that concentrates on developing, producing and touring new and established productions from and for Broadway, Off-Broadway and regional theaters, along with a roster of special attractions.
Founded: 2000

8509 EASTCOAST ENTERTAINMENT
3311 W Broad Street
Richmond, VA 23230
Phone: 804-355-2178
Fax: 804-353-3407
Toll-free: 800-277-6874
Web Site: www.eastcoastentertainment.com
Mission: Worldwide booking agency supplying talent throughout this country and overseas for a wide range of situations, including conventions and concerts, presidents and royalty, movies and television, bar mitzvahs and weddings.
Founded: 1976

Washington

8510 ROTH ARTS
PO Box 31120
Seattle, WA
Phone: 206-522-8151
Fax: 206-522-8141
e-mail: liz@rotharts.com
Web Site: www.rotharts.com
Management:
    Director: Elizabeth Roth
Mission: Booking and consulting performing arts agency representing remarkable American and international artists in theatre, contemporary dance and music.

Wisconsin

8511 ART FOR PETE'S SAKE!
1810 Sugar Place
De Pere, WI 54115
Phone: 920-336-9801
Fax: 920-964-1113
Toll-free: 800-788-0059
e-mail: ellen@artforpete.com
Web Site: www.artforpete.com
Management:
    Director: Ellen Rosewall
Mission: At Arts for Pete's Sake, we specialize in representing high quality, reasonably priced musicians and performing artists from Wisconsin. We work with performing arts series, festivals, fairs, schools, colleges, conventions, corporations and special events producers throughout Wisconsin, the Midwest and around the country.

8512 PERFORMING ARTISTS & SPEAKERS
732 W Main Street
Suite B
Lake Geneva, WI 53147

All listings are in alphabetical order by state, then city, then organization within the city.

Phone: 262-249-0700
Fax: 262-249-0773
Toll-free: 800-808-0917
e-mail: classact@iname.com
Web Site: www.class-act.com
Mission: Our goal is to enrich and broaden children's horizons through introduction to and participation in a large spectrum of art forms an opportunity which some children may never otherwise experience.

8513   OMICRON ARTIST MANAGEMENT
PO Box 11912
Milwaukee, WI 53211
Phone: 414-332-7600
Fax: 414-332-6473
e-mail: info@omicronarts.com
Web Site: www.omicronarts.com
Officers:
   President: Donald Sope
   VP: Brian McCreath
Mission: Works with over nationally know soloists, conductors, ensembles and institutions in classical music. Encourages artists to be knowledgeable decision-makers throughout their careers.
Founded: 1993

Associations

8514 ASCAP
One Lincoln Plaza
New York, NY 10023
Phone: 212-621-6407
Toll-free: 212-873-3133
e-mail: aalexander@ascap.com
Web Site: www.ascap.com
Account Service Manager: Krystal Jones
Director: Allen Alexander

8515 ACADEMY OF COUNTRY MUSIC
Suite 923
6255 W Sunset Boulevard
Hollywood, CA 90028-7410
Phone: 323-462-2351
Fax: 323-462-3253
Web Site: www.acmcountry.com
Executive Director: Fran Boyd
Involved in numerous events and activities promoting
country music. Presents annual awards.
4M Members Founded: 1964

**8516 ACCORDIAN FEDERATION OF NORTH
AMERICA**
16811 S Ardmore Avenue
Bellflower, CA 90706
Phone: 562-920-4888
President: Lola Wilson
VP: Sandy Martin
Executive Officer: Randy Martin
Executive Secretary: Priscilla
Martinez
Members are primarily teachers and music school owners.
The association's primary purpose is to encourage young
people to pursue their music study.
75 Members Founded: 1955 75 names

8517 ACCORDIAN TEACHERS GUILD
4949 Cherry Street
Kansas City, MO 64110
Phone: 816-235-2955
Fax: 816-235-5264
President: John Sommers
ATG members are accordian teachers and professionals.

**8518 AMERICAN ALLIANCE FOR THEATRE
AND EDUCATION**
ASU Department of Theatre
PO Box 872002
Tempe, AZ 85287-2002
Phone: 480-965-6064
Fax: 480-965-5351
e-mail: aate.info@asu.edu
Web Site: www.aate.com
Administrative Director: Christy M. Taylor
Members are artists, teachers and professionals who serve
youth theatres and theatre educational programs.
1000 Members Founded: 1986

**8519 AMERICAN ASSOCIATION OF
COMMUNITY THEATRE**
8402 Briar Wood Circle
Lago Vista, TX 78645-4118
Phone: 512-267-0711
Toll-free: 888-687-7838
Fax: 512-267-0712
e-mail: info@aact.org
Web Site: www.aact.org
Executive Director: Julie Angelo
President: Jill Patchin
Non-profit corporation fostering excellence in community
theatre productions and governance through community
theatre festivals, educational opportunity publications,
network, resources, and website.
1600 Members 6 per year Founded: 1986
Mailing list available for rent 10,000 names
Printed in on glossy stock

**8520 AMERICAN CHORAL DIRECTORS
ASSOCIATION**
PO Box 6310
Lawton, OK 73506-0310
Phone: 580-355-8161
Fax: 580-248-1465
e-mail: acda@acdaonline.org
Web Site: www.acdaonline.org
Executive Director: Dr. Gene Brooks
President: David Stutzenberger
A non-profit educational organization in the Choral area,
dedicated to providing information to members.
*19250 Members Founded: 1959 18300 names $60 per
M.*

**8521 AMERICAN COLLEGE DANCE
FESTIVAL ASSOCIATION**
Box 399
4423 Lehigh Road
College Park, MD 20740-1912
Phone: 301-405-8551
Fax: 301-405-8551
Executive Director: Diane DeFries
Works to provide regional and national visibility for dance
works produced in colleges and universities. Sponsors
biennial festival at John F. Kennedy Center for the
Performing Arts in Washington, D.C. and a scholarship
program.
200 Members Founded: 1973

8522 AMERICAN COLLEGE OF MUSICIANS
808 Rio Grande Street
Austin, TX 78701-2220
Phone: 512-478-5775
President: Richard Allison
Grants degrees and diplomas to worthy musicians.

8523 AMERICAN DANCE GUILD
Katya Pylyshenko Kolcio, Margot C. Lehman, author
PO Box 2006
Lenox Hill Station
New York, NY 10021
Phone: 212-932-2789
Web Site: www.americandanceguild.org

President: Marilynn Danitz
Non-profit membership organization; sponsors professional seminars, workshops, a student scholarship and other projects and institutes programs of national significance in the field of dance.
400 Members Founded: 1956 ISBN 0-934994-02-1

8524 AMERICAN DANCE THERAPY ASSOCIATION
2000 Century Plaza, Suite 108
10632 Little Patuxent Parkway
Columbia, MD 21044-3273
Phone: 410-997-4040
Fax: 410-997-4048
e-mail: info@adta.org
Web Site: www.adta.org
Newsletter Editor: Kathy Wallens
Founded in 1966; professional organization of dance movement therapists, with members both nationally and internationally; offers training, research findings, and a newsletter.
1.1M Members

8525 AMERICAN DISC JOCKEY ASSOCIATION
1964 Wagner
Pasadena, CA 91107
Phone: 626-844-3204
e-mail: adjanews@aol.com
Contact: Bruce Kessler
Assists and trains members, provides forums and conducts educational programs. Publishes bimonthly newsletter and holds an annual conference and seminar.
3000 Members

8526 AMERICAN FEDERATION OF MUSICIANS OF THE UNITED STATES AND CANADA
Suite 600
1501 Broadway
New York, NY 10036-5503
Phone: 212-869-1330
Fax: 212-764-6134
Web Site: www.afm.org
President: Steve Young
Secretary/Treasurer: Thomas Lee
Union Governance Coordinator: Jennifer Scheurich
Union representing over 100,000 professional musicians, performing in all genres of music.
120M Members
Printed in 4 colors on newsprint stock

8527 AMERICAN FEDERATION OF VIOLIN AND BOW MAKERS
No. 709
250 W 54th Street
New York, NY 10019
Toll-free: 800-633-2777
President: James McKean
Helps develop technical skills and knowledge. Conducts competitions, annual exhibition and publishes annual membership directory.
100 Members

8528 AMERICAN GUILD OF MUSIC
5354 Washington Street
Downers Grove, IL 60515-4905
Phone: 630-978-2696
Fax: 630-968-0197
Registered Agent: Elmer Herrick
Sponsors competitions, music contests, concerts, teacher workshops and displays of musical instruments and music.
325 Members

8529 AMERICAN GUILD OF MUSICAL ARTISTS
1727 Broadway
New York, NY 10019-5214
Phone: 212-265-3687
Fax: 212-262-9088
e-mail: AGMA@AGMANatl.com
Web Site: ww.musicalartists.org
President: Linda Mays
Executive Secretary: Sanford I. Wolff
Exclusive bargaining agent for all concert musical artists.
5.7M Members

8530 AMERICAN GUILD OF ORGANISTS
Suite 1260
475 Riverside Drive
New York, NY 10115-1260
Phone: 212-870-2310
Fax: 212-870-2163
e-mail: info@agohq.org
Web Site: www.agohq.org
Executive Director: James E. Thomashower
Dir of Development/Communications: F. Anthony Thurman
Editor: Anthony Baglivi
20000 Members Founded: 1896 25000 names $75 per M.

8531 AMERICAN HARP SOCIETY
6331 Quebec Drive
Hollywood, CA 90068-2831
Phone: 213-463-0716
Fax: 213-464-2950
Web Site: www.harpsociety.org
Executive Secretary: Dorothy Remsen
Improves the quality of the instrument and performance.
3.3M Members Founded: 1962

8532 AMERICAN INDIAN REGISTRY FOR THE PERFORMING ARTS
Suite 614
1717 N Highland Avenue
Hollywood, CA 90028-4403
Phone: 323-585-2202
American Indian association for performing artists.

8533 AMERICAN INSTITUTE OF ORGAN BUILDERS
PO Box 130982
Houston, TX 77219

Phone: 713-529-2212
Fax: 713-529-2212
Web Site: www.pipeorgan.org
Executive Secretary: Howard Maple
Sponsers training seminars, quarterly journal and annual convention for pipe organ builders and service technicians.
340 Members   350 names $250 per M.

**8534   AMERICAN KIDDIE RIDE
ASSOCIATION**
3800 Nicollet Avenue
Minneapolis, MN 55409-1304
Phone: 612-827-5588
Fax: 651-644-8295
Executive Director: Anita Bennett
Represents interests of manufacturers and operators of coin-operated rides.
72 Members Founded: 1990

**8535   AMERICAN MUSIC SCHOLARSHIP
ASSOCIATION**
Suite 1826
441 Vine Street
Cincinnati, OH 45202-2908
Phone: 513-421-2672
Fax: 513-742-3094
Executive Director: Gloria Ackerman
Seeks to expose young pianists, ages five to 30, to the influence of performances by great musicians.
2.5M Members Founded: 1956

**8536   AMERICAN MUSIC THERAPY
ASSOCIATION**
Suite 1000
8455 Colesville Road
Silver Spring, MD 20910-3315
Phone: 301-589-3300
Fax: 301-589-5175
e-mail: info@musictherapy.org
Web Site: www.namt.com
Executive Director: Dr. Andrea Farbman
A national organization whose mission is to advance the public awareness of music therapy benefits and increase accessibility to quality music therapy services.

**8537   AMERICAN MUSICIANS UNION
QUARTERNOTE**
8 Tobin Ct
Dumont, NJ 07628-3329
Phone: 201-384-5378
President: Ben Intorre
Association formed by a small group of musicians who chose to remain independent of the AFL-CIO merger of labor unions.
300 Members Founded: 1948 310 names

**8538   AMERICAN NATIONAL ACADEMY OF
PERFORMING ARTS**
10944 Ventura Boulevard
Studio City, CA 91604-3340
Phone: 818-763-4431
Administrative Director: Dorothy Barrett

Non-profit organization chartered by the state of California. All teachers offer their services without remuneration. A school teaching all the performing arts.
50 Members Founded: 1957

**8539   AMERICAN RECREATION EQUIPMENT
ASSOCIATION**
#395
407 2nd Avenue
Mason, OH 45040-1573
Phone: 513-423-9233
Fax: 513-398-2815
Executive Director: R.C. Fussner
Works to promote interests of amusement equipment manufacturers.
70 Members

**8540   AMERICAN SCHOOL BAND
DIRECTORS ASSOCIATION**
227 N First Street
Guttenberg, IA 52052-0696
Phone: 319-252-2383
Fax: 319-252-2500
e-mail: asbda@netins.net
President: Linda Fox-Miller
Office Manager: Dennis Hanna
Holds annual meetings in June. Membership dues: $75 active members, $65 affiliates, $65 associates, $25 retirees
1.3M Members Founded: 1952 1300 names

**8541   AMERICAN SOCIETY OF COMPOSERS,
AUTHORS AND PUBLISHERS**
1 Lincoln Plaza
New York, NY 10023-7129
Phone: 212-621-6000
Fax: 212-595-3342
e-mail: info@ascap.com
Web Site: www.ascao.com
Editor: Erik Philbrook
Association for songwriters, composers and music publishers.
120M Members Founded: 1914

**8542   AMERICAN SOCIETY OF COMPOSERS,
AUTHORS/ PUBLISHERS - WEST COAST**
3rd Floor
7920 Sunset Boulevard
Hollywood, CA 90046
Phone: 323-883-1000
Fax: 323-883-1049
America's first performing rights society.

**8543   AMERICAN SOCIETY OF MUSIC
ARRANGERS AND COMPOSERS**
PO Box 17840
Encino, CA 91416-7840
Phone: 818-994-4661
Fax: 818-994-6181
e-mail: tpi97@ix.netcom.com
Web Site: www.asmac.org
Director: Scherr Lillico

Professional society for arrangers, composers, orchestrators, and musicians. Monthly meetings with great speakers from the music industry.
400 Members Founded: 1938

8544 AMERICAN SOCIETY OF MUSIC COPYISTS
Times Square Station
Box 2557
New York, NY 10108
Phone: 212-222-3742
Fax: 212-961-9026
e-mail: asmc802@aol.com
Web Site: www.members.aol.com/asmc
President: Joe Muccioli
Supports music preparation and rights of the professionals in the industry.
100 Members Founded: 1961

8545 AMERICAN SYMPHONY ORCHESTRA LEAGUE
Suite 800
910 17th Street NW
Washington, DC 20006
Phone: 202-776-0212
Fax: 202-776-0224
e-mail: league@symphony.org
Web Site: www.symphony.org
President: Charles Otun
Advertising Manager: Laura Tucker
The national nonprofit service and educational organization dedicated to strengthening symphony and chamber orchestras. It provides artistic, organizational and financial leadership and service to orchestral conductors, managers, volunteers and staff.
3M Members Founded: 1942

8546 AMERICAN VIOLA SOCIETY
4600 Sunset Avenue
Butler University
Indianapolis, IN 46208
Phone: 317-283-9637
e-mail: dclark@butler.edy
Contact: Donna Clark

8547 AMUSEMENT AND MUSIC OPERATORS ASSOCIATION
Suite 300
1145 N Arlington Heights Road
Itasca, IL 60143-3171
Phone: 630-250-1430
Toll-free: 800-937-2662
Fax: 630-250-3533
e-mail: amoa@amoa.com
Web Site: www.amoa.com
Executive VP: Jack Kelleher
A trade association comprised of some 1,700 owners/operators, distributors and manufacturers of coin operated amusement, music and vending equipment.

8548 ASSOCIATED PIPE ORGAN BUILDERS OF AMERICA
PO Box 155
Chicago Ridge, IL 60415
Toll-free: 800-473-5270
President: Victor Schantz
Offers courses and marketing statistics; hosts monthly journal and annual meeting.
27 Members

8549 ASSOCIATION FOR THEATRE IN HIGHER EDUCATION
PO Box 4537
Boulder, CO 80306-4537
Phone: 303-440-0851
Toll-free: 888-284-3737
Fax: 303-440-0852
e-mail: info@athe.org
Web Site: www.hawaii.edu/athe
Administrative Director: Nancy Erickson
President: Kurt Dan
An organization of individuals and institutions that provides vision and leadership for the profession and promotes excellence in theatre education. ATHE consists of more than 2,000 members who represent education, retired colleagues and organizations creating, studying and teaching theatre.
1.9M Members Founded: 1986

8550 ASSOCIATION OF AMATEUR MAGICIANS
PO Box 265
Swampscott, MA 01907-0465
Phone: 978-921-2177
President: Thomas A. Roy
Association for amateur magicians.
16M Members Founded: 1988

8551 ASSOCIATION OF ARTS ADMINISTRATION EDUCATORS
525 West 120th Street
Columbia University
New York, NY 10027
Phone: 212-678-3271
e-mail: jj64@columbia.edu
Web Site: www.artsnet.org/aaae/
Program in Arts Adm: Joan Jeffri
The Association of Administration Educators (AAAE) is an international organization incorporated as a nonprofit institution within the United States. Its mission is to represent college and university graduate and undergraduate programs in the arts administration, encompassing training in the management of visual, performing, literary, media, cultural and arts service organizations.

8552 ASSOCIATION OF CONCERT BANDS
413 E 11th Avenue
Naperville, IL 60563-2801
Phone: 630-717-6717
Toll-free: 800-726-8720
Fax: 480-894-1986

Executive Director: Toni Ryon
Dedicated to the advancement of community and concert bands.
750 Members

8553 ASSOCIATION OF HISPANIC ARTS

4th Floor
250 W 26th Street
New York, NY 10001
Phone: 212-727-7227
Fax: 212-727-0549
e-mail: ahanews@latinoarts.org
Web Site: www.latinoarts.org
Deputy Executive Director: Delia Montalvo
Executive Director: Sandra M Perez
A multidisciplary organization which supports Latino arts organizations and individual artists with technical assistance. The organization facilitates projects and programs designed to foster the appreciation, growth, and well being of the Latino arts cultural community. It's quarter publication, AHA; Hispanic Arts News, features in depth articles on the local and national arts community, including artist profiles and a calendar of events.
Founded: 1975 5,000 names $80 per M.

8554 ASSOCIATION OF PERFORMING ARTS PRESENTERS

Suite 400
1112 16th Street NW
Washington, DC 20036
Phone: 202-833-2787
Fax: 202-833-1543
e-mail: artspres@artspresenters.org
Web Site: www.artspresenters.org
President/CEO: Sandra Gibson
COO: Jonathan Durnford

8555 BMI

Broadcast Music
320 W 57th Street
New York, NY 10019-3790
Phone: 212-586-2000
Fax: 212-582-5972
e-mail: webmaster@bmi.com
Web Site: www.bmi.com
President: Frances Preston
Corporate Relations: Robbin Ahrold
Secures the rights of songwriters/composers. Collects license fees for the public performance of music and pays royalties to its copyright owners.
Founded: 1940

8556 BIG BAND ACADEMY OF AMERICA

Milton Gerald Bernhart, Kelly Travel Service
Suite 516
6565 W Sunset Boulevard
Los Angeles, CA 90028-7217
e-mail: mbernhart@pacbell.net
Web Site: home.pacbell.net/mbernhar/
President: Milt Bernhart
Seeks to perpetuate the memory and sound of big bands and to introduce big band music to younger generations.
500 Members Founded: 1983

8557 BLUES FOUNDATION

49 Union Avenue
Memphis, TN 38103-3714
Phone: 901-527-2583
Fax: 901-529-4030
Executive Director: Howard Stovall
The goal of this organization is to develop a blues awareness program to educate Americans and people worldwide on the historical and musical value of blues music.
Founded: 1980

8558 CHAMBER MUSIC AMERICA

Chamber Music America
5th Floor
305 7th Avenue
New York, NY 10001
Phone: 212-242-2022
Fax: 212-242-7955
A national membership organization that offers programs, service, direct cash grant awards, technical assistance, publication, directories, educational programs, conferences and workshops, insurance programs, awards, advocacy, surveys and other specialized services.
10.5M Members Founded: 1979

8559 CHORUS AMERICA

Suite 310
1156 15th Street NW
Washington, DC 20005-1747
Phone: 202-331-7577
Fax: 202-331-2599
e-mail: chorusam@libertynet.org
Web Site: www.chorusamerica.org
President: Mary Peissler
Member Services Director: Kanre Richter
National service for orchestral choruses, independent choruses and professional choruses.
1100 Members Founded: 1954
Mailing list available for rent 7000 names
Printed in 2 colors on matte stock

8560 CIRCUS FANS ASSOCIATION OF AMERICA

PO Box 59710
Potomac, MD 20859-9710
e-mail: circus@inficad.com
Web Site: www.circusfans.org
Secretary/Treasurer: Irvin C. Mohler
Seeks to create an enthusiasm for the circus as an institution and preserve it for future generations.
2.5M Members Founded: 1926

8561 CIRCUS HISTORICAL SOCIETY

1954 Old Hickory Boulevard
Brentwood, TN 37027
Phone: 615-373-0946
Fax: 615-373-0946
Web Site: www.circusmodelbuilders.org
Secretary:
Information on the historical applications of the circus.
1.4M Members Founded: 1939

8562 CLASSICAL ACTION
Suite 1310
165 W 46th Street
New York, NY 10036
Phone: 212-997-7717
Fax: 212-997-7897
e-mail: classicalaction@bcefa.org
Web Site: www.classicalaction.org
Since 1993, Classical Action has provided a unified voice
for all those within the performing arts community to help
combat HIV/AIDS and the devastating effects of this
epidemic.

8563 COLLEGE MUSIC SOCIETY
202 W Spruce Street
Missoula, MT 59802-4202
Phone: 406-721-9616
Fax: 406-721-9419
e-mail: cms@music.org
Web Site: www.music.org
Executive Director: Robby D. Gunstream
Production Manager: Julie L. Johnson
The Society is a national service organization for college
conservatory and university music teachers.
8 Members Founded: 1959 30000 names $160 per M.
Printed in 1 color on matte stock

8564 CONDUCTORS GUILD
6219 N Sheridan Road
Chicago, IL 60660
Phone: 773-764-7563
Fax: 773-764-7564
e-mail: ConGuild@aol.com
Web Site: www.conductorsguild.org
Dedicated to encouraging the highest standards in the art
and profession of conducting. Founded in 1975.
1,900 Members

**8565 CONFERENCE OF NATIONAL PARK
CONCESSIONAIRES**
PO Box 29041
Phoenix, AZ 85038-9041
Fax: 602-208-6843
Executive Director: Rex Maughan
Acts as a liaison between private concessionaires in
United States national parks.
92 Members Founded: 1919

8566 CONGRESS ON RESEARCH IN DANCE
Department of Dance-SUNY College of Brockport
350 New Campus Drive
Brockport, NY 14420-2997
Phone: 716-395-2151
Fax: 716-395-5134
Office Administrater: Ginger Carlson
Publishes dance research journal two times a year, does
newletters 2 times a year, and publishes annual conference
proceedings.
900 Members Founded: 1965 750 names $75 per M.

**8567 COUNCIL OF DANCE
ADMINISTRATORS**
Department of Dance
Florida State University
Tallahassee, FL 32306
Phone: 850-216-1511
Fax: 850-644-1277
President: Prof. Sharon Vasquez
Members are administrators of dance departments in
educational institutions.
25 Members Founded: 1966

8568 COUNTRY MUSIC ASSOCIATION
1 Music Circle S
Nashville, TN 37203-4312
Phone: 615-244-2840
Fax: 615-726-0314
Web Site: www.CMAworld.com
Executive Director: Edwin Benson
Promotes and publicizes country music.
7M Members Founded: 1958

8569 COUNTRY RADIO BROADCASTERS
819 18th Avenue S
Nashville, TN 37203-3227
Phone: 615-327-4487
Fax: 615-329-4492
Executive Director: Paul Allen
Provides placement services, conducts a charitable
program, and offers professional development seminars.
Founded: 1970

8570 CREATIVE MUSICIAN COALITION
1024 W Willcox Avenue
Peoria, IL 61604-2675
Phone: 309-685-4843
Toll-free: 800-882-4262
Fax: 309-685-4878
e-mail: aimcmc@aol.com
Web Site: www.aimcmc.com
President: Ronald Wallace
A national organization that brings the world of new
music to its readers. Includes in depth music reviews,
informative artist interviews, interesting articles and
feature columns, and valuable resource material.
1000 Members Founded: 1984

8571 DANCE CRITICS ASSOCIATION
PO Box 1882
Old Chelsea Station
New York, NY 10011
Phone: 212-254-7905
Web Site: ww.criticaldance.com
Administrator: Kathy Hall
Encourages excellence in dance criticism through
education, research and the exchange of ideas.
250 Members Founded: 1974

8572 DANCE EDUCATORS OF AMERICA
PO Box 509
Oceanside, NY 11572-0509

Phone: 516-763-0400
Toll-free: 800-229-3868
Fax: 516-536-6502
Web Site: ww.deadance.com
Executive Director: Vickie Sheer
Promotes the education of teachers in the performing arts.
2M Members

8573 DANCE MASTERS OF AMERICA
PO Box 438
Independence, MO 64051-0438
Fax: 616-252-5501
Web Site: www.dma-national.org
Executive Secretary: Paul C. Zimmerman
Chap. at Large Pres.: Johann Meyer
An organization of dance teachers.
2.5M Members

8574 DANCE USA
Suite 820
1156 15th Street NW
Washington, DC 20005-1704
Phone: 202-833-1717
Fax: 202-833-2686
e-mail: danceusa@danceusa.org
Web Site: www.danceusa.org
Executive Director: Andrea Snyder
Provides a forum for the discussion of issues of concern to membersand a support network for exchange of information; also bestows awards.
400 Members Founded: 1982

8575 DRAMATISTS GUILD
Suite 701
1501 Broadway
New York, NY 10036-3909
Phone: 212-398-9366
Fax: 212-944-0420
Web Site: www.dramaguild.com
President: John Weidman
Comprehensive organization that deals solely with Broadway and off-Broadway producers, off-off-Broadway groups, agents, theatres and sources of grants.

8576 EDUCATIONAL THEATER ASSOCIATION
3368 Central Parkway
Cincinnati, OH 45225-2307
Phone: 513-421-3900
Fax: 513-559-0012
Web Site: www.etassoc.org
Executive Director: Ronald Longstreth
Managing Director: Jeffrey Leptak-Moreau
Theater educators working to increase support for theater programs in the educational system.
2.8M Members Founded: 1989

8577 FIRST BASS INTERNATIONAL
33 Essex Street
Hackensack, NJ 07601-5418
Phone: 201-489-4641
Fax: 201-489-5057
Editor: Joe Campagna

A national organization dedicated to the electric and acoustic bass player of all ages and backgrounds.

8578 FRITZ AND LAVINIA JENSEN FOUNDATION
9035-40 J.M. Keynes Drive
c/o Lendon Munday
Charlotte, NC 28262
e-mail: JensenFnd@aol.com
Web Site: www.jensenfoundation.org
Sponsors competitions.

8579 GINA BACHAUER INTERNATIONAL PIANO FOUNDATION
PO Box 11664
Salt Lake City, UT 84147
Phone: 801-521-9200
Fax: 801-521-9202
e-mail: gina@bachauer.com
Web Site: www.bachauer.com
Marketing Director: Tracey Turner
Executive Director: Kimberly Garvin
Produce a yearly piano international competition: artistmanagement

8580 GOSPEL MUSIC ASSOCIATION
1205 Division Street
Nashville, TN 37203
Phone: 615-242-0303
Fax: 615-254-9755
Web Site: www.gospelmusic.org
President: Frank Breeden
Senior Director Marketing: Rick Bowles
Since 1964, the GMA has been a widely recognized voice for Christian/Gospel music in all its forms and variations, dedicated to providing leadership, direction and unity for all facets of the gospel music industry. Through education, communication, information, promotion and recognition, the GMA is striving to help those involved in gospel music to work together in furthering the cause of Jesus Christ.
5000 Members Founded: 1964

8581 GUILD OF AMERICAN LUTHIERS
8222 S Park Avenue
Tacoma, WA 98408
Phone: 253-472-7853
Fax: 206-472-7853
e-mail: galhq@juno.com
Web Site: www.luth.org
Executive Director: Debra Olsen
Manufacturers and repairs stringed instruments; offers quarterly journal and triennial meeting.
3000 Members

8582 GUITAR FOUNDATION OF AMERICA
PO Box 1240
Claremont, CA 91711-1240
Phone: 909-624-7730
e-mail: gunnar@guitarfoundation.org
Web Site: www.guitarfoundation.org
General Director: Gunnar Eisel
Supports the serious studies of the guitar.

2M Members Founded: 1973

8583 INDEPENDENT MUSIC ASSOCIATION
215 Timberlane Drive
Palm Habor, FL 34683
Phone: 727-938-0571
e-mail: dgkmusic@netscape.net
President: Don Kulak
Seeks to increase radio play and distribution of
independent labels through marketing trade shows and
retail promotion. Provides discounts on industry services,
CD and cassette manufacturing, overnight shipping and
long-distance telephoning.
2.1M Members Founded: 1989

8584 INSTRUMENT SOCIETY OF AMERICA
PO Box 12277
Research Triangle Park, NC 27709
Phone: 919-549-8411
Fax: 919-549-8288
Web Site: www.isa.org

8585 INTERNATIONAL ASSOCIATION OF AMUSEMENT PARKS AND ATTRACTIONS
1448 Duke Street
Alexandria, VA 22314-3403
Phone: 703-836-4800
Fax: 703-836-4801
e-mail: convention@iaapa.org
Web Site: www.iaapa.org
Exhibit Manager: Marc Parsont
Exhibit Sales/Service Coordinator: Beth Baumgardner
CEO/President: Bret Lovejoy
Editor: Bill Stevenson
Production Manager: Duane Brewster
The largest international trade association for permanently
situated amusement facilities worldwide. The organization
represents over 5,000 facility, supplier and individual
members from more than 100 countries, including most
amusement parks and attractions in the US. IAAPA strives
to help members improve their efficiency, marketing,
safety, and profitability while maintaining the highest
possible professional standards. IAAOA runs the worlds
largest trade show and convention in the industry.
6500 Members Founded: 1918

8586 INTERNATIONAL ASSOCIATION OF ELECTRONIC KEYBOARD MANUFACTURERS
316 South Service Road
c/o Korg USA
Melville, NY 11747-3201
President: Mike Kovins
Makes electric keyboards and holds semiannual meeting.
14 Members

8587 INTERNATIONAL ASSOCIATION OF PIANO BUILDERS AND TECHNICIANS
3930 Washington
c/o Piano Technicians Guild
Kansas City, MO 64111

Phone: 816-753-7747
Fax: 816-931-0070
Web Site: www.ptg.org
Executive Director: David Hanzlick
Network of technical information. Publishes quarterly
newsletter; hosts biennial meeting.

8588 INTERNATIONAL CLARINET ASSOCIATION
PO Box 5039
Wheaton, IL 60189
Phone: 630-665-3602
Fax: 630-665-3848
e-mail: membership@clarinet.org
Web Site: www.clarinet.org
Membership Director: Elena M. Lance Talley
Seeks to focus attention on the importance of the clarinet
and to foster communication of the fellowship between
clarinetists.
3.3M Members Founded: 1990

8589 INTERNATIONAL COMPUTER MUSIC ASSOCIATION
Suite 330
2040 Polk Street
San Francisco, CA 91109
Phone: 650-493-9448
Fax: 650-493-8045
e-mail: icma@email.sjsu.edu
Web Site: www.computermusic.org
Supports the performance aspects of computer music;
publishes newsletter and holds annual conference.
700 Members

8590 INTERNATIONAL FEDERATION OF FESTIVAL ORGANIZATIONS
7085 Chappell Circle
Atlanta, GA 30360
Phone: 770-248-1097
Fax: 770-446-1603
e-mail: aims@america.net
Web Site: www.aimsintl.org
Executive Director: Todd Barber
Organizes events, publishes monthly bulletin, holds
annual conference.
480 Members

8591 INTERNATIONAL FESTIVALS AND EVENTS ASSOCIATION
PO Box 2950, Suite 302
115 E Railroad
Port Angeles, WA 98362-0336
Phone: 425-452-4695
Fax: 206-452-4695
e-mail: alexis@ifea.com
Web Site: www.ifea.com
President: Bruce Skinner
Network for planning events and exchange programs;
publishes quarterly magazine.
2400 Members

8592 INTERNATIONAL HORN SOCIETY
2220 N 1400 E
Provo, UT 84604-2150
Phone: 801-377-3335
Fax: 616-387-5809
Web Site: www.horndoggie.com/horn
Publisher: Johnny Pherigo
Editor: Katherine Thomson
A national organization that focuses on music industry news and information.

8593 INTERNATIONAL JUGGLERS' ASSOCIATION
PO Box 218
Montague, MA 01351-4133
Phone: 413-367-2401
Toll-free: 800-367-0160
Fax: 413-367-0259
e-mail: secretary@juggle.org
Web Site: www.juggle.org
Secretary/Treasurer: Richard Dingman
Festival Coordinator: Ginny Rose
3000 Members Founded: 1947

8594 INTERNATIONAL LASER DISPLAY ASSOCIATION
Suite B-23
4301 32nd Street W
Bradenton, FL 34205-2700
Phone: 941-758-6881
Fax: 941-758-1605
e-mail: ildadirect@aol.com
Web Site: www.laserist.org
Executive Director: Linda Hare
A nonprofit organization dedicated to advancing the use of laser displays, in the art, entertainment and education.
150 Members Founded: 1986

8595 INTERNATIONAL MAGIC DEALERS ASSOCIATION
Hank Lee's Magic
102 N Street
Medford, MA 02155-4239
Executive Director: Hank Lee
Provides a forum for dealers in equipment for magicians.
150 Members Founded: 1945

8596 INTERNATIONAL PIANO GUILD
PO Box 1807
808 Rio Grande Street
Austin, TX 78701-2220
Phone: 512-478-5775
Web Site: www.pianoguild.com
President: Richard Allison
A division of the American College of Musicians
Professional society of piano teachers and music faculty members. Sponsers national examinations.

8597 INTERNATIONAL PLANNED MUSIC ASSOCIATION
5900 S Salina Street
Syracuse, NY 13205

Phone: 315-469-7711
Fax: 315-469-8842
Information exchange; annual meeting.
200 Members

8598 INTERNATIONAL POLKA ASSOCIATION
4608 S Archer Avenue
Chicago, IL 60632-2442
Phone: 773-254-7771
Toll-free: 800-867-6552
Fax: 773-254-8111
Web Site: www.internationalpolka.com
President: Al Jelinek
Educational organization concerned with the preservation and advancement of polka music. Operates the Polka Music Hall of Fame and Museum, and presents the International Polka Fesitval every year during the complete first weekend of August.
8M Members Founded: 1968

8599 INTERNATIONAL SOCIETY FOR THE PERFORMING ARTS FOUNDATION
PO Box 909
17 Purdy Avenue, Suite 200
Rye, NY 10580-0909
Phone: 914-921-1550
Fax: 914-921-1593
e-mail: info@ispa.org
Web Site: www.ispa.org
CEO: Johann Zietsman
Bring global arts leaders together for acts engagements, exchange, interaction and advocacy.
500 Members Founded: 1948 500 names $500 per M.

8600 INTERNATIONAL SOCIETY OF FOLK HARPERS AND CRAFTSMEN
4110 Brandemere Way
Houston, TX 77066
Phone: 832-249-7885
Fax: 832-249-7885
e-mail: olunsf@swbell.net
Web Site: www.folkharpsociety.org
Secretary: Sylvia Fellows
Conducts technical and artistic programs and promotes craft exchange. *$26.00*
1200 Members Quarterly Founded: 1980

8601 INTERNATIONAL THEATRE EQUIPMENT ASSOCIATION
Suite 200
244 W 49th Street
New York, NY 10019-7400
Phone: 212-246-6460
Fax: 212-265-6428
Web Site: www.itea.com
Executive Director: Robert Sunshine
Fosters and maintains professional, business and social relationships among its members within all segments of the motion picture industry. Bestows annual Teddy award to manufacturer of the year and the annual Rodney award to dealer of the year.
110 Members Founded: 1971

8602 INTERNATIONAL THESPIAN SOCIETY

2343 Auburn Avenue
Cincinnati, OH 45219-2815
Phone: 513-651-3737
Fax: 513-559-0012
Executive Director: Ronald Longstreth
Advances theater arts in high school through publications, conferences, festivals and scholarships.
30M Members Founded: 1929

8603 INTERNATIONAL TICKETING ASSOCIATION

Suite 722
250 W 57th Street
New York, NY 10107
Phone: 212-581-0600
Fax: 212-581-0885
e-mail: info@intix.org
Web Site: www.intix.org
Show Manager: Ann Marie Gennardo
Deputy Director: Kathleen O'Donnell
Not-for-profit organizaiton whose purpose is to advance the success of the admission service industry and its members.
1200 Members Founded: 1979

8604 JACKIE PAUL ENTERTAINMENT GROUP

559 Wanamaker Road
Jenkintown, PA 19046-2219
Phone: 215-884-3308
Fax: 215-884-1083
President/CEO: Jackie Paul
Artist Management.

8605 JAZZ EDUCATION

PO Box 8031
Houston, TX 77288
Phone: 715-839-7000
Fax: 715-839-8266
e-mail: jazzed@jazzeducation.org
Web Site: www.jazzeducation.org
Executive Director: Bubbha Thomas
Development Officer: Zahia Raines
Festival Director: Richard Dabon
Nonprofit music organization providing worthwhile educational activities for school-aged youth in the field of music. Includes many subjects not covered by school systems. Promotes appreciation and understanding of Jazz.
Founded: 1970

8606 LEAGUE OF AMERICAN THEATRES AND PRODUCERS

226 W 47th Street
New York, NY 10036-1413
Phone: 212-764-1122
Toll-free: 888-292-9669
Fax: 212-719-4389
e-mail: league@broadway.org
Web Site: www.broadway.org
Executive Director: Harvey Sabinson

National trade association for the commercial theatre industry whose principal activity is negotiation of labor contracts and government relations.
275 Members Founded: 1930

8607 LITERARY MANAGERS AND DRAMATURGS OF THE AMERICAS

CUNY Grad Center
Box 355 CASTA
New York, NY 10036
Phone: 718-437-5462
Fax: 212-966-6940
Web Site: www.inda.org
President: Victoria Abrash
A national network of American literary managers and dramaturgs encouraging the emerging profession.
300 Members

8608 METROPOLITAN OPERA GUILD

6th Floor
70 Lincoln Center Plaza
New York, NY 10023-6577
Phone: 212-362-0068
Fax: 212-870-7695
Web Site: www.metguild.org
Seeks to promote greater understanding and interest in opera.
100M Members Founded: 1935

8609 MICRO-REALITY MOTORSPORTS

1500 SW 7th Street
Atlantic, IA 50022
Phone: 712-243-9035
Toll-free: 800-347-6977
Fax: 712-243-3552
e-mail: nsei@netins.net
Executive Director: Keith Namanny
Manufactures and promotes NASCAR micro-reality racing centers and speedshops, plus several other sports and entertainment/promotions.
294 Members Founded: 1986

8610 MID ATLANTIC ARTS FOUNDATION

Suite 401
201 N Charles Street
Baltimore, MD 21201-4199
Phone: 410-539-6656
Fax: 410-837-5517
Web Site: www.midatlanticarts.org
Executive Director: Alan W Cooper
Director Operations: Tom Gaeng
Director External Affarirs: Matthew Brown
Founded: 1979 30,000 names

8611 MUSIC CRITICS ASSOCIATION

7 Pine Ct
Westfield, NJ 07090-3444
Phone: 908-233-8468
Fax: 908-233-8468
Manager: Albert H. Cohen
Improving standards of quality in the music industry to the broadcast media, magazine and newspaper industries.
220 Members Founded: 1957

8612 MUSIC DISTRIBUTOR ASSOCIATION
Hershman Musical Instrument Company
Floor 5
38 W 21st Street
New York, NY 10010-6906
Phone: 212-691-8920
e-mail: assnhdqs@aol.com
Web Site: www.musicdistributors.org
Executive VP: Jerome Hershman
A trade association of 160 manufactures, importers,
wholesalers of musical instruments and accessories,
domestic and international selling to the trade only
160 Members Founded: 1939

8613 MUSIC DISTRIBUTORS ASSOCIATION
#5
38 W 21st Street
New York, NY 10010-6906
Phone: 212-691-8920
Fax: 212-675-3577
e-mail: assnhdqs@aol.com
Executive VP: Jerome Hershman
A trade association of 160 manufacturers, importers,
wholesalers of musical instruments and accessories,
domestic and international selling to the trade only
160 Members Founded: 1939

8614 MUSIC INDUSTRY CONFERENCE
1806 Robert Fulton Drive
c/o Music Educators National Conference
Reston, VA 20191
Phone: 703-860-4000
Fax: 703-860-1531
Web Site: www.menc.org
President: Earl Anderson
Instrument manufacturers and other suppliers to the music
industry.
450 Members

8615 MUSIC LIBRARY ASSOCIATION
Suite 180
8551 Research Way
Middton, WI 53562
Phone: 608-836-5825
Fax: 703-556-9301
e-mail: mla@areditions.com
Web Site: www.musiclibraryassoc.org
President: James Cassaro
Promotes growth and establishment in the use of music
libraries, musical instruments and musical literature.

8616 MUSIC PERFORMANCE TRUST FUNDS
Suite 202
1501 Broadway
New York, NY 10036-5501
Web Site: www.mptf.org
Trustee: Martin Paulson
Foundation allocates money for the promotion of black
music and the general public. The concerts must be free
of charge and have no admittance restrictions.

**8617 MUSIC PUBLISHERS ASSOCIATION OF
THE UNITED STATES**
1562 First Avenue
New York, NY 10017-4014
Phone: 212-327-4044
e-mail: mpa-admin@mpa.org
Web Site: www.mpa.org
President: John Shorney
Administrator: Christine Hoffman
Encourages understanding of the copyright laws and
works to protect musical works against infringements and
piracy.
65 Members

**8618 MUSIC TEACHERS NATIONAL
ASSOCIATION**
Suite 505
441 Vine Street
Cincinnati, OH 45202-2811
Phone: 513-421-1420
Toll-free: 888-512-5278
Fax: 513-421-2503
e-mail: mtnanet@mtna.org
Web Site: www.mtna.org
Director Meetings/Special Projects: Jennifer Martin
This is a nonprofit organization of independent and
collegiate music teachers committed to furthering the art
of music through teaching, performance, composition and
scholarly research.
*24000 Members Founded: 1876 24,000 names $85 per
M.*

8619 MUSIC WOMEN INTERNATIONAL
PO Box 776
Shreveport, LA 71162
Phone: 615-860-4084
Fax: 615-860-6910
e-mail: mwiboss@aol.com
Supports educational programs for woman in the music
industry; publishes quarterly newsletter; holds quarterly
convention.
600 Members

**8620 MUSICAL BOX SOCIETY
INTERNATIONAL**
2752 Shaftesbury Drive NW
Canton, OH 44708-8921
Web Site: www.mbsi.org/
Secretary: Marguerite Fabel
Publisher: Rosanna Harris
Collectors and dealers of antique music boxes and other
mechanical and automatic musical instruments from
seventeen countries.
2.8M Members Founded: 1949

8621 MUSICIANS CLUB OF NEW YORK
Apartment 19G
20 W 64th Street
New York, NY 10023
Phone: 212-799-4448
Fax: 212-799-4448

Provides annual competition, awards, recitals, concerts, receptions. Membership open to all professional musicians and music lovers.

8622 MUSICIANS FOUNDATION
200 W 55th Street
New York, NY 10019-5200
Phone: 212-239-9137
Web Site: www.musiciansfoundation.org
Executive Director: Brent Williams
Representing interests on the condition and social welfare of professional musicians and their families.

8623 NAMM - INTERNATIONAL MUSIC PRODUCTS ASSOCIATION
5790 Armada Drive
Carlsbad, CA 92008
Phone: 619-438-8001
Toll-free: 800-767-6266
Fax: 760-438-7327
Web Site: www.namm.com
President/CEO: Joe Lemond
Offers professional development seminars; sells musical instruments and allied products.
7700 Members

8624 NATIONAL ACADEMY OF SONGWRITERS
Suite 1023
6255 W Sunset Boulevard
Hollywood, CA 90028-7411
Phone: 323-463-2146
Fax: 213-463-2146
e-mail: nassong@lainet.com
Managing Director: Daniel A. Kirkpatrick
A non-profit organization acting as a resource base for songwriters, putting them in contact with publishing companies and the industry.
3M Members Founded: 1974

8625 NATIONAL ASSOCIATION MUSIC MERCHANTS MUSIC PRODUCTS ASSOCIATION
5790 Armada Drive
Carlsbad, CA 92008-4372
Phone: 760-438-8001
Toll-free: 800-767-6266
Fax: 760-438-7327
e-mail: tradeshow@namm.com
Web Site: www.namm.com
Director Trade Shows: Kevin Johnstone
Non-profit organization for the music products industry.

8626 NATIONAL ASSOCIATION FOR DRAMA THERAPY
15245 Shady Grove Road
Rockville, MD 20850-3222
Phone: 301-208-8787
Fax: 301-990-9771
e-mail: nadt@mgmtsol.com
Executive Director: Beth W. Palys

Members are professionals trained in theatre arts, psychology and psychotherapy who use drama/theatre processes as therapy.
325 Members Founded: 1979

8627 NATIONAL ASSOCIATION OF AFRICAN-AMERICAN MUSICIANS
PO Box 43053
11551 S Laflin Street
Chicago, IL 60643
Phone: 773-568-3818
Fax: 773-779-1325
e-mail: negro_musicians@hotmail.com
Web Site: www.nanm.8m.com
Executive Secretary: Ona B. Campbell
Promotes the advancement of all types of music.
2.5M Members Founded: 1919

8628 NATIONAL ASSOCIATION OF BAND INSTRUMENT MANUFACTURERS
Fifth Floor
40 W 21st Street
New York, NY 10010-6906
Phone: 212-924-9175
Fax: 212-675-3577
e-mail: assnhdqs@aol.com
Executive VP: Jerome Hershman
A trade association of band instrument manufacturers, importers and distributors including accessories selling to the trade only.
34 Members Founded: 1920

8629 NATIONAL ASSOCIATION OF COLLEGE WIND AND PERCUSSION INSTRUCTORS
Division of Fine Arts
Truman State University
Kirksville, MO 63501
Phone: 660-785-4442
Fax: 660-785-7463
Web Site: www.nacwpi.org
Executive Secretary/Treasurer: Richard Weerts
Teachers of wind and percussion instruments in American colleges and universities.
1400 Members Founded: 1951

8630 NATIONAL ASSOCIATION OF PERFORMING ARTS MANAGERS AND AGENTS
#133
459 Columbus Avenue
New York, NY 10024
Phone: 212-799-5308
Fax: 212-580-5438
e-mail: bcolton@napama.org
Web Site: www.napama.org
National not-for-profit trade association founded in 1979, dedicated to promoting the professionalism of its members and the vitality of the performing arts.

8631 NATIONAL ASSOCIATION OF PROFESSIONAL BAND INSTRUMENT REPAIR TECHNICIANS
PO Box 51
Normal, IL 61761-4009
Phone: 309-452-4257
Fax: 309-452-4825
Web Site: www.napbirt.org
Executive Director: Chuck Hagler
Promotes technical integrity in the craft. Surveys tools and procedures to improve work quality. Makes available emergency repair of band instruments. Provides placement services.
1500 Members Founded: 1976

8632 NATIONAL ASSOCIATION OF SCHOOLS OF MUSIC
Suite 21
11250 Roger Bacon Drive
Reston, VA 20190-5248
Phone: 703-477-0700
Fax: 703-437-6312
Web Site: www.arts-accrediting.org/nasm
Executive Director: Samuel Hope
Editor: David Bading
Postsecondary accreditation of music programs.
550 Members Founded: 1924

8633 NATIONAL ASSOCIATION OF THEATRE OWNERS
Suite 340
4605 Lankershim Boulevard
North Hollywood, CA 91602
Phone: 818-506-1778
Fax: 818-506-0269
e-mail: nato@mindspring.com
Web Site: www.natoonline.org
VP/Executive Director: Mary Ann Grasco
Communication Director: Jim Kozak
Advertising Director: Mary dela Cruz
Professional trade association serving the business intervals of theatre owners domestically and around the world. Assist theatre owners work with picture distribution and issues such as new technologies, legislation, marketing and first amendment. Publish monthly magazine and annual encyclopedias.
Printed in on glossy stock

8634 NATIONAL BALLROOM AND ENTERTAINMENT ASSOCIATION
2799 Locust Road
Decorah, IA 52101-7600
Phone: 563-382-4769
e-mail: nbea@oreota.net
Web Site: www.nbea.com
Executive Director: John Matter
Provides exchange for owners and operators of ballrooms.
450 Members Founded: 1947

8635 NATIONAL BAND ASSOCIATION
PO Box 121292
Nashville, TN 37212-1292

Phone: 615-385-2650
Fax: 615-385-2650
Web Site: www.nationalbandassoc.org
Secretary: L. Howard Nicar, Jr.
Sponsors clinics and other educational functions for band directors.
3M Members Founded: 1960

8636 NATIONAL COSTUMERS ASSOCIATION
3038 Hayes Avenue
Fremont, OH 43420
Phone: 419-334-4098
Toll-free: 800-622-1321
Fax: 419-334-7372
Web Site: www.costumers.org
Secretary: Gegg K. Kerns
Seeks to establish and maintain professional and ethical standards of business in the costume industry.
400 Members Founded: 1923

8637 NATIONAL COUNCIL OF MUSIC IMPORTERS AND EXPORTERS
5th Floor
38-44 W 21st Street
New York, NY 10010-6906
Phone: 212-924-9175
Fax: 212-675-3577
e-mail: ASSNHDQS@aol.com
Web Site: www.musicdistributors.org
Executive VP: Jerome Hershman
Importers and exporters of musical instruments and accesories.
60 Members

8638 NATIONAL DANCE ASSOCIATION
1900 Association Drive
Reston, VA 20191-1502
Phone: 703-476-3436
Fax: 703-476-9527
e-mail: nda@aahperd.org
Web Site: www.aaperd.org/nda
Executive Director: Barbara Hernandez, PhD
A nonprofit service organization dedicated to increasing knowledge, improving skills and encouraging sound professional practices in dance education while promoting and supporting creative and healthy lifestyles through high quality dance programs.
3M Members Founded: 1932

8639 NATIONAL ENDOWMENT FOR THE ARTS
1100 Pennsylvania Avenue NW
Washington, DC 20506
Phone: 202-682-5400
e-mail: webmgr@arts.endow.gov
Web Site: www.artsendow.gov
Chairman: William Ivey
Staff Assistant: Daniel Beattie
The National Endowment for the Arts, an investment in America's living heritage, serves the public good by nurturing the expression of human creativity, supporting

the cultivation of community spirit, and fostering the recognition and appreciation of the excellence and diversity of our nation's artistic accomplishments.

8640 NATIONAL FEDERATION OF MUSIC CLUBS
1336 N Delaware Street
Indianapolis, IN 46202-2415
Phone: 317-638-4003
Fax: 317-638-0503
Executive Director: Melinda Ullrich
Dedicated to finding and fostering young musical talent, promoting and encouraging the performance of American music.
200M Members

8641 NATIONAL MUSIC PUBLISHERS' ASSOCIATION
711 Third Avenue
New York, NY 10017
Phone: 212-370-5330
Fax: 212-953-2384
Web Site: www.nmpa.org
President: Edward Murphy
Publishes a quarterly newsletter and holds an annual meeting.
600 Members

8642 NATIONAL OPERA ASSOCIATION
Northwestern University
711 Elgin Road
Evanston, IL 60208-0804
Phone: 806-651-2857
Fax: 847-491-5260
Web Site: www.noa.org
Executive Secretary: Jeffrey E. Wright
To advance the appreciation, composition and production of opera.
350 Members Founded: 1955

8643 NATIONAL PIANO TRAVELERS ASSOCIATION
Sawkill Road
c/o Charles Ramsey Company
Kingston, NY 12402-1464
Phone: 845-338-5751
Fax: 914-338-5751
President: Bob Smith
Buys and sells pianos.
110 Members

8644 NEW ENGLAND THEATRE CONFERENCE
360 Huntington Avenue
Boston, MA 02115-5005
Phone: 617-373-2000
Fax: 617-424-9275
Web Site: www.netconline.org
Editor: Corey Boniface
President: Roger Shoemaker
Managing Director: Clinton D. Campbell

Non-profit educational corporation founded to develop, expand and assist theatre activity in community, educational and professional levels in New England.
1M Members Founded: 1950

8645 NEW MUSIC DISTRIBUTION SERVICE
7th Floor
598 Broadway
New York, NY 10012-9205
Phone: 212-925-2121
Fax: 212-925-1689
President: Timothy Marquand
Distributors of contemporary music.

8646 NORTH AMERICAN ASSOCIATION OF VENTRILOQUISTS
PO Box 420
Littleton, CO 80160-2302
Phone: 303-346-6819
Toll-free: 800-250-5125
Web Site: www.maherstudios.com/naav.htm
President/CEO: Clinton Detweiler
Disseminates information on ventriloquists and their activities.
1.7M Members Founded: 1940

8647 NORTHWEST FESTIVALS ASSOCIATION
2457 Ingra
c/o P.G. Martin
Anchorage, AK 99508-3945
Managing Director: P.G. Martin
Promotes ideas exchange, conducts workshops, offers management seminars, publishes annual directory, holds annual meeting and symposium.
156 Members

8648 OPERA AMERICA
Suite 810
1156 15th Street NW
Washington, DC 20005
Phone: 202-293-4466
Fax: 202-393-0735
e-mail: Frontdesk@operaamerica.org
Web Site: www.operaam.org
Opera America serves and strengthens the field of opera by providing a variety of informational, technical, and administrative resources to the greater opera community. Its fundamental mission is to promote opera as exciting and accessible to individuals from all walks of life.

8649 ORATORIO SOCIETY OF NEW YORK
881 Seventh Avenue, Suite 504
Carnegie Hall
New York, NY 10019
Phone: 212-247-4199
Competition Chairman: Janet Plucknett

8650 ORGANIZATION OF AMERICAN KODALY EDUCATORS
1612 29th Avenue S
Moorhead, MN 56560
Fax: 701-241-7051

Executive Director: Glenys Wignes
Members are music teachers interested in the Kodaly approach to music education.
1700 Members Founded: 1976

8651 OUTDOOR AMUSEMENT BUSINESS ASSOCIATION

Suite 1045A
1035 S Semoran Boulevard
Winter Park, FL 32792
Phone: 407-681-9444
Toll-free: 800-517-6222
Fax: 407-681-9445
e-mail: oaba@aol.com
Web Site: www.oaba.org
President: Robert W. Johnson
Promotes interest of the outdoor amusement industry.
4M Members Founded: 1965

8652 PERCUSSIVE ARTS SOCIETY

701 NW Ferris Avenue
Lawton, OK 73507-5442
Phone: 580-353-1455
Fax: 580-353-1456
e-mail: percarts@pas.org
Web Site: www.pas.org
Executive Director: Michael Kenyon
Marketing/Publications: Teresa Peterson
A music service organization promoting percussion education, research, performance and appreciation throughout the world. Offers two print publications, a website at www.pas.org, the Percussive Arts Society International Headquarters/Museum and the annual Percussive Arts Society International Convention. *$85.00*
7000 Members Bimonthly Founded: 1961 5,400 names

8653 PIANO MANUFACTURERS ASSOCIATION INTERNATIONAL

4020 McEwen Street, Suite 105
c/o Donald W. Dillon
Dallas, TX 75244
Phone: 972-233-9107
Fax: 972-490-4219
e-mail: dwdillon@aol.com
Web Site: www.pianonet.com
Executive Director: Donald Dillon
Manufacturers and suppliers of pianos and parts; holds annual trade show.
20 Members Founded: 1991

8654 PIANO TECHNICIANS GUILD

3930 Washington Avenue
Kansas City, MO 64111-3538
Phone: 816-753-7747
Fax: 816-531-0070
e-mail: ptg@ptg.org
Web Site: www.ptg.org
CAE, Executive Director: Dan W. Hall
Conducts technical institutes at conventions and seminars. Promotes public education in piano care. Bestows awards. Publishes monthly technical journal by subscriptions.
4000 Members Founded: 1957 4000 names

8655 PRODUCTION EQUIPMENT RENTAL ASSOCIATION

PO Box 55515
Sherman Oaks, CA 91413-0515
Phone: 818-906-2467
Fax: 818-906-1720
Executive Director: Edwin S. Clare
Members are rental companies who supply production equipment to the entertainment industry.
125 Members

8656 PRODUCTION MUSIC LIBRARY ASSOCIATION

747 Chesnut Ridge Road
Chesnut Ridge, NY 10977
Phone: 845-356-0895
Fax: 914-356-0895
President: Michael Nurko
Sets guidelines for use of production music; holds annual meeting.
20 Members

8657 PROFESSIONAL WOMEN SINGERS ASSOCIATION

PO Box 884
New York, NY 10024
Phone: 212-969-0590
Fax: 520-395-2560
e-mail: infowomensingers.org
Web Site: www.pwsa.homestead.com
President: Phyllis Fay Farmer
1st VP: Elissa Weiss
2nd VP: Beatrice Broadwater
Secretary: Claudia Crouse
Treasurer: Mary Lou Zobel
Non-profit networking organization for professional women singers.
40 Members Founded: 1982

8658 RETAIL PRINT MUSIC DEALERS ASSOCIATION

Suite 320, LB 120
13140 Coit Road
Dallas, TX 75240
Phone: 972-233-9107
Fax: 972-490-4219
Web Site: www.printmusic.org
Executive Director: Madeleine Crouch
275 Members Founded: 1976

8659 RHYTHM AND BLUES/ROCK AND ROLL SOCIETY

PO Box 1949
New Haven, CT 06509-1949
Phone: 203-924-1079
Director: William J. Nolan
Educational, charitable association on African American music culture.
54M Members Founded: 1974

8660 ROUNDALAB
4825B Valley View Avenue
Yorba Linda, CA 92886-3645
Toll-free: 800-346-7522
Fax: 714-572-0931
Web Site: www.roundalab.org
Executive Secretary: Patricia Rardin
A professional international society of individuals who
teach round dancing at any phase.
1500 Members Founded: 1977

**8661 SAN FRANCISCO BALLET
ASSOCIATION**
455 Franklin Street
San Francisco, CA 94102
Phone: 415-861-5600
Fax: 415-861-2684
e-mail: sfbmail@sfballet.org
Web Site: www.sfballet.org
Chairman: F. Warren Hellman
Secretary: Susan S. Briggs
Artistic Director: Helgi Tomasson
Executive Director: Arthur Jacobus
To provide a repertoire of classical and contemporary
ballet; to provide educational opportunities for
professional dancers and choreographers; to excel in
ballet, artistic direction and administration.

8662 SCREEN ACTORS GUILD
5757 Wilshire Boulevard
Los Angeles, CA 90027
Phone: 323-954-1600
Fax: 323-549-6656
Web Site: www.sag.org
National Executive Director/CEO: A. Robert Pisano
Labor union affiliated with AFL-CIO which represents
actors in film, television and commercials.
85M Members Founded: 1933

8663 SOCIETY FOR ASIAN MUSIC
Cornell University-Department of Asian Studies
Lincoln Hall at Cornell University
Ithaca, NY 14853-2502
Phone: 607-255-5049
Fax: 607-254-2877
Web Site: www.asianmusic.skidmore.edu
Treasurer: Marty Hatch
Members are academics and others with an interest in the
performing arts of the Middle East, South, East and
Southeast Asia, in their social and historical contexts.
600 Members Founded: 1959

**8664 SOCIETY FOR THE PRESERVATION OF
VARIETY ARTS**
7011 Franklin Avenue
Hollywood, CA 90028-8637
Phone: 310-306-2326
President: Milt Larsen
Dedicated to the preservation of the variety show and its
related arts.
2.5M Members Founded: 1975

8665 SOCIETY OF AMERICAN MAGICIANS
PO Box 510260
Saint Louis, MO 63151-0260
Web Site: www.magicsam.com
President: Steve Corbitt
VP: Joe Hardin
Founded to promote and maintain harmonious fellowship
among those interested in magic as an art, to improve
ethics of the magical profession, and to foster, promote
and improve the advancement of magical arts in the field
of amusement and entertainment. Membership inclides
professional and amateur magicians, manufacturers of
magical apparatus and collectors.
5.5M Members

**8666 SOCIETY OF PROFESSIONAL AUDIO
RECORDING SERVICES**
PO Box 770845
Memphis, TN 38120
Phone: 901-747-3111
Toll-free: 800-771-7727
e-mail: spars@spars.com
Web Site: www.spars.com
Executive Director: Larry Litman
Members are individuals, companies and studios
connected with the professional recording industry.
200 Members Founded: 1979 7,200 names

**8667 SOCIETY OF STAGE DIRECTORS AND
CHOREOGRAPHERS**
Suite 1701
1501 Broadway
New York, NY 10036-5601
Phone: 212-391-1070
Toll-free: 800-511-5204
Fax: 212-302-6195
e-mail: info@ssdc.org
Web Site: www.ssdc.org
Executive Director: Barbara Hauptman
An independent labor union representing directors and
choreographers in American theatre.
1700 Members Founded: 1959

8668 SONGWRITERS GUILD OF AMERICA
1500 Harbor Boulevard
Weehawken, NJ 07087-6732
Phone: 201-867-7603
Fax: 201-867-7535
e-mail: songnews@aol.com
Web Site: www.songwriters.org
Executive Director: Lewis M. Bachman
Provides agreements between songwriters, composers and
publishers.
4500 Members Founded: 1931

**8669 SOUTHEASTERN THEATRE
CONFERENCE**
University of North Carolina at Greensboro
PO Box 9868
1217 W Bessemer Avenue
Greensboro, NC 27429-0868

Phone: 336-272-3645
Fax: 336-272-8810
e-mail: setc@setconline.net
Web Site: www.setc.org
Executive Director: Elizabeth Baun
Office Manager: April Marshall
Purpose is to connect people interested in theatre arts to opportunity including employment, education and networking annual convention first working in march; Professional auditions each September; publications; and year round job search.
3600 Members Founded: 1949

8670 SOUTHERN ARTS FEDERATION
Suite 808
1800 Peachtree Street NW
Atlanta, GA 30309
Phone: 404-874-7244
Fax: 404-873-2148
Web Site: www.southarts.org
Executive Director: John W Talbott
Chief of Staff: Stacy Melich
Manager Comm./Marketing/Advocacy: David Batley
In partnership with nine state arts agencies: promotes and supports arts regionally, nationally and internationally; enhances the artistic excellence and professionalism of Southern Arts Organizations and artists; serves the diverse population of the south.

8671 THEATER AUTHORITY
Suite 640
6464 W Sunset Boulevard
Los Angeles, CA 90028-8008
Phone: 323-462-5761
Fax: 323-462-1930
Presides over theatrical agencies and performing arts organizations.

8672 THEATRE BAY AREA
Theatre Bay Area
Suite 375
870 Market Street
San Francisco, CA 94102-3002
Phone: 415-430-1140
Fax: 415-430-1145
e-mail: tba@theatrebayarea.org
Web Site: www.theatrebayarea.org
Interim Executive Director: Richard Smith
Business/Operations: Pete Ratajczak
Serving more than 400 member theatre companies and 3,000 individual members in the San Francisco Bay Area and Northern California, Theatre Bay Area provides monthly classes, workshops, events, information and publications. Also publishes callboard, a monthly theatre industry magazine. *$61.00*
3,000 Members Founded: 1976
Circulation: 5,000 $65 per M.

8673 THEATRE COMMUNICATIONS GROUP
4th Floor
355 Lexington Avenue
New York, NY 10017-6695

Phone: 212-697-5230
Fax: 212-983-4847
e-mail: tcg@tcg.org
Web Site: www.tcg.org
Executive Director: Ben Cameron
President: Kent Thompson
VP: David Henry Hwang
VP: Judith O. Rubin
Treasurer: Paula Tomei
Fosters cooperation, information sharing and interaction among members; maintains library.

8674 THEATRE DEVELOPMENT FUND
21st Floor
1501 Broadway
New York, NY 10036-5601
Phone: 212-768-1818
e-mail: info@tdf.org
Web Site: www.tdf.org
Executive Director: Henry Guettel
Not-for-profit service organization. Provides support for every area of the dance, music and professional theatre field. Founded 1968.

8675 THEATRE EDUCATION ASSOCIATION
3368 Central Parkway
Cincinnati, OH 45225-2307
Phone: 512-559-1996
Fax: 512-559-0012
Executive Director: Ronald L. Longstreth
Founded to advance quality theatre on high school level.

8676 THEATRE LIBRARY ASSOCIATION
149 West 45th Street
Shubert Archive
New York, NY 10036
President: Susan Brady
VP: Kevin Winkler
Executive Secretary: Maryann Chach
Treasurer: Paul Newman
This nonprofit, educational organization is involved in collecting, preserving, and encouraging the use of theatrical and performing arts materials of all kinds from all periods. Members include librarians, scholars, curators, archivists, performers, writers, designers and historians.
500 Members Founded: 1937

8677 THEATRICAL MUTUAL ASSOCIATION
326 W 48th Street
New York, NY 10036-1314
Phone: 212-399-0980
Fax: 212-315-1073
Executive Director: Angelo Leuzzi
Provides disability, sickness and death benefits for persons in the theatrical or amusements enterprises.

8678 UNITED STATES AMATEUR BALLROOM DANCERS ASSOCIATION
PO Box 128
New Freedom, PA 17349-0128

Phone: 717-235-6656
Toll-free: 800-447-9047
Fax: 717-235-4183
e-mail: usabdacent@aol.com
Web Site: www.usabda.org
President: Archie Hazelwood
Non-profit organization working to promote ballroom dancing, both as a recreational activity and as a competetive sport.
20M Members Founded: 1965

8679 UNITED STATES AMATEUR DANCERS ASSOCIATION

4216 Babcock Avenue
Studio City, CA 91604-1509
Phone: 818-255-0161
Treasurer: Arthur Miller
Presides over amateur dancers in the U.S.
250 Members Founded: 1968

8680 UNITED STATES INSTITUTE FOR THEATRE TECHNOLOGY

6443 Ridings Road
Syracuse, NY 13206-1111
Phone: 315-463-6463
Toll-free: 800-938-7488
Fax: 315-463-6525
e-mail: info@office.usitt.org
Web Site: www.usitt.org
Public Relations/Marketing Manager: Barbara El Lucas
Sales Manager: Michelle L. Smith
The association of design, production and technology professionals in the performing arts and entertainment industry whose mission is to promote the knowledge and skills of its members. International in scope, USITT draws its board of directors from across the US and Canada. Sponsors projects, programs, research, symposia, exhibits, and annual conference. Disseminates information on aesthetic and technical developments.
3600 Members Founded: 1960

8681 WASHINGTON OPERA GUILD

Suite 104
2600 Virginia Avenue NW
Washington, DC 20566-0001
Phone: 202-295-2420
Fax: 202-295-2479
Editor: Eleanor Forrer
Information on the opera productions at the Kennedy Center by the Washington Opera.

8682 WESTERN FAIRS ASSOCIATION

Suite 210
1776 Tribute Road
Sacramento, CA 95815-4495
Phone: 916-927-3100
Fax: 916-927-6397
e-mail: wfa@fairsnet.org
Web Site: www.fairsnet.org
Executive Director: Stephen J Chambers
Assistant Executive Director: Laura C Trout

National association for fairground owners, managers and workers. Also includes government regulations, fair vendors and service providers.
2,500 Members Founded: 1922 1000 names

8683 WOMEN IN THE ARTS FOUNDATION

Suite 2G
1175 York Avenue
New York, NY 10021-7169
Editor: Erin Butler
Publisher: Roberta Crown
Fights discrimination against women artists with membership of women visual artists and exhibitions
150 Members Founded: 1941

8684 WORLD MUSIC CONGRESSES

8000 York Road
Towson University, Administration Building 423
Baltimore, MD 21252-0001
Phone: 410-704-3451
Fax: 410-704-4012
e-mail: hbreazeale@towson.edu
Web Site: www.towson.edu/worldmusiccongresses
Executive Director: Helene Breazeale
Associate Director: Sergei Zverev
1997-2010 World Cello Congresses's II-V, 2004 The First World Guitar Congress and 2008 World Guitar Congress II. Celebrations of music with international gatherings, of the world's greatest musicians, composers, conductors, instrument manufacturers students, and music lovers from around the globe.
Founded: 1995 11,500 names $100 per M.

8685 WORLD WATERPARK ASSOCIATION

PO Box 68825
Lenexa, KS 66215
Phone: 913-599-0300
Fax: 913-599-0520
e-mail: wwa@waterparks.com
Web Site: www.waterparks.com
President/CEO: Al Turner
Provides forum for exchange of ideas related to water amusement park industry.
1.1M Members Founded: 1981

Newsletters

8686 AMU QUARTERNOTE

Ben Intorre, Editor, author
American Musicians Union
8 Tobin Ct
Dumont, NJ 07628-3329
Phone: 201-384-5378
Musicians union providing services to professional musicians, vocalists and band managers. Accepts advertising. *$5.00*
4 pages Quarterly Since: 1975
Circulation: 330
Printed in 2 colors on matte stock

8687 ACADEMY OF COUNTRY MUSIC NEWSLETTER
Academy of Country Music
Suite 923
6255 W Sunset Boulevard
Hollywood, CA 90028-7410
Phone: 323-462-2351
Fax: 323-462-3253
Publisher: Fran Boyd
Devoted exclusively to the country music industry.
12 pages   Monthly
Circulation: 4,500

8688 AMERICA'S SHRINE TO MUSIC MUSEUM NEWSLETTER
America's Shrine to Music Museum
414 E Clark Street
Vermillion, SD 57069-2307
Phone: 605-677-5306
Fax: 605-677-5073
e-mail: smm@usd.edu
Web Site: www.usd.edu/smm/
Publisher: Andre P. Larson
Newsletter offering information for enybody interested in
the history of musical instruments and the music industry.
$35.00
Printed in 4 colors

8689 AMERICAN DANCE
PO Box 2006
Lenox Hill Station
New York, NY 10021
Phone: 212-932-2789
e-mail: adg2@mai.idt.net
Executive Director: Margot Lehman
Contains articles on member news, dance, and education.
4x Year   Since: 1956
Circulation: 300

8690 AMERICAN GUILD ASSOCIATE NEWS
American Guild of Music
5354 Washington Street
Downers Grove, IL 60515-4905
Phone: 630-978-2696
Fax: 630-968-0197
Publisher: Elmer Herrick
Offers information and news for professionals in the
music profession.
Quarterly

8691 AMERICAN INSTITUTE OF ORGAN BUILDERS
Burton Tidwell, author
PO Box 130982
Houston, TX 77219-0982
Phone: 713-529-2212
Web Site: www.pipeorgan.org
Features technical articles, and the annual convention
includes supplier exhibits, technical lectures and tours to
area organs. Accepts advertising. *$12.00*

360 pages   Quarterly Since: 1974
Circulation: 600
Mailing list available for rent
Printed in on glossy stock

8692 AMERICAN MUSIC CENTER OPPORTUNITY UPDATE
American Music Center
Suite 1001
30 W 26th Street
New York, NY 10010-2011
Phone: 212-366-5260
Fax: 212-366-5265
e-mail: center@amc.net
Web Site: www.amc.net
Editor: G. Genova
A timely, comprehensive listing of opportunities for
composers and performers of new music, including
commissioning programs, funding sources, calls for
scores, competitions, job openings, and more. *$55.00*
Circulation: 2,600

8693 AMERICAN MUSICAL INSTRUMENT SOCIETY
2220 N 1400 E
Provo, UT 84604-2150
Phone: 801-378-3279
Web Site: www.amis.org
President: Harrison Powley
Editor: Thomas G. MacCracker
Manager: Peggy F. Bird
History of musical instruments. *$5.00*
16 pages   TriAnnual
Circulation: 800

8694 AMERICAN MUSICOLOGICAL SOCIETY NEWSLETTER
American Musicological Society
Room 201
201 S 34th Street
Philadelphia, PA 19104-6313
Phone: 215-898-8698
Fax: 215-573-3673
e-mail: ams@sas.upenn.edu
Web Site: www.ams-net.org
Editor: Susan Jackson
Society news for professionals in the music industry. The
society also publishes a journal three times a year.
25 pages   2x Year

8695 AMERICAN SCHOOL BAND DIRECTORS ASSOCIATION - NEWSLETTER
American School Band Directors Association
227 N First Street
Guttenberg, IA 52052-0696
Phone: 319-252-2383
Fax: 319-252-2500
e-mail: asbda@netins.net
Web Site: www.asbda.com
Publisher: Dennis Hanna
Editor: Al Johnston

6 pages   Quarterly
Circulation: 1300
Printed in 2 colors on matte stock

8696   AMERICAN SOCIETY OF MUSIC ARRANGERS AND COMPOSERS
PO Box 17840
Encino, CA 91416-7840
Phone: 818-994-4661
Fax: 818-994-6181
e-mail: tpi97@ix.netcom.com
Web Site: www.asmac.org
Director: Scherr Lillico
Information on composers, orchestrators, and musicians.
4-8 pages   Quarterly
Circulation: 1,000
Printed in on matte stock

8697   AMERICAN VIOLA SOCIETY-NEWSLETTER
4600 Sunset Avenue
Butler University
Indianapolis, IN 46208
Phone: 317-283-9637
e-mail: cforbes@utarlg.uta.edu
Web Site: www.americanviolasociety.org
President: Peter Slowick
Editor: Kathryn Steely
Treasurer: Ellen Rose
Newsletter devoted exclusively to professional viola musicians.
Monthly

8698   BLUE HOT
International Bluegrass Music Association
1620 Fredrica Street
Owensboro, KY 42303-4201
Phone: 270-684-9025
Fax: 270-686-7863
e-mail: ibma@ibma.org
Web Site: www.ibma.org
Editor/Production Manager: Nancy Cardwell
Blue Hot includes bluegrass radio and sales charts, information for buyers and distributors.
4 pages   Monthly   Since: 1996
Printed in 3 colors on glossy stock

8699   BLUEGRASS MUSIC NEWS
Kentucky Music Educator's Association
PO Box 65
Calvert City, KY 42029
Phone: 254-398-8340
Fax: 270-395-7156
e-mail: jimfern@ldd.net
Web Site: www.kmea.org/default.asp
Editor: Hazel O. Carver
Executive Secretary: Jim Fern
Offers articles that focus on music education. *$10.00*
Quarterly
Circulation: 2,000

8700   BOOMBAH HERALD
15 Park Boulevard
Lancaster, NY 14086-2510
Editor: Loren D. Geiger
Articles on band music composers, concert, circus, military bands. Record reviews of abnd music. 1 Printed arrangement for band. *$10.00*
BiAnnual   Since: 1973

8701   BOOSEY AND HAWKES NEWSLETTER
Boosey And Hawkes
35 E 21st Street
New York, NY 10010-7200
Phone: 212-358-5300
Fax: 212-473-5301
Web Site: www.boosey.com
Publisher: Steven Swartz
News on composers and their music.
8 pages   Monthly

8702   BROADSIDE
Theatre Library Association
149 W 45th Street
New York, NY 10023-7410
Publisher: Alan Pally
Makes theatre information available to all.
Monthly

8703   CARTOON WORLD
Hartman Associates
8210 S Street
Lincoln, NE 68506-6538
Phone: 402-483-6849
Publisher: George Hartman
Newsletter for amateur and professional artists and cartoonists. Prints 5-15 new markets in each issue. Accepts advertising. *$50.00*
26 pages   Monthly
Circulation: 300 Audited
Printed in on newsprint stock

8704   CASINO CHRONICLE
Casino Chronicle
PO Box 740465
Boynton Beach, FL 33474-0465
Phone: 561-732-6117
Fax: 561-477-3082
e-mail: casinoron@aol.com
Editor/Publisher: Ben A. Borowsky
Focuses on the gaming industry; emphasis is on Atlantic City, although includes nationwide coverage. *$175.00*
Weekly   Since: 1983

8705   CASINO JOURNAL'S NATIONAL GAMING SUMMARY
Casino Journal Publishing Group
5240 S Eastern Avenue
Las Vegas, NV 89119-2306
Phone: 702-733-7195
Fax: 702-253-6804
Editor: Adam A. Fine
Publisher: Glenn Fine
Review of activity in the gaming industry. *$198.00*

Weekly Since: 1993

8706 CIRCUS REPORT
Circus Report
525 Oak Street
El Cerrito, CA 94530-3699
Phone: 510-525-3332
Publisher: Don Marcks
Features circus related articles and stories as well as reviews and general information about the circus. *$40.00*
20 pages Weekly Since: 1972
Circulation: 2,100
Printed in 1 color

8707 CIRCUS WEEK
101 NE 45th Street
Miami, FL 33137-3419
Publisher: Tony Major
Covers news and events in the circus industry. *$20.00*
8 pages Monthly

8708 COMEDY WRITERS' NEWSLETTER
PO Box 23304
Brooklyn, NY 11202-3304
Phone: 718-855-5057
Editor/Publisher: Robert Makinson
Useful information for comedy writers in regard to creation and marketing. *$5.00*
SemiAnnual

8709 CONTEMPORARY RECORD SOCIETY NEWS
724 Winchester Road
Broomall, PA 19008-3431
Phone: 215-702-3600
Fax: 610-544-5921
e-mail: crsnews@erols.com
Web Site: www.erols.com/crsnews
Publisher: David Meyer
Editor: John Perotti
Society news for professionals in the music industry. *$45.00*
SemiMonthly
Circulation: 90,000

8710 COUNTRY DANCE AND SONG SOCIETY NEWS
17 New S Street
Northampton, MA 01060-4073
Phone: 413-268-7426
Fax: 413-268-7471
Web Site: ww.cdss.org
Newsletter devoted to English and Anglo-American folk dances and music and song. *$10.00*
BiMonthly
Circulation: 3,500

8711 DANCE NOTATION BUREAU NEWSLETTER
Suite 202
151 W 30th Street
New York, NY 10001
Phone: 212-564-0985
Fax: 212-904-1426
e-mail: notation@mindspring.com
Web Site: www.dancenotation.org
Executive Director: Ilene Fax
Dance news for consumers and professionals. *$40.00*
4 pages 2-3x/Year Newsletter
Circulation: 350
Printed in 2 colors on matte stock

8712 DANCE ON CAMERA JOURNAL
Dance Films Association
Suite 907
48 W 21st Street
New York, NY 10010-6806
Phone: 212-727-0764
Fax: 212-727-0764
e-mail: dfa5@juno.com
Web Site: www.dancefilmsassn.org
Editor: Deirdre Towers
The only service organization in the world dedicated to both the dance and the film community. *$25.00*
BiMonthly Since: 1956

8713 DANCE ON CAMERA NEWS
Dance Films Association
Floor 3
31 W 21st Street
New York, NY 10010-6806
Phone: 212-727-0764
Publisher: Deirdre Tower
Includes news of association and its members, new films and videotapes, list of films, and distributors, shown at yearly Dance on Camera Festival. *$20.00*
BiWeekly
Circulation: 200

8714 DANCEDRILL
Suite 310
3101 Poplarwood Court
Raleigh, NC 27604-1010
Phone: 919-872-7888
Fax: 919-872-6888
Publisher: Susan Wershing
Editor: Kay Crawford
Publication informs member of dance drill teams and their directors.
4x Year

8715 DRAMATISTS GUILD NEWSLETTER
234 W 44th Street
New York, NY 10036-3909
Phone: 212-398-9366
Fax: 212-944-0420
Editor: Jeff Zadroga
The Guild's Newsletter notifies members of Guild activities and news of immediate interest to playwrights, composers and lyricists.
10 pages 8x Year
Circulation: 6,500

8716 EARLY KEYBOARD STUDIES NEWSLETTER
Westfield Center for Early Keyboard Studies
1 Cottage Street
Easthampton, MA 01060-2901
Phone: 413-527-7664
Fax: 413-527-7089
e-mail: info@westfield.org
Publisher: Lynn Edwards
Newsletter providing information to professional keyboard musicians. *$30.00*
12 pages Monthly

8717 EARLY MUSIC NEWSLETTER
NY Recorder Guild
197 New York Avenue
Dumont, NJ 07628-2533
Web Site: www.priceclan.wm/nyrecorderguild/
Publisher: Eleanor Brodkin
Calendar of concerts and reviews. *$20.00*
10 pages Monthly

8718 EDUCATIONAL THEATRE NEWS
Southern California Educational Theatre Assn
9811 Pounds Avenue
Whittier, CA 90603-1616
Phone: 310-338-3097
Fax: 562-947-6333
Publisher: Lee Korf
News coverage in theatre activities. *$3.00*
BiWeekly
Circulation: 3,100

8719 ENTERTAINMENT MARKETING LETTER
EPM Communications
3rd Floor
160 Mercer Street
New York, NY 10012-3208
Phone: 212-941-0099
Fax: 212-941-1622
e-mail: imayer@epmcom.com
Web Site: www.epmcon.com
Publisher: Ira Mayer
Covers marketing techniques used in the entertainment industry, and by others who link their goods and services marketing through entertainment properties. *$449.00*
BiWeekly Since: 1988
Printed in on matte stock

8720 EQUITY NEWS
Actors Equity Association
165 W 46th Street
New York, NY 10036-2501
Phone: 212-719-9570
Fax: 212-921-8454
Editor-In-Chief: Dick Moore
Contains information for actors and stage managers.
9x Year Since: 1913
Circulation: 40,000
Printed in on newsprint stock

8721 FORD FOUNDATION LETTER
Ford Foundation
320 E 43rd Street
New York, NY 10017-4890
Phone: 212-573-5000
Fax: 212-351-3677
Publisher: William Rust
Offers a comprehensive overview of the Foundation's activities in the world of the performing arts.

8722 FORUM
ISPAA
6065 Pickerel Drive NE
Rockford, MI 49341-9052
Phone: 616-874-5703
Fax: 616-874-5723
Publisher: Michael Hardy
Accepts advertising.
12 pages Annual

8723 GMA TODAY
Gospel Music Association
1205 Division Street
Nashville, TN 37203-4011
Phone: 615-242-0303
Fax: 615-254-9755
Web Site: www.gospelmusic.org
Editor: Marks Ross
A quarterly newsmagazine of the contemporary Christian and gospel music industry.
24 pages BiMonthly
Circulation: 5,600

8724 GENE LEES JAZZLETTER
PO Box 240
Ojai, CA 93024-0240
Phone: 805-646-0835
Fax: 805-640-0253
Editor/Publisher: Gene Lees
Journal music history. *$60.00*
Monthly Since: 1981

8725 GIRL GROUPS GAZETTE
Department Net
PO Box 69A04
West Hollywood, CA 90069-0066
e-mail: gayboylaca@yahoo.com
Editor/Publisher: Louis Wendruck
For fans of girls groups and female singers of the 1960's and 70's including photos, discographies, records, t-shirts, postcards, and videos. *$20.00*
Quarterly Since: 1988

8726 HORN CALL
International Horn Society
8180 Thunder Street
Juneau, AK 99801-9114
Phone: 907-789-5477
Fax: 907-790-4066
e-mail: exec-secretary@hornsociety.org
Web Site: www.hornsociety.org
Editor: Jeff Snedeker
Executive Secretary: Heidi Vogel

Includes news, research, historical papers, pedagogy, biographies, music and record reviews and more pertaining to the Horn.
$35.00
100 pages 3x Per Year Since: 1971
Circulation: 3600 3600 names $70 per M.
Printed in 4 colors on glossy stock

8727 HOT LINE NEWS
Musicians National Hot Line Association
277 E 6100 S
Salt Lake City, UT 84107-7302
Phone: 801-268-2000
Publisher: Marvin Zitting
Newsletter on groups needing musicians and gigs and musicians wanting to join a group. Accepts advertising.
4 pages BiWeekly

8728 IN THEATER
Parker Publishing & Communications
#2605
1501 Broadway
New York, NY 10036-5601
Phone: 212-719-9777
Fax: 212-719-4477
e-mail: intheater@aol.com
Publisher: Michael Parker
Offers the reader a behind-the-scenes perspective of how a show is technically conceived, rehearsed and staged. Regular departments center on drama and musical reviews, listings of shows in major cities and columnist opinions. *$78.00*
Weekly
Circulation: 71,068

8729 IN THE GROOVE
Michigan Antique Phonograph Society
60 Central Street
Battle Creek, MI 49017-3704
e-mail: pgstewart@aol.com
Publisher: John Whitacre
Editor: Phil Stewart
Editor: Eileen Stewert
Each month 700+ worldwide members of the Michigan Phonograph Society regularly read feature articles, book and software reviews, letters to the editor, free classified and paid advertising in its newsletter. *$20.00*
Monthly
Circulation: 800

8730 INFOMEDIA'S DISCLIST
Infomedia
PO Box 304
Novi, MI 48376-0304
Fax: 248-340-2444
Publisher: Terry Pochert
Audio compact disc news and new release information.
$40.00
Monthly
Circulation: 1,700

8731 INTERNATIONAL BLUEGRASS
International Bluegrass Music Association
207 E 2nd Street
Owensboro, KY 42303-4201
Phone: 270-684-9025
Toll-free: 800-GET-IBMA
Fax: 270-686-7863
e-mail: ibma1@occ-uky.campus.mci.net
Web
Site: www.ibma.org
Editor/Production Manager: Nancy Cardwell
Editor: Nancy Cardwell
International Bluegrass provides you with information on new recordings, new festivals, new radio shows, industry focuses feature articles. *$25.00*

8732 INTERNATIONAL POLKA ASSOCIATION NEWSLETTER
International Polka Association
4145 S Kedzie Avenue
Chicago, IL 60632-2442
Phone: 773-254-7771
Toll-free: 800-867-6552
Fax: 773-254-8111
President: Al Jelinek
A newsletter published by the International Polka Association to inform and update members about events and news.
BiMonthly Since: 1968
Circulation: 1500

8733 INTERNATIONAL TICKETING ASSOCIATION
Suite 722
250 W 57th Street
New York, NY 10107
Phone: 212-581-0600
Fax: 212-581-0885
e-mail: info@intix.org
Web Site: www.intix.org
President: Patricia Spira
Deputy Director: Kathleen O'Donnell
Special Projects: AnnMarie Gennardo
An international organization of systems and technology advances for the admission's service industry.
8x Year Since: 1979
Printed in 4 colors on glossy stock

8734 INTIX NEWSLETTER
Box Office Management International
Suite 722
250 W 57th Street
New York, NY 10107
Phone: 212-581-0600
Fax: 212-581-0885
e-mail: info@intrix.org
Web Site: www.intix.org
Publisher: Patricia Spire
Editor: Laura-Ilene Harding
Systems and technology advances for ticketing industry.
Since: 1981
Printed in on glossy stock

8735 JAZZ REPORT
357 Leighton Drive
Ventura, CA 93001-1556
Phone: 416-537-2813
Web Site: www.jazzreport.com
Publisher: Paul Affeldt
Jazz news. *$3.00*
Monthly

8736 JOURNAL OF RESEARCH IN MUSIC EDUCATION
MENC: National Association for Music Education
1806 Robert Fulton Drive
Reston, VA 20191-4348
Phone: 703-860-4000
Fax: 703-860-4826
Web Site: www.menc.org
Editor: Cornelia Yarbrough
Covers research in music education and music history; both empirical and qualitative studies are included, and these cover a broad range of topics, under the above listed subjects *$32.00*
Since: 1953   3,000 names
Printed in on matte stock

8737 LHAT BULLETIN
League of Historic American Theatres
Suite 923
1511 K Street NW
Washington, DC 20005-1403
Phone: 877-627-0833
Fax: 202-393-2141
Web Site: www.lhat.org
Publisher: Tara Schroeder
Covers topics relevant to the restoration and use of historic theatres. Features include in-depth articles on some aspect of historic theatre restoration and management, a profile of a historic theatre and a question and answer column. Accepts advertising.
12 pages   Monthly

8738 LAUGHTER WORKS
Laughter Works Seminars
PO Box 1076
Fair Oaks, CA 95628-1076
Phone: 916-863-1592
Fax: 916-608-0776
e-mail: JimPelley@aol.com
Web Site: www.laughterworks.com
Editor: Jim Pelley
Seminars and keynote speeches on humor in the workplace. *$18.00*
6000 pages   Quarterly   Since: 1988
Circulation: 10,000
Printed in on matte stock

8739 LEAD BELLY LETTER
Lead Belly Society
PO Box 6679
Ithaca, NY 14851-6679
Phone: 607-273-6615
Fax: 607-273-4816
e-mail: sk86@cornell.edu

Editor: Seanf. Killeem
Foster appreciation and celebration of the music of Lead Belly. *$17.00*
12 pages   Quarterly Since: 1990
Circulation: 3000

8740 LINCOLN CENTER CALENDAR OF EVENTS
Lincoln Center
70 Lincoln Center Plaza
New York, NY 10023-6548
Phone: 212-875-5388
Fax: 212-875-5414
Web Site: www.lincolncenter.org
Editor: Sunny Levine
Two month listing of all events at Lincoln Center.
BiMonthly
Circulation: 100,000

8741 LYONS TEACHER NEWS
Lyons
2415 Industrial Parkway
Elkhart, IN 46516-5499
Editor: Charlotte Cikowski
Music education products.
12 pages   Monthly Since: 1940

8742 MAGIC-UNITY-MIGHT
Society of American Magicians
PO Box 510260
Saint Louis, MO 63151-0260
Phone: 314-846-5659
Fax: 314-846-5659
Publisher: Richard Blowers
Educational teaching publications. *$25.00*
60 pages   Monthly

8743 MANAGING TRAVEL & ENTERTAINMENT
Institute of Management & Administration
5th Floor
29 W 35th Street
New York, NY 10001-2299
Phone: 212-244-0360
Fax: 212-564-0465
e-mail: subserve@ioma.com
The report covers new technologies, T and E processing strategies, techniques and software, legal issues, how to get the most from third party service providers, gives readers sample company T and E policies they can use in their operations, and current methods for finding fraud in T and E reports.

8744 MARKETING THROUGH MUSIC
Rolling Stone Magazine
1290 Avenue of Americas
New York, NY 10104
Phone: 212-484-1616
Fax: 212-644-8982
Editor: David M. Rheins
$50.00
Monthly Since: 1986

8745 MISTER LUCKY
Coconut Grove
626 Connecticut Street
San Francisco, CA 94107-2835
Phone: 415-776-1616
Fax: 415-282-4394
e-mail: coconutg@wco.com
Editor: Steve Sando
Jazz-centric music reviews and cocktail culture. *$15.00*
Quarterly Since: 1993

8746 MONTHLY GUIDE OF BROOKLYN ACADEMY OF MUSIC
Brooklyn Academy of Music
30 Lafayette Avenue
Brooklyn, NY 11217-1430
Phone: 718-636-4194
Fax: 718-636-2116
Web Site: www.bam.org
Publisher: John Latham
Music news and Academy activities.
Monthly

8747 MUSIC FOR THE LOVE OF IT
67 Parkside Drive
Berkeley, CA 94705-2409
Phone: 510-654-9134
Fax: 510-654-4656
e-mail: tedrust@musicfortheloveofit.com
Web Site: www.musicfortheloveofit.com
Publisher: Ted Rust
An enthusiastic forum for musical amateurs. *$24.00*
26 pages BiMonthly Since: 1988
Circulation: 1,200
Printed in on matte stock

8748 NATIONAL CAVES NEWSLETTER
National Caves Association
RR 9 Box 106
Mc Minnville, TN 37110-9809
Phone: 931-668-2396
Fax: 931-688-3988
Publisher: Barbara Munson
A full-color directory brochure, CAVES AND CAVERNS, is published annually for free distribution to show cave owners and operators.
6 pages BiMonthly
Circulation: 130

8749 NEW YORK CITY BALLET NEWS
New York City Ballet Guild
Lincoln Center
NY State Theatre
New York, NY 10023
Phone: 212-675-7023
Fax: 212-870-4244
Publisher: Diane Kuhl
Articles, news and updates on the company.
TriAnnual
Circulation: 5,000

8750 NEW YORK OPERA NEWSLETTER
Suite 5
155 Maplewood Avenue
Maplewood, NJ 07040-0278
Phone: 973-378-9549
Fax: 973-378-2372
e-mail: tnyon@aol.com
Publisher: David D. Wood
Managing Editor: Karen Pond
Publication written for opera singers. *$48.00*
11x Year Since: 1986
Circulation: 4,100

8751 NEWSLETTER
Institute for Studies in American Music
Brooklyn College
Brooklyn, NY 11210
Phone: 718-951-5655
Fax: 718-951-6140
Publisher: H. Wiley Hitchcock
Editor: K. Robert Schwarz
Covers all aspects of American music, classical and popular. Accepts advertising.
16 pages

8752 NEWSLETTER OF THE INSTITUTE FOR STUDIES IN AMERICAN MUSIC
Institute for Studies in American Music
2900 Bedford Avenue
Brooklyn College
Brooklyn, NY 11210
Phone: 718-951-5655
Fax: 718-951-4858
Director: Carol J. Oja
Associate Editor: Ray Allen
Contains articles, research reports, book and record reviews and more on all aspects of American music. Accepts advertising.
16 pages Monthly

8753 NOTES A TEMPO
West Virginia Music Educators
Hall of Fine Arts
West Liberty, WV 26074
Phone: 304-843-4079
Fax: 304-336-8285
Editor: Edward Wolf
Music and music education with emphasis on music education in West Virginia. *$3.00*
10 pages 7x Year
Circulation: 1,200

8754 PFA FESTEVENTS
15 Enon Way
Pittsburgh, PA 15203-1207
Fax: 412-621-2209
Publisher: Dennis Huber
Covers touring attractions, variety and animal acts, vaudeville and all types of artistic performances. *$20.00*
6 pages Quarterly

8755 PAST TIMES: NOSTALGIA ENTERTAINMENT NEWSLETTER
PO Box 661
Anaheim, CA 92815-0661
Phone: 714-870-8013
Fax: 714-527-5845
Publisher: Jordan R. Young
Covers movies, actors, radio programs, music, popular culture and media of the 1920's through the early 1950's. *$10.00*
Quarterly
Circulation: 5,000

8756 PEDAL STEEL NEWSLETTER
Pedal Steel Guitar Association
PO Box 20248
Floral Park, NY 11002-0248
Phone: 516-616-9214
Fax: 516-616-9214
e-mail: bobpsgal@pb.net
Web Site: www.psga.org
Editor: Doug Mack
VP, Marketing: John DeMaille
Dedicated to the art of playing pedal steel guitar. Every issue contains tablature arrangements of songs for the steel guitar as well as coming events, record reviews, product reports and news concerning the instrument. *$25.00*
16 pages 10x Year Since: 1973
Circulation: 1500

8757 PEN/LENS PRESS
PEN/LENS Press
Suite 280
142 N Milpitas Boulevard
Milpitas, CA 95035
e-mail: plp@jps.net
Web Site: www.infopoint.com
Publisher: Jim Halto
Devoted to the string instrument craftsman. *$12.95*
Monthly

8758 PERFORMING ARTS INSIDER
Richmond Shepard And David Lefkowitz
Box 62
Hewlett, NY 11557-0062
Phone: 516-295-1511
e-mail: totalpost@totaltheuter.com
Publisher: David Lefkowitz
Editor: David
Author: Richmond Shepard
Gives detailed current and advance notice of all areas of performing arts.theatre, opera, cabinet, dance running and coming into New York up to a year in advance, and lists plays running in major U.S. cities, Canada and England. *$160.00*
BiWeekly Since: 1944
Circulation: 2,000
Printed in on matte stock

8759 PROJECT TROUBADOR
Soho Service Corporation
48 Greene Street
New York, NY 10023-2663

Phone: 212-925-7575
Fax: 212-334-4511
Editor: Louise Lindenmeyr
Editor: Eliot Osborn

8760 RIDIM/RCMI NEWSLETTER
Research Center For Music Iconography
33 W 42nd Street
New York, NY 10036
Phone: 212-642-2709
Fax: 212-817-1992
Publisher: Zdravko Blazekovic
Interdisciplinary research on depictions of performing arts in artworks. *$25.00*
32 pages BiWeekly
Circulation: 300

8761 RAG TIMES
Maple Leaf Club
5560 W 62nd Street
Los Angeles, CA 90056-2008
Web Site: www.ragtime.com
Publisher: Richard Zimmerman
Devoted to ragtime. *$9.00*
10 pages Monthly

8762 ROOTS AND RHYTHM NEWSLETTER
#2216
2321 Verna Ct
San Leandro, CA 94577-4205
Phone: 510-526-8373
Fax: 510-614-8830
e-mail: roots@hooked.net
Web Site: www.rootsandrhythm.com
Publisher: Bill Buster
Lists, reviews and makes available for sale, recordings of blues, rhythm and blues, rockabilly, country, folk, ethnic, nostalgia and jazz music. Each newsletter reviews about 400 items and lists another 500 without reviews.
BiMonthly
Circulation: 10,000
Printed in 2 colors on newsprint stock

8763 SONG OF ZION
Jackman Music Corporation
PO Box 1900
Orem, UT 84059-1900
Toll-free: 800-323-1049
Fax: 801-225-0851
e-mail: jackmanmc@aol.com
Publisher: Jerry R. Jackman
Editor: David R. Naylor
Articles of interest to LDS (Mormon) choir directors, singers, organists and music administrators. Music, book reviews, news, obituaries, how-to articles, limited advertising by invitation only.
16 pages Monthly

8764 SONGWRITER'S & LYRICISTS NEWSLETTER
Songwriters Club of America
PO Box 23304
Brooklyn, NY 11202-3304

Publisher: Robert Makinson
Useful information in regard to songwriter lyric writer and marketing.
SemiAnnual

8765 SPOTLIGHT
American Association of Community Theatre
8402 Briar Wood Circle
Lago Vista, TX 78645-4118
Phone: 512-267-0711
Toll-free: 866-687-2228
Fax: 512-267-0712
e-mail: info@aact.org
Web Site: www.aact.org
Publisher: Julie Angelo
Editor: Sheila Nickels
News and updates on issues pertinent to community theatre. *$2.00*
24 pages BiMonthly Since: 1986
Circulation: 1600 10,000 names $180 per M.
Printed in on matte stock

8766 TRAX DJ MUSIC GUIDE
TRAX Entertainment
111 N La Cienega Boulevard
Beverly Hills, CA 90211-2206
Fax: 310-659-7856
Edtior: Michael Love
Publisher: Jeff Fishman
New music charts for DJs and related news features.
$13.00
BiMonthly Since: 1985

8767 TECHNICAL BRIEF
Yale School of Drama
222 York Street
New Haven, CT 06511-4804
Phone: 203-436-1095
Fax: 202-432-1550
Publisher: Bronislaw Sammler
Editor: Laraine Sammler
Written for professionals by professionals, this newsletter offers a dialogue between technical theatre practitioners from the performing arts who share similar problems. The succinct articles and mechanical drawings represent the best solutions to recurring technical problems. *$14.00*
TriAnnual
Circulation: 600

8768 THEATRE EVENTS GUIDE
111 W 72nd Street
New York, NY 10023-3242
Publisher: Peter Moumousis
Information for New York City entertainment fields.
Monthly

8769 VARIETY DEAL MEMO
Baskerville Communications Corporation
2455 Teller Road
Thousand Oaks, CA 91320-2218
Phone: 805-499-9734
Fax: 805-499-9656

Editor: Meredith Amdur
Publisher: Tim Baskerville
Global theatrical and post-theatrical rights and markets.
$497.00
BiMonthly

8770 VOICE OF CHORUS AMERICA
Karen Richtar
Suite 401
1811 Chestnut Street
Philadelphia, PA 19103-3703
Fax: 215-563-2431
e-mail: chorusam@libertynet.org
Web Site: www.libertynet.org/~chorus
Editor: Fred Leise
$30.00
Quarterly
Circulation: 7,000
Mailing list available for rent 7000 names
Printed in 2 colors on matte stock

8771 WOMEN IN THE ARTS BULLETIN
Women in the Arts Foundation
1175 York Avenue
New York, NY 10021-7169
Phone: 212-751-1915
Publisher: Erin Butler
Gallery information and reviews.

Magazines & Journals

8772 1001 WAYS TO REWARD EMPLOYEES
Everyone wants to be appreciated. Studies indicate that employees find your personal recognition more motivational than money. Yet managers are often too busy to give many employees the recognition they crave.
$16.00
275 pages Paperbound ISBN 1-563053-39-x

8773 2002 RESOURCE GUIDE
A great desk reference to Arts Presenters Business Members artists rosters. Full of information current to the 2002 conference, the Annual Members Conference Resource Guide is conveniently persented in alphabetical-by-organization order. *$39.00*
Paperbound

8774 ABEL
Abel News Agencies
Apartment 3C
300 W 17th Street
New York, NY 10011-5005
Editor: Peter Abel
Covers the general entertainment industry. *$75.00*
32 pages Monthly

8775 ADVANCE! ACB MAGAZINE
Association of Concert Bands
Suite 102
2533 S Maple Avenue
Tempe, AZ 85282-3559

Toll-free: 800-726-8720
Fax: 480-894-1986
Web Site: www.afn.org/encore
Association news of the music industry.
Quarterly

8776 AFTERTOUCH - NEW MUSIC DISCOVERIES
Creative Musician Coalitie
1024 W Willcox Avenue
Peoria, IL 61604-2675
Phone: 309-685-4843
Toll-free: 800-882-4262
Fax: 309-685-4878
e-mail: aimcmc@aol.com
Web Site: www.aimcmc.com
Editor: Ronald Wallace
A magazine for music lovers who would like to experience new sights and sounds and would like to keep their fingers on the pulse of the music industry. *$5.00*
100 pages Annual Since: 1984
Circulation: 10,000

8777 AMERICAN ASTROLOGY
71002 W Butler Pike
Ambler, PA 19002
Phone: 215-643-6385
Fax: 212-889-7933

8778 AMERICAN CHEERLEADER
Lifestyles Publications
Apartment 2AA
350 W 50th Street
New York, NY 10019-6693
Fax: 212-988-0621
Publisher: Micheal Weiskopf
Editor: Julie Davis
A magazine which focuses on different aspects of cheerleading with articles on topics from looking good for competitions to celebrity cheerleaders. *$3.00*
Circulation: 40,000

8779 AMERICAN CHORAL DIRECTORS ASSOCIATION
PO Box 6310
Lawton, OK 73506-0310
Phone: 580-355-8161
Fax: 580-248-1465
e-mail: acda@acdaonline.org
Web Site: www.acdaonline.org
Executive Director: Dr. Gene Brooks
Non-profit music-education organization whose central purpose is to promote excellence in choral music through performance, composition, publication, research and teaching.
96 pages 10x Year Since: 1959
Circulation: 19948
Printed in 4 colors on glossy stock

8780 AMERICAN MUSIC
University of Illinois Press
1325 S Oak Street
Champaign, IL 61820-6903

Phone: 217-333-0950
Toll-free: 866-244-0626
Fax: 217-244-9910
e-mail: journals@uillinois.edu
Web Site: www.press.uillinois.edu/journals/am.html
Editor: David Nicholls
Advertising Manager: Clydette Wantland
The only publication devoted exclusively to all aspects of American music and music in America. Of interest to academic and professional audiences as well as to a broad spectrum of non-professional music enthusiasts. *$50.00*
128 pages Quarterly Since: 1983
Circulation: 1,650
Mailing list available for rent 1,650 names $100 per M.
Printed in
2 colors on glossy stock

8781 AMERICAN MUSIC TEACHER
Music Teachers National Association
Carew Tower, Suite 505
441 Vine Street
Cincinnati, OH 45202-2811
Phone: 513-421-1420
Toll-free: 888-512-5278
Fax: 513-421-2503
e-mail: mtnanet@mtna.org
Web Site: www.mtna.org
Publisher: Gary L. Ingle
Managing Editor: Marcie Gerrietts Lindsey
Features articles on musicology, music, materials and literature reviews as well as piano, organ, voice and string instrument theory for members of the Music Teachers National Association.
BiMonthly Since: 1951
Circulation: 25,000
Printed in 4 colors on glossy stock

8782 AMERICAN MUSICAL INSTRUMENT SOCIETY JOURNAL
Shrine to Music Museum
414 E Clark Street
Vermillion, SD 57069-2307
Phone: 605-677-5306
Fax: 605-677-5073
Web Site: www.vsd.edu/smm
Editor: Arthur Lawrence
A journal focusing on the music industry. *$35.00*
Circulation: 1,000

8783 AMERICAN ORGANIST
American Guild of Organists
Suite 1260
475 Riverside Drive
New York, NY 10115-0122
Phone: 212-870-2310
Fax: 212-870-2163
e-mail: info@agohq.org
Web Site: www.TheAmericanOrganist.com
Editor: Anthony Baglivi
Most widely read journal devoted to organ and choral music in the world. *$48.00*
96 pages Monthly Since: 1967
Circulation: 25,000 25,000 names $75 per M.
Printed in on matte stock

8784 AMERICAN THEATER
355 Lexington Avenue
New York, NY 10017-6603
Phone: 212-697-5230
Fax: 212-983-4847
e-mail: at@tcg.org
Web Site: www.tcg.org
Publisher: Terence Nemeth
Editor: Jim O'Quinn
Issues include stages, features, people, in print, trends, media.
6x Year
Circulation: 23,000

8785 AMERICAN THEATRE MAGAZINE
TCG
355 Lexington Avenue
New York, NY 10017
Phone: 212-697-5230
Fax: 212-983-4847
e-mail: tcg@tcg.org
Web Site: www.tcg.org

8786 AMERICAN VIOLA SOCIETY JOURNAL
American Viola Society
PO Box 97408
Baylor University
Waco, TX 76698
Phone: 254-710-6499
Fax: 254-710-3574
e-mail: kathryn_steely@baylor.edu
Editor: Kathryn Steely
Music industry publication. *$35.00*
88 pages   3x Year Since: 1984
Circulation: 1,500

8787 AMUSEMENT BUSINESS
VNU Business Media
Suite 300
49 Music Square W
Nashville, TN 37203-3232
Phone: 615-321-4290
Fax: 615-327-1575
Web Site: www.amusement business.com
Managing Editor: Doug Campbell
Publisher: Karen Oertley
Marketing/Promotions Manager: Keith Wright
Serves the management of more than 10,000 mass
entertainment and amusement facilities. *$129.00*
Weekly Since: 1894   : online

8788 AMUSEMENT TODAY
Amusement Today
PO Box 5427
Arlington, TX 76005-5427
Phone: 817-460-7220
Fax: 817-265-6397
Publisher: Gary Slade
Keeps decision makers in the amusement industry
up-to-date with current events, business, international
developments and new attractions at amusement parks and
waterparks.

Monthly
Circulation: 16,000

8790 ANCHORAGE PRESS PLAYS
International Agency of Plays for Young People
PO Box 2901
Louisville, KY 40201
Phone: 502-583-2288
Fax: 502-583-2281
e-mail: applays@bellsouth.net
Web Site: www.applays.com
Publisher: Marilee Miller
Plays for young audiences/creative education text books
ISSN 0876-02

8791 APPLAUSE MAGAZINE
Publishing House
1245 Champa Street
Denver, CO 80204-2154
Phone: 303-893-4000
Toll-free: 800-641-1222
Fax: 303-575-0080
e-mail: sdrake@dcpa.org
Web Site: www.denvercenter.org
Publisher: Wilbur Flachman
Editor: Sylvie Drake
8-10x Year Since: 1988
Circulation: 105,000
Printed in 4 colors on glossy stock

8793 ARTS ALIVE
Box 204
3140-B Tilghman Street
Allentown, PA 18104
Phone: 610-398-5660
Fax: 610-398-5663
Since: 1977
Circulation: 18,000

8796 ASIAN MUSIC
Cornell University-Department of Music
Lincoln Hall at Cornell University
Ithaca, NY 14853-2502
Phone: 607-255-5049
Fax: 607-254-2877
Web Site: www.asianmusic.skidmore.edu
Editor: Marty Hatch
Magazine of Cornell's Department of Asian Studies.
Concerned with the performing arts of the Middle East
and Asia. *$40.00*
200 pages   2 Per Year Since: 1969
Circulation: 600
Printed in on matte stock

8797 ASIAN PACIFIC AMERICAN JOURNAL
Suite 10A
16 W 32nd Street
New York, NY 10001
Phone: 212-494-0061
Fax: 212-228-7718
e-mail: desk@aaww.org
Web Site: www.aaww.org
Editor: Hanya Yanagihara

8798 ASSOCIATION OF PERFORMING ARTS PRESENTERS BULLETIN
Suite 400
1112 16th Street NW
Washington, DC 20036-4820
Phone: 202-833-2787
Fax: 202-833-1543
e-mail: ehilburn@artspresents.org
Web Site: www.artspresents.org
Editor: Gayle Stamler
Publication Coordinator: Ellen Hilburn
Performing arts presenters learn about up and coming artists; political and economical issues, trends in fundraising, arts education, etc. *$42.00*
misc pages BiMonthley Since: 1989
Circulation: 2300+

8800 AUDREY SKIRBALL-KENIS PLAY COLLECTION
630 W 5th Street
Los Angeles, CA 90071
Phone: 213-228-7327
Fax: 213-228-7339
Web Site: www.askplay.org
Project Director: Tom Harris

8801 AUTOHARPOHOLIC
LAD Publications
PO Box 1787
Elkins, WV 26241-1787
Fax: 415-467-1509
Editor: Becky Blackley
Covers information of interest to autoharp players. *$14.50*
Quarterly
Circulation: 2,000

8802 BMI MUSICWORLD
BMI
3rd Floor
320 W 57th Street
New York, NY 10019-3790
Phone: 212-244-1677
Fax: 212-582-5972
e-mail: hlevitt@bmi.com
Web Site: www.bmi.com
Editor: Robbin Ahrold
Circulation Director: Dana Nicolella
Performing rights organization. Articles of interest to the songwriting community
Circulation: 75m

8803 BACK STAGE
BPI Communications
770 Broadway
New York, NY 10003-8901
Phone: 646-654-5711
Fax: 646-654-5744
e-mail: showard@backstage.com
Web Site: www.backstage.com
Publisher: Steve Elish
Editor: Sherry Eaker

Contains industry news, reviews, features, interviews and audition notices. Special sections highlight reports from regional correspondents, columns on dance, cabaret, comedy and monthly listings of films starting in New York. *$84.00*
Weekly
Circulation: 30,000

8804 BAKER'S PLAYS
Box 699222
Quincy, MA 02269-9222
Phone: 617-745-0805
Fax: 617-745-9891
Web Site: www.bakersplays.com
General Manager: Kurt Gombar

8805 BALLOONS & PARTIES TODAY
PartiLife Publications
65 Sussex Street
Hackensack, NJ 07601-4105
Phone: 201-441-4224
Fax: 201-342-8118
e-mail: info@balloonsandparties.com
Web Site: www.balloonsandparties.com
Publisher: Mark Zettler
Editor: Andrea Zettler
Director of Sales: Carolyn Cardaci
Targeted, informative and practical ideas for the event decorating industry. Motivates readers to produce professional, innovative party services. *$29.95*
48 pages BiMonthly Since: 1986
Circulation: 8,000 7000 names $100 per M.
Printed in 4 colors on glossy stock

8806 BILLBOARD
BPI Communications
14th Floor
1515 Broadway
New York, NY 10036-8901
Phone: 646-654-5500
Fax: 212-536-5358
e-mail: hlander@billboard.com
Web Site: www.billboard-online.com
Publisher: Howard Lander
Contents provide news, reviews and statistics for all genres of music, including radio play, music video, related internet activity, and retail updates. Editorial features interviews and profiles of musicians and producers, and discusses upcoming music events, both national and international. *$265.00*
Weekly
Circulation: 40,502

8807 BLITZ
PO Box 48124
Los Angeles, CA 90048-0124
Fax: 323-962-1811
Web Site: ww.blitzmag.com
Editor: Mike McDowell
A rock magazine for thinking people. *$15.00*
Quarterly
Circulation: 5,000

8808 BLUEGRASS UNLIMITED
9514 James Madison Highway
Warrenton, VA 20137-0111
Phone: 540-349-8181
Fax: 540-341-0011
Web Site: www.bluegrassmusic.com
Editor: Peter V. Kuykendall
Covers traditional country and bluegrass music. *$20.00*
Monthly
Circulation: 21,540

8809 BOMB MAGAZINE
Betsy Sussler
Suite 905
594 Broadway
New York, NY 10012-3233
Phone: 212-431-3943
Fax: 212-431-5880
e-mail: info@bombsite.com
Web Site: www.bombsite.com
Publisher/Editor: Betsy Sussler
Managing Editor: Nell McClister
Editor: Rachel Kushner
Focuses on contemporary art, literature, theater, film, music. *$4.95*
112 pages   Quarterly Since: 1981
Circulation: 60,000
Printed in 4 colors on matte stock

8811 BOSTON SOUND CHECK
William Restuccia Jr.
Suite 301
389 Main Street
Malden, MA 02148
Phone: 781-388-7749
Fax: 781-388-1817
e-mail: info@bostonsoundcheck.com
Web Site: www.bostonsoundcheck.com
Managing Editor: Debbie Catalano
Managing Editor: Matt Robinson

8812 BOXOFFICE
RLD Communication
Suite 100
155 S El Molino Avenue
Pasadena, CA 91101
Phone: 626-396-0250
Fax: 626-396-0248
e-mail: editorial@boxoffice.com
Web Site: www.boxoffice.com
Editor-in-Chief: Kim Williamson
Main Editor: Christine Jones
Sr Editor: Francesca Dinglaram
$40.00
Monthly
Circulation: 6,000
Printed in on glossy stock

8813 BROADWAY PLAY PUBLISHING
56 E 81st Street
New York, NY 10028-0202

Phone: 212-772-8334
Fax: 212-772-8358
e-mail: BroadwayPl@aol.com
Web Site: www.broadwayplaypubl.com

8814 BUSCANDO AMOR
Lancer Productions
Suite 213
1241 S Soto Street
Los Angeles, CA 90023
Phone: 323-881-6515
Fax: 323-881-6524
e-mail: teleguia@aol.com
Publisher: John DiCarlo
Editor: Elizabeth DiCarlo
Office Manager: Lorena Mata
Weekly Since: 1986
Circulation: 100,000
Printed in 4 colors on newsprint stock

8815 CCM MAGAZINE
CCM Communications
3rd Floor
104 Woodmont Boulevard
Nashville, TN 37205-2207
Phone: 615-386-3011
Fax: 615-386-3380
Web Site: www.ccmmagazine.com
Editor: Matt Turner
Managing Editor: Tracey Bumps
Christian music magazine with industry news, artist interviews, tour listings, and more *$19.95*
75-85 pages   Monthly Since: 1978
Circulation: 50,000 47,000 names
Printed in on glossy stock

8816 CMJ NEW MUSIC REPORT
21st Floor
810 7th Avenue
New York, NY 10019
Phone: 646-485-6600
Toll-free: 800-265-9559
Fax: 646-557-0029
e-mail: cmj@cmj.com
Web Site: www.cmj.com
Publisher: Robert K. Haber
Articles on the alternative music scene and new release reviews geared toward college radio programmers. *$295.00*
Weekly

8818 CALLALOO
University of Virginia, Box 400121
322 Bryan Hall, Department of English
Charlottesville, VA 22904-4121
Phone: 804-924-6637
Fax: 804-924-6472
e-mail: callaloo@virginia.edu
Web Site: www.people.virginia.edu/~callaloo
Editor: Charles H. Rowell

8819 CALLBOARD

Theatre Bay Area
Suite 375
870 Market Street
San Francisco, CA 94102-3002
Phone: 415-430-1140
Fax: 415-430-1145
e-mail: tba@theatrebayarea.org
Web Site: www.theatrebayarea.org
Executive Editor: Belinda Taylor
Editor-in-Chief: Karen McKeritt
Author: Belinda Taylor
Provides trade information for professionals in the Bay
Area. *$5.50*
Monthly
Circulation: 5,000
Printed in 2 colors on matte stock

8820 CAMPUS ACTIVITIES TODAY

Cameo Publishing Group
917 Calhoun Street
Columbia, SC 29201-2307
Phone: 803-254-1040
Fax: 803-254-5798
Provides information on music for activities directors on
college campuses.

8821 CANADIAN THEATRE REVIEW

University of Toronto Press
5201 Dufferin Street
Toronto, Ontario M3H-5T8
Phone: 416-667-7810
Fax: 416-667-7881
e-mail: journals@utpress.utoronto.ca
Web Site: www.utpjournals.com
Focuses on Candian theatre. *$35.00*
4x Year Magazine/Journal Since: 1974
Circulation: 1,500
Mailing list available for rent $250 per M.

8823 CARNEGIE HALL STAGEBILL

Stagebill
7th Floor
144 E 44th Street
New York, NY 10017-4031
Phone: 212-286-0475
Editor: Charles Buccieri
Covers performances in Carnegie Hall.
Monthly

8824 CAROUSEL NEWS & TRADER

Walter L. Loucks
Suite 206
87 Park Avenue W
Mansfield, OH 44902-1612
Phone: 419-529-4999
Fax: 419-529-2321
e-mail: cnsam@aol.com
Web Site: www.carousel.net/trader
Author: Walter L. Loucks
Articles devoted to the collecting , restoring and selling of
carousel art. *$29.00*
Annual

8825 CASINO JOURNAL

GEM Communications
Suite 207 A
1771 E Flamingo Road
Las Vegas, NV 89119-5157
Phone: 702-794-0718
Fax: 702-794-0799
e-mail: casino@mail.idt.net
Web Site: www.worldgaminglive.com
Publisher: Pamela Sandbulte
GEM's mission is to be the primary information source for
the key decision makers in the worldwide casino, lottery,
parimutuel, bingo and emerging internet wagering markets.
Monthly
Circulation: 13034

8826 CASINO OPS

CJPG
5240 S Eastern Avenue
Las Vegas, NV 89119
Phone: 702-736-8886
Fax: 702-736-8889
Publisher: Glenn Fine
Dedicated to the efficient and effective operation of casino
and other gaming ventures.
Quarterly
Circulation: 15000

8827 CHAMBER MUSIC MAGAZINE

Chamber Music America
Floor 5
305 7th Avenue
New York, NY 10001-6008
Phone: 212-242-2022
Fax: 212-244-2776
Publisher: Leonard R. Levine
The journal of the professional chamber music field. Its
articles are aimed to professionals, amateurs, arts
administrators, concert presenters, educators and music
lovers. *$28.00*
BiMonthly
Circulation: 10,000

8828 CHILDRENS ENTERTAINMENT BUSINESS

Marquee Communications
PO Box 824
Dover, NJ 07802-0824
Publisher: William Webber
News on childrens entertainment professionals. *$15.00*
Circulation: 5,000

8829 CHINESE MUSIC

Chinese Music Society of North America (CMSNA)
PO Box 5275
Woodridge, IL 60517-0275
Phone: 630-910-1551
Fax: 630-910-1561
e-mail: syshen@megsinet.net
Web Site: www.chinesemusic.net
Executive Director: Prof. Yuan-Yuan Lee

Chinese Music is the only journal in the world devoted wholly to the study of the music and acoustics of China, and their relationship to those of other regions of the world. Chinese Music covers all phases of research and performance activities in Chinese music. It provides a forum for original papers concerned with musicology, musical life, composition, acoustics, analysis, orchestration, musicians, global interactions, intercultural studies, and musical instruments. *$28.00*
Quarterly
Circulation: 13,500
Mailing list available for rent
Computerized version available: Internet

8830 CHINESE MUSIC SOCIETY OF NORTH AMERICA
PO Box 5275
Woodridge, IL 60517-0275
Phone: 630-910-1551
Fax: 630-910-1561
Web Site: www.chinesemusic.net
Director: Dr. Yuan- Yuan Lee
Publishes a magazine in hardcover and paperback. *$53.75*
Quarterly Since: 1976 ISBN 1-880464-07-1
Circulation: 21,083

8831 CHORAL JOURNAL
American Choral Directors Association
PO Box 6310
Lawton, OK 73506-0310
Phone: 580-355-8161
Fax: 580-248-1465
e-mail: chojo@acdaonline.org
Web Site: www.acdaonline.org
Editor: Carroll Gonzo
Author: Wesley Coffman
The official publication of the American Choral Directors Association. Articles that embrace both scholarly and practical approaches to understanding issues affecting choral directors and their craft. Prints reviews of octavos, compact discs, and books related to choral music. Members of the association teach choral music in public and private schools as well as in colleges and universities. *$55.00*
88 pages 10 X Year Since: 1959
Circulation: 20,000
Mailing list available for rent 18500 names

8832 CLARINET
International Clarinet Society
University of North Texas
Denton, TX 76203
Phone: 630-665-3602
Fax: 940-565-4919
Web Site: www.clarinet.org
Editor: James Gillespie
Contains articles in wide variety of areas written by performers and scholars. *$25.00*
Quarterly
Circulation: 3,000

8833 CLAVIER
Instrumentalist Company
200 Northfield Road
Northfield, IL 60093-3390
Phone: 847-446-5000
Fax: 847-446-6263
Publisher: James Rohner
Editor: Judy Nelson
For pianists, organists and piano teachers. *$19.00*
48 pages 10x Year Since: 1962
Circulation: 16,000

8834 CLOSE UP MAGAZINE
Country Music Association
1 Music Circle S
Nashville, TN 37203-4312
Phone: 615-244-2840
Fax: 615-242-4783
e-mail: apatterson@cmaworld.com
Web Site: www.cmaworld.com
Editor: Athena Patterson
Profiles of country music artists, variouis songwriters and industry news.
40 pages Bi-Monthly
Circulation: 8,000

8835 CLUB MODEL MAGAZINE
Aquino Productions
PO Box 15760
Stamford, CT 06901-0760
Fax: 203-967-9952
Publisher: Andres Aquino
Editor: Elaine Hallgren
For those involved in all aspects of the modeling industry: models, photographers, fashion designers and executives, agents, pageant directors, and makeup artists. *$4.00*
Circulation: 105,000

8838 CONFRONTATION
English Department
C.W. Post College of Long Island University
Greenvale, NY 11548
Phone: 516-299-2720
Fax: 516-299-2735
e-mail: mtucker@liu.edu
Editor: Martin Tucker

8839 CONTACT QUARTERLY JOURNAL OF DANCE AND IMPROVISATION
PO Box 603
Northampton, MA 01061-0603
Phone: 413-586-1181
Fax: 413-486-1181
Web Site: www.contactimprov.net
Editor: Lisa Nelson
Editor: Nancy Stark Smith
2x Year
Circulation: 2,000

8840 CONTEMPORARY CHRISTIAN MUSIC
CCM Communications
3rd Floor
104 Woodmont Boulevard
Nashville, TN 37205-2207
Phone: 615-386-3011
Toll-free: 800-333-9643
Fax: 615-386-3380
Web Site: www.ccmcom.com
Publisher/President: John W. Styll
Managing Editor: April Hefner
Consumer magazine for fans of contemporary Christian music. *$21.95*
Monthly
Circulation: 100,000

8841 CONTEMPORARY MUSIC REVIEW
Harwood Academic Publishers
270 8th Avenue
New York, NY 10011-1619
Phone: 212-473-7616
Fax: 212-645-2459
Web Site: www.gbhap.com
Covers music composition. *$63.00*

8842 COUNTRY DANCE & SONG
Country Dance & Song Society
PO Box 338
Haydenville, MA 01039-0338
Phone: 413-268-7426
Fax: 413-268-7471
Scholarly journal concerning English and Anglo-American folk dance, music and song.
Annual
Circulation: 3,000

8843 CREEM
Alternative Media
28 W 25th Street
New York, NY 10010-2705
Phone: 818-985-7273
Fax: 212-647-0236
Editor: Mark J. Petracca
Publisher: Susan Traub
Covers all aspects of the music industry and focuses on the contemporary scene. *$3.50*
10x Year
Circulation: 200,000

8844 CUE MAGAZINE
PO Box 2027
Burlingame, CA 94011-2027
Phone: 650-348-8004
Fax: 650-348-7781
e-mail: cue@sirius.com
Web Site: www.cue-online.com
Publisher: Pat Henry
Includes information on the leaders and companies, news releases and a calendar of events for the film, video, multimedia, television, radio and talent industry. *$24.00*
Monthly
Circulation: 5M

8845 CUE SHEET
Society for the Preservation of Film Music
PO Box 93536
Los Angeles, CA 90093-0536
Phone: 818-248-5775
Fax: 818-248-8681
Editor: Leslie T. Zador
News on the art of composing for films.
Quarterly
Circulation: 300

8846 DJ TIMES
Testa Communications
25 Willowdale Avenue
Port Washington, NY 11050-3779
Phone: 516-767-2500
Fax: 516-767-9335
Publisher: Vincent Testa
Editor: Jim Tremayne
Colorful tabloid magazine dedicated to professional mobile and club DJs. Specialized music sections, new product departments for sound and lighting, record reviews, business columns, informative entertainer profiles, and more. *$30.00*
60 pages Monthly Since: 1968
Circulation: 20,000

8847 DAILY VARIETY
Cahners Business Information
Suite 120
5700 Wilshire Boulevard
Los Angeles, CA 90036
Phone: 323-857-6600
Fax: 323-932-0393
e-mail: news@variety.cahners.com
Web Site: www.variety.com
Publisher: Gerry Byrne
Focuses on film, television, video, cable, music and theater. Includes coverage of financial, regulatory and legal matters pertaining to the entertainment industry. *$187.00*
24 pages Daily Since: 1933
Circulation: 27,916

8848 DANCE CHRONICLE
Marcel Dekker
Floor 4
270 Madison Avenue
New York, NY 10016-0671
Phone: 212-696-9000
Toll-free: 800-228-1160
Fax: 212-685-4540
e-mail: journals@dekker.com
Web Site: www.dekker.com
Editor: George Dorris
Studies in dance and the performing arts. *$465.00*
TriAnnual ISSN 0147-2526
Circulation: 450

8849 DANCE EDUCATORS OF AMERICA WORKSHOPS AND COMPETITION
PO Box 607
Pelham, NY 10803-0607

Phone: 914-636-3200
Fax: 914-636-5895
Offers information, competition news and workshops for persons interested in dance.
Annual

8850 DANCE MAGAZINE

Suite 203
111 Myrtle Street
Oakland, CA 94607
Phone: 570-839-6060
Fax: 510-839-6066
Web Site: www.dancemagazine.com
Publisher: Barbara Paice Karlan
VP, Marketing: Robert Berner
Circulation Director: Sondra Weintraub
Production Manager: Amanda Alic
The dance world's most prestigious and authoritative monthly magazine providing national and international coverage of what's happening in dance. For dance professionals, students, teachers and audiences. *$34.95*
204 pages Monthly Since: 1927
Circulation: 55,000
Mailing list available for rent
Printed in 4 colors on glossy stock

8851 DANCE RESEARCH JOURNAL

Congress on Research in Dance/SUNY Dance Dept.
College at Brockport
State University of New York
Brockport, NY 14420
Phone: 716-395-2590
Fax: 716-395-5413
e-mail: gearlsin@brovkport.edu
Web Site: eordance.org
Editor: Julie Malnig
Published twice a year by the Congress on Research in Dance, this journal carries scholarly articles, book reviews, lists of books and journals received, and reports of scholarly conferences, archives and other projects of interest to the field. *$65.00*
100+ pages BiAnnual Since: 1968
Circulation: 850
Mailing list available for rent 750+ names $75 per M.

8852 DANCE SPIRIT

Suite 420
250 W 57th Street
New York, NY 10107
Phone: 212-265-8890
Fax: 212-265-8908
Web Site: www.dancespirit.com
President: Michael Weiskopf
Associate Publisher: Mary-Evelyn Holder
Publication consists of dance training and instruction from tap to ballet to jazz.
10x Year Since: 1997
Circulation: 75,000

8853 DANCE TEACHER NOW

SMW Communications
3020 Beacon Boulevard
West Sacramento, CA 95691-3436

Phone: 916-372-0510
Fax: 916-373-0232
Editor: K.C. Patrick
A magazine for professional dance educators, senior students, and other professionals on practical information for the teacher and/or business owner, economic and historical issues related to the profession. Profiles of schools, methods and people who are leaving their marks on dance. Stories must be thoroughly researched; query first. No puff pieces. *$24.00*
9x Year
Circulation: 6,000

8854 DANCE/USA JOURNAL

Dance/USA
Suite 820
1156 15th Street NW
Washington, DC 20005-1704
Phone: 202-833-1717
Fax: 202-833-2686
e-mail: danceusa@danceusa.org
Web Site: www.danceusa.org
Publisher: Andrea Snyder
Editor: Libby Smigel
The journal features articles on issues of importance to the dance community; news stories relating to arts and dance; essays from leaders in the dance field; notes on changes, transitions and opportunties in the field; calendar of up coming events; and highlights of Dance/USA sponsored events. *$40.00*
32 pages Quarterly Since: 1982
Circulation: 900+
Printed in 2 colors on glossy stock

8855 DANCING USA

Dot Publications
14160 Coral Sea Street NE
Ham Lake, MN 55304-7233
Phone: 763-757-6605
Toll-free: 800-290-1307
Fax: 612-757-6605
e-mail: ballroom@dancingusa.com
President: LeAnn Bamford
VP: Patti Johnson
Techniques and tips from experts to broaden your dance styles. Practice the steps from each issue, with inspiring stories that spark romance. Enliven relationships, learn better communication on the dance floor, and get the latest information on expert source dance videos, CDs, tapes, music reviews, and dance step history. *$21.97*
BiMonthly
Circulation: 20,000

8856 DESCANT

Toronto, Ontario
Box 314, Station P
CANADA M5S 2S8
Phone: 416-593-2557
Web Site: www.descant.on.ca
Managing Editor: Nathan Whitlock
Editor: Karen Mulhallen

8857 DIAPASON

Scranton Gillette Communications
Suite 200
380 E Northwest Highway
Des Plaines, IL 60016-2282
Phone: 847-298-6622
Fax: 847-390-0408
Web Site: www.thediapason.com
Editor: Jerome Butera
An international journal dealing with organ, harpsichord, carillon and church music. *$25.00*
28 pages   Monthly   Since: 1909
Circulation: 5,000

8859 DOWN BEAT

Maher Publications
102 N Haven Road
Elmhurst, IL 60126-3357
Phone: 630-941-2030
Fax: 630-941-3210
Editor: Frank Alkyer
Information on jazz and blues music. *$26.00*
Monthly
Circulation: 88,253

8860 DRAMA REVIEW

MIT Press
5 Cambridge Center
Cambridge, MA 02142-1493
Phone: 617-253-2889
Fax: 617-577-1545
e-mail: journals-orders@mit.edu
Web Site: mitpress.mit.edu
Publisher: Sarah Muzzy
Editor: Richard Schechner
A journal of performance studies. *$30.00*
Quarterly
Circulation: 4,750

8861 DRAMATIC PUBLISHING COMPANY

Box 129
311 Washington Street
Woodstock, IL 60098
Phone: 815-338-7170
Fax: 815-338-8981
e-mail: plays@dramaticpublishing.com
Web Site: www.dramaticpublishing.com
Editor: Linda Habjan

8862 DRAMATICS

International Thespian Society/Educational Theatre
2343 Auburn Avenue
Cincinnati, OH 45219-2815
Phone: 513-421-3900
Fax: 513-421-7077
e-mail: info@edta.org
Web Site: www.edta.org
Editor: Don Corathers
Edited for high school theatre student and teachers, Dramatics features new playscripts, interviews with theatre professionals, practical articles on acting, directing design and other aspects of theatre production, and college and career information. Annual special issues offer comprehensive and summer theatre work and study opportunities. *$20.00*
52 pages   Monthly   Since: 1929
Circulation: 36,000 $100 per M.
Printed in 4 colors

8863 DRAMATISTS PLAY SERVICE

440 Park Avenue S
New York, NY 10016
Phone: 212-683-8960
Fax: 212-213-1539
e-mail: postmaster@dramatists.com
Web Site: www.dramatists.com
President: Stephen Sultan

8864 DRUM BUSINESS

Modern Drummer Publications
12 Old Bridge Road
Cedar Grove, NJ 07009-1288
Phone: 973-239-4140
Fax: 973-239-7139
e-mail: mdinfo@moderndrummer.com
Web Site: www.moderndrummer.com
Publisher: Ronald Spagnardi
Associate Publisher: Kevin Kearns
Articles containing interviews with prominent drum retailers, reports on the world's leading percussion industry manufacturers, discussions with industry leaders, and reporting on all major industry trade shows.
36 pages   Monthly   Since: 1993
Circulation: 5000

8866 ELECTRONIC MUSICIAN

PRIMEDIA
Suite 12
6400 Hollis Street
Emeryville, CA 94608-1086
Phone: 510-653-3307
Fax: 510-653-5142
Web Site: www.emusician.com
Editor: Steve Eppenheimer
The #1 magazine for musicials recording and producing music in a home personal studio. *$24.00*
120 pages   Monthly   Since: 1986
Circulation: 72,000

8868 ENCORE PERFORMANCE PUBLISHING

Box 692
Orem, UT 84057
Phone: 801-225-0605
President: Michael C. Perry

8869 ENTERTAINMENT, PUBLISHING AND THE ARTS HANDBOOK

Clark Boardman Company
155 Pfingsten Road
Deerfield, IL 60015
Editor: John David Viera
Editor: Stephen Breimer

Provides information on the latest development in the expanding legal field of entertainment, publishing, and the arts. The articles focus on such issues as books, copyrights, right-of-publicity and more. *$79.50*
Annual

8871 FUNWORLD

IAAPA
1448 Duke Street
Alexandria, VA 22314-3403
Phone: 703-836-4800
Fax: 703-836-4801
e-mail: iaapa@iaapa.org
Web Site: www.iaapa.org
Editor: Michail Moran
Production Manager: Sherrie Ophof
For the amusement park and attraction industry. Published by the International Association of Amusement Parks and Attractions. *$4.00*
Circulation: 8,700

8872 FAIR DEALER

Western Fairs Association
Suite 210
1776 Tribute Road
Sacramento, CA 95815-4495
Phone: 916-927-3100
Fax: 916-927-6397
e-mail: wfa@fairsnet.org
Web Site: www.fairsnet.org
Editor: Laura C Trout
Offers information for fairground owners, managers and workers. *$35.00*
Quarterly
Circulation: 2,500
Printed in on glossy stock

8873 FAIRS & EXPOS

PO Box 985
Springfield, MO 65801-0985
Phone: 417-862-5771
Fax: 417-862-0156
e-mail: iafe@fairsandexpos.com
Web Site: www.fairsandexpos.com
Publisher: Max Willis
Advertising: Steve Sierer
Contains articles, news and information about the fair industry. *$30.00*
10x
Circulation: 3,250
Printed in on glossy stock

8874 FAMILY ENTERTAINMENT CENTER

International Association of Amusement Parks
1448 Duke Street
Alexandria, VA 22314-3403
Phone: 703-836-4800
Fax: 703-836-4801
Publisher: Rick Henderson
Editor: Sevena Leigh
Profiles and business analysis of and smaller amusement attractions including mini-golf courses, go-cart tracks, action parks, skating rinks, game arcades, family entertainment centers, and other unique leisure attrations.

8875 FESTIVALS

International Festivals and Events Association
PO Box 2950
Port Angeles, WA 98362-0336
Phone: 360-457-3141
Fax: 360-452-4695
Web Site: www.ifea.com
President: Bruce Skinner
Emphasizes profitable events through coverage of promotion and marketing, legal issues, and industry trends. Includes articles written by suppliers.
Quarterly
Circulation: 4000

8876 FIRST BASS

First Bass International
33 Essex Street
Hackensack, NJ 07601-5418
Fax: 201-489-5057
Editor: Joe Campagna
Directed to the electric and acoustic bass player of all ages and backgrounds. *$14.95*
Quarterly
Circulation: 86,000

8877 FLUTE TALK

Instrumentalist Company
200 Northfield Road
Northfield, IL 60093-3390
Phone: 847-446-5000
Fax: 847-446-6263
Editor: Diana Kodner
A magazine for flute teachers. *$16.00*
10x Year
Circulation: 12,000

8879 FREELANCE PRESS

Box 548
Dover, MA 02030
Phone: 508-785-8250
Fax: 508-785-8291
Managing Editor: Narcissa Campion
Editorial Assistant: Barbara Sanyer

8880 FRIDAY MORNING QUARTERBACK ROCK REPORT

Building F-36
1930 E Marlton Pike
Cherry Hill, NJ 08003
Phone: 856-424-9114
Fax: 856-424-6943

8882 FULL EFFECT!

Rob Group
PO Box 478
Guilford, CT 06437-0478
Fax: 203-775-1931
Editor: Steve Korte
Covers soul and rap music. *$14.95*
BiMonthly
Circulation: 225,000

8884 GIG MAGAZINE
9th Floor
460 Park Avenue S
New York, NY 10016-7315
Phone: 212-378-0400
Fax: 212-378-2149
e-mail: gig@psn.com
Web Site: www.gigmag.com
Publisher: Paul Gallo
Editor: Craig Anderton
Monthly
Circulation: 80,000

8885 GOSPEL TODAY
Suite 205
761 Old Hickory Boulevard
Brentwood, TN 37027
Phone: 615-376-5656
Toll-free: 800-472-6731
Fax: 615-376-0882
e-mail: gospeltodaymag@aol.com
Web Site: www.gospeltoday.com
Publisher: Teresa Hairston
Advertising Sales: James Nowlin
Distribution/Circulation: Shannon Warren
Gospel Today is America's Leading Christian Lifestyle
Magazine, serving consumers who enjoy reading about the
positive and progressive people, places and developments
in the Christian community. This magazine is forgoing
new ground culturally, historically, and sociologically, by
offering a positive outlook on high profile Christians,
including those in entertainment, professional sports,
ministry/church leadership and music.
$20.00
67 pages 8x Year Since: 1989
Circulation: 50,000 18,000 names $90 per M.
Printed in 4 colors

8886 GOSPEL VOICE
PO Box 682427
Franklin, TN 37068-2427
Phone: 615-851-1841
Toll-free: 888-323-3378
Fax: 615-851-9189

8887 GUITAR ONE
Cherry Lane Magazines
11th Floor
6 E 32nd Street
New York, NY 10016
Phone: 212-561-3000
Fax: 212-251-0840
e-mail: guitarshop@worldnet.att.net
Web Site: www.guitarmag.com
Editor in Chief: Troy Nelson
Information on everything from the guitar equipment
evaluations to news on the latest trends and technological
developments to special insider pieces covering the sound
secrets of today's top players.
BiMonthly
Circulation: 105000

8888 GUITAR REVIEW
Albert Augustine Limited
151 W 26th Street
New York, NY 10001
Phone: 917-661-0220
Fax: 917-661-0223
e-mail: mail@guitarreview.com
Web Site: www.guitarreview.com
Editor: Rose Augustine
Scholarly articles related to the classical guitar. *$28.00*
48 pages Quarterly Since: 1946
Circulation: 4000

**8889 GUITAR FOR THE PRACTICING
MUSICIAN**
Cherry Lane Music Company
11th Floor
6 E 32nd Street
New York, NY 10016-5415
Fax: 914-937-0614
Editor: Lorena Alexander
Supplies transcriptions to today's best-selling songs.
$27.50
Monthly
Circulation: 999,999

8890 HARMONIZER
6315 3rd Avenue
Kenosha, WI 53143-5101
Phone: 262-653-8440
Toll-free: 800-876-7467
Fax: 262-654-4048
Choral music

8891 HEUER PUBLISHING COMPANY
Box 248
Cedar Rapids, IA 52406
Phone: 319-364-6311
Fax: 319-364-1771
e-mail: editor@hitplays.com
Web Site: www.hitplays.com
Editor/Publisher: C. Emmett McMullen

8892 HIT PARADER
Suite 211
210 Route 4 E
Paramus, NJ 07652-5103
Phone: 201-843-4004
Fax: 201-843-8636

8893 HITMAKERS MAGAZINE
Hot Sheet Publishing
PO Box 2239
Orinda, CA 94562
Phone: 925-253-7862
Fax: 818-883-1097
e-mail: hitmakers@hitmakers.com
Web Site: www.hitmakers.com
Publisher: Barry Fiedel
Includes charts and listings on faces and places in the
music industry, street sheet and special interviews.
$295.00

Weekly
Circulation: 3,000

8894 HOLLYWOOD REPORTER
5055 Wilshire Boulevard
Los Angeles, CA 90036-4396
Phone: 323-525-2000
Fax: 323-525-2377
Web Site: www.hollywoodreporter.com
Covers the full spectrum of craft and commerce in the entertainment industry.

8897 I. E. CLARK PUBLICATIONS
Box 246
Schulenburg, TX 78956-0246
Phone: 979-743-3232
Fax: 979-743-4765
e-mail: ieclark@cvtv.net
Web Site: www.ieclark.com
Editorial Department: Donna Cozzaglio

8898 IMAGO MUSICAE
Duke University Press
PO Box 90660
Durham, NC 27708-0660
Phone: 919-687-3600
Fax: 919-688-4574
International yearbook of music, Volumes I & II. *$62.95*
Annual

8899 IMPACTO MUSICAL
Revista
Suite 150
13550 SW 88th Street
Miami, FL 33186
Phone: 305-408-9801
Fax: 305-408-8386
e-mail: marisol@resista-impacto.com
Web Site: www.revista-impacto.com
Editor: Marisol Lopez
Advertising Manager: Johnnie Eljack
Christian music magazine
6x/year
Circulation: 25,000

8900 IN FOCUS
National Association of Theatre Owners
Suite 340
4605 Lankershim Boulevard
North Hollywood, CA 91602-1875
Phone: 818-506-1778
Fax: 818-506-3674
e-mail: infocusmagazine@mindspring.com
Web Site: www.infocusmag.com
Editor-in-Chief: Jim Kozak
Advertising Director: Mary dela Cruz
Director of Communications: James Kozak
Assistant
Executive Director: Elaine Ceniceroz
A magazine for the business needs of theatre owners and operators from around the world. $75.00 subsription cost for foriegn countries. We also publish an Encyclopedia of Exhibition for an annual cost of $100.00. *$60.00*

Monthly Since: 2001
Printed in 4 colors on glossy stock

8901 INK NINETEEN
Suite 6
830 N Wickham Road
Melbourne, FL 32935
Phone: 321-253-0290
Fax: 321-259-8880

8903 INSTRUMENTALIST
Instrumentalist Company
200 Northfield Road
Northfield, IL 60093-3390
Phone: 847-446-5000
Fax: 847-446-6263
Managing Editor: Matthew R. Baumer
For school and college band directors. *$24.00*
100 pages Monthly Since: 1945
Circulation: 20,000
Printed in 4 colors

8904 INTERNATIONAL BLUEGRASS
International Bluegrass Music Association
1620 Frederica Street
Owensboro, KY 42301
Phone: 270-684-9025
Toll-free: 888-438-4262
Fax: 270-686-7863
e-mail: ibma@ibma.org
Web Site: www.ibma.org
IBMA works together for high standards of professionalism, a greater appreciation for our music, and the success of the world-wide bluegrass community. *$25.00*
20 pages BiMonthly
Printed in on n stock

8905 INTERNATIONAL GAMING AND WAGERING BUSINESS
BMT Commodity Corporation
24th Floor
530 Fifth Avenue
New York, NY 10036-5101
Phone: 212-302-4200
Fax: 212-302-0007
e-mail: bmt@bmktny.com
Publisher: Paul Dworin
Focuses on business strategy, legislative information, food service and promotional concerns.
Monthly
Circulation: 25000

8906 INTERNATIONAL MUSICIAN
American Federation of Musicians
Suite 600
1501 Broadway
New York, NY 10036-5503
Phone: 212-869-1330
Fax: 212-764-6134
e-mail: info@afm.org
Web Site: www.afm.org
Editor: Thomas F. Lee

Covers musicians and articles relating to them in the
United States and Canada. *$25.00*
20 pages   Monthly   Since: 2000
Circulation: 110,000

**8907   INTERNATIONAL READERS' THEATRE
PUBLISH-ON-DEMAND SCRIPT
SERVICE**
Blizzard Publishing
Winnipeg
73 Furby Street
Canada   MB R3C 2A2
Phone: 207-775-2923
Toll-free: 800-694-9256
Fax: 204-775-2947
e-mail: irt@blizzard.mb.ca
Web Site: www.blizzard.mb.ca/catalog
Production Coordinator: David Fuller

**8908   INTERNATIONAL SOCIETY FOR THE
PERFORMING ARTS-FORUM**
International Society for The Performing Arts
PO Box 909
17 Purdy Avenue, Suite 200
New York, NY 10580-0909
Phone: 914-921-1550
Fax: 914-921-1593
e-mail: info@ispa.org
Web Site: www.ispa.org
CEO: Johann Zietsman
Newsletter and membership directory included with
membership to International Society for the Performing
Arts.
6x/Year
Circulation: 500

8909   INTERVIEW MAGAZINE
Brant Publications
575 Broadway
New York, NY 10012
Phone: 212-941-2800
Fax: 212-941-2885
Publisher: Sandra Brant
Editor-in-Chief: Ingrid Sischy
Conversations with celebrities, designers, artists, etc.
$2.95
Monthly   Since: 1969
Circulation: 185,615

8910   JAM MAGAZINE
618 Wymore Road
Winter Park, FL 32789
Phone: 407-767-8377
Fax: 407-767-0533

8911   JAZZ EDUCATION JOURNAL
International Association for Jazz Education
PO Box 724
Manhattan, KS 66505-0724
Phone: 785-776-8744
Fax: 785-776-6190
e-mail: info@iaje.org
Web Site: www.iaje.org

Editor: Antonio Garcia
Publisher: William McFarlin
To promote the understanding and appreciation of jazz and
its heritage, provide leadership to educators regarding
curricula and
performance. *$55.00*
BiMonthly Journal   Since: 1968
Circulation: 8,000
Printed in on glossy stock

8912   JAZZ NOTES
PO Box 4487
Saint Paul, MN 55104-0487
Phone: 763-531-0411
Fax: 763-537-4819

8913   JAZZ WORLD
World Jazz Society
PO Box 777
New York, NY 10108-0777
Web Site: www.jazzsociety.com
Editor: Jan A. Byrczek
A publication covering the world of jazz music. *$35.00*
BiMonthly
Circulation: 6,000

8914   JAZZTIMES
5th Floor
8737 Colesville Road
Silver Spring, MD 20910-3921
Phone: 301-588-4114
Fax: 301-588-5531
e-mail: jtimes@aol.com
Web Site: www.jazztimes.com
Publisher: Glenn Sabin
$23.95
10x Year
Circulation: 86,000

8915   JERSEY JAZZ
PO Box 410
Brookside, NJ 07926-0410
Phone: 973-543-2039
Toll-free: 800-303-6557
Fax: 973-543-2039

**8916   JOURNAL OF ARTS MANAGEMENT,
LAW, SOCIETY**
1319 19th Street NW
Washington, DC 20036-1802
Phone: 202-296-6267
Toll-free: 800-365-9753
Fax: 202-296-5149
e-mail: jamis@heldref.org
Managing Editor: Elisabeth A. Graves
Editorial Director: Douglas J. Kirkpatrick
Covers of policy, management, marketing, finance. *$47.00*
4x Year   Since: 1970
Circulation: 437

8917 JOURNAL OF COUNTRY MUSIC
4 Music Square E
Nashville, TN 37203-4321
Phone: 615-416-2001
Fax: 615-255-2245

8918 JOURNAL OF MUSIC THEORY
Yale University
PO Box 208310
Department of Music
New Haven, CT 06520
Phone: 203-432-2985
Fax: 203-432-2983
e-mail: jmt.music@yale.edu
Web Site: www.yale.edu/jmt/
Publisher: David Clampitt
Editor: Eric Drott
Music theory academic journal *$44.00*
SemiAnnual Since: 1958
Circulation: 1,700

8919 JOURNAL OF MUSIC THERAPY
American Music Therapy Association
Suite 1000
8455 Colesville Road
Silver Spring, MD 20910-3315
Phone: 301-589-3300
Fax: 301-589-5175
e-mail: info@musicaltherapy.org
Web Site: www.musictherapy.org
Editor: Jayne Standley, PhD, MT.BC
Research in the area of music therapy and rehabilitation, a
forum for authoratative articles of current music therapy
research and theory, use of music in the behavioral
sciences, book reviews, and guest editorials. *$120.00*
Quarterly
Circulation: 6,000 6 M names

**8920 JOURNAL OF MUSICOLOGICAL
RESEARCH**
Gordon and Breach Science Publishers
270 8th Avenue
New York, NY 10011-1619
Phone: 510-642-4247
Fax: 212-645-2459
Web Site: www.gbhap.com
Statistical summaries and research reports on the study of
music. *$91.00*
Quarterly

8921 JOURNAL OF MUSICOLOGY
University of California Press, Journals Division
Suite 203
2000 Center Street Way
Berkeley, CA 94704-1223
Phone: 510-643-7154
Fax: 510-642-9917
e-mail: journals@ucop.edu
Web Site: www.ucpress.edu
Editor: John Nadas
Circulation Director: Kathi Young
Advertising Manager: Marge Dean
A review of music history and analysis. *$37.00*

Quarterly
Circulation: 1,450

8922 JUGGLER'S WORLD MAGAZINE
PO Box 443
Davidson, NC 28036-0443
e-mail: bigiduz@davison.edu
Web Site: www.juggling.org
Editor: Bill Giduz
Interviews, current events and information on juggling.
$20.00
Quarterly
Circulation: 3,000

8923 JUICE SOUND, SURF SKATE MAGAZINE
Suite D
52 Market Street
Venice, CA 90291
Phone: 310-399-5336
Fax: 310-399-8687

8924 JUKEBOX COLLECTOR MAGAZINE
2545 SE 60th Ct
Des Moines, IA 50327-5099
Phone: 515-265-8324
Fax: 515-265-1980
Editor: Rick Botts
Focuses on collectors of jukeboxes from the 40's, 50's,
and 60's. There are approximately 150 jukeboxes for sale
each month, along with show events information. Accepts
advertising. *$33.00*
36 pages Monthly Since: 1977
Circulation: 1800

8925 LASERIST
International Laser Display Association
Suite B-23
4301 32nd Street W
Bradenton, FL 34205-2700
Phone: 941-758-6881
Fax: 941-758-1605
e-mail: ildadirect@aol.com
Web Site: www.laserist.org
Editor: David Lyte
Executive Director: Linda Hare
Magazine of the laser entertainment and display industry.
$19.95
Quarterly
Circulation: 2,000

8926 LEONARD MUSIC JOURNAL
Pergamon Press
660 White Plains Road
Tarrytown, NY 10591-5104
Phone: 914-524-9200
Fax: 914-333-2444
Addresses the role of science and technology in
contemporary music. *$35.00*

8927 LIGHTING DIMENSIONS
Primedia Business
9800 Metcalf Avenue
Overland Park, KS 66212

Phone: 913-341-1300
Fax: 913-967-1898
e-mail: inquiries@primediabusiness.com
Web Site: www.intertec.com
Publisher: Jacqueline Tien
Editorial Director: David Barbour
Trade publication for lighting professionals in film, theatre, television, concerts, clubs, themed environments, architecctural, commercial, and industrial lighting. Sponsors of the LDI Trade Show and the Broadway Lighting Master Classes.

8929 LIVE SOUND! INTERNATIONAL
Huge Press
#222
4741 Central
Kansas City, MO 64112-1533
Phone: 913-677-8688
Fax: 913-677-6621
e-mail: amclean@livesoundint.com
Web Site: www.livesoundint.com
Publisher: Mark Herman
Editor: Anthony McLean
The editorial focus is Performance Audio and Event Sound. Contains audio production techniques, new products, equipment applications and associated commercial concerns. *$25.00*
7x Year
Circulation: 20,000
Printed in on glossy stock

8930 LIVING BLUES
University of Mississippi
Room 301
Hill Hall
University, MS 38677-9999
Phone: 662-915-5742
Fax: 662-915-7842

8931 LOTTERY BUSINESS
GEM Communications
17 High Street
Norwalk, CT 06851
Phone: 203-852-1340
Fax: 203-852-6746
Web Site: www.worlgaminglive.com
GEM's mission is to be the primary information source for the key decision makers in the wordwide casino, lottery, parimutuel, bingo, and emerging internet wagering markets.

8932 MBI MUSIC BUSINESS INTERNATIONAL
United Business Media
1 Ten Plaza
New York, NY 10119
Phone: 212-714-1300
Fax: 212-279-2969
e-mail: james@dotmusic.com
Web Site: www.unm.com
Publisher: Steve Redmond
Editor: James Poletti

Leading international music business trade magazine. Coverage of the international music industry, profiles and interviews, detailed reports on developed and emerging music markets, surveys of how new media is affecting the business. *$195.00*
BiMonthly
Circulation: 10,000

8936 MID-ATLANTIC EVENTS MAGAZINE
Suite 700
1080 N Delaware Avenue
Philadelphia, PA 19125-4330
Phone: 215-426-7800
Toll-free: 800-521-8588
Fax: 215-426-9720
e-mail: editor@eventsmagazine.com
Web Site: www.eventsmagazine.com
Publisher: Jim Cohn
Associate Editor: Richard Kupka
96 pages   6x Year Since: 1987
Circulation: 26,000
Printed in 8 colors on glossy stock

8937 MIX
PRIMEDIA
#12
6400 Hollis Street
Emeryville, CA 94608-1086
Phone: 510-653-3307
Fax: 510-653-5142
Web Site: www.mixonline.com
Publisher: Jeffrey Turner
Editor: George Petersen
Geared to professionals and aspiring professionals in the music industry, articles include recording engineering and production industry news, product reviews, and information concerning audio recording. *$46.00*
210 pages   Monthly Since: 1977
Circulation: 50,255

8938 MUSIC
Maher Publications
PO Box 906
102 N Haven
Elmhurst, IL 60126-2970
Phone: 630-941-2030
Fax: 630-941-3210
Editor: Mike Matrey
Information including industry news, retailer profiles, new products, business management and merchandising features. *$19.95*
Monthly
Circulation: 8,949

8939 MUSIC & SOUND RETAILER
Testa Communications
25 Willowdale Avenue
Port Washington, NY 11050
Phone: 516-767-2500
Fax: 516-767-9335
e-mail: testa@testa.com

8940 MUSIC ROW
PO Box 158542
1231 17th Avenue S
Nashville, TN 37215-8542
Phone: 615-321-3617
Fax: 615-329-0852
e-mail: news@musicrow.com
Web Site: www.musicrow.com
Editor/Publisher: David M. Ross
Music business industry reporters and critics review
records, music videos, and current news items, as well as
the discovery of hot new talent. *$159.00*
14x Year
Circulation: 5,000

8941 MUSIC TRADES MAGAZINE
Music Trades
80 W Street
Englewood, NJ 07631
Phone: 201-871-1965
Fax: 201-871-0455
Web Site: www.musictrades.com
Publisher: Paul Majeski
Leading magazine serving music retailers throughout
North America.

8942 MUSIC AND SOUND RETAILER
Testa Communications
25 Willowdale Avenue
Port Washington, NY 11050-3779
Phone: 516-767-2500
Fax: 516-767-9335
Publisher: Vincent Testa
Associate Publisher: Eric Young
Editor: Jeff Casey
Monthly newsmagazine for musical instrument and sound
product sellers, directed toward store managers, owners,
and floor sales personnel. Monthly survey of hottest-
selling products. *$18.00*
80 pages Monthly Since: 1984
Circulation: 11347
Printed in on matte stock

8943 MUSICAL MERCHANDISE REVIEW
50 Brook Road
Needham, MA 02494
Phone: 781-453-9310
Toll-free: 800-964-5150
Fax: 781-453-9389

8944 NATIONAL SQUARES
National Square Dance Convention
Apartment 2
6768 S E Street
Indianapolis, IN 46227-2250
Phone: 562-988-2275
Fax: 562-490-3425
e-mail: sbaysinger@juno.com
Web Site: earthlink.net/~zebrow
Editor: Floyd Lively
Editor: Clare Lively
General Chairman: Steve&Sharon Baysinger

A national square dance magazine published by the
National Executive Committee of the National Square
Dance Convention. *$5.00*
55 pages Quarterly
Circulation: 3,000

8945 NEW ENGLAND THEATRE JOURNAL
New England Theatre Conference
360 Huntington Avenue
Boston, MA 02115-5005
Phone: 617-373-2000
Fax: 617-424-9275
Operations Manager: Corey Boniface
Editor: Stuart Hecht
Scholarly and general educational articles about theatre;
overview of regional companies. *$10.00*
Circulation: 700

8946 NEW ON THE CHARTS
Music Business Reference
70 Laurel Pl
New Rochelle, NY 10801-7105
Phone: 914-632-3349
Fax: 914-633-7690
e-mail: info@note.com
Web Site: www.note.com
Publisher/Editor: Leonard Kalikow
A music business information service for professional use
only. *$225.00*
40 pages Monthly Since: 1976
Circulation: 5,000

8947 NIGHTLIFE MAGAZINE
990 Motor Parkway
Central Islip, NY 11722-1001
Phone: 631-435-8890
Fax: 516-435-8925
e-mail: nynl@aol.com
Publisher: Michael Cutino
Editor-In-Chief: Fran Petito
$2.50
Monthly
Circulation: 125,000

8948 NO COVER MAGAZINE
Suite 218
1935 Camino Vida Roble
Carlsbad, CA 92008
Phone: 760-602-0246
Fax: 760-602-0270

8949 NOUVEAU MAGAZINE
Barbara Tompkins
5933 Stoney Hill Road
New Hope, PA 18938-9602
Phone: 215-794-5996
Fax: 215-794-8305
e-mail: nouvo@comcast.net
Publisher: Barbara E. Tompkins
Editor: Barbara E. Tompkins
Features theater reviews.

140 pages 1x Month Since: 1981
Circulation: 11,000
Printed in on matte stock

8950 OFFBEAT

Suite 200
421 Frenchmen Street
New Orleans, LA 70116-2022
Phone: 504-944-4300
Toll-free: 877-944-4300
Fax: 504-944-4306
e-mail: editor@offbeat.com
Web Site: www.offbeat.com
Publisher/Editor: Jan Ramsey
Managing Editor: Joseph L. Irrera
Consumer-oriented music magazine focusing on New Orleans and Louisiana music. Regular columns on Cajun music, zydeco, traditional and contemporary jazz, brass band (Mardi Gras second-line music), New Orleans R & B, Louisiana and delta blues, Gospel, modern and roots rock and our internationally-appreciated culture and cusine. Information on music fairs and festivals in the region is given. *$2.95*
96 pages Monthly Since: 1988 ISSN 1090-0810
Circulation: 50,000
Printed in 4 colors on newsprint stock

8951 OPERA AMERICA NEWSLINE

Opera America
Suite 810
1156 15th Street NW
Washington, DC 20005-1704
Phone: 202-293-4466
Fax: 202-393-0735
e-mail: frontdesk@operaamerica.org
Web Site: www.operaamerica.org
Information Service Manager: Betsy Archetti
Publications Coordinator: Katherine Enle
Interview, articles, and brief reports on events in the opera field and other news that affects it. This magazine is a compendium of information from a variety of sources, including opera companies, Congress, the National Endowment for the Arts, the American Arts Alliance and other art organizations. Also covers opera activities, legislation and includes audition notices, awards,and positions available. *$40.00*
24 pages 10 x Per Year
Circulation: 2,000 : html

8952 OPERA JOURNAL

National Opera Association
West Texas State University
Canyon, TX 79016-0001
Fax: 806-656-2076
Editor: Robert Hansen
Articles and reviews on opera. *$20.00*
Quarterly
Circulation: 1,000

8953 OPERA MONTHLY

That New Magazine
4th Floor
28 W 25th Street
New York, NY 10010-2705

Fax: 212-727-9321
Reviews and interviews for the opera lover. *$25.00*
Monthly Circulation: 5,000

8954 PERFORMING ARTS

Performing Arts Network
Suite 350
10350 Santa Monica Boulevard
Los Angeles, CA 90025-5075
Phone: 310-551-1115
Fax: 310-551-1939
e-mail: info@performingartsmagazine.com
Web Site: www.performingartsmagazine.com
Editor-in-Chief: David Bowman
A publication aimed at the performing arts industry.
50 pages Monthly Since: 1965
Circulation: 750,000
Printed in 4 colors on glossy stock

8956 PERFORMING ARTS INSIDER MAGAZINE

Total Theatre
PO Box 62
Hewlett, NY 11557-0062
Phone: 516-295-1511
e-mail: totalpost@totaltheater.com
Author: Richmond Shepard
Gives detailed current and advance notice of all plays running and coming into New York up to a year in advance, and lists plays running in major U.S. cities, Canada and England. *$260.00*
BiWeekly Since: 1944
Circulation: 2,000

8957 PERFORMING ARTS MAGAZINE

Suite 350
10350 Santa Monica Boulevard
Los Angeles, CA 90025-5075
Phone: 310-551-1115
Fax: 310-551-1939
e-mail: info@performingartsmagazine.com
Web Site: www.performingartsmagazine.com
Editor Chief: David Bowman
Program book publisher.
12x Per Year Since: 1965
Circulation: 500K

8958 PIANO GUILD NOTES

American College of Musicians
808 Rio Grande Street
Austin, TX 78701
Phone: 512-478-5775
Fax: 512-478-5843
e-mail: ngpt@aol.com
Web Site: www.pianoguild.com
President: Richard Allison
Editor: Pat McCabe-Leche
Music industry publication focusing on Piano Guild members and activities. *$15.00*
Quarterly
Circulation: 11,000
Printed in 2 colors

8959 PIANO QUARTERLY
String Letter Publishing
255 W End Avenue
San Rafael, CA 94901
Phone: 415-485-6946
Fax: 415-485-0831
Editor: David Lusterman
Surveys piano literature and methods. *$20.00*
64 pages Monthly Since: 1952

8960 PIANO TECHNICIANS JOURNAL
Piano Technicians Guild
3930 Washnigton
Kansas City, MO 64111-3538
Phone: 816-753-7747
Fax: 816-531-0070
e-mail: ptg@unicom.net
Web Site: www.ptg.org
Publisher: Dan W. Hall
Advertising Manager: Shawn Bruce
Communications Manager: Joe Zeman
Covers technical issues and other business matters of the Piano Technicians Guild.Tuning and piano rebuilding and technical topics.
$95.00
60 pages Monthly Since: 1960
Circulation: 4200 4,000 names
Printed in 4 colors on glossy stock

8961 PITCH PIPE
Sweet Adelines International
PO Box 470168
Tulsa, OK 74147-0168
Phone: 918-622-1444
Toll-free: 800-992-7464
Fax: 918-665-0894
e-mail: Joey@sweetadelineintl.org
WebSite: www.sweetadelineintl.org
Publisher/Editor: Joey Mechelle Stenner
Official publication of Sweet Adelines International, the world's largest singing performance and music education organization for women. Publication features news and educational articles about and for our members. Accepts advertising.
36-50 pages Quarterly Since: 1947
Circulation: 30,000
Mailing list available for rent 30M names
Printed in 4 colors on
glossy stock

8962 PLAY METER
Skybird Publishing Company
PO Box 24170
6600 Fleur De Lis Drive
New Orleans, LA 70184
Phone: 504-488-7003
Toll-free: 888-473-2373
Fax: 504-488-7083
e-mail: news@playmeter.com
Web Site: www.playmeter.com/pmhome
Editor: Valerie Cognevich
Circulation Editor: Renee Pierson
Production Manager: Jane Nisbet

Covers the industry every month with the new product descriptions, interviews with the movers and shakers in the coin - operated entertainment industry, news, company profiles, trends, family entertainment center information, tax tips, game reviews from players, tournament and leauge updates, international news and more. *$25.00 Monthly*

8963 PLAYBACK
ASCAP
1 Lincoln Plaza
New York, NY 10023
Phone: 212-621-6322
Fax: 212-362-7328
Editor: Erik Philbrook
BiMonthly
Circulation: 100,000

8964 PLAYBILL - BOSTON
2nd Floor
332 Congress Street
Boston, MA 02210-1217
Phone: 617-423-3400
Fax: 617-423-7108
Publisher: Philip S. Birsh
Editor: Rita Fucillo
Features local and national theater news.
Monthly
Circulation: 118,000

8965 PLAYBILL - NEW YORK
11th Floor
52 Vanderbilt Avenue
New York, NY 10017-3808
Phone: 212-557-5757
Fax: 212-682-2932
e-mail: bobcharles@playbill.com
Web Site: www.playbill.com
Publisher: Philip S. Birsh
Editor: Judy Samelson
Theater publication providing cast names and information about Broadway play's.
Monthly Since: 1984
Circulation: 1,129,00

8966 PLAYBILL - PHILADELPHIA
5th Floor
3401 N I Street
Philadelphia, PA 19134-1442
Phone: 972-425-1155
Fax: 214-425-1155
Publisher: Philip S. Birsh
Editor-In-Chief: Joan Alleman
Theater magazine.
Monthly Since: 1945
Circulation: 180,000

8967 PLAYBOARD
3-11720 Voyager Way
Richmond,BC, V6x3g9, BC

Phone: 604-278-5881
Fax: 604-278-5813
e-mail: theatre@direct.ca
Web Site: plaboardmag.com
Publisher: Alan Slater
An informative guide to the live arts, theatre and broadway shows in the greater Vancouver area.
Monthly Since: 1965
Circulation: 35,000

8968 PLAYS, DRAMA MAGAZINE FOR YOUNG PEOPLE

Kalmbach Publishing Company
PO Box 1612
21027 Crossroads Circle
Waukesha, WI 53187-1612
Phone: 262-796-8776
Fax: 262-796-1142
Web Site: www.playsmag.com
Editor: Elizabeth Preston
Includes eight to ten royalty-free one-act plays, arranged by age level. Modern and traditional plays for the celebration of all important holidays and occasions. Adaptable to all cast sizes with easy to follow instructions for settings and costumes. A complete source of original plays and programs for school-age actors and audiences. *$30.00*
7x Year Since: 1940
Circulation: 8,000
Printed in on matte stock

8969 POLLSTAR

4697 W Jacquelyn Avenue
Fresno, CA 93722-6413
Phone: 559-271-7979
Toll-free: 800-344-7383
Fax: 209-271-7979
e-mail: info@pollstar.com
Web Site: www.pollstar.com
Editor-In-Chief: Gary Bongiovanni
Advertising Manager: Brad Snavely
Publication provides contact directories for talent agencies.
Weekly Since: 1981
Circulation: 18,000

8970 POLLSTAR: CONCERT HOTWIRE

4697 W Jacquelyn Avenue
Fresno, CA 93722-6413
Phone: 559-271-7900
Fax: 559-271-7979
Web Site: www.pollstar.com
Marketing Director: Gary Smith
Director Advertising: Paul Fountaine
For 20 years, Pollstar has provided music business professionals with the most reliable and accurate source of worldwide cocert tour schedules, ticket sales results, music industry contact directories, trade news and unique specialized data services. *$339.00*
48 Weekly Issues Since: 1982
Printed in 4 colors on matte stock

8973 PRE-VUE ENTERTAINMENT

National Pre-Vue Network
7825 Fay Avenue
La Jolla, CA 92037-4252
Phone: 858-454-1276
Fax: 760-542-0114
Publisher: Penny Langford
Movie-goers guide to the movies.
Circulation: 204,053

8974 PRELUDE

400 Cumberland Street
Ottawa, Ontario K1N-8X3
Phone: 613-241-7888
Fax: 613-241-3112
Publsiher: Stephen Ball
Managing Editor: Marc Choma
Covers music, theater, and dance.

8976 PREVUE

Mediascene, Mediascene Preview
Box 974
Reading, PA 19601
Phone: 610-371-4574
Fax: 212-888-3602
Publisher: James White
Advertising: Barbara Hanes
$4.00
Circulation: 250,000

8977 PRO AUDIO REVIEW

IMAS Publishing
PO Box 1214
Falls Church, VA 22041-0214
Phone: 703-998-7600
Fax: 703-820-3245
e-mail: par@imaspub.com
Web Site: www.proaudioreview.com
Publisher: John Gatski
Corporate Director Marketing: Sheryl Unangst
National Sales Manager: Alan Carter
Reviews of the latest new equipment written by audio professionals in the field, from bench tests checking the specs, to new product announcements. *$3.95*
Monthly Since: 1995
Circulation: 30,000 30,000 names $145 per M.

8978 PRO SOUND NEWS

United Business Media
1 Ten Plaza
New York, NY 10119
Phone: 212-714-1300
Fax: 212-378-2160
e-mail: pro@psn.com
Web Site: www.prosoundnews.com
Senior Editor: Frank Wells
Coverage of recording studios, sound companies, and post production facilities, as well as discussing the live sound. *$30.00*
Monthly
Circulation: 24,343

8980 PROMENADE
Promenade Magazine
6th Floor
20 E 49th Street
New York, NY 10017-1023
Phone: 212-888-3500
Fax: 212-888-3602
Publisher: James White
$4.00
Circulation: 225,000

8983 PUNCTURE
PO Box 14806
Portland, OR 97293-0806
Phone: 503-232-1649
Fax: 503-777-4627

8984 QUARTERNOTE
American Musicians Union
8 Tobin Court
Dumont, NJ 07628
Phone: 201-384-5378
Editor: Carol Intorre
Covers issues concerning union musicians. *$5.00*
Quarterly
Circulation: 150

8985 RAY GUN
Suite 204
2812 Santa Monica Boulevard
Santa Monica, CA 90404-2410
Phone: 310-315-1501
Fax: 310-315-1525
e-mail: webmaster@raygun.com
Web Site: www.raygun.com
Publisher: Seth Seaberg
Editor: Randy Bookasta
$18.95
Monthly

8986 RECREATIONAL BUSINESS OPPORTUNITIES
Weisner Publishing, LLC
7009 S Potomac Street, #200
Englewood, CO 80112-4034
Phone: 303-397-7600
Fax: 303-397-7619
Web Site: www.recreationalbusiness.com
Publisher: Whitney Crosby-Newman
Accurate market information to brokers, buyers and sellers showcasing recreational businesses and properties for sale.
$15.00
Quarterly
Circulation: 14,000

8987 REPLAY MAGAZINE
Replay Publishing
PO Box 7004
Tarzana, CA 91357-7004
Phone: 818-776-2880
Fax: 818-776-2888
e-mail: editor@replaymag.com
Web Site: www.replaymag.com

Publisher: Ed Adlum
Circulation: Ingrid Milkes
Advertising Director: Barry Zweben
Publication for the coin-operated entertainment industry.
$65.00
200 pages   Monthly   Since: 1975
Circulation: 4,300

8988 REQUEST
10400 Yellow Circle Drive
Minnetonka, MN 55349-9102
Phone: 952-931-8490
Toll-free: 800-325-0075
Fax: 612-931-8490
e-mail: staff@requestline.com
Web Site: www.requestline.com
Publisher: Karen Weium
Assistant Editor: Amy Welvoda
$12.95
Monthly
Circulation: 500,000

8989 REVIEW
STS Press
5645-E General Washington Drive
Alexandria, VA 22312-2403
Phone: 703-642-5758
Fax: 703-642-5838
Publisher: L.T. Bolt
Editor: Terri Corcoran
Features reviews of performing and visual arts. *$12.00*
24 pages   Monthly   Since: 1971
Circulation: 5,000
Printed in 1 color on newsprint stock

8990 REVOLUTION
Johnathan Simpson Blint
150 N Hill Drive
Brisbane, CA 94005
Phone: 415-468-4684
Fax: 415-468-4686
e-mail: jsimpson-bint@imaginemedia.com
Web Site: www.planetrevolution.com
Managing Editor: Jason Black
Executive Editor: Jason Brookes

8991 RHYTHM MAGAZINE
Suite 204
928 Broadway
New York, NY 10010-6008
Phone: 212-253-8869
Toll-free: 800-464-2767
Fax: 212-253-8892

8992 ROCKET
2028 5th Avenue
Seattle, WA 98121-2505
Phone: 206-728-7625
Fax: 206-728-8827
e-mail: rocketsea@aol.com
Web Site: www.musicuniverse.com
Publisher: Dennis Erokan
Editor: Steve Duda

2x Month
Circulation: 80,000

8993 ROCTOBER

#617
1507 E 53rd Street
Chicago, IL 60615
Phone: 773-288-5448
Fax: 773-288-5443

8994 ROLLER COASTER

American Coaster Enthusiasts News
Suite 115
5800 Foxridge Drive
Mission, KS 66202-2333
Phone: 913-262-4512
Fax: 913-262-0174
e-mail: webmaster@aceonline.org
Web Site: wwwaceonline.org
Publications Director: Tim Baldwin
Editor/Director: Tom Rhodes
Features news about roller coasters all over the world, roller coaster openings and preservation of coasters and all news associated
with roller coasters.
32-40 pages Quarterly
Printed in 4 colors on glossy stock

8995 SCRYE

Krause Publications
700 E State Street
Iola, WI 54990
Phone: 715-445-2214
Fax: 715-445-4087
Editor: John Jackson Miller
The guide to collectible card games. *$24.00*
132 pages BiMonthly
Printed in 4 colors on glossy stock

8996 SHAKESPEARE BULLETIN

Lafayette College
English Department
Easton, PA 18042-1781
Phone: 610-330-5245
Fax: 610-330-5606
e-mail: lusardij@lafayette.edu
Web Site: www.shakespeare-bulletin.org
Co-Editor: James P Lusardi
Co-Editor: June Schlueter
Covers performance criticism and scholarship on Shakespeare and Renaissance drama. *$20.00*
48 pages Quarterly Since: 1982
Circulation: 1,000
Printed in on matte stock

8997 SHEET MUSIC MAGAZINE, STANDARD PIANO- GUITAR EDITION

Music Group
333 Adams Street
Bedford Hills, NY 10507

Phone: 914-244-8500
Fax: 914-244-8560
e-mail: sheetmusic@yestermusic.com
Web Site: www.sheetmusicmagazine.com
Managing Editor: Kirk Miller
The actual reproduction of popular songs, both words and music, feature articles on various aspects of musical performance and interest for various types of musicians, and self improvement features for keyboard and fretter instrument players. *$18.97*
BiMonthly
Circulation: 50,000

8998 SHOW MUSIC

PO Box A
East Haddam, CT 06423-0466
Phone: 860-873-8664
Fax: 860-873-2329
e-mail: rklink@goodspeed.org
Web Site: www.showmusic.org
Managing Editor: Ryan Klink
Editor-in-Chief: Max O. Preeo
Internationally aclaimed by professionals and fans as the premier magazine covering musical theatre around the world, Show Music combines insightful interviews ans reviews of productions, recordings, videos and books.
$25.00
80 pages Quarterly
Circulation: 5,000
Mailing list available for rent 5000 names $130 per M.
Printed in 4 colors on
glossy stock
Computerized version available

8999 SHOWBIZ MAGAZINE

800 S Valley View Boulevard
Las Vegas, NV 89107-4411
Fax: 702-382-1089
Editor: Jim McGlasson
A total entertainment and weekly television schedule. Features articles on celebrities, shows, a restaurant guide, complete art gallery and show listings with a gaming section.
Weekly
Circulation: 142,000

9000 SINGING NEWS

330 University Hall Drive
Boone, NC 28607-6118
Phone: 828-264-3700
Fax: 828-264-4621
e-mail: singnews@world.std.com
Web Site: www.singingnews.com
Publisher: Maurice Templeton
Editor: Terry Keaksey
Managing Editor: Danny Jones
Circulation Director: Jamie Tedder
A fan and trade magazine that serves the southern gospel music industry. Accepts advertising. *$20.00*
132 pages Monthly Since: 1969
Circulation: 200,000

9001 SISTER 2 SISTER
Sister 2 Sister
Suite 205
9301 Annapolis Road
Lanham Seabrook, MD 20706-3152
Phone: 301-270-5999
Fax: 301-270-0085
Publisher: Jamie Foster
Editor: Mamie Lee Foster
African American fan magazine of Americas hottest entertainment industry's movies, music and television celebrities. *$3.00*

9002 SLOT MANAGER
GEM Communications
17 High Street
Norwalk, CT 06851
Phone: 203-852-1340
Fax: 203-852-6746
Web Site: www.worldgaminglive.com

9003 SONDHEIM REVIEW
PO Box 11213
Chicago, IL 60611-0213
Phone: 773-275-4254
Toll-free: 800-584-1020
Fax: 773-275-4254
e-mail: info@sondheimreview.com
Web Site: www.sondheimreview.com
Publisher: Ray Birks
Editor: Paul Salsini
$5.95
32 pages Quarterly Since: 1994
Circulation: 4,0000 6,000 names $105 per M.
Printed in on glossy stock

9004 SOUTHWESTERN MUSICIAN/TEXAS MUSIC EDUCATOR
Dennis Brothers Printers, Lubbock,TX
PO Box 140465
Austin, TX 78714-0465
Phone: 512-452-0710
Fax: 512-451-9213
e-mail: rfloyd@tmea.org
Web Site: www.tmea.org
Editor/Executive Director: Robert Floyd
Author: Robert Floyd
The magazine has 10 issues per year. $15 subscription rate. Annual TMEA membership of $50 includes magazine.
22
10x Year Since: 1938
Circulation: 9,500
Mailing list available for rent 10,000 names
Printed in 4 colors

9005 SPECTRUM
110 S Jefferson Street
Dayton, OH 45402-1810
Phone: 937-220-1600
Fax: 937-220-1642
Web Site: www.thinktv.org

Publisher: Dave Mikesell
Editor: Barb Compton-Keene
Monthly
Circulation: 23,000

9006 STAGE DIRECTIONS
PO Box 18869
Raleigh, NC 27619
Phone: 919-872-7888
Toll-free: 800-362-6765
Fax: 919-872-7888
e-mail: stagedir@aol.com
Web Site: www.enews.com/magazines/stage
Publisher: Susan M. Wershing
Managing Editor: Neil Offen
Practical guide for regional,community, and college theater groups. *$26.00*
10x Year Since: 1988
Circulation: 7,000

9007 STAGES
Curtains
Apartment 5A
301 W 45th Street
New York, NY 10036-3825
Fax: 201-836-4107
Editor: Frank Scheck
The national theatre magazine. *$20.00*
Monthly
Circulation: 35,000

9009 STAR BEACON
Earth Star Publications
PO Box 117
Paonia, CO 81428-0117
Phone: 970-527-3257
Fax: 970-527-2433
e-mail: earthstar@tripod.net
Web Site: www.earthstarpublications.com
Editor: Anne Miller
Unique source of information on UFO's, earth changes, latest sightings, conference news and reports, health/healing, spirituality, book reviews, art, poetry, astrology and meta physics.
Monthly
Circulation: 500

9010 SWEET SWING BLUES ON THE ROAD
Here are jive-talking cat daddies in the Amen Cadence, gorgeous and mysterious women in the Sweet Refrain, exotic vistas in the Bridge, and in the Chorus musicians, like J-Master on piano, who live the music the way they play it. *$14.00*
192 pages Paperbound ISBN 1-560251-55-7

9011 SYMPHONY MAGAZINE
American Symphony Orchestra League
5th Floor
33 W 60th Street
New York, NY 10023
Phone: 212-262-5161
Fax: 202-783-7228
Hyslop: Chester Sandra

The official magazine of the American Symphony Orchestra League, provides news, features and commentary about American symphony orchestras and increases public awareness of the value of orchestras, their repertoire, and their service to the community. *$35.00*
BiMonthly
Circulation: 17,000

9012 TCI: THEATRE CRAFTS INTERNATIONAL
PRIMEDIA Intertec-Communications & Entertainment
32 W 18th Street
New York, NY 10011-4612
Phone: 212-229-2965
Fax: 212-229-2084
e-mail: jackietien@intertec.com
Web Site: www.etecnyc.net
Publisher: Jacqueline Tien
Provides information on staging, production, costuming, makeup, sound, architecture, lighting design, and related stage technology, includes information on administration and management, as well as presenting detailed casebooks and how-to's on all aspects of theatre technology.
$40.00
11x Year
Circulation: 16,500

9013 TD&T
6443 Ridings Road
Syracuse, NY 13206-1111
Phone: 315-463-6463
Toll-free: 800-938-7488
Fax: 315-463-6525
e-mail: info@office.usitt.org
Web Site: www.usitt.org
Public Relations/Marketing Manager: Barbara El Lucas
Sales Manager: Michelle L. Smith
For professionals in theatre design and technology.

9014 TEACHING THEATRE
3368 Central Parkway
Cincinnati, OH 45225-2307
Phone: 513-559-1996
Fax: 513-559-0012
Editor: James Palmarini
Quarterly

9015 TECHNICAL BRIEF
Yale School of Drama
222 York Street
New Haven, CT 06511-4804
Phone: 203-436-1095
Fax: 203-432-8336
Editor: Bronislaw Sammler
Editor: Don Harvey
Written by professionals for professionals, providing a dialogue between technical practitioners from the several performing arts. The succinct articles, complete with mechanical drawings, represent the best solutions to recurring technical problems.

9018 TELEGUIA USA
Lancer Productions
Suite 213
1241 S Soto Street
Los Angeles, CA 90023
Phone: 323-881-6515
Fax: 323-881-6524
e-mail: teleguia@aol.com
Publisher: John DiCarlo
Editor: Elizabeth DiCarlo
Office Manager: Lorena Mata
Weekly Since: 1986
Circulation: 100,000
Printed in 4 colors on newsprint stock

9019 TEXAS MUSIC MAGAZINE
700 W 6th Street
Austin, TX 78701-2708
Phone: 512-472-6630
Fax: 603-687-9749

9020 THEATER MAGAZINE
Yale School of Drama
222 York Street
New Haven, CT 06511-4804
Phone: 203-436-1095
Fax: 203-432-8336
Editor: Erika Munk
Business Manager: Laraine Sammler
Publishes the most noted American and International critics, playwrights and scholars. Each issue contains essays, a major new playscript, reports from abroad, interviews, photographs, and theater and book reviews.
$22.00
TriAnnual Since: 1968
Circulation: 2,500
Mailing list available for rent 1.5M names
Printed in 1 color on matte stock

9021 THEATRE BILL
Jerome Press
2nd Floor
332 Congress Street
Boston, MA 02210-1217
Phone: 617-423-3400
Fax: 617-423-7108
Publisher: Rita K. Fucillo
Associate Editor: Rita A. Fucillo

9022 THEATRE DESIGN & TECHNOLOGY
6443 Ridings Road
US Institute for Theatre Technology
Syracuse, NY 13206-1111
Phone: 315-463-6463
Toll-free: 800-938-7488
Fax: 315-463-6525
e-mail: info@office.usitt.org
Web Site: www.usitt.org
Editor: David Rodger
Art Director: Deborah Hazelett
Focuses on developments in technical theater. *$48.00*
Quarterly Since: 1965
Circulation: 4,000

9023 THEATRE JOURNAL
Johns Hopkins University Press
2715 N Charles Street
Baltimore, MD 21218
Toll-free: 800-548-1784
Fax: 410-516-6968
e-mail: jlorder@jhupress.jhu.edu
Web Site: www.press.jhu.edu/press
Editor: Susan Bennett
Co-Editor: David Roman
One of the most authoritative and useful publications of theatre studies available today. Theatre Journal features social and historical studies, production reviews, and theoretical inquiries that analize dramatic texts and production. *$20.00*
Quarterly
Circulation: 3,327

9024 THEATRE TOPICS
2715 N Charles Street
Baltimore, MD 21218
Phone: 410-516-6990
Toll-free: 800-548-1784
Fax: 410-516-6968
e-mail: jlorder@hupress.jhu.edu
Web Site: www.press.jhu.edu
Editor: Harley Erdman
The first theatre publication devoted to issues of concern to practitioners, Theatre Topics focuses on performance studies, dramaturgy, and theatre pedagogy. *$20.00*
2x Year Since: 1990
Circulation: 1900

9025 TOASTMASTER
Toastmasters International
PO Box 9052
Mission Viejo, CA 92690-9052
Phone: 949-858-8255
Fax: 949-858-1207
Web Site: www.toatmasters.org
Editor: Suzanne Frey
Associate Editor: Kelly Ann LaCascia
Publishes educational articles on the subject of communication in general and public speaking in particular. Accepts advertising.
$20.00
32 pages Monthly Since: 1933
Circulation: 185,000
Printed in 4 colors on glossy stock

9026 TUNING IN
American Association for Music Therapy
Suite 1000
8455 Colesville Road
Silver Spring, MD 20910
Phone: 301-589-3300
Fax: 301-589-5175
Web Site: www.namt.com
Educational information and news on music therapies.
Quarterly

9027 US INSTITUTE FOR THEATRE TECHNOLOGY
Suite 5A
10 W 19th Street
New York, NY 10011-4206
Phone: 212-852-1000
Fax: 212-924-9343
Editor: Cecelia Fielding
Advertising/Sales: Helen Willard
An organization on the construction of theatres, technical developments and education information.

9028 USITT SIGHTLINES
6443 Riding Road
Syracuse, NY 13206-1111
Phone: 315-463-6463
Toll-free: 800-938-7488
Fax: 315-463-6525
e-mail: info@office.usitt.org
Web Site: www.usitt.org
Editor: Barbara E R Lucas
16-28 pages 11x Year Since: 1960
Circulation: 3,500
Printed in on matte stock

9029 URB MAGAZINE
Suite 1012
1680 N Vine Street
Los Angeles, CA 90028-8838
Phone: 323-993-0291
Fax: 323-466-1207

9030 URBAN NETWORK
SFX Multimedia Group
120 N Victory Boulevard
Burbank, CA 91502-1852
Phone: 818-843-5800
Fax: 818-843-4888
e-mail: urbnet@networkmags.com
President: Miller London
Album reviews, personality profiles, news from radio stations, and the latest music sales. *$375.00*
Weekly
Circulation: 1,200

9031 VIDEOGAMES
LFP
Suite 900
8484 Wilshire Boulevard
Beverly Hills, CA 90211-3221
Phone: 323-651-5400
Fax: 323-651-3525
$3.00
Circulation: 101,839

9032 VIRTUAL REALITY WORLD
Mecklermedia Corporation
20 Ketchum Street
Westport, CT 06880-5908
Phone: 203-341-2806
Fax: 203-454-5840
Editor in Chief: Sandra Heisel
Production Director: Sandra Huggard

Covers developments and use of virtual reality in the areas of entertainment, design, military use, networking and medical use.
Circulation: 30,000

9034 WHAT'S NEW FOR FAMILY FUN CENTERS

Adams Business Media
Suite 1150
250 S Wacker Drive
Chicago, IL 60606
Phone: 312-977-0999
Fax: 312-977-1042
Web Site: www.coach@aip.com
Product tabloid for the industry, presenting a virtual trade show of products in each issue.

9035 WHITE TOPS

Circus Fans Association of America
PO Box 59710
Potomac, MD 20859-9710
e-mail: mohlerbros@aol.com
Entertainment magazine aimed at circus fans.
BiMonthly
Circulation: 2,100

9037 YOUR FLESH QUARTERLY

PO Box 25764
Chicago, IL 60625-0764
Phone: 773-583-8148
Fax: 773-583-8178
e-mail: yourflesh@att.worldnet.net

9038 YOUTH THEATRE JOURNAL

American Alliance for Theatre and Education
PO Box 872002
Arizona State University, Dept. of Theatre
Tempe, AZ 85287-2002
Phone: 480-965-6064
Fax: 480-965-5351
e-mail: aate.info@asu.edu
Web Site: www.aate.com
Administrative Director: Christy Taylor
A journal covering research in the field of children and youth theatre world. *$25.00*
Annual 900 names $150 per M.

Trade Shows

9039 AMERICAN ASSOCIATION OF MUSIC THERAPY

PO Box 80012
Valley Forge, PA 19484-0012
15 booths. October

9040 AMERICAN CHORAL DIRECTORS ASSOCIATION DIVISIONAL CONVENTIONS

American Choral Directors Association
PO Box 6310
Lawton, OK 73506
Phone: 580-355-8161
Fax: 580-248-1465
e-mail: acda@acdaonline.org
Web Site: www.acdaonline.org
Executive Director: Gene Brooks
Seminar and over 50 exhibits of choral music, equipment, supplies and services. Check for your area.
1000 Attendees Biennial Since: 1959

9041 AMERICAN DANCE GUILD

PO Box 2006
Lenox Hill Station
New York, NY 10021
Phone: 212-932-2789
e-mail: julia@americandanceguild.org
Web Site: www.americandanceguild.org
Executive Director: Karen Deaver
Trade show for dance professionals and those who offer products and supplies to the industry. 10 booths.
200 Attendees July

9042 AMERICAN GUILD OF ORGANISTS, REGIONAL CONFERENCE

Suite 1260
475 Riverside Drive
New York, NY 10115
Over 20 exhibits and a workshop for professional, amatuer and student organists.
Biennial

9043 AMERICAN HARP SOCIETY NATIONAL CONFERENCE

6331 Quebec Drive
Hollywood, CA 90068-2831
Phone: 213-463-0716
Fax: 213-464-2950
Executive Secretary: Dorothy Remsen
Workshop and over 20 exhibits for professional, amateur and student harpists.
300 Attendees Annual Since: 1962

9044 AMERICAN INSTITUTE OF ORGANBUILDERS

PO Box 130982
Houston, TX 77219-0982
Phone: 713-529-2212
Editor: Howard Maple
Annual convention includes supplier exhibits, technical lectures and tours to area organs. 20 booths.
300 Attendees October

9045 AMERICAN MUSIC CONFERENCE

5790 Armada Drive
Carlsbad, CA 92008-4608

Phone: 760-438-9124
Toll-free: 800-767-6266
Fax: 760-438-7327
e-mail: sharonn@roman.com
Web Site: www.amc-music.com
President: Michael Faulhaber
Association represents the public relations and research arm of the music industry. The only organization promoting the benefits of music, music making and music education to the general public.
275 Attendees Since: 1947
Printed in 2 colors on glossy stock

9046 AMERICAN MUSIC THERAPY ASSOCIATON ANNUAL CONFERENCE
Suite 930
8455 Colesville Road
Silver Spring, MD 20910
Phone: 301-589-3300
Fax: 301-589-5175
e-mail: conference@musictherapy.org
Web Site: www.musictherapy.org
Seminar and 80 exhibits of publications, musical insturments, books, learning aids and recordings.
1500 Attendees Annual Since: 1950

9047 AMERICAN MUSICAL INSTRUMENT SOCIETY
414 E Clark Street
Vermillion, SD 57069-2307
Fax: 605-677-5073
Web Site: www.amis.org
President: Harrison Powley
10 booths.
April

9048 AMERICAN MUSICOLOGICAL SOCIETY ANNUAL CONVENTION
University of Pennsylvania
201 S 34th Street
Philadelphia, PA 19104
Phone: 215-898-8698
Toll-free: 888-611-4267
Fax: 215-573-3673
e-mail: ams@sas.upenn.edu
Web Site: www.ams.net.org
Executive Director: Robert Judd
A society of professional musicologists and university educators. The annual meetings are held in the fall each year; 2000: Toronto; 2001: Atlanta; 2002: Columbus; 2003: Houston. *$45.00*
1200 Attendees Annual Since: 1948

9049 AMERICAN ORFF-SCHULWERK ASSOCIATION NATIONAL CONFERNCE
American Orff-Schulwerk Association
PO Box 391089
Cleveland, OH 44139-8089
Phone: 440-543-5366
Fax: 440-543-2687
e-mail: info@avsa.org
Web Site: www.aosa.org
Executive Director: Cindi Wobig

110 exhibits of music, music books, software, insturments, and gifts in addition to National Conference of 2000+ music educators. 2002 conference - Las Vegas, NV.
2400 Attendees November Since: 1969

9050 AMERICAN SOCIETY FOR AESTHETICS ANNUAL CONFERENCE
PO Box 1881
404 Cudahy Hall, Marquette University
Milwaukee, WI 53201-1881
Phone: 414-228-7831
Fax: 414-228-7889
e-mail: asastcar@vms.csd.mu
Web Site: www.aestheticsonline.org
Seminar, conference, and exhibits related to the study of the arts, all disiplines.
500 Attendees Annual Since: 1942

9051 AMERICAN SYMPHONY ORCHESTRA LEAGUE NATIONAL CONFERENCE
5th Floor
33 W 60th Street
New York, NY 10023
Phone: 212-262-5161
Fax: 212-262-5198
e-mail: league@symphony.org
Web Site: www.symphony.org
Show Manager: Stephen Alter
80 booths incorporating all facets of classical music industries including industry suppliers, music publishers and computer technology.
1500 Attendees June

9052 AMUSE WORLD
Glahe International
PO Box 2460
Germantown, MD 20875-2460
Phone: 301-515-0012
Fax: 301-515-0016
e-mail: glahe@glahe.com
Exhibits of amusement machinery and related articles.

9053 AMUSEMENT COIN MACHINE EXPO
Association of American Amusement Machines
Suite 201
450 E Higgins Road
Elk Grove Village, IL 60007
Phone: 847-290-9088
Toll-free: 800-546-3300
Fax: 800-546-3300
e-mail: wtglasgow@aol.com
Web Site: www.asishow.com
President: William T. Glasgow Sr.
150 booth exposition features coin-operated amusement games and related products.
6M Attendees March

9054 AMUSEMENT INDUSTRY EXPO
I-X Center
6200 Riverside Drive
Cleveland, OH 44135

Phone: 216-265-2619
Toll-free: 800-870-3976
Fax: 216-265-2621
e-mail: events@i-xcenter.com
Web Site: www.i-xcenter.com
Assistant Show Manager: Brian Hopkins
Supplies and products for the amusement industry.
4100 Attendees Annual Since: 1995

**9055 AMUSEMENT SHOWCASE
INTERNATIONAL**
Association of American Amusement Machines
Suite 201
450 E Higgins Road
Elk Grove, IL 60007
Phone: 847-290-9088
Toll-free: 800-546-3300
Fax: 800-546-3300
Web Site: www.asishow.com
President: William T. Glasgow Sr.
Amusement industry exhibition.
Annual

**9056 AMUSEMENT AND MUSIC OPERATORS
ASSOCIATION CONVENTION**
Amusement & Music Operators Association
Suite 202
450 E Higgins Road
Elk Grove Village, IL 60007
Phone: 847-290-5320
Fax: 847-290-0409
e-mail: amoa@amoa.com
Web Site: www.amoa.com
Annual show of 250 companies. Exhibits of
coin-operated arcade, video and gaming machines, games,
juke boxes, stuffed toys, records and jewelry.
8000 Attendees Annual Since: 1948

**9057 ASSOCIATION OF COLLEGE UNIONS
INTERNATIONAL PROF. CONFERENCE**
Suite 200
120 W 7th Street
Bloomington, IN
Phone: 812-855-8550
Fax: 812-855-0162
e-mail: marcanne@indiana.edu
Web Site: www.indiana.edu/nacui
Member Services: Mary Ann Cannon
100 exhibits of graphic supplies, recreation equipment,
computer hardware & software, furnishings, entertainment
and speaker bureau information, food service equipment,
and more related information and supplies.
1000 Attendees Annual Since: 1951

9058 BAND ORCHESTRA CLINIC MIDWEST
Midwest Clinic
Suite 2
1920 Waukegan Road
Glenview, IL 60025-2229
Fax: 847-729-4635
e-mail: info@midwestclinic.org
Show Manager: Barbara Buehlman

Exhibits are composed of music accessories and other
related aspects in the music world.
10M Attendees December

9059 CHORUS AMERICA TRADE SHOW
Suite 310
1156 15th Street NW
Washington, DC 20005
Phone: 202-331-7577
Fax: 202-331-7599
e-mail: service@chorusamerica.org
Web Site: www.chorusamerica.org
Director Member Services: Jack Reiffer
Containing 25 booths and 25 exhibits.
500 Attendees June 700 names
Printed in 2 colors on matte stock

**9060 COLLEGE MUSIC
SOCIETY/ASSOCIATION FOR
TECHNOLOGY IN MUSIC**
College Music Society
202 W Spruce Street
Missoula, MT 59803
Phone: 406-721-9616
Fax: 406-721-9419

9061 COUNTRY RADIO SEMINAR
Country Radio Broadcasters
819 18th Avenue S
Nashville, TN 37203
Phone: 615-327-4487
Fax: 615-329-4492
e-mail: info@crb.org
Web Site: www.crb.org
Executive Director: Paul Allen
100 booths.
2300 Attendees February/March

9062 EVENTS! EXPO
Shore Varrone
Suite 200
6255 Barfield Road NE
Atlanta, GA 30328-4332
Toll-free: 800-241-9034
Fax: 770-252-4436
VP Trade Shows: Russ Eisenhardt
Brings together every facet of the events industry.
Exhibitors include major sporting and entertainment
events, event sponsors, festivals, arts, and charitable
events. 175 exhibitors in total.
4M Attendees October

**9063 FLORIDA MUSIC EDUCATORS
ASSOCIATION CLINIC /CONFERENCE**
Florida Music Educators Association
207 Office Plaza Drive
Tallahassee, FL 32301
Phone: 850-878-6844
Fax: 850-942-1793
60000 Attendees

9064 FOLK ALLIANCE
Folk Alliance
Suite 501
1001 Connecticut Avenue NW
Washington, DC 20036
Phone: 202-835-3655
1500 Attendees

9065 FORUM
ISPAA
6065 Pickerel Drive NE
Rockford, MI 49341-9052
Phone: 616-874-5703
Fax: 616-874-5723
Executive Director: Michael Hardy
95 booths.
400 Attendees December

9066 GOSPEL MUSIC WEEK
Gospel Music Association
1205 Division Street
Nashville, TN 37203-4011
Phone: 615-242-0303
Fax: 615-254-9755
Web Site: www.gospelmusic.org
Director/Event Management: David Votta
Annual trade show presented by the GMA, a widely
recognized voice for gospel music in all its forms and
variations, dedicated to providing leadership, direction and
unity for all facets of the gospel music industry.
Convention features approximately 65 exhibitors.
3,000 Attendees April Since: 1964
Circulation: 2,000

9067 GOSPEL MUSIC WORKSHOP AMERICA
3908 W Warren Avenue
Detroit, MI 48208-1824
Phone: 313-898-6900
Fax: 313-898-4520
Web Site: www.gmwa.org
Convention Manager: Marc Smith
275 booths.
16M Attendees August

9068 HARMONY INTERNATIONAL
PO Box 470168
Tulsa, OK 74147-0168
Phone: 506-459-8443
Toll-free: 888-871-7762
Show Manager: Peggy Pryor
30 booths.
8M Attendees October

9069 HORN CALL TRADE SHOW
International Horn Society
PO Box 6111
WVU College of Creative Arts
Morgantown, WV 26506-6111
Fax: 907-790-4066
e-mail: exec-secretary@hornsociety.org
Web Site: www.hornsociety.org
Show Manager: Esa Tapani
Advertising Agent: Paul Austin

Features recitals, lectures, reading sessions, and 50
exhibits in Lahti, Finland.
450 Attendees August 3600 names $70 per M.

**9070 IAAPA ORLANDO CONVENTION &
TRADE SHOW**
Int. Association of Amusement Parks & Attractions
1448 Duke Street
Alexandria, VA 22314
Phone: 703-836-4800
Fax: 703-836-4801
e-mail: mparsont@iaapa.org
Web Site: www.iaapa.org
VP Exhibitions: David K. Lee
Exhibit Manager: Marc Parsont
Amusement and theme park information, supplies and
equipment.
30000 Attendees November 6000+ names

9071 ILDA CONFERENCE
International Laser Display Association
Suite B-23
4301 32nd Street W
Bradenton, FL 34205-2700
Phone: 941-758-6881
Fax: 941-758-1605
e-mail: ildadirect@aol.com
Web Site: www.laserist.org
Containing 25 exhibits.
November

9072 IMEA STATE CONVENTION
IMEA/Indiana Music Educators Association
Ball State University School of Music
Mucie, IN 47306
Phone: 219-759-2561
12000 Attendees

**9073 INTERNATIONAL ASSOCIATION JAZZ
EDUCATION CONVENTION**
International Association of Jazz Educators
PO Box 724
Manhattan, KS 66502
Phone: 785-776-8744
Fax: 785-776-6190
e-mail: info@iaje.org
Web Site: www.iaje.org
Executive Producer: Steve Baker
Largest annual gathering of the global jazz community
7000 Attendees January

**9074 INTERNATIONAL ASSOCIATION OF
AMUSEMENT PARKS & ATTRACTIONS
CONVENTION**
Int'l Association of Amusement Parks & Attractions
1448 Duke Street
Alexandria, VA 22314-3403
Phone: 703-836-4800
Fax: 703-836-4801
e-mail: convention@iaapa.org
Web Site: www.iaapa.org

Conventions Director: David Leeel
Exhibit Manager: Marc Parsont
Convention Sales/Services: Beth Baumgardener
The world's largest tradeshow geared to the amusement park and attraction industry, running the gamut of exhibitions from high tech, to games, rides, food and beverage and much more. IAAPA showcases products and services for amusement parks, water parks, family enterainment centers, zoos, aquariums, museums—any company in the business of entertainment. Upcoming shows: November 2002-2004, Orange County Convention Center, Orlando, Florida USA
30M Attendees November Since: 1918

9075 INTERNATIONAL ASSOCIATION OF JAZZ EDUCATORS CONFERENCE
International Association of Jazz Educators
PO Box 724
Manhattan, KS 66502-2815
Fax: 785-776-6190
e-mail: iaje@aol.com
Web Site: www.iaje.org
Conference Coordinator: Bill McFarlin
Annual show of 125 manufacturers, suppliers and distributors of music, musical instruments, accessories, apparel, electronics, travel information and other services for musicians and educators.
5000 Attendees

9076 INTERNATIONAL DANCE ASSOCIATION IDEA CONVENTION
6190 Cornerstone Ct E
San Diego, CA 92121-4701
Phone: 858-784-3700
Fax: 858-535-8234
Convention Director: Noel Schartier
Clothing and footwear, exercise products, equipment and services. 200 booths.
4M Attendees July

9077 INTERNATIONAL DANCE EXERCISE ASSOCIATION IDEA CONVENTION
6190 Cornerstone Center E
San Diego, CA 92121-4701
Phone: 858-784-3700
Fax: 561-535-8979
Convention Director: Patricia Howard Jones
200 booths including exhibits on aerobic and dance exercise clothing and footwear.
1.5M Attendees March/May

9078 INTERNATIONAL NEW AGE TRADE SHOW
KJ Expositions
Suite 209
7200 E Hampden Avenue
Denver, CO 80224
Phone: 303-757-5969
2500 Attendees

9079 INTERNATIONAL STEEL GUITAR CONVENTION
9535 Midland Boulevard
Saint Louis, MO 63114-3314
Fax: 314-427-0516
President: Dewitt Scott, Sr.
65 booths that provide entertainment from steel guitarists and various instruments including the bass guitar.
3M Attendees Labor Day

9080 INTERNATIONAL TICKETING ASSOCIATION
INTIX
Suite 722
250 W 57th Street
New York, NY 10107-0799
Phone: 212-581-0600
Fax: 212-581-0885
e-mail: info@intix.org
Web Site: www.intix.org
President: Patricia Spira, CAE
Special Projects: Ann Marie Gennardo
Deputy Director: Kathleen O'Donnell
Not-for-profit association whose purpose is to advance the success of the admission service industry and its members.
$195.00
1500 Attendees January Since: 1980

9081 LEISUREXPO
Leisure Mini Golf & Entertainment Center Show
920 Honeysuckle Lane
Wynnewood, PA 19096-1667
Fax: 610-448-4630
Show Manager: Al Barry
Annual show of 250 manufacturers, distributors and suppliers of arcade games, food and beverage, mini golf, consultants, insurance facility suplies, go carts, laser tag, simulators, souvenir merchandise, amusement rides.
6800 Attendees

9082 MAGIC KIDS
MAGIC International
Suite 303
6200 Canoga Avenue
Woodland Hills, CA 91367
Phone: 818-593-5000
Fax: 310-593-5020
Web Site: www.magiconline.com
MAGIC Kids is the largest, most prestigious children's apparel, accessories and footweat event in the United States. This event contains boys' and girls' products in sizes layette to 'tween, powerful advertising and sponsorhsip opportunities, year round marketing, advertising and promotion.
90000 Attendees February

9083 MAGICIANS ALLIANCE EAST STATES
127 York Street
Gettysburg, PA 17325-1933
Secretary/Treasurer: Pierre Fountaine
15 booths.
250 Attendees August/September

9084 MENC STATE MUSIC EDUCATORS ASSOCAITION MEETING
Bobbie Smith
4110 Tralee Road
Tallahassee, FL 32308
Phone: 941-853-6146
Fax: 941-853-6130

9085 MENC STATE MUSIC EDUCATORS ASSOCIATION MEETING
Thomas Mosher
998 Ridge Avenue
Manasquan, NJ 08736
Phone: 732-528-1144
1000 Attendees

9086 MENC STATE MUSIC EDUCATORS ASS. MEETING
Norvil Howell
304 W Christopher
Clovis, NM 88101
Phone: 505-763-7019
Fax: 505-793-7452
1500 Attendees

9087 MENC STATE MUSIC EDUCATORS ASSOCIATION MEETING
Deena Lawley
272 N 600 W
Valparaiso, IN 46383
Phone: 207-876-4625

9088 MENC STATE MUSIC EDUCATORS ASSOCIATION - MEETING
Thomas Dean
3 Sewart Center
Dover, DE 19904
Phone: 302-672-1554
Fax: 302-674-3650
60 Attendees

9089 MIDWEST INTERNATIONAL BAND & ORCHESTRA CLINIC
Midwest International Band & Orchestra Clinic
1503 Huntington Drive
Glenview, IL 60025
Phone: 847-729-4629
Fax: 847-729-4635

9090 MUSIC EDUCATORS EASTERN DIVISION CONFERENCE
Music Educators National Conference
1806 Robert Fulton Drive
Reston, VA 20191
Phone: 703-860-4000
Fax: 703-291-5464

9091 MUSIC INDUSTRY CONFERENCE
1902 Association Drive
Reston, VA 20191-1502

Music forum.
April

9092 MUSIC TEACHERS NATIONAL ASSOCIATION NATIONAL CONFERENCE
Music Teachers National Association
Suite 505
441 Vine Street
Cincinnati, OH 45202-2811
Phone: 513-421-1420
Toll-free: 888-512-5278
Fax: 513-421-2503
e-mail: mtnant@mtna.org
Web Site: www.mtna.org
Director Meetings: Jennifer Martin
Annual conference for independent and collegiate music teachers. Containing 150 booths and 80 exhibits.
2000 Attendees March
Circulation: 23,289 23,289 names $90 per M.

9093 MUSIC TEACHERS NATIONAL ASSOCIATION CONVENTION
Music Teachers National Association
Suite 505
441 Vine Street
Cincinnati, OH 45273
Phone: 513-421-1420
1700 Attendees

9094 NAMM INTERNATIONAL MUSIC MARKET
National Association of Music Merchants
5790 Armada Drive
Carlsbad, CA 92008
Phone: 760-438-8001
59500 Attendees

9095 NAMM INTERNATIONAL MUSIC PRODUCTS ASSOCIATION
5790 Armada Drive
Carlsbad, CA 92008-4608
Phone: 760-438-8001
Toll-free: 800-767-6266
Fax: 760-438-7327
e-mail: tradeshow@namm.com
Web Site: www.namm.com
July

9096 NATIONAL ASSOCIATION MUSIC MERCHANTS WINTER MARKET
5140 Avenida Encinas
Carlsbad, CA 92008-4372
Phone: 760-438-8001
Toll-free: 800-767-6266
Fax: 760-438-7327
Web Site: www.namm.com
President: Joe Lamond
Show Manager: John Vincent
600 booths of musical instruments and accessories.
32M Attendees January

9097 NATIONAL ASSOCIATION MUSIC MERCHANTS SOUND EXPO
5140 Avenida Encinas
Carlsbad, CA 92008-4372
Phone: 760-438-8001
Toll-free: 800-767-6266
Fax: 760-738-7327
Web Site: www.namm.com
President: Joe Lamond
Show Manager: John Vincent
800 booths featuring displays of musical instruments and accessories.
30M Attendees June

9098 NATIONAL ASSOCIATION OF MUSIC MERCHANTS SUMMER SESSION
National Association of Music Merchants
5790 Armada Drive
Carsbad, CA 92008
Phone: 760-438-8001
Fax: 760-438-3483
e-mail: info@namm.com
Web Site: www.namm.com
20000 Attendees

9099 NATIONAL ASSOCIATION OF MUSIC MERCHANTS INTERNATIONAL MUSIC MARKET
National Association of Music Merchants
5790 Armada Drive
Carlsbad, CA 92008-4608
Phone: 760-438-8001
Toll-free: 800-767-6266
Fax: 760-438-7327
e-mail: kevin@namm.com
Web Site: www.namm.com
Trade Shows Director: Kevin Johnstone
Annual show of musical instruments and accessories, acoustical equipment and sheet music publications. 1,100 exhibitors.
65000 Attendees January

9100 NATIONAL ASSOCIATION OF PASTORAL MUSICIANS NATIONALO CONVENTION
National Association of Pastoral Musicians
225 Sheridan Street NW
Washington, DC 20011
Phone: 202-723-5800
4000 Attendees

9101 NATIONAL ASSOCIATION OF RECORDING MERCHANDISING
Suite 120
9 Eves Drive
Marlton, NJ 08053-3130
Phone: 856-596-2221
Fax: 859-596-3268
e-mail: still@narm.com
Web Site: www.narm.com
Director of Meetings/Conventions: Linda M. Still
150 booths covering all areas of the recording industry. 2000 trade show in San Antonio, Texas.
3M Attendees February/March

9102 NATIONAL OPERA ASSOCIATION CONFERENCE
National Opera Association
PO Box 60869
Canyon, TX 79016
Phone: 806-651-2857
Fax: 806-651-2958
e-mail: rhansen@mail.wtamu.edu
Web Site: www.noa.org
Executive Secretary: Robert Hansen
Editor: Robert Thieme
Annual conference and exhibits of opera related equipment, supplies and services. Quarterly publications of the Opera Journal, articles pertaining to opera productions and singer/actor training.
130 Attendees Annual Since: 1954 1M names $75 per M.

9103 NATIONAL SQUARE DANCE CONVENTION
Apartment 2
6768 SE Street
Indianapolis, IN 46227-2250
Phone: 317-635-4455
Web Site: www.sqdancing.com
Editor: Floyd Lively
250 booths and 250 exhibitors.
20M+ Attendees June

9104 NEW ENGLAND THEATRE CONFERENCE
Northeastern U. 360 Huntington Ave
Cushing Hall # 221, 102 The Fenway
Boston, MA 02115
Phone: 617-424-9275
Fax: 617-424-1057
e-mail: info@NETConline.org
Web Site: www.NETConline.org
Executive Director: Tara McCarthy
Conference for theater professionals.
800+ Attendees November Since: 1952
Circulation: 50Booths

9105 NEW MUSIC SEMINAR
#G29
332 Bleecker Street
New York, NY 10014-2980
This show features 97 booths of the most concentrated group of professionals in the music industry.
8M Attendees June

9106 NEW YORK STATE SCHOOL MUSIC ASSOCIATION WINTER CONFERENCE
New York State School Music Association
2165 Seaford Avenue
Seaford, NY 11783

Phone: 416-409-0200
Toll-free: 888-697-7621
Fax: 516-409-6033
e-mail: nyssmaexec@aol.com
Web Site: www.nyssma.org
Executive Administrator: Dr. Bert Nelson
4500 Attendees December

9107 NORTHEAST PERFORMING ARTS CONFERENCE
Suite 205
277 Linden Street
Wellesley, MA 02482
Phone: 781-235-3771
Toll-free: 877-272-3771
Fax: 781-235-1055
e-mail: info@nepac.org
Web Site: www.nepac.org

9108 OPERA AMERICA
Suite 810
1156 15th Street NW
Washington, DC 20005
Phone: 202-293-4466
Fax: 202-393-0735
Web Site: www.operaam.org
30 booths.
275 Attendees February

9109 PIANO TECHNICIANS GUILD ANNUAL CONVENTION
Piano Technicians Guild
3930 Washington
Kansas City, MO 64111
Phone: 816-753-7747
Fax: 816-531-0070
e-mail: ptg@ptg.org
Web Site: www.ptg.org
Show Manager: Shawn Bruce
Executive Director: Dan Hall
Trade show of pianos and tools/supplies used by piano tuners and rebuilders.
1,000 Attendees June

9110 PINBALL EXPO
Pinball Expo/Flip Out Pinball Tournament
2671 Youngstown Road SE
Warren, OH 44484-4404
Phone: 330-369-1192
Toll-free: 800-323-3547
Fax: 330-369-6279
e-mail: brkpinball@aol.com
Web Site: www.pinballexpo.org
Chairman: Robert Berk
Annual show of 25 manufacturers and related suppliers of pinball machines and supplies. Containing 70 booths and 25 exhibits.
1000 Attendees October

9111 SANDRA FRIDY
MENC: The National Association for Music Education
1806 Robert Fulton Drive
Reston, VA 20191-4348

Phone: 703-860-4000
Toll-free: 800-336-3768
Fax: 703-860-4000
e-mail: sandraf@menc.org
Web Site: www.menc.org
Exhibits Manager: Sandra Fridy
300 booths featuring music education products and sciences
5M Attendees April 65,000 names

9112 SHOWEST
Suite 706
116 N Robertson Boulevard
Los Angeles, CA 90048-3110
Phone: 310-657-7724
Fax: 310-657-4758
Executive Director: Herbert Burton
272 booths exhibiting theater equipment and concession offerings for the theater industry.
292 Attendees March Since: 1975

9113 SHOWBIZ EXPO
Live Time
2459 Panorama Terrace
Los Angeles, CA 90039-2537
Phone: 323-668-1811
Fax: 323-668-1033
Co-Producer: Nalini Lasiewicz
150 booths providing a unique environment for the film and video production communities.
5.5M Attendees September

9114 SHOWBIZ EXPO WEST
Live Time
2459 Panorama Terrace
Los Angeles, CA 90039-2537
Phone: 323-668-1811
Fax: 323-668-1033
Co-Producer: Nalini Lasiewicz
400 booths for the film and video professions.
22M Attendees June

9115 SOUTH DAKOTA IN - SERVICE MUSIC CONFERENCE
Corliss Johnson
PO Box 2212
South Dakota State University
Brookings, SD 57007
Phone: 605-688-5188
Fax: 605-688-4307
e-mail: Corliss_Johnson@sdstate.edu
Web Site:
www3.sdstate.edu/academics/artsandscience/music
300 Attendees

9116 SQUARE ROUND DANCE FESTIVAL MIDSOUTH
5263 S Germantown Road
Memphis, TN 38141-8527
Fax: 901-385-2064
Chairman: Bill Tinnaro
10 booths.
1M Attendees November

9117 TEXAS MUSIC EDUCATORS ASSOCIATION ANNUAL CLINIC/CONVENTION
Texas Music Educators Association
Box 140465
Austin, TX 78714-0465
Phone: 512-452-0710
Fax: 512-451-9213
e-mail: tkelly@tmea.org
Web Site: www.tmea.org
Exhibits Manager: Tesa Kelley
20M Attendees February
Circulation: 10,500

9118 THEATREFEST
Theatre Bay Area
Suite 375
870 Market Street
San Francisco, CA 94102-3002
Phone: 415-430-1140
Fax: 415-430-1145
e-mail: tba@theatrebayarea.org
Web Site: www.theatrebayarea.org
Manager: Dale Albright
A place for actors, acting students, theatre teachers, theatre companies, and volunteers of services to network. 90+ booths.
500+ Attendees May

9119 US INSTITUTE FOR THEATRE TECHNOLOGY ANNUAL CONFERENCE & STAGE EXPO
6443 Ridings Road
USITT
Syracuse, NY 13206-1111
Phone: 315-463-6463
Toll-free: 800-938-7488
Fax: 315-463-6525
e-mail: info@office.usitt.org
Web Site: www.usitt.org
Sales Manager: Helen Willard
Public Relations/Mktg. Manager: Barbara E.R. Lucas
More than 150 sessions, seminars and workshops plus a three-day exposition featuring cutting edge design and technology for theater and live performing arts.
3.5M Attendees March

9120 UNITED STATES INSTITUTION FOR THEATRE TECHNOLOGY CONFERENCE
Reed Exhibition Companies
255 Washington Street
Newton, MA 02458-1637
Fax: 617-630-2222
International Sales: Elizabeth Hitchcock
The only event which draws the top production, design and technical theatre professionals from across the country.
3M Attendees March

9121 WFSB TV 3 FESTIVAL FOR KIDS
North East Promotions
274 Silas Deane Highway
Weatherfield, CT 06109
Phone: 860-529-2123
Fax: 860-529-2317
e-mail: info@northeastpromo.com
Web Site: www.northeastpromo.com
VP: Joe Gonsalves
VP Sales/Marketing: Kristie Gonsalves
The Festival for Kids will be full of fun rides, commercial and non profit exhibits that both parents and kids will visit to obtain information on services and products that are available to them. WFSB TV3 and Infinity Broadcasting will have an area that will have interactive and informative fun for all attendees.
25000 Attendees February

9122 WORLD WATERPARK ASSOCIATION
PO Box 14826
Shawnee Mission, KS 66285-4826
Phone: 913-599-0300
Fax: 913-599-0520
e-mail: wwa@waterparks.com
Web Site: www.waterparks.org
Convention Manager: Marc McNeal
Director of Show: Patty Miller
320 booths: exhibits include waterpark attractions, water quality equipment and apparel.
2000 Attendees October

9123 WORLD OF BLUEGRASS
International Bluegrass Music Association
1620 Frederica Street
Owensboro, KY 42301
Phone: 270-684-9025
Toll-free: 888-GET-IBMA
Fax: 270-686-7863
e-mail: ibma@ibma.org
Web Site: www.ibma.org
Executive Director: Dan Hays
Special Projects Coordinator: Nancy Cardwell
Member/Convention Services: Jill Snider
Containing 100 booths.
1,800 Attendees October

Directories & Databases

9124 ACB NATIONAL DIRECTORY OF BANDS
Association of Concert Bands
Suite 102
2533 S Maple Avenue
Tempe, AZ 85282-3559
Toll-free: 800-726-8720
Fax: 480-894-1986
Association news of the music industry.
Annual

9125 AMC NEWS
American Music Conference
5790 Armada Drive
Carlsbad, CA 92008-4608
Phone: 760-431-9124
Fax: 760-438-7327
Web Site: www.amc-music.com
Editor: Pat Page
Production Manager: Amy Edgington
Since: 1947
Circulation: 500
Printed in 2 colors on glossy stock

9126 ACADEMY PLAYERS DIRECTORY
8949 Wilshire Boulevard
Beverly Hills, CA 90211-1907
Phone: 310-247-3058
Fax: 310-550-5034
e-mail: players@oscars.org
Web Site: www.playersdirectory.com
Editor: Keith W. Gonzales
Casting directory published every four months and distributed to the casting departments, directors, executives and others concerned with the employment of motion picture and commercial talent. Also available on-line
Since: 1937   Internet

9127 ACTOR'S PICTURE/RESUME BOOK
Theatre Directories
PO Box 510
Dorset, VT 05251-0510
Phone: 802-867-2223
Toll-free: 800-390-2223
Fax: 802-867-0144
e-mail: theatre@sover.net
Web Site: www.theatredirectories.com
Author: Jill Charles
Create a picture/resume for theatre, film, commercials and TV. *$16.95*

9128 AMERICAN CASINO GUIDE
Casino Vacations
PO Box 703
Dania, FL 33004-0703
Phone: 954-989-2766
Toll-free: 800-741-1596
Fax: 954-966-7048
e-mail: info@americancasinoguide.com
Web
Site: www.americancasinoguide.com
President: Steve Bourie
Publisher: Michelle Bourie
A guide to every casino/resort, riverboat and Indian casino in the United States. *$75.00*
464 pages Annual Since: 1992   ISBN 1-883768-11-X
Printed in 1 color

9129 AMERICAN MUSICAL INSTRUMENT SOCIETY MEMBERSHIP DIRECTORY
University of South Dakota
414 E Clark Street
Vermillion, SD 57069-2307

Phone: 605-677-5306
Fax: 605-677-5073
Directory of services and supplies to the industry.
80 pages Biennial

9130 AMERICAN SOCIETY OF COMPOSERS, AUTHORS AND PUBLISHERS - EAST COAST
1 Lincoln Plaza
New York, NY 10023-7129
Phone: 212-621-6000
e-mail: info@ascap.com
Web Site: www.ascap.com
President/Chairman: Marilyn Bergman
Vice Chairman: Cy Coleman
Secretary: Arthur Hamilton
Treasurer: Arnold Broido
Membership list of composers, authors and other artists nationwide.
125 pages

9131 AMERICAN SOCIETY OF COMPOSERS, AUTHORS AND PUBLISHERS
American Soc. of Composers, Authors & Publishers
1 Lincoln Plaza
New York, NY 10023-7129
Phone: 212-621-6000
Fax: 212-595-3342
Editor: Erik Philbrook
About 20,000 music publishers and their divisions and affiliates.
Annual

9132 ASSOCIATION OF PERFORMING ARTS PRESENTERS MEMBERSHIP DIRECTORY
Suite 400
1112 16th Street NW
Washington, DC 20036-4820
Phone: 202-833-2787
Fax: 202-833-1543
Presenters and arts management agencies in the United States and Canada are listed. *$122.00*
115 pages Annual

9133 AUDARENA STADIUM INTERNATIONAL GUIDE
BPI Communications
PO Box 24970
Nashville, TN 37202-4970
Phone: 615-321-4250
Fax: 615-327-1575
Web Site: www.amusementbusiness.com
Editor: Randy Tierney
Directory of over 6,500 arenas, stadiums, exhibit halls and amphitheatres in the US, Canada and overseas. *$65.00*
Annual Circulation: 9,000

9134 AUDITIONS & SCENES FROM SHAKESPEARE
Theatre Directories
PO Box 510
Dorset, VT 05251-0510
Phone: 802-867-2223
Toll-free: 800-390-2223
Fax: 802-867-0144
e-mail: theatre@sover.net
Web Site: www.theatredirectories.com
Author: Jill Charles
This book will direct an actor, student or teacher to every playable monologue and scene in Shakespeare's canon. *$12.95*

9135 BASELINE
5th Floor
30 Irving Place
New York, NY 10003
Phone: 212-254-8235
Fax: 212-529-3330
e-mail: info@baseline.hollywood.com
Web Site: www.pkbaseline.com
VP Marketing: Linda Brown
This large database offers access to information on the U.S. entertainment industry, with an emphasis on films, television and theater. Files included in this database range from Names, Titles and Rights to Polls, Mail and Video Sales/Rentals.
Full-text

9136 BLUEGRASS RESOURCE DIRECTORY
International Bluegrass Music Association
1620 Fredrica Street
Owensboro, KY 42301
Phone: 270-684-9025
Toll-free: 888-GET-IBMA
Fax: 270-686-7863
e-mail: ibma@ibma.org
Web Site: www.ibma.org
Executive Director: Dan Hays
Provides contacts and info on various companies involved in the Bluegrass music scene. *$25.00*
88 pages   Annual

9137 CAVALCADE OF ACTS AND ATTRACTIONS
Amusement Business
49 Music Square W
Nashville, TN 37203-3213
Phone: 615-329-0555
Fax: 615-327-1575
Web Site: www.amusementbusiness.com
Publisher: Karen Oertley
Associate Publisher: Tom Powell
Directory of personal appearance artist (musical and theatrical), touring shows, carnavals and other specialized entertainment such as fireworks firms, rodeos, etc. Also contains listings of booking agents, personal managers, promoters and producers. *$75.00*
350 pages   Annual, December
Circulation: 7,000

9138 CELEBRITY ACCESS-DIRECTORY: HOW AND WHERE TO WRITE THE RICH & FAMOUS
Celebrity Access Publications
Suite A241
20 Sunnyside Avenue
Mill Valley, CA 94941-1928
Phone: 415-389-8133
e-mail: support@addall.com
Web Site: www.addall.com
Author: Thomas Burford
Editor: Catherine Burford
Directory of Hollywood's finest. *$21.95*
333 pages   Annual   ISBN 0-961975-85-7

9139 CELEBRITY BULLETIN
Celebrity Service
Suite 819
250 W 57th Street
New York, NY 10107-0885
Phone: 212-757-7979
Fax: 212-582-7701
Web Site: www.celebrityservice.com
New York edition offering information on arrivals of celebrities in the vicinity. *$1750.00*
4 pages   BiWeekly

9140 CHAMBER MUSIC AMERICA MEMBERSHIP DIRECTORY
70 Lincoln Ctr Plaza
New York, NY 10023
Phone: 212-875-5776
Contact: Marlissa Monroe
Directory of services and supplies to the industry. *$20.00*
96 pages   Annual

9141 COMEDY USA INDUSTRY GUIDE
Laughing Matters
Apartment 3D
226 E 29th Street
New York, NY 10016
Phone: 212-929-8609
Offers valuable information on comedians, comedy agents, publicists, talent coordinators and television comedy clubs. *$59.95*
300 pages   Annual
Circulation: 2,500

9142 COMICS RETAILER
Krause Publications
700 E State Street
Iola, WI 54990
Phone: 715-445-2214
Fax: 715-445-4087
Web Site: www.krause.com/comics/cr/
Publisher: Mark Williams
Editor: John Jackson Miller
An essential tool for the professional comic retailer and the serious collector. Each issue provides comics retailers and professionals with marketing information, industry news and practical how to tips on selling comics, roleplaying games, anime, and related items.
$29.95

68 pages   Monthly   Since: 1992
Printed in 4 colors on glossy stock

9143   COMMUNITY THEATRE DATABASE
8402 Briar Wood Circle
Lago Vista, TX 78645
Phone: 512-267-0711
Fax: 512-267-0712
e-mail: info@aact.org
Web Site: www.aact.org
Editor: Julie Angelo
The database includes addresses for about 6,000
community theatre organizations in the USA. Only
available to members.
6,000 names $180 per M.

9144   COMPLETE CATALOGUE OF PLAYS
Dramatists Play Service
440 Park Avenue S
New York, NY 10016-8050
Phone: 212-683-8960
Fax: 212-213-1539
e-mail: postmaster@dramatists.com
Web Site: www.dramatists.com
Editor: Bradley G. Kalos
Lists all plays licensed by the Dramatists Play Service.
Annual Circulation: 35,000

9145   COMPLETE DIRECTORY OF RECORDS, TAPES AND VIDEOS
Sutton Family Communications & Publishing
Company
11565 Ridgewood Cir
Seminole, FL 33772-4115
Phone: 727-391-6709
Fax: 727-397-1888
Editor: Theresa Sutton
General Manager: Lee Sutton
Print-out from database of wholesalers, manufacturers,
distributors, importers and close-out houses. Data base is
up-dated daily.
$39.50
100+ pages

9146   CONTEMPORARY DRAMATISTS
St. James Press/Gale Research
27500 Drake Road
Farmington Hills, MI 48331
Phone: 313-961-2242
Toll-free: 800-877-GALE
Fax: 313-961-6741
Over 450 living dramatists who are writing or have
written in the English language are profiled. *$135.00*
843 pages

9147   CONTEMPORARY MUSIC ENSEMBLES: A DIRECTORY
American Music Center
Suite 1001
30 W 26th Street
New York, NY 10010-2011

Phone: 212-366-5260
Fax: 212-366-5265
e-mail: center@amc.net
Web Site: www.amc.net
Editor: Eero Richmond
A directory of over 350 Americans ensembles which have
demonstrated a commitment to performing contemporary
American music. Includes instrumental and/or vocal
chamber groups of two or more performers, one to a part.
$15.00

9148   COSTUME DESIGNERS GUILD DIRECTORY
Suite 309
13949 Ventura Boulevard
Sherman Oaks, CA 91423-3570
Phone: 818-905-1557
Fax: 818-905-1560
Directory of services and supplies to the industry. *$17.90*
200 pages   Annual Circulation: 5,000

9149   DANCE DIRECTORY
American Alliance for Health Phys. Ed. Rec. Dance
1900 Association Drive
Reston, VA 20191-1502
Toll-free: 800-213-7193
Fax: 703-476-9527
Web Site: www.aahperd.org
Includes dance class offerings in programs from two and
four year colleges and universities, high schools and
professional studios in the United States, Canada and
Australia. *$14.95*
Biennial

9150   DANCE MAGAZINE COLLEGE GUIDE
Dance Magazine
Suite 203
111 Myrtle Street
Oakland, CA 94607
Phone: 510-839-6060
Fax: 510-839-6066
e-mail: danceguide@dancemagazine.com
Web Site: www.dancemagazine.com
Dance Magazien College Guide is the source for
information on college and university dance programs.
Includes over 170 undergraduate and graduate programs,
updated yearly with descriptions, audition dates, contact
information and more

9151   DANCE MAGAZINE-SUMMER DANCE CALENDAR ISSUE
Dance Magazine
Floor 10
33 W 60th Street
New York, NY 10023-7905
Phone: 212-245-9050
Toll-free: 800-331-1750
Web Site: www.dancemagazine.com
A list of dance workshops and special programs for
students are listed. *$3.95*
Annual Circulation: 100,000

9152 DANCE/USA MEMBERSHIP DIRECTORY
Dance/USA
Suite 820
1156 15th Street NW
Washington, DC 20005-1704
Phone: 202-833-1717
Fax: 202-833-2686
e-mail: danceusa@danceusa.org
Membership listing.

9153 DINNER THEATRE: A SURVEY AND DIRECTORY
Greenwood Publishing Group
PO Box 5007
88 Post Road W
Westport, CT 06881-5007
Phone: 203-226-3571
Toll-free: 800-225-5800
Fax: 203-750-9790
Web Site: www.greenwood.com
Listings of dinner theaters, including in-depth profiles are offered in this comprehensive directory. *$59.95*
160 pages ISBN 0-313284-42-3

9154 DIRECTORY OF FAIRS, FESTIVALS & EXPOSITIONS
Amusement Business
49 Music Square W
Nashville, TN 37203-3213
Phone: 615-329-0555
Fax: 615-327-1575
Web Site: www.amusementbusiness.com
Publisher: Karen Oertley
Associate Publisher: Tom Powell
Directory of over 4,500 arenas, auditoriums, stadiums, exhibit halls and ampitheaters worldwide, as well as listings of companies offering services and supplies to the industry. *$.90*
350 pages Annual, January
Circulation: 7,000

9155 DIRECTORY OF FUNPARKS & ATTRACTIONS
Amusement Business
49 Music Square W
Nashville, TN 37203-3213
Phone: 615-329-0555
Fax: 615-327-1575
Web Site: www.amusementbusiness.com
Publisher: Karen Oertley
Associate Publisher: Tom Powell
Guide to over 2,600 amusement/theame parks, water parks, tourist attractions, zoos, kiddielands and family entertainment centers worldwide. *$60.00*
130 pages Annual, October Circulation: 8,000

9156 DIRECTORY OF HISTORIC AMERICAN THEATRES
Greenwood Publishing Group
PO Box 5007
88 Post Road W
Westport, CT 06880-4208
Phone: 203-226-3571
Toll-free: 800-225-5800
Fax: 203-750-9790
Web Site: www.greenwood.com
Directory of theaters built between 1800 and 1915. *$75.00*
367 pages ISBN 0-313248-68-0

9157 DIRECTORY OF MUSIC LIBRARIES AND COLLECTIONS IN NEW ENGLAND
A-R Editions
Suite 180
8551 Research Way
Middleton, WI 53562
Phone: 608-836-5825
Web Site: www.musiclibraryassoc.org
Libraries and collections of music and musical literature in the New England states are listed. *$8.50*
105 pages

9158 DIRECTORY OF RECORD AND CD RETAILERS
Power Communication Group
38 Hance Street
Wharton, NJ 07885-2019
Fax: 973-361-2924
Over 1,000 record and compact discs stores are profiled. *$14.95*
370 pages

9159 DIRECTORY OF SCENERY, COSTUMES, MUSICAL MATERIALS AND TITLE PROJECTIONS
Opera America
Suite 810
1156 15th Street MW
Washington, DC 20005
Phone: 202-293-4466
Fax: 202-393-0735
e-mail: Frontdesk@operaamerica.org
Web Site: www.operaam.org
Directory for the entertainment industry of pre production manufacturers and suppliers. *$25.00*
68 pages Biennial

9160 DIRECTORY OF THEATRE TRAINING PROGRAMS
Theatre Directories
PO Box 510
Dorset, VT 05251-0510
Phone: 802-867-2223
Toll-free: 800-390-2223
Fax: 802-867-0144
e-mail: theatre@sover.net
Web Site: www.theatredirectories.com
Editor: Barbara Ax

Offers valuable information on colleges, universities and conservatories offering theater study programs at graduate and undergraduate levels. *$34.50*
280 pages   Biennial   ISBN 0-933919-50-6   580 names

9161   DIRECTORY OF TRADITIONAL MUSIC
International Council for Traditional Music
2960 Broadway
Columbia University, Department of Music
New York, NY 10027
Phone: 212-695-0680
Individuals and institutions interested in traditional music are offered.
120 pages   Biennial

9162   DRAMATICS MAGAZINE - SUMMER THEATRE DIRECTORY
International Thespian Society
2343 Auburn Avenue
Cincinnati, OH 45219-2815
Phone: 513-651-3737
Fax: 513-421-7077
e-mail: info@edta.org
Web Site: www.edta.org
A list of study and performance opportunities in summer schools and summer theatre education programs. *$3.50*
Annual Circulation: 35,000

9163   DRAMATIST'S SOURCEBOOK
Theatre Communications Group
4th Floor
355 Lexington Avenue
New York, NY 10017-6695
Phone: 212-697-5230
Fax: 212-983-4847
e-mail: tcg@teg.org
Web Site: www.tcg.org
Executive Director: Ben Cameron
Lists over 400 theaters that consider new plays for production, festivals and awards and more for the entertainment industry. Over 1,000 listings. 17,000 individual members. *$18.95*
360 pages   Annual   Since: 1980   ISBN 1-559361-75-1
Circulation: 6M

9164   DRAMATISTS GUILD QUARTERLY-DIRECTORY ISSUE
Dramatists Guild
11th Floor
234 W 44th Street
New York, NY 10036-3909
Phone: 212-944-3700
Fax: 212-944-0420
This comprehensive issue is dedicated to Broadway and off-Broadway producers, off-off-Broadway groups, agents, theatres and sources of grants.
Annual

9165   EPM ENTERTAINMENT MARKETING SOURCEBOOK
EPM Communications
160 Mercer Street
New York, NY 10012-3208
Phone: 212-941-0099
Fax: 212-941-1622
e-mail: info@cpmcom.com
Web Site: www.epmcom.com
Over 4,600 media companies, sponsors and retailers that provide products and services to entertainment marketers. *$295.00*
Annual   ISBN 1-885747-36-5
Printed in on matte stock

9166   ENTERTAINMENT MARKETING LETTER
EPM Communications
160 Mercer Street
New York, NY 10012-3208
Phone: 212-941-0099
Fax: 212-941-1622
Database covering marketing techniques used in the entertainment industry. *$319.00*
Monthly

9167   FEEDBACK THEATREBOOKS AND PROSPERO PRESS
Feedback Theatrebooks & Prospero Press
PO Box 220
Nasheag Point Road
Brooklin, ME 04616
Phone: 207-359-2781
Fax: 207-359-5532
Directory of services and supplies to the industry. Specialists in Pre-World War I American Plays (histories, anthologies, single plays). *$14.95*
208 pages

9168   GOSPEL MUSIC NETWORKING GUIDE
Gospel Music Association
1205 Division Street
Nashville, TN 37203-4011
Phone: 615-242-0303
Fax: 615-254-9755
e-mail: GMAToday@aol.com
Web Site: www.gospelmusic.org
Editor: Jackie Chapman
Comprehensive listing of all facets of the gospel music industry — artists, record companies, agents, managers and music publishers.
$37.95
Circulation: 6,000

9169   GREY HOUSE PERFORMING ARTS DIRECTORY
Grey House Publishing
PO Box 860
185 Millerton Road
Millerton, NY 12546
Phone: 518-789-8700
Toll-free: 800-562-2139
Fax: 518-789-0545
e-mail: books@greyhouse.com
Web Site: www.greyhouse.com
Publisher: Leslie Mackenzie
Editor: Laura Mars-Proietti

Current information on over 7,700 dance companies, instrumental music programs, opera companies, choral groups, theatre companies, performing arts series and performing arts facilities. Gives mailing addresses, phone and fax numbers, e-mail addresses, web sites, mission statements, key management contacts, facilities, seating capacity, season, attendance and more. Includes hundreds of performing arts associations, magazines, newsletters, trade shows, directories, data bases, industry web sites.
$220.00
1,104 pages   ISBN 1-930956-03-7

9170 INTERNATIONAL AMUSEMENT INDUSTRY BUYERS GUIDE

Amusement Business
49 Music Square W
Nashville, TN 37203-3213
Phone: 615-329-0555
Fax: 615-327-1575
Web Site: www.amusementbusiness.com
Publisher: Karen Oertley
Associate Publisher: Tom Powell
Complete source book containing comprehensive listings of manufacturers, importers and suppliers of all types of rides, games and merchandise, plus food and drink equipment and suppliers. *$60.00*
130 pages   Annual, October
Circulation: 8,000

9171 INTERNATIONAL BUYER'S GUIDE OF THE MUSIC RECORD-TAPE INDUSTRY

Billboard Directory Central
Nashville, TN
Phone: 615-321-4277
Worldwide music business to business directory. *$75.00*
Annual

9172 INTERNATIONAL DIRECTORY & BUYERS GUIDE

International Association of Amusement Parks
1448 Duke Street
Alexandria, VA 22314-3403
Phone: 703-836-4800
Fax: 703-836-4801
e-mail: iaapa@iaapa.org
Web Site: www.iaapa.org
Editor: Michael Moran
Publisher: William Stevenson
Directory of amusement park and attraction industry and related topics.

9173 INTERNATIONAL DIRECTORY OF THE PERFORMING ARTS

Commonwealth Business Media
10 Lake Drive
Hightstown, NJ 08520-5397
Phone: 609-371-7700
Toll-free: 800-221-5488
Fax: 609-371-7879
e-mail: info@musicalamerica.com
Web Site: www.musicalamerica.com
President/CEO: Alan Glass

The international information center of the performing arts industry

9174 INTERNATIONAL RECORDING STUDIO AND EQUIPMENT DIRECTORY

Billboard Directory Central
Nashville, TN
Phone: 615-321-4277
International recording studies, equipment, and manufacturers are listed worldwide. *$50.00*
100 pages   Annual

9175 INTERNATIONAL TALENT AND TOURING DIRECTORY

Billboard Directory Central
Nashville, TN
Phone: 615-321-4277
A worldwide reference source for talent, talent agents, promoters and products and venues. *$85.00*
Annual Circulation: 5,000

9176 KEYBOARD TEACHERS ASSOCIATION INTERNATIONAL

Dr. Albert DeVito
361 Pin Oak Lane
Westbury, NY 11590-1941
President: Dr. Albert DeVito
Music teachers and those related to keeping members updated as to activity going on in music world.
Quarterly Since: 1963

9177 LOUISIANA MUSIC DIRECTORY

Suite 200
421 Frenchmen Street
New Orleans, LA 70116-2022
Phone: 504-944-4300
Toll-free: 877-944-4300
Fax: 504-944-4306
e-mail: editor@offbeat.com
Web Site: www.offbeat.com
Publisher/Editor: Jan Ramsey
Managing Editor: Joseph L. Irrera
Only privately-published directory of Louisiana musical resources in the nation. Contains over 7,000 listings of music businesses, including such categories as attorneys, recording studios, media, publishers, festivals and fairs, clubs and venues, managers, web services, musician services and instructors and much more. Also listings of over 3,500 band and musicians, with contact phone number and e-mail addresses, along with booking agent information. *$2.95*
140 pages   Monthly ISSN 1072-4427
Printed in 4 colors on newsprint stock

9178 MONEY FOR PERFORMING ARTISTS

American for the Arts
1 E 53rd Street
New York, NY 10022-4200
Phone: 212-223-2787
Toll-free: 180-032-1451
Fax: 732-225-1562
Web Site: www.artsusa.org

Offers information on organizations that sponsor grants, fellowships, artists' residences, competitions and technical assistance for professional artists. *$18.95*
240 pages   Since: 1991   ISBN 0-915400-96-0

9179 MUSIC LITERATURE INTERNATIONAL

International RILM Center
Room 1009
33 W 42nd Street
New York, NY 10036-8003
Phone: 607-225-7126
Fax: 212-642-2642
Offers information on more than 120,000 citations, with abstracts, to significant literature on music and music performances.
Bibliographic

9180 MUSIC-IN-PRINT SERIES

Musicdata
PO Box 12380
Philadelphia, PA 19119-0380
Phone: 215-248-3530
Fax: 215-248-3531
e-mail: musicdat@voicenet.com
Web Site: www.voicenet.com/~musicdat
A series of master catalogs of printed music published throughout the world. The 34 volume set of reference works is constantly updated and at present includes sacred choral, secular choral, organ, classical vocal, orchestral, string, classical guitar and woodwind.

9181 MUSICAL AMERICA INTERNATIONAL DIRECTORY OF THE PERFORMING ARTS

Commonwealth Business Media
10 Lake Drive
Heightstown, NJ 08572
Phone: 609-371-7783
Toll-free: 800-221-5488
Fax: 609-371-7879
Web Site: www.musicalamerica.com
international listings of dance and vocal groups, facilities and business and management services.

9182 MUSICAL AMERICA'S LIST RENTAL PROGRAM

10 Lake Drive
Hightstown, NJ 08520
Phone: 609-371-7877
Toll-free: 800-221-5488
Direct access to Musical America's leading buyers of talent. 15,000 listings.

9183 NYC/ON STAGE

Theatre Development Fund
1501 Broadway
New York, NY 10036-5601
Phone: 212-221-0013
Theater, dance, and music companies and performing arts centers in New York City.
100 pages   Biennial

9184 NATIONAL OPERA ASSOCIATION MEMBERSHIP DIRECTORY

PO Box 60869
Canyon, TX 79016
Phone: 703-790-3393
Web Site: www.noa.org
A membership directory. *$45.00*
40 pages   Annual
Circulation: 800

9185 NATIONWIDE MUSIC RECORD INDUSTRY TOLL FREE DIRECTORY

CDE
PO Box 310551
Atlanta, GA 31131-0551
A dirctory of the record industry players. *$50.00*
50 pages   Annual
Circulation: 5,000

9186 ORION BLUE BOOK: GUITARS AND MUSICAL INSTRUMENTS

Orion Research Corporation
Suite 330
14555 N Scottsdale Road
Scottsdale, AZ 85254-3487
Phone: 480-951-1114
Web Site: www.bluebook.com/appraisals
A directory of guitars and musical instruments. *$149.00*
Annual

9187 ORION BLUE BOOK: PRO SOUND 2002

Orion Research Corporation
Suite 330
14555 N Scottsdale Road
Scottsdale, AZ 85254-3487
Phone: 480-951-1114
Toll-free: 800-844-0759
Fax: 480-951-1117
e-mail: orion@bluebook.com
Web Site: www.bluebook.com
List of manufacturers of high-end professional sound equipment.
Annual

9188 ORION BLUE BOOK: VINTAGE GUITAR

Orion Research Corporation
Suite 330
14555 N Scottsdale Road
Scottsdale, AZ 85254-3487
Phone: 480-951-1114
Toll-free: 800-844-0759
Fax: 480-951-1117
e-mail: orion@bluebook.com
Web Site: www.bluebook.com
List of manufacturers of classic guitars.
Annual

9189 PERFORMING ARTS CAREER DIRECTORY

Gale Research
27500 Drake Road
Farmington Hills, MI 48331

Toll-free: 800-877-GALE
Fax: 313-961-6741
Over 350 organizations are listed that are directly related to the performing arts industry. *$29.95*
300 pages   Cloth

9190 PERFORMING ARTS MAJORS COLLEGE GUIDE

Arco Publishing
Floor 16
15 Columbus Circle
New York, NY 10023-7707
Phone: 212-373-7799
Toll-free: 800-858-7674
Fax: 212-373-8642
Editor: Carole Everette
More than 260 college and conservatory programs in dance, drama, or music. *$20.00*

9191 PERFORMING ARTS RESOURCES

Theatre Library Association
Room 513
111 Amsterdam Avenue
New York, NY 10023-7410
Publishes rare historical documents and out-of-print works in the field which might otherwise be lost to scholarship. International in scope, recent editions of this directory have covered management issues in performing arts collections, the performing arts in nineteenth and twentieth-century periodicals and the Drew-Barrymore acting dynasty. This annual publication is distributed to all members as part of their membership dues.
Annual

9192 PLAYS AND PLAYWRIGHTS

International Society of Dramatists
1638 Euclid Avenue
Miami Beach, FL 33139-7744
Phone: 305-882-1864
Offers valuable information on over 1,000 dramatists producing works in English. *$29.95*
200 pages   Annual
Circulation: 10,000

9193 RECORD RETAILING DIRECTORY

Billboard Directory Central
Nashville, TN
Phone: 615-321-4277
Web Site: www.billboard.com
Profiles over 7,000 independent and chain store music retailers in the United States, American Samoa, Guam and Puerto Rico.
$99.00
250 pages   Annual

9194 REGIONAL THEATRE DIRECTORY

Theatre Directories
PO Box 510
Dorset, VT 05251-0510

Phone: 802-867-2223
Toll-free: 800-390-2223
Fax: 802-867-0144
e-mail: theatre@sover.net
Web Site: www.theatredirectories.com
General Manager: Barbara Ax
Employment in US regional and dinner theatres. *$19.95*
Annual ISBN 9-339194-33-   400 names $180 per M.

9195 SCRIPTWRITERS MARKET

Film Makers Publishing
Suite 306
8033 W Sunset Boulevard
West Hollywood, CA 90046-2427
Literary agents, film producers, television producers and directors are listed. *$39.95*
200 pages   Annual
Circulation: 10,000

9196 STARS IN YOUR EYES...FEET ON THE GROUND

Theatre Directories
PO Box 510
Dorset, VT 05251-0510
Phone: 802-867-2223
Toll-free: 800-390-2223
Fax: 802-867-0144
e-mail: theatre@sover.net
Web Site: www.theatredirectories.com
Author: Jill Charles
This book can assess, direct or re-direct your focus on your teen career in the arts. *$16.95*

9197 STERN'S DIRECTORY

Dance Magazine
Suite 203
111 Myrtle Street
Oakland, CA 94607
Phone: 510-839-6060
Fax: 510-839-6066
e-mail: stern@dancemagazine.com
Web Site: www.dancemagazine.com
Stern's Directory the premier source for dance field contacts

9198 STERN'S PERFORMING ARTS DIRECTORY

Dance Magazine
33 W 60th Street
New York, NY 10023-7905
Phone: 212-245-9050
Toll-free: 800-458-2845
Fax: 212-956-6487
Publisher: Robert D. Stern
Editor: Allen McCormack
The 'Yellow Pages' of dance and classical music provides easy to use categorical listings of dance companies, choreographers, college dance programs, artist management agencies, service organizations and merchandise. *$65.00*
Annual Circulation: 8,000

9199 STUDENT'S GUIDE TO PLAYWRITING OPPORTUNITI ES
Theatre Directories
PO Box 510
Dorset, VT 05251-0510
Phone: 802-867-2223
Toll-free: 800-390-2223
Fax: 802-867-0144
e-mail: theatre@sover.net
Web Site: www.theatredirectories.com
Author: Jill Charles
Profiles in-depth college and university programs and developmental programs for the student with an interest in Playwriting. *$16.95*

9201 THEATRE PROFILES
Theatre Communications Group
Room 401
355 Lexington Avenue
New York, NY 10017-6695
Phone: 212-661-1225
Theater reviews and statistics. *$21.95*
240 pages Biennial

9202 VENDING TIMES BUYERS GUIDE AND DIRECTORY ISSUE
Vending Times
1375 Broadway
New York, NY 10018-7001
Phone: 212-444-6000
Fax: 212-221-3311
e-mail: info@vendingtimes.com
Web Site: www.vendingtimes.com
Editor: Tim Sanford
Managing Editor: Nick Montano
President/Publisher: Victor Uvay
Lists of manufacturers and suppliers of equipment and products used by vending machine industry operators, including product venders,
juke boxes, pinball and other games; industry trade associations. *$35.00*
Annual June
Circulation: 17,558

9203 WHO'S WHO IN ENTERTAINMENT
Marquis Who's Who/Reed Reference Publishing
121 Chanlon Road
New Providence, NJ 07974-1544
Phone: 908-464-6800
Fax: 908-464-3553
A list of the industry's finest. *$235.00*
702 pages

9204 WHOLE ARTS DIRECTORY
Midmarch Arts Press
Apartment 8A
300 Riverside Drive
New York, NY 10025-5239
Phone: 212-666-6990
Fax: 212-865-5510
Directory of services and supplies to the industry. *$12.95*
175 pages Triennial Since: 1987 ISBN 0-960247-67-x
Printed in on matte stock

9205 YELLOW PAGES OF ROCK
Album Network
120 N Victory Boulevard
Burbank, CA 91502-1852
Phone: 818-955-4000
Fax: 818-955-8048
$90.00
400 pages Annual

Industry Web Sites

9206 HOME.PACBELL.NET/MBERNHAR/
Milton Gerald Bernhart, Kelly Travel Service
Seeks to perpetuate the memory and sound of big bands and to introduce big band music to younger generations.

9207 HTTP://AISLESAY.COM
Aislesay
e-zine that reviews professional productions in major American cities and Canada.

9208 HTTP://ASA.AIP.ORG
Acoustical Society of America
Information of interest to sound designers.

9209 HTTP://BACKSTAGE.COM
Backstage.com
For actors and writers.

9210 HTTP://BALLETDANCE. MININGCO.COM
Ballet/Dance
Ballet and dance information.

9211 HTTP://COME.TO/THEBALLET
Come to the Ballet
Information, book reviews and links.

9212 HTTP://DIR.ALTAVISTA.COM
Alta Vista
From home page, click on Arts and Entertainment, then Arts and Culture. Choose Theater, Musical Theater or Dance.

9213 HTTP://DIR.HOTBOT.LYCOS.COM/ARTS
Hotbot
Arts and Entertainment has Performing Arts and Theatre division.

9214 HTTP://DIR.WEBRING.YAHOO.COM/RW
Yahoo! Webring
For theatre information, use search engine.

9215 HTTP://DIR.YAHOO.COM/ARTS/ PERFORMING_ARTS
Yahoo!: Performing Arts

9216 **HTTP://DMOZ.ORG/ARTS**
Open Directory Project
Theatre and Dance sites.

9217 **HTTP://FRONTPAGE.SHADOW.NET/ USA829FL**
United Scenic Artists
For entertainment industry designers and artists.

9218 **HTTP://LIBWEB.UNCC.EDU/ REF-ARTS/ THEATER**
UNCC.edu
Theatrical website guide.

9219 **HTTP://MANIAC.DEATHSTAR.ORG/ GROUPS/ROS**
Ring of Steel
Theatrical combat/stunt group provides information on weapons, fight choreographers and groups.

9220 **HTTP://MEMBERS.AOL.COM/ AWORLDLINK**
Actors World Link
Actors can display headshot, resume and web address for a nominal fee.

9221 **HTTP://MEMBERS.AOL.COM/ MSJ1140/INDEX.HTML**
Shan's
Costume and theatre history.

9222 **HTTP://MEMBERS.AOL.COM/THEGOOP/ GAFF.HTML**
Gaff Tape Webring
Tech theatre.

9223 **HTTP://MILIEUX.COM/COSTUME**
Milieux.com
Costume information and resources.

9224 **HTTP://MUSE.JHU.EDU/JOURNALS**
Project Muse
Directory of journals, including 'The Drama Review,' 'Theatre Topics,' 'Theatre Journal' and 'Theatre.'

9225 **HTTP://PLAYWRIGHTS.ORG**
Playwrights Center of San Francisco
Stages readings of plays by members.

9226 **HTTP://SHAKESPEARE.PALOMAR.EDU**
Shakespeare.palomar.edu
Scholarly Shakespeare resources online.

9227 **HTTP://THEATRE-LINK.COM**
Scott's Theatre-Link.com
Theatre-related sites.

9228 **HTTP://VL-THEATRE.COM**
WWW Virtual Library
Links to theatre and drama resources. Updated daily.

9229 **HTTP://WWAR.COM**
World Wide Arts Resources
Links to Theatre and Dance.

9230 **WW.DEADANCE.COM**
Dance Educators of America
Promotes the education of teachers in the performing arts.

9231 **WW.MUSICALARTISTS.ORG**
American Guild of Musical Artists
Exclusive bargaining agent for all concert musical artists.

9232 **WWW.CMAWORLD.COM**
Country Music Association
Promotes and publicizes country music.

9233 **WWW.PERFORMINGARTS.NET/ LINKS/I-NLINKS.HTML**
Performing Arts Online

9234 **WWW.TALKINBROADWAY.COM**
Talkin' Broadway
Theatrical events and information on anf off Broadway and other selected geographical locations.

9235 **WWW.AACT.ORG**
American Association of Community Theatre
Non-profit corporation fostering excellence in community theatre productions and governance through community theatre festivals, educational opportunity publications, network, resources, and website.

9236 **WWW.AAPERD.ORG/NDA**
National Dance Association
A nonprofit service organization dedicated to increasing knowledge, improving skills and encouraging sound professional practices in dance education while promoting and supporting creative and healthy lifestyles through high quality dance programs.

9237 **WWW.AATE.COM**
American Alliance for Theatre and Education
Members are artists, teachers and professionals who serve youth theatres and theatre educational programs.

9238 **WWW.ABSOLUTEWRITE.COM**
Absolute Write
Advice for writers, including playwrights.

9239 **WWW.ABTT.ORG.UK/TRAIN/ WORKIN.HTML**
Abtt.org
Describes the responsibilities and functions of all backstage workers.

9240 WWW.ACDAONLINE.ORG
American Choral Directors Association
A non-profit educational organization in the Choral area, dedicated to providing information to members.

9241 WWW.ACMCOUNTRY.COM
Academy of Country Music
Involved in numerous events and activities promoting country music. Presents annual awards.

9242 WWW.ACTORSEQUITY.ORG/ HOME.HTML
Actors Equity Association
Labor union affiliated with AFL-CIO which represents actors in film, television and commercials.

9243 WWW.ACTORSITE.COM
Actor Site
Audition and other information.

9244 WWW.ACTORSOURCE.COM
Actorsource
Extensive information and resources for actors.

9245 WWW.ACTORSTHEATRE.ORG
Actors Theatre of Louisville
Supports new playwrights. For information on entering a play, click Humana Festival.

9246 WWW.ADTA.ORG
American Dance Therapy Association
Founded in 1966; professional organization of dance movement therapists, with members both nationally and internationally; offers training, research findings, and a newsletter.

9247 WWW.AFM.ORG
American Federation of Musicians of the United States and Canada
Union representing over 100,000 professional musicians, performing in all genres of music.

9248 WWW.AFVBM.COM
American Federation of Violin and Bow Makers
Strives to elevate professional standards of craftmanship and ethical conduct among members. Helps members develop technical skills and knowledge.Research and study organization.

9249 WWW.AGOHQ.ORG
American Guild of Organists

9250 WWW.AIMCMC.COM
Creative Musician Coalition
A national organization that brings the world of new music to its readers. Includes in depth music reviews, informative artist interviews, interesting articles and feature columns, and valuable resource material.

9251 WWW.AIMSINTL.ORG
International Federation of Festival Organizations
Organizes events, publishes monthly bulletin, holds annual conference.

9252 WWW.AMERICANDANCEFESTIVAL.ORG

American Dance Festival
American Dance Festival offers classes and workshops, auditions and scholarships.

9253 WWW.AMERICANDANCEGUILD.ORG
American Dance Guild
Non-profit membership organization; sponsors professional seminars, workshops, a student scholarship and other projects and institutes programs of national significance in the field of dance.

9254 WWW.AMERICANTHEATERWEB.COM
American Theater Web
Theater news and events.

9255 WWW.AMOA.COM
Amusement and Music Operators Association
Exhibits of coin-operated arcade, video and gaming machines, games, juke boxes, stuffed toys, records and jewelry.

9256 WWW.ANGELFIRE.COM/OR/COPYRIGHT 4PRODUCERS
Angelfire.com
Copyright information for amateur theatre producers.

9257 WWW.ANSWERS4DANCERS.COM
Answers for Dancers
Dance Magazine sponsors this site.

9258 WWW.ARTS-ACCREDITING.ORG/NASM
National Association of Schools of Music
Postsecondary accreditation of music programs.

9259 WWW.ARTSENDOW.GOV
National Endowment for the Arts
The National Endowment for the Arts, an investment in America's living heritage, serves the public good by nurturing the expression of human creativity, supporting the cultivation of community spirit, and fostering the recognition and appreciation of the excellence and diversity of our nation's artistic accomplishments.

9260 WWW.ARTSLYNX.ORG
Artslynx
International Arts Resources. Links to theatre, dance, music.

9261 WWW.ARTSLYNX.ORG/JOBS.HTM#TTHE ATRE
Artslynx
Theatre Employment Resources section.

9262 WWW.ARTSLYNX.ORG/THEATRE/COSTUME.HTM
Artslynx
Resources in costume history.

9263 WWW.ARTSLYNX.ORG/THEATRE/DESIGN.HTM
Artslynx
Links about design, including lighting, costume, makeup, masks, scenery and sound, as well as stage management and theatre engineering/architecture.

9264 WWW.ARTSLYNX.ORG/THEATRE/INDEX.HTM
Artslynx
Artslynx International Theatre Resources.

9265 WWW.ARTSNET.ORG/ATHEE
Theatre Management Journal

9266 WWW.ARTSNET.ORG/AAAE/
Association of Arts Administration Educators
The Association of Administration Educators (AAAE) is an international organization incorporated as a nonprofit institution within the United States. Its mission is to represent college and university graduate and undergraduate programs in the arts administration, encompassing training in the management of visual, performing, literary, media, cultural and arts service organizations.

9267 WWW.ARTSNET.ORG/CAMT
Center for Arts Management and Technology
Mission is to link artists with tomorrow's technology.

9268 WWW.ARTSNET.ORG/INDEX.HTML
Artsnet
Offers access to ArtSites directory and culture/arts sites.

9269 WWW.ARTSPRESENTERS.ORG
Association of Performing Arts Presenters
Celebrates rich and diverse performing arts to the public.

9270 WWW.ARTSTABILIZATION.ORG
National Arts Stabilization
Offers training and technical assistance to arts organizations.

9271 WWW.ARTSWIRE.ORG/CURRENT/JOBS.HTML
Arts Wire
Employment openings in the arts.

9272 WWW.ARVOTEK.NET/~PROPS
Proptology
Journal of props professionals.

9273 WWW.ASCAO.COM
American Society of Composers, Authors and Publishers
Association for songwriters, composers and music publishers.

9274 WWW.ASHLAND.NET/MADRONE/TSOUND_RING.HTML
Theatre Sound Designer and Composer Ring
Resources and suppliers.

9275 WWW.ASMAC.ORG
American Society of Music Arrangers and Composers
Professional society for arrangers, composers, orchestrators, and musicians. Monthly meetings with great speakers from the music industry.

9276 WWW.BACHAUER.COM
Gina Bachauer International Piano Foundation
Produce a yearly piano international competition: artistmanagement

9277 WWW.BACKSTAGE.COM
Backstage.com
Click on Casting to find job listings for actors, staff and tech.

9278 WWW.BACKSTAGE.COM/BACKSTAGE/INDEX.JSP
Backstage.com
Resource for actors.

9279 WWW.BACKSTAGEJOBS.COM
Theatre Design and Technical Jobs Page
Employment opportunities.

9280 WWW.BACKSTAGEWORLD.COM
Backstage World
Post your resume and search for design and technical job opportunities worldwide.

9281 WWW.BILLBOARD.COM
The ultimate music industry research tool and information source. The Member Service databased is state of the art electronic information service, enabling users to efficiently access onformation from a variety of music industry databases via the World Wide Web.

9282 WWW.BMI.COM
BMI
Secures the rights of songwriters/composers. Collects license fees for the public performance of music and pays royalties to its copyright owners.

9283 WWW.BROADWAY.ORG
League of American Theatres and Producers
National trade association for the commercial theatre industry whose principal activity is negotiation of labor contracts and government relations.

9284 WWW.CADVISION.COM/SDEMPSEY/ICWPHMPG.HTM
International Centre for Women Playwrights

9285 WWW.CARYTRIVANOVICH.COM/ACAD.ASP
American Academy of Mime
Teaching, promoting and encouraging the study of mime.

9286 WWW.CASEWEB.COM/ACTS/INDEX.HTML
Arts, Crafts and Theater Safety
ACTS is a nonprofit corporation specializing in providing safety and health services for the arts.

9287 WWW.CATF.ORG
Contemporary American Theater Festival

9288 WWW.CHORUSAMERICA.ORG
Chorus America
National service for orchestral choruses, independent choruses and professional choruses.

9289 WWW.CIRCUS.WEB.COM
Circus Fans Association of America
Seeks to create an enthusiasm for the circus as an institution and preserve it for future generations.

9290 WWW.CIRCUSFANS.ORG
Circus Fans Association of America
Seeks to create an enthusiasm for the circus as an institution and preserve it for future generations.

9291 WWW.CIRCUSMODELBUILDERS.ORG
Circus Historical Society
Information on the historical applications of the circus.

9292 WWW.CLARINET.ORG
International Clarinet Association
Seeks to focus attention on the importance of the clarinet and to foster communication of the fellowship between clarinetists.

9293 WWW.CLASSICALACTION.ORG
Classical Action
Provides a unified voice for all those within the performing arts community to help combat HIV/AIDS.

9294 WWW.COMPUTERMUSIC.ORG
International Computer Music Association
Supports the performance aspects of computer music; publishes newsletter and holds annual conferance.

9295 WWW.CONDUCTORSGUILD.ORG
Conductors Guild
Dedicated to encouraging the highest standards in the art and profession of conducting. Founded in 1975.

9296 WWW.CONTACTIMPROV.NET
Contact Improv
Improvisation for dancers.

9297 WWW.COSTUME-CON.ORG
Costume Connections

9298 WWW.COSTUME.ORG
International Costumers' Guild

9299 WWW.COSTUMEGALLERY.COM
Costume Gallery

9300 WWW.COSTUMERS.ORG
National Costumers Association
Seeks to establish and maintain professional and ethical standards of business in the costume industry.

9301 WWW.COSTUMES.ORG
Costumer's Manifesto
Online book, information and links.

9302 WWW.COSTUMESOCIETYAMERICA.COM/WELCOME
Costume Society of America

9303 WWW.CREATIVEDIR.COM/HTML/18.HTML
Creativedir.com
Diectory of suppliers for costumes, sets, special effects and stunts.

9304 WWW.CRITICALDANCE.COM
Dance Critics Association
Encourages excellence in dance criticism through education, research and the exchange of ideas.

9305 WWW.CSULB.EDU/~JVANCAMP/COPYRIGH.HTML
Csulb.edu
Copyrighting choreographic works.

9306 WWW.CSUSA.ORG/FACE/INDEX.HTM
Friends of Active Copyright Education
Playwrights should click on Words, then Copyright Basics.

9307 WWW.CULTUREFINDER.COM
CultureFinder.com
Lists arts events for major cities around the country.

9308 WWW.CULTURENET.CA/USITT
United States Institute for Theatre Technology
The association seeks to enhance its members' knowledge and skills.

9309 WWW.CYBERDANCE.ORG
Cyber Dance

Collection of links to modern dance and classical ballet resources.

9310 WWW.DANCEART.COM/EDANCING
Danceart.com
Discusses eating disorders in the field of dance.

9311 WWW.DANCENOTATION.ORG
Dance Notation Bureau
Notation basics, Notated Theatrical Dances Catalogue and links.

9312 WWW.DANCEONLINE.COM
Dance On-Line
Dance news and information.

9313 WWW.DANCEPAGES.COM
Dance Pages.com
Offers resources to dance teachers.

9314 WWW.DANCER.COM/DANCE-LINKS
Dance Links
Links to many dance sites.

9315 WWW.DANCEUSA.ORG
Dance USA
Provides a forum for the discussion of issues of concern to membersand a support network for exchange of information; also bestows awards.

9316 WWW.DMA-NATIONAL.ORG
Dance Masters of America
An organization of dance teachers.

9317 WWW.DRAMAGUILD.COM
Dramatists Guild
Comprehensive organization that deals solely with Broadway and off-Broadway producers, off-off-Broadway groups, agents, theatres and sources of grants.

9318 WWW.DRAMALEAGUE.ORG
Drama League
Seeks to strengthen American theatre through the nurturing of stage directors.

9319 WWW.DRAMATURGY.NET
Dramaturgy.net
Site for dramaturgs, whose function is to revise a play as an editor revises a novel.

9320 WWW.DRAMATURGY.NET/ DRAMATURGY
Dramaturgy.net
Information and insight from working dramaturgs.

9321 WWW.DRAMEX.ORG
Dramatic Exchange
For anyone interested in plays.

9322 WWW.DTW.ORG
Dance Theater Workshop

9323 WWW.ELIZREVIEW.COM
Elizabethan Review
Scholarly journal on Elizabethan topics, with Shakespeare information and links.

9324 WWW.EPERFORMER.COM
eperformer.com
Auditions, agents and resources for actors and dancers.

9325 WWW.ETASSOC.ORG
Educational Theater Association
Theater educators working to increase support for theater programs in the educational system.

9326 WWW.ETECNYC.NET/DEFAULT.HTML
Entertainment Technology Online
For employment in design and technical theatre, click on Classifieds. Also offers resources and buyers guides for theatrical lighting.

9327 WWW.ETECNYC.NET/LD.HTML
ETEC: Lighting Dimensions Magazine
Articles on how to use light creatively in opera, dance, theatre and other entertainment areas.

9328 WWW.FAIRSNET.ORG
Western Fairs Association
For fairground owners, managers and workers.

9329 WWW.FOLKHARPSOCIETY.ORG
International Society of Folk Harpers and Craftsmen
Conducts technical and artistic programs and promotes craft exchange.

9330 WWW.GEOCITIES.COM/BROADWAY/2938 /HOME.HTML
Society of Prop Artisan Managers

9331 WWW.GEOCITIES.COM/ BROADWAY/3738
Stage Technician's Page
Basic information and links.

9332 WWW.GEOCITIES.COM/ BROADWAY/5222
World of Mime Theatre
Education and information on the art of mime.

9333 WWW.GEOCITIES.COM/ HOLLYWOOD/LOT/4759
Soc. of Amateur & Prof. Spec. Effects Makeup Art.
Nonprofit organization of theatrical and film special effects and makeup artists.

9334 WWW.GMN.COM
Global Music Network
Go backstage, watch rehearsals, listen to performances of classical and jazz artists.

9335 WWW.GOLDMIME.COM
Goldston Mime Foundation: School for Mime
Holds summer seminars and workshops.

9336 WWW.GOSPELMUSIC.ORG
Gospel Music Association
Dedicated to providing leadership, direction and unity for all facets of the gospel music industry. Through education, communication, information, promotion and recognition, the GMA is striving to help those involved in gospel music.

9337 WWW.GREYHOUSE.COM
Grey House Publishing
The Grey House Performing Arts Directory is the most comprehensive resource covering the Performing Arts. This important directory provides current information on over 8,000 Dance Companies, Instrumental Music Programs, Opera Companies, Choral Groups, Theater Companies, Performing Arts Series and Performing Arts Facilities.

9338 WWW.GUITARFOUNDATION.ORG
Guitar Foundation of America
Supports the serious studies of the guitar.

9339 WWW.HANDSON.ORG/IDEAS.HTML
Interactive Drama for Education and Awareness in the Schools (IDEAS)
Offers school-based drama artist-in-residency programs for students with disabilities.

9340 WWW.HARADA-SOUND.COM/ SOUND/HANDBOOK
Kai's Sound Handbook
Information for sound designers.

9341 WWW.HARPSOCIETY.ORG
American Harp Society
Improves the quality of the instrument and performance.

9342 WWW.HAWAII.EDU/ATHE
Association for Theatre in Higher Education
An organization of individuals and institutions that provides vision and leadership for the profession and promotes excellence in theatre education. ATHE consists of more than 2,000 members who represent education, retired colleagues and organizations creating, studying and teaching theatre.

9343 WWW.HENIFORD.NET/1234
Small Cast One-Act Guide Online
List of short plays.

9344 WWW.HOLLYWOOD.COM
National Association of Theatre Owners
Supports theatrer owners; publishes a monthly magazine. Largest motion picture exhibition trade organization in the world.

9345 WWW.HORNDOGGIE.COM/HORN
International Horn Society
A national organization that focuses on music industry news and information.

9346 WWW.IAAPA.ORG
Int'l Association of Amusement Parks & Attractions
For permanently situated amusement facilities worldwide.

9347 WWW.IAEKM.ORG
International Association of Electronic Keyboard Manufacturers

9348 WWW.IATSE-LOCAL1.ORG
Union of Stage Employees: Local One, IATSE
Union includes the Theatrical Sound Designers Association.

9349 WWW.IATSE.LM.COM
Intl. Alliance of Theatrical Stage Employees
Represents entertainment industry artisans, craftspersons and technicians.

9350 WWW.IBMA.ORG
World of Bluegrass
IBMA; working together for high standards of professionalism, a greater apprciation for our music, and the success of the world-wide bluegrass community.

9351 WWW.IFEA.COM
International Festivals and Events Association
Network for planning events and exchange programs; publishes quarterly magazine.

9352 WWW.IMPROVAMERICA.COM
Improv Across America
State-by-state information on improvisational companies.

9353 WWW.INDA.ORG
Literary Managers and Dramaturgs of the Americas
A national network of American literary managers and dramaturgs encouraging the emerging profession.

9354 WWW.INTERNATIONALPOLKA.COM
International Polka Association
Educational organization concerned with the preservation and advancement of polka music. Operates the Polka Music Hall of Fame and Museum, and presents the International Polka Fesitval every year during the complete first weekend of August.

9355 WWW.INTIX.ORG
International Ticketing Association

Not-for-profit organizaiton whose purpose is to advance the success of the admission service industry and its members.

9356 WWW.ISA.ORG
Instrument Society of America

9357 WWW.ISPA.ORG
International Society for the Performing Arts Foundation
Supports international cooperation, facilitates networking and enhances professional dialogue.

9358 WWW.ITEA.COM
International Theatre Equipment Association
Fosters and maintains professional, business and social relationships among its members within all segments of the motion picture industry. Bestows annual Teddy award to manufacturer of the year and the annual Rodney award to dealer of the year.

9359 WWW.IWAYNET.NET/~PHANTOM/THEAT RELINKS
Tech Theatre Links

9360 WWW.JENSENFOUNDATION.ORG
Fritz and Lavinia Jensen Foundation
Sponsors competitions.

9361 WWW.JUGGLE.ORG
International Jugglers' Association

9362 WWW.LASERIST.ORG
International Laser Display Association
Dedicated to advancing the use of laser displays, in the art, entertainment and education.

9363 WWW.LATINOARTS.ORG
Association of Hispanic Arts
A multidisciplary organization which supports Hispanic arts organizations and individual artists with technical assistance. The organization facilitates projects and programs designed to foster the appreciation, growth, and well being of the Latino cultural community. It's quarter publication, AHA; Hispanic Arts News, features in depth articles on the local and national arts community, including artist profiles and a calendar of events.

9364 WWW.LE-US.COM/LGTMATH.HTM
Stage Lighting Math
Lighting designers will find math formulas here.

9365 WWW.LIB.COLUM.EDU/ COSTWAIS.HTML
Costume Image Database
Access costume images.

9366 WWW.LIB.OHIO-STATE.EDU/ OSU_PROFILE/TRIWEB
Lawrence and Lee Theatre Research Institute
Research materials on the performing arts.

9367 WWW.LIGHT-LINK.COM
Lightsearch.com
Lists of lighting equipment suppliers.

9368 WWW.LMDA.ORG
Literary Managers and Dramaturgs of the Americas
Voluntary membership organization.

9369 WWW.LUTH.ORG
Guild of American Luthiers
Manufacturers and repairs stringed instruments; offers quarterly journal and triennial meeting.

9370 WWW.LYCOS.COM
Lycos
Click Arts and Entertainment, then Dance, Theatre or Performing Arts.

9371 WWW.LYONSLPGAS.COM/ SEWSCAPE/COSTUME.HTML
Lyonslpgas.com
Design and sewing resources for costumers.

9372 WWW.MAGICSAM.COM
Society of American Magicians
Founded to promote and maintain harmonious fellowship among those interested in magic as an art, to improve ethics of the magical profession, and to foster, promote and improve the advancement of magical arts in the field of amusement and entertainment. Membership inclides professional and amateur magicians, manufacturers of magical apparatus and collectors.

9373 WWW.MAHERSTUDIOS.COM/ NAAV.HTM
North American Association of Ventriloquists
Disseminates information on ventriloquists and their activities.

9374 WWW.MAKEUPMAG.COM
Make-Up Artist Magazine
Make-up artist magazine online.

9375 WWW.MARQUISE.DE/WEBRING/ COSTUMERING.HTML
Costume Webring

9376 WWW.MEMBERS.AOL.COM/ASMC
American Society of Music Copyists
Supports music preparation and rights of the professionals in the iindustry.

9377 WWW.MENC.ORG
Music Industry Conference

Instrument manufacturers and other suppliers to the music industry.

9378 WWW.METGUILD.ORG
Metropolitan Opera Guild
Seeks to promote greater understanding and interest in opera.

9379 WWW.MIDATLANTICARTS.ORG
Mid Atlantic Arts Foundation

9380 WWW.MILIEUX.COM/COSTUME/ SOURCE.HTML
Costume Source
Provides online sources for materials, costumes, accessories and books.

9381 WWW.MPA.ORG
Music Publishers Association of the United States
Encourages understanding of the copyright laws and works to protect musical works against infringements and piracy.

9382 WWW.MPTF.ORG
Music Performance Trust Funds
Foundation allocates money for the promotion of black music and the general public. The concerts must be free of charge and have no admittance restrictions.

9383 WWW.MTISHOWS.COM
Music Theatre International
Scripts, cast recordings, study guides, production slides and other resources.

9384 WWW.MTNA.ORG
Music Teachers National Association
This is a nonprofit organization of independent and collegiate music teachers committed to furthering the art of music through teaching, performance, composition and scholarly research.

9385 WWW.MUSIC.ORG
College Music Society
The Society is a national service organization for college conservatory and university music teachers.

9386 WWW.MUSICALAMERICA.COM
Musicalamerica.com
Late-breaking industry news, full search capabilities, immediate interaction between Presenter and Artist Manager/Artist.

9387 WWW.MUSICALARTISTS.COM
Musical Artists Performers and Teachers
Place your picture, bio and recording on the internet.

9388 WWW.MUSICDISTRIBUTORS.ORG
National Council of Music Importers and Exporters
Importers and exporters of musical instruments and accesories.

9389 WWW.MUSICIANSHEALTH.COM/ CPAA.HTM
Chiropractic Performing Arts Association
To educate amateur and professional entertainers, musicians and dancers about reaching optimum health potential through natural, drug-free, conservative chiropractic care.

9390 WWW.MUSICLIBRARYASSOC.ORG
Music Library Association
Promotes growth and establishment in the use of music libraries, musical instruments and musical literature.

9391 WWW.MUSICMESSAGE.ORG
Music Message Network
Founded by pianist Donna Stoering to create a network between musicians and their audiences, via global benefit concerts for music education, outreach projects and retreat centers for musicians.

9392 WWW.NACWPI.ORG
National Association of College Wind and Percussion Instructors
Teachers of wind and percussion instruments in American colleges and universities.

9393 WWW.NADT.ORG
National Association for Drama Therapy
Promotes the profession of Drama Therapy.

9394 WWW.NAMM.COM
NAMM - International Music Products Association
Offers professional development seminars; sells musical instruments and allied products.

9395 WWW.NAMT.COM
American Music Therapy Association
A national organization whose mission is to advance the public awareness of music therapy benefits and increase accessibility to quality music therapy services.

9396 WWW.NAPAMA.ORG
National Association of Performing Arts Managers and Agents
National not-for-profit trade association founded in 1979, dedicated to promoting the professionalism of its members and the vitality of the performing arts.

9397 WWW.NAPBIRT.ORG
National Association of Professional Band Instrument Repair Technicians
Promotes technical integrity in the craft. Surveys tools and procedures to improve work quality. Makes available emergency repair of band instruments. Provides placement services.

9398 WWW.NATIONALBANDASSOC.ORG
National Band Association
Sponsors clinics and other educational functions for band directors.

9399 WWW.NATOONLINE.ORG
National Association of Theatre Owners
Professional trade association serving the business intervals of theatre owners domestically and around the world. Assist theatre owners work with picture distribution and issues such as new technologies, legislation, marketing and first amendment. Publish monthly magazine and annual encyclopedias.

9400 WWW.NBEA.COM
National Ballroom and Entertainment Association
Provides exchange for owners and operators of ballrooms.

9401 WWW.NETCONLINE.ORG
New England Theatre Conference
Non-profit educational corporation founded to develop, expand and assist theatre activity in community, educational and professional levels in New England. Holds annual auditions.

9402 WWW.NETSWORD.COM/ STAGECOMBAT.HTML
Netsword
Lessons on stage combat.

9403 WWW.NEWPLAYSFORCHILDREN.COM
New Plays Online
Plays for children and young adults.

9404 WWW.NMPA.ORG
National Music Publishers' Association
Publishes a quarterly newsletter and holds an annual meeting.

9405 WWW.NOA.ORG
National Opera Association
To advance the appreciation, composition and production of opera.

9406 WWW.NTCP.ORG
Non-Traditional Casting Project
Promotes inclusive practices in television, theatre and film.

9407 WWW.NYPL.ORG/RESEACH/LPA/ LPA.HTML
New York Public Library for the Performing Arts
Primary research collection.

9408 WWW.NYTIMES.COM
New York Times on the Web
Arts and Theatre contains play reviews.

9409 WWW.OABA.ORG
Outdoor Amusement Business Association
Promotes interest of the outdoor amusement industry.

9410 WWW.ONSTAGE.ORG
Onstage: The Actor's Resource
For professional actors.

9411 WWW.OOBR.COM
Off-Off-Broadway Review

9412 WWW.OPENCASTING.COM
Open Casting
Bulletin board containing auditions, crew calls, casting notices and links.

9413 WWW.OPERAAM.ORG
Opera America
Opera America serves and strengthens the field of opera by providing a variety of informational, technical, and administrative resources to the greater opera community. Its fundamental mission is to promote opera as exciting and accessible to individuals from all walks of life.

9414 WWW.PAS.ORG
Percussive Arts Society
Promotes drums and percussion through a viable network of performers, teachers, students, enthusiasts and sustaining members. Offers publications, a worldwide network of the World Percussion Network, the Percussive Arts Society International Headquarters/Museum and the annual Percussive Arts Society International Convention.

9415 WWW.PEN.ORG
PEN: American Center
Site of the international literary community organization.

9416 WWW.PERFORMANCE-DESIGN.COM
Design Image Online
For lighting, scene, sound and costume designers.

9417 WWW.PIANOGUILD.COM
International Piano Guild
A division of the American College of Musicians Professional society of piano teachers and music faculty members. Sponsers national examinations.

9418 WWW.PIANONET.COM
Piano Manufacturers Association International
Manufacturers and suppliers of pianos and parts; holds annual trade show.

9419 WWW.PIPEORGAN.ORG
American Institute of Organ Builders
Sponsers training seminars, quarterly journal and annual convention for pipe organ builders and service technicians.

9420 WWW.PLASA.ORG
Professional Lighting and Sound Association

9421 WWW.PLAYBILL.COM
Playbill.com

9422 WWW.PLAYWRIGHTSHORIZONS.ORG
Playwrights Horizon

At home page click arrow. On next page click working with PH. You will see Writing Submissions.

9423 WWW.PLAYWRIGHTSPROJECT.COM
Playwrights Project
Promotes literacy, creativity and communication skills in young people through drama-based activities.

9424 WWW.PLAYWRIGHTSWORKSHOP.ORG
Playwright's Workshop

9425 WWW.PRESS.JHU.EDU/PRESS/ JOURNALS/PAJ
A journal of performance and art.

9426 WWW.PRESS.JHU.EDU/PRESS/ JOURNALS/TJ
Theatre Journal

9427 WWW.PRESS.JHU.EDU/PRESS/ JOURNALS/TT
Theatre Topics

9428 WWW.PRINTMUSIC.ORG
Retail Print Music Dealers Association

9429 WWW.PROPPEOPLE.COM/ INDEX.SHTML
Proppeople.com
Online home for props professionals.

9430 WWW.PTG.ORG
International Association of Piano Builders and Technicians
Network of technical information. Publishes quarterly newsletter; hosts biennial meeting.

9431 WWW.REAL.COM/REALGUIDE/ INDEX.HTML
Timecast RealGuide: Live
Provides information on business, music, news, sci/tech, showbiz and sports.

9432 WWW.REDBIRDSTUDIO.COM/AWOL/ ACTING2.HTML
Acting Workshop On-Line: AWOL
Information on breaking into the acting business.

9433 WWW.RENFAIRE.COM/LANGUAGE/ INDEX.HTML
Renfaire.com
Lessons on proper Elizabethan accents.

9434 WWW.RHODES.EDU
Theatre Resources: Rhodes
List of sites includes Drama Resources, Technical Resources and Theatre Home Pages.

9435 WWW.RIGGING.NET
Rigger's Page
Technical information on stage rigging equipment.

9436 WWW.ROUNDALAB.ORG
Roundalab
A professional international society of individuals who teach round dancing at any phase.

9437 WWW.SAFD.ORG
Society of American Fight Directors
Promotes safety in directing staged combat and theatrical violence.

9438 WWW.SAG.ORG
Screen Actors Guild
Labor union affiliated with AFL-CIO which represents actors in film, television and commercials.

9439 WWW.SAPPHIRESWAN.COM/DANCE
Dance Directory
Dance resources.

9440 WWW.SAVAGESHAKESPEARE.COM
Savage Shakespeare
Shakespeare discussions.

9441 WWW.SCILS.RUTGERS.EDU/ ~CYBERS/HOME.HTML
Women of Color, Women of Words
African-American women playwrights.

9442 WWW.SCRIPTSEEKER.COM
Scriptseeker.com
Links playwrights with producers.

9443 WWW.SDHS.ORG
Society of Dance History Scholars
Dance history and links to organizations, funding and libraries.

9444 WWW.SETC.ORG
Southeastern Theatre Conference
Annual conventions include auditions.

9445 WWW.SFBALLET.ORG
San Francisco Ballet Association
To provide a repertoire of classical and contemporary ballet; to provide educational opportunities for professional dancers and choreographers; to excel in ballet, artistic direction and administration.

9446 WWW.SIUE.EDU/ITDA
International Theatre Design Archive
Designs for costumes, lighting and scenery.

9447 WWW.SONGWRITERS.ORG
Songwriters Guild of America

Provides agreements between songwriters, composers and publishers.

9448 WWW.SOUTHARTS.ORG
Southern Arts Federation
Serve as the leadership voice to increase the regional, national and international awareness and prominence of Southern arts. Create mechanisms and partnerships to expand local, regional, national and international markets for Southern arts.

9449 WWW.SPARS.COM
Society of Professional Audio Recording Services
Members are individuals, companies and studios connected with the professional recording industry.

9450 WWW.SPOLIN.COM
Spolin Center
Information on improvisational theatre.

9451 WWW.SSDC.ORG
Society of Stage Directors and Choreographers
An independent labor union representing directors and choreographers in American theatre.

9452 WWW.STAGE-DIRECTIONS.COM
Stage Directions Magazine
The practical and technical side of theatrical operations.

9453 WWW.STAGEPLAYS.COM/ MARKETS.HTM
Playwrights Noticeboard
Information on contests, publishing and production opportunities.

9454 WWW.STETSON.EDU
McCoy's Guide to Theatre and Performance Studies

9455 WWW.STUDYWEB.COM/LINKS/ 5032.HTML
Studyweb: Theatre Behind the Scenes
Designed for classes. Rated according to grade level.

9456 WWW.SUMMERTHEATER.COM
Directory of Summer Theater in the United States
Search for summer theater opportunities by alphabetized listings or geographic region.

9457 WWW.SUNDANCE.ORG
Sundance Institute
Information on the Sundance Theatre Laboratory summer workshop for directors, playwrights, choreographers, solo performers and composers. For information on submitting a play, click Theatre Program on home page.

9458 WWW.SYMPHONY.ORG
American Symphony Orchestra League

The national nonprofit service and educational organization dedicated to strengthening symphony and chamber orchestras. It provides artistic, organizational and financial leadership and service to orchestral conductors, managers, volunteers and staff.

9459 WWW.TCG.ORG
Theatre Communication Group
Supports alliances among playwrights, theatres and communities. Promotes not-for-profit theatre and offers resources to jobseekers. Offers financial support to designers and directors through its Career Development Program.

9460 WWW.TDF.ORG
Theatre Development Fund
Not-for-profit service organization. Provides support for every area of the dance, music and professional theatre field. Founded 1968.

9461 WWW.TELEPORT.COM/~BJSCRIPT/ INDEX.HTM
Essays on the Art of Dramatic Writing
Essays on writing a screenplay, play or novel.

9462 WWW.TELEPORT.COM/~CDEEMERS/ SCRWRITER.HTML
Screenwriters and Playwrights Homepage

9463 WWW.TELEPORT.COM/~MJGALLAG
Teleport.com
Information for sound designers.

9464 WWW.THEATERSERVICESGUIDE.COM
Theater Services Guide
Employment information for stage managers, actors and technicians. Also provides information on commercial suppliers.

9465 WWW.THEATRE-LINK.COM/ CASTING.HTML
Scott's Theatre-Link.com
Casting and Contact Services offers many links.

9466 WWW.THEATRE-RESOURCE.COM
Theatre Resource
Career and employment information.

9467 WWW.THEATRE-SOUND.COM/TSINDEX. HTML
Theatre Sound Design Directory

9468 WWW.THEATREBAYAREA.ORG
Theatre Bay Area
Serving more than 400 member theatre companies and 3,000 individual members in the San Francisco Bay Area and Northern California, Theatre Bay Area provides monthly classes, workshops, events, information and publications.

9469 WWW.THEATRECRAFTS.COM
Theatrecrafts.com
The glossary provides definitions for more than 800 theatrical terms.

9470 WWW.THEATREJOBS.COM
Theatrejobs.com
Online job placement. Festival listings, summer stock, assistantships, apprenticeships, fellowships and internships.

9471 WWW.THEATRELIBRARY.ORG/LINKS
Performing Arts Links
General resources including applied and interactive theatre, performing arts data service and art sites. Digital librarian includes
glossary of technical theatre terms.

9472 WWW.THEATRELIBRARY.ORG/LINKS/INDEX.HTML
Theatrelibrary.org
Master categories are Theatre, Dance, Cinema and Reviews.

9473 WWW.THECASTINGNETWORK.COM/WEBRING.HTML
Casting Network.com
By and for actors.

9474 WWW.THEPLAYS.ORG
Electronic Literature Foundation
William Shakespeare's plays online.

9475 WWW.TOP20PERFORMINGARTS.COM/
Top 20 Performing Arts
Performing arts websites

9476 WWW.TOWSON.EDU/WORLDMUSICCONGRESSES
World Music Congresses
1997-2010 World Cello Congresses's II-V, 2004 The First World Guitar Congress and 2008 World Guitar Congress II. Celebrations of music with international gatherings, of the world's greatest musicians, composers, conductors, instrument manufacturers students, and music lovers from around the globe.

9477 WWW.TOY-TMA.COM/INDEX.HTML
Toy Manufacturers of America
For toys, games and hobby decoration manufacturers and their representatives.

9478 WWW.UNC.EDU/DEPTS/OUTDOOR
Institute of Outdoor Drama
Summer jobs for all theatrical personnel.

9479 WWW.UPS.EDU/PROFESSIONALORGS/DRAMATURGY
Dramaturgy Northwest

Relevant information for all dramaturgs.

9480 WWW.URTA.COM
University/Resident Theatre Association
Coalition of theatre training programs. Sponsors unified auditions.

9481 WWW.USABDA.ORG
United States Amateur Ballroom Dancers Association
Non-profit organization working to promote ballroom dancing, both as a recreational activity and as a competetive sport.

9482 WWW.USITT.ORG
United States Institute for Theatre Technology
The association of design, production and technology professionals in the performing arts and entertainment industry whose mission is to promote the knowledge and skills of its members. International in scope, USITT draws its board of directors from across the US and Canada. Sponsors projects, programs, research, symposia, exhibits, and annual conference. Disseminates information on aesthetic and technical developments.

9483 WWW.VARIETY.ORG
Variety
e-version of the show business newspaper.

9484 WWW.VCU.EDU/ARTWEB/PLAYWRITING
Playwriting Seminars

9485 WWW.VPA.NIU.EDU/THEATER/AWEB1.HTM
Scenic Collection
Resources for scenic designers.

9486 WWW.WATERPARKS.COM
World Waterpark Association
Provides forum for exchange of ideas related to water amusement park industry.

9487 WWW.WOMENSINGERS.COM
Professional Women Singers Association
Non-profit networking organization for professional women singers.

9488 WWW.WRITERSGUILD.COM
Writers Guild of America
List of Agents and information on Mentor program.

9489 WWW1.PLAYBILL.COM
Theatre Central
Links to theatre.

9490 WWW1.PLAYBILL.COM/PLAYBILL
Playbill Online
Listings for Broadway and off Broadway theatre productions. Also guides for sites, including summer stock, national touring shows and

regional theatres worldwide.

9491 **WWW2.HAWAII.EDU/ATHE**
Association for Theatre in Higher Education
Promotes quality in theatre education.

9492 **WWW3.SK.SYMPATICO.CA/ERACHI/**
Drama Teacher's Resource Room

D

Q

R

V

W

X

Y

Z

A

Aalex Ragotzy, Penelope, 3087
Aarestad, Margaret, 6208
Aaron, Gregory, 260
Aaron, Jeffrey, 2171
Aaron, Jon, 8411
Aaron, Sandie, 6592, 6593
Abate, Hank, 7851
Abate, Stephen, 101, 2495
Abbas, Chad, 6668
Abbate, Allison, 374
Abbitt, Jerry, 2472
Abbott, Bob, 1224
Abbott, Carol, 5237
Abbott, Chuck, 2997
Abbott, Gail, 3915
Abdel-Ra'oof, Wali, 1231
Abdella, Carolyn, 1367
Abdul-Hanson, Toni, 4125
Abel, James K., 2283
Abel, Jan, 3633
Abel, Yves, 2215
Aberlin, Robert E, 535
Abernathky, Joe, 7122
Abildsoe, Deborah, 4270
Abillio, David, 133
Abington, Michael, 8108
Abler, Tim, 5765
Ables, Jane F, 5399
Abraham, Valerie, 371
Abraham, Vivan, 944
Abrahamsen, Daniel, 8431
Abrahamsen, Gerri, 8431
Abramowitz, Roy, 1698
Abrams, Aly, 3188
Abrams, Linda, 1426
Abrams, Marilyn, 2843
Abrams, Richard, 1498
Abramson, Lynn, 6102
Acevedo, David, 2466
Achabal, Julie, 266
Acker, Mark, 6594
Ackerley, Dr. Julian M, 1895
Ackerman, Bob, 1638
Ackerman, Jerry, 4141
Ackerman, Mark, 2825
Ackert, Stephen, 1015, 4298, 4313
Adamcik, Robert, 1773
Adams, Abigail, 3307, 3705, 4944
Adams, Alan D, 4181
Adams, Bettie S, 8206, 8207
Adams, Betty, 8307
Adams, Beverly, 1803
Adams, Brandon, 8346
Adams, Catherine, 2340
Adams, Chris, 667
Adams, Daria, 857, 4143
Adams, David, 3582
Adams, Dean, 2633, 4289
Adams, Donna, 3193
Adams, Elissa, 3130
Adams, Fred C, 3879, 5576
Adams, Gail V, 857, 4143
Adams, George, 1099
Adams, Herb, 1449
Adams, Jennifer F, 2371
Adams, John, 600
Adams, John W, 2874
Adams, Joielle, 1826
Adams, Jolene, 2429
Adams, Judith, 4623
Adams, Leigh Anne, 3158
Adams, Lyn, 3641
Adams, Lynea, 2684
Adams, Maxey, 8247
Adams, Maxey D., 8243
Adams, Meredith, 2290
Adams, Michael, 857, 4143
Adams, Pat, 6570
Adams, Paul, 3370
Adams, Randy, 2462, 2479

Adams, Sam, 1876
Adams, Susan H, 223
Adams, Yvonne, 2390
Adams III, Thaddeus A, 1581
Adcock, Elizabeth, 1388
Addaman, Linda, 6614
Addison, Debbie, 3904
Addison, Mary, 6804
Adducci, Denise M, 4428
Addy, G Keith, 1647
Addy, Obo, 71
Adelberg Rudow, Vivian, 4635
Adelson, Larry, 284
Aderente, David R, 1311
Adkins, Adala, 6804
Adkins, Thomas, 3782
Adkins, Tracey, 5876
Adkins, William, 1348
Adkison, Jen, 6358
Adler, Bob, 868
Adler, Courtney, 3181
Adler, Jeff, 2768
Adler, Joseph, 2686
Adler, Lisa, 2768
Adler, Sol, 4995
Adrian, Renae, 5647
Aduddell, Monique, 4482
Aester, Dale, 6449
Affron, Beatrice Jona, 629
Agar, Eunice, 1294
Agresti, Ben, 3813
Aguila, Miguel del, 864
Aguilar, Sylvester, 855
Aguilar, Violeta, 31
Aguilar-Thompson, Peggy, 4216
Agustin, Sandy, 4743
Ahem, Dan, 1224
Ahmad, Rosemary, 1773
Ahn, Jooyong, 1212
Ahrens, Dick, 2460
Ahrens, Elizabeth, 4744
Ahrold, Robbin, 7373
Aibel, Anthony, 1017
Aibel, Douglas, 3471
Aiken, Mary, 2902
Ainslie, Lauri, 6482
Ainsworth, Reg, 3900
Aitken, Donna, 6857
Aito, Suguru, 3397
Aja, Ron, 3371
Ajkun, Chiara, 417
Ajkun, Leonard, 417
Ajlouny, Jr, Joseph S, 6939
Akina, Henry G, 2022
Akins, Thomas N, 1168
Akiyama, Kazuyoshi, 1557
Alameida, Joseph, 4172
Albanese, John, 3452
Alber, Jennifer, 2863
Albers, Judith, 6982
Albers, Kathly, 1107
Albert, Philip, 2792
Albert, Sharon, 2792
Albert-Loewenberg, Susan, 2572
Alberti, Patricia, 8327
Albertie, Dante, 3291
Alberts, Elizabeth, 3159
Albrecht, Jerry, 1176
Albright, Mary, 6371
Albright, Raymond, 8357
Albright/Dieterl, Jane, 8294
Albritton, Susan, 3825
Albulario, David TR, 1904
Alcorn, Clayton, 3309
Alcott, Matt, 7730
Alder, Jac, 3832
Alder, Jennifer, 6817
Alderman, Lisa, 3904
Alderson, Danon, 505
Alderson, Nan, 2681
Aldredge, Russell, 368
Alegant, Marci, 5245

Alem, Ziad, 1224
Aleskie, Mary Lou, 836, 5526
Alexander, Allen, 7371
Alexander, Andrew, 2852
Alexander, Benjamin, 2280
Alexander, Carol, 2701
Alexander, Jacinthia, 3258, 3265
Alexander, Jeanne, 1650
Alexander, Jeffrey, 5189
Alexander, John, 1952, 1986
Alexander, Ken, 848
Alexander, Michael, 4124
Alexander, Steve, 3672
Alexander Griffin, Janet, 2660
Alfandre, Dominique, 642
Alfaro, Manny, 3381
Alfonso, Estelle, 411
Alfonso, Sebrina Maria, 1038
Alford, Alex, 3809
Alford, Alex B, 3808
Alford, David, 3794
Alford, Jesse, 2618
Alford, Marcus R, 262
Alford, Warmer, 6555
Alford, Warner, 6764
Alfton, Dennis, 7011
Aliev, Eldar, 301
Allan, Betty, 7579
Allan, Doug, 4936
Allan, Paul, 3289
Allar, Barry, 3952
Allard, Dr. Michael A, 934
Allard, Roger, 3072
Allardice, Bruce, 467, 3432
Allbritten, James, 2251
Allcorn, Ed, 1775, 5507
Allen, Amy, 3191
Allen, Bob, 5868
Allen, Christine, 611
Allen, Dalis, 5539
Allen, Darlene, 817
Allen, David, 7945
Allen, Dennis R, 7360
Allen, Faye, 2758, 2773, 6443
Allen, Geraldine, 2470
Allen, Gloria Marinacc, 1883
Allen, James, 2121
Allen, Janet, 2919
Allen, Jerry D, 3740
Allen, Joan, 1447
Allen, Joe, 5334
Allen, Joyce, 1843
Allen, Judith, 7523
Allen, LaRue, 556
Allen, Mary, 1373
Allen, Patrick, 2212
Allen, Rebecca, 2749
Allen, Ronald G, 1935
Allen, Russel P, 2014
Allen, Sanford, 4947
Allen, Sharon, 219
Allen, Todd Eric, 219
Allen Alford, Janie, 4
Allen Baxter, Karen, 3748
Allen Fiske, Dr. Richard, 875
Allen Sawyer, Marilyn, 888
Allen, III, Dr. Robert T, 5657
Allen-Farley, Anita, 2789
Allenbach, Brent, 5588
Allison, Joan, 1782
Allman, Elizabeth, 1870
Allred, Dr. Brady R, 2285
Alltop, Stephen, 1129, 5739
Ally, Barbara, 6260
Alme, Joseph T, 1598, 2255
Almoite, Irene, 31
Almonor, Anesta, 2443
Aloe, Verna, 1175
Alonzo, Adam, 8120
Alper, Bryna, 6085
Alper, Joel, 1258
Alphonsestephenson, Maestro, 1415

Alrey, AC, 1659
Alsedek, Anne L, 3696
Alsedek, Donald, 2482
Alsedek, Donald L, 3696
Alsina, Ramon, 2196
Alsop, Mafia, 1508
Alsop, Marin, 1509, 4209
Alstyne, Chris Van, 7479, 7480
Alter, Dennis, 2280
Alterman, Barry, 405
Altman, Lou, 2832
Altman, Peter, 3179
Altman, Thom, 2752
Altmann, Yvonne, 2231
Alva, Santos, 333
Alvarado, Elisa Marina, 2538
Alvarado, Linda, 1338
Alvarcz, Aracelly, 2433
Alvarez, Barry, 8294
Alvarez, Emma, 1044
Alvarez, Jackie, 2609
Alvarez, Steven, 4026
Alvarez-Brake, Mariana, 228
Alves, Dennis, 1262
Alvidrez, Jan, 3276
Alvord, Dr Buster, 716
Alzado, Peter, 3675
Amado, David, 1382
Amador, Rosi, 1278, 8380
Amano, Karen, 2530
Amara, Lucine, 2172
Amaral, Joesph, 3033
Amaral, Joseph, 3033
Amaral, Russ, 5860
Amarose, Caito, 5380
Amato, Anthony, 2202
Ambrose, Jane, 5602
Ambush, Benny, 5653
Ament, Istvan, 706
Ames, Chris, 2773, 6443
Ames, Karen, 902
Ames, Kirsten, 7447
Amey, Kevin, 361
Amicarella, Toni, 3349
Amirkhanian, Charles, 4191
Ammmen, Richard, 4743
Ammon, Sandra, 1874
Amo, Mark, 1447
Amodio, Pamela, 4271
Amos, David, 890
Amos Jr., James H., 1935
Amrein, John, 1139
Amster, Clara, 5207
Amsterdam, Mark Russell, 1479
Amsterdam, Susan, 1479
Amudd, John, 3389
Amundson, Steven, 1357
Anagnost, Dino, 1514
Anang, Amma, 717
Anang, Kofi, 717
Anastasio, Robert, 4316
Anaya, Dulce, 224
Andato, Vanessa, 401
Anderegg, Dr. David, 1294
Anderko, Connie, 2850
Anderle, Jeff, 2834
Anders, Patricia, 1874
Andersen, Derek, 7156
Andersen, Ib, 9
Andersen, Sarah J, 8286
Anderson, Addell, 3095
Anderson, Amy, 806
Anderson, Ben, 4867
Anderson, Bettie, 1801
Anderson, Blair, 3093
Anderson, Bob, 7143
Anderson, Bradley D, 2382
Anderson, Carolyn, 3487
Anderson, Chilton, 4921
Anderson, Chris, 2134
Anderson, Dan, 3813, 7993
Anderson, David, 8303, 8305

Anderson, Dewey, 1031, 4324, 4325, 4326
Anderson, Dianne, 1296, 4683
Anderson, Donna Gay, 4585
Anderson, Doug, 2203
Anderson, Ed, 7869
Anderson, Edgar A, 3058
Anderson, Eric, 5373
Anderson, Eva, 320
Anderson, Gary, 3095, 7166
Anderson, Glenn, 2632
Anderson, Grant, 1273
Anderson, Helane, 8447
Anderson, James, 3304
Anderson, Jeanette, 351, 4579
Anderson, Jennifer, 3914
Anderson, Jennifer D, 3915
Anderson, John, 4084
Anderson, Joy Rayman, 1197
Anderson, Kent, 611
Anderson, Larry, 8275
Anderson, Lawrence P, 5428
Anderson, Leonard A, 2893
Anderson, Lisa, 2267
Anderson, Marion, 5924
Anderson, Marjorie, 7330
Anderson, Marvin, 7354
Anderson, Mary, 3120
Anderson, Michele, 159, 4206
Anderson, Monique, 3948
Anderson, Noonie, 341
Anderson, Paula, 3145, 8275
Anderson, Rhonda Jo, 3761
Anderson, Robert P, 7178
Anderson, Ron, 2782
Anderson, Sandie, 4250
Anderson, Sandra, 7793
Anderson, Stephen C, 4219
Anderson, Steven C, 3602, 3603
Anderson, Thelma, 5375
Anderson, Thomas, 1085
Anderson, Virginia, 8231, 8232, 8233, 8235
Anderson, Waldie, 1064
Anderson, Walter E, 3010
Anderson, Wendy, 2438
Andoe, Bill, 7740
Andorf, Erica, 2942
Andrade, Bea, 1925
Andre, David, 942
Andreassi, James, 2622
Andreini, Lynn, 1145
Andres, Clay, 194
Andres, Dennis J, 6628
Andrew, Collie, 7829
Andrews, Bill, 2788
Andrews, Carol, 670
Andrews, Douglas, 4320
Andrews, Eric, 5724, 8273
Andrews, Gail, 5568
Andrews, Ginny, 2885
Andrews, Kenneth, 1558
Andrews, Linda Z, 355
Andrews, Mark, 1800
Andrews, Mike, 5584
Andrews, Susie, 2741
Andrews, Whit, 3565
Andringa, Mel, 4528
Andrucki, Judith W, 1233, 2075
Andrucyk, Stanley, 4880
Angelico, Andria, 388
Angelini, Marcello, 608
Angell, Dianna, 3510
Angermeier, Tom, 2911
Angiel, Brenda, 114
Angle, Steven, 7491
Anglen, Reginald, 7650
Ankele, Jason, 3825
Ankele, Nina, 1931
Ankrom, David, 3874
Ankrom, Robert, 3539
Anmed, Sharon, 6440
Ann Klaus, Jean, 3603
Annas, Alicia, 2505

Ansbacher, Charles A, 4661
Ansley, Joe, 3
Ansley, Shepard B, 2014
Ansnes, Cris, 1481
Ansotegui, Dan, 266
Ansotegui, Toni, 266
Antenucci, Steve, 3149
Anthony, Carmen, 3390
Anthony, David, 5994
Anthony, Deborah, 619
Anthony, Dr. Sofia, 1299
Anthony, Jesse, 4086
Anthony, Jesse W, 4147, 5310
Anthony, Kathy, 4145
Anthony, Mary, 512
Anthony, Peter, 2597
Anthony, Shpritz, 2497
Anthony, Vincent, 2763
Antinori, Ronald R., 2014
Anton, Sara, 953, 4241
Antonelli, Cynthia, 2905
Antoni, Recardo, 792
Antonio, Lou, 2453
Antoniou, Theodore, 1261
Antonson, Sara, 3980
Antunez, Oskar, 5
Anzalotti, Cynthia, 4688
Aody, G Keith, 5236
Aoyama, Barron, 304
Apitz, John, 3159
Apone, Carl, 5382
Appel, Libby, 3651, 5285
Appelhof, Dr. Ruth, 3311
Appels, Jonathon, 454
April, Paula, 7038
Aquiline, Carlyn Ann, 3728
Aracena, Beth, 5636
Aragon, Antonio, 7263
Araujo, Maria, 1429
Arbesfeld, Bobbie, 7232
Arceneaux, George E, 4589
Archambealt, Kevin, 3804
Archer, Leslie, 3509
Archer, Richard A, 4205
Archer, Rickard, 3875
Archer Adams, Brenda, 1492
Arciniegas, Diego, 3037
Arcudi, Evelyn R, 2232
Arden, Ron, 2900
Ardizzone, Matthew, 8386
Arend, Arlene, 1977
Arends, Mildred, 2049
Arens, Fred, 98
Arey, Dana, 635
Arie-Gaifman, Hanna, 7439
Arisco, David, 2685
Arkenberg, Scott, 2033
Arlt, Lewis, 3332
Armistead, Elizabeth, 6569
Armitage, Donald L, 2251
Armore, Anthony, 1699
Armour, Thomas, 234
Armstrong, Anton, 2140
Armstrong, Drew, 6359
Armstrong, Helen, 4291
Armstrong, Nicholas, 1464
Armstrong, Sharon, 3795
Arnaiz, Lara, 47
Arnett, Kevin, 3083
Arnold, Anita G, 5272, 7719
Arnold, Bonnie, 1033
Arnold, Bruce, 7491
Arnold, Michael, 7883
Arnold, Soozie, 4255
Arnold, Tara, 6971
Arnoult, Philip, 3016
Aronson, Maure, 4672
Arpino, Gerald, 275
Arrington, Beth, 4332
Arrington, Kevin, 5806
Arrington, Mary, 679
Arrowsmith, Judy, 4332

Arsove, Priscilla, 732
Artenian, Rich, 8183
Arthur, Chistopher, 2918
Arthur, Janice, 6690
Arthur, Ken, 3465
Arthur, Mary A, 1864
Artiach, Miren, 266, 2025
Artistic Advisor, David Drummond, 373
Artistic Director, Jay Fishman, 1354
Artists, Baylin, 631
Arturo Diemecke, Enrique, 842
Arunasalam, Chitra, 1924
Aruny, Donita, 4270
Arvay, WJ, 3754
Arzewski, Cecilia, 1073
Asalde, Yrene, 6026
Asbell, David, 6144
Asch, Sunny Charla, 79, 80, 4119
Ascione, Gerard J, 1024, 1997
Asen, Rita, 1510
Ash, Roy L., 1916
Ash, William, 1379
Ashbaker, Susan, 2280
Ashburner, Richard, 2156
Ashby, Hollis, 4088, 5947
Ashby, Jay, 5381
Ashby, Marty, 5381
Ashe, Kevin, 7251
Ashens, Robert, 2272
Asher, Ronald J, 1422
Ashford, James, 2733, 6411
Ashler, Ret Adm Philip, 1065
Ashley, Bruce, 2887
Ashley, Eli D., 5708
Ashley, Karl, 1035
Ashley, Mary Ellen, 3418
Ashley, Rebecca, 465
Ashton, Heather, 3236
Ashton, John, 5722
Ashton, Jon, 3589
Ashton, Judy, 3947
Ashton, Patricia, 1052
Ashwander, Lindy, 4011, 5807
Askew, Penny, 602
Assaf, Dennis G, 1227, 4594
Assante, Claudio, 460
Assenheimer, Paul, 1648
Assink, Brent, 902
Astolfi, Cher, 4296
Astrachan, Margot, 1516
Aswegan-Thornhill, Carol, 6641
Atherton, David, 886, 4178
Atherton, J Scott, 3684
Atkins, Nicolette, 847
Atkinson, Bill, 673
Atkinson, Emily, 3750
Atkinson, Eve, 5329
Atkinson, Susan D, 3687
Atkinson, Tim, 1065
Atkinson, Timothy, 8120, 8121
Aubel, Leo, 2834
Auberger Jr, Donald C, 1615
Aubrey, Daniel, 3259
AuBuchon, Kathleen J, 1107
Auderhalt, Xandra, 585
Auer, Elizabeth, 4334
Auerbach, Marvin, 376
Auger, Giselle A, 4625
Aukin, Daniel, 3449
Aulderheide, Lawrence, 1646
Ault, Chris, 7180, 7181
Auman, Barry, 1579
Auman, Elizabeth, 2860
Aune, Gregory, 4554
Aurand, Ellie, 2275
Aurell, Skip, 7126
Aurisch, Helga, 1801
Austen, Linda Jane, 5873
Austin, Alan, 5531
Austin, Dr. James, 5527
Austin, Jeffrey, 2081
Austin, Kelli, 6601

Austin, Larry, 1489
Austin, Lyn, 3408
Austin, Marilyn, 3841
Austin, Mary K, 632
Austin, Robert Carter, 1798
Autin, Holly O, 4101
Autry, Timothy, 7898
Avans, Ronald D, 5809
Aven, Jerry, 3855, 5529
Averill, Evelyn, 1971
Avery, Jennifer, 2849, 2856
Avery, Kenneth P, 2391
Avery, Tricia, 3818
Avisar, Eytan, 169
Avital, Samuel, 178, 2579
Avitsur, Monica, 1537, 5047
Avni, Rau, 3391
Avril, Franck, 1691, 5302
Ax, Barbara, 3896, 5603
Axtell, Jamie, 2816
Ayala, Juan, 1904
Ayazi, Sara, 4187
Ayers, Jim, 3929
Aykal, Gurer, 1793
Ayoung, Patrick, 418
Ayres-Frederick, Linda B, 2522
Azer, Karen, 1720
Azevedo, Ann, 2617

B

B. Swope, Jr, Mrs. Herbert, 5409
Baad, Debbie, 1928
Baad, Mike, 1928
Baar, Rachael, 6712
Baarsvick, Richard, 339
Babbitt, David P, 1940
Babbitt, Milton, 5321
Babbitt, Samuel, 3749
Babcock, Linda M, 1821
Babin, Andrea, 2070
Babin, L Randolph, 2305
Babin, Sarajean, 1365
Baccellieri, Rich, 7173
Bach, Bobbi, 1956
Bach, Timothy, 891, 900, 4182
Bachand, Bill, 5861
Bachelor, Louise, 2960
Bacher, Kenneth, 4041
Bacher, Steve, 3811
Back, Lyle, 7540
Backer, Paul, 4152
Backes, Sarah, 6058
Backmon, James, 2221
Bacon, Bobby, 1065
Bacon, Louise, 2113
Bacon, Paul, 3230
Bacon, Sarah, 5013
Bader, Alicia, 2656
Bader, C Ulrich, 1017
Bader, Hannah, 4198
Badgett, Darlene, 4939
Badhan, Raj, 2497
Badu-Younge, Zelma, 245
Bae, Ik-Hwan, 1461
Baer, Miriam Reitz, 4250
Baff, Ella, 327, 4656
Bagan, Merwyn, 7189
Bagish, Bernard, 848
Bago, Dan, 7662
Bagwell, James, 2057
Bagwell, Keith, 5796
Baham, Patricia, 2986
Bahiri, Medhi, 463
Bahr, Jill Eathorne, 647
Bahr, Michael, 3879, 5576
Baierlein, Ed, 2588
Bailen, Sarah, 611
Bailey, Ann, 3777
Bailey, Bob, 2788
Bailey, Chad, 1354

Bailey, Erin, 4324
Bailey, Grady S, 567
Bailey, Mark, 984, 1976
Bailey, Mary K, 585
Bailey, Robert, 2273
Bailey, Stephen, 1982
Bailey, Steve, 3873
Bailey, William C, 2327
Bailey Timm, Faye, 3922
Baileyts, Erin, 4325
Bailly, Jean, 1042
Bain, Agnes M, 407, 3302, 4939
Bain, Donald K, 4247
Bain, Donnalee, 1867
Bain, Gay, 2940, 6418
Bair, Sheldon, 1252
Baird, Connie, 3522
Baird, M Rex, 1406
Baird, Thomas, 433
Baites, William, 6439
Baitzel, Edgar, 1916
Bajuk, Laura, 911
Bak, Anne, 349, 2125
Baker, Adele, 1411
Baker, Angie, 2794
Baker, Ann Meier, 1986
Baker, Ann T, 2963
Baker, Anna, 654
Baker, Art, 941
Baker, Barbie, 1837
Baker, Ben, 3059
Baker, Brian, 1492
Baker, Carol, 5571
Baker, Cassandra E, 6460
Baker, Cymthia, 1519
Baker, Daniel, 2919
Baker, Deb, 5356
Baker, Fred, 5514
Baker, Hub, 5517
Baker, Keith Alan, 2668
Baker, Mark, 4124
Baker, Melissa, 7066
Baker, Pam, 1117
Baker, R Palmer, 482
Baker, Raymond, 6254
Baker, Richard, 4802
Baker, Robert, 6926
Baker, Robert Hart, 978
Baker, Scott, 2536
Baker, Stacy, 3237
Baker, Stephen, 1353
Baker, Tommy, 7916
Baker, Tyrone, 78
Baker-Haines, Janice, 305
Balaban, Rachel, 642
Balanchine, George, 528
Balcher, Frances, 1583
Balchunas, Heather, 3039
Baldenhofer, Chris, 831
Balderose, George, 8492
Baldet, Jean Louis, 2680
Baldonieri, Amy, 1720
Baldwin, Anne, 899
Baldwin, Constance, 975
Baldwin, Daniel, 1192
Baldwin, Elaine, 726
Baldwin, Eleanor, 684
Baldwin, George, 4525
Baldwin, Melissa, 1232
Baldwin, Pat, 1786
Baldwin, Patricia, 2544
Baldwin, Ron, 2934, 6661
Balentine, Douglas, 3862
Balentine, Susan, 3862, 5537
Baley, Virko, 1406
Balgeman, Thomas, 3992
Balkin, Richard, 1476
Balko, Harris L, 5780
Ball, Amy, 3865
Ball, Betsy, 1447
Ball, Bob, 2026
Ball, Dana, 423

Ball, Leland, 2493
Ball, Peggy, 1666, 5263
Ball, Steve, 3055
Ball, Teri, 2545
Ballam, Michael, 2323
Ballard, Brownie, 6361
Ballard, Cindy, 6202
Ballard, Doris, 3230
Ballard, H Byron, 3520
Ballard, Jodee, 885
Ballas, Debi, 2780
Ballentine, Thomas, 4430, 4443
Baller, Ann, 7344
Ballesteros, Joe, 6143
Ballew, III, William V, 1793
Ballinger, June, 3268
Ballone, Dale, 3101, 6956
Ballou, Joan, 3904
Balmer, Stephanie, 16
Balogh, Lajos, 1696
Balogh, Rebbeca M, 3615
Baloghn, Lajos, 1342
Balph, Judy, 2749
Balsamo, Rita, 7478, 7479, 7480
Baltar, Joseph, 4608
Balter, Alan, 5171
Balzano, Richard, 4936
Bammert, Carl, 6965
Banazek, Matt, 3309
Bandelato, Michael, 1827, 5596
Banerdt, Vonnie, 829
Baney, David, 2283
Banks, Eric, 2338
Banks, James C, 1081
Banks, Jean, 7373
Banks, Tom, 4788
Bankston, Thomas, 2262
Banno, Joe, 2667
Bannon, Steve, 3202
Banta, Jody, 2978
Banta, Joyce, 6632
Banta, Martha, 3315, 4965
Banwart, Sidney, 1142
Barabas, Gabor, 3247, 4881
Barabas, SuzAnne, 3247, 4881
Barathan, Viein, 1488
Barauskas, Madeline, 2698
Barbarita, Michael C, 1743
Barbaro, Dr. Cosmo A, 5331
Barbash, Lillian, 1470, 4955
Barber, Kim, 3232
Barber, Michael R, 6416
Barber, Myrt, 6389
Barber, Nathan, 4729
Barberio, Steve, 3123
Barbieri, Carol, 1929
Barbour, Ashley S, 2968
Barbre, Beth, 616
Barckhoff, Greg, 6435
Barclay, Barbara, 2097
Barclay, Barbara M., 1941
Barclay, Jud, 4554
Barclay, Margaret, 1461
Barclay, Neil, 7980
Barclay, Steven, 8341
Barcly, Barbara, 1502
Bard, Dr. Karlyn, 5592
Bardellini, Keith, 2394
Bardenstein, Ruth, 6913
Barefoot, Carolyn, 8193
Barenboim, Daniel, 1116, 1119
Barenboim, Thomas S, 3033
Barese, Jan, 6265
Barger, JP, 1264
Bargiel, Diane, 5341
Bargman, Theresa, 3173
Barile, Caitlin, 6311
Barilla, Anthony, 3856
Barimo, Millicent, 2012
Barkdoll, Holly, 3573
Barker, Alain, 4492
Barker, Elaine, 1769

Barker, Joan, 2180
Barker, Juliay, 8437
Barker, Vick, 7731
Barker-Henwood, Catherine, 792
Barkes, Tom, 2927
Barkhymer, Lyle, 1661
Barko, Stephen B, 1019
Barlow, Dr. John, 3762
Barnard, Robert, 9
Barnea, Dr. Uri, 1387
Barnea, Uri, 2159
Barnell, Robert J, 5176
Barnes, Dr. Arthur, 841
Barnes, Jack, 2955
Barnes, Jessica, 1767
Barnes, Jill, 698
Barnes, Karen L, 1489
Barnes, Mark, 8299
Barnes, Milton, 6990
Barnes, Pat, 3787
Barnes, Philip, 2150
Barnes, Sue, 3777
Barnet, David, 1387
Barnett, Carol, 5462
Barnett, Carrie, 4568
Barnett, Nancy, 2706, 2707
Barnett, R Joseph, 2011
Barnett, Robby, 200
Barnhart, Frank A, 3604
Barnhart, J Kent, 3180
Barnhart, Mitch, 7752
Barnicle, Andrew, 2423
Barnum, Sibyl, 611
Baron, Henry Scott, 3701
Baron, Leonard, 7798
Baron, Suzanne, 7798
Barr, Daniel, 2774
Barr, Eric, 2487
Barr, Margaret, 1638
Barra, Donald, 822
Barras, Rhon, 4588
Barrese, Rocco S, 1489
Barrett, Dave, 901
Barrett, Dean, 7092
Barrett, Ellie, 229
Barrett, Gayle, 2606
Barrett, Jeanne, 4883
Barrett, Kevin, 3230, 6326
Barrett, Leigh, 2854
Barrett, Louise, 7247
Barrett, Marsha, 4299
Barrett, Michael, 5582
Barriz, Albert, 6913
Barroga, Jeannie, 2462
Barron, Alice, 2122, 4717
Barron, Maida, 6842
Barrons, Molly, 127
Barrus, Andrew, 3892
Barrus, JaccSon, 3892
Barry, Carole, 6657
Barry, Grace, 275
Barry, Jerome, 4304
Barry, Jolee, 3205
Barry, Linda, 2370
Barry, Mike, 7168
Barston, Gilda, 4487
Barstow, Barbara, 1426
Barstow, Bill, 1786
Bartczak, Janice, 4049
Bartee, Dr. Neale King, 13, 788, 2381
Barth, Margaret M, 1742
Barthelemy, Paul, 1702
Barthelman, Barbara, 2750
Barthelmes, Alix, 2231
Bartholomew, David, 2340
Bartholomew, Judith W, 4205
Bartholow, Timothy, 6428
Bartlett, Ken, 248
Bartlett, Michael, 902
Bartlett, Wendy, 1922
Bartoli, Anna, 4685
Bartolini, Louis, 915

Barton, Blair, 2496
Barton, Dave, 2542
Bartruff, Jim, 3154
Bartsch, Jim, 1353
Bartz, Paul, 8464, 8508
Barudin, Stuart, 1433
Basbas, Louise, 5038
Basch, Sarah, 3582
Basden, Millie, 2502
Basehore, Vicky, 5971
Bashaw, Mary, 3705
Baskett, Shirley, 190
Basney, Nyela, 1808, 2319
Basom, Rita, 5787
Bass, EE, 5314
Bass, Robert, 2209
Bass, Sherman, 7970
Basse, Jayne, 5498
Basset, Ralph, 6893
Bassett, Debbie, 564
Bassett, Emma, 4939
Bassett, Lynn, 691
Bassin, Joel, 3477
Bassler Sullivan, Alice, 6
Bastos-Klein, Eveliny, 2002
Batdorf, Kay L, 4512
Bate, Judy, 2684
Bateman, Danny, 1161
Batemen, Ray H, 7213
Bates, Andrea, 1270
Bates, Ann, 369
Bates, Betty, 250
Bates, Jeff, 6585
Bates, Linda, 3878
Bateson, Kathleen P, 5432
Batjer, Margaret, 847
Battali, Kathy, 4040
Battan, Suzette, 777
Batterson, Brett, 2124
Battle, De Ama, 339
Battle, Jr, George A, 5161
Bauch, Ronnie, 4853
Bauch, Esquire, Robert, 4009
Bauchens, Robert, 8368
Bauchman, Bob, 2940
Bauchman, Robert, 6418
Baudoin, James, 6451
Bauer, Bob, 7605, 7611
Bauer, David, 6608
Bauer, Gail, 3090
Bauer, Harold, 1133, 2046
Bauer, Lindsay, 190
Bauer, Victor, 1430
Bauers, John, 2589
Baum, Jeff, 954, 4241
Baum, Marlyn, 3447
Baum, Maude, 395
Bauman, Wayne, 2063
Baumeister, Randy, 6636
Baumgart, Jr, Warren W, 2837
Baumgartner, Ted, 241
Baun, Barbara, 3739
Baune, Terrie, 904
Bavaria, Edward C, 2006
Baxter, Sandra, 1631
Bay, John, 3071
Bay, Peter, 612, 1689, 1779, 3661, 4242, 5299
Bayer, Daniel, 3589
Bayes, Jack, 807
Bayes, Sammy Dallas, 3487
Bayley, David, 3943
Baylin, Marc J, 8485
Baylor, Cecil, 7670
Baynter, , 2178
Bazirjian, BA, Stephanie, 4180
Beach, Christopher, 7462
Beach, Doug, 4457
Beach, Milo C, 4306
Beadle, Robert, 2990
Beadle, Tony, 1262
Beal, Mark, 6538
Beal, Tandy, 166

Beale, Jennifer, 2567
Beals, Meghan, 3430
Bean, Janet R, 4427
Beane, Frank, 1241, 2078
Beard, Beth, 8249
Beard, Beverly, 2990
Beard, Gary, 2299
Beard, Paul S, 5518
Bearley, Cynthia, 309
Beaser, Robert, 1495
Beasley, Kelly, 2689
Beattie, Michael, 1218
Beatty, Matt, 6648
Beatty, Max, 2948
Beaubeaux, James, 2399
Beauchamp, Bill, 2971
Beaudry, Suzanne, 745
Beaugard, Theresa, 7221
Beaumont, Andre, 2651
Beauvais, Corinne, 901
Beaven, Robert G, 572
Beaver, Kathy, 3500
Beaver, Mary L, 2890
Becerra, Rodney, 3859
Becher, Amy, 201
Bechtle, Nancy H, 902, 1946
Bechtolsheim, Catherine Von, 1843
Beck, Carl, 3220
Beck, Crafton, 1027, 1365, 1648
Beck, Ellie, 3285
Beck, Isha Manna, 3400
Beck, James, 6371
Beck, James F, 2704
Beck, Marilyn, 265
Beck, Tom, 8275
Beck Johnson, Lani, 2620
Beck Jr, Howard, 3929
Beckenbach, Bill, 3616
Becker, AS Micky, 754
Becker, Bill, 6398
Becker, Wendy, 8220
Becker, William L, 6399
Becker, OSB, Father Bruno, 5308
Beckett, Tom, 6268, 6269
Beckham, Rosemary, 3648
Beckley, Barbara, 2394
Beckman, Chris, 8093
Beckman, Jack B, 8093
Beckman Ross, Tonya, 3617
Beckmann, Nancy, 4792
Beckos, Barbara, 3510
Bedford, Danella, 217
Bedford, Dr. Clark, 2292
Bedford, John, 606
Bednaiz, Karen, 2272
Bednarek, James, 6859
Bedovich, Christine, 2497
Beebx, George, 3112
Beekman, Betty, 2613
Beeler, Kathryn, 7976
Beeman, Doug, 3352
Beeman, Frances, 3092
Beene, Meg, 655
Beeny, Suzanne, 2183, 2696
Beer, Samantha A, 2322
Beerman, Burton, 5180
Beers, John H, 4272
Beers, John H., 983
Beers, Larry, 3478
Beesley, Karine, 872
Beggs, Patricia K, 2257
Begley, Doris, 2019
Begovich, Christine, 2497
Behmke, Jay M, 831
Behnke, Anne, 4115
Behonek, John, 2225
Behrends, Alan, 4768
Behrns, Pat, 7166
Beilein, John, 8199
Beilina, Nina, 1499
Beinecke, John B, 3399
Beirne, Christine, 864

Belansky, Gail, 871
Belber, Robert, 7286
Belbruno, John, 984
Beles, Craig, 5697
Belfy, Jeanne, 1095, 4414
Belgrave, Nigel, 6909
Belilove, Hank, 3869
Belilove, Jim, 504
Belilove, Lori, 504
Belin, Susan S, 1711
Belkin, Robert A, 3472
Belknap, Norton, 535
Bell, Caitlin, 4638
Bell, Candace, 2761
Bell, Daivd, 6286
Bell, Dr. Richard, 1377
Bell, Gary, 2185
Bell, Jack, 3226
Bell, Janine, 709
Bell, Lee, 6420
Bell, Mu'afrida, 904
Bell, Muriel, 2117
Bell, Robert, 1660, 2117
Bell, Sandra, 486
Bell, Sandy, 6718
Bell, Stuart, 5142
Bell, Susan, 5721
Bell, Vanessa, 5538
Bell-Hanson, Jeffery, 1329
Bellamy, Lou, 3162
Bellas, Steve, 6397
Beller, Hava Kohav, 3393
Bellinger, Barbara P., 974
Bellinger, Samuel J, 3336
Bellingham, Sandra, 369
Bellrichard, Cindy, 3117
Belo, Paul, 3914
Belsky, Joel, 3589
Beltran, Victoria, 1876
Beltz, Steve, 3621
Belz, Jason M, 8447
Bemelmans, Norman, 5159
Bemis, Stephen T, 8386
Ben-Dor, Gisele, 920
Benac, William P, 3830
Benachowski, Edwin R, 833
Benachowski, Marilyn, 833
Benbow, Anne, 3253
Benda, Jean, 3003, 3237
Bendall, JoEllen, 1169
Bender, Eric, 563
Bendett, David, 927
Bendix, Richard, 3959
Benedette Snyder, Patricia D, 3511
Benell, Keri, 182
Benenson, Claire B, 4995
Benezra, Steve, 3523
Benfield, Knolan, 3561
Bengston, Paul, 2560
Benham, Verna, 684
Beninato, Barbara L, 1083
Benitez, Cecilio, 393
Benitez, Joseph, 5017
Benitez, Maria, 393
Benjamin, Chuck, 3025
Benjamin, Eric, 1653, 5171
Benjamin, Jan, 4356
Benner, Lynnette, 1490
Bennett, Cameron, 5226
Bennett, Dale, 1810
Bennett, Diane Tobin, 2971
Bennett, Dick, 8294
Bennett, Dr. Cameron, 5225
Bennett, Elizabeth, 2420
Bennett, Karen, 402
Bennett, Kate, 4640
Bennett, Lauren E, 8466
Bennett, Lori, 2983
Bennett, Mike, 6553
Bennett, Neil, 823
Bennett, Robert, 1334, 7880
Bennett, Rodger, 5513

Bennett, Suzanne, 3476
Bennett, Tom, 1765
Bennett, Willis, 5616
Benninga, Carla, 2730
Bennion Feeney, Krista, 894
Benoist, Joan, 2168
Benoit, David, 802
Bensel, Mary, 6341
Bensignor, Jane, 627
Benstein, Julianne, 627
Bent, Kim, 3898
Bentley, Jeff, 7539
Bentley, Jeffrey J, 362
Bentley, John, 1608
Benton, Judy, 254
Benton, Louisa, 3462
Benton, Patrick, 3168
Berberian, George, 1029, 4323
Berdahl, James, 1958, 4230
Berez, Jay Allen, 388
Berg, Harriet, 343
Berg, Nancy, 5735
Berg, Paul, 2882, 4473
Berg, Ron, 2122, 4717
Berg, Stu, 2453
Berger, Chuck, 1948
Berger, Jesse, 378
Berger, Larry, 994
Berger, Sidney, 3853
Berger, Sidney L, 3855, 5529
Bergeret, Albert, 2225
Bergeron, Ann A, 3121
Bergeron, Julian, 1410
Bergman, Cathy, 305
Bergmans, Chad Eric, 2840
Bergstrom, Mary Jo, 1679
Berier, Jacques, 187
Berkeiser, Will, 7497
Berkenblit, Dr. Daniel, 5086
Berkenstein, Catherine, 2831
Berkenstock, Dr. James, 1131
Berkow, Jay, 3899
Berkowitz, Patricia, 900
Berliet, Nathalie, 519
Berlin, Ernest, 4355
Berlovitz-Desbois, Barbra, 3148
Berman, Erica C, 1637
Berman, Harris A, 4662
Berman, Howard, 2424
Berman, Laura, 344
Berman, Mitchell, 1211
Berman, Patricia, 1488
Berman, Ruth, 1258
Berman PhD, Rabbi Donna, 6254
Bermingham, John, 1876
Berna, Linda, 4430, 4442, 4443
Bernal, Pedro, 182
Bernard, Allan, 993
Bernardi, Rich, 209
Bernardi, Robert J, 6789
Bernegger, Sandra, 1545, 1546, 2235
Bernegger, Sandra P, 566
Berner, Barbara, 2157
Berner, Jennifer, 5685
Berner, Joseph L, 2006
Bernet, Glenn, 4808
Berney, Tim, 3641
Bernfield, Susan, 3417
Bernhardt, Elise, 465, 498, 7400
Bernhardt, Robert, 1218, 1766, 2297
Bernstein, Jini, 6002
Bernstein, Leonard, 1522
Bernstein, Sue Renee, 8405
Bernzen, Avril Marie, 2050
Bero-Johnson, Jamie, 5325
Berrier, Kristen, 8193
Berry, Chris, 1869

Berry, Debra, 4751
Berry, Dr. Richard, 5549
Berry, Duper, 2993
Berry, Gus, 3944
Berry, Jim, 5911
Berry, John, 2904
Berry, Sharon W, 1240
Berry, Jr, Stafford C, 573
Berryhill, Andrew, 1346
Bersen, Amy, 8080
Berseth, John, 1709
Bershad, Jack R, 2280
Berson, Marc E., 7232
Bertacci, Franco, 1422
Bertani, Steve, 3194
Bertaux, Betty, 2091
Berthelsdorf, Mildred, 1699
Berthelsdorf, MD, Mildred, 1699
Bertley, Terrie, 181
Bertnik, Nancy, 6550
Bertoni, Al, 6392
Bertrand, Blaine, 3814
Bertsch, Anneke, 1036
Berube, Ernest D, 4856
Berube, Rick, 3448
Berven, Wynn, 1966
Besa, Tina, 127
Besanko, John, 8169
Besen, Robert, 8425
Beshore, Rebecca, 4238
Bess, David, 3975, 5723, 8270, 8271
Bessett, Gary, 3046
Bessey III, Earle, 6814
Best, Grant, 2189
Best, Judi, 6616
Best, Patricia, 2631
Best, Paul, 58
Best, Reverend David, 3395
Beste, Jeff, 5184
Beston, Dr. Rose Marie, 5078
Betanzos, Odon, 3508
Bethany, Dr. Adeline, 5387
Bethea, Charles Henry, 4830
Bethel, Charles, 3140
Bethelsen, Maren, 5049
Bethune, Brian D, 3631
Bethune, Zina, 58
Betley, Marge, 3160, 3493
Bettinson, Greg, 2326
Betts, Kathleen, 4317
Betts, Roland H, 4125
Betz, Beth Ann, 5595
Betz, Beth-Ann, 2329
Betzer, Susan, 1066
Beucke, Maria, 3214
Beusmann, Bob, 2139
Beutel, Paul, 3806
Bevan, Ted B, 3840
Bevans Gillett, Mary, 3112
Bever, Steve, 6691
Bever, Susan, 1163
Bevis, Sharon, 4378
Bevning, Joyce, 3145
Bewley, James, 4187
Bewley, Thomas, 345
Bewtel, Paul, 7979
Beyer, Duane, 4705
Beyers, Ann Marie, 280
Beyrau, Sheri, 3919
Beznos, Lois R, 1318
Bialand, Leif, 1058
Bialburn, Jodi, 442
Bianchi, Laurie, 6106
Bianco, Marie R, 908
Bichards, , 3372
Bichel, Steven D, 3758
Bickel, Jerry, 2742
Bickel, Nancy, 1710
Bicknell, Marcus, 5017
Biddle, Wendy, 1331
Biddle, William, 6925
Biebesheimer, Jerome, 4070

Biederwolf, Robert I, 5758
Bieganski, Ron, 2835
Biemot, Linda, 1459
Bierny, Dr. Jean Paul, 782, 4057
Bierny, Dr. Jean-Paul, 774
Biesanz, Katja, 614
Biggerstaff, Ken, 2941
Bigler, Jeff, 1269
Bilancio, Francis, 3104
Biles, Anita, 7944
Biles, Richard, 8345, 8429
Bill, Pastor Earl, 2392
Billeci, Celesta, 4207
Billerbeck, Ronda, 5681
Billick, Dean, 7990, 7991
Billig, Etel, 2886
Billings, Jim, 1964
Billmann, Sara, 2120, 4709
Bilotti, Richard, 1433
Bilsky, Steve, 7835
Bilyea, Julie K, 4558
Bindman, Rosalyn, 1527
Bingham, Mark, 7335
Bingham, Marla, 5575
Bingham, Wendy, 4198
Binns, Ralph, 2323
Bintinger, Thomas P., 1414
Birdman, Beatrice, 982
Birdsong, Alexa, 5008
Birdsong, Ronnie, 5921
Birdsong-James, Jacque, 6058
Biris, Dino, 2813
Birkhauser, Robert, 3986
Birks, Frederick P, 1021
Birman, Robert, 896
Birman, Robert A, 1195
Birmingham, Ron, 4090
Birmingham, Tom, 2696, 3983
Birnbaum, Neilnda, 1033
Birtles, Rod, 1274
Bishoff, Murray, 4799
Bishop, Rita, 1838
Bishop, Toby J, 1117
Bisignano, John, 6367
Bissett, Colin, 3523
Bither, Philip, 1355, 3151
Bitner, Barbara, 4411
Bittel, Michael, 4350
Bitting, Angelyn S, 7515
Bitting, Lisa, 4516
Bitz, Kim Patrick, 2819
Bivins, Wally, 3207
Bjaland, Leif, 1001
Bjerke, Vicki, 2062
Bkakacj, Tua, 6216
Bla, Jeaneane KO, 3180
Blachere, Brigitte, 4316
Blachly, Michael, 4334, 6347
Black, Anne, 1621, 2306, 5197, 5198
Black, Delores, 2305
Black, Diane, 341
Black, F Scott, 3013
Black, Freddie, 7
Black, Kathy, 698
Black, Linda C, 2097
Black, Oliver, 2692
Black, Ruth, 4685
Black, Sandra, 2052
Black, Shekena, 6154
Black, Susan, 8166
Blackaby, Anita, 7806
Blackburn, David, 4777
Blackburn, Sheila, 3814
Blackledge, Barbara, 3700
Blackman, Amy, 474
Blackman, Gary, 3252
Blackman, Gary W, 8398
Blackman, Mark, 3252
Blackman, Mark A, 8398
Blackman, Rachel, 1288
Blackmon, Mark Robert, 3017
Blackstone, Douglas, 5332

Blackweider, Stephen, 2053
Blackweldor, Stephen, 1152, 2054
Blackwell, Frank, 1094
Blackwell, Susan, 1634
Blackwood, Randall, 7120
Blackwood, Sandra, 2019
Blades, Marika, 3448
Blafield, Robert P, 2111
Blaha, Jeffrey, 3182
Blaine, Martha, 1671
Blair, Chris, 2764
Blair, Ellen L, 2232
Blair, Grace, 2315
Blair, Jena L, 3620
Blair, Meredith, 8427
Blair, Patricia, 268
Blair, Robert, 6908
Blaizely, Doris, 2572
Blake, Laurence, 93
Blake, Mark, 6746
Blakely, Claude W, 3758
Blakemore, Donna, 140
Blakey, Carolyn, 2060
Blakistone, Olive, 2557
Blakistone, Tom, 2557
Blalock, Roger, 6634
Blanc, George, 4100
Blanchard, Linda, 4753
Blanchard, Sonya, 312
Blanco, Carol, 444
Blanco, Gabriella, 1509
Blanco, R Michael, 444
Blanco, Sheila, 6751
Blandy, Susan, 1560
Blank, Dave, 6653
Blankenship, Karen, 5434
Blanker, Larae, 3764
Blanton, James, 1456
Blanton, Sonnet, 3284
Blattner, Sharon, 4201
Blaufuss, Patricia, 2636
Blaum, Bryan, 8061
Blauvelt, Betsy, 3918
Blaylock, Suzy, 3823
Blazey, Darla, 4509
Bleakley, Nancy, 5346
Bledsoe, Alyce, 810
Bledsoe, Jerry H, 3933, 5666
Bleeke, Evelyn, 2183
Bleiweis, Phyllis, 4371
Blenn, John, 5100
Blevins, Jennifer, 3544
Bley, Jonathan, 5071
Bligandi, Phil, 4113
Bliss, Sally A, 364
Bliss, Shirley, 698
Block, Dr. Glenn, 1208
Block, Gail S, 476
Block, Glenn, 1383
Block, Jean, 3276
Blocker, Brandt, 6769
Blodgett, Dana, 1865
Bloemendaal, Joyce, 4542
Bloom, Lawrie, 4647
Bloom, Nicolaus, 4622
Bloom, Olga, 1461
Bloom, Roberta, 6226
Bloom, Russell, 5396, 5397
Bloom, Steve, 1091
Bloom, Wallace, 7579
Bloomfield, Gregg, 3109
Bloomgarden, Jennifer L, 1399
Blossom, Beverly, 441
Blount, Rhoda, 1736
Bluestein, Frank, 3776
Bluestone, Stanton J, 5763
Blum, Charles, 2922
Blum, Gregory, 2786
Blum, Irene Harriet, 2668
Blumberg, Judy, 482
Blumenthal, Alan, 3680
Blumenthal, Amy, 572

Blumethal, Steve, 3680
Blumstein, Dorothy, 4990
Blunck, Russ, 7767
Bluner, John, 964
Blus, Larry, 5289
Boals, Dr. Frank M, 1104
Boals, Gregory, 902, 1946
Boatman, Anthony C, 1096
Boatman, Linda, 3822
Boatright, Jo, 1789
Boburka, Robert D, 2827
Boccabella, Anthony V, 2174
Bochette, Jeanne, 218
Bock, Phil, 3275
Bockrath, Bob, 5829
Bocook, Susan, 1760
Bodan, , 3684
Bode, Dr Robert, 1844
Bodell, Bill, 6972
Boden, Matt, 2500, 6100
Bodenstein, Ira, 284
Bodig, Joyce, 5019
Bodine, Joanne, 1931
Bodine, Veronica, 3621
Bodley, Muriel, 1558
Bodovitz, Joseph, 2463
Bodwitch, Christine, 7220
Boehlke, Bain, 3140
Boehm, Gari, 691
Boehm, Marc, 7853
Boehmer, Gretchen, 1698
Boemer, Carmel, 39
Boerlage, Frans, 1919
Boespflug, George, 6005
Boevers, Eileen, 2876
Bogardus, Ray, 1715
Bogart, Anne, 3333
Bogash, Carol, 4316
Bogenrief, Richard, 1202
Boggess, Sarah, 5095
Boggioni, Josh, 3414
Boggs, Cindy, 3558
Bogle, Gary, 2128
Bogomolny, Robert L, 1502
Boheme, Irene, 5091
Bohmann, Jeffrey, 3990
Bohnen, Joyce, 2107
Bohyer, John, 4822
Boland, Sue, 1933
Bolduc, Sue, 4864
Bolen, Bob, 3840
Bolin, John, 7886
Bolle, James, 4859
Bollenbacher, Sandy, 1174
Bolling, Elana, 5223
Bollinger, Michael, 3170, 7071
Bolt, Cheryl, 7539
Bolton, Fred C, 1254
Bolton, John, 6732
Bolzer, Bill, 2779
Bombac, JB, 4268
Bombaci, Joseph, 4268
Bonamico, Joseph, 5242
Bonamico, Margaret M, 3622, 5242
Bonanno, Russell E, 3293
Bond, Elizabeth, 2220
Bond, Laura, 3869
Bond, Robert, 1724
Bond, Yari, 1501
Bondi, John C, 7888
Bondurant, Janet, 3564, 7253
Bonelli, Dr. Eugene, 5499
Bonelli, Emilio, 1727, 5363
Bonenfant, Timothy, 1406
Bonham, Bill, 3425
Bonifas, Barry, 4144
Bonino, Dr. MaryAnn, 4129
Bonis, Fred, 3399, 3472
Bonnefoux, Jean-Pierre, 409, 572
Bonnell, Diane, 1446
Bonnell, Steve, 6079
Bonner, Janet, 932, 933

Bonner, Jeb, 1916
Bonnet, Leslie, 1924
Bonney, Betty, 8382
Bonolow, Bob, 344
Bonta, Martha, 1503
Bontrager, Charles, 1384
Bontwood, Johanna, 2669
Bonus, Alex, 4439
Bonville, Sandra, 4626
Bonzo, Barbara, 813
Booher, Mark, 2550, 6151
Bookman, Theodora, 1487, 4988
Bookwalter, Elaine, 2058
Boone, Charles S, 8198, 8199
Boone, Matt, 1049
Boone, Vicky, 3807
Booth, Elizabeth, 2198
Booth, Jack, 2700
Booth, Lisa, 8448
Booth, Melanie, 1889
Booth, Susan V, 2761
Booth, Tod, 2700
Borack, Eugene, 883
Boram, Carrie, 895
Boratgis, Marta, 985
Borchert, Mary Ann, 756
Borda, Deborah, 849, 4114
Bordein, Tim, 8258
Borden, Steve, 915
Borders, Stephany, 4113
Bordner, Laura, 1162
Borek, Thomas, 459
Boren Heinze, Cheryll, 754
Borenstein, Eric, 1306
Borer, Lennky, 5306
Borey, Sonny, 6769
Borgelt, Bruce B, 1406
Boris, Charry, 2636
Boriskin, Ronnie, 975, 4674
Bork, Charlotte, 3777
Borkovitz, Mary, 5403
Born, Alfred, 6208
Born, Nancy, 102
Bornhoeft, Jamie, 828
Bornhoeft, Robert, 828
Bornt-Ledeboer, Bernice, 5096
Borodofsky, Ted, 6733
Borowski, June, 2709
Borromeo, Venustiano, 3283
Borron, Dave, 3116
Borrup, Tom, 4743
Borsnold, David, 1162
Borstel, John, 325
Bortolotti, Steve, 2885
Borton, Deborah, 2609
Borton, Terry, 2609
Bosanquet, N. Thompson, 1295
Boschi, Phoebe, 4926
Bosen, John, 3237
Boslau, Olinda, 3215
Bost, Donna, 608
Boswell, Mary, 4852
Boswell, Michelle, 2928
Boswell, Partridge, 2167
Boswell, William, 5352, 7814
Bosworth, Bonnie, 7865
Botsford, Andrea, 6149
Botstein, Leon, 1496
Bott, David, 915
Botte, Michael, 4662
Bottles, Scott, 847
Botto, Louis, 1941
Bottomley, Kevin, 3033
Bottoms, Heather, 3773
Botwinick, Michael, 7504
Boucher, Lucretia, 8033
Boud, Jan, 1767
Boue, Renate, 381
Boue, Renate A, 3253
Bouifas, Barry, 923
Bouley, Lisa, 8437
Boulez, Pierre, 1116

Bouman, Liz, 7088
Boume, Jeff, 8176
Bourdette, Phil, 942
Bourgeois, Edward, 1885
Bourk, James, 7670
Bourla, Dan, 836
Bourne, Bill, 1928
Bourne, Lowell, 1182
Bove, Frank, 708
Bove, Janina, 708
Bowden, David, 1159, 1182
Bowen, Gwen, 186
Bowen, Jeff, 4504, 6613
Bowen, John, 2085
Bowen, Linnell R, 6817
Bower, Marilyn, 4491
Bowers, Bill, 3208
Bowers, Karen, 2810
Bowers, Lucy, 387
Bowers, Martha, 406
Bowers Coleman, Ginny, 3252
Bowers, PhD, James Lewis, 888
Bowes, Paulette, 4695
Boweyer, Ann Marie, 2005, 3703
Bowles, Bill, 1938
Bowles, Paul, 8202
Bowles, William, 1947
Bowley, Jim, 1865
Bowling, Gayle, 3970
Bowling, Scott, 2948
Bowman, David, 8104
Bowman, Jamie, 1982
Bowman, Liz, 7089
Bowman-Moore, Andrea, 2081
Bowser, Barbara, 1072, 4386
Bowser, Bryan, 7593
Bowser, Chris W, 7120
Bowsher, John, 5014
Box, Michael, 5569
Boxill PhD, Nancy A, 4388
Boxley, Johnna, 8247
Boxman, Joyce, 1170
Boyce, Alice, 4729
Boyce, Kelcey, 611
Boyce, Sandra, 5123
Boyd, Carl, 1634
Boyd, Charles/Chief, 3645
Boyd, Dr. Bradford M, 47
Boyd, Gregory, 3851, 8057
Boyd, Joe, 6397
Boyd, Jon, 1313
Boyd, Julianna, 3070
Boyd, Melinda, 3994
Boydstun, Chree, 5535
Boye Christense, Charlotte, 698
Boyer, M Christopher, 3962
Boyer, Michael, 6364
Boyer, Mike, 6362
Boyer, Scott, 703
Boyett, Carl, 855
Boykin, Glynda, 1791
Boykins, Clarence, 5886, 5887, 5888, 5889, 5890
Boylan, Llyena, 1722
Boylan, Mary John, 3049
Boylan, Paul, 3086
Boyle, David, 4940
Boyle, Dennis, 2171
Boynton, James, 6453
Boynton, Rick, 2877
Boys, Penny, 793
Boyse, Carol, 5261
Bozzi, Jim, 6283
Brace, Peg, 3112
Brackett, Brett, 3539
Brackins, C Anne, 1773
Bracy, Alecia, 7517
Bradac, Thomas F, 2476
Bradburd, Douglas, 3079
Bradbury, Susan M, 2904
Braddock, Steven, 3081
Braden, Elizabeth, 2278
Braden, Jan, 1399

Braden, Kale, 2496
Bradford, Ann, 2383
Bradford, Barlow, 2325
Bradford, Barlow D, 1823
Bradford, Chris, 168
Bradford, Kirk, 2309
Bradford, Maria, 3193
Bradham, Sharon, 1138
Bradley, Ann, 6034
Bradley, Bob, 6718
Bradley, Gary, 3693
Bradley, Gene M, 1966
Bradley, Karen, 499
Bradley, Robert, 3218
Bradley, Scott, 2975
Bradlin, Deborah, 3597
Bradshaw, Frank, 6754
Bradshaw, John, 3954
Brady, Donna, 562
Brady, Dorothy, 2606
Brady, Gerald, 935
Brady, Jim, 1795
Brady, Karen, 4559
Brady, Kevin, 3305
Brady, Pat, 1916
Brady, Robyn, 3688, 5323
Brady, Tom, 3054
Brady Donohue, Therese, 326
Bradyck, John, 1895
Braford Whitteg, Amy, 353
Bragan, Peter, 6358
Bragg, Oceola, 384
Brainin, Risa, 2549
Bram, Jeff, 1066
Bramhall, Robyn, 904
Brancato, Joe, 3507
Branch, Cynthia, 1757
Branch, Donna, 1078
Branch, John, 8096
Branch, John Watusi, 3322
Brand, Elaine, 3447
Brand, Kenneth, 2291
Brand, Morris A, 1713
Brandle, Cindy, 271
Brandon, Carl, 2166
Brandon, Michelle, 3430
Brandt, Barbara, 2910
Brandt, Julliane, 1182
Brandys, Victoria, 8355
Branfield, Judy, 1769
Brantingham, Kim, 647
Brashear, Craig, 542
Brashear, William R, 4714
Brassil, Kris, 7249
Bratcher, Freddick, 226
Bratton, Evangeline, 5787
Bratton, Jim, 3859
Bratton, Shelley, 5114
Brauchli, Bernard, 1275
Brauer, Robert, 2220
Braum, Jeff D, 953
Braun, Claire, 2653
Braun, Douglas, 3631
Braun, Edgar, 796
Braun, Edgar J, 794, 1899
Braun, Elaine, 1255
Braun, Joyce, 3591
Braun, Ksthleen, 1867
Braun, Laurel, 5067
Braun, Stacy, 5440
Braunlich, Helmut, 1011
Brause, Jay, 2363
Bravermau, Barbara, 194
Bray, Ed, 2847
Bray, Mary Ann K, 1083
Bray, Michael, 2800
Bray, Sheilds-Collins, 1789
Brayton, John, 1895
Brazakis, Debora, 1316
Brazier, Bob, 5818
Breaux, Chip, 5390
Breazeale, Dr. Helene, 4637

Breckner, Scott, 6936
Breckner, Scott H, 6937
Breder, Caroline, 2707
Breder Watts, Caroline, 2706
Breed, John, 729
Breen, Riza, 3219
Breig, Jim, 6399
Brennan, Ed, 1539
Brennan, Tom, 7821
Brennen, Maryann, 175
Brenner, Alan, 4096
Brenner, Janis, 484
Brent, Bill, 4597
Breskin, Efrem, 5073
Breslin, Frances, 566, 1545
Breslin, Frnaces, 1546, 2235
Breslin, Marc, 4231
Bresner, Carol, 3429
Brett, Carol, 6812
Brevig, Per, 984
Brevoort, Gregg W, 3246
Brewer, Denise, 4819
Brewer, Johnny, 749
Brewer, Judy, 885
Brewer, Ralph, 6835
Brewer, Sheila, 3558
Brewington, Scott, 3539
Brewster, Cornelia, 1558
Breyo, John, 7472
Brezer, Lawrence, 497
Brezer, Laz, 497
Briane, Mireille, 621
Briansky, Oleg, 621
Briccetti, Joan T, 3189
Briccetti, Mary, 876
Brickford, Jewella, 556
Brickley, Michael, 5738
Bricmmeier, Mel, 1939
Bridenstine, Art, 3956
Bridgeforth, Pamela, 7207
Bridges, Scott A, 8365
Bridgewater, Laura, 692
Brien, Patrick, 4007
Brierre, Guy, 314
Briggs, David, 7539
Briggs, Donald, 7441
Briggs, John, 3772
Briggs, Julie, 2445
Briggs, Kim, 1116
Briggs, Lisa, 1935
Briggs, Mary, 2172
Briggs, Norma, 732
Briggs, Patricia, 2478
Briggs, William, 1213
Bright, Nancy Lou, 511
Brigtman, Stacy, 1916
Brill, Linda, 1636
Brillhart, Jeffery, 2284
Brim, Martha, 5425
Brincefield, John, 3557
Brindag, Wayne, 3733
Brindisi, Michael, 3119
Brininger, Betsy, 8170
Brink, Jennifer, 1096
Brink, Jim K, 5858
Brink, Robert, 1290
Brinkmeyer, Kurt, 6148
Brinn, Mildred C, 423
Briody, Katheleen, 3710
Brisk, Barry, 877
Bristol, Brynn, 3842
Bristor, Katherine, 500
Brite, Nem, 462
Britton, Barbara, 3540, 3541
Britton, Charlotte, 8488
Broad, Jay, 3425
Broadhead, Ann, 2298
Brock, Carol, 4552, 6674
Brock, Cynthia, 691
Brock, Jim, 1638
Brock, Kathy, 7101, 7103, 7124
Brock, Kenneth, 1306

Brock, Robert, 2963
Brockman, Charles, 2799
Brockmeier, Matthew, 270
Brocksieck, Kevin, 2952
Brocksieck, Nicole, 2952
Brockway, Adrienne, 3426
Brockway, Amie, 3327, 3426
Brockway, Christi, 832
Broderick, Valerie, 1527
Brodeur Ludwig, Maria, 4878
Brodsky, Gisela, 4319
Brodsky, Giselle, 1026
Brodsky, Jack, 1026
Brodsky, Norris, 4638
Brody, Paul R, 2520
Broh, Michael, 4003
Brohan, Paul, 2868, 2869, 4460
Bromacki, GP, 7321
Broman, John, 4395
Bromley, Lynn, 3944
Bronfman, Matthew, 4995
Bronner, Gwethalyn, 4462
Bronson, Jerry, 2122, 4717
Bronstein, Fred, 1400, 1401
Brooke, Karen, 1189
Brooks, Alfred, 2584
Brooks, Barbara, 4096
Brooks, Ben, 1687
Brooks, Bonnie, 272
Brooks, Cathy, 6837
Brooks, Elizabeth, 3565
Brooks, Geoffrey, 6000
Brooks, Glen O, 3837
Brooks, Greg, 101, 2495
Brooks, Keith, 1781
Brooks, Marae, 5486
Brooks, Marty, 6255
Brooks, Robin, 596
Brooks, Rosetta, 213
Brooks, Ruth, 5722
Brooks Hopkins, Karen, 4936
Brooks Williamson, Adrienne, 316
Brooks-Bruzzese, James, 1054
Brookshire, Alexandra A, 1850
Brophy, Judith, 1985
Broschart, Elizabeth E, 1652
Brosius, Peter C, 3130
Brosivs, Peter C, 3012
Brosowsky, Bert, 2349
Brosvik, Steven R, 1811
Brothers, Cassie, 4067
Brotman, Jill, 1624
Brott, Boris, 937
Broughton, Johanna, 3085
Broussard, Jacqueline, 803
Broussard, Mike, 6752
Brover, Becky, 103
Browand, John, 1763
Browell, Douglas, 3614
Brower, Bruce, 1710
Brown, Abena Joan, 2833
Brown, Abena Joan P, 2833
Brown, Amy B, 8245
Brown, Angela, 5082
Brown, Beth, 390
Brown, Bob, 6106
Brown, Bobbie, 1877, 5254
Brown, Bonnie, 2243
Brown, Charles, 1147
Brown, D David, 718
Brown, Dave, 5849
Brown, David, 474, 519, 747, 1985, 2955
Brown, David N, 1985
Brown, David R, 8017
Brown, Deborah, 3840
Brown, Denise, 7944
Brown, Dr. Bruce, 4974
Brown, Dr. Larry, 3793
Brown, Elliot, 3426
Brown, Eric J, 7606
Brown, F Reed, 3187
Brown, Fred, 901

Brown, George, 2068
Brown, Glenda, 677
Brown, Greg, 5535
Brown, Hearth, 8260
Brown, Jean, 6272
Brown, Jeff, 6006
Brown, Jerry Lee, 2044
Brown, Jim, 7662
Brown, Joan Myers, 631
Brown, John, 1890, 6417
Brown, Joshua, 3617, 5203
Brown, Kara, 2971
Brown, Karen, 5653
Brown, Kenneth, 5140
Brown, Kristy, 1333
Brown, Lee, 3101, 6956
Brown, Lenora Inez, 3254
Brown, Leslie A, 1664
Brown, Lila, 5081
Brown, Melissa, 3505
Brown, Morgan, 8209
Brown, Morley, 807
Brown, Patrick, 5264
Brown, Peter, 87
Brown, Peter H, 1885
Brown, Randy L, 6598
Brown, Ray, 611
Brown, Richard, 1933, 4945
Brown, Ricklin, 729
Brown, Robert A, 3722
Brown, Ryan, 4213, 4314
Brown, Sabrina, 5615
Brown, Sandra, 8306
Brown, Shelley, 3692
Brown, Staci, 7259
Brown, Stacy A, 2910
Brown, Stephanie, 582
Brown, Susan, 2618, 6036
Brown, Tom, 3101, 6956
Brown, Tony, 3141
Brown, Trisha, 556
Brown, Vanessa, 677
Brown Cornett, Nancy, 1081
Browne, Dr. Bruce, 2077
Browne, Jeanne, 1661
Browning, April, 4438
Browning, Helene, 561
Browning, Molly, 2303
Browning, Robert, 5056
Browning, Robert H, 561
Browns, Anna Lisa, 1538
Broyles, Chuck, 6689, 6691
Brozozowska, Phyllis, 590
Bruce, Alice, 4662
Bruce, Dolores, 5920
Bruce, Eloise, 3260
Bruder Munafo, MJ, 3074
Bruek, Sonja, 1881
Bruffee, Matthew, 455
Bruffy, Jason, 5191
Bruker, Davenport, 2019
Brumbaugh, Mary, 8182
Brumit, J Scott, 2106
Brummel, Susan, 2158
Brundies, Steve, 4531
Brunelle, Philip, 2136, 4758
Bruning, Linda, 3131
Brunkow, Wonda, 2946
Brunner, Karen, 3798
Bruno, Carol, 4166
Bruns, Gary, 1805
Brunschmid, Robert, 3305
Brunsell, Leslie, 1863
Brunson, Jamie, 3718
Brustad, Wesley O, 6105
Brustein, Robert, 3040
Bruwmostt, Bob, 4268
Bry, Kevin, 2884
Bryan, Dave, 7836
Bryan, Victoria, 2543
Bryan, Wayne, 2951
Bryant, Alice Jane, 7457

Bryant, Barbara, 8232
Bryant, Del R, 7373
Bryant, Dr. William, 1584
Bryant, Paul A, 5626
Bryant, Peter, 6862
Bryant, Robert, 1575
Bryce, Alan, 7119
Bryenton, John, 2973
Bucci, Tony, 3732
Buccola, Keith, 1230
Buch, Rene, 1124, 3439
Buchan, Kimberly, 6641
Buchenholz, Marilyn, 2631
Buchhauser, Tom, 1870
Buchmann, Molly, 312
Buchner, Nadine, 108
Buchwalter, Charles, 4824
Buck, Dawn, 3168
Buck, Evan, 2341
Buck, JoAnn, 5187
Buck, Naomi, 1046
Buck, Roseann, 3628
Buck, Rueben, 3794
Buckelew, Sally, 5969
Buckholz, Carol, 1314
Buckley, John, 6858
Buckley, Robert A, 2217
Buckner, LJ, 3176
Buckwalter, Ian, 1987
Bucz, Bruce, 5978
Buday, Kathleen, 6982
Buddeke, Kate, 2812
Budzyna, John, 6891
Buelow, Carol, 732
Buerns, Bill, 1791
Buescher, Mary Beth, 1174
Buff, Gary, 2185
Buffett, Susie, 3222
Buffington, Robert E, 2600
Buffum, Brad, 3216
Bugli, David, 1402
Bugli, Elinor, 1402
Bujeaud, Mark, 3948
Bujnoski, Joanne, 2005, 3703
Bujones, Fernando, 231
Bulan, Diane, 2948
Bulenburg, Ralph, 5766
Bull, Bergen, 1708, 5309
Bullard, Sally S, 3705
Bullard, Therese, 346
Bullard II, Roland K, 1733
Bullin, Christine, 1941
Bullock, Gayle, 42
Bumby, Brian D, 5010
Bump, Charles, 2332
Bumstedd, John, 1300
Bunch, Dan, 3850
Bundy, James, 2625
Bundy, Rob, 3858
bunge, Eric L, 3125
Bunge ood, Eric L, 3125
Bunker, Gail, 5587
Bunker, Julie B, 5893
Bunker, Paul R, 1605, 4281
Bunn, Andrew, 1090, 4409
Bunnell, Judy, 3959
Buoy, Jean, 2632
Buoy, Larry, 2632
Burbach, Trisha, 1966
Burch-Pesses, Michael, 1686
Burchet, Emmy Lou, 2245
Burchfield, Donna Faye, 5117
Burchinal, Kenneth, 4549
Burchmore, John, 4257
Burck, Christina, 2451
Burd, Mary, 7944
Burden, Bessie, 3095
Burden, Marianna, 1449
Burdett, Patricia, 2679
Burdick, Alan, 785
Burdick, Brad, 3936
Burdick, Cathie, 5094

Burg, Michael, 2522
Burger, David, 2303
Burger, Katie, 7026
Burger, Michelle, 1338
Burgess, Dana Tai Soon, 208
Burgess, Elisabeth, 3920
Burgess, Hunter, 7095
Burgess, Suzanne, 3557
Burgoine, Nigel, 600
Burgraff, Michael, 7002
Burian, Laura, 806
Burke, Barbara, 8321
Burke, Charles, 1343
Burke, Dermot, 589
Burke, James, 5008
Burke, John J, 3273
Burke, Ken, 2473
Burke, Morgan, 6633, 6634
Burke, Sean, 3337
Burke, Sue, 2111
Burke, Susan, 760
Burke, Thomas, 2520
Burke, Victoria, 254
Burkett, Andrew, 7248
Burkett, Genie, 1585
Burkhalter, Linda, 1648
Burkhardt, Richard, 5157
Burkharht, Allison, 2896
Burkhart, Laura, 364
Burkholter, Chris, 8074
Burkot, Jerry, 6920
Burkot, Louis, 2166
Burks, Douglas, 3824
Burks, Kathy, 3824
Burleson, D Cal, 6609
Burling, David, 3281
Burlingham, Johanna, 1512
Burlow, Andy, 1344
Burman, Howard, 2425
Burman, Troy, 320
Burman-Hall, Linda, 922, 4210
Burmester, Robert W., 2097
Burmin, Peter, 993
Burnell, Diana, 2566
Burner, Dr. Victor, 4156
Burness, Judy, 4212
Burnett, Angela, 3790, 7949
Burnett, Anthony, 4301
Burnett, Ellen, 2632
Burnett, Gary, 3208
Burnett, Kathleen, 47
Burnett, Marc, 2887, 4478
Burnett, Steven, 5924
Burnett Jr, Robert B, 4497
Burnett, Jr, Zaron W, 2770
Burnett, Jr., Zaron, 2770
Burnette, Dr. Sonny, 4571
Burnham, Dianne, 2617
Burns, Brett, 5966
Burns, Cheryl, 642
Burns, Jerry, 3522
Burns, Jessie, 971
Burns, John, 2914
Burns, Miriam, 1668
Burns, Pat, 3641
Burns, Paul, 2303
Burns, R Jamesson, 4921
Burns, Susan, 1317
Burns, Victoria, 8357
Burr, Amanda, 4112
Burr, harles, 2123
Burrey, Felicia A, 1262
Burrill, Christopher, 5998
Burrows, Lee, 4137
Burrows, Thomas, 7320
Burrus, John, 1215
Burt, Willie, 573
Burtless, Chris, 2006
Burton, Cathy, 6605
Burton, Colleen, 1039
Burton, James, 3593
Burtrand, Blaine, 3814

Burtzel, Joan, 4195
Burwell, Ronald, 3322
Bury, John R, 1998
Busa, Steve, 3146
Busackijno, Barbara, 3380
Buschlen, Eric, 4750
Bush, Bonita J, 1251
Bush, Brenda, 1255
Bush, Ellen, 2698
Bush, Estelle, 2471
Bush, Lucille A, 1459
Bushell Jr, Robert G, 3896
Bushlow, Lisa, 3318
Buskirk, Mary, 3973
Buss, Sue J, 4829
Bussell, Julie, 1952
Bussey, Amy, 3770
Bussiki, Marcelo, 1781
Bustamante, Jose Luis, 667
Bustillo, Zelma, 436
Bustos, Valerie, 2593
Buswellk, Richard, 2948
Butcher, Carolyn, 2545
Butera, Robert J, 1733
Buterbauch, Vicki, 2304
Butiu, Precious, 3956
Butler, Charles, 4066
Butler, Chris, 4887, 7231
Butler, Dick, 2878
Butler, Elizabeth, 5170
Butler, Gloria, 779
Butler, Jonathan, 2171
Butler, Louise, 1435
Butler, Maureen, 4495
Butler, Rebecca, 5388
Butler, Sandra, 1316
Butler, Steve, 365
Butler, Susan L, 2668
Butler, Winston, 2444
Butt, Peter, 140
Butt, Randy, 8163
Butterman, Michael, 2184
Buttram, Jan, 3336
Buttram, Joan, 243
Buttram, Susan, 5696
Butz, Ellen C, 7297
Buvinger, Dr. Margaret S, 5267
Buxton, Donald C, 4647
Buzby, Susan, 2344
Bye, Donna, 298
Byer, Diana, 529
Byers, Vicki, 4175
Byers, Walter G., 1309
Byess, Steven, 1082
Bymes, Dan P, 6617
Bynum, Jr, Dr. Leroy E, 6424
Byral, Keven, 6617
Byrd, Tamara, 1
Byrne, Brooke, 126
Byrne, Laura, 2081
Byrne, Mary Jane, 3078
Byrne, Teresa, 1942
Byrnes, Katie, 6821
Byrnes, Mollie, 1296, 4683
Byron, Lee, 7350
Byron, Richard, 3804
Byus, Roz, 3012

C

Cabe, Lucy C, 5920
Cabrera, Hilda, 2206
Caccam, Juanita, 31
Cacciotti, Tony, 3335
Cacioppo, Robert, 2695
Cademenos, Anne, 1266
Cadenhead, Ian, 2631
Cadore, Austin, 3358
Cadorette, Lisa, 7789
Cady, Drew, 888
Cafferty Ross, Suzanne, 1741

Caffery, Steven J, 3969
Caffrey Gabriel, Lynn, 914
Cage, Timothy, 2213
Cagle, Benny, 5920
Cagle, Wanda, 6448
Cahill, Keri Ellis, 3049
Cahill, Mary, 2651
Cahill, Peter, 1433
Cahn, Marcia, 2871
Cai, Lily, 115
Cain, Brenda, 3099
Cain, Danielle, 2553
Caine, Robert, 2469
Caine, Sunny, 2469
Calabrese, Cynthia, 7512
Calabrese, Michael, 3631
Calandra, Dale, 2883
Calandra, Dr. Denis, 2747
Caldarella, Lisa, 770
Calder, Tom, 6824
Calderon, Yolando Nora, 600
Caldwell, Barbara, 7478
Caldwell, Dale, 3254
Caldwell, Damon, 2612
Caldwell, David, 4498
Caldwell, Dr. Hansonia, 849
Caldwell, George, 3950
Caldwell, Lauren, 6349
Caldwell, Raymond, 3864, 5542
Caleshu, Jennifer, 2509
Calhoon, Patrick M, 6410
Calhoun, Eva, 6341
Califano, Cheryl, 2603
Calkins, Jeffrey E, 7463
Callahan, Ryan, 2436
Callahan, Shannon, 2920
Callen, James, 3433
Calocerinos, Nancy B, 3494
Caltvedt, Siri, 1201
Calvert, Chad, 2245
Calvert, Pamela, 3311
Calvin, Darrell, 4352
Calvin, Sandra, 130, 4184
Calvin, Sandra J, 8347
Camacho, Tara, 6733
Camargo, Rick, 3859
Cambariere, Peter, 3591
Cambron, Ed, 1033
Camera, Rev. Kathleen L, 3425
Cameron, Clark, 3395
Cameron-Webb, Gavin, 3304
Caminiti, Robert, 2172
Camp, Joanne, 3430
Camp, Libby, 5543
Camp, Philip, 5544
Campanelli, Joe, 919
Campanero, Connie, 3531
Campbell, Ann S, 1935
Campbell, Barbara, 6482
Campbell, Charlene, 1129
Campbell, David, 12
Campbell, Diane, 2026
Campbell, Dr. Jeffery I, 4056
Campbell, Gary, 4779
Campbell, Ian D, 1935
Campbell, James, 1932
Campbell, Jeff, 6740
Campbell, Jim, 4701
Campbell, Kasi, 3019
Campbell, Krista, 7587, 7663
Campbell, Neil, 8234
Campbell, Patrick J, 943
Campbell, Patrick M, 7490
Campbell, Paul, 3054
Campbell, Philip, 3922
Campbell, Sandy, 4572
Campbell, Scott, 2369
Campbell, Suzy, 4046
Campbell, Thomas, 7026
Campion, Geoff, 8302
Campo, Steve, 2614
Campopiano, Remo, 5410

Canada, Tonya, 3456
Canady, George, 2784
Canan, Laurel A, 5743
Canarina, John, 1194
Cancro, Larry, 6858
Candee III, William, 482
Canedo, Dana, 4588
Canfield, James, 616
Canfield, Nanette, 7593
Canning, Kathie, 6397
Cannon, Anthon, 832
Cannon, C Christopher, 2280, 2281
Cannon, Kristine, 3118
Cannon, Pat, 569
Cantarella Culpo, Madeline, 338
Canter, Jim, 6456
Canterbury, Patricia, 2496
Cantler, William, 3404
Cantoni, Linda, 2193
Cantoni, Marie, 2193
Cantrell, Brent, 5459
Cantwell, Don, 647
Cantwell, Patricia, 647
Canty, Dean R PhD, 5548
Caparelli, Tony, 86
Capasso, Michael, 2210
Capaz, Caresa, 2509
Caples, Richard J, 500
Capone, William J, 8421
Caporale, Anthony C, 5122
Cappala, Anna, 6283
Capparella, Donald, 3796, 5469
Carabajal, Dia, 3285
Carafelli, GA, 3719
Caraher, James, 2056
Caravaglia, Doris, 8345, 8429
Card, Deborah R, 1850
Cardenes, Andres, 971
Cardona, Cora, 3829
Cardoni, John, 7855
Cardy, Kathryn, 8410
Careefix, Jack, 6484
Caremichael, Nancy, 744
Caretto, Lisa, 6092, 8342
Carey, Alison, 2437
Carey, Christopher, 3027
Carey, James, 2432
Carey, Jon, 7767
Carey, Tama M, 622
Carey, Thomas, 2267
Carey, Toni, 1727, 5363
Cargill, Clinton, 3369
Cargill, John, 4046
Carhart, Glenda, 98
Carhart-Hensly, Glend, 98
Carignan, Steve, 4524, 6641
Carino, Glenda, 2365
Carl, Jim, 3531
Carl, Katherine, 5014
Carless, Timothy, 902
Carlin, Drew, 3275
Carling, Thomas, 1496
Carlisle, Eilleen, 2553
Carlo, Chris De, 2551
Carlo, Dr. Thomas J, 1649
Carlon, Kirsten R, 7315
Carlon, Pete, 7976
Carlson, Bruce, 4767
Carlson, Ed, 2251
Carlson, Eric A, 3598
Carlson, Gloria, 5777
Carlson, Margaret, 583
Carlson, Marian, 1681
Carlson, Nancy, 1449
Carlson, Trevor, 514
Carlucci, Aileen, 6817
Carlucci, David E, 7655
Carlucci, Joseph, 1780
Carmichael, Cary, 6466
Carmichael, Steve, 4468
Carmola, Joe, 3578
Carnevali, Patricia, 5345, 7811

Carney, Kathy, 3343
Carney, Philip M, 3059
Carney, Rober E, 7213
Carney, Timothy, 2024
Carobine, Anthony, 4930, 7294
Caron, Jim, 3208
Caron, Nancy, 3208
Carpenter, Ar, 1037
Carpenter, Dale R, 2691
Carpenter, David, 8432
Carpenter, Deborah, 2691
Carpenter, Emma Lee, 2736
Carpenter, Gery, 7141, 7142
Carpenter, JD, 5713
Carpenter, Karen, 2499
Carpenter, Ken, 2251
Carpenter, Steve, 3376
Carr, Carolyn, 1316
Carr, David, 2502
Carr, George H, 3592
Carr, Jennifer, 4638
Carr, John, 819, 1316
Carr, Kathlene, 3286
Carr, Kenneth H, 1024, 1997
Carr, Lonne, 858
Carr, Michael, 281
Carr, Shary, 937
Carreras, Denyse, 2886
Carrington, Mark, 4315
Carroll, Ed, 6874
Carroll, Elaine C, 1481
Carroll, Gerald P, 2245
Carroll, James FL, 5349
Carroll, Joanne P., 5349
Carroll, Stuart, 102
Carroll, Susan, 102
Carroll, Thomas, 3265
Carroll, Tom, 7208
Carroll, William, 2247
Carroway, Melvin, 2058
Carsey, Richard, 3998
Carson, Dr. William S, 4526
Carter, Angela, 5150
Carter, Angela V, 373
Carter, Brad, 2942
Carter, Brenda, 6381
Carter, Cassandra, 4474
Carter, Chris, 3958, 7517
Carter, Danby, 309
Carter, Jill, 3948
Carter, Larry, 8399
Carter, Lois, 2705
Carter, M Erwin, 4388
Carter, Ray, 3280
Carter, Selina, 1595, 2253
Carter, Shirley, 2312, 5515
Carter, Sonja, 265
Carter, Sonta, 265
Carter, Stephen, 3958
Carter, Steve, 1230
Carter, Walter F, 1291
Carter Beane, Douglas, 3369
Carter Covington, Claudia, 3528
Carter PhD, Lolita D, 31
Carter-West, Cynthia, 8188
Cartier, Carol, 1698
Cartmill, Joyce, 3216
Carto, Dr. Thomas J, 1650, 3619
Carton, Gary, 6977
Carton, Shirley, 6977
Cartwright, Kathy, 6508, 6509
Caruso, Emily, 4
Caruso, Peter, 5818
Carvajal, Carlo, 153
Carvajal, Carlos, 152
Carver, James C, 3103
Carver, Lucinda, 823
Cary, Richard, 3057
Casanta, Phil, 4152
Case, Deborah, 685
Case, Del, 4080
Case, Rose, 7000

Case, Stacey B, 140
Caselli, Anthony, 3090
Casey, David, 3512
Casey, Deborah, 2628
Casey, Joyce, 3597
Casey, Madison, 4250
Casey, Mrs. Eugene B, 1995
Casey, Stephen, 3712
Casey Wells, John, 7799
Cash, Marsha, 2974
Cashin, Kathryn, 237
Cashman, Bob, 7302
Caskie, Wendy, 3682
Casl, Karyn, 2467
Casper, George, 8133
Cassanova, Marcia, 2991
Cassaro, James P, 8297
Cassell, Jim, 8329
Cassidy, James R, 1220
Casso, Alan, 2114
Castaldi, Peter, 424
Castellani, David, 2414
Castellino, Bill, 3106
Castilla, Rene, 1803
Castillo, Eugene F, 881
Castle, Tom, 991
Castleman, Charles, 1549
Castracane, Audrey, 3681
Castro, Alpha, 2632
Castronovo, Robdert, 7213
Castronovo, Robert, 7212
Caswell, James Michael, 1824
Caswell, Ruth, 5696
Catalano, Marie Lou, 3345
Cates, George E, 1771
Catlett, Jack, 919
Cato, Marcus, 2549
Cattanach, John, 3194
Caulk, Martha, 4328
Caulker, Ferne, 739
Cauthen, Caroline, 7535
Cavallaro, Nicholas, 697
Cavanaugh, Jan, 2005, 3703
Cavanaugh, John S, 373
Cave, Rick, 1826
Cavendish, Thomas, 2000
Cayea, Christiane, 3352
Cazzolla, Paul, 2940
Ceasare, Denise, 7862
Cecconi, Jr, Warren R, 1021
Cecsarini, David, 3996
Celeste Humphries, Elizabeth, 670
Celli, Andrea, 395
Center, Brigitte, 392
Center, Donna, 3797
Centrella, Maria, 6151
Cepeda, Adela, 275
Cerato, Sara A, 2280
Cerchio, Robert, 6506
Cermack, Jim, 3153
Cerone, David, 1623
Cerritelli, Rhoda, 557
Cervenak, Anna, 1711
Cervone, Thomas A, 3782
Cesar, Kamala, 505, 5032
Chace, Amanda, 1271
Chace Jr, Arnold B, 3750
Chacin, Javier, 2685
Chacko, Joyce, 4433
Chaffin, John, 7949
Chaffin, John P, 3790
Chaiken, Barry, 3042
Chaimson, Judie, 3027
Chain, Harry, 1477
Chait, Andrea, 432
Chait, Matt, 2436
Chalfant, Margaret, 5269
Chalsty, John S, 3399
Chamber S, Gerald, 2019
Chamberlain, Chris, 3795
Chamberlain, Jeanne, 5777
Chamberlain, Richard C, 5328

Chamberlin, Alice P, 2993
Chamberlin, Chris, 3794
Chambers, Alan, 2844
Chambers, David Kirk, 3891
Chambers, Denise, 6628
Chambers, Mary Jane, 5895, 5896
Chambers, Raymond G., 7232
Chamblee, James, 1581
Chambord, Jacqueline, 5018
Chamness, Lisa, 7926
Champagne, Mario, 931
Chan, Kim, 4318
Chan, Lilly, 447
Chan, Oiman, 1504
Chan, Wing-Chi, 1012
Chance, Angela, 3565
Chancellor, Dorine, 4047
Chancey, Tina, 1833
Chandler, Barbara, 7034
Chandler, C, 1572
Chandler, Paul, 5454
Chandler, Ray, 7035
Chandler, Tessa, 8484
Chandley, Dr. Paul, 5155
Chang, Tisa, 3427
Chang, Tony, 1198
Chang, Tsuan-Nien, 1504
Chang, Wendy, 2023
Chang-Barnea, Anne, 1395
Channel, Suzanne, 4840
Chanter, Pam, 929
Chao, Mei-yuan, 3454
Chaparro, Javier, 1781
Chapin, Frances White, 5677
Chaplik Harris, Linda, 275
Chaplin, Diane, 4877
Chapman, Aara, 3623
Chapman, Benson J., 1525
Chapman, Jim, 6632
Chapman, Joe, 4395
Chapman, Lonny, 2470
Chapman, Pete, 7168
Chapman, Wes, 1
Chappell, Drew, 2532
Chappell, John, 1985
Chappell, Ross, 3466
Chappell, Wallace, 423
Charles, Gerard, 586
Charlop, Vivian, 4956, 7334
Charon, Susan, 1693
Charry, Yoni, 3919
Chart, Joseph, 1494
Chase, Alison, 200
Chasitz, Robbie, 3049
Chastain, Steve, 7891
Chatal, Ed, 8077
Chatterjea, Ananya, 434
Chaudhri, Javade, 836
Chaudry, Art, 7090
Chaussee, Andrea, 4463
Chaves, Frank, 280
Chavez, Raul, 2498
Chavez, Robert, 1613
Chavies, Judge Michael, 2710
Chaya, Masazumi, 421
Cheadle, Nancy, 661
Cheberenchic, Bethne, 1741
Checchia, Anthony, 1731
Checchia, Anthony P, 1730, 5368
Checketts, David W, 7407
Cheever, Jean, 3430
Chelesvig, Jeffrey L, 6651
Cheline OSB, Father Paschal, 5308
Chelminski, Sarah Jane, 194, 2628
Chemaly, Ed, 3405
Chemiavsky, Anne, 2097
Chen, Dr. Donald, 1148
Chen, Francis W, 1944
Chen, HT, 450
Chen, Mei-Ann, 1702
Chen, Stella, 868
Chenault, Marilyn, 2749

Chenault, Roxanne, 939
Chenette, Jonathan, 4538
Chenevey, Paul, 1714
Cheney Rhoades, Gretchen, 1337
Cheng, Mariette, 4970
Chereskin, Alvin, 514
Cherniak, Renee, 6025
Cherniak, Susan, 539
Chernin, Megan, 4172
Cherry, John W, 976, 1969
Cherry, Yvonne, 1974
Cherryholmes, Diana, 4975
Cherryholmes, Diana J, 4976
Cherwien, David, 2134
Chesbrough, Herbert A, 1552, 3503, 7472
Chester, Emily, 652
Chestnut, Madge, 4575
Cheverino, Debra, 823
Chi, Jacob, 970
Chiang, Andrew, 375
Chiao-Ping, Li, 743
Chichmanian, Tania, 206
Chick, Kathleen, 4673
Chiesa, Bill, 7134
Chila, Doreen, 3367
Chilberg, Marty, 3959
Chilcot, Helen, 1720
Childers, Martin, 2975
Childs, Casey, 3434
Childs, Kendall, 1196
Childs, Lucinda, 507
Chilers, Mike, 8017
Chille, Alan, 7870
Chilton, Carol, 7126
Chin, Amy, 451
Chin, Deanne, 992, 4283
Chin, Debbie, 4084
Chin, Melissa, 2498
Chin, Paul B, 5944
Ching-ming, Ciu, 3454
Chiodo, Louis, 3480
Chiong, Ruby Pearl B, 31
Chipman, John, 1136
Chirco-Coontz, Sue, 1857
Chisholm, Dan, 4822
Chishti, Muzaffar, 3427
Chmpion, Elizabeth, 4107
Chobaz, Dr. Raymond, 1035
Chojnicki, Virginia, 3080
Chong, Alan, 6862
Chong, Ping, 3374, 3432
Chookasezian, John, 35
Chookasian, John, 37
Chotard, Dr. Ann, 5920
Chow, Elaine, 4157
Chow, Lisa R, 8, 11
Choy, Al, 2438
Choy, Colleen, 4428
Chrisman, Neil, 4936
Christ, Ann, 3770
Christ, Maggie, 438
Christ, Maureen, 4212
Christen, Tim, 3986
Christensen, Carl, 4176
Christensen, Carol, 807
Christensen, June, 5535
Christensen, June M, 1459
Christensen, Lee, 4070
Christensen, Lynda, 8152
Christensen, Mac, 1823, 2325
Christensen, Mahlon, 1841
Christensen, Russ, 352, 7765
Christenson, Chris, 153
Christenson, Patrick J, 7178
Christian, Skip, 3128
Christiansen, Clay, 2325
Christie, Alfred, 3231
Christie, Dave, 6995
Christie, Michael, 4235
Christman, M Kaye, 3982
Christner, Tom, 970
Christophel, Susan, 3789

Christopher, Sybil, 3499
Christopher, Virginia, 5483
Christy, John G, 1733
Chruchill, Ben, 163
Chuckerman, Jill, 2850
Chudnick, Phyllis, 2171
Chuma, Yoshiko, 547
Chung, II-Ryun, 758
Chung, Riku, 7584
Church, Jeff, 3176
Church, Phyllis, 1887
Church, Ron, 6624
Church, Tony, 2585
Churchill, Angeline, 1785
Churchill, Dan, 1189
Churchill, Deb, 7091
Churchill, Mark, 1268, 1284
Ciak, Kent, 1865
Ciarlillo, Marjorie Ann, 5200
Cieply, Jeff, 8283
Cilley, Brock, 4100
Cintron, Becca, 3918
Cion, Shira, 1924
Cioruttoli, Robert, 7862
Cisneros, Ron, 8342
Ciszewski, John, 6918
Citron, Bea, 4350
Civilette, Kurt, 1447
Clagett, Kay, 971
Clair, Cynthia, 4276
Claisen, Artie, 3819
Clancy, Heather, 1366
Clancy, Nancy, 1443
Clapp, Constance L, 3399
Clapp, Deb, 2623
Clare, Karen, 940
Claridge, Jon Palmer, 5618, 5619
Clark, Bob, 876
Clark, Carolyn, 379
Clark, Dave, 5282
Clark, Dennis, 2873
Clark, Derek, 3054
Clark, Donna, 420
Clark, Dr. Leroy, 2711
Clark, Elaine, 697
Clark, Ernest, 1303, 4698
Clark, Gaby, 4016
Clark, Harry, 981
Clark, Jaci, 7660
Clark, James, 3870
Clark, James A, 3510
Clark, Jan, 3578
Clark, Janet, 2660, 4305
Clark, Jeff, 6854
Clark, Jim, 2828, 7674
Clark, Jocelyn, 758, 4032
Clark, John, 4933
Clark, John C, 4707
Clark, Judy, 3843
Clark, Julie, 7587
Clark, Karen, 7684
Clark, Kathryn, 2509
Clark, Kelly, 7741
Clark, Leslie, 8492
Clark, Marianne, 3773
Clark, Marilyn, 5501
Clark, Mark E, 2321
Clark, Mary Higgins, 3425
Clark, Mary Jane, 4249
Clark, Nancy, 7790
Clark, Paul M, 2794
Clark, Peter, 1409
Clark, Ray, 1660
Clark, Richard C, 1494
Clark, Rod, 3985
Clark, Rodrigo Durte, 2512
Clark, Ron, 2933
Clark, Simon H, 847
Clark Helzer, Katherine, 3373
Clark Ph.D, Donald, 5375
Clark Smith, Carolyn, 3352, 8426
Clarke, Beth, 303

Clarke, Bill, 7526
Clarke, Lucy, 6277, 6279
Clarke, Tracey, 3030
Clarke, William, 2004
Clary, Barbara, 3286
Clausen, Christopher, 4082
Clauss, Dennis, 1858
Claussen, Diane, 2828
Clausson, Marilyn, 2993
Clay, Ben G, 888
Clay, Carl, 3353
Clay, Ken, 6721
Clayton, Ellen, 2081
Clayton, Thomas F, 1161
Cleage, Pearl, 2770
Cleage, Pearle, 2770
Cleary, Robert E, 731
Cleary Griffiths, Sally, 1635
Cleland, Charles, 1016
Clemens, Stephanie, 288
Clement, Barbara, 1304
Clement, Linda, 1765
Clement, Tamara R, 1229
Clement Ghni, Judith, 689
Clements, Bernadette, 219
Clemons-Rodgers, Christy, 5721
Clemons-Rodgers, Christy, 5721
Clendenen, Bob, 4223
Clephane, Connie, 4291
Clephane, Thoams, 4291
Clervi, Paul, 4784
Cleve, George, 893, 4185
Cleveland, BJ, 3803
Cleveland, Carol, 5051, 7441
Cleveland, Janet, 3095
Cleveland, Rose Ann, 6832
Cleven, Gary, 3985
Cliff, Jim, 1060
Cline, Ed, 6828
Cline, Edward E, 6829
Cline, Jesse, 3707
Cline, Judith, 5655
Cline, Kathleen, 6
Cline, Susan, 5017
Clinger, Cliff, 7178
Clinkenbeard, Donna, 4519
Clint, Jane, 684
Clinton, Angeline, 7517
Clinton, Suzanne, 6733
Clinton, Tom, 3099
Clooten, Lucas, 756
Close, Bill, 4135
Close, Roy, 3145
Clough, Peter, 7494
Clouts, Alexander W, 1850
Clover, Lisa, 132
Clowes, Kevin, 5950
Cluckerman, Jill, 2850
Cluff, Cheryl Ann, 3886
Clure, Randall, 3984
Clurman, Judith, 2224
Clutter, William B, 5134
Clysdale, Matthew, 3104
Coar, Constance, 5405
Coash, Tom, 3910
Coates, George, 2514
Coates, Mark, 6864
Cobb, Joe, 1838
Cobb, Steve, 5898
Cobbs, Dr. Paul-Elliot, 1855, 5709
Cobia, Dennis H, 695
Cobler, John, 1198
Cobrda, Pauline, 3539
Cochran, April S, 2974
Cochran, B Barnett, 5241
Cochran, Grant, 1884
Cochran, Kevin, 2409
Cochran, Linda, 3600
Cochran, Michael L, 2974
Cochran Heath, David, 2399
Cock, Christopher M, 2061
Cockburn, Marilyn, 1810

Cockburn, Mrs. Harold, 5559
Cockrell, Ginny, 1
Cockrell, Lila, 5558
Cocuzza, Peter, 2865
Codd, Barbara, 18, 3313
Coddington, Paul, 940
Cody, Carol, 86
Cody, Jeff, 3781
Coe, John G, 5787
Coe, NancyBell, 1958
Coenig, George, 8059
Coffee, Sara, 406
Coffey, Richard, 1974
Coffey, Tamara, 2977
Coffield, Philip, 3170
Coffin IV, Jed, 929
Coffman, Mara, 1741
Coghill, John, 1974
Cogswell, Ann, 2160
Cohan, Muriel, 306
Cohen, Andrew, 4135
Cohen, Ann, 1229
Cohen, Dr. Erik, 2536
Cohen, Edward S, 1525
Cohen, Gary, 3244
Cohen, Herbert A, 1260
Cohen, Jeff, 6900
Cohen, Joel, 2093
Cohen, Judith, 5695
Cohen, Miles, 1731
Cohen, Oscar, 8423
Cohen, Rachel, 58, 59, 8336
Cohen, Ralph Alan, 3930
Cohen, Rusty, 3012, 3130
Cohen, Sanford, 5137
Cohen, Sara, 3918
Cohen, Sue, 3582
Cohen, Warren, 778
Cohen Jr, Benjamin J, 4205
Cohler, Jonathan, 1270
Cohn, George L, 3074
Cohn, Marjorie, 2866
Colanna, Tom, 3014
Colbenson, Mark, 3157
Colbert, MM, 734
Colbourn, Chris, 8384
Colburn, Brian, 2480, 6071
Colby, David, 3982
Colby, Fred, 108
Colby, Janice, 379
Colby, Laura, 8484
Cole, C Carroll, 4431
Cole, Cecil S, 1037
Cole, Laura, 1828, 5597
Cole, Mary, 340
Cole, Richard, 2514
Cole, Robert W, 4083, 4088, 5947
Cole, Robin, 394
Cole, Ronald, 105
Cole, Skip, 2999
Cole, Thomas H, 2469
Cole, William, 1595, 2253
Cole, Jr., Dr. Olen, 5131
Colegrove, Kathryn, 2764
Coleman, Ann, 1349
Coleman, Barbara, 2880
Coleman, Bill, 2955
Coleman, Bobbi L, 1030
Coleman, Chris, 3671
Coleman, Elinor, 473
Coleman, FR, 2880
Coleman, Jennifer, 7195, 7196
Coleman, Kevin, 4886
Coleman, Michael, 1295
Coleman, RJ, 2820
Coler, Douglas, 2429
Coles, Carol, 2914
Coletti, Pamela, 1156, 1756
Coley, Al, 3490
Coley, Melissa, 5025, 5055
Colf, Howard, 4211
Colglazier, Phillip, 2914

Collazo, Steven, 6373
Colledge, Jacqueline, 692
Collett, Robert L, 1850
Colley, Bryan, 2948
Colley, Lynn A, 3198
Colliander, Esquire, John, 3237
Collier, Katherine, 971
Collier, Mary, 2012
Collier, Winston, 1608
Collins, Cathleen, 7297
Collins, Cindy, 837
Collins, Dick, 5106
Collins, Don, 8064
Collins, Elizabeth, 580
Collins, John W, 5627
Collins, Judy, 6690
Collins, Kai, 2509
Collins, Laurie, 3632
Collins, Leon, 2026
Collins, Lloyd, 1030
Collins, Lyman, 7514
Collins, Mary, 8488
Collins, Michelle, 1115
Collins, Russell, 6913
Collins, Walter, 876
Collmann, Larry, 2315
Collver, Larry, 7765
Colon, Miriam, 3437
Colon Lespier, Alvan, 3292
Colosa Lucas, Stacey, 2767, 4387
Colosimo, Murry, 1443
Colpitts, Phyllis, 8320
Colquhoun, Michael, 2194
Colson, John F, 1762
Coltman, Felicity, 1777, 5476
Colvig, Lane, 684
Colwell, Denis, 1743
Combes, Alison, 1896
Combs, Mike, 8249
Combs-Ballard, Rebecca, 5612
Comeau, L Renee, 1935
Comess, Linda, 3818
Comly, Mark, 3685
Commanday, David, 1142
Commander, Teri, 708
Commeret, Lorraine, 318
Common, Lori, 7684
Common, Ross, 1390
Commons, Dede, 2058
Compton, Casey, 3501
Compton, Melinda, 3188
Compton, Patricia, 2166
Compton, Tyson, 6705
Comstock, Allan, 1204
Comtois, Liza, 3956
Conabi, Mick, 6592
Conant, Dawn, 2416
Conant, Nancy, 1480
Conant, Robert, 1480, 4968
Conati, Mick, 6593
Conaty, Michael J, 384
Conaway, Robert, 8277
Conboy, Ron, 2523
Concra, Joseph, 2237
Condit, Philip M, 3952
Condon, Dwayne, 1915
Condon, Frank, 2496
Cone, Laurie, 5430
Confessore, Chris, 744
Congdon, Richard, 1186
Conjura, Vivienne, 3520
Conklin, Chaunce, 2875
Conley, Alexandra, 3449, 7435
Conley, James P, 5848
Conlisk, Elizabeth, 7650
Conlon, James, 5189
Conn, Bill, 2665
Connally, Susan Beil, 689
Connaughton, Kelly, 816
Connell, Robert, 1457
Conner, Bill, 5210
Conner, CC, 680

Conner, Kaye Ellen, 1159
Conner, William, 6267
Conners, Jeanne, 1657
Connery, Nancy R, 1236, 4613
Connor, Susan R, 2346
Conquist, Robert L, 1647
Conrad, Gordon, 1300
Conrad, Richard, 2606
Conrow, William, 108
Conroy, Dorthy, 7492
Conry, Randal, 8125
Consolo, Frank, 5402
Constable, Robert C, 4365
Constance, Lawrence A, 2169
Constantine, Mark, 5667
Conte, John, 2622
Conti, Louis, 5031
Contino, Bobbie, 5128
Contino, Flora, 2049
Contri, Larry, 2349
Conway, Paul B, 3555
Conway, Robert, 2074
Conway, Scott, 5555
Coogan, Sean, 2403
Cook, Alisa, 3506, 5089
Cook, Camille, 1240
Cook, David, 897
Cook, Diane, 1718
Cook, Douglas, 5461
Cook, Elaine, 1215
Cook, Ginger O, 658
Cook, Gregg, 7805
Cook, H Richard, 1103
Cook, HR, 6693
Cook, Jeff Holland, 1650
Cook, Jennifer, 4256, 6630
Cook, Kevin, 6373
Cook, Kim, 144, 2529
Cook, Quarrier, 4917
Cook, Renee, 378
Cook, Richard G, 3161
Cook, Sandra, 648
Cook, Thomas, 1315
Cook-Glover, Rosemarie, 803
Cooke, M Todd, 1731
Cool, Michael, 7238
Cooley, Pamela, 5064, 5066
Cooley, William, 338
Coolich, Stephanie, 6106
Coombs, Rene,, 4973
Coon, Susan, 5121
Coon, Susan L, 5119
Coons, Carol, 5058
Coons, William, 5058
Cooper, Barry, 2982
Cooper, Cheryl, 2915
Cooper, Connie, 5701
Cooper, David, 2145
Cooper, Dianne L, 1615
Cooper, Edward, 8190
Cooper, Frank, 4506
Cooper, Grant, 1557, 4026
Cooper, Lonnie EJ, 6236
Cooper, Marlene, 6304
Cooper, Paula, 1465
Cooper, Philip, 5156
Cooper, Rachel, 5000
Cooper, Sean, 5258
Cooper, Steve, 3300
Cooper, Suzanne, 7980
Cooper Albright, Ann, 597
Cooper Hilton, Donna Lynn, 4265
Cope, Daniel, 1027
Cope, Shirley, 5433
Copeland, Nathan, 4385
Copeland, Rene, 3794
Copeland, Scot, 3795
Copos, Carolyn, 5228
Coppaway, Craig, 3689
Copper, Don, 2834
Coppock, Ada, 3722
Coppock, Bruce, 1362

Coppola, Agustin, 2433
Coppola, Anton, 2168
Coppola, Arthur, 1416
Coppola, Camille, 2201
Coppom, John T, 966
Cora, Edgardo, 662
Corbett, Sally, 4390
Corbett-Barnes, Joanne, 8346
Corbin, R Richard, 1485, 4982
Corcoran, Anthony, 7457
Corcoran, Christine, 1351
Corcoran, Kathleen, 1286
Corcoran, Rosemary, 3616
Cord, Jeanette, 1727, 5363
Corday Kozberg, Joanne, 6034
Cordick, Edward, 1027
Cordill, Naomi, 1228
Corey, Dean, 834, 4116
Corham, Albert C, 3293
Corley, Dr. Sheila, 5862
Corley, Richard, 3986
Corman, Joel, 1291
Cornelison, Gayle, 2566
Cornelius, Marti, 6629
Cornell, Allen D, 2749, 2940, 6418
Cornell, Anne, 7654
Cornell, Heather, 508
Cornish, Brett, 6554
Cornwall, Ramon, 1457
Correa, J Gerrard, 1032
Correa, Marie, 6563
Corrick, Jeffery, 3474
Corrie, Sarah, 7556
Corrigan, Barbara V, 2815
Corrigan, Thom, 5137
Corsette, Bob, 3512
Corsi, Fred, 7126
Cortelyou, Don, 2816
Cortes, Sara, 933
Cortes, Jr, Pedro, 3128
Cortese, Alda, 3705
Cortese, Federico, 1266
Cortese, Glen, 1033
Cortez, Hernando, 455, 583
Corto, Diana, 2204
Cortright, Joanna, 7012
Cortwright, Tomnt, 1676
Corvino, Andra, 476
Corvino, Ernesta, 476
Corwin, John, 2861
Corwin, Mike, 7751
Cory, Anna May, 4038
Cory, Richard, 2128
Cosby, Dorothy, 2533
Cosnow, Iris, 1135
Cossa, Joanne, 5049
Costa, Jorge, 6121
Costantini, Valerie, 3019
Costanza, Ellen, 359
Costello, Christy, 2767, 4387
Costello, John, 3918
Costello, Mark, 2755
Costello, Pat, 3425
Costello, Steve, 5764
Costello, Suzanne, 596
Cota, Joe, 6804
Coteus, Carol, 702
Cotnoir, Tracy, 8504
Cotter, Patti, 4521
Couch, Guy, 4061
Couch, Suzanne, 3191
Couchin, Alice, 5334
Coughlan, Pauline, 2878
Coulmas, Nancy, 3684
Coulson, Penny, 2582
Coulter, Flossie, 4136
Coulter, Ken, 4136
Coulter, Martha, 2948
Coulter, Mindy, 658
Coulthard, Anita, 5628
Coune, Jac, 6795
Countryman, Dr. John, 2715

Counts, Dr. Michael L, 2377
Counts, Paulett S., 4939
Counts, Philip, 5922
Courely, Richard S, 908
Couret, Kerion, 2980
Courier, Nora, 955
Courson, Graig, 8017
Courtney, Janice, 4769
Cousar, Kathryn, 3688, 5323
Coutin, Noreen, 1433
Covalinski, Rik, 1152, 2053, 2054
Covault, Jim, 3838, 3844
Covelli, John, 1459
Coven, Richard, 4499
Coverdale, Thad, 1260
Covington, Jr, Howard E, 1581
Covitz, Aviva, 2572
Covrest, Keiron, 4585
Cowan, Christina, 6481
Cowan, Phil, 8248
Cowart, Steed, 4148
Cowee, Bill, 3224
Cowell, Carin, 3920
Cowen, Phyllis, 6570
Cowherd, Tara M, 1400
Cowles, Elizabeth, 1852
Cowles, Sage F, 514
Cowperthwaite, Janet, 892
Cox, Alice, 3970
Cox, Alice C, 1
Cox, Bud, 1647
Cox, David M, 4253
Cox, Donnie, 6766
Cox, Douglas, 5610
Cox, Joanne B, 4357
Cox, Joy, 7514
Cox, Katharine, 8261
Cox, Lee, 4096
Cox, Martha, 1055
Cox, Nikki, 576
Cox, Paul, 5201
Cox, Tommy, 2781
Coyle, Nan Coyle, 6359
Coyle, Peter, 3533, 5120
Cozzalio, Dawna, 4227
Cpsbu, Goma, 1218
Crabb, Chuck, 6586
Crabb, Harry, 99, 2489
Crabtree, Dawn, 2967
Crabtree, Elizabeth, 2121
Crabtree, Jim, 3772
Crabtree, Larry, 430
Craff, Pat, 3608
Craft, Chris, 5238
Craft Jr, Robert H, 3681
Crager, Adora, 2172
Cragin Brittan, Kathleen, 1269
Craig, Avard, 3048, 6875
Craig, Carol, 2932
Craig, Laura, 1711
Craig, Marilyn, 3645
Craig, Mimi, 3386
Craig, Thomas F, 3
Craioveanu, Mihai, 1326
Cramer, Trevor, 1056, 1057, 1058, 1059, 1060, 1061,
    1063, 4366, 4370
Crandace, Leo, 5092
Crane, Adam, 1767
Crane, David A, 1615
Crane, Hyla, 2622
Crane, Morton, 1034
Cranfill, Jerry, 2332
Cranford, Ereka, 7521
Crappa-Hurley, Andrea, 647
Crawford, Allyson, 1640
Crawford, Carol I, 2271
Crawford, Dr. JC, 5776
Crawford, Eddie, 6740
Crawford, Ereka, 7520
Crawford, Iain, 2910
Crawford, John R, 3615
Crawford, Jonnell, 4427

Crawford, Lisa, 1579
Crawford, Lynn, 5211
Crawford, Marilyn, 1953
Crawford, Rick C, 4076
Crawford, Sonni, 6629
Crawford, Sue, 1110
Crawford, Thomas, 993
Creach, Terry, 456
Creamer, III, Anthony B., 514
Creed, Betsy, 4585
Crellin, Justin, 4167, 4168
Cremata, Alfonso, 2712
Cremeens, Timothy, 286
Crenshaw, Catherine Sloss, 4009
Creswell, Brooke, 1857
Crewdson, Arlene, 2845
Crews, Brad, 3882
Crews, Ell, 4187
Crippen, Mary, 776
Cripps, Lori, 4088
Criscuolo, Lou, 3563
Crisp, Lynette, 8113
Criss, Jr, C. William, 4195
Cristofer, Michael, 3288
Cristofori, Jon, 12
Cristofori, Marilyn, 264
Criswell, Rick, 2744
Crocker, Dr. Ron, 1393
Crocker, Joe, 2251
Crocker, Warner, 3918
Crockett, Amy, 776
Croghan, Jack, 7127
Croitoroo, Paul, 437
Croken, Peter, 3251
Cromer, Jr, a Harrison, 240
Crommelin-Ball, Priscilla, 5
Cromwell, Caron, 1841
Crone, David, 2176
Cronin, Robert Jay, 3373
Cronk, Daniel, 4712
Crook, David, 3557
Crooker, Kasson E, 5227
Crooks, Ian, 2609
Cropp, Harold N, 3125
Cropp, John, 6718
Crosby, Danshia, 3017
Crosby, Pamela, 3794
Crosby, S, 4924
Cross, Dr. Gavin, 4527
Cross, Mildred Morton, 3095
Cross, Nancy, 6634
Cross, Robert W, 5647
Crouch, Richard L, 3732
Crouse, Janan, 202
Crouse, Lisa D, 6585
Crout, Stephen, 1994
Crow, Genevia, 5547
Crow, Marlon, 5449
Crow, Pat, 7993
Crow, Terry, 2155
Crow, Todd, 4618
Crowden, John, 4567
Crowe, Davis, 2760
Crowe, George, 2516
Crowe, Jack, 2884
Crowell Sawyer, Cathey, 3973
Crowley, Cassandra, 578
Crowley, Esther, 7189
Crown, A. Steven, 284
Cruernsey, Stew, 6805
Crum, Michael E, 7520, 7521
Crump, Amy, 5140
Crumpton, Roger, 7080
Cruszewski, Jeff, 3615
Cruz De Jeses, Enrique, 420
Cruzan, Carol, 3782
Cubbage, Linda, 1666, 5263
Cuccaro, Chris, 6909
Cuddy, Mark, 3493
Cue, Nancy Bell, 1626
Cuesta, Carlo, 3145, 3841
Cueva, Roberto, 1933

Culbersom, Pam, 2790
Culbert, John, 2830
Culbertson, Lloyd, 284
Culbertson, Myrna, 4546
Culkin, Daniel J, 1299
Cull, Christopher, 2645
Cullen, Teresa, 294
Culligan, Janine, 8261
Cullinane, Dennis, 6614
Cullum, Bonnie, 3811
Culp, Jennifer, 892
Culpo, John, 338
Culshaw, Denise, 1351
Culver, Daniel, 1144
Cumbo, Willie A, 7570
Cumitz, Hagnette, 2097
Cummings, Jolie, 226
Cummins, Jean, 3597
Cummins, Sharon, 6643, 6644, 6645
Cummis, Clive S., 7232
Cunico, Pete, 6648
Cuningham, Joesph, 1549
Cunningham, Hannah, 2070, 4594
Cunningham, John, 6484, 8232, 8235
Cunningham, Merce, 514
Cunningham, Merte, 966
Cunningham, Michael, 2031
Cunningham, Ron, 103
Cura, Barry Van, 654
Curcio, Richard, 3272
Curcio, Vincent, 2648
Curl, Bill, 6770
Curl, Joe, 8074
Curl, Sid, 6817
Curley, Geoffrey, 2849
Currie, Fergus G, 2882, 4473
Currier, Robert, 2541
Currier, Summer, 1880
Curro, Sally, 4915
Curry, Alice O., 1159
Curry, Eddie, 2917
Curry, Joan, 6126
Curry, Michael, 2666
Curry, Michael P, 5633
Curry, Richard, 3581
Curtis, Chris, 2602
Curtis, Elyse, 3356
Curtis, Gregory, 2982
Curtis, Jane Lawrence, 8364
Curtis, Martha, 711
Curtis, Norman, 3356
Curtis, Patti, 7221
Curtis PhD, Elyse, 3356
Curtiss, Brain, 2602
Curtiss, Jane Lawrence, 425, 1497
Cushing-Reid, Anne, 1616
Cuson, Roger, 4296
Custanza, Kathy, 2532
Custer, John, 5414
Cutforth, Tyler, 2214
Cutrone, Signe, 1363
Cutter MD, Phillip D, 1296, 4683
Cyrus, Edgar, 3056
Cyrus, Jim, 4997
Czaplinski, Lane, 5699

D

D'Addio, Dan, 1002
D'Agostino, Linda, 3305
D'Agostino, Tina, 4688
D'Alamberte, Sandy, 2008
D'Alessandro, Ed, 5697
d'Amboise, Jacques, 449, 522
D'Amico, Grace, 371
D'Amico, Julian, 3549
D'amour, Shelly, 166
D'Angelo, Patrick J, 6129
D'Angelo, Robert B, 8292
D'Anna, Dorothy, 3752
D'Antuono, Eleanor, 379

D'Arcy, Richard, 3305
D'Rivera, Paquito, 1424
da Costa, Carlos, 8488
Daab, James, 3925
Dabney, Lewis S, 1264
Dabon, Richard, 5528
Dacey, Ben, 6805
Dackow, Dr. Sandra, 1718
Daehler, Carl, 7682
Dagen, D'Ann Reed, 3840
Dahl, Dan, 5174
Dahlberg, Anders, 1331
Dahlin, Marshall, 7354
Dahlinger Fair, Catherine, 326
Daigle, Steven, 2266
Dailey, Michael, 2856
Daino, Muriel, 381
Dale Weary, Marca, 622
Dalena, David A, 4662
Daley, Bob, 1098
Daley Uebelhoer, Joan, 300
Dalis, Irene, 1949
Dallas, Walter, 3718
Dallin, Heidi J, 3049
Dally, Lynn, 65
Dalrymple, James, 4301, 6298
Dalton, J Truman, 2341
Dalvit, Lewis, 1768
Daly, Kevin R, 3012
Daly, Maureen, 2962
Damangne, Tammy, 6750
Dame, Benjamin B, 7566, 7567
Dameron, Allan, 718
Damp, Norma, 2750
Damron, Sandra, 1961
Danch, Michael J, 6621, 6622
Danenhauer, Bob, 7166
Dang, Tim, 2438
Daniel, Carol, 2785
Daniel, Meg, 3379, 5023
Daniel, T, 295, 296, 2897, 2898
Daniel, Jr, Isaac, 1025
Daniele, Graciela, 3399
Daniels, David, 2146
Daniels, Erica, 2855
Daniels, Fred, 3504
Daniels, Jeff, 3090
Daniels, Lewis A, 4890
Daniels, Myra Janco, 1046
Daniels, Priscilla, 1872
Daniels, Roger, 3877
Daniels, Sean, 2764
Daniels, Shelia, 3963
Daniels, Susan, 3072
Daniels Nowells, Julie, 5142
Daniels, CPA, Wesley, 3276
Danielson, Neil, 1361
Danilian, Sergei, 8418
Danis, Ann, 1750
Danis, Susan J, 2006
Dannenberg, Roger, 1739
Danner, Frank, 1883
Danner, Vincent L, 1771
Dannick, Jeff, 7280
Dannies, Robert, 989
Dante, Sharon E, 197
Danzig, Janice, 2695
Danziger, Howard, 3871
Daoust, Deborah K, 1846
Darby, Brian, 7492
Darby, Lorrin, 2160
Darby, Melanie, 1074
Darden, Patricia, 3922
Darling, Martha A, 1309
Darling, Jr, Nelson J, 1264
Darlington, Madge, 3809
Darmise, Richard, 3465
Darnell, Ddkjennifer, 6106
Darr, Patt, 6307
Darrow, Peter, 8386
Darrow, Robert K., 2991
Darsie, Jann, 208

Darwin, Donna, 7943
Das, Chitresh, 116
Dash, Jayne, 5705
Dattagupta, Ran Jan, 6443
Dattagupta, Ranjan, 2773
Dattilo, Michael, 1431
Daugherty, Brannen, 2816
Daughety, R Morgan, 5160
Daughtey, Dr. Michael, 5138
Daughtridge, Emily E, 576
Davalos, Rudy, 7264, 7266
Davenny Wyner, Susan, 1300
Davenport, Cindy, 3202
David, Cristian E, 3726
David, Pat, 3107, 6976
Davidman, Aaron, 2531
Davidoff, Judith, 1520
Davidson, Aviva, 465
Davidson, Barry, 1436
Davidson, Charles, 5535
Davidson, David, 2308, 2445
Davidson, Della, 121
Davidson, Gordon, 2431, 2447
Davidson, Paula, 7000
Davidson, Tippen, 2689, 4324, 4325
Davidson, Virginia S, 2227
Davidson, Warren, 1723
Davies, Dennis Russell, 1495
Davies, Greg, 6640
Davies, Jane, 3672
Davies, Molly, 498
Davies, Rick, 4735
Davies, Sandra, 3606
Davis, Al, 3053
Davis, Alan, 1158
Davis, Aurea, 2294
Davis, Barbara, 7504
Davis, Carl, 5518
Davis, Carol, 2225
Davis, Chuck, 573
Davis, Cydney, 3915
Davis, David E, 798
Davis, Deborah C, 3567
Davis, Doralene, 2283
Davis, Evie, 4187
Davis, Frederic H, 2969
Davis, Gregory A, 6753
Davis, Heather, 1889
Davis, Helen B, 105
Davis, Isabelle, 1037
Davis, Jack, 2374, 7073
Davis, Jackie, 1072, 4386
Davis, Janet, 2063
Davis, Jerome, 3552
Davis, Jillian, 3592
Davis, Jim, 3672
Davis, Katheryn, 6821
Davis, Kay L, 50
Davis, Lawrence, 1500
Davis, Ljuba, 798
Davis, Luane, 3386
Davis, Lynwood, 168
Davis, Marcia, 2012
Davis, Mary K, 1982
Davis, Milton, 2833
Davis, Montgomery, 3993
Davis, Patricia, 27
Davis, Paul, 1761
Davis, Paula J, 5964
Davis, Peter, 3446
Davis, Priscilla, 2394
Davis, Quint, 4600
Davis, Rick, 5629
Davis, Ron, 172
Davis, Ruth, 7309
Davis, Sandra, 5009
Davis, Sarah K, 5458
Davis, Scottie, 3445
Davis, Sir Andrew, 2038
Davis, Sir Colin, 1522
Davis, Susan, 5088
Davis, Sybil, 4033

Davis, Teddy, 783
Davis, Terry, 7265
Davis, Therese, 2068
Davis Jones, Lori, 6749
Davis, III, Charles, 756
Davis-Tucker, Joyce, 5523
Davoust, Jean, 1815
Davydova, Carol, 2497
Dawe, Dr. Lloyd A, 603
Dawes, Carol, 8154
Dawn, Karalee, 3448
Daws, Russell, 4374
Dawson, George, 2878
Dawson, Terry, 3832
Dawson, Verlina, 3717
Dawson CPA, Donna, 600
Day, Dan, 3825
Day, H Corbin, 744
Day, Iris, 686
Day, Kate, 3552
Day, Mary, 214
Day, Susan, 8382
Daye, Christine, 4732
Daykin, Judith E, 4936, 7381
Daykin, Judith E., 4936
Dayley, Jo, 1098
Dayley, K Newell, 8146
de Abruna, Laura, 5392
de Azcarraga, Dolores, 424
De Bernard, Johnnie, 3089
de Bievre, Micheline, 1273
de Bouteiller, Yves, 26
De Brier, Donald, 832
De Feis, Frederic, 3310
de Figols, Anne, 2196, 5642
de Fontaine, Didier, 899
De Francis, Karen, 5007
de Grasse, Gretchen, 1856
de Jong, Jennifer, 1781
De La Roza, Maria, 231
De Laurentis, Semina, 2641
De Lavallade, Carmen, 492
De Leon De Vega, Sonia Marie, 850
de Luna, Patricia, 42
de Ment, Ted, 374
De Michele, John, 888
de Montebello, Philippe, 5035
De Paola, Donna, 4224
De Poorter, Christine, 1878
De Renzi, Victor, 2006
de St. Aubin, Jean, 2849
de Veer, Ilse, 2214
de Velder, Anne, 6953
De Walle, Thomas, 1115
de Warren, Robert, 233
De Wayne, Dan, 5956
De Young, Bill, 340
Deaderick, Lesley D, 7650
Deal, Chris, 7095
Deal, Karen, 1108
Deal, Karen Lynne, 661
Deal, Melvin, 205
Dean, Bill, 1813
Dean, Dr. Maria, 4527
Dean, Jay, 1364, 2147, 2148
Dean, Joe, 6738
Dean, Margo, 674
Dean, Molly, 5529
Dean, Stan, 6404
Dean, Tim L, 5930
Dean Mainer, Leslie, 892
Deane, Diane, 5253
Deane, Robilee F, 857, 4143
Dearing, Janice, 3305
Dearling, Kevin, 7994
DeAtley, Kathleen, 4170
Deaton, Jimmy, 3167
Deaver, Susan, 4938
Debiak, Gail, 3054
DeBoer, Kathleen, 6718
DeBolt, Ben, 1927
DeBree, Lynn, 3733

DeCaprio, Gene, 5359
Decheimer, Roy, 3318
Decima, Karlee, 4124
Decker, Chip, 3526
Decker, Ed, 2520
Decker, Tray, 3720
Declert, Alain, 5552
Declert, Alain G, 8104
Decurtins, Russ, 7908
DeDee, Ted, 7958
Deegan, Judy, 4704
Deely, Anita, 2861
Deener, Larry, 1215
Deering, Lynn H, 581
Deering, Sidney, 720
Deerwater, Raven, 2460
Deeter, Jasper, 3706
DeFazi, Dr. Joseph, 4900, 7244
Defillippo, Gene, 6873
Deforrest, Michael, 3286
DeFranco-Brown, Diane, 92
DeFries-D'Albert, Beverly, 4434
DeGarmo, Penny, 1312
Degerness, Marv, 2254
deGraauw, Linda, 6448
Degroff, Anne, 971
Dehaan, Kelly, 2328
Dehart, Deborah, 2655
Deiker, Joseph, 7072
Deissler, Mary, 1267, 2096
Deissler, Walter, 942
Del Colletti, David, 2930
Del Conte, Andrea, 429
Del Gobbo, George, 1079
del Mazo, Angelique, 2686
Del Rossi, Angelo, 3251
Del Sesto, Janice, 2094
Delaney, Carla, 3683
Delaney, Christine, 2123
Delaney, Derek, 1731, 5368
Delaney, Jim, 6859
Delaney, Shannon, 931
Delanghe, Gay, 340
delaPena, Karin, 2545
DeLeone, Carmon, 579, 1141, 1651
Delfs, Andreas, 1362
Delgado, Anthony, 6373
DelGrosso, Kim, 693
DeLio, Carla, 2861
Delisi, Daniel, 1206
Delisle, Eric, 6531
Delk, Marilyn, 5230
Della-Vechia, Guido, 3765
Dellaripa, Jr, Victor J, 6249
Delliger, Todd, 2428
Dellinger, Steve, 2245
DelMarcelle, Charlie, 3708
DeLoach, Katherine, 2019
DeLorenzo, Hazel M., 1692
DelRosario, Roger R, 723
Deluca, Bernie, 6307
DeLuca, Bobby, 6006
Delury, Cecilia, 2493
DelValle, Jonah, 217
DeMain, John, 1951
Demarco Goor, Anita, 4714
Demas, Carol, 3066
Demeter, Ellen, 1261
Demeter, George, 1261
DeMetrick, Linda, 2565
Deming, Karen, 1457
Deminster, Larry, 4931
Demke, Dave, 3672
Demler, Susan, 8447
Demos, Nick, 3640
DeMoss, Virginia, 2426
Dempsey, Bob, 4027
Dempsey, Katie, 1083
Dempsey, Marilyn, 2330
Dempsey, Mark, 1961
Dempsey, Micheal J, 2550
Dempster, Curt, 3372

Demson, Martha, 2414
Deneau, Andrew L, 67
Denet, Chuck, 930
Denevan, Dion, 3764
Dengler, Nancy J, 630
Denhard, August, 1845
Denhard, Gus, 5693
DeNigro, Nicole E, 1445
Denisola, Joe, 2549
Denison, Scott B, 6182
Denmark, Leon, 7232
Denne, Carolyn, 278
Dennin, Steve, 6259
Denning, Ed, 5100
Dennis, Don, 6997
Dennis, Dr. Allan, 1136
Dennis, John, 1948
Dennis, Karen, 1136
Dennis, Kim, 5538
Dennis, Patricia, 3121
Dennis, Reid W., 1944
Dennison, EW, 6729
Dennison, John, 803
Densmore, Ginny, 1064
Dent, Jennifer, 3107
Denton, Dean, 5296
Denton, Nina, 729
Denton, Sharon, 760
Dentzel, Paul A, 4146
Deodorff, Beth Ann, 1255
DePreist, James, 1697
der Hoeven, Bill van, 1567, 5103
der Weiden Bejamin, Dr. Wieke Van, 1182
Deranleau, Shirley, 3964
Derda, Denise, 876
Derderian, Pat, 1338
Derivan, Miriam, 5073
Derr, Matthew, 337
Derryberry, Griff, 878
Derstine, Sharon R, 1727, 5363
DeRuggiero, Sal, 642
Dervisa, Ashia, 3411
Desalvo, Steve, 7893
DeSantis, Deborah, 1964
Deschere, Karen, 2032
Desens, Joan, 2162
Desio, Alfred, 60, 76
Desjardins, Marilyn, 6918
Desola, Carla, 21
DesRochers, Rick, 3018
Desroches, Jack, 3046
Desrosiers, Ted E, 3074
DeStefano, Frank, 5342
Destefano, Todd, 6026
Destocki, Robert, 6572, 8307
Detamore, Betty, 2717
DeTroy, Douglas, 3512
Detweiler, Carol, 3487
Deuel, Carolyn, 5786
Deuschle, Connie, 2905
Deuter, Patti, 899
Deutsch, Margery, 1874
Deveau, David, 1296, 4683
DeVere, Rollin, 3579
Devereux, Fr. Thomas, 3704
Deville, Pam, 6753
Devin, Richard M, 2578, 4236
Devine, Maryann, 2277
Devine, Scott, 6779
DeVisser, Joan, 808
DeVivo, Elizabeth J, 2735
Devon, R., 7413
Dew, John, 3112
Dewar, Janet L, 2668
Dewhurst, Stephen, 5014
Dewit, Dortha, 1190
Dewitt, Adam, 2849
DeWitt, Rufus, 2506
DeWolf, Anne, 6896
di Palma, Susana, 3128
Diamond, Amanda, 2394
Diamond, Becky, 1980

Evans, Charles Jones, 790
Evans, Clifton, 1800
Evans, Dale, 6550
Evans, Eva, 4167, 4168
Evans, John H, 1714
Evans, Linda, 2808
Evans, Lois, 847
Evans, Lydia, 1473
Evans, Steve, 4121
Evans, Susan, 1965
Evans, Terri, 4325
Evans-Jones, Caitlin, 8398
Evens, John, 5916
Everett, David J., 3099
Everett, Dr Mark A, 1671
Everett, Dr. H Dean, 1671
Everitt, John, 2270, 5279
Evert, Elizabeth, 3797
Evert, Susana, 593
Evert, Timothy, 593
Evert, Tom, 593
Evert Jr, Lawrence L, 593
Evleshin, Catherine, 3667
Ewalt, James B Ewalt, 6636
Ewalt, Mark E, 6636
Ewan-Kroeger, JoAnne, 5971
Ewanus, Donald S, 8267
Ewell, Maryo, 4247
Ewen, John G, 1973
Ewen, Malcolm, 3902
Ewers, Anne, 2327
Ewing, Brad, 966
Ewing, Dr. Ray G, 4781
Ewing, Iris, 5696
Ewing, Lawrence, 119
Exoo, Henk, 2139
Eyerdan, Debbie, 2710
Eylar, Leo, 867
Eyring, Teresa, 3012, 3130

F

Facci, Marc, 1676
Fackel, Josef, 4471
Fagan, Garth, 567
Fagan, Patrick, 7317
Fagan, Polly, 7297
Fagan, Tabby, 7611
Fager, Brenda, 3850
Fager, Judie, 691
Fahey, Mark, 2485
Fahle, Kathleen A, 3048, 6875
Fahringer, James, 813
Faiella, Ida, 4923
Faine, Audrey, 901
Fairchild, Dan, 8309
Fairchild, Jeannine, 2448
Faircloth, Janice, 4405
Fairservis, Teviot, 2607
Faison, Ade, 3410
Faison, Nabi, 3410
Faison, Shirley, 3410
Faker, Brian, 5702
Faktor, Viktoria, 6122
Falardo, Vincent, 311
Falco, Art J, 3595
Falco, Dara, 3370
Fale, Debra, 5776
Faley, Freda, 689
Falgiano, Rob, 7320
Falk, Elizabeth, 2233
Falk, Larry, 7981
Falk, Libby, 1384
Falky, Stephen, 2304
Falland, Rachel, 1186
Fallat, Andrew, 3952
Fallon, Dan, 3810
Falls, Gregory A, 3952
Falls, Robert, 2836
Fambrough, Douglas, 4636
Famrom, Ron, 8082

Fan, Sylvia, 3427
Fanelli, Jacqueline, 8466
Fanik, Blanche, 5781
Fankhauser, Teresa, 4800
Fanning, Dave, 4344
Fanning, Wendy, 5788
Fantini, Paul, 7231
Farago, Annke, 5367
Faraone, Cheryl, 3897
Farber, Dave, 4152
Farber, Dr. Stuart, 4598
Farco, Denise, 4872
Farer, Lian, 4887
Faridany, Nana, 805, 4093
Farina, Joe, 3723
Farley, Bill, 800
Farley, Robert J, 2789
Farm, Lis, 7758
Farmer, Joy, 6491
Farmer, Martha P, 3930
Farnbaugh, Danielle, 1483
Farnks, CE Bud, 1936, 2507
Faro, Gretchen, 1654
Faron, Sally R, 4367
Farquhar, Robin R, 3537
Farr, Susan, 1249, 4642
Farr, Susie, 6832
Farrah, Jen T, 2220
Farrand, Chelle, 1370
Farrell, Carol, 2998
Farrell, Dan, 7122
Farrell, Dawn, 3600
Farrell, Wayne, 2736
Farrelly, Wallace, 4107
Farrer, John, 791, 1450
Farrier, Van, 3072
Farrow Raines, Wendy, 2658
Fastabend, Jeanne Maddox, 618
Fathauer, Ted, 756
Fattman, George, 7856
Faue, Larry, 6720
Faue, Larryy, 6719
Faulkner, Curtis, 4810
Faulkner, Scott, 1407
Faulkner Jr, Grady L, 2618
Faure, Laura, 317, 4616
Faust, Betty M, 4067
Faust, Laura, 1772
Faust, William F, 1712, 5733
Favara, Annette, 3972
Favre, Niels, 7208
Fawcett, Linda K, 922, 4210
Fay, David, 6253
Fay, Kathleen, 4659, 4668
Fayman, Danah, 108
Fazekas, Sandra, 7320
Fazenbaker, Alexa, 3972
Fazzini, Susan, 2124
Fead, Barbara, 1033
Fearing, Don, 5518
Fearn, Pam, 3747
Featherman, David, 2120, 4709
Featherman, Jo-Ann M, 8386
Feder, Phyllis, 7413
Federick, Dan, 940
Federico, Robert, 3439, 3451
Fedie, Dan, 311
Fee, Charles, 2804, 4415
Fee, Charlie, 5205
Feeling, Gene, 6227
Feeney, James, 1883
Fehr, Cinnie, 1985
Fehr, Deborah, 4699
Feigel, Naomi, 1819
Feingold, Ed, 1266
Feinour, Ted, 3929
Feinsod, Arthur, 2930
Feld, Barbara, 5173
Feld, Eliot, 438
Felder, David, 4940
Felder, Elaine, 1117
Felder, Harvey, 1854

Feldman, Anita, 565
Feldman, Charles, 7373
Feldman, David, 3325
Feldman, Edgar, 1285
Feldman, Erika, 3462
Feldman, Heidi, 2846, 4440
Feldman, Howard, 7156
Feldman, Len, 4030
Feldman, Michael, 1534
Feldman, Richard, 5432
Feldman, Susan, 4935
Feldman, Toba, 5216
Feleppe, Virginia, 4729
Felix, Jessica, 4111
Felkel, Monica J, 8466
Feller, Bart, 376
Fellows, Ardelle, 4081
Fellows, David, 3033
Fellows, DeWayne, 1146
Fellows, Kathryn, 762
Felt, Kelli Shana, 5433
Felt, Ruth A, 4195
Feltman, Joel, 3365
Feltsman, Vladimir, 4994
Fenandez, Robert I, 3841
Fender, George, 2003, 3700
Fendrich, Sharon, 822
Fenger, Dan, 360
Fenley, Molissa, 518
Fennel, Mike, 7783
Fennelly, Brian, 5054
Fennessey, Bob, 7753
Fentress, Duke, 3553
Fentroy, Ruth, 48
Ferdland, Elliot, 2816
Ferguson, Ann, 2005
Ferguson, Brad, 1671
Ferguson, Erick, 4155
Ferguson, Richard, 2919
Feriend, Carmen, 12, 4054
Ferlo, Joseph A, 8295
Fern, Dr. Terry, 5107
Fernandaz-Haegg, Cristina, 1290
Fernandes, Erin, 3874
Fernandez, Belen, 446
Fernandez, Segundo, 1065
Ferra, Max, 3385
Ferranti Ferguson, Heather, 298
Ferrara, Cheryl, 2695
Ferrara, Mary, 2449
Ferraro, David, 1771
Ferre, Loren, 6695
Ferrell, Dr David M, 5078
Ferrell, Edward, 1570
Ferrelli, Ellen, 7199
Ferrelli, Tony, 7199
Ferri, Rita, 6146
Ferriera, Linda, 5083
Ferris, Chris, 1319
Ferris, Christina, 4723, 6942
Ferris, Harry, 371
Ferris, Julie, 2941
Ferris, Lesley, 3601
Ferro, Kathy, 3509
Ferry, Martha, 504
Fessenden, Charles, 4886
Fetertag, Dan, 3618
Fether, Harriet, 5566, 8127
Fetler, David, 1548, 1550
Fetsch, Ann, 955
Fetta, Frank, 815, 1913, 4165
Fetterman, Bob, 2689
Fettkether, Louis, 1186
Fetty, Byran, 3578
Feuchtenberger, Pat, 8506
Feuer, Willie, 192
Fey, Lorenne, 2759
Fickle, Nora, 5334
Field, Crystal, 3458
Field, Eliot, 438
Field, Johnathan, 2259
Fielding, Tamara, 3482, 3483

Fields, Allen, 350
Fields, Craig, 2335
Fields, James, 655
Fields, Joan, 1708, 5309
Fields, Laura, 2824
Fields, Mark, 7217
Fields, Michael, 2393
Fields, Michael D, 1373
Fields, Patricia, 7528
Fierce, Douglas E, 5484
Fierce, Hughlyn F, 1513
Figols, Alberto, 2196, 5642
Figueredo, Marie, 1424
Figueroa, Guillermo, 1447
Fijolo, Alberto, 5642
Filer, Barbara, 2059
Filer, Randall, 3037
Fillmer, Leslie, 1, 745
Filstrup, Scott, 2271
Fimer, Ann, 2822
Finch, Vance, 4859
Finchter, Nina, 118
Finck, Leslee, 369
Fine, Arlene, 5584
Fine, Bernard J, 4697
Fine, Franklin M, 933
Fine, Lew, 5584
Fine, Rachel, 4198
Fine, Stacy, 3904
Fineman, Carol, 3262, 3263, 4896
Finger, Dr. Ellis, 5330
Fingerote, Paul S, 4142
Fink, Donald, 6208
Finkel, Alan, 2572
Finkelberg, Jessica, 4874, 7216
Finkelman-Gividen, Nicki, 2265
Finks, Ellen, 5348
Finlaw, Jack, 1965
Finley, Gillian, 42
Finn, Dale, 2199
Finn, Jim, 3366
Finn, Kay, 3324
Finn, Robert, 1622
Finnegan, Mick, 2602
Finneran, Alan, 2526
Finnerty, Mary, 3161
Finnerty, Patty, 2236
Finney, Daniel, 490
Finney Jr, R Terrell, 3583
Fioccola, Joe, 3520
Fiol, Stephen, 2042
Fiorello, Sally, 3819
Fiorello, Sarah Jayne, 3824
Fiorito, Geoff, 2427
Fioritto, John, 1634
Fiorrato, Hugo, 528
Fiqueroa, Phillip, 3829
Firedman, Jerry, 6122
Firman, Linsay, 3449
Fiscella, Edward P, 3229
Fischelis, Mea, 5697
Fischer, Barry, 322
Fischer, Daryl, 3099
Fischer, David, 1066
Fischer, Herman, 2722
Fischer, Kenneth C., 4709
Fischer, Mark, 1048
Fischil, Charles, 4045
Fish, Maria, 5613
Fishback, Rachel, 2901
Fishburn, Joan E, 1564
Fisher, Ann, 19
Fisher, Bill, 3204, 7133
Fisher, Cindy, 8321
Fisher, Claresa, 1519
Fisher, Corey, 2531
Fisher, David, 8005
Fisher, Douglas, 2008
Fisher, Emily L, 1182
Fisher, Eve, 5444
Fisher, Joe, 7535
Fisher, John L, 1024, 1997

Fisher, Karen, 6481
Fisher, Larry, 3280
Fisher, Marc, 2849
Fisher, Marianne M, 3696
Fisher, Philip, 1161
Fisher, Randy, 4350
Fisher, Rick, 2151
Fishkin, Larry, 4203
Fishman, Carol, 3446
Fishman, Jack, 842
Fishman, Karen, 2039
Fishman Davis, Lenore, 1444
Fisk, Lynette, 2402
Fisk, Robert, 1920
Fisk, Sarah, 930
Fisner, John F, 6267
Fistler, Jack, 3137
Fitchuk, Kathy, 5749
Fitts, Debbie, 3528
Fitzgerald, Clyde, 2252
Fitzgerald, James F., 1051
Fitzgerald, Virginia, 2105
Fitzpatrick, Bridget, 5391
Fitzpatrick, James L., 1935
Fitzpatrick, John H., 1264
Fix, Scott, 3914
Flagg, Adrienne, 3672
Flagg-Pitts, Laura, 605
Flaherty, Tess, 1864
Flam, Karen, 3729
Flanahan, Don, 7266
Flarup, Tam, 8294
Flatt, Adam, 957, 959
Flatt, Robyn, 3819
Flaum, Peggy, 1515
Flaum, Stuart, 1027
Flax, John, 3096
Fleck, Wanda, 1462
Fleder, Mark, 1445
Fleeter, Nancy, 423
Fleisch, Marsha, 7255
Fleischer, Mary, 3466
Fleischer, Randall Craig, 754, 761, 1542, 7460
Fleischer, Jr, Arthur, 498
Fleischmann, Ernest, 4150
Fleishaker, Leonid, 1505
Fleisher, Leon, 1018
Fleisher, Mark, 644
Fleitz, Deborah L, 5181
Fleming, Barbara, 2121
Fleming, Carolann, 4447
Fleming, Irving A, 766
Fleming, JoAnne, 2858
Fleming, Marc, 4887
Flesher, Gina, 5264
Fleshler, Clementina, 1467
Fletcher, Kathleen, 5412
Fletcher, Leslie, 4392
Fletcher, Mark, 8168
Fletcher, Steve, 927
Fletcher, Todd J, 5043
Fletcher-Kilmer, Janelle A, 5788
Fleur, Ryan, 1279
Flinchum, Doug, 3929
Flint, Jere, 1073, 1074
Flint, Karen, 1005
Flint, Mark, 2019
Flood, Greg, 2665
Flood, Matthew E, 1489
Flood, Megan, 355
Flook, Darlene, 2933
Flook, Steve, 4002
Flor, Craig, 7013
Flores, Ramon A, 3278
Florescu, William, 2236
Florio, Ermanno, 680
Florip, Daniel, 2121
Florko, Brian, 8048
Flournoy, Spencer, 2553
Floyd, Nancy J, 3046
Floyd-Archibald, Robbye, 3857
Fluck, Jonathan, 3386

Fluger, Martin, 3337
Flugum, Ron, 755
Flummerfelt, Joseph, 2179, 5422
Flummerfrlt, Joseph, 649, 1758, 3753
Flusser, Beth, 5040, 5050
Flynn, Bob, 3944
Flynn, Brigid, 1121, 2846, 4440
Flynn, Elizabeth, 455
Flynn, Joan M, 6825
Flynn, Patrick, 879
Flynn, Vivian, 3861
Flynn Peterson, Kathleen, 3130
Fofel, Jessica, 340
Fofonoff, Meg, 3065
Fogarty, Sharon, 3401
Fogel, Charlotte, 412
Fogel, Henery, 1119
Fogel, Henry, 1116
Fogg, Anthony, 1263
Fogle, Ann B, 3754
Foglia, Sophia, 1477
Fogliane, Sophia, 4930
Fokine, Irine, 386
Foley, Beatrice, 6641
Foley, Bob, 8199
Foley, Delia, 570
Folger, Marvin, 3561
Folin, Paul, 4760
Folk, Bill, 6540
Folk, Jim, 7625
Folkers, Linda, 720
Folse, Bart, 2214
Foltz, Jamie, 2867
Foltz, Roger, 4836
Fomin, Pavel, 233
Fonda, Carol, 447
Fonda, Jeanne D, 1752
Fong, Robert King, 2496
Fong, Willy, 856
Fonseca, Bryan, 2920
Foody, Jan, 309
Foran, Kathleen, 3137
Forbes, Natalie, 1738
Forbrich, Joe, 2853
Ford, Anthony L, 6450
Ford, Bev, 3621
Ford, Jerry, 8101
Ford, Joshua S, 6311
Ford, Kelly, 2383
Ford, Kristen, 7351
Ford, Linda Marie, 3823
Ford, Matthew, 5340
Ford, Michael, 7774
Ford, Michael T, 311
Forde, Jane, 4862, 7202
Fordham, Jim, 1176
Foreman, George, 4570
Foreman, Laura, 501
Foreman, Richard, 3424
Forette, Kim M, 7492
Forman, Tony, 3986
Forrest, Cheryl, 608
Forrest, Donald, 2393
Forrest Helmuth, Paula, 1184
Forrester, Gretta, 3192
Forshee, Debbi, 7941
Forster, T, 728
Forsyte, John E, 917
Forsythe, Eric, 2939
Fort, Martha, 3619
Forte, Dan, 4975
Forte, James, 4655
Fortney, Dr. Pat, 1394
Fortune, Susan, 5294
Foss, Ed, 612, 1689, 3661, 5299
Foss, Lukas, 4925
Fosse, Stephanie, 1404
Foster, Heidi, 4693
Foster, Holly, 1412
Foster, Jeremy S, 38
Foster, Ken, 2375, 4058
Foster, Mark, 1915

Foster, Michelle, 2941
Foster, Randy, 3922
Foster, Senja, 993
Foster, Steven, 890
Foster, Thomas M, 2463
Foster Weya, Mary, 2796
Foulds, Michael, 2369
Fountain, Robin, 1748
Fourtier, Serge, 5471
Foust, Amanda, 2271
Foust, Diane, 1074
Fowler, Dr Gregory, 1678
Fowler, G William, 3868
Fowler, Liz, 4362
Fowler, Susan R, 3698
Fowler, Terry, 5142
Fowler, Tobin, 1496
Fowler, Vicki, 3880
Fowler Slade, Frances, 2178
Fowlkes, H Lee, 5165
Fox, Barry, 8289, 8290
Fox, Charlotte, 1885
Fox, Dani, 2669
Fox, Edward A, 423
Fox, Evarts, 6482
Fox, Jean, 2031
Fox, Jonathan, 3264
Fox, Michael A, 6614
Fox, Patricia, 592
Fox, Sheila, 582
Fox, Steve, 7942
Fox Hillard, Claire, 1367
Fox, Jr, William H, 790
Foxx, Tina, 5132
Fraher, David, 3129
Frahm, Laraine, 231
Fraider, Steven, 4115
Frain, David, 2951
Fraley, Robert, 4858
Franano, Susan, 781
France, Bill, 7124
France, Hal, 1048, 2162
Francett, Barbara, 381
Francis, Ceciclia M, 5763
Francis, Dan, 5902
Francis, Debra, 3882
Francis, Jay, 5588
Francis, Vickie, 3584
Francis, Wayne, 4152
Francis Wada, Toshimasa, 1286
Francuz, Liliane, 5787
Frandina, Joe, 7456
Franez, Louis, 1445
Frani, Massimiliano, 1821
Frank, David, 4003
Frank, Howard, 1045
Frank, Janie, 3838
Frank, Jeff, 3808
Frank, Kathie M, 3971
Frank, Michael, 8369
Frank, Nola, 2015
Frankel, Simon J, 4187
Frankenfield, Chet, 2427
Frankey, Cindy, 1983
Frankl, Marika, 949
Franklin, Al, 3709
Franklin, Cary John, 776, 1350
Franklin, Derek, 6769
Franklin, Douglas, 589
Franklin, Frederic, 679
Franklin, Jane, 702
Franklin, Joseph, 1737
Franklin, Luanne A, 2966
Franklin, Melane, 1366
Franklin, Toni, 5419
Franks, Becky, 5895
Frano Stockman, Jacqpea, 670
Fransto, Hector, 3872
Frantz, Eric, 2971
Frantz, Patrick, 27
Franz, Robert, 1218
Franzen, Dale, 2552

Fraschilla, Fran, 7264, 7266
Fraser, Bridget, 268
Fraser, John, 1381
Fratti, Mario, 3425
Frauntelle, Eric, 1985
Frazier, Lynn, 2383
Frazor, Terence, 1804
Freck, Scott, 1586
Freddy, Halli, 1967
Fredeman, JC, 5808
Frederick, Bridget, 5943
Frederick, Larry, 3216
Frederick, Rebecca, 2654
Frederick, Sue, 3980
Frederickson, Alan P, 4251
Fredmann, Martin, 182
Fredricks, Rita, 2645
Fredricks, Tom, 4209
Fredrik, Burry, 2645
Free, Katharine B, 2446
Free, Sherry, 4606
Freed, Jennifer, 3886
Freedberg, Richard, 3076
Freedland, Kathy R, 870
Freedman, Deborah, 446
Freedman, Robert, 438, 6321
Freeman, Alan, 7944
Freeman, Isadore, 4876
Freeman, Joann, 4713
Freeman, John A, 6542
Freeman, Judy, 259
Freeman, Lee, 1075
Freeman, Mac, 6225
Freeman, Nathan Ross, 3566
Freeman, Paul, 1115
Freeman, Roxanne, 6766
Freeman, Virginia Ray, 576
Freemarl, Alan, 7942
Freese, Leon, 7017
Freestone, Bruce K, 2597
Freiberg, Richard, 8303, 8305
Freking, Debra, 7126
Fremaux, Sylvain, 5301
Fremont, Felecia, 7088
Fremont-Alexiou, Felicia, 7089
Fremont-Smith, Anne, 1289
French, Bryan, 7001
French, Catherine, 1896
French, Cheryl, 3369
French, Donna, 5787
French, James, 1094
French, Pam, 1322
French, Ruthann, 4715
French, Tom, 12
Frenz, Dr. Terren, 7611
Frenzel, Andrea, 3128
Freriotti, Jo Ann, 7855
Freundel, Carl, 3013
Frew-Waters, Pati, 7190
Frewen, Peter, 1233, 2075
Frewen, Ray, 2885
Frey, Adam L, 899
Frey, Brian, 6440
Frey, Jonathan, 351
Frey, Mary, 5733
Frey, Rick, 2493
Friberg, Eric G, 649, 1758, 3753, 5422
Frick, Elaine, 682
Fricke, Heinz, 1014
Fridrich, Tom, 6817
Fridy, Scott, 5617
Fried, Lawrence J, 1811
Friedenberg, David, 1850
Friedlander, William, 1713
Friedman, Barbara B., 446
Friedman, Beatrice, 1058, 4366, 4370
Friedman, Carole, 1271
Friedman, Cheri E, 2602
Friedman, Dan, 3357
Friedman, Jay, 1140
Friedman, Leslie, 128
Friedman, Peggy, 5053

Friedman, Richard, 2892
Friedman, Robert, 137, 8350
Friedson, Adam, 57
Frierson, Scott, 3758
Friesen-Carper, Dennis, 1183
Fritz, Barry, 2637
Fritz, Joanie, 3400
Fritz, Richard, 7791
Fritz Blank, Chef, 2283
Fritz-Logrea, Beth, 564
Froehlich, Brenda, 2649
Froehlich, Rose, 2532
Froman, Abe, 915
Froncek, Michael C, 2536
Froot, Dan, 3368
Froso, Raymond, 3066
Frost, Christy, 6644, 6645
Frost, Jack L, 4370
Frost, Judy, 2550
Frost, Richard I, 3686
Frost, Sue, 4266, 6250
Frost Heard, Heidi, 4909
Frost6, Judy, 6151
Frousto, Hector, 687
Fruchter, Danny S, 3705
Frugoli, Donna, 1295
Fry, Andrea, 2769
Fry, Charles, 1137
Fry, Keener, 8321
Fry, Tim, 993
Frydel Kim, Irene, 2202
Fryling, Robert, 627
Fryman, Hubert, 3711
Fryman, Louis, 3726
Fu, Christopher, 856
Fuchs, F John, 1485, 4982
Fuehrer, Kris, 4820
Fuerstner, Fiona, 740
Fuesy, Margaret, 6414
Fugate, Judith, 463
Fuhrman, Michael J, 7801
Fukuhara Arthurs, Lynn, 2438
Fulgham, Jeffery R, 6290
Fullen, Ruth, 3608
Fuller, Albert, 5022
Fuller, David, 3390
Fuller, Elizabeth, 2482
Fuller, Linda, 2024
Fuller, Rex, 1965
Fuller, Sarah D., 2969
Fuller, Susan, 1129
Fuller Lett, Nanacy, 940
Fullmer, Terry, 3735
Fulmer, Paul, 2276
Fultz, Audrey, 4541
Funderburk, Liz, 7903
Funfgeld, Greg, 5315
Funk, Eric, 1390
Funk, Gary, 1390
Funk, Lori, 3398
Furey Esq, Michael K, 379
Furham, Ardis, 2254
Furland, Bob, 6991
Furlong, Danny, 32
Furlong, Jim, 3382
Furman, Ty, 3708
Furniss, Judy, 1142
Furr, William P, 1586, 3023
Furshpan, Roy, 5935
Furstenberg, Barbara, 1092
Furumoto, Kimo, 1861
Fusaris, Kurt, 2606
Fusaro, Ruby, 1842
Fusco, Erin, 1117
Fuscomeese, Gigi, 6011
Fuson, Rick, 4504, 6613
Fussaro, Dianne, 2276
Fyodorov, Deborah, 6843

G

Gaal, Stephen J, 1290
Gabb, Carolyn S, 2756
Gabbert, John, 8169
Gabel, Audrey, 6664
Gabel, Ed, 775
Gabel, Theresa, 858
Gabel, PhD, Sarah, 2842
Gabhard, Tom, 8163
Gable, Jane, 5313
Gabriel, Nancy, 8442
Gabriel, Norma, 358
Gabriels, Jane, 399
Gacioch, Jim, 4931
Gaddy, Rupert, 3760
Gaffney, Floyd, 2506
Gaffney, Mary Beth, 735
Gaffney, Thomas G, 3545, 5136
Gaffney, Tom, 3841
Gage, Nancy, 2258
Gage, Richard, 1136
Gagliano, Patrick, 3760
Gagne, Kathleen, 6908
Gagne, Roland, 5514
Gahan, Joan, 7873
Gahan, Rachel, 2208
Gaifman, Hanna, 1538
Gaigalas, Laima, 4240
Gailmann, Greg, 8152
Gaines, Barbara, 2823
Gaines, Dr. Robert A, 2359
Gaines, Jeff, 7950
Gajewski, Piotr, 1258
Gajewslei, Piotr, 1013
Galante, Marco, 503
Galasso, David, 2493
Galatz, Eric, 3140
Galazzi, Marcia, 3066
Galban, Margarita, 2433
Galbraith, Scott, 3633
Galbreath, Woody, 8180, 8181
Gale, John, 1661
Galeota, Jay, 1027
Galey, Ramona, 2091
Galicia, Albert, 5996
Galindo, Louis, 945
Gallagher, Art, 2649
Gallagher, Jean, 5674
Gallagher, Jerry, 7487
Gallagher, John, 3706
Gallagher, Marie, 5371
Gallagher, Mark, 6290
Gallagher, Nancy N, 6255
Gallagher, Sheila, 8461
Galland, Jack, 964
Gallant, Thomas, 4892
Gallas, Robert, 6518
Gallas, Stephanie, 3501
Gallegos, Debra, 2593
Galles, Cynthia, 2426
Galligan, David, 7027
Gallion, Steve, 858
Gallman, Ronald, 903
Gallo, Steve, 7203
Gallogly, John, 2453
Galuppo, Dante, 1001
Galvez, Frank, 310
Gamache, John, 3942
Gamage Tucker, Meg, 2919
Gambill, Larry, 3549
Gambini, Lindsay, 1441
Gamble, John, 576
Gambone, Ralph M, 1025
Gamer, Jack, 8211
Gandy, Tasha, 649, 1758, 3753, 5422
Ganem, Shirley, 3238
Gangemi, Marie, 2232
Gann, Julie, 4427
Gannon, Jason, 1904
Gansky, Gary, 2280

Ganun, Alan, 4895
Ganus, Dr. Clifton L, 4072
Gapko, Laurie F, 5737
Garay, Mary Beth, 2322
Garber, William, 3842
Garber-Cohen, Francine, 2193
Garberson, Jeffrey B, 4122
Garbo, Bernard, 2825
Garcia, Al Beto, 1783, 5495
Garcia, Anthony J, 2593
Garcia, David, 2705
Garcia, Donaldo, 4899
Garcia, Irene, 1447
Garcia, Maria, 245
Gardels, David, 2162
Gardenhire, Charles, 182
Gardinel, Pam, 230
Gardiner, Gayle, 383
Gardiner, Sheila, 988
Gardner, Elaine, 408
Gardner, Jack, 1229
Gardner, Jeannette, 8437
Gardner, Jeffrey L, 6894
Gardner, Marcia, 3908
Gardner, Marie, 1961
Gardner, Pam, 8064
Gardner, Robert, 350
Gardnine, Robert K., 1676
Garfield, Leslie J, 1525
Garlock, Dr. Scott, 4461
Garmendia, Terrie, 1044
Garner, Kathleen, 1882
Garner, Richard, 2767, 4387
Garnes, Lori, 7273
Garnn, Kimberly, 1821
Garofolo, Claudia, 4594
Garonzik, Sara, 3722
Garrard, Mimi, 517
Garrett, David A, 4506
Garrett, Stacy, 7272
Garrett, Stephine, 1366
Garrett, Walter, 5803
Garrick, J Joshua, 4379
Garrin, Richard, 1950
Garrison, Brian, 3272
Garrison, Kelly, 4129
Garritson, Dr. Maric, 4458
Garrity, Rachel, 1832
Garstka, Jeff, 1213
Garton, Deirdre Wilson, 731
Garton Edie, Diane, 2345
Garuer, Wendy, 6628
Garvey, Dominic, 2996
Garvey, Kevin, 1168
Garvey, Tara, 4688
Garvin, Emily, 6817
Garvin, Janet, 1943
Garwood, David, 3701
Gary, Ellen M, 5920
Gasbarre, Roberta, 2659
Gaspardo, Cindy, 6539
Gasper, David W, 1755
Gasper, Mary M, 6785
Gasport, Etta, 735
Gassaway, JB, 5500
Gassen, Jerome J, 1177
Gassner, David, 2466
Gately, Timothy F, 4256
Gates, J. Robert, 1309
Gates, John, 876, 885
Gates, Laura D, 275
Gathers, Greg, 3236
Gatto, Angelo, 1253
Gatto, Marharet, 1253
Gatz, Jill, 1207
Gatz, Joni, 2847
Gaub, Eugene, 4953
Gaubatz, Kathy, 1029, 4323
Gaupp, Natalie, 3838, 3844
Gause, Leland V, 1022
Gavin, Ellen, 2511
Gawinski, Neil A, 4754

Gay Anderson, Donna, 2980
Gaydos, Gary, 3174
Gaylard, Timothy, 1835
Gayley, Oliver G., 498
Gaylin, David, 2334
Gaylin, Jed, 1417
Gaylor, Gregory, 8325
Gaynor, Maureen, 101, 2495
Gaynor LaPat, Beth, 5368
Geary, Robert, 4158
Gebara, Marsha, 4165
Geddeis, Peter, 2272
Geddes, Lila, 2323
Gedeon, Jean, 620
Gee, Renouard, 458
Geer, Ellen, 2567
Geer, Sarah, 4944
Geers, Robert, 4244
Geers, Robert T, 6201
Geeting, Daniel, 4221
Gehr, Jennifer, 2829
Gehrke, Dilbert E, 6662
Geidt, Jan, 3041
Geiger, Cindy, 351
Geile, Cindy, 2026
Geiogamah, Hanay, 112
Geisler, Barry H, 8169
Geiss-Robbins, Suzanne, 4291
Geist, Dr. Joseph, 4783
Gelbart, Norman, 1924
Gelblum, Seth, 3415
Gelfand, Michael, 1603
Gelfand, Michael D, 5260
Gellar, Marc, 3377
Gelleerd, Judith, 1139
Geller, Michael, 1495
Gellis, Herb, 905
Gelman, Linda, 3358
Geltner, Beverley, 4709
Geltner, Beverly, 2120
Gemar, Jan, 2063
Genn, Charla, 437
Gennaro, Michael, 2855
Genochio, Jerry, 3525
Genovese, Terry M, 6400
Gens, Terri, 4132
Gentile, Rebecca, 3607
Gentry, Anne, 1256
Gentry, Brad, 7073
Gentry, Lucy, 3948
Genualdi, Robert, 977
George, April, 2553
George, David, 1819
George, James, 2982
George, Roberta, 4407
George, Scott, 8361
George, Teady, 1809, 2320
George, Vance, 1946
George, Wayne, 2736
Gerber, Barbara, 2509
Gergerich, Tom, 8299
Gerhart, Douglas, 888
Gerig, Vern, 1598, 2255, 3032
Gerking, Tim, 1689
Gerland, Dr. Oliver, 2580
Gerlt, Michelle, 3202
Germain, James St, 703
Germain, Kelly, 3589
Germann, Kathleen, 3391
Gerould, Robert C, 99, 2489
Gerould, Rosemarie, 99, 2489
Gerritson Brauer, Sasha, 2044
Gershenfeld, Mitchell, 6066
Gershunoff, Naxim, 1050
Gersmann, Joel, 3985
Gersten, Fredrick, 5789
Gersten, Jenny, 4699
Gersten Luckman, Sharon, 421
Gessel, Arnold, 1732
Gessler, Tom, 4372
Gestring, Brian, 380
Getchell, Les, 8491

Getman, Tim, 6311
Getmick, Pamela, 2109
Getto, Elissa, 2634
Getty, Carrie, 2808
Getty, Daniel, 1309
Getty, Sarah, 2105
Geyer, Richard A, 8303
Geyer, Richards A, 8305
Geyser, Amy, 3996
Gfaller, Joe, 2773, 6443
Gherty, Mark J, 8286
Ghin, Vadim, 515
Ghion, Keith, 8428
Giacobbe, Joseph, 313
Giacobbe, Maria, 313
Giagmi, Ann, 4123
Giaimo, Kathryn A, 3508
Giangiulio, Richard, 1788
Gianni, Jodi, 1470, 4955
Giannini, Richard, 7048, 7050
Giannini, Richard C, 7049
Gianotti, Marilyn, 1907
Giantonio, John, 6409
Giardina, Joseph, 3462
Giatas, Ted, 6066
Gibb, Keren, 3
Gibbons-Brown, Karen, 299
Gibbs, Barbara, 6088
Gibbs, Dr. Andrew, 2379
Gibbs, Jimmy, 1576
Gibert, Mervin, 2460
Gibney, Gina, 481
Gibson, Beth, 1074
Gibson, Camille, 2049
Gibson, Cecile, 314
Gibson, Elizabeth, 792
Gibson, Eric, 2270, 5279
Gibson, Frances, 5519
Gibson, Kenny, 6730
Gibson, Mara, 4940
Gibson, Mark, 1612
Gibson, Rob, 4403, 5028
Gibson, Susan Davis, 651
Gibson, Timothy, 3882
Gibson-Brehon, Dawn, 6368
Gideons, Rod, 2340
Gidley, Margaret, 2293
Gidwitz, John, 1244, 4630
Gies, Ken, 7091
Giese, Jeff, 265
Giesen, Mary, 5778
Giffen, Linda, 5489
Giffin, Marie, 3058
Gifford, James, 5098
Gilad, Yehuda, 1414
Gilardi, Susan Johann, 2463
Gilbert, David, 979, 1437
Gilbert, Elizabeth, 3058
Gilbert, Sally, 5512
Gilbert, Tricia, 3474
Gilbertson, Carole, 932
Gilbertson, Rhonda, 756
Gilbreath, John, 5694
Gilchrist, Reed, 4097
Gilcrease, Lynn, 2963
Gildan, Laurie, 2706
Gildea, Patricia, 5313
Giles, Charlotte, 5720
Giles, Diane, 6574
Giles, Melissa, 1838
Gilette, Robin, 3470
Gilfus, John, 3496
Gilgore, Laurence, 1977
Gilgus, Mark, 3176
Giliotto, Maria T, 1733
Gilkey, Leslie, 1390
Gill, Diane, 4738
Gill, Dr. Michael, 5776
Gill, E Benton, 1353, 7014
Gill, Margaret G, 140
Gill-Doleac, Sue, 211
Gillan, Maria M, 4894

Gillane, Jackie, 1230
Gillen, Pete, 8168
Gillespy, Clark, 2349
Gillette, Michael, 8182
Gilley, J Wade, 5719
Gillfillan, Jack, 2014
Gilliam, Joshua M, 5142
Gilliam, Ryan, 3368
Gillispie, John, 8261
Gillum, Linda, 2829
Gilmartin, Kevin, 6912
Gilmartin, Matthew, 1927
Gilmer, Martha, 1116
Gilmore, Geoff, 3888
Gilmour, Matt, 7102
Gilreath, Nena, 246
Gilstrap, Kenneth, 4814
Gimbel, Anne E, 844
Gime, Cherie, 7690
Gimenez, Jana, 1262
Gindrele, Jerry, 1741
Gingelli, Patricia, 929
Ginwala, Cyrus, 1769
Gionfriddo, Gina, 3434
Giordano, Chris, 6785
Giordano, Delta, 3136
Giordano, Nan, 284
Giordano, Philip, 1977
Giordano, Sam, 6785
Giovando, John W, 1451, 4260
Giovannetti, Claire, 1942
Giovanni, Greg, 3716
Girouard, Peggy, 677
Giroux, Leigh, 3370
Gisselman, Margo, 3119
Gitchell, David D, 6685
Gittleman, Neal, 1640
Giudice, Angelina, 3903
Giudicessi, Joy, 6656
Giunta, Joseph, 1193
Giusti, Tom, 3608
Givan, Julianne, 6236
Giza, Tom, 2793
Gizzi, Vincent, 6336
Gladchuk, Chet, 8065, 8074
Gladden, Dean, 7618
Gladden, Dean R, 3591
Gladstone, Josh, 3311
Glaesemann, Joyce, 1397
Glann, Kimberley, 2448
Glaser, Amy, 3892
Glass, Barry, 156
Glass, Philip, 498
Glass, Ronald R., 1676
Glasscock, Tom, 1320, 4724
Glasscok, Tom, 4723, 6942
Glaudini, Steven A, 2486
Glaze, Debbie, 2077
Glaze, Gary, 4711
Glazebrook, Bob, 6528
Glazer, Charlie, 3903
Glazer, Jeffrey S, 582
Glazer, Norma, 1605
Gleasner, Gregg, 902
Gleason, Bobby, 8082
Gleason, Larry, 303
Gleason, Velma, 2315
Gleen, Pleas, 7261
Gleeson, Patricia M, 3034
Glendinning, Elizabeth P, 1731
Glenn, Cynthia, 4172
Glenn, Laura, 191
Glenn, Neil, 3528
Glenn, Ruth, 4025
Glenn, Tim, 733
Glenn-Lewin, JoAnn, 6290
Glick, Charles R., 807
Glick, Robert, 4917
Glick, Vern, 910
Glidden, Elizabeth, 776
Glidewell, Rae, 5900
Gliman, Phil, 3316

Glines, John, 3376
Glist, Kothi, 2699
Globenfelt, Jack, 7301
Globerman, Evie, 4200
Glover, CR, 3860
Glover, Jane, 2039
Gloyeski, Lynn, 1577
Glymph, Joseph, 1118
Glynn, Jr, Robert D, 1946
Gnage, Marie, 3258, 3265
Gnam, Adrian, 1081
Gobrick, Joanne, 3310
Gockley, David, 2314
Goddar, Matty B, 6423
Goddard, Jennifer, 726
Godfrey, Elizabeth, 20
Godfrey, Margaret, 2948
Godfrey, Pamela, 1242
Godfrey, Susan, 1742
Godfrey, Virginia, 2698
Godman, Kate, 3956
Godward, William W, 1944
Godwin, Ralph, 1592, 3028
Goede, Gordon, 2406
Goeden, Sherrie, 1400
Goehring, Jerry, 2613
Goepfert, Robert C, 7285
Goetsch, Lara, 2859
Goetz, Linda, 38
Goff, Mark, 6631
Goforth, Renea, 308
Gofuken, Mirna, 918
Gogol, Peter, 3747
Gohn, Kay, 6632
Goin, Bob, 7605, 7611
Goins, Luther, 2824
Golay, Ardis, 3766, 3767
Gold, Gene, 2794
Gold, Michele, 3363
Gold, Rob, 3109
Goldberg, Alan P, 1454
Goldberg, Barry, 1525
Goldberg, Joel, 3795
Goldberg, Linda C, 2081
Goldberg, Michael, 3988
Goldberg, Moses, 2972
Goldberg, Nancy, 6841
Goldberg, Naomi, 70
Goldberg, Paul, 1418
Goldberger, Ariel, 3948
Goldberger, Cindy, 667
Golden, Chuck, 419
Golden, Eugene, 4131
Golden, Judy, 3843
Goldenberg, Helyn, 1121
Goldhirsch, Sheri, 3481
Golding, Margot, 899
Goldkamp, Joseph A., 2293
Goldman, Douglas, 4198
Goldman, Dr. Fran, 2189
Goldman, Fran, 1767
Goldman, John D, 1946
Goldman, Lawrence P, 7232
Goldman, Robert T, 3338
Goldman, Sherwin, 2223
Goldsmith, Richard, 1501
Goldsmith, William, 3600
Goldspiel, Alan, 4602
Goldstein, Barry, 4634
Goldstein, David Ira, 2374
Goldstein, John, 2790
Goldstien, Jo, 7255
Goldwater, Bobby, 6042
Gollop, LaVerne, 1815
Golston, David, 3182
Golub, Spencer, 3745
Gomer, Wes, 2318
Gomes, Lisa, 6174
Gomez, Ileana, 6382
Gomez, Judy, 232
Gomez, Robert, 2433
Gomez, Vicki, 3869

Gonce, Nancy C, 4013
Gonda, Brad, 2031
Goner, Brian, 1872
Gonzales, Fernando, 3859
Gonzales, Hymie, 5886, 5887, 5888, 5889, 5890
Gonzales, Kelly, 612, 1689, 3661, 5299
Gonzales, Regina, 1828, 5597
Gonzalez, Adrian, 104
Gonzalez, Annabella, 432
Gonzalez, Rene, 2010
Gonzalez, Rene J, 2746
Gonzalez, Rolando, 1791
Good, Art, 4092
Good, James, 3684
Good, Karen, 2718
Goodchild, James, 1734
Goode, Joe, 124
Goode, Kenneth A, 1615
Goodloe, Mark, 3286
Goodman, Darryl, 2833
Goodman, Eve, 1741
Goodman, Jodi, 4669
Goodman, Kirk, 6358
Goodman, Leonard, 7413
Goodman, Martha, 3795
Goodman, Michael, 2387
Goodman, Richard, 1898
Goodman, Rob, 3991
Goodrich, Jerry, 2304
Goodwill, James, 627
Goodwin, John Daly, 2222
Goras, Rose, 2123
Gorden, Suzanne, 7550
Gordley, Deb, 1196
Gordley, Rich, 1196
Gordon, Ain, 467
Gordon, Andrea, 2513
Gordon, Bill, 3930
Gordon, Bruce, 7
Gordon, David, 467
Gordon, Deborah, 2843
Gordon, Derek, 4308
Gordon, Gabriel, 1429
Gordon, Joel, 1585
Gordon, Joyce, 2132
Gordon, Leila, 5649
Gordon, M., 1999
Gordon, Marjorie, 1999
Gordon, Mark Robert, 3365
Gordon, Michael, 5001
Gordon, Michael S, 917
Gordon, Nicholas, 4286
Gordon, Priscilla, 5642
Gordon, Seth, 3434
Gordon Shydko, Maria, 447
Gordon Shydlo, Maria, 447
Gore, Jeannie, 3974
Gore, Kristi, 3276
Gorecki, Kate, 1017
Gorelick, Richard, 6821
Gorman, David, 2617
Gorman, Michael, 5640
Gormley-Chapman, Margaret, 5153
Goss, Karen, 2020, 6458
Gosse, Jodi, 4466
Gosselin, Jeffrey R, 1233, 2075
Gosule, John, 4036
Gotch, Lou Ann, 578
Gotesman, Victor, 2634
Gothoni, Ralf, 1846
Goto, Bruce T, 3952
Goto, Makiko, 758
Gottfried Arnhold, Jody, 436
Gottlieb, Harriet, 3267
Gottsacker, Tom, 1872
Gottschalk, Chuck, 1046
Gotwald, Mercedes, 3308
Goudimiak, Oleg, 624
Goudy, David, 1796
Gould, Betty, 3610
Gould, Deborah L, 2244
Gould, Dr. Charlene, 7086

Gould, Gwen, 1482
Gould, John B., 1692
Gould, Paul, 6849
Gould, Walter, 1909
Gould Sugden, Alisa, 4085
Goulet, James F, 3080
Gourley, Richard S, 908
Govan, Michael, 5014
Govanucci, Renee, 5381
Govatos, Barbara, 4296
Gow, John, 5529
Grabar, John, 2606
Grabel, Naomi, 3725
Graber, Alysia, 3914
Graber, Paula, 58
Grabowski, John, 3339
Grace, Elizabeth, 4250
Grace, J, 1280
Grace, Matthew D, 2121
Grace, Sylvia, 837
Gracie, Nancy, 4638
Gracieux, Vincent, 3148
Graczyk, Ed, 3603
Grady, Barbara, 42
Graf, Buddy, 2728
Graf, Carol, 2728
Graff, Julie, 4782
Graff-Falzon, Patricia, 2400
Graffagna, Juliana, 1924
Grafos, Tania, 92
Graham, Bettie J, 1021
Graham, Col. Lowell E, 1009
Graham, Colin, 2155
Graham, Duane, 1882
Graham, Frank, 1390
Graham, Jo Ann, 646
Graham, John, 1086
Graham, John M, 5478, 7983
Graham, Kerry, 3797
Graham, Niki, 5848
Graham, Nora, 848
Graham, Paul Stuart, 2424
Graham, Stephen, 3426
Graham, Wallace A, 7472
Graham Glann, Dr. Jann, 3575
Graham Hughes, Jeffrey, 577
Grainger, Melissa R, 3303
Gramann, Fred, 1587
Granados, Gabriela, 424
Grande-Weiss, Robert, 2544
Graney, Matt, 6333
Graney, Pat, 719
Granger, Eric, 7944
Granger, John Larry, 923
Granito, Joe, 7660
Grannan, Riley, 611
Grant, Benjamin L, 1024, 1997
Grant, Debbie, 5110
Grant, Michael, 2851
Granum, Fred, 616
Granville, Patty, 5521
Grapes, David, 3797
Grapey, Marc, 2834
Grasey, Jerry W, 7828
Grasing, Nancy, 1001
Grassby, Betse, 971
Grasseschi, Steven, 6908
Grasty Lata, Celia, 2246
Gratch, Susan, 2450
Grau, Evelyn, 5661
Gravagno, Carole Haas, 1733
Graves, David, 747
Graves, Nicholas M, 2391
Graves, Robert, 2894
Gray, Acia, 669
Gray, Brian, 7530
Gray, David, 384
Gray, Delia, 2824
Gray, Dian, 1359
Gray, Dr. Stephen, 2824
Gray, Harold, 1700
Gray, Jennifer, 6641

Gray, John, 278
Gray, Kathy T, 7562
Gray, Margaret, 603
Gray, Patricia, 1016, 4048
Gray, Perien, 1567, 5103
Gray, Peter C, 3091
Gray, Rick, 5142
Gray, Roger, 603
Gray, Ron, 3633
Grayson, Hope, 7877
Greason, Kathy, 2997
Greaves, Nicole, 5322
Greco, Philip, 6579
Gredy, Mimi, 373
Greedom, Thomas, 1676
Greeley, Mike, 3621
Green, Andrew, 1547, 5077, 7465
Green, Ann, 4735
Green, Bill, 3822
Green, Carol, 3077
Green, Caroline Klempe, 1179
Green, Christine, 3545, 5136
Green, David, 144
Green, Diane, 3178
Green, Erika, 3333
Green, Gretchen, 3394
Green, J Ernest, 1242
Green, Jay, 5864
Green, Jennifer, 1837
Green, John, 2159
Green, Laura Gayle, 8297
Green, Lauren, 1665
Green, Leonard I, 1916
Green, Leslie C., 914
Green, Marianne, 2906
Green, Mary Woodmansee, 2274
Green, Randy, 6550
Green, Richard, 4749
Green, Rose4, 1033
Green, Sharon, 1768
Green, Shelly, 1576
Green, Tod, 2517
Green, Vicki, 7054
Greenawald, Sheri, 1938
Greenbaum, Ron, 2732
Greenberg, Hon Mel, 3080
Greenberg, Matthew, 2029
Greenberg, Shira, 389
Greenberg, Steve, 7852
Greenberg, Vanessa, 6172
Greenblatt, Michael, 4864
Greenburg, Bernard A., 1916
Greenburg, Martin, 4402
Greene, Andrew M, 2107
Greene, Jane, 155
Greene, Joanne, 2076
Greene, Kathleen, 3393
Greene, Jr, Frank S, 6129
Greenhalgh, Jo, 2344
Greenhill, Manuel, 8352
Greenhill, Matthew, 8352
Greenhill, Mitchell, 8352
Greenlaw, Michelle, 1739
Greenwald, Sheri, 1945
Greenway, Sandra L, 3828, 5502
Greenwood, Jean, 5782
Greenwood, Juanita P, 4251
Greer, Julie, 1760
Greer, Laura, 4388
Grefe, Tamara, 1339
Grega-Pikul, Alicia, 3736
Gregg, Willaim, 3548
Gregory, Diana, 4396
Gregory, Graig, 2309
Gregory, Greg, 6765
Gregory, Herold, 2325
Gregory, Lisa, 3076
Gregory, Roy, 7920
Gregovitz, Vic, 7837
Greig, Rick E, 5553
Greil, Steven J, 7958
Grein, Jenna, 8436

Haim, Patricia Ann, 1692
Haimes, Todd, 3443
Haines, Marty, 5672
Hainsworth, Chris, 2861
Hair, Ray, 5505
Haire, James, 2509
Hairston, Jay, 5178
Haist, Dean, 1398
Haist, Dean W, 1394
Hakenberg, Stefan, 4032
Hakoshima, Yass, 3253
Halberstam, Michael, 2874
Halboupis, John, 3492
Halbreich, Kathy, 1355, 3151
Halbritter, Judy, 1710
Halbstein, Sandra, 699
Halcrow, Jennifer, 3148
Hale, Alisa, 6764
Hale, Andrena, 3416
Hale, Gay, 4334
Hale, Marie, 240
Hale, Mary Ann, 241
Hale, Ruth J, 4254
Hale, Sally, 3892
Halen, David, 1381
Haley, Carolann, 2132
Hall, Adam, 1986
Hall, Ann, 105
Hall, Betty, 4826
Hall, Billy, 8128
Hall, Craig, 4351
Hall, Donna, 2780
Hall, Doug, 6357
Hall, Dr. William D, 1905, 1926
Hall, Dwight, 6203
Hall, Gary, 3215
Hall, Joel, 274
Hall, Katy, 608
Hall, Kevin, 5864
Hall, Michael, 2679
Hall, Miche, 2524
Hall, Noah, 3449
Hall, Randy, 1598, 2255
Hall, Roger, 942
Hall, Steve, 6632
Hall, Tom, 2081
Hall, Wilhelmina, 1069
Hall, William, 1906
Hall III, John E, 817
Hallen, Mark, 3719
Haller, D Joe, 3158
Hallett, Tom, 1116
Halliday, Janis, 3852
Halligan, Sherry, 5282
Hallinan, Hugh, 6245
Hallinan, Richard, 6245
Hallman, Susan, 2407
Halloran, Catherine, 729
Halpert, Carrie, 1985
Halquist, Don, 391
Halsell, George, 1103
Halsted, Carole E, 4205
Halteman, Susan, 6628
Halterman, H Lee, 86
Halton, Barbara, 5104
Haltrop, Bob, 806
Halverson, Mike, 3295
Halverson, Paul, 3137
Halverson, Rhonda L, 1020
Halverson, Steve, 1037
Haman, Lisa, 1349
Hamblen, Susan, 4088
Hamburger, Anne, 3371
Hamburger, Richard, 3821
Hamby, Doug, 319
Hamel, Ernest, 1992
Hamel III, John J, 1434
Hamer, Bill, 6553
Hamernik, Tom, 4454
Hamiliton, Rick, 6330
Hamilton, Craig Robert, 2281
Hamilton, Del, 2758, 2773, 6443

Hamilton, Ed, 3837
Hamilton, Frankie, 5909
Hamilton, Jean, 1017
Hamilton, Jenny R, 314
Hamilton, Jim, 6684
Hamilton, Kathy, 3779
Hamilton, Lisa, 305
Hamilton, Martha, 1628
Hamilton, Michael, 3194
Hamilton, Stephen, 3499
Hamilton, Steve, 2955
Hamilton, Tom, 5955
Hamitlon, Marie G, 3276
Hamlin, Jeff, 3399, 3472
Hamlin, Larry Leon, 3566
Hamm, Sam, 4940
Hamman, Ralph, 3079
Hammann, Ralph, 3079
Hammerli, Angela, 4607
Hammerstad, John, 1698
Hammond, David, 3525
Hammond, Jared, 3804
Hammond, Paul, 5274, 7585
Hammond, Susan, 3964
Hammond, Tony, 1934
Hammoney, Dimity, 5672
Hamner, W. Easley, 1279
Hamor, Jane, 4860
Hampton, Gray, 1861
Hampton, Jamey, 613
Hampton, Neal, 4691
Hanani, Yehunda, 4675
Hancock, Curt, 1945
Hancock, Joe, 1221
Hancock, John, 1852
Hancock, Larry, 1949
Hancock, Mariko, 5598
Hand, Kevin, 753
Hand III, Elbert O, 2039
Handelman, Carol, 1922
Handlan, Robin R, 6398
Handley, Lawrence M, 1292, 4680
Handman, Wynn, 3347, 7369
Handorf, Jerry, 3584
Handy, Patricia, 1456
Hanes, Howard, 2176
Hanfor, Pat, 301
Hangen, Bruce, 1287, 2076
Hanger, Howard, 1568
Hanies, Andrew, 3963
Hanka, Stephen, 1818
Hankins, R Bruce, 3939
Hanks, Tom, 6890
Hanks, Zach, 3914
Hanna, Marsha, 3611
Hannabass, Gary, 8201
Hannay, Allison, 260
Hanrahan, Greg, 6531
Hanreddy, Joe, 3995
Hanscom, Judy L, 2994
Hanselman, David, 5735
Hansen, Bea, 5334
Hansen, Caroline, 1461
Hansen, Chris, 7035
Hansen, David, 3590
Hansen, Dr. Robert, 663
Hansen, Harold, 6694
Hansen, Holden, 7545
Hansen, Kathy, 5861
Hansen, Neil, 5790
Hansen, Ralph, 693
Hansen, Trudy, 4873
Hansey, Sue, 1189
Hanson, Armin, 3570
Hanson, Brian, 1981
Hanson, Faith, 4859
Hanson, Francis, 697
Hanson, George, 781
Hanson, Les, 2456
Hanson, Lisa, 3908
Hanson, Nathan, 6740
Hanson, Randy, 3539

Hanson, Robert, 1128
Hanson, Sarah, 1871
Hanson, Tom, 8307
Hanson, Troy, 6086
Hanthorn, Dennis, 2347
Hanvik, Jan Michael, 510
Happ, Michael, 2813
Happe, Dave, 2941
Harada, Ricki, 2590
Harberd, Pat, 6502
Harbour, Nancy M, 5837
Harclerode, Albert, 767
Harclerode, Bert, 4050
Harcourt, Chris, 4155
Harder, Lillian U, 7881
Hardesty, Kevin, 2964, 2965
Hardie, Peter, 3964
Hardin, David, 1069
Hardin, Ed, 5106
Harding, Adrian, 1004
Hardman, Chris, 2555
Hardman, Scott, 3962
Hardy, Bruce, 8080
Hardy, John, 3904
Hardy, Peter, 2765
Hardy, Tom, 588
Hare, William, 820
Hargrove, Gwen, 5501
Harris, Jessie L, 7052
Harlan, Mark, 5883
Harland, Robert, 8283
Harle, Jim, 1242
Harley, Margot, 3338
Harley, Rob, 6947
Harlow, Leslie, 5585
Harman, Wier, 2760
Harmon, Jo Ann, 2155
Harmon, John, 995
Harmon Gardner, Kathleen, 8152
Harms, Benjamin, 1482
Harms, Tim, 6609
Harnish, Jim, 2322
Harp, James, 2082
Harpel Kehler, Elizabeth, 423
Harper, Beverly A, 1733
Harper, Clifford D, 6023
Harper, Deborah, 446
Harper, Jackie, 8099
Harper, Mary, 3564, 7253
Harper, Sandy, 2362
Harper, Steve, 8238
Harrell, Celeste, 279
Harrell, Richard, 1947
Harrelson, Sharon, 3838
Harrer, Debra, 2145
Harriamn, Suzie, 3804
Harries, Jean, 817
Harrigan, Anne, 1174, 1259
Harrill, Stephen, 5143
Harriman, Richard, 4795
Harrington, David, 892
Harrington, John, 6858
Harris, Albert, 3463
Harris, Angela, 3857
Harris, Arnie, 2824
Harris, Barbara, 2876
Harris, Bernadette, 588
Harris, Beverly, 1017
Harris, Christine, 740
Harris, David M, 1587
Harris, Ed, 7995
Harris, Elizabeth, 3589
Harris, Eve, 2960
Harris, Jay, 3473
Harris, JB, 2894
Harris, Laura, 3742
Harris, Lizzie, 3240
Harris, Mike, 1778
Harris, Patricia, 4842
Harris, Patricia L, 1404
Harris, Paulette D, 4939
Harris, Scott, 924

Harris, Tim K, 7505
Harris, Winifred R, 30
Harris, Yvonne, 6256
Harrison, Alan, 4017
Harrison, Amy, 511, 1249, 4642
Harrison, Cheryl, 629
Harrison, Constance, 1770
Harrison, Joanne, 817
Harrison, Kim, 2963
Harrison, Majors, 862
Harrison, Marylin, 4350
Harrisr, Nancy, 4138
Harrity, Michael, 2565
Harrod, Beth Miller, 4250
Harrod, Chris, 3640
Harsh, Edward, 1503
Harshaw, Jason W, 4265
Harsta, Kathryn, 1646
Hart, Alison, 317, 4616
Hart, Daniel, 1636, 5211
Hart, Daniel J, 955
Hart, J Erik, 4335, 6356
Hart, Juliet, 2859
Hart, Lizanne, 5015, 7413
Hart, Luke, 2358
Hart, Mark, 1029, 4323
Hart, Phil, 5573
Hart, Sharon, 6985
Harth, Robert, 7378
Harth-Bedoya, Miguel, 1795
Hartkern, David, 4887
Hartley, Carol, 2824, 4723, 6942
Hartley, David, 5804
Hartley, Heather, 272
Hartley, Marty, 231
Hartman, Bruce, 3919
Hartman, Mike, 2909
Hartnett, Bill, 3181
Hartzell, Lance, 7020
Hartzell, Linda, 3959
Harvard, Bernard, 3726
Harvey, Ann, 3441
Harvey, Cameron, 2417, 3879, 5576
Harvey, Cy, 957
Harvey, David, 2848
Harvey, Gertrude, 5706
Harvey, Jennifer, 2315
Harvey, Margarete, 1874
Harvey, Mark, 3121
Harvey, Raymond, 1332
Harvey, Stuart C, 5668
Harveycutter, Carey, 8202
Harvill, Robert, 1224
Harwood, Kathy, 2534
Haschke, Nicki, 2888
Haskell, C Conrad, 2341
Haskins, James, 3721
Haslam, Kevin, 7168
Hasler, Jim, 861
Haslun, Robert A, 2101
Haslun, Ursula R, 2101
Hasner, Kelly, 2941
Hassa, Linda, 7221
Hassan, Mary T, 3922
Hasse, Marie, 4341
Hassel, Beverly, 5769
Hassel, Dan, 3220
Hassett, Tim, 7214
Hassig, John, 8309
Hassle, John, 546
Hastings, Brian, 7837
Hastings, Mary, 5004
Hastings, Randy, 3183
Hasty, Laurie, 7114
Hatch, Dick, 3066
Hatch, Mary, 6539
Hatcher, Lucia Corsiglia, 239
Hatfield, Richard, 841
Hathorn Jr, Byron, 3903
Hatim, Mohammed, 2229
Hatton, Betsy, 1693
Haugan, Kristine, 1916

Hauge, Kevin R, 2532
Hauge, Peter, 2242
Haugen, Glenda, 2254
Hausam, Wiley, 7396
Hausch, Mary, 6349
Hauschild, Doug, 7660
Hauser, Anothony, 6073
Hauser, Dan, 6918
Hauser, Jacqueline, 6073
Hauser, Michael, 3128
Hauser, Ralph, 6073
Hauser Jasmin, Heidi, 352
Hausman, Jane, 1377
Hausman, William, 1296, 4683
Hausmann, Dr. Charles, 2316
Hava-Robbins, Nadia, 97
Havarek, Wayne, 368
Havemeyer, Robert, 2238, 2239
Haven, Barbara, 8432
Havener, Jaqueline, 1990
Haver, Steven J, 5718
Haver, Susan, 2946
Havercroft, Joan, 964
Haviaras, Steve, 2124
Havlik, Dorothy, 3770
Havranek, Donna, 397
Havranek, Sara, 397
Havwood, Amy, 4661
Hawery, Alan, 2112
Hawken, Leila, 201
Hawken, Susan, 3159
Hawkey, Christina, 5894
Hawkins, Adrienne T, 330
Hawkins, Andrew, 2259
Hawkins, Claudie D, 7987
Hawkins, Heather, 5792
Hawkins, Joy, 2703
Hawkins, Lois, 2072
Hawkins, Penelope, 887
Hawkins, Staci, 6323
Hawkins, Steven, 7095
Hawks, Richard, 4427
Hawley, Anne, 6862
Hawley, L/Col Robert J., 1021
Hawley, Patricia A, 4929
Hawn, Thomas R, 593
Hawpt, Paulette, 2643
Hawryliw, Neil, 6974
Hawthorne, Randal, 3215
Hawthorne, Susan, 3930
Hay, Frank, 655
Hay, Melinda, 1458
Hayashi, Edwin K, 6476
Hayashi, Noel, 1527
Haycook, Bill, 3083
Haycox, Rolanda, 1170
Hayden, Carol, 8299
Hayden, Lynne, 3306
Hayden, Robert, 4212
Hayes, Alison, 2768
Hayes, Andy, 2478
Hayes, Carol M, 2665
Hayes, Charlotte, 3014
Hayes, David, 2283
Hayes, Dr. Michelle, 176
Hayes, Eileen, 2163
Hayes, Jackie, 2516
Hayes, Scott, 3612
Hayes, Stephen R, 3913
Hayley, Barbara, 2989
Hayllar, Ben, 1733
Hayman, Mark, 8466
Haymes, Lisa, 3856
Haynes, Beth, 2779
Haynes, Helen, 5319
Haynes, Peter, 1240
Hays, Melissa, 4681
Hayward, Ellen, 2347
Hayward, Tom, 2964
Hazatrd, Sarah Lynn, 3328
Hazelip, Pat, 2960
Hazelwood, Matthew, 1312

Hazlet, Carolee, 3185
Hazzard, Wayne, 120
Hcapma, Jefferson, 3779
Head, Julia, 2121
Headlee, Nancy, 4239
Headrick, Samuel, 1261
Heakey, Maureen, 3037
Healey, John, 3915
Healey, Roberta, 4970
Hearn, Page, 2826
Heath, Richard, 893, 4185
Heath, Robert, 1029, 4323
Heatherington, Alan, 1137
Heatherington, Gayle, 1137
Heaton, Richard, 2955
Heberling, Dan, 3628
Hecht, Dick, 8299
Hecker, Julie, 888
Heckman, Kevin, 2854
Heckscher, Martin A, 1733
Hedblom, CW4 Bruce J, 1360
Hedding, Dale, 764
Hedgepeth, Linda, 920
Hedgepeth, Tim, 4774
Hedges, Mollie, 808
Hedges, Susan, 797
Hedges-Peerman, Kelly, 2702
Hedlund, Roger, 1877
Hedstrom, Cynthia, 4277
Heeley, John, 3914
Heffelfinger, Peter, 8225
Heffner, Kenneth, 1032
Heffner, Richard, 3752
Heffner, Virginia E, 5183
Heffner Hayes, Dr. Michelle, 4349
Hefty, Noel, 176
Hege, Daniel, 1207, 1557
Heideman, Lisa, 1020
Heider, George H, 2162
Heidrich, Eckhard, 298
Heidt, Jack, 2632
Heidtke, Brian, 3430
Heidtke, Brian J, 423
Height, George, 7521
Heilbron, Gail, 304
Heilbut, Francis L, 4998
Heilenbrond, Harry, 4200
Heim, Father Jack, 1617, 1619, 1620, 5192, 5193, 5195, 5196
Hein, Janice, 3688, 5323
Heinemann, Dr. Harry, 1477
Heins, Donna, 3525
Heins, Tim, 3146
Heinze, Joan I, 3686
Heise, Frank, 6485
Heiser, Mark, 4088
Heitikko, Betty, 1603
Heitman, Teri, 99, 2489
Hejl, Patsy, 5519
Helander, Danelle, 177
Helfrich, Paul, 1860
Helfter, Susan, 4129
Heling, Kevin, 4002
Hellard, Ellen, 2968
Heller, Rosalie, 4914, 7271
Heller Zorn, Franny, 498
Hellerich, Jean, 108
Hellman, Bonnie, 1739
Hellman, F Warren, 140
Hellman, Shari, 5228
Hellman, Sheila, 4908
Helm, Charles, 7649
Helm, Linda, 1213
Helmerich, Jonathan, 2271
Helmers, Carl, 1410
Helmick Jr, Carl N, 4169
Helmly, Linda, 647
Helpenstell, Cheryl, 1843
Helsing, Dawn, 6821
Helsinger, Jim, 4353
Heltman, Gregory, 1453, 2187
Heltne, Dan, 4818

Helton, Kim, 8074
Helweg, Richard, 2821
Helzberg, Shirley Bush, 1373
Hemat, David Von, 644
Hemenway, Anne, 3361
Hemingway, Jason, 1384
Heminover, Lillian, 2832
Hemiston, Connie, 4789
Hemker, Paul, 2060
Hendckson, Marlene, 4821
Henderson, Criss, 2823
Henderson, David, 3446
Henderson, Glenna, 663
Henderson, Jo Ann, 4016
Henderson, Mark, 4606
Henderson, Skitch, 1524
Henderson, T Scott, 3241
Henderson, Yvonne, 1880
Henderson Hale, Jane, 4870
Hendricks, Beverly, 1068
Hendricks, Lesley, 646
Hendrickson, Chris, 3107
Hendrickson, Peter A, 2131
Hendrix, Bettye W, 4067
Henke, Robert L, 1645, 1653
Henks, Rick, 1370
Henley, Larry, 7177
Hennigan, Phyllis, 2431, 2447
Henniger, Rai, 6203
Henning, Daniel, 2412
Henning, Kevin S, 6922
Henningsen, Charlie, 7625
Henock, Dee, 3254
Henrichsen, Kari, 6129
Henrickson, John, 2309
Henry, Alvin A, 140
Henry, Christine, 3871
Henry, Ed, 7208
Henry, Gregg, 2663, 4297
Henry, Helen, 5366
Henry, Judi, 8082
Henry, Mary Pat, 363
Henry, Mike, 3809
Hensley, Charlie, 3922
Hensley, Iris, 257
Hensley, Martha, 684
Hensley, Nancy Turner, 2671
Henson, Cherly, 3379, 5023
Henson, Colonel Eben, 2957
Henson, Holly, 2957
Henson, Robby, 2957
Henson, Robin, 1928
Henzler, Martha Claire, 2251
Hepburn, Charles, 3505
Hepple, David, 1243
Herald, Marjorie, 2919
Herbert, F John, 4528
Herbert, Jim, 140
Herbert, Kathy, 6137
Herbert, II, James H, 140
Herbst, Cynthia B, 8408
Herbst, George, 2753
Herbst, Jeffrey, 3982
Herbst, Scott, 3150
Herendeen, Ed, 3977, 5726
Herman, Debra, 1065
Herman, Harold, 2371
Herman, Susie, 176
Herman Barlow, Janet, 7637
Herman-Barlow, Janet, 7636
Hermann, Jeffrey, 2365
Hermanto, Wilson, 801
Hermiller, Anne, 3612
Hernandez, Amalia, 57
Hernandez, Christie, 3829
Hernandez, Kin, 5018
Hernandez, Rhonda, 3228
Hernandez, Rusty, 2816
Hernandez, Sandra, 4198
Herndon, Lynda, 1477
Herold, Abastasia, 824
Herold, Heather, 4396

Herold, Jordi, 3063
Herr, Eric M, 3161
Herr, Linda, 2627
Herrera, Gilbert, 6695
Herrick, Menilyn T, 245
Herriford, Pam, 6710
Herring, Beverly, 3275
Herring, Howard, 1045, 4983, 4984, 7355
Herring, Linda, 7441
Herrington, Alisa L, 8421
Herriott, David, 3
Herrlinger, Berton, 1613
Hermann, Judi, 6817
Herron, Clifford, 6391
Herron, Isom, 1560
Herron, Royce, 2395
Herschensohn, PhD, Michael, 5697
Hersey, Marilyn, 2645, 2979
Hersh, Jaye, 4152
Herskovits, David, 3456
Herz, Michael, 3337
Herzig, David, 1599
Herzog, Floyd R, 4932
Hesler, D Corey, 8291
Hess, Craig, 3831
Hess, Neil, 663
Hess, Ralph, 4046
Hess, Richard, 3583
Hesselink, Dr. K Chung, 836
Hesselman, Jim, 2971
Hesselroth, Loisd, 1351
Hesser, Karl, 2002
Hester, Richard, 4668
Heston, Vicki, 1906
Hestter, Dale, 6450
Hetrick, Charles, 1177
Hettinger, Beverly, 2582
Hettinger, John, 7199
Hetzel, Dr. Marilyn, 2591
Heuer, Robert, 2002
Heusinkveld, Mindy, 2943
Hewitt, Frankie, 2661
Hewitt, William B, 649, 1758, 3753, 5422
Heydenburg, Patrick, 3725
Heydt, Mary Beth, 731
Heyman, Duane, 1883
Heyman, Richard, 3222
Hibberd, Vikki, 5886, 5887, 5888, 5889, 5890
Hibbs, Marie, 1178
Hibbs, Micki, 2784
Hibshman, Dan, 2569
Hick, Joe, 5504
Hicken, Leslie W, 1759
Hickes, Denice, 3796, 5469
Hickey, Michael, 2766
Hickey, Michael E, 2766
Hickey, Patricia, 5739
Hicklin, Jennifer, 2956
Hickman, Tim, 7080
Hickman, Timothy L, 7078, 7079
Hicks, Ann, 368
Hicks, Chas, 575
Hicks, Joe, 5562
Hicks, Robert B, 2009
Hiclklin, Kat, 2423
Hiczewski, Marta, 7313
Hidalgo, Michael, 2790
Hiddlestone, John, 2635
Hides, Sue, 7088
Hiendlmayr, Jackie, 2742
Hiendlmayr, Richard, 974
Hier, Susan, 6971
Hieronymus, Theodore, 5240
Higby, Sha Sha, 24
Higginbotham, Joe, 3623
Higgins, Kelly, 7915
Higgins, Ruth, 2844
Higginson, Pam, 3882
High, Steve, 6691
Hihn, Richard R, 5085
Hilbert, Mira, 3070
Hilburger, Jimmy, 2117

Hildabrant, Rebecca, 2072
Hilgeman, Carol, 4027
Hill, Dick, 7173
Hill, Ellen, 1435
Hill, Eric, 3073
Hill, Erin, 1777, 5476
Hill, Jess, 2856
Hill, Jessi D, 2854
Hill, John-Edward, 3075, 4692
Hill, Lloyd N, 7056
Hill, Mars, 3282
Hill, Meg, 5072
Hill, Patrick, 7579
Hill, Patsy, 232
Hill, Richard, 2938
Hill, Sharon, 7956
Hill, Stan, 2135
Hillard, Claire Fox, 1069
Hilliard, Sarah, 2794
Hilliker, Thomas, 1321
Hillman, Ira, 3017
Hillman, Marie, 2012
Hillman, Rita, 4936
Hills, Ernie, 4173
Hillyard, Fabbey, 6218
Hilmy, Stephen, 1782
Hilsmier, William, 2265
Hilson, Paul, 2702
Hilton, Bonnie, 1089
Hilton, Katherine, 1242
Himberg, Phillip, 3888
Himes, Ron, 3193
Hinchliffe, Robin, 6136
Hinckley, Kristen, 2606
Hinds, Andrew, 1967
Hinds, Sims, 7555
Hinds, Thomas, 752
Hine, Roy, 2932
Hiner, Lawrence, 1602
Hines, Leslie, 1221
Hines, Lynn, 3107, 6976
Hines, Mindy, 3850
Hinkebein, Adrienne, 1218
Hinkle, Loren, 1705
Hinkley, Laura, 1180
Hinners, Jennifer, 5737
Hinrichs, Jay, 7090
Hinrichsen, Greg, 4108, 5985
Hinton, Keith D, 1998
Hinton, Patricia, 4345
Hinton, Patricia M, 4345
Hintz, Gail, 2156
Hippensteel, Carl, 2811
Hirabayashi, PJ, 909
Hirabayashi, Roy, 909
Hird, Tom, 4110
Hirokawa, Erika, 3427
Hiroshima, Terri, 3954
Hirsch, Ellen, 3430
Hirsch, Melissa, 3869
Hirschman, Dale, 1519
Hirschtritt, Joel, 1508
Hirsh, Jonathan, 1293
Hirshberg, Jane, 325
Hirshman, Karl, 4931
Hirst, R Dennis, 5579
Hirzano, Michiko, 5027
Hitchcock, Dennis, 2889
Hitchcock, Linda, 898
Hitchings, Carolyn, 7101, 7103
Hite Jacob, Karen, 1570
Hitt, David, 5483
Hitt, W C, 4069
Hittinger, Hollie, 257
Ho, Sally, 856
Ho, Suet May, 332
Hoak, Tanya, 5897
Hoang, Jennifer, 2100
Hobart, Max, 1260, 1302
Hobner, Antje, 8450
Hobson, Ian, 1151
Hochoy, David, 302

Jackson, Andrew, 3594
Jackson, CMSgt. Daisy, 1009
Jackson, Dr. Eugene R, 2357
Jackson, Dr. Floyd Grant, 1692
Jackson, Earl G, 1882
Jackson, Isaiah, 1279
Jackson, Jean, 2080
Jackson, Jeff, 1180
Jackson, Jim, 2911, 6450
Jackson, John, 4078
Jackson, Julie, 2582
Jackson, Kelly, 3649
Jackson, Linda, 2103
Jackson, Mary Jo, 3202
Jackson, Mary K, 1880
Jackson, Michele T, 1767
Jackson, Neal, 1984
Jackson, Ralph N, 7373
Jackson, Robert H, 1605
Jackson, Roberta, 339
Jackson, Ron, 303
Jackson, Sara, 3139
Jackson, Sherry, 3841
Jackson, Susan, 303
Jackson, Thomas E, 6683
Jackson, Tim, 4142, 6148
Jackson, Tom, 1185
Jackson, V Charles, 1915
Jackson-Forsyth, Elena, 2271
Jackson-Grimes, Capucine, 7206
Jackson-Harmon, Tammy, 6291
Jacob, Judy, 710
Jacob, Karen Hite, 1570
Jacob, Sue, 3621
Jacobey, Linda, 2183, 2696
Jacobowitz, Diane, 403
Jacobs, April, 2180
Jacobs, Claudia, 1410
Jacobs, Ellen, 3451
Jacobs, Jake, 3848
Jacobs, Johann, 694
Jacobs, Marc, 6129
Jacobs, Paul, 836
Jacobs, Rea, 4959, 4960
Jacobs, Susan, 6909
Jacobs Hanigan, Marcy, 58
Jacobson, Denny P, 1469
Jacobson, James, 3089
Jacobson, Joshua, 2107
Jacobson, Leslie B, 2675, 3907
Jacobson, Ruth Ellen, 1793
Jacobson Randolph, Marsha, 3854
Jacoby, Ginny, 1248
Jacoby, Mike, 7243
Jacoby, Sandy, 5705
Jacumin, Johnny, 7888
Jaeger, Lois, 4756
Jaffe, David B, 2643
Jaffe, Doug, 2572
Jaffe, Elise, 535
Jaffe, Jeff, 1659
Jaffe, Jerry, 3458
Jaffe, Peter, 933
Jaffe, Robert M, 4172
Jaffee, Mary S, 1272
Jaffee, Michael, 1541
Jagoditz, Joseph F, 5188
Jahi, Runako, 2833
Jahn, Chris, 2685
Jahn, Kerry, 3922
Jahnke, Joel, 3205
Jahnou, Kerry, 3922
Jakobson, Ellen, 3430
Jam, Burke, 4821
James, David, 3871
James, David F, 4952
James, Eugene, 478
James, Jaffrey, 8409
James, Janell, 5584
James, Jefferson, 580
James, Jeffrey, 514
James, Lana, 3202

James, Lance C, 2390
James, Lori, 7177
James, Oscar, 3256
James, Rachel, 580
James, Randy, 376
James, Richard L, 8153
James, Ruby, 4606
James, Terry, 2877
Jameson, Yvonne, 3182
Jamieson, Brandan, 2234
Jamieson, Brendan, 1536
Jamieson, Paul, 4377
Jamison, Judith, 418, 421
Janco Daniels, Myra, 6388
Jane Ward, Sarah, 3920
Janicki, Steven G, 6374
Janisch, Dr. Joseph, 2342
Jankowski, John, 7478
Jannikrtner, Donna, 2019
Janowicz, Carol, 4738
Jansa, Beth, 2778
Jansen, Debra, 3494
Jansons, Mariss, 1740
Jantzen, Rhonda, 2582
Janz, Deborah, 8313
Jaqua, Mary, 4363
Jaquay, Cheryl, 2928
Jaramillo, Jesse, 304
Jaray, Istvan, 1720
Jardanhazy, Lisa, 2333
Jarden, Charles, 2192
Jares, Terry, 8368
Jarjisian, Catherine, 7593
Jarjisian, Dr. Catherine, 1607
Jaroslow, Risa, 543
Jarrell, J Calvin, 2865
Jarrett, Jennifer, 600
Jarrett, Lori, 8478
Jarriel, Janet, 8373
Jarski, Christine, 265
Jarvi, Neeme, 1317
Jaskela, May Lou, 1603
Jasmin, Heidi, 352
Jaudon, Jon, 8163
Jauregui, Art, 15
Jaynes, Carl H, 3395
Jeannette, Gertrude, 3378
Jecklin, Lois, 8374
Jeenkins, Dr. Robert, 2537
Jefcoate, Colin, 731
Jeffcoat, Joe, 3374
Jeffers, Tinay, 1595, 2253
Jeffery, Diane, 4861
Jeffords, Jr, Walter M., 1552, 3503
Jeffrey, Chad, 7249
Jeffrey, Diane, 7237
Jeffries, Gayle, 2190
Jeffries, John Peter, 2127
Jekowsky, Barry, 874, 1408
Jelinek, Dr. Mark, 1448
Jemison-Keisker, Lynn, 2323
Jenkins, Charla, 6679
Jenkins, Connie, 3759
Jenkins, David, 8017
Jenkins, DeVida, 7829
Jenkins, Diane, 1843
Jenkins, Doanld P, 1961
Jenkins, Graeme, 2307
Jenkins, J Mark, 140
Jenkins, JT, 4904
Jenkins, Lainey, 5826
Jenkins, Margaret, 129
Jenkins, Ron, 2619
Jenkins, Ronald J, 2261
Jenkins, Steve, 1653
Jenkins, Willard, 5206
Jenkins Williamson, Barbara, 5161
Jenkner, Helmut, 4636
Jenks, Donna, 2949
Jenneman, Eugene, 6982
Jenneman, Eugene A, 6981
Jennings, Amelia, 2477

Jennings, Chris, 3750
Jennings, Christina, 1608
Jennings, James, 3348
Jennings, Joseph, 1941
Jennings, Judy, 8201
Jennings, Robert, 6447
Jennings, Vicki, 4539
Jennings-Roggensack, Colleen, 4052
Jensen, Beth, 5675
Jensen, Carolyn, 2060
Jensen, Eric, 3884
Jensen, Hans, 4000
Jensen, J Peter, 1950
Jensen, Randy, 5578
Jensen, Rebecca, 7248
Jensen, Sandy, 3884
Jensen, Walter, 5881
Jepson, James, 1908
Jerome, Chuck, 3570
Jeske, Charlie, 7581
Jessee, John, 3929
Jessen, Christian A, 4195
Jessop, Craig, 2325
Jessup, Richard, 3656
Jeter, John, 786
Jett, Donna, 807
Jewison, Becky, 6624
Jeynes, Carl H, 7369
Jhank, Cheryl L, 6585
Jimison, Kevin, 7973
Jinbo, Michael, 1237, 1746
Jipson, Jim, 2723
Jiranek, David, 3390
Jo, Whitney, 3786
Jo Zollar, Jawole Willa, 557
Jobel, George, 1411
Jobin, David, 3728
Jobin, Sara, 819
Joe, Glenda, 5530
Joergenson, Lea, 1987, 1988
Joffe, Linda, 1056, 1057, 1059, 1060, 4370
Jogner, Dwight, 2135
Johansen, Pam, 759
Johanson, Charles, 2409
Johanson, Robert, 3251
John, Katherine St, 696, 1820, 5589
John, Shallan, 7710
Johngren, Jane, 4945
Johns, Peter, 7035
Johnsen, Christie, 2982
Johnson, Allen, 4343, 6372, 6373
Johnson, Alvis, 6718
Johnson, Arabella, 4300
Johnson, Barbara, 1679
Johnson, Becki, 2694
Johnson, Ben, 4709
Johnson, Beth, 5116
Johnson, BJ, 2140, 4765
Johnson, Brian, 3938
Johnson, C Nicholas, 308
Johnson, Carl, 1196
Johnson, Carla, 1381
Johnson, Charles, 1799
Johnson, Charmaine, 5754
Johnson, Colin, 3880
Johnson, Craig, 1741
Johnson, Dale, 2133
Johnson, Deborah, 1248
Johnson, Dieneke, 1258
Johnson, Don, 6102
Johnson, Dori, 1110
Johnson, Dr. Corinne, 6650
Johnson, Dr. James, 1392
Johnson, Dr. Warletta, 2824
Johnson, Eileen, 1108
Johnson, Elle, 62
Johnson, Erika, 8346
Johnson, Gail, 5501
Johnson, Gordon, 4824
Johnson, Gordon J, 762, 1389
Johnson, Greg, 3209, 5916
Johnson, Harry, 3083

Johnson, Hewitt V, 1442
Johnson, James A, 4309
Johnson, James M, 1524
Johnson, Jean, 3795
Johnson, Jeff, 6613
Johnson, Joann Taylor, 808
Johnson, Jody, 963
Johnson, Kallin, 6909
Johnson, Kathy, 5572
Johnson, Ken, 1960
Johnson, Kevin, 1077, 4391
Johnson, Khalil, 6435
Johnson, Kristen, 3044
Johnson, Lauren, 2877
Johnson, Lia, 2395
Johnson, Lucille Lewis, 502
Johnson, Mark G, 3874
Johnson, Maroene, 3584
Johnson, Michael, 3214, 5113
Johnson, Miles, 323
Johnson, Mimi, 3424
Johnson, Misty, 3857
Johnson, Murphree, 3378
Johnson, Nancy, 3768
Johnson, Nick, 5792
Johnson, North, 7538
Johnson, Patrick, 1365
Johnson, Paul A, 7576
Johnson, Priscilla, 5346, 5347
Johnson, Reverdy, 3281
Johnson, Rich, 4530
Johnson, Richard A, 4506
Johnson, Robert, 1523
Johnson, Roy, 1598, 2255, 3032
Johnson, Ruth, 5642
Johnson, Sam, 5123
Johnson, Sandy, 3118
Johnson, Sarah, 465
Johnson, Scott E, 7531
Johnson, Sheila, 2184
Johnson, Stephen, 5046
Johnson, Sue, 5346
Johnson, Susan, 2694
Johnson, Thomas P, 6661
Johnson, Thomas Peter, 2934
Johnson, Virgina, 1442
Johnson, Walter, 7321
Johnson, Warren H, 3219
Johnson, William H, 5824
Johnson Klein, Kathleen, 225
Johnson, Jr, Franklin P, 1944
Johnson, Jr, Joseph S, 5467
Johnson-Hamilton, Joyce, 943
Johnston, Alex, 1496
Johnston, Angela, 1874
Johnston, David C, 2803
Johnston, Rick, 2246
Joiner, Dr. Thomas, 1582
Jolink, Terry, 3083
Jolivet, Claire, 956, 4245
Jolly, Linda Lee, 7695
Jonas, Lauren, 173
Jonason, Susan, 1234
Jones, Allison, 3337
Jones, Alun, 311
Jones, Amy, 4152
Jones, Andrea, 4170
Jones, April, 3529
Jones, Betty, 6746
Jones, BJ, 2892
Jones, Brain, 3700
Jones, Brenda, 7110
Jones, Bret, 7708
Jones, Brian, 6227
Jones, Brock, 8188
Jones, Cathy, 4634
Jones, Cliffie, 5206
Jones, David Allen, 171
Jones, De Ann S, 3553
Jones, Dennis, 2558
Jones, Dianne, 8316
Jones, Dr. Martin, 4781

Jones, Dr. Roger, 1228
Jones, Elliot, 2282
Jones, Eric, 7005
Jones, Gary, 6225
Jones, Guy, 3080
Jones, Jo-Ann, 4957
Jones, Joan, 3514
Jones, Joela, 2258
Jones, John D, 1880
Jones, Julia, 4146
Jones, Karen, 1641
Jones, Kay, 749
Jones, Kim, 7721
Jones, Krystal, 7371
Jones, Kurt, 3210
Jones, Latal, 7052
Jones, Lisa, 6876
Jones, Mark W, 490
Jones, Martha, 4662
Jones, Millicent, 4195
Jones, Neal, 3387
Jones, Pam, 5924
Jones, Paula, 4124
Jones, Phil, 1843
Jones, Renata, 1937
Jones, Robert C, 1017
Jones, Rocky R, 6554
Jones, Roy, 7624
Jones, Russ, 2933
Jones, Sabra, 3406
Jones, Sara, 2558, 6157
Jones, Sarah, 1966
Jones, Sharon, 807
Jones, Sheri, 2818
Jones, Stacey, 4065
Jones, Stephanie, 12
Jones, Susan, 611
Jones, Timothy, 2065
Jones, Vel, 7172
Jones, Victoria, 6876
Jones, Walton, 2421
Jones, Wendy, 1676
Jones, William, 3553
Jones III, Dr. Bob, 3757
Jones, III, DeWitt C, 2101
Joneshill, Larry, 7089
Jonker-Burke, Sarah, 3321
Jonnes, Michael, 1298
Jopke, LeAnn, 4754
Jordahl, Trish, 772
Jordan, Alan, 1829
Jordan, Bob, 8017
Jordan, Bruce, 2843
Jordan, Cheryl, 823
Jordan, Desiree K, 5557
Jordan, Eleonor, 5150
Jordan, Julie-Ann, 968
Jordan, Kim, 8111
Jordan, Mark, 3618
Jorden, Cule, 4901
Jordin, Melanie, 5909
Jordy, Deborah, 6187
Jorgensen, Jackie, 4797
Jorgensen, Judy, 1873
Jorgenser, Kathy, 4826
Jorgenson, Jerry, 7273
Joseph, Frances, 4041
Joseph, Judy, 6338
Joseph, Michael, 1673
Josephson, Karen, 193
Jost, Jack, 4366
Joy, Christopher, 8485
Joyal, Debbie, 4390
Joyce, Dudley, 1856
Joyce, Kathryn, 761
Joyce, Michael, 3703
Joyner, Alexis, 5124
Joyner, Rob, 6026
Jubelirer, Dr. Steve, 5715
Judd, James, 1033, 4327
Judice, Sandy, 3855, 5529
Judin, Joy, 5548

Judisch, David, 2062
Judy, George, 3879, 5576
Judy, Molly, 2752
Juergensen, Tim, 1147
Juetty, Sue, 2068
Juhrend, Albert, 4070
Julian, Donna P, 6819
Julian, Fred, 7003
Julian, Kim, 2760
Julian, Lorraine, 803
Juliano, Richard, 7208
Julka, Mary Liz, 1864
Jundt, M. Joahn, 3132
June, Mike, 8403
Jungels, Aaron, 643
Jungels, Therese, 643
Jupin, a Alexandra, 8363
Jurczyk, Annie, 3992, 3995
Jurgens, Ronald, 4366, 4370
Juska, Phillip, 629
Jussel, Richard, 3214
Justice, Richard, 2780
Justice, William, 875
Justo, Hannah, 652
Jutagir, Hattie K, 3399, 3472

K

Ka'ai, Malla, 2023
Kaats, Rod, 7455
Kacenjar, Leonard, 1807
Kacinski, Kathi, 2997
Kaddar, Yoan, 3331
Kaduri, Arie, 4333
Kaehler, Frank, 922
Kaelin, Michelle, 2971
Kager, Stephen J, 7257
Kahan, James, 1139
Kahane, Jeffrey, 847, 912, 4202
Kahler, Jim, 7624
Kahlert, Helmut, 1361
Kahn, Elizabeth, 498
Kahn, Gina, 986
Kahn, Hannah, 188
Kahn, Kevin, 6211
Kahn, Michael, 2666
Kahn, Paul, 8384
Kahne, Roberta, 2013
Kai, Njia, 4719
Kaikkonen, Gus, 3235, 3441
Kaine, Paul, 661
Kaiser, Amy, 1381, 2156, 3430
Kaiser, James F, 4626
Kaiser, Keith, 153
Kaiser, Roy, 629
Kajima, Fusao, 1105
Kakuk, Charles, 3996
Kalajian, Jan, 58
Kalam, Tonu, 1805
Kalberg, Sheldon, 2185
Kaler, Ilia, 1551
Kaler, Lenore P, 3603
Kali, Pearl, 3095
Kalkbrenner, Jim, 7110
Kalkor, Dr. Alan, 1585
Kallish, Jan, 2815, 6513
Kalmanash, Bobbi, 2533
Kalmijn, Vera, 887
Kalmu, Geoffrey M, 4909
Kalogeras, Alexandros, 1261
Kalonia, Catherine, 6277, 6279
Kalson, Dorothy, 1470, 4955
Kaltenbach, Janet, 2177
Kalver, Gail, 273
Kamgar, Moira, 98
Kaminski, Shanna, 2119
Kaminsky, Laura, 5692
Kammerdiner, Lori, 2942
Kanaga, Sarah R, 2110
Kanayama, Takao, 1017
Kanazawa, Chris, 2795

Kancianic, Phil, 6831
Kandall, Hazel, 535
Kane, Daniel, 233
Kane, Darrel, 7754
Kane, Elissa, 5066
Kane, John, 1156, 1756, 6874
Kane, Richard, 1463
Kane, Tom, 5975
Kaney, Georgia, 4324
Kang, Emil, 1317
Kanoff, Scott, 3810
Kantar, Ned, 8389
Kantor, Herbert C, 3393
Kao, Henry, 1429
Kapelinski, Ken, 7919
Kapell, Lesli, 449, 522
Kaper, Dr. Hans, 4426
Kaper, Dr. Hans G, 4453
Kaper, Hans G, 4454
Kapito, Robert S, 3328
Kaplan, Lewis, 1236, 1493, 4613, 4614
Kaplan, Melvin, 8504
Kaplan, Norma, 5619
Kaplan, Shari, 6267
Kaplan, Stanley H, 1463
Kaplan, Van, 3840
Kapp, Rich, 6613
Kapp, Richard, 1469
Kappel, Mark, 8449
Kappel, Victoria, 5059
Karabin, Mike, 7687
Karac, Tom, 6417
Karadin, Kenneth, 4358
Karakula, Jane, 3057
Karas, Edie, 807
Karbank, Steve, 1371
Kardan, Sel, 4636
Karidoyanes, Steven, 1295
Karima, Laila, 2413
Karlin, Jan, 873
Karlson, Eileen, 2180
Karmi, Laura, 358
Karnopp, Adam, 5441
Karnosh, Patricia, 1653
Karp, Nancy, 132
Karp, Steve, 2636
Karpus, Janet, 2129, 4737
Karseu, Kathryn, 2141
Karwan, Judy, 3577
Kary, Sarah, 3054
Kasch, Marya, 1908
Kashuba, Chris, 3027
Kaslewicz, Holly, 4197
Kasowitx, Lori A., 4995
Kass, Jeff, 5462
Kass, Linda, 1636
Kastelic, Patty, 4029
Kasten, Garry, 621
Kaster, Steven, 140
Kastle, Margaret, 2279
Kastner, Simmie, 3552
Katnolos, Ellen A, 7440
Katona, Cathy, 2667
Katsahnias, Tom, 1178
Katseanes, Kory, 1826
Kattelman, Karey, 3584
Katz, David, 2079, 2117
Katz, Donalee, 8437
Katz, Gerry, 2102
Katz, Helene, 1470, 4955
Katz, Irwin, 4350
Katz, Joel, 8193
Katz, Pamela, 1522
Katz, Sherman, 2667
Katz, Steven, 4880
Katzenmeyer, John, 5205
Kauble, Susan, 611
Kaufaman, Mark, 6770
Kauffman, Thom, 6854
Kauffman, Welz, 4465
Kaufman, Elaine, 7413
Kaufmann, Jane, 668

Kaufmann, Marcia, 5683
Kauk, Cindy, 4825
Kaukonen, Brenda, 5228
Kaushagen, Ingrid Joy, 4816
Kautzman, Chavon, 3206
Kauvar, Joanne, 6226
Kavafian, Ida, 1451
Kavanaugh, Dr. Patrick, 5637
Kavanaugh, Scot W, 6976
Kawash, Stephen E, 3971
Kay, Albert, 571
Kay, Kenneth, 3522
Kay, Linda, 793
Kaye, Marvin, 3425
Kaye, Michael, 2088
Kaye, Saralee, 3425
Kaylor, Kaylor, 8446
Kayser, Denise, 4650
Kazan, Frances, 498
Kazanjian, John, 3957
Keagle, Karen, 3476
Kearns, Gail M, 45
Kearns, Lauren W, 45
Kearns, Patrick Alan, 2600
Keary, David, 356
Keating, Wayne, 2070, 4594
Kechley, David, 4698
Keck Combs, Nina, 5612
Keden, H. Michael, 974
Keefer, Krissy, 118
Keegan, Brian, 7670
Keegan, Henry T, 1021
Keel, Ellen, 4653
Keelan, Hugh, 1712
Keeler, Janet E, 1650
Keeley, Dawn, 2796
Keeley, Michael, 4382
Keenan, Cecilie, 2876
Keenan, John, 2084
Keenan, Robert, 861
Keene, Dennis, 2242
Keene, Howard, 2955
Keene, James, 4832
Keffer, J Lindsay, 8028
Keffer, Lindsay, 8028
Kehl, Bill, 966
Keicher, Roger, 3303
Keimach, Brad, 829
Kein, Karl, 761
Keiser, Anne, 1985
Keith, Brian, 6448
Keith, Daryle, 6609
Keith, David, 823
Keith, Dennis, 42
Keith, Kathleen, 4273
Kelin, II, Daniel A, 2797
Kellachan, Dan, 5100
Kellar, Holly J, 1332
Keller, Barrie, 3061
Keller, Joel E, 1760
Keller, Werner, 1901
Kellerman, Tiffany, 3871
Kellett, Brett, 13, 788, 2381
Kelley, Brian, 2689
Kelley, Debbie, 1104
Kelley, Dorothea, 1786
Kelley, Joan, 3907
Kelley, John, 1865
Kelley, Kathleen, 2111
Kelley, Robert, 170, 2462, 2479
Kelley, Steve, 2066
Kellogg, Cal Stewart, 1889
Kellogg, Jan, 5762, 8298
Kellogg, Paul, 2223
Kelly, Alexi, 8234
Kelly, Ann, 701
Kelly, Barbara, 1982
Kelly, Cynthia K, 1459
Kelly, Joe, 4863
Kelly, Kristina, 1056, 1057, 1059, 1060, 4370
Kelly, Laura, 3270
Kelly, Leonard, 3708

Kelly, M Wade, 1221
Kelly, Mary, 2064
Kelly, Mike, 7660
Kelly, Monica, 1241, 2078
Kelly, Nicole, 5545
Kelly, Owen, 3597
Kelly, Rebecca, 542
Kelly, Sue, 829
Kelly, Tony, 2530
Kelm, John, 1948
Kelsay, Kelly E, 3639
Kelso, Amy, 2872
Keltner, Karen, 1935
Kembles, Ray, 2578, 4236
Kemp, Dan, 1762
Kemp, Judy, 2867
Kemp, Kara, 3778
Kemp, Nancy, 4034, 5844
Kemp, Randy, 5080
Kemph, Richard, 1600
Kemphouse, Randy, 241
Kemson, J, 1280
Kenaston, Kimberly, 1707
Kendall, Christopher, 6831
Kendall, Kay, 214
Kendall, Paulette, 2408
Kenderdine, Henry, 5332
Kendrick, Donald, 1908
Kenerup, Amy, 7639
Keninll, Rohana, 5045
Kenmelley, John, 2333
Kenna, Michael, 7329
Kennan Hough, Claudia, 2223
Kennard, John, 2120, 4709
Kennedy, Alfred D, 2014
Kennedy, Barbara, 42
Kennedy, Bill, 6749
Kennedy, Charry, 7170
Kennedy, Courtney, 259
Kennedy, Daniel, 4173
Kennedy, Diane, 2262
Kennedy, Dione, 7661
Kennedy, Dr. F Scott, 2074
Kennedy, John Dale, 4483
Kennedy, Margert, 587
Kennedy, Padraic M, 4646
Kennedy, Pat, 7770
Kennedy, Patrick, 6636
Kennedy, Paul, 7
Kennedy, Rod, 5540
Kennedy, Steve, 3175
Kenner, Doug, 1380
Kenney, Brad, 3080
Kenney, Micheal, 223
Kennison, Scott, 2087
Kenny, Daryl, 3893
Kenny, Shelia, 2966
Kent, Dennis, 832
Kent, Dennis M., 849
Kent, George, 2294
Kent, Sidney E, 1232
Kent, Terri, 3615
Kenton, Carolyn, 1405
Kenworthy, Jane, 1838
Kenyan, Thomas, 4291
Kenyon, Dr. Paul, 4179
Kephart, Charles, 2947
Kerbel, Sherman B, 6828
Kerley, Jean, 387
Kerlin, Bill, 2710
Kern, Diane, 2079
Kern, Jerome, 957
Kern, Kathy, 7763
Kern, Marty, 7882
Kernaghan, Maryellen, 8422
Kernodle, Jr, John R, 1581
Kerr, Donna, 1661
Kerr, Joseph, 3949, 5691
Kersey, Don, 3715
Kersey, Wade, 2797
Kersh, Nunally, 649, 1758, 3753, 5422
Kersh, Tricia, 2179

Kershaw, Jeff, 6738
Kershaw, Stewart, 718
Kershow, Jeff, 6737
Kerslake, Glen, 3507
Kersnar, David, 2841
Kertess, Klaus, 556
Keshishian, Moira, 3205
Kessick, Steve, 8260
Kessler, Karen Gail, 3742
Kessler, Martin, 1606
Kessler, Melvin P, 1025
Kessler, Michael, 5349
Kessler, Patricia, 5256
Ketcham, Lisa, 2281
Ketchum, Ellen, 5984
Ketner, Robert C., 1581
Ketrow, Sara, 376
Ketterer, James P, 1480
Kettering, Lance M, 7120
Key, Fred, 1809, 2320
Key, Tom, 2779
Keyes, Dave, 569
Keyes, Jack, 3994
Keyes, Jeff, 3145
Keyes, Jeffrey, 4671
Keysevling, Judith, 1873
Keyworth, Robin M, 2145
Khalifa, Jayne, 3162
Khan, Ricardo, 3254
Kharatian, Roudolf, 206
Kharfen, Michael, 3027
Khaury, Andre, 22
Khochayan, Vahe, 1407
Khuner, Jonathan, 1898
Kibbe, Adam, 6871
Kibblewhite, Lisa, 3641
Kichner, Chuck, 5697
Kickhaefer, Scott, 1210, 2950
Kickle, Lynn, 6538
Kidd, James, 5632
Kidd, Linda, 3647
Kidd, Onalee, 2961
Kidder, George H., 1264
Kidwell, Linda, 2369
Kiedrowski, Jay, 3132
Kieffer, Vicki, 2635
Kielty, Linda, 7004
Kiely, Damon, 2813
Kiesel, David, 2978
Kieser, Bob, 4820
Kieser, John, 902
Kiesler, Kenneth, 1150, 1311
Kiester, Kenneth, 1412
Kikta, Tammey, 6575
Kilbourn, Jennifer, 7274
Kilduff, Karl, 7810
Kiley, Clare, 8185
Kiley, Clare M, 3917
Kiley, Paul, 1295
Kilgore, Stephen, 4694
Kilgus, James, 1759
Killeen, Tracy, 5096
Kilpatrick, Annette, 1718
Kilwien, Richard, 8082
Kim, David, 1749, 5407
Kim, Kwang-Wu, 5510, 5511
Kimball, Carma, 1844
Kimball, Ellen, 5446
Kimball, Joan7, 1735
Kimball III, Leland P, 1983
Kimbell, Jon, 3033
Kimbrell, Marketa, 3323
Kimbrough, Karen, 6683
Kimsey, James V, 1995
Kincaias, Tess, 2789
Kincaid, Jack, 3219
Kinch, John, 7993
Kinch, John P, 3813
Kincke, Dee Ann, 5476
Kincman, Laurie, 107
Kindall, Kara V, 3794
King, Alonzo, 111

King, Barbara, 2847
King, Betty, 2303
King, Brian, 3616
King, Cathleen, 2536
King, Chip, 4008
King, Curtis, 5501
King, Cynthia, 1978
King, Dexter, 6486
King, Dr. Dennis, 5765
King, James, 421, 7367
King, Jayne, 165
King, John, 498
King, Katherine, 1691, 5302
King, Kelley, 8493
King, Mertedith, 2534
King, Mike, 6635
King, Prof. Gordon, 4562
King, Randall, 2536
King, Robert, 4207
King, Stephen P, 3973
King, Theresa, 5581, 5582
King, Tim, 1218
King, W. Davies, 2546
King, William V, 4146
King Jr, Woodie, 3411, 3416
King Shepherd, Doris, 1215
Kinglsey, Catherine, 430
Kingsley, Catherine, 430
Kingsley, Robert, 430
Kingston, Bob, 2940
Kingston, Robert, 6418
Kingston, Susan, 1151
Kinne, Mary, 7499
Kinney III, J Patrick, 2114
Kinnison, Sharon, 2971
Kinsey III, James W, 4229
Kinsman, Brad, 6934
Kinstle, Bob, 2968
Kipe, Andrew, 1240
Kipp, Robert A, 1373
Kippenberger, Terry, 8391
Kirby, S Dillard, 4883
Kirchdoerffer, Ed, 4874, 7216
Kirck, Robin, 895
Kirhser, Fran, 504
Kirk, Kim, 3841
Kirkpatrick, Libby, 1964
Kirkpatrick, Tom, 2654
Kirkwood, James, 1476
Kirkwood, Judy A, 1177
Kirlcham, Carol, 5569
Kirousis, Kyle, 8108
Kirshbaum, Shirley, 8447
Kirsner, Steve, 6127
Kirstein, Lincoln, 528
Kirtland, John, 266, 2025
Kiser, Kristie, 681
Kisling, Jeremy, 2967
Kissell, Ted, 7660
Kissler, John, 1894, 3506, 5089
Kistler, David, 3219
Kitchen, Gail, 3505
Kitchen, Heather, 2509
Kitchen, Nicholas, 1292, 4680
Kitson, John, 3773
Kitterman, Susan, 1163
Kitts, Lynn, 1582
Kitzes, Joseph, 1139
Kizaur, Matthew, 3631
Kjelgaard, Roberta, 229
Klaas, Brian, 3009
Klaczak, Paul, 7605, 7611
Klande, Tim, 7000
Klapper, David, 2919
Klassen, Glenn, 1312
Klausner, Florence, 2166
Kleeper, Barbara, 3116
Kleiman, Rose, 2918
Klein, Carole, 824
Klein, Demetrius, 225
Klein, Dr. Lonnie D, 1449
Klein, Eri, 1463

Klein, Julie, 3607
Klein, Sabrina, 5943
Klein, Scott Richard, 3638
Klein, Stephen, 3732
Kleindorfer, Candace, 2886
Kleinfeld, Lauren, 2738, 6416
Kleinmann, James, 142
Kleinmann, James A, 2463
Kleinmann, Kurt, 3826
Kleinsasser, Alan, 829
Kleis, John, 3981
Kleiser, David, 4936
Klemme, Katie, 2870
Klenjoski, Regina, 49
Klepperich, Bob, 7032
Klett, Terry, 3940
Kliewer, Mary, 3865
Kligerman, Beth, 2852
Klimash, Dr. Victor A, 1336
Klimko, Justin, 3095
Kline, Joan, 3841
Kline, Norman, 3499
Kline, Randall, 901, 4197
Kline, Randell, 901
Kliner, Bob, 964
Kling, Hannes, 836
Kling, Leroy T, 996
Klinger, Lori, 588
Klinger, Nan, 588
Klingler, Eugene, 6683
Klitsner, Rhoda, 1956
Kloecker, Paul V, 827
Klood, Martin, 877
Kloppenburg, Bernie, 6828
Klotz, Paul, 1881
Kluger, Joseph H, 1733
Klugherz, Laura, 4970
Klugman, Marcia, 2224
Klussner, Alexis, 2031
Klynsma, Don, 2941
Knabel, Wayne, 5171
Knapp, Angela, 663
Knapp, Barry G, 4234
Knapp, Gunnar, 755
Knapp, Maggie, 3838
Knapp, Mary, 3929
Knapp, Mary C, 3929
Knee, Bill, 7335
Kneissl, Bill, 3448
Knepper, Joan L, 3713
Kniep, Linda, 2064
Knight, Casey, 4046
Knight, Laura, 2003
Knight, Terri, 7944
Knighton, Maurine, 4934
Knittle, Carolyn, 2063
Knoch, Cherly, 5394
Knoedler, Vicky, 737
Knoedler, William, 737
Knoepfel, Gerald, 5781
Knoles, Amy, 811
Knopp, Charlene, 2735
Knopp, James, 6987
Knopp, Seth, 5610
Knorr, Sharon, 5306
Knott, Don, 6630
Knott, Paula, 1221
Knouse, Kelly, 2276
Knowles, Charles, 233
Knowles, Diane, 158
Knowles, Dr. Lawrence J, 6834
Knowles, Jack, 1764
Knowles, Katherine, 4646
Knowles, Sharon, 2160
Knox, James B, 3087
Knox, Kenny, 2873
Knox, Marilyn, 3610
Knox, Steve, 2802
Knutson, Barbara, 3660
Ko, Benjamin, 931
Kober, Dieter, 1114
Koch, Arend-Julius, 1786

Koch, David, 423
Kocha, Amy L, 5741
Kodadek, Ellen, 7481
Koehler, James, 6531
Koehner, Anne, 3770
Koenig, Rodney, 1801
Koenig, Ron, 6971
Koenig, Victoria, 78
Koenning, Vick, 8321
Koerner, Debby, 4779
Koerper, Ronn, 3625
Koetters, Florence, 1613
Koffin, Nancy, 2635
Koffler, Abby, 6318
Koffler, Abby C, 6318
Kogan, Deen, 3724
Koganrson, Pavel, 1826
Koge, Jonas, 694
Kohashi, Cheryl, 1092
Kohberger, Ken, 7197
Kohl, Deborah, 2113
Kohl, Lawrence, 911
Kohler, Kristina, 904
Kohler, Marie, 3997
Kohler-Hall, Kristine, 1124
Kohlstedt, Marian, 4195
Kohn, Gloria, 4806
Kohn, Michael, 3769
Kohr, Poykon, 1452
Kohrs, Dave, 6640
Kok, Andrea, 588
Kokoskie, Douglas S, 7235, 7236
Kokun, Mike, 6106
Kolb, Margaret, 2252
Kolchinsky, Dr. Camilla, 868
Koldenhoven, James, 1200
Kolek, John, 6098
Kollmar, Dorothy, 1034
Kolowich, Michael E, 2114
Kolson, Rob, 2814
Komaiko, Libby, 2832
Komar, Veronica, 2127
Komdat, Mark, 244
Komlyn, Lorie, 337
Komro, Joseph, 1361
Konar, Sandra, 4180
Kondak, Ann, 1324
Kondek, Charles, 2959
Kondziolka, Michael, 2120, 4709
Kongsgaard, John, 884
Konneker, Dr. Wilfred R., 1381
Konowitz, Suzanne, 1496
Kontnik, Virginia, 188
Kontos, Lydia, 7413
Kooken, Dan, 2334
Koolbeck, Tammky, 6643
Koonsman, Ann, 1795
Kopelman, Roberta, 1304
Kopf, Judy, 4950
Kopp, Patrick W, 2397
Koppel, Tina, 3069
Kopple, Alexander, 978
Korb, Kristi L, 4798
Kordel, John, 1514
Kordenbrock, Jackie, 7604
Kordes, Gesa, 1182, 4492
Kordos, Richard S, 6085
Korelitz, Ruthy, 5189
Koresh, Alon, 628
Koresh, Nir, 628
Koresh, Roni, 628
Korf, Anthony, 1532
Korican, Nina, 1278
Korkmas, Marguerite, 1803
Korney, Cornelia, 1923
Korngold, Samuel, 1106
Kornstein, Jamie, 3895
Koropeckyj-Cox, Matt, 4334
Korsmo, John, 3994
Korth, Mike, 7981
Korzec, Patricia, 879
Koshak, John, 865, 866

Koslow, Milton, 726
Koslow, Philip, 756
Koston, Dina, 1018
Kostusiak, Thomas, 7312
Kotchik, Jim, 7782, 7783
Kotik, Peter, 1465
Kotler, Milton, 1021
Kotze, Mike, 2045
Kouma, Cecelia, 2502
Kourilsky, Francoise, 3470
Kovac, Kim Peter, 6304
Kovacic, Tony, 7639
Kovacs, Rudy, 6494
Kovar, Joshua, 7793
Kowalewski, Rich, 2520
Kowalski, Peggy, 7836
Kozadayev, Sergey, 293
Kozlov, Leonid, 379
Krabach, Larry, 3107, 6976
Kraff, Dr. Michelle, 5544
Kraft, Anne, 2736
Kraft, Debra L, 3025
Kraft, Dr. James, 5637
Kraft, John, 4901
Kraft, Kathleen, 795
Krajewski, Michael, 1447
Kramarcyzk, Nancy, 6971
Kramberg, Ross, 535
Kramer, Christine, 4638
Kramer, Lori, 3663, 3666, 3668, 7773
Kramer, Mickey, 2340
Kranicke, Michaelle, 282
Kranitz, Tobie, 2773, 6443
Kransberg-Talvi, Marjorie, 1846
Krantz, Allen, 3709
Krantz, Ken, 1161
Krantz, Roberta F, 4903
Krape, William E, 2016
Krashan, Matt, 721
Krashan, Matthew, 716, 8240
Krasnoo, Eric, 7212
Krasny, Peter, 3408
Krassovska, Nathalie, 286
Kraus, Joe, 1395
Krause, Arthur B., 1373
Krause, Bill, 2335
Krause, Gloria, 2200
Krause, JoAnne, 1874
Krause, Melissa, 1987
Kraushaar, John F, 3493
Krauss, Donna, 2308
Krebs, Amy K, 5357
Krebs, Eric, 2441, 3418
Krebs, Paul, 7594, 7595
Krebs, S. Warren, 3058
Kreeger, Julian H, 1041
Kreider, Dr. Paul, 1403
Kreider, Jim, 5295
Kreider, Paul, 1406
Kreiling, Samuel R, 778
Kreiman, Kerry L, 675
Kreinberg, Steven, 7834
Kreitz, Joesph, 996
Krekhofer, Catherine, 2347
Kreloff, Dr. Hersel, 776
Krempasky, Stephen F, 7807
Kreston, Jeannette, 1117, 5742
Kreuger, Timothy, 4239
Kreuscher, Wayne, 302
Kreutz, Charlotte, 3408
Kreutzberg, James D, 6967
Kreutzer, Leah, 385
Krey, Peggy, 8295
Krezwick, Richard, 6859
Krichels, Andrew, 662
Kridler, Douglas F, 5210
Kriegel, I Stanley, 1463
Kriegel, I. Stanley, 4936
Krieger, Abbe, 1519
Krieger, Barbara Zinn, 3471
Krieger, David, 5073
Krieger, Mitchell, 1951

Krieger PhD, Leslie H, 223
Kriegsmann, Thomas O., 8452
Krienitz, Cherie, 682
Krinitsky, Ann, 793, 931
Krinsky, Robert D, 522
Krist, Andrea, 3616
Kriston, Julie, 7329
Krivin, Dr. Martin, 4907
Krivin, Martin, 4906
Krizer, Jodi Pam, 421
Krohley, Anne, 380
Krohn, Chesley, 3858
Krohnengold, Jay, 1943
Kroll, Mark, 4658
Kromm, Leroy, 808
Kroneberg, Cynthia, 2287
Krosnck, Evelyn, 1433
Krott, Joel, 1425
Krueger, John, 6193
Krum, Roger, 944
Krumbine, Rovbert, 5115
Krupa, Roger, 7554
Kruse, Jon, 1698
Krywosz, Ben, 3160
Kuba, Samuel, 3697
Kuchar, Theodore, 825, 952, 4239
Kucirko, Peter, 1215
Kuehn, David L, 918
Kuehn, Kathy, 6187
Kuehn, DMA, David L, 4205
Kuepper, Jeff, 5759
Kuharksy, Merry, 653
Kuharsky, Andrew, 653
Kuhi, Mary Ellen, 1353
Kuhlman, Jessica, 8504
Kuhlman, Kevin, 3515
Kuhlman, Yvonne, 4532
Kuhn, Gay, 3706
Kuhn, Irwin, 661
Kuhn, Marni, 8426
Kuhn, Sharon L, 5958
Kujawsky, Dr. Eric, 878
Kujawsky, Eric, 878
Kukier, Donald, 2125
Kukuk, Jack, 4047
Kulas, Matthew, 8504
Kulkarni, Subhash, 2070, 4594
Kumar, Mythili, 148
Kumery, Jerri, 572
Kumral, Lale, 2557
Kunellis, Andy, 2800
Kuniners, Nathan, 1258
Kunitomi, Darrell, 2448
Kunkel, David S, 1839
Kunkel, III, John P, 7706
Kunstadter, Geraldine, 438
Kunze, Kathryn, 3084
Kunzel, Erich, 1046
Kunzel, Karen, 86
Kuppler, Karl, 2049
Kuppman, Walter, 1142
Kupsco, Beth, 1589, 2250
Kuras, Jeffrey, 3086
Kurens, Larry, 823
Kurichh, Kathy, 3023
Kurl, Ken, 8017
Kurland, Phyllis, 4961
Kurland, Ted, 8378
Kurnick, Judith, 1733
Kurtz, Andrew M, 1055
Kurtz, Jamie, 1711
Kushigian, Elise, 6603
Kushigian, Elise J, 4503
Kushner, Nancy, 8405
Kushner, William, 1223
Kushnick, Eleanor, 2258
Kuske, Barclay, 3309
Kussmann, K, 1229
Kussmann, Kenneth K, 1229
Kutt, Amy, 2126
Kutulas, Janet, 1924
Kuuth, Lucinda, 1971

Kuykendall, Jeff, 3275
Kuzma, Jennifer, 7636
Kuzmanko, J Larry, 5376
Kwan, Paul, 2521
Kwok, Glen, 1169
Kyasky, Lynelle, 4291
Kyle, Barry, 2979
Kyler, Tricia, 2948
Kymptom, Howard, 2084
Kypros, Callt, 343
Kyte, Jennifer, 4677
Kyzmir, Anne K, 3303

L

La Bonne, Pamala L, 3386
La Coque, Louis, 1155, 4489
La Mee, Maurice, 2582
La Rosa, Ricard de, 1530, 5044
Labedz, Jr, Chester S, 2293
LaBella, Frank, 7497
Laboda DMD, Gerald, 2695
LaBombard, Chad, 4688
LaBonte, Renee, 1054
LaBrake, Randolph W, 7321
LaBruyere, Dr. Louise, 2070
Labuta, Joe, 1313
LaCamera, Lisa, 5659
Lacatell, Kate, 2113
LaCause, Elizabeth, 1554, 7481
Lacer, Lorene, 3814
Lacey, Cassandra, 5643
Lachiusa, Laurie, 408
LaCorte, Jerome, 5234
LaCourse, Donald, 351
Lacy, Ellen, 1792
Lacy, Lucile, 4015
Lacy, Nancy, 6307
Laczko, Brian J, 2661
Ladd, Kate, 5955
LaDew, Lisa, 644
Ladner, Benjamin, 6296
LaDouceur, Philip A, 7707
Ladr, Sue, 2114
Laffitte, Ron, 5460
Laffoon, Don, 2543
Lafler, Donald, 919
LaFleur, Mark, 2612
LaFollette, Amanda, 2834
Lafond, James F, 4318
LaFontaine, Kim, 7975
Lagg-May, Susan, 1057, 1059, 1060, 4370
Lago, Randolph del, 2690
Lagos, Marta, 4718
Lagrade, Naurice L, 6779
LaGruth, Anthony, 1438
LaGuardia, Jr, Vincent C, 961
LaGue, Lydia, 739
Laguni, Andrea, 847
Lahaie, Lawrence, 7160
Lahti, Dianne, 1603
Laich, Walter, 1778
Laifer, Matthew, 8450
Laing, Susan, 1139
Laing, Vashti, 1044
Laird, Michael, 3242
Lake, Barbara, 2005
Lake, J Bryan, 5496
Lake, Jody G, 8143
Lake, Michael, 2691
Lake, Ralph, 5462
Lake, SSG Robert A, 1360
Lakey, Arnold, 7562
Lakoff, Evelyn, 887
Lam, Amy W, 4662
LaMarca, Priscilla, 1954
LaMarca, Stephen, 1542, 7460
Lamb, Barbara, 4278
Lamb, David, 3300
Lamb, Roberta Pearle, 2115
Lamb Scudiery, Yvonne, 7243

Lambert, Cliff, 6630
Lambert, Dr. Richard, 5637
Lambert, Karen, 2020
Lambert, La Doyce, 3868
Lambert, Prentis, 1586
Lambert, Rebekah, 1683
Lambert, Sally E, 45
Lameier, Mark, 8459
Lamere, Gloria, 3504
Lamette, Bill, 7092
Lamette, William, 7091
LaMette, William H, 7088
Lamhut, Phyllis, 538
Lamitola, Mike, 2613
Lamkin, Dr. Fletcher M, 7081
LaMonaca, Mary, 1388
Lamort, Robert, 1710
LaMorte, Dan, 534, 2820
Lampert, Judith, 1150
Lampert, Rachel, 3319
Lamphere, Carla, 1313
Lampitelli, Jude, 2796
LaMuro, Leslie, 5784
Lamy, Larry, 1895
Lanahan, Jim, 3363
Lancaster, Bob, 2953
Lancaster, Dona, 2953
Lancaster, Linda, 4577
Lancaster, Mike, 1798
Lancia, David J, 635
Land, Pat, 3564
Landa, Harvey, 2498
Landau, Barbara G., 2220
Landau, Edna, 8442
Landesmann, Margaret, 697
Landess, Susan E, 3905
Landeverk, Wayne, 1702
Landgraf, Heidi, 86
Landon, Mark, 1104
Landovsky, John, 263
Landow, Brett, 2066, 2949
Landry, Drew, 1410
Landsman, Dennis, 307
Landsman, Kathy, 307
Landstreet, Susan, 3307, 4944
Lane, Andrew, 1068
Lane, Jack, 3194
Lane, Louis, 1368
Lane, Marcia, 2775
Lane, Margaret, 3954
Lane, Margaret Mary, 8261
Lane, Peter B, 7828
Lane, Richard, 694
Lane Carroll, JJ, 300
Lane Christilles, Karen, 6678
Laney, Rachel, 5109
Laney, Roachel, 7508
Lang, Amanda, 8298
Lang, Brien, 3747
Lang, David, 5001
Lang, Ellen, 2347
Lang, Mark E, 3377
Lang, Pearl, 536
Langbehn, Marilyn, 3964
Langdon, Robert B, 2775
Lange, Abby, 3230
Lange, Sandra A, 8303, 8305
Langevin, Diane, 5606
Langford, Rebecca, 2733
Langley, Bill, 7088
Langley, Dee, 351
Langley, Jeff, 2488
Langley, Robert F, 2220
Langlitz, Harold N., 1552, 3503
Langner, Phillip, 3335
Langone, Kenneth G, 1051
Langstaff, Kay, 972, 4258
Langton, Bryan, 1058, 4370
Lanham, Lou Ann, 8257
Lanham, Mark, 611
Lankay, Cristina, 3258, 3265
Lankford, Marie, 691

Lann, Nonie, 2394
Lanners, Bunny, 4394
Lannicielle, Bill, 7335
Lansbury, Edgar, 3338
Lantz, Dr. Gordon D, 1676
Lantz, Jere, 2141
Lantz, Jo, 6976
Lantz, Marjorie, 619
Lanzilotti, Louise, 2797
Lanzisera, Philip, 1342
Lapenieks Rosenberg, Sarma, 16
Lapidas, Jerry, 2689
Lapidus, Dr. Ira, 4699
Lapinel, Catherine, 2664
Lappin, Bob, 1051
Lappin, W Robert, 1051
Lapslay, James, 770
Laredo, Jaime, 1829
Larew, Don, 3569
Large, Larry D, 4389
Largess, William, 2670
Laribee, Nancy, 7280
Larimore, David, 7921
Larkin, Bob, 7000
Larkin, Regina, 492
Larmore, Stephen, 1380
LaRocco, Claire, 3973
Larr, Adam, 5996
Larsen, Georganne, 1248
Larsen, Honey, 2730
Larsen, Jim, 5630
Larsen, Karen, 3039
Larsen, Robert L, 2064
Larsen, Steven, 1110, 1146
Larson, Andr,, 7912
Larson, Dale, 5777
Larson, Dr. David, 5416
Larson, James, 3221, 3222
Larson, Kenneth A, 1975
Larson, Leonard, 7161
Larson, Linda, 4757
Larson, Nicki, 2159
Larson, Priscilla, 5535
Lasansky, Enrique, 775
Laskin, Emily, 5990
Lassiter, Joe, 1
Lassiter, Tina S, 4300
Lastkey, Kim, 3936
Laszloffy, Jerome, 986
Lata, Matthew, 2008
Latimer, Chip, 2690
LaTorella, Anthony, 3472
Latorre, Frank P, 6807, 6808
LaTorre, Frank P, 6809
Laturno, Nancy S, 886, 4178
Lau, Clara, 1790
Laubacher, Susan, 257
Lauderdale, Joe, 2423
Lauer, Deidre, 3592
Laughead, Scott, 3328
Laughlin, Eugene, 6683
Laughman, Henry, 2402
Lauren, Ellen, 3333
Lauridsen, Morten, 1915
Laurie, Jonathan, 804
Laurie, Marilyn, 528
Lauritzen, Sharon, 6172
Lautenberger, Fran, 2364
Lauterbach, Gregg, 1456
Lavallee, Kari Ann, 641
Lavaway, Mark, 7889
Lave, Roy, 2427
Lavelle, Jim, 2730
Lavelli, Lucinda, 582
Lavely, Chip, 3084
Lavery, James G, 7554
Lavey, Martha, 2855
Lavietas, Robert, 1579
Lavy, Marc D, 1255
Law, Bill, 1356
Law, Donna, 3879, 5576
Law, Harold, 3802

Law, Paula, 4354
Law, Reggie, 3798
Lawerence, Abigail, 93
Lawler, Frank, 1930
Lawless, Sarah, 3281
Lawlol, Deborah, 2440
Lawrence, Beth, 7888
Lawrence, Blake, 3370
Lawrence, Donna, 2174
Lawrence, Fred, 2245
Lawrence, John, 4214
Lawrence, Margaret, 4850
Lawrence, Paula, 5027
Lawrence Rivera, Jon, 2452
Laws, Jennifer, 3965
Lawson, Eric, 1199
Lawson, Joanne, 2222
Lawson, John, 2222
Lawson, Michael, 1424
Lawson, Robert, 3240
Lawson-Haith, Juanita, 5129
Lawson-Whitney, Windy, 7175
Lawton Brown, Katharine, 4806
Laxalt, Mrs. Paul, 2661
Laycock, Mark, 1434
Laycock, Mark A, 1185
Layne, Dr. J, 1630
Layne, Helene, 4350
Layton, Jon, 3990
Layton, Richard, 1182
Lazar, Joel, 1257
Lazarus, Michael, 901
Lazenberg, William, 5311
Lazorcik, Dave, 1715
Lazorcik, David, 5336
Lazzari, OSB, Boniface V, 5682
Le Blanc, Christopher J, 3059, 6890
Le Serere, Sue, 144
Leach, Alan, 1365
Leach, Howard H., 1944
Leach, Kate, 5406
Leahy, Carol, 3027
Leahy, Larry, 632
Leahy, Mike, 8384
Leahy, Sharon, 591
Leal, Consatnce, 594
Leal, Joann, 4717
Leal, Joann P, 2122, 6924
Leaming, Jim, 2812
Leary, Mike, 7960
Lease, Diane M, 594
Leavitt, Diane, 2871
Leb, Mary, 5721
LeBar, David, 1178
Lebarron, Kathy, 6592
Lebdetter, Jason, 6106
Lebeau, Jim, 7466
LeBlanc, Denis, 754
Lebo, Amy, 7217
Lebo, Ester, 2863
LeBouef, Jane, 4729
LeBreton, Cynthia, 314
LeCompte, Elizabeth, 3477
Ledbetter, Robert Mark, 1368
Ledbetter, Susan, 369
Leddy, Thomas, 871
Lederkramer, Ron, 6026
Ledford, Jim, 3693
Ledney, Gerald, 5402
Lee, Bill, 6931
Lee, Bruce, 3879, 5576
Lee, Charlotte C, 3743
Lee, Doc, 3762
Lee, Dr. Yuan-Yuan, 1153
Lee, Ella W, 5202
Lee, Grace E, 2222
Lee, Gregory, 7127
Lee, Heather, 2449
Lee, Irene S, 261
Lee, James L, 7992
Lee, Jonathan, 6026
Lee, Josephine, 2030

Lee, Kathleen, 7088, 7091
Lee, Kathy, 4121
Lee, Kristen, 8485
Lee, Larry E, 1676
Lee, Leeheng, 3454
Lee, Ralph, 3501
Lee, Robert, 434
Lee, Robert M, 2349
Lee, Sandy, 527
Lee, Stanley, 910
Lee, Terri, 6683
Lee, Young Jean, 3449
Lee, Dean, Carole A, 5522
Lee, Jr, George, 1786
Leedom, Kenneth, 8416
Leeestma, Heidi Holst, 3099
Leemon, Dick, 3069
Leeper, Stephanie, 617
Leeping, Richard, 1869
Lees, Brian E., 6817
Lees, Larry, 8428
Leese, Joseph De, 2298
Leet, Richard, 6664
Leeth, Arthur, 699
Leevers, Carol, 3570, 7265
Lefebvre, Pat, 1282
Lefebvre, Patricia, 1044
Lefton, Esquire, Ira, 627
Leggett, Douglas, 4027
Lehan-Siegel, Pamela, 610
Lehman, David, 5338
Lehman, Howard, 5777
Lehman, Katherine, 1774
Lehman, Kathy, 5324
Lehman, Ross, 2876
Lehmann, Carter, 3032
Lehmann, Hattie Jo, 7143
Lehmann, Jay, 793
Lehmann, Scott, 999
Lehnert, Oswald, 951
Lehr, Dr Lester E, 809
Lehrman, Matt, 5873
Leib, Tom, 582
Leibeusperger, Robert L, 1609
Leibman, Ed, 3420
Leibson, Andrea, 326
Leick, Darla, 5758
Leid, Kelly, 6216
Leifer, Mel, 460
Leifheit, Lex, 2642
Leigh, Barbara, 3994
Leighton, Birta, 6110
Leighton, Paula, 3280
Leighton Smith, Lawrence, 990
Leinbach, Connie, 5389
Leininger, Tom, 1648
Leipold, Louisa, 1980
Leishner, Jane, 5574
Leiter, Martha, 4368
Leith, Helen, 964
Leiweke, Tim, 6042
Lelauren, Susan, 3875
Lelbach, Bill, 3312
Lemak, MD, Lawrence J, 4009
LeMasters, S, 728
Lemer, Marc, 5872
Lemle, Robert, 7407
Lemmon, Jack R, 265
Lemmon, Ron, 266
Lemoine, Chris, 2112
Lemoine, Jerry, 6358
Lemon, Ralph, 457
Lemon, W Tucker, 1838
Lemus, Maria, 226
Lendaro, Melody, 6123
Leney-Midkiff, Ruth, 340
Leniado-Chira, Joseph, 980
Lenicheck, Ed, 958
Lenix-Hooker, Catherine J, 3256
Lenn, Sarah, 3117
LeNoire, Rosetta, 3344
Lent, Richard, 4744

Lente, Diane Van, 2885
Lentino, Joanne, 7171
Lents, Steve, 3658
Lentz, Lamar, 8104
Lenz, Ron, 4779
Leon, Steven, 2555
Leonard, Angela Jo, 3022
Leonard, Arlene, 4529
Leonard, Connie, 2448
Leonard, Gayle, 7126
Leonard, June, 390
Leonard, Kelly, 2852
Leonard, Kristen, 423
Leonard, Randy, 2007
Leonard, Reid, 3557
Leonetti, Mario E, 1910
Lepisko, Vladimir, 400
Leporati, Douglas, 4606
Lepscomb, JR, Jim, 3584
Lerber, Joel, 3328
Lerian, Steve, 8223
Lerian, Steven, 3953
Lerman, Mark, 7868
LeSarron, Kathy, 6593
Lesenger, Jay, 409, 2195
Lesicko, Dan, 2154
Lesley, Lana, 3809
Leslie, Charles, 7980
Leslie, Christine, 152, 153
Leslie, Dottie, 4945
Leslie, High, 6964
Lesnik, Peter, 6013
Less, Alicia D, 1802
Less, Mitchell R., 2710
Lessard, Martin, 3237
Lesser, Felice, 479
Lesser, Henry, 1921
Lesser, Peter, 7281
Lester, Bronwyn, 1757
Lester, G Ron, 2532
Lester, Gideon, 3040, 3041
Lester, Julia, 1679
Lester, William, 7011
Leszczewicz, Cher, 1558
Lethone, Evelyn, 93
Letner, Jenny, 4
Lettiere, Dominic J, 2750
Leuchter, Hope, 4370
Leuschel, Jani, 1789
Levene, Leslie, 1459
Levenfus, Mark, 3338
Levengood, Barney, 6614
Levenson, Jeffrey, 822
Levenson, Leon, 3027
Leventhal, Max, 2761
Leverette, Adrienne, 1691
Leveridge, Cindy, 1215
Levi, Yoel, 1073
Levin, Allen J, 5353
Levin, Cynthia, 3182
Levin, James, 3592
Levin, Jill, 6311
Levin, John, 3929
Levin, Kathi R, 6304
Levin, Larry, 2813
Levin, Michael, 1797
Levin, Steven A, 1051
Levine, Dena, 4624
Levine, Jesse, 994
Levine, Joel, 1673
Levine, Mary, 564
Levine, Steve, 3755
Levine Pizano, Jessica, 4292
Levinson, Amy, 2441
Levinson, Debby, 179
Levinson, Robert E, 1033
Levinson, Tia, 554
Levit, Ben, 3714, 5362
Levitch, Edward, 798
Levitz, Shari M, 1489
Levy, Anne, 1894
Levy, Bob, 108

Levy, David, 1304
Levy, Elsi, 1477
Levy, Ira, 1083
Levy, Karen E, 5645
Levy, Marc D, 1187
Levy, Maria L, 1973
Levy, Michael, 702, 3225
Levy, Mike, 7090
Levy, Morton, 1033
Levy, Philip, 376
Levy, Simon, 2440
Lewandowski, Randy, 6609
Lewey, David, 2878
Lewis, Bill, 2810
Lewis, Blanche, 8370
Lewis, Dale, 5052
Lewis, Del, 6866
Lewis, Dora, 2102
Lewis, Dr. J Reilly, 1019
Lewis, Drenda, 3848
Lewis, Edward, 3066
Lewis, Gail, 2294
Lewis, Irene, 3011, 6821
Lewis, J Reilly, 1984, 1993
Lewis, Jason, 3965
Lewis, Jennifer, 3564
Lewis, John, 1338
Lewis, June, 460
Lewis, Marc, 3425
Lewis, Mark, 6581, 7783
Lewis, PM, 980
Lewis, Ralph, 3337, 3431
Lewis, Ramsey, 4465
Lewis, Richard, 2493
Lewis, Robert A, 3513
Lewis, Skip, 2728
Lewis, Trivian, 888
Lewis, Walter, 1343
Lewis, Wayvle, 5835, 5836
Lewis, Wilbur Watkin, 2180
Lewitin, Margot, 3475
Lewyckyi, Taras, 624
Ley, William A, 6931
Leyden, Norman, 1697
Li, Tim, 1366
Li, Xiao-Lu, 1225
Liachowitz, Irvin R, 5393
Libby, Christopher, 3998
Liberatore, Marianne, 4293
Liberatori, Victoria, 3262, 3263, 4896
Libin, Paul, 3359, 7380
Libman, Stephen B, 635
Libonati, Daren, 7175, 7178
Lichenstein, Elly, 2481
Lichtenstein, Alan N, 3094
Lickteig, Steve, 3011
Liddell, Alan, 3258, 3265
Liddicoat, Joan, 100
Liden, Katherine, 5740
Lidstone, Meredith, 4265
Lidvall, Christine, 678
Lieberman, Donna, 3479
Lieberman, Leonard, 7232
Lien, Hsien-Liang, 1146
Lienau, Rudy, 8292
Lienhard, Paul, 3641
Lieto, Suzanne, 5332
Liffick, Cynde, 5652
Liftson, Marvia, 1469
Ligateng, Dr. Linda, 4808
Lighffoot, Kay, 3787
Light, John, 2498, 3929
Light, Mark, 2262, 7661
Lightcap, JoAnn R, 1713
Lightfoot, Roslyn L, 3256
Lightfoot, William, 951, 3552
Lightfoot, William C, 952
Lignelli, Ron, 6301
Ligon, Claude M, 4645
Lilien, Dr. David, 1232
Lilienthal, Sallie, 1362
Liljeberg, Robert, 3543

Lilley, Clarence C, 3257
Lillie, Jana, 3893
Lillie, Robert, 2062
Lilly, Michael W, 2341
Lilly, Jr, David, 353
Lim, Thomas, 450
Lima, Ilona, 3370
Limondjian, Hilde Annik, 5035
Lin, Ann, 115
Lin, Kun-Yang, 512
Lin O'Donnell, Anita, 601
Linares, Thomas, 4794
Linchon, Victoria, 3458
Lincoln, Amy, 3678
Lincoln, Deborah, 1409
Lind, Louis, 4155
Lind, Mary Joyce, 305
Lindahl, Kristina, 499
Lindbeck, Marjorie, 1915
Lindberg, Jeffrey, 1662
Lindberg, Nancy, 5707
Lindberg, Timothy, 2027, 2233
Lindbergh, Kristina, 564
Lindblom, Ronald A, 3731
Linden Martin, Cindy, 6208
Lindenauer, Paul, 4163
Lindenmeyr, Louise, 4284
Linder, Edward L, 3732
Linder, Martha, 1039
Linder, Steve, 832
Lindgren, Robert, 572
Lindholm, Eric, 814
Lindner, Dan, 1831
Lindner, David, 764
Lindorff, Joyce, 5355
Lindsay, Shaylor, 2105
Lindsay, Stephen, 8458
Lindsey, Gary, 8347
Lindsey, Iris, 7
Lindsey, Joanna, 2694
Lindsley, Clyde, 5404
Lindstrom, Amy, 2141
Lindstrom, Cindy, 36
Lindstrom, Lori, 3
Line, Rita, 1644, 2263
Ling, Christopher H, 8330
Ling, Teresa, 5661
Lingener, Kevin, 2553
Lingle, Cherie, 3699
Link, Kristin, 878
Link, Lisa, 1777
Link Edwards, Lisa, 5476
Linkous, Lee, 2748
Linn, Irena, 659
Linn, Susan, 6559
Linnell, Sherry, 2398
Lino, Christopher, 3885
Linsler, Connie F, 1033, 5171
Lint, Shirley, 2915
Linton, Jeffrey, 582
Linton, Judy, 937
Linton, Meg, 6146
Linzee, Jill, 5697
Lionberger, Justine, 2062
Lipari, Peter, 1134
Lipkin, Seymour, 4611
Lipman, Susan, 1121, 2846, 4440
Lipp, Robert I, 528
Lippe, Randy, 6926
Lippert, Robert, 825
Lippincott, Alexandria, 4646
Lipsey, Elliott, 3358
Lipshie, Jean, 1470, 4955
Lipsky, Arie, 1309, 1602
Lipsky, David, 3348
Lipton, Lini, 4995
Lipuma, Kathryn M, 3448
Lisa, Jeanine, 3804
Lisi, Michele, 528
Liske, Pete, 7693
Liss, Judith, 3428
Listokin, Ophrah, 7246

Liston, Betty, 1370
Liston, Craig, 6952
Litfin, Michael, 2478
Litoff, Mel, 4972
Litoff, Phyllis, 4972
Litt, Susan, 376
Little, Anne, 7571
Little, Carol, 1803
Little, Charles, 1084
Little, Frank, 4487
Little, Meery, 8307
Little, Sabrina, 272
Littlejohn, Christina, 751
Littlepage, Craig, 8168
Littles, Ernest M, 461
Littman, Mara, 2094
Littman, Tom, 5534
Littman, Wendy, 868
Litvin, Mark, 7386
Litvin, Mrk G, 7381
Litwin, Sharon, 1229
Lively, Dr. Judy, 5862
Livingston, Amanda, 1852
Livingston, Barbara, 2993
Livingston, Derek Charles, 2573
Livingston, Loretta, 66
Livingston, Mike, 6733
Livingstone, Pamela, 3542
Livollen, Kathleen, 6814
Lizenbery, Gregg, 164
Llewellyn, Grant, 1267, 2096
Lloveras, Sonia, 2415
Lloyd, B. Michl, 1406
Lloyd, Bob, 3238
Lloyd, David, 8382
Lloyd, Elinor, 829
Lloyd, Joe, 5862
Lobrano, Sue, 357
LoBue, Louis, 2978
Lock, Lisa K, 27
Locke, Steve, 8082
Lockert, Robin, 4087
Lockett, Bonnie, 1898
Lockhart, Keith, 1262, 1826
Lockwood, Marianne C, 1527
Lockwood, Marriane C, 1534
Lockwood, Steven Kent, 3161
Lockwood, William W, 3261
Lockwood Blais, P, 7328
Loder, Jim, 3952
Loebel, David, 1771, 4811
Loeffler, Barbara, 5343
Loehr, Lynn, 1583
Loehrlein, Evelyn, 748
Loewen, Debra, 741
Loewith, Jason, 2867
Loewy, Andrea, 4592
Loewy, Peter, 3250
Lofdahl, Will, 4913, 7270
Lofthouse, Karen, 6291
Loftin, Dennis, 1189
Loftin, Mark, 4927
Loftin, Stephen A, 5186
Lofy, Heidi, 8299
Logan, Dennis, 6074
Logan, Gaylon, 6110
Logan, Patricia E, 4741
Logan, Terri, 1180
Logan III, Joseph, 2335
Logefeil, Pegge, 1911
Logrea, Jean, 564
Logue, Frank, 2622
Lohrey, Gina, 768, 4051
Loker, Elizabeth, 1020
Lokken, Lawrence, 1035
Lombard, Mary Frances, 1990
Lombardo, Rick, 3060
Lombardy, Lisa, 1388
LoMonaco, Dr. Martha, 2610
Loncto, Nancy, 6172
London, Dr. Edwin, 1622
Long, Carolyn, 1830

Long, Charles, 2337
Long, Curtis, 1006, 1640
Long, Daniel, 2322
Long, Eleanor, 1829
Long, Flo, 7045
Long, Hugh W, 1229
Long, Joe, 1779
Long, Kathy, 4113, 5988
Long, Kenny, 7667
Long, Kevin, 706
Long, Rocky, 7264, 7266
Long, Shara, 1670
Long, Wayna, 6444
Longest, Karen, 3745
Longfield, Ross, 1414
Longhi, Kym, 3141
Longhurst, John, 2325
Longman, Stanley V, 2757
Longo, Peter, 1416
Longo, Vince, 3052
Longstreth, Clara, 2221
Lonick, Deb, 4001
Lonn, Ginny, 8328
Lonn, Jerry, 8328
Loomis, John, 2665
Loomis, Kathleen, 7798
Loomis, Shirley, 4096
Loos, Jon, 7911
Lopes, Bernadette, 6109
Lopez, Abel, 2662
Lopez, Consuelo, 1804
Lopez, Elmo, 1804
Lopez, Raquel, 118
Lopez, Soledad, 3508
Lopresti, Joseph, 5205
Lorang, Dianne, 369
Lord, Barbara Beck, 219
Lord, Carolyn, 448
Lord, Stephen, 2094, 2155
Lord, Sue, 4046
Loren, Bonnie, 3435
Lorentzen, Patsy L, 373
Lorenz, Jacqueline, 3954
Lorenz, Tom, 7156
Lorenzen, Sherry, 2961
Lorimore, David, 7922
Lorraine, Ted, 906
Lorre, Gary, 1679
Lortel, Lucille, 2648
Losche, Keri, 2497
Losey, Ryan, 1266
Louch, Annette, 6550
Loudermilk, Wanda, 4074
Loughran, Una, 613
Lourie, Frances, 998
Lovaglia, Toni, 5529
Love, Ed, 1398
Love, Edith, 3821
Love, Jim, 2496
Love, Paula, 3640
Love, Reve, 7262
Love, Ruth, 2298
Love, Wil, 3694
Lovell, David, 1870
Loving, Bruce, 5721
Lovinggood, David, 2600
Lowder, Michael, 5146
Lowe, Philip, 5525
Lowensberg, Jaime, 1792
Lowenstein, Amy, 3910
Lowentritt, Henry, 1230
Lowery, Eugene, 7381
Lowman, William, 4115
Lowr, Linda, 914
Lowrie, Gerald M, 2661
Lowry, Greg, 7944
Lowry, Lee Manwaring, 2727
Lowry, Sara Jane, 3729
Lozano, Danilo, 946, 4228
Lozano, Raul, 2538
Lubell, Rachel, 544
Lubovitch, Lar, 500

Lubsen, Jr, Walter H, 1019
Luca, Sergiu, 5297
Lucas, Ashley, 1976
Lucas, Bob, 103, 3632
Lucas, Cynthia, 155
Lucas, Darren, 7516
Lucas, James, 2534
Lucas, Katie, 5209
Lucas, Waverly, 246
Luce, Mike, 6482
Lucero, Amarante L, 667
Lucero, Larry, 964
Luchowski, Alicia, 209
Luchsinger, Ron, 2166
Lucia, Olga, 3600
Luckey, Joe, 5334
Luckow, Lynn DW, 1941
Lucky, Dr. Harrell, 2317
Luczak, Nancy, 5747, 5748
Ludlow, Morgan, 3886
Ludwig, Richard, 7209
Luebbert, Heidi, 360
Lueben, Becky, 3118
Luedders, Jerry D, 859
Lueger, Susan, 3995
Lufkin Weiss, Suzanne, 4610
Luiggi, Kimberly, 2114
Luka, MD, Norman, 1445
Luley, Gail, 2289
Lum, Eileen, 2021
Luna, Sonia, 927
Lunch, David, 2369
Lund, Benjamin, 6800
Lund, Cecilia, 1101
Lund, Karen, 3962
Lund, Susan, 3158
Lund, Tom, 3204, 7133
Lundberg, Susan, 1596
Lundy, Anne, 8060
Lundy, Larry, 735
Lunser, Leo, 3006
Lunsford, Martha, 8260
Lupo, Lelsie, 6987
Lupone, Robert, 3404
Lupp, Barbra, 5222
Luquire, Dr. Wilson, 747
Lusco, C Matthew, 4009
Luse, Don, 5113
Lusk, Don, 3643
Luskin, Evan R, 2152
Lussier, Henry, 3041
Lustig, Graham, 384
Luther, Christina, 2941
Luther, Hope, 1058
Luther, Robert, 4030
Lutwak, Mark, 2797
Lutz, Paula M, 7100
Lutz, Tony, 4546
Luukko, Peter, 5365, 7826
Lux, Daniel, 689
Luxner, Michael, 1126
Lyall, Robert, 2072, 2127, 2298
Lybeck, Greg, 8252
Lyddon-Hattan, Lana, 305
Lydum, Chip, 8238, 8239
Lyell, Kathy, 357
Lyle, Dianne, 5129
Lyle, Jacqueline, 4590, 6754
Lyle, Shawn F, 3279
Lyman, Burt, 7005
Lyman, Perry, 190
Lyman Geotz, Jean, 5053
Lyn, Janaea Rose, 321
Lynam, Mary, 8399
Lynch, Brian, 4472
Lynch, Dennis M, 5670
Lynch, Florence, 975
Lynch, Jeanne, 2303
Lynch, Jeffrey, 3572
Lynch, Jim, 6814
Lynch, Mike, 1381
Lynch, Molly, 42

Lynch, Patrick J, 6026
Lynch Jex, Jori, 1659
Lyndes, Catherine, 3903
Lyndon, Donlyn, 892
Lyne, Dr. Greg, 1867
Lynn, Barry, 730
Lynn, Doug, 7697
Lynn, Enid, 190
Lynn, Fred A, 5208
Lynn, James, 3348
Lynn, Jim, 1037
Lynn, Judy, 722
Lynn, Nancy, 4204
Lynn, Robert, 4048
Lynnell, Laureen H, 1882
Lyon, David, 1380
Lyon, Pro, 642
Lyons, Brad, 2881
Lyons, Kit, 3752
Lyons, Robert, 3423

M

Ma, Rong-Hong, 8466
Maack, Linda, 1397
Mabini, Fernie, 8033
Mably, Mary, 298
Mabry, George, 2301
Macal, Zdenek, 1430, 4888
MacAllister, PE, 2058
Macatsoris, Christofer, 2277
Macchiarini, Marianella, 2517
MacDiarmid, Katherine, 176
MacDonald, Eleanor, 2113
MacDonald, Jeannette, 3682
MacDonald, Jennifer, 5620
MacDonald, John, 2670
MacDonald, Rae, 1901
MacDonald, Robert, 4342
MacDuffil, Robin, 7280
Mace, Jerilee M, 2064
Mace, Katherine, 7748
Macewicz, Diane, 1127
MacGillivary, Thomas, 764
Mach, Jean, 868
Machado, Paul, 4257
Macias, Mike, 4076
MacIntyre, Donald-Mac, 2918
Mack, Brooke, 942
Mack, Carl, 187
Mack, Doris, 5395
Mack, Frank, 4883
Mack, Sharon, 1323
MacKay, Charles R, 2155
MacKay-Galbraith, Janet, 4428
Mackeigan, Rich, 6949
MacKeigan, Rich, 6950
MacKenzie, David, 612, 1689, 3661, 5299
MacKenzie, Jennifer, 710
Mackey, Eileen, 2112
Mackey, Jennifer, 1982
Mackey, Roberta, 3304
Mackie, Richard, 1868
MacKinnon, J Allan, 1888
Mackintosh, Steve, 570
MacLachlan, Nancy, 823
Maclay, John, 2212
MacLean, Calvin, 2882, 4473
MacLean, Heather, 4035
Maclean, Lyla, 4462
MacLean, Malcolm, 2132
Macleod, Judy, 7732
MacLeod, Michael, 989
MacNeill, Loree, 3212
MacNish, Linda, 3306
Macor, Chris, 2590
MacPhearson, Iain, 3773
MacPherson, Bruce, 8103
MacPherson, Don, 3774
MacPherson, Pat, 3774
MacQhie, Catriena, 5169

Macris, Peter, 3487
Macugenroth, Steve, 2496
Madden, Elisabeth, 5203
Madden, J. Robert, 5483
Madden, Linda, 1961
Madden, Tiffany, 7831
Maddox, Jane, 3660
Maddox, Joyce, 6019
Maddux, Jennifer, 4573
Madigan, Leslie, 3564, 7253
Madkour, Christopher, 5605
Madnick, Ellie, 2463
Madoni, Pat, 4000
Madore, Paul, 2112
Madsen, Marshall, 7005
Madsen, Nancy, 3175
Madson, Heidi, 2340
Maerhofer, John, 6837
Maes, Kathy, 2594
Maess, Jeff, 1170
Maffongelli, Ralph, 4002
Magee, Irma A, 7491
Magee, Linda, 1691, 5302
Magendanz, Dr. Jon, 1563
Magers, Shannon, 4016
Mages, William, 2857
Magette, Patricia, 4235
Maggio, Michael, 2836
Maghiochetti, Joe, 1660
Maginnis, Tara, 2366
Magpiong, Bret, 4172
Magruder, Jim, 3011
Magruder, Kate, 2569
Maguire, Kate, 4689
Maguire, Matthew, 3361
Maguire, Michael, 4916
Mahon, Maxine, 104
Mahon, Nan, 2496
Mahoney, Eva, 3412
Mahoney, Leanne, 4775
Mahood, James, 1818
Mahraun, Daniel, 4554
Mahrdt, Margie, 3067
Maidenberg, Sharon, 4187
Maifeld, Kevin, 2585, 3959
Main, Alice Lee, 1960
Maine, Pat, 411
Maiorano, Robert, 194, 2628
Maisonet, Elba, 2832
Maister, Nigel, 3496
Majikina, Aiko, 69
Majkowski, Kurt, 3980
Major, Leon, 2094
Makofsky, Jimmy, 3607
Makowski, Stan, 7316
Malan, Danielle, 3667
Malan, Roy, 972, 4258
Malashock, John, 107
Malashock, Nina, 107
Malaty, Jean-Philippe, 392, 394
Maldonado, Gregory, 926
Malecaech, Ruth, 3401
Maleczech, Ruth, 3401
Malfitano, Frank, 4720, 4721, 6933
Malin, Tova, 5610
Malina, Arnie, 1827, 5596, 8156, 8157
Malina, Judith, 3400
Malina, Stuart, 1579, 1716
Malinova, Margarita, 4946
Malinowski, Barbara, 2515
Malins, Susan, 3657
Malitz, Morton, 4713
Malizia, Lester, 2689
Malkovich, III, Dr. Mark P, 5409
Malkovich, IV, Mark, 5409
Mallalieu, Stephen, 7334
Mallen, Thomas, 847
Mallette, David, 676
Mallette, Lisa, 2566
Mallin, Heidi, 6614
Mallory, Desiree, 4117

Malloy, Jeffrey P., 2509
Malloy, Sue, 2928
Mallquist, Carol, 4291
Malmed, Leslie, 561
Malmstrom, Laurie, 2504
Maloff, Peter, 379
Malone, Doug, 7888
Malone, Fran, 4000
Malone, Giles, 6322
Malone, Ryan, 5266
Maloney, Dauphne, 3618
Maloney, Kathy, 1241, 2078
Maloney, Mary, 2393
Maloney, Richard, 2093
Maloof, Jim, 289
Malottke, Brenda, 2155
Maluso, Mark S, 8442
Manager, Reynold Fauci, 7229
Mancinelli-Cahill, Margaret, 7280
Mancuso, Jim, 1091
Mancuso, Kim, 3031
Mancuso, Susan, 2292
Mandel, Catherine, 3073
Mandel, Michael, 3280
Mandel, PhD, Jerry E, 5961
Mandelbaum, Marvin, 2107
Mandella, Teresa, 933
Mandeville, Patricia, 1829
Mandia, Albert W, 2277
Mandicott, Bill, 4649
Mandler, Susan, 200
Mandt, Robert, 7335
Manduzzi, James, 6929
Manetta, Edward J, 7353
Maneval, Philip, 1731, 5368
Manfinger, Dan, 5966
Mangels, Tonya, 7090
Mangelsdorf, Margaret, 2048
Mangili, Jan, 2558
Manguard, Carol, 3307
Manildi, Anna, 5687
Manion, Diane, 5609
Manji, KC, 941
Mankin, Dan, 3946
Mann, Emily, 3261
Mann, George T, 4331
Mann, John, 3090
Mann, Jonathan, 7380
Mann, Mark, 3600
Mann, Theodora, 4030
Mann, Theodore, 2204, 3359, 7380
Mannard, Suzanne, 7277
Manning, Maura Elizabeth, 2884
Manning, Roger, 2901
Manos, Christopher B, 2777
Manos, George, 1015, 4298, 4313
Manos, Nicholas F, 2777
Manrique, Anthony S, 1904
Mans, Lorenzo, 3385
Mansfield, Paul, 4910
Manson, Anne, 1373
Manson, III, Lawrence C, 437
Manspeaker, Kathryn, 4168, 6080
Mantner, Fred, 2451
Manuel, Barbara B, 2110
Manwarren, Matthew, 5427
Manwell, Penny, 2725
Manze, Andrew, 4668
Maples, Steven, 5809
Maragon, Donald, 2292
Marble, Jennifer, 1412
Marcanio, Jerry, 3050
Marcante, Mark, 3458
Marceau, Kathryn, 830, 4109
March Romanovsky, Paula, 1939
Marchant, Greg, 6486
Marchant, Susan, 4560
Marchant, Tyler, 3434
Marchese Sidoti, Catherine, 8414
Marchewka, Bob, 4863
Marchiel, Paul, 3465
Marchini, Italo, 2175

Marcoux, Tina, 3236
Marcus, Ann, 3667
Marcus, Leslie, 3433
Marcy, Kirk, 5684
Mardsen Fox, Ana, 641
Marek, Reverend Walter, 3113
Marek, Vladimir, 688
Marenchin, Ron, 1602
Mares, Liz, 967
Maresca, Rosalia, 2012
Margolin, Isabel, 3274, 7254
Margolis, Craig, 710
Margolis, Karl, 3141
Margolis, Laura, 3316
Marguiles, Vicki, 8466
Margulies, Michael, 3130
Margulies, Vicki, 5015, 7413
Marha, Tony, 4751
Mariarty, Kevin, 3318
Maric, Jena, 974
Marier, Cheryl, 1690
Marietta, Robert, 3019
Marinaccio, Mike, 7295
Marino, Catherine, 4995
Marino, Nancy, 3251
Marino, Peter, 1747, 5398
Marino, Sandy, 3688, 5323
Marion, Michael, 5857
Marion, William, 1405
Maritn, Dana, 2335
Mark, Julie, 6128
Mark, Peter, 2333
Mark, Susan, 5087
Markey, Donovan, 2585
Markey, Michael, 3223, 4834
Markham, Judith, 1406
Markou, Kypros, 1316
Markov, Kypros, 1713
Marks, David, 2304
Marks, Dick, 7886
Marks, Kristin, 194, 2628
Marks, Lorraine, 1420
Marks, Ron, 3809
Marks, Victoria, 75
Markuson, Cira P, 5065
Markwalter, Zoe, 4995
Markward, Dr. Edward, 1753, 1754
Markward, Edward, 2293
Marlock, Walter, 6066
Marlowe, Ina, 2870
Marlyn Singer, Audrey, 2465
Marmor, Martin, 5584
Marpe, James, 997
Marquardt, Tom, 6817
Marqulies, Michael, 3012
Marr, Doug, 3218
Marr, Laura, 3218
Marra, Jr, Robert A, 1260
Marrero, Kyle, 2005, 2184
Marri, Richard A, 1435
Marroguin, Sharon, 669
Mars, Rockland, 2902
Marsalis, Wynton, 1513, 5028
Marsden, Barbara Ann, 641
Marsden, Herci, 641
Marsden Fox, Ana, 641
Marsh, Frazier, 2969
Marsh, Julian, 3256
Marsh, Melinda, 1658
Marsh, Micheal, 2091
Marsha, Jeff, 7312
Marshall, Angela, 3789
Marshall, Bradford, 647
Marshall, Cathleen, 373
Marshall, Corrina, 4198
Marshall, Craig, 2940, 6418
Marshall, Dennis, 679
Marshall, Douglas, 3725
Marshall, Frederick, 2918
Marshall, Galen, 1950
Marshall, Kelli, 1729
Marshall, Kevin, 2697

Marshall, L Gerald, 1553
Marshall, Lois, 1437
Marshall, Margo, 679
Marshall, Nancy J, 5498
Marshall, Scott, 2953
Marshall, Susan, 554
Marshall, Tom, 2653
Marsten, David, 857, 4143
Martell, Fredrick, 2226
Martell, Sharon, 3669
Marten, Ethan, 3919
Marten, James, 1272
Marten, Richard, 3919
Martin, Carol, 2604
Martin, Carter, 586
Martin, Chris, 2808
Martin, Craig, 2514
Martin, Danita, 13, 788, 2381
Martin, Dennis, 1987, 1988
Martin, Dorrell, 681
Martin, Dr Alice, 2854
Martin, Eff W., 1946
Martin, Elisa, 3050
Martin, Floyd, 4071
Martin, Jill, 2565
Martin, John, 7664
Martin, John W, 2695
Martin, Judith, 3428
Martin, Kathryn, 836, 4120
Martin, Kenneth, 527
Martin, Lynda, 1074
Martin, Martha, 1920
Martin, Mary, 4555, 6676
Martin, Myron, 4843
Martin, Nancy, 6126
Martin, Nicholas, 3035, 6861
Martin, Panda, 2392
Martin, Richard, 4556
Martin, Richard P, 6683
Martin, Rick, 2530
Martin, Robert, 1502, 3412
Martin, Ron, 3643, 5271
Martin, Russ, 1856
Martin, Sharon, 1231
Martin, Steve, 2373, 6202
Martin, Sue, 5379
Martin, Sue N, 5380
Martin, Terry, 3801
Martin, Virginia D, 2331
Martin, William C, 4145
Martin, William H, 2001
Martin-Mintz, Deborah, 3535
Martin-Wilkins, Danita, 13, 788, 2381
Martindale, Diane, 2210
Martinez, Diana, 2891, 4427
Martinez, Francisco, 171
Martinez, Rebecca, 3667
Marting, Kristen, 3380
Marting, Kristin, 3380
Martins, Peter, 528
Martint, Marya, 5006
Marty, David, 4727, 4755
Martyn Zike, Steven, 1188
Marver, James D, 140
Marvin, Jameson, 2100
Mascette Brandt, Susan, 3493
Maschka, Dennis, 6993
Masini, Jim, 2850
Maso, Michael, 3035, 6854, 6861
Mason, Ann F, 1742
Mason, Francis, 511
Mason, Martha, 3042
Mason, Mary Ellen, 2876
Mason, William, 2038
Mason Gregg, Lynette, 690
Masonson, Norman, 835
Massaro, John, 1889
Massengale, Joni, 3512
Massengale, Shirley, 207
Massenkoff, Nikolai, 130, 4184
Massey, Andrew, 1685
Massey, Peter, 2681

Massod, Al, 1710
Mastalski, Elaine, 3693
Mastenbrook, Ellen, 333
Masterson, Marc, 2969
Masterson, Veronica, 2516
Masur, Kurt, 1522
Mata, Ray, 8252
Mata, Tony, 3624
Matan, Debbie, 3598
Matczynski, Leonard, 4660
Matheke, Susan, 192
Matheny, Jane, 3973
Matheny, Jerry, 3599, 3684
Matheny, K Robert, 5255
Mather, Randy, 3940
Mathes, Malcolm, 3659, 5296
Mathes, Scott, 858
Matheson, Nancy, 166
Mathews, Kurt, 883
Mathews, Marguerite, 3236
Mathews, Paul, 8299
Mathews, Renee, 390
Mathews, Sharon, 312
Mathias, Dick, 8168
Mathis, Paige, 2016
Mathison, John, 7753
Mathys, Elena, 4233
Matin, Beatrice, 1692
Matison, Katie, 1846
Matlick, Barbara, 3653
Mato, Nancy, 4354
Matson, L, 1280
Matsunaga, Heather C, 69
Mattaliano, Christopher, 4729
Matter, Charles E, 7472
Matter, Linda, 3697
Matteson, Bill, 1376
Matteson, Steve, 2322
Matthews, Benjamin, 2229
Matthews, Bill, 5810
Matthews, Craig, 1463
Matthews, Ingrid, 1849
Matthews, John, 3802
Matthews, Mark, 1377
Matthews, Paula D, 8297
Matthews, Virginia, 784, 5902
Mattison, Donald C, 1134
Matton, Annie, 1852
Mattoon, Bill, 2604
Mattox, Hoyt T, 5535
Matyas, Charles, 1112
Mauceri, John, 832, 2291, 4114
Maughan, Kent, 3180
Mauk, Shelley A, 3619
Mauldin, Dr. Walt, 5450
Maull, George Marriner, 1442
Maur, Elsie von, 1189
Mauro, Micheal, 2091
Mautha n, Geraldine, 5546
Max, Darla, 3719
Max, Doug, 6231, 6233
Maxey, William, 1330
Maxwell, Carla, 490
Maxwell, Hugh, 3618
Maxwell, Linda, 167
Maxwell, Martha Ellen, 1771
Maxwell, Meghan, 4480
Maxwell, Mihael D, 2356
May, Bettina, 492
May, Bobby, 8072
May, Eldonna, 1313
May, Linda, 4359, 4826, 6407
May, Thomas D, 1262
May-Lagg, Susan, 4366
Mayer, Diane, 2978
Mayer, Janice, 8444
Mayer, Stuart, 6931
Mayes, Doug, 1771
Mayes, Jennie, 5969
Mayes, Joseph, 1732
Mayes, Randy, 5784
Mayes-Smith, Susan, 3228

Mayfield, Maryhelen, 574
Mayleas, William, 1933
Mayne, Joseph, 1867
Mayo, Anna Y, 4174
Mayo, Sonje, 662
Mayon, Dan M, 2438
Mayor, Mara, 4316
Mays-Floyd, Dawn, 5133
Mazern, Leonard, 4713
Mazon, Janusz, 257
Mazonson, Eric, 2105
Mazuca, Roland, 5557
Mazur, Joe, 7622
Mazza, Lynne S, 1451
Mazzeo, Cindy, 715
Mazzolini, Tom, 4192
Mazzonelli, Joan, 2844, 6529
McAdams, Beverly, 5140
McAdams, Charles, 1386
McAdams, Lorraine, 383
McAdams-Connor, Kenna, 383
McAfee, Kathy, 663
McAfee Weakley, Janet, 2155
McAlister, Meredith, 5543
McAllister, Kevin, 6593
McAllister, Robert, 4239
McAlwain, Joe, 8223
McAmis, Craig, 940
McAniss, Edward J, 1915
McAnuff, Des, 2420
McArver, R Dennis, 1832
McBeth, Christopher, 2327
McBride, Don, 3616
McBride, Howard, 3087
McBride, Karen, 6933
McBride, Mary, 3371
McBride, Patricia, 572
McBride, Rebecca, 6575
McCabe, RoseAnne, 4370
McCabe, Terry, 2862
McCafferty, Tom, 5948
McCalhoah, Colleen, 3970
McCall, John, 6574
McCall, Sean, 2934, 6661
McCance, Martha, 2790
McCann, Gregory, 589
McCarl, F James, 635
McCarthy, Jim, 5269
McCarthy, Joe, 3224, 7169
McCarthy, Kevin, 7335
McCarthy, Linda, 6750
McCarthy, Steven, 3762
McCarty, Bill, 3168
McCarty, Steve, 8095
McCasland, Debbie, 5871
McCauley, Esquire, Richard G., 4646
McCay, Harold, 6566
McCellain, Roberta, 881
McClain, Joseph, 2303
McClain, Steve, 8321
McClamy, Gerry, 3594
McClanahan, Susan, 2120
McClatchey, Ethel, 848
McClaugherty, John L, 1860
McCleery, Dan, 3055
McClements, Nancy, 732
McClenan, Julie, 4270
McClendon, Nancy, 3814
McClintock, Darby, 1882
McClintock, Thomas C, 5289
McCloskey, Sharon, 8163
McClure Mautinko, Victoria, 3924
McCluremahood, Sandra, 3817
McClusky, Lynette, 1161
McColgan, Judy, 2074
McCollum, Ken, 809
McCollum, Mary Lou, 304
McCollum, Michael, 1162
McCollum, Timothy, 1871
McComb, Sharon, 5474
McConkey, Carey, 3105
McConnaughey, Shelly, 6616

Mears, Cliff, 3618
Mears, Karen Kelly, 1711
Mechetti, Fabio, 1037, 1852
Meckel, Peter, 1902
Medak, Susan, 2391
Meddick, Tom, 6279
Meder, Deborah M, 3685
Medina, Derek, 2563
Medina, Joe, 3875
Medler, Marcy Chiasson, 1371
Medrano, Hugo, 2662
Medved, Danita, 3992
Medved, Paul, 3992
Medvitz, James T, 917
Meegan, Mardie, 2884
Meehan, Daivd, 7336
Meehan, David, 7332
Meehan, Kathleen, 7353
Meek, Don, 4113
Meeker, M David, 5875
Meena, James, 2245
Megginson, Julie, 1070, 4384
Megna, Scott, 6082
Mehenett, Pam, 5205
Mehler, Leilane G, 1990
Mehrberg, Randy, 284
Mehta, Navroj, 935
Meier, Ann, 1993
Meier, Gustav, 974
Meier, Johanna, 3765
Meier, Spencer, 187
Meigs, Jaon, 1137
Meiki, Kendra, 316
Melby Phaneuf, Cindy, 4834
Melchior, Sharon, 1213
Mele, Kathy, 3428
Melichar, Jill, 703
Melilo, Joseph V, 4936
Mellen, Andrew J., 3364
Melnick, Dan, 5034
Melnick, Jacqueline, 1297
Melnick, Peter, 7980
Meloccaro, Lynne, 1496
Melone, Roger, 1447
Melrose, Claudia, 733
Melstrom, Laurie, 1314
Melvin, Sue, 6804
Menarchik, Douglas, 1781
Menard, Glenn, 6773
Menashe, Marlinda, 7279
Mench, 1st Lt. Michael, 1009
Menchaca, Louis A, 5760
Mendelsohn, Joann, 1849
Mendelson, Marianne, 378
Mendelson, Melinda, 857, 4143
Mendes, Sue, 3795
Mendes, William, 6113
Mendoz, Marian, 338
Mendro, Donna, 1789
Meneely, Veronica, 6817
Meneer, Christine, 599
Menefee, Ken, 2914
Menendian, Michael, 2847
Menezes, Bill, 7198
Meng, Rosie, 5538
Mengers, Kay, 5361
Menichino Parou, Debbie, 626
Menner, Vera, 5189
Mennino, Mary-Therese, 7188
Mennino, MT, 4847
Menz Werble, Katherine, 1020
Merced, Jorge, 3292
Mercer, Gwenn, 5483
Mercer, Jane, 4568
Merchant, Elaine, 3621, 5239
Merck, Al, 831
Merckens, Meg, 2934, 6661
Meredith, Jeff, 3932
Meredith, Mary Ellen, 3645
Merell, Lucy, 760
Mericott, Douglas, 1045
Merit, Adrienne, 4836

Merkley, Marty, 409, 1468, 4942
Merletti, Lew, 7615
Mermell, Barbara, 568
Merriam, Jr, Burton, 5386
Merrick, Bruce C, 2969
Merrill, Dee, 7517
Merrill, Lisa B, 3993
Merrill, Susan, 2123
Merrill-Buttzak, Lisa B, 3056
Merrins, James, 1473
Merritt, Jennifer, 5319
Merritt, Laura, 1447
Merritt, Robert, 1979
Merritt, Susan, 1074
Mers, Kaye E, 954
Merson, Barbara, 1481
Merten, Melissa, 3860
Mery, James G, 8115
Mery, Jim, 8108
Merz, Jan, 3968
Merz, Jesse, 3968
Merz, Peter, 357
Mester, Jorge, 872
Metallo, Vincent, 2177
Metre, Cheryl Van, 660
Mettar, Jennifer, 679
Mettard, Janet, 389
Mettetal, Carla, 7066
Metz, Douglas, 1021
Metz, John, 4280
Metzgar, Rae, 5011
Metzger, Margery, 1726
Metzger, Philip, 1726
Mewborne, Dr. Mark, 47
Meyer, Anita, 1405
Meyer, Denise, 4269
Meyer, Joe, 2139
Meyer, Kurt, 3985
Meyer, MW, 4427
Meyer, Paul, 2499
Meyer, Terry, 5078
Meyerer, Shannon, 3215
Meyers, Ann, 1769
Meyers, Betty, 2258
Meyers, Bob, 5675
Meyers, D Lynn, 3582
Meyers, Karen, 4226
Meyers, Nancy, 4912
Meyers, Paul, 3795
Meyers, Vicki, 2059
Meyrose, Tom, 7592
Mezger, Melissa, 8017
Mica, Alan, 1459
Michael, Hermann, 764, 765
Michael, Shawn, 2465
Michael Gold, Dr. Edward, 1559
Michael Hanvik, Jan, 7424
Michaels, Cary, 5560
Michalec, Mychaelyn, 7649
Michalson, Jay, 5284
Michel, Aimee K, 2987, 4601
Michel, Robin, 4198
Michie, Donald, 1867
Mickelsen, Rob, 3352
Mickelson, Joan, 3152
Miclon, Mike, 4621
Micotto, Steve, 2858
Middledorf, Harriet, 4096
Middleton, Sharon, 3993
Midgley, Judith, 806
Midkiff, Robert, 2796
Mier, Dorothea, 410
Miers, Don, 6366
Migala, Lucyna, 276, 2034, 2035, 2036
Mihalick, Denise, 5402
Mike, Louise, 3378
Mikelick, Kathryn, 595
Mikkelson, Dawn, 3145
Miksa, Cindy, 6053
Mikula, Deborah E, 4708
Milanov, Rossen, 1421
Milarch, Carla, 3085

Milarsky, Jeffrey F, 1507
Milbrandt, Dr. Lanny, 2791, 4406
Milder, Larry, 1626
Milenski, Michael, 1912
Miler, Paul, 7095
Miles, C, 2204
Miles, Julia, 3476
Miles, Lisette, 5577
Miles, Philip, 871
Miles-Burger, Deidre, 6909
Milgrein, Philip L, 4995
MILK, FLORENCE, 415, 1491
Mill, Neil, 2559
Millan, Bruce E, 3092
Millard, Stephen, 5497
Millay, Mike, 6367
Millen, Christine M, 3448
Miller, Allison, 6061
Miller, Barry, 2735
Miller, Bebe, 440
Miller, Beth, 6209, 6219
Miller, Betty Jo, 7144
Miller, Brad, 616
Miller, Bruce, 3924
Miller, Bruce J, 2687
Miller, Carlane, 3631
Miller, Carley, 1872
Miller, Carrie A, 10
Miller, Chad, 1167
Miller, Christopher, 8222
Miller, Clayton, 3549
Miller, Connie, 2352
Miller, Curt, 6636
Miller, Darren, 7297
Miller, David, 1506
Miller, David Alan, 1454
Miller, Deb, 5350
Miller, Don, 4043
Miller, Dr. Greg, 5247
Miller, Dr. James, 8078
Miller, Elizabeth M, 6207
Miller, Ellwood, 1699
Miller, Erica, 7798
Miller, Ernest, 320
Miller, George, 3679
Miller, Grace, 413
Miller, Jane, 4744
Miller, Jean, 3896
Miller, Jeffrey S, 2399
Miller, Joan, 486
Miller, JoEllen, 2917
Miller, John J, 1428
Miller, Jonathan, 2029
Miller, Jonathan Seth, 3041
Miller, Kara L, 3598
Miller, Karen, 3160
Miller, Kathaleen, 6891
Miller, Ken, 1332
Miller, Kris J, 7970
Miller, Lani, 3672
Miller, Linda, 6733
Miller, Lloyd, 696, 1820, 5589, 5593
Miller, Luann, 2946
Miller, Lucy, 1502, 5338
Miller, Lynn, 2915
Miller, Mae, 993
Miller, Marie, 1204
Miller, Mary, 634, 1260
Miller, Melvin, 5803
Miller, Michael A, 3055
Miller, Milton J, 1999
Miller, Mindy, 1169
Miller, Pamela G, 4242
Miller, Pat, 2242, 2776
Miller, Patte, 6939
Miller, Peggy, 5490
Miller, Ralph E, 2348
Miller, Rich, 6908
Miller, Robert, 869
Miller, Robert C, 2236
Miller, Robert W, 914
Miller, Ronnie, 7060

Miller, Russell, 2205
Miller, Sandra, 4240
Miller, Steve, 6949, 6950
Miller, Susan, 4187
Miller, Sydney, 651
Miller Casey, Donna, 4172
Miller Saunders, Rebecca, 1570
Miller-Michelson, Jonna, 3208
Millern, Greg, 3157
Milligan, Sharon, 2402
Millman, Howard J, 2732, 4364
Mills, Alicia, 1985
Mills, Alvin, 925
Mills, Bart, 5238
Mills, David, 2916, 3836
Mills, David A, 2451
Mills, David D, 5509
Mills, Gail, 4848
Mills, Grant, 1402
Mills, Kelley, 575
Mills, Michael M., 2283
Mills, Norma, 5142
Mills, Pamela, 2980, 4585
Mills, Stephen, 664
Milne, Dorothy, 2839
Milone Williams, Lucia, 3220
Milspaw, Roberts, 1741
Mimick, Ron, 1399
Mina, Manelo, 2713
Minadakis, Jasson, 5191
Minard, Deborah, 3640
Minasi, Mark, 5097
Mincey, Mike, 6727
Minde, Stefan, 1704
Minderman, Dean, 3191
Miner, Ellen, 6053
Mingo, Theresa, 407
Minner, DC, 5273
Minner, Selby, 5273
Minning, Gail, 324
Minst, Winthrop, 1272
Mintz, Gary, 6172
Mioi, Margaret M, 1502
Mirageas, Evans, 1264
Miranda, Michael, 4126
Miranda, Regina, 499
Mirich-Spear, Helene, 815
Mirikitani, Cora, 64
Mirrione, Jim, 3362
Mische, Erich, 7034
Mischel, Hal L, 6731
Misenheiner, Christa, 5146
Mishu, Fuad, 2298
Miskinis, Mark, 5350
Mitalis, Christina, 6354
Mitchell, Arthur, 461
Mitchell, Cheri, 586
Mitchell, CJ, 1121
Mitchell, Clyde, 1711
Mitchell, David, 2309
Mitchell, Donna, 3748
Mitchell, Elizabeth, 1000
Mitchell, Henry, 1586, 3023
Mitchell, Janet, 794, 796, 1899
Mitchell, Judith, 6420
Mitchell, Katherine, 1
Mitchell, Kathryn, 7969
Mitchell, Ken, 5151
Mitchell, Kevin, 4964
Mitchell, Michael, 3702
Mitchell, Michael D, 2275
Mitchell, Patricia, 832
Mitchell, Paul, 427
Mitchell, Roy, 6693
Mitchell, Rusty, 4001
Mitchell, Ruth, 259
Mitchell, Steve, 5805
Mitchell, Steven V, 635
Mitchell, Todd, 7091
Mitchell, Tom, 4735
Mitchell, Tracey E, 2005
Mitchelson, Bill, 3478

Mitchko, Janet, 2993
Mitchum, Cindy, 6399
Mittelman, Arnold, 2710
Mitze, Marnie, 6046
Mitze, Teri Solomon, 3992
Miura, Naoyuki, 5039
Mixon, Emily, 4771
Miyamura, Henry, 1089
Moats, Kyle, 6718
Moats, Maria L, 3683
Moats, Michael E, 3683
Mobley, Penne, 6788
Mocek, Rita, 3189
Moe, Karen, 3118
Moehlenkamp, Betty Sue, 5641
Moehring, Albert E, 1572
Moehring, Jim, 7612
Moehring, Patricia, 1572
Moeller, Laura, 4786
Moffat, Lynn, 3422
Moffatt, Michael, 2918
Moghrabi, Diana, 3557
Mohoney, Ruth, 1473
Mohylsky, Katherine, 1612
Molano, Alvaro, 367
Molden, Jennifer, 6632
Molina, Carlos, 1043
Molina, Jose, 491
Molinaro-Blonigan, Bryan, 6668
Mollicone, Henry, 827
Molloy, Honour, 3478
Molloy, Peggy, 258
Molnar, Jane, 2818
Molsen, Anita, 6174
Monaghan, Kate, 2656
Monaghan, Megan, 3145
Monahan, Julie, 2647
Monahan, Thomas P, 3754
Moncer, Anne S, 5719
Monchant, Jessica, 209
Moncrief, Clare, 2987, 4601
Monder, Steven, 1615, 5189
Monestere, Noralee, 915
Monetti, Marta, 7783
Monnier, Liz, 300
Monroe, Diane, 1008
Monroe, Jensen, 7329
Monroe, Kendyl K, 3395
Monroe, Mary, 4334
Monroe, Parker E, 894
Monroe, Polly, 1889
Monroe, Richard, 2116
Monroe, Robert, 2072
Monson, Judy, 1402
Montague, Gray, 533
Montana, Robert, 2064
Montanari, John, 4685
Montanaro, Tony, 6812
Monte, Bonnie J, 4883
Monte, Elisa, 474, 519
Monteith, James, 1450
Montejano, Vivian, 5533
Montera, Melissa, 4983, 7355
Montero, Lucia, 310
Montes, Lola, 40
Montes, Victoria, 173
Monteux, Claude, 1237
Monteux-Barendse, Nancie, 1237
Montfort, Matt, 43
Montgomery, Bob, 7039
Montgomery, Buddy, 862
Montgomery, Charla, 862
Montgomery, Chris, 5859
Montgomery, David, 862
Montgomery, Gary D, 4044
Montgomery, J Sherwood, 1933
Montgomery, Sara, 3705
Montier, Judith Service, 4388
Montoya, Rosa, 138
Monts, Lester, 2120, 4709
Montville, William, 1810
Moody, Dwain, 2353

Moody, Gloria N, 744
Moody, Joan, 4332
Moodyes, Robert, 764
Moon, Beata, 549
Moon, Jean F, 4646
Moon, Lee, 8321, 8324
Moon, Lisa, 611
Moon, Marjorie, 3294
Moon, Roger, 2954
Mooney, Kenneth, 3893
Mooney, Kevin, 2729
Mooney, Robert, 3441, 3474
Moore, Alan G, 1439
Moore, Benjamin, 3961
Moore, Brian, 3725
Moore, Charles R, 1788
Moore, Charlie, 3142
Moore, Chris, 6750
Moore, Connie, 6616
Moore, Dave, 1767, 6211
Moore, Dick, 4268
Moore, Douglas B, 1303
Moore, Dr Brain, 1397
Moore, Dr. Chet, 4164
Moore, Ezekial J, 4606
Moore, Faryce, 402
Moore, Heather, 3280
Moore, J Chris, 5250, 5251
Moore, James C, 3493
Moore, Jim, 4563
Moore, John, 2322, 4807, 7517
Moore, Judith, 1333
Moore, Karen E, 2110
Moore, Kathleen H, 722
Moore, Ken, 3660
Moore, Kevin, 3611
Moore, Linda G, 1150
Moore, Myrtle, 803
Moore, Rita, 1289
Moore, Sharon, 7549
Moore, Sharon D, 2016
Moore, Sharon Herr, 7552
Moore, Sonia, 3345
Moore, Thomas, 319
Moore, Thurston, 3785
Moore, Wiley, 2833
Moorer, Stephen, 4095, 4096
Moorhouse, Linda V, 1609, 1610
Moorman, Lisa, 8201
Moorman, Shaun W, 3575
Moots, Erin K, 3275
Moquin, Andrew, 5672
Moquin, George, 4643, 4644
Morales, Phoebe, 1669, 5270
Morales Matos, Jamie, 1643
Morales-Matos, Jamie, 1656
Moran, Ellen, 424
Moran, Eve, 2825
Moran, Jim, 3091
Moran, Lisa Dupaul, 697
Morant, Trente, 1925
Moravec, Dorothea, 1887
Morca, Teo, 220
Mordan, David, 1720
Mordaunt, Ninetter S, 3275
Mordine, Shirley, 277
Moreau, Donna, 3370
Moredock, George, 6276
Moreno, Rolando, 2713
Morer, Paul, 2441
Morey, Charles, 3885
Morgan, Ben, 2817
Morgan, Daniel, 698
Morgan, David L., 2919
Morgan, Deb & Jerry, 2941
Morgan, Eli, 6058
Morgan, Ian, 3414
Morgan, Jim, 78, 1861, 3480
Morgan, Marjorie, 3042
Morgan, Michael, 861, 863, 882
Morgan, Rhoan, 3318
Morgan, Robin, 139

Morgan, Tammy, 3892
Morgan, Victoria, 579
Morganstern, Shirley, 1604
Morgenstern, Gil, 5108
Morgenstern, Sheldon, 5129
Moriarty, John, 1963
Moricz, Michael, 635
Morin, Lindsey, 2460
Morise, Kristina, 957
Moroney, Ross, 5538
Morphet, Tom, 4030
Morr, Judy, 5961
Morrell, Gareth, 2258
Morrelli, Marietta, 2636
Morrill, Dr. Michael J, 1215
Morrill, Pamela, 1306
Morris, Aaron, 226
Morris, B Matt, 5433
Morris, Bonnie, 3136
Morris, Brad, 6609
Morris, Charlotte, 5313
Morris, Clark, 4795
Morris, Dave, 3597
Morris, David, 3511
Morris, Dr. Calvin, 2824
Morris, Duane, 7136
Morris, Enoch, 7121
Morris, Eric, 2967
Morris, Ginger, 3804
Morris, Heather, 5880
Morris, Jeannine, 5255
Morris, Jennifer, 8381
Morris, Jeremiah, 2469
Morris, Jeremy M, 3102
Morris, Jim, 4690
Morris, Justine, 5787
Morris, Ken, 1074, 2309
Morris, Mark, 405
Morris, Marley, 2566
Morris, Millie, 3698
Morris, Pat, 703
Morris, Sandy, 1368
Morris, Susan Waring, 3475
Morris, Terry, 2042
Morris, WS, 5541
Morrison, Chris, 1407
Morrison, Cynthia, 1843
Morrison, Fred, 1117
Morrison, Lawan, 713
Morrison, Marcia K, 4929
Morrison, Sandy, 4350
Morrison, Sarah, 584
Morrison, Scott, 379
Morrison, Sharon, 3962
Morrison, William L., 1045
Morrissey, Charles, 2292
Morrissey, Kahtleen, 7131
Morrissey, Michael, 5784
Morse, Gretchen, 1333
Morse, Steve, 3112
Morss, Anthony, 2172
Mortan, MD, William, 5920
Morten, Ivonne, 2699
Mortensen, Joann, 4047
Mortensen, Robert E, 2283
Mortimer, Glenn, 990
Morton, Bill, 5920
Morton, Dr. Paul, 4591, 4596
Morton, Ivory X, 6110
Morton, Mae, 2878
Morton, Paul, 4592
Morton, Susan M, 1081
Morton, Virginia D, 2114
Morton, Wyant, 4221
Mosakowski, Susan, 3361
Mosce, Diane, 2402
Moscone, Jonathan, 4084
Moseley, Charles, 7247
Moseley, Chuck, 3561
Moser, Chris, 2766, 5334
Moser, Paul, 597
Moses, Jane, 629

Moses, John, 2749
Moses, Jon, 2940
Moses, Jon R, 6418
Mosey, Susan, 4719
Mosher, Mala Yee, 3472
Moshtaghi, Eleni, 691
Mosier, Cj, 6226
Mosier, Diane K, 34
Mosier, Diane K, 4105
Mosler, Diane K, 4105
Mosley, Alta, 6392
Mosley, Dr. Loma, 5709
Mosley, Dr. Loma L, 1855
Mosley, George, 1196
Moss, Dean, 498
Moss, Robert, 3510
Moss, Sam, 244
Moss, Sandy, 4046
Moss, Vanessa, 1116
Mossbrucker, Tom, 392, 394
Mostaroy, Marc, 5343
Mostovoy, Marc, 1729
Mote, Tonya, 2593
Moudy, Amy, 2014
Mouledoux, John, 2400
Moultan, Stuart, 3804
Mouser, Elizabeth, 3751
Mouwad, Jerry, 3488
Mowbray, Maria, 1115
Moxley, Noel, 1857
Moye, Darrell, 3065
Moye, Stacie, 3065
Moyer, Dr. Brigitte, 4082
Moyer, Lavinia, 3091
Moynihan, Mike, 3994
Moyse, Blanche Honegge, 2329
Mucci, Michael, 1268
Mudd, Tom, 2973
Mueller, Ivan, 1635
Mueller, Jim, 3980
Mueller, Karen, 1321
Mueller, Katrina, 5846
Mueller, Midge, 5289
Mueller, Paul, 2226
Mueller, Paul F, 1972
Mueller, Renee, 6482
Mueller Grace, Elizabeth, 4249
Muir, Diane L, 233
Muirhead, Janice, 2647
Mulcahy, Bob, 7234
Mulder, Joan, 6965
Mulderick, Ed, 1230
Mulgrew, Anne-Marie, 627
Mulholland, Dana, 6798
Mulka, Dr. John S, 5318
Mullane, Susan, 5631
Mullen, Betty H, 1862
Mullen, Dennis, 162
Mullen, Gina, 4661
Mullen, Rick, 6677
Mullen, William, 4918
Mullenberg, Bettie, 2416
Muller, Elly, 6853
Muller, Jennifer, 485
Mullholland, Michelle, 144
Mullich, Elizabeth, 1159
Mulligan, David A, 3956
Mullins, Dora M, 1839
Mullins, John, 2168
Mulroney, Jack, 2280
Mulroney, John P, 2281
Muncaster, Carol Anne, 103
Mundiler, Janine, 5988
Mundinger, John, 1390
Mundwiler, Janine, 4113
Muni, Nicholas, 5190
Munilasis, Nicholas, 2257
Munkittrick, Alain, 2618
Munn, Charles, 5453
Munn, Susan, 1176
Munoz, Oliver, 14
Munoz, Roberto, 635
Munro, Pat, 3214

Munroe, Shirley Ann, 1450
Munsell, Robert, 1005
Munson, John, 2847
Munson, William G, 7456
Munt, Maxine, 2584
Muntean, Rick, 7816
Mura, Debbie, 3247, 4881
Murdoch, Alexandra, 2886
Murdoch, Colin, 900, 4182
Murdock, Christine, 5458
Murdock, Colleen, 4707
Murphey, Margaret Anne, 1368
Murphree, Marie, 2158
Murphy, Amy L, 3678
Murphy, Brad, 7136
Murphy, Dan, 3676, 6881
Murphy, David, 2385
Murphy, Donix, 2665
Murphy, Donna, 2112
Murphy, Elizabeth, 568, 3248
Murphy, Gary, 1916
Murphy, Hugh, 433
Murphy, J Austin, 2294
Murphy, Mark, 7341
Murphy, Michael G, 1935
Murphy, Robert, 1147, 4484
Murphy, Robyn, 2956
Murphy, Tim, 7973, 8197
Murphy, Vincent, 2776
Murray, Amy, 7650
Murray, Ann, 4435, 6683
Murray, Barbara, 2548
Murray, Bruce, 4024
Murray, Chris, 1236, 4613
Murray, Cope, 3238
Murray, Gibbs, 3239
Murray, Jon, 2649
Murray, Kathleen, 373
Murray, Kevin, 3912
Murray, Krista, 4553
Murray, Lindsay, 6182
Murray, Michael, 3075
Murray, Raymond, 1066
Murray, Rich, 8168
Murray, Robert, 4578
Murray III, James, 1374
Murrow, Gene, 1511
Muse, Mary, 7144
Musgrave, Suzanne, 5659
Music, Lyn, 5880
Muspratt, Kirk, 1178
Musselman, Sean, 235
Musser, Margaret, 4735
Musson, Renee, 6350
Must, Miriam, 3146
Muszynski, Michael, 1068
Muti, Lorenzo, 1589, 2250
Muze, Barbara, 4322
Mwanger, Mary, 2402
Myatttt, Jonathon N, 1934
Myer, Linda, 3076
Myers, Bob, 2959
Myers, C William, 233
Myers, Carolyn, 2914
Myers, Clair, 3696
Myers, Don L, 4972
Myers, Dr. Gerald E, 5117
Myers, Ed, 5215
Myers, Gerald, 8082
Myers, Ginny, 4060
Myers, Holly I, 2870
Myers, Ken, 1962, 3660
Myers, Kenneth, 1961
Myers, Kevin, 78
Myers, Lois, 2904
Myers, Michael E, 2866
Myers, Michal, 134
Myers, Milton, 631
Myers, Rick, 2941
Myers, Robert, 4511
Myers, Steve, 392
Myers, Willie, 8316

Myers, Yvonne, 3522
Myers-Morgan, Pam, 3823
Myhre, Barbara, 2026
Myhre, Mona L, 769
Mylin, Rich, 5968, 6027, 6036
Myrls, Shirley, 3325

N

Nachtwey, Kathy, 1864
Nada, Sherif A, 2094
Nadeau, Joseph P, 2151
Nadel, Jim, 4217
Nadel, Sybil, 3427
Nadelman, Manny, 2190
Nadler, Paul, 1034
Nadzadi, Rebecca, 5712
Nafe, Rick, 6417
Nafziger, Kenneth, 5636, 5675
Nagano, Kent, 792, 1916
Nagashina, Jackie, 187
Nagelhout, Gary, 411
Nagle, Cynthia, 3285
Nagy, Martin W, 5252
Nahat, Dennis, 150
Nahulu, Nola A, 2023
Naiditch, Beverley, 1595, 2253
Nail, Nancy, 3180
Nair, Corinne, 8386
Nair, Garyth, 2182
Naishtat, Sandy, 611
Najar, Leo, 1339
Nakada, Ruth, 8354
Nakahara, Ron, 3427
Nakasians, Stacy, 644
Nally, Donald, 2281
Nance, Andrew, 2520
Nanko, Lorraine C, 2191
Nanna, Marylouise, 1466, 4941
Nanon, Patricia N, 3047
Narramore Moody, Gloria, 8444
Narver, Allison, 3954
Nash, Edward, 7245
Nash, Florence, 2246
Nash, Jennifer, 2503
Nash, Juanita, 4738
Nash, Mark, 3895
Nash, Royston, 1306
Nassicera, John, 5603
Nassif, Dr. S Joseph, 6422
Nassif, S Joseph, 2754
Nassif, PhD, S Joseph, 2753
Nassivera, John, 3896
Nataker, Leon, 1933
Natarajan, Meena, 3143
Nath, John W, 6696
Nations, Chris, 5880
Natochenny, Professor Lev, 4958
Natter, John T, 1880
Natter, Patricia, 2685
Nause, Allen, 3664
Navaroli, Al, 827
Navarro, Marge, 960
Nave, JL, 1224
Navias, Geoffrey, 3509
Nazzaro, Dennis, 976, 1969
Neace, Larry, 7658
Nead, Ben, 779
Neal, Gwendolyn, 4939
Neal, Susan, 3502
Neale, Alasdair, 903, 915, 4424
Near, Timothy, 2535
Neary, Paul, 735
Neblett, Wil, 2503
Nees, David, 5784
Neese, Linda, 6668
Neff, Larry, 892
Neff, Tina, 3633
Negley, Marvin, 4529
Negrete, Kim, 4112
Nehring, Larry, 3617, 5203

Neibaur, Sesan, 1098
Neidig, Rick, 1982
Neier, Yvette, 438
Neiger, Gary A, 6075
Neikrug, Marc, 4917
Neil, Terri, 4377
Neill, Jackie, 3244
Neilly, Adam, 1583
Neilson, Alan, 1588
Neilson, Margaret, 1382
Neiss, Edgar, 6434
Neisser, Judy, 1121
Neisser, Judys, 2846, 4440
Nelson, Chrissy, 177
Nelson, Christine, 3142
Nelson, David, 1391
Nelson, Eleanor, 1304
Nelson, Esther, 2197
Nelson, Geoffrey, 3599
Nelson, Gwen W, 3106
Nelson, Janice, 2991
Nelson, Jennifer L, 2657
Nelson, Lindsey, 4114
Nelson, Lisa, 7830
Nelson, Madeline, 2044
Nelson, Mary Ann, 2186
Nelson, Michael A, 1931
Nelson, Pamela, 5742
Nelson, Paul, 5608
Nelson, Rose, 2533
Nelson, Ross, 2435
Nelson, Sandie, 3930
Nelson, Willie, 6397
Nelson, Winnie, 3815
Nelson Nash, Denise, 4155, 6069
Nemac, Lucy, 4174
Nemec, Chris, 2299
Nemeth, Grey, 2281
Nemeth, Lynne, 4646
Nemiroff, Steve, 4874, 7216
Nerenhausen, Mark, 6335
Ness, Mildred, 390
Nestor, Erin, 719
Nestvold, Karen, 1849
Nethercott, Robert, 3286
Netherton, Nancy, 4073
Netter, D Terence, 4336
Neu, Georgia, 3225
Neu, Robert R, 1353
Neubauer, Brenda, 4776
Neuberger, Emily, 2871
Neuchterlein, Dot, 2061
Neuert, Natalie, 5602
Neufeld, Ken, 3304
Neujahr, James, 1864
Neumann, Frederick, 3401
Neumann, Michael, 883
Neumever, Josh, 3589
Neuon, Donald, 1901
Neustadter, Kathryn, 4149
Neustein, Robin, 423
Neuzel, Larry, 309
Nevarez, Glenda, 3837
Nevenschwander, Janet, 3875
Neville-Andrews, John, 4735
Nevins, E. Marc, 285
Nevins, BA, Rhoda, 4180
Nevitt, Cindy, 2908
Nevola, Gabriel, 1416
New, Lea, 3660
New, Sherry, 9
Newberg, Joan, 4172
Newberger, Sheri, 1443
Newberry, Bill, 3841
Newberry, Susan, 5149
Newcastle, Mimi, 4303
Newcomb, Garlan, 5334
Newcomb, Janet, 4948
Newcomb, Kenneth, 7247
Newcomb, Lynn, 2300
Newcomer, Lee, 6520
Newell, Beck, 3207

Newell, Charles, 2828
Newell, Douglas, 1667
Newell, Lloyd, 2325
Newell, Marylaide, 4332
Newell, Ron, 3597
Newland, Julie, 2045
Newlin, Helen, 1370
Newlin, James C, 573
Newman, Carole K, 535
Newman, Fred, 3357
Newman, Jennifer, 395
Newman, Jow, 2916
Newman, Judith, 228
Newman, Michael, 4891
Newman, Nancy, 7828
Newman, Rosalind, 459
Newman, Stacey, 1795
Newman, Suzanne F, 1081
Newport, Bari, 2695
Newsom, Jon, 4311
Newson, Dr. Mary Ellen, 1166
Newton, Bill, 6918
Newton, CM, 6713, 6718
Newton, Roger, 6376
Neyman, Rob, 5877
Ng, Kok-Koon, 1153
Nibley, Robert M., 1702
Nice, Carter, 4081
Nicholas, Diane, 1377
Nicholas, Stephanie, 7728
Nichols, G Arwen, 3968
Nichols, Jackie, 3786, 3788
Nichols, Jason, 5419
Nichols, Jellymmeison, 964
Nichols, Lan, 5158
Nichols, Lynn, 2578, 4236
Nichols, Nick, 6129
Nichols, Terry, 2448
Nichols, Trey, 2445
Nichols, Wade, 3338
Nichols, II, Humphrey T., 974
Nichols-Kitchell, Cindy, 99, 2489
Nicholson, Dr. Barbara, 7646
Nicholson, Melanie A., 3254
Nicholson, Paul, 3651, 5285
Nicholson, Jr, Norman C, 4662
Nickel, Jerri, 3868
Nickle, Scott, 6828
Nickles, Larry, 3214
Nickols, Beverly, 7120
Nicks, Lisa, 470
Nicola, James C, 3422
Nics, Helen, 876
Niebauer, Joyce, 5327
Niederberg, Richard, 2564
Niehaus, Patricia J, 2157
Niehaus, Tim, 5735
Niekrasz, Virginia L, 32
Nielson, Abe, 7753
Niemann, John, 5902
Niemann, Tom, 4710
Nienhouse, Brenda S, 4730
Nierenberg, Roger, 997
Niesen, Jim, 3388
Niessner, Madelyn, 1419
Nile, Jamie, 7297
Niles, Barb, 776
Niles, Nicholas H, 1711
Nilsen, Andrea, 8289, 8290
Nilsen, Janis, 5129
Nimcham, Teresa, 1804
Nirenberg, Ken, 2695
Nisbet, Wyck, 2383
Nishikawa, Lane, 2513
Nishimuta, Tracy, 818
Nissien, Mikko, 328
Nitsch, Paul, 1574
Nitter, Susanne, 3037
Niven, Doug, 2997
Nixa, Diane, 7232
Nixon, Darryl, 883
Nixon, David, 585

Nixon, Kay, 608
Nixon, Pennie, 883
Nizer, Mark, 8431
Noack, Lori, 1708, 5309
Noah, Libby, 3564, 7253
Noah, Mike, 6840
Nobbe, PhD, Stephan, 7391
Noble, Bree, 1951
Noble, Gail, 588
Noble, Sherri, 6367
Nocek, Bob, 7862
Nocera, Mia, 641
Nocks, Nancy S, 3608
Nocks, Ronald E, 3608
Nocon, Nannette, 3493
Nodal, Adolfo, 4123
Nodler, Jason, 3856
Noe, Kevin, 1739
Noel, Buddy, 181
Noel, Craig, 2499
Noel Fiorino, Paul, 180
Noerr, Beverly, 4165
Nofziger, Sarah, 720
Nolan, Carl J, 3246
Nolan, Keith, 430
Nolan, Richard P, 7643
Nolan, Victoria, 2625
Nolan-Long, Clare, 2818
Noland, Lynn, 2978
Nolen, Terrence J, 3678
Noll, William, 2017
Nolte, Alicia, 360
Nolte, Carol, 458
Nolte, Pamela, 3962
Nolte, Scott, 3962
Noltemy, Kim, 1262
Noon, Rosemary, 6903
Noonan, Ed, 7143
Norcdahl, Sandy, 6641
Nordcum, Samuel, 865
Nordeen, Kate, 4725
Nordgren, Carol, 987, 4276
Nordstrom, Harry, 4764
Noren-Iacovino, Mary-Jo P., 2232
Norfleet, James, 3254
Norlander, Angela, 2547
Norman, Beth, 3176
Norman, Jeffrey, 7232
Noroian, Sharyl, 2111
Norris, Lynet, 3137
Norris II, Harold, 463
North, Carol, 3189
North, Mark, 4521, 6636
North, Moira, 482
Northcutt, Tim, 1171
Northrup, Pam, 3924
Northway, JD, 825
Norton, Ann, 2670
Norton, Candace, 1582
Norton, David, 1818
Norton, Dennis, 3698, 5462
Norton, John, 3918
Norton, Laura, 4031
Norton, Peter, 3448
Norton, Rachel, 3472
Norwood, Philip W, 2245
Notara, Darrell, 638
Notara, Sally, 638
Noteboom, Lowell J, 1362
Nothnagle Reese, Margaret, 6663
Nottage, James, 6605
Nottingham, Sue, 4823
Notz, Joanne, 2857
Nova, Giuseppe, 4163
Novak, Dan, 2037
Novak, Mary, 1873
Novo, Celia, 8407
Novoa, Tony, 5556
Novoil, Jennifer, 679
Novosel, John, 6495
Nowak, Michael, 913
Nowaker, Jr, Edward J, 847

Nowell, Sean, 3354
Nowers, Roy, 6643, 6644, 6645
Nowytski, Natalie, 351
Noyalas, Christy, 7837
Noyes, David, 1376
Noyes, Roger, 5987
Ntiri, Dr. Daphne W, 4722
Nugent, Virgina, 3159
Nunes, Alycs M, 808
Nurasz, Huroco, 3428
Nusbaum, Alan S, 3340
Nussbaum, Jeff, 5024
Nussdorfer, David, 1333
Nutt, Patricia, 1045
Nutter, Bill, 7248
Nuzzolo, Laura, 5100
Nyheim, John A, 2277
Nyman, Brent, 2323
Nys, Jim, 7143

O

O'Brian, Mary Beth, 2942
O'Brien, Jack, 2499
O'Brien, James P, 5874
O'Brien, Keith, 1461
O'Brien, Kevin J, 6122
O'Brien, Mary Beth, 2942, 6668
O'Brien, Nancy, 1291
O'Brien, Peggy, 3189
O'Brien, Ron, 6487
O'Brien, Terrence, 3307, 4944
O'Brien, Tom, 6874
O'Brien, III, James F, 3089
O'Bryan, Michelle, 187
O'Connell, Daniel, 7700
O'Connell, Dennis, 3573
O'Connell, Jim, 5783
O'Connell, Peter, 3309
O'Connell, Rev. Dianne, 2363
O'Connell, Richard, 2866
O'Connell, Timothy J, 7660
O'Conner, Linda, 1983
O'Conner, Ron, 3337
O'Connor, Jerry P, 3882
O'Connor, Jim, 2933
O'Connor, Tom, 1452
O'Dell, David, 2345
O'Dell, Susan, 1522
O'Donnell, Gail, 2654
O'Donnell, James, 4838
O'Donnell, James F, 3191
O'Donnell, Jane, 812, 4098
O'Donnell, Lois, 2063
O'Donnell, Rich, 1378, 4803
O'Donovan, Brian, 2114
O'Grady, Brian, 6905
O'Hagan, John, 2805
O'Hara, Dennis, 1229
O'Hara, Kathleen, 144
O'Hara, Michele, 616
O'Keefe, Claudia, 3973
O'Leary, E Colin, 3359, 7380
O'Leary, Sr. Michele, 3730
O'Malley, Bill, 1142
O'Malley, Peter, 3007
O'Malley III, Charles A, 989
O'Neal, Dennis, 3220
O'Neal, Hank, 501
O'Neal, John, 2984
O'Neal, Judi, 4008
O'Neal, Judy, 1883
O'Neal, Steve, 7101
O'Neil, James, 4619
O'Neil, Kathleen, 179
O'Neil Frank, Molly, 3448
O'Neill, Dick, 2982
O'Neill, Scott, 1826
O'Neill, Vincent, 3299
O'Neill, PhD, Rosary H, 2988
O'Neill-Butler, Marjorie, 3899

O'Neill-Butler, Robert, 3899
O'Niel, Craig, 6399
O'Reilly, Anita, 3021
O'Reilly, Terry, 3401
O'Rourke-Smith, BJ, 2416
O'Shaughnessy, Ferris, 1115
O'Shaughnessy, Harry, 7335
O'Shaughnessy, Paul, 3054
O'Sullivan, Susan, 2565
Oakes, Carlton, 6489, 6490
Oakes, Yvette, 3875
Oakley, Kirsten, 26
Oberfelder, Jody, 487
Oberg, David, 1446
Oberheu, Jerry, 6668
Oberman, Gabriel, 2801
Oberrecht, Becky, 1884
Oberschelp, Deborah, 2031
Obuchowski, Sara, 929
Ochs, Carol, 3334
Odegard, Dale, 7906
Odom, Dr. Gale, 4603
Oek, Robert, 3048, 6875
Oelker, Kity, 6371
Oesch, Michael, 3631
Offerman, Patricia, 3241
Officer, Lisa C, 1384
Offut, Treva, 498
Offutt, Treba, 7400
Ogle, James, 1096
Oglesby, Donald, 1029, 4323
Ohlsen, Miki, 642
Ohnmacht, Mark W, 1984
Ohyama, Heiichiro, 919
Oien, Fred, 7904
Okashiro, Chitose, 1530, 5044
Okeru, Maury, 349
Oki, Lauie, 3959
Okun, Maury, 1341, 4748
Olah, Janos Zsolt, 25
Olan, Ben, 2451
Olans, Stephen, 1622, 4064
Olans, Steven A, 1411
Olbrich, Tom, 7747
Oldfield, Jane, 6545
Oldham, Barbara, 1531
Oldham, Sandy, 1161
Oldham, Susanne, 6299
Oldham Jr, Kenneth A, 1020
Oldis, Patricia, 3565
Olds, Dirk, 2189
Oler, Lee, 776
Oliansky, Patricia, 823
Olin, Matt, 3528
Oliver, Amy, 751
Oliver, Barbara, 2389
Oliver, Bill, 4582
Oliver, Kathryn, 1693
Oliver, Russ, 6358
Olivera, Pascal, 291
Oliverson, Cathy, 4207
Olivier, Larry, 1613
Ollis, Richard, 7119
Ollman, Sue, 1128
Olmstead, Laurie, 776
Olmsted, Daniel H, 1414
Olsen, Barb, 7141, 7142
Olsen, Barbara, 5763
Olsen, Beth, 328
Olsen, Carol, 763
Olsen, Jan, 1103
Olsen, Janeen, 3651, 5285
Olsen, Kathleen, 5075
Olsen, Kathy, 5074
Olsen, Lori, 6979
Olsen, Merritt, 3763, 3943
Olsen, Paul, 2224
Olsen, Rowena, 6685
Olsen, Tom, 8302
Olsen Potts, Kristen, 89
Olshan, Alan, 535
Olson, Carl, 1397

Olson, Danette, 5252
Olson, Dr. Robert, 969
Olson, Lance, 4886, 6857
Olson, Marina, 2942
Olson, Marne, 929
Olson, Michelle, 1677
Olson, Robert, 1375, 4234
Olson, Shirley, 7273
Olson, Todd, 3797
Olsson, Dr. Milton, 1329
Oltman, Dwight, 5177
Oludaja, Bayo, 4796
Oman, Norman, 2056
Omilami, Afemo, 2772
Omilami, Elizabeth, 2772
Omodt, Jeff, 858
Ondov, Nancy, 1451
One, Darryl, 855
Onorato, Sharon, 6908
Oorchard, Joseph, 975
Opertner, Geoffery, 4901
Opiela, Ellen, 3301
Oppenheim, Alyne, 77
Oquendo, Christi, 4470
Orange, Catherine B, 3008
Orange, Jr, Rodney, 3008
Orbach, Evelyn, 3114, 3115
Orbach, Pearl, 3114
Orchard, Joseph, 4674
Orchard, Robert J, 3040, 3041
Orcholski, Jim, 7942
Ordover, Jerald, 1465
Oresicovich, Mark S, 3975, 5723, 8270, 8271
Oreskovich, Mark, 8274
Oreskovick, Mark, 8270
Organisak, Paul, 329, 636
Orgel, Frank, 6425
Orgeron, Marie, 1225
Orkin, Milton, 1743
Orlando, Angelo A, 4872
Orlando, Richard T, 2534
Orloff, Carole, 1680, 5300
Ormai, Ted, 5349
Ormes, Vance, 3773
Orr, Asley, 1861
Orr, Carin, 3786
Orr, Terrence S, 635
Orrios, Angel Gil, 3508
Orscheln, Wayne, 6710
Orselli, Lisa, 4138
Orsillo, Mike, 3565
Ort, Don, 1786
Orthmann, Trevor, 1421
Ortmann, Jefferey, 2862
Ortner, Richard, 4657
Ortolano, David, 6195
Osborn, Eliot, 4284
Osborn, George D, 4987
Osborn, J Marshall, 2344
Osborn, Jack D, 3581
Osborn, Marilyn J, 1615
Osborn, Thomas, 820, 852
Osborne, Allan, 3562
Osborne, Bo, 3523
Osborne, David, 2124
Osborne, Donald E, 8344
Osborne, Doug, 1409
Osborne, Douglas, 1409
Osborne, Jay, 663
Oshust, Mike, 6438
Osinski, Michael, 2867
Ostapink, Marta, 4681
Ostberg, Ed, 1486, 4985
Ostby, Trudy, 1856
Ostling, Jr, Dr. Acton, 1217
Ostman, Jessica, 4769
Ostrander, Thomas W, 436
Ostrich, Lisa, 2336
Ostrom, Don M, 7340
Ostrow, Carol, 3351
Ostrow, Elizabeth, 1527
Ostrow, Maynard, 927

Oswald, David, 5765
Otake, Eiko, 472
Otake, Koma, 472
Otake, Miko, 541
Otrembiak, Randall, 4462
Ott, Mike, 1696
Ott, Sharon, 3961
Otten, Dave, 4341
Otteni, David, 5150
Ottman, Dwight, 1607
Otto, Ellen, 5171
Otto, Roberta J, 1295
Oumansky, Valentina, 74
Ovellet, Renee, 7428
Ovens, Dr. Douglas, 5312
Overton, Cindy Lee, 2730
Overton, David, 4739
Oviatt, Larry, 93
Ovitsky, Steven A., 5763
Owen, Dee, 3220
Owen, Jean, 1590
Owen, Michael, 337
Owen, Moris, 4831
Owen, William B, 2966, 6714
Owen Lyles, Desiree, 6733
Owener, Dr. Jean, 3026
Owens, Anne, 5851
Owens, Barbara D, 5126
Owens, Charles, 983, 4272
Owens, Haynes, 4
Owens, Judson H, 2390
Owens, Katherine, 3833
Owens, Mitchell, 1854
Owews, Jen, 2603
Oxton, Sara, 351
Ozawa, Seiji, 1264
Ozerman, Rhonda, 2252
Ozmun, Ralph, 3789

P

Paben, Mark Charles, 1846
Pabst, Michelle, 99, 2489
Pacana, Nicolas, 260
Pace, Annamaria, 8459
Pace, Richard A, 2232
Pacey, Jane, 1109
Pachecano, Sophia, 419
Pachella, Andriana, 2121
Paciorek, Larry Patch, 1624
Packard, Jill, 816
Packer, Mark E, 4873
Packer, Tina, 3055
Pacuba, Katherine, 446
Pacylowski, Anita, 652
Padula, Roberta, 2293
Padwe, Gerald, 1984
Paffrath, Mark, 5771
Pafumi, Debbie, 6896
Page, G Troy, 3556
Page, John, 5365
Page, Robert, 2286
Pagella, Heather, 2667
Pahnke, Amy, 698
Paige, Alvin, 4687
Painter, David Lee, 2809
Painter, Jan, 1967
Pak, Jung-Ho, 888
Paki, Lisa, 330
Palacios, Hector, 3508
Palao, Sally, 3486, 5061
Paleau, Regina, 7243
Palermo, James W, 4436
Palermo, Peter, 4198
Palin, JoDee, 3205
Palin, Meredith, 3456
Palleja-Vissicchio, Evelyn, 633
Palma, Michael, 3437
Palmbush, Steve, 5675
Palme, Natalie, 4663
Palmer, Barbara, 7100

Palmer, Bob, 8292
Palmer, Cathy, 5702
Palmer, David, 227
Palmer, John, 8234
Palmer, Lynn K, 3253
Palmer, Nicholas, 1221
Palmer, Nicolas, 1710
Palmer, Richard, 2161
Palmer, Stephen, 4744
Palmer, Susan, 8007
Palocz, Henry, 1556
Palrea, Mike, 6249
Palreiro, Donna, 7873
Paluch, Tom, 2139
Palumbo, Adrianne, 6896
Palumbo, Benjamin L, 4318
Pandolfi, Judy, 8493
Panella, Victoria, 3887
Panettalalt, Lisa, 6986
Panetti, Joan, 992, 4283
Panfel, Jillian C, 7414
Pangman, Marylee, 3506, 5089
PanGriff, Gabin, 2409
Panico, Stephanie, 6265
Panis, Alleluia, 127
Panitz, Harriet, 4636
Panky-Mebane, Deborah, 4633
Pannabecker, Jameser, 3026
Panoff, Kathleen, 5651
Pansch, Dave, 743
Pansch, Ralf, 6538
Pansky, Miroslav, 2343
Pantano, Mary, 3081
Pantazelos, Janice, 4433
Pantely, Harold J, 2630
Pantely, Susan P, 2630
Panttaja, Micki, 267
Paolin, Jack, 1419
Paones, Dr. Irwin, 4089
Papa, Phyllis, 374
Paparella, Lynn, 5614
Pape, LaVon, 3213
Papian, Sharon, 7040
Paponis, Dena M, 2444
Pappas, Gwen, 1353
Pappas, Harry, 6567
Pappas, Roberta, 4036
Pappas, Ted, 3732
Pappin, Diana, 1180
Paradis, Timothy, 4624
Paradise, Paul, 1427
Parch, Jerry, 3891
Pareles, Julie, 7306
Parent, Matthew, 3266
Parfet, RT, 6961
Parish, RJ, 3175
Parisi, Barbara, 3297
Parisi, Diane, 3885
Park, Tom, 2841
Park, Jr, John N, 1733
Parke, David, 6735
Parker, Alan, 2267
Parker, Carrie, 3117
Parker, Cheryl, 1051
Parker, Elizabeth C, 2208
Parker, Elwreta, 5272
Parker, Jim, 5825
Parker, Kathy, 4732
Parker, Keith, 2667
Parker, Larry D, 3276
Parker, Mark Edward, 2269, 3642
Parker, Scott, 1826
Parker, Scott J, 3524
Parker, Ted, 99, 2489
Parker, Tina, 3825
Parker-Bass, Harriet, 4424
Parker-Brass, Myran, 332
Parkhill, Barry, 8168
Parkhill, Tom, 3783
Parkhurst, John C, 3494
Parkinson, Coleridge, 1120
Parkinson, III, John, 498

Parkman, Pam, 1806
Parks, Demetrice, 6453
Parks, Gary, 749
Parks, Jeffrey A, 5316
Parks, Justin, 2402
Parks, Loretta J, 7268
Parks, Monica, 1522
Parks, T Gordon, 964
Parmelee, Bill, 3556
Parmerlee, Craig, 1170
Parnell, Rachel M, 1588
Parodi, Terri, 1079
Parolari, Kim, 6109
Parou, Debbie, 626
Parr, Grace M, 4921
Parr, Rick, 8032
Parran, Teeko, 2437
Parrella, Ellen, 4282
Parrella, Nancianne, 2179
Parrilla, Max, 3873
Parris, Miki, 2318
Parris-Bailey, Linda, 3781
Parrish, Debbie, 232
Parrish, Greg, 693
Parrish, Phyllis, 693
Parrone, Donna M, 3200
Parry, Greg, 2006
Parry, John, 6602
Parry, Jude, 2714
Parsonnet, Victor, 1430
Parsons, Anne, 528
Parsons, David, 533
Parsons, Estelle, 3340
Parsons, Jefff, 6333
Parsons, Joan, 4831
Parsons, John T, 1024, 1997
Partington, Rex, 3904
Partis, Jeanette, 1458
Partlon Strauss, Cathleen, 1169
Partridge, Allen, 2757
Partridge, Laura, 7993
Partusch, C Noelle, 6
Pascal Escher, Alice, 315
Pashigan, Kathy, 2367
Pasion, Rodney, 1924
Paskalian, Arlene, 8421
Paskoff, Arnold, 2081
Passalacqua, Dominic, 570
Pasternack, Barbara, 3465
Pasterneck, Michael, 3297
Pastilong, Ed, 8272
Pastrana, Jose, 7221
Pastreich, Michael, 1128
Pastrick, Nora Ann, 5358
Patacca, Pam, 7675
Patches, John I, 6804
Pate, Andy, 5538
Pate, Maldwyn, 497
Patel, Jamshed, 1874
Patenaude, Libby, 229
Paterson Mills, Grusha, 925
Patmon, Jr, Charles W, 2402
Patrelle, Frances, 464
Patrelle, Francis, 359
Patrick, Bob, 1895, 3507
Patrick, David, 2879
Patrick, Judy, 904
Patrick, Pamela, 1292, 4679, 4680
Patrick, Penny, 3803
Patrik, Janaki, 495
Patrone, Brian, 8488
Patrone, Edward N, 8488
Patt, Robert D, 7597
Patterson, Brandon, 573
Patterson, Camille, 3556
Patterson, Elizabeth C, 2110
Patterson, Greg, 4789
Patterson, Jan, 4676
Patterson, Karen, 3276
Patterson, Kraig, 5005
Patterson, Kurtne, 709
Patterson, Pat, 7710

Patterson, Richard, 4190
Patterson, Sarah, 3782
Patterson, Trinette, 1201
Patterson, Yole, 1419
Patton, Kirk, 5903
Patton, Maureen M, 5520
Patton, Phillip, 2960
Paukert, Karel, 5201
Paul, Andrew S, 3730
Paul, Christopher, 3072
Paul, Dorit S, 4506
Paul, Frank, 1715
Paul, James, 5287
Paul, Jessica, 2062
Paul, Jim, 8034
Paul, John, 5298
Paul, Karen, 1792
Paul, Pamela, 3336
Paul, Robert, 3591
Pauley, Kim R, 726
Pauley, Marlene, 1351
Paulin, Dorothy, 3490
Paulin, WM, 4146
Paulson, Thom, 4734
Pausher, Robert, 1459
Pautza, Sabin, 1432
Pavlacka, Ron, 286
Pavlik, Ann, 2784
Pawlowski, Roman, 1004
Paxson, H Douglas, 2281
Payant, V Robert, 1407
Payn, Dr. William A, 1587
Payne, Peggy Green, 1672
Payne, Thomas, 6670
Payne, Tony, 4486
Payson, Priscilla R, 202
Peace, Annalisa, 5557
Peace, Paula, 1071
Peacock, Margaret, 13, 788, 2381
Peak, Cynthia S, 366
Peakes, John, 3105
Peakes, Judith, 3105
Pear, Russ, 6718
Pearce, Mark, 3445
Pearce, Pelham G, 1963
Pearce, William, 1596
Pearlman, Cid, 172
Pearlman, Jeanne, 5377
Pearlman, Martin, 1271
Pearlman, Richard, 2037
Pearlman, Sondra, 3669
Pearson, Alexandra, 886, 4178
Pearson, Barry, 2042
Pearson, Karen, 858
Pearson, Norris A, 7492
Pearson, Raquel, 2485
Pearson, Ron, 5426
Pearson, Rose, 3841
Peart, Annette J, 4530
Pease, Jim, 767, 4050
Peceri, Michael, 1034
Pechar, Thomas, 6821
Peck, Michele, 7126
Peckett, Donna, 735
Peckumn, Debra, 4533
Pedaci, Brain, 3590
Pedersen, Leif-Ivar, 2339
Pederson, Steve, 7847, 7853
Peditto, Chris, 3384
Peditto, Paul, 3384
Pedretti, Michael, 3741
Pedretti, Michael A, 4875
Pedroso, Dr. Angelina, 2832
Peeling, Dianne, 3684
Peeples, Wiliam, 3552
Peer, Charles, 101, 2495
Peet, Nancy, 5078
Pegg, Valerie, 4733
Peierls, Ronald, 3489
Peiffer, Chris, 7691
Peiner, Jordan, 39
Peirez, David H, 1489

Peirson, Nathan, 2399
Pelc, Stanley, 540
Pell, Barry, 621
Pell, Jonathon, 2307
Pell, Robin, 447
Pellegrino, Lauren, 8431
Pellon, Karen, 5623
Pelloquin, Andrea, 5777
Pelster, Jolette M, 3176
Pelton, Darla, 7574
Peltz, Charles, 1478
Peluso, Ron, 3159
Pena, Mario, 3396
Penberthy, Beverly, 3425
Pence, Brad, 2520
Pendleton, Curtis, 912, 4202
Pendleton, Moses, 199
Penezic, Robert A., 933
Penfield, Jane, 1974
Penhoet, Stephen, 51
Penington, Gary, 6229
Penn, Dr. Pat, 2785
Penn, Laura, 3956
Pennewell, Karen, 3107
Pennington, Cyndee, 6403
Pennington, David, 8123
Penny, Anne, 2918
Penny, Jennifer, 368
Penny, Mary, 1953
Penovi, Cameron, 2690
Pensinger Witman, Kim, 2336
Penterman, Carol, 2300
Pentilla, Roy, 1333
Penway, Anne, 2039
Penza, Marie, 1554
Peoples, Nancy, 704
Peoples Halio, Marcia, 4296
Pepmueller, Calla Ann, 4909
Pepper, Cam, 7732
Peraino, Dan, 8384
Percival, Jon, 7890
Pereira, Tony, 8234
Perez, Fernando, 3859
Perez, Jorge D, 2832
Perez, Rudy, 72
Perez, Sandra, 2685
Pergament, Lori, 639
Pergolizzi, Frank, 6749
Perick, Christof, 1573
Perillo, James E, 6265
Perkins, Cecil, 7743
Perkins, David, 2818
Perkins, Jerry R, 5465
Perkins, Lew, 6278
Perkovich, Lori, 59, 8336
Perlman, Nancy, 474
Perlo, Carla, 209
Perloff, Carey, 2509
Perlstein, George, 1110
Perman, Gerald, 1992
Pernetti, Gina, 103
Perreca, Michael, 3329
Perreovlt, Mark, 1291
Perret, Peter, 1595, 2253
Perrin, Ben, 5498
Perrin, Gregory, 2303
Perry, Byron W, 3322
Perry, Dan, 2696
Perry, David R, 3954
Perry, Glenn C, 4198
Perry, Jacqueline, 1366
Perry, Jess, 1941
Perry, Joan, 1864
Perry, Margaret, 667
Perry, Martina, 1465
Perry, Paul, 4036, 4144
Perry, Randall, 5343
Perry, Robert, 424
Perry, Shaunielle, 3411
Persico, Denise, 4872
Person, Garth, 2816
Persson, Diane, 1176

Reichlin, Louise, 60, 68
Reicin, Edward C, 2044
Reid, Alice, 412
Reid, Ann, 1458
Reid, Beverly, 1174
Reid, Charles, 3838
Reid, Clark, 311
Reid, Jim, 8199
Reid, Karen, 6574
Reid, Larry, 4039
Reid, Nancyen, 1841
Reid, Rufus, 4906, 4907
Reifel, Charles, 1019
Reifsnyder, David, 6581
Reilly, Elizabeth, 2413
Reilly, Judith, 4933
Reilly, Katharine, 3883
Reilly, Lisa, 7478
Reilly, Shannon, 6693
Reilly, Teresa, 295, 2897
Reiman, Sue Ellen, 3636
Reinach, Richard, 7943
Reineccius, Richard, 2516
Reinecke, Virginia, 4639
Reines, M Seth, 2893
Reing, Tom, 3721
Reinhard, Johnny, 4996
Reinhart, Charles, 5117
Reinhart, Julia, 2234
Reinhart, Marylinn, 6592
Reinhart, Stephanie, 5117
Reinhold, Donald, 5792
Reinis, Hillary, 3577
Reinis, Jonathan, 3577
Reinmiller, George C, 1702
Reinschmidt, Laura, 360
Reinschmidt, Matthew, 360
Reiser-Memmer, Michelle, 4943
Reisinger, Laura, 3989
Reiss, Anne, 3262, 3263, 4896
Reiss, Scott, 1833
Reissig, Shirley, 6685
Reiter, Fran, 3420
Reiter, Linda, 2853
Reither, Pat, 5705
Reitmair, Dawn, 964
Rejto, Peter, 782, 4057
Relyea, Deanna, 6911
Remaly, Glad, 4717
Remington, Greg, 7264, 7266
Remmel, Lee, 8283
Remond, Jim, 1624
Renal, Celia, 1980
Renberg, Julie, 4807
Rende, Carol, 1012
Rendon, III, Nicholas, 162
Renehan, M Smokey, 5877
Renick, Kyle, 3479
Renkopf, Brian, 6440
Renner, Daniel, 2592
Rennich, Christen, 7911
Rennick, Dean, 8302
Rennie, Lorraine, 249
Rennie, Thomas, 703
Reno, Rick, 6714
Renz, Frederick, 1511, 2211
Renz, Kim Edward, 5448
Rernington, Ralph, 2664
Rescia, Richard R, 2102
Retenbach, Paul R., 3091
Retrum, Jo Jean, 742
Rettman, Zeke, 2413
Reuhl, Doug, 1868
Reuing, Johnathan, 3370
Reuler, Jack, 3142
Reuss, David, 7495
Reuter, Laurel, 5167
Reuter, Paul, 7114
Reutlinger, Sally, 3286
Reuymer, Leslieen, 300
Revel, Darrell, 2349
Reveles, Nicolas M, 1935

Revels, Jeff, 2720
Reverand, II, Cedric D, 5788
Revzen, Joel, 1473, 2103
Rexford, Heidi, 1710
Reyer, Jim, 4931
Reyes, Richard E, 3859
Reyes, Samuel, 628
Reynes, Roberta, 5088
Reynes, Wendy W., 1117
Reynolds, Andrea, 5191
Reynolds, Brett, 3481
Reynolds, Carla, 3813
Reynolds, Cindy, 3954
Reynolds, Clara, 7993
Reynolds, David, 447
Reynolds, Debbie, 5563
Reynolds, Dudley, 1
Reynolds, H. Robert, 1341
Reynolds, Henry, 4707
Reynolds, James, 7658
Reynolds, James B, 1615
Reynolds, Jeff, 7888
Reynolds, Jennifer, 202
Reynolds, Kurt, 2861
Reynolds, Molly, 2453
Reynolds, Noreenor, 338
Reynolds, Patrick, 1641
Reynolds, Phil, 272
Reynolds, Rina, 2159
Reznik, Todd, 41
Reznikov, Hanon, 3400
Rhamstine, John, 8231, 8235
Rhea, Martha, 4561
Rhee, Byung-Hyun, 1772
Rhine, Anthony, 6145
Rhodes, Amy, 8435
Rhodes, Cynthia, 965
Rhodes, David W, 4553
Rhodes, Kevin, 1298, 7758
Rhodes, Lawrence, 493
Rhodes, Marian, 7122
Rhodovi, Marilyn, 1242
Rhoton, Nick, 2759
Riazantsev, Vladimir, 134
Ribant, Alan, 3090
Ribeau, Dr. Sydney, 3575
Ribenborm, Myriam, 1029, 4323
Ricca, Bobbi, 2393
Riccardi, Gilda, 446
Ricci, Roberta, 2236
Ricciuti, Holly, 7380
Rice, Bobby, 5830
Rice, David, 4475
Rice, Ellis, 1404, 4842
Rice, Ernest, 4366
Rice, Homer, 6437
Rice, Keith W, 181
Rice, Martin R, 3561
Rice, Patton, 2149
Rice, Philip O, 1083
Rice, Shannon, 6914, 6915, 6916
Rich, Andrea, 4127
Rich, Craig, 582
Rich, Gayle, 2114
Rich, Geoffrey, 3414
Rich, Jeff, 585
Rich, Millie, 1289
Rich, Mimi, 2618
Rich, Nancy, 3551
Richard, Ellen, 3443
Richard, Julie, 5429
Richard, M John, 7232
Richard, Stephen, 2658
Richards, David, 2044
Richards, Dr. John, 1342
Richards, Dr. John K, 1696
Richards, Edward, 886, 4178
Richards, Evan, 1870
Richards, Innes, 1053
Richards, Innis, 927
Richards, James E, 1385
Richards, Jamie, 3372

Richards, Jeff, 3944, 6804
Richards, Judy, 7700
Richards, Martha, 3073
Richards, Mary P, 4296
Richardson, Catherine, 919
Richardson, Jenny, 6769
Richardson, Jon, 1659, 5858, 7522
Richardson, Leslie, 663
Richardson, Lynne, 3830
Richardson, Michael, 2380
Richardson, Sarah, 3809
Richardson, Steve, 3148
Richardson, Susan, 6636
Richardson, Tad, 8234
Richardson, W Mack, 1181
Richman, Frances S, 1874
Richman, Gerald W., 2220
Richman, James, 1785
Richman, Stephen E, 1873, 5763
Richmond, Barry Alan, 3460
Richmond, Grady Lee, 2429
Richmond, Rosemary, 4997
Richmond-Cullen, Dr. Catherine, 455
Richter, Al, 2696
Richter, Jaralee, 5751
Richter, Martha, 2696
Richter, Nicole, 82
Richter, Pat, 8293, 8294
Richter, Robert A, 4279
Rickbone, Catherine, 4550
Ricke, Alan, 6352
Ricks, Murray, 5505
Riddelll, Jean, 1987
Riddick, Deveaux, 703
Riddle, Jack, 2076
Riddle, Mary Ann, 3209
Ridenhour, Gail, 3776
Ridenour, Stacy, 1332
Rider, Rhonda, 4693
Rider, Wendell, 893, 4185
Ridley, Anthony, 3868
Ridout, Kyle, 6619
Ried, Cindy, 412
Riedel, David T., 2293
Riedling, Patrick, 2066
Riegel, Marcia, 2866
Riegel, Megan, 7894
Riehart, Ruth, 686
Riemann, Lyndie, 144
Rienecke, Wayne, 945
Ries, Renee C, 1843
Riesenbach Esq, E Gerald, 3722
Rigerman, Marilyn, 2684
Rigg S, Jaon, 632
Riggs, Bill, 1613
Riggs, Dr. Robert, 4778
Riggs, Dudley, 3164
Riggs, Tommy, 6691
Rigler, Denise, 5108
Riherd, Mark, 3362
Riker, Kathleen, 98
Rile, Joanne, 1719, 8486
Rile, John R, 8486
Rile, Jonh R, 8486
Rilette, Ryan, 2982
Riley, Brian, 3755
Riley, Dale, 683
Riley, Deborah, 209, 210
Riley, Emily, 2059
Riley, John L, 1454
Riley, Kate, 4004
Riley, Rebecca Hill, 1151
Riley, Richard, 4978
Riley, Sean, 144, 2529
Riley, Sharon, 8504
Rilley, Michael, 5210
Rilling, Helmuth, 1684, 5290
Rinaldi, Denise, 159, 4206
Rinaldi, Michele, 159, 4206
Rinaldo, Moon, 4208
Rinderknecht, Margarit, 843
Rindfleisch, Andrew, 1622

Root, Robert T, 2369
Roots, Desiree, 5650
Roper, Berry, 392
Roque, Jaime, 233
Rorie, Carolyun, 2141
Rosario, Burt, 2470
Rose, Celeste, 3655
Rose, JD, 7352
Rose, Jerome, 5033
Rose, Kathy, 496
Rose, Kevin, 7765
Rose, Laura Love, 644
Rose, Leslie, 6817
Rose, Mary, 3419
Rose, Michael, 5371
Rose, Peggy, 2524
Rose, Phyllis, 539
Rose, Richard, 3904
Rose, Zoe, 2164
Rosean, Christopher, 286
Roseland, Chad, 1182
Rosen, Freda, 428
Rosen, Ilene, 3369
Rosen, Ivy, 539
Rosen, Jenice, 799
Rosen, Michael, 8459
Rosen, Richard, 3874
Rosen, Robert, 3148
Rosen, Todd, 3351
Rosenbaum, Dr. Arthur, 1558
Rosenbaum, Edie, 2238
Rosenbaum, Harold, 2239
Rosenbaur, Edie, 2239
Rosenberg, Carol Weiss, 4516
Rosenberg, Joel, 395
Rosenberg, Lana Kay, 598
Rosenberg, Laura S, 787, 4068, 4069
Rosenberg, Lawrence, 16
Rosenberg, Michael S, 3369
Rosenberg, Pamela, 1944
Rosenberg, Richard, 787, 4068, 4069
Rosenberg, Robert C, 1463
Rosenberg, Steve, 5216
Rosenblum, Ann, 8402
Rosenblum, M Edgar, 3462
Rosenblum, Mark, 230
Rosenblum, Mark C, 1414
Rosenblum, Paul, 4983, 7355
Rosenbluth, Susan, 2442
Rosenboom, David, 939, 4223
Rosenbuam, Harold, 2238, 2240
Rosenfield, Jack, 3180
Rosenfield, Jim, 886, 4178
Rosenhagen, Lisa, 2597
Rosenholtz, Ellen, 7830
Rosenstock, Susan L, 1636
Rosenthal, Ann, 457, 8452
Rosenthal, Debbie, 4350
Rosenthal, Herbert, 145
Rosenthal, Judy, 2180
Rosenthal, Linda, 759
Rosenthal, Prue, 2120
Rosenthal, Richard I., 1711
Rosentnal, Pruuueu, 4709
Rosentrater, Jill, 6236
Rosetti, Patricia, 7855
Rosewall, Ellen, 8511
Roshchakovsky, Ksenia, 7636
Rosmarin, Annalisa, 4305
Rosoff, Robert B, 1478
Ross, Alice, 1488
Ross, Bertam, 512
Ross, Bruce, 4920
Ross, Cassie W, 1021
Ross, David, 7073
Ross, James, 6831
Ross, Jane Rooks, 1332
Ross, Jeanette, 1079
Ross, Jennifer, 144
Ross, John G, 1583
Ross, Keith, 3860
Ross, Leslie, 822

Ross, Michael, 2623, 3011
Ross, Mike, 4485, 6575
Ross, Murray, 6325
Ross, Nancy, 804, 4332
Ross, Robert, 4566
Ross, Terri, 3281
Ross, Tom, 2389, 3452, 5514
Ross, Zoraba Q, 7646
Rossall, Gina, 47
Rossberg, Karen, 7139
Rossi, Armand, 4270
Rossi, Bob, 6321
Rossi, Deborah C, 4334
Rossi, Lana, 882
Rossi, Richard Robert, 1111
Rossi-Copeland, Carolyn, 3395
Rossler, Jennifer, 6085
Rostan, Mark, 3561
Rote, Carey, 5494
Roth, Ari, 6311
Roth, Daryl, 3399
Roth, Don, 1381, 1958, 4230
Roth, Elizabeth, 8510
Roth, Judy, 1104
Roth, Mayda, 5385
Roth, Virginia, 1705
Rothaar, Sarah, 4518
Rothaar, Sarah C, 1183
Rothamer, Jill, 4446
Rothbard, Michael, 7347
Rothenberg, Michael G, 4993
Rothenberg, Sarah, 5526
Rothman, Carole, 3446
Rothman, George, 1507, 1532
Rothman, Greta, 3404
Rothman, Janlee, 1331
Rothman, Rob, 1030
Rothmann, Lola, 1645, 5172
Rothmann, MD, Bruce F, 1645
Rothrock, Leilani M, 1889
Rothschild, Luke, 4135
Rothsciller, Lisa, 2829
Rothstein, Sidney, 996, 1745
Rotman, Dr. Harold, 1567, 5103
Rottenberg, Herman, 419
Roucher, Jerry, 1062
Roudenbush, Cecilia, 4047
Rougeau, Weldon, 1115
Rouggieri, Alex, 1817
Roulette, Cindy L, 4170
Roundnev, Dmitri, 6522
Rouse, Allison, 4242
Rouse, Charles, 4868
Rouse, James J, 2658
Rouse, Terrie, 244
Roush, Philip S., 3194
Rousseau, Charles R, 6844
Rousselot, Doris, 1809, 2320
Routh, Paloma, 1889
Routt, Jean, 2623
Rowan, Jean, 3475
Rowe, Alan, 2330
Rowe, Bill, 7118
Rowe, Dan, 3238
Rowe, GF, 3920
Rowe, Ken, 5501
Rowe, Ray, 6667
Rowe, Tim, 7684
Rowell, Barry, 3337
Rowell, David, 3881
Rowen, Carol, 2469
Rowitz, Scott, 6209, 6219
Rowlette, Jeanne, 4707
Rowley, Hillary, 6329
Rowley, Wesley, 7548
Rowsey, RL, 2807
Roy, Cathy, 4874, 7216
Roy, Phyllis, 3050
Roy, Thomas, 3690
Royak, Jamie, 1934
Royall, Richard, 5552
Royall, Richard R, 8104

Royston, Bill, 5303
Rozin, Seth, 3721
Rubardt, Peter, 1053
Rubarth, Clara Jane, 2380
Ruben, Bruce, 2224
Rubenstein, Ed, 7891
Rubenstein, Eric, 2871
Rubenstein, Jerry G, 1731
Rubin, Anne K., 4707
Rubin, Holli, 2742
Rubin, Joanne, 2091
Rubin, Mark, 5191
Rubin, Scott, 6609
Rubin, Sylvia, 1435
Rubino, Caroline, 5101
Rubsam, Henning, 549
Rucciay, Fernando, 1433
Rudd, Wiss, 1797
Rude, Leslie, 1222
Rude, Ron, 5736
Ruderman, Marcia, 3033
Rudiakov, Ariel, 5607
Rudiakov, Michael, 5606
Rudie, Evelyn, 2551
Rudie, Robert, 5480
Rudley, Carolyn, 3973
Rudolph, Ellen, 7438
Rudsill, Guy, 2252
Rudy, Kippy, 3004
Ruen, David, 3125
Ruenzel, Neil, 991
Ruffer, Greg, 2003
Ruffin, Sylvester L., 3805, 5477
Rugolo, Edith, 801
Ruigomez, Christopher W, 1262
Ruiz, Cookie, 664
Ruiz, Kara, 8485
Ruiz, Victor, 3833
Rukark, Joel K, 3415
Rulfs, Marcia, 410
Rumley, Susan, 889
Rumohr, Floyd, 3295
Rumsey, Mark, 786
Rund, Robert, 4879, 7219
Rungis, Sniedze, 3104
Runice, Linda, 3217
Runnicles, Donald, 1073, 1944
Runyan, Daniel, 3104
Runyan, Dr. William, 962
Runyon, Marlene, 1192
Rupe, Robin, 1447
Rupp, Mark, 2914
Ruppenthal, Todd J, 2041
Ruscetti, Rosanna, 6306
Rush, David, 6696
Rush, John, 121
Rush, Sam, 3064
Rush, Stephen, 340
Rush, Tracey, 1195
Rushin, Dana, 1675
Rushton, Lia, 1
Ruskin, David, 754
Ruskin, Nicole, 3446
Rusnak, G. Alan, 2072
Rusnock, Joseph, 570
Russell, Anne, 1772
Russell, Anthony, 465
Russell, Ben, 7501
Russell, Bob, 3493
Russell, Dr. Timothy, 1639
Russell, Dr. William B., 2956
Russell, Francia, 718
Russell, Jill, 5017, 5026
Russell, Mark, 1878, 3510, 7425
Russell, Martin, 5017, 5026
Russell, Mary M, 6236
Russell, Paul, 2402
Russell, Peter, 1965
Russell, Richard, 1995, 5313
Russell, Sheryl, 2402
Russell, Steve, 1881
Russell, Tal, 4039

Russell, Timothy, 771
Russell, Vick, 6618
Russell, Vicki, 3170
Russell Jr, Robert R, 3754
Russenberger, Sally, 5286
Russo, John, 1610
Russo, Joseph, 1003
Russo, Robert, 7407
Russo, William, 3433
Rust, Catherine, 4878
Rutenberg, Peter, 1914
Ruth, Thomas, 808
Ruthenbeck, Lorin, 1349
Rutherford, Jody, 199
Rutherford, Mary J, 1671
Ruthven, Andrew, 3857
Rutkowski, Joan, 1953
Rutkowski, Rebecca, 877
Rutland, John, 1386
Ruttenberg, Stan, 4234
Rutter, Martha, 701
Ruvolo, Ally, 4821
Rux, Macksene, 5580
Ryan, Arthur E., 7232
Ryan, Benita, 1725
Ryan, Debbie, 8168
Ryan, Denise, 1158
Ryan, G Jeremiah, 3258, 3265
Ryan, George, 3255
Ryan, Grace, 1673
Ryan, Jamie, 7033
Ryan, Jim, 2423
Ryan, Judy, 3570, 7265
Ryan, Lawrence, 6272
Ryan, Nancy, 6683
Ryan, Vincent J, 8421
Rybak, Greg, 3158
Ryberg, William A, 1321
Ryder, Linda, 2150
Rylyk, Andrew, 701
Ryno, W Douglas, 8416
Rysczek, Michael, 2841
Rystrom, Nancye, 1351
Ryvkin, Valery, 1953

S

S Balliet, Franklin, 5311
S Jones, Rhett, 3748
Saadeh, Sean, 6106
Saar, David, 2373
Saario, Terry T., 1362
Sabatini, Jane, 1001
Sabella, Marilyn, 4423
Sabellico, Richard, 3391
Sabie, Jennyk, 311
Sabin, Phyllis B, 4740
Sabo, Jonathan, 4510
Sabota, Andrea, 8394
Sacarahs, Deborah, 7793
Sacharow, Lawrence, 3288
Sachs, Dana, 2605
Sachs, Joel, 5048
Sachs, Stephen, 2440
Sackett, Laurie, 3773
Sackett, Linda, 3616
Sacks, Ruth, 2332
Sackstein, Dr. Rosalina, 4348
Sadeh, Eitan, 829
Sadewhite, James, 1436
Sadlek, Lance, 6647
Sadler, Tom, 5880
Saetta, Mary Lou, 1455
Sagan, Nate, 5898
Sagawa, Susan, 5671
Sagisi, Sandra, 4413
Saglimbene, Andrea, 6933
Sagon, Patrica B, 1985
Saibel, Natalie, 2524
Saint, David, 3255
Saisselin, Numa, 7243

Saisselin, Numa C, 7479, 7480
Saker, James R, 4836
Saks, Toby, 5701
Saladrigas, Stephen, 6668
Salamone, Vincent, 7310
Salamun, Betty, 738
Salamunovich, Paul, 1915
Salascruz, Marisel, 367
Salazar, Daniel, 982
Salchow, William, 4967
Saldana, John, 2372
Salerno, Lee, 1304
Salimpout, Suhaila, 22
Salina, Sue, 3623
Salinas, Ben, 3813
Saline, Carol, 3722
Salisbury, Holly, 4574
Salisbury, Meredith P, 4977
Salisbury, Robert, 6190
Salmen, Sharyn, 963
Salomon, Frank, 5045, 8436
Salomon, Frank E, 1529
Salonen, Esa-Pekka, 849, 4114
Salovey, Todd, 4177
Salter, Johnathan, 1532
Saltzman, H Royce, 1684, 5290
Salvaggio-Walker, Sandie, 1582
Salzenstein, Alan, 2845
Salzer, Anne, 3236
Salzer, Deborah, 2502
Salzman, Jaquee, 4001
Salzman, Jeanne, 4886
Salzman, Marth, 773
Salzman, Tom, 2679
Salzwedel, Erik, 1579
Samardza, Catherine, 202
Samay, Lawrence R, 1720
Samborski, Craig, 7001
Sammis, III, Jesse F, 1829
Samoff, Marjorie, 3723
Sampite, Chris, 6767
Samson, Bruce, 1702
Samson, Suzanne, 1414
Samuel, Gail, 832, 849
Samuel, Tunde, 3410
Samuel, Wendy, 3366
Samuels, Janie, 1232
San Diego, Armando, 691
Sanchez, Grace, 4433
Sanchez, Mario Ernesto, 2713
Sanchez, Mark T, 1448
Sand, Barbara, 5696
Sand, Julia, 3140
Sandack, Susan, 697
Sandberg, Dr. Hershel, 1324
Sandek, Barbara, 3465
Sander Higgins, Stacey, 3252
Sanderling, Stefan, 1066
Sanders, Ann Meade, 1331
Sanders, Barry A, 849
Sanders, Donald T, 4681
Sanders, Dudley W, 2783
Sanders, Jamie, 289
Sanders, Jeanette, 564
Sanders, Jeffri, 773
Sanders, John, 6106
Sanders, Lynda, 5535
Sanders, Ron, 3663, 3666, 7773
Sanders, Wayne, 2229
Sanders, Wendy, 3304
Sanderson, Brian, 7026
Sandersr, Ron, 3668
Sandison, Norma J, 6908
Sandkamp, Anthony, 3435
Sandler, Deborah, 2066
Sandor, April, 3708
Sandoud, Liz, 2549
Sandoval, Gema, 174
Sandoval, Robbie, 7931
Sandretto Hull, Jennifer, 2532
Sandridge, Laura, 3557
Sands, Jr, Resita M, 1120

Sanferrare, Bob, 1300
Sanfilippo, Phyllis, 736
Sanford, Mike, 861
Sanford, Tim, 3433
Sankey, Jean, 1714
Sankovich, Dennis, 3629
Sankowich, Lee, 2463, 6182
Sanner, Laura, 5538
Sanner, Lois, 1126
Sannuto, John, 3297
Sansone, Laurie, 4893
Santa, Brock, 374
Santana, Carlota, 446
Santarelli, Marilyn, 7862
Santer, Don, 3568
Santiago, Joseph, 7175
Santo, Amen, 113
Santora, Mischa, 1613
Santora, Philip J, 2767, 4387
Santoro, Angelo, 1618
Santoro-Au, Lynette, 5253
Santos, Amy, 507
Santos, Charles, 3830
Santos, Jose, 162
Sanville, Guy, 3090
Sapp, Celia, 1882
Sara, Elizabeth C, 1990
Sarasvati, Bala, 242
Sarathy, Vijaya, 707
Saravati, Bala, 243
Sarch, Kenneth, 5354
Sardou Klein, Mitchell, 843
Sargent, Dean Peter, 7117
Sarmir, Patricia, 186
Sarver, David, 588
Saslav, Ann, 5550
Sasser, John, 2044
Sassi, Rebekah A, 3726
Sasso, Lauryn, 7868
Satchell, Reho, 631
Saternow, Pauline, 7700
Satisky, Marvin, 1027
Sato Ambush, Benny, 2513, 3927
Satrang Hoel, Roger, 2137, 2138
Satter, Michelle, 3888
Satterfield, Ann, 1039
Satterfield, Pamela, 744
Satz, Linda, 886, 4178
Sauage, James, 1333
Sauer, Sharonian, 2176
Sauers, Tim, 4447
Saul, Randal L, 1384
Saul, Tom, 2788
Saunders, Anne, 4285, 4288
Saunders, Bert, 807
Saunders, De Bare, 1001
Saunders, Denise D, 6303
Saunders, Jacqueline, 4150, 4151
Saunders, John, 8202
Saunders, Kevin J., 2014
Saunders, Shelley, 3959
Saunders, Steve, 4627
Saunders Grayson, June, 7517
Sauro, Karen, 3146
Sauter, David, 3101, 6956
Sauter, Tom, 1582
Savage, Laura Q, 1182
Savage, William U, 153
Savarise, Lyn, 7586
Savarise, Terry, 6531
Savathphoun, Friday, 2514
Savelson, Kenny, 5001
Saver, Susan, 1775
Savia, Alfred, 1048
Savod, Bob, 7516
Sawada, Shohei, 792
Sawallisch, Wolfgang, 1733
Sawnson, Jill K, 3805, 5477
Sawyer, A, 1337
Sawyer, Suzanne, 4012
Saxer, Robert J, 219
Saxon, Ellen, 4886

Saybrook, David, 2170
Sayles, Edward, 3286
Sayyad, Banafsheh, 175
Sberro, Joan, 2003
Scaglione, Louis, 1734
Scalamoni, Sam, 2995
Scales, Robert, 6045
Scales, Robert R, 2455
Scallen, Tom, 3138
Scanlon, Michael, 7249
Scannell, Cheryl, 701
Scarlata, Estela, 2433
Scarlato, Amy, 1147
Scartelli, Dr. Joe, 5648
Scavuzzo, Jennifer H, 1726
Scerbo, Richard, 6831
Schaack, Tom Van, 7488
Schacherbauer, Michael, 3614
Schackne, Dr. HM, 1630
Schaefer, Gary, 2978
Schaefer, Gretchen, 3922
Schaefer, John Paul, 2333
Schaefer, Matt, 1459
Schaeffer, Allison, 376
Schaeffer, Eric D, 3908
Schaeffer, Nancy, 3819
Schafer, Dr. Ronald E, 1717
Schaffer, Barbara, 2622
Schaffer, Karl, 164
Schaffer, Lois, 536
Schaffer, Sandra, 1073
Schaffhausen, Dick, 2928
Schairer, Laura, 1889
Schakel, Mary, 3100, 6953
Schaldweiler, John, 1117
Schalek, Marsha, 3568
Schalf, Jim, 6704
Schall, Karin, 3399
Schallig, Nicole, 2497
Schambelan, Ike, 3457
Schantz, Ellen, 1168
Schantz, Jack, 1624
Schanwald, Steve, 6531
Scharer, Fr. Dennis, 2050
Schario, Christopher, 2993
Scharres, John, 2055
Scharres, John H, 2899
Schattschneider, Dr. Adam J, 5179
Schatzlein, Dale, 354, 4759
Schaubert, Bethany J, 1160
Schaus, Susie, 3618
Scheele, Birgitte, 346
Scheele, Rebecca, 2132
Scheers, Amy, 358
Schehr, Kevin, 3202
Scheib, Charles W, 1233, 2075
Scheible, William, 1431
Scheibler, Kevin, 6921
Scheidler, Catherine, 3672
Scheidler, Martha, 6550
Scheil, Chuck, 3542
Schein, David, 2835
Scheinuk, Veronica Porteo, 2071
Schelhammer, Robert, 2730
Schelkopf, Mary M, 4826
Schelkopf, Mary M., 4826
Schell, Steve, 4334
Schempf, Kevin, 1608
Schendel, Kaye, 5774
Schenkman, Bryon, 1849
Schenly, Paul, 4954
Scher, Scott, 5697
Scherer, Danieele, 632
Schermerhorn, Elizabeth, 412
Schermerhorn, Kenneth, 1772
Schertzinger, Stephen, 3962
Schesiuk, Volodymyr, 1334
Scheuer, Walter, 535
Schickler, Peter, 2794
Schiele, Cheryl, 1461
Schieman, Sue, 1634
Schience, Jane, 5705

Schiffmacher, Jennifer, 2187
Schildcrout, Jordan, 3342
Schilke, Melissa Z, 2618
Schilling, Darren, 4115
Schilling, Falko, 3901
Schiosser, Leo, 7682
Schirle, Joan, 2393
Schirm, Ted, 2183, 2696
Schiro, Henry A, 907
Schisgall Currier, Lesley, 2541
Schlachter, Rosemary, 3584
Schlaker, Tom, 7127
Schlath, Raymond M, 3318
Schlefer, James R, 7379
Schlegel, Jane, 2919
Schlegel, Rudi, 1075
Schlei, Marlys, 189
Schleicher, Donald, 1189
Schlenker, John, 2474
Schleuse, Paul, 2214
Schloegel, Peggy, 1363
Schmechel, Dan V, 2145
Schmeling, Pete, 1865
Schmelzle, Alan, 7088
Schmid, Norbert, 8400
Schmid-Salm, Birgit, 8400
Schmidt, Anita, 1784
Schmidt, Bernard, 453, 516, 520, 525, 560
Schmidt, Bernard G, 519
Schmidt, Daniel, 4242
Schmidt, Gordon P, 344
Schmidt, Judy, 1920
Schmidt, M Judith, 3125
Schmidt, Marlene, 2604
Schmidt, Sarah, 3175
Schmidt, Stanley, 2161
Schmidt, Steven J, 1358, 4766
Schmitt, Keith, 4981
Schmitz, Linda Marty, 5755
Schmuck, Tobin, 2213
Schnabel, Tom, 4114
Schnake, Ken, 5212
Schneider, Bekki Jo, 2908
Schneider, Cindi, 1425
Schneider, Jack, 1949
Schneider, Mike, 6609
Schneider, Peggy, 1110
Schneider, Steve, 7085
Schnell, Anna, 7001
Schnell, Kim T, 1081
Schnepp, Mary, 885
Schnur, Joel, 2878
Schoeder, Collen, 1406
Schoedinger, Janet, 3189
Schoeffler, a Diane, 1710
Schoeffler, A. Diane, 1658
Schoen, Jerry, 326
Schoenberg, Deborah, 3037
Schoenbrun, Jodi, 3404
Schoephoerster, Kristin, 1351
Schofield, 1st Lt. Donald, 1009
Schofield, Christine, 5624
Schofield, Susan R.S., 446
Scholl, Dale, 100
Scholle, Mary, 3994
Scholze, Elizabeth, 2632
Schon, Robyn, 8201
Schonike, Scott, 7005
Schoof, RoseAnn, 55
Schoonover, Kevin, 7339
Schornbrun, Jody, 3471
Schors, Wendy, 2999
Schotten, Yizhak, 971
Schrade, Randolph RA, 4952
Schrade, Robert, 4952
Schrade, Robert W, 4952
Schrade, Rolande Y, 4952
Schrade, Rorianne C, 4952
Schrade-James, Robelyn, 4952
Schraff, Paul, 2796
Schraft, Micah, 3364
Schray, Alison Y, 5224

Schreiner, Bob, 1368
Schreiner, Craig, 737
Schrickel, William, 1352
Schroeder, Sue, 252
Schrub, Andre-Michel, 5129
Schubert, Barbara, 1124, 1132
Schubert, Barbara S, 577
Schubert OSFS, Gerard J, 3688
Schubert, OSFS, Gerard J, 5323
Schuessler, Nina, 3078
Schuland, Richard A, 7754
Schuldmann, Sanda, 981
Schuldmann, Sandra, 779
Schuler, Peg, 3434
Schuler Hint, Kristin, 1933
Schulfer, Roche, 2836
Schulingkamp, Miriam, 2982
Schulkind, Marcus, 331
Schull, Ronald K, 2967
Schuller, Gunther, 5706
Schulte, Erika, 1012
Schultz, Caron, 1388
Schultz, Dave, 6358
Schultz, J Bernard, 3975, 5723, 8271
Schultz, Lisa, 705
Schultz, Reverand Blaine, 4548
Schultz, Todd, 1935
Schulz, Eva, 2190
Schulz, Tom, 7136
Schulze, Dr. Otto, 1166
Schulze, Dr. Richard, 1166
Schulze, Theodora, 1166
Schumach, August, 1896
Schumacher, Bruce, 6609
Schumacher, Jane, 5415
Schumacher, Max B, 6609
Schumacher, Paul, 3167
Schumacher, Wesley John, 1067
Schuman Silver, Jo, 2527
Schumann, Laura E, 1652
Schurr, Carl, 3694
Schussel, Rick, 527
Schutt, Carl, 3694
Schutz, Michelle, 2100
Schutz, Will, 2829
Schwab, Cynthia H, 4787
Schwab, Sarah, 2346
Schwartz, Bob, 7826
Schwartz, Carol, 153
Schwartz, Carolyn, 1962
Schwartz, Dr. Daniel, 985
Schwartz, Ellen, 3509
Schwartz, Frederic W, 4441
Schwartz, Lilly, 7831
Schwartz, Melissa, 5877
Schwartz, Susan M, 1623
Schwartz, Tim, 2180
Schwarz, Eric, 4661
Schwarz, Gerard, 5037
Schwarz, Horace W, 1731
Schwarz, Mary, 5217
Schwei, Barbara, 112
Schweikand, Linda, 1819
Schweizer, Eric, 1987
Schweizer II, Al, 2332
Sciabica, Chris, 7805
Scianna, Dominic, 7353
Sciarratta, Patrick, 3354
Sciarretto, John, 3027
Scippione, Don, 2259
Sciro, Cherrie, 4602
Scism, Anita K, 5906
Sckolnik, David, 185
Sclar, Gary, 3042
Scofield, Elizabeth, 7793
Scolamiero, Michael, 629
Scorby, Don, 3663, 3666, 3668, 7773
Scott, Brian A, 7567
Scott, Cliff, 3368
Scott, David, 2313
Scott, Deborah, 3285
Scott, Douglas, 250

Scott, Edd, 5306
Scott, Garland, 2660
Scott, Jamie, 1714
Scott, Jo Ryman, 4029
Scott, John E, 7733
Scott, John T., 2984
Scott, Kathy, 1196
Scott, Lauren, 2209
Scott, Rebecca L, 3340
Scott, Richard, 1397
Scott, Richard L, 370
Scott, Rick, 3220
Scott, Ron, 5979
Scott, Sean, 2392
Scott, Stefanie, 3366
Scott, Steven, 3237
Scott, Toby, 7858
Scott, William Fred, 2014
Scott Jussila, Nicolai, 1953
Scribner, Norman, 1985
Scribner, William, 1460
Scripps, Douglas, 1308
Scrivens, Connie O, 7888
Scrofani, Robert, 1977
Scroggs, William, 7516
Scruggs, David, 7931
Scruggs, Tammy S, 5625
Scudder, June, 3787
Scuffle, Kate, 3679
Scurci, Dan, 1650
Seabeck, Joe, 3955
Seacord, Alana, 2026
Seagrave, Fran, 5491
Seagren, Stan, 4002
Seale, Kitty, 4
Seaman, Christopher, 1046
Seaman, Mark, 5482
Seamons, Darla, 2323
Searcy, Joe, 2974
Seat, Charles, 3646
Seaton, David D, 4846
Seaver, Patrick, 1951
Seaver, Richard, 1916
Seawell, Angela, 1581
Seay, Dr. Donald W, 2721
Sebena, Jane, 2367
Sebens, Tod, 2367
Secor, Jonathan, 6892
Secrist, Alice, 2426
Secttor, Stuart, 6623
Sedley, Aimee, 3043
Sedore, Shirley, 411
Seeberg, Mary, 3982
Seefeldt, Chris, 5779
Seekatz, Kathleen, 761
Seekins, Deborah, 6804
Seelig, Dr. Timothy, 2309
Seevak, Elinor A, 3338
Sefton, David, 6043
Segal, Uriel, 409, 1218, 1468
Segal-Mill, Barbara, 2559
Segall, Aviva, 1399
Segall, Cissy, 3861
Segell, Kerri, 392
Seggerman, Yvonne, 3750
Segul, Betty, 6381
Sehr, Heidi, 1765
Seibel, Klauspeter, 1229
Seidel, Kathryn, 2720
Seil, Ronald, 1496
Seiler, James J, 2170
Seipter, Harvey, 1528
Seitz, David, 3672
Seitz, Tom, 5816, 5817
Sekhran, Ajay, 7015
Sekon, RP, 2848
Sekulow, Gary, 2790
Selby, Denise, 3107, 6976
Self, Bette, 5142
Self, Sandy, 2973
Self, Sharee, 5818
Selid, Wood, 6709, 6710

Selig, Helen, 4069
Seliga, Hap, 5916
Seligson, Gary, 1272
Sell, Justin, 6640
Sell, Lisette, 4187
Sellers, Barbara, 2401, 2585
Sellers, Laura, 7526
Seltzer, Norm, 3027
Selvey, Alta, 1674, 5278
Selvey, Barbara, 652
Selvey, Susan, 7167
Selzer, Josh, 3029
Semanitzky, Mischa, 4248
Sendzimer, Jane, 1001
Seneca, Matthew, 2283
Senft, Deborah, 1469
Senftem, Penny, 6684
Senior, Kimberly, 2849
Seow, Hsien, 1976
Sepico, Daniel, 1306
Serafica, Maria, 51
Serating, Arthur, 1472
Seres, Sarah, 1870
Serifica, Maria, 51
Serpa, Valerie J, 4841
Serquinia, Julie, 2395
Serrand, Dominique, 3148
Serrano, Elana, 83
Serrano, Hector M, 5509
Serrz, Renny, 3742
Sertich, Tony, 6943
Sessions, Ann, 3980
Sessions, Sally, 5484
Setapen, James, 1776
Sethness, Ann, 582
Setzer, Doug, 7247
Setzer, Marc, 1572
Setzer, Marc S, 2244
Seuell, Shawn, 3093
Sever, Micki, 2532
Severinson, Doc, 764
Sevy, Bruce K, 2585
Sewell, Andrew, 1211, 1869
Sewell, Ronald F, 1159
Sewlyn, Amanda, 3377
Sexton, Bonnie, 3558
Sexton, Mark, 6349
Seybolt, Cynthia, 8504
Seyer, David, 3610
Seyffer, Gene, 2685
Seymour, Libby, 5127
Sforzini, Mark, 1032
Sgro, Joe, 6909
Shabal, Denah, 3796, 5469
Shackelford, John, 194, 2628
Shackelford, Lee, 3764
Shade, C Edwin, 3267
Shadier, Bob, 3972
Shadler, Sandy, 3972
Shadley, Sherry, 3568
Shadur, Kimberly, 2064
Shafer, John, 7068, 7069
Shafer, Robert, 1896
Shafer, Scott, 1648
Shaff, Richard, 6123
Shaffer, Frank, 1774
Shaffer, Kathleen, 656
Shaffer, Larry, 7730
Shaffer, Martha, 2150
Shaffer, Susan, 2663
Shaffner, Joe, 7670
Shafman, Arthur, 491, 3461, 8419
Shagan, Rena, 554
Shagan Associates, Rena, 3209
Shahan, William Justin, 1260
Shaheed, Margie, 6876
Shain, Paul, 2344
Shakarian, Ropen, 1842
Shaley, Geoffrey C, 4096
Shallue, Shana, 5731
Shalom, Anna, 424
Shalwitz, Howard, 2671

Shames, Jonathan, 1877, 5704
Shamie, Eric, 3070
Shamlian, Bill, 3054
Shamlian, Linda, 2736
Shanahan, Kim, 1648
Shane, Molly A, 302
Shangrow, George, 2339
Shank, Carolyn, 5658
Shank, Terrence, 2716
Shanley, Douglas, 4370
Shanley, Kelley, 6335
Shanley, Steve, 4526
Shannon, Jerome, 1882
Shannon, Paddy, 1967
Shannon, Patricia R, 3600
Shannon, Peggy, 2497
Shannoni, Jerome, 1881
Shapiro, Barry R, 1489
Shapiro, Bonnie, 3043
Shapiro, Daavid, 1810
Shapiro, Ethel, 1638
Shapiro, Mark, 2214
Shapiro, Nina, 894
Shapiro MD, Sandor S, 1731
Sharir, Yacov, 667
Sharn, Deborah, 8391
Sharp, Dale, 2242
Sharp, Shannon, 6358
Sharp, Steve, 6066
Sharp, Tom, 1136
Sharpan, Susan, 2997
Sharpe, Carla, 6876
Sharpe, Larry, 5678
Sharpe, Melissa, 7268
Sharrett, Charles R, 7694
Sharrock, P Susan, 3603
Shary, Mark, 1638
Shasberger, Michael, 6208
Shauf, Karen, 1710
Shaver, John, 3799
Shavitz, Peter, 5049
Shaw, Annette, 1602
Shaw, Arthur, 1679
Shaw, David, 2849
Shaw, Kevin, 6364
Shaw, Robert, 2015
Shay, Anthony, 56
Shay, Ira, 5476
Shay, Mike, 5787
Shay, Ora, 1777
Shea, Patrick, 2636
Shea, Robert, 4854
Shea, Sheila, 7685
Shea, William, 2654
Sheaffer, Charles, 1920
Sheaffer, Karen, 1715
Shealy, Laura, 5423
Shearer, Coleen, 5286
Sheble, Gerald, 303
Shedd, Betsy, 4
Sheehan, Jason, 3054
Sheehan, Kate, 2525
Sheeley, Michael K, 1034
Sheels, Harriet, 3060
Sheenan, Jr, Edward, 1720
Sheets, Dr. Thomas, 1905
Sheffer, Ismiah, 5049
Sheffer, Jonathan, 1512
Sheffield, Elizabeth, 927
Sheffield, John, 7611
Sheffield, Simone, 4154
Shehee, Virginia, 1232
Sheiburne, Mercyla, 1809, 2320
Sheing, Tina M., 2653
Sheingold, Rick, 2819
Sheir, Rebecca, 3481
Shelburne, Norman, 7
Shelby, Bryan, 3107
Sheldon, Richard, 1917
Shelhorn, Donald, 2258
Shell, Gary, 7563
Shelley, Sarah, 141, 4193, 4199

Shelley, Stephen, 692
Shelley Evans, Muriel, 705
Shellman, Nick, 3948
Shelly, Sarah, 145
Shelt, Christopher, 4773
Shelton, Chris, 3966
Shelton, Claudia, 746
Shelton, Debbie, 2761
Shelton, Lara, 13, 788, 2381
Shelton, Lillian Britt, 5164
Shelton, Linda, 7397
Shelton, Richard, 770
Shelton-Mason, Joan, 599
Shen, Dr. Sin-yan, 1153, 1154
Shen, Heidi, 3825
Shepard, Joan, 2616
Shepard, Noel C, 3598
Sheperd, Sheri, 1905
Shephard, Edson, 3112
Shephard, Eric, 3865
Shepherd, Anne, 7110
Shepherd, Daneta, 3604
Sheppard, Al, 7143
Sheppard, Barbara S, 6058
Sheppard, Dr. Kenneth, 2304
Sheppard, Ellen, 2285
Shepperd, Teresa, 2349
Sheptak, Gracia, 2291
Sher, Bartlett, 3956
Sheran, Nancy Idaka, 734
Sherba, John, 892
Sherber, Aaron, 2085
Sherer, Tom, 2111
Sheridan, Roseann, 4003
Sherling, Steve, 8459
Sherling, Steven, 8459
Sherman, Brenda, 3900
Sherman, David, 2699
Sherman, Donna, 4638
Sherman, Howard, 2642, 2643, 7498
Sherman, Joan, 8385
Sherman, Joanna, 3354
Sherman, Leslie, 933
Sherman, Val, 3413
Sherr, Rebecca, 3956
Sherrod, Deborah, 578
Sherwood, David, 7888
Sherwood, Virginia, 2683
Shewell, Hazel, 4144
Shields, Dr. Ron, 3575
Shields, Michelle, 1949
Shields, Timothy, 3995
Shiffman, Carol, 5688, 5689, 5690
Shiffman, Merle E, 292
Shiffman, Steve, 5933
Shifrin, David, 1691, 5302
Shiley, Kim, 2278
Shimada, Toshiyuki, 1240
Shindle, Elaine, 2112
Shine, Stephanie, 5703
Shine, Susan, 4983, 7355
Shineflug, Nana, 271
Shinn, Carmelita, 3641
Shinner, Sandy, 2860
Shiomi, Rick, 3147
Shiplet, Donna, 390
Shipley, Yvette, 320
Shiraishi, Poppo, 541
Shire, Marlene, 2493
Shirky, John, 6976
Shirley, Bobbie, 7926
Shives, Missy, 3026
Shivley, Karissa, 7650
Shkolnick, Rachel, 7163
Shoaff, John, 1162
Shobe, Mary Lu, 7684
Shockley, Dr. Pam, 955
Shoemake, Anne, 5117
Shoemaker, Dan, 3526
Shoemaker, Lilia, 589
Shoemaker, Suzanne, 1092
Sholemson, David, 8378

Shollenbarger, Kay, 7259
Shoptaw, Carrie, 4790
Shorin, Maryann, 2735
Short, Carol, 5505
Short, Donald J, 3033
Shoss, Deb, 2965
Shoup, John, 2905
Shoup, Robert, 2334
Shrader, Dr. Steven, 1774
Shrader, Steven, 5473
Shrider, Sharon, 6631
Shroder, DL, 3398
Shubert, Roy A, 5372
Shughart, Lyle, 3697
Shuler, Jyl, 3879, 5576
Shulman, Ivan, 848
Shultz, Jr, Bud-Emmerson, 1104
Shuman, Trish, 4318
Shumate, Al, 3923
Shumway, Beth, 607
Shurr, Buff, 5521
Shuster, Dianna, 1948, 6129
Shutze, Cindy, 6923
Sibley, Thomas E, 2249
Sicilia, Domenick B, 6291
Sicilian, Peter, 2189
Siciliani, Alessandro, 1636
Sides, Shawn, 3809
Sidon, Frederick, 1953
Sieberling, David, 1569
Siebert, Cynthia, 1371
Siebrecht, Kyle, 1848
Siegal, Adam, 3472
Siegel, Ethel, 425, 1497
Siegel, Glenn, 4652
Siegel, Marc, 610
Siehl, John, 5220, 7662
Siemssen, Judy, 3663, 3666, 3668, 7773
Siena, Jane, 1016
Sienko, Mary, 7030
Siever, David T, 6230
Siff, Ira, 2216
Sifuentes, Maria Elva, 28
Sigel, Steve, 6272
Sigler, Mike, 3684
Sigler, Richard, 58
Sigman, Janice, 6632
Sigmon, Susan, 4393
Sigurdson, Sandi, 913
Siiq, Penelope, 173
Sikora, Michelle, 4213, 4314
Silber, Merry, 1999
Silberblatt, Steven, 86
Silbiger, Kathy, 1575
Silipigni, Alfredo, 2174
Silipigni, Maestro Alfredo, 2174
Sill, Andrews, 1806
Sill, Sara, 8466
Silon, Alan, 1639
Silow, Alan, 929
Silva, Chris, 1542, 7460
Silver, Dan, 750
Silver, Ruth, 1964
Silverstein, Liz, 425, 1497, 8371
Simanjuntak, Michiko, 482
Simmervillo, Jean, 93
Simmons, Beverly, 1506
Simmons, Bill, 2918
Simmons, Carter, 1874
Simmons, Deidre, 2275
Simmons, Jeffrey T, 1821
Simmons, Kenneth, 2833
Simmons, Michael, 1732
Simmons, Peter, 1236, 4613
Simmons, Scott, 1352
Simmons, William, 1147
Simolij, Mariusz, 1725
Simon, Barbara, 8428
Simon, Brad, 8428
Simon, David, 2451
Simon, David G, 882
Simon, Mary, 2875

Simon, Stacy, 392
Simon, Stephen, 1020
Simone, Denise, 2807
Simone, Giovanni, 2172
Simone, John, 7488
Simone, Tex, 7488
Simons, Annette, 926
Simons, Betsy, 3307, 4944
Simons, Dennis, 1232
Simons, Diane, 3843
Simons, Johnny, 3843
Simons, Katie, 3167
Simons, Russ, 7950
Simpkins, Al, 3717
Simpkins, James, 1846
Simpson, Alissa, 5228
Simpson, Charles, 4242
Simpson, Geraldine, 3630
Simpson, Jim, 3351
Simpson, John, 2528
Simpson, Judy, 5404
Simpson, Marcy, 3742
Simpson, Robert L, 2313
Sims, Deborah, 2503
Sims, Larry, 1080
Sims, Laura, 3782
Sinclair, Dr. John V, 4379, 4381
Sinclair, George, 1931
Sinclair, James, 1003
Sinclair, Kathleen, 12
Sinder, Michael, 8432
Sinel, Norman, 1020
Singer, Deborah, 3614
Singer, Isabelle G, 991
Singer, Ken, 1829
Singer, Matt, 2534
Singer, Paulette, 426, 2205
Singer, Valerie, 2534
Singh, Shelley, 8232
Singleton, Jacki, 2854
Singleton, Jim, 1781
Singleton, JL, 7870
Singleton Schmidt, Andrea, 1840
Sink, Christopher, 3055
Sinn, Rose, 1373
Sinta, Donald, 1310
Sioman, Scott, 4343
Sipp, Jerry, 3558
Sirama, Malini, 707
Sircar, Mary, 4488
Sirna, Denise, 4872
Sirota, Brett, 8458
Sirovatka, Stephanie, 8287
Sisemore, Tommy, 6781, 6783
Sisson, Rhonda, 4486
Sistek, Linda, 3117
Sistron, Charlotte, 631
Sites, Cindy L, 423
Sitton, Carl, 81
Situ, Gang, 115
Sitzer, Kathleen, 7109
Sizemore, Brad, 3558
Sjoerdsma, Dr. RD, 1866, 5745
Sjoerdsma, Richard, 5746
Skala, Gary, 2816
Skalicky, LaRana, 185
Skeehan, Sean, 3851
Skeeman, Sean, 8057
Skiles, Christa, 3581
Skiles, David L, 5764
Skiles, Scott, 3598
Skinner, Al, 6874
Skinner, Anita Sims, 1648
Skinner, Corby, 3204, 7133
Skinner, Cris, 2382
Skinner, Dr. Lynn J, 4417
Skinner, Howard, 966
Skinner Wells, Janet, 871
Skirball-Kenis, Audrey, 1916
Skoney, Robert C, 7956
Skov, Kent, 2556
Skrabalak, Duane, 2189

Sotolongo, Jose, 6378
Soucy, Martha M, 373
Soukup, Gregory, 847
Soukup, Patty, 390
Soussan, Russell, 6777
South, Dave, 7999
South Clemans, Katrina, 711
Southard, AnneMarie, 1282, 8382
Southard, Laurel, 3318
Southard, Scott, 1282, 8382
Southwell-Sander, Peter, 2027
Sowell, Johnny, 7940
Sowers, Richard, 1156, 1756
Spada, Ida, 2749
Spain PhD, Anthony, 1127
Spallone, Elaine, 2245
Spangenberg, Gail, 529
Spangler, Beth, 8188
Spanhauer, Charles, 5781
Spann-Swallwood, Carolyn, 4900, 7244
Spano, Robert, 1073, 1463
Sparger, Dr. a Dennis, 2154
Sparger, Lori, 2933
Sparhawk, Don, 4420, 6499
Sparks, Barbara, 1296, 4683
Sparks, Don, 156
Sparks, John, 6529
Sparks, Kevin, 4581
Sparks, WF, 1368
Sparrow, John, 1073
Sparrow, Thomas W, 5796
Sparrow, Tom, 5795
Spath-Mercado, Evelyn, 4900, 7244
Spaulding-Gaston, Aubra, 2374
Spaven, Kerry, 1351
Spear, Victor, 4212
Spears, Lisa, 7611
Spector, Wendy, 1290
Speer, Alexander, 2969
Speers, David, 1893
Speirs, Jim, 2806
Spejewski, Eugene, 3798
Spellens, Dan, 6010
Spence, Laurie, 1376
Spence, Mike, 8033, 8039
Spence, Sten, 5557
Spencer, Dr. Michael, 932
Spencer, Gerard H., 1309
Spencer, Kevin, 3916
Spencer, Marty, 5882
Spencer, Michael, 932
Spencer, Rebecca, 3593
Spencer, Scott, 3616
Sperry, Jeffrey K, 1600, 1601
Sperry, Paula, 2595
Sperry, Sandra, 1554
Spetzer, Bonnie, 3685
Spielberg, Genevieve, 8402
Spielberger, Christine, 1949
Spieler, Sandy, 3137
Spierman, Ben, 2190
Spierman, Michael, 2190
Spieth, Cathy, 868
Spieth, Donald, 1722
Spiga, Carlos, 818
Spigner, Dolly, 652
Spillman, Robert, 950, 4232
Spinosa, Amy, 1069
Spiotto MFA, Bob, 4971
Spira, Robert, 3652
Spires, H Edward, 2646
Spitz, Richard, 1800
Spitznagel, Frank, 3358
Spivack, Dara, 1399
Sprague, Carol, 7853
Sprague, Jid, 4699
Sprenger PhD, Craig M, 5955
Sprick, Andrea, 394
Sprinkle, Jim, 6222
Sproles Mock, Kara, 651
Sproul, Robert, 1718
Spry, III, Granville H, 1586

Spurlock, Daniel, 1219, 2068
Spurlock, Rebecca, 1876
Spurrier, PhD, James J, 2931
Squires, Catherine, 1147
Squires, Joan H, 765
Squires, Stephen, 1147
Squires, Steven, 1122
Sramek, Jean M, 3120
Srirama, Malini, 707
Srnold, Malcolm, 2000
Sroka, Elliot, 4969
Sroka, Scott L, 3303
St Clair, Neil, 3548
St John, Jenny, 9
St. Clair, Carl, 917
St. John, Anita, 5216
St. John, Katherine, 696, 1820, 5589
St.John, Winnie, 858
Staab, Jane, 3038
Staab, Len D, 4525
Staats, Cheryl, 950, 4232
Staats, Terri, 1889
Stabenow, Amy, 5378
Stabenow, Steve, 2942, 6668
Staber, Judy, 5088
Stack, Barbara, 863
Stack, Kenneth, 3001
Stackell, Joe, 3401
Stackhouse, Holly, 1722
Stacy, Sharone, 3327
Stadler, Tim, 2876
Stadsklev, Joan, 4346
Stafford, Lisa, 4588
Stafford Wilson, Peter, 1658, 1661
Stafura, Paul, 7846
Stafura, Paul G, 1744
Staggs, Charlie, 5919
Stahl, Barbara, 7691
Stahl, David, 1757
Staiger, Ron, 7573
Stair, Mary, 3006
Stakenas, Carol, 5013
Staley, Dr. Grant B, 5420
Staley, Jim, 1533
Stalheim, Kevin, 1875
Stallworth, Steve, 7178
Stalvey, Dorrance, 4127, 4128, 4133
Stamoulis, Lorraine, 2557
Stamper, Robin, 2164
Stanberry, Marty, 3200
Stanbery, Paul, 1614, 1618, 1644, 2263
Stander, Patricia, 90
Standish, Thomas K, 1973
Stangelberger, Georg, 1892
Staniloff, Fran, 2172
Staniloff, Stan, 2172
Staniunas, John, 6679
Stanke, Ann, 2344
Stanko, Tracy, 3222
Stanley, NJ, 3740
Stansbury, George W, 5485
Stansell, Fritz, 3113
Stanton, Don, 2416
Stanton, Jane, 2616
Stanton, Robin, 3965
Stantoon, Phil, 8199
Stapin, Scott, 7193
Stapp, Olivia, 1957
Star, Patty, 2361
Starck, Tamra, 573
Stark, Derrick, 651
Stark, Diane, 6764
Stark, Douglas, 2917
Stark, Peter, 231
Stark, Sharon, 3156
Stark, Tony, 1011
Starkman, Stephen, 1543
Starks, Rosie, 2933
Starling, Darline, 4170
Starling, Kimberly, 3003
Starnes, Ron, 2296
Staroff, Larry, 3395

Starr, Helen, 311
Starr, John, 3352
Starrett, Jon, 7625
Starrett, Mary, 8125
Starrett, William, 651
Starrs, John, 693
Startzman, Lorna, 6608
Starzman, Jane, 577
Staton, Chris, 7221
Statz, Cathy, 3980
Stauber, Steven, 4002
Stauffer, Michael, 6581
Stava, Keith, 2333
Stavnes, Diane, 7141, 7142
Steadham, Charles, 8359
Steadman, Jan, 716, 721
Stearns, Nancy, 2743
Stearns, Roland B, 7297
Stebley, Jay, 126
Stedman, Peri, 8447
Steed, Christian, 670
Steel, George, 3392
Steel, James, 8286
Steele, Barry, 439
Steele, Christopher, 2412
Steele, D Bryan, 695
Steele, Dana, 3238
Steele, Helen, 3238
Steele, Jan, 5265
Steele, Jonathan E, 4373
Steele, Pamela, 4505
Steele, Robert, 637
Steele], David, 1613
Steelman, Rachel, 2246
Steen, Anita I, 3722
Stefanac, David, 3683
Stefanac, Meg, 3683
Steffee MD, William, 1605
Steffek Blaske, Mary, 1309
Steffen, Randy, 3510
Steffens, Margaret, 2582
Steffes, Carl K, 5041
Steffey, 1st Lt. Chad, 1009
Steffy, Don, 6608
Stegall, Joel, 5163
Stehlik, Milos, 2831
Steichen, MD, James B, 1168
Steigler, Lou R, 4682
Steigman, Stephen, 4793
Stein, Barbara S, 2685
Stein, Bonnie, 547
Stein, Daniel, 23
Stein, David, 1477
Stein, Dean K, 1502
Stein, Dr Lawrence, 2685
Stein, Eugene P., 1916
Stein, Joan, 3426
Stein, Paulette, 6990
Stein, Richard, 2423
Stein, Rick, 5058
Stein, Robert, 6083
Steinberg, Barrie, 8436
Steinberg, Mark, 227
Steinbrenner, Jan, 5088
Steineker, Helen, 752
Steiner, Christian, 1492
Steiner, Dr. Frances, 810, 869
Steiner, Gail, 3241
Steiner, Randall, 2914
Steiner, Sheri, 971
Steiner, Steve, 3241
Steiner, Susan, 3578
Steiner, Urs Leonhardt, 898
Steinfield, Joseph D, 4662
Steinman, Esquire, Harvey B., 4646
Steinzor, Curt, 408
Steitler, Dr. Wallace, 7862
Steivel, Bruce, 371
Stem, N David, 1859
Stende, Dave, 3568
Stengle, Diane, 1453, 2187
Stensrud, William R, 1935

Stephan, Bill, 6493
Stephens, Darlene, 413, 712
Stephens, Dennis, 757
Stephens, Doris, 5412
Stephens, Elizabeth, 888
Stephens, Grethen L, 5175
Stephens, John, 2778
Stephens, Michael, 4084
Stephens, Thomas, 4884
Stephenson, Alphonse, 1415
Stephenson, Authur H, 6808
Stephenson, David B., 4029
Stephenson, John, 1069
Stepner, Daniel, 975
Steptoe, Eugene, 6110
Stern, Diane, 5583
Stern, Ed, 3581
Stern, Erik, 164
Stern, Jay, 3358
Stern, Joe, 2430
Stern, Marc I, 1916
Stern, Marcus, 3041
Stern, Mary K., 3012
Stern, Michael, 5454
Sternberg, Alicia, 3876
Sternberg, Donna, 168
Sternberg, Patricia, 3328
Sternberg, Ruth, 3750
Sternenberg, Phil, 2180
Sterner, Scott, 2571
Sterrenberg, Elsie, 769
Stetta, Jane, 1349
Stettner, Enid, 4991
Steven, Cara, 4155
Stevens, Adrian, 1951
Stevens, Byam, 3045
Stevens, Delores, 1299
Stevens, Diane, 1810
Stevens, Erik Joe, 6234
Stevens, Fern M, 2775
Stevens, Greg, 2769
Stevens, John H, 2775
Stevens, Jonn H, 2775
Stevens, Katie, 4006
Stevens, Keith, 1834, 3235
Stevens, Kenji, 1091
Stevens, Les, 2536
Stevens, Mark, 3075
Stevens, Michael J, 8094
Stevens, Pamela, 151
Stevens, Roger L, 4309
Stevens, Terry, 1720
Stevenson, Ben, 680
Stevenson, Eric, 1896
Stevenson, Hunter, 2409
Stevenson, Joseph, 5375
Stevenson, Josiah, 1264
Stevenson, Sara, 355
Stevenson, W Jerome, 3637
Stewart, Allison E, 1377
Stewart, Anna, 1839
Stewart, Barbara D, 2014
Stewart, Carol, 4544
Stewart, Caroline B, 3758
Stewart, Dr. Rowena, 1736
Stewart, Edna, 2439
Stewart, Edward, 318
Stewart, Ellen, 3394
Stewart, Greg, 8252
Stewart, Gussie, 4195
Stewart, Jacques, 3239
Stewart, Janet J, 5292
Stewart, Kathie, 1655
Stewart, Kathryn, 357
Stewart, L Jean, 1839
Stewart, Leslie, 916
Stewart, Mary, 7208
Stewart, Mary E, 4871
Stewart, Nancy, 1162, 2609
Stewart, Natalie, 805, 4093
Stewart, Nick, 2439
Stewart, Rev., 700

Stewart, Scott A, 1076
Stewzut, Anita, 3004
Sthrner Traum, Lynda, 3408
Stibbe, Sue, 2340
Stich, Jennifer, 7316
Stickel, Peter, 1300
Stickler, Martha, 5903
Stidfole, Arthur, 1737
Stieber, Richard, 1798
Stiham, Scott, 6804
Stike, John R, 1592, 3028
Stiles, Diane, 3357
Stiles, Mary, 904
Stilfeman, Leslie, 1508
Still, Chuck, 2940, 6418
Still, Donna, 631
Stiller, Lisa, 2095
Stillman, Heidi, 2841
Stilson, Joyce, 3298
Stilwagner, Frank, 8223
Stilwell, Sandra, 2695
Stilwill, Charles, 2942, 6668
Stilwill, Patricia, 2942
Stimack, Anthony, 3409
Stimack, Marilyn, 3409
Stimpert, Karen, 2256
Stimpson, Andy, 2119
Stimson, Susan, 4987
Stip, Catherine, 2416
Stirling Munro, Cristina, 671
Stites, Fred, 4124
Stitt, Jan, 4027
Stitt, Katea, 4302
Stock, David J, 2532
Stockard, Matt, 343
Stocks, Melanie, 7136
Stocks, Melanie J, 7135
Stockton, David, 2725
Stofft, Pat, 3762
Stokes, Ellen, 4638
Stokes, Harvey, 1839
Stoll, Carmen J, 1020
Stollmack, Noele, 2347
Stolz, Don, 3122
Stolz, Mark, 4341
Stolzfus, Eric, 4628
Stone, Carol, 4870
Stone, Chris, 2617
Stone, Christine, 1066
Stone, Donnan, 144
Stone, Dorothy, 811
Stone, Howard, 4261
Stone, Jason, 5100
Stone, Leonard, 1066
Stone, Mark, 6086
Stone, Maureen, 1942
Stone, Philip, 3293
Stone, Ronald G., 1045
Stone, Sayard, 988
Stone, Shawn, 629
Stone, Susan, 5206
Stoneking, Barry B, 574
Stoner, Gyda, 4427
Stool, Ann, 5503
Stoors, Bob, 2966
Stopa, Jean, 4987
Storey, Bonnie, 693
Storey, Bruce, 4246
Storment, JR, 2800
Stott, Sherrill, 984
Stotts, Michael, 3255
Stoughton Marafino, Teresa, 3701
Stout, Carol, 569
Stout, S., 728
Stover, Darrell, 7527
Stover, Paula, 3640
Stowell, Kent, 718
Stowell Jr, Don, 3569
Strader, Peter, 2735
Strafacci, Barry J, 7779
Strain, Charlene, 1230
Strait, Margie, 7321

Strand, Darlene, 4729
Strand, Vicky, 7757
Strang, Rebecca, 3073
Strange, John-Michael, 2991
Strange, Laurie, 1841
Strange, Peter S, 1615
Strangfeld, Jack, 2180
Stranix, John, 6307
Strasacci, Barry, 7777
Strasberg, David, 2574
Strasheim, James, 1396
Strassler, Robert B, 975
Straub, Joyce, 237
Straughn Pratt, Suzanne, 3015
Straus Cullman, Joan, 3399
Strause, Nancy, 585
Strauss, Fred E, 5078
Strauss, Iris Lynn, 1935
Strauss, Jana, 1463
Strauss, Melinda, 1433
Strauss, William, 756
Straw, James B, 2280
Straw, Marcy, 4084
Strazza, Preston, 4424
Street, Stacey, 874
Streeter, Carol, 173
Streeter, Jim, 6990
Strein, Bill, 3027
Strelow, Eric T, 2343
Stressing, Jo Lynn, 3325
Stribling, Lafayette, 7052
Strickland, Steve, 2383
Strickland, Ted, 7945
Strickler, Beulah, 4106
Strickler, Gary, 6856
Strickler, John, 1209
Strickler, John Wesley, 1363
Strider, Julie, 4511, 6617
Stried, Robert, 6346
Strimennos, Sarah, 299
Stringer, Dr. Mary Ann, 4772
Strode, Dr. Thomas, 2118
Stroebel, Pamela, 275
Strohmeyer, Donna, 5564
Strokosch, Caitlin, 2028
Strollo Holbrook, Toni, 1068
Stroman, Susan, 3399
Strong, Craig, 7277
Strong, John, 1486, 4985
Strongren, Richard, 2102
Stroud, Ken, 93
Stroup, Daniel, 5046
Strubbe, Sandra, 2242
Strubhar, Lita, 2317
Struble, George, 1706
Struck, Ben, 3351
Strul, Hellene, 4350
Strunsky, Jean, 2391
Struthers, Kevin A, 4310
Stuart, Ann, 446
Stuart, Annie, 6182
Stuart, Betsy, 3971
Stuart, Paul, 5902
Stubblefield, Barbara, 1856
Stubbs, David, 6690
Stubbs, Frank, 4758
Stuber, Karen, 8281
Stubner, Heidi, 4962
Stubs, Lydia, 6948
Stucker, Susan, 1430
Stucki, Steve, 2144
Stucki, Steven, 2144
Studard, Leslie, 8008
Studdard, Les, 5500
Studley, Julien, 568
Stuhlreyer, Gus, 2761
Stumacher, Eric, 1410
Stump, Terry Lee, 2959
Stumpf, Thomas, 2104
Sturgell, James F, 2688
Sturgeon, Jeff, 6367
Sturgill, Mike, 612, 1689, 3661, 5299

Sturgis, Jack, 4822
Sturgis, Jeff, 697
Sturm, Robert, 5637
Sturtevant, Sara, 3854
Stussi, Doug, 1673
Styren, Celia, 3206
Suarez, Michelle J, 6505
Suczek, Alexander, 1324
Sudbrink, Bridgette, 5470
Sudik, Nancy F, 976, 1969
Sueoka, Ryan, 2796
Sugar, Richard, 1136
Suju, Ludwig, 715
Sukenik, Phil, 1710
Sulahian, Nancy, 1915
SulKowski, Pioir, 5920
Sulley, Chena, 3566
Sullivan, Bill, 973
Sullivan, Dan, 2750
Sullivan, Daniel, 3399
Sullivan, David, 5371
Sullivan, J R, 5576
Sullivan, Jerry, 2725
Sullivan, Joseph, 45
Sullivan, JR, 3879
Sullivan, Karl, 2862
Sullivan, Laura L, 5404
Sullivan, Michele, 1927
Sullivan, Nancy, 4244
Sullivan, Pam, 2030
Sullivan, Paul H, 6980
Sullivan, Robert E., 1944
Sullivan, Sean, 7622
Sullivan, Taimur, 5016
Sumbroff, Gayle, 3176
Sumey, Doug, 2970, 4576
Summer, Maryann, 3318
Summers, Barbara, 5233
Summers, David, 819
Summers, Liz, 5132
Summers, Patrick, 2314
Summerville, Dr. Suzanne, 1886, 4030
Summerville, Thomas, 846
Sumpter, Teresa, 1201
Sumtter, Micheal, 7154
Sunday, Rob, 7851
Sundel-Schoenwald, Rebecca, 2254
Sundquist, Cindy, 5286
Suplee, Ray, 2735
Suprina, Joffrey Scott, 250
Sur, Jennifer, 2114
Surber, Sharon, 7242
Surles, Georgina, 263
Surslen, Sera, 1484, 4980
Sutcliff, Dennis, 593
Suter, William P, 2631
Sutherford, Robin, 972, 4258
Sutherland, L Frederick, 3705
Sutherland, Margaret, 1699
Sutherland, Melanie, 3341
Sutowski, Thor, 139
Suttle, Cyndi, 764
Sutton, Dick, 1798
Sutton, Jeff, 3578
Sutton, Susan, 2946
Sutton, Vern, 1897
Sutton Self, Sandra, 1078
Suydam, John, 6759
Suydam, Johnny, 6758
Suzeau, Patrick, 306
Svedlow, Dr. Andrew J, 5435
Svejkosky, Susan, 3194
Swadling, Jeff, 2122, 4717
Swaha, Leslie, 17
Swain, Angela, 5123
Swain, Margaret, 2049
Swain, Mitch, 1638
Swain, William, 2049
Swain Brownlee, Elizabeth, 6446
Swanborn, Edwin, 2107
Swanglier, Tom, 7579
Swango, Carol, 5262

Swank, Jan D, 3762
Swank, Jill, 3762
Swanner, Tom, 101, 2495
Swansen, Samuel, 1727, 5363
Swanson, Clifton, 912, 4202
Swanson, Dana, 3079
Swanson, Dr. Thomas L, 1345
Swanson, Dwight, 3846
Swanson, Kris, 5770
Swanson, Maureen, 1846
Swanson, Patrick, 2114
Swantak, Andrew, 621
Swartwout, Glen, 2794
Swartz, F Randolph, 627
Swartz, Micheal, 1397
Swartz, Nita, 1449
Swattn, Chuck, 2309
Swayze, Marsha, 101, 2495
Sweat, John E, 1081
Swedberg, Robert, 2003
Sweed, Diann, 3875
Sween, Doug, 3157
Sweeney, Jillian, 447
Sweeney, Mike, 5978
Sweet, Alice, 5189
Sweet, Chad, 3309
Sweet, Lee, 6019
Sweet, Roger, 4859
Sweetser, Sandy, 7015
Sweezey, C Otis, 2865
Sweibel, Robert, 3033
Swenson, Paula, 304
Swenson, Penelope, 1259
Swenson, Wendy, 36
Swerling, Jeremy A, 1125
Swicker, Shelia, 2449
Swift, James A, 930
Swiger, Celia, 1798
Swiggart, Barbara, 5277
Swiggart, James, 1897
Swihart, Tom, 299
Swindell, Jeanette, 1666, 5263
Swirsky, Marvin, 3552
Switzer, Kathleen, 1933
Switzler, Jonne-Marie, 800
Swofford, Patti Hannan, 5246
Swoope, Janice, 1577
Swyer, Edward P., 7472
Syak, Patricia C, 1664
Syer, Fontaine, 2654
Sykes, Jeffrey, 2345
Sylvester, Mark, 3726
Symington, Jennifer, 3072
Symonds, Alan, 6871
Syroney, Jeffery, 3592
Syrotiak, David, 3894
Szablewski, Laurie R, 1271
Szakacs, Jim, 3595
Szczeciana, Anita, 2709
Szczepkowski, Michael, 6869
Szczesiul, Mary Lou, 2916
Szlasa, David, 2529
Szlaza, David, 144

T

Tabbitas, Julie, 5062
Taccone, Tony, 2391
Tack, Stephanie, 485
Tada, Steve, 760
Taft, Dr. Burns, 1955
Taft, Dr. E Burns, 4224
Taft, Steve, 6642
Taggart, Sylvia, 1980
Taheosian, Lisa, 126
Tait, Lane, 3862, 5537
Takei, Kei, 497
Takemoto, Susan, 3954
Taki, Tomio, 1508
Talasek, JD, 4312
Talbert, Les, 1815

Talbut, Greg, 7073
Tallchief, Maria, 286
Tallman, Donald, 6208
Tally, Lou, 2691
Tam, Sherman, 5306
Tamarkin, Kate, 808
Tamayo, Mami, 4316
Tamberlane, John, 1463
Tamburrit, Lawrence J, 1430
Tamez, Jonathan, 3809
Tamm, Olive, 2294
Tammes, Eric, 5773
Tammi, John KV, 6953
Tamulevich, David, 8403
Tanaka, Ted T, 802
Tang, David J, 2278
Tang, Dr. Jordan, 1222, 1767
Tanguay, Marc, 642
Tani, Anne, 1241, 2078
Tanis, Carol, 1321
Tannenbaum, David, 1106
Tanner, Jessica, 1266
Tapia, John, 2885
Tarble, Sherrie, 3165
Taribassi, Maria, 3384
Tarjan, Karen, 2851
Tarshis, Jay, 2854
Tarver, Helga, 2658
Tassaro, Alicia, 1178
Tassos, Michael, 726
Tate, Tom, 1449
Tate-Opel, Justine, 2184
Tatesian, Lisa, 1410
Tatge, Pamela, 6260
Tatich, Lea Evelyn, 5140
Tatum, Douglas, 3177
Tatum, Michelle, 168
Tatum, Richard, 2563
Taubert, Uwe, 3452
Taubman, William, 5777
Taurins, Diane, 7159
Tautvydas, Nida, 1959, 6189
Tavera, Deidre, 6253
Tavernier, David M, 5431
Taxman, Barbara, 4835
Taylor, C Rene, 709
Taylor, Chip, 3522
Taylor, Darlene, 3619
Taylor, David, 187
Taylor, Delia, 2667
Taylor, Ferren, 2460
Taylor, Holly, 7691
Taylor, Jackie, 2817
Taylor, James, 1563, 1622
Taylor, Jan, 5281, 5283
Taylor, Janet L, 5186
Taylor, Johy, 3556
Taylor, Jonathan, 1481
Taylor, Julie, 1116
Taylor, Mark, 632
Taylor, Michael, 5426
Taylor, Monika, 964
Taylor, Nanette, 2449
Taylor, Patricia, 3476
Taylor, Paul, 535
Taylor, Queenie, 4198
Taylor, Rob, 4199
Taylor, Rowan, 948
Taylor, Rozalynn, 3539
Taylor, Scott, 5021
Taylor, Stacy, 1143
Taylor, Susan, 1816
Taylor, Thomas, 2967
Taylor, Tom, 2901
Taylor, Tracey, 3335
Taylor, Wayne C, 1023, 1996
Taylor, William, 339
Taylor, William B., 1373
Taylor Schuman, Trish, 1995
Taylor Swain, Jenni, 5906
Taylor-Smith, Jennifer, 3798
Tcherkassky, Mariannaen, 635

Tchivzhel, Edvard, 1162, 1760
Teager, William, 2265
Teague, Thomas S, 5456
Team, Nancy, 2246
Tedesco, Margaret, 4187
Tedesco, Michael, 2557
Teel, Mike, 3409
Teel, Skipp, 608
Teer, Barbara Ann, 3410
Teeter, Lara, 2045
Teft, Pat, 5736
Teinowitz, Nancy, 274
Teixeira, Kristen, 8382
Teixeria, Kristen, 1282
Tekulsky, Mike, 4203
Telford, Kay, 7161
Tellalian, Robert S, 974
Teller, Deborah, 3413
Teller, Ryan, 3390
Temirkanov, Yuri, 1244
Temirkanov, Yurird, 2083
Temple, Nancy, 3425
Temple, Reggi, 5916
Temple, Riley K, 2658
Templeton, Larry, 7057, 7062
Templeton, Loyd, 5464
Templeton, Tom, 2582
Ten Eyck, Bill, 7208
Teng, Yu-chiung, 1504
Tenley, Karrie, 956, 4245
Tenuta, James C, 288
Tenzin, Lobsang, 261
Tepper, Frances, 7345
Teraspulsky, Leopold, 1297, 4686
Terekhov, Miquel, 604
Teresa Abalos, Maria, 31
Terrell, Bobbie, 885
Terry, Cori, 347
Terry, Ed, 3008
Terry, Maxine, 3989
Terry, Michael, 4712
Terry, Phillip, 2682
Terry-Morgan, Elmo, 3748
Teske, Melissa, 290
Tesley, Bernard, 3404
Tessitore, Antonio, 2215, 2216
Tessler, Allan, 5792
Teter, Dane, 938
Teter, Samantha, 6597
Teter, Jr, Harry, 2665
Tetreanlt, Paul, 3851
Tetreault, Paul, 8057
Tew, William, 2332
Thaggard, David P, 7545
Thakar, Markand, 1346
Thatcher, Graham, 351
Thatcher, Paula, 7760
Thatcher, Sue, 6608
Thayer, Ronald, 4895
Thayer, Tom, 3771
Thein, Dr. Anthony, 5168
Theis, Audrey, 2084
Theriault, Candy, 7178
Theryoung, Richard, 4900, 7244
Theting, Ella, 1416
Theusen Gell, Nancy, 255
Thibault, Beth, 3093
Thielen, Mark, 1039
Thielen, Tom, 229
Thielman, Jim, 7689
Thigpen, Jim, 3755
Thigpen, Kay, 3755
Thoburn, Christina, 4709
Thoma, Melissa, 5920
Thomae-Morphew, Susan, 8055
Thomas, AC, 2866
Thomas, Augusta Read, 1116
Thomas, Beverly, 8391
Thomas, Bill, 1522, 5468, 7962
Thomas, Bob, 3335
Thomas, Candyce, 4259
Thomas, Carolyn, 2908

Thomas, Charles E, 6682
Thomas, Cynthis A., 3026
Thomas, David, 2790, 6827
Thomas, Dennis E, 8175
Thomas, Devin, 1351
Thomas, Evelyn, 85
Thomas, George, 1732
Thomas, Joan, 1332
Thomas, John, 6086
Thomas, Juames, 2189
Thomas, Judyth, 6953
Thomas, Keith, 1715
Thomas, Kristina, 5709
Thomas, Laurie, 4665
Thomas, Marilyn, 1743
Thomas, Mark, 1711, 2870
Thomas, Marni, 18
Thomas, Michael Tilson, 902
Thomas, Mike, 8168
Thomas, Nancy, 1881
Thomas, Patricia, 8210
Thomas, Patricia M, 4638
Thomas, Paula, 4243
Thomas, Philip S, 7232
Thomas, Richard L, 4242
Thomas, Roger, 7578, 7580
Thomas, Ronald, 1272, 4269
Thomas, Steven, 1564
Thomas, Susan, 5458
Thomas, Tom, 5675
Thomas, Vanessa, 631
Thomas, Venessa, 631
Thomas, Wendy, 388
Thomas, Wesley, 4395
Thomas, William D, 7636
Thomason, Scott, 616
Thomley, Sandy, 6950
Thompsom, Doug, 3830
Thompson, Alan, 2058
Thompson, Anna M, 7025
Thompson, Argo, 2553
Thompson, Barbara, 632, 4412
Thompson, Barry, 2468
Thompson, Betty, 1800
Thompson, Buddy, 2290
Thompson, Diane, 2955
Thompson, Donna, 1230
Thompson, Dr. Norma, 1294
Thompson, Ed, 2328
Thompson, Edgar J, 1825
Thompson, Emily Anne, 3770
Thompson, ES Whitney, 4668
Thompson, George, 214, 916
Thompson, Herbert, 5343
Thompson, J Lynn, 2775
Thompson, J. Lynn, 2266
Thompson, Jeanie, 8362
Thompson, Jena, 698
Thompson, Jennifer, 1877
Thompson, Jim, 4225
Thompson, Jocelyn, 2243
Thompson, John, 5707
Thompson, Kate, 3238
Thompson, Kent, 4017
Thompson, Kerby, 3309
Thompson, Lisa, 3062
Thompson, Mary, 6948
Thompson, Michael, 4500, 6398
Thompson, Myrtis, 1962
Thompson, Owen, 3436
Thompson, Richard L., 2661
Thompson, Robert D, 3637
Thompson, Robin, 2223
Thompson, Scott, 3804
Thompson, Shel, 1733
Thompson, Sheldon, 3722
Thompson, Steven B, 4537
Thompson, Thomas M., 3732
Thompson, TK, 6889
Thompson, Walter, 2755
Thompson-Cantu, Katya, 2322
Thompson-Moore, Ella, 402

Thompston, Dennis M, 3734
Thomson, Donna, 4945
Thomson, Judith, 2870
Thomson, Melissa, 2103
Thomson, Susan, 2154
Thomson Kretschmer, Dr. Joan, 1515
Thorn, Elisabeth, 412
Thornburg, Phyllis, 186
Thorne, Francis, 1495
Thorne, Gordon G, 3062
Thornton, Bobbie, 1105
Thornton, Doug, 6770
Thornton, Flora, 1916
Thornton, Patricia, 691
Thornton, Paul A, 3226
Thorp, Bo, 3535
Thorpe, Ken, 4008
Thorpe, Tracy, 4008
Thorsell, W Kellogg, 1698
Thorson, Jon, 4424
Thorson, Martin, 1856
Thorton, Doug, 6773
Thorton, Liesl, 3997
Thouveny Doyle, Francoise, 36
Threadgill, Susan, 3805, 5477
Throndill, Margaret, 5711
Throne, Tracy, 2230
Throp, Mike, 4666
Thuesen, Barbara W, 413
Thuesen Gell, Nancy, 256, 413
Thuesen RDE, Barbara W, 413
Thur, Paul, 8279
Thurell, Lisa Andrea, 731
Thurman, Erik, 6663
Thurman, Keith, 3171
Thurman, Scott, 6777
Thurston, Cloris, 663
Thuyer, Joel, 3004
Tiano, Cheryl, 4127
Tiboris, Peter, 5036
Tick, Carolyn, 5412
Tick, Michael, 2979
Tickler, Mike, 2380
Tieber, Helen, 1789
Tiebout, Bobbie, 2632
Tiedemann, Pat, 2859
Tiedtice, John M, 4379
Tiedtke, John, 4381
Tielking, Mary Evelyn, 2335
Tiemeyer, Christian, 1187
Tiff, Natasha, 969
Tiffany, Edwin P, 4661
Tighe, Joan, 1050
Tighe, John, 1050
Tikham, Allen, 1117
Tiknis, Michael, 6966
Tilghman, Romalyn, 156
Tilley, Susan, 4376
Tilson-Thomas, Michael, 1045
Tilton, Barbara, 1981
Tilton, Carly, 3260
Tilton, Mary, 4492
Timmins, Marissa, 2114
Timmons, Kathleen, 6705
Tindall, Karen, 4332
Tines, Paul J, 6284
Tingey, Diane, 655
Tingle, Chip, 860
Tingley, Tracy, 8394
Tinker, Bruce, 3097
Tinsley, Toni, 3608
Tippel, Matthew, 2056
Tipson, Baird, 1658
Tirbak, Peter, 2024
Tischler, Rachel, 3360
Tivnan, Brian T, 3082
Tizzie, Peter, 4268
Tjaden, Karen, 2124, 5915
Tkach, Tom, 7265
Tobey, Marta, 893, 4185
Tobias, Nina, 4752
Toch, Ed, 710

Toci, Dee R, 4046
Todaro, Bobbi, 6148
Todd, David, 748
Todd, Dina, 4868
Todd, Karin A, 1435
Todd, Lou, 1772
Todd, Shelley, 6728
Todd, Shelly, 6730
Todd, Tom, 1740
Toeplitz, Gideon, 1740
Toff, Ruth, 1481
Tofteland, Curt L, 2970, 4576
Tognoli, Era, 2168
Toirac, Margarita, 3396
Tokar, Chris, 1511
Tolbert, Cathy, 2264
Tolbert, Scott, 7329
Tolen, Tallie, 1452
Toliver, Linda, 2458
Tolj, Donald, 298
Tollett, Gerald J, 5533
Tolloti, Patricia, 1653
Tollson, Robert, 5870
Tolokan, Toby, 1171
Tomaro, Robert, 1863
Tomas, Nancy, 1882
Tomascak, Lawrence, 6264
Tomassi, Noreen, 4999
Tomasson, Helgi, 140
Tomaszek, Michael, 1889
Tomei, Paula, 2400
Tomer, Limor, 1456
Tomilson Hill, J, 3399
Tomkalski, Don, 7732
Tomkins, Leslie, 5582
Tomlinson, Janis, 4299
Tomlinson, John, 535
Tomlinson, Linda, 4723, 6942
Tomlinson, Rebecca, 6364
Tomlinson, Tom, 6383
Tomov, George, 571
Tompkins, David, 231
Tompkins, Glenn, 6634
Tompkins, Kathy, 4729
Tompkins, Susan, 1405
Tompkins O'Neill, Zoura, 94
Toney, Bobbie, 735
Toohey, Bill, 7929
Toohey, Christopher, 861
Toohey, John, 1795
Toomey, Helen, 1990
Topchik, David, 3465
Topilow, Carl, 954, 1604, 4241
Topp, Bobb, 3211
Topper, Paul, 1581
Toqawa, Jill, 136
Torbeck, Vanessa, 579
Torbert, Max L, 8318
Torbin, Becky, 635
Torchia-Sizemore, Kathleen, 1903
Torgerson, Arlene, 8209
Torgerson, Jeff, 3989
Torijan, Sandra, 340
Tornow, Ted, 6646
Torok, Leslie, 2905
Torralva Alonso, Maria Elenz, 687
Torrano, Sharon, 152
Torre, Paul, 4723, 6942
Torree, Nathan, 5858
Torrelva Alonso, Marie Elena, 3872
Torres, Adam, 1361
Torres, Donna, 446
Torres, Mark, 2994
Torres, Robert, 7993
Torres Webbe, Serena, 2370
Torrey, Janice, 4421
Torri, Erika, 6000
Tortolano, Dr. William, 5600, 5601
Tosch, Mary, 4449
Totten, Cynthia, 2737
Totten, John, 1128
Toultant, William, 4145

Toups, Joe, 1229
Tourangeau, Frank, 2818
Tourigny, Roxana, 5408
Towers, Charles, 3056
Towner, Tracey, 3112
Townsend, Brendon, 1812
Townsend, Don, 2298
Townsend, Erik Buck, 1920
Townsend, Erika, 1920
Townsend, Helen, 2631
Townsend, Lorraine, 6529
Townsend, Pat, 5492
Tracey, Fred, 5971
Trachtman, Susan, 744
Tracy, Christine, 5926
Tracy, Michael, 200
Tracy, Rick, 6131
Trafford, Ed, 1071
Trahan, Susan, 6641
Train, Simon, 6392
Tranter, Charles R, 3738
Trapnell, Susan, 3132
Trapp, Phillip R, 2391
Trask, Sally, 1349
Traska, Susan, 1876
Traub, Claudia, 7868
Traub, Denise M, 5767
Traub, John P, 1948
Trauber, Stephen, 5535
Traughber, Jan, 6538
Traum, Richard, 2716
Traupman-Carr, Carol, 5317
Trautman, Carl O., 3194
Trautman, Mark, 2173
Travaline, Barbara, 1419
Travaline, Philip, 1419
Traveis, Albert J, 1289
Travers, Beverly, 5982
Travers, Kerry, 5675
Traxler, Denise, 5228
Traynor, Jane, 3570, 7265
Traynor, John, 3570
Treadway, John, 3167
Treen, Mary Beth, 25
Trefzger, Lynn, 8431
Trego, Jim, 8129
Treiger, Betty Lou, 5701
Tremayne, Kristy, 2941
Trenkle, Swede, 6691
Trent, Pamela, 390
Tresansky, F. Victoria, 1990
Tressel, Jim, 7700
Treuer, Mary, 3120
Treuhaft, Alec C, 8442
Trevens, Janine Nina, 3453
Trevino, Esther, 5569
Trevino, Victor, 3397
Trevor, Kirk, 1167
Trexell, Brad, 1944
Tribbey, Stuart N., 1876
Trifiro, Dorian, 989
Trifle, Carol, 3488
Trilling, Whitney, 8347
Trimble, Pat, 2749
Trimble, Rick, 1798
Trimis, Antigone, 145, 4199
Trinca, Carl E, 78
Trinkle, Steven, 1585
Trinkoff, Donna, 3344
Trives, Nathaniel, 927
Trizila, Jo, 5538, 8079
Troland, Charles, 2335
Trombka, Candace, 608
Trombly, Robert, 3591
Trost, Chris, 2132
Trott, Stephen S, 1096
Trott, Steve, 1097
Trotta, Thomas, 974
Trotter, Laura, 4107
Trotter, Porrin, 2782
Trotter, Terri, 5906
Troup, BP, 1280

Trout, Mark, 5921
Trowbridge, Marcella, 2618
Troxler, George, 5125
Truax, Brandon, 2918
Truax, John F, 682
Truax, Nan, 3822
Truckenbrod, Phillip, 8357
Trudeau, George, 5099
TrudellIseler, Vicki, 4735
Truebllod, Mark, 4204
Truelove, Mike, 8062
Truex, Judy, 5455
Truex, Kathi, 5566
Trugdeau, John, 5433
Truild, Julia, 2689
Truitt, Jennifer, 257
Truitt, Steve, 5518
Truitt, Suzanne, 6713
Trujillo, Joyce, 8038
Trunzo, Robert, 8300
Truong, Cammy, 2551
Truskot, Joseph, 808
Trust, Sam, 4094
Truvillion, Vanessa, 274
Truyell, Diana, 1645
Tsafoyannis, John, 3150
Tsao, Joe, 8174
Tseitlin, Michael, 4161, 4162, 4163
Tseng, Muna, 521
Tu, Chi-Tsao, 3454
Tu, Johnny, 4124
Tubb, Billy, 7265
Tubey, Marta, 940
Tucci, Albert D, 2376
Tuceling, Barbara, 4316
Tucker, Billie, 2201
Tucker, Charlotte, 1402
Tucker, Claire, 661
Tucker, Curtis, 2060, 2265
Tucker, Earl, 2228, 5042
Tucker, Eric, 3749
Tucker, JoAnne, 378
Tucker, Joyce, 2605
Tufts, Robert R., 1946
Tuggle, Jerry, 7948
Tujillo, Melissa, 4053
Tukloff, Scott, 2536
Tuma, Dorothy, 4833
Tuomey, Ann, 7381
Turbyfil, John, 2333
Turbyne, Will, 5191
Turchen, Barry, 4146
Turley, Pauline, 3387
Turnbull, Dr. Walter J, 2206
Turnbull, Horace, 2206
Turnbull, Ramona, 1388
Turner, Carolyn, 1586, 3023
Turner, Christian, 2399
Turner, David, 3315, 4965
Turner, H Woodruff, 2291
Turner, James, 4736
Turner, Kathleen, 8197
Turner, Lorna, 3795
Turner, Todd, 7960, 7961
Turner, Tracey, 1821
Turoff, Robert, 2734
Turpin, Jacquie, 1883
Turrell, Wendy, 1600
Turrell, Wendy A, 1601
Turrentine, CMSgt. Julianne, 1991
Tutterow, Russ, 2822
Tuttle, JB, 7980
Tuttle, Lynn, 1892
Tuttle, Mo, 5529
Twiss, Linda, 3150
Twohig, Kevin J, 8245
Tyler, Brian, 3697
Tyler, Cheever, 2622
Tyler, Leslie, 127
Tyler, Sally, 5535
Tyler, Scott, 5916
Tyler, Summer, 7591

Tyler, Suzanne, 6803
Tylor, Paul, 1085
Tylor-Morris, Rebie, 5826
Tymon, Beborah, 7302
Tyree, Alan, 1370
Tyree, Jane, 216
Tyree, Priscilla, 5150
Tyrrell, Louis, 2706, 2707
Tyson, Steven, 2824
Tyson, Susan, 701

U

Ubell, Shirley, 450
Uchida, Christy, 1121, 2846, 4440
Udagawa, Yoichi, 1304, 1305
Udden, Rebecca Greene, 3857
Ueefe, Anne, 2645
Ugarte, Salvador, 2712
Uher, Fene, 1765
Uhlaender, Barbara, 1779
Uhler, J Thomas, 1034
Uhlman, Ed, 4910
Ulibarri, Linda, 7263
Ullestad, Kevin, 4429
Ullestard, Kevin, 6507
Ullyette, Laurel, 3286
Ulrich, Sally, 1485, 4982
Ulrich, Tom, 1343
Ulvested, Glen, 5443
Ulwelling, Kay, 4248
Umanoff, Nancy, 405
Umbarger, Julie, 3140
Umberger, Steve, 3528
Undeland, Anne, 3068
Underwood, Cindy, 7126
Underwood, Denny, 2901
Underwood, Jill, 3125
Unger, Francie, 5818
Unger, Marcia, 593
Ungrangsee, Bundit, 1757
Uniatowski, Dr. Joanne, 5199
Unrein, Laurie, 4418
Upchurch, Jennifer, 3296
Updegraff, Jean, 1905, 1906
Uprichard, Laurie, 466, 557
Upton, Barb, 977
Urban, Al, 4793
Urban, Sheri, 741
Urbanowski, Alexandra, 2535
Urbis, Richard, 5488
Uribe, Dawn, 861
Urquhart, Sandra L, 1953
Urquidi, Rhonda, 6492
Urton, Dan, 1144, 2051
Uryasz, Steve, 8082
Usher, Joann, 2135
Utter, Anne, 2294

V

Vaalburg, Virginia, 1981
Vacca, Michele L, 2827
Vaccaro, Sal, 4983, 7355
Vadney, Mark, 4864
Vagis, Judith A, 766
Vahle, Cindy, 3195
Vail, Martha, 1605
Vail, Robin, 1576
Vail, Walt, 3706
Vail, Walter, 3724
Vaillant, Caroline, 2166
Valacich, Carolyn, 1389
Valdez, Ernest, 5978
Valdez, Luis, 2539
Vale, E Merritt, 1595, 2253
Valencia, Veronica, 7259
Valenta, George, 2119
Valente, Barbara, 2485
Valentina, Edith, 2343

Valentine, Alan D, 1772
Valentine, Bill, 5916
Valk, Kate, 3477
Valladeres, Leo, 4168
Valle, Laura, 1196
Valliere, Roland E, 1373
Van Ausdal, Francis, 1679
Van Berg, Diane, 960
Van Bergen, Kathleen, 1381
Van Blancom, Julie W, 1983
van Boer, Bert, 5673
van Boer, Bertil, 8213
Van Boxtel, Faye, 2536
Van Damme, Sven, 439
Van Der Kamp, Steve, 6963
Van Der Zaag, Glenda, 839
Van Dyke, Jan, 575
Van Dyke Roudnev, Mary, 6522
Van Fleteren, Roger, 1
van Hamel, Martine, 526
Van Hemert, Lettie, 3215
Van Hook, Kenny, 3773
Van Kleeck, Marty, 3848
Van Leer, Tim, 6173, 6678
Van Loo, Scott, 5184
Van Osdel, DDS, Virginia, 823
Van Patten, Mauriel, 4361
Van Pelt, Jovonna, 3039
Van Pelt, Nita, 1696
Van Rysdam, Jennifer, 7314
Van Sant, Gus, 5306
Van Slyke, Linda, 1545, 1546, 2235
Van Straaten, Thomas, 1502
Van Voorst, Tracy, 3157
Van Wickler, Cate, 3686
Van Winkle Campbell, Sandra, 3782
Vanausdall, John, 6605
Vanaver, Livia, 568
Vanberg Wolff, George, 2520
Vance, Craig, 1399
Vance, Kathleen, 1399
Vance, Tom, 3527
Vance, Jr, Cyrus R, 1850
Vance-Watkins, Lequita P, 5612
Vande Berg, Leah, 1908
Vande Hey, Jean, 1865
Vanden Wyngaard, Julianne, 4703
Vandenberg, Diane, 1966
Vandenberg-Suju, Christina, 715
VanDenburg, RH, 4242
Vandergrift, Barbara, 4457
Vandermaten, Ann, 3153
Vandermaten, John, 3153
Vanderpool, Neil, 592
Vandervelde, Mike, 6947
Vanderyacht, Darcie, 7765
VanDeVeen, Ron, 7214
Vanison-Blakely, Dolores, 420
Vann, Karen S, 4321
Vann, Marvin, 8183
Vann, Stephen, 1512
VanOsch, Michael, 2768
Vanska, Osmo, 1353
VanStone, Molly, 2123
Vapnek, Dianne, 161
Varano, Tom, 8406
Vargo, Robert, 3634
Vari, John, 3231
Varineau, John, 1322
Varner, Allen D, 4517
Varney, Raye, 2773, 6443
Vaslev, Susan, 3677
Vasterling, Paul, 661
Vaughan, Anne, 3245
Vaughan, David, 999
Vaughan, George M, 1810
Vaughan, Jeff, 3938
Vaughan, Mark D, 3183
Vaughan, Mary K, 1810
Vaughan Scott, Dr. Mona, 2392
Vaughn, Michael, 7517
Vautar, James L, 5344

Vazquez, Jose, 3508
Veater, Claire, 1029, 4323
Vega, Dianne, 2538
Vega, Kay, 3659
Veintimilla, Pablo, 1046
Velasquez, Ben, 5896
Velasquez, Carol, 729
Velloff, Kittianne, 3786
Veloso, Michael J, 1265
Veloudos, Spiro, 3036, 3037
Veloz, Frank, 1949
Venanzi, Henri, 1951
Vendice, William, 1919
Venekamp, Jeff, 7911
Vener, Andre C, 914
Vener, Victor, 914
Venman, Bill, 2092
Vennerbeck, Eric, 2443
Vento, Art, 6481
Ventre, Philip T, 1000
Venzago, Mario, 4630
Vera, John, 933
Vera, Nella, 3351
Verbsky, Franklin, 1471
Verbsky, Marilyn, 1471
Verdeyen, Jacqueline, 3752
Verdier, Paul, 2415
Verenezi, Claire, 5088
Vergilio, Rosie, 7828
Vermillion, Jeani, 6977
Vernael, Gina, 3595
Vernick, Clifford, 4918
Vertosick, Suzanne M, 2286
Verville, Timothy, 1670
Vesely, Alison C, 4475
Vestal, Charlie R, 7567
Vestal, Robby, 5543
Vezner, Tony, 2896
Vhl, Dustin L, 4002
Vialet, Debra L, 4979
Vicari, Mary Ellen, 2191
Vick, Nancy, 993
Vickerman, John, 1242
Vickers, F Norman, 1052
Vickery, William, 789
Vickrey, Dr. Jim, 4021
Victor, Jane, 4451
Victor Bordo, Guy, 1180
Viebranz, Cristin, 365
Viebrock, Lois, 3202
Viera, Jelon, 462
Viertel, Thomas, 2642, 2643
Vigessa, Delores, 1388
Vigil, Cynthia, 187
Vigilant, Michael, 4720, 6933
Villalobos, Cesar, 333
Villani, Frank, 5556
Villanueva, Joesfa, 162
Villanueva, Josefa, 162
Villasana-Ruiz, Rosario, 123
Villaume, Beth, 1362
Villaume, Emmanuel, 649, 1758, 3753, 5422
Villella, Edward, 379
Villeua, Edward, 230
Vilmik, Elizabeth, 5049
Vincent, Jim, 273
Vincent, Johnell, 1809, 2320
Vincent Davis, Paul, 3039
Viniard, Mark, 7890
Vinogradov, Oleg, 80
Viorica, Stela, 28
Vipperman, Dick, 3929
Virgin, Jan, 302
Virkhaus, Taavo, 748
Visocky, Donna, 963
Visscher, William, 922
Vitaich, Roger, 4113, 5988
Vitale, Katherine B, 1081
Vitale, Ted, 3067
Vitek, Thomas, 1141
Vivirito, Dale, 3628
Vizolis, Andris, 1291

Vlassis, Dennis, 2706
Vmphress, Jessica, 2855
Vockey, Denton, 3839
Vodnoy, Robert, 1340
Voeks, Keith E, 6970
Voelker, Brian, 2859
Vogel, Anna, 8328
Vogelstein, John L, 528
Vogl, Joe, 6984
Vogt, John, 4481
Vokolek, Dana, 8432
Volk, Bill, 1110
Volkmen, Chris, 7119
Vollmer, Erich, 4983, 7355
Volpe, Mark, 1264, 4678
Volstad, Paul, 904
von der Schmidt, Jeff, 873
Von Eschen, Lynn, 7027
Von Frankencerg, Carlosc, 6083
von Heidecke, Kenneth, 286
von Hochstetter, Georg, 8400
Von Hoffmann, Betty, 3194
von Tempsky, Frances A, 2803
von Wurtzler, Dr. Aristid, 1521
Vonk, Hans, 4801
Vorhis, Patricia, 1837
Vorrasi, John, 2040
Vorsanger, Fred, 5905
Vosburgh, David, 3634
Voss, Kelly, 2928
Voss, Muriel, 4530
Voss, Ray, 4530
Voss, Ron, 2074
Voss, Zannie Giraud, 3532
Vossbrink, David, 1922
Voth, Pam, 3202
Vought, Nancy, 5318
Voyles, Lisa, 4476
Vriens, Taylor, 1821
Vrieze, Kory, 1774, 5472
Vulgamore, Allison, 1073
Vumbaco, Brenda J, 985
Vystrcil, Karel, 910

W

W. Radcliffe, Richard, 979
Waalkes, Ruth, 1249, 4642
Waber, Art, 8474
Wacholz, JC, 1139
Wachowski, Phillip, 1676
Wachtel, Linda, 1139
Wachter, Sheryl, 1384
Wada, Francis, 1286
Wade, Ann, 4291
Wade, Bob, 6200
Wade, Charles, 1073
Wade, Dawn, 819
Wade, Dr. Janice E, 1203
Wade, Dr. Jere D, 2568
Wadhams, John, 1979
Wadler, Michael, 2394
Wadley, Susan, 3509
Wadsworth, Kim, 3405
Wadsworth, Pebbles, 7980
Wadsworth, Susan, 5057, 8466
Wagan, Sixto, 8063
Wagar, Jeannine, 4064
Wagar, Paul, 2563
Wager, Timothy, 2166
Waggoner, Marion, 3580
Wagman, Laurie, 2280
Wagner, Amy, 3390
Wagner, Andrea, 5702
Wagner, Barbara, 1215
Wagner, Christine, 7798
Wagner, Howard V, 4668
Wagner, Jeannine, 1918
Wagner, Julie, 6828
Wagner, Kaye, 5738
Wagner, Lisa, 4543

Wagner, Lois, 4218
Wagner, Pat, 6661
Wagner, Roger, 1915
Wagner, Shirley, 2948
Wagner, Vincent, 5102
Wagoner, Bob, 8188
Wagy, Hillary, 1082
Wahamaki, Kirk M, 6972
Wahl, Dyno, 4422
Wahlberg, Sonja, 3140
Waickman, Kit, 3148
Wainio, Jeanne, 7698
Wainstein, Michael, 2949
Wait, Charles V, 1552, 3503
Wait, Gregory, 1921
Wakefield, Al, 5612
Wakely, Judith, 4408
Wakeman, Kelly, 4931
Walakovits, Edward, 1726
Walbel, Tim, 3938
Walbolt, Margo, 2682
Walczak, Jim, 7907
Walden, Josh, 793
Walden, Leigh, 3775
Walder, Diane, 5697
Waldo, Elisabeth, 4146
Waldo, Elizabeth, 4146
Waldschmidt, Linda, 289
Wales, Lorraine, 5229
Waliyaya, Shadiyah, 3322
Walker, Andrew, 4341
Walker, Bill, 6769
Walker, Charles D, 2207
Walker, Dan, 2575, 3085
Walker, David, 3840
Walker, Debbie J, 6006
Walker, Edward, 1673
Walker, Eric, 6975
Walker, Ethel Pitts, 2508
Walker, Faye, 709
Walker, Fred, 7581
Walker, James, 1474, 1475
Walker, James L, 3761
Walker, January, 4336
Walker, Jeffry, 6258
Walker, Jim, 2928
Walker, John, 5859
Walker, John T, 7680
Walker, Johnny, 7658
Walker, Judith, 1178
Walker, Judith H, 3909, 5622
Walker, Katheryn, 3408
Walker, Kay, 4332
Walker, Philip, 1567, 5103
Walker, Phillip E, 2508
Walker, Rich, 4456
Walker, Robert C, 3102
Walker, Todd, 8382
Wall, Betty, 1799
Wall, Elizabeth W, 2141
Wall, John, 1300
Wall, Kendall B, 7528
Wallace, Angela, 1470, 4955
Wallace, Bruce, 4152
Wallace, Lorraine, 1985
Wallace, Marilyn, 4152
Wallace, Reed M, 1592
Wallace, Sandra, 762
Wallace, Steven W, 7718
Waller, Richard, 1621, 5197, 5198
Waller, Rosemarie, 4212
Waller, Winifred, 3802
Walley, Patti, 8391
Wallis, Kathy, 4339
Wallnau, Carl, 4878
Waln, Kathleen H, 2484
Walsh, Diane, 5087
Walsh, Freda, 6287
Walsh, Helena, 4494
Walsh, Jack, 4937
Walsh, John Powel, 4805
Walsh, Karen, 2344

Walsh, Liz, 3725
Walsh, Paul, 2509
Walsh, Robert, 4855
Walsh, Sharon, 1454, 4922
Walter, Deanne M, 1990
Walter, Michele, 1837
Walter, PhD, Elaine R, 1990
Walters, Carole, 3099
Walters, CJ Chapman, 4844
Walters, Doris, 5827
Walters, Dr. Teresa, 4885
Walters, Ellen, 2154
Walters, Gary D, 7239
Walters, Jr, Charles A, 5659
Walton, Emma, 3499
Walton, Kacky, 5462
Walton, Mark, 583
Walton, William, 2608
Walvoord, Kay, 1327
Walz, Philip L, 5395
Wampler, Ralph M, 7657
Wandruff, Dorothy, 2460
Wang, I Fu, 2129
Wang, Shou-lai, 3454
Wang, Ya-Hui, 1601
Wankel, Edward E., 1470, 4955
Wanlass Szalla, Megan, 3333
Wanner, Dan, 5031
Wanpler, Karen, 7657
Want, Hsu, 3454
Wantroba, Kim, 2606
Warburg, Joan M, 3338
Ward, Bonnie, 106, 1936, 2507
Ward, Bonnie J, 2506
Ward, Buzz, 3581
Ward, Carolyn T, 4882
Ward, Don, 1936, 2507
Ward, Donna, 1787
Ward, Harry, 3684
Ward, Herbert, 1088
Ward, Jacqueline, 1088
Ward, Jeff, 6795
Ward, Joan, 1458
Ward, Kevin, 590
Ward, Laura, 3545, 5136
Ward, Patrick, 3707
Ward, Renee, 5129
Ward, Steven, 1688
Ward, Tammie, 4309
Ward, Thomas P, 582
Ward, William D, 2454
Wardell, Brandon, 2867
Warder, Jo Anna, 3762
Ware, Thomas, 2480, 6071
Warfield, Benjamin, 1976
Warfield, Todd, 3298
Warg, Dane, 7015
Warga, Tim, 7687
Warhol, Mark, 1352
Warland, Dale, 2145
Warmflash, Stuart, 3377
Warne, Katherine M, 5204
Warner, Dena, 5924
Warner, Doug, 2460
Warner, Irene, 4350
Warner, Kate, 2779
Warner, Sara T, 203
Warnick, Kevin, 3890
Warnke, Marsha, 368
Waroff, John, 2551
Warrell, Bill, 4302
Warren, Don, 2604
Warren, Gina, 7937
Warren, Jean S, 2355
Warren, Jim, 3930
Warren, Joel, 7455
Warren, John, 2518
Warren, Lee, 7726
Warren, Moorea, 1948
Warren, Norm, 3578
Warren, Rita, 1577
Warren, Russell, 8082

Warshaw, Marya, 401
Warshawski, Evy, 4654, 4707
Wartella, Brad, 3970
Wartella, Nicholas, 1470, 4955
Washburn, Nan, 880, 1338
Washington, Ajene, 3378
Washington, Erwin, 41
Washington, J Barry, 3256
Washington, Jennifer J, 1113
Washington, Jesse, 4222
Washington, Pat, 2030
Wassergord, Dale, 3180
Wasserman, Elliot H, 2910
Wasserman, Peter, 1075
Wasserman, Rena, 2457
Wasserman, Shoshanna, 3641
Watanabe, June, 154
Waterfall, Julia L., 1889
Waters, Byron, 8082
Waters, Neville, 4301
Waters, Shirley, 2628
Waters, Sylvia, 418
Waters, Willie, 1973
Watkins, Dawn, 5130
Watkins, Penny, 5719
Watkins, Robert, 703
Watkins, Thaddeus, 6123
Watley, Dennise, 7085
Watley, Matt, 7055
Watson, Barbara, 3011
Watson, Kip, 6365
Watson, Larry, 5973
Watson, Lisa L, 2769
Watson, Lola, 2752
Watson, Paul, 45
Watson, Walter, 1645
Watt, Jim, 6950
Watterson, Ralph, 3843
Watton, Janet, 5611
Wattrick, Lou Anne, 4728
Watts, John, 6554
Watts, Linda, 1099
Wax, David M, 1755
Way, Em, 3798
Waye, Avril K, 4700
Waymire, Nichole, 301
Wayte, Alan, 832, 849
Wead, Carol, 1414
Weatherington, Jim, 2887
Weathers, Rosemary, 1615
Weaver, Earl D, 3195
Weaver, Jerry, 5635
Weaver, Jessica, 3843
Weaver, Jim, 8163, 8165
Weaver, Justin, 4204
Weaver, Martha, 1770
Weaver, Michael, 3965
Weaver, Susan, 1800
Weaver Miller, Trudy, 4684
Weaver Smith, Barbara, 2916
Webb, Donald A, 1232
Webb, Dr. John, 5568
Webb, Terry, 5238
Webber, Christine, 1205
Webber, Len, 5289
Webber, Mary, 1894
Weber, Betsy, 2316
Weber, Bill, 822
Weber, Denny, 955
Weber, Dr. Ronald B, 4360
Weber, Eugene, 5185
Weber, Matt, 1791
Weber, Michael, 2924
Weber, Paul, 5106
Weber, Richard, 1596
Weber Federico, Robert, 1124
Weberg, Loyld, 1890
Webre, John, 103
Webre, Septime, 214, 4646
Webster, Chris, 1929
Webster, Douglas, 482
Webster, Ellen, 3641

Webster, Lynne, 1082
Webster, Nick, 1477
Webster, Obie, 7919
Webster, Richard R, 1130, 4459
Webster, Rick, 202
Webster Latshaw, Sunshine, 202
Wechsler, Martin, 7397
Weckesser, John, 7274
Wedin, Sharon, 4153
Wedseltoft, Jorgen, 6068
Weed, April, 1410
Weeda, Linn, 755
Weeden, Mary, 1485, 4982
Weekly, Joyce, 5546
Weeks, Jacqueline, 4865
Weesk, Jon, 3137
Wegher, Michael, 6113
Wegmann, Linda, 6769
Wehman, Rollin, 3913
Wehman, Rollin E, 3913
Wehrle, John, 1766, 2297
Weichei, Cindy, 929
Weidemann, Tom, 7329
Weidman, Kim, 667
Weigel, Jay, 6768
Weil, Ben, 3896
Weil, Bruno, 805, 4093
Weil, Christopher, 886, 4178
Weil, James, 2637
Weil, Joan, 5863
Weil, John, 3189
Weil, Richard, 2049
Weil, Suzanne, 514
Weiland, Don, 6820
Weiland, Martin J, 2307
Weilbaecher, Danial, 4599
Weiler, Robert, 6981
Weiler, Susan, 4672
Wein, George T, 5030
Wein, Marge, 2352
Weinand Esquire, Jerry, 3733
Weinberger, Barbara, 3826
Weiner, Earl D, 3338
Weiner, Jane, 470
Weiner, Louis, 4183
Weiner, Melanie, 3472
Weinert, Richard S, 5010
Weingarten, Robert I, 832, 849
Weinkle, Susan, 4366
Weinraub, Melanie, 3399
Weinstein, Alan, 5656
Weinstein, David, 1533
Weinstein, Ellen, 449, 522
Weinstein, Mark, 2291
Weinstein, Stanley, 8397
Weinstock, Janell, 1615
Weintraub, Aviva, 7394
Weintraub, Jason, 1468
Weir, Debi, 2312, 5515
Weir, James, 3846
Weirich, Robert, 5087
Weis, Liza, 1739
Weisenburger, Perk, 6556
Weiser, Charles, 1745
Weiskel, Catherine, 1266
Weisman, Walter, 3888, 3889, 3891
Weiss, Debra, 563
Weiss, Ellen, 3465
Weiss, Harriet, 3722
Weiss, Jurgen, 3042
Weiss, Nancy, 2087
Weiss, Pam, 90
Weiss, RJ, 4340
Weiss, Sandra, 1135
Weiss, Scott, 732
Weissberg, Franklin, 4936
Weissman, Neile, 3450
Weitz, Roger, 2031
Weitzman, Ron A, 807
Welborn, Robin, 7531
Welch, Barbara, 7270
Welch, David M, 1266

Welch, Doris Fritz, 1266
Welch, George, 2326
Welch, Maranne Purcell, 3729
Welch, Mia, 588
Welch, Paula, 3978
Welch, Richard, 2934, 6661
Welch, Roger, 2806
Weldon, Virginia, 1381
Welk, Lois, 7326
Wellbaum, Ray F, 1263, 1264
Wellbourne, Jr, Dr. Sullivan, 5131
Weller, Harold L, 1405
Weller, Henry, 3003
Weller, Kirk, 4395
Weller, Mary, 2091
Wellert, Michael, 3208
Welles, Joana, 2047
Wellin, Thomas, 1596
Wellman, Ron, 7565
Wellmann, Frank, 7670
Wells, Barbara, 5653
Wells, Chris, 2410
Wells, Christine, 1295
Wells, David, 5750
Wells, E Warner, 3754
Wells, Jeff, 4427
Wells, Joan, 7208
Wells, John, 5333
Wells, Kermit, 2048
Wells, Larry, 1696
Wells, Palmer, 6464
Wells, Palmer D, 2787
Wells, Pat, 3885
Wells, Philippe, 3042
Wells, Rex, 963
Wells, Steve, 6198
Wells, Steven, 4237
Welniak, Randy, 8324
Welsh, George, 8168
Welsh, John, 1841
Welsh, John D, 1773
Welsh, Melody, 1219
Welter, Bonnie, 1863
Welter, Philip, 2142, 2143
Weltman, Alexis, 181
Weltner, Karen, 3176
Welty, Karl, 3948
Welty, Peg, 6341
Wenger, Philip R, 2275
Wenger, Sheri Grace, 7877
Weninger, Jill, 7891
Weninger, John W, 8279
Wente, Charles, 2265
Wenthen, Fred, 1539
Wentworth, Kenneth, 8410
Wenzel, Kenneth J, 29
Wenzel, Pete, 8260
Werblin, Dr. Alan, 862
Werch, Shifra, 2044
Werder, Tom, 388
Werlinich, Lucille, 1469
Wermuth, Dr. Robert, 750
Wermuth, Robert A, 5763
Werner, Ellen, 4611
Werner, Joseph, 1551
Werner, Noel, 4902
Werner, Ray, 3730
Werner, Tobias, 5661
Wernick-Cassell, Linda S, 1010
Wernimont, Kathleen, 1186
Werstler, Gregory, 2813
Werth, Ernest, 3107, 6976
Wertheim, James, 5017
Werthemier, Esquire, Spencer, 631
Wertz, Ellen, 4476
Wertzer, Carla, 2963
Werz, Andreas, 826
Wesenburger, Perk, 6557
Wesler, Ken, 1729
Wesler, Kenneth A, 1982
Wesley, Barbara, 1920
Wessel, Kenn, 3940

Wesson, Ed, 5824
West, Don, 4817
West, George, 1409
West, Jessica, 2787
West, Judy, 4516
West, Kathleen, 1879
West, Katie, 5369
West, Lance, 5717
West, Lance A, 8264
West, Lori, 4113, 5988
West, Martha, 1590
West, Morgayne, 539
West, Stacy, 365
West, Steve, 7956
West Muir, Vita, 4274, 4275
Wester, Alica, 292
Westerfield, Richard, 744
Western, Rick, 2761
Westerwick, Bob, 1966
Westheimer, Richard, 5191
Weston, Elsie, 822
Weston, Elsie V, 822
Westrope, Daniel, 1128
Westwater, James, 8481
Westwood, Donald, 2230
Wetherber, Charles, 5225
Wethers, Shane, 7026
Wetli, Peg, 3124, 3158
Wettach Esquire, Thomas, 3733
Wetter, Margaret, 8231, 8233
Wetz, Gary, 7765
Wetzel, Brooke, 3903
Wetzel, Todd E, 4520
Wexchler, Malcolm, 3376
Whaley, Dawn Ellen, 976, 1969
Wham, Robert, 3798
Wheatley III, Kenneth, 4069
Wheeland, Charles, 1186
Wheeland, Ronnell, 3145
Wheeldon, Jeannie B, 2596
Wheeler, Dic, 2618
Wheeler, Douglas H, 4318
Wheeler, Jedediah, 8434
Wheeler, Mindy, 5484
Wheeler, Ronald, 1677
Wheeler, Scott, 1265
Wheelock, Tina, 7660
Whelan, Anita, 1155, 4489
Whelan, Christine, 7318
Whelan, Patrick, 3645
Whelihan, Paul, 3271
Whidby, Nannette, 232
Whidden, Shannon, 1889
Whiddon, Jerry, 3017
Whimper, Carl, 5869
Whisler, Garold, 2149
Whisler, W Scott, 6053
Whitaker, Don, 1177
Whitaker, Jean M, 573
Whitaker, John, 5114
Whitaker, Kathy, 241
Whitcare, Hunt, 3903
Whitcomb, Margo, 2509
Whitcomb, Zafra, 3347
White, Andrew, 3782
White, Barry, 5462
White, Bob, 757
White, Burton, 2796
White, Carolyn, 4710
White, Chris, 1484, 4980
White, Coral, 1764
White, D Patton, 247
White, David R, 7385
White, Donny, 8178, 8179
White, Dr. Leslie, 3362
White, Felicia, 672
White, Janet, 7144
White, Janis, 6814
White, Jeffrey G, 1340
White, Jodi, 556
White, Joel, 7302
White, Joyce, 5903

White, Keith, 6566
White, Leah, 2929
White, Linda, 3846, 5498
White, LuAnn, 2063
White, Lyla L, 2480
White, Lyla L., 6071
White, Lynn, 1767
White, Malissa, 5676
White, Mary T, 1663
White, Matthew, 5483
White, Melanie, 7143
White, Molly, 2671
White, Pat, 3416
White, Ryan, 6083
White, Sandy, 1861
White, Steven, 1880
White, Teresa A, 2833
White, Thalia, 3345
White, Vicki, 5683
White-Spunner, Jon, 3684
White-Spunner, Merv, 1881
White-Thomson, Ian, 1916
Whitehead, John, 650
Whitehill, Angela, 699
Whitehill, David, 865
Whitehill, James, 699
Whiteman, Ray, 7879
Whitener, William, 361, 362
Whiteside, George, 3042
Whiteway, Phil, 3924
Whitfield, David, 1068
Whitfield, Suan, 306
Whiting, Martin R, 6921
Whiting, Suzethe, 3241
Whitler, Kelli, 4464
Whitler, Kellye, 6549
Whitley, Holly, 3770
Whitley, Ran, 5112
Whitlock, Bobbi, 1180
Whitlock, David, 3766
Whitlock, Dr. Keith, 5862
Whitlock, Kendra, 764
Whitlock, Mary, 1876
Whitlock, R David, 3767
Whitman, Robert F, 8386
Whitmarsh, Kelly, 5518
Whitmer, Lou, 1599
Whitmore, John, 7103
Whitney, Cornelius, 1552, 3503
Whitney, John, 3929
Whitney, John C, 1049
Whitney, Linda, 3948
Whitney, Penny, 955
Whitsted, Don, 3020
Whitt, Ruth Ellen, 5565
Whitt-Lambert, Connie, 3834
Whittaker, Jetta, 760
Whitten, Kay, 825
Whittlsey, Betsy, 2178
Whittman, Loretta, 8203
Whittry, Diane M, 1709
Wicke Davis, Kelli, 640
Wickel, Shannon, 689
Wicker, Russell J, 7560
Wicks, Debra, 3109
Wicks, Stephen, 6804
Widdon, Caroline W, 1830
Widemann, John, 3258
Width, Tom, 3911
Wied, Douglas B, 933
Wiedermann, John, 3265
Wiegand, Mona, 1047
Wiegraffe, Merrell, 7108
Wiegraffe, Merrill, 7125
Wiemken, Robert, 1735
Wiender, Lynn, 1405
Wiener, Matthew, 2370
Wiensch, Adam J, 2346
Wier, Richard, 2819
Wiese, Rochelle, 5288
Wiesen, Ruth, 234
Wiess, Marjorie, 3616

Wietzke, Phoebea, 4744
Wifler, Raymond C, 1864
Wiggins, Cathy, 6358
Wiggs, Keith, 1527
Wight, Nathan, 5862
Wigstrom, Amy, 6500
Wigtil, Laurie, 4762
Wigton, Norm, 4037
Wijsmuller, Mary, 3272
Wikle, Sarah D, 2014
Wikswo, Quintan, 142
Wilbrecht, Dick, 2139
Wilbur, Roy, 5371
Wilcosky, James E., 1605
Wilcox, Agnes, 3191
Wilcox, Ericka, 8383
Wilcox, Fran, 1819
Wilcox, Mark, 3669
Wilcox-Burton, Maggie, 2158
Wilcox-Smith, Tamara, 3412
Wilder, Bruce, 1739
Wilder, Glenn, 2196, 5642
Wilder, Jim, 2628
Wilder, Michael, 6857
Wildges, John D, 6414
Wildman, Esquire, Thomas R, 983, 4272
Wilenius, Heidi, 3379, 5023
Wiley, Bert, 1584
Wiley, David, 1838, 5668
Wiley, Ella, 2392
Wiley, Jackson, 1172
Wiley, Mike, 2180
Wiley, Steve, 4222
Wiley Pickett, Kyle, 760
Wilford, Ronald A, 8430
Wilhelm, Robert, 1635
Wilhelm, Roberta, 3222
Wilhelmi, Butch, 6540
Wilhelmus, Tom, 2910
Wilhite, Jim, 3672
Wilhoit, Mel R, 5452
Wilinson, Donna M., 2155
Wilis, Danette A, 5659
Wilker, Laurence J, 4309
Wilker, Lawrence J, 6304
Wilkes, Dan, 6691
Wilkes, Pegi, 7683
Wilkins, Christopher, 955, 1811
Wilkins, Gary, 8060
Wilkins, Helen, 714
Wilkins, Jaci, 4424
Wilkins, John, 714
Wilkins, Thomas, 1032
Wilkinson, Gary, 2654
Wilkinson, Jane, 1309
Wilkinson, John, 4746
Wilkinson, Martha, 7949
Wilkinson, Scott, 3835
Wilks, Carolyn, 206
Will, Tracy, 3985
Willaims, Bruce, 4129
Willberg, Mack, 2325
Wille, Steve, 6086
Willeke, Linda, 6664
Willems, Conny, 314
Willems, Stephen, 3404
Willems, Tristan, 8409
Willemssen, Ann, 355
Willenbrink, Bob, 2378
Willet, Susan, 1466, 4941
Willets, Laurie, 295, 296, 2897, 2898
Willett, Lance, 1190, 1191
Willett, Lance O, 1189
Willey, Katherine, 2102
Willey, Marty, 4650
William Kuhs, George, 1112
Williams, Alison, 2478
Williams, Amy, 4940
Williams, Anita, 1841, 2788
Williams, Ann M, 672
Williams, Ben, 3640
Williams, Bill, 7956

Wood, Leon, 804
Wood, Margaret, 190
Wood, Marla, 389
Wood, Pamela, 2311
Wood, Paul L, 1173
Wood, Sandy, 1221
Wood, Shannon, 3792
Wood, Wendell P, 3033
Wood Bertrand, Lynn, 7512
Wood III, Ira David, 3556
Wood, Jr, Lawrence B, 5644
Wood-Price, Mrs. William, 5409
Woodard, Steve, 3050
Woodbridge, Edward, 326
Woodbridge, Ron, 7775, 7783
Woodcockne, Jim, 7126
Woodey, Emmutt, 6837
Woodham, Leigh, 6315, 6316
Woodhouse, Sam, 2504
Woodland, Jr, Naaman J, 5483
Woodruf, Judith, 657
Woodruff, Dr. Ernest, 7096
Woodruff, Louise, 1295
Woodruff, Robert, 3040, 3041
Woodruff, Sarah Beth, 5149
Woods, Darren, 2310
Woods, Martha, 8410
Woods, Prenza, 5557
Woods, Sue, 1861
Woodside, Lyndon, 2232
Woodward, Ervin C, 4122
Woodward, Geirgine, 840
Woodward, Geoffrey, 3928
Woodward, Jeffrey, 3261
Woodward, Sandy, 1710
Woodward-Morris, Suzie, 2463
Woodworth, Mary Ann, 2019
Woolbright, Normadien, 573
Wooldridge, Charlotte, 327, 4656
Wooley, Larry, 1881
Woolf, Steven, 3192
Woolridge, Dave, 99, 2489
Wooten, Alice, 5627
Wooten, Jim, 1363
Wooten, John, 3270
Wootton, Robert, 1115
Worboys, Bill, 3777
Worby, Joshua, 1434
Worcester, William, 927
Word, Jim, 6769
Woreman, Bernie, 5211
Working, Thomas, 1326
Workman, Harold, 6719, 6720
Workman, Linda, 1602
Worland, Len, 2602
Worley, Ernestine, 3564, 7253
Worrell, Mimi, 650
Worthen, Ellis C, 1822
Worthington, Douglas, 6040
Worthington, Wendy E, 3705
Woske, Lira, 4200
Wotta, Craig, 6917
Wozniak, Amy, 3713
Wozniak, Edward, 6272
Wray, Chuck, 4739
Wray, Robin, 3709
Wredegreen, Sandy, 2883
Wreen, Peggy, 5049
Wregand, Amy, 1870
Wren, Jody, 2745
Wrenn, Nancy, 1815
Wright, Ardis, 8091
Wright, Charles W, 4059
Wright, Detra J, 1081
Wright, Dr. Nathan A, 3378
Wright, Ed, 4110
Wright, Gary, 2467
Wright, Gregory, 6321
Wright, Jason S, 1776
Wright, Jim, 989
Wright, Julia, 1602
Wright, Lee, 2130

Wright, Mary, 3682
Wright, Matthew, 6478
Wright, Michael, 3996
Wright, Rebecca, 336, 3522
Wright, Sarah, 751, 1881
Wright, Tom, 1889
Wright, William, 6938
Wright Maurer, Holly, 1570
Wrighthouse, Mike, 4490
Wrigley, John, 1473
Writz, Cassandra, 300
Wroe, David, 1445
Wrong, Paul, 227
Wrubel, Austin S, 8447
Wu, Dennis, 4198
Wu, Eva, 3565, 7256
Wu, Hsing-Kuo, 3454
Wu, Jing-jyi, 3454
Wu, Nancy, 5012
Wu, Pamela, 2510
Wuepper, Ken, 4745
Wunsch, Renate, 806
Wurdack, Hope, 3195
Wurdeman, Carrie, 219
Wyant, Gladys, 4397
Wyatt, Charles, 5417
Wyatt, Doug, 1942
Wyatt, Nancy, 1837
Wyatt, Robert, 6901
Wyckoff, Laurel, 1737
Wyer, Dr. Peter, 5069
Wyle, Noah, 2412
Wyley, Kay, 2582
Wyman, Donna, 653
Wyman, Karen Ilyse, 6348
Wynkoop, Rodney, 2246
Wynn, J. H., 5103
Wynn, JH, 1567
Wynne, Judy, 8182
Wynne, Laurie, 1045
Wyse, Cynthia, 5117
Wyse, Gary, 7692

X

Xu, Joy, 290

Y

Yaeger, George, 1775
Yaelisa, , 146
Yaffe, Micheal, 201
Yagura, Terry, 4220
Yakstis, Gary, 6277, 6279
Yampolsky, Victor, 5739
Yan, Amy, 2475
Yancey, Rex, 2885
Yanci, Ricardo, 2025
Yancy, Ricardo, 266
Yang, Christina, 7400
Yang, Xiaoliang, 451
Yannatos, Dr. James, 1276
Yarborough, Joe, 8193
Yarbrough, Kathy, 744
Yarbrough, Robert, 2824
Yardbrough, John, 6343
Yarenhuk, Marcella, 5722
Yates, Becky, 786
Yates, Christopher, 5686
Yates, Debra, 1117
Yatfe, Michael, 1002
Ybarguen-Stockman, Pamela, 670
Ybarra, Patricia, 3424
Yeager, Derryl, 693
Yeamans, Nancy, 615
Yearley, Graham, 3015
Yefchak, George, 905
Yeh, John Bruce, 295, 2897
Yeh, Terence, 1504
Yeh, Tsung, 1181

Yekovich, Robert, 1593, 5162
Yeoman, Kathy, 2928
Yerger, Jenae, 3838
Yerger, KellyLee, 1718
Yerger, MaryLee, 1718
Yerman, Dan, 2681
Yestadt, James, 770
Yetter, Erich, 289
Yeung, Peter, 42
Yianilos, Bea, 2699
Ying, Phillip, 1502
Ying Pang, Ching, 867
Yoder, Lonelle, 3602
Yoder, Stephanie, 2905
Yoder, Timothy, 2905
Yoeng, Alan, 2781
Yoffe, Jane, 3054
Yoga, Joseph, 3310
Yoho, Terri, 5748
Yokouchi, Susan, 1092
Yokoyama, Brian, 4226
Yoo, Jay S, 8416
York, Diane, 2076
York, John, 3603
York, Scott, 2318
Yorto, Terri, 5747
Yost, Donald C, 2915
Yost, Emily, 5951
Yost, William A, 7500
Younan, Anne, 2435
Young, Aaron, 3888, 3889
Young, Becky, 1079
Young, Bill, 443
Young, Christine, 498
Young, Cynthia, 93
Young, Frank M, 3861
Young, Haven, 3167
Young, Jack, 3688, 5323
Young, John WK, 3754
Young, Karen, 2649
Young, Karey, 8504
Young, LouAnn, 297
Young, Matt, 7119
Young, Michael, 7091
Young, Patricia, 4224
Young, Patty, 1079
Young, Peter, 2636
Young, Sue, 5536
Young, Tami, 3865
Young, Tim P, 744
Young, Wallace, 2984
Young, Wendy T, 1839
Young Schrade, Rolande, 4952
Young, III, HG, 5725
Youngblood, Agnes, 1026
Youngblood, Anges, 4319
Youngdahl, Jon T, 1025
Youngerman, Suzanne, 1533
Youtsey, Phil, 7522
Ypma, Dr. Nancy, 4469
Ypung, David, 6122
Ysaguiree, Trevor, 2413
Ysuguirre, Angel, 2867
Yu Fong, Kuang, 3320
Yukevich, Gerald, 3074
Yung, Eleanor, 434
Yuoung, Kathy, 604
Yuritic, Alice, 1182
Yurkanin, Mark, 5374

Z

Zaback, Jerry, 3498
Zabel, Bruce, 1864
Zabel, William D, 3399
Zacek, Dennis, 2860
Zach, Jane, 4827
Zachary, Luccio, 2168
Zachary, Nedra, 799, 1900
Zachary, Richard, 3461
Zack, George, 1215

A

A.R.T New Stages, 3041
Aaron Davis Hall, 2229, 7367
Aaron Deroy Theatre, 3115
Aasu Fine Arts Auditorium, 4401
Abbeville Opera House, 7874
Abbot Pennings Hall of Fine Arts, 5734
Abe Lebewohl Park, 5040
Abilene Civic Center, 1775, 7964
Abilene Civic Center: Exhibit Hall, 7965
Abilene Civic Center: Theater, 7966
Abravanel Hall, 1824
Academic Hall Auditorium, 4781
Academy of Music, 1733, 1734, 2277, 2278, 2281,
    2283, 5372, 7822
Academy of Music: Hall, 7823
Academy of Music: Main Auditorium, 7824
Academy Playhouse, 3066, 6893
Academy Theatre: First Stage, 6430
Academy Theatre: Lab, 6431
Academy Theatre: Phoebe Theatre, 6432
Ackerman Auditorium, 5451
Actors Studio, 3340
Actors' Gang Theater, Actors' Gang El Centro, 2410
Actors' Theatre, 3675
Acts' One Reid Street Theatre, 2981
Adams Center Theatre for the Performing Arts, 4021
Adams Event Center, 7144
Adams Memorial Stage, 3879, 5576
Adams Memorial Theater, 4699
Adams Theatre, 5956
Addison Centre Theatre, 3818
Adelphi Academy, 3293
Adelphi University, 492
Adelphia Stadium, 7948
Adirondack Lakes Center for the Arts, 7297
Adler Theatre, 1189,1190, 1191, 2936
Administration Auditorium, 4072
Administration Building, 3081
Admiral Theatre, 1841
Adobe Theatre, 3275
Adrian College, 6910
Aea Summer Musical Theatre, 2997
African-American Cultural Center: Paul Robeson Hall,
    7311
Afrikan Poetry Theatre, 3322
Afro-American Cultural Center, 7517
Agency for the Performing Arts, 6016
Agnes Scott College, 6453
Aia Actor's Studio, 5951
Aiken Community Playhouse, 3751
Aillet Stadium, 6781
Airpra Theatre, 2389
Ak-Sar-Ben Future Trust, 7161
Akron Civic Theatre, 588, 7582
Aksarben Coliseum, 7162
Alabama Shakespeare Festival, 4017
Alabama Shakespeare Festival - Festival Stage, 5822
Alabama Shakespeare Festival - Octagon, 5823
Alabama Theater, 1880
Alamodome, 8108
Alaska Center for the Performing Arts, 6, 754, 755,
    1884, 1885, 5837
Alaskaland Civic Center, 1887, 5839
Albano Ballet and Performing Arts Center, 6252
Albany James H Gray Sr: Civic Center, 6423
Albany Municipal Auditorium, 6424
Albany State University Department of Fine Arts, 6424
Albert Iva Goodman, Owen Bruner Goodman Theater,
    2836
Albert J. Lupin Experimental Theatre, Dixon Hall, 2989
Albert Lea City Arena, 6991
Albert Lea Civic Theater, 6992
Albert Lupin Experimental Theatre, Dixon Hall, 6778
Albert Taylor Hall, 4550
Alberta Bair Theater for the Performing Arts, 2159,
    7133
Albright College Chapel, 5390
Albright College Theatre, 5390
Albuquerque Convention Center, 7260
Albuquerque Sports Stadium, 7261

Alcazar Theatre, 2515, 6109
Alcorn State University Athletic Complex, 7056
Alex Box Stadium, 673
Alex Theatre, 828, 829, 5984
Alex Theatre Glandale, 847
Alexander Auditorium, 4564
Alfond Arena, 6802
Alfred University: Merrill Field, 7290
Alhambra Dinner Theatre, 2700, 6353
Alhambra Theatre, 4573
Alice Busch Opera Theater, 2197
Alice Statler Hall, 7348
Alice Tully Hall, 1503, 1505, 1532, 2215, 4147
Allaert Hall, 6647
Allen County War Memorial Coliseum, 6598
Allen Fieldhouse, 6677
Allenberry Playhouse, 3686
Alley Theater (Pavilion, Circle Forum), 2469
Alley Theatre, 3851, 8057
Alley Theatre: Hugo V Neuhaus Arena Stage, 8070
Alley Theatre: Large Stage, 8058
Alliance Theatre, 2014, 2761
Allstate Arena, 6567
Alltel Arena, 5857
Alltel Stadium, 6354
Alma Thomas Theater, 5522
Aloha Stadium, 6476
Alsc Playhouse, 2449
Alumni Auditorium, 5466
Alumni Bowl Stadium, 5836
Alumni Coliseum, 6735
Alumni Hall, 1752, 6815
Alumni Stadium, 6803
Alva Public Library Auditorium, 7709
Alverno College, 8298
Alvina Krause Theatre, 3684
Alys Robinson Stephens Performing Arts Center, 5797
Alys Stephens Center, 1, 744
Aman Arena, 7925
Amarillo Civic Center, 1776, 7970
Amarillo Civic Center: Arena, 7971
Amarillo Civic Center: Music Hall, 7972
Ambassador Theatre, 7368
America West Arena, 5859
America's Shrine To Music Museum, 7912
American Airlines Arena, 6376
American Concert Hall, 1523
American Legion, 7711
American Place Theatre, 7369
American Stage Company Theatre, 2727
American Stage in Residence, Fairleigh Dickinson
    University, 3266
American Theater Company, 2813
American Theatre, 5633, 7104
American University - Mcdonald Recital Hall, 6294
American University - New Lecture Hall, 6295
Ames City Hall Auditorium, 1185, 6635
Amherst Middle School, 1564
Amherst Regional High School Auditorium, 2092
An Authentic Replica of An Elizabethan Theatre, 3868
Anaheim Convention Center, 5931
Anaheim Convention Center - Arena, 5932
Anb Community Hall, 4033
Anderson Auditorium, 4543
Anderson Center at Bingham University, 1459
Anderson Center for Performing Arts, 4931
Anderson Theater, 218, 5064
Andrew Jackson Hall, 2300
Andy Griffith Playhouse, 5144
Andy Kerr Stadium, 7341
Angelle Hall Auditorium, 4592
Angelo State University Auditorium, 8105
Angels Gate Cultural Center, 6136
Angus Bowmer Theatre, 3651, 5285
Ann Goodman Recital Hall, 5015
Annenberg Center for the Performing Arts, 627
Annenberg Theatre, 6067
Annie Russell Theatre, 2753, 4379
Anniston Museum of Natural History, 5794
Apollo Theatre, 7370
Appalachian State U Department of Athletics: Kidd
    Brewer Stadium, 7508

Appalshop Theatre, 2977
Appel Farm Arts and Music Center, 7215
Arcadia Stage/Studio Theatre, 3678
Arch-Opera House of Sandwich, 2052, 6568
Arco Arena, 6086
Arden Playhouse, 6087
Ardrey Auditorium, 761, 4039, 4040, 5848
Arena in Oakland and Network Associates Coliseum,
    6057
Arena Players, 6818
Arena Players Repertory Theater, 3310
Arena Theatre, 3643, 3858
Arena Theatre (Fichandler & Kreeger), 2658
Arie Crown Theatre, 6510
Ariel Theatre, 7666
Arizona Stadium University of Arizona, 5883
Arizona State University - Gammage Auditorium, 5878
Arizona State University Activity Center, 5879
Arizona State University West, 770
Arizona State University: Sundome Center, 5877
Arizona Western College, 5894
Arkansas Art Center Theater, 2382
Arkansas Repertory Theatre, 2383
Arkansas River Valley Arts Center, 5926
Arkansas Tech University - Witherspoon Arts Arena,
    5927
Arlene Schnitzer Concert Hall, 1696, 1702
Arlington Center for the Performing Arts, 6142
Arlington Theatre, 920, 4204
Armand Hammes Auditorium, 1011
Armstrong State College Fine Arts Auditorium, 6468
Arneson River Theatre, 8109
Arnold Hall Theater, 4259
Arnold Hall Theater - United States Air Force, 6199
Arnold T. Olson Chapel, 4451
Arrowhead Stadium, 7085
Art Complex at Duxbury, 6878
Art Museum, 5246
Artemus W. Ham Hall, 1403
Artemus West Ham Concert Hall, 2163
Arthur Ashe Stadium, 7332
Artist's Theatre, 839
Artists Civic Theatre and Studio, 6757
Arts and Science Center for Southeast Arkansas, 5922
Arts Center, 2046
Arts Center of the Ozarks, 5929
Arts Consortium Studio Theatre, 7599
Arts Council Theatre, 3565
Arts District Theater, 3821
Arts Hall, 192
Arts in Education: Capital Region Center, 7279
Arts in the Parks: Portable Stage, 6996
Arvada Center for the Arts and Humanities, 6187
Asbury First Methodist Church, 1550
Ascap, 7371
Asheville Civic Center, 7506
Ashland Community College Auditorium, 4566
Ashmore Fine Arts Auditorium, 6404
Ashtabula Arts Center, 7586
Ashtabula Campus, 1603
Askanase Auditorium, 3569
Assembly Hall, 5591, 6507, 6586
Association of American Theatre for Youth, 2942
Association of Performing Arts Presenters, 566
Astoria High School Auditorium, 618
Astrodome, 8059
Athenaem, 6000
Athenaeum Music & Arts Library, 6000
Athenaeum Theatre, 2044, 2857, 6511
Athens School of Ballet, 241
Atherton Auditorium, 6164
Atlanta Civic Center- Theatre Auditorium, 6433
Atlantic Center for the Arts, 6390
Atlantic Theater Mainstage, Black Box, 3349
Atlas Theatre, 4007
Atwood Center Ballroom, 4769
Atwood Stadium, 6941
Auditorium Theater - Denver Performing Arts
    Complex, 6207
Auditorium Theatre, 187, 275, 2815, 6512, 6513
Augusta Civic Center, 6790
Augusta Civic Center - Arena, 6791

Nichols Pennell Theatre, 2874
Nightingale Concert Hall, 1407
Nikos Stage, 4699
Nippert Stadium, 7605
Nmsu Performance Center, 1449
Noank, 4280
Nob Hill Masonic Center, 6119
Nord Theatre, 2985
Nordstrom Recital Hall, 1846
Norfolk Scope Cultural and Convention Center, 8188
Norris Center for the Performing Arts, 6085
Norris Cultural Arts Center, 1147, 6572
Norris Theatre for the Performing Arts, 869
North American Folk Enthusists and Dance Alliance, 566
North Carolina Blumenthal Performing Arts Center, 572, 1573, 5114, 7523
North Carolina Museum of Art, 7550
North Carolina Performing Arts Center, 2245
North Carolina School of the Arts - Roger, 7568
North Carolina State University Center Stage, 7552
North Carolina State University: Carter Finley Stadium, 7551
North Carolina State University: Reynolds Coliseum, 7553
North Charleston Performing Arts Center, 7897
North Hennepin Community College, 6999
North Hollywood High School, 1923
North Iowa Community Auditorium, 6665
North Junior High School, 1416
North Scottsdale, 4036
North Shore Center for the Performing Arts, 2892
North Shore Music Theatre, 3033
Northeastern Junior College Theatre, 6244
Northeastern University Center for the Arts, 6866
Northeastern University: Parsons Field Stadium, 6867
Northern Michigan University: Superior Home, 6965
Northland Pines High School, 5735, 8280
Northrop Memorial Auditorium, 354, 4759
Northshore Center for the Performing Arts, 6570
Northside Theatre, 2518
Northwest Lounge, 4815
Northwest Missouri State University, 7096
Northwestern College, 6666
Northwestern University: Dyche Stadium, 6542
Norton Center for the Arts, 6711
Norton Hall, 409, 2195, 4942
Norton Simon Museum, 873
Norwalk Concert Hall, 995, 1971
Notre Dame Stadium, 6622
Noyes Cultural Arts Center, 2867, 2871

O

O'Donnell Auditorium, 1394
O'Laughlin Auditorium, 4513
O'Neill Center, 6249
O'Reilly Theater, 3732
O'Rourke Center, 2845
O'Shaughnessy Auditorium, 2144
Oak Acres Amphitheatre, 3843, 8043
Oak Ridge High School Auditorium, 1773, 5471
Oak Ridge Playhouse in Jackson Square, 3798
Oakdale Theatre, 6283
Oakland-Alameda County Arena & Network Associates Coliseum, 6061
Oakmont Auditorium, 4212
Oberlin Conservatory, 1655
Occidental College - Thorne Hall, 6035
Occidental Community Church, 4149
Ocean Center, 4325, 6330
Odeum Sports & Expo Center, 6579
Odyssey Theatre, 2451
Ogdensburg Free Academy, 3486
Ogunquit Playhouse, 3003, 6801
Ohio State University, 1637
Ohio State University Wexner Center for the Arts, 7649
Ohio State University: Stadium Ii Theatre, 7647
Ohio State University: Thurber Theatre, 7648
Ohio State Univesity: Ohio Stadium, 7650

Ohio Theatre, 582, 585, 1636, 2261, 3342, 3423, 5210, 7688
Ohio Theatre Playhouse Square Center, 5205
Ohio University: Patio Theater, 7588
Ohio University: School of Music, 7589
Okaloosa-Walton Community College, the Arts Center, 6391
Oklahoma City University, 7722
Oklahoma City University: Burg Theatre, 7723
Oklahoma City University: Kirkpatrick Auditorium, 7724
Oklahoma City Zoo Amphitheatre, 7725
Oklahoma Panhandle State College: Carl Wooten Stadium, 7713
Oklahoma Summer Arts Institute, 7726
Okoboji Summer Theatre, 7076
Old Bastrop Opera House, 3812, 7984
Old Chief Theatre, 3118
Old City Hall, 3542
Old Colony Players Amphitheater, 3561
Old Creamery Theatre, 6661
Old First Church, 1945, 4189
Old Globe, 2499
Old Jail Art Center, 7969
Old Log Theatre, 3122
Old Opera House Company, 8254
Old Rock School, 3561
Old Towne Hall, 3576
Old Trinity Centre, 2973
Old Wharling Church, 1299
Olin Hall, 5656
Olive Swann Porter Hall, 4394
Oliver T. Joy Mainstage, 3215
Olmstead Theatre, 492
Olson Auditorium, 5060
Olympic Center, 7360
Olympic Velodrome/California State University, 5954
Omaha Civic Auditorium, 7160
Omaha Civic Auditorium: Music Hall, 7164
Omaha Community Playhouse, 3220
Omni Auditorium, 2000
Omni Auditorium - Broward Community College, 6324
One World Theatre, 7978
Ontological at St. Mark's Theater, 3424
Open Air Pavilion, 3983
Open Air Theatre, 7812
Open Eye: New Stagings, 7421
Opera, 3394
Opera House, 2122, 4086
Opera, Theatre, Concerts, 6796
Opperman Music Hall, 2008
Orange Bowl Stadium, 6382
Orange County Convention Center, 6397
Orange County Performing Arts Center, 834, 917, 1905, 1951, 1952, 5961
Orchard Hill Church, 2292
Orchard Road Christian Church, 961
Orchestra Hall, 1117, 1317, 1318, 1351, 1353, 1796, 2032, 2132, 7014
Orchestra Hall at Symphony Center, 1119
Ordway Center for the Performing Arts, 1362, 7027
Ordway Music Theatre, 2132, 2133, 4767, 7029
Ordway Music Theatre: Mcknight Theatre, 7028
Oregon Ridge Dinner Theatre, 3010
Oregon Shakespeare Festival: Angus Bowmer Theatre, 7744
Oregon Shakespeare Festival: Black Swan Theater, 7745
Oregon Shakespeare Festival: Elizabeth Station, 7746
Oregon State University: Gill Coliseum, 7751
Oriole Park at Camden Yards, 6828
Orkney Springs Pavilion, 5670
Orlando Centroplex, 6398
Orlin D. Trapp Auditorium, 1152, 2054
Oroville State Theater, 6063
Orpheum Theatre, 656, 764, 1401, 1229, 2162, 6120, 6775, 7165, 7422, 7943
Orpheum Theatre Foundation, 5863
Orrie De Nooyer Auditorium, 7218
Orvis Auditorium, 1090, 1092, 4409
Oscar Meyer Theatre, 1868, 2344
Osceloa County Stadium & Sports Complex, 6366

Osceola Center for the Arts, 6365
Osh Kosh Civic Auditorium, 1876
Otero Junior College - Humanities Center Theatre, 6238
Otis A. Singletary Center for the Arts Concert Hall, 4574
Ottawa Municipal Auditorium, 6687
Otterbein College, 1661
Ouachita Baptist University: Department of the Arts, 5899
Outdoor Theatre Complex, West Campus of Century College, 3166
Outdoor, Stanley-Sinsheimer-Glen Theater, 2549
Ovens Auditorium, 7524
Overland Theatre, 2948
Owen Theatre, 3548
Owensboro Sportscenter City of Owensboro, 6731
Oxnard Civic Auditorium, 937, 6064
Oxnard Performing Arts and Convention Center, 6065
Ozark Civic Center, 5827

P

P&C Stadium, 7488
P.E. Monroe Auditorium, 1583
Pabst Theatre, 3992, 8304
Pac Mainstage Theatre, Pac Concert Hall, 5673
Pacific Bell Park, 6121
Pacific Conservatory of the Performing Arts, 6151
Pacific Grove Middle School, 808
Pacific University, 7760
Pacific University: Tom Miles Theatre, 7761
Pack Place, 5104
Paducah Community College Fine Arts Center, 6734
Page Auditorium, 3533, 5117, 5119, 5120
Painted Bride, 7830
Palace at Auburn Hills, 6918
Palace Civic Center, 7671
Palace of Fine Arts, 145, 4199
Palace of Fine Arts Theatre, 6122
Palace Performing Arts Center, 7285
Palace Theatre, 578, 594, 1411, 1454, 1638, 1713, 2635, 2961, 3126, 3621, 5210, 6266, 7423, 7673, 7804
Palace Theatre and Music Hall, 1412
Palace Theatre of the Arts, 195, 997, 1977
Palestine Civic Center Complex, 8098
Palm Beach Community College, 6369
Palm Beach Community College, Glades Campus, 6316
Palm Springs Desert Museum: Annenberg Theater, 6067
Palmer Auditorium, 4279
Palmer College, 6487
Palo Alto Children's Theatre, 2478
Pan American Center, 7270
Pan American Musical Art Research, 7424
Pan American University Fine Arts Auditorium, 1791
Panida Theatre, 2810, 4423
Panola Playhouse, 7066
Pantages Centre, 725, 1855
Pantages Theater, 724, 1853, 1854, 2340, 5708
Paper Mill Playhouse, 3251, 7226
Paradise Theatre, 3944
Paramount Arts Center, 1105, 6705
Paramount Center for the Arts, 704, 3770, 7457
Paramount Theatre, 861, 1187, 2168, 2302, 4525, 6062, 6644, 6979, 7979
Paramount Theatre, Asbuty Park, 1413
Pardington Hall, 5060
Paris Junior College, 8100
Park College: Alumni Hall Theatre, 7098
Park College: Graham Tyler Memorial Chapel, 7093
Park Hill South School Auditorium, 1374
Park Place Hotel, 6983
Park Theatre Performing Arts Centre, 7251
Parker Playhouse, 6337
Parker School Auditorium, 2800
Parrish Auditorium, 5231
Pasadena Civic Auditorium, 872, 6070
Pasadena Playhouse - Mainstage Theatre, 6071
Passavant Memorial Center, 1714
Patriot Hall, 5438

St. Ambrose University, 4481
St. Andrews Lutheran Church, 1488
St. Andrews Presbyterian Church, 838
St. Anne's Chapel, 5298
St. Barnabas Presbyterian Church, 1784
St. Cecelia Cathedral, 4833
St. Francis Auditorium, 4918
St. James Church, Great Barrington, 4675
St. James-By-The-Sea, 887
St. John Auditorium, 1198
St. John Theatre Stage, 2990
St. John Vianney Church, 767, 4050
St. John's Lutheran Church, 1385
St. John's United Methodist Church, 1446
St. John's University, 7353
St. John's University (Festival Site), 4544
St. Johns Presbytarian Church, 4087
St. Joseph Auditorium, 4536
St. Joseph's Historic Foundation/Hayti Heritage Center,
 7527
St. Lawrence University: Augsbury Center, 7321
St. Mark's Church, 213
St. Mark's Episcopal, 1942
St. Martin's, 1570
St. Mary's, 1570
St. Mary's Cathedral, 1704
St. Mary's Hall, 1747, 5398
St. Patrick's Church, 4188
St. Paul's Chapel & Trinity Church, 2228, 5042
St. Paul's Episcopal Church-Westfield, 1444
St. Pauls By-The-Sea Episcopal Church, 4339
St. Peter's Church, 5722
St. Philip Neri Church, 1692
St. Philip's in the Hills Episcopal Church, 773, 4056
St. Stephen's Sanctuary, 5374
Stabler Arena, 7791
Stadium Theatre Performing Arts Center, 7873
Stage West, 2370, 3838
Stage-Theater-Arts Center, 5126
Stages Repertory Theatre, 8075
Stages Theatre, 2415
Staller Center, 1489
Staller Center for the Arts, 5090
Stambaugh Auditorium, 5259, 7699
Stambaugh Stadium, 7700
Stamford High School, 998
Stanford University - Annenburg Auditorium, 6158
Stanford University - Braun Recital Hall, 6159
Stanford University - Camble Recital Hall, 6160
Stanford University - Coverly Auditorium, 6161
Stanford University - Dinkelspiel Auditorium, 6162
Stanford University - Memorial Auditorium, 6163
Stanley Performing Arts Center, 5099, 7496
Stanly County Agri-Civic Center, 7505
Staples Center, 6042
Star Plaza Theatre, 1178
Starlight Bowl, 1936, 2507
Starlight Theater, 6108
State Museum of Pennsylvania, 7806
State Theatre, Olympia, Washington and the
 Governor's, 5695
State Univerity of New York College at Brockport:
 Tower Fine Arts Center and Hartwell Hall, 7299
State University of New York, 1473, 1481
State University of New York at Buffalo: Department
 of Theatre & Dance, 7318
State University of New York at Purchase, 1972
State University of New York College-Brockport, 7300
State University of New York-Albany: Arena, 7287
State University of New York-Albany: Main Theatre,
 7288
State University of New York-Albany: Recital Hall,
 7289
State University of New York-Binghampton: Anderson
 Center for the Arts, 7296
State University of New York-Fredonia: Michael C
 Rockefeller Arts Center, 7337
State University of New York-Oneonta, 1540
Stauford Center for the Arts, 1970
Steadman Theatre, 5354
Steinman Hall of Fine Arts, 5712
Stella Boyle Smith Concert Hall, 4071

Stephen C O'Connell Center, 6350
Stephen F Austin State University: Homer Bryce
 Stadium, 8095
Stephen Foster State Folk Culture Center, 6421
Stephens Auditorium, 4521
Steppenwolf Theater, 2855
Sterling & Francine Clark Art Institute, 6905
Sterling Auditorium, 4945
Sterling Centennial Auditorium, 6573
Stern Grove, 1945
Sternberger Auditorium, 5130
Stevens Center, 5162
Stiemke Theater, 3996
Stillwater Community Center, 7728
Stillwell Theatre, 1082
Stocker Arts Center, 5227
Stockton Performing Arts Center, 7238
Stranahan Theater, 600
Strand Theatre, 2168, 3756, 7221
Strand Theatre of Shreveport, 6788
Strand-Capitol Performing Arts Center, 7864
Strathmore Hall Arts Center, 6839
Strauss Performing Arts Center, 4836
Stuart Theatre, 3745
Stude Concert Hall, 5534
Student Center Auditorium, 4395
Student Union Ballroom, 4419
Subplot Theatre, 3347
Sue Bennett College Auditorium, 4575
Suffolk Community College, 4933
Suffolk County Community College: Shea Theatre,
 7475
Sullivan County Community College, 2200
Sullivan Street Playhouse, 7436
Summerlin Performing Arts Center, 3225
Summit Middle School, 1436
Summit Senior High School, 1436
Sumter County Cultural Center, 7902
Sun Bowl, 8039
Sun Devil Stadium, 5880
Sun Entertainment, 5848
Sun Theatre, 3213
Sun Valley Center for the Arts and Humanities, 6500
Sundome Center for the Performing Arts, 770, 4052
Sunken Gardens, 921
Sunny Hills High School Performing Arts Center, 4106
Sunset Center, 5952
Sunset Concert Pavilion, 5046
Sunset Playhouse, 3981
Sunset Theatre, 808
Supper Club, 7437
Surdna Foundation, 7438
Susquehanna Township Middle School, 1717
Sweet Briar College: Babcock Auditorium, 8203
Swope Music Hall, 5394
Sylvia & Danny Kaye Playhouse, 5056
Symphony Hall Tanglewood, 1264
Synod Hall, 1742
Syracuse Area Landmark Theatre, 7489
Syracuse University: Carrier Dome, 7490

T

T.G. Field Auditorium, 1805
Tabernacle at Temple Square, 1823, 5591
Tacoma Actors Guild, 3966
Tacoma Dome, 8249
Tad Gormley Stadium, 6777
Tampa Bay Performing Arts Center, 2010, 2746
Tanglewood, 1263, 4678
Tannery Pond, 1492
Taos Community Auditorium, 4921
Target Center, 7015
Tarrant County Convention Center, 1795
Tawes Fine Arts Center, 4644
Tawes Theater, 4640
Td Waterhouse Centre, 6399
Teatro Dallas, 3829
Technical High School Auditorium, 2143
Tecumseh Civic Auditorium, 6980
Ted Menn Concert Hall, 2135

Ted Shawn Theatre, 327, 4656
Temple Beth El, 1313
Temple Civic Theatre, 8124
Temple Hoyne Buell Theatre, 182
Temple Israel, 4294, 5715
Temple Sanctuary, 4350
Temple Square, 1824
Temple Theatre, 3558
Temple Theatre Company, 7559
Temple University, 7834
Tennessee Performing Arts Center, 1772, 3794, 3797,
 5467, 7958
Tennessee Performing Arts Center: Andrew Jackson
 Hall, 7959
Tennessee State University: Charles M Murphy Athletic
 Center, 7947
Tennessee Tech University: Hooper Eblen Center, 7921
Tennessee Theater, 660, 1913, 7933
Tennessee Williams Fine Arts Center, 1038
Tennessee Williams Theatre, 6364
Tennis Center at Crandon Park, 6360
Terrace of Alger House, 4728
Terrace Theater, 842, 1911, 1912
Terrace Theater of the Kennedy Center, 1992
Terrace Theatre, 5057
Terry Concert Hall, 4336
Texas Christian University: Amoin G Carter Stadium,
 8049
Texas Christian University: Ed Landreth Auditorium,
 8045
Texas Hall, 5475
Texas Stadium, 8080
Texas Tech University Center: Allen Theatre, 8089
Texas Tech University School of Music, 8090
Texas Wesleyan College: Fine Arts, 8046
Texas Woman's University: Redbud Theatre, 8025
Thalia Mara Hall, 357, 1365
Thalian Hall Center for the Performing Arts, 3563,
 7564
Thanksgiving Square: Chapel of Thanksgiving, 8023
Thanksgiving Square: Courtyard at Thanksgiving, 8024
The Alberta Bair Theater for the Performing Arts, 1387
The Ames City Auditorium, 303
The Ann & Richard Barshinger Center, 5350
The Art Emporium, 1331, 2129
The Arts Council Theatre, 3564
The Baptist Temple, 2341
The Barnstormers Theatre, 3238
The Bijou Theater, 3784
The Bilingual Foundation of the Arts Theatre, 2433
The Britt Gardens, 612, 3661, 5299
The Bushnell Hall, 190
The Carlson Center, 307
The Carnegie Music Hall, 1738
The Carriage Club of Charlotte, 2244
The Center Theatre, 2575, 5386
The Chapel, Western Reserve Academy, 1645
The Cherry Lane Theatre, 3367
The Chorus of Westerly Performance Hall, 2294
The Civic Center Music Hall, 3640
The Cleveland Play House, 1605
The College of Williamsburg, 3933, 5666
The Commons, 4497
The Concert Hall, Callifornia State University, Fresno,
 826
The Crest Theater, 809
The Dance Center of Columbia College, 277
The Dance Hall, 580
The Dance Place, 210
The Delaware Theatre Company, 2654
The Edith Oliver Theatre, 2643
The Elizabethan Theatre at the Folger, 4305
The Embers, 1659
The Empire Theatre, 3926
The Ensemble Studio Theatre, 3372, 3854
The Ethical Society, 1379
The Fine Arts Council Hall, 5789
The Folly Theater, 2151
The Former Bullocks Wilshire, 4129
The Forum, 1716
The Found Theatre, 2426
The Grand 1894 Opera House, 5520

X

Y

Z

Alabama

Anniston
Anniston Museum of Natural History, 5794

Auburn
Auburn University Theatre, 2348
Beard Eaves Memorial Coliseum, 5795
Joel H Eaves Memorial Coliseum, 5796

Birmingham
Alabama Ballet, 1
Alabama Symphony Orchestra, 744
Alys Robinson Stephens Performing Arts Center, 5797
Birmingham Children's Theatre, 2349
Birmingham International Festival, 4009
Birmingham Music Club, 1879
Birmingham-Jefferson Civic Center - Theatre, 5801
Birmingham-Jefferson Convention Complex - Concert Hall, 5799
Birmingham-Jefferson Convention Complex - Theatre, 5800
Birmingham-Jefferson Convention Complex: Arena, 5798
Birmingham-Southern College Theatre, 5802
Boutwell Municipal Auditorium, 5806
Garden Variety Shakespeare, 2350
Independent Presbyterian Church-November Organ Recital Series, 4010
Legion Field Stadium, 5803
Opera Birmingham, 1880
Red Mountain Chamber Orchestra, 745
Samford University, 5804
Uab Arena, 5805
University of Alabama, Birmingham: Department of Theatre, 2351

Decatur
Princess Theatre Center for the Performing Arts, 5807
Princess Theatre Professional Series, 4011

Dothan
Dothan Civic Center, 5808
Southeast Alabama Community Theatre, 2352
Southeast Alabama Dance Company, 2

Double Springs
Looney's Tavern Productions, 2353

Enterprise
Coffee County Arts Alliance, 4012

Florence
University of North Alabama: Department of Communications & Theatre, 2354
Wc Handy Music Festival, 4013

Gadsden
Gadsden Symphony Orchestra, 746

Gulf Shores
City of Gulf Shores Entertainment Series, 4014

Huntsville
Broadway Theatre, 2355
Huntsville Ballet Company, 3
Huntsville Chamber Music Guild, 747
Huntsville Opera Theater, 1881
Huntsville Symphony Orchestra, 748
Huntsville Youth Orchestra, 749
Milton Frank Stadium, 5810
Oakwood College Arts & Lectures, 4015
Panoply Arts Festival, 4016
Von Braun Civic Center, 5811
Von Braun Civic Center - Arena, 5812
Von Braun Civic Center - Concert Hall, 5813
Von Braun Civic Center - Exhibit Hall, 5814
Von Braun Civic Center - Playhouse, 5815

Jacksonville
Paul Snow Memorial Stadium, 5816
Pete Mathews Coliseum, 5817

Mobile
Mobile Chamber Music Society, 750

Mobile Civic Center, 5818
Mobile Civic Center - Arena, 5819
Mobile Opera, 1882
Mobile Symphony, 751
Mobile Theatre Guild, 5820
Saenger Theatre, 2356
University of South Alabama, 2357
Usa Saenger Theatre, 5821

Montevallo
University of Montevallo: Division of Theatre, 2358

Montgomery
Alabama Dance Theatre, 4
Alabama Shakespeare Festival, 4017
Alabama Shakespeare Festival - Festival Stage, 5822
Alabama Shakespeare Festival - Octagon, 5823
Auvrun University Montgomery Theatre, 2359
Garret Coliseum, 5824
Jasmine Hill Arts Council, 4018
Joe L Reed Acadome, 5825
Montgomery Ballet, 5
Montgomery Civic Center, 5826
Montgomery Symphony Orchestra, 752

Opelika
Opelika Arts Association, 4019

Ozark
Ozark Civic Center, 5827

Selma
Selma Community Concert Association, 4020

Troy
Troy State University-Lyceum Series, 4021

Tuscaloosa
Arts Council of Tuscaloosa Fanfare, 4022
Bama Theatre Performing Arts Center, 5828
Bryant Denny Stadium, 5829
Coleman Coliseum, 5830
Horizons Performing Arts Series, 4023
Tuscaloosa Symphony Orchestra, 753
University of Alabama - Concert Hall, 5831
University of Alabama - Gallaway Theatre, 5832
University of Alabama - Huey Recital Hall, 5833
University of Alabama - Morgan Auditorium, 5834
University of Alabama School of Music Celebrities, 4024
University of Alabama, Tuscaloosa: Department of Theatre and Dance, 2360

Tuskegee
Alumni Bowl Stadium, 5836
Logan Hall, 5835

Alaska

Anchorage
Alaska Center for the Performing Arts, 5837
Alaska Dance Theatre, 6
Alaska Light Opera Theatre, 1883
Anchorage Community Theatre, 2361
Anchorage Concert Association, 4025
Anchorage Concert Chorus, 1884
Anchorage Festival of Music, 4026
Anchorage Opera Company, 1885
Anchorage Symphony Orchestra, 754
Anchorage Youth Symphony, 755
Eccentric Theatre Company, 2362
Out North Contemporary Art House, 2363
University of Alaska, Anchorage: Department of Theatre and Dance, 2364
William a Egan Civic and Convention Center, 5838

Douglas
Perseverance Theatre, 2365

Fairbanks
Alaskaland Civic Center, 5839
Fairbanks Arts Association, 4027
Fairbanks Choral Society and Children's Choir, 1886
Fairbanks Concert Association Master Series, 4028

Fairbanks Light Opera Theatre, 1887
Fairbanks Summer Arts Festival, 4029
Fairbanks Symphony Association, 756
North Star Ballet, 7
Red Hackle Pipe Band, 757
University of Alaska - Charles W. Davis Concert Hall, 5840
University of Alaska, Fairbanks: Theatre Department, 2366

Haines
Chilkat Center for the Arts, 5841
Haines Arts Council, 4030
Lynn Canal Community Players, 2367

Homer
Kenai Peninsula Orchestra String Festival, 4031
Pier One Theatre, 5842

Juneau
Centennial Hall Convention Center, 5843
Crosssound, 4032
Jocelyn Clark, 758
Juneau Arts & Humanities Council, 4033
Juneau Jazz and Classics, 759
Juneau Oratorio Choir, 1888
Juneau Symphony, 760

Kodiak
Kodiak Arts Council, 4034, 5844

Sitka
Sitka Centennial Building, 5845
Sitka Summer Music Festival, 4035

Arizona

Carefree
Desert Foothills Musicfest, 4036

Chandler
Chandler Center for the Arts, 5846

Coolidge
Pinal County Fine Arts Council: Arts in the Desert, 4037

Cottonwood
Verde Valley Concert Association, 4038

Flagstaff
Coconino Center for the Arts, 5847
Flagstaff Festival of the Arts, 4039
Flagstaff Symphony Orchestra, 761
J Lawrence Walk-Up Skydome, 5849
Northern Arizona University: Theatre Division, School of Performing Arts, 2368
Northern Arizona University Spectrum Series, 4040
Sun Entertainment, 5848

Fountain Hills
Patricia Alberti Performing Artists Management, 8327

Glendale
Glendale Community College Performing Arts Center, 5850
Glendale Public Library, 5851

Grand Canyon
Grand Canyon Music Festival, 4041

Kingman
Mohave Community College, 5852

Litchfield Park
West Valley Fine Arts Council, 4042

Little Rock
Barton Coliseum, 5853

Mesa
Crossroads Performance Group, 8
Mesa Community Center, 5856
Mesa Community Center - Amphitheatre, 5854
Mesa Community Center - Centennial Hall, 5855

Mesa Symphony Orchestra, 762

North Little Rock
Alltel Arena, 5857

Paradise Valley
Paradise Valley Jazz Party, 4043

Peoria
Peoria Sports Complex, 5858
Theater Works, 2369

Phoenix
Actors Theatre of Phoenix, 2370
America West Arena, 5859
Arizona Exposition & State Fair, 4044
Arizona Opera, 1889
Ballet Arizona, 9
Bank One Ball Park, 5860
Celebrity Theatre, 5861
Grand Canyon University, 5862
Grounding Point Dance Company, 10
Orpheum Theatre Foundation, 5863
Orpheus Male Chorus of Phoenix, 1890
Phoenix Bach Choir, 1891
Phoenix Boys Choir, 1892
Phoenix Chamber Music Society, 763
Phoenix Civic Plaza, 5864
Phoenix Civic Plaza - Convention Center and Stage,
    5865
Phoenix Civic Plaza - Exhibition Halls, 5866
Phoenix Civic Plaza - Grand Ballroom, 5867
Phoenix Stages, 5868
Phoenix Symphony, 764
Southwest Arts & Entertainment, 4045
Theatre Division, 2371

Pine Bluff
Golden Lion Stadium, 5869
Hestand Stadium, 5870

Prescott
Prescott Fine Arts, 4046
Yavapai College, 5871
Yavapi Symphony Association, 765

Safford
Gila Valley Arts Council, 4047

Scottsdale
Encore Attractions, 8328
Ragtyme-Jazztyme Society, 4048
Rawhide Pavilion & Rodeo Arena, 5872
Scottsdale Arts Festival, 4049
Scottsdale Center for the Arts, 5873
Scottsdale Community College, 5874
Scottsdale Symphony Orchestra Association, 766

Sedona
Chamber Music Sedona, 767
Sedona Chamber Music Society & Festival, 4050
Sedona Jazz On the Rocks, 768, 4051

Sierra Vista
Cochise College, 5875
Sierra Vista Parks and Leisure Services, 5876

Sun City
Sun Cities Chamber Music Society, 769
Symphony of the West Valley, 770

Sun City West
Arizona State University: Sundome Center, 5877

Tempe
Arizona State University - Gammage Auditorium, 5878
Arizona State University Activity Center, 5879
Arizona State University Public Events, 4052
Arizona State University Symphony Orchestra &
    Chamber Orchestra, 771
Arizona State University Theatre, 2372
Childsplay, 2373
Desert Dance Theatre, 11
Michelob Cool Summer Jazz Series, 4053
Sun Devil Stadium, 5880

Thatcher
Eastern Arizona College- Community Orchestra, 772

Tsaile
Navajo Dine College, 5881

Tubac
Tubac Center of the Arts, 5882

Tucson
Arizona Early Music Society, 773
Arizona Friends of Chamber Music, 774
Arizona Opera, 1893
Arizona Stadium University of Arizona, 5883
Arizona Theatre Company, 2374
Catalina Chamber Orchestra, 775
Civic Orchestra of Tucson, 776
Desert Voices, 1894
Greater Oro Valley Arts Council, 4054
Hi Corbett Field, 5884
Mckale Memorial Center, 5885
Philharmonia Orchestra of Tucson, 777
Pima Community College for the Arts, 4055
Southern Arizona Symphony Orchestra, 778
St. Philip's in the Hills Friends of Music, 4056
Tucson Arizona Boys Chorus, 1895
Tucson Convention Center, 5886
Tucson Convention Center - Arena, 5887
Tucson Convention Center - Exhibition Hall, 5888
Tucson Convention Center - Leo Rich Theatre, 5889
Tucson Convention Center - Music Hall, 5890
Tucson Convention Center - Theatre, 5891
Tucson Jazz Society, 779
Tucson Philharmonia Youth Orchestra, 780
Tucson Symphony Orchestra, 781
Tucson Winter Chamber Music Festival, 782, 4057
Uapresents Centennial Hall, 2375
University of Arizona - Centennial Hall, 5892
University of Arizona - Crowder Hall, 5893
University of Arizona Presents, 4058
University of Arizona School of Theatre Arts, 2376

Washington
Washington Chorus, 1896

Yuma
Arizona Western College, 5894
Ray Kroc Baseball Complex, 5895
Yuma Ballet Theatre, 12
Yuma Civic and Convention Center - Yuma Room,
    5896

Arkansas

Anchorage
George M Sullivan Sports Arena, 5897
Uaa Sports Arena, 5898

Arkadelphia
Ouachita Baptist University: Artists Series, 4059
Ouachita Baptist University: Department of the Arts,
    5899

Batesville
Lyon College Theatre Department, 2377

Beebe
Arkansas State University at Beebe, 783

Blytheville
Ritz Civic Center, 5900

Clarksville
Walton Arts and Ideas, 4060

Conway
University of Central Arkansas Public Appearances,
    4061
University of Central Arkansas Theatre Program, 2378

El Dorado
El Dorado Municipal Auditorium, 5901
South Arkansas Arts Center, 5902
South Arkansas Symphony, 784

Eureka Springs
Eureka Springs Jazz Festival, 4062
Inspiration Point Fine Arts Colony, 4063

Fairbanks
Carlson Center, 5903

Fayetteville
Fine Arts Concert Hall, 5904
North Arkansas Symphony, 4064
Symphony Society of North Arkansas, 785
University of Arkansas at Fayetteville: Department of
    Drama, 2379
University of Arkansas Bud Walton Arena, 5905
Walton Arts Center, 5906

Fort Smith
Fort Smith Civic Center - Exhibition Hall, 5907
Fort Smith Civic Center - Theater, 5908
Fort Smith Convention Center, 5909
Fort Smith Little Theatre, 2380, 5910
Fort Smith Symphony, 786
Kay Rogers Park, 5911
Westark College Season of Entertainment, 4065
Westark Community College - Breedlove Auditorium,
    5912

Harrison
North Central Arkansas Concert Association, 4066

Helena
Warfield Concerts, 4067

Holiday Island
Opera in the Ozarks at Inspiration Point, 1897

Hot Springs
Hot Springs Convention and Visitors' Bureau, 5913
Hot Springs Music Festival, 4069
Hot Springs Music Festival Chamber Orchestra, 4068
Hot Springs Music Festival Symphony Orchestra, 787

Jonesboro
Forum, 5914
Foundation of Arts, 13, 788, 2381, 5915
Fowler Center at Arkansas State University, 4070

Little Rock
Arkansas Arts Center Children's Theater, 2382
Arkansas Reperatory Theatre, 2383
Arkansas Symphony Orchestra, 789
Artspree, 4071
Ballet Arkansas, 14
Ray Winder Field, 5916
Robinson Center Music Hall, 5917
University of Arkansas at Little Rock: Department of
    Theatre and Dance, 2384
University of Arkansas-Little Rock, 5918
War Memorial Stadium, 5919
Wildwood Park for the Performing Arts, 5920

Magnolia
Southern Arkansas University Theatre & Mass
    Communications Department, 2385
Wilkins Stadium, 5921

Mountain Home
Twin Lakes Playhouse, 2386

Pine Bluff
Arts and Science Center for Southeast Arkansas, 5922
Pine Bluff Convention Center, 5923
Pine Bluff Convention Center - Arena, 5924
Pine Bluff Convention Center - Auditorium, 5925
Pine Bluff Symphony Orchestra, 790

Russellville
Arkansas River Valley Arts Center, 5926
Arkansas Tech University - Witherspoon Arts Arena,
    5927
John E Tucker Coliseum, 5928

Searcy
Harding University Concert & Lyceum Series, 4072

Downey
Downey Symphony Orchestra, 820

Drake Stadium
Event Facilities Management Office, 5968

El Cajon
Christian Community Theater, 2402
East County Performing Arts Center - Theatre, 5969
Samahan Filipino American Performing Arts, 31

El Centro
Imperial Valley Symphony, 821
Southwest Performing Arts Theatre, 5970

Encinitas
San Diego Chamber Orchestra, 822

Encino
Los Angeles Mozart Orchestra, 823

Escondido
California Center for the Arts-Escondido, 5971
Welk Resort San Diego Theatre, 2403

Eureka
Redwood Coast Dixieland Jazz Festival, 4103
Redwood Concert Ballet, 32

Fairfield
Fairfield City Arts, 4104

Ferndale
Ferndale Repertory Theatre, 2404

Fontana
Fontana Civic Auditorium, 5972
Fontana Performing Arts Center, 5973

Foster City
American Repertory Theatre Ballet, 33

Fremont
Fremont Symphony Orchestra, 824
Smith Center for the Fine and Performing Arts, 5974

Fresno
Bulldogs Stadium, 5975
California State University, Fresno: Theatre Arts Department, 2405
California State University-Fresno, 5976
California State University-Fresno, Wahlberg, 5977
Central California Ballet, 34
Chookasian Armenian Concert Ensemble, 35
Fresno Ballet, 36
Fresno Convention Center, 5978
Fresno Philharmonic, 825
John Chookasian International Folk Ensemble, 37
Lively Arts Foundation, 4105
Philip Lorenz Memorial Keyboard Concerts, 826
Ratcliffe Stadium, 5979
Theatre Three Repertory Company, 2406
Tower Theatre for the Performing Arts, 5980
Warnor's Theater, 5981

Fullerton
California State University, Fullerton: Department of Theatre and Dance, 2407
Fullerton Civic Light Opera, 1907
Fullerton Friends of Music, 4106
Fullerton Professsional Artists in Residence, 4107
Muckenthaler Cultural Center, 5982
Plummer Auditorium, 5983
Vanguard Theatre Ensemble, 2408

Garden Grove
Grove Theatre Center, 2409

Gilroy
South Valley Symphony, 827

Glendale
Alex Theatre, 5984
Glendale Symphony, 828
Glendale Youth Orchestra, 829

Glendora
Citrus College Haugh Performing Arts Center, 4108, 5985

Gold River
Sacramento Choral Society and Orchestra, 1908

Granada Hills
Spotoma, 8334

Guerneville
Russian River Jazz Festival, 830, 4109

Half Moon Bay
Bach Dancing and Dynamite Society Group, 38

Hayward
California State University-Hayward - Main Theatre, 5986
California State University: Hayward, 4110
Chabot College Performing Arts Center, 5987

Healdsburg
Healdsburg Jazz Festival, 4111
Russian River Chamber Music, 831

Hemet
Ramona Bowl Amphitheatre, 5988
Ramona Hillside Players, 4112
Ramona Pageant Association, 4113

Hermosa Beach
Albert Mcneil Jubilee Singers of Los Angeles, 1909

Hoboken
Island Heart Artists, 8335

Hollywood
Actors' Gang Theater, 2410
American Academy of Dramatic Arts/Hollywood, 2411
Blank Theatre Company, 2412
Casa Italiana Opera Company, 1910
Complex, 5989
Diavolo, 39
Hollywood Bowl, 5990
Hollywood Bowl Orchestra, 832
Hollywood Bowl Summer Festival, 4114
Hollywood Palladium, 5991
Hudson Theatre, 2413
James a Doolittle Theatre, 5992
John Anson Ford Theatres, 5993
Lola Montes & Her Spanish Dancers, 40
Open Fist Theatre Company, 2414
Stages Theatre Center, 2415

Huntington Beach
Golden West College - Mainstage Theatre, 5995
Golden West College Community Theatre, 5994
Huntington Beach Playhouse, 2416

Idyllwild
Idyllwild Arts-Academy & Summer Program, 4115

Indian Wells
Indian Wells Desert Symphony, 833

Inglewood
Great Western Forum, 5996
Lula Washington Dance Theatre, 41

Irvine
Ballet Pacifica, 42
Bren Events Center, 5997
Eclectic Orange Festival, 4116
Irvine Barclay Theatre, 5998
Philharmonic Society of Orange County, 834
Uci Cultural Events, 4117
University of California-Irvine - Village Theatre, 5999
University of California-Irvine: School of the Arts (Drama), 2417

Julian
Julian's Live Dinner Theatre, 2418

Kelseyville
Kids 4 Broadway, 2419

Kentfield
Ancient Future: #1 Net World Music Ensemble, 43
Marin Community College Symphony, 835
Sapphira, 44

Kings Beach
Tahoe Jazz Festival, 4118

La Canada
Celebrity Presentations, 4119

La Crescenta
Bodytalk, 45

La Jolla
Athenaeum Music & Arts Library, 6000
La Jolla Chamber Music Society, 836
La Jolla Chamber Music Society's - Summerfest La Jolla, 4120
La Jolla Playhouse, 2420
La Jolla Symphony & Chorus Association, 837
Mandell Weiss Performing Arts Center, 6001
Museum of Contemporary Art, San Diego, 6002
Sherwood Auditorium, 6003
University Events Office, 4121
University of California-San Diego - Mandeville, 6004
University of California-San Diego: Department of Theatre and Dance, 2421

La Mirada
Biola University, 6005
La Mirada Theatre for the Performing Arts, 6006
Tom Bozigian, 46

LaVerne
University of Laverne, 2422

Laguna Beach
Laguna Playhouse, 2423, 6007

Laguna Hills
Mozart Classical Orchestra, 838

Laguna Niguel
Laguna Chamber Music Society, 839

Lancaster
Antelope Valley Ballet, 47

Lawndale
Ruth Fentroy, 48

Livermore
Concert in the Vineyards, 840
Del Valle Fine Arts Concert Series, 4122
Livermore-Amador Symphony, 841

Long Beach
California Repertory Company, 2424
California State University, Long Beach: Department of Theatre, 2425
Found Theatre, 2426
Jordan Theatre, 6008
Long Beach Civic Light Opera, 1911
Long Beach Community Playhouse - Stage, 6009
Long Beach Convention and Entertainment Center, 6010
Long Beach Opera, 1912
Long Beach Playhouse - Studio Theatre, 6012
Long Beach Playhouse: Mainstage and Studio Theatres, 6011
Long Beach Symphony Orchestra, 842
Regina Klenjoski Dance Company, 49
Rhapsody in Taps, 50
Richard & Karen Carpenter Performing Arts Center, 6013
Woodrow Wilson High School, 6014

Los Altos
Bus Barn Stage Company, 2427
Peninsula Symphony Orchestra, 843

Los Altos Hills
Robert C Smithwick Theatre, 6015

Colorado

Enfield
Enfield Cultural Arts Commission, 4267

Essex
Hot Steamed Jazz Festival, 4268

Fairfield
Fairfield County Chorale, 1971
Fairfield University: Department of Visual &
Performing Arts, 2610
Greater Bridgeport Symphony Youth Orchestra, 977
Quick Center for the Arts, 6251

Greenwich
Connecticut Philharmonic Orchestra, 978
Greenwich Choral Society, 1972
Greenwich Symphony Orchestra, 979
Symphony On the Sound, 980

Guilford
Chestnut Hill Concerts, 4269
Shoreline Arts Alliance, 4270

Hartford
Albano Ballet and Performing Arts Center, 6252
Artists Collective, 2611
Bushnell Center for the Performing Arts, 6253
Chamber Music Plus, 981
Charter Oak Cultural Center, 6254
Connecticut Classical Guitar Society, 982
Connecticut Opera, 1973
Dance Connecticut, 190
First Night Hartford, 4271
Hartford Civic Center, 6255
Hartford Office of Cultural Affairs, 6256
Hartford Stage Company, 2612
Hartford Symphony Orchestra, 983
Horace Bushnell Memorial Hall, 6257
National Theatre of the Deaf, 2613
Talcott Mountain Music Festival, Summer Series, 4272
Theaterworks, 2614
Trinity College Theatre and Dance Department, 2615
Trinity College: Austin Arts Center, 6258
Woodland Concert Series, 4273
Works, 191

Ivoryton
River Rep at Ivoryton Playhouse, 2616

Litchfield
Litchfield Jazz Festival, 4274
Litchfield Performing Arts Series, 4275

Manchester
Manchester Musical Players, 2617
Manchester Symphony Orchestra/Chorale, 984

Mashantucket
Mashantucket Pequot Museum & Research Center, 6259

Meriden
Meriden Symphony Orchestra, 985

Middletown
Center for the Arts, 6260
Dances for 2, 192
Oddfellows Playhouse, 2618
Wesleyan University Theater Department, 2619

New Britain
Central Connecticut State University: Department of Theatre, 2620
Connecticut Choral Artists (Concora), 1974
Greater New Britain Opera Association, 1975
Hole in the Wall Theatre, 2621
New Britain Symphony Orchestra, 986

New Canaan
Silvermine Guild Art Center Series, 4276
Silvermine Guild Chamber Music Series, 987

New Haven
Connecticut Chamber Orchestra, 988
Elm Shakespeare Company, 2622

Ingalls Rink, 6261
International Festival of Arts & Ideas, 4277
Long Wharf Theatre, 2623, 6262
Long Wharf Theatre - Stage Ii, 6263
Lyman Center, 6264
New Haven Jazz Festival, 4278
New Haven Symphony Orchestra, 989
New Haven Veterans Memorial Coliseum, 6265
Palace Theatre, 6266
Philharmonia Orchestra of Yale, 990
Sacred Dance Guild, 193
Shubert Theater, 6267
Southern Connecticut State University: Department of Theatre, 2624
Yale Baseball Stadium, 6268
Yale Bowl, 6269
Yale Repertory Theatre, 2625, 6270
Yale Russian Chorus, 1976
Yale School of Drama, 2626

New London
Connecticut College - Palmer Auditorium, 6271
Connecticut College Department of Theatre, 2627
Connecticut College: On Stage, 4279
Connecticut Early Music Festival, 4280
Eastern Connecticut Symphony, 991
Garde Arts Center, 6272
Summer Music, 4281

New Milford
Connecticut Conservatory of the Performing Arts, 2628
Conservatory of the Performing Arts, 194

Newtown
Newtown Friends of Music, 4282

Norfolk
Greenwoods Theatre at Norfolk, 2629
Norfolk Chamber Music Festival/Yale Summer School of Music, 992, 4283

Norwalk
American Classical Orchestra, 993
Norwalk Symphony Orchestra, 994
Norwalk Youth Symphony, 995

Oakville
Clockwork Repertory Theatre, 2630

Ridgefield
Ridgefield Playhouse for Movies & the Performing Arts, 6273
Ridgefield Symphony Orchestra, 996

Salisbury
Project Troubador, 4284

Sharon
Falcon Ridge Folk Festival, 4285
Music Mountain, 4286
Northwest Corner Young Artists Series, 4287
Tri-Arts at the Sharon Playhouse, 2631
Winterhawk - Bluegrass & Beyond, 4288

Sherman
Sherman Players, 2632
Sherman Playhouse, 6274

Simsbury
Centennial Theater Festival, 2633, 4289

South Norwalk
Theatre Project Consultants, 2634

Southington
Southington Community Theatre, 6275

Stamford
Connecticut Ballet Theatre, 195
Connecticut Grand Opera and Orchestra, 1977
Palace Theatre of the Arts, 2635
Pro Arte Chamber Singers of Connecticut, 1978
Rich Forum, 6276
Stamford Symphony Orchestra, 997
Stamford Theatre Works, 2636
Young Artists Philharmonic, 998

Zig Zag Ballet, 196

Stony Creek
Puppet House Theatre, 2637

Storrs
Connecticut Repertory Theatre, 2638
Jorgensen Center for the Performing Arts, 6277
Sports Complex, University of Connecticut, 6278
University of Connecticut - Harriet S. Jorgen Center, 6280
University of Connecticut: Department of Dramatic Arts, 2639
University of Connecticut: School of Fine Arts, 6279
Willimantic Orchestra, 999

Stratford
Stratford Festival Theater, 2640, 4290

Torrington
Coe Park Civic Center, 6281
Nutmeg Conservatory for the Arts, 197
Warner Theatre, 6282

Wallingford
Oakdale Theatre, 6283
Paul Mellon Arts Center, 6284
Wallingford Symphony Orchestra, 1000

Warren
Mask Messengers, 198

Washington Depot
Armstrong Chamber Concerts, 4291
Gami/Simonds, 8356
Momix, 199
Pilobolus Dance Theatre, 200

Waterbury
Seven Angels Theatre, 2641
Waterbury Symphony Orchestra, 1001

Waterford
Eugene O'neill Theater Center, 2642
National Theater Institute, 2643

West Hartford
Connecticut Concert Opera, 1979
Connecticut Youth Symphony, 1002
Hartt School, 201
Hartt School Concert Series, 4292
Lincoln Theater, 6285
Phillip Truckenbrod Concert Artists, 8357
Sports Center: University of Hartford, 6286
University of Hartford: Department of Art History, Cinema, Drama, 2644

West Haven
Orchestra New England, 1003

Westport
Fairfield County Stage Company, 2645
Levitt Pavilion for the Performing Arts, 6287
South Shore Music, 4293
Temple Israel of Westport Series, 4294
Westport Community Theatre, 2646, 6288
Westport Country Playhouse, 2647, 6289
White Barn Theatre, 2648

Wilton
Wilton Playshop, 2649

Delaware

Bear
Diamond State Chorus of Sweet Adelines, 1980

Dover
Kent County Theatre Guild, 2650
Schwartz Center for the Arts, 6290

Georgetown
Possum Point Players, 2651

1431

Newark

Bob Carpenter Center, 6291
Delaware Dance Company, 202
Madrigal Singers of Wilmington, 1981
Mid-Atlantic Ballet, 203
Newark Symphony Orchestra, 1004
University of Delaware Performing Arts Series, 4295
University of Delaware: Department of Theatre, 2652

Wilmington

Artists Theatre Association, 2653
Brandywine Baroque, 1005
Delaware Chamber Music Festival, 4296
Delaware Symphony Association, 1006
Delaware Theatre Company, 2654
Dickinson Theatre Organ Society, 1007
Grand Opera House, 1982, 6292
Mid-Atlantic Chamber Music Society, 1008
Opera Delaware, 1983
Playhouse Theatre, 6293
Russian Ballet Centre, 204
Shoestring Productions Limited, 2655
Wilmington Drama League, 2656

District of Columbia

African Continuum Theatre Company (Actco), 2657
African Heritage Dancers & Drummers, 205
American College Theater Festival, 4297
American Music Festival, 4298
American University - Mcdonald Recital Hall, 6294
American University - New Lecture Hall, 6295
American University Theatre Program, 2672
Catholic University of America: Theatre Department, 2673
Center for Movement Theatre, 2674
Arena Stage, 2658
Arka Ballet, 206
Arts in the Academy, National Academy of Sciences, 4299
Bender Arena, 6296
Capitol Ballet Company, 207
Cathedral Choral Society, 1984
Charles E Smith Center, 6313
Charlin Jazz Society, 1010
Children's National Medical Center, New Horizons Program, 4300
Choral Arts Society of Washington, 1985
Chorus America, 1986
Constitution Hall, 6297
Contemporary Music Forum, 1011
Commodores, 1022
Country Current, 1023, 1996
Cruisers, 1024, 1997
Dana Tai Soon Burgess & Company, 208
Dance Place, 209
DC Armory, 6298
DC Sports & Entertainment Commission, 4301
DC Youth Orchestra Program, 1012
Deborah Riley Dance Projects, 210
Discovery Theater, 2659
District Curators, 4302
Dumbarton Concert Series, 4303
Embassy Series, 4304
Folger Consort, 6299
Folger Shakespeare Library, 2660
Folger Theatre, 4305
Ford's Theatre Society, 2661
Freer Gallery of Art, Bill & Mary Meyer Concert Series, 4306
Gala Hispanic Theatre, 2662
Gallaudet Dance Company, 211
Gaston Hall, 6300
George Washington's Series at Mount Vernon College, 4307
George Washington University: Department of Theatre and Dance, 2675
George Washington University Symphony Orchestra, 1013
Georgetown University Office of Performing Arts, 6301

Gw's Lisner Auditorium, 6306
Hall of Nations Black Box Theatre, 6302
Howard University Cramton Auditorium, 6303
Howard University Department of Theatre Arts, 2676
Imagination Celebration - Kennedy Center Performances for Young People, 4308
John F Kennedy Center for the Performing Arts, 6304
Kennedy Center American College Theatre, 2663
Kennedy Center Annual Open House Arts Festival, 4309
Kennedy Center Opera House Orchestra, 1014
Kennedy Center/Mary Lou Williams Women in Jazz Festival, 4310
Library of Congress, 6305
Library of Congress Chamber Music Concert Series, 4311
Living Stage, 2664
Lois Howard & Associates, 8358
Maida Withers Dance Construction Company, 212
Master Chorale Chamber Singers, 1988
Master Chorale of Washington, 1987
Mci Center, 6307
National Academy of Sciences Concerts, 4312
National Conservatory of Dramatic Arts, 2677
National Gallery of Art/Concert Series, 4313
National Gallery Orchestra, 1015
National Musical Arts, 1016
National Symphony Orchestra Association, 1017
National Theatre, 2665
Opera Lafayette, 4314
Opera Music Theater International, 1989
Phillips Collection Sunday Afternoon Concert Series, 4315
Sea Chanters, 1998
Shakespeare Theatre, 2666, 6308
Smithsonian Institution - Baird Auditorium, 6309
Smithsonian Institution - Carmichael Auditorium, 6310
Smithsonian Institution: the Smithsonian Associates, 4316
Society of the Cincinnati Concerts at Anderson House, 4317
Source Theatre Company, 2667
St. Mark's Dance Studio, 213
Studio Theatre, 2668
Summer Opera Theatre Company, 1990
Theater Chamber Players, 1018
Theater J, 6311
United States Air Force Band, 1009
United States Air Force Singing Sergeants, 1991
United States Navy Band, 1025
Vocal Arts Society, 1992
Vsa Arts, 2669
Warner Theatre, 6312
Washington Bach Consort, 1019, 1993
Washington Ballet, 214
Washington Chamber Symphony, 1020
Washington Concert Opera, 1994
Washington Opera, 1995
Washington Performing Arts Society, 4318
Washington Stage Guild, 2670
Washington Symphony Orchestra, 1021
Woolly Mammoth Theatre Company, 2671

Florida

Anna Maria

Island Players, 2678
Island Players Theatre, 6314

Aventura

Classical Ballet School of Vladimir Issaev, 215
Miami International Piano Festival, 1026, 4319

Avon Park

South Florida Community College Cultural Series, 4320

Belle Glade

Dolly Hands Cultural Arts Center, 6315
Palm Beach Community College, Glades Campus, 6316

Blountstown

Wt Neal Civic Center, 6317

Boca Raton

Boca Ballet Theatre, 216
Boca Pops Orchestra, 1027
Caldwell Theatre Company, 2679
Century Village Theatres, 6318
Chamber Music South, 1028
Florida Atlantic University: Department of Theatre, 2680
Piccolo Opera Company, 1999
University Center Auditorium, 6319

Bradenton

Manatee Players/Riverfront Theatre, 2681

Bunnell

Flagler Auditorium, 6320

Clearwater

City Players, 2682
Clearwater Jazz Holiday, 4321
Ruth Eckerd Hall, 6321
Showboat Dinner Theatre, 2683

Cocoa

Cocoa Expo Sports Center, 6322
Cocoa Village Playhouse, 6323

Cocoa Beach

Surfside Players, 2684

Coconut Creek

Omni Auditorium - Broward Community College, 6324
Wynmoor Recital Hall, 6325

Coconut Grove

Momentum Dance Company, 217

Coral Gables

Actors' Playhouse at the Miracle Theatre, 2685
Festival Miami, 4322
Gablestage, 2686
Miami Bach Society/Tropical Baroque Music Festival, 1029, 4323
University of Miami: Department of Theatre Arts, 2687

Coral Springs

Coral Springs City Center, 6326

Daytona Beach

Central Florida Cultural Endeavors, 4324
Daytona Beach Community College - Theatre Center, 6327
Daytona Beach Symphony Society, 1030
Daytona Playhouse, 2688, 6328
Florida International Festival, 4325
Florida International Festival Featuring the London Symphony Orchestra, 1031, 4326
Jackie Robinson Ball Park, 6329
Ocean Center, 6330
Peabody Auditorium, 6331
Seaside Music Theater, 2689

Delray Beach

Delray Beach Playhouse, 2690, 6332

Dunedin

Pinellas Youth Symphony, 1032

Eustis

Bay Street Players, 2691

Fellsmere

Mesa Park, 6333

Fort Lauderdale

Bailey Concert Hall, 6334
Beethoven By the Beach, 4327
Broward Center for the Performing Arts, 6335, 6338
Coral Ridge Presbyterian Church Concert Series, 4328
Florida Philharmonic Orchestra, 1033
Fort Lauderdale Broadway Series / Parker Playhouse, 4329
Fort Lauderdale Children's Theatre, 2692

Fort Lauderdale Stadium, 6336
Gold Coast Opera, 2000
One Way Puppets, 2693
Opera Guild, 2001
Parker Playhouse, 6337
Ptg-Florida/Parker Playhouse, 6339
War Memorial Auditorium, 6340

Fort Myers
Barbara B Mann Performing Arts Hall, 6341
Broadway Palm Dinner Theatre, 2694
Florida Arts Concert Series, 4330
Florida Repertory Theatre, 2695
Fort Myers Community Concert Association Series,
    4331
Fort Myers Harborside, 6342
Gulfcoast Dance, 218
Peninsula Players, 2696
Southwest Florida Symphony Orchestra & Chorus
    Association, 1034
William H Hammond Stadium, 6343
William R Frizzell Cultural Centre & Claiborne & Ned
    Foulds Theatre, 6344

Fort Pierce
Saint Lucie County Civic Center, 6345

Fort Walton
First Arts Series, 4332

Fort Walton Beach
Northwest Florida Ballet, 219

Gainesville
Blade Agency, 8359
Curtis M Phillips Center for Performing Arts, 6347
Gainesville Symphony Orchestra, 1035
Harn Museum: University of Florida, 6348
Hippodrome State Theatre, 6349
Morca Dance Theater, 220
Stephen C O'connell Center, 6350
University of Florida: Department of Theatre, 2697

Hialeah
Ballet Etudes, 221

Hollywood
Golden Thespians, 2698
Hollywood Playhouse, 2699
Nyk Productions, 4333
Scott Evans Productions, 222
Young Circle Park and Bandshell, 6351

Homestead
Homestead Sports Complex, 6352

Indialantic
Melbourne Chamber Music Society, 1036

Jacksonville
Alhambra Dinner Theatre, 2700, 6353
Alltel Stadium, 6354
Delius Festival, 4334
Florida Ballet at Jacksonville, 223
Florida National Pavilion, 6355
Florida Theatre, 6356
Florida Theatre Performing Arts Series, 4335
Gator Bowl, 6357
Jacksonville Ballet Theatre, 224
Jacksonville Symphony Orchestra, 1037
Jacksonville University Master-Class & Artists Series,
    4336
Kuumba Fest, 4337
Ritz Theatre and La Villa Museum, 2701
Sam Wolfson Baseball Park, 6358
Veterans Memorial Coliseum, 6359
Wjct Jacksonville Jazz Festival, 4338

Jacksonville Beach
Beaches Fine Arts Series, 4339

Key Biscayne
Tennis Center at Crandon Park, 6360

Key Largo
South Florida Center for the Arts, 6361

Key West
Florida Keys Community College, 6362
Key West Council On the Arts Series, 4340
Key West Players, 2702
Key West Symphony, 1038
Red Barn Theatre, 2703, 6363
Tennessee Williams Theatre, 6364

Kissimmee
Osceloa County Stadium & Sports Complex, 6366
Osceola Center for the Arts, 6365

Lake Buena Vista
Walt Disney Wide World of Sports, 6367

Lake Worth
Demetrius Klein Dance Company, 225
Duncan Theatre, 6368
Palm Beach Community College, 6369

Lakeland
Bach Festival of Central Florida, 4341
Branscomb Memorial Auditorium, 6370
Florida Southern College, 6342
Florida Southern College - Buckner Theatre, 6371
Florida Southern College: Department of Theatre Arts,
    2704
General Motors Place, 6372
Imperial Symphony Orchestra, 1039
Lakeland Center, 6373
Lakeland Center Entertainment Series & Broadway
    Series, 4343

Largo
Suncoast Dixieland Jazz Classic, 4344

Lynn Haven
Kaleidoscope Theatre, 2705

Madison
North Florida Community College, 4345

Manalapan
Florida Stage, 2706
Theatre Club of the Palm Beaches, 2707

Marathon
Marathon Community Theatre, 2708

Marianna
Chipola Junior College Series, 4346

Melbourne
Brevard Symphony Orchestra, 1040
King Center for the Performing Arts, 6374
Melbourne Auditorium, 6375
Melbourne Civic Theatre, 2709

Miami
American Airlines Arena, 6376
Coconut Grove Playhouse, 2710
Dade County Auditorium, 6377
Florida Grand Opera, 2002
Florida International University: Department of Theatre
    and Dance, 2711
Freddick Bratcher & Company, 226
Friends of Chamber Music of Miami, 1041
Golden Panther Sportsplex, 6378
Gusman Center for the Performing Arts, 6379
James L Knight Center, 6380
Key West Music Festival, 4347
Las Mascaras Theatre, 2712
Maximum Dance Company, 227
Miami Arena, 6381
Miami Chamber Symphony, 1042
Miami Civic Music Association Series, 4348
Miami Classic Guitar Society, 1043
Miami Dade Community College, 4349
Miami Dance Theatre, 228
Orange Bowl Stadium, 6382
Performing Arts Center of Greater Miami, 6383
South Florida Youth Symphony, 1044

Teatro Avante, 2713
Temple Beth Am Series, 4350

Miami Beach
Concert Association of Florida Series, 4351
Florida Dance Association, 229
Gold Coast Theatre, 2714
Jackie Gleason Theater, 6384
Miami City Ballet, 230
New World Symphony, 1045
Performing Arts Society of South Florida, 4352

Mobile
Mobile Civic Center - Exposition Hall, 6385
Mobile Civic Center - Theatre, 6386

Monticello
Monticello Opera House, 6387

Mount Berry
Berry College Theatre Program, 2715

Mount Dora
Icehouse Theatre, 2716

Naples
Naples Philharmonic Orchestra, 1046
Philharmonic Center for the Arts, 6388

New Port Richey
Center for the Arts at River Ridge, 6389

New Smyrna Beach
Atlantic Center for the Arts, 6390

Niceville
Okaloosa-Walton Community College, the Arts Center,
    6391

North Fort Myers
Lee Civic Center - Arena, 6393
Lee Civic Center - Small Theater, 6394

North Miami Beach
Victory Park Auditorium, 6395

Ocala
Central Florida Symphony, 1047

Orange Park
Orange Park Community Theatre, 2717

Orlando
Bob Carr Performing Arts Center, 6396
Mark Two Dinner Theater, 2718
Orange County Convention Center, 6397
Orlando Ballet, 231
Orlando Centroplex, 6398
Orlando Opera, 2003
Orlando Philharmonic Orchestra, 1048
Orlando-Ucf Shakespeare Festival, 4353
Peyton & Day Entertainmnet, 8360
Td Waterhouse Centre, 6399
Theatre-In-The-Works, 2719
Ucf Arena, 6400
Ucf Civic Theatre, 2720
University of Central Florida Orchestra, 1049
University of Central Florida: Department of Theatre,
    2721
Valencia Community College - Black Box Theatre,
    6401
Valencia Community College - Performing Arts, 6402

Osprey
New Century Artists, 8361

Palatka
Siegel Artist Management, 8362

Palm Beach
Greater Palm Beach Symphony Association, 1050
Palm Beach Pops, 1051
Society of the Four Arts, 4354

Palm City
Treasure Coast Concert Association, 4355

Robert W Woodruff Arts Center: Alliance Theatre, 6441
Robert W Woodruff Arts Center: Symphony Hall, 6442
Schwartz Center for Performing Arts at Emory, 4390
7 Stages, 2758, 2773, 6443
Six Flags Over Georgia, 2774
Southeastern Savoyards, 2775
Spelman College Fresh Images Chamber Music Series, 1077, 4391
Theater Emory, 2776
Theater of the Stars, 2777
Theatre Gael, 2778
Theatrical Outfit, 2779
Troika Balalaikes, 2018
Turner Field, 6444
World Artists, 8367

Augusta
Augusta Opera Association, 2019
Augusta Players, 2780
Augusta Symphony Orchestra, 1078
Augusta/Richmond County Civic Center Complex, 6445
Greater Augusta Arts Council, 4392
Imperial Theatre, 6446

Carrollton
Maurice K Townsend Center for the Performing Arts, 6447
West Georgia Theatre Company Summer Classic, 2781

Cedartown
Cedartown Civic Auditorium, 6448

Clarkston
Georgia Perimeter College Guest Artist Series, 4393

Columbus
Columbus Civic Center, 6449
Columbus Symphony Orchestra, 1079
Memorial Stadium, 6450
Rivercenter for the Performing Arts, 6451
Springer Opera House, 2782
Three Arts Theatre, 6452

Covington
Arts Association in Newton County, 4394

Dahlonega
North Georgia College & State University Music Series, 4395

Decatur
Agnes Scott College, 6453
Agnes Scott College: Department of Theatre and Dance, 2783
Charne Furcron, 251
Neighborhood Playhouse, 2784
Piccadilly Puppets Company, 2785
Rosalee Shorter, 253
Several Dancers Core, 252

Duluth
Gwinnett Performing Arts Center, 6454

Ellijay
Gilmer Arts & Heritage Association Series, 4396

Gainesville
Arts Council, 4397
Gainesville Ballet, 254
Gainesville Symphony Orchestra, 1080

Jekyll Island
Jekyll Island Amphitheater, 6455
Jekyll Island Soccer Complex, 6456

LaGrange
Lagrange Ballet, 255
Theatre Plus, 256

Macon
Grand Opera House, 6457
Grand Opera House Season at the Grand, 2020
Grand Opera House-A Performing Arts Center, 6458
Macon Concert Association, 4398

Macon Symphony Orchestra, 1081
Music Mercer Series, 4399
Wesleyan College - Porter Auditorium, 6459

Madison
Madison: Morgan Cultural Center, 6460

Marietta
Cobb County Civic Center, 6461
Cobb County Civic Center - Jennie T. Anderson, 6462
Cobb County Civic Center - Romeo Hudgins Memorial Center, 6463
Cobb Symphony Orchestra, 1082
Georgia Ballet, 257
Parenthesis Theatre Club, 2786
Pegalomania Molloy, 258
Ruth Mitchell Dance Company, 259
Theatre in the Square, 2787, 6464

Morrow
Spivey Hall, 6465

Moultrie
Colquitt County Arts Center, 6466

Mount Vernon
Brewton-Parker College Fine Arts Council, 4400

Perry
Perry Players, 2788

Rome
Rome City Auditorium, 6467
Rome Symphony Orchestra, 1083

Roswell
Georgia Ensemble Theatre, 2789
Orchestra Atlanta, 1084

Savannah
Armstrong Atlantic State University, 4401
Armstrong State College Fine Arts Auditorium, 6468
Savannah Civic Center, 6469
Savannah Civic Center - Arena, 6470
Savannah Civic Center - Theatre, 6471
Savannah Concert Association, 4402
Savannah Music Festival, 4403

Statesboro
Georgia Southern University - Puppet Theatre, 6472

Stockbridge
Festival Ballet Company, 260

Stone Mountain
Art Station Theatre, 2790

Thomaston
Thomaston-Upson Arts Council Performing Series, 4404

Thomasville
Thomasville Cultural Center Auditorium, 6473
Thomasville Entertainment Foundation, 4405

Tucker
Dekalb Symphony Orchestra, 1085
Mystical Arts of Tibet, 261

Valdosta
Jekyll Island Musical Theatre Festival, 2791, 4406
Lowndes/Valdosta Arts Commission, 4407
Valdosta State College - Sawyer Theatre, 6474
Valdosta State College - Whitehead Auditorium, 6475
Valdosta Symphony Orchestra, 1086

Woodstock
Jazz Dance Theatre South, 262

Young Harris
Southern Appalachian Stages, 2792

Hawaii

Fort Shafter
Army Entertainment Program, 2793

Hilo
Hawaii Concert Series, 4408
Hilo Community Players, 2794

Honolulu
Aloha Stadium, 6476
Chamber Music Hawaii, 1087
Diamond Head Theatre, 2795
Hawaii Chamber Orchestra Society, 1088
Hawaii Ecumenical Chorale, 2021
Hawaii Opera Theatre, 2022
Hawaii State Ballet, 263
Hawaii Theatre, 2796
Hawaii Youth Symphony Association, 1089
Honolulu Academy of Arts, 6477
Honolulu Chamber Music Series, 1090, 4409
Honolulu Children's Opera Chorus, 2023
Honolulu Dance Theatre, 6478
Honolulu Symphony Orchestra, 1091
Honolulu Theatre for Youth, 2797
Kimu Kahua Theatre, 2798
Men Dancing-Gregg Lizenbery Dance Pioneers, 264
Neal S Blaisdell Center, 6479
Oahu Choral Society, 2024
Saint Louis Center for the Performing Arts -, 6480
University of Hawaii at Manoa, 1092
University of Hawaii Series, 4410

Kahului
Maui Arts & Cultural Center, 6481
Maui Community College Series, 4411

Kailua
Windward Theatre Guild, 2799

Kamuela
Halau Hula Ka No'eau, 4412
Kahilu Theatre, 6482
Waimea Community Theatre, 2800

Kapaa
Kauai International Theatre, 2801

Laie
Brigham Young University: Hawaii Performance Series, 4413
Mckay Auditorium at Brigham Young University, 6483

Pearl City
Leeward Community College Theatre, 2802

Wailuku
Maui Academy of Performing Arts, 2803
Maui Philharmonic Society, 1093
Maui Symphony Orchestra, 1094

Idaho

Boise
Ballet Idaho, 265
Bank of America Centre, 6484
Biotzetik Basque Choir, 2025
Boise Chamber Music Series, 1095, 4414
Boise Master Chorale, 2026
Boise Philharmonic Association, 1096
Idaho Classical Guitar Society, 1097
Idaho Shakespeare Festival, 2804, 4415
Idaho Theater for Youth, 2805
Morrison Center for the Performing Arts, 6485
Oinkari Basque Dancers, 266
Opera Idaho, 2027
Pavilion at Boise State, 6486

Burley
Magic Philharmonic Orchestra, 1098

Caldwell
Caldwell Fine Arts Series, 4416

Coeur d'Alene
Coeur D'alene Summer Theatre/Carrousel Players, 2806

Urban Gateways Series: Center for Arts Education, 4447
Victory Gardens Theater, 2860, 6532
Wax Lips Theatre Company, 2861
Wilbur College Cultural Events Series, 4448
William Ferris Chorale, 2040
Windy City Performing Arts, 2041
Wisdom Bridge Theatre, 2862
Women's Theatre Alliance, 2863
Wrigley Field, 6533
Zephyr Dance, 282

Crystal Lake
Judith Svalander Dance Theatre, 283

Danville
Danville Symphony Orchestra, 1125

De Kalb
Egyptian Theatre, 6534
Northern Illinois University Fine Arts Series, 4449

Decatur
Decatur Civic Center, 6535
Decatur Civic Center - Arena, 6536
Decatur Civic Center - Theater, 6537
Millikin University Kirkland Fine Arts Center, 6538
Millikin University Opera Theatre, 2042
Millikin-Decatur Symphony Orchestra, 1126
Performing Arts Series for Students, 4450

Deerfield
Trinity College Artist Series, 4451

Des Plaines
Des Plaines Theatre Guild, 2864
Maine Township Community Concert Association, 4452
Northwest Symphony Orchestra, 1127

Downers Grove
Artists Showcase West, 4453
Downers Grove Choral Society, 2043
Downers Grove Concert Association Series, 4454

East Peoria
Illinois Central College Subscription Series, 4455

Edwardsville
Southern Illinois University-Edwardsville Series, 4456
University Theatre: Summer Show Biz, 2865

Elgin
Elgin Community College Visual & Performing Arts Center, 6539
Elgin Symphony Orchestra, 1128
Hemmens Cultural Center, 6540

Elk Grove
L'opera Piccola, 2044

Elmhurst
Elmhurst College Jazz Festival, 4457
Elmhurst Symphony Orchestra, 1129

Elsah
Principia College Concert Series, 4458

Evanston
Bach Week Festival in Evanston, 1130, 4459
Gus Giordano Jazz Dance Chicago, 284
Light Opera Works, 2045
Live Theatre, 2866
National/Louis University Library, 6541
Next Theatre Company, 2867
Northwestern University Summer Drama Festival, 2869, 4460
Northwestern University Theatre and Interpretation Center, 2868
Northwestern University: Dyche Stadium, 6542
Organic Theater Company, 2870
Pick-Staiger Concert Hall, 6543
Piven Theatre Workshop, 2871
Siegel Artist Management, 8371
Symphony Ii, 1131

Galesburg
Knox College: Eleanor Abbott Ford Center for the Performing Arts, 6544
Knox-Rootabaga Jamm Jazz Festival, 4461
Orpheum Theatre, 2872
Prairie Players Civic Theatre, 2873

Glen Ellyn
College of Dupage Arts Center, 6545
College of Dupage Arts Center - Mainstage, 6546
College of Dupage Arts Center - Studio Theatre, 6547
College of Dupage Arts Center - Theatre 2, 6548
Dupage Opera Theater, 2046
Dupage Symphony, 1132
Glen Ellyn Children's Chorus, 2047
New Philharmonic, 1133
Wheaton Symphony Orchestra, 1134

Glencoe
Chamber Music Society of the North Shore, 1135
Writers' Theatre Chicago, 2874

Goodfield
Conklin Players Dinner Theatre, 2875

Graylake
College of Lake County - Performing Arts Building, 4462

Greenville
Greenville College Guest Artist Series, 4463

Harrisburg
Southeastern Illinois College Cultural Arts Series, 4464
Southeastern Illinois College Visual & Performing Arts Center, 6549

Highland Park
Apple Tree Theatre, 2876
Ballet Entre Nous, 285
Ravinia Festival, 4465

Highwood
Midwest Young Artists, 1136

Homewood
Starry Nights Summer Concert Series, 4466

Indianapolis
Mystery Cafe Series, 4467

Joliet
Rialto Square Theatre, 6550

Lake Forest
Barat College Performing Arts Center Season, 4468
Lake Forest Symphony, 1137

Lebanon
Mckendree College Fine Arts Series, 4469

Libertyville
David Adler Cultural Center, 6551

Lincolnshire
Capitol International Productions, 8372
Marriott's Theatre in Lincolnshire, 2877

Litchfield
Encore Players, 2878

Macomb
Summer Music Theatre, 2879
Western Illinois University - Hainline Theatre, 6552
Western Illinois University Bca Performing Artist Series, 4470

Marion
Marion Cultural and Civic Center, 6553

Maywood
Coleman Puppet Theatre, 2880

Moline
Moline Boys Choir, 2048
Quad-Cities Jazz Festival, 4471
The Mark of Quad Cities, 6554

Monroe
Ewing Coliseum, 6555

Mount Vernon
Cedarhurst Chamber Music, 1138

Mt. Carroll
Timber Lake Playhouse, 2881

Naperville
Naperville-North Central College Performing Arts Series, 4472
Von Heidecke's Chicago Festival Ballet, 286

Normal
Hancock Stadium, 6556
Illinois Shakespeare Festival, 2882, 4473
Illinois State University Music Series, 4474
Illinois State University: Redbird Arena, 6557

Northbrook
Northbrook Symphony Orchestra, 1139
Sheely Center for the Performing Arts, 6558

Oak Brook
First Folio Shakespeare Festival, 4475
Natyakalalayam Dance Company, 287

Oak Park
Momenta, 288
Oak Park Festival Theatre, 2883
Symphony of Oak Park & River Forest, 1140
Village Players Theater, 2884

Oakbrook Terrace
Drury Lane Oakbrook Terrace, 2885

Palos Hills
Moraine Valley Community College Fine & Performing Arts Center, 6559

Park Forest
Freedom Hall: Nathan Manilow Theatre, 6560
Illinois Philharmonic Orchestra, 1141
Illinois Theatre Center, 2886, 6561

Peoria
Community Children's Theatre of Peoria Park District, 4476
Midwest Jazz Heritage Festival, 4477
Opera Illinois, 2049
Peoria Ballet, 289
Peoria Civic Center Broadway Theater Series, 2887, 4478
Peoria Players Theatre, 2888
Peoria Symphony Orchestra, 1142

Quincy
Muddy River Opera Company, 2050
Quincy Civic Music Association, 4479
Quincy Symphony Orchestra, 1143

River Forest
Dominican University Center Stage Guest Artist Series, 4480

River Grove
Richard Burton Performing Arts Center, 6562
Triton College Performing Arts Center, 6563

Rock Island
Augustana Choir, 2051
Augustana College - Centennial Hall, 6564
Augustana Symphony Orchestra, 1144
Circa '21 Dinner Playhouse, 2889
Quad City Arts, 4481

Rockford
Mendelssohn Club, 1145
Midway Theatre, 6565
New American Theater, 2890
Rock Valley College Lecture/Concert Series, 4482
Rockford Area Youth Symphony Orchestra, 1146
Rockford Dance Company, 290

Indiana

Kansas

Pella
Central College Community Orchestra, 1199

Sioux Center
Northwest Iowa Symphony Orchestra, 1200

Sioux City
Roberts Stadium, 6667
Sioux City Community Theatre, 2941
Sioux City Symphony Orchestra, 1201
Siouxland Youth Symphony Orchestra, 1202

Storm Lake
Buena Vista University Academic & Cultural Events Series, 4543

Waterloo
Hope Martin Theatre, 6668
Waterloo Community Playhouse & Black Hawk Childrens Theatre, 2942
Waterloo Riverfront Stadium, 6669

Waukee
Americafest: International Singing Festival for Women, 4544
Ladysing Festival for Women, 4545

Waverly
Wartburg College - Neumann Auditorium, 6670
Wartburg College Artists Series, 4546
Wartburg Community Symphony Orchestra, 1203

Kansas

Abilene
Great Plains Theatre Festival, 4547

Atchison
Community Concerts Association of Atchison Series, 4548

Augusta
Augusta Arts Council/Augusta Historical Theatre, 2943

Chanute
Chanute Community Theatre, 2944
Memorial Auditorium, 6671

Coffeyville
Coffeyville Community Theatre, 2945
Coffeyville Cultural Arts Council, 4549
Floral Hall, 6672

Concordia
Brown Grand Theatre, 2946

Dodge City
Dodge City Civic Center, 6673

Emporia
Emporia Arts Council Performing Arts/Concert/Children's Series, 4550
Emporia Symphony Orchestra, 1204

Goodland
Goodland Arts Council, 4551

Hays
Fort Hays State University Encore Series, 4552
Fort Hays State University-Felton Center, 6674
Hays Symphony Orchestra, 1205

Hesston
Hesston/Bethel Performing Arts Series, 4553

Hutchinson
Hutchinson Symphony Association, 1206
Kansas State Fair - Grandstand, 6675

Iola
Bowlus Fine Arts Center, 6676

Lawrence
Allen Fieldhouse, 6677
Cohan/Suzeau Dance Company, 306
Lied Center of Kansas, 6678

University of Kansas: Crafton-Preyer Theatre, 6679

Leavenworth
Saint Mary College - Xavier Hall Theatre, 6680

Lindsborg
Bethany College - Burnett Center, 6681
Messiah Festival of Music, 4554

Lola
Bowlus Cultural Attractions Series, 4555

Manhattan
Fred Bramiage Coliseum, 6682
Kansas State University - Mccain Auditorium, 6683
Kansas State University Mccain Performance Series, 4556
Manhattan Arts Center, 6684

McPherson
Mcpherson College - Brown Auditorium, 6685

Neodesha
Neodesha Arts Association, 6686

North Newton
Newton Mid-Kansas Symphony Orchestra, 1207

Ottawa
Ottawa Municipal Auditorium, 6687
Ottawa Municipal Auditorium Entertainment Series, 4557

Overland Park
Johnson County Community College, Carlsen Center, 6688
Kansas Regional Ballet, 307
Overland Park Arts Commission, 4558

Pittsburg
Carnie Smith Stadium, 6689
Memorial Auditorium and Convention Center, 6690
Pittsburg Arts Council, 4559
Pittsburg State University Solo & Chamber Music Series, 4560
Pittsburgh State University: Weede Arena, 6691

Salina
Salina Arts & Humanities Commission, 4561
Salina Bicentennial Center, 6692
Salina Community Theatre, 2947

Shawnee Mission
Barn Players Theatre, 2948
Youth Symphony Association of Kansas, 1208

Sterling
Sterling College Artist Series, 4562

Topeka
Kansas Expocentre, 6693
Topeka Civic Theatre & Academy, 2949
Topeka Jazz Festival, 4563
Topeka Performing Arts Center, 6694
Topeka Symphony, 1209
Topeka Symphony Chorus, 2065
Washburn University: Lee Arena, 6695

Valley Center
Kansas Coliseum, 6696

Wamego
Columbian Theatre: Museum & Art Center, 1210, 2950, 6697

Wellington
Wellington Memorial Auditorium, 6698

Wichita
Century Ii Civic Center - Convention Hall, 6699
Century Ii Civic Center - Exhibition Hall, 6700
Century Ii Civic Center - Theatre, 6701
Century Ii Convention & Performing Arts Center, 6702
Cessna Stadium, 6703
Friends University Miller Fine Arts Series, 4564
Music Theatre of Wichita, 2951
Tapestry Performing Arts, 2952

Wichita Community Theatre, 2953
Wichita Contemporary Dance Theatre, 308
Wichita State University Connoisseur Series, 4565
Wichita State University: Henry Levitt Arena, 6704
Wichita Symphony, 1211

Winfield
Horsefeathers & Applesauce Summer Dinner Theatre, 2954

Kentucky

Ashland
Artists in Concert Series, 4566
Paramount Arts Center, 6705

Bardstown
J Dan Talbott Amphitheatre, 6706
Stephen Foster Drama Association, 2955

Berea
Berea College Convocation Series, 4567
Phelps-Stokes Auditorium at Berea College, 6707

Bowling Green
Bowling Green-Western Symphony Orchestra, 1212
Capitol Arts Alliance, 4568
Capitol Arts Center, 6708
Diddle Arena, 6709
Fountain Square Players, 2956
Lt Smith Stadium/Western Kentucky University, 6710

Campbellsville
Central Kentucky Arts Series, 4569

Danville
Great American Brass Band Festival, 4570
Norton Center for the Arts, 6711
Pioneer Playhouse of Kentucky, 2957

Elizabethtown
Hardin County Playhouse, 2958

Falmouth
Kincaid Regional Theatre, 2959

Georgetown
Foust Artist Series, 4571

Glasgow
Far-Off Broadway Players, 2960

Greenville
Muhlenberg Community Theatre, 2961

Harrodsburg
Legend of Daniel Boone/James Harrod Amphitheatre, 2962

Hazard
Greater Hazard Area Performing Arts Series, 4572

Henderson
Henderson Fine Arts Center, 6712

Hopkinsville
Pennyroyal Arts Council Series, 4573

Horse Cave
Horse Cave Theatre, 2963

Lexington
Actors' Guild of Lexington, 2964
Actors' Theatre of Lexington, 2965
Broadway Live at the Opera House, 2966
Central Kentucky Youth Orchestras, 1213
Chamber Music Society of Central Kentucky, 1214
Commonwealth Stadium, 6713
Kentucky Ballet Theatre, 309
Lexington Ballet, 310
Lexington Center Complex, 6714
Lexington Children's Theatre, 2967
Lexington Opera House, 6715
Lexington Philharmonic Society, 1215
Singletary Center for the Arts, 6716

Gaithersburg
City of Gaithersburg Cultural Arts Division, 4650

Glen Echo
Adventure Theatre: Glen Echo Park, 3021
Institute of Musical Traditions, 2090

Glenwood
Maryland Youth Symphony Orchestra, 1253

Grantsville
Music at Penn Alps, 1254

Hagerstown
Maryland Symphony Orchestra, 1255
Maryland Theatre, 6836
National Tap Ensemble, 323

La Plata
College of Southern Maryland Fine Arts Center, 6837

Landover
Fedex Field, 6838

Largo
Capital Jazz Festival, 4651

Laurel
Petrucci's Dinner Theatre, 3022
Young Artists Theater, 3023

Mt. Rainier
Smallbeer Theatre Company, 3024

North Bethesda
Strathmore Hall Arts Center, 6839

Ocean City
Roland E Powell Convention Center, 6840

Olney
Olney Theatre Center, 3025

Owings Mills
Gordon Center for the Performing Arts, 6841

Riverdale
Prince George's Philharmonic, 1256

Rockville
Jewish Community Center of Greater Washington, 6842
Jewish Community Center Symphony, 1257
Metropolitan Ballet Theatre and Academy, 324
Montgomery College: Robert E Parilla Performing Arts Center, 6843
National Chamber Orchestra Society, 1258
Washington Jewish Theatre, 3026

Salisbury
Wicomico Youth and Civic Center, 6844

Silver Spring
Silver Spring Stage, 3027

Takoma Park
Liz Lerman Dance Exchange, 325

Timonium
Baltimore Chamber Orchestra, 1259

Towson
Children's Chorus of Maryland, 2091
F Scott Black's Dinner Theatre, 3028
Towson State University: Fine Arts Center, 6845
Towson State University: Stephens Auditorium, 6846

Westminster
Theatre On the Hill, 3029

Massachusetts

Amherst
Amherst Ballet, 326
Annie Tiberio Agency, 8375
Bright Moments Festival, 4652

Music at Amherst Series, 4653
University of Massachusetts: Concert Hall, 6848
University of Massachusetts: Fine Arts Center, 6847
Valley Light Opera, 2092
William D Mullins Memorial Center, 6849

Ann Arbor
Ann Arbor Summer Festival, 4654

Arlington
Electric Symphony Festival, 4655
Underground Railway Theater, 3030

Ashfield
Pilgram Theater Research & Performance Collaboration, 3031

Becket
Jacob's Pillow Dance Festival: School/Archives/Community Programs, 327, 4656

Belmont
Belmont Dramatic Club, 3032

Berkley
Marge Guillarducci Agency, 8376

Beverly
North Shore Music Theatre, 3033
North Shore Philharmonic Orchestra, 1260

Boston
Alea Iii, 1261
Boston Ballet, 328
Boston Camerata, 2093
Boston Center for the Arts: Cyclorama, 6850
Boston Center for the Arts: the National Theatre, 6851
Boston Children's Theatre, 3034
Boston Conservatory, 4657
Boston Lyric Opera Company, 2094
Boston Opera House, 6852
Boston Pops Orchestra, 1262
Boston Symphony Chamber Players, 1263
Boston Symphony Orchestra, 1264
Boston University Early Music Series, 4658
Boston University Theatre, 6854
Boston University Theatre: Main Stage, 6855
Boston University: Nickerson Field, 6856
Boston University: School of Fine Arts, 6853
Cantata Singers, 2095
Charles River Concert Series, 4659
Dance Umbrella, 329
Dinosaur Annex Music Ensemble, 1265
Ed Keane Associates, 8377
Emerson College: Emerson Majestic Theatre, 6857
Emmanuel Music Series, 4660
Fenway Park, 6858
First Night Boston, 4661
Fleetboston Celebrity Series, 4662
Fleetcenter, 6859
Greater Boston Youth Symphony Orchestras, 1266
Handel and Haydn Society, 1267, 2096
Harvard Musical Association in Boston, 4663
Harvard University: Harvard Stadium/Bright Arena, 6860
Huntington Theatre Company, 3035, 6861
Impulse Dance Company, 330
Isabella Stewart Gardner Museum, 6862
Jordan Hall at New England Conservatory, 6863
King's Chapel Concert Series, 4664
Kurland Associates, 8378
Lordly & Dame, 8379
Lyric Stage Company of Boston, 3036
Marcus Schulkind Dance Company, 331
Massachusetts Youth Wind Ensemble, 1268
Matthews Arena, 6864
Museum of Fine Arts Concerts & Performances, 4665
New England Conservatory, 6865
New England Philharmonic, 1269
Northeastern University Center for the Arts, 6866
Northeastern University: Parsons Field Stadium, 6867
Opera New England, 2097
Publick Theatre, 3037
Symphony Hall, 6868

Topf Center for Dance Education, 332
Wang Theatre, 6869
Wheelock Family Theatre, 3038

Braintree
Braintree Choral Society, 2098

Bridgewater
Bridgewater State College Program Committee, 4666

Brockton
Brockton Symphony Orchestra, 1270
Massasoit Community College Buckley Arts Center Performance Series, 4667

Brookline
Puppet Showplace Theatre, 3039

Cambridge
American Repertory Theatre, 3040, 3041
Boston Baroque, 1271
Boston Chamber Music Society, 1272
Boston Early Music Festival and Exhibition, 4668
Boston Globe Jazz & Blues Festival, 4669
Boston Musica Viva, 1273
Boston Philharmonic Orchestra, 1274
Cambridge Society for Early Music: Chamber Music Series, 1275
Harvard-Radcliffe Orchestra, 1276
Inca Son: Music and Dance of the Andes, 333
Jose Mateo's Ballet Theatre, 334
Klezmer Conservatory Band, 1277, 2099
Loeb Drama Center, 6870
Mandala Folk Dance Ensemble, 335
Mit Guest Artists Series, 4670
Music Amador, 8380
Musicamador, 1278
Pro Arte Chamber Orchestra, 1279
Radcliffe Choral Society, 2100
Radcliffe College: Agassiz Theater, 6871
Radcliffe College: Lyman Common Room, 6872
Regattabar Jazz Festival at the Charles Hotel, 4671
Snappy Dance Theater, 3042
World Music Festival, 4672

Carver
King Richard's Faire, 3043

Charlestown
Charlestown Working Theater, 3044

Chester
Miniature Theatre of Chester, 3045

Chestnut Hill
Boston College: Alumni Field Stadium, 6873
Siegel Artist Management, 8381
Silvio O Conte Forum/Boston College, 6874

Chicopee
Strawberry Productions, 3046

Chilmark
Yard, 3047

Concord
Concord Band, 1280
Concord Orchestra, 1281
Friends of the Performing Arts, 4673
St. Paul's School Ballet Company, 336

Dennis
Cape Playhouse, 3048, 6875

Dorchester
M Harriet Mccormack Center for the Performing Arts/Strand Theater, 6876

Dover
Festival Theatre, 6877

Duxbury
Art Complex at Duxbury, 6878

Fall River
Bristol Community College Arts Center, 6879

Williamstown
New Phoenix, 3079
Sterling & Francine Clark Art Institute, 6905
William College: Weston Field, 6906
Williams Chamber Players, 1303
Williams College Series, 4698
Williams College: Chapin Hall, 6907
Williamstown Theatre Festival, 4699

Wollaston
Quincy Symphony Orchestra, 1304

Worcester
Foothills Theatre Company, 3080
Mechanics Hall, 6908
Performing Arts School of Worcester, 6909
Salisbury Lyric Opera, 2116
Worcester Children's Theatre, 3081
Worcester Forum Theater, 3082
Worcester Music Festival, 4700

Yarmouth Port
Cape Ann Symphony Orchestra, 1305
Cape Symphony Orchestra, 1306

Michigan

Adrian
Adrian College, 6910
Adrian College Events Series, 4701
Adrian Symphony Orchestra, 1307
Opera! Lewanee, 2117

Albion
Albion Performing Artist & Lecture Series, 4702

Allendale
Grand Valley State University Arts at Noon Series, 4703

Alma
Alma College Performing Arts Series, 4704
Alma Symphony Orchestra, 1308
Community Theatre Association of Michigan, 3083

Alpena
Thunder Bay Arts Council, 4705
Thunder Bay Theatre, 3084

Ann Arbor
Ann Arbor Blues & Jazz Festival, 4706
Ann Arbor Dance Works, 340
Ann Arbor Summer Festival, 4707
Ann Arbor Symphony Orchestra, 1309
Boychoir of Ann Arbor, 2118
Comic Opera Guild, 2119
Dance Gallery Company, 341
Great Lakes Performing Artist Associates, 8386
Kerrytown Concert House, 6911
Michigan Association of Community Arts Agencies, 4708
Michigan Stadium, 6912
Michigan Theater, 6913
Musical Society of the University Series, 4709
Performance Network of Ann Arbor, 3085
Power Center for the Performing Arts, 6914
University Musical Society Choral Union, 2120
University of Michigan Dance Company, 342
University of Michigan Gilbert and Sullivan, 2121
University of Michigan School of Music: Michigan Youth Programs, 1310
University of Michigan Symphony Orchestras, 1311
University of Michigan: Mendelssohn Theatre, 6915
University of Michigan: Trueblood Theatre, 6916
University Productions: University of Michigan, 3086
Yost Ice Arena, 6917
Zajonc/Valenti, 8387

Auburn Hill
Palace at Auburn Hills, 6918

Augusta
Barn Theatre, 3087

Battle Creek
Battle Creek Civic Theatre, 6919
Battle Creek Symphony Orchestra, 1312
Co Brown Stadium, 6920
Kellogg Arena, 6921
United Arts Council Discovery Theatre, 6922

Bay City
Bay Arts Council, 4710
Bay City Players, 3088

Bay View
Bay View Music Festival, 4711

Benton Harbor
Lake Michigan College, Mendel Center for the Arts & Technology, 6923

Big Rapids
Ferris State University-Arts & Lectures Series, 4712

Birmingham
Birmingham-Bloomfield Symphony, 1313

Bloomfield Hills
American Artists Series, 4713
Cranbrook Music Guild Concert Series, 4714

Cadillac
Cadillac Symphony Orchestra, 1314
Gopherwood Concert Series, 4715

Calumet
Calumet Theatre Company, 3089

Cass City
Village Bach Festival, 4716

Cheboygan
Cheboygan Area Arts Council Concert Series, 4717
Cheboygan Area Arts Council/Opera House, 2122
Cheboygan Opera House: City Hall, 6924

Chelsea
Purple Rose Theatre Company, 3090

Clinton Township
Macomb Center for the Performing Arts, 6925
Macomb Symphony Orchestra, 1315

Coldwater
Tibbits Opera Foundation and Arts Council, 2123

Dearborn
Dearborn Orchestral Society / Dearborn Symphony, 1316

Detroit
Attic / New Center Theatre, 3091
Casa De Unidas Series, 4718
Cobo Arena, 6926
Comerica Park, 6927
Detroit Festival of the Arts, 4719
Detroit Repertory Theatre, 3092
Detroit Symphony Orchestra, 1317
Detroit Symphony Orchestra Hall, 6928
Fisher Theatre, 6929
Ford Detroit International Jazz Festival, 4720
Fox Theatre, 6930
Hilberry Theatre, Wayne State University, 3093
Joe Louis Arena, 6931
Madame Cadillac Dance Theatre, 343
Masonic Temple Theatre, 3094, 6932
Michigan Opera Theatre, 2124
Music Hall Center for the Performing Arts, 6933
Plowshares Theatre Company, 3095
Rackham Symphony Choir, 2125
Syracuse Jazz Festival, 4721
Theater Grottesco, 3096
United Black Artists: Usa Series, 4722
University of Detroit Mercy: Calihan Hall, 6934
Wayne State University: College of Fine, Performing & Communication Arts, 6935

East Lansing
Breslin Student Events Center, 6937

Michigan State University Wharton Center Presentations, 6938
Spartan Stadium, 6936

Farmington Hills
Chamber Music Society of Detroit, 1318
Community Center Farmington, 6940
1515 Broadway Performance Venue, 6939
Opera Lite, 2126

Flint
Atwood Stadium, 6941
Flint Institute of Music, 4723, 6942
Flint School of Performing Arts: Youth Ensembles, 1319
Flint Symphony Orchestra, 1320
Ima Sports Arena, 6943
Music in the Parks, 4724

Garden City
Maplewood Community Center, 6944

Gaylord
Gaylord Area Council for the Arts, 4725

Grand Haven
City of Grand Haven Community Center, 6945

Grand Rapids
Calvin College Fine Arts Center, 6946
Civic Theatre & School of Theatre, 3097
Community Circle Theatre, 3098
Deltaplex Entertainment & Expo Center, 6947
Festival of the Arts, 4726
Fountain Street Church, 6948
Grand Center: Auditorium, 6950
Grand Center: Devos Hall, 6949
Grand Rapids Ballet Company, 344
Grand Rapids Symphony, 1321
Grand Rapids Youth Symphony, 1322
Opera Grand Rapids, 2127
Reif Arts Council, 4727
St. Cecilia Music Society, 1323
Urban Institute for Contemporary Arts, 3099, 6951
Van Andel Arena, 6952

Grosse Pointe Farms
Grosse Pointe War Memorial, 4728
Pro Musica of Detroit, 1324

Hancock
Pine Mountain Music Festival, 4729

Hillsdale
Hillsdale College Community Orchestra, 1325

Holland
Holland Area Arts Council, 4730
Holland Chamber Orchestra, 1326
Holland Chorale, 2128
Holland Symphony Orchestra, 1327
Hope College Great Performance Series, 4731
Hope College Orchestra, 1328
Hope College Theatre Department, 6953
Hope Summer Repertory Theatre, 3100

Holly
Michigan Renaissance Festival, 4732

Houghton
Keweenaw Symphony Orchestra of Michigan Technological University, 1329
Mtu/Great Events Series, 4733

Interlochen
Interlochen Arts Festival, 4734
Interlochen Center for the Arts - Dendrinos Center, 6954
Interlochen Center for the Arts: Kresge Auditorium, 6955
Interlochen Dance Ensemble, 345

Ironwood
Ironwood Theatre, 3101, 6956

Minnesota

Ethnic Dance Theatre, 351
Greater Twin Cities Youth Symphonies, 1351
Guthrie Theater, 3132, 7007
Hauser Dance Company and School, 352
Hennepin Center for the Arts, 7008
Hidden Theatre, 3133
Historic Orpheum Theatre, 3134, 7009
Historic State Theatre, 3135, 7010
Hubert H Humphrey Metrodome, 7011
Illusion Theater, 3136
In the Heart of the Beast Puppet and Mask Theatre, 3137
International Theatres Corporation, 3138
Jackson Marionette Productions, 3139
Jungle Theater, 3140
Macphail Center for the Arts, 7012
Margolis Brown Theatre Company, 3141
Mariucci Arena, 7013
Metropolitan Symphony Orchestra, 1352
Minneapolis Park & Recreation Board-Summer Music in the Parks, 4757
Minnesota Chorale, 2132
Minnesota Dance Theatre, 353
Minnesota Opera, 2133
Minnesota Orchestra, 1353
Minnesota Sinfonia, 1354
Mixed Blood Theatre Company, 3142
National Lutheran Choir, 2134
Ned Kantar Productions, 8389
Northrop Dance Season, 354
Orchestra Hall, 7014
Pangea World Theater, 3143
Pillsbury House Theatre, 3144
Playwrights' Center, 3145
Plymouth Music Series of Minnesota, 4758
Red Eye, 3146
Target Center, 7015
Theater Mu, 3147
Theatre De La Jeune Lune, 3148
Theatre in the Round, 3149
Theatre in the Round Players, 7016
Troupe America, 3150
Twin Cities Gay Men's Chorus, 2135
University of Minnesota at Minneapolis Series, 4759
University of Minnesota: Sports Pavillion, 7017
Vocalessence, 2136
Walker Art Center, 1355, 3151, 7018
World Tree Puppet Theater, 3152
Zenon Dance Company and School, 355
Zorongo Flamenco Dance Theatre, 3128

Minnetonka
Allied Concert Services, 4760
Minnetonka Chamber Choir, 2137
Minnetonka Symphony Chorus, 2138

Moorhead
Concordia College Cultural Events Series, 4761
Fargo-Moorhead Symphony Orchestra and Association, 1356
Gooseberry Park Players, 3153
Minnesota State University Moorhead Series, 4762
Straw Hat Players, 3154

Morris
University of Minnesota Morris Cac Performing Arts Series, 4763

New Hope
New Hope Outdoor Theatre, 7019
Off-Broadway Musical Theatre, 3155

New Ulm
Concord Singers of New Ulm, 2139
Martin Luther College Lyceum, 7020

Northfield
Carleton College Concert Series, 4764
Saint Olaf Choir, 2140
Saint Olaf College Orchestra, 1357
St. Olaf College Artist Series, 4765

Owatonna
Little Theatre of Owatonna, 3156

Rochester
Mayo Civic Center, 7021
Mayo Civic Center: Arena, 7022
Mayo Civic Center: Auditorium, 7023
Mayo Civic Center: Theatre, 7024
Rochester Civic Music, 1358, 4766
Rochester Civic Theatre, 3157
Rochester Orchestra & Chorale, 2141

Saint Cloud
Minnesota Center Chorale, 2142
Quite Light Opera Company, 2143
St. Cloud State University Program Board Performing Arts Series, 4769
St. Cloud Symphony Orchestra, 1359

Saint Joseph
College of Saint Benedict - Benedicta Arts Center, 7025

Saint Paul
Climb Theatre - Creative Learning Ideas, 3158
College of St. Catherine: O'shaughnessy Auditorium, 7033
Dale Warland Singers, 2145
Dudley Riggs Instant Theatre Company, 3164
Fitzgerald Theater, 7026
451st Army Band, 1360
Great American History Theatre, 3159
Midway Stadium, 7032
Minnesota State Band, 1361
Nautilus Music Group, 3160
North Star Opera, 2144
Ordway Center for the Performing Arts, 7027
Ordway Music Theatre, 7029
Ordway Music Theatre: Mcknight Theatre, 7028
Pacific Composers Forum, 4770
Park Square Theatre Company, 3161
Penumbra Theatre Company, 3162
Rainbo Children's Theatre Company, 3163
Rivercenter, 7034
Roy Wilkins Auditorium at River Centre, 7030
Saint Paul Chamber Orchestra, 1362
Schubert Club International Artist Series, 4767
Xcel Energy Center, 7035

Saint Peter
Gustavus Adolphus College Artist Series, 4768
Gustavus Adolphus College: Schaeffer Fine Arts Center, 7031

White Bear Lake
Lakeshore Players, 3165
Lakeshore Playhouse, 7036
Shakespeare & Company, 3166

Mississippi

Bay Springs
Jazz in the Grove, 4771

Belzoni
Depot Theatre, 7037

Biloxi
Gulf Coast Opera Theatre, 2146
Gulf Coast Symphony, 1363
Mississippi Coast Coliseum, 7038
Saenger Theatre of the Performing Arts, 7039

Cleveland
Delta State University Bologna Performing Arts Center, 7040
Whistle Stop Playhouse, 7041

Columbus
Columbus Convention and Civic Center, 7042
Princess Theatre, 7043

Corinth
Coliseum Civic Center, 7044
Corinth Theatre-Arts, 3167

Greenwood
Leflore County Civic Center, 7045

Hattiesburg
Center for Opera & Music Theatre, 2147
Mannoni Performing Arts Center, 7046
Saenger Theatre, 7047
Southern Arts Festival Opera, 2148
University of Souther Mississippi: Reed Green Coliseum, 7050
University of Southern Mississippi College of the Arts, 4772
University of Southern Mississippi Symphony, 1364
University of Southern Mississippi: Mm Roberts Stadium, 7048
University of Southern Mississippi: Pete Taylor Baseball Park, 7049

Indianola
Indianola Little Theatre, 7051

Itta Bena
Mississippi Vally State University, 7052

Jackson
Ballet Mississippi, 356
Belhaven College Preston Memorial Series, 4773
Belhaven College: Girault Auditorium, 7053
Jackson Municipal Auditorium: Thalia Mara Hall, 7054
Mississippi Arts Commission, 4774
Mississippi Opera Association, 2149
Mississippi Symphony Orchestra, 1365
Mississippi Veterans Memorial Stadium, 7055
Mississippi Youth Symphony Orchestra, 1366
New Stage Theatre, 3168
Puppet Arts Theatre, 3169
Usa International Ballet Competition, 357
World Performance Series: Thalia Mara Foundation, 4775

Lorman
Alcorn State University Athletic Complex, 7056

Mathiston
Wood College: Theatre, 7058

McComb
State Theatre, 7059

Meridian
Meridian Community College-Theatre, 7060
Meridian Symphony Orchestra, 1367

Natchez
Natchez Opera Festival, 4777

Oxford
University of Mississippi: Fulton Chapel, 7064
University of Mississippi: Meek Auditorium, 7063
University of Mississippi: Studio Theatre, 7065

Sardis
Panola Playhouse, 7066

Tupelo
Tupelo Coliseum, 7067
Tupelo Symphony Orchestra Association, 1368

University
University of Mississippi Artist Series, 4778
University of Mississippi: Cm Tad Smitgh Coliseum, 7068
University of Mississippi: Vaugh-Hemingway Stadium, 7069

Yazoo City
Triangle Cultural Center, 7070

Missouri

Arrow Rock
Arrow Rock Lyceum Theatre, 3170
Lyceum Theatre, 7071

Boonville
Friends of Historic Boonville Performing Arts, 4779
Missouri River Festival of the Arts, 4780

Montana

Bigfork
Bigfork Center for the Performing Arts, 7132
Bigfork Summer Playhouse, 3203

Billings
Alberta Bair Theater, 3204
Alberta Bair Theatre for the Performing Arts, 7133
Billings Symphony Orchestra & Chorale, 2159
Billings Symphony Society, 1387
Metrapark, 7134
Red Lodge Music Festival, 4814
Yellowstone Chamber Players, 1388

Bozeman
Associated Students of Montana State University, 4815
Montana Ballet Company, 369
Montana Shakespeare in the Parks, 3205
Montana State University Sports Facilitites: Breenden
    Field House, 7135
Reno H Sales Stadium/Montana State University, 7136
Vigilante Theatre Company, 3206

Dillon
Dillon Community Concert Association, 4816

Great Falls
Four Seasons Arena, 7137
Great Falls Civic Center Theater, 7138
Great Falls Symphony Association, 1389
Montana Chorale, 2160
Montana State Fair & Four Seasons Arena, 7139
Montana Traditional Jazz Festival, 4817

Havre
Havre Community Concert Association, 4818
Montana State University Northern Showcase, 4819

Helena
Aleph Movement Theatre, 3207
Carroll College: Theatre, 7140
Helena Civic Center: Auditorium, 7141
Helena Civic Center: Ballroom, 7142
Helena Symphony Society, 1390
Myrna Loy Center, 7143

Kalispell
Flathead Valley Festival, 4820

Missoula
Adams Event Center, 7144
Missoula Children's Theatre, 3208
Missoula Symphony Association, 1391
Montana Repertory Theatre, 3209
University of Monatana-Missoula: Grizzili Stadium,
    7145
University of Montana Performing Arts Series, 4821
University of Montana: Montana Theatre, 7146
Young Audiences of Western Montana Series, 4822

Sheridan
Old Timers Concert Series, 4823

Whitefish
Flathead Festival of the Arts, 4824
Whitefish Theatre Company, 3210

Nebraska

Albuquerque
Northern Lights Management, 8392

Alma
Harlan County Arts Council, 4825

Bassett
Bassett Arts Council, 4826

Beatrice
Community Players, 7147

Bellevue
Bellevue Little Theatre, 3211, 7148

Bladen
Bladen Opera House, 7149

Chadron
Chadron State College: Memorial Hall, 7150

Columbus
Columbus Friends of Music Association, 4827

Crawford
Post Playhouse Incorporated, 3212

Fremont
Midland Lutheran College Concert: Lecture Series,
    4828

Gothenburg
Gothenburg Community Playhouse, 3213
Gothenburg Community Playhouse: Sun Theatre, 7151

Hastings
Hastings Symphony Orchestra, 1392

Kearney
Kearney Area Symphony Orchestra, 1393
Kearney Community Theatre, 3214, 7152
University of Nebraska: University Theatre, 7153
Unk Sports Center, 7154

Lincoln
Abendmusik Series, 4829
Lied Center for Performing Arts, 7155
Lincoln Civic Orchestra, 1394
Lincoln Community Playhouse, 3215
Lincoln Friends of Chamber Music, 1395
Lincoln Symphony Orchestra, 1396
Lincoln Youth Symphony, 1397
Nebraska Jazz Orchestra, 1398
Nebraska Repertory Theatre, 3216
Pershing Center, 7156
University of Nebraska at Lincoln Lied Center Season,
    4830
University of Nebraska-Lincoln: Bob Devaney Sports
    Center, 7158
University of Nebraska-Lincoln: Kimball Recital Hall,
    7159
University of Nebraska-Lincoln: Lincoln Memorial
    Stadium, 7157

McCook
Heritage Days Festival, 4831

Omaha
Ak-Sar-Ben Future Trust, 7161
Aksarben Coliseum, 7162
Brownville Concert Series, 4832
Cathedral Arts Project Series, 4833
Center Stage, 3217
Circle Theatre, 3218
Clarion Chamber Chorale, 2161
Grande Olde Players Theatre Company, 3219
Jewish Community Center of Omaha, 7163
Nebraska Shakespeare Festival, 4834
Nebraska Theatre Caravan, 370
Omaha Area Youth Orchestras, 1399
Omaha Civic Auditorium: Music Hall, 7164
Omaha Community Playhouse, 3220
Omaha Symphony, 1400
Omaha Symphony Chamber Orchestra, 1401
Omaha Theater Company for Young People, 3221
Omaha Theatre Company for Young People, 3222
Opera Omaha, 2162
Orpheum Theatre, 7165
Shakespeare On the Green, 3223
Tuesday Musical Concert Series, 4835
University of Nebraska at Omaha, 7166
University of Nebraska at Omaha Music Series, 4836

Scottsbluff
West Nebraska Arts Center, 7167

Seward
Concordia University Concert Series, 4837

Wayne
Wayne State College Special Programs Black & Gold
    Series, 4838
Wayne State College/Athletic Department, 7168

Nevada

Boulder City
Boulder City Arts Council, 4839

Carson City
Brewery Arts Center, 3224, 7169
Carson City Symphony, 1402
Nevada Arts Council, 4840

Fallon
Churchill Arts Council, 4841

Las Vegas
Actors Repertory Theatre, 3225
Caesars Palace, 7170
Chamber Music Southwest, 1403
Charleston Heights Arts Center, 7171
Las Vegas Civic Symphony, 1404
Las Vegas Convention and Visitors Authority, 7172
Las Vegas Little Theatre, 3226
Las Vegas Philharmonic, 1405
Mgm Grand Garden, 7173
Nationwide Entertainment Services, 8393
Nevada Ballet Theatre, 371
Nevada Opera Theatre, 2163
Nevada Symphony Orchestra, 1406
Nevada Theatre Company, 3227
Reed Whipple Cultural Arts Center, 4842, 7174
Sam Boyd Stadium, 7178
Thomas & Mack Center, 7175
University of Nevada-Las Vegas: Artemus Ham, 7176
University of Nevada-Las Vegas: Performing Arts
    Center, 7177
University of Nevada: Las Vegas Master Series, 4843

Reno
Centennial Coliseum: Reno Sparks Convention, 7179
Lawlor Events Center, 7180
Mackey Stadium, 7181
Nevada Festival Ballet, 372
Nevada Opera Association, 2164
Pioneer Center for the Performing Arts, 7182
Reno Chamber Orchestra, 1407
Reno Little Theater, 7183
Reno Philharmonic, 1408
Theater Coalition/The Lear Theater, 3228
University of Nevada-Reno: Church Fine Arts, 7184
University of Nevada-Reno: Lawlor Events Center,
    7185
University of Nevada: Reno Performing Arts Series,
    4844

Virginia City
Nevada Shakespeare Festival, 4845
Piper's Opera House, 7186

New Hampshire

Blackwood
Mainstage Center for the Arts, 3229

Claremont
Claremont Opera House, 2165, 7187

Concord
Capitol Center for the Arts, 7188
Community Players of Concord, 3230
Friends of the Concord City Auditorium, 7189
Keiser Concert Series, 4846
Nevers' 2nd Regiment Band, 1409
William H Gile Trust Fund Concert Series, 4847

Deerfield
New Hampshire Shakespeare Festival, 4848

Durham
University of New Hampshire, 7190
University of New Hampshire Celebrity Series, 4849
University of New Hampshire-Durham - Hennessy Center, 7192
University of New Hampshire-Durham: Bratton Recital Hall, 7191
Whittemore Center, 7193

East Sullivan
Apple Hill Center for Chamber Music, 1410

Hampton
Hampton Playhouse, 3231
Hampton Playhouse Theatre Arts Workshop, 7194

Hanover
Dartmouth College Hopkins Center Performing Series, 4850
Memorial Stadium/Dartmouth College, 7195
Opera North, 2166
Thompson Arena, 7196

Henniker
New England College Cultural Events Series, 4851

Keene
Colonial Theatre, 7197
Redfern Arts Center On Brickyard Pond, 7198

Laconia
Belknap Mill Society, 4852

Lancaster
Skyline Music Agency, 8394

Lebanon
Lebanon Opera House, 2167

Lincoln
Ncca Papermill Theatre, 7199
Papermill Theatre/North County Center for the Arts, 3232

Littleton
North Country Chamber Players Summer Festival: Music in the White Mountains, 4853

Manchester
New Hampshire Philharmonic Orchestra, 1411
New Hampshire Symphony Orchestra, 1412
Saint Anselm College Performing Arts Series, 4854

Meredith
Lakes Region Summer Theatre, 3233

Nashua
American Stage Festival, 4855
Nashua Community Concert Association, 4856

New London
Colby-Sawyer College, 4857
New London Barn Playhouse, 7200
Summer Music Series, 4858

North Conway
Eastern Slope Inn Playhouse, 7201
Mount Washington Valley Theatre Company, 3234

Peterborough
Monadnock Music, 4859
Peterborough Players, 3235

Plymouth
Plymouth Friends of the Arts Series, 4860
Plymouth State College Silver Cultural Arts Center Silver Series, 4861

Portsmouth
Ballet New England, 373
Friends of the Music Hall Concert Series, 4862
Harbor Arts Jazz Night: Portsmouth Jazz Festival, 4863
Music Hall, 7202
Pontine Movement Theatre, 3236
Prescott Park Arts Festival, 4864
Seacoast Repertory Theatre, 3237

Rindge
Franklin Pierce College Crimson-Grey Cultural Series, 4865

Tamworth
Barnstormers, 3238

Waterville Valley
Waterville Valley Foundation Summer Festival, 4866

Whitefield
Weathervane Theatre, 3239

Wilton
Andy's Summer Playhouse, 3240

Wolfeboro
Great Waters Music Festival, 4867

New Jersey

Absecon
Atlantic Contemporary Ballet, 374

Allenhurst
Metro Lyric Opera, 2168

Asbury Park
Asbury Park Jazz Festival, 4868
Monmouth Symphony Orchestra, 1413

Basking Ridge
Colonial Symphony, 1414

Bay Head
Orchestra of St. Peter By the Sea, 1415

Bayonne
Bayonne Veterans Memorial Stadium, 7203

Beach Haven
Surflight Theatre, 3241

Belleville
Great George Festival, 4869

Bergenfield
North Jersey Choral Society, 2169

Blairstown
Blair Academy, 7204

Bloomfield
Bloomfield Mandolin Orchestra, 1416

Bridgeton
Bay Atlantic Symphony, 1417

Caldwell
Caldwell College: Student Union Building, 7205

Camden
Rutgers-Camden Center for the Arts, 7206
Walt Whitman Cultural Arts Center, 7207

Cape May
Cape May Jazz Festival, 4870
Cape May Music Festival, 4871
Cape May Stage, 3242
Mid-Atlantic Center for the Arts, 7208
Middle Township Performing Arts Center, 7209

Chatham
Solid Brass, 1418

Cherry Hill
Philharmonic of Southern New Jersey, 1419

Closter
Lois Scott Management, 8395

Cranford
Cranford Dramatic Club, 3243
Cranford Dramatic Club Theatre, 7210
New Jersey Intergenerational Orchestra, 1420

Demarest
Aureus Quartet, 2170

Dover
Dover Little Theatre, 7211

East Brunswick
Philomusica Choir, 2171

East Rutherford
Continental Airlines Arena, 7214
Giants Stadium, 7212
Meadowlands/New Jersey Sports & Exposition Authority, 7213

Edison
Edison Arts Society, 4872
Plays-In-The-Park, 3244

Elmer
Appel Farm Arts and Music Center, 4873, 7215

Englewood
John Harms Center for the Arts, 4874, 7216

Ewing
College of New Jersey: Celebration of the Arts, 4875

Fair Lawn
Aviv Productions, 8396

Fort Lee
Nai-Ni Chen Dance Company, 375
Verismo Opera/New Jersey Association of Verismo Opera, 2172

Glassboro
Rowan University: Glassboro Center for the Arts, 7217

Hackensack
Fair Lawn Summer Festival, 4876
Orrie De Nooyer Auditorium, 7218
Soundfest Chamber Music Festival, Colorado Quartet, 4877

Hackettstown
Centenary College Performing Arts Guild, 4878

Haddonfield
Haddonfield Symphony, 1421

Hampton
Stanley Weinstein, 8397

High Bridge
New Globe Theater, 3245

Highland Park
Randy James Dance Works, 376

Highstown
Community Arts Partnership Series With Peddie School, 4879
Richard L Swig Arts Center, 7219

Hillsborough
Raritan Valley Chorus, 2173

Hoboken
Lyric Theatre, 1422

Holmdel
Am Productions Series, 4880
Holmdel Theatre Company, 3246

Jersey City
Attic Ensemble, 377
Avodah Dance Ensemble, 378
Liberty Science Center, 7220
New Jersey City University Orchestra, 1423

Lakewood
Strand Theatre, 7221

Lawrenceville
Rider University: the Yvonne Theater, 7222

Livingston
New Jersey Ballet Company, 379

Long Branch
New Jersey Repertory Company, 3247, 4881

Madison
Arts Council of the Morris Area, 4882
Drew University: Bowne Theatre, 7223
New Jersey Shakespeare Festival, 4883
Playwrights Theatre of New Jersey, 3248

Mahwah
Ramapo College of New Jersey: Berrie Center for
   Performing and Visual Arts, 7224

Manasquan
Algonquin Arts, 4884

Maplewood
New Jersey Dance Center, 380

Martinsville
Simulations, 3249

Medford
Culture Hall of Medford New Jersey, 7225

Metuchen
Forum Theatre, 3250

Millburn
Paper Mill Playhouse, 3251, 7226

Montclair
Artspower National Touring Theatre, 3252, 8398
New Jersey Music Society, 1424
Renate Boue Dance Company, 381
St. John's Renaissance Dancers, 382
Yass Hakoshima Mime Theatre, 3253

Montvale
Supreme Talent International, 8399

Moorestown
West Jersey Chamber Music Symphony & Society,
   1425

Morristown
Academy of Saint Elizabeth Performing Arts Series,
   4885
Artists International Management, 8400
Community Theatre, 7227
Morris Museum, 7228
William G Mennen Sports Arena, 7229

Mount Laurel
National Ballet of New Jersey, 383

Murray Hill
New Jersey Youth Symphony, 1426

Neptum
Paradise Chamber Orchestra, 1427

New Brunswick
American Repertory Ballet, 384
Crossroads Theatre Company, 3254
George Street Playhouse, 3255
Lkb Dance, 385
Rutgers Arts Center, 7230
Rutgers University Concert Series, 4886
State Theatre, 7231
State Theatre/New Brunswick Cultural Center, 4887

Newark
Cathedral Basilica of the Sacred Heart Concert Series,
   1428
Greater Newark Orchestra, 1429
New Jersey Performing Arts Center, 7232
New Jersey State Opera, 2174
New Jersey Symphony Orchestra, 1430
New Jersey Symphony Orchestra Amadeus Festival,
   4888
Newark Museum Association, 4889

Newark Performing Arts Corporation/Newark
   Symphony Hall, 3256
Newark Symphony Hall, 7233
Theatre of Universal Images, 3257

North Branch
Theatre of Raritan Valley Community College, 3258

Ocean City
Ocean City Pops, 1431

Ocean Grove
Annual Ocean Grove Choir Festival, 4890

Oldwick
Raritan River Concert Series, 4891
Raritan River Music Festival, 4892

Paramus
Ars Musical Chorale & Orchestra, 2175
Pro Arte Chorale, 2176

Passaic
Julius Forstmann Library Second Sunday Series, 4893

Paterson
Passaic County Community College Series, 4894

Pemberton
Foundation Theatre, 3259

Piscataway
Louis Brown Athletic Center, 7234
Rutgers University: Rutgers Athletic Center, 7235
Rutgers University: Rutgers Stadium, 7236

Plainfield
Crescent Concerts, 4895
Plainfield Symphony Orchestra, 1432

Plymouth
Silver Cultural Arts Center, 7237

Pomona
Stockton Performing Arts Center, 7238

Princeton
American Boychoir, 2177
Creative Theatre, 3260
Greater Princeton Youth Orchestra, 1433
Jadwin Gymnasium, 7239
Mccarter Theatre, 3261, 7240
Princeton Pro Musica Chorus & Orchestra, 2178
Princeton Repertory Company, 3262
Princeton Shakespeare Festival, 3263, 4896
Princeton Symphony Orchestra, 1434
Princeton University Concerts, 4897
Princeton University: Richardson Auditorium in
   Alexander Hall, 7241
Westminster Choir, 2179
Young Audiences of New Jersey, 4898

Rahway
Union County Arts Center, 7242

Readington
Sail Productions, 8401

Red Bank
Count Basie Theatre, 7243
Two River Theatre Company, 3264

Ridgewood
Irine Fokine Ballet Company, 386
Ridgewood Gilbert and Sullivan Opera Company, 2180
Ridgewood Symphony Orchestra, 1435

Ringwood
Ringwood Friends of Music Series, 4899

Rutherford
Williams Center for the Arts, 4900, 7244

Somerville
Raritan Valley Community College: Nash TheatreY,
   7245
Theatre at Raritan Valley Community College, 3265

South Orange
Broadway Center Stage, 387

Stanhope
Waterloo Foundation for the Arts Series, 4901

Summit
Central Presbyterian Church Brown Bag Concert
   Series, 4902
Community Opera, 2181
Genevieve Spielberg, 8402
Summit Chorale, 2182
Summit Symphony, 1436

Teaneck
American Stage Company, 3266
Bergen Philharmonic Orchestra, 1437
Teaneck New Theatre, 3267

Tenafly
Jcc On the Palisades, 7246

Toms River
Garden State Philharmonic Symphony Orchestra, 1438
Garden State Philharmonic Symphony Youth Orchestra,
   1439
Ocean County College Fine & Performing Arts
   Select-A-Series, 4903

Trenton
Greater Trenton Symphony Orchestra, 1440
New Jersey State Museum Auditorium, 7247
Passage Theatre Company, 3268
Patriots Theater at the War Memorial, 7248
Sovereign Bank Arena, 7249
The War Memorial Theatre, 3269

Union
Carolyn Dorfman Dance Company, 388
Kean College of New Jersey: Wilkens Theatre, 7250

Union City
Park Theatre Performing Arts Centre, 7251

Upper Montclair
Montclair State College: Memorial Auditorium, 7252
Theatrefest, 3270
Unity Concerts of New Jersey, 1441

Vauxhall
Jette Performance Company, 4904

Verona
Pushcart Players, 3271

Vineland
Cumberland Players, 3272

Warren
Philharmonic Orchestra of New Jersey, 1442

Wayne
Jazz It Up Festival, 4905
Orchestra at William Paterson College, 1443
William Paterson College: the Jazz Room Series, 4906
William Patterson University, 7253
Willowbrook Jazz Festival, 4907
Ym-Ywha of North Jersey Cultural Arts Series, 4908

West Long Branch
Shadow Lawn Summer Stage, 3273

West Orange
Jcc Metrowest, 7254
Jewish Community Center of Metropolitan New Jersey,
   7255
Maurice Levin Theater, 7256
Maurice Levin Theater Season, 3274

Westfield
Arbor Chamber Music Society, 1444
Choral Arts Society of New Jersey, 2183
Westfield Symphony Orchestra, 1445

Westwood
Drake & Associates/Tam, 8403

St. John's University, 7353

Jamaica Estates
New York Street Theatre Caravan, 3323

Jamestown
Arts Council for Chautauqua County, 4981
Jamestown Concert Association, 1485, 4982
Lucille Ball Little Theatre Building, 7354

Katonah
Caramoor Center for Music and the Arts, 4983, 7355
Caramoor International Music Festival, 4984
Venetian Theatre, 7356

Kingston
Coach House Players, 3324
Ulster Performing Arts Center, 7357

Lafayette
Contemporary Theatre of Syracuse, 3325

Lake George
Lake George Dinner Theatre, 3326, 7358
Lake George Jazz Weekend, 1486, 4985

Lake Luzerne
Luzerne Chamber Music Festival, 4986

Lake Placid
Lake Placid Center for the Arts-Theater, 7359
Olympic Center, 7360

Lancaster
Lancaster New York Opera House, 7361

Lewiston
Artpark, 4987

Lindenhurst
Studio Theatre, 7362

Little Falls
Mohawk Valley Center for the Arts, 7363

Lockport
Kenan Center, 7364

Locust Valley
Beethoven Festival, 1487, 4988
Long Island Baroque Ensemble, 1488

Long Island City
Laguardia Performing Arts Center, 7365

Mamaroneck
Emelin Theatre for the Performing Arts, 4989, 7366

Margaretville
Open Eye Theater, 3327

Massapequa
Oyster Bay Arts Council Distinguished Artists Concerts, 4990

Massapequa Park
Jeffrey James Arts Consulting, 8409

Medusa
International Piano Festival at Williams, 4991

Melville
Chamber Music Festival of the East, 4992
Long Island Philharmonic, 1489

Millbrook
Nomadics, 1490

Monticello
Periwinkle National Theatre, 3328

Mount Kisco
Mount Kisco Concert Association, 4993

Mt. Vernon
Jonathan Wentworth Associates Limited, 8410

Naples
Bristol Valley Theater, 3329

Narrowsburg
Delaware Valley Opera, 2200

New Berlin
Del-Se-Nango Olde Tyme Fiddlers Association, 415, 1491

New Hyde Park
Eglevsky Ballet, 416

New Lebanon
Tannery Pond Concerts, 1492
Theater Barn, 3330

New Paltz
New Paltz Summer Repertory Theatre, 3331
Piano Summer at New Paltz, 4994

New Rochelle
Ajkun Ballet Theatre, 417
Fleetwood Stage, 3332
New Rochelle Opera, 2201

New York
A.V. Productions and Theatre Guild, 3335
Aaron Concert Artists, 8411
Aaron Davis Hall, 7367
Abaca Productions, 8412
Abc Associated Booking Corporation, 8413
Abingdon Theatre Company, 3336
Aboutface Theatre Company, 3337
Acting Company, 3338
Acting Studio, 3339
Actors Studio, 3340
Actors' Alliance, 3341
Adobe Theatre Company, 3342
Aeolian Artists International Management, 8414
Aeolian Chamber Players, 1493
Affiliate Artists, 1494
Agency Group, 8415
Ailey, 418
Ailey Ii, 418
Albert Kay Associates, 8416
Allan Albert Productions Incorporated, 3343
Allnations Dance Company, 419
Alpha-Omega Theatrical Dance Company, 420
Alvin Ailey American Dance Theater, 421
Amanda Mckerrow, 422
Amas Musical Theatre, 3344
Amato Opera Theatre, 2202
Ambassador Theatre, 7368
American Ballet Theatre, 423
American Bolero Dance Company: Carnegie Hall, 424
American Center for Stanislavski Theatre Art, 3345
American Chamber Opera Company, 2203
American Composers Orchestra, 1495
American Ensemble Company, 3346
American Festival of Microtonal Music, 4996
American Indian Community House Series, 4997
American Landmark Festivals, 4998
American Opera Music Theater, 2204
American Place Theatre, 3347, 7369
American Symphony Orchestra, 1496
American Tap Dance Orchestra, 425, 1497
American Theatre of Actors, 3348
American-International Dance Theatre, 426
American-International Lyric Theatre, 2205
Amy Horowitz Solo Dance, 427
Amy Pivar Projects, 428
Andrea Del Conte Danza Espana, 429
Anglo-American Ballet, 430
Anik Bissonnette, 431
Annabella Gonzalez Dance Theater, 432
Anthony George Artist Management, 8417
Apollo Theatre, 7370
Apollo's Banquet, 433
Ardani Artists Management, 8418
Arthur Shafman International, 8419
Artist Management, 8420
Arts International, 4999
Arts Management Group, 8421
Arts4all, 8422
Ascap, 7371
Asia Society, 5000

Asian American Dance Theatre, 434
Associated Booking Corporation, 8423
Association for the Advancement of Creative Arts, 1498
Atlantic Theater Company, 3349
Bachanalia Chamber Orchestra, 1499
Baker Field, 7372
Ballet Galaxie, 435
Ballet Hispanico of New York, 436
Ballet Manhattan, 437
Ballet Tech, 438
Bang On a Can, 5001
Barrow Group, 3350
Basketball City, 5002
Bat Theatre Company, 3351
Battery Dance Company, 439
Bebe Miller Company, 440
Bell Atlantic Jazz Festival, 5003
Bernard Schmidt Productions, 8424
Besenarts, 8425
Beverly Blossom and Company, 441
Big League Theatricals, 8426
Big League Theatricals, Inc., 3352
Bill T. Jones/Arnie Zane and Company, 442
Bill Young & Dancers, 443
Black Spectrum, 3353
Blanco & Blanco, 444
Bloomingdale School of Music, 1500
Bloomingdale School of Music Concert Series, 5004
Bmi (Broadcast Music), 7373
Bond Street Theatre Coalition, 3354
Booking Group, 8427
Booth Theatre, 7374
Bopi's Black Sheep/Dance By Kraig Patterson, 5005
Boys Choir of Harlem, 2206
Brad Simon Organization, 8428
Bridge State of the Arts, 3355
Bridgehampton Chamber Music Festival, 5006
Broadhurst Theatre, 7375
Broadway Theatre, 7376
Broadway Tomorrow, 3356
Brooks Atkinson Theatre, 7377
Cami, 445
Canterbury Choral Society, 2207
Carlota Santana Spanish Dance Company, 446
Carnegie Chamber Players, 1501
Carnegie Hall Corporation, 7378
Carol Fonda and Company, 447
Carolyn Lord and Company, 448
Castillo Theatre, 3357
Cathedral Arts, 5007
Celebration Team of National Dance Institute, 449
Center for Traditional Music & Dance, 7379
Central Park Summerstage, 5008
Chamber Music America, 1502
Chamber Music Society of Lincoln Center, 1503
Chen and Dancers, 450
Chicago City Limits, 3358
Children's Aid Society Chorus, 2208
Chinese Folk Dance Company, 451
Chinese Music Ensemble of New York, 1504
Christine Camillo, 452
Cia Vincente Saez, 453
Circle in the Square, 7380
Circle-In-The-Square, 3359
Circum Arts, 8429
City Center, 7381
City Center of Music and Drama, 7382
City Symphony Orchestra of New York, 1505
Clarion Music Society, 5009
Classic Stage Company, 3360
Classical Quartet, 1506
Collegiate Chorale, 2209
Columbia Artists Management, 8430
Columbia University Orchestra, 1507
Columbia University: Wien Stadium, 7383
Company Appels, 454
Concert Artists Guild New York Recital Series, 5010
Concert Socials, 5011
Concerts at the Cloisters, 5012
Concordia, 1508
Concordia Orchestra, 1509

Penn Yan
Yates Performing Arts Series, 5070

Pine Bush
Musical Concerts at the Burlingham Inn, 5071

Pleasantville
Music at Port Milford, 5072
Summit Music Festival, 5073

Port Jefferson
Theatre Three Productions, 3489
Theatre Three Productions: Mainstage, 7458
Theatre Three Productions: Second Stage, 7459

Port Washington
Anita Feldman Tap/Tapping Music, 565
Ireland On Stage, 8468

Potsdam
Community Performance Series, 5074
Crane School of Music Annual Spring Festival of the Arts, 5075

Poughkeepsie
Bardavon 1869 Opera House, 7460
Clearwater's Great Hudson River Revival, 5076
Hudson Valley Philharmonic, 1542
Mid-Hudson Civic Center, 7461
New Day Repertory Company, 3490
Powerhouse Theater at Vassar, 3491

Purchase
Purchase College, Suny: the Performing Arts Center, 7462

Rhinebeck
Chamber Music at Rodef Shalom With Stephen Starkman & Friends, 1543
Rhinebeck Chamber Music Society, 1544

Richfield Springs
Mamadou Diabate, 1545
Matapat, 1546, 2235
On Queue Performing Artists, 566, 8469

Rochester
Blackfriars Theatre, 3492
Blue Cross Arena, 7463
Eastman Philharmonia, 1547
Eastman School of Music, 5077, 7465
Eastman School of Music Kilbourn Hall, 7464
Frontier Field, 7466
Garth Fagan Dance, 567
Geva Theatre, 3493
Greece Symphony Orchestra, 1548
Nazareth College Arts Center Series, 5078
Nazareth College: Nazareth Arts Center, 7467
Poetry in Motion, 8470
Pyramid Arts Center, 7468
Quartet Program, 1549
Roberts Wesleyan College, 5079
Rochester Broadway Theatre League, 3494
Rochester Chamber Orchestra, 1550
Rpo Summermusic, 5080
Society for Chamber Music in Rochester, 1551
Theatre On the Ridge, 3495
University of Rochester Theatre Program, 3496
University of Rochester-River Campus: Strong Theatre, 7469

Rome
Capitol Civic Center, 7470
Capitol Theatre Summerstage, 3497

Ronkonkoma
Broadhollow Players Limited, 3498

Rosendale
Vanaver Caravan, 568

Rye
Rye Arts Center, 7471

Sag Harbor
Bay Street Theatre, 3499

Salem
Fort Salem Theatre, 3500
Mettawee Theatre Company, 3501
Music From Salem, 5081

Saranac
Hill & Hollow Music, 5082

Saranac Lake
Adirondack Festival of American Music, 5083
Pendragon Theatre, 3502

Saratoga Springs
Freihofer's Jazz Festival at the Saratoga Performing Arts Center, 5084
Lake George Opera Festival, 2236
Saratoga Performing Arts Center, 1552, 3503, 7472
Skidmore Music Department Series, 5085

Scarsdale
Empire State Pops: Symphony and Chamber Orchestra, 1553

Schenectady
Proctor's Theatre, 3504, 7473
Schenectady Civic Players, 3505, 7474
Schenectady Light Opera Company, 2237
Schenectady Museum: Union College Concert Series, 5086

Selden
Suffolk County Community College: Shea Theatre, 7475

Skaneateles
Skaneateles Festival, 5087

Sloatsburg
Pat Cannon's Foot & Fiddle Dance Company, 569

South Salem
Canticum Novum Singers, 2238
New York Virtuoso Singers, 2239
Westchester Oratorio Society, 2240

Southampton
Long Island University: Fine Arts Theatre, 7476

Spencertown
Spencertown Academy Performing Series, 5088

St. Bonaventure
Reilly Center Arena, 7477

Staten Island
Center for the Arts at the College of Staten Island, 7478
Center for the Arts at the College of Staten Island: Lecture Hall, 7479
Center for the Arts at the College of Staten Island: Recital Hall, 7480
Snug Harbor Cultural Center, 7481
Staten Island Symphony, 1554
Veterans Memorial Hall, 7482

Sterling
Sterling Renaissance Festival, 3506, 5089

Stony Brook
Sports Complex, 7483
State University of New York at Stony Brook Concert Series, 5090

Stony Point
Penguin Repertory Company, 3507

Sunnyside
Rosewood Chamber Ensemble, 1555
Thalia Spanish Theatre, 3508

Syracuse
Civic Center of Onondaga County, 7484
Civic Center of Onondaga County: Carrier Theatre, 7485
Civic Center of Onondaga County: Crouse-Hind Hall, 7486
Civic Morning Musicals, 5091

Cultural Resources Council of Syracuse, 5092
Mulroy Civic Center at Oncenter, 7487
Open Hand Theater, 3509
P&C Stadium, 7488
Prestige Agency, 8471
Syracuse Area Landmark Theatre, 7489
Syracuse Friends of Chamber Music, 1556
Syracuse Opera, 2241
Syracuse Society for New Music, 5093
Syracuse Stage, 3510
Syracuse Symphony Orchestra, 1557
Syracuse Symphony Youth Orchestra, 1558
Syracuse University: Carrier Dome, 7490

Tallman
Rockland Summer Institute - Orchestral & Chamber Music Studies, 1559

Ticonderoga
Ticonderoga Festival Guild, 5094

Troy
Friends of Chamber Music of Troy, 1560
Hudson Valley Community College Cultural Affairs Program, 5095
Knickerbacker Recreational Facility and Ice Arena, 7491
New York State Theatre Institute, 3511
Rensselaer Newman Foundation Chapel and Cultural Center, 7493
Rensselaer Polytechnic Institute: Houston Field House, 7492
Troy Chromatic Concerts, 5096
Troy Chromatics Concerts, 1561
Troy Savings Bank Music Hall, 7494

Tuxedo
New York Renaissance Faire, 3512

Uniondale
Nassau Symphony Society, 1562
Nassau Veterans Memorial Coliseum, 7495

Utica
A Good Old Summer Time's Genesee Street Festival, 5097
Broadway Theatre League of Utica, 3513
Chamber Music Society of Utica, 1563
Mohawk Valley Community College Cultural Events Series, 5098
Mohawk Valley Ballet, 570
Munson-Williams-Proctor Arts Institute, 5099
Stanley Performing Arts Center, 7496
Utica Memorial Auditorium, 7497

Wappingers Falls
Bennett Morgan & Associates Limited, 8472

Waterford
Eugene O'neill Theater Center, 7498

Watertown
Jefferson Community College, 7499
Watertown Lyric Theater Productions, 3514

West Point
Us Military Academy: Eisenhower Hall Theatre, 7500
Us Military Academy: Mishie Stadium, 7501

Westbury
Westbury Music Fair, 5100

Westfield
Das Puppenspiel Puppet Theater, 3515

Westport
Arts Council for the Northern Adirondacks, 5101

White Plains
Street Theater, 3516

Williamsville
Amherst Symphony Orchestra, 1564

Woodbury
Chamber Players International, 1565

Marion
Foothills Community Theatre, 3547

Mars Hill
Moore Auditorium, 7541
Southern Appalachian Repertory Theatre, 3548

Misenheimer
Pfeiffer University Artist Series, 5143

Mooresville
Mooresville Community Theatre, 3549

Morganton
City of Morganton Municipal Auditorium, 7542

Mount Airy
Mount Airy Fine Arts Center, 7543
Surry Arts Council, 5144

Murfreesboro
Chowan College: Mcdowell Columns Auditorium, 7544

Pembroke
University of North Carolina at Pembroke: Givens
   Performing Arts Center, 7545

Pittsboro
Unto These Hills, 3550

Raleigh
Actors Comedy Lab, 3551
Arts Ncstate, 5145
Artsplosure: 2003 Spring Jazz & Art Festival, 5146
Bti Center for the Performing Arts: Aj Fletcher Opera
   Theater, 7546
Bti Center for the Performing Arts: Meymandi Concert
   Hall, 7547
Burning Coal Theatre Company, 3552
Eastcoast Entertainment, 8479
First Night Raleigh, 5147
Js Dortin Arena, 7548
Ncsu Center Stage, 7549
North Carolina Arts Council, 5148
North Carolina Museum of Art, 7550
North Carolina State University Center Stage, 7552
North Carolina State University: Carter Finley Stadium,
   7551
North Carolina State University: Reynolds Coliseum,
   7553
North Carolina Symphony, 1586
North Carolina Theatre, 3553
Pine Cone-Piedmont Council of Traditional Music,
   5149
Raleigh Boychoir, 2249
Raleigh Civic Center Complex, 7554
Raleigh Ensemble Players, 3554
Raleigh Entertainment & Sports Arena, 7555
Raleigh Little Theatre, 7556
Raleigh Ringers, 1587
Raleigh Symphony Orchestra, 1588
Side By Side, 3555
Theatre in the Park, 3556, 7557
United Arts Council of Raleigh and Wake County, 5150

Rocky Mount
Tar River Choral & Orchestral Society, 1589, 2250

Salisbury
Catawba College: College Community Center, 7558
Piedmont Players Theatre, 3557
Salisbury Symphony Orchestra, 1590

Sanford
Temple Theatre Company, 3558, 7559

Smithfield
Johnston Community College On Stage Concert Series,
   5151

Snow Camp
Snow Camp Historical Drama Society, 3559

Southern Pines
Arts Council of Moore County, 5152
Sandhills Little Theatre, 3560

Spindale
Isothermal Community College Performing Arts
   Center, 7560

Swannanoa
Swannanoa Chamber Music Festival, 5153

Tarboro
Edgecombe County Arts Council, 5154

Troy
Messiah 2000, 5155

Tryon
Paddywhack, 1591
Tryon Concert Association Subscription Series, 5156
Tryon Fine Arts Center, 7561

Valdese
Old Colony Players, 3561

Whiteville
Southeastern Community College Performing Arts
   Series, 5157

Wilkesboro
Walker Events, 7562

Williamston
Martin Community Players, 3562

Wilmington
Cape Fear Blues Festival, 5158
Legion Stadium, 7563
Opera House Theatre Company, 3563
Thalian Hall Center for the Performing Arts, 7564
University of North Carolina at Wilmington, 5159
Wilmington Symphony Orchestra, 1592

Wilson
Barton College Concert, Lecture & Convocation
   Committee Series, 5160

Wingate
Noel Musical Artist Series, Jesse Ball Dupont Fund,
   5161

Winston-Salem
Bowman Gray Stadium, 7566
Children's Theatre Board, 3564
Lawrence Joel Veterans Memorial Coliseum, 7567
Little Theatre of Winston-Salem, 3565
North Carolina Black Repertory Company, 3566
North Carolina School of the Arts - Roger, 7568
North Carolina School of the Arts Symphony Orchestra,
   1593
North Carolina School of the Arts: School of Music
   Performance Series, 5162
Piedmont Chamber Singers, 2251
Piedmont Opera Theatre, 2252
Reynolds Memorial Auditorium, 7569
Salem College Concert Series, 5163
Wake Forest University Secrest Artists Series, 5164
Wake Forest University Symphony Orchestra, 1594
Winston-Salem Piedmont Triad Symphony Association,
   1595, 2253
Winston-Salem State University, 7570
Winston-Salem University: Ce Gaines Complex, 7571

Yadkinville
Yadkin Players, 3567

Yanceyville
Caswell County Civic Center, 7572
Caswell Performing Arts Series, 5165

North Dakota

Bismarck
Bismarck Civic Center: Arena, 7573
Bismarck Civic Center: City Auditorium, 7574
Bismarck-Mandan Orchestral Association, 1596

Fargo
Fargo-Moorhead Community Theatre, 3568

Fargo-Moorhead Opera Company, 2254
Fargodome, 7576
Little Country Theatre, 3569
North Dakota State University Lively Arts Series, 5166
University of North Dakota: Festival Concert Hall,
   7577

Fort Totten
Fort Totten Little Theatre, 3570

Grand Forks
Greater Grand Forks Symphony Orchestra, 1597
Hyslop Sports Center, 7578
North Dakota Museum of Art Concert Series, 5167
University of North Dakota, 7580
University of North Dakota: Chester Fritz Auditorium,
   7579

Jamestown
Jamestown Civic Center, 7581

Mayville
Mayville State University (Nd) Fine Arts Series, 5168

Minneapolis
Medora Musical, 3571

Minot
International Music Camp, 1598, 2255
Minot Symphony Association, 1599

Ohio

Ada
Ohio Northern University Artist Series, 5169

Akron
Akron Civic Theatre, 7582
Akron Symphony Orchestra, 1600
Akron Youth Symphony Orchestra, 1601
Carousel Dinner Theatre, 3572
Children's Concert Society of Akron, 5170
Ej Thomas Performing Arts Hall, 7583
Greater Akron Musical Association, 5171
James a Rhodes Arena, 7584
Music From Stan Hywet, 5172
Ohio Ballet, 577
Tuesday Musical, 5173
University of Akron: Akron Rubber Bowl, 7585
University of Akron: Ej Thomas Hall Series, 5174

Ashland
Ashland Symphony Orchestra, 1602

Ashtabula
Ashtabula Arts Center, 7586
Ashtabula Chamber Orchestra, 1603

Athens
Dairy Barn Cultural Arts Center, 7587
Ohio University Performing Arts Series, 5175
Ohio University: Patio Theater, 7588
Ohio University: School of Music, 7589

Barberton
Magical Theatre Company, 3573, 7590

Batavia
Uc Clermont College: Calico Theatre, 7591

Bay Village
Huntington Playhouse, 7592
Huntington Theatre, 3574

Beachwood
Cleveland Pops Orchestra, 1604
Ohio Chamber Orchestra, 1605
Suburban Symphony Orchestra, 1606

Bellefontaine
Logan County Community Concerts, 5176

Berea
Baldwin Wallace College: Kulas Musical Arts, 7593
Baldwin-Wallace Bach Festival, 5177

Carnegie-Mellon Concerts, 5378
Carnegie: Lecture Hall, 7843
Carnegie: Museum of Art Theatre, 7844
Carnegie: Music Hall, 7845
City Theatre Company, 3728
Dan Kamin, 8489
Dance Alloy, 632
Duquesne University Tamburitzans, 7846
First Friday at the Frick Concert Series, 5379
First Fridays at the Frick Concert Series, 5380
Fitzgerald Fieldhouse, 7847
George Balderos, 8490
Heinz Hall for the Performing Arts, 7848
Joan Sherman Artist Management, 8491
Labco Dance, 633
Manchester Craftsmen's Guild, 5381, 7849
Mary Miller Dance Company, 634
Mellon Arena, 7850
Mendelssohn Choir of Pittsburgh, 2286
Music for Mt. Lebanon, 5382
Music Tree Artist Management, 8492
Opera Theater of Pittsburgh, 2287
Pittsburgh Ballet Theatre, 635
Pittsburgh Camerata, 2289
Pittsburgh Chamber Music Society, 1738
Pittsburgh Civic Arena, 7851
Pittsburgh Civic Light Opera, 2290
Pittsburgh Clo, 2288
Pittsburgh Dance Council, 636
Pittsburgh International Children's Theater, 3729
Pittsburgh Irish & Classical Theatre, 3730
Pittsburgh New Music Ensemble, 1739
Pittsburgh Opera, 2291
Pittsburgh Playhouse of Point Park College, 3731
Pittsburgh Public Theater, 3732
Pittsburgh Symphony Orchestra, 1740
Pittsburgh Youth Symphony Orchestra Association, 1741
Pnc Park, 7852
Point Park College Guest Artists Series, 5383
Prime Stage, 3733
Renaissance and Baroque Society of Pittsburgh, 1742
River City Brass Band, 1743
Tamburitzans Folk Ensemble, 1744
Three Rivers Arts Festival, 5377
University of Pittsburgh Concert Series, 5384
University of Pittsburgh: Pitt Stadium, 7853
Veronica's Veil Players, 3734
Y Music Society of the Jewish Community Center, 5385

Pottstown
Hill School Center for the Arts Lively Arts Series, 5386

Radnor
Cabrini College, 5387

Reading
Albright College Concert Series, 5388
Berks Jazz Festival, 5389
Rajah Theatre, 7854
Reading Community Players, 3735
Reading Symphony Orchestra, 1745
Star Series Association, 5390

Scranton
Northeastern Theatre, 3736
Scranton Community Concerts, 5391
Scranton Cultural Center at the Masonic Temple, 7855

Selinsgrove
Susquehanna University Artist Series, 5392

Shamokin
Central Community Concerts, 5393

Shawnee-on-Delaware
Shawnee Playhouse, 3737

Slippery Rock
Slippery Rock University - Performing Arts Series, 5394

Somerset
Laurel Arts/The Philip Dressler Center, 7856

State College
Central Pennsylvania Festival of the Arts, 5395
Nittany Valley Symphony, 1746
Pennsylvania Dance Theatre, 637

Stroudsburg
Notara Dance Theatre, 638

University Park
Bryce Jordan Center, 7857
Music at Penn's Woods, 5396, 5397
Penn State University Beaver Stadium, 7858
Penn State University: Center for the Performing Arts, 7859
Pennsylvania Centre Stage, 7860

Villanova
Villanova University Chamber Series, 1747, 5398

Warren
Struthers Library Theatre, 3738

Warrendale
Pittsburgh Concert Chorale, 2292

West Chester
Farrel Stadium, 7861

Wexford
Saltworks Theatre Company, 3739

White Mills
Wildflower Music Festival, 5399

Wilkes-Barre
Fm Kirby Center for the Performing Arts, 7862
King's College Experiencing the Arts Series, 5400
Wilkes University: Dorothy Dickson Darte Center, 7863

Williamsport
Arena Summer Theatre, 3740
Williamsport Community Concert Association, 5401
Williamsport Symphony Orchestra, 1748

Windber
Arcadia Performing Arts, 5402

Yardley
Lower Makefield Society for the Performing Arts, 5403
Movement Theatre International, 3741

York
Greater York Youth Ballet, 639
Strand-Capitol Performing Arts Center, 7864
Strand-Capitol Performing Arts Center Series, 5404

Rhode Island

Barrington
Kelli Wicke Davis/Shoda Moving Theatre, 640

Bristol
Concerts By the Bay, 5405

East Greenwich
Cultural Organization of the Arts, 5406

Kingston
Kingston Chamber Music Festival at Uri, 1749, 5407
New England Presenters: University of Rhode Island Great Performances, 5408
University of Rhode Island Fine Arts Center, 7865
University of Rhode Island Symphony Orchestra, 1750

Lincoln
State Ballet of Rhode Island, 641

Matunuck
Theatre-By-The-Sea, 3742

Newport
Astors Beechwood Mansion, 3743

Island Moving Company, 642
Newport Music Festival, 5409

Providence
As220, 7866
Brown Stadium, 7867
Brown Summer Theatre, 3744
Brown University Orchestra, 1751
Brown University Theatre, 3745
Capitolarts Providence Cultural Affairs, 5410
Convergence 2000 Arts Festival: Workshop With Ts Thomas, 5411
Everett Dance Theatre, 643
Festival Ballet Providence, 644
First Night Providence, 5412
Groundwerx Movement Center, 645
Looking Glass Theatre, 3746
Newgate Theater, 3747
Perishable Theatre, 7868
Providence Civic Center, 7869
Providence Division of Public Programming Departments, 5413
Providence Performing Arts Center, 7870
Rhode Island Chamber Music Concerts, 1752
Rhode Island Civic Chorale & Orchestra, 1753
Rhode Island Civic Chorale and Orchestra, 2293
Rhode Island College Symphony Orchestra, 1754
Rhode Island College: Performing Arts Series, 5414
Rhode Island Philharmonic Orchestra and Music School, 1755
Rites and Reason, 3748
Sandra Feinstein-Gamm Theater, 3749
Trinity Arts Center, 7871
Trinity Repertory Company, 3750
Veterans Memorial Auditorium, 7872

Westerly
Chorus of Westerly, 2294

Woonsocket
Stadium Theatre Performing Arts Center, 7873

South Carolina

Abbeville
Abbeville Opera House, 7874

Aiken
Aiken Community Playhouse, 3751
University of South Carolina: Aiken Etherredge Center, 5415

Anderson
Anderson College: Rainey Fine Arts Center, 5416
Anderson Symphony Orchestra, 1756
Civic Center of Anderson, 5417

Beaufort
Byrne Miller Dance Theatre, 646
University of South Carolina-Beaufort, 5418

Camden
Fine Arts Center of Kershaw County, 7875

Charleston
Charleston Ballet Theatre, 647
Charleston Concert Association, 5419
Charleston Symphony Orchestra, 1757
Citadel Fine Arts Series, 5420
Dock Street Theatre, 7876
Footlight Players, 3752
Footlight Players Theatre, 7877
Gaillard Municipal Auditorium, 7878
Johnson Hagood Stadium, 7879
Mcalister Fieldhouse, 7880
Piccolo Spoleto Festival, 5421
Robert Ivey Ballet, 648
Spoleto Festival Usa, 649, 1758, 3753, 5422

Clemson
Clemson University: Brooks Center for the Performing Arts, 7881
Clemson University: Clemson Memorial Stadium, 7882

Clemson University: Littlejohn Coliseum, 7883

Clinton
Presbyterian College, 5423

Columbia
Carolina Ballet, 650
Carolina Productions, Performing Arts Commission, 5424
Columbia City Ballet, 651
Columbia College Sosoho Performance Series, 5425
Columbia Stage Society at Town Theatre, 3754
Koger Center for the Arts, 5426, 7884
Trustus, 3755
University of South Carolina: Carolina Coliseum, 7886
University of South Carolina: Drayton Hall, 7887
University of South Carolina: Longstreet Theatre, 7885
Williams-Brice Stadium/University of South Carolina, 7888

Florence
Florence Civic Center, 7889
Francis Marion University Artists Series, 5428

Ft. Hill
Charlotte Knights Baseball Stadium, 7890

Georgetown
Swamp Fox Players, 3756

Greenville
Bi-Lo Center, 7891
Bob Jones University Concert, Opera & Drama Series, 3757
Carolina School of Ballet, 652
Carolina Youth Symphony, 1759
Centre Stage-South Carolina, 3758
Furman University: Mcalister Auditorium, 7892
Greenville Ballet, 653
Greenville Municipal Stadium, 7893
Greenville Symphony Orchestra, 1760
Magicmusic Productions, 8493
Metropolitan Arts Council, 5429
Peace Center for the Performing Arts, 7894
Warehouse Theatre, 3759

Greenwood
Greenwood Civic Center, 7895
Greenwood-Lander Performing Arts, 5430

Hartsville
Center Theater, 7896
Hartsville Community Concert Association, 5431

Hilton Head Island
Arts Center of Coastal Carolina, 5432

Mt. Pleasant
Eastcoast Entertainment, 8494, 8495

Myrtle Beach
Coastal Concert Association, 5433

Newberry
Newberry College Theatre, 3760
Newberry Opera House, 2295

North Charleston
North Charleston Performing Arts Center, 7897

Orangeburg
South Carolina State University, 7898

Pawleys Island
Group H Entertainment, 8496

Rock Hill
Arts Etc, 5434
Winthrop College: James F Byrnes Auditorium, 7899
Winthrop University College of Visual & Performing Arts, 5435

Spartanburg
Arts Partnership of Greater Spartanburg, 5436
Converse College Sinfonietta, 1761
Music Foundation of Spartanburg Concert Series, 5437

Spartanburg Memorial Auditorium: Arena, 7900
Spartanburg Memorial Auditorium: Theatre, 7901

Sumter
Fine Arts Council of Sumter Performing Arts Series, 5438
Sumter County Cultural Center, 7902

Tigerville
North Greenville College: Fine Arts Series, 5439

York
Mccelvey Center of York, 7903

South Dakota

Aberdeen
Aberdeen Community Concert Association, 5440
Aberdeen Community Theatre, 3761

Brookings
Brookings Chamber Music Society, 1762
Coughlin Alumni Stadium, 7904
South Dakota Art Museum, 7905
South Dakota State University Civic Symphony, 1763
South Dakota State University Student Activities, 5441

Custer
Black Hills Playhouse, 3762

De Smet
Laura Ingalls Wilder Pageant Society, 5442

Huron
Huron Arena, 5443

Madison
Madison Area Arts Council, 5444

Mitchell
Corn Palace, 7906

Pierre
Pierre Community Concerts Association, 5445

Rapid City
Black Hills Community Theatre, 3763
Black Hills Symphony Orchestra, 1764
Rushmore Plaza Civic Center, 7907

Sioux Falls
Sioux Falls Arena, 7908
Sioux Falls Coliseum, 7909
Sioux Falls Community Playhouse, 3764, 7910
South Dakota Symphony, 1765
Washington Pavilion of Arts & Science, 7911

Spearfish
Black Hills Passion Play, 3765
Matthews Opera House Society, 3766, 3767

Vermillion
America's Shrine To Music Museum, 7912
University of South Dakota: Dakota Dome, 7915
University of South Dakota: Slagle Auditorium, 7913
University of South Dakota: Warren M Lee Center, 7914

Watertown
Town Players, 3768

Yankton
Lewis & Clark Theatre Company, 3769

Tennessee

Athens
Athens Area Council for the Arts, 5446

Bristol
Theatre Bristol, 3770
Viking Hall Civic Center, 7916

Chattanooga
Ballet Tennessee, 654

Chattanooga Ballet, 655
Chattanooga Boys Choir, 2296
Chattanooga Symphony and Opera, 1766
Chattanooga Symphony and Opera Association, 2297
Riverbend Festival, 5447
Roland Hayes Concert Hall, 7917
Tivoli Theatre, 7918
University of Tennessee at Chattanooga, 5448
University of Tennessee-Chattanooga: Utc Mckenzie Arena, 7919

Clarksville
Austin Peay State University, 5449
Dunn Center, 7920
Roxy Theater, 3771

Cleveland
Lee University Presidential Concert Series, 5450

Collegedale
Southern Adventist University, 5451

Cookeville
Tennessee Tech University: Hooper Eblen Center, 7921
Tulane University, 7922

Cordova
Ballet Memphis, 656

Crossville
Cumberland County Playhouse, 3772

Dayton
Bryan College Department of Music, 5452

Etowah
Etowah Arts Commission, 5453

Franklin
Pull-Tight Players, 3773

Gatlinburg
Sweet Fanny Adams Theatre & Music Hall, 3774

Germantown
Germantown Community Theatre, 3775
Germantown Performing Arts Centre, 5454
Herschel Freeman Agency, 8497
Poplar Pike Playhouse, 3776

Jackson
Aman Arena, 7925
Jackson Arts Council, 5455
Jackson Civic Center, 7923
Jackson Symphony Association, 1767
Jackson Theatre Guild, 3777
Lambuth College: Lambuth Theatre, 7924

Jefferson City
Carson-Newman College Concert-Lecture Series, 5456

Johnson City
East Tennessee State University Performing Arts, 5457
Freedom Hall Civic Center, 7926
Johnson City Area Arts Council, 5458
Johnson City Symphony Orchestra, 1768
Milligan College: Derthick Theatre, 7927
Milligan College: Seeger Chapel Concert Hall, 7928
Mini Dome, 7929
Tennessee Association of Dance, 657

Kingsport
Kingsport Symphony Orchestra, 1769

Knoxville
Actors Co-Op, 3778
Arts & Culture Alliance of Greater Knoxville, 5779
Bijou Theatre, 3780
Bijou Theatre Center, 7930
Carpetbag Theatre, 3781
City Ballet, 658
Clarence Brown Theatre Company, 3782
Jubilee Community Arts, 5459
Knoxville Civic Auditorium and Coliseum-Auditorium, 7931
Knoxville Opera Company, 2298

Knoxville Symphony Orchestra, 1770
Neyland Stadium, 7932
Tennessee Children's Dance Ensemble, 659
Tennessee Stage Company, 3783
Tennessee Theater, 7933
Theater Knoxville, 3784
Thompson-Boling Arena, 7934
University of Tennessee at Knoxville: Cultural Arts, 5460
University of Tennessee Music Hall, 7935

Lebanon
Cumberland University Auditorium, 7936

Madison
Tennessee Players, 3785

Martin
University of Tennessee at Martin Arts Council, 5461
University of Tennessee-Martin: Skyhawk Arena, 7937

Maryville
Appalachian Ballet Company, 660
Maryville College, 7938

Memphis
Circuit Playhouse, 3786
Concerts International, 5462
Ewing Children's Theatre, 3787, 7939
Liberty Bowl Memorial Stadium, 7940
Lindenwood Concerts, 2299
Memphis Cook Convention Center Complex, 7941
Memphis in May International Festival, 5463
Memphis Symphony Orchestra and Youth Symphony Orchestra, 1771
Mid-South Coliseum, 7942
Orpheum Theatre, 7943
Playhouse On the Square, 3788
Pyramid Arena, 7944
Rhodes College: Mccoy Visiting Artist Series, 5464
Theatre Memphis, 7945

Morristown
Morristown Theatre Guild, 3789
Theatre Guild, 7946

Murfreesboro
Middle Tennessee State University, 5465
Tennessee State University: Charles M Murphy Athletic Center, 7947

Nashville
Adelphia Stadium, 7948
Chaffin's Barn, 7949
Chaffin's Barn - a Dinner Theatre, 3790
Class Act Entertainment, 8499
Corporate Magic, 3791
Darkhorse Theater, 3792
David Lipscomb University Theater, 3793
David Lipscomb University: Music Department, 5466
Friends of Music, 5467
Gaylord Entertainment Center, 7950
Grand Ole Opry House, 7951
Greer Stadium, 7952
Howard C Gentry Complex, 5468
Langford Auditorium, 7953
Mockingbird Public Theatre, 3794
Nashville Ballet, 661
Nashville Children's Theatre, 3795
Nashville Convention Center, 7954
Nashville Jewish Community Center, 7955
Nashville Municipal Auditorium, 7956
Nashville Opera Association, 2300
Nashville Shakespeare Festival, 3796, 5469
Nashville Symphony, 1772
Nashville Symphony Chorus, 2301
Ryman Auditorium, 7957
Tennessee Dance Theatre, 662
Tennessee Performing Arts Center, 7958
Tennessee Performing Arts Center: Andrew Jackson Hall, 7959
Tennessee Repertory Theatre, 3797
Vanderbilt Stadium, 7960
Vanderbilt University: Great Performances, 5470

Vanderbilt University: Memorial Gym, 7961
W.J. Hale Stadium, 7962
William Morris Agency, 8498

Oak Ridge
Oak Ridge Civic Music Association, 5471
Oak Ridge Playhouse, 3798
Oak Ridge Symphony Orchestra, 1773

Pigeon Forge
Dixie Stampede, 3799

Sewanee
Sewanee Festival Orchestras / Sewanee Music Festival, 1774
Sewanee Summer Music Festival, 5472
University of the South: Performing Arts Series, 5473

Townsend
Life of Christ Passion Play, 3800

Tullahoma
South Jackson Civic Center, 7963

Watertown
Watertown Jazz Festival, 5474

Texas

Abilene
Abilene Civic Center, 7964
Abilene Civic Center: Exhibit Hall, 7965
Abilene Civic Center: Theater, 7966
Abilene Opera Association, 2302
Abilene Philharmonic Association, 1775

Addison
Watertower Theatre, 3801

Albany
Aztec, 7967
Fort Griffin Fandangle Association, 3802
Fort Griffin Fandangle Outdoor Theatre, 7968
Old Jail Art Center, 7969

Amarillo
Amarillo Civic Center, 7970
Amarillo Civic Center: Arena, 7971
Amarillo Civic Center: Music Hall, 7972
Amarillo Symphony, 1776
Lone Star Ballet, 663

Arlington
Ballpark in Arlington, 7973
Theatre Arlington, 3803, 7974
University of Texas at Arlington, 5475
University of Texas at Arlington: Maverick Stadium, 7976
University of Texas at Arlington: Theatre Arts, 7975

Austin
Austin Chamber Music Center, 1777
Austin Chamber Music Festival, 5476
Austin Classical Guitar Society, 1778
Austin Lyric Opera, 2303
Austin Musical Theatre, 3804
Austin Shakespeare Festival, 3805, 5477
Austin Symphony Orchestra Society, 1779
Austin Theatre Alliance, 3806
Ballet Austin, 664
Chorus Austin, 2304
Deborah Hay Dance Company, 665
Frank C Erwin Jr Special Events Center, 7977
Frank Erwin Center/University of Texas-Austin, 5478
Frontera, 3807
Holden & Arts Associates, 8501
Johnson/Long Dance Company, 666
New Texas Music Works, 5479
One World Theatre, 7978
Paramount Theater for the Performing Arts, 7979
Project Interact - Zachary Scott Theatre Center, 3808
Rude Mechanicals, 3809
Salon Concerts, 5480
Sharir Dance Company, 667

State Theater Company, 3810
Stillpoint Dance, 668
Tapestry Dance Company, 669
University of Texas at Austin Performing Arts Center, 7980
University of Texas at Austin: Darrell K Royal-Texas Memorial Stadium, 7981
University of Texas at Austin: Texas Memorial Stadium, 7983
University of Texas at Austin: Theatre Room, 7982
Vortex Repertory Company, 3811

Bastrop
Bastrop Opera House, 3812
Old Bastrop Opera House, 7984

Bay City
Bay City Festival Arts Association, 5481
Festival Arts Association, 5482

Beaumont
Beaumont Civic Center Complex: Exhibit Hall, 7985
Beaumont Civic Center Complex: Julie Rogers Theatre, 7986
Beaumont Civic Opera, 2305
Beaumont Music Commission, 5483
Civic Center Complex, 7987
Lamar University Proscenium, 7988
Lamar University Studio Theatre, 7989
Lamar University: Cardinal Stadium, 7990
Montagne Center, 7991
Symphony of Southeast Texas, 1780
Young Audiences of Southeast Texas, 5484

Beeville
Coastal Bend College, 7992

Bellaire
Discovery Dance Group, 670

Belton
University of Mary Hardin: Baylor Lyceum, 5485

Big Spring
Big Spring Cultural Affairs Council, 5486

Brenham
Arts Council of Washington County, 5487

Brownsville
Camille Lightner Playhouse, 7993
Camille Players, 3813
University of Texas at Brownsville, 5488

Brownwood
Brownwood Coliseum, 7994

Bryan
Brazos Valley Symphony Orchestra, 1781
City of Bryan Parks and Recreation, 5489

Canyon
Kimbrough Memorial Stadium, 7995
Pioneer Amphitheatre, 7996
Texas Musical Drama, 3814
West Texas State University: Branding Iron Theatre, 7997

College Station
G Rollie White Coliseum, 7998
Kyle Field, 7999
Stagecenter, 3815
Texas A&M University Opera & Performing Arts, 2306
University Center Theatre Complex and Conference Center, 8000

Conroe
Montgomery County Performing Arts Series, 5490

Corpus Christi
Bayfront Plaza Convention Center: Auditorium, 8001
Cathedral Concert Series, 5491
Corpus Christi Ballet, 671
Corpus Christi Chamber Music Society, 1782
Corpus Christi Community Concert, 5492
Del Mar College Student Cultural Programs, 5493

Wassermann Piano Festival, 5579

Manti
Manti Temple Grounds Amphitheatre, 8140
Mormon Miracle Pageant, 5580

Moab
Canyonlands Arts Council, 5581
Moab Music Festival, 5582

Ogden
Eccles Community Art Center, 8141
Peery's Egyptian Theater, 3881
Perry's Egyptian Theatre, 3882
Val a Browning Center for the Performing Arts, 8142
Weber State University Cultural Affairs, 5583
Weber State University: Dee Events Center, 8143

Park City
Fidelity Investments Park City Jazz Festival, 5584
Park City International Music Festival, 5585

Provo
Brigham Young University Harris Fine Arts Center, 8146
Brigham Young University Cougar Stadium, 8145
Brigham Young University Performing Arts Series, 5586
Brigham Young University: Marriott Center, 8144
Utah Classical Guitar Society, 1818

Saint George
Dixie College Celebrity Concert Series, 5587
Dixie College Fine Arts Center Arena Theatre, 8148
Dixie College Fine Arts Center Proscenium Theatre, 8149
Dixie College: Fine Arts Center, 8147
Tuacahn Center for the Arts, 3890

Salt Lake City
Ballet West, 694
Capitol Theatre, 8150
Chamber Music Society of Salt Lake City, 1819
Clog America, 695
Delta Center, 5588
Eastern Arts International Dance Theater, 696, 1820, 5589
Emily Company, 3883
Gina Bachauer International Piano Competition & Festival, 5590
Gina Bachauer International Piano Foundation, 1821
Granite Youth Symphony, 1822
Off Broadway Theatre, 3884
Oratorio Society of Utah, 2324
Orchestra at Temple Square, 1823
Pioneer Theatre Company, 3885
Plan - B Theatre Company, 3886
Repertory Dance Theatre, 697
Ririe Woodbury Dance Company, 698
Salt Lake Acting Company, 3887
Salt Lake Mormon Tabernacle Choir, 2325
Salt Lake Symphonic Choir, 2326
Salt Lake Symphony, 1824
Sundance Institute, 3888
Sundance Theatre Program, 3889
Symphony Hall, 8151
Temple Square Concert Series, 5591
University of Utah: Department of Music, 1825
University of Utah: Jon M Huntsman Center, 8153
University of Utah: Kingsbury Hall, 8152
Utah Opera Company, 2327
Utah Symphony, 1826
Utah Symphony Chorus, 2328
Westminster College, 5592
World Arts/Noon Concerts Series, 5593

Sundance
Sundance Children's Theatre, 3891

Wellsville
Utah's Festival of the American West, 5594

West Valley City
Hale Centre Theatre at Harman Hall, 3892

Vermont

Barre
Barre Opera House, 8154

Bennington
Davis Rowe Artists, 8503
Oldcastle Theatre Company, 3893

Brattleboro
Brattleboro Music Center, 2329
National Marionette Theatre, 3894
New England Bach Festival, 5595

Burlington
Burklyn Ballet Theatre, 699
Burlington Discover Jazz Festival, 1827, 5596
Burlington Memorial Auditorium, 8155
Flynn Center for the Performing Arts, 8156
Flynn Theatre for the Performing Arts, 8157
Melvin Kaplan, 8504
University of Vermont: Recital Hall, 8158
Vermont Mozart Festival, 1828, 5597
Vermont Stage Company, 3895
Vermont Symphony Orchestra, 1829
Vermont Youth Orchestra, 1830

Castleton
Castleton State College Performing Arts Series, 5598

Chester
Green Mountain Festival Series, 5599

Colchester
Music in a Great Space, 5600
St. Michael's College Concerts, 5601
University of Vermont: George Bishop Lane Series, 5602

Dorset
American Theatre Works, 3896
Dorset Theatre Festival, 5603

Irasburg
Warebrook Contemporary Music Festival, 5604

Manchester
Festival of the Arts, 5605

Manchester Center
Manchester Music Festival, 5606, 5607

Middlebury
Middlebury College Concert Series, 5608
Middlebury College: Theatre Program, 8159
Potomac Theatre Project, 3897

Montpelier
Banjo Dan and the Mid-Nite Plowboys, 1831
Lost Nation Theater, 3898
Onion River Arts Council: Celebration Series, 5609

Orwell
Abbey Music Management, 8505

Pittsfield
Green Mountain Guild, 3899

Putney
Yellow Barn, 8160
Yellow Barn Music Festival, 5610

Randolph
Chandler Center for the Arts, 5611
Chandler Music Hall and Cultural Center, 8161

Rutland
Crossroads Arts Council, 5612
Killington Music Festival, 5613

Saint Johnsbury
Catamount Film and Arts Company, 3900

Saxtons River
Saxtons River Playhouse, 3901

Stowe
Stowe Performing Arts, 5614

Wells River
North Country Chorus, 2330

Weston
Weston Playhouse, 3902

White River Junction
Northern Stage, 3903

Woodstock
Pentangle Council On the Arts and the Woodstock Town Hall Theatre, 5615

Virginia

Abingdon
Barter Playhouse/Theatre House, 8162
Barter Theatre - State Theatre of Virginia, 3904

Alexandria
Alexandria Recital Series, 5616
Kathy Harty Gray Dance Theatre, 3905
Metrostage, 3906

Annandale
Fairfax Symphony Orchestra, 1832
International Children's Festival, 5617
Rev. J. Bruce Stewart, 700

Arlington
Arlington Cultural Affairs Division, 5618
Arlington Dance Theatre, 701
Arlington's Arts Al Fresco & the Innovators, 5619
Hesperus, 1833
Horizons Theatre, 3907
Jane Franklin Dance, 702
Opera Theatre of Northern Virginia, 2331
Signature Theatre, 3908

Asheland
Concert Ballet of Virginia, 703

Blacksburg
Virginia Tech Union Lively Arts Season, 5620
Virginia Tech University: Burruss Auditorium, 8164
Virginia Tech University: Casell Coliseum, 8165
Virginia Tech University: Lane Stadium, 8163

Bluefield
Feuchtenberger Management, 8506

Bridgewater
Bridgewater College Lyceum Series, 5621

Bristol
Bristol Ballet Company, 704

Charlottesville
Ashlawn-Highland Summer Festival, 3909, 5622
Marsjazz Booking Agency, 8507
Offstage Theatre, 3910
Saint Anne's-Belfield School Summer Music Academy, 8166
Scott Stadium, 8167
Tuesday Evening Concert Series, 5623
University of Virginia: University Hall, 8168

Chester
John Tyler Community College, 5624

Colonial Heights
Swift Creek Mill Playhouse, 3911

Covington
Alleghany Highlands Arts Council/Performing Arts, 5625

Danville
Averett University Concert-Lecture Series, 5626
Danville Area Association for the Arts & Humanities, 5627

Washington

Ellensburg
Jazz in the Valley, 5678

Enumclaw
Enumclaw Arts Commission, 5679

Everett
Everett Civic Auditorium, 8219
Everett Parks and Recreation Dept., 8220
Everett Theatre, 3940
Village Theatre, 3941

Federal Way
Aria Dance Company, 715
Knutzen Family Theatre - City of Federal Way, 3942

Friday Harbor
San Juan Community Theatre and Arts Center, 3943
San Juan Jazz, 5680

Gig Harbor
Paradise Theatre, 3944

Hoquiam
7th Street Theatre, 8221

Issaquah
Village Theatre, 3945

Kent
Kent Civic and Performing Arts Center, 8222
Kent Parks & Recreation, 5681

Kirkland
Kirkland Performance Center, 8223

Lacey
Abbey Church Events, 5682

Leavenworth
Icicle Creek Chamber Festival, 5683

Longview
Columbia Theatre for the Performing Arts, 3946
Mcclelland Arts Center, 8224

Lynnwood
Lynnwood Jazz Festival, 5684

Mercer Island
Mercer Island Arts Council, 5685

Metaline Falls
Cutter Theatre, 3947

Mt. Vernon
Lincoln Theatre Center, 8225

Oak Harbor
Whidbey Playhouse, 8226

Olympia
Evergreen State College Evergreen Expressions, 5686
Harlequin Productions, 3948
Olympia Symphony Orchestra, 1843
South Puget Sound Community College, 8227
Washington Center for the Performing Arts, 8228

Port Angeles
Juan De Fuca Festival of the Arts, 5687

Port Townsend
Dance Festival: Centrum Festival, 5688
Jazz Port Townsend: Centrum Festival, 5689
Port Townsend Blues Heritage Festival: Centrum Festival, 5690

Pullman
Beasley Performing Arts Coliseum, 3949
Pullman Summer Palace, 3950
Washington State University, 5691

Raymond
Raymond Theater, 3951

Redmond
Chaspen Opera Theatre, 2337

Richland
Mid-Columbia Symphony, 1844

Seattle
A Contemporary Theatre, 8229
Act Theatre, 3952
Bathhouse Theatre, 3953, 8230
Cornish College: Cornish Series, 5692
Early Music Guild International Series/Recitals, 5693
Early Music Guild of Seattle, 1845
Earshot Jazz Festival, 5694
Empty Space Theatre, 3954
Esoterics, 2338
Governors Chamber Music Series, 5695
Hyperion Theatre, 3955
Intiman Theatre Company, 3956
Keyarena at Seattle Center, 8231
Ladies Musical Club, 5696
Marion Oliver Mccaw Hall, 8232
Meany Theatre, 716
Mercer Arena at Seattle Center, 8233
New City Theater, 3957
Northwest Chamber Orchestra, 1846
Northwest Folklife Festival, 5697
Northwest Puppet, 3958
Ocheami, 717
Olympic Music Festival, 5698
On the Boards, 5699
One Reel, 5700
Orchestra Seattle & Seattle Chamber Singers, 2339
Pacific Northwest Ballet, 718
Pat Graney Company, 719
Philadelphia String Quartet, 1847
Puget Sound Chamber Music Society, 1848
Radost Folk Ensemble, 720
Roth Arts, 8510
Safeco Field, 8234
Seattle Baroque, 1849
Seattle Center, 8235
Seattle Center Opera House, 8236
Seattle Chamber Music Festival, 5701
Seattle Children's Theatre, 3959
Seattle International Children's Festival, 5702
Seattle Mime Theatre, 3960
Seattle Repertory Theatre, 3961, 8237
Seattle Shakespeare Festival, 5703
Seattle Symphony Orchestra, 1850
Seattle Youth Symphony Orchestra, 1851
Seattle Youth Symphony Orchestra's Marrowstone Music Festival, 5704
Taproot Theatre Company, 3962
Theater Schmeater, 3963
University of Washington: Hec Edmundson Pavilion, 8239
University of Washington: Husky Stadium, 8238
University of Washington: Meany Hall for the Performing Arts, 8240
World Series, 721

Seaview
Water Music Festival, 5705

Sequim
Performing Company of Pioneer Dance Arts, 722

Shoreline
Filipiniana Arts and Cultural Center, 723

Spokane
Avista Stadium, 8241
Connoisseur Concerts Association, 5706
Gonzaga University: Gene Russell Theatre, 8242
Joe Albi Stadium, 8243
Metropolitan Performing Arts Center, 8244
Pinesong/Spokane Falls Community College, 5707
Spokane Arena, 8245
Spokane Civic Theatre, 3964
Spokane Convention Center, 8246
Spokane Interplayers Ensemble, 3965
Spokane Opera House, 8247
Spokane Symphony Orchestra, 1852

Tacoma
Broadway Center for the Performing Arts, 5708
Cheney Stadium, 8248
Evergreen Music Festival: Tacoma Youth Symphony Association, 5709
Pacific Lutheran University Program Board, 5710
Tacoma Actors Guild, 3966
Tacoma City Ballet, 724
Tacoma Dome, 8249
Tacoma Opera Association, 2340
Tacoma Performing Dance Company, 725
Tacoma Philharmonic, 1853
Tacoma Symphony Orchestra, 1854
Tacoma Youth Symphony, 1855
University of Puget Sound Cultural Events, 5711

Vancouver
Old Slocum House Theatre Company, 3967

Walla Walla
Walla Walla Symphony, 1856
Whitman College: Cordiner Hall, 8250

White Salmon
Columbia Gorge Repertory Theatre, 3968

Yakima
Capital Theatre, 8251
Capitol Theatre, 3969
Yakima Symphony Orchestra, 1857
Yakima Valley Sundome, 8252
Yakima Youth Orchestra, 1858

West Virginia

Beckley
Theatre West Virginia, 3970

Bethany
Bethany College, 5712

Bluefield
Bluefield State College, 5713

Buckhannon
West Virginia Wesleyan College Atkinson Auditorium, 8253

Charles Town
Old Opera House Company, 8254

Charleston
Charleston Ballet, 726
Charleston Chamber Music Society, 1859
Charleston Civic Center, 5714, 8255
Charleston Civic Chorus, 2341
Geary Auditorium, 8256
Jewish Cultural Series, 5715
Kanawha Players, 3971
Laidley Field Athletic Recreational Center, 8257
Montclaire String Quartet, 1860
Watt Powell Stadium, 8258
West Virginia State College Capitol Center, 8259
West Virginia Symphony Chorus, 2342

Glenville
Glenville State College Cultural Affairs Commission, 5716

Huntington
Cam Henderson Center, 5717
Huntington Chamber Orchestra, 1861
Huntington Civic Arena, 5718, 8260
Huntington Museum of Art Amphitheatre, 8261
Huntington Museum of Art Auditorium, 8262
Keith-Albee Theatre, 8263
Marshall Artists Series, 5719
Marshall Athletics, 8264
Marshall University: Joan C Edwards Playhouse, 8265
Marshall University: Smith Recital Hall, 8266
Veterans Memorial Field House, 8267

Institute
West Virginia State College, 5720

West Virginia State College Theatre, 8268

Keyser
Apple Alley Players, 3972

Lewisburg
Carnegie Hall, 5721, 8269
Greenbrier Valley Theatre, 3973

Logan
Aracoma Story, 3974

Morgantown
College of Creative Arts: Choral Recital Hall, 8270
Fairmont Chamber Music Society, 5722
Lyell B Clay Concert Theatre, 5723, 8271
Montaineer Field, 8272
Vivian Davis Michael Laboratory Theatre- College of
    Creative Arts, 3975
West Virginia Public Theatre, 3976
West Virginia University Coliseum, 8273
West Virginia University Creative Arts Center, 8274
Wvu Arts Series, 5724

Parkersburg
Mid Ohio Valley Ballet Company, 727
Parkersburg Wheeling Ballet Company, 728
West Virginia University at Parkersburg, 5725

Shepherdstown
Contemporary American Theater Festival, 3977, 5726
Performing Arts Series at Shepherd, 5727

South Charleston
Appalachian Youth Jazz-Ballet Company, 729
Charleston Community Music Association, 5728

Wellsburg
Brooke Hills Playhouse, 3978

West Liberty
West Liberty College Concert Series, 5729

Wheeling
Capitol Music Hall, 8275
Oglebay Institute, 5730
Wheeling Civic Center, 8276
Wheeling Island Stadium, 8277
Wheeling Symphony, 1862

Wisconsin

Appleton
Lawrence University: Music-Drama Center, 8278
Performing Arts at Lawrence, 5731

Baraboo
Al Ringling Theatre Lively Arts Series, 3979
Al Ringling Theatre: Lively Arts Series, 5732

Beloit
Beloit College Performing Arts Series, 5733
Beloit Janesville Symphony Orchestra, 1863

Cedarburg
Cedarburg Performing Arts Center, 8279

De Pere
Art for Pete's Sake!, 8511
St. Norbert College Performing Arts, 5734

Eagle River
Headwaters Council for the Performing Arts, 5735
Northland Pines High School, 8280

Eau Claire
Chippewa Valley Theatre Guild, 3980
Eau Claire Regional Arts Center, 5736
University of Wisconsin at Eau Claire Artists Series,
    5737
Wl Zorn Arena, 8281

Egg Harbor
Birch Creek Music Center, 8282
Birch Creek Music Performance Center, 5738

Elm Grove
Sunset Playhouse, 3981

Ephraim
Peninsula Music Festival, 5739

Fish Creek
American Folklore Theatre, 3982
Door Community Auditorium Series, 5740
Peninsula Players, 3983

Fond du Lac
Fond Du Lac Symphonic Band, 1864

Green Bay
Brown County Civic Music Association, 5741
Green Bay Symphony Orchestra, 1865
Lambeau Field, 8283
Pamiro Opera Company, 2343
University of Wisconsin: Weinder Center for the
    Performing Arts, 8285
University of Wisconsin:P Brown County Arena, 8284

Green Lake
Green Lake Festival of Music, 5742

Hazelhurst
Northern Lights Playhouse, 3984

Hudson
Phipps Center for the Arts, 8286

Janesville
Janesville Concert Association, 5743

Jefferson
Council for the Performing Arts, 5744

Kenosha
Carthage Chamber Music Series, 1866, 5745
Carthage College Arts & Lecture Series, 5746
Kenosha Symphony Association, 1867
University of Wisconsin at Parkside, 8287

Kohler
Distinguished Guest Series, 5747
Kohler Foundation, 5748

La Crosse
Great River Festival of Arts, 5749
Great River Jazz Fest, 5753
Mitchell Hall Gymnasium, 8288
Pump House Regional Arts, 5750
University of Wisconsin at La Crosse Lectures, 5751
Viterbo University Bright Star Season, 5752

Ladysmith
Flambeau Valley Arts Association, 5754
Lynn Dance Company, 730

Lake Geneva
Performing Artists & Speakers, 8512

Madison
Broom Street Theater, 3985
Camp Randall Stadium, 8289
Capital City Jazz Fest, 5755
Kanopy Dance Theatre, 731
Kohl Center, 8290
Madison Area Technical College, Mitby Theater, 8291
Madison Blues Festival, 5756
Madison Civic Center, 8292
Madison Opera, 2344
Madison Repertory Theatre, 3986
Madison Scottish Country Dancers, 732
Madison Symphony Orchestra, 1868
Madison Theatre Guild, 3987
Melrose Motion Company, 733
Mm Colbert, 734
Opera for the Young, 2345
Tapit/New Works, 735
University of Wisconsin: Sports Center, 8293
University of Wisconsin: University Fieldhouse, 8294
Willow: a Dance Concern, 736
Wisconsin Chamber Orchestra, 1869
Wisconsin Union Theater, 3988

Wisconsin Youth Symphony Orchestras, 1870

Manitowoc
Capitol Civic Centre, 8295
Silver Lake College, 8296
Silver Lake College Guest Artist Series, 5757

Marshfield
Marshfield-Wood Community Symphony, 1871
University of Wisconsin Lectures and Fine Arts, 5758

Menasha
Fox Valley Symphony, 1872
University of Wisconsin Center - Fox Valley, 5759

Menomonie
Mabel Tainter Memorial Theater, 3989

Mequon
Concordia University Wisconsin, 5760

Merrill
Merrill Area Concert Association, 5761

Middleton
Mesoghios Dance Troup, 737
Music Library Association, 8297

Milwaukee
Acacia Theatre, 3990
Alverno College, 5762, 8298
Artist Series at the Pabst, 5763
Bel Canto Chorus, 2346
Betty Salamun's Dancecircus, 738
Bradley Center, 5764
Cardinal Stritch University School of Visual and
    Performing Arts, 5765
Early Music Now, 5766
First Stage Children's Theater, 3991
Florentine Opera Company, 2347
Great American Children's Theatre Company, 3992
Ko-Thi Dance Company, 739
Marcus Center for the Performing Arts, 8299
Miller Park, 8300
Milwaukee Area Technical College: Cooley
    Auditorium, 8301
Milwaukee Ballet, 740
Milwaukee Chamber Theatre, 3993
Milwaukee County Stadium, 8302
Milwaukee Public Theatre, 3994
Milwaukee Repertory Theater, 3995
Milwaukee Symphony Orchestra, 1873
Milwaukee Theatre, 8303
Milwaukee Youth Symphony Orchestra, 1874
Next Act Theatre, 3996
Omicron Artist Management, 8513
Pabst Theatre, 8304
Present Music, 1875
Renaissance Theaterworks, 3997
Skylight Opera Theatre, 3998
Theatre X, 3999
Us Cellular Arena, 8305
Wild Space Dance Company, 741
Wisconsin Conservatory of Music, 5767

Minocqua
Lakeland Performing Arts Association, 5768

Monona
Dance Wisconsin, 742

Monroe
Monroe Arts Center, 8306

Oregon
Li Chiao-Ping Dance, 743

Oshkosh
Grand Opera House, 8307
Oshkosh Symphony Orchestra, 1876
University of Wisconsin at Oshkosh Chamber Arts
    Series, 5769

Platteville
Pioneer Field, 8308

Wyoming

A

Abel, 8774
Academy of Country Music, 8515
Academy of Country Music Newsletter, 8687
Academy Players Directory, 9126
ACB National Directory of Bands, 9124
Accordian Federation of North America, 8516
Accordian Teachers Guild, 8517
Actor's Picture/Resume Book, 9127
Advance! ACB Magazine, 8775
AfterTouch - New Music Discoveries, 8776
AMC News, 9125
America's Shrine to Music Museum Newsletter, 8688
American Alliance for Theatre and Education, 8518
American Association of Community Theatre, 8519
American Association of Music Therapy, 9039
American Astrology, 8777
American Casino Guide, 9128
American Cheerleader, 8778
American Choral Directors Association, 8520, 8779
American Choral Directors Association Divisional
    Conventions, 9040
American College Dance Festival Association, 8521
American College of Musicians, 8522
American Dance, 8689
American Dance Guild, 8523, 9041
American Dance Therapy Association, 8524
American Disc Jockey Association, 8525
American Federation of Musicians of the United States
    and Canada, 8526
American Federation of Violin and Bow Makers, 8527
American Guild Associate News, 8690
American Guild of Music, 8528
American Guild of Musical Artists, 8529
American Guild of Organists, 8530
American Guild of Organists, Regional Conference,
    9042
American Harp Society, 8531
American Harp Society National Conference, 9043
American Indian Registry for the Performing Arts, 8532
American Institute of Organ Builders, 8533, 8691
American Institute of Organbuilders, 9044
American Kiddie Ride Association, 8534
American Music, 8780
American Music Center Opportunity Update, 8692
American Music Conference, 9045
American Music Scholarship Association, 8535
American Music Teacher, 8781
American Music Therapy Association, 8536
American Music Therapy Associaton Annual
    Conference, 9046
American Musical Instrument Society, 8693, 9047
American Musical Instrument Society Journal, 8782
American Musical Instrument Society Membership
    Directory, 9129
American Musicians Union Quarternote, 8537
American Musicological Society Annual Convention,
    9048
American Musicological Society Newsletter, 8694
American National Academy of Performing Arts, 8538
American Orff-Schulwerk Association National
    Confernce, 9049
American Organist, 8783
American Recreation Equipment Association, 8539
American School Band Directors Association, 8540
American School Band Directors Association -
    Newsletter, 8695
American Society for Aesthetics Annual Conference,
    9050
American Society of Composers, Authors and
    Publishers, 8541, 9131
American Society of Composers, Authors and
    Publishers - East Coast, 9130
American Society of Composers, Authors/ Publishers -
    West Coast, 8542
American Society of Music Arrangers and Composers,
    8543, 8696
American Society of Music Copyists, 8544
American Symphony Orchestra League, 8545
American Symphony Orchestra League National
    Conference, 9051

American Theater, 8784
American Theatre Magazine, 8785
American Viola Society, 8546
American Viola Society Journal, 8786
American Viola Society-Newsletter, 8697
AMU Quarternote, 8686
Amuse World, 9052
Amusement and Music Operators Association, 8547
Amusement and Music Operators Association
    Convention, 9056
Amusement Business, 8787
Amusement Coin Machine Expo, 9053
Amusement Industry Expo, 9054
Amusement Showcase International, 9055
Amusement Today, 8788
Anchorage Press Plays, 8790
Applause Magazine, 8791
Arts Alive, 8793
ASCAP, 8514
Asian Music, 8796
Asian Pacific American Journal, 8797
Associated Pipe Organ Builders of America, 8548
Association for Theatre in Higher Education, 8549
Association of Amateur Magicians, 8550
Association of Arts Administration Educators, 8551
Association of College Unions International Prof.
    Conference, 9057
Association of Concert Bands, 8552
Association of Hispanic Arts, 8553
Association of Performing Arts Presenters, 8554
Association of Performing Arts Presenters Bulletin,
    8798
Association of Performing Arts Presenters Membership
    Directory, 9132
Audarena Stadium International Guide, 9133
Auditions & Scenes from Shakespeare, 9134
Audrey Skirball-Kenis Play Collection, 8800
Autoharpoholic, 8801

B

Back Stage, 8803
Baker's Plays, 8804
Balloons & Parties Today, 8805
BASELINE, 9135
Big Band Academy of America, 8556
Billboard, 8806
Blitz, 8807
Blue Hot, 8698
Bluegrass Music News, 8699
Bluegrass Resource Directory, 9136
Bluegrass Unlimited, 8808
Blues Foundation, 8557
BMI, 8555
BMI Musicworld, 8802
Bomb Magazine, 8809
Boombah Herald, 8700
Boosey and Hawkes Newsletter, 8701
Boston Sound Check, 8811
Boxoffice, 8812
Broadside, 8702
Broadway Play Publishing, 8813
Buscando Amor, 8814

C

Callaloo, 8818
Callboard, 8819
Campus Activities Today, 8820
Canadian Theatre Review, 8821
Carnegie Hall Stagebill, 8823
Carousel News & Trader, 8824
Cartoon World, 8703
Casino Chronicle, 8704
Casino Journal, 8825
Casino Journal's National Gaming Summary, 8705
Casino Ops, 8826
Cavalcade of Acts and Attractions, 9137
CCM Magazine, 8815

Celebrity Access-Directory: How and Where to Write
    the Rich & Famous, 9138
Celebrity Bulletin, 9139
Chamber Music America, 8558
Chamber Music America Membership Directory, 9140
Chamber Music Magazine, 8827
Childrens Entertainment Business, 8828
Chinese Music, 8829
Chinese Music Society of North America, 8830
Choral Journal, 8831
Chorus America, 8559
Chorus America Trade Show, 9059
Circus Fans Association of America, 8560
Circus Historical Society, 8561
Circus Report, 8706
Circus Week, 8707
Clarinet, 8832
Classical Action, 8562
Clavier, 8833
Close Up Magazine, 8834
Club Model Magazine, 8835
CMJ New Music Report, 8816
College Music Society, 8563
College Music Society/Association for Technology in
    Music, 9060
Comedy USA Industry Guide, 9141
Comedy Writers' Newsletter, 8708
Comics Retailer, 9142
Community Theatre Database, 9143
Complete Catalogue of Plays, 9144
Complete Directory of Records, Tapes and Videos,
    9145
Conductors Guild, 8564
Conference of National Park Concessionaires, 8565
Confrontation, 8838
Congress on Research in Dance, 8566
Contact Quarterly Journal of Dance and Improvisation,
    8839
Contemporary Christian Music, 8840
Contemporary Dramatists, 9146
Contemporary Music Ensembles: A Directory, 9147
Contemporary Music Review, 8841
Contemporary Record Society News, 8709
Costume Designers Guild Directory, 9148
Council of Dance Administrators, 8567
Country Dance & Song, 8842
Country Dance and Song Society News, 8710
Country Music Association, 8568
Country Radio Broadcasters, 8569
Country Radio Seminar, 9061
Creative Musician Coalition, 8570
Creem, 8843
Cue Magazine, 8844
Cue Sheet, 8845

D

Daily Variety, 8847
Dance Chronicle, 8848
Dance Critics Association, 8571
Dance Directory, 9149
Dance Educators of America, 8572
Dance Educators of America Workshops and
    Competition, 8849
Dance Magazine, 8850
Dance Magazine College Guide, 9150
Dance Magazine-Summer Dance Calendar Issue, 9151
Dance Masters of America, 8573
Dance Notation Bureau Newsletter, 8711
Dance on Camera Journal, 8712
Dance on Camera News, 8713
Dance Research Journal, 8851
Dance Spirit, 8852
Dance Teacher Now, 8853
Dance USA, 8574
Dance/USA Journal, 8854
Dance/USA Membership Directory, 9152
DanceDrill, 8714
Dancing USA, 8855
Descant, 8856
Diapason, 8857

Y

Online Database

The Grey House Performing Arts Directory is also available in an Online Database. Using this comprehensive Online Database you can access over 7,400 Performing Arts Organizations & Facilities including 600+ Dance Companies, 1,300+ Instrumental Music Programs, 600+ Theaters, 1,500+ Series & Festivals and 1,800+ Facilities, with access to 9,700 industry contacts by name, 2,900 e-mail addresses and over 2,800 web sites. Using the Online Database you can search by Organization or Facility Name, Contact Name, Performance Type, Attendance, Profit or Non-Profit Status and much more to quickly and easily locate the contact information you're looking for. Your subscription to this unique and rich resource for the arts puts at your fingertips the most comprehensive database of the Performing Arts available today. Try our FREE SEARCH now and then subscribe today for full access all year long. Visit www.greyhouse.com or call (800) 562-2139 for more information.

Mailing List Information

This directory is available in mailing list form on mailing labels or diskettes. Call (800) 562-2139 to place an order or inquire about counts. There are a number of ways we can segment the database to meet your mailing list requirements.

Licensable Database on Disk

The database of this directory is available on diskette in an ASCII text file, delimited or fixed fielded. Call (800) 562-2139 for more details.

---

www.greyhouse.com

Clicking on www.greyhouse.com takes you through our complete list of Business, Statistics, Demographics, Health and Education Directories and Reference Works. The site is fully illustrated and provides complete details on each product along with easy ordering capability.

Grey House Publishing
Business Directories

The Directory of Business Information Resources, 2002

With 100% verification, over 1,000 new listings and more than 12,000 updates, this 2002 edition of *The Directory of Business Information Resources* is the most up-to-date source for contacts in over 98 business areas – from advertising and agriculture to utilities and wholesalers. This carefully researched volume details: the Associations representing each industry; the Newsletters that keep members current; the Magazines and Journals - with their "Special Issues" - that are important to the trade, the Conventions that are "must attends," Databases, Directories and Industry Web Sites that provide access to must-have marketing resources. Includes contact names, phone & fax numbers, web sites and e-mail addresses. This one-volume resource is a gold mine of information and would be a welcome addition to any reference collection.

"This is a most useful and easy-to-use addition to any researcher's library." –The Information Professionals Institute

2,500 pages; Softcover ISBN 1-930956-75-4, $250.00 ◆ Online Database $495.00

Nations of the World, 2003 A Political, Economic and Business Handbook

This completely revised Third Edition covers all the nations of the world in an easy-to-use, single volume. Each nation is profiled in a single chapter that includes Key Facts, Political & Economic Issues, a Country Profile and Business Information. This 2003 edition has been completely updated with the latest Political and Economic data including changes since September 11, 2001 and now reflects the most current information on Politics, Travel Advisories, Economics and more. You'll find such vital information as a Country Map, Population Characteristics, Inflation, Agricultural Production, Foreign Debt, Political History, Foreign Policy, Regional Insecurity, Economics, Trade & Tourism, Historical Profile, Political Systems, Ethnicity, Languages, Media, Climate, Hotels, Chambers of Commerce, Banking, Travel Information and more. Five Regional Chapters follow the main text and include a Regional Map, an Introductory Article, Key Indicators and Currencies for the Region. Noted for its sophisticated, up-to-date and reliable compilation of political, economic and business information, this brand new edition will be an important acquisition to any public, academic or special library reference collection.

"A useful addition to both general reference collections and business collections." –RUSQ

1,700 pages; Softcover ISBN 1-930956-00-2, $135.00

Research Services Directory, 2001 Commercial & Corporate Research Centers

This Eighth Edition provides access to well over 7,000 independent Commercial Research Firms, Corporate Research Centers and Laboratories offering contract services for hands-on, basic or applied research. Each entry provides the company's name, mailing address, phone & fax numbers, key contacts, web site, e-mail address, as well as a company description and research and technical fields served. Four indexes provide immediate access to this wealth of information: Research Firms Index, Geographic Index, Personnel Name Index and Subject Index.

"An important source for organizations in need of information about laboratories, individuals and other facilities." –ARBA

1,309 pages; Softcover ISBN 1-891482-82-3, $395.00 ◆ Online Database $850.00

The Directory of Venture Capital Firms, 2003

This brand new Sixth Edition has been extensively updated and broadly expanded to offer direct access to over 2,800 Domestic and International Venture Capital Firms, including address, phone & fax numbers, e-mail addresses and web sites for both primary and branch locations. Entries include details on the firm's Mission Statement, Industry Group Preferences, Geographic Preferences, Average and Minimum Investments and Investment Criteria. You'll also find details that are available nowhere else, including the Firm's Portfolio Companies and extensive information on each of the firm's Managing Partners, such as Education, Professional Background and Directorships held, along with the Partner's E-mail Address. *The Directory of Venture Capital Firms* offers five important indexes: Geographic Index, Executive Name Index, Portfolio Company Index, Industry Preference Index and College & University Index. With its comprehensive coverage and detailed, extensive information on each company, *The Directory of Venture Capital Firms* is an important addition to any finance collection.

"The sheer number of listings, the descriptive information provided and the outstanding indexing make this directory a better value than its principal competitor, Pratt's Guide to Venture Capital Sources. Recommended for business collections in large public, academic and business libraries." –Choice

1,300 pages; Softcover ISBN 1-930956-77-0, $350.00 ◆ Online Database $889.00

To preview any of our Directories Risk-Free for 30 days, call (800) 562-2139 or fax to (518) 789-0556

The Directory of Mail Order Catalogs, 2003

Published since 1981, this Seventeenth Edition features 100% verification of data and is the premier source of information on the mail order catalog industry. Details over 12,000 consumer catalog companies with 44 different product chapters from Animals to Toys & Games. Contains detailed contact information including e-mail addresses and web sites along with important business details such as employee size, years in business, sales volume, catalog size, number of catalogs mailed and more. Four indexes provide quick access to information: Catalog & Company Name Index, Geographic Index, Product Index and Web Sites Index.

"This is a godsend for those looking for information." –Reference Book Review
"The scope and arrangement make this directory useful. Certainly the broad coverage of subjects is not available elsewhere in a single-volume format." –Booklist

1,700 pages; Softcover ISBN 1-891482-73-4, $250.00 ◆ Online Database $495.00

The Directory of Business to Business Catalogs, 2003

The completely updated 2003 *Directory of Business to Business Catalogs*, provides details on over 6,000 suppliers of everything from computers to laboratory supplies… office products to office design… marketing resources to safety equipment… landscaping to maintenance suppliers… building construction and much more. Detailed entries offer mailing address, phone & fax numbers, e-mail addresses, web sites, key contacts, sales volume, employee size, catalog printing information and more. Jut about every kind of product a business needs in its day-to-day operations is covered in this carefully-researched volume. Three indexes are provided for at-a-glance access to information: Catalog & Company Name Index, Geographic Index and Web Sites Index.

"Much smaller and easier to use than the Thomas Register or Sweet's Catalog, it is an excellent choice for libraries… wishing to supplement their business supplier resources." –Booklist

800 pages; Softcover ISBN 1-891482-69-6, $165.00 ◆ Online Database $325.00

Thomas Food and Beverage Market Place, 2002/03

Thomas Food and Beverage Market Place is bigger and better than ever with thousands of new companies, thousands of updates to existing companies and two revised and enhanced product category indexes. This comprehensive directory profiles over 18,000 Food & Beverage Manufacturers, 12,000 Equipment & Supply Companies, 2,200 Transportation & Warehouse Companies, 2,000 Brokers & Wholesalers, 8,000 Importers & Exporters, 900 Industry Resources and hundreds of Mail Order Catalogs. Listings include detailed Contact Information, Sales Volumes, Key Contacts, Brand & Product Information, Packaging Details and much more. *Thomas Food and Beverage Market Place* is available as a three-volume printed set, a subscription-based Online Database via the Internet, on CD-ROM, as well as mailing lists and a licensable database.

8,500 pages, 3 Volume Set; Softcover ISBN 1-930956-95-9, $495.00 ◆ CD-ROM ISBN 1-930956-33-9, $695.00 ◆ CD-ROM & 3 Volume Set Combo ISBN 1-930956-34-7, $895.00 ◆ Online Database $695.00 ◆ Online Database & 3 Volume Set Combo, $895.00

The Grey House Safety & Security Directory, 2003

The Grey House Safety & Security Directory is the most comprehensive reference tool and buyer's guide for the safety and security industry. Published continuously since 1943 as Best's Safety & Security Directory, Grey House acquired the title in 2002. Arranged by safety topic, each chapter begins with OSHA regulations for the topic, followed by Training Articles written by top professionals in the field and Self-Inspection Checklists. Next, each topic contains Buyer's Guide sections that feature related products and services. Topics include Administration, Insurance, Loss Control & Consulting, Protective Equipment & Apparel, Noise & Vibration, Facilities Monitoring & Maintenance, Employee Health Maintenance & Ergonomics, Retail Food Services, Machine Guards, Process Guidelines & Tool Handling, Ordinary Materials Handling, Hazardous Materials Handling, Workplace Preparation & Maintenance, Electrical Lighting & Safety, Fire & Rescue and Security. The Buyer's Guide sections are carefully indexed within each topic area to ensure that you can find the supplies needed to meet OSHA's regulations. Six important indexes make finding information and product manufacturers quick and easy: Geographical Index of Manufacturers and Distributors, Company Profile Index, Brand Name Index, Product Index, Index of Web Sites and Index of Advertisers. This comprehensive, up-to-date reference will provide every tool necessary to make sure a business is in compliance with OSHA regulations and locate the products and services needed to meet those regulations.

1,500 pages, 2 Volume Set; Softcover ISBN 1-930956-71-1, $225.00

To preview any of our Directories Risk-Free for 30 days, call (800) 562-2139 or fax to (518) 789-0556

Universal Reference Publications
Statistical & Demographic Reference Books

The Value of a Dollar – Millennium Edition

A guide to practical economy, *The Value of a Dollar* records the actual prices of thousands of items that consumers purchased from the Civil War to the present, along with facts about investment options and income opportunities. The first edition, published by Gale Research in 1994, covered the period of 1860 to 1989. This second edition has been completely redesigned and revised and now contains two new chapters, 1990-1994 and 1995-1999. Each 5-year chapter includes a Historical Snapshot, Consumer Expenditures, Investments, Selected Income, Income/Standard Jobs, Food Basket, Standard Prices and Miscellany. This interesting and useful publication will be widely used in any reference collection.

"Recommended for high school, college and public libraries." –ARBA

493 pages; Hardcover ISBN 1-891482-49-1, $135.00

Working Americans 1880-1999
Volume I: The Working Class, Volume II: The Middle Class, Volume III: The Upper Class

Each of the volumes in the *Working Americans 1880-1999* series focuses on a particular class of Americans, The Working Class, The Middle Class and The Upper Class over the last 120 years. Chapters in each volume focus on one decade and profile three to five families. Family Profiles include real data on Income & Job Descriptions, Selected Prices of the Times, Annual Income, Annual Budgets, Family Finances, Life at Work, Life at Home, Life in the Community, Working Conditions, Cost of Living, Amusements and much more. Each chapter also contains an Economic Profile with Average Wages of other Professions, a selection of Typical Pricing, Key Events & Inventions, News Profiles, Articles from Local Media and Illustrations. The *Working Americans* series captures the lifestyles of each of the classes from the last twelve decades, covers a vast array of occupations and ethnic backgrounds and travels the entire nation. These interesting and useful compilations of portraits of the American Working, Middle and Upper Classes during the last 120 years will be an important addition to any high school, public or academic library reference collection.

"These interesting, unique compilations of economic and social facts, figures and graphs will support multiple research needs. They will engage and enlighten patrons in high school, public and academic library collections." –Booklist (on Volumes I and II)

Volume I: The Working Class ◆ 558 pages; Hardcover ISBN 1-891482-81-5, $135.00
Volume II: The Middle Class ◆ 591 pages; Hardcover ISBN 1-891482-72-6; $135.00
Volume III: The Upper Class ◆ 567 pages; Hardcover ISBN 1-930956-38-X, $135.00

Working Americans 1880-1999 Volume IV: Their Children

This Fourth Volume in the highly successful *Working Americans 1880-1999* series focuses on American children, decade by decade from 1880 to 1999. This interesting and useful volume introduces the reader to three children in each decade, one from each of the Working, Middle and Upper classes. Like the first three volumes in the series, the individual profiles are created from interviews, diaries, statistical studies, biographies and news reports. Profiles cover a broad range of ethnic backgrounds, geographic area and lifestyles – everything from an orphan in Memphis in 1882, following the Yellow Fever epidemic of 1878 to an eleven-year-old nephew of a beer baron and owner of the New York Yankees in New York City in 1921. Chapters also contain important supplementary materials including News Features as well as information on everything from Schools to Parks, Infectious Diseases to Childhood Fears along with Entertainment, Family Life and much more to provide an informative overview of the lifestyles of children from each decade. This interesting account of what life was like for Children in the Working, Middle and Upper Classes will be a welcome addition to the reference collection of any high school, public or academic library.

600 pages; Hardcover ISBN 1-930956-35-5, $135.00

Weather America, A Thirty-Year Summary of Statistical Weather Data and Rankings, 2001

This valuable resource provides extensive climatological data for over 4,000 National and Cooperative Weather Stations throughout the United States. *Weather America* begins with a new Major Storms section that details major storm events of the nation and a National Rankings section that details rankings for several data elements, such as Maximum Temperature and Precipitation. The main body of *Weather America* is organized into 50 state sections. Each section provides a Data Table on each Weather Station, organized alphabetically, that provides statistics on Maximum and Minimum Temperatures, Precipitation, Snowfall, Extreme Temperatures, Foggy Days, Humidity and more. State sections contain two brand new features in this edition – a City Index and a narrative Description of the climatic conditions of the state. Each section also includes a revised Map of the State that includes not only weather stations, but cities and towns.

"Best Reference Book of the Year." –Library Journal

2,013 pages; Softcover ISBN 1-891482-29-7, $175.00

To preview any of our Directories Risk-Free for 30 days, call (800) 562-2139 or fax to (518) 789-0556

The Environmental Resource Handbook, 2002

This brand new first edition is the most up-to-date and comprehensive source for Environmental Resources and Statistics. Section I: Resources provides detailed contact information for thousands of information sources, including Associations & Organizations, Awards & Honors, Conferences, Foundations & Grants, Environmental Health, Government Agencies, National Parks & Wildlife Refuges, Publications, Research Centers, Educational Programs, Green Product Catalogs, Consultants and much more. Section II: Statistics, provides statistics and rankings on hundreds of important topics, including Children's Environmental Index, Municipal Finances, Toxic Chemicals, Recycling, Climate, Air & Water Quality and more. This kind of up-to-date environmental data, all in one place, is not available anywhere else on the market place today. This brand new title is a must-have for all public and academic libraries as well as any organization with a primary focus on the environment.

"...the intrinsic value of the information make it worth consideration by libraries with environmental collections and environmentally concerned users." –Booklist

998 pages; Softcover ISBN 1-930956-04-5, $155.00 ◆ Online Database $300.00

Profiles of America, 2002 A Statistical Guide to All U.S. Cities, Towns and Counties

Profiles of America is the only source that pulls together, in one place, statistical, historical and descriptive information about almost every place in the United States in an easy-to-use format. This award winning reference set, now in its second edition, compiles statistics and data from over 30 different sources – the latest census information has been included along with more than nine brand new statistical topics. This Four-Volume Set details over 40,000 places, from the biggest metropolis to the smallest unincorporated hamlet, and provides statistical details and information on over 50 different topics including Geography, Climate, Population, Vital Statistics, Economy, Income, Taxes, Education, Housing, Health & Environment, Public Safety, Newspapers, Transportation, Presidential Election Results and Information Contacts or Chambers of Commerce. Profiles are arranged, for ease-of-use, by state and then by county. Each county begins with a County-Wide Overview and is followed by information for each Community in that particular county. The Community Profiles within the county are arranged alphabetically. *Profiles of America* is a virtual snapshot of America at your fingertips and a unique compilation of information that will be widely used in any reference collection.

A Library Journal Best Reference Book
"An outstanding compilation." –Library Journal

3,200 pages; Four Volume Set; Softcover ISBN 1-891482-80-7, $500.00

The Comparative Guide to American Suburbs, 2001

The Comparative Guide to American Suburbs is a one-stop source for Statistics on the 2,000+ suburban communities surrounding the 50 largest metropolitan areas – their population characteristics, income levels, economy, school system and important data on how they compare to one another. Organized into 50 Metropolitan Area chapters, each chapter contains an overview of the Metropolitan Area, a detailed Map followed by a comprehensive Statistical Profile of each Suburban Community, including Contact Information, Physical Characteristics, Population Characteristics, Income, Economy, Unemployment Rate, Cost of Living, Education, Chambers of Commerce and more. Next, statistical data is sorted into Ranking Tables that rank the suburbs by twenty different criteria, including Population, Per Capita Income, Unemployment Rate, Crime Rate, Cost of Living and more. *The Comparative Guide to American Suburbs* is the best source for locating data on suburbs. Those looking to relocate, as well as those doing preliminary market research, will find this an invaluable timesaving resource.

"Public and academic libraries will find this compilation useful...The work draws together figures from many sources and will be especially helpful for job relocation decisions." – Booklist

1,681 pages; Softcover ISBN 1-930956-42-8, $130.00

America's Top-Rated Cities, 2003

America's Top-Rated Cities provides current, comprehensive statistical information and other essential data in one easy-to-use source on the 100 "top" cities that have been cited as the best for business and living in the U.S. This handbook allows readers to see, at a glance, a concise social, business, economic, demographic and environmental profile of each city, including brief evaluative comments. In addition to detailed data on Cost of Living, Finances, Real Estate, Education, Major Employers, Media, Crime and Climate, city reports now include Housing Vacancies, Tax Audits, Bankruptcy, Presidential Election Results and more. This outstanding source of information will be widely used in any reference collection.

"The only source of its kind that brings together all of this information into one easy-to-use source. It will be beneficial to many business and public libraries." –ARBA

2,500 pages, 4 Volume Set; Softcover ISBN 1-891482-79-3, $195.00

To preview any of our Directories Risk-Free for 30 days, call (800) 562-2139 or fax to (518) 789-0556

America's Top-Rated Smaller Cities, 2002

A perfect companion to *America's Top-Rated Cities*, *America's Top-Rated Smaller Cities* provides current, comprehensive business and living profiles of smaller cities (population 25,000-99,999) that have been cited as the best for business and living in the United States. Sixty new, never-before profiled cities make up this 2002 edition of *America's Top-Rated Smaller Cities*, all are top-ranked by Population Growth, Median Income, Unemployment Rate and Crime Rate. In addition to this new selection procedure, city reports reflect the most current data available on a wide-range of statistics as well. Each includes a Background of the City, an Overview of the State Finances and statistical details on Employment & Earnings, Household Income, Unemployment Rate, Population Characteristics, Taxes, Cost of Living, Education, Health Care, Public Safety, Recreation, Media, Air & Water Quality and much more. *America's Top-Rated Smaller Cities* offers a reliable, one-stop source for statistical data that, before now, could only be found scattered in hundreds of sources. This volume is designed for a wide range of readers: individuals considering relocating a residence or business; professionals considering expanding their business or changing careers; general and market researchers; real estate consultants; human resource personnel; urban planners and investors.

"Provides current, comprehensive statistical information in one easy-to-use source...
Recommended for public and academic libraries and specialized collections." –Library Journal

1,072 pages; Softcover ISBN 1-930956-67-3, $160.00

Crime in America's Top-Rated Cities, 2000

This volume includes over 20 years of crime statistics in all major crime categories: violent crimes, property crimes and total crime. *Crime in America's Top-Rated Cities* is conveniently arranged by city and covers 76 top-rated cities. *Crime in America's Top-Rated Cities* offers details that compare the number of crimes and crime rates for the city, suburbs and metro area along with national crime trends for violent, property and total crimes. Also, this handbook contains important information and statistics on Anti-Crime Programs, Crime Risk, Hate Crimes, Illegal Drugs, Law Enforcement, Correctional Facilities, Death Penalty Laws and much more. A much-needed resource for people who are relocating, business professionals, general researchers, the press, law enforcement officials and students of criminal justice.

"Data is easy to access and will save hours of searching." –Global Enforcement Review

832 pages; Softcover ISBN 1-891482-84-X, $155.00

The American Tally, 2002

This important statistical handbook compiles, all in one place, comparative statistics on all U.S. cities and towns with a 10,000+ population. *The American Tally* provides statistical details on over 3,000 cities and towns and profiles how they compare with one another in Population Characteristics, Education, Language & Immigration, Income & Employment and Housing. Each section begins with an alphabetical listing of cities by state, allowing for quick access to both the statistics and relative rankings of any city. Next, the highest and lowest cities are listed in each statistic. These important, informative lists provide quick reference to which cities are at both extremes of the spectrum for each statistic. Unlike any other reference, *The American Tally* provides quick, easy access to comparative statistics – a must-have for any reference collection.

"A solid library reference." –Bookwatch

500 pages; Softcover ISBN 1-930956-29-0, $125.00

The Comparative Guide to American Elementary & Secondary Schools, 2002/03

The only guide of its kind, this 2002/03 edition of the award winning Comparative Guide to American Elementary and Secondary Schools has been broadly expanded to offer a snapshot profile of every public school district in the United States serving 1,500 or more students – more than 5,900 districts are covered, that's almost 2,000 more than the previous edition. Organized alphabetically by district within state, each chapter begins with a Statistical Overview of the state. Each district listing includes contact information (name, address, phone number and web site) plus Grades Served, the Numbers of Students and Teachers and the Number of Regular, Special Education, Alternative and Vocational Schools in the district along with statistics on Student/Classroom Teacher Ratios, Drop Out Rates, Ethnicity, the Numbers of Librarians and Guidance Counselors and District Expenditures per student. Brand New to this edition, *The Comparative Guide to American Elementary and Secondary Schools* provides important ranking tables, both by state and nationally, for each data element. For easy navigation through this wealth of information, this handbook contains a useful City Index that lists all districts that operate schools within a city. These important comparative statistics are necessary for anyone considering relocation or doing comparative research on their own district and would be a perfect acquisition for any public library or school district library.

"This straightforward guide is an easy way to find general information. Valuable for academic and large public library collections." –ARBA

2,355 pages; Softcover ISBN 1-930956-93-2, $125.00

To preview any of our Directories Risk-Free for 30 days, call (800) 562-2139 or fax to (518) 789-0556

Sedgwick Press
Health Directories

The Complete Directory for People with Disabilities, 2003

A wealth of information, now in one comprehensive sourcebook. Completely updated for 2003, this edition contains more information than ever before, including thousands of new entries and enhancements to existing entries and thousands of additional web sites and e-mail addresses. Plus, the chapters on Camps and Rehabilitation Facilities have been extensively updated and a brand new chapter on Sub-Acute Rehabilitation Facilities has been added to this edition. This up-to-date directory is the most comprehensive resource available for people with disabilities, detailing Independent Living Centers, Rehabilitation Facilities, State & Federal Agencies, Associations, Support Groups, Periodicals & Books, Assistive Devices, Employment & Education Programs, Camps and Travel Groups. Each year, more libraries, schools, colleges, hospitals, rehabilitation centers and individuals add *The Complete Directory for People with Disabilities* to their collections, making sure that this information is readily available to the families, individuals and professionals who can benefit most from the amazing wealth of resources cataloged here.

"No other reference tool exists to meet the special needs of the disabled in one convenient resource for information." –Library Journal

1,200 pages; Softcover ISBN 1-930956-69-X, $165.00 ◆ Online Database $215.00 ◆ Online Database & Directory Combo $300.00

The Complete Directory for People with Chronic Illness, 2001/02

Thousands of hours of research have gone into this completely updated 2001/02 edition – several new chapters have been added along with thousands of new entries and enhancements to existing entries. This widely-hailed directory is structured around the 90 most prevalent chronic illnesses – from Asthma to Cancer to Wilson's Disease – and provides a comprehensive overview of the support services and information resources available for people diagnosed with a chronic illness. Each chronic illness has its own chapter and contains a brief description in layman's language, followed by important resources for National & Local Organizations, State Agencies, Newsletters, Books & Periodicals, Libraries & Research Centers, Support Groups & Hotlines, Web Sites and much more. This directory is an important resource for health care professionals, the collections of hospital and health care libraries, as well as an invaluable tool for people with a chronic illness and their support network.

"A must purchase for all hospital and health care libraries and is strongly recommended for all public library reference departments." –ARBA

1,152 pages; Softcover ISBN 1-930956-63-7, $165.00 ◆ Online Database $215.00 ◆ Online Database & Directory Combo $300.00

The Complete Learning Disabilities Directory, 2002

The 2002 Complete Learning Disabilities Directory is the most comprehensive database of Programs, Services, Curriculum Materials, Professional Meetings & Resources, Camps, Newsletters and Support Groups for teachers, students and families concerned with learning disabilities. This information-packed directory includes information about Associations & Organizations, Schools, Colleges & Testing Materials, Government Agencies, Legal Resources and much more. For quick, easy access to information, this directory contains four indexes: Entry Name Index, Subject Index and Geographic Index. With every passing year, the field of learning disabilities attracts more attention and the network of caring, committed and knowledgeable professionals grows every day. This directory is an invaluable research tool for these parents, students and professionals.

"Due to its wealth and depth of coverage, parents, teachers and others... should find this an invaluable resource." -Booklist

848 pages; Softcover ISBN 1-930956-36-3, $145.00 ◆ Online Database $195.00 ◆ Online Database & Directory Combo $280.00

The Complete Mental Health Directory, 2002

This is the most comprehensive resource covering the field of behavioral health, with critical information for both the layman and the mental health professional. For the layman, this directory offers understandable descriptions of 25 Mental Health Disorders as well as detailed information on Associations, Media, Support Groups and Mental Health Facilities. For the professional, *The Complete Mental Health Directory* offers critical and comprehensive information on Managed Care Organizations, Information Systems, Government Agencies and Provider Organizations. This comprehensive volume of needed information will be widely used in any reference collection.

"... the strength of this directory is that it consolidates widely dispersed information into a single volume." –Booklist

800 pages; Softcover ISBN 1-930956-06-1, $165.00 ◆ Online Database $215.00 ◆ Online & Directory Combo $300.00

To preview any of our Directories Risk-Free for 30 days, call (800) 562-2139 or fax to (518) 789-0556

Older Americans Information Directory, 2002/03

Completely updated for 2002/03, this Fourth Edition has been completely revised and now contains 1,000 new listings, over 8,000 updates to existing listings and over 3,000 brand new e-mail addresses and web sites. You'll find important resources for Older Americans including National, Regional, State & Local Organizations, Government Agencies, Research Centers, Libraries & Information Centers, Legal Resources, Discount Travel Information, Continuing Education Programs, Disability Aids & Assistive Devices, Health, Print Media and Electronic Media. Three indexes: Entry Index, Subject Index and Geographic Index make it easy to find just the right source of information. This comprehensive guide to resources for Older Americans will be a welcome addition to any reference collection.

"Highly recommended for academic, public, health science and consumer libraries..." –Choice

1,200 pages; Softcover ISBN 1-930956-65-7, $165.00 ◆ Online Database $215.00 ◆ Online Database & Directory Combo $300.00

The Complete Directory for Pediatric Disorders, 2002/03

This important directory provides parents and caregivers with information about Pediatric Conditions, Disorders, Diseases and Disabilities, including Blood Disorders, Bone & Spinal Disorders, Brain Defects & Abnormalities, Chromosomal Disorders, Congenital Heart Defects, Movement Disorders, Neuromuscular Disorders and Pediatric Tumors & Cancers. This carefully written directory offers: understandable Descriptions of 15 major bodily systems; Descriptions of more than 200 Disorders and a Resources Section, detailing National Agencies & Associations, State Associations, Online Services, Libraries & Resource Centers, Research Centers, Support Groups & Hotlines, Camps, Books and Periodicals. This resource will provide immediate access to information crucial to families and caregivers when coping with children's illnesses.

"Recommended for public and consumer health libraries." –Library Journal

1,120 pages; Softcover ISBN 1-930956-61-4, $165.00 ◆ Online Database $215.00 ◆ Online Database & Directory Combo $300.00

The Complete Directory for People with Rare Disorders, 2002/03

This outstanding reference is produced in conjunction with the National Organization for Rare Disorders to provide comprehensive and needed access to important information on over 1,000 rare disorders, including Cancers and Muscular, Genetic and Blood Disorders. An informative Disorder Description is provided for each of the 1,100 disorders (rare Cancers and Muscular, Genetic and Blood Disorders) followed by information on National and State Organizations dealing with a particular disorder, Umbrella Organizations that cover a wide range of disorders, the Publications that can be useful when researching a disorder and the Government Agencies to contact. Detailed and up-to-date listings contain mailing address, phone and fax numbers, web sites and e-mail addresses along with a description. For quick, easy access to information, this directory contains two indexes: Entry Name Index and Acronym/Keyword Index along with an informative Guide for Rare Disorder Advocates. The Complete Directory for People with Rare Disorders will be an invaluable tool for the thousands of families that have been struck with a rare or "orphan" disease, who feel that they have no place to turn and will be a much-used addition to the reference collection of any public or academic library.

"Quick access to information... public libraries and hospital patient libraries will find this a useful resource in directing users to support groups or agencies dealing with a rare disorder." –Booklist

726 pages; Softcover ISBN 1-891482-18-1, $165.00

Sedgwick Press
Education Directories

Educators Resource Directory, 2003/04

Educators Resource Directory is a comprehensive resource that provides the educational professional with thousands of resources and statistical data for professional development. This directory saves hours of research time by providing immediate access to Associations & Organizations, Conferences & Trade Shows, Educational Research Centers, Employment Opportunities & Teaching Abroad, School Library Services, Scholarships, Financial Resources, Professional Consultants, Computer Software & Testing Resources and much more. Plus, this comprehensive directory also includes a section on Statistics and Rankings with over 100 tables, including statistics on Average Teacher Salaries, SAT/ACT scores, Revenues & Expenditures and more. These important statistics will allow the user to see how their school rates among others, make relocation decisions and so much more. *Educators Resource Directory* will be a well-used addition to the reference collection of any school district, education department or public library.

"Recommended for all collections that serve elementary and secondary school professionals." –Choice

1,000 pages; Softcover ISBN 1-59237-002-0, $145.00 ◆ Online Database $195.00 ◆ Online Database & Directory Combo $280.00

To preview any of our Directories Risk-Free for 30 days, call (800) 562-2139 or fax to (518) 789-0556

Sedgwick Press
Hospital & Health Plan Directories

The HMO/PPO Directory, 2003

The HMO/PPO Directory is a comprehensive source that provides detailed information about Health Maintenance Organizations and Preferred Provider Organizations nationwide. This comprehensive directory details more information about more managed health care organizations than ever before. Over 1,100 HMOs, PPOs and affiliated companies are listed, arranged alphabetically by state. Detailed listings include Key Contact Information, Prescription Drug Benefits, Enrollment, Geographical Areas served, Affiliated Physicians & Hospitals, Federal Qualifications, Status, Year Founded, Managed Care Partners, Employer References, Fees & Payment Information and more. Plus, five years of historical information is included related to Revenues, Net Income, Medical Loss Ratios, Membership Enrollment and Number of Patient Complaints. Five easy-to-use, cross-referenced indexes will put this vast array of information at your fingertips immediately: HMO Index, PPO Index, Other Providers Index, Personnel Index and Enrollment Index. *The HMO/PPO Directory* provides the most comprehensive information on the most companies available on the market place today.

"Individuals concerned (or those with questions) about their insurance may find this text to be of use to them." -ARBA

600 pages; Softcover ISBN 1-930956-91-6, $250.00 ◆ Online Database, $495.00 ◆ Online Database & Directory Combo, $600.00

The Directory of Hospital Personnel, 2003

The Directory of Hospital Personnel is the best resource you can have at your fingertips when researching or marketing a product or service to the hospital market. A "Who's Who" of the hospital universe, this directory puts you in touch with over 150,000 key decision-makers. With 100% verification of data you can rest assured that you will reach the right person with just one call. Every hospital in the U.S. is profiled, listed alphabetically by city within state. Plus, three easy-to-use, cross-referenced indexes put the facts at your fingertips faster and more easily than any other directory: Hospital Name Index, Bed Size Index and Personnel Index. *The Directory of Hospital Personnel* is the only complete source for key hospital decision-makers by name. Whether you want to define or restructure sales territories… locate hospitals with the purchasing power to accept your proposals… keep track of important contacts or colleagues… or find information on which insurance plans are accepted, *The Directory of Hospital Personnel* gives you the information you need – easily, efficiently, effectively and accurately.

"Recommended for college, university and medical libraries." -ARBA

2,500 pages; Softcover ISBN 1-930956-72-X, $275.00 ◆ Online Database $545.00 ◆ Online Database & Directory Combo, $650.00

The Directory of Health Care Group Purchasing Organizations, 2003

This comprehensive directory provides the important data you need to get in touch with over 1,000 Group Purchasing Organizations. By providing in-depth information on this growing market and its members, *The Directory of Health Care Group Purchasing Organizations* fills a major need for the most accurate and comprehensive information on over 1,000 GPOs – Mailing Address, Phone & Fax Numbers, E-mail Addresses, Key Contacts, Purchasing Agents, Group Descriptions, Membership Categorization, Standard Vendor Proposal Requirements, Membership Fees & Terms, Expanded Services, Total Member Beds & Outpatient Visits represented and more. Five Indexes provide a number of ways to locate the right GPO: Alphabetical Index, Expanded Services Index, Organization Type Index, Geographic Index and Member Institution Index. With its comprehensive and detailed information on each purchasing organization, *The Directory of Health Care Group Purchasing Organizations* is the go-to source for anyone looking to target this market.

"The information is clearly arranged and easy to access…recommended for those needing this very specialized information." –ARBA

1,000 pages; Softcover ISBN 1-59237-001-2, $325.00 ◆ Online Database, $650.00 ◆ Online Database & Directory Combo, $750.00

The Directory of Independent Ambulatory Care Centers, 2002/03

This first edition of *The Directory of Independent Ambulatory Care Centers* provides access to detailed information that, before now, could only be found scattered in hundreds of different sources. This comprehensive and up-to-date directory pulls together a vast array of contact information for over 7,200 Ambulatory Surgery Centers, Ambulatory General and Urgent Care Clinics, and Diagnostic Imaging Centers that are not affiliated with a hospital or major medical center. Detailed listings include Mailing Address, Phone & Fax Numbers, E-mail and Web Site addresses, Contact Name and Phone Numbers of the Medical Director and other Key Executives and Purchasing Agents, Specialties & Services Offered, Year Founded, Numbers of Employees and Surgeons, Number of Operating Rooms, Number of Cases seen per year, Overnight Options, Contracted Services and much more. Listings are arranged by State, by Center Category and then alphabetically by Organization Name. Two indexes provide quick and easy access to this wealth of information: Entry Name Index and Specialty/Service Index. *The Directory of Independent Ambulatory Care Centers* is a must-have resource for anyone marketing a product or service to this important industry and will be an invaluable tool for those searching for a local care center that will meet their specific needs.

986 pages; Softcover ISBN 1-930956-90-8, $185.00 ◆ Online Database, $365.00 ◆ Online Database & Directory Combo, $450.00

To preview any of our Directories Risk-Free for 30 days, call (800) 562-2139 or fax to (518) 789-0556